PHARMACOLOGY
for WOMEN'S HEALTH

Edited by

TEKOA L. KING, CNM, MPH

Associate Professor
Department of Obstetrics, Gynecology,
and Reproductive Sciences
University of California at San Francisco
San Francisco, California

Deputy Editor
Journal of Midwifery & Women's Health

MARY C. BRUCKER, CNM, PHD

Professor and Director of Graduate Program
Baylor University
Louise Herrington School of Nursing
Dallas, Texas

JONES AND BARTLETT PUBLISHERS

Sudbury, Massachusetts

BOSTON   TORONTO   LONDON   SINGAPORE

World Headquarters
Jones and Bartlett Publishers
40 Tall Pine Drive
Sudbury, MA 01776
978-443-5000
info@jbpub.com
www.jbpub.com

Jones and Bartlett Publishers Canada
6339 Ormindale Way
Mississauga, Ontario L5V 1J2
Canada

Jones and Bartlett Publishers International
Barb House, Barb Mews
London W6 7PA
United Kingdom

Jones and Bartlett's books and products are available through most bookstores and online booksellers. To contact Jones and Bartlett Publishers directly, call 800-832-0034, fax 978-443-8000, or visit our website, www.jbpub.com.

Substantial discounts on bulk quantities of Jones and Bartlett's publications are available to corporations, professional associations, and other qualified organizations. For details and specific discount information, contact the special sales department at Jones and Bartlett via the above contact information or send an email to specialsales@jbpub.com.

The authors, editor, and publisher have made every effort to provide accurate information. However, they are not responsible for errors, omissions, or for any outcomes related to the use of the contents of this book and take no responsibility for the use of the products and procedures described. Treatments and side effects described in this book may not be applicable to all people; likewise, some people may require a dose or experience a side effect that is not described herein. Drugs and medical devices are discussed that may have limited availability controlled by the Food and Drug Administration (FDA) for use only in a research study or clinical trial. Research, clinical practice, and government regulations often change the accepted standard in this field. When consideration is being given to use of any drug in the clinical setting, the health care provider or reader is responsible for determining FDA status of the drug, reading the package insert, and reviewing prescribing information for the most up-to-date recommendations on dose, precautions, and contraindications, and determining the appropriate usage for the product. This is especially important in the case of drugs that are new or seldom used.

Production Credits
Publisher: Kevin Sullivan
Acquisitions Editor: Emily Ekle
Acquisitions Editor: Amy Sibley
Associate Editor: Patricia Donnelly
Editorial Assistant: Rachel Shuster
Associate Production Editor: Lisa Cerrone
Marketing Manager: Rebecca Wasley
V.P., Manufacturing and Inventory Control: Therese Connell
Composition: diacriTech
Cover Design: Scott Moden
Cover Image: © Bruno Sinnah/Dreamstime.com
Printing and Binding: Courier Stoughton
Cover Printing: Courier Stoughton

Library of Congress Cataloging-in-Publication Data
Pharmacology for women's health / [edited by] Tekoa L. King, Mary C. Brucker.
　　p. ; cm.
　Includes bibliographical references and index.
　ISBN-13: 978-0-7637-5329-0 (pbk.)
　ISBN-10: 0-7637-5329-7 (pbk.)
　1. Gynecologic drugs. 2. Women—Diseases—Chemotherapy. I. King, Tekoa L. II. Brucker, Mary C.
　[DNLM: 1. Pharmacological Processes. 2. Genital Diseases, Female—drug therapy. 3. Pregnancy Complications—drug therapy. 4. Women's Health.
　QV 38 P3197 2011]
　RG131.P43 2011
　615'.1082—dc22

2009043589

6048

Printed in the United States of America
13 12 11 10 09　10 9 8 7 6 5 4 3 2 1

Table of Contents

Chapter 10   Complementary and Alternative Therapies.......228
*Wendell Combest, Austin J. Combest,
and Juliana van Olphen Fehr*

Section III   *Essential Drug Categories* 247

Chapter 11   Anti-Infectives....................................249
*Tekoa L. King, Anne Marie Mitchell,
Barbara J. Lannen, and Marie Daly,
with acknowledgment to Lori A. Spies*

Chapter 12   Analgesia and Anesthesia...........................310
Tekoa L. King and Elissa Lane Miller

Introduction

Most books about drugs fall into one of two categories—they either focus on basic pharmacology, rich with information about pharmacokinetics and pharmacodynamics, or they address pharmacotherapeutics with an emphasis on conditions and indicated treatments. The former provides in-depth information that, unfortunately, is often detached from actual practice, making it difficult for a reader to retain and later use. The pharmacotherapeutics approach helps the clinician link a condition and drug together, but frequently does not provide enough information for future decision making as postmarketing adverse effects become apparent or similar new agents emerge.

Pharmacology for Women's Health is specifically designed for the healthcare provider who cares for women. This book addresses both basic pharmacology and pharmacotherapeutics and is divided into six distinct but complementary sections. The first section, "Introduction to Pharmacology," begins with an overview of modern pharmacology and continues with chapters that provide the basic framework needed by a clinician. For some readers, this content may be new; for others it will provide a needed review.

Recognition that some agents are used for reasons other than treating a pathologic condition provided the rationale for clustering chapters into the second section, "Lifestyle and Preventive Healthcare Practices." The chapters in this section explore drugs used to prevent disease, such as vitamins and minerals; habits that confer increased risks, such as smoking, and drugs to aid withdrawal; weight loss agents; and general information about use of drugs involved with substance abuse.

Some agents reside within one drug category, such as anti-infectives or hormonal agents, but are used to treat a wide variety of conditions. Medications such as these can be used for their therapeutic effects or for their side effects (e.g., the use of antihistamines for sedation). Detailed discussion of the identical antibiotic indicated for a respiratory, urinary, or dermatologic infection would be redundant information for readers and writers alike if reviewed in each separate chapter. Therefore, selected drug classifications, namely anti-infectives, analgesics and anesthetics, antihistamines, and steroidal hormones, comprise the chapters in this section. Although few in number, these chapters include a large amount of needed material about these classes of drugs, and when specific ones are mentioned for pharmacotherapeutic reasons in other chapters, the reader will be able to refer to this section for detailed information. Due to the common use of these types of agents, this section is titled, "Essential Drug Categories."

The largest number of chapters is found in the next section, "Pharmacotherapeutics for Common Conditions." In these chapters, evidence-based information about treatment of women with conditions ranging from the common cold to cancer can be found. All chapters are focused on care provided by primary care professionals. When appropriate, agents that have management variations based on gender, age, or reproductive state are so discussed.

Reproduction, contraception, and gynecologic conditions, as well as pregnancy and breastfeeding are addressed in the last two sections, "Gynecology" and "Pregnancy and Lactation." Women experience profound physiologic changes over the course of adult life. These changes affect pharmacotherapeutics and are therefore a primary consideration prior to prescribing medications. Thus, it is appropriate that we honor these transitions with separate chapters.

All the chapters in this book start with a glossary of terms used in that chapter. Most chapters include cases that illustrate clinical use of the agents reviewed. Every effort has been made to verify that the information presented is current and accurate. This book is not intended to be a replacement for appropriate health care, and although physiology often is included for the reader to better understand use of pharmacologic agents, this book is not designed to provide detailed physiology of pathologic conditions, diagnosis, and nonpharmacologic treatments.

"My drug rep brings great pizza. I always support her by prescribing her products."

WOMEN'S HEALTHCARE PROVIDER IN PRACTICE

"As long as a student knows the name, dose, and contraindications for at least one or two drugs for a specific condition, they can practice safely."

FACULTY TEACHING A GRADUATE CLINICAL
PHARMACOLOGY COURSE

"I can always look it up when I'm in practice."

STUDENT

Acknowledgments

The above comments illustrate why this book is needed. As the amount of drug information available explodes, individuals find themselves overwhelmed and sometimes unprepared to identify the appropriate intervention in a clinical situation. This text is dedicated to women, with the hope that they all receive the care that they need and deserve, especially when pharmacologic agents are indicated.

Many colleagues cautioned us upon undertaking the editing of this text. More than once we heard that writing a textbook was as onerous as a prolonged labor. Yet for us, this was a labor of love. Although we encountered some speed bumps along the way, the "birth" was not preterm and it has been a joyful pregnancy. Overall, the process was stimulating, probably in large part because of our editing partnership. During the writing we adopted each other and each other's families. We also benefited from a wide network of old and new friends and colleagues. We were fortunate to have a fabulous group of authors and reviewers who shared their time and expertise so liberally. The University of California at San Francisco and Baylor University enabled us to obtain the needed resources and obscure references. Colleagues, including Deanne Williams, Francie Likis, Judy Lott, Catherine Rosser, and Mary Ann Faucher

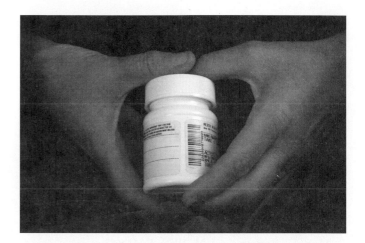

understood the bags under our eyes after late-night editing and frequently gave therapeutic comments.

Family members provided support and understanding. Our heartfelt thanks to Bill Fawley, Nancy Jo Reedy, Kya Fawley, Linda Cady, Todd Fawley, and Ted Brucker. These family members all saw more of our computers than they ever anticipated. For the one who said, "When will that book be done?" when the computer emerged one evening in the midst of a Mediterranean cruise, and for the one who said, "What year will that book be done?" . . . here it is.

Contributors

Susan A. Albrecht, RN, PhD, FAAN
Associate Professor, Associate Dean
University of Pittsburgh School of Nursing
Pittsburgh, Pennsylvania

Nancy Botelho, RN, FNP-BC
Nurse Practitioner Center for Women's
  Gastrointestinal Services
Women & Infants Hospital
Adjunct Faculty Member
Department of Nursing, University of Rhode Island
Providence, Rhode Island

Mary C. Brucker, CNM, PhD, FACNM
Professor, Associate Dean
Baylor University Louise Herrington School
  of Nursing
Dallas, Texas

Lawrence Carey, PharmD
Associate Director, Academic Coordinator
Physician Assistant Program
Philadelphia University
Philadelphia, Pennsylvania

Nancy A. Carroll, RNC, WHNP-BC, MS
Women's Health Nurse Practitioner
Maine Center for Reproductive Health
South Portland, Maine
Coastal Women's Healthcare
Scarborough, Maine

Donna D. Caruthers, RN, PhD
Assistant Professor
University of Pittsburgh School of Nursing
Pittsburgh, Pennsylvania

Austin J. Combest, MBA, PharmD
Drug Development, Clinical Research Fellow
University of North Carolina Eshelman School of
  Pharmacy
Chapel Hill, North Carolina

Wendell Combest, PhD
Professor of Pharmacology
Bernard J. Dunn School of Pharmacy Shenandoah
  University
Winchester, Virginia

Robin Webb Corbett, RNC, PhD
Associate Professor
East Carolina University
Greenville, North Carolina

Marie Daly, MSN, FNP-BC
Clinical Faculty
Baylor University Louise Herrington School of Nursing
Dallas, Texas

Susan E. Davis Doughty, RN, WHNP-BC, MSN
Owner, Cofounder
New England WomenCenter
South Portland, Maine

Cathy L. Emeis, CNM, PhD
Assistant Professor
Nurse–Midwifery Program
Oregon Health & Science University School of Nursing
Portland, Oregon

Jason Farley, NP, MPH, PhD
Assistant Professor
Johns Hopkins University School of Nursing
Adult NP
Johns Hopkins AIDS Service
Baltimore, Maryland

William P. Fehder, RN, CRNA, PhD
Clinical Associate Professor
Boston College William F. Connell School of Nursing
Boston, Massachusetts

Juliana van Olphen Fehr, CNM, PhD, FACNM
Associate Professor, Nurse–Midwifery Coordinator
Shenandoah University
Winchester, Virginia

Vivian Gamblian, RN, MSN
Lecturer, Coordinator
Simulation Laboratory
Baylor University Louise Herrington School of Nursing
Dallas, Texas

Barbara W. Graves, CNM, MN, MPH, FACNM
Director
Midwifery Education Program
Baystate Medical Center
Springfield, Massachusetts

Jessica A. Grieger, BSc(hons), PhD
Postdoctoral Research Fellow
The Pennsylvania State University
University Park, Pennsylvania

Barbara Hackley, CNM, MS
Associate Professor
Yale University School of Nursing
New Haven, Connecticut

Thomas W. Hale, PhD
Professor
Department of Pediatrics
Texas Tech University School of Medicine
Amarillo, Texas

Ashley Hanahan, CRNP, MSN, MPH
Nurse Practitioner
Veterans Administration Medical
    Center Baltimore
Baltimore, Maryland

**Jennifer G. Hensley, CNM, WHNP-BC,
    LCCE, EdD**
Coordinator
Nurse–Midwifery Option
University of Colorado Denver College of Nursing
Denver, Colorado

Therese M. Horan, MSN
Graduate Student Research Assistant
Seattle University
Seattle, Washington

Cecilia Jevitt, CNM, PhD
Associate Professor
University of South Florida College of Nursing
Tampa, Florida

Ruth Johnson, CNM, MSN, MPA
Advanced Practice Psychiatric Nurse, Certified
    Nurse–Midwife
Massachusetts General Hospital
Wellesley, Massachusetts

Vijaya Juturu, PhD, FACN
Consultant, Nutritionist, Adjunct Faculty
United Bio-Med, Inc.
Dobbs Ferry, New York

Heather I. Katcher, RD, PhD
Clinical Research Coordinator
Washington Center for Clinical Research
Washington, DC

Joyce King, CNM, PhD, FACNM
Clinical Assistant Professor
Nell Hodgson Woodruff School of Nursing,
    Emory University
Atlanta, Georgia

Tekoa L. King, CNM, MPH, FACNM
Associate Clinical Professor
University of California at San Francisco
San Francisco, California

Mary Beth Koslap-Petraco, DNP, MS,
PNP-BC, CPNP
Coordinator—Child Health
Suffolk County Department of Health Services
Hauppauge, New York
Clinical Assistant Professor
Stony Brook University School of Nursing
Stony Brook, New York

Jan M. Kriebs, CNM, MSN, FACNM
Assistant Professor, Director of Midwifery
University of Maryland School of Medicine
Baltimore, Maryland

Penny M. Kris-Etherton, RD, PhD
Distinguished Professor of Nutrition
The Pennsylvania State University
University Park, Pennsylvania

Barbara J. Lannen, CNM, MS
NMW/WHNP Faculty
Wayne State University College of Nursing
Detroit, Michigan

Emily E. Weber LeBrun, MD
Fellow in Female Pelvic Medicine and Reconstructive
Medicine
University of Massachusetts Memorial Medical Center
Worcester, Massachusetts

Judith A. Lewis, RN, WHNP, PhD, FAAN
Professor Emerita
Virginia Commonwealth University School
of Nursing
Richmond, Virginia

Frances E. Likis, CNM, NP, DrPH
Editor-in-Chief
Journal of Midwifery & Women's Health
Associate Director of Graduate Studies
Institute for Medicine and Public Health
Vanderbilt University
Nashville, Tennessee

Judy Wright Lott, NNP-BC, DSN, FAAN
Dean, Professor of Nursing
Baylor University Louise Herrington School
of Nursing
Dallas, Texas

Nancy K. Lowe, CNM, PhD, FACNM, FAAN
Professor, Chair
Division of Women, Children, and Family Health
University of Colorado Denver College of Nursing
Denver, Colorado

Laura Manns-James, CNM, MSN, WHNP-BC
Course Faculty
Frontier School of Midwifery and Family Nursing
Hyden, Kentucky

Hayley Mark, RN, MPH, PhD
Assistant Professor
Johns Hopkins University School of Nursing
Baltimore, Maryland

Jane Mashburn, CNM, MN, FACNM
Clinical Associate Professor
Nell Hodgson Woodruff School of Nursing, Emory
University
Atlanta, Georgia

Brian Meadors, PharmD
Clinical Pharmacist
Baylor Health Care System
Fort Worth, Texas

Elissa Lane Miller, CNM, FNP-C, PhD
Nurse Practitioner
Searcy Clinic for Women
Searcy, Arizona
Adjunct Professor
Arkansas State University Department of Nursing
Jonesboro, Arizona

Angela R. Mitchell, APRN-BC, MSN, DNP
Family Nurse Practitioner
Mecklenburg Medical Group: Gastroenterology
Charlotte, North Carolina

Anne Marie Mitchell, CNM, WHNP, PhD
Associate Professor
Oakland University
Rochester, Michigan

Cindy L. Munro, RN, ANP, PhD, FAAN
Professor of Adult Health
Virginia Commonwealth University School
of Nursing
Richmond, Virginia

Patricia Aikins Murphy, CNM, DrPH, FACNM
Professor, Annette Poulson Cumming Presidential
Endowed Chair in Women's and Reproductive Health,
Executive Director of Clinical Graduate Programs
University of Utah College of Nursing
Salt Lake City, Utah

Patrick J. M. Murphy, PhD
Assistant Professor
Seattle University College of Nursing
Seattle, Washington

Michael W. Neville, PharmD, BCPS
Clinical Associate Professor
University of Georgia
Athens, Georgia

Katharine K. O'Dell, CNM, PhD
Assistant Professor
University of Massachusetts Memorial Medical Center
Worcester, Massachusetts

Laura Williford Owens, PharmD
Chief of Pharmacy Services
Carolina Family Health Centers, Inc.
Wilson, North Carolina

Nancy Jo Reedy, CNM, MPH, FACNM
Director of Midwifery Services
Texas Health Care, PLLC
Fort Worth, Texas

Mary Ann Rhode, CNM, MS
Exempla Certified Nurse–Midwives
Exempla Healthcare at Saint Joseph Hospital
Denver, Colorado

Lillie Rizack, CNM, MSN
Associate Program Director
Philadelphia University
Philadelphia, Pennsylvania

Mary Ellen Rousseau, CNM, MS, FACNM
Professor
Yale University School of Nursing
New Haven, Connecticut

Rebekah L. Ruppe, CNM, DNP
Assistant Professor of Clinical Nursing
Columbia University School of Nursing
New York, New York

**Kerri Durnell Schuiling, CNM, WHNP-BC,
PhD, FACNM**
Associate Dean, Director
Northern Michigan University School of Nursing
Marquette, Michigan

Barbara Peterson Sinclair, MN, RNC, OGNP, FAAN
Professor Emerita
California State University, Los Angeles School of Nursing
Los Angeles, California

Lori Smith, CRNP, MSN
Clinical GYN, Oncology Nurse Practitioner
Hospital of the University of Pennsylvania, Jordan Center
for Gynecologic Cancer
Philadelphia, Pennsylvania

Lori A. Spies, RN, FNP-C, MS
Coordinator of Family Nurse Practitioner Program,
Mission Coordinator, Lecturer
Baylor University Louise Herrington School of Nursing
Dallas, Texas

Marianne (Teri) Stone-Godena, CNM, MSN
Lecturer, Director of Nurse–Midwifery Specialty
Yale University School of Nursing
New Haven, Connecticut

Shirley A. Summers, MSW
Chief Operating Officer
Behavioral Health Services Inc.
Gardena, California

Nell Tharpe, CNM, CRNFA, MS
Adjunct Faculty
Philadelphia University
Philadelphia, Pennsylvania

Reviewers

Diane J. Angelini, CNM, EdD, FACNM, FAAN
Cinical Associate Professor and Director
Midwifery
Warren Alpert Medical School of Brown University
Providence, Rhode Island

Mary K. Barger, CNM, MPH, PhD, FACNM
Assistant Professor
Department of Family Health Care Nursing
University of California–San Francisco
San Francisco, California

Joanne Bigness, CNM, FNP-C, PhD
Faculty and Course Coordinator Pharmacology
   and Primary Care IV
Frontier School of Midwifery and Family Nursing
Hyden, Kentucky

Sharon M. Bond, CNM, APRN-BC, PhD
Assistant Professor
Medical University of South Carolina College of Nursing
Charleston, South Carolina

Mary Ellen Bouchard, CNM, MS
Staff Nurse–Midwife
InovaCares Clinic for Women, Inova
   Health Systems
Falls Church, Virginia

**Barbara Camune, CNM, WHNP-BC,
   DrPH, FACNM**
Clinical Associate Professor, Director
Nurse–Midwifery & Women's Health Nurse
   Practitioner Programs
University of Illinois–Chicago
Chicago, Illinois

Patricia W. Caudle, CNM, FNP-BC, DNSc
Faculty
Frontier School of Midwifery and Family Nursing
Hyden, Kentucky

**Jeannette Crenshaw, RN, IBCLC, LCCE,
   NEA-BC, MSN**
Family Educator
Texas Health Presbyterian Hospital of Dallas
Dallas, Texas
Graduate Faculty
Nursing Administration Program, University of
   Texas–Arlington
Arlington, Texas

Steven Deville, RN
Family Nurse Practitioner Student
Baylor University Louise Herrington School
   of Nursing
Dallas, Texas

Shareen Y. El-Ibiary, PharmD, BCPS
Associate Professor of Pharmacy Practice
Midwestern University College of Pharmacy—Glendale
Glendale, Arizona

Janet L. Engstrom, CNM, WHNP-BC, PhD, FACNM
Chair
Women, Children, and Family Nursing
Rush University
Chicago, Illinois

Jenifer O. Fahey, CNM, MSN, MPH
Assistant Professor
University of Maryland School of Medicine
Baltimore, Maryland

Cindy Farley, CNM, PhD, FACNM
Associate Program Director, Coordinator of Graduate
    Studies
Midwifery Institute of Philadelphia University
Yellow Springs, Ohio

Mary Ann Faucher, CNM, PhD
Associate Professor
Baylor University Louise Herrington School of Nursing
Dallas, Texas

Sarah Feddema, PharmD, BCPS
Assistant Professor (Clinical)
Department of Pharmacotherapy
University of Utah College of Pharmacy
Salt Lake City, Utah

Marilynn C. Frederiksen, MD
Associate Professor
Clinical Obstetrics and Gynecology
Feinberg Medical School of Northwestern University
Chicago, Illinois

Debra K. Goodwin, RD, PhD
Assistant Professor
Jacksonville State University
Jacksonville, Alabama

Barbara Hackley, CNM, MS
Associate Professor
Yale University School of Nursing
New Haven, Connecticut

Brandon T. Jennings, PharmD
Assistant Professor (Clinical) of Pharmacotherapy
University of Utah College of Pharmacy
Salt Lake City, Utah

Cynthia Jensen, RN, CNS, MSN
Clinical Nurse Specialist
Intensive Care Nursery
University of California–San Francisco
    Children's Hospital
San Francisco, California

Cecilia Jevitt, CNM, PhD
Associate Professor
University of South Florida College of Nursing
Tampa, Florida

Angela Kedzior, MD
Pediatric Psychiatrist
MMC at South Bronx Health Center for Children &
    Families
Bronx, New York

Joyce King, CNM, PhD, FACNM
Clinical Assistant Professor
Nell Hodgson Woodruff School of Nursing Emory
    University
Atlanta, Georgia

Karen King, CNM, MSm, MSN
Certified Nurse–Midwife
Arlington Women's Center
Potomac Falls, Virginia

Ruth A. Lawrence, MD
Professor
Departments of Pediatrics and Obstetrics
    and Gynecology
University of Rochester
Rochester, New York

Frances E. Likis, CNM, NP, DrPH
Editor-in-Chief
Journal of Midwifery & Women's Health
Associate Director of Graduate Studies
Institute for Medicine and Public Health
Vanderbilt University
Nashville, Tennessee

Jane Mashburn, CNM, MN, FACNM
Clinical Associate Professor
Nell Hodgson Woodruff School of Nursing Emory
    University
Atlanta, Georgia

Katherine W. Morgan, WHNP, ANP, MS, DNP
Associate Professor (Clinical)
University of Utah College of Nursing
Salt Lake City, Utah

Jacquelin S. Neatherlin, RN, CNRN, PhD
Professor and Interim Graduate Director
Baylor University Louise Herrington School
    of Nursing
Dallas, Texas

Michael W. Neville, PharmD, BCPS
Clinical Associate Professor
University of Georgia
Athens, Georgia

Katharine K. O'Dell, CNM, PhD
Assistant Professor
University of Massachusetts Memorial
    Medical Center
Worcester, Massachusetts

Kathryn Osborne, CNM, PhD
Faculty
Frontier School of Midwifery and Family Nursing
Hyden, Kentucky

Debra S. Penney, CNM, MS, MPH
Associate Professor (Clinical)
University of Utah College of Nursing
Salt Lake City, Utah

Susan Rawlins, RN, WHNP-BC, MS
Director of Education
National Association of Nurse Practitioners
    in Women's Health
Pottsboro, Texas

Mary Ellen Rousseau, CNM, MS, FACNM
Professor
Yale University School of Nursing
New Haven, Connecticut

Ailey A. Runyon, RN, FNP-C, MSN
Assistant Professor
Concordia University Wisconsin
Mequon, Wisconsin

Sharon Myoji Schnare, CNM, FNP, MSN, FAANP
Clinical Instructor Department of Family and Child
    Nursing
University of Washington–Seattle School of Nursing
Seattle, Washington

**Kerri Durnell Schuiling, CNM, WHNP-BC,
    PhD, FACNM**
Associate Dean, Director
Northern Michigan University School of Nursing
Marquette, Michigan

Barry E. Schwarz, MD
Professor Obstetrics and Gynecology
University of Texas Southwestern Medical School
Dallas, Texas

Maureen T. Shannon, CNM, FNP, PhD
Associate Professor, Frances A. Matsuda
    Chair in Women's Health
University of Hawaii–Manoa School of
    Nursing & Dental Hygiene
Honolulu, Hawaii

Juanita Elaine Sidawi, MD
Staff Anesthesiologist
NorthStar Anesthesia PA
Ft. Worth, Texas

Kathleen Rice Simpson, RNC, PhD, FAAN
Perinatal Clinical Nurse Specialist
St. John's Mercy Medical Center
St. Louis, Missouri

B.J. Snell, CNM, PhD, FACNM
Associate Professor, Director
Women's Health Care Concentration
California State University–Fullerton Department
    of Nursing
Fullerton, California
Certified Nurse–Midwife
Beach Cities Midwifery & Women's Health Care
Laguna Hills, California

Jason Trahan, PharmD
Manager Clinical Pharmacy Services
Baylor All Saints Medical Center
Ft. Worth, Texas

Dwight Utzman, PharmD, BCPS
Health Sciences Assistant Clinical Professor
University of California–San Francisco School
    of Pharmacy
San Francisco, California

Carol A. Verga, CNM, ARNP, MS, MSN
Certified Nurse–Midwife
Private Practice
Seattle, Washington

Susan Wysocki, WHNP-BC, FAANP
President and CEO
National Association of Nurse Practitioners
    in Women's Health
Washington, DC

Jerome Yankowitz, MD
Professor, Director
Division of Maternal–Fetal Medicine Department
    of Obstetrics & Gynecology
University of Iowa College of Medicine
Iowa City, Iowa

Introduction to Pharmacology

Pharmacologic agents are ubiquitous in today's society, and pharmacotherapeutics is an essential component of primary care practice. The four chapters in this section are dedicated to basic information about drugs. The chapter titled "Modern Pharmacology" reviews the clinical context that prescribing takes place in today, including regulation, taxonomy, and general use. "Principles of Pharmacology" describes the pillars in the foundation of pharmacology, including pharmacokinetics and pharmacodynamics. The chapter titled "Pharmacogenomics" introduces a 21st-century approach that will soon be an essential consideration prior to prescribing many drugs. This chapter reviews information about genetics that influence the clinical effects of pharmacologic agents. Prominent among this information is the discussion of drug–drug (or herb) interactions that are secondary to drug metabolism by the CYP450 enzymes. The CYP450 enzymes exhibit many genetic variations that cause some drugs to not be therapeutic and others to have exaggerated toxic responses. The future may well encompass a genetic assessment prior to customized prescribing. The last chapter in this section, "Adverse Drug Reactions, Toxicology, and Poisoning," addresses adverse effects of drugs in more detail, including toxic effects and poisonings. All of the chapters in this section have clinical examples to illustrate the importance of the pharmacologic principles in practice.

1

Modern Pharmacology

Mary C. Brucker

 Chapter Glossary

Abbreviated new drug application (ANDA) An application in the FDA process usually reserved for facilitating an existing agent onto the market (e.g., current prescription drug to over-the-counter status).

Adverse drug event (ADE) Harm caused by use of a drug. Includes harm from the drug itself and harm that occurs from using the drug that could be secondary to increasing or decreasing the dose or discontinuing the drug.

Adverse drug reaction (ADR) Response to a drug that is noxious and unintended and that occurs at doses normally used for prophylaxis, diagnosis, or therapy of disease or for the modification of physiologic function.

Approved drug In the United States, the FDA must approve a substance as a drug before it can be marketed. The approval process involves several steps including preclinical laboratory and animal studies, clinical trials for safety and efficacy, filing of a new drug application by the manufacturer of the drug, FDA review of the application, and FDA approval/rejection of application.

Behind the counter (BTC) Drugs that are sold without prescription, but that are subject to some restrictions such as proof of identity because of potential risks. For example, pseudoephedrine may be used as an ingredient for production of methylamphetamine.

Bioequivalent Pharmacologically equivalent.

Black box warning One method that the FDA uses to identify unusual harm associated with an agent. Often it is added to package inserts after postmarketing studies find unexpected risks.

Blockbuster drug A pharmaceutical whose sales exceed $1 billion annually.

Brand name A trademarked name assigned to a drug by the manufacturer. Some brand names are similar to the generic name (e.g., pseudoephedrine/Sudafed); others suggest their indications for use (e.g., Tamiflu is used for treatment of influenza).

Chemical name Although rarely used by prescribers and consumers, the chemical name of a drug describes the chemical composition of the agent.

Clinical trial A research study to answer specific questions about vaccines, new therapies, or new ways of using known treatments. Clinical trials are used to determine whether new drugs or treatments are both *safe* and *effective*. Trials occur in four phases following preliminary laboratory and animal studies.

Combined drug intoxication (CDI) See polypharmacy. Poisoning or overdose associated with use of multiple agents.

Compounding Mixing or combining ingredients to produce a pharmaceutical agent.

Contraindication Condition that specifies who should not take the drug.

Controlled substances Pharmaceuticals as listed in schedules found in US Law 21 U.S.C. §802(32)(A). These agents include both opiates as well as nonopiates, but generally have a high risk of addiction, often without valid medicinal use. An example is heroin.

Co-pay Fee assessed for a drug in addition to the costs paid by a drug benefit plan.

Dangerous drugs Definition depends upon legislative locale. Often indicates any drug that is obtained only by prescription.

Delegated prescriptive authority Ability to prescribe linked to collaboration with a prescriber who has full legal authority. An example is a physician who delegates authority to prescribe to a physician assistant.

Designer drugs Drugs created based on sophisticated technology. Often these agents manipulate the chemistry to decrease untoward side effects.

Direct-to-consumer (DTC) Advertising of selected drugs placed in popular media and directed to the general public as opposed to providers in peer-reviewed journals.

Dispense (furnish) The process of giving a drug to the consumer.

Drug (medication or pharmaceutical) A chemical substance that brings about changes in a biologic system through its chemical action(s).

Drug recall Removal of a pharmaceutical agent from the marketplace. May be voluntary or mandatory.

Efficacy The maximum ability of a drug or treatment to produce a result regardless of dose. A drug passes efficacy trials if it is effective at the dose tested and against the illness for which it is prescribed. In the procedure mandated by the FDA, Phase II clinical trials gauge efficacy and Phase III trials are used for confirmation in larger groups.

FDA warnings Identification and dissemination of information about potential conditions associated with major adverse effects.

Formulary List of approved or available drugs. Often used by insurance companies to identify agents that will be reimbursed or paid for by the insurer.

Generally recognized as safe and effective (GRAS/E) Often used to describe why an agent is sold over the counter.

Generic name A formulation that contains the same active ingredients found in the original brand formulation and is bioequivalent.

Investigational new drug (IND) Designation for an agent that may become a drug for clinical trials. The federal government regulates this process.

Medication error Mishap that occurs during prescribing, transcribing, dispensing, administering, adhering to, or monitoring a drug.

Multiple drug intake (MDI) Synonym for polypharmacy.

Negative formulary A list of drugs for which generic drugs cannot replace brand name drugs.

New drug application (NDA) Application by which a potential agent is registered as part of the process for approval. For example, a company must have an NDA filed in order to engage in clinical trials.

Off-label use A drug prescribed or used for conditions other than those approved by the FDA.

Orphan drugs Agents that are indicated for rare conditions.

Over-the-counter (OTC) Pharmaceuticals sold without prescriptions; if some restrictions are required, then the OTC agent also may be called a behind-the-counter (BTC) drug.

Pharmacoeconomics Field of study that identifies, measures, and evaluates the costs of drug therapy to healthcare systems and society.

Pharmacogenomics The study of how variations in the human genome affect the response to medications.

Pharmacology The study of how drugs interact with a living organism in order to produce a change in physiologic functioning.

Pharmacotherapeutics Use of drugs to treat or prevent illness or disease.

Phase I trials Studies to determine the distribution, metabolism, and pharmacologic actions of drugs in humans, to determine the side effects associated with increasing doses, and to evaluate for evidence of effectiveness. These trials typically include healthy participants.

Phase II trials Controlled clinical studies conducted to evaluate the effectiveness of the drug for a particular indication or indications in patients with the disease or condition under study, and to determine the common short-term side effects and risks.

Phase III trials Expanded controlled and uncontrolled trials after preliminary evidence suggesting effectiveness of the drug has been obtained. These trials are intended to gather additional information to evaluate the overall benefit–risk relationship of the drug and provide an adequate basis for physician labeling.

Phase IV trials Postmarketing studies to delineate additional information including the drug's risks, benefits, and optimal use.

Placebo Agent that has no active ingredients.

Polypharmacy The practice of treating individuals using multidrug regimens; this term generally is accepted to mean administration of five or more drugs. Polypharmacy may be the result of drug treatment for multiple comorbidities, complex disease processes, lack of concordance between multiple practitioners, illicit drug use, and use of medication to treat side effects of other pharmacologic agents. May also be referred to as multiple drug intake (MDI) or, in the case of poisonings and overdoses, as combined drug intoxication (CDI).

Positive formulary A list of drugs that can be replaced with generic formulations when dispensed per pharmacist or consumer choice.

Precaution A condition that may suggest increased risk for adverse drug reactions by use of the drug compared to the general population; however, the risk is not to such a degree that the condition is considered a contraindication. Plural: A list of these conditions.

Pregnancy categories An FDA drug classification system to identify the relative risk of drug use during pregnancy.

Prescriptive authority Legal ability to prescribe drugs, medical devices, etc.

Safety The level of a drug's known adverse effects.

Side effect Physiologic response unrelated to the desired drug effect.

Therapeutic index The dose range between the minimum therapeutic dose and the dose that initiates a toxic reaction.

Society and Health

All societies have major concerns, both collectively and among individual members, about the maintenance of health and treatment of diseases. Over the millennia, a wide variety of interventions have been used for either or both of these objectives. Even today, interventions such as spiritual care, manipulation of body positions, variations in nutrition, and types of exercise still are the topics of research studies and are often the primary treatments for some medical conditions. However, the use of pharmaceuticals has become one of the most, if not *the* most, common treatment for medical disorders today. But concerns about adverse drug reactions, cost, and even potential lack of effectiveness are among the problems involving modern pharmaceuticals. The Chapter Glossary provides definitions of terms used in the discussion of drugs in society today. First however, a brief review of history is in order.

History of Pharmaceuticals

Details of the historical origins of use of botanicals, herbals, or other types of medications remain shrouded in the past. Early records suggest that traditional Chinese medicine included liberal use of such agents. From the Indian subcontinent, Ayurvedic medicine combined medications with surgical procedures as early as 1000 BC. Hippocrates, the great Greek physician, was also a herbologist, advocating multiple botanical treatments, many of which remain on the market today.

During the Middle Ages in Europe, herbs were integral agents for treatment of diseases. Some of the spices brought back from the Crusades were said to have attributes of magical healing. In the 1500s, apothecaries were found in various European towns, and by the 1600s, botanists and herbalists, such as the Englishman Nicholas Culpeper, were codifying use of herbs and publishing their findings and recommendations. Gradually, the use of botanicals became accepted as an expected intervention when health was threatened or disease was evident.

A new industry was born with the advent of patent medicines and potions in the 1800s.[1] Ironically, patent medicines were not copyrighted, but tended to be composed of secret ingredients under a trademarked name. Lydia Pinkham's Vegetable Compound included a number of herbs contained in alcohol. While she engaged in marketing the product to women for treatment of menstrual pain and disorders, she also accrued a personal fortune from widespread sales.

Other older remedies continue to live in today's over-the-counter market, albeit with different ingredients, including Carter's Little Liver Pills, Luden's Cough Drops, and Fletcher's Castoria. The soft drink Coca-Cola was originally marketed as a patent medicine. Use of patent medicines was a logical strategy to treat common diseases in an era in which healthcare providers were unregulated and many provider-prescribed strategies tended to have harmful effects such as those associated with the liberal use of heavy metals. Most patent medicines were not harmful in regular doses, although their effectiveness could be subject to debate.

The 19th century was midwife to the birth of today's major pharmaceutical houses. Between 1830 and the turn of the 20th century, the following groups began wholesale production of drugs: Schering and Merck in Germany; Hoffman-LaRoche in Switzerland; Burroughs Wellcome in England; and Abbot, Smith Kline, Parke-Davis, Eli Lilly, Squibb, and Upjohn in the United States. Other important companies such as Bayer (Germany); Ciba–Geigy and Sandoz (Switzerland); and Pfizer (United States) were first founded as producers of organic chemicals during the same time frame, and later moved into the area of pharmacology.[1]

The 20th Century

If the 19th century were one of creation and growth of the modern pharmaceutical industry, the 20th century was one of explosion and controversy. Pharmaceuticals moved into the role of being agents used for health promotion as well as for treatment of disease. Vaccines were lauded as an example of primary prevention of disease. The Great Race of Mercy, or the trip from Seward to Nome, Alaska, occurred in order to provide antitoxin to children who were threatened by a diphtheria epidemic in the 1920s. This pharmaceutical event is commemorated every spring by the famous Alaskan Iditarod Trail Sled Dog Race and promotes a positive connotation to the use of medications. Today, the vast majority of states report that close to 90% of children entering school have the recommended routine immunizations, although controversy exists regarding types of vaccines, timing, and potential adverse effects.[2] Vaccines, including controversies about their current use, are discussed in Chapter 6.

During the 1900s, it became clear that not all pharmaceuticals were innocuous. Reports of drug adverse effects, allergic reactions, drug interactions, and resistance to microbes began to populate the literature, especially in the last half of the century. Former US First Lady Eleanor Roosevelt died in 1962 of complications of tuberculosis, and a subsequent analysis a half century later noted that drug resistance was a major factor in her death.[3] Inadvertent or intentional overdoses from combining prescription drugs became infamous because of the deaths of celebrities such as Marilyn Monroe and Elvis Presley, and, in the 21st century, Heath Ledger. The ease of availability of medications with potent **side effects** is a current topic in the pharmaceutical literature and popular press. Combining different agents has become such an issue that it is alternatively referred to by some as **polypharmacy**, **combined drug intoxication** (CDI), or **multiple drug intake** (MDI).

Thus, it was predictable that regulation of pharmaceuticals came of age in the 1900s. This was the century in the United States when laws were passed in an attempt to protect the public in a variety of areas. Some drugs were removed from the prescription and/or over-the-counter market, although they were relatively few, especially compared to the number of new drugs introduced in the same century.

The United States Food and Drug Administration

The US Food and Drug Administration's mission is one of protection of the public by assuring the country that drugs, biologic products, medical devices, and other agents are safe, effective, and secure. In 1938, the United States Federal Food, Drug, and Cosmetic Act was passed, establishing the Food and Drug Administration (FDA) as a governmental body regulating aspects of pharmaceuticals. This act has undergone many modifications from changes in minor rules to major revisions of the act itself, changes that continue today as Congress oversees the work of the FDA. The origins of the FDA first began in 1906 with the passage of the Pure Food and Drug Act, also known as the Wiley Act. This legislation was designed to provide regulatory oversight to prevent manufacture,

sale, and transportation of adulterated, misbranded, or poisonous foods, drugs, medicine, or liquors. The second reason for the FDA was to create an agency that would regulate transport of these agents. In 1938, the Wiley Act was replaced with the Federal Food, Drug, and Cosmetic Act. Since 1938, this legislation has been amended several times, primarily to expand the oversight of the federal government.

The Kefhauver-Harris Amendment of 1962 was passed in response to the discovery of the teratogenic effects of thalidomide and required the additional evidence of safety and effectiveness of pharmaceuticals that are the essence of these standards today.[4] More recent additions have authorized regulation of bioterrorism agents, requirements for enrollment into clinical trials, and expansion of authority to assess postmarketing **safety** of drugs. Drug safety is paramount for the FDA. Among the myriad of activities of the current FDA are monitoring drug claims, especially those advertised to consumers; establishing standards for drug testing; and awarding approval for new pharmaceuticals, or those prescription medications that companies desire to move to over-the-counter status. These activities will be discussed in more detail later in the chapter and also in Chapter 4.

In 1997, an amendment to the Federal Food Drug and Cosmetic Act was passed that established a Web site registry (www.ClinicalTrials.gov) for clinical trials that is open to the public. Only drugs that were to be used for life-threatening conditions were required to register on this site. However, in other ways, the 1997 amendment eased FDA oversight of drugs. Drug approval could be based on one RCT and confirmatory evidence, a fast-track approval process was established whereby drug approval could be granted based on surrogate endpoints, and pharmaceutical companies were allowed to disseminate **off-label uses** of their drugs to healthcare providers.

However, following the Institute of Medicine's publication of *To Err is Human* in 1999, prevention of medication errors has taken center stage among the strategies promoted to provide safe health care. Experts from many disciplines have strategies that include different patient identification methods when a person is hospitalized; incorporation of "time-outs" during procedures, including those involving anesthesia; promotion of electronic prescribing to decrease misreading drug or dose; recommendations to avoid sound-alike brand names; simplification of packaging; and education of patients so that they know their medications and can personally advocate for the correct administrations.

In 2006, the Institute of Medicine published a report titled *The Future of Drug Safety*. This report included 25 recommendations for improving the process of overseeing drug development from the preapproval process through postmarketing evaluations. A primary theme of this report was the recommendation that the FDA authority be expanded and strengthened in order to protect the public from **adverse drug events**.

Building on this work, the Food and Drug Administration Amendments Act of 2007 (H.R. 3580) expanded the FDA's authority in many ways (Table 1-1). Today the FDA has expanded authority to monitor and regulate the safety of marketed drug products by requiring drug manufacturers to conduct postapproval studies or clinical trials if the FDA becomes aware of new safety information. In addition, the FDA can require postapproval changes to drug labels that address safety issues such as the risk for **adverse drug reactions**. The 2007 amendment also gives the FDA authority to review **direct-to-consumer** television advertisements prior to their dissemination; the FDA can now assign civil monetary penalties if advertisements are determined to be false or misleading.

This new ability to mandate postapproval changes to drug labels is well intended, albeit often difficult to implement. In order to provide an informed consent, comprehensive information must be available about the benefits and adverse effects of the medication in question. Beneficial effects often are more likely to be available than the risks. Most drug studies use a randomized controlled trial (RCT) approach, a methodology that is particularly useful to demonstrate if an intervention is beneficial, but is less useful for identifying adverse effects. RCTs tend to be small in number; limited to enrollees who are either healthy, as in the case of contraceptive studies, or have a single diagnosis; and are conducted for a relatively short period of time. In reality, the effects of drugs women use are rarely completely evaluated in RCTs. Therefore, agents may come onto the market, only to be removed within a few years as unexpected risks emerge. Large observational studies have been found to increase identification of risks, and although they do not have the rigor of an RCT, they can be combined with the results of RCTs in order to help the provider obtain more complete information on risks and benefits necessary for the person being informed.

The United States Pharmacopeia

An agency that works closely with the FDA is the United States Pharmacopeia (USP). The mission of the USP is to establish public standards in order to assure consumers regarding quality, safety, and benefit of medicines and foods through a unique process of public involvement and use of volunteers. However, unlike a federal agency such as the FDA, the USP is a nongovernment, not-for-profit, public health organization. This organization is approximately a century older than the FDA, and by the end of the 1800s, it had been mandated to be used by all state boards of pharmacy. USP standards enable drugs to be assessed for purity, potency, and consistency. Although the USP standards are US based, they are recognized and used in more than 100 countries. USP standards are published in the *United States Pharmacopeia–National Formulary* and applied to prescription and over-the-counter medications. Should there ever be a dispute regarding purity or identity, the methods found in the USP for evaluation of purity, potency, assay/bioassay, etc., would be the legally binding ones.

Although the development of standards and verification of purity and quality are the most well known of USP's activities, several other activities exist. These additional functions include development of healthcare information that is unbiased about drugs; administration of the Medication Errors Reporting Program (MedMark), an online program for the reporting of medication mistakes and

Table 1-1 The 2007 Amendments to the Federal Food Drug and Cosmetic Act

Amendment Provision	Description
Clinical trial registries expanded to include new drugs	All clinical trials evaluating any drug or biologic or medical device must be registered with www.ClinicalTrials.gov. The information on this Web site is available to the public and the drug manufacturer is required to maintain updated status about the clinical trial.
Required disclosure of study results	All clinical trials must disclose study results to the registry and results data bank section of www.ClinicalTrials.gov.
Postapproval safety studies may be required	To date, postapproval studies have been voluntary. Now, if the FDA has information about possible safety concerns, the agency can require that a postapproval study be conducted.
Safety labeling changes	The 2007 amendment gives the FDA authority to mandate a change to a drug label that describes safety information.
Risk evaluation and mitigation strategy (REMS)	The FDA may require that a drug manufacturer submit a REMS plan that specifies how a drug will be monitored to determine that benefit continues to outweigh risk as the drug is disseminated.
Technologies to ensure safety in the drug supply chain	The FDA is required to develop standards and methods to identify and validate effective technologies that will ensure the safety of the drug supply chain. This is designed to ensure that drugs marketed in the United States are free of contaminates, adulteration, or misbranding.

adverse drug effects; and a drug quality and information project to promote international drug safety.

Although the FDA is essential to pharmaceutical regulation and scrutiny, the sheer number of other organizations involved in aspects of drugs illustrates the complexity involved in use of pharmaceuticals today. The private sector, as exemplified by pharmaceutical companies and manufacturers of medical goods, also are major stakeholders. The USP belongs to the public section, although it is nongovernmental. Other governmental bodies intimately involved with drugs in the United States include the Centers for Disease Control and Prevention (CDC, recommendations for care), Drug Enforcement Administration (DEA, regulation of controlled substances), Federal Communications Commission (FCC, regulation of advertising for over-the-counter drugs), as well as state governments, which usually control prescriptive authority.

Legalized Prescriptive Authority

Prescriptive authority was afforded to physicians, veterinarians, dentists, and podiatrists by law in all states during the 1900s. During the same time frame, pharmacists were authorized to fill prescriptions and dispense drugs. In the last few decades of the 20th century and the first years of the 21st century, physician assistants, midwives, nurses in advanced practice, and psychologists have received full or limited prescriptive authority by most legislative entities. These professionals, as well as pharmacists, continue to seek expansion of legal authority in most areas.

Controversy continues to exist regarding individual rights versus societal good in the use, cost, and potential rationing of drugs. Other issues have emerged about both definitions and connotations of use of various terms used in pharmacology, some terms as basic as the definition of the word *drug*.

▌ The Definition of a Drug

Pharmacology is a word derived from the Greek meaning the study of drugs. Most sources basically define pharmacology more precisely as the study of how drugs interact with a living organism in order to produce a change in physiologic functioning. Any agent, substance, or medication that is used for medicinal purposes is a pharmaceutical. Although there appears to be general consensus on the definition of *pharmacology*, one of the great difficulties in the discussion of pharmaceuticals in modern society is existence of multiple connotations regarding the basic term *drug*. Within one context, *drug* connotes use of an illegal substance (e.g., cocaine)

and is associated with substance abuse; yet not all drugs are illicit. The FDA has been attempting to label tobacco as a drug for purposes of regulation; although tobacco, like alcohol, is a licit agent.[5,6] Prescriptive pharmaceuticals as well as **over-the-counter** (OTC) agents also are termed drugs and are subject to regulation by the FDA. Nutritional supplements are viewed as drugs by most consumers, although they are not regulated as such in the United States.[7] Therefore, it is wise to clarify how terms are used. For this chapter, a **drug** is a chemical substance that brings about changes in a biologic system through its chemical action. The terms *pharmaceuticals*, *medications*, and *drugs* will be used interchangeably. Illicit or recreational drugs will be noted as such to promote clarity. Other chapters, particularly Chapter 2 and Chapter 4, will provide more in-depth definitions in terms specific to pharmacology and toxicology.

Other terms add to the confusion. Many of these terms are intertwined with legal vocabulary. For example, because the United States is composed of more than 50 legal jurisdictions, variety in legal language exists. In some states or territories, the term **dangerous drugs** describes any agent that is limited to use by prescription only, including some prenatal vitamins. In other areas, the term is a synonym for **controlled substances**, or pharmaceuticals that are closely regulated especially because of increased risk of addiction.

The Naming of Drugs

Individual drugs also can be confusing since every agent can have multiple names. Each agent has a **chemical name**, or a precise term describing it. The chemical name often is abbreviated or truncated into the **generic name**. Today there often is an active attempt to share a suffix with other pharmaceuticals in the same drug category in an attempt to simplify relationships. For example, angiotensin-converting enzyme (ACE) inhibitors used for hypertension tend to end in *pril*, such as *captopril* and *lisinopril*. In addition to chemical name and generic names, patented trade names, or **brand names** also exist. These brand names are the ones most frequently remembered by consumers due to advertising. Sometimes brand names sound alike, which may contribute to consumer confusion. For example, the brand Celebrex is an analgesic, whereas the sound-alike Celexa is an antidepressant.

Due to the confusion involved with the lexicon of pharmaceuticals, the public may have conflicted opinions about such agents. Most men and women appreciate individual agents, especially if they have had positive therapeutic experiences with them. However, a small group may recoil from common use of pharmaceuticals because of the aforementioned issues, as well as factors such as adverse effects and/or the feeling that they are unnatural interferences in the body.

Cost of Drugs in Modern Society

Most persons in the United States have found the cost of prescription and nonprescription drugs has increased radically over the last 2 decades, particularly as such pharmaceuticals have become ubiquitous. The study of the costs and consequences of drug therapy to healthcare systems and society is called **pharmacoeconomics**. In today's healthcare settings, pharmacoeconomic methods can be applied for effective management of drug products, individual treatment, medication policy determination, and resource allocation.

Law described the use of pharmaceuticals in the modern world as part of the medicalization of society, or the belief that any condition, trivial or serious, can and should be treated with a drug instead of other interventions, especially nutrition and exercise.[8] The United States is the largest market in the world for prescription drugs, with consumption of up to 75% of the top selling agents and one in four individuals taking prescription agents.[9] Tracking of medical expenditures for prescription drugs provides some insight into the costs. In 2007, the United States Agency for Healthcare Research and Quality reported that from 1997 to 2004, total expenditures for outpatient prescription drugs increased from $72.3 billion to $191.0 billion, or an increase of 160%.[10] Citizens of the United States tend to pay more for the same drug than people in most other countries, much of it out of pocket,[11] although it can be argued that availability of the wide array of agents is richer than in most areas of the world and the disparity may be explained at least in some part due to variations in cost of living.

More than $16.1 billion has been estimated to be spent for over-the-counter treatments during the 2007 calendar year. This amount, although extreme by most parameters, is likely to be an underestimate of real costs, as it did not include sales from the megastore, Wal-Mart.[12]

In an era in which the majority of personal bankruptcies are related to medical costs, the costs of drugs have a visible and important economic role. Medical expenses are in large part out-of-pocket costs, including those for drugs that are not covered by insurance policies, even when a person has health insurance.[13] Consumers in the United States are not the only persons concerned about expenditures for prescription and over-the-counter drugs. These costs are important to the economy of the country as a whole. It is likely that the cost of drugs directly influences

healthcare inflation, which has risen more than twice as much as regular inflation from 2006 to 2007.[14]

Costs of drugs often are blamed on high profits gained by pharmaceutical houses. In the *Fortune 500* list published in 2008, eight pharmaceutical companies were in the top 200 companies with high profits and revenues. Pfizer lost both revenue and significant profits during 2007, perhaps due at least in part to difficulty with its brand-name product, varenicline (Chantix), a smoking cessation medication that has received negative press due to adverse side effects. Conversely, Abbott posted profits twice as high as the year before, possibly due to double-digit increases in uses of drugs that it marketed for treatment of Crohn's disease and treatment of migraines.[15]

The Role of Health Insurance Plans

Healthcare insurance also is involved in pharmaceuticals. The first modern major American commercial health plan is attributed to a vice president of Baylor University who was responsible for the Baylor College of Medicine, School of Nursing, College of Dentistry, and hospital in Dallas. In 1929, he developed a plan for teachers that guaranteed coverage for 21 days of hospital care at an annual rate of $6, and he used a blue cross for the symbol. Healthcare plans are predominantly offered as part of employment. As healthcare plans became the norm, their coverage expanded from catastrophic hospital care to include preventive care, ambulatory services, and, more recently, drug benefits.

Drug benefits were added by commercial insurances in an attempt to curtail costs and add benefits to their subscribers. It has been estimated that in 1960, more than 95% of pharmaceuticals were paid for by individuals, whereas 30 years later, more than 50% were paid by insurance plans, and that number has increased with Medicare coverage.[16]

Although there is not one single uniform process, most insurers have consumers pay a **co-pay** or an amount that varies by whether or not the agent is on the **formulary**, or the list of drugs approved by the company. A formulary generally lists the most common agents, usually in a generic form. Uncommon and thereby expensive drugs may be covered with additional documentation specific to the individual and the condition. Often, pharmaceutical companies have negotiated favorable charges for common drugs directly with these insurers. However, as an unintended consequence, it has been found that co-pays may decrease the use of drugs, especially by individuals who use them to treat chronic conditions.[17]

Medicare and Medicaid

Medicare and Medicaid are types of public insurance partially funded by either the federal government or a combination of state and federal governments. Medicare is primarily for the elderly, and Medicaid (or its state equivalent such as MediCal) is primarily for those who are deemed to meet eligible criteria that demonstrate that they are unable to pay for healthcare costs and unable to obtain healthcare insurance. Medicare is completely a federal program, whereas Medicaid is state managed, and the states contribute to paying for the program. The program pays for the drugs; individuals usually do not have a co-pay if they are on Medicaid and the drug is Medicaid approved. Over-the-counter agents are not reimbursed for persons on Medicaid, although the generic equivalent written as a prescription may be covered.

A Medicare prescription drug plan was enacted in 2003, with implementation in 2006. This plan followed the Medicare terminology: Medicare Part A reimburses hospitals, Medicare Part B reimburses providers, and the new plan, Medicare Part D, is a drug benefit. Medicare Part D is administered by private insurance companies, who in turn are reimbursed by the federal government. Almost 2000 separate Part D plans exist, and the numbers and types have some regional variations. There have been complaints about the complexity of the system, including variations in amount of co-pay and amount of deductibles; controversy about the amount that must be paid before benefits are available for some (a so-called doughnut hole); lack of standardization of covered medications; legal inability of Medicare to negotiate for lower rates, as the Veterans Administration does; and the general need for subscribers to be computer literate to access information about benefits and manage enrollment. However, early indications suggest that part D may decrease the numbers of individuals who forgo needed medications in order to save money.[18]

Some pharmacies and pharmaceutical companies have special programs that offer some cost relief as well as attract customers. Several large companies now offer specially priced prescriptions for selected agents (e.g., $4 per prescription) and some companies will provide drugs under special circumstances for specific individuals if a provider contacts the company directly.

Cost-Saving Strategies

In addition to seeking the most inexpensive sales outlet for the agent and using drug benefits if available, a few other options exist. Often a tablet at twice the dose is not twice the price; and the provider may be able to educate an individual on how to split a tablet. This action is not possible for capsules, extended release agents, or some other formulations. Generic brands, which are discussed later, are identical agents as brand names, yet cost less. For those with chronic conditions, a prescription for 90 days generally is less costly than three 30-day refills, and it often has a lower co-pay for those with drug benefits. Lastly, individuals should not only continue medications such as antimicrobials until the prescription is finished, but they should also be aware of when therapies may no longer be warranted so that they do not have to pay for drugs unnecessarily.

Most Popular Drugs in the United States

Every year, a list of the drugs for which the most prescriptions have been filled in the United States is disseminated. For several years, the top of the list encompassed drugs for both health promotion (e.g., statins) and for treatment of medical disorders (e.g., antimicrobials). Pharmaceuticals, like other consumables, particularly are subject to changes associated with publicity. For example, after widespread media coverage revealed that the Women's Health Initiative found routine use of hormone therapy by perimenopausal/menopausal women did not reduce cardiac risk and had adverse effects, the popularity of the brand-named product Premarin (conjugated equine estrogens) dropped from number 1 in 1999 to number 68 on the 2007 list.

Medical expenditures for over-the-counter agents and herbal/botanical treatments are more difficult to estimate. Secondary analysis of the 2002 national survey by Gardiner revealed more than 20% of Americans use a botanical or herbal remedy; 72% who do so concurrently use prescription agents, and more than half never tell their healthcare provider.[20] Such widespread use of these agents must be associated with major costs, although they are difficult to estimate.

Creation of New Drugs

Originally drugs were developed largely based on empirical observations of the effects purported to occur after ingestion of plant substances. Later, newer drugs were developed using anecdotal information about the effects of older drugs. Some agents used for one disorder have been found to have side effects that are advantageous as a treatment for another disorder. For example, antihistamines have become FDA approved for treatment of motion sickness or insomnia, not because of their basic therapeutic effect to treat histamine attacks, but because of their side effects. Another example is the drug terbutaline that originally was developed for treating persons with asthma. This agent also is used as a uterine tocolytic because of its effect on the uterus. Since terbutaline is not FDA approved for use as a tocolytic, use in this fashion is called off-label use.

New drugs have been developed based upon biologic targets. Some sources call these **designer drugs**, although confusion with this term may exist as it is also used in the context of substance abuse to designate combining a variety of agents to create a new illicit drug. This confusion again illustrates some of the difficulty in creating a terminology for modern drugs.

Designer drugs directed toward a specific biologic target may be developed to bind to and inhibit key molecules involved in a disease or pathologic event. For example, the selective estrogen receptor modulator raloxifene (Evista) is chemically similar to tamoxifen citrate (Nolvadex), but does not have the latter's risk for inducing endometrial cancer. Synthetic drugs are only one of the common drug sources. Others include plants or botanicals; animal derivations, including humans, for such agents as insulin; minerals; and engineered agents such as antimicrobials.

The study of **pharmacogenomics** is providing insight into how and why certain drugs do not behave uniformly for all consumers and it heralds potential gene therapy in the area of designer drugs for the treatment of many diseases in the future.[21] Additional information about pharmacogenomics is found in Chapter 3.

Stakes are high as manufacturers in the United States operate with a capitalistic approach and desire for financial gain to support their companies. Approximately 25 novel drugs are marketed each year, but not all are profitable. All manufacturers seek a **blockbuster drug**, or an agent producing more than $1 billion in annual revenues. Pfizer has such an agent currently with their brand of atorvastatin, Lipitor. This pharmaceutical agent amassed more than $8 billion in revenues in 2007.[19] Yet development and marketing of a new drug is a complex and expensive process. Since an increasing number of agents are designer drugs as described previously, there are years involved in research and development. In addition, attention to pharmacogenomics and personalization of drugs may limit the potential marketplace for any single agent, causing the development of blockbuster drugs to become ever more elusive.

Marketing Drugs

The Pharmaceutical Research and Manufacturers of America (PhRMA) is the trade association for pharmaceutical companies in the United States. This group's mission is to encourage public policies that promote discovery of pharmaceutical agents that help individuals. As such, it is one of the largest lobbyists in the country, spending millions annually. Over the years there has been strong criticism regarding the marketing of various pharmaceuticals to healthcare providers. Some physicians were given financial gifts in recognition of their prescribing practices. A nonprofit group, No Free Lunch, was developed to encourage prescribers to be wary of marketing strategies from pharmaceutical groups that include free drug-labeled paraphernalia, continuing education, and food.

In 2002, PhRMA released a marketing code in response to criticism of how pharmaceuticals are marketed to healthcare providers, and a revision will be implemented in 2009 that recommends major changes in the promotion of products. For example, even pens and pads with the name of the drugs are to be strictly limited or stopped; dinners or other activities for prescribers and family members are curtailed; and independent continuing education sponsored by pharmaceutical companies will be promoted separate from marketing. PhRMA feels that these changes will enhance the professionalism of the group and diminish concerns about the organization.

Legal Regulation of Prescriptive Authority

Although the creation of new drugs appears to be the privy of private industry, regulation is a major consideration in the development of drugs. In the United States, legal jurisdictions may be federal, state, or other groups. In general, the federal government usually is involved in pharmaceuticals through the FDA. The FDA has regulatory authority for prescription, nonprescription, and nondrug agents such as medical devices and infant formula. State or other jurisdictions regulate or license prescribers.

Prescriptive Authority

Physicians, veterinarians, dentists, and podiatrists generally are recognized prescribers in all states and territories. However, they are legally entitled to prescribe only in the state or location in which they are recognized. Physicians usually have no limitation as to type of prescriptions, but veterinarians, dentists, and podiatrists often are limited according to their scopes of practice. Within the last few decades, other prescribers have emerged in most states. Pharmacists have presented claims that they can be safe prescribers and should be integral members of the healthcare team. The burgeoning array of psychoactive agents has led to some governmental agencies recognizing psychologists and other mental health professionals as prescribers. Primary care providers such as physician assistants, nurse practitioners, midwives, and others now have prescriptive authority, although it usually is limited to scopes of practice and often is **delegated prescriptive authority** from a prescribing physician, which is more limited than full prescriptive authority.

Discussion has occurred regarding the state-based approach to prescriptive authority.[22] In the mid-1900s, it was logical to assume that a written prescription would be hand carried to the local pharmacy, where it was filled. Today it is common for a prescriber to electronically transmit a new prescription to a pharmacy, even if the pharmacy is just a few blocks away. But that pharmacy, even if close in proximity to the prescriber, also is likely to be a branch of a large conglomerate. Although the prescriber is authorized in one state, the individual may just as easily receive her medication from another branch, in another state, where she is vacationing more than 1500 miles away from the office of the prescriber. Moreover, the role of Internet pharmacies involves issues of legality. US pharmacies can operate online assuming the agents are FDA approved and a legal prescription is available. However, there are a number of reports of Internet pharmacies based out of the country, which do not require a prescription and illegally mail pharmaceuticals, including those not FDA approved, to individuals in the United States. Under these circumstances, such transport is considered illegal. These discussions add to the controversy as to whether or not it is time for a federal prescriptive authority to be developed.

Prescribing Controlled Substances

One example of prescriptive authority closely intertwined with federal laws is the prescription of drugs that are considered to have a high risk for addiction. Controlled substances are agents, both opiates and nonopiates, that are regulated by the US federal government. These agents generally are categorized according to schedules as found in Table 1-2.[23,24] Prescribers must have legal state authority to prescribe and also possess a number issued by the Drug Enforcement Administration (DEA) to prescribe controlled substances. Originally, prescribers were provided DEA numbers that began with the letter A, and since those numbers have been exhausted, most now start with the letter B. It is anticipated that the letter C will be the prefix in the near future. For physician assistants, nurses in advanced practice, midwives, and others, the DEA number begins with the letter M. The number of types of drugs that these healthcare professionals prescribe may be limited by a state according to state-devised schedules. DEA numbers are computer generated from a mathematical equation so that the sum of certain digits plus twice the sum of the remaining ones produce the final digit in the number. This complex system was devised in an attempt to enable pharmacists to identify forgeries. In reality, the equation can be found on the Internet,

Table 1-2 Schedules for Controlled Substances

Schedule	Description	Example
I	The drug or other substance has a high potential for abuse. The drug or other substance has no currently accepted use in treatment in the United States. There is lack of accepted safety for use of the drugs or other substance under medical supervision.	Heroin
II	The drug or other substance has a high potential for abuse. The drug or other substance has a currently accepted medical use in treatment in the United States. Abuse of the drug or other substance may lead to severe psychological or physical dependence.	Methadone, morphine
III	The drug or other substance has less potential for abuse than the drugs or other substances in schedules I and II. The drug or other substance has a currently accepted medical use in treatment in the United States. Abuse of the drug or other substance may lead to moderate or low physical dependence or high psychological dependence.	Amphetamines
IV	The drug or other substance has a low potential for abuse relative to the drugs or other substances in schedule III. The drug or other substance has a currently accepted medical use in treatment in the United States. Abuse of the drug or other substance may lead to limited physical dependence or psychological dependence relative to the drugs or other substances in schedule III.	Phenobarbital
V	The drug or other substance has a low potential for abuse relative to the drugs or other substances in schedule IV. The drug or other substance has a currently accepted medical use in treatment in the United States. Abuse of the drug or other substance may lead to limited physical dependence or psychological dependence relative to the drugs or other substances in schedule IV.	Acetaminophen with codeine

Source: United States Public Law 2007 December.[24]

and busy pharmacists have little time to do the necessary calculations, but the system continues.

Drug Testing and Approval

Drug testing and approval is regulated at the federal level.[23,24] Figure 1-1 provides a visual overview of the process. The FDA has several centers, including the Center for Drug Evaluation and Research, and it is through the Center for Drug Evaluation and Research that the FDA regulates the drug testing and approval processes. The following is a general description of how a new drug is studied, although some exceptions may occur.

An **investigational new drug** (IND) application is a legal method by which federal approval may be obtained to transport pharmaceuticals or medical devices to areas in which they may be used in **clinical trials**. These trials are financially supported by both the pharmaceutical company and the US National Institutes of Health. Ideally, clinical trials are randomized, double blinded, and placebo controlled.

Placebos (derived from Latin for *I will please*) are agents that have no active ingredients. The original intention was to provide an inactive agent to a control group of subjects and compare findings to another group of subjects who took an active pharmaceutical. It was theorized that only individuals taking an effective pharmaceutical would demonstrate change. However, the placebo effect has been found to be strong for subjective reports of both therapeutic effects and adverse effects. For example, women taking placebos for perimenopausal hot flashes commonly report an improvement of more than 30%, albeit less than the improvement with estrogen. In addition to use of placebos in drug testing, it would be helpful to have new drugs compared to current drugs in terms of safety and **efficacy**. In reality, these studies are rarely if ever conducted. It may be hypothesized that pharmaceutical companies are hesitant to risk comparisons to products from other manufacturers and certainly do not wish to incur the risk of comparison to their own current products, in which case at least one of their own products will perform less well than another.

When used in a clinical trial, the pharmaceutical agent is deemed to be part of a **new drug application** (NDA). In the past there has been criticism that companies may undertake multiple clinical trials to study one drug and only release data from those that successfully demonstrated effectiveness or safety. Currently, clinical trials are to be registered before data are obtained in an attempt to promote transparency.

Clinical Drug Trials

Three distinct phases of clinical testing are required for any NDA. Establishment of drug safety is a major factor involved in the testing. **Phase I trials** are designed to determine basic pharmacokinetics of the new drug. When established drugs are being proposed for new indications, previous studies may be used. Animal testing and in vitro models are still in active use. However, computer modeling and other technological modalities for evaluating the metabolism or toxicity of a drug have also been developed. Application of genomics, proteomics (the study of the

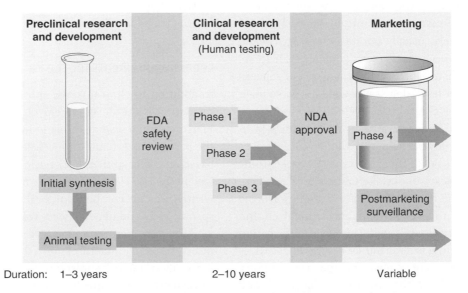

Figure 1-1 Steps required by the FDA for reviewing a new drug. *Source:* Reprinted with permission from Hanson GR et al. 2003.[23]

structure and functions of proteins), and computational approaches now allow scientists to predict the metabolites of molecules. These molecules are based on an agent's chemical structure, more accurately predict the pharmacodynamic activity of a drug and its metabolites, and integrate these predictions with human cell signaling and metabolic processes and networks. Toxicogenomic data can be included in this process.[25]

Once a promising pharmaceutical agent has been developed, toxic and therapeutic doses are determined. Animal testing is initially performed to evaluate drug safety, including determination of the dose range that results in adverse or toxic side effects. Animal testing protocols typically use two or more species in an attempt to control for interspecies differences in pharmacokinetics. The results of animal testing are used to determine the doses used in preliminary human testing and may be described in the drug product labeling or human trial documents. Unfortunately, cross-species pharmacokinetics are not consistent, and the results of animal testing are not always predictive of human response to a pharmaceutical agent.

Dose–response relationships describe the required dose and frequency of dosing based on the **therapeutic index** for a drug in a specific population (such as pregnant women, neonates, or nonpregnant reproductive-aged women). The therapeutic index is the dose range between the therapeutic dose and the toxic dose. Development of the therapeutic index determines the potential therapeutic value and safety of a drug. Increasing the dose of a drug with a narrow therapeutic index (e.g., theophylline) increases the probability of drug toxicity. Factors such as body mass index, metabolic rates, and genetics affect the therapeutic index for an individual. Human participants in Phase I studies are healthy individuals, usually adults of average weight and without chronic diseases. Persons younger than 18 are included only in pediatric focused trials, an area of concern for contraceptive studies. Adolescents aged 17 or younger are excluded from the clinical trials, yet women in this age range frequently need and use contraceptive products.

Phase II trials employ participants who have the disease or condition for treatment. Thus, they may have a chronic illness. **Phase III trials** are undertaken after there is indication of effectiveness in the smaller phase II studies. During Phase III, greater numbers of participants are involved, and risks and benefits are established. The basic information needed for drug labeling is determined during Phase III.

Phases I–III also are called preapproval studies. Controversy exists about the inherent subjectivity and difficulty involved in comparing the risks to the benefits in Phase III studies as compared to the risks and benefits

found in studies of the drug after it enters the general marketplace when larger numbers of persons are exposed, and uses in real life, such as taking it with other foods and drugs, are analyzed.[26]

Phase IV trials are known as postmarketing studies. No matter how rigorous Phase I–III studies are, wide postmarketing may reveal unexpected results. For example, if a Phase III trial had 3000 participants, but a major adverse effect occurs once in 10,000 individuals; postmarketing may be the only venue in which this adverse effect will be revealed. Also, drug–drug interactions may be first identified in postmarketing studies that include individuals who are taking other drugs as well as the one being evaluated. The 2007 FDA Amendment Act strengthened this section by increasing reporting of drug adverse effects, and it is anticipated that additional attention will be paid to this area in the future.

Untoward events or responses identified during the drug preapproval process are considered adverse drug reactions (a type of adverse drug event) when there is a reasonable possibility of association between the adverse event and the pharmaceutical agent. (See Chapter 2 for detailed information on adverse drug reactions.) During the postmarketing period, adverse reactions are adverse events that occur within the accepted therapeutic dose range of approved pharmaceutical agents. Adverse drug reactions may also occur between a drug and nonpharmaceutical agents such as synthetic chemicals, naturally occuring substances in the environment, or nutriceuticals. Serious adverse drug reactions may precipitate a life-threating illness or death that may be expected (dose related) or unexpected (idiosyncratic). These serious adverse effects also may be included in drug trial documents or product labeling.

Legal Requirements for the Package Insert

In addition to clinical trials, another important aspect of regulation is the development of the package insert. The FDA determines what information is to be contained in the package insert, and on occasion will mandate changes based on newer studies. Package inserts were first standardized in the late 1960s. One of the first package inserts to be written was for combination oral contraceptives in which specific risks and benefits were required to be included.

Although there is a standard format for the package insert, some manufacturers deviate slightly such as changing some of the titles into lower literacy to make it easier to read by those expected to use the agent. Among the required components are the brand/generic name of the drug; description of chemical structure, formulation, route of administration as well as inactive ingredients; clinical pharmacology, usually containing a synopsis of the clinical trials; approved indications; **contraindications**; warnings, including serious side effects; precautions, especially for drug–drug interactions; adverse drug reactions, including those that might be considered trivial; drug abuse and dependency potential; overdose; recommended dose; and how the agent is supplied, including constraints for storage. Since 2006, package inserts also must include "Highlights," a section that summarizes risks and benefits; a table of contents; the date of initial approval; and contact information (Web address and toll-free telephone number) to promote easier reporting of adverse reactions.[27]

Precautions may appear on package inserts and are different than contraindications. A contraindication specifies who should not take the drug. Persons who are allergic to a drug have a contraindication to its use because adverse reactions are very likely. However, precautions indicate that the drug should be used carefully by specific individuals who may be at a higher risk for an adverse effect than the general population. The transdermal contraceptive patch, marketed as Ortho Evra, has a precaution for women who weigh more than 90 kg or 198 pounds.[28] This precaution exists because there was some evidence that contraception is decreased among women who are heavier, although the strength of association is difficult to assess from the original studies, as participation was limited to women who were of a healthy weight or at least no more than 35% over the optimal weight.[28] Therefore, currently there are no strong data to mandate labeling a contraindication, but the precaution is included, which means the provider should discuss the situation with a woman who weighs more than 90 kg and is considering using the contraceptive transdermal patch.

FDA Warnings

FDA warnings are identification of areas of potential major consequences, both for individuals and for the manufacturer. After a drug is approved and marketed, the FDA continues to have a role. The manufacturer is legally required to review and report any adverse drug reaction to the FDA that is reported to the company. Unexpected serious reactions are to be reported within 15 days, the others on a quarterly basis as long as the drug is being marketed. The FDA also solicits direct reports from consumers and providers through a program called MedWatch. This system includes an online voluntary reporting form, which can be completed on the FDA Web site. Based on reports received, the FDA may choose to issue additional warnings as an addition or substitution to the initial package insert

warnings. When warnings are issued, they are placed on the FDA Web site and publicized through press releases; they may also be explained in letters directly sent to prescribers and included in the package inserts.

Postmarketing, large numbers of consumers are involved and the drugs are used in real-life situations that include the possibility of potential drug–drug, drug–food, or drug–herb interactions. Additional studies that demonstrate unexpected hazards may ensue. For example, in 1999, Merck and Company received approval to market a drug, Vioxx, their brand name for rofecoxib. Rofecoxib is a nonsteroidal anti-inflammatory drug (NSAID) that did not induce gastrointestinal irritation, a common side effect with the other NSAIDs available at the time. Subsequent studies suggested rofecoxib (Vioxx) was associated with increased risks of cardiovascular events.[29] There was a flurry of editorials questioning details about the original clinical trials after publication of one of these studies. One study in particular, sponsored by Merck, was conducted with the intention of assessing rofecoxib (Vioxx) for the additional indication of prevention of colorectal polyps, but it was terminated prematurely when it became apparent that the relative risk for myocardial infarctions and stroke were increased almost 100% among individuals on Vioxx compared to those taking the placebo (RR = 1.92; 95% CI, 1.19–3.11; P = .008).[29] Although the FDA was in discussion about the implications of these findings, Merck withdrew the drug from the marketplace, making FDA warnings moot.[29]

When a prescription drug is found to be associated with serious adverse reactions, including life-threatening risks, the FDA can require its strongest warning, or a **black box warning**. A black box warning is named such since there is a black border around the text of the warning in the package insert, and on the FDA Web site/publications. An example of a black box warning is the one mandated by the FDA for medroxyprogesterone acetate in oil (Depo-Provera). In 2004, such a warning was added to this contraception, advising women and providers that there was sufficient data to identify a relationship between prolonged use of the drug and loss of bone density. The new recommendation contained within the black box was that women should not use the agent for more than 2 years continuously unless other contraceptive methods were inadequate.

The most severe action that the FDA can take is to issue a **drug recall** from the market. Drug recalls or withdrawals are almost exclusively due to safety issues. As mentioned with Vioxx, some withdrawals are voluntary by the pharmaceutical company. A report in 2001 by the US General Accounting Office noted that the majority of drugs withdrawn between 1997 and 2001 had more pronounced adverse effects for women than men.[30] For some drugs, they are withdrawn from the market in the United States, but remain available in other countries or on the Internet.

Regulation of Direct-to-Consumer Advertising

Prior to 1997, the vast majority of pharmaceutical marketing in the United States consisted of educating healthcare professionals directly through visits by pharmaceutical representatives and exhibits at conferences or indirectly through advertisements in journals. However, controversy about marketing existed even at that time. A 1992 study with a group of experts using the FDA criteria of the time evaluated more than 100 drug ads and found that greater than 40% had misleading claims and 44% were deemed inadequate to be the sole source of information.[31]

In 1997, changes in the FDA regulations fostered advertising directly to consumers, an action only legalized in the United States and New Zealand.[32] Direct-to-consumer (DTC) ads are to follow the new FDA criteria and the organization has regulatory power over the content regarding prescription drugs. There are three types of DTC advertisements. The most common type is product claim advertisements, which include the brand name, indications, risks, and benefits. This type of DTC must conform to FDA criteria. Help-seeking advertisements or disease awareness communications discuss the condition, but do not name the drug and, therefore, are not regulated by the FDA. Reminder advertisements simply list the brand name, dose, or cost. They do not make claims or discuss indications and thus are also exempt from FDA regulation. Advertising for over-the-counter drugs is under the purview of the Federal Trade Commission.

DTC initially was advocated as an attempt to better educate consumers and ultimately promote appropriate use of medications. Manufacturers potentially could argue for some shared responsibility with a so-called well-educated consumer.[33] A review of a decade of such advertising found that DTC was firmly entrenched in US media, with the estimate that the average American sees 16 hours every year of these ads on television alone.[32] But it also was associated with problems such as potential overuse of medications; medicalization of common discomforts; and expenditures of more than $40 billion annually.[34] In 2005, the five most common DTC requests from consumers were related to prescription agents advertised for treatment of impotence, anxiety, arthritis, menopausal symptoms, and allergies.[35]

Over the years, the FDA has required some ads to be withdrawn. An ad for Viagra showing a "devilish" man falsely claimed that it could result in the same degree of sexual activity of years past. The manufacturer of Lamisil had to change the implication that it always was a totally successful treatment for nail infection. Claritin ads were changed to include risks as well as benefits. Yet some questions exist as to whether or not the FDA is doing enough to stop inaccurate or incomplete advertising. In 2008, the president-elect of the American Medical Association testified to a subcommittee of Congress that the FDA needed to more vigorously enforce the regulations, especially since there was some suggestion that the elderly and people of color were more susceptible to DTC.[36] However, there are no indications that DTC will be prohibited.

The Role of the Pharmacist

During the Middle Ages, the role of the apothecary was well established. These healthcare professionals were the forerunner of today's pharmacists. They read prescriptions and filled them with the appropriate remedy. Many of the treatments required mixing, or **compounding**. These providers developed the apothecary system of weights and measures, including the use of drams, scruples, and other terms replaced today primarily by the metric system. As the role evolved, most apothecaries entered the profession with a background in chemistry; hence they also were called dispensing chemists by some.

In order to be legally recognized as a pharmacist in the United States today, one must have graduated from a recognized program and received a doctor of pharmacology (Pharm D) degree. Pharmacists increasingly work collaboratively in hospital settings and in some areas have or are attempting to obtain a degree of prescriptive authority.[7] Pharmacists fill prescriptions, **dispense** the drugs (sometimes termed **furnish**), and counsel the individuals obtaining the agent. Counseling is an important aspect of the pharmacist's role today; it includes advising individuals taking either prescription or nonprescription drugs or both, particularly regarding how to safely take the agent(s); signs/symptoms of therapeutic as well as adverse effects; and the information about the emerging body of evidence on drug–drug, drug–food, and/or drug–herb interactions.

Drug Samples

Samples of agents, usually prescription drugs, are commonly found in ambulatory facilities. Healthcare providers should be aware if they are legally allowed to dispense these samples. Although some professionals claim that sampling allows the medically uninsured an alternative path for access to necessary agents, studies have found that sampling is a method of marketing, encouraging individuals to continue on a specific pharmaceutical for the course of the condition or disease, or health promotion.[37]

In addition to prescription drugs, several other types of agents exist. These include over-the-counter agents, generic agents, and even orphan drugs, all of which are discussed next.

Categories of Drugs

Not all drugs require a prescription, and not all prescription-only drugs are brand-name formulations made by large pharmaceutical companies. The various categories of drugs include over-the-counter, generic, orphan, and compounded agents.

Over-the-Counter Drugs

As opposed to drugs that require a legal prescription prior to purchase, over-the-counter (OTC) agents are pharmaceuticals that may be purchased by a consumer at a supermarket, airport, or other commercial site. Originally, prescription drugs were only available at the counters of pharmacies or apothecaries. Over-the-counter agents were found at the counters of general stores, hence the term. OTC agents are most commonly used for reasons or conditions that are usually considered minor and not an indication for medical consultation. OTC products rarely need detailed drug monitoring or have a major risk of addiction. Both OTC and prescription drugs are regulated by the FDA, although advertising of OTC agents is regulated by the Federal Communications Commission rather than the FDA. There are more than 80 drug categories of OTC agents, and millions are spent on these pharmaceuticals annually.

In the early 1970s the FDA called together panels of experts in order to evaluate the OTC agents at that time.[23] The FDA desired to reassure the public that all OTC drugs were both safe and effective. This was a major undertaking, as more than 300,000 products were available as OTC products and the number of ingredients was more than 1000. Eventually it was decided that the ingredients only would be assessed. An OTC monograph system was devised so that the drugs determined to be **generally recognized as safe and effective** (GRAS/E) could remain on the market and not need to obtain an NDA, although options could be used should the manufacturer desire. Few pharmaceutical companies choose to expend the time and financial commitment associated with an NDA. Therefore, most

of the OTC products available today are well established pharmaceuticals. Aspirin is likely to be the most recognizable of the OTC agents. All OTC agents have specific labeling regulations including name, indication, dosing, warnings, and information for healthcare providers.

Although most OTC drugs have been available for years, the last few decades have seen a number of pharmaceuticals that have moved from prescription-only to OTC status. After a drug has been available by prescription and has an established record of safety, and usually when the patent is about to expire, manufacturers may seek to obtain permission to move the agent to the OTC market. Although the manufacturer may sell the agents more cheaply on the OTC market than by prescription, more drugs are sold overall and they have an opportunity to develop a brand following. Consumers tend to like OTC agents because of the decreased cost of the drugs when on the open market, as well as the provision of various self-care therapies. Antisecretory antihistamines originally used for ulcer treatment and marketed for OTC treatment of heartburn (pyrosis) such as cimetidine (Tagamet) moved from prescription-only status to OTC in 1995. Other popular drugs that are now OTC include nonsedating antihistamines like loratadine (Claritin) and cetirizine hydrochloride (Zyrtec). Discussion has ensued regarding the possibility of more agents being switched, especially statins, because some other countries have done so or are considering such a change.[38]

Because of either the length of time/wide availability of the OTC agents or the scrutiny involved with prescription agents before they became OTC, few problems have been noted with OTC drugs. One notable exception was the FDA mandate in 2000 to withdraw phenylpropanolamine (PPA), a common ingredient in both cold remedies and weight loss agents. It is of note that PPA was found not only to be associated with hemorrhagic stroke, but this risk was higher in women compared to men. In 2007, manufacturers voluntarily removed OTC cough and cold remedies for infants after the FDA released information about both the ineffectiveness of the agents and the risk of overdose.

Another OTC agent, pseudoephedrine, has initiated a new term, **behind the counter** (BTC). Pseudoephedrine remains an OTC agent, because no prescription is needed to purchase it. However, this drug can be used with other substances to produce methamphetamine for illicit use. Moving it from an easily accessible open shelf to a location behind the pharmacy counter allows a pharmacist or other individual to obtain identification and record each purchase. The intention is that abuse could be tracked, yet consumers who legitimately wish to use the drug can continue to do so.

Generic Drugs

Generic drugs are pharmaceuticals that contain the same active ingredients found in the original brand formulation. More than 60% of prescriptions are filled with generic drugs.[39] Generics must be demonstrated to be **bioequivalent**, or have identical pharmacokinetics and pharmacodynamics. These drugs usually emerge after patent protections for the original brands have expired, usually 7–12 years after first commercial production or 20 years after the first application for FDA consideration. According to the 1984 Drug Price Competition and Patent Term Restoration Act (Hatch-Waxman Act) an applicant desiring to market a generic agent files an **abbreviated new drug application** (ANDA) with the FDA. Scientific materials that support the bioequivalence of the generic to the brand are presented, and when the ANDA is approved, the **approved drug** is added to the FDA Approved Drug Products list (sometimes called the *Orange Book*) with an annotation to illustrate the equivalency. Prior to 1984, manufacturers of generics had to conduct the same testing that the pharmaceutical companies performed for the original brand-named drug, making generics rare on the marketplace because of the cost of these studies.

In the majority of states, when a pharmacist fills a prescription, that professional may substitute a generic drug for the equivalent brand name. Although generics are bioequivalent, some prescribers choose to note that no substitution is allowed and in that case the pharmacist must furnish the brand-name agent. Several states have codified these actions in a formulary, either negative or positive. A **positive formulary** is a list of drugs for which generics may be substituted; a **negative formulary** is one in which the list indicates brand names for which generics may not be substituted. Lanoxin and Synthroid are two brand names commonly under a negative formulary, although most research suggests bioequivalence with the generic forms.

Although generic drugs cost a manufacturer far less than the costs paid by the original manufacturer, profit margins also are likely to be lower. When a generic drug is released, it is accepted that it has the same dosing, route of administration, effectiveness, risks, benefits, and indications as the original drug. An FDA project, the Generic Initiative for Value and Efficiency (GIVE), was initiated in 2007 in an attempt to decrease the time involved in the generic drug approval process.

Orphan Drugs

Occasionally there is a relatively rare medical condition (affecting fewer than 200,000 individuals) that can be treated by a pharmaceutical agent. The drugs used to treat these rare conditions, called **orphan drugs**, are the antithesis of blockbuster drugs and may cost too much to interest most pharmaceutical houses. Some incentive is provided to companies that will develop and manufacture orphan drugs, including selected federal grants, as well as an exclusive 7-year period on the marketplace. In the future, pharmacogenomics may increase the number of orphan drugs.

Compounded Formulations

In years past, pharmacists mixed together pharmaceutical compounds instead of filling a prescription with pills sealed in blister packs. The process of mixing a pharmaceutical remedy, especially for a specific individual, is known as compounding. Although few pharmacists practice compounding today, the number appears to be growing. Some of the reasons for this growth are to avoid inactive ingredients that may be allergens such as glutin; transform solid formulations into more easily swallowed liquids; and produce bioidentical hormones, which are formulations of hormones that have varying potencies. Discussion of such therapies can be found in Chapter X. However, there are regulatory issues involved in compounding.

Compounding pharmacies are regulated in the same manner as other pharmacies. Moreover, there have been arguments that large compounding pharmacies are becoming indistinguishable from pharmaceutical companies. Based on that argument, compounds should be evaluated in the same way that new drugs are assessed. In 2006, a court ruling from US District Court for the Western District of Texas found that compounding pharmacies are not under FDA regulation. However, upon appeal in 2008, the United States Court of Appeals for the Fifth Circuit rejected that finding and issued a judgment that compounded drugs should be subject to similar regulations by the FDA for new drugs. Currently there is discussion of potential pursuit to the Supreme Court. In any case it is likely that the controversy about FDA regulation of compounding will continue for some time.

Special Populations

Clinical Trials and Women

Until the 1990s, women of childbearing age frequently were excluded from clinical drug trials due to their potential for pregnancy and the related risk of inadvertent embryonic or fetal exposure to drugs. The disadvantage of this exclusion is that even commonly prescribed drugs frequently have never been evaluated for the presence of gender-related adverse effects or appropriate dosing for women.

Statistically, women have a higher incidence of adverse drug reactions than men.[40,41] For this reason, since the 1991 inception of the US Office of Women's Health, researchers have been encouraged to include of women as participants in clinical drug trials and analyze trial data by gender. Inclusion of women as participants in clinical trials offers researchers the opportunity to evaluate gender-related differences that influence disease prevalence, presentation, and response to pharmacologic therapy. Analysis of these differences provides insight into the biologic processes that contribute to gender differences in disease presentation and the responses to pharmacologic therapies. Understanding these differences offers new direction for future research.

Pregnancy and the FDA

In 1980, the FDA published a description of five categories that ranked the risk of teratogenic effects of pharmaceutical agents to be used in drug labeling. This list of five discrete **pregnancy categories** can be found in Table 1-3 and is unique to the United States. Other countries have either similar categories or use a narrative approach to describe information available about the drugs. Contrary to popular belief, the FDA does not assign the category to a specific drug. Instead, the manufacturer generally uses the FDA categorization and assigns the letter. Because of the degree of evidence that the FDA requires, few drugs fall into Pregnancy Category A. Most agents that are commonly used are in Pregnancy Category B. Pregnancy Category C is the most problematic of the categories because it actually contains two separate concepts. The agent may be categorized as FDA Pregnancy Category C because there have been reports of teratogenicity in animals. For example, glucocorticosteroids are Pregnancy Category C because rabbits have demonstrated embryotoxic and fetotoxic effects after exposure to the drug, although no such findings have been reported in humans. However, far more common than animal teratogenicity is the other concept in Pregnancy Category C—namely, lack of information. It is for this reason that most drugs fall into Pregnancy Category C; and it is because of this vagueness that the categorization system is problematic. Critics have been advocating a new system for several decades primarily because of the difficulty determining what the teratogenic risk is for drugs in Pregnancy Category C.

The current categories can also mislead healthcare providers because teratogenic risk does not necessarily increase as the categories move from A to X. Pregnancy Categories C, D, and X are based on risk weighed against

Table 1-3 Current FDA Categorization for Drug Use During Pregnancy

FDA Pregnancy	Description
A	Adequate, well-controlled studies in pregnant women have not shown an increased risk of fetal abnormalities.
B	Animal studies have revealed no evidence of harm to the fetus; however, there are no adequate and well-controlled studies in pregnant women. or Animal studies have shown an adverse effect, but adequate and well-controlled studies in pregnant women have failed to demonstrate a risk to the fetus.
C	Animal studies have shown an adverse effect and there are no adequate and well-controlled studies in pregnant women. or No animal studies have been conducted and there are no adequate and well-controlled studies in pregnant women.
D	Studies, adequate well-controlled or observational, in pregnant women have demonstrated a risk to the fetus. However, the benefits of therapy may outweigh the potential risk.
X	Studies, adequate well-controlled or observational, in animals or pregnant women have demonstrated positive evidence of fetal abnormalities. The use of the product is contraindicated in women who are or may become pregnant.

Source: Federal Regist 1980.[43]

benefits, which means a particular drug labeled FDA Pregnancy Category C may engender the same risks that a drug labeled FDA Pregnancy Category X engenders but have more benefits.[42]

The last two categories are relatively clear. Both categories D and X are used to label agents that are associated with human teratogenicity. However, an FDA Pregnancy Category D may be recommended for use by pregnant women because the risk of nontreatment outweighs the risk of the teratogenic effects. For example, many antiepileptic drugs may be continued during pregnancy in spite of the risk of known congenital anomalies such as cleft palate with the assumption that surgical repair of a cleft palate is less of a threat to the fetus/newborn than prolonged anoxic events associated with seizures. Pregnancy Category X is reserved for the few agents that are known teratogens for which either alternative nonteratogenic agents exist, or that treat conditions that are not serious. Acne is an example of a condition that is not life threatening, but retinoids can cause lifelong congenital effects to the intrauterine conceptus and should never be used by pregnant women.

In 2008, a new system for the pregnancy and lactation section of drug labeling was proposed. The proposed system omits the letter categories in the FDA pregnancy categories. If this system is adopted as presented, there will be three separate sections that include information using a narrative format. "Fetal Risk Summary," the first section, will address effects of the drug on a human fetus or animal fetus. The data are to specifically include known risks. For example, the following statement might appear in this section of the labeling, "Human data indicate that drug *A* increases the risk of limb deformities." The second section, "Clinical Considerations," will review known information about exposure prior to the woman recognizing she is pregnant; risks of not treating the disease this specific drug is used for, including potential teratogenic effects associated with the untreated condition; dosing information; and additional information about complications in a separate section, "Data," that will consist of detailed data about the studies used to develop the fetal risk summary. The pregnancy section of the label would also include whether or not a pregnancy exposure registry exists.

An additional new feature is the proposed addition of drug information in the section on lactation. Prior to this suggested rule, there was no federal categorization of the risk to newborns from drugs used by a woman who is breastfeeding. It should be noted that this proposed rule only addresses drugs under FDA regulation and does not include nutritional supplements, pesticides, or other chemicals.

As this chapter is being written, it is unclear if the proposed rule will be adopted as is, modified in some way, or rejected out of hand. Even if a new system for FDA categorization of drugs for pregnant and lactating women is adopted, it will take years for all current pharmaceutical labeling to be changed. Therefore, throughout this text, the current, or 1979 FDA categories are used.[43]

Clinical Trials and the Elderly

Current rules regarding clinical drug trials necessitate that the published reports include the demographics of the subjects, including age, gender, and racial/ethnic backgrounds. Clearly, age is a major factor that must be involved in analysis because older individuals are more likely than younger persons to have a history of previous exposures to pharmaceuticals, multiple pathologic conditions; biologic variations in pharmacokinetics, and use other agents (i.e., to be a polypharmacy user). Polypharmacy includes over-the-counter or herbal/botanical formulations. Multiple agents increase the risk of drug–drug or drug–herb and drug–food interactions. Therefore, the elderly are not restricted from participation in clinical trials and should be encouraged to enroll.

Medication Errors

In 1999, the US Institute of Medicine released a study estimating that more than 90,000 individuals die in hospitals annually due to errors in the delivery of care.[44] Among these errors are many that are associated with pharmaceuticals, which are termed **medication errors**.

Approximately 7000 deaths occur annually in the United States specifically due to medication errors, almost exclusively among prescription drugs. More than 1.5 million people experience side effects, adverse drug events, or adverse drug reactions, costing approximately $3.5 billion each year.[45] Although these effects have been estimated in the hospital to occur with fewer than 0.5% of medication orders, more than a quarter of them were considered preventable.[44] Adverse drug events in ambulatory facilities may even be higher. A study by Gandhi and colleagues in 2003 surveyed more than 1000 individuals who had received a prescription within the previous 4 weeks. They found 13% of respondents had an adverse drug effect, far higher than those reported in the Institute of Medicine studies, and estimated that 20% of those were preventable.[46]

A suggested intervention to decrease medication error is to use computerized ordering or electronic charting. Illegibility increases the risk of a person receiving the wrong drug or dose. E-prescribing, or electronic prescribing, was recognized in the 2003 Medicare Prescription Drug Improvement and Modernization Act, but rates of implementation have been estimated to be as low as 5%.[47]

How to Write a Prescription

A standard prescription contains several components. A prescription should include the name, credentials, and contact information for the prescriber; the name and identifying information for the person for whom the prescription is written; the superscription or Rx insignia (derived from an abbreviation for the Latin for *recipe* or *take*); the inscription or generic name of the drug with dose; the subscription or directions to the individual filling the prescription; the signature, which is from the Latin *signetur* or "let it be labeled," that details how the person for whom the drug is intended should use it; and lastly it should be signed by the authorized prescriber. Today it is recommended that all prescriptions are written in English with no or minimal abbreviations. In particular, most

Latin abbreviations should be avoided, as they often can be misinterpreted. For example, *qod* indicates every other day, but can be misread as *qid*, resulting in eight administrations over a 48-hour period, as opposed to one. Some abbreviations exist in common usage and may continue to be seen, including in texts. These standard abbreviations include *PO* (for oral administration or by mouth); *bid, tid, qid* (for twice daily or three or four times daily, respectively); *prn* (for as needed); as well as metric abbreviations such as *mg* and *mL* for milligrams and milliliters. Many facilities commonly have a list of acceptable abbreviations for charting as well as prescriptions. Box 1-1 lists recommendations to decrease medication errors when writing a prescription, and Figure 1-2 illustrates the components of a sample prescription.

Box 1-1 Recommendations to Decrease Medication Errors when Writing a Prescription

Use

Both numbers as words and numerals (e.g., 60 [sixty] tablets)

Clear writing, print in ink, or type

Correct spelling (especially in an era of drugs with similar names)

English whenever possible instead of Latin

Specific times (e.g., 8 AM) if possible

Standard format, especially on preprinted blanks

The most common formulation (e.g., 500 mg instead of 0.5 g)

A zero prefix with decimals less than 1 (e.g., 0.5 mg)

The abbreviation *mL* instead of *ccs* because *mL* is less likely to be misread

Avoid

Trailing zeros in decimals (e.g., 5.00)

Unusual measurements such as teaspoons, tablespoons, pints, ounces, drams, grains, minims

Vagueness (e.g., *prn*—at minimum, write "as needed *for pain*")

The Advent of Rational Prescribing

Due to the complexity and seriousness involved with prescribing the appropriate agent for an individual, a rational approach has been advocated.[48] Several definitions exist for rational prescribing, as well as various examples. In general, rational prescribing includes the following four goals: (1) maximizing effectiveness of an agent; (2) minimizing side effects and risks; (3) minimizing cost; and (4) customizing the agent for an individual.[49] Customization today includes consideration of an individual's lifestyle, insurance drug benefits (if any), and desire. For example, use of an injectable pharmaceutical may be a problem for a woman with severe arthritis in her hands. When prescribing a statin for a mature woman, it would be wise to ask if her partner also is taking a statin. If so, the prescriber should consider using the same drug for the woman with the assumption that the couple may drug share, even though all individuals are warned not to do so. The two individuals also may share knowledge about the drug and be more likely to remember the name and dosing of the agent.

The prescriber should keep in mind that rational prescribing is PERSON centered. The acronym *PERSON* denotes pragmatics, effectiveness, route/dose, safety, options, and needs/desires. *Pragmatics* is described above with the example of prescribing a statin that already is used in the home. The homeless have no access to refrigerators, and, therefore, prescribing a drug for a person with diabetes that requires a low temperature for storage is irrational. *Effectiveness* is essential. If an agent is not effective, then it should not be prescribed at all. The effect desired also should be considered, such as, is it meant to be curative, prophylactic, or simply to reduce symptoms or act palliatively. *Route* and dose need to be considered. Although most drugs have wide therapeutic indices for safety, toxicity and poisonings still can occur, especially if doses or pathologic issues such as kidney or liver dysfunction, especially with the elderly, are not taken into account. Toxicity is discussed in detail in Chapter 4. Some individuals are unable to swallow and need transdermal, topical, or parental agents. *Safety*, like effectiveness, is an essential consideration. The potential adverse effects and contraindications must be weighed against the disease condition, whether present or potential. Medications for women in special populations such as pregnancy and lactation should be carefully considered. Interactions between the agent and other drugs, herbs, or foods need to be addressed. *Options* include consideration of other pharmaceutical agents as well as

Mary Breckinridge, CNM Certified Nurse-Midwife UCSF Women's Health UC # 54321 NPF: 1234-789	Kate Smith MD Obstetrician/Gynecologist UCSF Women's Health BNDD No. AS345678 CA Lic. No. F28765

Name: Jenny Jones   Age: 24

Address: 326 Orange Vale Road, Fair Oaks, Ca   Date: 10-10-2009

℞   Metronidazole 500 mg tablets
            sig: twice daily for 7 (seven) days
            disp: 14 (fourteen)

Indication: Bacterial vaginosis

Refills: ⓪ 1 2 3 4 5

Allergies: None

Dispense as written ☐

Label: English ☒ Spanish ☐ Other _____

Mary Breckinridge
_____
Signature

Figure 1-2 Sample prescription.

nonpharmaceutical agents like exercise and nutrition. Less costly generics should be possible agents. Knowledge of the marketplace enables a prescriber to know when it is less expensive to prescribe a generic than buy it over the counter, or when agents are covered by drug benefits. *Needs and desires* of the woman also should be considered. Some women will accept a prescription for a suppository but never fill it because of personal distaste for the procedure. A woman may request a scopolamine patch just in case for a planned cruise or prefer a certain kind of packaging for ease of use.

Monitoring is an important additional component in rational prescribing. The response of the individual helps determine future treatments. For example, optimally a drug should result in a positive therapeutic response. However, adverse effects may dictate a modification of the drug regimen, and toxic effects may require complete discontinuation. Irrational prescribing is never intended, but often occurs because our healthcare system today is both complex and busy. Intentional engagement of the goals and approaches to rational prescribing is of value to the entire modern society.

Ethics and Prescribing Drugs

By definition, ethical dilemmas have no simple answer. Much of the discussion about ethical use of drugs concentrates on isolated specifics such as **pharmacotherapeutics**, or use of a drug as treatment for specific conditions. However, just as drugs have an important role in economics, they also have major ethical implications. It is beyond the scope of this chapter to explore ethics and drug use in detail. However, the healthcare professional should consider how to personally approach a variety of issues including prescribing for one's family; prescribing for oneself; selling nutritional supplements or other nonprescription items within one's office; use of placebos; support of selling agents overseas that are not marketed in the United States because of lack of effectiveness or risk of adverse effects; providing free samples of drugs; or acceptance of gifts from pharmaceutical companies, regardless of how minor the cost might be.[37,50,51] The interested reader is referred to recent reviews of this topic.[52,53,54]

Conclusion

Drugs are ubiquitous in modern society. Many medications have provided health, help, and hope for women. Unfortunately, some agents also have resulted in harm. Medicalization of conditions often has led women to seeking pharmaceuticals as first-line treatment, whether or not other options may be as effective and even safer. To promote the health of modern society, drugs should be addressed in a rational, legal, and ethical manner.

References

1. Daemmrich A, Bowden ME. A rising drug industry. Chem Eng News 2005;83(25):28–42.
2. Centers for Disease Control and Prevention. Vaccination coverage among children entering school: United States 2005–06 school year. MMWR 2006;55 (41);1124–6.
3. Lerner BH. Revisiting the death of Eleanor Roosevelt: was the diagnosis of tuberculosis missed? Int J Tuberc Lung Dis 2001;5(12):1080–5.
4. Oats JA. The science of drug therapy. In: Brunton LL, Lazo JJ, Parker KL, eds. Goodman & Gilman's the pharmacological basis of therapeutics. New York: McGraw-Hill; 2006:117–36.
5. Brandt AM. FDA regulation of tobacco: pitfalls and possibilities. N Engl J Med 2008;359(5):444–8.
6. Curfman GD, Morrissey S, Drazen JM. The FDA and tobacco regulation. N Engl J Med 2008;359:1056–7.
7. Abood RR. Pharmacy practice and the law. 5th ed. Sudbury, MA: Jones and Bartlett, 2008.
8. Law J. Big pharma. New York: Carroll & Graf; 2006.
9. National Center for Health Statistics. Health, United States, 2004, with chartbook on trends in the health of Americans. Hyattsville, Maryland: Government Printing Office, 2004.
10. Stagnitti MN. Trends in outpatient prescription drug utilization and expenditures, 1997 and 2004. Rockville, MD: Agency for Healthcare Research and Quality; 2007 April. 6 p. MEPS Statistical Brief No.168.
11. Danzon PM, Furukawa MF. Prices and availability of pharmaceuticals: evidence from nine countries. Health Aff 2003;3:521–36.
12. Consumer Healthcare Products Association. OTC retail sales 1964–2007. Available from: *www.chpa-info.org/content.aspx?id=115&pid=77&cc=6* [Accessed September 22, 2008].
13. Himmelstein DU, Warren E, Thorne D, Woolhandler S. Illness and injury as contributors to bankruptcy. Health Aff 2006;25(2):74–83.
14. Poisal JA, Truffer C, Smith S, Sisko A, Cowan C, Keehan S, et al. Health spending projections through 2016: modest changes obscure Part D's impact. Health Aff 2007;26(2):242–53.
15. Fortune 500: Our annual ranking of America's largest corporations. Fortune 2008 May:21.
16. Lyles A, Palumbo FB. The effect of managed care of prescription drug costs and benefits. Pharmacoeconomics 1999;15:129–40.
17. Wagner TH, Heisler M, Piette JD. Prescription drug co-payments and cost-related medication underuse. Health Econ Policy Law 2008;3:51–67.
18. Madden JM, Graves AJ, Zhang F, Adams AS, Briesacher BA, Ross-Degnan D, et al. Cost-related medication nonadherence and spending on basic needs following implementation of Medicare Part D. JAMA 2008;299(16):1922–8.
19. Lamb E. Top 200 prescription drugs of 2007. Pharm Times 2008;(5):20–3.
20. Gardiner P, Graham R, Legedza AT, Ahn AC, Eisenberg DM, Phillips RS. Factors associated with herbal therapy use by adults in the United States. Altern Ther Health Med 2007;13(2):22–9.
21. Wilke RA, Rief DM, Moore JH. Combinatorial pharmacogenetics. Nat Rev Drug Discov 2005;4(11):911–8.
22. Gerber DJ. Prescriptive authority: global markets as a challenge to national regulatory systems. Houston J Int Law 2004;26:287.
23. Hanson GR, Venturelli PJ, Fleckenstein AE. Drugs and society. Sudbury, MA: Jones and Bartlett, 2006.
24. United States Public Law Title 21 Code of Federal Regulations (CFR) Part 1300 to 21 CFR §1308.
25. Ekins S, Andreyev S, Ryabov A, Kirillov E, Rakhmatulin EA, Sorokina S, et al. A combined approach to drug metabolism and toxicity assessment. Drug Metab Dispos 2006;34:495–503.
26. Fleming TR. Identifying and addressing safety signals in clinical trials. N Engl J Med 2008;359(13):1400–2.
27. FDA. Two guidances for industry on the content and format of labeling for human prescription drug and

biological products. Federal Regist 2006; Docket Nos. 2OOOD–1306.

28. Audet MC, Moreau M, Koltun WD, Walbaum AS, Shangold G, Fisher AC, et al. Ortho Evra/Evra 004 study group. Evaluation of contraceptive efficacy and cycle control of a transdermal contraceptive patch vs. an oral contraceptive: a randomized controlled trial. JAMA 2001;285(18):2347–54.

29. Bresalier RS, Sandler RS, Quan H, Bolognese JA, Oxenius B, Horgan K, et al. Adenomatous polyp prevention on Vioxx (APPROVe) trial investigators. Cardiovascular events associated with rofecoxib in a colorectal adenoma chemoprevention trial. N Engl J Med 2005;352(11):1092–102.

30. Heinrich J. Drug safety: most drugs withdrawn in recent years had greater risks for women. Washington DC: United States General Accounting Office, 2001. GAO 01–286R.

31. Wilkes MS, Doblin BH, Shapiro MF. Pharmaceutical advertisements in leading medical journals: experts' assessments. Ann Intern Med 1992;116(11):912–9.

32. Frosch DL, Krueger PM, Hornick RC, Cronholm PF, Barg FK. Creating demand for prescription drugs: a content analysis of television direct-to-consumer advertising. Ann Fam Med 2007;5(1):6–13.

33. Mello MM, Rosenthal M, Neumann PJ. Direct-to-consumer advertising and shared liability for pharmaceutical manufacturers. JAMA 2003;289:477–81.

34. Donohue JM, Cevasco M, Rosenthal MB. A decade of direct-to-consumer advertising of prescription drugs. N Engl J Med 2007;357:673–81.

35. Berndt ER. To inform or persuade direct-to-consumer advertising of prescription drugs. N Engl J Med 2005;352:325–8.

36. US House Committee on Energy and Commerce. Testimony 2008. Available from: *http://energycommerce.house.gov/cmte_mtgs/110-oi-hrg.050808.DTC.shtml* [Accessed January 8, 2009].

37. Cutrona SL, Woolhandler S, Lasser KE, Bor DH, McCormick D, Himmelstein DU. Characteristics of recipients of free prescription drug samples: a nationally representative analysis. Am J Public Health 2008;98(2):284–9.

38. Cohen JP, Paquette C, Cairns CP. Switching prescription drugs to over the counter. BMJ 2005;330;39–41.

39. Frank RG. The ongoing regulation of generic drugs. N Engl J Med 2007;357(20):1993–7.

40. Gomes ER, Demoly P. Epidemiology of hypersensitivity drug reactions. Curr Opin Allergy Clin Immunol 2005;5:309–16.

41. Zopf Y, Rabe C, Neubert A, Gassmann KG, Rascher W, Hahn EG, et al. Women encounter ADRs more often than do men. Eur J Clin Pharmacol 2008 Oct; 64(10):999–1004.

42. Doering PL, Botthby LA, Cheok M. Review of pregnancy labeling of prescription drugs: is the current system adequate to inform of risks? Am J Obstet Gynecol 2002;187:337–9.

43. Federal Regist 1980;44: 37434–67.

44. Kohn LT, Corrigan JM, Donaldson MS. To err is human: building a safer health system. Washington, DC: National Academy Press, 2000.

45. Dunham DP, Makoul G. Improving medication reconciliation in the 21st century. Curr Drug Safety 2008;3(3):227–9.

46. Gandhi TK, Weingart SN, Borus J, Seger AC, Peterson J, Burdick E, et al. Adverse drug events in ambulatory care. N Engl J Med 2003;348(16):1556–64.

47. McGarth D. E-prescribing. J Med Pract Manage 2008;24(1);50–2.

48. Flockhart DA, Usdin-Yasuda S, Pezzullo JC, Knollmann BC. Teaching rational prescribing: a new clinical pharmacology curriculum for medical schools. Naunyn Schmeidebergs Arch Pharmacol 2002;336(1):33–43.

49. Thomas LJ, Coleman JJ. The medic's guide to prescribing: rational prescribing. Student BMJ 2007;15:133–68.

50. Adams J. Prescribing: the ethical dimension. Nurse Prescriber 2006;1(7); e22–4.

51. Cutrona SL, Woolhandler S, Lasser KE, Bor DH, McCormick D, Himmelstein DU. Characteristics of recipients of free prescription drug samples: a nationally representative analysis. Am J Public Health 2008;98(2):284–9.

52. Crigger NJ. Pharmaceutical promotions and conflict of interest in nurse practitioner's decision making: the undiscovered country. J Am Acad Nurse Pract 2005;17:201–212.

53. American Medical Association Journal of Ethics. Virtual mentor 2006;8:357–436. Available from: *http://virtualmentor.ama-assn.org/2006/06/toc-0606.html* [Accessed January 8, 2009].

54. Santoro MA, Gorrie TM. Ethics and the pharmaceutical industry. Cambridge, NY, Cambridge University Press, 2005.

2

"Before a man can be in any capacity to speak on any subject, 'tis necessary he be acquainted with it."
JOHN LOCKE (1632–1704), *SOME THOUGHTS CONCERNING EDUCATION*

Principles of Pharmacology

Laura Williford Owens, Robin Webb Corbett, and Tekoa L. King

Chapter Glossary

Absorption Movement of drug particles from GI tract to systemic circulation by passive absorption, active transport, or pinocytosis.

Adverse drug reaction Any noxious, unintended, and undesired effect of a drug that occurs at doses used in humans for prophylaxis, diagnosis, or therapy.

Affinity The degree of attraction between a drug and a receptor. The greater the attraction, the greater the extent of binding.

Agonist A drug that stimulates a response when bound to a receptor.

Agonist-antagonist A drug that has agonist properties for one opioid receptor and antagonist properties for a different type of opioid receptor.

Antagonist Drugs that prevent a response when bound to a receptor.

Bioavailability Percentage of administered drug available to target tissues.

Bioequivalence Two products are bioequivalent if their bioavailabilities fall within 80–125% of the reference drug. If two products are bioequivalent, one can be substituted for the other.

Biotransformation Chemical changes a substance undergoes in the body.

Blood–brain barrier Characteristic of the capillaries surrounding the brain that creates a natural barrier to the exchange of drugs between the systemic circulation and the circulation in the central nervous system.

Chronobiology (chronopharmacology) Synonym for chronopharmacology or use of knowledge of circadian rhythms to time administration of drugs for maximum benefit and minimal harm.

Clearance The measure of the body's ability to eliminate a drug.

Competitive antagonist Drug or ligand that reversibly binds to receptors at the same receptor site that agonists use (active site) without activating the receptor to initiate a reaction.

Cytochrome P450 (CYP450) Generic name for the family of enzymes that are responsible for most drug metabolism reactions.

Dissolution Disintegration of solid drugs (tablets) into small particles in the GI tract to dissolve into a liquid.

Distribution Process by which a drug becomes available to body fluids and body tissues.

Dose–response relationship (or dose–response curve) The change in response caused by different doses of a drug. Dose–response curves help determine safe doses for drugs.

Drug–drug interaction Modification of effect of a drug when administered with another drug.

Drug–food interaction Altered drug effect when certain foods or liquids are taken at the same time or in close proximity to a drug.

Drug–herb interactions Altered drug effect when certain herbs are taken at the same time or in close proximity to a drug.

Efficacy The potential maximum therapeutic response.

Elimination Removal of most drugs or their metabolites whereby they are changed to a water-soluble form, which is primarily removed via the kidneys; lesser routes include liver, bile, feces, saliva, lungs, sweat, and breast milk.

Enteric coated Drug coating to prevent release and absorption of a drug in the stomach.

Excretion Elimination of a drug from the biologic system.

Extended release (sustained release or slow release) Drug is designed to release over an extended period of time.

Extensive metabolizer A person with a normal response to the standard dose of a specific drug.

First pass metabolism (first pass effect) Drug metabolism that occurs as a drug passes through the intestinal lumen, portal vein, and liver prior to getting to the target organ. Also known as hepatic first pass.

G protein coupled receptor Type of cell membrane receptor. The drug binds with a receptor, which binds with guanosine triphosphate (GTP) and activates an effector (enzyme).

Half-life The time it takes for one-half of the drug concentration to be eliminated from the body (t½).

Inducer A drug that stimulates production of the enzyme, which, in turn, rapidly metabolizes the substrate drug and can cause a decreased therapeutic effect.

Inhibitor A drug that prevents production of the enzyme, which, in turn, decreases metabolism of the substrate drug and can cause an increased plasma level and therefore an increased therapeutic effect or perhaps adverse effects.

Inverse agonist A drug that binds to receptors that have an intrinsic or basal activity, which results in antagonism of this basal activity and down-regulation of the receptor's effect. Antihistamines are inverse agonists.

Ligand The drug or chemical that binds to a specific receptor.

Lipophilic Drugs having a high affinity for fat.

Loading dose Large, initial drug dose administered.

Maximum effect Maximum drug effect. Varies by drug.

Metabolism Change in drug, primarily by the liver, into metabolites that are able to be eliminated.

Noncompetitive antagonist Drug or ligand that reversibly binds to a receptor at a site different from the active site used by agonists in which this binding causes a structural change that inhibits the agonist from binding to the active site. Thus they do not compete for the active binding site.

Partial agonist Drug molecule that elicits a partial pharmacologic response.

Peak levels The highest plasma drug concentration.

Pharmacodynamics The study of drug concentration and the recipient's response. The drug's effects, including the duration and the magnitude of the response in relationship to the drug dose.

Pharmacoepidemiology Study of the use of and effects of drugs in large groups of people.

Pharmacogenetics Study of drug action (efficacy and toxicity) that varies as a result of genetically determined factors.

Pharmacogenomics The study of how variations in the human genome affect the response to medications.

Pharmacokinetics Process of drug absorption, distribution, metabolism, and elimination.

Pharmacovigilance Science and study of detection, assessment, and prevention of adverse drug effects or drug-related issues.

Phase I reaction The first half of enzymatic metabolism that makes a drug water soluble so it can be excreted. Oxidation, hydrolysis, and/or reduction reactions.

Phase II conjugation reaction The second half of the drug metabolism process that makes the drug polar and finalizes the changes that make it water soluble.

Poor metabolizer A person with a CYP450 enzyme polymorphism who does not metabolize a specific drug as expected. Higher than normal plasma levels can occur.

Potency The concentration at which the drug elicits 50% of its maximal response.

Prodrug A biologically inactive or partially active drug that is changed as a result of the body's metabolism to an active drug.

Protein binding The fraction of total drug in the plasma that is bound to plasma proteins.

Receptor A protein or molecular complex that, when bound to a ligand (drug), either initiates a physiologic response or blocks the specific response that receptor normally stimulates.

Sensitivity The concentration of a drug required to induce 50% of the maximum effect. Sensitivity is determined by measuring the blood concentration of a drug and assessing the individual's response.

Side effect Physiologic response unrelated to the desired drug effects that occur with therapeutic doses of the medication. Side effects may be beneficial, and if they are negative, the negative effects are not a threat to health and usually resolve spontaneously. In some studies, side effects are reported as a type of adverse effects.

Steady state Concentration of drug in the systemic circulation that will be achieved when the drug is administered at a constant state.

Therapeutic effect Desired physiological or psychological response to a drug.

Therapeutic equivalence Two different drugs are therapeutically equivalent if they are pharmaceutically equivalent (contain same active ingredient at same dose) and they have the same clinical effect with regard to both safety and efficacy when administered under specified conditions. The FDA has criteria for determining therapeutic equivalence.

Therapeutic index Guideline that estimates the margin of safety of a drug through the use of a ratio that measures the effective dose in 50% of persons and/or animals and the lethal dose in 50% of subjects.

Therapeutic range (therapeutic window) Plasma drug concentration between the minimum effective concentration in the plasma for obtaining the desired drug action and the mean toxic concentration.

Threshold dose The lowest dose that initiates the desired response.

Toxicology Study of poisons, detection, effects, and treatment.

Ultrarapid metabolizer A person who metabolizes specific drugs more rapidly than most based on genetic polymorphisms in the CYP450 enzyme family.

Volume of distribution The relationship between the dose of the drug administered and the serum concentration after administration.

Xenobiotic A chemical found in an organism that is not normally produced or expected to be present. Drugs can be xenobiotics, but the term is more frequently used to refer to toxins and poisons.

Introduction

During life, the average woman will most likely take numerous medications, including prescription and nonprescription, and perhaps some natural medicinal substances such as herbs or other dietary supplements. These chemicals, via their action on physiologic processes, can be used to produce therapeutic benefit but can also cause toxic effects. This chapter reviews basic pharmacologic principles as applied to women's health.

The Nature of Drugs

Before a drug can elicit a physiologic response, the drug must be absorbed into the body and transported from a site of administration to the site of action. In most cases the chemical (or drug) interacts with a specific target or **receptor** in the biologic system. There are several different types of receptors in the body. Many of them are located on the cell membrane (Figure 2-1). For a drug to possess the ability to produce medical benefits, it must have the appropriate size, electrical charge, shape, and composition to interact with a receptor and produce an effect. Interestingly, most receptors in the body exist naturally as targets for endogenous chemicals (e.g., epinephrine, serotonin, estrogen). Thus, drugs used for medical purposes have some structural similarity to our own natural chemicals. Lastly, the chemical should be able to leave the biologic system (through elimination or inactivation) in a reasonable amount of time so that the drug's actions are not inappropriately long or permanent.

Drugs can be solid, liquid, or gaseous at room temperature. This physical nature of the chemical often determines the best route that the drug should be administered. Examples of routes of administration include intravenous (IV), intramuscular (IM), subcutaneous (SQ), inhalation or transdermal (TTS), and examples of enteral administration include oral (PO), rectal (PR), and

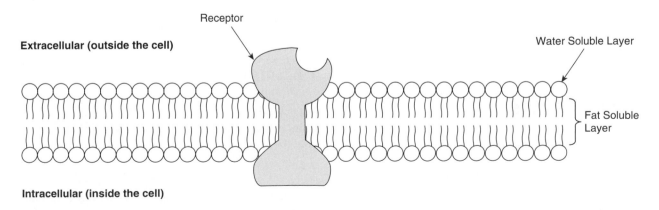

Figure 2-1 Cell membrane receptor.

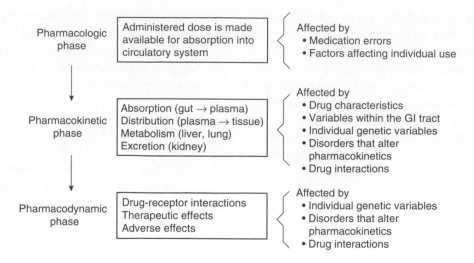

Figure 2-2 Factors that determine the intensity of drug responses.

sublingual. Routes of administration vary depending on the physiochemical properties (molecular weight, fat or water solubility, degree of ionization, etc.) of the drug. Furthermore, different routes may require different doses and dosage forms, which can then change the potential for certain side effects.

In considering all the aforementioned factors, it is difficult to conceptualize how safe and efficacious drugs are developed and utilized for their beneficial effects in the human body. The multitude of changes a drug undergoes between administration and stimulating an intended response can be divided into two major categories. **Pharmacokinetics** refers to the action the drug has on the body and **pharmacodynamics** refers to physiologic effects the drug has on body function (Figure 2-2). It is imperative that clinicians have a firm understanding of the basic principles of pharmacology in order to appropriately administer medications, monitor for anticipated effects and adverse reactions, and communicate as needed with women and their families as well as other healthcare team members.

Pharmacokinetics

Pharmacokinetics is the study of how a body processes a drug. More specifically, pharmacokinetics focuses on the kinetics of drug **absorption**, **distribution**, **metabolism**, and **excretion**. This study of the kinetics of drugs involves both experimental and theoretical approaches. Pharmacokinetics is a scientific study that involves

biologic sampling and analysis. Theoretical approaches involve the development of models that predict drug disposition after administration.

What may be more applicable to the clinician is the application of clinical pharmacokinetics. Clinical pharmacokinetics incorporates known pharmacokinetic principles of drug absorption, distribution, metabolism, and excretion but is based on the woman's disease state and takes into consideration individual-specific factors. A commonly seen example is when a laboratory measures a person's serum or plasma drug level. This numerical drug level is combined with knowledge of the disease state and conditions that influence the distribution of a particular drug. Kinetic principles can then be applied and used to modify the drug dose and therefore drug serum levels to produce desirable changes in the individual's disease state. Drugs in which serum plasma levels are drawn for clinical decision making include magnesium sulfate, vancomycin, theophylline, phenobarbital, lithium, and digoxin.

Absorption

After a drug is administered, it should be able to reach its intended site of action. This requires that the drug be absorbed into the blood from its site of administration (Table 2-1). Drugs can be absorbed via passive diffusion, active diffusion, or pinocytosis. Most drugs rely on passive diffusion. When a drug has a structure similar to a physiologic compound that moves across cell membranes via active transport, it is likely to be transported via active

Table 2-1 Absorption Speed of Various Drug Formulations

Type of Formulation	Absorption Rate
Oral Formulations	Fastest
Liquids, syrups, and elixirs	
Suspensions	
Powders	
Capsules	
Tablets	
Coated tablets	
Enteric coated tablets	Slowest
Parenteral Formulations	Fastest
Intravenous (IV)	
Intramuscular (IM)	
Subcutaneous (SC)	
Intrathecal (IT)	
Epidural	Slowest

Source: Adapted from Guttierrez K 2008.[48]

transport as well. Penicillin moves into the circulatory system via active transport. Macromolecules such as insulin and protein drugs access the circulatory system via pinocytosis.

Role of pH

Most drugs are weak organic acids or bases that exist in either an ionized or un-ionized form. Acidic drugs are in an un-ionized form that is lipid soluble (lipophilic), and therefore they diffuse easily across the phospholipid bilayer cell membrane. Basic drugs are in an ionized form and are water soluble (hydrophilic). These drugs cannot get through the cell membrane into the intracellular compartment easily. The pH in the gastrointestinal tract also affects this process because the proportion of the un-ionized form of a drug that is present is dependent on the pH of the environment. The stomach is acidic, and therefore, drugs that are acidic and un-ionized will readily be absorbed in the stomach. Conversely, the pH in the small intestine is more basic, and weak bases are absorbed more readily in this environment.

Oral Administration

Administering drugs orally is the preferred route of administration because it is considered safe, inexpensive, and convenient compared to other routes. Orally administered drugs (typically as tablet or capsule forms) must disintegrate into smaller particles and dissolve in the gastrointestinal tract (GI) to be absorbed. In addition, passage through the GI tract must alter the chemical characteristics of drugs that rely on passive diffusion so they become un-ionized and lipid soluble.

Even though the oral route generally is considered the preferred route, it does possess several disadvantages the clinician must consider (Figure 2-3). Some drugs have limited absorption due to how their chemical characteristics work in the environment of the GI tract (e.g., water solubility), low pH of gastric acid (which can increase absorption in some cases), destruction of the drug molecule by gastric enzymes, differences in gastric emptying rates, or adverse reactions such as vomiting due to gastric irritation. Infants and older persons have less gastric acidity, which, in general, decreases drug absorption. Food also influences the absorption of drugs, and the effect of food in the stomach when a drug is ingested is very drug-specific. Food–drug interactions are discussed in detail later in this chapter.[1] Some drugs are best taken with food to minimize gastrointestinal irritation while other drugs' absorption may be impeded by food. Also, specific foods may enhance drug absorption. For example, women with HIV should take efavirenz (Sustiva) with food because high-fat meals increase the absorption of efavirenz.[2]

Some drugs are **enteric coated** to prevent disintegration and absorption in the stomach with subsequent absorption in the less acidic small intestine. In addition, **extended release** (also known as **sustained release** or **slow release**) drugs may have compressed multiple coatings to allow release of the drug over time. These preparations are designed to produce slow, uniform absorption of the drug for 8 hours or longer. The advantages of the coated preparations compared to their immediate release counterparts include a reduction in the frequency of administration of the drug, maintenance of a therapeutic effect for a prolonged period of time, and decreased incidence and/or intensity of both undesired effects and nontherapeutic blood levels of the drug. Often, these drugs are designated by abbreviations such as *CR* (controlled release), *LA* (long acting), or *SR* (sustained release). To add to this confusion, extended release is the term recommended by the US Pharmacopeia, but extended release formulations can be labeled *XL*, *XR*, or *ER* depending on the choice of the pharmaceutical company marketing the drug.[3] Drugs that are labeled to indicate they work over a prolonged period of time should not to be crushed, chewed, or scored (broken).

First Pass Effect

After an orally administered drug enters the body, it passes through the intestine, intestinal wall, the portal

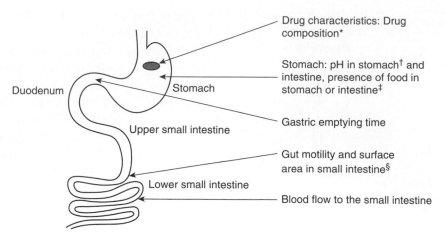

*Various aspects of the drug's chemical characteristics will affect absorption. For example, enteric coating will slow absorption, and drugs that are lipid-soluble will be absorbed more rapidly.

†Presence of antacid in the stomach will change the pH. This increases absorption of basic drugs and decreases absorption of acidic drugs.

‡Food that is in the stomach or intestine can either facilitate or interfere with drug absorption.

§The small intestine has the greatest surface area, which is why most drugs are absorbed in the small intestine.

Figure 2-3 Factors that affect absorption of drugs.

blood system, and the liver before it enters the systemic circulation. Most drugs undergo metabolic changes during this trip via interaction with the following: (1) bacterial enzymes in the intestine, (2) other enzymes present in the gastrointestinal lumen, (3) cytochrome 450 enzymes (CYP450 enzymes) present in the cells of the intestinal wall (discussed later), and (4) CYP 450 enzymes in the liver. This metabolism is called **biotransformation** because the structure of the drug is altered chemically. The process is referred to as the **first pass metabolism** or the **first pass effect**.[4,5] As a result of first pass metabolism, an amount of the drug dose fails to enter the systemic circulation and is not available to travel to the intended site of action, thus reducing the drug's bioavailability (Figure 2-4). Estrogen, for instance, is extensively metabolized during the first pass through the liver. Alternate routes of administration for estrogen compounds have been devised to decrease the amount of drug needed to accommodate the first pass effect. Some drugs are recycled through the enterohepatic circulation back to the liver, and when this occurs there is an increased risk that their toxic effects will occur.[6]

Drugs enter the liver via the portal vein and hepatic artery with the metabolized drug returning to the body via the hepatic vein. Some drugs, such as digoxin

(Digitek, Lanoxin) are recycled via bile excretion and reenter the gastrointestinal system where they are reabsorbed into the portal circulation. To decrease drug levels and toxicity, binding agents such as sodium polystyrene sulfonate (Kayexalate) may be given to bind with the recycled drug in order to block reabsorption in the GI tract. Drugs administered by routes other than oral may bypass the portal system and thereby also bypass the first pass effect.

In summary, determinants of drug absorption following oral administration include properties that affect **dissolution** such as dosage forms, pH in the stomach and small intestine, and the size of the active drug. The next determinant is gastric emptying time; stability of the drug at a specific pH; the effect of food, antacids, or other drugs; and disease processes that might exist in the GI tract. Thirdly, intestinal motility affects the time a drug is presented to the gastric lumen cells and, occasionally, drug degradation by microflora in the gut. Next, chemical properties of the drug such as how lipophilic it is affect drug passage through the gut wall, and some drugs are metabolized by the intestinal endothelium. Finally, the extent to which a drug is metabolized via the first pass effect will dictate the dose that must be used for oral administration.

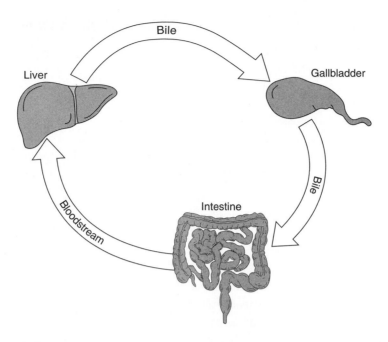

Figure 2-4 Hepatic first pass metabolism.

Parenteral Administration

Drugs administered by parenteral routes (intravenous, subcutaneous, or intramuscular) bypass the GI tract. Bypassing the GI tract allows for a more rapid, extensive, and predictable drug absorption. Also, the drug's effective dose is likely to be delivered to the site of intended action more accurately. In the case of an emergency situation (e.g., the person who is to receive the drug is unconscious or unresponsive) the parenteral route is often used as a necessity. In the case of subcutaneous and intramuscular administration, the drug creates a depot under the skin and is absorbed into the systemic circulation by simple diffusion. The rate of absorption for these routes is limited by the area of the absorbing capillary membranes and by the solubility of the substance in the interstitial fluid. A subcutaneous injection can only be used for drugs that are not irritating to tissue; otherwise, severe pain, necrosis, and tissue sloughing may occur. The rate of absorption following subcutaneous injection of a drug often is sufficiently constant and slow to provide a sustained effect. This slow and constant rate is used and altered intentionally, as seen with insulin. In this case, altering particle size, protein complex, and pH can provide short (3 to 6 hours), intermediate (10 to 18 hours), and long-acting (18 to 24 hours) preparations (see Chapter 18 for information on insulin preparations).

Drugs in aqueous solution are absorbed rapidly after intramuscular injection. This rate can be altered if the rate of blood flow surrounding the injected area is increased, as can happen with local heating (e.g., a hot bath), massage, or exercise. All of the above measures increase vasodilatation that, in turn, increases drug absorption into the systemic circulation. A slow, constant absorption from the intramuscular site can be achieved if the drug is injected in solution in oil vehicles, and antibiotics often are administered in this manner. Because a drug molecule is injected directly into the systemic circulation with intravenous administration, 100% bioavailability is achieved. There is no first pass effect, and there are no barriers (e.g., skin) to drug absorption with this route. The drug delivery is controlled and achieved with an accuracy and immediacy not possible by any other route. With intravenous administration, the person receiving the drug must be monitored closely, and once the drug is administered there is often no retreat. Drugs that cannot be administered intravenously include drugs in an oily vehicle, drugs that precipitate blood constituents or hemolyze erythrocytes, and drug combinations that result in the formation of precipitates.

Sublingual Administration

Sublingual administration occurs when a drug is placed under the tongue and absorbed into the blood. The sublingual route is used as a convenient route that bypasses the first pass effect. The venous drainage from the mouth is to the superior vena cava; this protects the drug from rapid first pass metabolism. Nitroglycerin is absorbed rapidly through the sublingual route.

Transdermal Administration

Transdermal administration refers to the administration of a drug molecule through the skin for absorption into the bloodstream. This administration intends for the drug to reach the systemic circulation to cause its action rather than remaining locally at the site of administration (i.e., topically). Transdermal preparations are developed to deliver a consistent drug dose over a day or a period of days. Not all drug molecules can readily penetrate intact skin, but when drug molecules are able to penetrate, the amount that does penetrate depends on the surface area over which the drug is applied and on lipid solubility because the epidermis behaves as a lipid barrier. Transdermal administration can be convenient for some individuals, and this dosage form has become more popular. Controlled-release topical patches that have become increasingly available include nicotine for tobacco-smoking withdrawal, scopolamine for motion sickness, nitroglycerin for angina pectoris, estrogen for menopausal therapy, and estrogens plus progestins for contraception. Systemic absorption of drugs occurs much more readily through abraded, burned, or denuded skin because the dermis is freely permeable. Also, when the skin is inflamed (causing an increase in cutaneous blood flow) drug molecules are more permeable through the skin layer. Toxic effects can be seen if highly lipid-soluble drug molecules are applied to skin that is not intact, so one must avoid transdermal administration in this situation. Conversely, lotion and ointments on the skin tend to impair drug transfer through a transdermal administration.

Rectal Administration

When a drug is administered rectally, the drug molecule is absorbed into either the systemic circulation or placed to induce a localized effect (as in the case of hydrocortisone suppositories for hemorrhoids). The potential for first pass metabolism is less than that when an oral dose is given because approximately 50% of the drug that is absorbed from the rectum will bypass the portal system. However, rectal absorption often is irregular and incomplete, and many drugs can cause irritation of the rectal mucosa.

Pulmonary Administration

Some drugs are inhaled and absorbed through the pulmonary epithelium and mucous membranes of the respiratory tract. Systemic absorption of drug molecules through this route is typically rapid due to the lungs' large surface area. Advantages of this route of administration include rapid absorption of a drug molecule into the blood, avoidance of first pass metabolism, and local application of the drug at the desired site of action in the case of pulmonary disease such as asthma. Inhaled drugs are often administered by nebulizer or a metered dose inhaler that can create aerosols of small particles. For example, albuterol (Proventil) may be administered by inhaler for individuals experiencing an acute asthma attack. More than one treatment may be required, depending upon the severity of the attack and the person's response to the drug.

Topical Administration

When the drug is intended for local action (e.g., administration of eye drops for glaucoma) it is administered topically. Drug absorption through this route is continuous, although it has a slower onset of action. Systemic absorption is unlikely but does increase if the drug molecule is applied to mucous membranes. An example of topical administration includes ophthalmic drugs, which may be drops or an ointment such as erythromycin ointment (Ilotycin) that often is administered to newborns in the first few hours after birth to prevent ophthalmic neonatorium. Another example includes otic drugs (ear drops), which may be given to treat infections or to facilitate removal of cerumen or a trapped object placed by a toddler or small child. Both ophthalmic and otic drugs require diligence in identifying the correct eye/ear for administration, appropriate positioning of the individual for otic drug administration, and administration techniques specific to the drug medium.

In summary, factors that affect absorption are important considerations for the clinician because the drug must reach its intended site of action before it can begin to produce a change in the biologic system. However, in the end, the clinician is primarily concerned with bioavailability rather than the absorption of the drug. **Bioavailability** is a term used to indicate the fractional extent to which a dose of drug reaches its site of action when it is administered by any route.

Distribution

Following a drug's administration and subsequent absorption into the systemic circulation, the drug then distributes

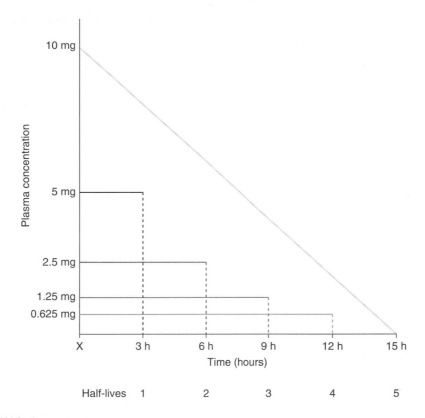

Figure 2-5 Elimination half-life determination.

itself into interstitial and intracellular fluids by passive mechanisms such as diffusion or by specific drug transport mechanisms. Distribution of the drug varies depending upon multiple factors, including the size of the drug molecule, affinity for aqueous and lipid tissues, tissue permeability, systemic circulation, protein binding, and pH. These factors collectively determine the rate of delivery and potential amount of drug distributed into tissues. There are two main phases of distribution. The first phase is that which most of the well perfused organs (e.g., liver, kidney, and brain) receive most of the drug. During the second phase of distribution, the less well perfused organs receive concentrations of drug. These less well perfused organs include muscle, most viscera, skin, and fat. This second distribution phase may require minutes to several hours before the concentration of drug in tissue is in equilibrium with that in blood. There are several clinically important pharmacokinetic processes that occur as a drug is distributed.

Steady State

A term often used when discussing absorption and administration of drugs is **steady state**. This term refers to a concentration of a drug in the systemic circulation that will eventually be achieved when a drug is administered at a constant rate. When a drug reaches this point, the rate of drug elimination (discussed later) will equal the rate of drug availability (or absorption).[7] This concept is often used in calculations of drug dose and interval between doses (Figure 2-5).

Half-Life

Half-life refers to the time it takes for the plasma concentration or the amount of drug in the body to be reduced by 50% (or one half). Half-life is important because it determines the time required to reach steady state and the dosage interval. Steady state is usually reached after 4–5 half lives and **elimination** also takes approximately 4–5 half-lives (Figure 2-6).

Another important concept when considering drug administration is loading dose. A **loading dose** is one or a series of doses that may be given at the onset of therapy with the aim of achieving the target plasma concentration rapidly. This dose, or series of doses, is used to rapidly obtain a steady state when the treatment of the individual necessitates a quick therapeutic response.

Another common term found when discussing drug distribution is **volume of distribution**. This concept refers to the apparent volume (V_D) in which the drug is dissolved. In other words, the V_D relates to the concentration of drug in plasma and the amount of drug in the body. The volume

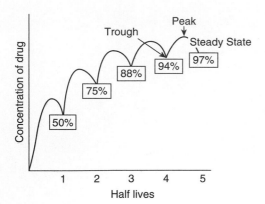

Figure 2-6 Steady state after repeated drug dosing.

of distribution does not have a true physiologic meaning in terms of an anatomic space. However, it often is used to calculate the loading dose of a drug that will immediately achieve a desired steady-state drug level[2] because it refers to the relationship between the dose of the drug administered and the serum concentration after administration.

Plasma Protein Binding

Protein binding is perhaps the most important factor when a drug is distributed in the systemic circulation. Plasma protein binding refers to the fraction of total drug in the plasma that is bound to plasma proteins. Many drugs bind to proteins in plasma (Figure 2-7). More than 60 proteins exist in plasma that can bind to drugs, yet the most common protein that binds to drugs is albumin. Albumin is a major carrier for acidic drugs, and the protein α_1-acid glycoprotein binds drugs that are basic in nature. The amount of drug that is bound to plasma proteins is determined by the drug concentration in the systemic circulation, the affinity of the binding sites on the protein for the drug, and the number of binding sites. This concept is important because only the unbound (free) drug can distribute to its intended site of action; a drug's response is related to the free rather than the total circulating plasma drug concentration. The binding of drug to protein is readily reversible, lasting only a half of a millisecond and is continually shifting from bound to unbound status.[6]

Binding sites are not unlimited and may become saturated. When this phenomenon occurs there is an increased risk for drug toxicity as drugs not bound to plasma proteins are pharmacologically active. For drugs that are normally highly protein bound, small changes in the extent of binding can produce a large change in the amount of unbound drug, and hence drug effect. Factors that can cause a change in

the extent of protein binding include myocardial infarction, surgery, neoplastic disease, rheumatoid arthritis, and burns. These factors actually increase the amount of circulating protein and thus lead to increased drug binding and a decrease in pharmacologic effect. Additionally, conditions such as hypoalbuminemia, liver disease, and renal disease can decrease the amount of circulating plasma protein. With this situation, plasma concentration of free drug is increased and drug efficacy and toxicity can be enhanced.

Converse to the protein-binding concept, many drugs accumulate in tissues at higher concentrations than those in the extracellular fluids and blood. This concept may be a result of active transport into the tissue, but more commonly it is a result of tissue binding. Tissue binding is often reversible. When a large fraction of drug is tissue bound, it may serve as a reservoir that prolongs drug action in that same tissue or at a distant site reached through the circulation.

Caution must be exercised in some situations with drugs that are highly protein bound. An aminoglycoside antibiotic, gentamicin (Garamycin) has a high affinity for kidney tissue, and it can cause local toxicity to the kidney if drug levels become too high (Figure 2-8).

Other examples of tissue binding include drugs that are **lipophilic**, which have a high affinity for fat and for bone.[8] Highly lipid soluble drugs can be stored in fat tissues, which results in fat becoming a drug reservoir. Fat is a relatively stable reservoir because it has low blood flow. Bone is another tissue that has tissue binding, and drugs can accumulate in bone by adsorption onto the bone crystal surface with eventual incorporation into the crystal lattice. Using bone as a tissue reservoir can be used as a therapeutic advantage for the treatment of osteoporosis. Alendronate (Fosamax) binds tightly to crystals in mineralized bone matrix. However, unlike naturally occurring pyrophosphates, alendronate is resistant to degradation and thus stabilizes the bone matrix.

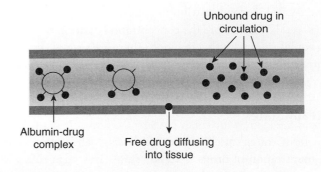

Figure 2-7 Protein binding of drugs.

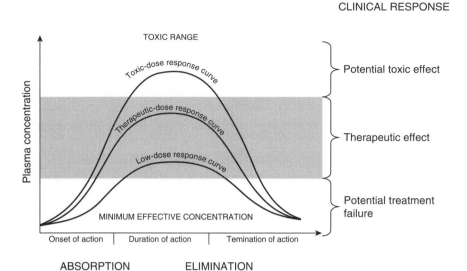

CLINICAL RESPONSE

Figure 2-8 Time course of a single dose.

The Blood–Brain Barrier

The distribution of drugs into the central nervous system (CNS) from the blood is unique. The endothelial cells in the capillaries surrounding the brain are packed very tightly together, which disallows passive transport of materials in the blood out into the surrounding cerebral tissue. This **blood–brain barrier** creates a natural barrier to the exchange of drugs between the blood and the brain.[9] A drug must be able to travel *through* the cell to penetrate this barrier. In the rest of the body, the drug is able to pass between endothelial cells because the cells are not joined as tightly. For a drug to be able to pass into the brain it must be highly lipophilic; the more lipophilic a drug is the more likely it is to pass through the blood–brain barrier.

Another natural drug barrier is the placenta. This organ is fundamentally the organ of exchange between the mother and fetus. The placenta was once viewed as an absolute barrier to drugs to the developing fetus and an agent of protection from other agents that might cause anomalies, but today it is well known that this view is completely inaccurate. The fetus is exposed to some extent to all drugs taken by the mother. Lipid solubility, the extent of plasma binding, and degree of ionization of weak acids and bases are important general determinants in drug transfer across the placenta. Additionally, export transporters are present in the placenta and function to limit fetal exposure to potentially toxic agents. Additional information about the use of drugs in pregnancy can be found in Chapter 35.

Metabolism

Termination of drug effect by the body is usually achieved by metabolism and excretion. Drug metabolism refers to the process by which a drug is chemically converted in the body to a metabolite. This transformation is usually enzymatic, and the enzymes responsible are mainly located in the liver. Other tissues such as kidney, lung, small intestine, and skin also contain enzymes that metabolize drugs. These reactions are classified as either **phase I reactions** or **phase II conjugation reactions**.[10]

The two-step process of phase I and phase II reactions make the drug molecule more water soluble so the drug can be excreted via the kidney. Phase I reactions are oxidation, hydrolysis, or reduction reactions. These reactions generally result in the loss of pharmacologic activity. Phase II conjugation reactions involve conjugation to form glucuronides, acetates, or sulfates. Both types of reactions play a major role in diminishing the biologic activity of a drug.

For most drugs, this metabolism results in a pharmacologically inactive compound; however, there are a few drugs that are transformed in the body to metabolites that have pharmacologic activity. These drugs are referred to as **prodrugs**. For example, valacyclovir (Valtrex) is not an effective antiviral drug, but its active metabolite, acyclovir, is active against herpes virus.[11] Prodrugs are being developed intentionally to improve drug stability, increase systemic drug absorption, or to prolong the duration of drug activity.

Drug Interactions

When drugs are metabolized into inactive metabolites that are excreted, all is well. However, there are multiple ways drug metabolism can result in adverse health consequences. Therefore, a review of these mechanisms is in order.

The Cytochrome P450 Enzymes

The **cytochrome P450** (CYP450) enzyme family is the name for the group of enzymes that are responsible for the majority of drug metabolism reactions.[7,12] The name P450 was chosen because these enzymes are bound to membranes within mitochondria or endoplasmic reticulum within the cell (cyto) and contain a heme pigment that absorbs a wave of light at 450 nm when exposed to carbon monoxide. Each enzyme name reflects a family, subfamily, and then an individual number (Table 2-2). CYP2D6 is number 6 in the subfamily "D" in the "2" family.[12]

Currently, 57 different CYP450 enzyme genes have been identified, yet only 6 of the resultant enzymes are responsible for the majority of drug metabolism in humans.[13] Three types of CYPs (CYP1, CYP2, and CYP3) predominate in the metabolism of most commonly used

pharmaceuticals. The various ways these enzymes act is perhaps the most interesting and most important set of processes that prescribers of drugs must know in order to practice prescribing drugs safely. Table 2-3 gives examples of the clinically important consequences of CYP450 enzyme function and interactions. Note that a few drugs appear to influence metabolism of many other drugs. Cimetidine (Tagamet) is an inhibitor for several CYP450 enzymes, whereas rifampin (Rifadin) is an inducer for several CYP450 enzymes.

Each CYP450 enzyme is encoded by a specific gene, and we each have two alleles that determine expression of enzymatic activity. There are multiple forms (polymorphisms)

Table 2-2 Cytochrome P450 Enzymes Naming Convention

Designation	Meaning	Examples of Specific Enzymes in Family
CYP	Cytochrome P450 enzyme	
CYP1	Family designation	CYP2, CYP3, CYP4
CYP1A	Subfamily A	CYP1B, CYP1C
CYPY1A1	Individual enzyme within subfamily	CYP1A2
CYP1A1*1A	Allelic variant of the individual enzyme	CYP1A1*1B

Table 2-3 Clinical Examples of CYP450 Enzyme Interactions

CYP450 Enzyme Activity	Drug–Drug Interaction	Clinical Implication
Inducer	Carbamazepine (Tegretol) and ethynyl-estradiol containing contraceptives	Carbamazepine induces CYP34A4, and CYP34A4 metabolizes ethinyl-estradiol containing contraceptives in the intestinal lumen during first pass metabolism. When more CYP34A4 is made, more contraceptive is metabolized, which results in lower plasma levels of the contraceptive and decreased efficacy of the contraceptive.
Inhibitor of active metabolite	Fluoxetine (Prozac) and tramadol (Ultram)	Fluoxetine inhibits CYP2D6, which converts tramadol to its active metabolite. Thus concomitant use of these two drugs can decrease the analgesic effect of tramadol.
Inhibitor	Erythromycin (E-mycin) and theophylline (Theo-Dur)	Erythromycin inhibits CYP3A, which metabolizes theophylline. Elevated blood levels of theophylline can cause seizures and arrhythmias.
Poor metabolizer	Amitriptyline (Elavil)	Amitriptyline is metabolized by CYP2D6. Persons who do not have sufficient CYP2D6 do not metabolize amitriptyline and have higher plasma levels of the drugs metabolized by this enzyme (e.g., tricyclic antidepressants).
Ultrarapid metabolizer	Codeine	Persons who have extra CYP2D6 rapidly metabolize codeine into its active metabolite (morphine) and can have an increased analgesic effect. The FDA has a warning on use of codeine by nursing mothers because ultrarapid metabolizers can have increased amounts of morphine in breast milk, and there is one case report of an infant death from an overdose of morphine that was in breast milk.
Racial and ethnic polymorphism	Tricyclic antidepressants	African Americans are more likely to be poor metabolizers of CYP2C19. This results in a better response to tricyclic antidepressants, but an increased risk for adverse effects as well.
Drug induces CYP450 enzyme that also metabolizes it	Carbamazepine (Tegretol)	Carbamazepine is an inducer of the same CYP450 enzyme that metabolizes it. Thus doses must be started lower and gradually increased to get a therapeutic response.
CYP450 enzyme metabolizes prodrug into active metabolite	Codeine	Codeine is metabolized by a CYP450 enzyme into its active metabolite, which is morphine.
CYP450 enzyme metabolizes drug into hepatotoxic metabolite	Acetaminophen (Tylenol)	CYP1A2 converts acetaminophen into a toxic metabolite. Overdoses of acetaminophen can cause overproduction of this metabolite, which then causes liver failure.

of each allele, and their clinical expression as a metabolizer for a specific drug ranges from absent to highly efficient.[14] (See Chapter 3 for more information on pharmacogenomics.) Thus, depending on genetic makeup, an individual can be an **ultrarapid metabolizer** for drugs that are metabolized by a specific CYP450 enzyme, she can have any of several degrees of normal metabolizing ability, in which case she is referred to as an **extensive metabolizer**, or she can even be a **poor metabolizer** if the two alleles inherited have little metabolizing ability. Secondly, there are sex differences as well. CYP3A activity is higher in women, whereas CYP1A2 activity is higher in men.[15,16] Third, there are racial and ethnic differences. For example 7% of persons who are Caucasian are poor metabolizers of drugs dependent on CYP2D6, which metabolizes many of the beta-blockers, opioids, and antidepressants. Similarly, 2–7% of persons who are African American are also poor metabolizers of these drugs.[17]

Once individual, sex, and ethnic variations are accounted for, the CYP450 enzymes get to work and their function can be significantly affected by other drugs, food, herbs, and even vitamin supplements (Table 2-4).

Drug–Drug Interactions

Drug–drug interactions refer to a modification of an expected drug response due to an exposure to another drug or substance at approximately the same time. The risk of drug–drug interactions increases with multiple drug therapy, multiple prescribers, problems with taking drugs on schedule, and advancing age. When two drugs are administered that have the same clinical effect, an additive effect can occur. Additive effects of drugs that cause central nervous system sedation can at the extreme cause unconsciousness. Most commonly, drug–drug interactions occur when two drugs are coadministered and are metabolized or have affinity to the same CYP450 enzyme. Drugs are typically classified as **inhibitors** or **inducers** of enzymatic activity. When the two drugs are coadministered, Drug *A* can inhibit the enzyme's activity and not allow the metabolism of Drug *B*. This results in an increase in the serum concentration of Drug *B* and subsequent risk of toxicity by Drug *B*. Conversely, administration of Drug *A* may induce the enzyme activity and increase the metabolism of Drug *B*, decreasing the serum concentration and the pharmacologic activity of Drug *B*. The effect of inducers is slower than the effect of inhibitors because it takes a while to increase the number of the relevant CYP enzymes. Since most of these drug–drug interactions are due to CYP450 enzymes, it becomes important to determine the identity of the CYP450 enzyme that metabolizes a particular drug,

to research the effects of the drug–drug interaction, and to educate individuals when coadministering drugs that are metabolized by the same enzyme.[11]

Coadministering drugs with known drug–drug interactions can be done intentionally in clinical practice. An example of this intentional coadministration can be found in the treatment of those who are HIV infected. Ritonavir (Norvir), a strong inhibitor of the CYP450 enzymes, is commonly coadministered with atazanavir (Reyataz), thus increasing plasma levels and the HIV activity of atazanavir. The ritonavir acts to boost the levels of atazanavir drug concentration.[18] Two different drugs can also be put together in one combination formulation to minimize drug interactions and facilitate patient adherence. For example, individuals with human immunodeficiency virus (HIV) and acquired immunodeficiency syndrome (AIDS) had a medication regimen that required taking 30 medications daily prior to the development of highly active antiretroviral therapy combination drugs that now allows them to take significantly fewer pills.[19]

Drug–drug interactions can also occur when two drugs are given concomitantly and interact via the pharmacokinetic or pharmacodynamic processes. For example, when phenytoin (Dilantin) is given with salicylates (aspirin), the plasma levels of free phenytoin increase because the salicylates compete for plasma protein binding. Phenytoin has a very narrow therapeutic index and increased levels can reach toxic levels quickly, resulting in ataxia, nystagmus, or increased seizure activity.

P-glycoprotein Drug Interactions

P-glycoproteins (P-gp) are a family of proteins that function as efflux transporters. Fueled by ATP, these proteins transport drugs and **xenobiotics** out of cells. They are found in the plasma membranes of epithelial cells in the intestinal tract, liver, kidney, brain capillaries, and placenta. It appears that their function may be to transport harmful substances out of the body and prevent them from crossing the blood–brain barrier. P-glycoprotein activity is increased or decreased by a number of endogenous and environmental stimuli. Although their physiologic function is not fully elucidated, it is clear that they play a physiologic role in drug absorption, distribution, and elimination. In a similar fashion to the CYP450 system, some drugs are substrates (inducers) and others are inhibitors of the P-glycoproteins. Thus, P-glycoprotein inhibition results in increased plasma levels of a specific drug, and conversely, P-glycoprotein induction results in more rapid elimination and decreased plasma levels of the drug in question. For example,

Table 2-4 Examples of CYP450 Enzymes That Frequently Metabolize Drugs and Their Pharmacologic Effects*

Inhibitors[†]—Generic (Brand)	Inducers[‡]—Generic (Brand)	Substrates[§]—Generic (Brand)
CYP1A2		
Fluoroquinolones: ciprofloxacin (Cipro), clarithromycin (Biaxin) Oral contraceptives Others: amiodarone (Cordarone), cimetidine (Tagamet), erythromycin (E-mycin), fluvoxamine (Luvox), isoniazid (INH)	Carbamazepine (Tegretol), insulin, phenobarbital (Luminal), phenytoin (Dilantin), primidone (Mysoline), rifampin (Rifadin), tobacco	Antidepressants: amitriptyline (Elavil), clomipramine (Anafranil), clozapine (Clozaril), desipramine (Norpramin), fluvoxamine (Luvox), imipramine (Tofranil) Antipsychotics: haloperidol (Haldol) Other: amitriptyline (Elavil), caffeine, theophylline (Theo-Dur)
CYP2C9		
Anti-infectives: fluconazole (Diflucan), isoniazid (INH), metronidazole (Flagyl), ritonavir (Norvir), trimethoprim/sulfamethoxazole (Septra) Other: amiodarone (Cordarone), cimetidine (Tagamet), fluoxetine (Prozac), fluvoxamine (Luvox)	Carbamazepine (Tegretol), phenobarbital (Luminal), phenytoin (Dilantin), primidone (Mysoline), rifampin (Rifadin)	Carvedilol (Coreg), celecoxib (Celebrex), diazepam (Valium), glipizide (Glucotrol), glyburide (Micronase), ibuprofen (Advil, Motrin), irbesartan (Avapro), losartan (Cozaar)
CYP2C19		
Fluoxetine (Prozac), fluvoxamine (Luvox), isoniazid (INH), modafinil (Provigil) , omeprazole (Prilosec), ritonavir (Norvir), topiramate (Topamax)	Carbamazepine (Tegretol), phenobarbital (Luminal), phenytoin (Dilantin), rifampin (Rifadin)	Omeprazole (Prilosec), phenobarbital (Luminal), phenytoin (Dilantin)
CYP2D6		
Amiodarone (Cordarone), cimetidine (Tagamet), diphenhydramine (Benadryl), fluoxetine (Prozac), paroxetine (Paxil), quinidine, ritonavir (Norvir), sertraline (Zoloft)	No significant inducers	Antidepressants: amitriptyline (Elavil), clomipramine (Anafranil), desipramine (Norpramin), doxepin (Sinequan), fluoxetine (Prozac), imipramine (Tofranil), paroxetine (Paxil), venlafaxine (Effexor) Antipsychotics: haloperidol (Haldol), risperidone (Risperdal), thioridazine (Mellaril) Beta-blockers: carvedilol (Coreg), metoprolol (Lopressor), propranolol (Inderal) Opiates: codeine, tramadol (Ultram) Other: donepezil (Aricept), ondansetron (Zofran)
CYP3A4		
Azole fungals: fluconazole (Diflucan), itraconazole (Sporanox), ketoconazole (Nizoral) Anti-infectives: clarithromycin (Biaxin), ciprofloxacin (Cipro), erythromycin (E-mycin), isoniazid (INH), metronidazole (Flagyl), ritonavir (Norvir) Other: amiodarone (Cordarone), cimetidine (Tagamet), diltiazem (Cardizem), verapamil (Calan)	Carbamazepine (Tegretol), St. John's wort, dexamethasone, phenobarbital (Luminal), phenytoin (Dilantin), protease inhibitors, rifampin (Rifadin)	Alprazolam (Xanax), amlodipine (Norvasc), atorvastatin (Lipitor), cyclosporine (Sandimmune), diazepam (Valium), estradiol (Estrace), simvastatin (Zocor), sildenafil (Viagra), verapamil (Calan), zolpidem (Ambien)

* This table is not comprehensive as new information is being identified on a regular basis.
[†] These drugs inhibit the metabolism of substrates by these CYP450 enzymes.
[‡] These drugs induce production of the CYP450 enzyme, which causes increased metabolism of the substrate.
[§] The plasma levels of these drugs are increased by inhibitors and decreased by inducers of the specific CYP450 enzyme responsible for their metabolism.
Source: Adapted from Lynch et al. 2007[12]; Johns Cupp M et al. 1998.[47]

St. John's wort is a potent inducer of P-glycoprotein; when St. John's wort is given concomitantly with digoxin (Lanoxin), the plasma levels of digoxin decrease because the augmented intestinal P-glycoprotein activity effectively keeps digoxin out of the systemic circulation.

Drug–Food Interactions

Drug metabolism can also be influenced by diet (**drug–food interactions**). Foods can affect drug bioavailability via these two mechanisms: (1) decreased oral bioavailability via interference with absorption, and (2) increased bioavailability via inhibition of CYP3A in the cells of the intestinal wall. This second mechanism increases plasma levels of the drug metabolized by CYP3A and can precipitate adverse effects or toxicities.[20]

Components in grapefruits and grapefruit juices (naringin and furanocoumarins) are potent inhibitors of CYP3A[13,21,22] (Box 2-1). Medications that have a narrow therapeutic index or low oral bioavailability are most likely to have adverse reactions if they are metabolized by CYP3A and taken within 48 hours of ingesting grapefruit

Box 2-1 The Grapefruit Juice Story

In 1989, a group of researchers used grapefruit juice to mask the taste of alcohol in a study that was evaluating possible interactions between alcohol and felodipine (Plendil), a calcium channel blocker used to treat hypertension. The study participants had increases in plasma felodipine levels that were unrelated to alcohol or known felodipine pharmacokinetics. The culprit was the grapefruit juice!

Grapefruit has a number of constituents that inhibit the function of CYP3A4 enzymes in the cells of the intestinal lumen. Because CYP3A4 metabolizes many drugs before they get into the systemic system, inhibition of CYP34A can cause increased plasma levels of drugs, adverse effects, and toxicity. How much grapefruit juice does it take? Is it just the juice or does a grapefruit eaten for breakfast have the same effect? What about different types of grapefruit? Here is the story:

Grapefruit juice irreversibly inhibits CYP34A, so new enzymes must be synthesized before normal function is restored. Thus 30% of the inhibitory effect is still present 24 hours after ingestion of a single 8-oz glass of normal strength grapefruit juice. It is recommended that medications affected by grapefruit juice not be taken until 72 hours after the last glass of grapefruit juice. Unfortunately for grapefruit juice lovers, the effect is the same if they drink white, pink, or ruby red.

Table 2-5 Examples of Grapefruit Juice–Drug Interactions

Drug Generic (Brand)	Clinical Effect of Increased Serum Concentration of Drug when Taken with Grapefruit Juice
Antiarrhythmics	
Amiodarone (Cordarone)	Thyroid, pulmonary, or liver injury. Cardiac athymias, prolonged QT syndrome, bradycardia
Quinidine	*Torsades de pointes*
Benzodiazepines	
Diazepam (Valium)	Increased CNS depression
Midazolam (Versed)	Increased CNS depression
Triazolam (Halcion)	Increased CNS depression
Calcium channel blockers	
Felodipine (Plendil)	Flushing, peripheral edema, headaches, hypotension, tachycardia
Nicardipine (Cardene)	Flushing, peripheral edema, headaches, hypotension, tachycardia
Nimodipine (Nimotop)	Flushing, peripheral edema, headaches, hypotension, tachycardia
Verapamil (Covera-HS)	Flushing, peripheral edema, headaches, hypotension, tachycardia
CNS depressants	
Buspirone (BuSpar)	Increased adverse effects of buspirone
Carbamazepine (Tegretol)	Increased adverse effects of carbamazepine
Clomipramine (Anafranil)	Increased effect of clomipramine
Sertraline (Zoloft)	Increased adverse effects of sertraline
Immunosuppressants	
Cyclosporine (Neoral)	Increased plasma levels of cyclosporine
Tacrolimus (Protopic)	Increased plasma levels of tacrolimus
Statins	
Atorvastatin (Lipitor)	Increased levels of atorvastatin can cause rhabdomyolysis.
Lovastatin (Mevacor)	Increased levels of lovastatin can cause rhabdomyolysis.
Pravastatin (Pravachol)	Increased levels of pravastatin can cause rhabdomyolysis.
Simvastatin (Zocor)	Increased levels of simvastatin can cause rhabdomyolysis.

juice. Table 2-5 provides a list of drugs that have a clinically significant interaction with grapefruit juice.[23]

Another clinically important drug–food interaction is the hypertensive crisis that can occur when persons taking monamine oxidase (MAO) inhibitors eat protein-rich foods (often those aged, fermented, pickled, or smoked) that are high in tyramine.[1] Table 2-6 lists additional important food–drug interactions.[24-26]

Drug–Herb Interactions

Drug–herb interactions are particularly difficult to assess. Most herbal products obtained over the counter are unregulated because they are considered dietary supplements and not recognized as drugs.[27] Therefore, there is wide variation in the pharmaceutically active compounds in different herbal preparations. Nonetheless, adverse effects are known to occur when specific herbs and drugs are taken concomitantly. For example, patients taking warfarin (Coumadin) can have increased bleeding if they take Salvia miltiorrhiza (danshen) or garlic preparations.[25,26]

Some of the most well-known herb–drug interactions are associated with use of St. John's wort.[28] This herb has purported effectiveness in helping persons with depression become less depressed. However, placebo trials of St. John's wort have been inconclusive and meta-analyses have concluded that it might be effective for mild depression only.[29] In addition, St. John's wort decreases

Table 2-6 Examples of Clinically Important Drug–Food Interactions*

Drug Generic (Brand)	Foods	Mechanism of Action	Clinical Implications
Angiotensin-converting enzyme inhibitors (ACE inhibitors)	High-potassium foods such as bananas, oranges, legumes, meats, salt substitutes	ACE inhibitors spare potassium so the addition of food high in potassium can cause toxicity.	Bradycardia and potential cardiac arrest
Digoxin	High-fiber products such as bran, pectin, bulk laxatives	Decreases absorption of digoxin.	Insufficient digoxin effect
MAO inhibitors	Absolute: aged cheese, aged and cured meat, sausage, banana peel, fava bean pods, Marmite or yeast extracts, sauerkraut, soy sauce, tap beer Moderate: red and white wine, bottled or canned beer	Monoamine oxidase found in the GI tract inactivates tyramine. Tyramine can cause hypertension when absorbed into the systemic system.	Severe hypertensive reaction
Quinolones, antifungals, and tetracyclines	Dairy products, calcium supplements, calcium-fortified orange juice, antacids, iron-containing vitamins	The drugs bind to iron and calcium in the GI tract and form a compound that is excreted without entering the systemic system.	Decreased absorption of the antibiotic
Theophylline (Theo-Dur)	High-fat meal	High-fat meals increase absorption of theophylline.	Theophylline toxicity: nausea, vomiting, headache, irritability
Warfarin (Coumadin)[†]	Alcohol		More than three drinks/day increases effect of warfarin
	Foods with vitamin K must be used with consistency: broccoli, brussels sprouts, turnip greens, kale, spinach	Large amounts of vitamin K interfere with the effect of warfarin.	Inadequate anticoagulation

* This table is not comprehensive as new information is being identified on a regular basis.
[†] Warfarin has multiple drug–drug, drug–food, and drug–herb interactions.
Source: Adapted from Rapaport MH 2007[24]; Gardner DM et al. 1996.[25]

the plasma levels of many drugs including midazolam (Versed), digoxin, warfarin (Coumadin), and theophylline (Theo-Dur).[30] It has also caused breakthrough bleeding when taken concomitantly with oral contraceptives and may interfere with the contraceptive effectiveness.[31,32]

Drug-Induced Toxicity

Finally, some metabolites of drugs are toxic to the liver or to the kidney. In some instances tests for liver function are required either before therapy with a specific drug is started or during therapy as a way to monitor liver function. The direct toxic effects of drugs or their metabolites on liver and/or kidney function are discussed in more detail in Chapter 4.

▍Excretion

Drug excretion is the way the body terminates drug action. Drug excretion refers to the elimination of a drug molecule or its metabolite from the biologic system. Drugs are primarily excreted via the kidneys, though some excretion does occur via saliva, feces, sweat, and mammary glands.

Excretion of drugs in breast milk is important not because of the amounts eliminated, but because the excreted drugs are potential sources of unwanted pharmacologic effects on the nursing infant.

Excretion of drugs and metabolites in the urine involves three distinct processes: glomerular filtration, passive tubular reabsorption, and active tubular secretion. All drugs that are low molecular weight and not bound to protein are filtered in the glomerulus into the glomerular filtrate. Lipid soluble drugs move back into the blood via passive tubular reabsorption, but ionized hydrophilic drugs remain in the urine. Some drugs are actively secreted from the circulatory system into the proximal tubule. Penicillin-G is a good example of a drug that is eliminated via tubular secretion. Probenecid (Benemid) is given to block this mechanism and increase plasma levels of penicillin. Finally, the pH of the urine affects elimination.

Weak acids are excreted more easily in alkaline urine and slower when the urine is more acidic. The converse is true for drugs that are weak bases. Changes in overall renal function will affect drug dosage levels. When deciding on initial doses for drugs that are eliminated renally, the renal function should be assessed for the person who will be taking the drug. A common, useful way to do this is to measure the serum creatinine concentration and convert this value into an estimated creatinine clearance. For example, gentamicin (Garamycin) is excreted via the kidney, and it can be toxic to proximal tubule cells. Therefore, when gentamicin is given in large doses or for a prolonged period of time, kidney failure can occur. As the kidney fails, less gentamicin is excreted, which predisposes one to additional kidney damage.[33]

Clearance

Clearance is the measure of the body's ability to eliminate a drug. This measure is often used in pharmacokinetic calculations, and it does not identify the mechanism or process of elimination (e.g., this calculation does not consider if the drug is eliminated by metabolic processes or excretion). This measure is the most important pharmacokinetic parameter because it determines the steady-state concentration for a given dosage route. The mechanisms of drug elimination are complex, but collectively, drug elimination from the body may be quantified using the concept of drug clearance.

Pharmacodynamics

Dose–Response Relationship

Pharmacodynamics is the study of the relationship between the concentration of a drug in the systemic circulation and the response obtained, often termed the **dose–response relationship**. A **dose–response curve** can be drawn by plotting the concentration of the drug on the X-axis and the response on the Y-axis. The **threshold dose** is the lowest dose at which a desired response is noted. The same dose of a drug often results in different plasma concentrations among individuals. This difference is secondary to individual differences in pharmacokinetic parameters. For instance, the onset, intensity, and duration of response an individual experiences are dependent upon both the dose of the drug administered and the pharmacokinetics of the drug in that individual.

Two important parameters can be calculated in drawing dose–response relationship curves for particular drugs. **Potency** is the concentration at which the drug elicits 50% of its maximal response. **Efficacy** is the maximal response produced by the drug. A clinical example of a study of pharmacodynamics is recording changes in blood pressure when a woman is being treated with antihypertensive medications. According to this concept, there is a

drug receptor located within the target organ tissue. When a drug molecule finds and attaches to the receptor target, it forms a complex with that target that causes the biologic response, which is the specific mechanism of action of that drug.

Drug–Receptor Interactions: The Role of Cell Membrane Receptors

In order for a clinician to make rational therapeutic decisions, the prescriber must understand how drug–receptor interactions underlie the relationship between dose and response. A receptor is the cell component that interacts with drugs to produce psychophysiologic effects. Drug receptors are often proteins, and common examples include receptors for hormones, growth factors, transcription factors, and neurotransmitters; the enzymes of crucial metabolic or regulatory pathways; proteins involved in transport; secreted glycoproteins; and structural proteins. Receptors are the governing agent in determining the dose for any drug. Specifically, it is the **affinity**, or propensity of a drug to bind with a specific receptor, that determines the drug concentration necessary to achieve the desired effect. Drugs have a specific affinity for a particular chemical group or cellular component. Drug binding will either increase or decrease the rate of the biologic response controlled by that specific receptor. Note it does not change the physiologic activity but either enhances or blocks it.

There are four common receptor systems, which are: (1) embedded enzyme, (2) ligand-binding ion channel, (3) G protein coupled receptor, and (4) the nuclear receptors that are on the nuclear or mitochondrial membrane called transcription factor (Figure 2-9). The receptor of a cell membrane-embedded enzyme extends across the cell membrane with the ligand-binding area located on the cell surface and the site for the enzyme activity on the intracellular portion of the receptor. The response time of these receptors is usually within seconds. Insulin and atrial natriuretic factor are endogenous **ligands** that affect target cells via this signaling mechanism.[33] Ligand-binding ion channels are similar to the embedded enzymes in that the ion channels cross the cell membrane. These receptors control the flow of ions into and out of the cell. The ligand-binding domain is specific for a precise ion (e.g., calcium). With binding of the ligand to the receptor, the channel opens, allowing ions to flow into or out of the cell. Responses in this system commonly occur in milliseconds. The neurotransmitter acetylcholine and the amino acid glycine act through this receptor family.[33]

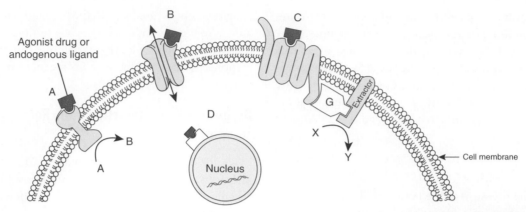

(A) Embedded enzyme: When a drug binds to the extracellular domain of this receptor, an enzymatic intracellular domain function is activated or inhibited. (B) Ligand binding ion channel: The drug binds to the extracellular portion of this transmembrane protein complex, which causes it to change shape and alter conductance. (C) G protein-coupled receptors are also known as seven transmembrane domain receptors. When the extracellular domain of this receptor is bound by a drug, a G protein in the intracellular space is activated to stimulate an effector mechanism. (D) Transcription factor: A lipid-soluble drug crosses the cell membrane and binds to an intracellular or nuclear receptor.

Figure 2-9 Four receptor types.

The **G protein coupled receptor** family is the largest group of cell surface receptors, and approximately 30% of the drugs used today interact with these receptors (Box 2-2). Therefore, these receptors are of particular import in pharmacology.[34] The G protein coupled receptor has three parts, the receptor, the G protein, and the effector or the second messenger. These receptors may be located on the cell surface or in a pocket accessible from the cell surface. Ligands bind to the receptors on the exterior portion of the cell membrane. Intracellularly, the bound receptors act as a catalytic enzyme. The second messenger then interacts with intracellular components. The G protein stimulates the enzyme adenyl cyclase to change ATP to cyclic AMP or cAMP intracellularly with subsequent activation of protein kinases and cellular reactions. Drugs acting via a G protein coupling receptor include beta blockers and antiasthma drugs.[35,36]

In contrast, transcription factors are intracellular receptors and have a longer response time. Lipid-soluble ligands cross the cell membrane to reach these receptors located in the cell nucleus on DNA where the transcription factors regulate protein synthesis. Therefore, activation of these receptors stimulates the transcription of messenger RNA templates for protein synthesis. With transcription factors there is a response time from hours to days. Steroid hormones, such as estrogen and progesterone, act through these intracellular receptor sites.[36]

Agonists, Partial Agonists, and Antagonists

Agonists are drugs that elicit a pharmacologic response when interacting with the receptor. Agonists shift the equilibrium between the active and inactive forms of the receptor in the direction of the active form—by binding the active form more avidly (i.e., they induce a conformational change in the receptor that leads to a maximal effect), they drive the physiologic response in the direction of activation. Insulin and dobutamine of examples of drugs acting as agonists. Affinity refers to the degree of attraction between a drug and receptor. Drugs with high affinity bind more extensively to the receptor than a drug with less affinity. A **partial agonist** is a drug molecule that elicits a partial pharmacologic response when bound to a specific receptor. Partial agonists have only a slightly higher affinity for the active receptor than for the inactive form, so they display some agonist activity but interfere with the function of a full agonist. Buspirone (BuSpar), which is used to treat general anxiety disorder, is a partial agonist. **Agonist-antagonists** are similar to partial agonists in that they have an effect that is not as potent as full agonist stimulation. These drugs affect receptors that have different forms, and they act as an agonist at one form and as an antagonist at another. Butorphanol (Stadol) blocks the effect of morphine at the mu opioid receptor but stimulates the kappa opioid receptor. The net result is analgesia that is not as potent as the effect obtained with morphine.

An **antagonist** is a drug molecule that inhibits the action of an agonist when binding to the receptor and has no effect on the agonist itself. Antagonists may have high affinity for the receptor, but they do not activate the receptor when bound to it. Though antagonists do not initiate a response, they prevent activation of the receptor by an agonist, and therefore they have a pharmacologic effect. The physiologic response to drugs acting as antagonists is dependent upon the presence of an agonist. For example, antihistamines and naloxone (Narcan) are examples of antagonists. Diphenhydramine (Benadryl), an antihistamine, is effective only in response to histamine activated-receptors that occurred as a response to a specific allergen.

Antagonists can be competitive or noncompetitive. A **competitive antagonist** occurs when the antagonist has equal affinity for both the active and inactive conformations of the receptor and competes with an agonist for binding to the active form of the receptor. Ligands with the highest affinity will bind with the receptor. If there is an equal affinity, then the ligand in the highest concentration will bind with the receptor. In contrast, **noncompetitive antagonists** bind with a part of the receptor away from the usual site to which an agonist binds. This causes a structural or functional change in the receptor that inactivates it, so agonist binding at the usual site fails to stimulate the expected physiologic response. The response

to competitive antagonists is reversible, and large enough amounts of the agonist may surmount the inhibitory effect, whereas the effect of noncompetitive antagonists is usually irreversible.

The attractive feature of this model is that it explains **inverse agonists** rather well. If there is a basal tendency of the receptor to be in the active state then these active receptors will demonstrate a tonic, basal effect even in the total absence of agonist ligands binding to them! If one adds an inverse agonist with a preference for the inactive receptor, the equilibrium shifts to the left, and the tonic agonist effect is reversed!

Therapeutic Effect

All pharmacologic responses must have a maximum effect. The **maximum effect** is defined as the point at which no further response is achieved regardless of drug concentration. If the clinician increases the dose of a drug for a specific woman but this does not lead to further clinical response, it is likely that the maximum effect has been reached. There is one other possible explanation: Some target organs may be more or less sensitive to the drug being administered. **Sensitivity** refers to the drug concentration required to produce 50% of maximum effect. Therefore, it is important to note the drug dose required for the **therapeutic effect**. For some drugs, there is a narrow **therapeutic range** (or **therapeutic window**). The therapeutic range is the plasma concentration of the drug that produces the desired action without toxicity. Hence, a therapeutic range is between a minimal effective drug dose and the toxic concentration. Lithium (Eskalith), a drug frequently prescribed for women with bipolar disorder, has a narrow therapeutic range of 0.6–1.2 mEq/L with toxic concentrations at serum levels greater than 1.5 mEq/L.

Drugs also must be evaluated for the **therapeutic index** (Figure 2-10). The therapeutic index is the ratio of lethal doses in 50% of the population (LD_{50}) over the median minimum effective dose (ED_{50}) in 50% of subjects.[6] The therapeutic index is a quantitative measure of the safety of a drug. A drug has a narrow therapeutic index (NTI) if the difference between the minimum effective concentration and minimum toxic concentration is less than 2 fold. The FDA has named approximately 25 drugs as having a narrow therapeutic index (NTI) (Table 2-7). The higher the number of the therapeutic index, the safer the drug. Lower therapeutic index numbers are associated with an increased risk of toxicity.

The therapeutic index sets the stage for considering **bioequivalence**. Bioequivalence is determined by comparing

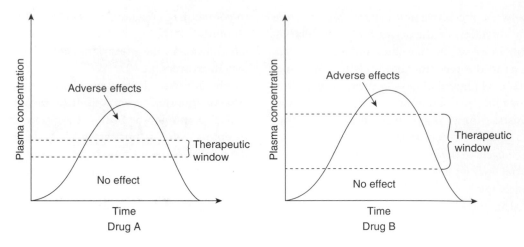

Figure 2-10 Therapeutic window and therapeutic index.

Table 2-7 Drugs with a Narrow Therapeutic Index

Drug Generic (Brand)	Drug Generic (Brand)
Amphotericin B (Amphotec)	Lithium (Eskalith)
Aminophylline	Metaproterenol sulfate (Alupent)
Carbamazepine (Tegretol)	Minoxidil (Rogaine)
Clindamycin (Cleocin)	Phenytoin sodium (Dilantin)
Clonidine (Catapres)	Prazosin hydrochloride (Minipress)
Digoxin (Lanoxin)	Primidone (Mysoline)
Dimercaprol	Procainamide hydrochloride (Procanbid)
Ethinyl estradiol/progestin oral contraceptives	Quinidine sulfate
Guanethidine sulfate	Theophylline (Theo-Dur)
Gentamicin (Garamycin)	Tricyclic antidepressants
Isoproterenol sulfate (Isuprel)	Warfarin (Coumadin)
Levothyroxine (Synthroid)	Valproic acid (Depakene)

Source: Food and Drug Administration: Center for Drug Evaluation and Research (CDER). Guidance for industry: immediate release solid oral dosage forms.

the mean bioavailability of two drug products in multiple samples. If the mean bioavailability of one drug is within 80–125% of another drug, the two are determined to be bioequivalent and can be substituted for each other. However bioequivalence does not guarantee **therapeutic equivalence** because bioavailability is dependent on multiple individual factors. For example, an elderly woman with renal compromise may have a pharmacodynamic profile that allows her to metabolize one formulation of digoxin (Lanoxin) to obtain a therapeutic plasma level, but another formulation may cause her to have subtherapeutic plasma levels. If the prescriber does not want the pharmacy to substitute one drug for another

that has been determined to be bioequivalent, the words "no substitution" must be written on the prescription.

When drugs with a narrow therapeutic index are being administered intravenously, the trough level should be drawn just before the next dose, or approximately 8 to 12 hours after the last dose. In contrast, when gentamicin sulfate (Garamycin) is being administered, blood levels are obtained for **peak levels** 30 minutes after the intravenous infusion ends and trough levels are obtained just before the next dose. The drug dose may be adjusted according to the levels obtained. It is important to note that peak and trough levels vary with the drug.

Pharmacotherapy

Understanding pharmacokinetics and pharmacodynamics is important in achieving a desired beneficial effect with minimal adverse effects. The pharmacokinetic processes of absorption, distribution, metabolism, and excretion determine how rapidly, in what concentration, and for how long the drug will appear at the target organ. The pharmacodynamic concepts of maximum response, therapeutic index, and sensitivity determine the magnitude of the effect at a particular concentration. Knowing the relationship between drug concentrations and effects allows the clinician to take into account the various features of an individual that make them different from the average individual in responding to a drug.

Pharmacotherapeutics refers to the clinician applying drug knowledge of the benefits and risks of drug therapy to individual care. In addition to pharmacokinetics and pharmacodynamics, other determinants of drug therapy include the age or gender of the person receiving the drugs, past and present health status, family history, lifestyle behaviors, and drug compliance. The following factors must be considered when selecting and monitoring drug therapy.

The Effects of Age

There are clearly a number of factors about drugs that influence drug dose, absorption, and efficacy; however, there also are numerous factors about the biologic system that influence drug therapy. Newborns and children generally require lower drug doses secondary to their size and their immature hepatic and renal systems. Drugs cannot be metabolized or excreted as effectively due to the immature liver and kidneys, respectively. Conversely, older women also may require a decreased dose and are at greater risk for toxicity due to the decreasing efficiency of hepatic metabolism and excretion associated with aging of the hepatic and renal systems. The lowered level of enzyme activity slows the rate of drug elimination, causing higher plasma drug levels per dose compared to young adults. Also, certain diseases such as impaired renal and liver conditions mandate dosage adjustments.

Gender Differences in Drug Metabolism

Metabolic differences between the sexes have been noted for a number of drugs. This suggests that hormonal activity might affect the activity of certain CYP450 enzymes. For example, women metabolize diazepam (Valium), prednisolone (Orapred), caffeine, and acetaminophen (Tylenol) slightly faster than their male counterparts. Conversely, men metabolize propranolol (Inderal), chlordiazepoxide (Librium), lidocaine, and some steroids faster than women. Gender differences in drug metabolism may relate to several factors. Women are generally smaller in stature and weight than men; consequently, when women are prescribed a dosage standard for men, they are often found to have an increase in drug concentration. In addition, individual differences in water and fat content may affect drug metabolism, as some drugs are more soluble in water or fat.

Health Status

Both illness and some normal changes in health status can affect the pharmacokinetics and pharmacodynamics of a given drug. During pregnancy, a woman's reduced gastrointestinal motility and increased gastric pH affect drug absorption. Drug distribution in pregnancy may change because the maternal plasma volume increases by 50%. Serum albumin binding capacity is decreased during pregnancy, which results in an increase in unbound drug. Maternal hormones can affect drug metabolism by enhancing or inhibiting metabolism of various drugs. Drug excretion may also be affected due to the increase in renal blood flow (see Chapter 35 for more information on pregnancy).

A woman with liver disease and tuberculosis will be unable to take some of the antitubercular drugs due to their hepatic toxicity. This is because the liver is the major organ involved in metabolism and elimination of drugs in the biologic system. Congestive heart failure decreases hepatic blood flow by reducing cardiac output, which alters the extent of drug metabolism.

An alteration in albumin production (the body's major drug-binding protein) can alter the fraction of bound to unbound drug. Thus, a decrease in plasma albumin can increase the fraction of unbound (free) drug, which then becomes available to exert more of a pharmaceutical effect. The reverse is true when plasma albumin increases.

Family History

Drug action may vary as a result of genetic factors. For example, there are several families of CYP450 enzymes that have demonstrated genetic variations. Essentially, the metabolism rate of certain drugs can be slower or faster in some individuals based on genetic determinants. There are individuals who are poor metabolizers because a certain CYP450 enzyme is slower in them than those in the general population.[37] These individuals exhibit impaired metabolism of several drugs, including beta-blockers, antiarrhythmics, opioids, and antidepressants, and this places these individuals at risk for adverse drug reactions.

The effort to optimize a person's response to drug therapy based on his/her DNA, is called pharmacogenetics. **Pharmacogenetics**,[6] which is often used interchangeably with the term **pharmacogenomics**, is the study of the impact of genetic polymorphisms on drug response.[7] For example, individuals with Down syndrome are hypersensitive to atropine sulfate (Sal-Tropine).[6] Additional information about pharmacogenomics can be found in Chapter 3.

Lifestyle Behaviors

Lifestyle behaviors also are linked to pharmacodynamics and pharmacokinetics. For example, a woman who is prescribed a barbiturate, a drug that causes sedation and drowsiness, and who also ingests alcohol may have a drug–drug interaction that will enhance the sedative effect. Therefore, individuals need to be questioned frequently and directly with exacting questions such as, "How much alcohol do you drink a day, and what do you drink?" rather than "Do you drink alcohol?" Women also need to be carefully questioned regarding self-medication with over-the-counter drugs, herbs, and dietary supplements. Any and all of these substances may interfere with a prescribed drug's effectiveness. For example, a pregnant woman with nausea and vomiting self-medicates with the herb, ginger. Generally in small and moderate doses, ginger may be helpful for some pregnant women, but for those pregnant women who are at high risk for hemorrhage, ginger inhibits platelet aggregation, thereby increasing their potential for bleeding.[38]

Individuals should also be questioned about their use of illegal substances. The use of illegal substances in addition to prescribed medications can result in acute toxicity. When a person who is taking heroin also takes a barbiturate, the combined sedative effect can result in a coma. Appropriate treatment is contingent upon the correct identification of the toxic substance. Illegal drug use is found in every age group, ethnicity, and socioeconomic status, so all individuals should be questioned.

The Role of Polypharmacy

When a person is taking several medications due to multiple medical problems, the chance that a drug–drug interaction will occur increases. Since individuals may be taking from 10 to 15 medications at a time and fail to report all these drugs to their varied healthcare providers, the potential for drug–drug interactions often is high.[39]

Drug Compliance

Ultimately, therapeutic success depends on the individual actually taking the drug according to the prescribed dosage regimen. A former surgeon general of the United States, C. Everett Koop, once made the point that drugs do not work if people do not take them. This statement is remarkably accurate, and inability to follow the prescribed dosing schedule is a major reason for therapeutic failure, especially in the long-term treatment of disease using antihypertensive, antiretroviral, and anticonvulsant agents. When no special efforts are made to address this issue with the people for whom the drugs are prescribed, only approximately 50% of them follow the prescribed dosage regimen.[40] Pharmacoadherence is the extent to which a person adheres to a medication regimen as agreed upon with his or her healthcare professional.[40] Measures of pharmacoadherence include direct, indirect, and subjective indexes. Direct

measures may include biochemical assays as serum iron or total iron binding capacity levels for patients with iron deficiency anemia who are prescribed ferrous sulfate (Feosol). Indirect measures would include pill counts. In addition, common side effects associated with specific drugs need to be explored to determine if they are present and resulting in an individual not taking the drug. For example, subjective measures would include women with obsessive compulsive disorder who may be treated with the drug clomipramine hydrochloride (Anafranil). A metabolic side effect is weight gain, so a woman may not take the medication due to this side effect.[41] Therefore, common side effects need to be explored by the clinician by asking questions such as, "Have you had any problems with the medication or noticed any changes since you began taking this medication?" Taking the time to discuss the medications will elicit this information, and, if side effects are present, other drugs may be prescribed for the primary problem whose side effect profile does not include the aforementioned side effect. Much attention and focus should be committed to health education.

Adverse Drug Reactions

According to the World Health Organization, an **adverse drug reaction** is "any noxious, unintended, and undesired effect of a drug that occurs at doses used in humans for prophylaxis, diagnosis, or therapy,"[42] and it implies a causal relationship between use of the drug and the noxious event. Virtually any drug can have adverse effects. In this textbook, the term *adverse drug reaction* is used to denote unwanted negative consequences that are serious and may or may not be predictable. **Side effects** is the term used to refer to predicted effects that occur with therapeutic doses of the medication. Side effects usually resolve spontaneously. They may be beneficial, but if they are negative, the negative effects are not a threat to health and do not require stopping the medication. In some studies, side effects are reported as a type of adverse effects. Adverse effects are discussed in more detail in Chapter 4.

Pharmacovigilance[2] is the science and activities relating to the detection, assessment, understanding, and prevention of adverse effects or any other drug-related problems. It refers to the continual monitoring for unwanted effects and other safety-related aspects of marketed drugs.

Poisoning can result from exposure to excessive doses of any chemical, with medicines being responsible for most childhood and adult poisonings. The pharmacokinetic characteristics of drugs taken in overdose may differ from those observed following therapeutic doses. Preventive measures, such as child-resistant containers, have reduced mortality in young children. **Toxicology** refers to the branch of pharmacology that deals with the nature, effects, and treatments of poisons. Additional information about toxicology and drug toxicity can be found in Chapter 4.

Research in Pharmacology

Pharmacoepidemiology is a discipline that provides valuable information about the health and cost outcomes of drugs, devices, and biologics, particularly after their approval for clinical use. It is defined as the study of the use of and effects of drugs in large numbers of people. Drugs newly released to the public are monitored for adverse effects different than reported in clinical trials and for morbidity and mortality. As a result, some drugs are withdrawn for use after being approved by the FDA.

Chronobiology/Chronopharmacology

Chronobiology or **chronopharmacology** is the study of pharmacokinetics as related to circadian rhythms or temporal changes. Variations in metabolism may differ by time of day, as well as by the age of the individual. In particular, the elderly may evidence changes in metabolism associated with time of day.[43] It has been suggested that use of drugs may be safer as well as more effective if timing of drug administration is considered.[44]

Intriguing studies exist regarding the use of aspirin during pregnancy and chronopharmacology. Although large studies have failed to find any positive effects of aspirin (ASA) on the risk of preeclampsia, studies that account for the time that the drug is administered have found a decrease in hypertension. Hermida and colleagues reported a study of 341 women at high risk for preeclampsia. These women were divided into six groups based on whether or not they received ASA or a placebo and the time at which the agent was administered (upon wakening, 8 hours after wakening, or at bedtime). No women (0%) developed preeclampsia if they received ASA at bedtime, although 17.9% of cohorts receiving placebos were diagnosed with the condition, as well as more than 10% of those who received ASA at other times (p > 0.001).[45] More studies need to be performed in the area of chronopharmacology.

Conclusion

As identified by the Institute of Medicine, in a 7-day period, four out of five adult Americans take prescription medications, over-the-counter medications, and supplements.[46] In its report, *Preventing Medication Error: Quality Chasm Series*, medication errors have been found to be a significant cause of morbidity and mortality. Providers of women's health care have the responsibility to have an initial understanding of pharmacodynamics and pharmacokinetics for the drugs they order or administer. These professionals need to be cognizant of multiple factors: age, gender, ethnicity, underlying health status, lifestyle behaviors that influence a drug's action, and effects. Routes and timing of drug administration vary dependent upon the drug and the woman's general health status. Monitoring for drug interactions with food, herbs, and other drugs[47] and for adverse reactions is an important intervention. In addition, drug administration and responses vary across the life span, with pregnancy, lactation, pediatrics, and geriatrics demanding special vigilance. Health education requires assessment of literacy, knowledge, and concerns, as well as the synergy of multidisciplinary healthcare members working together to provide the best care possible for women.

References

1. Kirk JK. Significant drug–nutrient interactions. Am Fam Physician 1995;51:1175–8.
2. Smith PF, DiCenzo R, Morse GD. Clinical pharmacokinetics of non-nucleoside reverse transcriptase inhibitors. Clin Pharmacokinet 2001;40:893–905.
3. Berman A. Reducing medication errors through naming, labeling, and packaging. J Med Syst 2004; 28:9–29.
4. Routledge PA, Shand DG. Presystemic drug elimination. Ann Rev Pharmacol Toxicol 1979; 19:447–68.
5. Kato M. Intestinal first-pass metabolism of CYP34A substrates. Drug Metab Pharmacokinet 2008;23:87–94.
6. Buxton IL. Pharmacokinetics and pharmacodynamics. In Brunton LL, Lazo JS, Parker KL. Goodman and Gilman's the pharmacological basis of therapeutics, 11th ed. New York: McGraw-Hill, 2006: p. 1–39.
7. DiPiro J, Talbert R, Yee G, Matzke G, Wells B, Posey M. Pharmacotherapy: a pathophysiologic approach, 6th ed. New York: McGraw-Hill, 2005:54.

8. Dobson P, Kell DB. Carrier-mediated cellular uptake of pharmaceutical drugs: an exception or the rule? Nat Rev Drug Discov 2008;7:205–20.

9. Cecchelli R, Brezowski V, Lundquist S, Culot M, Renftel M, Dehouck MP, et al. Modelling of the blood-brain barrier in drug discovery and development. Nat Rev Drug Discov 2007;650–61.

10. Wilkinson JN, Mottett IK, Hardman JG. Modes of drug elimination. Anesth Intensive Care Med 2008;9:362–65.

11. Li F, Maag H, Alfredson T. Prodrugs of nucleoside analogues for improved oral absorption and tissue targeting. J Pharm Sci 2008;97:1109–34.

12. Lynch T, Pice M. The effect of cytochrome P450 metabolism on drug response, interactions and adverse effects. Am Fam Phys 2007;76:391–6.

13. Wilkinson G. Drug metabolism and variability among patients in drug response. N Engl J Med 2008;352(21):2211–21.

14. Tomaszewski P, Kubiak-Tomaszewska G, Tukaszkiewicz J, Pachecksa J. Cytochrome P450 polymorphism-molecular, metabolic, and pharmacogenetic aspects. III. Influence of CYP genetic polymorphism on population differentiation of drug metabolism phenotype. Acta Pol Pharm 2008;65:319–20.

15. Scandlyn MJ, Stuart EC, Rosengren RJ. Sex-specific differences in CYP450 isoforms in humans. Expert Opin Drug Metab Toxicol 2008;4:413–24.

16. Gandhi M, Aweeka F, Greenblatt RM, Blaschke TF. Sex differences in pharmacokinetics and pharmacodynamics. Ann Rev Pharmacol Toxicol 2004;44:499–523.

17. Bernard S, Neville KA, Nuugyen AT, Flockhart DA. Interethnic differences in genetic polymorphisms of CYP2D6 in the US population and clinical implications. Oncologist 2008;11:126–35.

18. Von Hentig N. Atazanavir/ritonavir: a review of its use in HIV therapy. Drugs Today 2008;44:103–32.

19. Hammer SM, Eron JJ, Reiss P, Schooley RT, Thompson MA, Walmsley S, et al. Antiretroviral treatment of adult HIV infection: 2008 recommendations of the International AIDS Society–USA Panel. JAMA 2008;300:555–70.

20. Genser D. Food and drug interactions: consequences for the nutrition/health status. Ann Nutr Metab 2008;52:29–32.

21. Dahan A, Altman H. Food–drug interaction: grapefruit juice augments drug bioavailability-mechanism, extent and relevance. Euro Clin Nutr 2004;58:1–8.

22. Fuhr U. Drug interactions with grapefruit juice: extent, probable mechanism and clinical relevance. Drug Saf 1998;18:251–72.

23. Sica DA. Interaction of grapefruit juice and calcium channel blockers. Am J Hypertens 2006;19:768–73.

24. Rapaport MH. Dietary restrictions and drug interactions with monoamine oxidase inhibitors: the state of the art. J Clin Psychiatry 2007;68[suppl 8]:42–6.

25. Gardner DM, Shulman KI, Walker SE, Tailor SA. The making of a user friendly MAOI diet. J Clin Psychiatry 1996;57:99–104.

26. Foster BC, Arnason JT, Briggs CJ. Natural health products and drug disposition. Annu Rev Pharmacol Toxicol 2005;45:203–26.

27. Hu Z, Yang X, Ho PC, Chan SY, Heng PW, Chan E, et al. Herb-drug interactions: a literature review. Drugs 2005;65:1239–82.

28. Linde K, Berner MM, Kriston L. St John's wort for major depression. Cochrane Database Syst Rev 2008 Oct 8;(4):CD000448.

29. Izzo AA. Drug interactions with St. John's wort (Hypericum perforatum): a review of the clinical evidence. Int J Clin Pharmacol Ther 2004;42:139–48.

30. Madabushi R, Frank B, Drewelow B, Derendorf H, Butterweck V. Hyperforin in St. John's wort drug interactions. Eur J Clin Pharmacol 2006;62:225–33.

31. Murphy PA, Kern SE, Stanczyk FZ, Westhoff CL. Interaction of St. John's Wort with oral contraceptives: effects on the pharmacokinetics of norethindrone and ethinyl estradiol, ovarian activity and breakthrough bleeding. Contraception 2005;71(6):402–8.

32. Martinez-Salgado C, Lopez-Hernandez FJ, Lopez-Novoa JM. Glomerular nephrotoxicity of aminoglycosides. Toxicol Appl Pharmacol 2007;223:86–98.

33. Hogg RC, Raggenbass M, Bertrand D. Nicotinic acetylcholine receptors: from structure to brain function. Rev Physiol Biochem Pharmacol 2003;147:1–46.

34. Hill SJ. G protein coupled receptors: past, present and future. Br J Pharmacol 2006;147:S27–S37.

35. Hausch F. Betablockers at work: the crystal structure of the B_2 adrenergic receptor. Angew Chem Int Ed 2008;47:3314–6.

36. Giguère V. Steroid hormone receptor signaling. In Bradshaw RA, Dennis EA. Handbook of cell signaling. Philadelphia PA: Elsevier, Academic Press, 2003: p. 57–9.

37. Haile CN, Kosten TA, Kosten TR. Pharmacogenetic treatments for drug addiction: alcohol and opiates. Am J Drug Alcohol Abuse 2008;34:355–81.

38. Nurtjahja-Tjendraputra E, Ammit AJ, Roufogalis BD, Tran VH, Duke CC. Effective anti-platelet and COX-1 enzyme inhibitors from pungent constituents of ginger. Thromb Res 2003;111(4–5):259–65.

39. Tousi B. Movement disorder emergencies in the elderly: recognizing and treating an often-iatrogenic problem. Cleve Clin J Med 2008;75:449–57.

40. Chisholm-Burns MA, Spivey, C. Pharmacoadherence: a new term for a significant problem. Am J Health Syst Pharm 2008;65(7):661–7.

41. Maina G, Albert U, Salvi V, Bogetto F. Weight gain during long-term treatment of obsessive-compulsive disorder: a prospective comparison between serotonin reuptake inhibitors. J Clin Psychiatry 2004 October;65(10):1365–71.

42. World Health Organization. International drug monitoring: the role of the hospital. Technical report series no. 425. Geneva, Switzerland: World Health Organization, 1966.

43. Bruguerolle B. Clinical chronopharmacology in the elderly. Chronobiol Int 2008;25(1):1–15.

44. Ohdo S. Changes in toxicity and effectiveness with timing of drug administration: implications for drug safety. Drug Saf 2003;26(14):999–1010.

45. Hermida RC, Ayala DE, Iglesias M. Chronopharmacology of aspirin: administration-time dependent effects on the incidence of complications in women at high risk for preeclampsia. Am J Hypertens 2002;15:109A.

46. Institute of Medicine. Preventing medication errors: quality chasm series. Washington, DC: Institute of Medicine, 2006.

47. Johns Cupp M, Tracy TS. Cytochrome P450: new nomenclature and clinical implications. Am Fam Physician 1998;57:107–15.

48. Guttierrez K. Pharmacotherapeutics, 2nd ed. St. Louis: Saunders Elsevier, 2008: p. 44.

3
Pharmacogenomics

Judith A. Lewis and Cindy L. Munro

"It is placed beyond doubt that for the formation of the new embryo a perfect union of the elements of both reproductive cells must take place. How could we otherwise explain that among the offspring of the hybrids both original types reappear in equal numbers and with all their peculiarities?"

GREGOR MENDEL, EXPERIMENTS IN PLANT
HYBRIDIZATION, 1865

⬧ Chapter Glossary

Chromosome The self-replicating genetic structure of cells containing the cellular DNA that bears in its nucleotide sequence the linear array of genes.

Gene The fundamental physical and functional unit of heredity. A gene is an ordered sequence of nucleotides located in a particular position on a particular chromosome that encodes a specific functional product.

Genetics The study of inheritance patterns of specific traits.

Genomics The study of all of the genes in an organism's makeup, including their interaction with the environment.

Genotype The genetic constitution of an organism, as distinguished from its physical appearance (its phenotype).

Mutation Difference in DNA sequence. The difference between a mutation and a polymorphism is in the frequency of occurrence; mutations occur in less than 1% of the population.

Penetrance The extent to which a genetically determined condition is expressed in an individual.

Pharmacogenetics The study of the consequences of genetic variations in drug handling that affect individual response. These are usually rare individual differences.

Pharmacogenomics The study of the interaction of an individual's genetic makeup and response to a drug.

Phenotype The observable traits or characteristics of an organism. Examples include weight or the presence or absence of a disease. Phenotypic traits are not necessarily genetic, although they may result from an interaction between a genotype and the environment.

Polymorphism Difference in DNA sequence. The difference between a mutation and a polymorphism is in the frequency of occurrence; polymorphisms occur in greater than 1% of the population.

Single nucleotide polymorphism (SNP—pronounced "snip") DNA sequence variations that occur when a single nucleotide (A, T, C, or G) in the genome sequence is altered.

Source: Adapted from Genome Glossary[3]; Wolpert CM et al. 2005[36]; Lashley FR 2007.[37]

▌ Introduction

In 2003, on the 50th anniversary of the publication of Watson and Crick's landmark article describing the molecular structure of DNA,[1] the National Institutes of Health held a conference in Bethesda, Maryland, to announce the completion of the sequence of the human genome.[2] Along with the celebration of the completion of this massive undertaking—notably ahead of schedule and under budget—the conference laid the cornerstones of the postgenomic era in health care. **Pharmacogenomics**, or the science of the interaction of an individual's genetic makeup and response to a drug,[3] was acknowledged as one of the genomic applications that holds the greatest promise to transform the practice of health care in the 21st century. Pharmacogenomics, genetics, and genomics all are intertwined, but they also differ slightly. Definitions of various terms in pharmacogenomics can be found in the chapter glossary.

In the late 1850s, an Austrian priest named Gregor Mendel performed experiments on plants and founded modern **genetics**, or the study of the inheritance pattern of a single trait.[3] Mutations in single **genes** are well known to cause disorders such as cystic fibrosis, sickle cell anemia, Tay-Sachs disease, or Huntington disease. There are recognizable patterns of Mendelian inheritance responsible for these conditions, which, while serious, are relatively rare. For example, cystic fibrosis, although the most common autosomal recessive inherited condition among Whites, has an incidence of 1 in 3200 live births; and the frequency is less among African Americans and Asian Americans.[4] Many conditions appear to be controlled by multiple genes acting together; thus, they are not in congruence with Mendelian patterns for a single gene alone. For example, Mendelian genetics do not fully address why the degree of expression varies among individuals, with some having significant disease and others mild conditions. This degree of genetic **penetrance** is likely to be associated with the relationship between **genotype** and environment.

In contrast to genetics, **genomics** is a relatively new science and is defined as a study of all of the genes in an organism's makeup, including their interaction with the environment. There is a level of complexity in the study of genomics many times magnified beyond the original study of genetics. Examples of conditions that are included in the study of genomics include common disorders such as diabetes, cancer, and hypertension. Some have posited that every condition affecting human health and illness has both a genetic and an environmental component. Some conditions, such as cystic fibrosis, have a relatively large genetic component and a smaller environmental component, but if one looks at differences in the course of the illness among individuals with similar genotypes and different environmental variables, it is clear that the **phenotype**, or expression of the illness, varies among affected individuals. Conditions such as human immunodeficiency virus (HIV) have a relatively large environmental component and a smaller genetic component. This relationship between environment and genetics can help explain why two individuals who are both exposed to the HIV virus may have different outcomes. It is possible that one of these individuals might not even become infected while the other does. Even if both are infected, differences may exist in the severity and course of the disease.[5]

One of the findings of the Human Genome Project is that, as humans, 99.9% of the genetic code is identical from individual to individual. It is the 0.1% from which individual variations arise. Interestingly, there is more within-group variation among races than there is between-group variation. Race alone is not a sufficient explanation for some of the responses to illness that have been attributed to it in the past. Although it has been argued previously that diversity is simply a social construction,[6] population differences in gene frequency among subgroups of the population have been identified. For example, Ashkenazi Jews are significantly more likely to be carriers of several disorders, including Tay-Sachs disease, cystic fibrosis, Canavan disease, familial dysautonomia, Fanconi anemia, and Gaucher's disease, than are other populations. Members of this group also are more likely to carry the cancer susceptibility genes BRCA-1 and BRCA-2 mutations that put them at greater risk for inheritable breast and ovarian cancer.

Not all of the differences among individuals cause disease. Some of the differences in the genetic code are normal variations, or **polymorphisms**. In contrast, **mutations** are rare events, occurring in less than 1% of the population; polymorphisms are a variation that occurs in more than 1% of the population, such as ABO blood groups or Rh blood factors. The latter variation can be a **single nucleotide polymorphism** (SNP) (Figure 3-1). The analysis of SNPs will be the undergirding of understanding human variation in responses to pharmaceuticals.[7]

Pharmacogenomics

Pharmacogenomics is a branch of pharmacology that applies knowledge of the whole genome to use of pharmaceuticals, especially as related to therapeutic, side, and toxic effects. As more information about pharmacogenomics becomes available, consideration of a person's genotype will be increasingly important in selection of optimal therapeutic agents and modification of drug doses for individuals.[8,9]

Clinical Implications of Pharmacogenomics

Polymorphisms in the genes can lead to individual differences in the effectiveness and/or toxicity of medications. It has been a dream of every provider to be able to offer a drug that is precisely targeted, specifically dose calibrated, and chosen to avoid adverse effects for an individual with a known condition.[10] This dream may become a reality within the next generation.[11] Even if advanced knowledge of pharmacogenomics can only decrease the incidence or severity of adverse drug reactions, new rational prescribing can have a significant

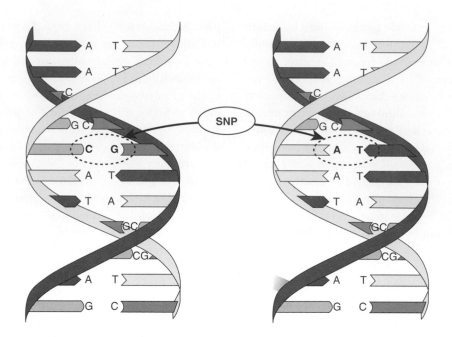

Figure 3-1 A single nucleotide polymorphism is a change of a nucleotide at a single base-pair location on DNA. *Source:* Adapted with permission from David Hall.

positive influence on drug-related morbidity, mortality, and costs, especially because these reactions have been linked to approximately 7% of all hospitalizations.[12,13] Figure 3-2 provides an illustration of pharmacologic treatment in the clinical arena based on recognition of genetic profile.

To date, the majority of pharmacogenomic research has been conducted in the area of drug metabolism.[14] However, other areas of research importance are emerging. For example, gene targets are under study. Studies also are exploring genetic reasons individuals fail to respond to common therapies, such as vaccine failures.[15]

Genomic Differences in Pharmacokinetics

Drug Metabolism

For many medications, genotype can predict whether an individual will be a poor (slow) metabolizer, an intermediate metabolizer, an extensive metabolizer, or an ultrametabolizer (ultra rapid) for a given medication. Poor metabolizers have significantly elevated plasma concentrations of drugs and a greater risk of toxicity than extensive or ultrametabolizers. If a medication must be processed to an active metabolite in order to have an effect, poor metabolizers

may have a much poorer therapeutic response; conversely, maintaining therapeutic drug levels in ultrametabolizers may be difficult. In 2006, a case report was published about a mother who was an undiagnosed ultrarapid metabolizer for codeine. She took codeine for postpartum pain while also breastfeeding. Unfortunately, the ultrarapid metabolism resulted in an accumulation in metabolites, which passed through the breast milk to her infant, who later died of opiate poisoning.[16] Although this is a rare and extreme example, the ability to identify ultrametabolizers will enable pharmacotherapeutic interventions to be identified that are both safer and more effective.

The Cytochrome P450 Enzymes

Cytochrome P450 enzymes (CYPs) are a group of enzymes important in the area of pharmacogenomics. As noted in Chapter 2, polymorphisms of the genes encoding the CYP enzyme family are distributed differently among racial and ethnic groups, although heterogeneity within groups prohibits simple prediction of an individual's genotype by race or ethnicity. CYP interactions with specific medications may result in changes in activity of the drug (either reducing or enhancing activity) or changes in the concentration of the drug (reducing or enhancing elimination of the drug). For example, CYP2D6 is involved in metabolism of many commonly prescribed medications, including beta-blockers, some tricyclic antidepressants,

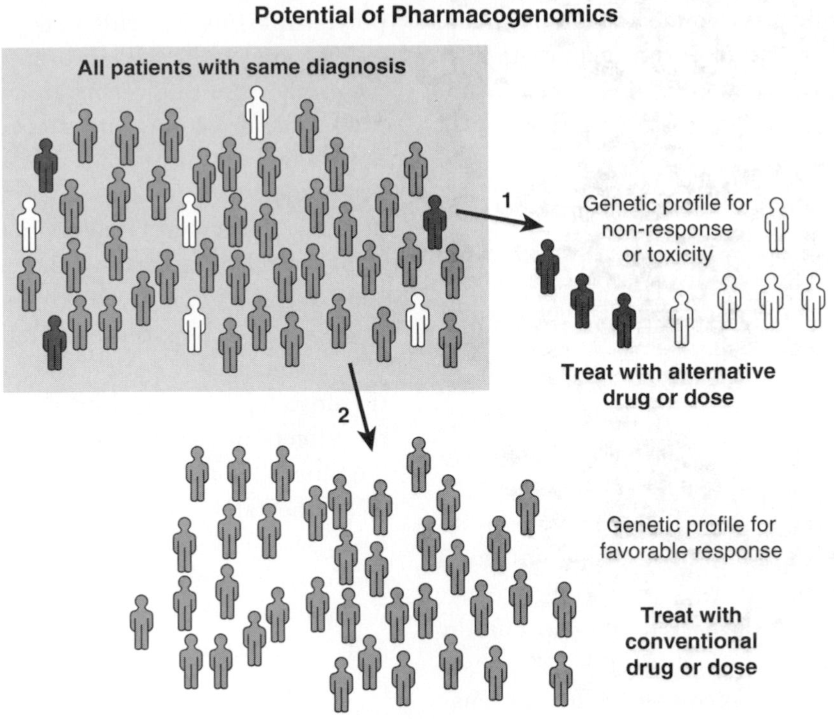

Potential of Pharmacogenomics

Figure 3-2 Potential of pharmacogenomics. *Source:* Reprinted with permission from Evans WE et al. 2001.[7]

selective serotonin reuptake inhibitors, and codeine.[8] Both CYP2D6*17 (more common in African Americans than in other groups) and CYP2D6*10 (more common in Asians than other groups) result in poor metabolism. A variation that involves duplication of CPY2D6 (resulting in as many as 13 copies of the gene) results in ultrametabolism.

Although much attention has been focused on CYPs, other enzymes are also critical in clinical effects of drugs and can serve as a prediction of severe adverse drug reactions.[17] For example, 10 common polymorphisms in vitamin K epoxide reductase complex subunit 1 (VKORC1) account for as much as 25% of the dose response to warfarin (Coumadin).[9] People can be grouped as likely to need high, intermediate, or low doses of warfarin to achieve a therapeutic effect based on their VKORC1 type. Other common polymorphisms that affect drug metabolism are listed in Table 3-1. In 2007 the FDA changed labeling on warfarin to reflect the need to consider genotype in drug dosing and administration.

Drug Transporters

In addition to the relationship between genotype and metabolism, other components of pharmacokinetics (i.e., absorption, distribution, and excretion) are involved

in pharmacogenomics. For example, transport proteins are essential agents for distribution of a number of therapeutic drugs. P-glycoprotein is an example of a protein with a role in excretion of metabolites into urine, bile, and the intestines. This protein also can decrease movement of various drugs such as digoxin and domperidone across the

Table 3-1 Examples of Selected Drug–Gene Interactions

Gene	Drug—Generic (Brand)	Nature of Interaction
VKORC1	Warfarin (Coumadin)	Polymorphism associated with variable response to the drug.
CYP2C9	Phenytoin (Dilantin), glipizide (Glucotrol), warfarin (Coumadin)	Polymorphism associated with variable response to these drugs.
CYP2D6	Codeine	Polymorphism associated with differential ability to convert codeine to morphine (codeine's active metabolite), resulting in individual differences in pain relief.
CYP3A	Erythromycin	Drug inhibits the activity of CYP3A and alters therapeutic and toxic levels of drugs metabolized by CYP3A (e.g., lovastatin, midazolam, and verapamil).
	St. John's wort	Drug increases the activity of CYP3A and alters therapeutic and toxic levels of drugs metabolized by CYP3A.

blood–brain barrier, and it limits accumulation of those agents in the brain. A single nucleotide polymorphism has been found to influence this transport protein's action for some individuals.[18]

Drug Targets

A key molecule involved in a particular metabolic or signaling pathway can be a drug target. Dozens of gene targets or receptors have been discovered. The genetic influence of these receptors is independent of changes associated with drug metabolism, or even transport. One example of drug targets concerns the use of beta$_2$ agonist drugs. Persons with genetic polymorphisms of the beta$_2$ adrenoreceptor have been found to have down-regulation or other previously unexpected reactions when they take these agents. Specific sequelae include susceptibility to agonist-induced desensitization as well as various untoward cardiovascular effects.[18]

Drug targets also provide the basis of some specifically developed drugs. These so-called designer drugs are usually thought of as prescription medications, but they may also be over-the-counter preparations or even botanicals. For example, studies of ginseng have identified a group of nuclear steroid hormone receptors in the ginseng that may be manipulated to create a variation of ginseng that might be more effective as a pharmacologic agent.[19]

Rapid Versus Slow Acetylator

As discussed in Chapter 2, drug metabolism occurs via phase I and phase II reactions that alter drugs from lipophilic to hydrophilic so they can be eliminated in urine. As part of this process, many drugs transfer an acetyl group from acetyl coenzyme A to the acceptor amine drug to form an amide. This process is catalyzed by the enzyme N-acetyltransferases (NAT). There are at least three polymorphisms of NAT that result in a person being a rapid versus a slow acetylator. Thus individuals who are slow acetylators have an increased risk for toxic reactions to drugs that are metabolized via this process such as isoniazid (INH), sulfonamides, hydralazine (Apresoline), caffeine, and clonazepam (Klonopin). The incidence of slow acetylator status is 10% in Koreans, 25% in Thai, 20% in Chinese, 10% in Japanese, 60% in Indians, 50% in Germans, 55% in Italians and Spanish.

▌ Pharmacogenomics and Gender

Genes encoding enzymes involved in drug metabolism are located on autosomes rather than sex **chromosomes**. Females and males in the same racial or ethnic group have similar distributions of particular polymorphisms. For this reason, the effects of gender on drug metabolism have often been assumed to result primarily from differences in average body size, renal excretion, and composition (body fat).[20] However, sex hormones can influence the expression and activity of drug metabolism enzymes.[21,22,23] Activity of CYPs and other liver enzymes are modulated by sex hormones. Thus, even if a woman and man have identical genes for CYP3A4, the amount and the activity of the CYP3A4 protein may differ in men versus women, resulting in different drug medication effects despite adjustment of the dose for body size. Research studies investigating the effects of sex hormones on drug metabolism are ongoing.

Women are more likely than men to develop adverse drug reactions, including cardiac arrhythmias associated with medications that prolong the QT interval (with some antihistamines, antibiotics, antiarrhythmics, and antipsychotics).[23] Two-thirds of reported drug-related arrhythmias occur in women. Long QT syndrome, the most common condition associated with adverse cardiac response to selected medications, is caused by mutations in the potassium-channel genes KCNQ1 and KCNH2. Although inheritance of the potassium-channel genes is generally considered autosomal dominant, for reasons not totally understood, there is a greater likelihood for mothers to transmit long QT syndrome to daughters than to sons.[24] There is also evidence that sex hormones modulate the response to medications that prolong the QT interval. Premenopausal women show greater QT prolongation during the menses and ovulation than at other phases of the menstrual cycle.[23] A female with the KCNQ1 or KCNH2 mutation may have a lower threshold for developing an adverse reaction than a male who has identical potassium-channel mutations, and in addition, her individual response to the medication may vary throughout her menstrual cycle.

Differences between females and males in response to pain medications have received a great deal of attention since the turn of the century. Drug metabolism effects related to CYP expression affect pain response, but differences in pain receptors also may be important. Men report a better response to ibuprofen than women do, despite similar pharmacokinetics.[22] Although opioid receptors are not sex linked, for example, some studies have reported that women have better analgesia and fewer side effects from kappa-receptor opiates than men do; with other studies reporting no sex difference in mu-receptor opiate effect.[22,25,26] It has been hypothesized that estrogen affects opioid kappa-receptor density and binding, but additional research is needed. See Chapter 12 for more details on analgesia and anesthesia.

Resources for Pharmacogenomics

Healthcare providers who have an understanding of genomics and the application of genomic science to pharmacology can be more effective prescribers. In 2000, the National Coalition of Health Professions Education in Genetics (NCHPEG), an interdisciplinary group, published core competencies that serve as the framework for the education of health professionals in the area of genetics. These core competencies were reviewed, updated, and republished in the fall of 2007.[27] Several obstetric and genetic healthcare professional associations have endorsed these competencies.[28] One of the competencies specifically targets understanding of pharmacogenomics and the need to match prescribed drugs to individual genomic profiles. This interdisciplinary group is working to ensure that resources are available for all clinicians to have the tools necessary to think genomically. Some groups, such as nursing, also have a set of separate but complementary competencies.[29] As the era of personalized pharmacologic care emerges, genetic testing may be appropriate to determine the most effective pharmacologic regimen, the expected response to the medication, the appropriate dosage regimen, or the proper way of monitoring drug effectiveness.

The Institute of General Medical Sciences has a subgroup dedicated to **pharmacogenetics**. The Pharmacogenetics Research Network is a nationwide collaboration of scientists studying the effect of genes on an individual's responses to a wide variety of medicines. The network has an interactive Web site that enables a clinician to explore the current state of knowledge about a specific drug or even a gene. Publications on in-depth bench science and articles that are relevant for clinicians are both available.[30]

In order to customize care, a person may need to have a personalized risk profile, individualized health promotion and disease prevention strategies, and pharmacologic regimens based on individual genomic patterns. Pharmaceutical companies are developing designer drugs, or medicines that reflect emerging genomic knowledge. One major concern is that of access. As pharmaceuticals become more individualized, it is expected that the already high cost of drugs in the United States will continue to increase. Health insurance, or the lack of adequate prescription coverage, may increase disparities in adverse health outcomes and limit opportunities for some subgroups on the basis of their genetics.

Controversies for the Future

Most of the studies currently being conducted relate to genotypes and drug effectiveness and adverse effects. However, several topics germane to the overall field of genetics also have profound implications for pharmacogenomics. For example, the issue of informed consent in an emerging area of clinical implications obviously can be problematic.[31] Although it may be anticipated that ordering a genotype can assist in making drug decisions, it also may open the proverbial Pandora's box when potential discrimination in terms of employment and health insurance are considered.[31]

Legal issues also have been discussed in regard to pharmacogenomics. Already there are patents issued for designer drugs that may be highly profitable not only for the manufacturers, but for the scientists involved in their discovery because of intellectual property laws. Liability associated with failure to genetically screen, or failure even to offer such screening before prescribing a medication may be on the horizon in the not-too-distant future.[32]

In the area of genetics as a whole, ethics now are recognized as a major thematic concern. Ethical dilemmas often occur when the needs of an individual differ from family opinion or social mores.[33] These dilemmas may occur within the area of pharmacogenomics as well as genetics as a whole. Ethical considerations are beyond the scope of this chapter, but should be acknowledged, and readers are encouraged to consider these factors when prescribing pharmaceuticals.

Conclusion

In the near future, the field of pharmacology undoubtedly will be deeply intertwined with expanding knowledge of pharmacogenomics. However, it would be premature to anticipate that widespread genotyping will be implemented within the next few years. More likely, such genotyping will occur sooner rather than later for persons with high-risk conditions and for drugs that are particularly difficult to manage with regard to adverse effects (e.g., meperidine) or achieving a therapeutic response (e.g., warfarin).

As knowledge continues to grow about drug metabolism and genotypes, there also will be an explosion in research in other pharmacogenomic areas, including excretion, absorption, drug targets, and others. Clinical challenges include the probability that identifying genetic and pharmacogenomic risk factors will precede the development of new therapies or interventions for prevention.[34] Thus, healthcare professionals may be faced with the ability to diagnose drugs that are genetically contraindicated for a specific individual, but without data identifying alternative options. In summary, clinicians need to be aware of the emerging information in pharmacogenomics. Eventually it will form one of the foundations of rational, genetically guided prescribing.[35]

References

1. Watson JD, Crick, FHC. Molecular structure of nucleic acids: a structure for deoxyribose nucleic acid. Nature 1953;171:737.

2. National Institutes of Health. From double helix to human sequence. Scientific symposium; April 14–15, 2003;Bethesda, MD.

3. Genome glossary. Available from: *www.ornl.gov/sci/techresources/Human_Genome/glossary* [Accessed October 7, 2007].

4. Telenti A, Zanger UM. Pharmacogenetics of anti-HIV drugs. Annu Rev Pharmacol Toxicol 2008;48:227–56.

5. Shulman LP. Cystic fibrosis screening. J Midwifery Womens Health 2005;50(3):205–10.

6. Lewis JA. The social construction of diversity [Editorial]. Issues Interdisciplinary Care 2001;3:175.

7. Evans WE, Johnson JA. Pharmacogenomics: the inherited basis for interindividual differences in drug response. Annu Rev Pharmacol Toxicol 2001; 41:101–21.

8. Wilkinson GR. Drug metabolism and variability among patients in drug response. N Engl J Med 2006;21:2211–21.

9. Service RF. Pharmacogenomics. Going from genome to pill. Science 2005;308:1858–60.

10. Shurin S, Nabel EG. Pharmacogenomics: ready for prime time? N Engl J Med 2008;358(10):1061–3.

11. Prows CA, Prows DR. Medication selection by genotype: how genetics is changing drug prescribing and efficacy. Am J Nurs 2004;104(8):60–71.

12. Eichelbaum M, Ingelman-Sundberg M, Evans WE. Pharmacogenomics and individualized drug therapy. Annu Rev Med 2006:27:119–37.

13. Phillips KA, Veenstra DL, Oren E, Lee JK, Sadee W. Potential role of pharmacogenomics in reducing adverse drug reactions: a systematic review. JAMA 2001;286(18):2270–9.

14. Weinshilboum R. Inheritance and drug response. N Engl J Med 2003;348(6):529–37.

15. McLeod HL, Evans WE. Pharmacogenomics: unlocking the human genome for better drug therapy. Annu Rev Pharmacol Toxicol 2001;41:101–21.

16. Koren G, Cairns J, Chitayat D, Gaedigk A, Leeder SJ. Pharmacogenetics of morphine poisoning in a breast-fed neonate of a codeine-prescribed mother. Lancet 2006;368:704.

17. Ingelman-Sundberg M. Pharmacogenomic biomarkers for prediction of severe adverse drug reactions. N Engl J Med 2008;358(6):637–9.

18. Evans WE, McLeod HL. Pharmacogenomics—drug disposition, drug targets and side effects. N Engl J Med 2003;348(6):538–49.

19. Yue PY, Mak NK, Cheng YK, Leung KW, Ng TB, Fan DT, et al. Pharmacogenomics and the Yin/Yang actions of ginseng: anti-tumor, angiomodulating and steroid-like activities of ginsengosides. Chin Med 2007;15(2):6.

20. Gandhi M, Aweeka F, Greenblatt RM, Blaschke TF. Sex differences in pharmacokinetics and pharmacodynamics. Annu Rev Pharmacol Toxicol 2004;44:499–523.

21. Anderson, GD. Sex and racial differences in pharmacological response: where is the evidence? Pharmacogenetics, pharmacokinetics, and pharmacodynamics. J Womens Health 2005;14:19–29.

22. Kaiser J. Gender in the pharmacy: does it matter? Science 2005;308:1572.

23. Anthony M, Berg MJ. Biologic and molecular mechanisms for sex differences in pharmacokinetics, pharmacodynamics, and pharmacogenetics: part I. J Womens Health Gend Based Med 2002;11:601–615.

24. Imboden M, Swan H, Denjoy I, Van Langen IM, Latinen-Forsblom PJ, Napolitano C, et al. Female predominance and transmission distortion in the long-QT syndrome. N Engl J Med 2006;355:2744–51.

25. Fillingim RB, Gear RW. Sex differences in opioid analgesia: clinical and experimental findings. Eur J Pain 2004;8:413–25.

26. Fillingim RB, Ness TJ, Glover TL, Campbell CM, Hastie BA, Price DD, et al. Morphine responses and experimental pain: sex differences in side effects and cardiovascular responses but not analgesia. J Pain 2005;6:116–24.

27. National Coalition for Health Professional Education in Genetics. Core competencies in genetics essential for all heath-care professionals. February 14, 2000. Available from: *www.nchpeg.org/* [Accessed August 23, 2007].

28. Engstrom JL, Sefton MG, Mattheson JK, Healy KM. Genetic competencies essential for health care professionals in primary care. J Midwifery Womens Health 2005;50:177–83.

29. Consensus Panel on Genetic/Genomic Nursing Competencies. Essential nursing competencies and curricula guidelines for genetics and genomics. Silver Spring, MD: American Nurses Association, 2006.

30. Shurin S, Nabel EG. Pharmacogenomics: ready for prime time? N Engl J Med 2008;358(10):1061–3.

31. Hampton T. Researchers draft guidelines for clinical use of pharmacogenomics. JAMA 2006;296(12):1453–4.

32. Rothstein MA. Pharmacogenomics: social, ethical, and clinical dimensions. Hoboken, NJ: Wiley-Liss, 2003.

33. Lea DH, Williams J, Donahue MP. Ethical issues in genetic testing. J Midwifery Womens Health 2005;50(3)234–40.

34. Hunter DJ, Khoury MJ, Drazen JM. Letting the genome out of the bottle: will we get our wish? N Engl J Med 2008;358(2):105–7.

35. Singh A, Emergy J. Pharmacogenomics—the potential of genetically guided prescribing. Aust Fam Physician 2007;36(10):820–4.

36. Wolpert CM, Singer ML, Speer MC. Speaking the language of genetics: a primer. J Midwifery Womens Health. 2005;50(3):184–8.

37. Lashley FR. Essentials of clinical genetics in nursing practice. New York: Springer, 2007.

Appendix Pharmacogenomic Resources

Genomic competencies for healthcare professionals	Web sites for genetics information
• Core competencies in genetics essential for all healthcare professionals. Available at *www.nchpeg.org*	• US Food & Drug Administration E15 terminology in pharmacogenomics. Available at *http://www.fda.gov/Cder/Guidance/8083fnl.pdf*
• Essential nursing competencies and curricula guidelines for genetics and genomics. Available at *www.genome.gov/Pages/Careers/HealthProfessionalEducation/geneticscompetency.pdf*	• National Human Genome Research Institute. Available at *www.genome.gov.* This site has valuable links to many important resources.
• Physician assistant competencies for genomic medicine: Where we are today and how to prepare for the future. Available at *www.genome.gov/25520786*	• Centers for Disease Control and Prevention. Available at *www.cdc.gov/genomics.* This site has a link to sign up for a weekly update that provides valuable information about the impact of current genetic research on disease prevention and public health.
	• GeneTests and its companion site, GeneClinics. Available at *www.geneclinics.org.* This site is sponsored by the University of Washington, with funding from the National Institutes of Health. It contains a current description of genetic conditions and genetic tests, including an international list of clinical laboratories and prenatal diagnostic centers.
	• The Genetic Alliance. Available at *www.geneticalliance.org.* This site is an international coalition of more than 600 organizations that represent the interests of people with genetic disorders. The purpose of this site is to educate both the public and healthcare professionals and to help people understand the impact of ethical, legal, and public policy sites. It is an excellent site to find referrals for individuals with genetic conditions.
	• Pharmacogenetics Research Network, a subgroup of the Institute of General Medical Sciences that is part of National Institutes of Health. Available at *www.pharmgkb.org.* This group is a national collaboration of scientists who study pharmacogenetics, and the site has interactive capability to answer a professional's questions about specific agents.

"All substances are poisons; there is none that is not a poison. The right dose differentiates a poison and a remedy."
PARACELSUS (1493–1541)

4
Adverse Drug Reactions, Toxicology, and Poisoning

Nell Tharpe and Tekoa L. King

Chapter Glossary

Adverse drug event (ADE) Harm caused by use of a drug. Includes injury from the drug itself or from increasing or decreasing the dose or discontinuing the drug.

Adverse drug reaction (ADR) Response to a drug that is noxious and unintended and that occurs at doses normally used for prophylaxis, diagnosis, or therapy of disease or for the modification of physiologic function.

Allergic reaction Immune response brought on by contact with or inhalation, consumption, or injection of substances called allergens.

Anaphylactoid reaction A severe, systemic reaction that occurs after the first exposure to a substance. Anaphylactoid reactions are not allergic or dependent on IgE. The substance itself causes this reaction.

Anaphylaxis Acute systemic severe Type I hypersensitivity reaction that is life threatening.

Antidote A substance or agent that counteracts or neutralizes the effect of a poison or toxin through binding with it (chemical antidote) or preventing intestinal absorption (mechanical antidote).

Bioaccumulation A functional biologic process where substances are taken up and stored faster than they are metabolized or excreted. This results in an increase in the concentration of a chemical within the organism over time, compared to the environmental concentration of the chemical. Physiologic bioaccumulation is the process by which we acquire many fat-soluble vitamins, minerals, and fatty acids.

Biologic agent Substance derived from living organisms, such as the botulism toxin, antivenin, and live virus vaccines.

Chelating agent Chemical that bonds with metal ions to reduce absorption, facilitate removal from tissues, and enhance excretion from the body.

Desensitization A method to reduce or eliminate a physiologic negative reaction. Most commonly used to treat penicillin allergy in persons who have a disorder that requires penicillin therapy.

Drug allergy Hypersensitivity reaction where activation of an immunologic mechanism is demonstrated, such as the presence of anaphylaxis, or cutaneous manifestations such as rash, hives, or the wheal related to allergen skin testing.

Drug overdose The act of accidental or deliberate administration of a dose of a drug beyond that of therapeutic value.

Hapten Combination of a drug with an intrinsic protein that forms a complex. This complex then becomes antigenic and induces a hypersensitivity response.

Hepatotoxicity Injury to the liver that is associated with impaired liver function caused by exposure to a drug or noninfectious agent.

Hypersensitivity reaction A state of altered reactivity wherein the body reacts to a foreign substance with an exaggerated immune response. Classified as Type I, II, III, or IV depending on the specific pathologic response.

Idiosyncratic reaction Unpredictable reaction that is uncommon and unexpected with any dose of a medication and is not within the known pharmacologic properties of the drug. Theoretical causes of idiosyncratic reactions include immune-mediated responses to reactive metabolites and genetic variations that alter metabolic processes, particularly those involving the liver.

Material data safety sheets (MSDS) Detailed information about commercially prepared chemicals and their effects on humans. The MSDS system was developed by OSHA to ensure consistent dissemination of chemical safety information across multiple industries. Individual MSDSs provide information on chemical properties, effects of exposure, recommendations for cleanup, and postexposure treatment. OSHA recommends that MSDSs follow the 16-section format established by the American National Standards Institute (ANSI) standard for preparation of MSDSs.

Photoallergic reaction An uncommon photosensitivity skin reaction that occurs in the presence of a photosensitizing drug and sunlight. Photoallergic reactions are immune mediated and typically present 24–72 hours following exposure to the agent/light combination. Photoallergic reactions may occur in the presence of a small amount of the agent and have a contact dermatitis-like appearance that may extend to nonexposed areas of the skin.

Phototoxic reaction A common cutaneous reaction with a rapid onset in persons exposed to a significant amount of a photosensitizing agent and sunlight. This reaction appears rapidly after exposure to the agent/light combination. An inflammatory response, phototoxicity appears as an exaggerated sunburn on sun-exposed skin. Blistering and hyperpigmentation may occur.

Poison Defined by the CDC as "any substance that is harmful to your body when ingested, inhaled, injected, or absorbed through the skin."

Prodrug A medication that is administered in an inactive form. Through metabolic processes, this agent undergoes chemical transformation to a pharmacologically active agent.

Toxicants Toxic agents that are inorganic, such as heavy metals, chemicals, and industrial effluent.

Toxicity Consequence of a does that is beyond the body's capability to metabolize under physiologic conditions.

An adverse effect produced by a drug that is detrimental to the participant's health.

Toxicology The scientific discipline in which the frequency and distribution of health effects related to pharmaceutical agents, chemical substances, physical agents, and radiation are studied.

Toxins Toxic agents produced by or occurring naturally in living organisms.

Type I hypersensitivity reaction True IgE-mediated allergic reaction.

Type II hypersensitivity reaction Cytotoxic reaction wherein IgG or IgM antibodies destroy cells containing antigens or haptens.

Type III hypersensitivity reaction Reaction in which soluble antigens not bound to cell surfaces (which occurs in Type II reactions) bind to antibodies and form complexes that are not easily cleared, and these complexes deposit in organs and induce an inflammatory response.

Type IV hypersensitivity reaction Delayed cell-mediated reaction.

Urticaria Often called hives; raised and circumscribed erythematous patches on skin that are highly pruritic.

Xenobiotics Chemicals that are found in biologic organisms that are not expected to be found in them, such as drugs and environmental pollutants. The biologic effects of many xenobiotic substances are due to the effects of the products of biotransformation or metabolites of the drug or substance.

Sources: Centers for Disease Control and Prevention. Poisoning in the United States: fact sheet; International Society for the Study of Xenobiotics.

Introduction

Women's health professionals prescribe medications for their clients on a regular basis. Medication side effects, **adverse drug reactions (ADRs)**, **adverse drug events (ADEs)**, and drug-related poisoning are potential consequences of prescription medication use. Knowledge of adverse outcomes is an integral component of the study of pharmacology.

Additionally, women's healthcare providers may be called upon to render opinions regarding the safety of occupational or environmental exposure to chemicals, biologic materials, and physical agents (e.g., energy sources, noise, and radiation). This is of particular urgency for women during puberty and the childbearing years, when exposure to chemical agents may result in significant **bioaccumulation** of reproductive **toxicants** that have the potential to diminish fertility and affect offspring. Environmental and occupational toxicants are associated with a range of disorders of great concern to parents including preterm birth, autism, attention deficit hyperactivity disorder, low birth weight, and developmental delays.[1,2] This chapter reviews adverse health outcomes that are secondary to pharmacologic preparations, including adverse drug reactions, drug overdose, anaphylaxis, and poisoning.

Epidemiology of Adverse Drug Reactions and Poisoning in the United States

In an analysis of all serious adverse drug events reported to the Food and Drug Administration (FDA) between 1998 and 2005, Moore et al. identified a total of 467,809 serious adverse drug event reports that were submitted to the FDA.[3] Serious drug events were defined as death, disability or birth defects, and other serious outcomes such as acute organ failure.[4] Reports of serious adverse outcomes and drug-related mortality increased nearly threefold during this reporting period. Interestingly, these adverse drug reactions were linked to relatively few new drugs. Out of a total of 1489 pharmacologic agents, 20% (n = 298) accounted for 87% (n = 467,808) of the adverse events. In considering this information, it is important to keep in mind that these statistics represent voluntary reports wherein a drug is suspected of causing or contributing to an adverse outcome, and therefore they are probably an underrepresentation of the true incidence of adverse drug events.

Adverse Drug Reactions in Women

Drug safety and postmarket surveillance systems seek to identify problems early in drug development and marketing. While some ADRs affect both women and men, others are specific to women and their offspring. Examples include thalidomide in the 1960s, and diethylstilbestrol (DES), which was prescribed from 1938 to 1971.

Overall, women use prescription drugs more than men do. As more studies examine the relationship between gender and adverse reactions to prescription drugs, it appears that women have a nearly twofold greater risk of experiencing an adverse reaction to drugs compared to men.[5] Of the 10 prescription drugs withdrawn from the market between 1997 and 2001, eight had more health risks for women than for men.[6] Approximately 59% of patients admitted to hospitals with drug-related reactions are female.[7] Compared to men, women are significantly more likely to present with drug-induced nephropathy or lupus-like syndrome. Further research is necessary to determine whether this relationship exists because women are physiologically more prone to develop adverse drug reactions than men or because women use more medications and also report adverse reactions more often than do men.[6,7]

Drug Exposure During Pregnancy

Adverse drug effects that occur during pregnancy are of particular concern as they can affect both the mother and the developing fetus. It has been estimated that as many as 10% of congenital anomalies may be attributed to environmental exposure to toxicants.[8] An estimated 59% of women are prescribed medication during pregnancy in addition to prenatal vitamins and mineral supplements.[8]

In one study, nearly one in five (19.4%) pregnant women was prescribed at least one agent classed as FDA Pregnancy Category C (15.8%), FDA Pregnancy Category D (5.2%), or DA Pregnancy Category X (3.9%). The majority of drugs were prescribed in early pregnancy (11.2%), followed by late pregnancy (8.2%), with the remainder (7.3%) occurring in the second trimester.

Overall, the drugs identified most often included albuterol (Accuneb, ProAir HFA, Proventil, Proventil HFA, Ventolin HFA), sulfamethoxazole/trimethoprim (Bactrim), ibuprofen (Advil), naproxen (Aleve, Anaprox, Naprosyn, and others), and oral contraceptives.[9] In addition, many pregnant women self-treat using over-the-counter medications, herbs, and dietary.[8]

Effects of Drug Exposure on the Fetus

The effects of toxicants on the developing fetus are influenced by numerous factors. Drugs normally considered safe in pregnancy may exhibit teratogenic effects if administered during embryonic development in unusually high doses or following chronic use. The genetic makeup (genotype) of both mother and fetus may affect the teratogenicity of a medication by affecting placental transport mechanisms and receptor binding affinity, and of course pregnancy itself changes many aspects of drug distribution, metabolism, and excretion.[8] Teratogenic effects from prescription drugs are described in more detail in Chapter 35.

Toxicology

Toxicology is the broad scientific discipline in which the frequency and distribution of health effects related to pharmacologic agents, chemical substances, physical agents, and radiation are studied. Toxicologists evaluate factors that modify the effects of **toxins** and toxicants on the biologic systems of individuals or populations and are instrumental in the development of preventive and safety practices to minimize exposures.[10]

The concept of toxicology has existed throughout the ages. Out of necessity, humans learned to identify plants that were safe to eat and to avoid poisonous flora and fauna. The long-term effects of chemical warfare used during World War I and nerve agents used during World War II highlighted the potentially devastating effects of environmental toxins and stimulated the development of the modern science of toxicology. Also at the time of World War I, scientists pioneered the development of numerous synthetic chemicals with the goal of producing commercial products to enhance numerous aspects of daily life. The 1935 DuPont chemical company slogan, "Better Things for Better Living . . . Through Chemistry," summarizes this time well. During the post-World War II years, significant advances in the prevention and treatment of disease were made possible due to the development of highly effective new pharmacologic agents. However, the extensive and often indiscriminate use of new chemicals, including drugs, ultimately revealed the toxic effects of many of these substances.

Rachel Carson is well known for her popular book, *Silent Spring* (Houghton Mifflin, 1962), which clearly portrays the alarming negative effects of widespread use of toxic compounds, such as dichloro-diphenyl-trichloroethane (DDT). Carson's work was the impetus behind the development of the environmental movement, and it contributed to the development of the scientific discipline of environmental toxicology. Ironically, while Carson was writing *Silent Spring*, she was diagnosed with breast cancer, one of the many disorders with a known link to exposure to environmental toxicants.[11]

Rachel Carson died at the age of 56, only 2 years after the publication of *Silent Spring*.

Environmental Toxicology

Environmental toxicology is the branch of toxicology that evaluates the harmful effects of toxins and **toxicants** that occur in the environment either naturally (e.g., the toxins present in certain mushrooms); through the dispersal of synthetic chemicals (e.g., spraying of pesticides or herbicides), or through discharge of industrial effluent and residential waste; and physical agents (e.g., radiation or noise). Contamination of water supplies by prescription medications disposed of into the sewer system, or landfill runoff, is an example of environmental toxins.

Environmental toxicants with deleterious effects on women and their offspring include lead and other heavy metals such as mercury, herbicides and pesticides, pharmacologics and veterinary medicines, personal care products, heat, and radiation.

Medical Toxicology

Medical toxicology is the subspecialty that focuses on the diagnosis, management, and prevention of poisoning and other adverse health effects due to medications, occupational and environmental toxins, and **biologic agents**. Medical toxicologists interface with providers of emergency medicine, occupational medicine, and poison control centers during the treatment of acute toxicant or toxin exposure.

Occupational Toxicology

The branch of toxicology that focuses on the presence and effects of toxins in the workplace is known as occupational toxicology. This branch establishes control measures to prevent or minimize exposure, as well as actively monitors for toxic effects of chemicals in the workplace. The Occupational Safety and Health Administration (OSHA) originated in 1971 to address safety issues in the workplace. The OSHA hazard communication standard requires that manufacturers develop safety data sheets for all hazardous materials. **Material safety data sheets** (MSDS) are designed to be informational tools for establishing occupational preventive safety practices, including procedures for spill cleanup and postexposure treatment recommendations. Employers are required to maintain MSDSs in a location easily accessed by employees for use as a reference tool in the event of an exposure.[12,13]

Unfortunately, many products contain multiple chemicals and the MSDS may not address all components of the product or provide adequate information regarding the effects of occupational exposure.

Mechanisms of Drug Toxicity

Chemical **toxicity** following the administration of a drug or medication may be the result of one or more of the following: (1) drug overdose or toxic effect, (2) drug interactions with herbal, food, or dietary supplements, or (3) drug–drug interactions. The effects of drug–drug interactions are discussed in Chapter 2. The focus in this chapter will be on toxicity that is secondary to effects of a drug or chemical substance. First, it is important to review factors that can affect drug toxicity.

Genetic Influences

The genes that encode drug-metabolizing enzymes developed long before the advent of modern drug therapy. Genetic variations in pharmacokinetics and drug disposition processes may lead to increased risk of ADRs. For example, phenylketonuria is a genetic inborn error of metabolism that results in failure to metabolize phenylalanine, which subsequently accumulates in toxic amounts.

The Role of the P450 Enzyme System

The hepatic enzyme CYP3A4 metabolizes more than 50% of currently available therapeutic drugs.[14] Polymorphisms frequently affect the cytochrome P450 system, which results in significant differences between individuals in either the phase I or phase II metabolic reactions of drugs[15] (Chapter 2). A genetic polymorphism may produce two enzymes that act simultaneously. Both may inactivate the drug; one may activate and the other inactivate the drug; or both may activate the drug. Any of these can alter the metabolism of the medication in that individual.

CYP3A4 is inhibited by a number of **xenobiotics** and commonly used drugs. This effect has resulted in some drugs being withdrawn from the market secondary to serious toxicity-related events.[14] Drug toxicity and the drug–drug interactions that occur due to the cytochrome P450 enzyme CYP3A4 are affected by multiple factors, including the amount of substrate, genetic polymorphisms, gender, and age.[16] In an attempt to minimize ADRs and drug toxicity, pharmaceutical companies are developing drugs that do not involve the cytochrome P450 enzyme system. These drugs have highly predictable pharmacokinetics and are not metabolized before they are excreted through the bile or kidney, thereby reducing their risk of adverse reactions secondary to metabolic pathways.[14]

Adverse Drug Reactions (ADRs)

Adverse drug reactions were defined by the World Health Organization in 1972 as noxious and unintended human response to a pharmacologic agent occurring at a dose normally considered therapeutic.[17] Adverse drug reactions can be related to the active component of the drug itself, or a reaction to the medication excipient or filler, metabolites of the drug, or contaminants from the manufacturing process.[18] ADRs are distinguished from ADEs, which include harm that is caused by errors in administration such as dose errors.

The FDA MedWatch Program: Reporting of Adverse Drug Reactions

The FDA has collected and analyzed drug-related adverse event data since 1998 through the FDA MedWatch program. This program has an adverse event reporting system (AERS) whereby the FDA collects postmarketing reports on ADRs, ADEs, and other medication errors that are voluntarily submitted or reported directly to the drug manufacturer.[3]

Clinician participation in data collection through reporting of suspicious or confirmed adverse drug reactions is an integral part of an AERS. In particular, postmarketing reporting of ADRs and ADEs provides an opportunity for the FDA and the drug manufacturer to evaluate the safety of medication for use in the general population (Box 4-1).

In an analysis of all serious ADRs and ADEs reported to the FDA between 1998 and 2005, the vast majority were expedited reports submitted by the manufacturer regarding new serious adverse events that occurred during the postmarketing period that were not previously included in product labeling (314,145 or 67%).[3] Data included adverse events related to abuse of prescription drugs and accidental or deliberate overdose.

Drugs associated with mortality included opiate analgesics such as oxycodone (OxyContin) and fentanyl (Duragesic); acetaminophen (Tylenol); nonsteroidal anti-inflammatory drugs (NSAIDs), including ibuprofen (Motrin), naproxen (Aleve), and others; and antidepressants. Drugs associated with disability or other serious

> ## Box 4-1　FDA MedWatch Program: Adverse Drug Reaction Reporting
>
> The adverse event reporting system (AERS) is a computerized database encompassing the FDA's postmarketing safety surveillance program for all approved drug and therapeutic biologic products. The goal of AERS is to improve public health through effective collection and analysis of safety reports.
>
> The FDA receives adverse drug reaction reports from manufacturers as required by regulation. Healthcare professionals and consumers send reports voluntarily through the MedWatch program. FDA staff use reports from AERS in conducting postmarketing drug surveillance and compliance activities and in responding to outside requests for information.
>
> Reports submitted to AERS are evaluated by clinical reviewers in the Center for Drug Evaluation and Research and the Center for Biologics Evaluation and Research to detect safety signals and to monitor drug safety. These evaluations form the basis for further epidemiologic studies when appropriate. As a result, the FDA may take regulatory actions to improve product safety and protect public health, such as updating a product's labeling information, sending out a "Dear Healthcare Professional" letter, or reevaluating an approval decision.
>
> Healthcare professionals can report adverse events through the FDA MedWatch program, safety information and adverse event and reporting system available at: *www.fda.gov/medwatch/index.html.*

Table 4-1 Types of Adverse Drug Reactions

Immune-Mediated Drug Reactions		Nonimmune-Mediated Drug Reactions	
Type	**Example**	**Type**	**Example**
Type I hypersensitivity (IgE-mediated)	Anaphylaxis from B-lactam antibiotic	*Predictable*	
		Pharmacologic side effect	Dry mouth from antihistamines
Type II hypersensitivity (cytotoxic)	Hemolytic anemia from penicillin	Secondary effect	*Candida* vaginal infection after taking antibiotics
Type III (immune complex)	Arthus reaction (local); serum sickness (systemic)	Drug toxicity	Hepatotoxicity from acetaminophen
Type IV hypersensitivity reaction (delayed-cell mediated)	Ampicillin rash	Drug–drug interactions	Seizure from taking theophylline and erythromycin
Specific T-cell activation	Morbilliform rash from sulfonamides	Drug overdose	Central nervous system depression from overdose of opiates
Fas/Fas ligand-induced apoptosis	Stevens-Johnson syndrome	*Unpredictable*	
		Pseudoallergic	Anaphylactoid reaction to radiocontrast dye
Other	Drug-induced lupus	Idiosyncratic	Hemolytic anemia in person with G6PD deficiency after taking aspirin
		Intolerance	Tinnitus after a single dose of aspirin

Source: Adapted with permission from Riedl MA et al. 2003.[5]

outcomes included estrogens, insulins, antidepressants, NSAIDs, and anticoagulants.[3]

Types of Adverse Drug Reactions (ADRs)

Adverse drug reactions are classified as resulting from either immune or nonimmune mechanisms (Table 4-1).

Nonimmune drug reactions are most commonly secondary to known pharmacologic effects and dose related. These ADRs can occur in anyone independent of individual susceptibility. Conversely, immune reactions are unpredictable, not related to the pharmacologic action of the drug, and generally occur in individuals who have an underlying susceptibility to **allergic reactions**. Immune reactions are a result of immunologic sensitivity to the pharmacologic agent.[19]

Nonimmune Drug Reactions

Nonimmune drug reactions can be either predictable secondary to the pharmacologic effects of the drug or its metabolites, or they can be unpredictable idiosyncratic or **anaphylactoid reactions**. Known side effects are technically a type of predictable nonimmunologic drug reaction, and these effects are addressed throughout this book in the sections on specific drugs. Drug overdoses, drug toxicity from toxic metabolites, and drug–agent interactions are classic examples of predictable nonimmune drug reactions that will be discussed in this chapter. Also discussed are anaphylactoid and pseudoallergic reactions, which are unpredictable nonimmune drug reactions.

The terms *anaphylactoid* and **anaphylaxis** deserve comment. Anaphylactoid reactions are the response to the substance itself and not an actual allergic response that involves the antibody–antigen interaction. True anaphylaxis is a "severe, potentially fatal, systemic allergic reaction that occurs suddenly after contact with an allergy-causing substance."[20] Anaphylaxis is always mediated by immunoglobulin E (IgE); however, the two reactions are indistinguishable clinically, which highlights one of the difficulties clinicians have in diagnosing and treating ADRs.

Dose-Dependent Drug Reactions

Dose-dependent reactions comprise 75–80% of all ADRs and are a result of predictable, nonimmunologic processes.[5] These reactions may result from intrinsic or extrinsic factors. Intrinsic factors include conditions that affect metabolic pathways, such as genetic variations affecting drug-metabolizing enzymes, while extrinsic factors include inadvertent or deliberate overdose and interactions between the medication and other ingested substances that result in toxic blood levels. Dose-dependent drug reactions are a result of the known pharmacologic action of the agent and typically are eliminated by reduction in dose or withdrawal of the pharmacologic agent.[5] The direct toxicity of a drug or agent is influenced by the dose, the frequency and duration of exposure, absorption and distribution, the mechanisms and processes of metabolism, the toxicity of drug metabolites, and the routes and speed by which the drug is eliminated from the body.

Toxic Metabolites

Some medications, known as **prodrugs**, are not actively therapeutic as administered; instead, metabolites of the original substance become the therapeutically active component of the drug. In other instances, in particular in the presence of renal or hepatic dysfunction, or genetic polymorphisms such as those that occur in the cytochrome P450 enzyme system, the process of metabolism may transform drugs or chemical agents to reactive species that cause cellular damage, toxicity, or both.[16]

Drug Overdose

A **drug overdose** occurs when the dose of a drug or a combination of drugs is cytotoxic. Drug overdose may occur when a dose above the therapeutic level is administered, during administration of a therapeutic dose to a person who has renal or hepatic compromise, through a drug–agent interaction that decreases metabolism of the drug, or when metabolic or genetic variations that decrease metabolism of the agent are present.

One of the most common causes of drug-induced liver disease is an overdose of acetaminophen (Tylenol).[21] The damage is caused by a metabolite N-acetyl-p-benzoquinone, which is normally detoxified during a phase II reaction. In the case of an overdose, the large amount of metabolite generated overwhelms the ability of the liver to detoxify it, and liver damage ensues.[5] Acetaminophen (Tylenol) is a common component of many over-the-counter cold products, and therefore, consumers may be unaware of how much they are ingesting (Figure 4-1).

Drug–Drug Interactions: The Case of Oral Contraceptives

Combination oral contraceptives (COCs) containing both estrogen and a progestin are prescribed by virtually every women's health practitioner and provide an excellent illustration of drug–drug interactions. Oral contraceptives can interact with medications and/or other substances as the drug being acted upon, or they might affect the metabolism of another drug. Ethinyl estradiol, the most common estrogen in OCs, is metabolized via the intestinal mucosa CYP3A4 during absorption and also in the liver CYP3A4, while progestins are not metabolized by the intestinal mucosa and have only minor first-pass hepatic metabolism.[22,23]

Women taking medications that increase circulating COC hormone levels may note nausea, hypertension, breast tenderness, migraine, or edema. Such drugs include acetaminophen (Tylenol), nefazodone (Serzone), and vitamin C.[22,23] In addition, grapefruit juice inhibits intestinal

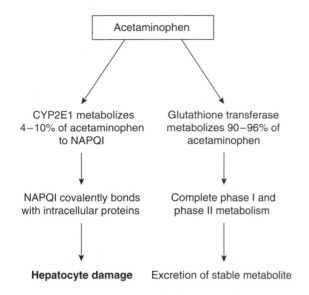

Figure 4-1 Mechanism of acetaminophen-induced hepatotoxicity.

The anaphylactoid reaction to aspirin is a good example of an idiosyncratic reaction. This reaction is variously called "aspirin allergy," "aspirin-induced-asthma," "aspirin-exacerbated respiratory disease (AERD)," and the "aspirin triad." Aspirin allergy induces either respiratory or skin reactions and occurs in 10% of adults with asthma and approximately 0.3% of the general population.[26] Symptoms of the respiratory version include profuse rhinorrhea, bronchospasm, periorbital edema, and flushing, which occur within a few hours of ingestion.

Aspirin and some first generation NSAIDs inhibit the enzyme COX-1, which produces prostaglandin E2 (PGE_2). PGE_2 prevents the release of histamines and synthesis of leukotrienes that cause bronchoconstriction. Thus, aspirin can facilitate the release of leukotrienes and cause bronchospasm in some individuals. It is not known why this reaction occurs in a small proportion of persons and not the majority. See Box 4-2 for a case study regarding such an occurrence.

CYP3A4, resulting in increased levels of circulating estrogen. While herbs such as cat's claw, chamomile, echinacea, and goldenseal act as inhibitors of CYP3A4, studies have not yet documented the clinical significance of the effect on hormone levels from use of these substances.[23]

Drugs that result in a clinically significant decrease in the concentration of circulating COC hormones in women, potentially leading to breakthrough bleeding or unintended pregnancy, include ampicillin (Omnipen, Polycillin, Principen), carbamazepine (Tegretol), nevirapine (Viramune), phenobarbital (Luminal), phenytoin (Dilantin), rifampin (Rifadin), and tetracyclines (doxycycline).[22,23] St. John's wort, an herb used for depression, induces CYP3A4, resulting in decreased efficacy of COCs. Paradoxically, administration of sulfamethoxazole/trimethoprim (Septra) may result in either decreased or increased circulating hormone levels in women taking COCs.[24]

Idiosyncratic Drug Reactions: Aspirin Allergy

Idiosyncratic drug reactions are dose independent, occur infrequently, and are highly unpredictable. Due to their infrequent nature and irreproducibility, they are challenging to study. Clinical reactions are unrelated to the pharmacologic properties of the drug and are thought to be pseudoallergic reactions to reactive metabolites that occur only in a small population of the individuals to whom the drug is administered.[25]

Box 4-2 The Story of an Idiosyncratic Drug Reaction

CR, a 22-year-old college student, was given minocycline (Minocin) for treatment of new onset pustular acne. Three weeks after CR started taking minocycline, she developed fever, a generalized rash, and arthralgia. CR was examined at her college health center and noted to have some lymphadenopathy. She had no known exposure to any infectious diseases and no history of allergic reactions.

CR was admitted to the hospital for observation and over the next day she developed angioedema and dyspnea. She had normal laboratory values that included complete blood count (CBC) and tests of liver function and renal function. She also had a normal chest X-ray and negative blood cultures. Tests for systemic lupus erythemoatosus, hepatitis, and other autoimmune disorders were all negative. It was determined that CR had a serum sickness-like reaction, which is a well known adverse effect of minocycline. CR was treated with steroids and the minocycline was discontinued. Her symptoms improved quickly and she was able to return to her normal activities 3 weeks after the initial onset of symptoms.

Immune Hypersensitivity Reactions

True **hypersensitivity reactions** comprise only 10–15% of adverse drug reactions.[13] The term **drug allergy** specifically refers to hypersensitivity reactions where activation of an immunologic mechanism occurs, such as anaphylaxis, cutaneous manifestations such as rash, hives, or wheal related to allergen skin testing.[13] Immune-mediated adverse reactions can occur rapidly, are frequently life threatening, and are a major cause of adverse drug reaction hospitalization and death. Drugs associated with severe hypersensitivity reactions include antibiotics, NSAIDs, radiologic contrast media, and neuromuscular blocking agents used during the administration of general anesthesia.

Substances with greater molecular weight and complex chemical structures, such as exogenous proteins (e.g., insulin), have a greater propensity for immunogenic hypersensitivity or allergic reactions. Other drugs with smaller molecular weight become antigenic by binding to endogenous proteins to form chemical-carrier complexes known as **haptens**. The hapten then has the antigenic properties that initiate the hypersensitivity immune response.[5,19]

Antibiotics are the most common etiology of mild and severe Type I hypersensitivity reactions and are particularly well known for their immunogenicity.[19,27] The drug most often implicated is amoxicillin (Amoxil), followed by ampicillin (Principen), sulfonamides, and cephalosporins.[5,19]

The four types of hypersensitivity reactions are listed in Table 4-2 and Figure 4-2. Histamine is thought to be the primary mediator of hypersensitivity reactions.[25] Individuals with hypersensitivity reactions frequently exhibit hives (urticaria) or rash, pruritus, wheezing, arthralgia, and localized edema. Hypotension, blistering of the skin, high fever, angioedema, or airway compromise signal the onset of a severe reaction.

Treatment with Epinephrine

Individuals with a history of serious hypersensitivity reaction are frequently prescribed an epinephrine auto-injector (EpiPen). This device is designed to provide a unit dose of 0.3 mg epinephrine 1:1000 in 3 mL via an auto-injector syringe that can be injected right through clothing to allow the individual to rapidly self-administer the drug intramuscularly immediately following exposure to a known allergen. Epinephrine is the agonist for alpha and beta adrenergic receptors that, when stimulated, initiate vasoconstriction, increased peripheral vascular resistance, increased cardiac contractility, relaxed respiratory smooth muscle, and decreased inflammatory response, all of which counter the histamine-initiated physiologic responses.[28]

Additional treatments for hypersensitivity reactions include corticosteroids to limit inflammatory response, bronchodilators to maintain airway function, and NSAIDs for pain relief. New preventive therapies under development and evaluation include immunotherapy with allergen extracts, administration of anti-IgE to individuals who have allergic asthma, and other immunomodulator treatments to preemptively modulate immune hypersensitivity reactions.[29]

Table 4-2 Gell and Coombs Classification of Types of Drug Hypersensitivity Reactions

Type	Mediators	Mechanism of Action	Timing of Reaction	Examples
Type I (immediate)	IgE antibodies	Fc portion of IgE antibody binds to mast cell and/or basophil and if FaB portion of IgE antibody binds to antigen that causes mast cell to release histamine, bradykinin, prostaglandins, leukotrienes	Minutes to hours after drug exposure	Anaphylaxis, urticaria, angioedema, bronchospasm, pruritus, vomiting, diarrhea
Type II (cytotoxic)	IgG and IgM	IgG or IgM antibodies directed at drug-hapten coated cells	Variable	Hemolytic anemia, neutropenia, thrombocytopenia
Type III (immune complex)	Drug-antibody complexes	Tissue deposition of drug-antibody complexes	1–3 weeks after drug exposure	Arthritis, nephritis, serum sickness, glomerulonephritis, vasculitis
Type IV (delayed, cell-mediated)	T-cell, cytokines	MHC presentation of drug molecules to T cells and subsequent cytokine and inflammatory mediator release	2–7 days after cutaneous drug exposure	Allergic contact dermatitis, maculopapular drug rash*

* This rash is suspected to be a Type IV reaction, but the mechanism has not been fully elucidated.
Source: Adapted with permission from Riedl MA et al. 2003.[5]

	Type I	Type II	Type III	Type IV		
Immune reactant	IgE	IgG	IgG	T_H1 cells	T_H2 cells	CTL
Antigen	Soluble antigen	Cell- or matrix-associated antigen	Soluble antigen	Soluble antigen	Soluble antigen	Cell- associated antigen
Effector mechanism	Mast-cell activation	FcR cells (phagocytes, NK cells)	FcR cells Complement	Macrophage activation	Eosinophill activation	Cytotoxicity
Example of hypersensitivity reaction	Allergic rhinitis, asthma, systemic anaphylaxis	Some drug allergies (e.g., penicillin)	Serum sickness, arthus reaction	Contact dermatitis, tuberculin reaction	Chronic asthma, chronic allergic rhinitis	Contact dermatitis

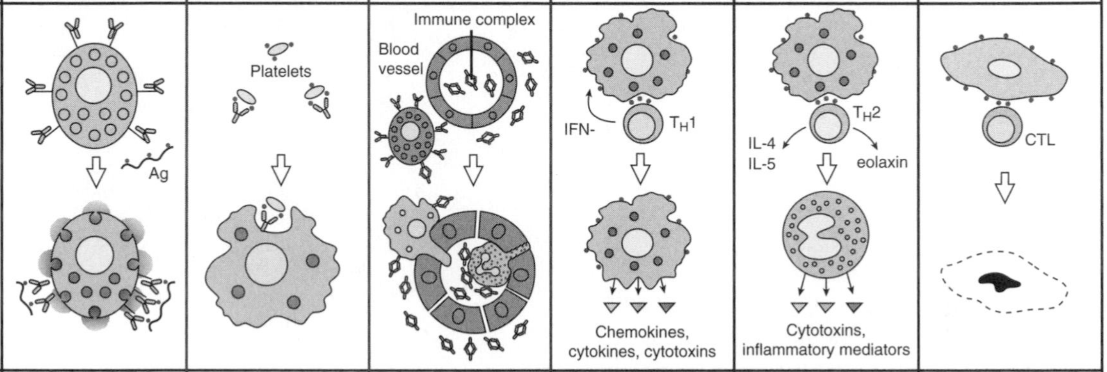

Figure 4-2 Four types of hypersensitivity reactions.
Source: Reprinted with permission from Janeway CA, Walport M, Shomchik M. The Immune System in Health and Disease. New York: Garland Publishing, 2001.

Type I Hypersensitivity Reactions

Type I hypersensitivity reactions are true IgE-mediated allergic reactions. As many as 70% of Type I reactions occur in females.[27] Immune sensitivity is enhanced by intermittent and repeated administration compared to continuous treatment. Immune sensitivity occurs most often following parenteral administration of medication; however, cutaneous exposure is also an important route of sensitization.

Following exposure to a specific allergen, the antibody IgE binds to mast cells. When the antigen (i.e., drug) reappears a second time, the IgE-bound mast cells release histamine, prostaglandins, and leukotrienes, which results in clinical manifestations within minutes to hours following exposure to the drug.[5,27] The amount and combination of pharmacologically active substances released contribute to the severity of the hypersensitivity reaction, which may range from mild (hay fever) or moderate (urticaria

and bronchial asthma) to severe (generalized anaphylactic shock or red man syndrome).

True penicillin allergy is a classic Type I hypersensitivity reaction. Persons who are allergic to penicillin who require penicillin therapy can undergo a process called **desensitization** whereby they are given very small amounts that are gradually increased to larger doses (in an inpatient setting) over several hours. This process makes the mast cells insensitive to the antibiotic and allows regular dosing once the desensitization process is completed.

Treatment of mild hypersensitivity reactions consists of stopping the offending agent and administering an antihistamine such as diphenhydramine (Benadryl).

Anaphylaxis

There is no standard definition or diagnostic criteria for anaphylaxis.[20] However, criteria have been proposed and are listed in Table 4-3. Acute anaphylaxis is characterized by respiratory difficulty and hypotension that require rapid administration of epinephrine and prompt emergency treatment to secure the airway and provide fluid management.[28] The dose of epinephrine for adults is 0.5 mL diluted to 1:1000 given intramuscularly and repeated every 5–15 minutes as needed. Once the individual is stable, follow-up evaluation may include skin testing or radioallergosorbent testing to positively identify the allergen(s). There are no contraindications to use of epinephrine to treat anaphylaxis (Figure 4-3).

Individuals at risk for anaphylaxis can carry epinephrine in an auto-injector. This device must be prescribed, and because it expires annually, the prescription must be renewed annually.

Type II Hypersensitivity Reactions

Type II hypersensitivity reactions are cytotoxic reactions wherein IgG or IgM antibodies tag cells enveloped by drug-hapten molecules and signal destruction of the cell. Examples of cytotoxic drug reactions include transfusion reactions, penicillin-induced hemolytic anemia, and thrombocytopenia from exposure to propylthiouracil (PTU). Treatment includes supportive care and monitoring, as well as administration of anti-inflammatory agents, immunosuppressive agents, and transfusion if necessary.[5]

Table 4-3 Criteria for Diagnosis of Anaphylaxis

Anaphylaxis is Highly Likely when Any One of the Following Criteria Are Fulfilled:

1. Acute onset of an illness (minutes to several hours) with involvement of the skin, mucosal tissue, or both (e.g., generalized hives, pruritus or flushing, or swollen lips, tongue, or uvula) *and at least one of the following:*
   a. Respiratory compromise (e.g., dyspnea, wheeze-bronchospasm, stridor, reduced PEF, hypoxemia)
   b. reduced BP or associated symptoms of end-organ dysfunction (e.g., hypotonia [collapses], syncope, incontinence)

2. Two or more of the following that occur rapidly after exposure to a *likely allergen for that patient* (minutes to several hours):
   a. Involvement of the skin-mucosal tissue (e.g., generalized hives, itch-flush, swollen lips, tongue, or uvula)
   b. Respiratory compromise (e.g., dyspnea, wheeze-bronchospasm, stridor, reduced PEF, hypoxemia)
   c. Persistent gastrointestinal symptoms (e.g., crampy abdominal pain, vomiting)

3. Reduced BP after exposure to a *known allergen for that patient* (minutes to several hours)
   a. Infants and children: low systolic BP (age specific) or > 30% decrease in systolic BP
   b. Adults: systolic BP of < 90 mm Hg or > 30% decrease in systolic BP from that person's baseline

Source: Reprinted with permission from Sampson HA et al. 2006.[20]

Type III Hypersensitivity Reactions

Type III hypersensitivity reactions are immune-complex reactions whereby drug-antibody complexes permeate tissues resulting in complement activation and a local or

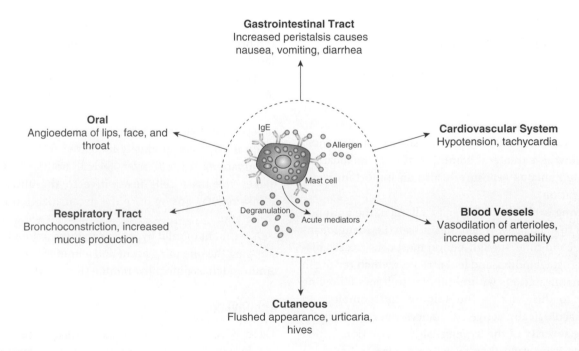

Gastrointestinal Tract
Increased peristalsis causes nausea, vomiting, diarrhea

Oral
Angioedema of lips, face, and throat

Cardiovascular System
Hypotension, tachycardia

IgE
Allergen
Mast cell
Degranulation
Acute mediators

Respiratory Tract
Bronchoconstriction, increased mucus production

Blood Vessels
Vasodilation of arterioles, increased permeability

Cutaneous
Flushed appearance, urticaria, hives

Figure 4-3 Mechanism of anaphylaxis.

systemic inflammatory response, such as serum sickness or drug-induced fever. Soluble antigens not bound to cell surfaces (which occurs in Type II reactions) bind to antibodies and form complexes that are not easily cleared. These complexes deposit in organs and induce an inflammatory response. Immune complex reactions generally occur 7–21 days following drug administration.[5,27] Type III reactions mimic disorders such as lupus and arthritis. For example, minocycline (Minocin) can induce a Type III reaction called "drug induced lupus." Laboratory evaluation includes erythrocyte sedimentation rate (ESR), C-reactive protein, and antinuclear antibodies.[5] Treatment includes supportive care and monitoring, as well as administration of anti-inflammatory agents.

Type IV Hypersensitivity Reactions

Type IV hypersensitivity reactions are delayed cell-mediated reactions that result in contact dermatitis. This type of reaction can occur following exposure to latex gloves, tuberculosis purified protein derivative (Mantoux) testing, and exposure to poison oak or poison ivy. In these reactions, interaction of T cells with molecules from the drug or substance results in cytokine and inflammatory mediator release approximately 2–7 days following exposure.[5] Type IV reactions are divided into three categories based on the specific immune response generated. Diagnosis is based on appearance, although patch testing may be performed following treatment to verify the allergen. Treatment consists of comfort measures and topical or systemic corticosteroid therapy as indicated.

Manifestations of Drug Toxicity

In clinical terms, it is sometimes more helpful to categorize adverse drug reactions by the organ system affected or syndrome that is elicited. This section reviews the common adverse drug reactions.

Drug-Induced Skin Eruptions

Cutaneous manifestations are the most frequent type of drug reaction and often the cardinal sign of drug toxicity or hypersensitivity.[19] Drug-induced eruptions are usually Type IV hypersensitivity reactions that develop several days or a few weeks after the initial exposure to the inciting agent, or mild Type I hypersensitivity reactions such as the classic "ampicillin rash." Symptoms include rash, hives or **urticaria**, and angioedema that appears after the drug

is discontinued. The most common drug-induced eruptions are drug-induced exanthem or rashes, which account for about 75% of all cutaneous drug reactions.[27] While drug-induced rashes occur in response to many medications, the most frequent is secondary to the administration of antibiotics or sulfa drugs. Rash typically presents with intense pruritus and the formation of spreading macular, papular, or morbilliform (measles-like) eruptions that begin in dependent areas and spread.[30] The morbilliform type is more frequently associated with Stevens-Johnson syndrome (SJS) and serum sickness, which are addressed later in this chapter.

If the rash is an IgE-mediated Type I hypersensitivity reaction, urticaria may occur as an isolated finding or as a precursor of acute anaphylactic reaction. The superficial lesions are typically raised, erythematous wheals with central pallor that are initially clearly defined and intensely pruritic. Urticaria, or hives, are often the initial sign of a reaction to agents such as penicillins, cephalosporins, sulfa drugs, local anesthetics, or latex that is mediated by cutaneous mast cells' release of histamine.[5] Non-IgE-mediated hives also occur, most frequently in response to angiotensin-converting enzyme (ACE) inhibitors, opiates, and anesthetic agents. An idiopathic form can worsen with exposure to aspirin, acetaminophen (Tylenol), or indomethacin (Indocin).

Angioedema, which is associated with ACE inhibitor administration, may occur independently or in association with urticaria. Angioedema involves the deep dermis and subcutaneous tissues and may cause laryngeal edema with resultant airway compromise.[5]

Fixed drug eruptions can occur following exposure to NSAIDs, including aspirin, tetracyclines and sulfonamides, the phenolphthalein found in some laxatives, and barbiturates. These eruptions appear as either eczematous plaques or bullous lesions, and when the individual is reexposed to the same antigen, lesions recur in the same (fixed) locations where they appeared during the initial attack.

Pemphigus is a rare form of skin drug eruption. Pemphigus is a blistering disease. The drugs most commonly involved are ACE inhibitors.[31]

A few drugs are specifically implicated in a rare, but serious drug-induced cutaneous reaction called drug-hypersensitivity syndrome, which is characterized by rash, fever, and internal organ involvement. Anticonvulsants appear to have a toxic metabolite that induces this disorder. Similarly, sulfonamide antibiotics cause drug-hypersensitivity syndrome via a metabolic pathway that produces toxic metabolites. Although approximately 2% of the population have the slow acetylator makeup, the incidence of drug-sensitivity syndrome is only 1 in 10,000 individuals exposed to sulfa antibiotics.[32] Other drugs that can cause this syndrome include allopurinol (Zyloprim), minocycline (Minocin), nevirapine (Viramune), and abacavir (Ziagen).

Diagnosis of drug eruptions is based on the appearance of the lesions, coupled with a history of recent drug administration. Consultation is based on the severity of the symptom profile and signs of systemic involvement, which may indicate the presence of a life-threatening disorder such as SJS or toxic epidermal necrolysis (TEN). Treatment involves discontinuing the offending drug and providing supportive care and comfort measures to avoid undue itching until the rash subsides. Topical antihistamines or corticosteroids are the first-line treatment. Systemic corticosteroids can be utilized as needed (Chapter 26).

Photosensitivity Reactions

Photosensitivity reactions occur when persons using photosensitizing agents such as medications and personal care products are exposed to ultraviolet light. Photosensitivity drug reactions include phototoxic and photoallergic reactions.

Phototoxic reaction presents as hypersensitivity to sun exposure, resulting in severe sunburn in exposed areas of the skin that may or may not itch. Antibiotics, NSAIDs, cardiovascular drugs, diuretics, antidepressants, antihistamines, and a few others can cause phototoxic reactions. Phototoxic reactions are a result of dose-related direct cellular damage caused by the photoactivated agent and usually develop within minutes or hours after exposure to the drug and light.[33] Phototoxic reactions can occur following use of tetracyclines (doxycycline, minocycline, and others), quinolones (ciprofloxacin), and NSAIDs (naproxen, ibuprofen, and others).

Photoallergic reactions are also drug-related light sensitivity. Photoallergic reactions are unpredictable immune-mediated reactions that typically occur 24–72 hours after exposure to the agent and light. The rash is eczematous and itchy. These reactions have a similar mechanism to contact dermatitis reactions, and appear as eczematous patches in exposed areas, which can extend to nonexposed skin.[33]

Hepatotoxicity

Drug-induced liver injury is the primary cause of the postmarketing withdrawal of prescribed drugs.[34] Although hepatoxicity is a rare occurrence, acetaminophen overdose was the leading cause of acute liver failure in the United States in 2008, and over 1000 drugs that cause **hepatotoxicity** have been identified.[21,35] Hepatotoxicity can be the result of an idiosyncratic response and altered metabolism

(e.g., isoniazid [INH] toxicity is secondary to the creation of toxic metabolites that directly harm hepatocytes) or the result of an immune reaction (e.g., acetaminophen [Tylenol] toxicity is the result of a metabolite-protein compound that stimulates an immune response) (Figure 4-1). Clinically, two kinds of drug-related hepatotoxicity occur: (1) the hepatocellular type, which presents with a marked elevation in alanine aminotransferase; and (2) the cholestatic type, which reveals an initial rise in serum alkaline phosphatase.[36]

An individual's risk of hepatotoxicity is affected by a multitude of factors. In particular, preexisting hepatic compromise, drug–agent interactions, and some genetic polymorphisms of the cytochrome P450 system can increase the risk of hepatotoxicity. Other associated factors include race, female gender, immune response, and chronic or acute alcohol intake.[37] Women develop hepatotoxicity much more often than men do.[21] Concomitant use of some complementary and alternative therapies, such as kava-kava, germander, and others can also contribute to hepatic injury.[38]

The pathophysiologic mechanisms may be related to the toxicity of the drug itself or highly reactive toxic metabolites that are either produced in excess or not reduced to nonreactive compounds.[34,36,39,40]

Drug-induced hepatitis can be acute or chronic in nature and can result in liver failure. Cirrhosis and hepatic cholestasis can also occur, with jaundice being prolonged in the presence of cholestasis.[31] Extrahepatic symptoms, such as fever, rash, or serum-sickness syndrome are not uncommon, particularly in individuals with immune-mediated hepatic injury. A significant decrease in serum transaminase levels within 7–10 days of stopping the drug aids diagnosis of drug-related hepatotoxicity.[39]

Prompt recognition allows for early laboratory testing and referral for evaluation and treatment. Prompt discontinuation of the offending agents is indicated. Referral for specialty care is indicated for individuals with severe hepatotoxicity. Treatment is based on symptoms and is largely supportive, although individuals with acute liver failure may require transplant.

Nephrotoxicity

Nephrotoxicity occurs as a result of renal excretion of drugs and toxic metabolites. In order to form urine, the kidney receives approximately 25% of the cardiac output, which exposes renal glomerular, tubular, and interstitial cells to large concentrations of drugs and their metabolites. As urine is concentrated in the kidney's proximal tubule, nephrotoxins accumulate and may result in site-specific nephrotoxicity. There are four drug-induced toxic renal syndromes: acute renal failure, chronic renal failure, nephritic syndrome, and renal tubular dysfunction.[41]

The mechanisms by which drug-related kidney damage occurs are numerous and include decreased renal perfusion, vascular or direct tubular injury, allergic interstitial inflammation, glomerular basement membrane injury, chronic interstitial injury, papillary necrosis, direct tubular toxicity, free radical injury, abnormal phospholipid metabolism, and intracellular calcium toxicity.[41]

A wide range of commonly administered prescription and over-the-counter drugs possess the potential for nephrotoxicity. Risk is elevated in the presence of preexisting renal compromise, low fluid volume, polypharmacy, bolus dosing, and drug interactions that increase circulating drug levels. Drugs that may contribute to nephrotoxicity include ACE inhibitors, acyclovir (Zovirax), cephalosporins, ciprofloxacin (Cipro), immunoglobulin, lithium (Lithobid), NSAIDs, penicillins, sulfonamides, rifampin (Rifadin), and valproic acid (Depakote).[41]

Prevention of nephritis consists of adequate circulating fluid volume and serial monitoring of renal function when indicated. Elevations in blood urea nitrogen (BUN) and creatinine indicate renal compromise. Withholding of the drug and prompt consultation for complete evaluation are indicated if laboratory indices of kidney function are abnormal.

Drug Fever

Drug fever is a nonspecific sign of drug toxicity that mimics numerous medical conditions. While fever is a predictable side effect of some medications and vaccines, it can also be the primary indicator of an adverse drug reaction. Drug fever occurs more commonly in individuals taking multiple medications, the elderly, and those infected with HIV.[42]

The physiologic mechanisms behind febrile reactions to pharmacologic agents are not well understood. Drug-related temperature elevations are associated with hypersensitivity (allergic) reactions, pharmacologic alterations in thermoregulatory mechanisms, alterations in skeletal muscle action and metabolism, idiosyncratic drug reactions, and as a direct result of drug pharmacokinetics.[42]

Febrile hypersensitivity reactions are most often associated with use of anticonvulsants, antibiotics, allopurinol (Zyloprim), and heparin. Antibiotics are associated with approximately one-third of drug-related fevers, and they often confuse the clinical picture by simulating a relapse of the underlying condition that prompted use of antibiotics,

thus prolonging exposure to antibiotic treatment if drug-induced fever is not considered as the cause.

Some drugs, such as thyroid replacement hormone (Synthroid), those with an anticholinergic effect (e.g., tricyclic antidepressants, antihistamines, and phenothiazines), and sympathomimetic agents, such as amphetamines, cocaine, and ecstasy, may disrupt physiologic thermoregulation of the body, resulting in temperature elevation that is secondary to increased heat production or diminished heat dissipation.[43]

Parenteral administration of medications may cause fever, which is secondary to contamination of the medication or site, a localized inflammatory response, or a response to the drug, as is common following administration of some vaccines. Fever may also occur in response to the pharmacologic properties of the drug itself, most commonly following oncology-related chemotherapy and treatment of conditions such as secondary or tertiary syphilis or brucellosis.

Treatment of drug fever consists of discontinuing the offending medication, providing supportive care, and administering appropriate therapy where such therapy exists (such as dantrolene sodium [Dantrium] for malignant hyperthermia).[43] Fever usually resolves in 72–96 hours following drug withdrawal. Treatment consists of fluid management, active cooling, and supportive care.

Malignant Hyperthermia

Malignant hyperthermia is a life-threatening condition that occurs in response to medications used during anesthesia induction and maintenance. It requires prompt recognition and rapid initiation of treatment to prevent excess morbidity or mortality. Febrile **idiosyncratic reactions**, while highly unpredictable, may have a familial or genetic basis such as malignant hyperthermia.

Stevens-Johnson Syndrome and Toxic Epidermal Necrolysis

Stevens-Johnson syndrome (SJS) and toxic epidermal necrolysis (TEN) are acute idiosyncratic hypersensitivity reactions that can occur spontaneously but are also associated with the administration of medications. The drugs with the highest incidence of SJS/TEN are trimethoprim-sulfamethoxazole (Bactrim) (1–3 reactions per 100,000 users), sulfadoxine/pyrimethamine (Fansidar-R) (10 reactions per 100,000 users) and carbamazepine (Tegretol) (14 reactions per 100,000 users).[44] Other drugs associated with SJS/TEN are NSAIDs, anticonvulsants, penicillins, and cephalosporins (Table 4-4). Approximately 35% of hospital admissions for SJS/TEN are coded as being drug related, with the highest mortality rate among individuals at or older than age 65 years.[30]

SJS and TEN are a spectrum of mucocutaneous bullous disorders. SJS has an estimated incidence of 0.4–1.2 persons per million per year and has approximately a 5% mortality rate.[27] TEN is a severe form of SJS, which presents with blistering and desquamation of the epidermis. TEN affects approximately 1.2–6 persons per million per year and has an overall mortality rate of 30%.[27,30] SJS typically presents with flu-like symptoms for 1–3 days, followed in hours or days by persistent fever, skin lesions (rash, blisters), blisters on mucous membranes, and ocular involvement.[45] Skin desquamation results in a burned appearance.

The pathophysiology of this syndrome is not well understood. SJS and TEN are considered an inflammatory hypersensitivity reaction resulting from a combination of T-cell mediated cytotoxic response to drug antigens and cell-mediated immune reaction.[36] Cell-mediated immune response results in cytokine release leading to a significant inflammatory reaction and apoptosis of epidermal cells.[45]

Diagnosis is based on symptoms. Treatment consists of discontinuation of suspected drug(s) in any individual with blisters or erosions following drug administration. Prompt admission to intensive care or a burn center is required for aggressive fluid management, pain control, antibiotic therapy, and wound care.

Table 4-4 Selected Drugs That Can Cause Stevens-Johnson Syndrome

Drugs Most Frequently Associated	Drugs Also Associated
Allopurinol (Zyloprim)	Cephalosporins
Amithiozone (Tibione)	Diclofenac (Voltaren)
Aminopenicillins	Ethambutol (Myambutol)
Barbiturates	Fenbufen (Lederfen)
Benoxaprofen (Oraflex)	Fluoroquinolones
Carbamazepine (Tegretol)	Ibuprofen (Advil)
Chlormezanone (Trancopal)	Ketoprofen (Orudis)
Cotrimoxazole (Septra)	Chlormezanone (Trancopal)
Phenylbutazone	Naproxen (Aleve)
Phenytoin (Dilantin)	Rifampin (Rifadin)
Piroxicam (Feldene)	Sulindac (Clinoril)
Sulfadoxine (Fansidar)*	Tenoxicam (Tilcotil)
Sulfadiazine (Diazin)	Tiaprofenic acid (Surgam)
Sulfasalazine (Azulfidine)	Thiabendazole (Mintezol)
	Vancomycin (Vanocin)

* sulfadoxine/pyrimethamine
Source: Adapted from Roujeau JC 1994.[44]

Long QT Syndrome

Prolongation of the QT interval (*torsades de pointes*) is a side effect of a number of structurally unrelated drugs. The clinical presentation is usually syncope (hypotension) and palpitations (tachycardia) that are self-limited, but this syndrome can cause seizure-like activity and sudden cardiac arrest.[46] Drug-induced prolonged long QT syndrome is more prevalent in individuals with the following risk factors: female gender, hypokalemia, bradycardia, polymorphisms of the sodium ion channels, naturally occurring long QT syndrome, treatment of cardiac symptoms with QT-prolonging drugs, and profoundly low magnesium levels.[47]

Female gender is a powerful predictor of drug-related long QT syndrome, especially when the physiologic factors that maintain normal polarization are altered, as occurs in congenital and acquired long QT syndromes.[47] Approximately 10–15% of persons who develop drug-induced long QT interval have genetic polymorphisms that result in subclinical long QT intervals.[46]

Drugs most commonly associated with long QT syndrome include cardiac drugs such as disopyramide (Norpace), dofetilide (Tikosyn), ibutilide (Corvert), procainamide (Pronestyl), quinidine (Quinora and others), sotalol (Betapace), and bepridil (Vascor). Clarithromycin (Biaxin), erythromycin (E-mycin and others), droperidol (Inapsine), methadone (Dolophine), antipsychotic agents, and other drugs have a small, but documented risk of long QT syndrome, which may be exacerbated by concurrent administration of drugs that inhibit drug-elimination mechanisms.[47]

Evaluation of the QT interval is used as a marker during drug development for the prediction of serious adverse drug effects, syncope, and sudden cardiac arrest. However, the number of participants in drug trials is often too low to effectively quantify the risk. Symptoms of long QT syndrome can be missed during preliminary drug trials when new drugs are administered to study participants with preexisting higher-than-average risk of sudden death, as changes in the QT interval occur secondary to disease states, and as physical manifestations of psychologic conditions such as psychosis.

In addition, current evidence postulates that 5–10% of individuals with drug-induced long QT syndrome have common polymorphisms that affect normal action potentials, leading to subclinical long QT syndrome.[47] Cardiac evaluation with ECG is frequently recommended prior to initiating a medication associated with long QT syndrome. This is particularly appropriate for women who have specific factors that significantly elevate the risk of long QT syndrome such as age older than 65 years, a family history of sudden death, use of medications that prolong the QT interval, and coadministration of pharmacologic agents that inhibit drug elimination mechanisms (e.g., erythromycin [E-mycin and others], clarithromycin [Biaxin], ketoconazole [Nizoral], itraconazole [Sporanox], amiodarone [Cordarone], quinidine [Quinora and others], antidepressants, and antiretroviral agents).[47]

Women who are prescribed medications that have the potential to prolong the QT interval should be instructed to return for ECG evaluation if worrisome symptoms such as palpitations or syncope develop, or if they have conditions that may lead to hypokalemia, such as vomiting or diuretic use. Treatment consists of cardiac monitoring, early defibrillation when indicated, correction of electrolyte imbalance, administration of intravenous magnesium sulfate, external or internal pacing as necessary, and supportive care.[46]

Drug-Induced Lupus

Drug-induced lupus is a drug-induced autoimmune disorder that is reversible following cessation of drug therapy.[48] Drug-induced lupus occurs in individuals on long-term therapy (> 1 month duration). It is more common in the elderly and has a 1:1 ratio between females and males.[49] Symptoms include malaise, fever, joint pain, and swelling. Although the mechanism responsible for this disorder is not definitively known, it is assumed that the offending drugs or a reactive metabolite blocks the innate process of tolerance, thereby facilitating production of autoantibodies, or the drug (or metabolite) creates a hapten that functions as an autoantibody.[49]

While a wide array of medications may cause drug-induced lupus, the drugs most often associated with the disorder are procainamide (Pronestyl) and hydralazine (Apresoline). In addition, quinidine (Quinaglute), isoniazid (INH), methyldopa (Aldomet), minocycline (Minocin), and chlorpromazine (Thorazine) are known to induce this disorder.[48,49] Other drugs that are considered probable causes of drug-induced lupus include anticonvulsants, statins, fluorouracil agents, terbinafine (Lamisil), antithyroid medications, and hydrochlorothiazide (HydroDIURIL).[49]

Testing for drug-induced lupus includes antinuclear antibody (ANA) testing, specific for reactivity with a histone-DNA complex.[48] Treatment consists of withdrawal of drug therapy followed by substitution of a medication not associated with drug-induced lupus. Mild constitutional symptoms are treated with NSAIDs, while severe presentation (serositis or renal dysfunction) is an indication for referral to a rheumatologist for systemic therapy.[48]

Serum Sickness

Serum sickness is an immune-complex hypersensitivity disorder (Type III) that results from exposure to a foreign protein antigen or hapten, such as following tetanus antitoxin or antirabies serum administration.[5] Bee stings and other drugs may also cause a serum-sickness-like reaction. Serum sickness was seen much more frequently in the mid-20th century when drug development was less precise and heterologous serum products were in use.

Serum sickness is characterized by fever, followed by rash, and accompanied by general malaise that includes headache, nausea and vomiting, and prominent polyarthralgia or polyarthritis that occur 8–14 days after the antigen exposure.[50] Thoughtful differential diagnosis is necessary, as this presentation is consistent with several infectious and autoimmune disorders. Consultation with an allergist or rheumatologist can be helpful.

Treatment for serum sickness consists of supportive care. As most of the medications associated with serum sickness are administered parenterally, time must be allowed for metabolism of the agent. Symptomatic relief may be obtained with administration of NSAIDs for pain control and antihistamines to relieve itching. Corticosteroids are reserved for those individuals with severe systemic symptoms.[50]

Thrombocytopenia

Bleeding and bruising following use of quinine for treatment of malaria was first reported in *Lancet* in 1865.[51] Although quinine is not used to treat malaria today, it continues to be used for the treatment of nocturnal muscle cramps, and thrombocytopenia continues to be a complication. The University of Oklahoma Health Sciences Center maintains an ongoing database and evaluation of drugs that cause thrombocytopenia and have at the time of this writing identified approximately 85 drugs that can cause thrombocytopenia.[52] Drugs that induce thrombocytopenia do so by various mechanisms.[53] Ultimately, antibodies stimulated by the drug or drug-platelet complex destroy platelets. The overall incidence of drug-induced thrombocytopenia is quite rare (10 cases per million population per year), but some drugs are more likely to cause this complication than others.

The drugs most often associated with drug-induced thrombocytopenia are quinine, platelet inhibitors such as abciximab (ReoPro), antirheumatic drugs such as gold salts, sulfonamide antibiotics such as trimethoprim-sulfamethoxazole (Bactrim), heparins, cimetidine (Tagamet), acetaminophen (Tylenol), diuretic agents such as chlorothiazide (Diuril), and some chemotherapeutic agents.[53]

Common Drug Toxicities

This section reviews dose-related toxicity of select commonly used over-the-counter and prescription medications to illustrate the potential for drug toxicity with all medications. While virtually any agent becomes toxic at high levels, some drugs have toxic effects at relatively low or therapeutic doses. Drug toxicity frequently targets specific organs, causing transient changes that can progress to irreversible damage.

Acetaminophen

Acetaminophen (Tylenol) was the most frequently dispensed analgesic in the United States in 2005.[54] Acetaminophen is a component in multiple combination over-the-counter formulations and prescription products in addition to acetaminophen-only products such as Tylenol. Therefore, elevated serum acetaminophen levels can be accidental or from deliberate ingestion of acetaminophen-containing products. In fact, acetaminophen toxicity accounted for 50% of the cases of acute liver failure in the United States in 2005.[55] In 2009, the FDA issued a new rule that requires all over-the-counter acetaminophen products to list a warning on the label about possible liver injury that can occur following large doses. Table 4-5 contains a partial list of over-the-counter and prescription formulations that contain acetaminophen.

The maximum recommended total adult daily dose of acetaminophen from all sources is 4 g (65 mg/kg for children).[56] Toxicity occurs when 10 g or more is ingested as a single dose and can occur at lower doses when individual characteristics that increase the risk of acetaminophen toxicity are present. For example, alcohol induces the CYP450 enzyme that metabolizes acetaminophen into the reactive metabolite that causes liver damage (Box 4-3).[57]

Acetaminophen-related hepatotoxicity occurs within 72 hours following acute overdose but can also occur following chronic, excessive acetaminophen use. The clinical presentation occurs in three distinct stages that develop rapidly from the presenting gastroenteritis (24 hrs), to subclinical hepatotoxicity (24–72 hrs), to fulminant hepatic failure (72–96 hrs).

The mechanism of action of acetaminophen toxicity is well known. As the normal pathway for acetaminophen

Table 4-5 Acetaminophen Content of Common Medications*

Over-the-Counter Preparations (Brand)	Acetaminophen Content (mg)
Actifed	325–500 mg
Alka-Seltzer	250–325 mg
Allerest	325–500 mg
Anacin	80–500 mg tablets, 1000 mg/mL, 160 mg/5 mL
Benadryl Allergy/Cold Tablets	500 mg
Comtrex	325–1000, 500 mg/5 mL, 500 mg/15 mL, 650 mg/oz, 1000 mg/oz, 1000 mg/5 mL
Coricidin D	325 mg
Drixoral	325–500 mg
Excedrin Migraine	250 mg
Midrin	325 mg
Percogesic	325–500 mg
Sinutab	325–500 mg, 1000 mg/oz
Sominex pain relief formula	500 mg
Sudafed sinus products	325–500 mg
TheraFlu	325–650 mg, 650–1000 mg/packet
Vicks DayQuil	325 mg/caplet
Vicks NyQuil	250 mg, 167 mg/5 mL, 1000 mg packet, 500 mg/15 mL, 325 mg/caplet
Prescription Medications	**Acetaminophen Content (mg)**
Darvocet-N50	325 mg
Darvocet-N100	650 mg
Darvocet-A500	500 mg
Endocet	325–650 mg
Esgic Plus	500 mg
Fioricet	325 mg
Lorcet	325–750 mg, 500 mg/15 mL
Lortab	325–500 mg, 500 mg/15 mL
Norco	325 mg
Percocet	325–660 mg
Tylenol No. 2, No. 3, No. 4	300 mg
Ultracet	325 mg
Vicodin	500 mg
Vicodin ES	750 mg
Vicodin HP	660 mg

* This list does not contain all OTC or prescription medications. Prescribers and consumers should read the label of any medication that is used for allergies, colds, coughs, fevers, or pain.

JT, a frequent social drinker, spent an afternoon on the beach with friends. The next morning she had a headache, which she thought was from being in the sun too long. JT took four extra-strength tablets (2 g) of acetaminophen (Tylenol), forgot to eat breakfast, and went to work. About 72 hours later, she developed acute liver failure. How did this happen?

Approximately 90% of acetaminophen is metabolized into sulfate and glucuronide metabolites that are nontoxic and eliminated via the kidney. However, approximately 4–6% of acetaminophen is metabolized via CYP2E1 into a toxic metabolite NAPQI, which, under normal circumstances, is rapidly altered by glutathione into the same nontoxic water-soluble metabolite produced via the primary metabolic system.

However, alcohol is a substrate for CYPE1 and increases the amount of CYPE1 twofold in persons who drink heavily. Alcohol also inhibits the production of glutathione. Thus the drinks JT had the day before on the beach created more CYP2E1 and depleted the enzyme responsible for converting acetaminophen to a nontoxic metabolite. The acetaminophen she ingested was metabolized preferentially by CYPE1, which created sufficient NAPQI to produce liver failure even though the dose was below the usual toxic dose.

This relationship between chronic alcohol use and liver toxicity at high therapeutic doses is controversial. However, in 1998, the FDA issued a warning that persons who drink more than three glasses of alcohol a day should consult their healthcare provider before using acetaminophen, and this warning is printed on the label of acetaminophen products.

metabolism becomes saturated, excess acetaminophen is metabolized through CYP450 enzymatic reactions that result in formation of toxic metabolites (Figure 4-1).[56]

Suspected or confirmed acetaminophen overdose is treated with acetylcysteine (Acetadote, Mucomyst), which is most effective when administered within 8 hours of overdose. Acetylcysteine prevents the toxic metabolite *N*-acetyl-*p*-benzoquinoneimine from binding to hepatocytes and thus prevents hepatotoxicity. Acetylcysteine

may be administered orally or intravenously and has been shown to pass through the placenta to the fetus.[58] Liver and kidney function are assessed serially through laboratory testing of electrolytes, creatinine clearance levels, prothrombin time, bilirubin, aspartate aminotransferase, and alanine aminotransferase.[59] Consultation with a medical toxicologist via a poison control center is indicated. With severe toxicity or late onset of treatment, liver failure requiring transplantation may occur.[60]

Acetaminophen also has multiple drug–drug interactions. Acetaminophen is a substrate for CYP2E1, and metabolism of this drug is therefore affected by drugs that are either inhibitors or inducers of this enzyme. Common drug–drug interactions for acetaminophen are listed in Table 4-6.

Calcium Channel Blockers and Beta-Blockers

Calcium channel blockers and beta-blockers are cardiovascular medications with a demonstrated potential for lethal cardiotoxicity. Both are commonly prescribed for the treatment of angina, hypertension, arrhythmia, and migraine. At therapeutic doses, these drugs alter cardiovascular function by modifying the transport of calcium ions across membranes in the myocardium and vascular smooth muscle. Systemic vasodilatation, reduced myocardial contractility,

Table 4-6 Selected Acetaminophen Interactions*

Elevated Risk of Hepatotoxicity	Decreased Analgesic Effect of Acetaminophen	Decreased Absorption of Acetaminophen
Alcohol	Barbiturates	Cholestyramine (Questran)†
Barbiturates	Carbamazepine (Tegretol)	Food intake
Carbamazepine (Tegretol)	Hydantoins (Dilantin)	St. John's wort
Cholestyramine (Questran)	Isoniazid (INH)	
Hydantoins (Dilantin)	Rifampin (Rifadin)	
Isoniazid (INH)	Sulfinpyrazone (Anturane)	
Nephrotoxicity		
Rifampin (Rifadin)		
Sulfinpyrazone (Anturane)		

* This table is not comprehensive as new information is being identified on a regular basis.
† Separate dosing by more than 1 hour.

and diminished sinoatrial and atrioventricular conduction are the therapeutic results. During cardiotoxicity secondary to drug overdose, the pharmacologic effects of these drugs results in profound hypotension, bradycardia, and conduction disturbances leading to cardiovascular collapse.[61] In addition, hyperglycemia may occur secondary to calcium channel blockade inhibition of insulin release. Lactic acidosis can also occur. Overdose of calcium channel blockers requires active cardiovascular support in an inpatient setting. Calcium channel blockers are both substrates and inhibitors of CYP3A4. Thus, they can inhibit their own metabolism, which increases plasma levels and can result in toxicity.

Nonsteroidal Anti-Inflammatory Drugs

Nonsteroidal anti-inflammatory drugs (NSAIDs) have analgesic, antipyretic, and anti-inflammatory properties and are popularly used for a multitude of indications, particularly among persons with arthritis and other inflammatory disorders. Even at nontoxic levels, NSAIDs can cause erosive tissue damage in the gastrointestinal (GI) tract, inhibit the function of platelets, and alter renal function. While toxicity of NSAIDs is more likely to occur with an excessive dose or prolonged use, toxicity also occurs in individuals administered therapeutic doses secondary to the known pharmacologic effects on physiologic function. The most common NSAID-related toxicities are nephrotoxicity and GI ulceration.

NSAIDs prevent prostaglandin synthesis by inhibiting the cyclooxygenase enzymes (COX-1 and COX-2) that convert arachidonic acid to prostaglandin.[62] COX-1 facilitates production of the prostaglandins that stimulate gastric mucus secretion (Chapter 12).[62] Thus, NSAID suppression of COX-1 increases the risk of gastric upset and gastric ulcer. While these effects are primarily associated with nonselective NSAIDs such as ibuprofen (Motrin) or naproxen (Aleve), which inhibit both COX-1 and COX-2, they can also occur following use of COX-2 inhibitors such as celecoxib (Celebrex).

Nephrotoxicity results in functional renal insufficiency secondary to the vasoconstrictive action of NSAIDs.[62] Constriction of renal arterioles leads to reversible renal ischemia and a diminished glomerular filtration rate. These effects are exacerbated in individuals with fluid deficits or preexisting renal compromise, particularly in persons over age 65 years.[62]

Acute tubulointerstitial nephritis secondary to NSAID therapy is twice as likely to occur in women as in men. Concomitant use of other nephrotoxic substances increases

the risk. Nephritis presents with hematuria, pyuria, proteinuria, and elevated serum creatinine levels. Nephritis and renal ischemia typically resolve spontaneously following discontinuation of the drug; however, infrequently persistent changes occur, leading to renal failure.[62]

Cardiotoxic effects associated with NSAIDs, in particular with COX-2 inhibitors, include mild elevations in blood pressure, increased risk of acute myocardial infarction, and stroke. Research indicates that cardiac risk appears to increase when the recommended NSAID dose is exceeded or the drug is used during long-term therapy.[63] Based on the individual's age and cardiac risk profile, the risk of acute myocardial infarction or stroke may offset the GI benefit of COX-2 inhibitors.

In women's health practice, NSAIDs are commonly recommended preemptively to ameliorate cramping dysmenorrhea. In the event of unanticipated pregnancy, exposure to NSAIDs, including aspirin, around the time conception or use during early pregnancy for more than 7 days may result in a significantly increased risk for spontaneous abortion.[64] Acetaminophen does not have this effect.

NSAIDs are not considered teratogens; however, evidence linking NSAIDs to facial clefts when used during fetal development is inconclusive. Although one study found an association between use of naproxen (Aleve) and facial clefts, this data has not been replicated.[65] Interpretation of data is confounded by the variable rates of facial clefts associated with racial and ethnic heritage, as well as several other commonly used medications, and variables such as maternal nutrition, gender of the fetus, and maternal exposure to social, environmental, or occupational toxins.

Antidepressant Toxicity

Antidepressants are among the most common prescription drugs for which overdose is reported to poison control centers. Initial improvement in symptoms of depression following use of an antidepressant can increase suicidal and self-harm behaviors, or the medication may be accidentally ingested.[66]

Overdose of tricyclic antidepressants rapidly leads to cardiotoxicity and neurologic compromise. Tricyclic antidepressants have a narrow therapeutic index, and toxicity is of concern when even a maximum single dose is exceeded.[67] Women are more likely to develop serious cardiac arrhythmias form tricyclic antidepressant overdose than men.[67] This tendency is exacerbated in the presence of additional risk factors such as preexisting heart disease, electrolyte imbalance, impaired hepatic function, and stimulant drug abuse. Myocardial sodium channels are blocked during overdose, leading to alterations in cardiac conduction.[67] Vascular resistance is diminished, resulting in profound hypotension. Coma or convulsions may also occur secondary to central nervous system depression.

Serotonin Syndrome

Selective serotonin reuptake inhibitors (SSRIs) have a wide therapeutic index. Unlike tricyclics, up to five times the usual dose of an SSRI may be taken without significant ill effects.[68] However, SSRIs do interact with a wide variety of agents, which can result in serious adverse effects.[68] High plasma levels of SSRIs can cause serotonin syndrome, wherein excess serotonergic activity in the central nervous syndrome very quickly causes a life-threatening constellation of symptoms (Chapter 25).

Serotonin syndrome can occur following a significant overdose or following a milder overdose in the presence of other medications such as meperidine (Demerol), tricyclic antidepressants, or lithium (Lithobid). Concentrations of serotonin become elevated following administration of agents that provide the amino acid L-tryptophan, limit metabolism of serotonin (i.e., MAO inhibitors, such as Nardil and Parnate), increase serotonin release (e.g., lithium [Lithobid], amphetamines, ecstasy), or inhibit serotonin reuptake (e.g., SSRIs, cocaine, meperidine [Demerol], dextromethorphan [DM, found in products such as Robitussin DM], venlafaxine [Effexor], trazodone [Desyrel], tricyclic antidepressants, and St. John's wort). In addition, serotonin receptor agonists (e.g., buspirone [BuSpar], lysergic acid diethylamide [LSD]), or dopamine agonists (l-dopa [levodopa]) can cause this syndrome.[68]

While serotonin syndrome is a life-threatening condition, prompt recognition and treatment typically results in resolution of symptoms within 24 hours. Treatment consists of discontinuing the offending agent(s), administration of activated charcoal for large or intentional overdose, and maintaining normothermia. Muscle rigidity, agitation, and seizures are treated if necessary with benzodiazepines such as alprazolam (Xanax), clonazepam (Klonopin), diazepam (Valium), and lorazepam (Ativan).[68]

▌ Poisoning

Poisoning is the result of accidental or deliberate overdose of pharmacologic substances, or exposure to toxic levels of nonpharmacologic chemical, biologic, or physical agents that results in organ impairment or injury, or systemic effects.[69]

Poisoning may occur from ingestion of household substances such as lead paint chips, solvents, or cleaners; inadvertent overdose of medication secondary to impaired renal or hepatic function; deliberate overdose of medications; poisoning related to dietary supplements; or excessive exposure to environmental or occupational toxins.[70]

Although half of all poisonings occur in children under 6 years of age, according to 2006 data from the American Association of Poison Control Centers, the majority of adult poisoning victims (58.4%), whether intentional or unintentional, were women age 20 or older. Fatalities from poisoning are essentially evenly distributed between males and females, with the overwhelming majority (72.9%) occurring in individuals between the ages of 20 and 59 years.[71]

In this report, the percentage of poisoning reported during pregnancy (0.37% [n = 8919]) comprised a small number of the total number of human poisonings. During pregnancy, the majority of documented poisonings occurred in the second trimester (37.4%), closely followed by first trimester poisoning (31.7%), with the remainder (29.8%) occurring in the third trimester. Nearly 75% of poisonings during pregnancy were unintentional.[71] Hence, women's health clinicians must remain alert to the risk of poisoning in all women under their care.

In 2006, there were 61 poison control centers in the United States serving a population of over 299 million people.[71] There were 2,403,539 human exposure calls reported, resulting in 8 reported exposures per 1000 people. More than 70% of these exposures were handled over the telephone by the poison control center and the exposed individual was not evaluated by a healthcare professional. Poisoning is not a reportable occurrence; therefore it is likely that individuals who were treated by healthcare professionals were not included in these numbers. The 2004 report on poisoning from the Institute of Medicine estimates that there are over 4 million **poison** exposures annually in the United States, resulting in over 30,000 fatalities.[70] Poison control centers in the United States are now linked to a real-time poison control database and surveillance system that is continually updated and offers callers current research-based poison exposure management guidelines relevant to clinical and medical toxicology.

Care of the Poisoning Victim

During evaluation of the suspected poisoning victim, the type of exposure and level of toxicity should be determined. Physical toxins include energy, noise, cold, heat, and radiation. Chemical toxicants include many household products, chemicals used in industry, and most pharmacologics. Biologic toxins include vaccines and pharmacologic products from plant or animal sources, as well as occupational or environmental exposure to the same.

Criteria for consultation and hospitalization will vary based on the agent, the age and health of the woman receiving care, and other factors. Prompt access to emergency medical care is indicated with signs of an acute allergic reaction, fever, and dermatologic manifestations of SJS or toxic erythema multiforme.

Care of the poisoning victim begins with rapid assessment of basic physiologic function (airway, breathing, state of consciousness) while determining the offending agent(s) and time elapsed since exposure. Primary therapy consists of interruption of poison absorption, provision of appropriate antidotal therapy if available, and facilitation of poison excretion.[69] Postexposure treatments are based on information and recommendations from poison control centers, MSDSs, and drug product information. Cutaneous, mucous membrane, or ocular exposures are treated with irrigation using copious amounts of water or normal saline. Oral ingestion of poisons is treated using a combination of adsorbing agents or binding agents, diluting agents, agents that enhance intestinal motility, and antidotal therapy when applicable, accompanied by supportive and advanced medical care as indicated.

Activated Charcoal and Sorbitol

Activated charcoal is considered first-line therapy for ingested poisons. Activated charcoal is an inert fine carbon powder that is both insoluble and nonabsorbable, with an extensive network of interconnecting pores. It acts by rapidly binding with (adsorbing) the chemical, thus limiting systemic absorption and toxicity. Activated charcoal is most effective when it is administered within 30 minutes following ingestion of the offending substance, before gastric absorption has occurred.[69]

The recommended dose of activated charcoal for adsorbable poison victims is 1 g/kg with a 1:10 ratio of toxicant to charcoal. A typical single adult dose is 25–100 g of activated charcoal mixed with water or sorbitol to form a slurry that is administered orally or via nasogastric tube. Sorbitol acts to enhance bowel motility, thereby facilitating elimination of the charcoal–poison complex and preventing constipation secondary to activated charcoal administration.

Ipecac Syrup

Due to its hyperemetic effects, ipecac syrup is no longer recommended as first-line therapy. Syrup of ipecac increases risk of aspiration pneumonitis and interferes with the actions of activated charcoal.

Gastric Lavage

Gastric lavage is no longer routinely recommended for treatment of poisoning either.[72] Gastric lavage is a time-consuming procedure that can delay administration of the more effective activated charcoal.

Whole Bowel Irrigation and Cathartics

Whole bowel irrigation and cathartics are forms of decontamination that rapidly empty the GI tract of bulky or coated toxic materials and foreign bodies such as drug packets, sustained-release medications, and batteries. Polyethylene glycol solution (Colyte, GoLYTELY) is administered to clear toxic substances not bound by activated charcoal. The adult dose is 2 liters/hr orally (or per nasogastric tube) until rectal effluent is clear. Whole bowel cleansing may reduce the binding capacity of activated charcoal; therefore, when indicated, polyethylene glycol solution is administered after the administration of activated charcoal.[69]

Specific Poison Antidotes

Antidotes are agents that are administered to counteract the effects of a poison or toxin. Antidotes act through inhibiting absorption, reversing the action of poisons, or neutralizing the poison. Pharmaceutical antidotes are agents that treat the toxic effects of specific drugs, such as naloxone (Narcan) for opioid overdose. Specific antidotes interact directly with the agent of overdose or poisoning, such as N-acetylcysteine (Acetadote, Mucomyst) for acetaminophen overdose, calcium gluconate for magnesium sulfate toxicity, or species-specific antivenin. Antidotes to common poisons are listed in Table 4-7.

Toxicity from Heavy Metals

Heavy metals are naturally occurring substances that contribute, in trace amounts, to healthy physiologic functioning. Excess amounts of heavy metals can result in alterations in central nervous system function and organ damage

Table 4-7 Antidotes to Common Poisons

Poison—Generic (Brand)	Antidote
Acetaminophen (Tylenol)	N-acetylcysteine
Anticholinergics	Physostigmine
Anticoagulants	Vitamin K_1, protamine
Benzodiazepines	Supportive care, flumazenil*
Beta-blockers	Glucagon
Calcium channel blockers	Calcium, glucagon
Cholinergics	Atropine, pralidoxime (organophosphate overdose)
Digoxin (Lanoxin)	Digoxin Fab antibodies
Iron	Deferoxamine
Isoniazid (INH)	Pyridoxine
Lead	BAL, EDTA, DMSA
Opioids	Naloxone†
Alcohols	Dialysis; experimental trials are underway on enzyme inhibitors
Tricyclic antidepressants	Sodium bicarbonate

* Use of flumazenil is contraindicated in the presence of tricyclic overdose or chronically habituated benzodiazepine users as it may precipitate seizures.
† Use of naloxone is contraindicated in persons hypersensitive to it and in certain situations wherein the individual is tolerant to opioid agonists/antagonists.
Disclaimer: This tool may not represent standard of care in your area. In case of emergency, consult a poison control center.
Source: University of Illinois at Chicago.[80]

and can affect normal growth and development. Chronic exposure may result in progressive physical, muscular, and neurologic conditions that mimic numerous other health conditions.

Iron Toxicity

Iron is necessary for hematologic function and is commonly administered as replacement therapy to treat anemia. The vast majority of iron overdoses occur in children less than 6 years old. Prenatal vitamins and iron supplements have a high concentration of iron per tablet, and therefore pose the greatest risk for overdose. Toxicity is related to the dose of elemental iron ingested and results in free-radical formation and lipid peroxidation.

Iron toxicity initially presents with the GI symptoms of nausea, vomiting, and abdominal pain within the first 6 hours after ingestion. Vomiting may be severe and lead to hypovolemic shock. With continued deterioration, shock ensues, accompanied by metabolic acidosis. Hepatic necrosis may occur within 96 hours after ingestion of a toxic dose of iron salts and may lead to fatal liver failure. Serum iron levels aid in quantifying the severity of the overdose with

results over 500 mcg/dL considered serious toxicity, and results over 1000 mcg/dL considered life threatening.[73]

Treatment consists of volume replacement, airway protection, prompt intravenous administration of deferoxamine (Desferal) for serious toxicity, and supportive care.[55] Deferoxamine is a **chelating agent** that binds with circulating ferric iron to form a water-soluble solution able to be excreted through the kidneys.

Adult Lead Poisoning

Lead is a naturally occurring elemental metal that was once used in many products such as paint, lead solder in food cans, and gasoline. Lead may still be found in commercial products such as hair dye, batteries, and fishing weights. Lead is a waste product of the steel and iron industries and is released into the atmosphere as a result of coal-based power generation.[74,75] Lead cannot be destroyed, and it is transferred continuously between air, water, and soil. As a result, in areas with elevated environmental lead concentrations, exposure may occur secondary to atmospheric exposure, ingestion of locally grown produce, or by contaminated soil, dust, and water supplies.[74]

The vast majority of adult lead poisoning is related to occupation, although environmental exposure does occur secondary to lead paint (most commonly in houses built prior to 1970) and imported products such as health remedies, spices, foods, pottery, and cosmetics.[75] In 1997, a case of adult lead poisoning was diagnosed in a Cambodian woman who was using a traditional Asian folk remedy for menstrual cramps.[76] This case of lead toxicity was identified through routine screening at a free lead-screening clinic because the patient did not report any symptoms.

Lead is absorbed through skin and mucous membranes, and it bioaccumulates in humans. Elevated blood lead levels inhibit enzyme function of multiple biochemical pathways due to lead's affinity to bind to biologically active molecules in the body. Lead stored in bones may contribute to lead toxicity in women with hypothyroidism, during postmenopausal bone resorption, and during pregnancy when it passes to the fetus.[74]

Elevated blood lead levels are most commonly diagnosed through screening because individuals with low levels of lead toxicity are typically asymptomatic. Effects of adult lead poisoning include neurologic damage, hypertension, and reproductive problems for both women and men. Lead screening recommendations include evaluation of blood lead levels in women with occupational or environmental exposure who are pregnant or planning pregnancy, women who exhibit pica, and those with low intake of dietary calcium.[76] Elevated lead levels in pregnant women may cause low birth weight, lower than usual head circumference, mental retardation, and impaired neurobehavioral development in their offspring.[74,75] Even low levels of lead poisoning have potential to affect the developing fetus, and women with elevated blood lead levels excrete lead in breast milk.

Blood lead levels should be less than 10 mcg/dL. For lead levels above 10 mcg/dL, removing exposure to the source is frequently adequate to reduce blood lead levels to the normal range. Lead exposure can be diminished through covering of lead-painted walls, regular damp dusting of surfaces, hand washing before meals, washing of all fruits and vegetables before use, and allowing tap water to run for 30 seconds before drinking.[74] For those individuals with persistent elevated blood lead levels, significant symptoms, or nonpregnant women with fertility concerns, chelating agents may be administered under the direction of a medical toxicologist.

Mercury Toxicity

Have you heard the phrase "mad as a hatter?" In the 19th-century hat-making industry, hatters were chronically exposed to mercury vapors during the felting process, and as a result many developed the mental and emotional changes of anxiety, memory loss, fearfulness, excitability, and the personality changes that are the symptoms of mercury toxicity.

The primary sources of exposure to mercury today are ingestion of fish that have a significant bioaccumulation of methylmercury (e.g., tuna, swordfish, walleye, and pike), occupational exposures, and amalgam dental fillings.[75] Minute amounts of mercury are used in the preservation of many pharmacologic products, most commonly ophthalmic and otic solutions, and some adult vaccines.

The preservative thimerosal is a mercury derivative postulated to contribute to autism and attention deficit hyperactivity disorder in young children through the administration of childhood vaccines in which it was used as a preservative. Thimerosal is no longer used in vaccines intended for children, but it does remain in some vaccines, such as the influenza vaccine, although thimerosal-free influenza vaccine is available and produced by one manufacturer.

Mercury toxicity results in intention tremor of the hands, inflamed gums and excessive salivation, and mental and emotional changes. Mercury vapor is easily absorbed through the lungs, while only small amounts are absorbed through the GI tract. Mercury is excreted via the GI tract, respiratory system (mercury vapor), and kidneys. Mercury accumulates in both the kidney and central nervous system, where it can cause nephrotoxicity and neurologic changes.[75]

While mercury toxicity in adults is now relatively uncommon, small amounts of mercury are harmful to the developing fetus. The bioaccumulation of mercury in fish is primarily in the methylmercury form, which is more toxic than elemental mercury, leading to recommendations that these fish be avoided.[77] Fetal exposure to very small amounts of methylmercury can cause impaired neurologic development, such as diminished ability in cognitive thinking, memory, attention, language, and fine motor and visual spatial skills.[75]

Mercury toxicity is determined through evaluation of blood and urine concentrations. Normal adult serum mercury levels are less than 5 mcg/L, with symptoms of toxicity becoming present at a concentration of about 100 mcg/L. Persons who eat a lot of fish may have up to four times the accepted level of blood mercury. Thiol-based chelating agents are used to treat confirmed mercury toxicity.

Endocrine Disruptors

Endocrine disruptors are synthetic chemicals that disrupt physiologic function through interference with normal hormone secretion or action. These chemicals mimic or block the action of hormones, resulting in developmental, neurologic, immune, and reproductive system aberrations.[78]

Exposure to endocrine disruptors may occur through the environment, such as drinking water contaminated with dioxin, polychlorinated biphenyls (PCBs), or dichloro-diphenyl-trichloroethane (DDT), or through the use of commercial products such as plastics, drugs, or cosmetics that contain preservatives such as paraben or ethylene oxide. Endocrine disruptors may be found in water, soil, and the atmosphere. Endocrine disruptors are lipophilic, and can accumulate in the fatty tissues of plants and animals, and ingested through the diet.

Many endocrine disrupting chemicals have significant estrogenic effects and bind to estrogen receptor sites. Genetic and environmental interactions associated with endocrine disruptors are postulated to contribute to the development of conditions such as breast cancer, infertility, endometriosis, immune disorders, childhood developmental and cognitive delay, and birth defects.[78] Due to their affinity to fatty tissues, effects of endocrine disruptors may be diminished in women with a lower body mass index (BMI).

Preventing Adverse Drug Reactions

Modifiable factors leading to ADRs and ADEs can be classed as either prescribing problems or adherence problems. These include inaccurate clinical diagnosis resulting in incorrect treatment; inaccuracy in the prescription process, such as incorrect spelling or dose, and errors in dispensing or administration; inappropriate self-medication with drugs or other substances; insufficient consumer education or understanding regarding drug therapy; noncompliance with recommended drug therapy; and drug interactions secondary to polypharmacy or coadministration with certain foods, herbs, or other substances. In addition, undiagnosed preexisting medical, genetic, or allergic conditions may contribute to ADRs.

In a prospective observational study examining the frequency, severity, and preventability of ADRs, Rivkin found that 7.5% (n = 21) of the admissions to a medical intensive care unit were related to ADRs.[79] Of the 21 ADRs analyzed, 86% were deemed to be preventable. Prevention would have resulted in significantly lower morbidity and mortality for the individuals involved, and considerable cost savings to the healthcare system. Drug interactions were considered 100% preventable and comprised 57% of the ADRs. In this population, aspirin was the most commonly implicated medication, and bleeding was the most common aspirin-related ADR admission diagnosis.[79]

Most studies of ADRs and ADEs evaluate the incidence of adverse events in hospitalized individuals or hospitalizations occurring secondary to drug-related adverse events. As a result, hospitals have set up internal systems aimed at preventing medication errors in the hospital setting. Practices such as unit-dose medications, limited-access medication carts, computer entry of medication orders, and integrated bedside documentation systems reduce medication errors and prevent adverse drug events. Clinicians who practice in the community setting frequently do not have the benefit of these systems.

Prevention of ADRs and ADEs in the outpatient setting relies on every individual participating in the drug prescription process acting correctly 100% of the time. The process of prescribing involves the clinician, the pharmacist, and the individual for whom the medication is prescribed. Often there are one or more other individuals, such as the office nurse, pharmacy staff, parent, or caregiver involved in the process as well. Correct prescribing and drug use requires accurate diagnosis, selection of an optimal and appropriate pharmacologic agent, assessment of potential for interactions with other agents, evaluation for genetic or physiologic variations or conditions that may affect drug metabolism, correct and legible prescription writing, developmentally and culturally appropriate medication instruction, accurate reading of the prescription, correct medication, dose, dispensing, and labeling, and lastly, compliance with recommended therapy by the individual.

Electronic prescribing in the outpatient setting is rapidly becoming an everyday part of practice. Electronic generation, transmission, and tracking of prescriptions is efficient and offers greater security than the paper-based system. Additionally, e-prescribing can offer greater safety through cross-referencing for drug interactions, correct doses, and patient-specific factors including prior ADRs. However, at this time the Drug Enforcement Administration does not allow e-prescribing for controlled substances, which comprise an estimated 20% of all prescriptions.

Patient education is another integral part of the prevention of adverse drug reactions and other events related to toxicity. Ongoing continuing education in pharmacology is an urgent necessity for women's health professionals to keep abreast of the rapid changes in this discipline. Information is constantly being updated regarding drug interactions, effects specific to women, and the effects of drugs during pregnancy and lactation. In spite of the best efforts at preventing ADRs and ADEs, no agent is deemed 100% safe. Therefore, all practitioners must be prepared to evaluate individuals who present with signs or symptoms of drug-related reactions or potentially toxic exposures.

Clinical Practice: Assessment of Risk for Toxicity

When assessing an individual for drug toxicity, a comprehensive health history includes obtaining relevant information regarding diet; use of supplements, nutraceuticals, and complementary or alternative therapies; and environmental or occupational exposure to toxins and toxicants.

Preventive evaluation for women at risk of exposure to occupational or environmental toxicants includes discussion of protective practices and equipment used, as well as exposure duration and frequency. Synergistic or additive effects may occur with the concomitant use of other substances such as alcohol, tobacco, prescription medication, recreational drugs, or drugs of abuse.

When evaluating toxicity risk for an exposed individual, information regarding the physical and chemical properties of the agent may be found through the manufacturer, drug resources, or the MSDS. The route of exposure (cutaneous, inhalation, ingestion, injection); duration and timing of exposure (minutes, hours, days); frequency of exposure (chronic versus acute exposure); and exposure to other substances are all additional factors that affect the risk of toxicity. Other factors that may contribute to risk include the individual's age, concurrent medical conditions, and social and cultural practices.

Laboratory testing frequently includes tests of endocrine and metabolic function, with hepatic and renal function tests and blood glucose levels performed as a baseline evaluation. Common tests for toxicity include serum drug levels, blood-lead levels, blood-alcohol levels, screening for drugs of abuse, cotinine testing for tobacco exposure, and radiographs in the presence of oral iron supplement ingestion.

Treatment is based on the agent and its potential for toxicity. Consultation with a poison control center or drug manufacturer is useful in determining the need for medical consultation or referral for treatment. Most drug exposures are not life threatening and may be evaluated and treated on an outpatient basis. More serious exposures or reactions require hospitalization.

Regardless of whether an individual is treated on an outpatient basis or hospitalized, it is essential that the clinician document care provided and toxicity- or drug-related adverse events in the medical record. ADEs are reported through MedWatch. Clinician reporting of ADRs helps build the database of information about drug reactions and provides invaluable data to determine drug safety, optimal doses, and identification of drug-related risk factors.

Drugs offer a multitude of effective therapies for chronic and acute conditions. With thoughtful consideration about the balance between therapeutics and drug toxicity or adverse reactions, women's healthcare providers can help women live healthier lives and engage in the stewardship of their health.

References

1. Braun JM, Froehlich TE, Daniels JL, Dietrich KN, Hornung R, Aulinger P, et al. Association of environmental toxicants and conduct disorder in US children: NHANES 2001–2004. Environl Health Perspect 2008;116:956–62.

2. Quackenbush R, Hackley B, Dixon J. Screening for pesticide exposure: a case study. J Midwifery Womens Health 2006;51:3–11.

3. Moore TJ, Cohen MR, Furberg CD. Serious adverse drug events reported to the Food and Drug Administration 1998–2005. Arch Internal Med 2007;167:1752–9.

4. Grenouillet-Delacre M, Verdoux H, Moore N, Haramburu F, Miremont-Salame G, Etienne G, et al. Life-threatening adverse drug reactions at admission to medical intensive care: a prospective study in a teaching hospital. Intensive Care Med 2007;33:2150–7.

5. Reidl MA, Casillas AM. Adverse drug reactions: types and treatment options. Am Fam Physician 2003;68:1781–90.

6. Heinrich J. US General Accounting Office. Drug safety: most drugs withdrawn in recent years had greater health risks for women. GAO-01–286R. Washington DC: US General Accounting Office, 2001.

7. Patel H, Bell D, Molokhia M, Srishanmuganathan J, Patel M, Car J, et al. Trends in hospital admissions for adverse drug reactions in England: analysis of national hospital episode statistics 1998–2005. BMC Clin Pharmacol 2007;7:9doi:10.1186/1472–6904-7–9.

8. Cragan JD, Friedman JM, Holmes LB, Uhl K, Green NS, Riley L. Ensuring the safe and effective use of medications during pregnancy: planning and prevention through preconception care. Matern Child Health J. 2006;10:S129–35.

9. Wen SW, Yang T, Krewski D, Yang Q, Nimrod C, Garner P, et al. Patterns of pregnancy exposure to prescription FDA C, D and X drugs in a Canadian population. J Perinataol 2008;28:324–30.

10. Woodland C, Wells PG. Principles of toxicology. In: Kalant H, Grant DM, Mitchell J, eds. Principles of medical pharmacology. Toronto: Saunders, 2007.

11. Coyle YM, Hynan LS, Euhus DM, Minhajuddin AT. An ecological study of the association of environmental chemicals on breast cancer incidence in Texas. Breast Cancer Res Treat 2005;92:107–14.

12. Bernstein JA. Material safety data sheets: are they reliable in identifying human hazards? J Allergy Clin Immunol 2002;110:35–8.

13. OSHA. Recommended format for material safety data sheets (MSDSs). 2004. Available from *www.osha.gov/dsg/hazcom/msdsformat.html* [Accessed July 31, 2008].

14. Zhou SF. Potential strategies for minimizing mechanism-based inhibition of cytochrome P450 3A4. Curr Pharm Des 2008;14:990–1000.

15. Wilke RA, Reif DM, Moore JH. Combinatorial pharmacogenetics. Nat Rev Drug Discovery 2005;4:911–8.

16. Zhou S, Chan E, Li X, Huang M. Clinical outcomes and management of mechanism-based inhibition of cytochrome P450 3A4. Ther Clin Manage 2005;1:3–13.

17. World Health Organization. International drug monitoring: the role of national centres. World Health Organ Tech Rep Ser 1972;498:1–25.

18. Cobert BL. Manual of drug safety and pharmacovigilance. Sudbury, MA: Jones and Bartlett, 2007.

19. Gruchappa R. Understanding drug allergies. J Allergy Clin Immunol 2000;105:S637–44.

20. Sampson HA, Muñoz-Furlong A, Campbell RL, Adkinson NF Jr, Bock SA, Branum A, et al. Second symposium on the definition and management of anaphylaxis: summary report. Second National Institute of Allergy and Infectious Disease/Food Allergy and Anaphylaxis Network symposium. J Allergy Clin Immunol 2006 February; 117(2):391–7.

21. Larson AM, Polson J, Fontana RJ, Davern E. Acetaminophen-induced acute liver failure: results of a United States multicenter, prospective study. Hepatology 2005;42:1364–72.

22. Zhang H, Cui D, Wang B, Han YH, Balimane P, Sinz M, et al. Pharmacokinetic drug interactions involving 17 alpha-ethinylestradiol: a new look at an old drug. Clin Pharmacokinet 2007;46:133–57.

23. Osterheld JR, Cosa K, Sandson NB. Med-Psych drug–drug interactions update: oral contraceptives. Psychosomatics 2008;49:168–75.

24. Uetrecht J. Idiosyncratic drug reactions: past, present, and future. Chem Res Toxicol 2008;21:84–92.

25. Johnson RF, Peebles RS. Anaphylactic shock: pathophysiology, recognition and treatment. Semin Respir Crit Care Med 2004;25:695–703.

26. Knowles SR, Drucker AM, Weber EA, Shear NH. Management options for patients with aspirin and nonsteroidal antiinflammatory drug sensitivity. Ann Pharmacother 2007;41:1191–200.

27. Gomes ER, Demoly P. Epidemiology of hypersensitivity drug reactions. Curr Opin Allergy Clin Immunol 2005;5:309–16.

28. McLean-Tooke AP, Bethune CA, Fay AC, Spickett GP. Adrenaline in the treatment of anaphylaxis: what is the evidence? BMJ 2003;327:1332–5.

29. Sicherer SH, Leung DY. Advances in allergic skin disease, anaphylaxis, and hypersensitivity reactions to foods, drugs, and insects in 2007. J Allergy Clinical Immunol 2008;121:1351–8.

30. Stern RS. Utilization of hospital and outpatient care for adverse cutaneous reactions to medications. Pharmacoepidem Drug Saf 2005;14:677–84.

31. Kaplan RP, Potter TS, Fox JN. Drug-induced pemphigus related to angiotensin-converting enzyme inhibitors. J Am Acad Dermatol 1992;26(2 Pt 2);364–6.

32. Knowles SR, Shear NH. Recognition and management of severe cutaneous drug reactions. Dermatol Clin 2007;25:245–53.

33. Dubakiene R, Kupriene M. Scientific problems of photosensitivity. Medicina 2006;42:619–24.

34. Lee WM. Drug induced hepatotoxicity. N Engl J Med 2003;349:474–85.

35. Makarova SI. Human N-acetyltransferases and drug-induced hepatotoxicity. Curr Drug Metab 2008;9:538–45.

36. Navarro VJ, Senior JR. Drug-related hepatotoxicity. N Engl J Med 2006;354:731–9.

37. Maddrey WC. Drug-induced hepatotoxicity: 2005. J Clin Gastroenterol 2005;39:S83–9.

38. Chitturi S, Farrell GC. Hepatotoxic slimming aids and other herbal hepatotoxins. J Gastroenterol Hepatol 2008;23:366–73.

39. Kaplowitz N. Drug-induced liver injury. Clin Infect Dis 2004;38:S44–8.

40. Hussaini SH, Farrington EA. Idiosyncratic drug-induced liver injury: an overview. Expert Opin Drug Saf 2007;6:673–84.

41. Guo X, Nzerue C. How to prevent, recognize, and treat drug-induced nephrotoxicity. Curr Drug Ther 2002;69:289–312.

42. Eyer F, Zilker T. Bench-to-bedside review: mechanisms and management of hyperthermia due to toxicity. Crit Care 2007;11:236.

43. Rusyniak DE, Sprague JE. Toxin-induced hyperthermic syndromes. Med Clin North Am November 2005;89:1277–96.

44. Roujeau JC, Stern RS. Severe adverse cutaneous reactions to drugs. N Engl J Med 1994;331:1272–85.

45. Garcia-Doval I, LeCleach L, Bocquet H, Otero XL, Roujeau JC. Toxic epidermal necrosis and Stevens Johnson syndrome: does early withdrawal of causative drugs decrease the risk of death? Arch Dermatol 2000;136:323–7.

46. Gupta A, Lawrence AT, Krishnan K, Kavinsky CJ, Trohman RG. Current concepts in the mechanisms and management of drug-induced QT prolongation and torsade de pointes. Am Heart J 2007;153: 891–9.

47. Roden DM. Drug-induced prolongation of the QT interval. N Engl J Med 2004;350:1013–22.

48. Borchers AT, Keen CL, Gershwin ME. Drug-induced lupus. Ann NY Acad Sci 2007;1108:166–82.

49. Vasoo S. Drug-induced lupus: an update. Lupus 2006;15:757–61.

50. Katta R, Anusuri V. Serum sickness-like reaction to cefuroxime: a case report and review of the literature. J Drug Dermatol 2007;6:747–8.

51. Vipan W. Quinine as a cause of purpura. Lancet 1865;2:37.

52. Li X, Swisher K, Vesely SK, George JN. Drug-induced thrombocytopenia: an updated systematic review. Drug Saf 2007;30:185–95.

53. Aster RH, Bougie DW. Drug-induced immune thrombocytopenia. N Engl J Med 2007;357:580–7.

54. Hersh EV, Pinot A, Moore PA. Adverse drug interactions involving common prescription and over-the-counter analgesic agents. Clin Therapeut 2007;29:24777–97.

55. Khashab M, Tector AJ, Kwo PY. Epidemiology of acute liver failure. Curr Gastroenterol Rep 2007;9:66–73.

56. Zagaria MA. Unintentional acetaminophen overdose: focus on prevention. Am J Nurse-Pract 2008;12:47–51.

57. Larson AM. Acetaminophen hepatotoxicity. Clin Liver Dis 2007;11:525–48.

58. Kanter MZ. Comparison of oral and IV acetylcysteine in the treatment of acetaminophen poisoning. Am J Health System Pharm 2006;63:1821–7.

59. Mazer M, Perrone J. Acetominophen-induced nephrotoxicity: pathophysiology, clinical manifestations, and management. J Med Toxicol 2008;4:2–6.

60. Fontana RJ. Acute liver failure including acetaminophen overdose. Med Clin N Am 2008;92:761–94.

61. DeWitt CR, Waksman JC. Pharmacology, pathophysiology and management of calcium channel blocker and beta blocker toxicity. Toxicol Rev 2004;23:223–38.

62. Bakris GL, Sidney RK. Renal dysfunction resulting from NSAIDs. Am Fam Physician 1989;40:199–204.

63. Rahme E, Watson DJ, Kong SX, Toubouti Y, LeLorier J. Association between naproxen NSAIDs, COX-2 inhibitors and hospitalization for acute myocardial infarction among the elderly: a retrospective cohort study. Pharmacoepidemiol Drug Saf 2007;16:493–503.

64. Li DK, Liu L, Odouli R. Exposure to non-steroidal anti-inflammatory drugs during pregnancy and risk of miscarriage: population based cohort study. BMJ 2003;327;368 doi:10.1136/bmj.327.7411.368.

65. Ericson A, Kallen BA. Nonsteroidal anti-inflammatory drugs in early pregnancy. Repro Toxicol 2001;15:371–5.

66. Jick H, Kaye JA, Jick SS. Antidepressants and the risk of suicidal behaviors. JAMA 2004;292:338–43.

67. Woolf AD, Erdman AR, Nelson LS, Caravati EM, Cobaugh DJ, Booze LL, et al. Tricyclic antidepressant poisoning: an evidence-based consensus guideline for out-of-hospital management. Clin Toxicol 2007;45:203–33.

68. Nelson LS, Erdman AR, Booze LL, Cobaugh DJ, Chyka PA, Woolf AD, et al. Selective serotonin reuptake inhibitor poisoning: an evidence-based consensus guideline for out-of-hospital management. Clin Toxicol 2007;45:315–32.

69. Woodland C. Poisonings and antidotal therapy. In Kalant H, Grant DM, Mitchell J, eds. Principles of medical toxicology. Toronto: Saunders, 2007.

70. Institute of Medicine Committee on Poison Prevention and Control. Forging a poison prevention and control system. Washington DC: National Academies Press, 2004.

71. Bronstein AC, Spyker DA, Cantilena LR, Green J, Rumack BH, Heard SE. The 2006 annual report of the American Association of Poison Control Centers' national poison data system (NPDS). Clin Toxicol 2007;45:815–917.

72. American Academy of Clinical Toxicology. Position paper: gastric lavage. J Toxicol Clin Toxicol 2004;42:933–43.

73. Matiwale T, Liebelt E. Iron: not a benign therapeutic drug. Curr Opin Pediatr 2006;18:174–9.

74. Agency for Toxic Substances and Disease Registry. Toxicological profile for lead 2007. Available from: *www.atsdr.cdc.gov/toxprofiles/tp13.html* [Accessed July 22, 2008].

75. Brodkin E, Copes R, Mattman A, Kennedy J, Kling R, Yassi A. Lead and mercury exposures: interpretation and action. Can Med Assoc J 2007;176:59–63.

76. CDC. Adult lead poisoning from an Asian remedy for menstrual cramps—Connecticut, 1997. MMRW 1999;48:27–29. Available from *www.cdc.gov/mmwr/preview/mmwrhtml/00056277.htm* [Accessed July 21, 2008].

77. Environmental Protection Agency. Health effects of mercury. 2007. Available from *www.epa.gov/mercury/effects.htm* [Accessed August 11, 2008].

78. Gore AC. Developmental programming and endocrine disruptor effects on reproductive neuroendocrine systems. Front Neuroendocrinol 2008;29(3):358–74.

79. Rivkin A. Admissions to a medical intensive care unit related to adverse drug reactions. Am J Health Syst Pharm 2007;64(17):1840–3.

80. University of Illinois at Chicago. Available at *www.uic.edu/com/er/toxikon/antidot.htm* [Retrieved July 21, 2008].

Appendix Additional Toxicology Resources for Clinicians

American Association of Poison Control Centers	This site offers poisoning prevention information, as well as patient management guidelines for commonly ingested substances.	*www.aapcc.org*
Center for Research on Occupational and Environmental Toxicology	An organization comprised of scientists, educators, and information specialists working at Oregon Health & Science University in Portland, Oregon, on occupational safety and health issues.	*www.croetweb.com/*
Centers for Disease Control and Prevention: Poisoning in the United States: Fact sheet	This quick reference sheet identifies those at greatest risk for poisoning as well as the most common substances implicated in poisoning incidents.	*www.cdc.gov/ncipc/factsheets/poisoning.htm*
Centers for Disease Control and Prevention National Center for Environmental Health		*www.cdc.gov/nceh/*
The Collaborative on Health and the Environment	This site offers a searchable database that summarizes links between chemical contaminants and approximately 180 human diseases or conditions.	*http://database.healthandenvironment.org/*
Cornell University: Poisonous plants information database		*www.ansci.cornell.edu/plants/*
Drug-induced thrombocytopenias		*http://w3.ouhsc.edu/platelets/DITP/Database_group/Database_group.htm*
Extoxnet	This site provides toxicology information briefs on a number of topics.	*http://extoxnet.orst.edu/tibs/ghindex.html*
FDA Center for Drug Evaluation and Research: Frequently asked questions	This site answers basic questions about how drug development and testing occur. A useful introduction to the topic.	*www.fda.gov/cder/about/faq/*
Haz-Map	A clinical research tool for the evaluation of occupational toxicology based on disease categories and agents.	*www.haz-map.com/toxicology.htm*
Information for healthcare providers on adult lead poisoning		*www.nyc.gov/html/doh/downloads/pdf/lead/lead-hcp-factsht.pdf*
National Capitol Poison Center		1-800-222-1222
OSHA lead information		*www.osha.gov/SLTC/lead/recognition.html*
Safety of medicines	A guide to detecting and reporting adverse drug reactions.	*http://whqlibdoc.who.int/hq/2002/WHO_EDM_QSM_2002.2.pdf*
Selected environmental toxins Web sites	This site offers quick links to several useful toxicology Web sites.	*http://library.med.utah.edu/ed/eduservices/handouts/Toxins_Web/toxin-urls.html*
A Small Dose Of . . .	This is an online toxicology resource. This site includes PowerPoint presentations and other teaching resources related to toxicology.	*www.asmalldoseof.org/index.php*
Toxicology/occupational health resources	This site provides links to many online resources related to toxicology.	*www.lib.berkeley.edu/PUBL/tox.html*
Women's Health USA	This site provides a wealth of information about the state of women's health in the United States.	*www.mchb.hrsa.gov/whusa_05/pages/toc.htm*

II

Lifestyle and Preventive Healthcare Practices

Habits can be either healthy or unhealthy. However, even so-called healthy habits are not universally positive. In the chapter, "Vitamins and Minerals," nutritional supplements are discussed. Evidence about the benefits of selected vitamins such as folic acid is described. Other dietary supplements, although perhaps not harmful, are costly and of questionable effectiveness. In addition, too much of a good thing may be bad; megavitamins and minerals can be harmful and sometimes even teratogenic.

The iconic example of primary health prevention is the use of immunizations. For many years, there were a relatively small number of vaccines, and they were primarily for children. Today the number of vaccines, especially for adolescents and adults, has increased, and so has the controversy about effectiveness and adverse effects. When individuals decide not to avail themselves of vaccines, the entire concept of herd immunity begins to unravel. The chapter titled "Immunizations" addresses these issues and provides national recommendations for regular vaccinations.

Two unhealthy situations have pharmacologic regimens that support efforts to regain health. "Drugs to Promote Optimum Weight" examines the myths and realities about drugs and weight loss. This chapter addresses the use of pharmacologic agents used to augment diet and exercise in an attempt to attain a healthy body mass index. Unfortunately, this topic is getting increasing attention in a society in which obesity is an emerging epidemic. Although there is no single magic drug, at the end of this chapter, the reader will have an understanding of the agents available and the uses for which they are effective.

Nicotine replacement therapies (NRTs) have demonstrated value for individuals who find it difficult to discontinue smoking. The plethora of over-the-counter gums, patches, and other options can be confusing. The chapter "Smoking Cessation" reviews available evidence on types of NRTs and reported effectiveness of the over-the-counter products and those that are prescription only.

Drugs also can be abused. The chapter titled "Substance Abuse" addresses licit agents such as alcohol, illicit drugs like cocaine and marijuana, and abuse of prescription drugs such as opiates. The latter, often euphemistically termed *recreational drugs*, are used by millions of Americans annually, and they are associated with multiple long-term adverse effects and even death. Treatments with other agents may pose trading one habit for another. The delicate balances involved in pharmacotherapeutic agents for individuals who abuse substances are examined in this chapter.

The last chapter in this section, "Complementary and Alternative Therapies," presents an overview of herbs and botanical products that should be considered as seriously as prescription drugs. Randomized clinical trials have shown that some of these agents have therapeutic effects. Some herbs and botanical products have adverse drug–herb interactions that are clinically significant. Alternatively, some widely used agents may be safe but of questionable efficacy.

All of these chapters present agents that may not commonly be found inscribed on a prescription pad. However, information about these drugs, both for good and bad, can be important considerations for clinicians who are writing on prescription pads as they care for women.

"Let thy food be thy medicine, and thy medicine be thy food."

HIPPOCRATES (460–377 BC)

5
Vitamins and Minerals

Jessica A. Grieger, Heather I. Katcher, Vijaya Juturu, and Penny M. Kris-Etherton

Chapter Glossary

Adequate intake (AI) The amount that sustains good health. Adequate intake is used for nutrients where there is not enough scientific evidence to set an official RDA or where no RDI has been established.

Daily value (DV) The percent of a particular vitamin or mineral that appears in one serving of the food based on a 2000-calorie daily diet. A measurement on food labels that lists the percentage of fat, calories, etc. based on recommended daily intakes per serving. Usually abbreviated on the label as "% Daily Values."

Dietary Reference Intake (DRI) A set of four nutrient-based reference values issued by the Institute of Medicine of the National Academies. Currently, the DRI recommendation is composed of AI, EAR, RDI, and UL. Not all nutrients have an established DRI.

Dietary supplement* Product taken by mouth that contains a dietary ingredient intended to supplement the diet. The dietary ingredients in these products may include vitamins, minerals, herbs or other botanical elements, amino acids, and substances such as enzymes, organ tissues, and metabolites. Dietary supplements can also be extracts or concentrates, and may be found in many forms, such as tablets, capsules, softgels, gel caps, liquids, or powders.

Estimated average requirements (EAR) Requirements expected to satisfy the needs of 50% of the individuals in a specified age group.

Functional food Food in which the concentrations of one or more ingredients have been manipulated or modified to enhance their contribution to a healthful diet. Also known as nutraceuticals.

Megadose An exceptionally large amount of a vitamin or mineral. The exact dose has not been defined, but a factor of 10, 100, or more times the usual dose has been used as the definition by various sources.

Nutraceutical Food or supplement that is marketed as having a beneficial effect on health. May include manipulation or modification of ingredients in order to attain this goal. Also known as functional food.

Preformed vitamin Usually applied to vitamin A; a vitamin found in animal sources or supplements and easily absorbed.

Provitamin Usually applied to plant-based vitamin A; a substance that can be converted into a vitamin through animal tissues. Similar to prodrug.

Recommended Dietary Allowance (RDA) The RDA was expanded in 1997 and became one measure in the guidelines outlined in the Dietary Reference Intake. When this occurred, the term was changed from RDA to RDI.

Reference (recommended) daily intake (RDI) The daily dietary intake level of a nutrient considered sufficient to meet the requirements of nearly all (97–98%) healthy individuals in each life-stage and gender group. The RDI is used to determine the recommended daily value (RDV), which is printed on food labels in the United States and Canada.

Tolerable upper intake level (UL) Amount used to caution against excessive intake of nutrients (like vitamin D) that can be harmful in large amounts.

Trace element Chemical element required in minute quantities by the body for normal function.

Vitamin Organic compound that the body needs in small quantities for normal growth and development and metabolic processes.

* Definition from the Dietary Supplement Health and Education Act of 1994.

Source: From National Academies of Sciences.[8]

Introduction

The belief that good nutrition is paramount to good health is a long-held credo. Hippocrates, touted as the father of modern medicine, recognized this principle, as evidenced in his quote at the beginning of the chapter. Historically, the focus of nutrition practice has been on meeting nutrient needs and preventing vitamin and mineral deficiencies. More recently, however, the emphasis of nutrition practice has shifted to the prevention of chronic diseases such as cardiovascular disease, diabetes, and cancer.

Nutrition experts have long emphasized the message of *food first,* or in other words, food before supplementation, because many of the nutrients found in food confer a wide range of remarkable health benefits. However, **dietary supplements** have become quite popular, and this trend has led to the emergence of **nutraceuticals** (also called **functional foods**) that are marketed as having a beneficial effect on health.[1] There are many instances where the scientific evidence is insufficient to support the health benefits presented on the labels of dietary supplements and/or nutraceutical food products. In addition, as science advances, questions are emerging concerning not only the benefits but also potential risks associated with these products. In some cases, evidence from clinical trials may indicate that the use of selected supplements should be recommended. However, when the data are lacking or where adverse effects have been reported, recommendations for their use are not warranted.

Dietary supplements include vitamins, minerals, herbs, and a broad category of other products added to foods or manufactured as food products. In some countries, dietary supplements are categorized as foods, and in other countries they are categorized as drugs. The purpose of this chapter is to provide an overview of **vitamins** and minerals, review the current evidence for use of popular dietary supplements, and provide guidance regarding appropriate recommendations for clinical practice. Herbal products are agents that have a very limited database and are outside the scope of this chapter. Recent reviews have been published,[2,3] and

additional information about herbal products can be found in Chapter X. Definitions of common terms used throughout this chapter can be found in the Chapter Glossary.

The majority of clinical studies evaluating the health effects of vitamins and minerals is based on epidemiologic studies reporting a lower risk of chronic disease among individuals with higher circulating levels or intakes of these micronutrients. Studies often do not report whether subjects were taking other supplements before and during the study, and there is little information addressing other variables that may modify the effects of supplements. For example, since food fortification has become popular, intakes of certain nutrients often exceed the Recommended Daily Intake (RDI). Therefore, it is important to understand the risk/benefit profile of multivitamin/mineral supplement use in real life. First however, a brief description of terms is in order.

Dietary Reference Intake Guidelines

The United States government has issued dietary guidance via the **Recommended Dietary Allowances** (RDA) since 1943.[4] These guidelines were originally designed as part of a World War II effort to assess how nutrition might affect national defense.[5] The original RDAs were based on amounts of essential vitamins and minerals that were necessary for prevention of a deficiency disease or for normal growth and development. The definition of RDA has been "the levels of intake of essential nutrients considered, in the judgment of the Food and Nutrition Board on the basis of available scientific knowledge, to be adequate to meet the known nutritional needs of practically all healthy persons."[6]

They are updated approximately every 5 years, and in 1997, the RDAs became part of an expanded system called the **Dietary Reference Intake** (DRI). The DRI is composed of **Estimated Average Requirements** (EAR), **Reference (Recommended) Daily Intake** (RDI), **Tolerable Upper Intake levels** (TUI), and **Adequate Intake** (AI).[7] The criteria for these values today are based on positive evidence that the nutrient is essential for a beneficial biologic function rather than the demonstration of clinical disorder.

The DRI guidelines used in the United States and Canada are developed by the Food and Drug Administration (FDA). They are intended for use by the general public; on food labels; for determining the composition of diets for school, prison, hospital, and nursing home menus; by industries developing new food products; and by healthcare policy makers or public health officials. The **Daily Value** (DV) is a fifth reference value that is printed on the nutrition facts label, which is part of all food labels. The DV is the percent of a particular vitamin or mineral that appears in one serving of the food based on a 2000-calorie daily diet.[8] The purpose of the DV is to make it easier for consumers to interpret food labels.

Supplements vs Food

The dietary supplement market is a rapidly growing economic sector. Data from the third National Health and Nutrition Examination Survey (NHANES III, 1999–2002) reported that approximately 55% of men and women ≥ 40 years of age in the United States reported using at least one dietary supplement.[8] Epidemiologic and clinical studies that have evaluated dietary supplements for the prevention or treatment of disease are inconsistent, often showing little or no benefit; and data assessing total mortality have found no reduced risk between persons who regularly take dietary supplements and those who do not take them.[9] Few studies have been designed specifically to assess the risk associated with different intake levels of single or multiple micronutrients. The media reporting of some benefits of supplements may influence the public's attitude about the use of these products. This is discussed in further detail in the sections on use of vitamins for prevention and treatment of specific diseases.

A food-based dietary pattern that meets current nutrient goals is recommended, as foods can deliver the full complement of nutrients and dietary factors that target a broad array of health benefits and risk reduction for chronic diseases. Although most Americans have access to a full range of foods, data from the 2001–2002 NHANES reported that only 10–11% of men and 7–8% of women met the EAR for vitamin A (12 mg/day; 18 IU).[4] Likewise, many persons do not get enough calcium or iron.[10,11]

Regulation of Nutrient Supplements in the United States

The FDA regulates dietary supplements under the Dietary Supplement Health and Education Act of 1994 (DSHEA). Under this act, the dietary supplement manufacturer is responsible for ensuring that a supplement is safe before it is marketed, and the FDA is responsible for taking action against any unsafe dietary supplement product after it reaches the market. In general, manufacturers do not need to register their products with FDA nor obtain FDA approval before producing or selling dietary supplements. However, manufacturers must make certain that the product label information is truthful and not misleading.

The postmarketing responsibilities of the FDA include monitoring safety, voluntary dietary supplement adverse event reporting, and establishing or updating rules for product information, such as labeling, claims, package inserts, and accompanying literature. Dietary supplement advertising is regulated by the Federal Trade Commission.

▌ Vitamins

Vitamins are organic compounds that are essential in small quantities for normal growth and development and metabolic processes but are not endogenously produced (except vitamin D) and therefore must be obtained from external sources. Box 5-1 discusses the naming of

---

▌ Box 5-1 Where Is Vitamin G? The Discovery and Naming of Vitamins

The first third of the 20th century was the age of discovery for vitamins. In the early 1900s, scientists were conducting various research studies, especially with animals, in which they discovered nutritionally limited diets resulted in various disease conditions. They noted that deficiencies such as rickets, beriberi, pellagra, and scurvy could be resolved by some unknown substance(s) found in food. Casmir Funk, a European biochemist, suggested that the active factors were vital amines and called them such. When it became apparent that these substances were not amino acids, vital or not, the name had become relatively common and eventually became shortened to *vitamin*.

Vitamins are named with alphabetical letters. Many individuals question why certain letters are missing. Some vitamins, such as vitamin G (riboflavin), vitamin H (biotin), and vitamin M (folic acid) were reclassified as part of the vitamin B complex. Others, such as vitamin F (essential fatty acids) and vitamin P (flavinoids), ultimately were found not to be vitamins at all. Vitamin J (catechol) and vitamin L_1 (anthranilic acid) were found to be protein metabolites. Vitamin K was named by German-speaking scientists who felt its association with coagulation (*koagulation*) warranted the specific letter.

vitamins. Vitamins primarily function as coenzymes in the conversion of macronutrients to energy and in building and maintaining body tissues and cell membranes; some vitamins are antioxidants and some promote immune function. Thirteen specific vitamins have been discovered to date and are divided into two categories: fat soluble and water soluble. Those vitamins from both groups that function as antioxidants are often combined into a third antioxidant group. Table 5-1 and Table 5-2 list the main functions of these vitamins, recommended intakes, and food sources. The Dietary Reference Intakes for vitamins can be found on the Web site of the Food and Nutrition Information Center of the United States Department of Agriculture. An overview of the essential vitamins and minerals is presented first followed by discussion of how these essential compounds are currently being used as pharmacologic agents.

Although there is controversy about use of vitamin supplements by healthy individuals, there are some conditions that are known to predispose to vitamin deficiency states. Persons who are elderly, vegans, alcoholic, on hemodialysis or parenteral nutrition, have

Table 5-1 Water-Soluble Vitamins with Action, Source, and Effect of Deficiency

Nutrient	Function	Selected Food Sources	Adverse Effects of Excessive Consumption*	Clinical Considerations
Thiamin (Vitamin B$_1$) Also known as aneurin	Coenzyme in the metabolism of carbohydrates and branched-chain amino acids.	Enriched, fortified, or whole-grain products; bread and bread products, mixed foods whose main ingredient is grain, and ready-to-eat cereals.	No adverse effects associated with thiamin from food or supplements have been reported.	Persons who may have increased needs for thiamin include those being treated with hemodialysis or peritoneal dialysis or individuals with malabsorption syndrome.
Riboflavin (Vitamin B$_2$)	Coenzyme in numerous redox reactions.	Organ meats, milk, bread products, and fortified cereals.	No adverse effects associated with riboflavin consumption from food or supplements have been reported.	None.
Niacin (Vitamin B$_3$)* Includes nicotinic acid amide, nicotinic acid (pyridine-3-carboxylic acid), and derivatives that exhibit the biologic activity of nicotinamide.	Coenzyme or cosubstrate in many biologic reduction and oxidation reactions—thus required for energy metabolism.	Meat, fish, poultry, enriched and whole-grain breads and bread products, fortified ready-to-eat cereals.	There is no evidence of adverse effects from the consumption of naturally occurring niacin in foods. Adverse effects from niacin-containing supplements may include flushing and gastrointestinal distress. The UL for niacin applies to synthetic forms obtained from supplements, fortified foods, or a combination of the two.	Extra niacin may be required by persons treated with hemodialysis or peritoneal dialysis or those with malabsorption syndrome.
Pantothenic Acid (Vitamin B$_5$)	Coenzyme in fatty-acid metabolism.	Chicken, beef, potatoes, oats, cereals, tomato products, liver, kidney, yeast, egg yolk, broccoli, whole grains.	No adverse effects associated with pantothenic acid from food or supplements have been reported.	None.
Pyridoxine (Vitamin B$_6$) Vitamin B$_6$ comprises a group of six related compounds: pyridoxal, pyridoxine, pyridoxamine, and 5'-phosphates (PLP, PNP, PMP).	Coenzyme in the metabolism of amino acids, glycogen, and sphingoid bases.	Fortified cereals, organ meats, fortified soy-based meat substitutes.	No adverse effects associated with vitamin B$_6$ from food have been reported. Sensory neuropathy has occurred from high intakes of supplemental forms.	None.
Biotin (Vitamin B$_7$)	Coenzyme in synthesis of fat, glycogen, and amino acids.	Liver, fruits, and meats.	No adverse effects of biotin in humans or animals were found.	None.

(continues)

Table 5-1 Water-Soluble Vitamins with Action, Source, and Effect of Deficiency (*continued*)

Nutrient	Function	Selected Food Sources	Adverse Effects of Excessive Consumption*	Clinical Considerations
Folate (Vitamin B₉)† Also known as folic acid, folacin, and pteroylpolyglutamate.	Coenzyme in the metabolism of nucleic and amino acids; prevents megaloblastic anemia.	Enriched cereal grains, dark leafy vegetables, enriched and whole-grain breads and bread products, fortified ready-to-eat cereals.	Masks neurologic complications among individuals with vitamin B_{12} deficiency. No adverse effects associated with folate from food or supplements have been reported.	In view of evidence linking folate intake with neural tube defects in the fetus, it is recommended that all reproductive-aged women should consume 400 mcg from supplements or fortified foods in addition to intake of food folate from a varied diet. Women should continue consuming 400 mcg from supplements or fortified food until the end of the periconceptional period—the critical time for formation of the neural tube.
Cobalamin (Vitamin B₁₂)	Coenzyme in nucleic acid metabolism; prevents megaloblastic anemia.	Fortified cereals, meat, fish, poultry.	No adverse effects have been associated with the consumption of the amounts of vitamin B_{12} normally found in foods or supplements.	Since 10–30% of older persons malabsorb dietary vitamin B_{12}, it is advisable for those older than 50 years to meet their RDA mainly by consuming foods fortified with vitamin B_{12} or a supplement containing vitamin B_{12}.
Ascorbic Acid (Vitamin C) Also known as dehydroascorbic acid (DHA).	Cofactor for reactions requiring reduced copper or iron metalloenzyme and as a protective antioxidant.	Citrus fruits, tomatoes, tomato juice, potatoes, brussels sprouts, cauliflower, broccoli, strawberries, cabbage, and spinach.	Gastrointestinal disturbances, kidney stones, excess iron absorption.	Individuals who smoke require an additional 35 mg/d of vitamin C over that needed by nonsmokers. Nonsmokers regularly exposed to tobacco smoke are encouraged to ensure they meet the RDA for vitamin C.

Note: For most vitamins, data on the adverse effects are limited and caution regarding high doses or long-term use may be warranted. Lack of reported effects does not assure total safety.

* Given as niacin equivalents (NE). 1 mg of niacin = 60 mg of tryptophan; 0–6 months = preformed niacin (not NE).

† Provided as dietary folate equivalents (DFE). 1 DFE = 1 mcg food folate = 0.6 mcg of folate from fortified food or as a supplement consumed with food = 0.5 mcg of a supplement taken on an empty stomach.

Table 5-2 Fat-Soluble Vitamins with Action, Source, and Effect of Deficiency

Nutrient	Function	Selected Food Sources	Adverse Effects of Excessive Consumption	Clinical Considerations
Vitamin A* Includes provitamin A carotenoids that are dietary precursors of retinol.	Required for normal vision, gene expression, reproduction, embryonic development, and immune function.	Liver, dairy products, fish, dark-colored fruits, and leafy vegetables.	Teratological effects, liver toxicity Note: From preformed vitamin A only.	Individuals with high alcohol intake, preexisting liver disease, hyperlipidemia, or severe protein malnutrition may be distinctly susceptible to the adverse effects of excess preformed vitamin A intake. β-Carotene supplements are advised only to serve as a provitamin A source for individuals at risk of vitamin A deficiency.
Vitamin D† Also known as calciferol.	Maintain serum calcium and phosphorus concentrations.	Fish liver oils, flesh of fatty fish, liver and fat from seals and polar bears, eggs from hens fed vitamin D, fortified milk products, and fortified cereals.	Elevated plasma 25 (OH) D concentration causing hypercalcemia.	Individuals on glucocorticoid therapy may require additional vitamin D.

(continues)

Table 5-2 Fat-Soluble Vitamins with Action, Source, and Effect of Deficiency *(continued)*

Nutrient	Function	Selected Food Sources	Adverse Effects of Excessive Consumption	Clinical Considerations
Vitamin E Also known as α-tocopherol.	A metabolic function has not yet been identified. Vitamin E's major function appears to be as a nonspecific chain-breaking antioxidant.	Vegetable oils, unprocessed cereal grains, nuts, fruits, vegetables, meats.	No adverse effects from vitamin E naturally occurring in foods. Adverse effects from vitamin E supplements hemorrhagic toxicity.[‡]	Individuals on anticoagulant therapy should be monitored when taking vitamin E supplements.
Vitamin K	Coenzyme during the synthesis of many proteins involved in blood clotting and bone metabolism.	Green vegetables (collards, spinach, salad greens, broccoli), brussels sprouts, cabbage, plant oils, and margarine.	No adverse effects with vitamin K from food or supplements have been reported. Because data on the adverse effects of vitamin K are limited, caution may be warranted.	Individuals on anticoagulant therapy should monitor vitamin K intake.

Note: For most vitamins, data on the adverse effects are limited and caution regarding high doses or long-term use may be warranted. Lack of reported effects does not assure total safety.

* Given as retinol activity equivalents (RAEs). 1 RAE = 1 mcg retinol, 12 mcg β-carotene, 24 mcg β-carotene, or 24 mcg β-cryptoxanthin. To calculate RAEs from REs of provitamin A carotenoids in foods, divide the REs by 2. For preformed vitamin A in foods or supplements and for provitamin A carotenoids in supplements, 1 RE = 1 RAE.

[†] 1 mcg calciferol = 40 IU vitamin D. The DRI values are based on the absence of adequate exposure to sunlight.

[‡] Applies to any form of α-tocopherol obtained from supplements, fortified foods, or a combination of the two.

had bariatric surgery, and those with inborn errors of metabolism that affect vitamin metabolism need to be evaluated carefully and often need specific vitamin supplements.

Antioxidant Vitamins

Antioxidants are substances that are capable of slowing or preventing oxidation. Oxidation reactions can generate free radicals that can damage cells. Antioxidant vitamins can be either water soluble or fat soluble. These vitamins protect against potential damage caused by the effects of reactive oxygen species on cellular tissues. Antioxidant vitamins include vitamin E (α-tocopherol), vitamin C (ascorbic acid), and vitamin A (retinol, β-carotene), which are primarily found in fruits and vegetables. Vitamin E also is found in vegetable oils, whole grains, and nuts and can be taken in its natural form (from the diet) or synthetic form (as a supplement). Vitamin E also modulates immune cell function through regulation of redox-sensitive transcription factors and affects production of cytokines and prostaglandins.[12] There is little evidence of toxic effects associated with β-carotene, which is the precursor and inactive form of vitamin A, vitamin E, and vitamin C.[7] However, high intakes of vitamin A can cause headaches, drowsiness, nausea, hair loss, dry skin, diarrhea, bone resorption, and amenorrhea. Very high doses of vitamin A have been found to be teratogenic.[13]

Fat-Soluble Vitamins

The fat-soluble vitamins are stored in body fat as well as the liver and other organs. Generally, fat-soluble vitamins pose a greater risk for toxicity (with the exception of vitamin E) than water-soluble vitamins when consumed in excess, since they can accumulate in tissue and are not excreted as rapidly as water-soluble vitamins.

Vitamin A

Vitamin A is a fat-soluble vitamin that exists in four forms, each with a different biologic function: retinal, retinol, retinoic acid, and retinyl ester, which is the storage form. Retinal is required for vision, while retinoic acid is the principal hormonal metabolite required for growth and differentiation of epithelial cells. Vitamin A is involved with the maintenance of mucous membranes, skin, bone, and hair, assists with vision at night, and also acts as an antioxidant. Vitamin A levels often are not adequate in average American diets.[7] The vitamin A that is found in supplements or food that comes from animals (e.g., liver, milk, egg yolks, butter) is **preformed vitamin** and can be absorbed as retinol. Vitamin A that is found in plants is called β-carotene, which is actually a **provitamin**. Provitamins are converted into a vitamin by animal tissues.

Vitamin A deficiency causes blindness, specifically impaired night vision and xerophthalmia.[14] In fact, the ancient Egyptians recognized that night blindness could be cured by eating liver. Vitamin A deficiency can occur secondary to inadequate intake of green and yellow vegetables or secondarily in persons who have malabsorption of lipids, low-fat diets, impaired bile production, or chronic exposure to oxidants such as cigarette smoke. This secondary deficiency syndrome occurs because vitamin A depends on fat and lipids for absorption.

Persons who abuse alcohol can develop vitamin A deficiency through an alcohol–vitamin interaction in the liver.[15] Alcohol stimulates increased catabolism of vitamin A via inducing a P450 enzyme. One of the enzymes responsible for metabolism of alcohol is also induced by alcohol. However, the same enzyme metabolizes retinol, and once stimulated by alcohol, the metabolism of vitamin A is enhanced as well.

Vitamin A toxicity was first noticed when arctic explorers ate polar bear liver, which has high amounts of vitamin A.[4] Very large amounts of any liver can cause vitamin A toxicity (called hypervitaminosis A), but the most common cause is an overconsumption of vitamin A supplements, or preformed vitamin A, rather than overconsumption of β-carotenes or provitamin A from plant sources. Research related to vitamin A toxicity has been primarily conducted in animals, with most studies being short term, focused on acute effects. Moreover, these studies often use intramuscular or venous injections of the agent. These conditions indicate that the study results cannot be extrapolated to physiologic conditions in humans.[16] Acute toxicity occurs when an individual ingests a **megadose**. Chronic toxicity results from the ingestion of high amounts of preformed vitamin A for months or years. Daily intakes of > 25,000 IU for more than 6 years and > 100,000 IU for more than 6 months are considered toxic, but there is wide interindividual variability, especially in regard to determining the lowest threshold required to elicit toxic effects.[17]

Among adults, symptoms of acute vitamin A toxicity include nausea and vomiting, increased cerebrospinal fluid pressure, headaches, blurred vision, and lack of muscular coordination. For women, observational studies have identified associations between chronic high intakes (> 1.5 g/day) of preformed vitamin A and bone loss and risk of osteoporosis leading to fractures, especially at the hip.[18] Supplemental intakes ≥ 25,000 IU by pregnant women may result in birth defects and is discussed in more detail later in the chapter.[19]

Vitamin D

Vitamin D's role in maintaining bone health is simply the most well known biologic function of this vitamin. Vitamin D receptors can be found in bone, immune cells, brain cells, breast, and colon. Although a detailed discussion of the biologic function of vitamin D is beyond the scope of this chapter, the interested reader can find this information in recent reviews.[20-22]

Epidermal 7-dehydrocholesterol converts UVB rays in the range of 290 nm to 310 nm into the previtamin necessary for making vitamin D_3. Next, a thermal reaction in the epidermis converts the previtamin into vitamin D_3, also named cholecalciferol. Vitamin D_3 is metabolized into 25(OH)D, also named calcifediol, in the liver. Calcifediol is the inert form of vitamin D and is stored in body fat for future use during long sunlight-limited winters. Finally, calcifediol is converted to 1,25-dihydroxyvitamin D (1,25[OH]2D), also named calcitriol, in the kidney. Calcitriol is the active hormonal form of vitamin D. Serum 25-hydroxyvitamin D (25[OH] D) is used to measure vitamin D levels.[23]

Few foods naturally contain vitamin D, with the notable exception of oily fish such as herring, sardines, and mackerel. Despite vitamin D fortification of foods in the United States, including milk and cereal, reported dietary intakes remain low.[24] More than 90% of the vitamin D requirement for most individuals comes from casual exposure to the sun.[25] Although many individuals are adequately exposed, low serum 25(OH)D levels (< 37 nmol/L) are prevalent in many age groups.[26]

Concern regarding sunlight exposure relates to its involvement in skin cancer. Among adults, application (2 mg/cm², i.e., 1 oz) of sunscreen over the majority of the body has been found to reduce vitamin D_3. However, sunlight exposure of 5–15 minutes between 10 AM and 3 PM each day during the spring, summer, and autumn appears sufficient to produce vitamin D.[25,27] Application of a sunscreen with a sun protection factor (SPF) of ≥ 15 is recommended to prevent the damaging effects of chronic, excessive exposure to sunlight if exposure beyond 5–15 minutes per day is planned.

Vitamin D deficiency results in rickets in children. In adults, vitamin D deficiency can cause osteomalacia and hyperparathyroidism.[20] Vitamin D supplements given in large doses generally have not been found to produce toxic effects. One study of 50 individuals with vitamin D deficiency, in which each study participant received a single intramuscular injection of 15,000 mcg vitamin D_3, reported that 4% became hypercalcemic (serum calcium > 2.65 mmol/L).[28] Thus, a concern of toxicity does exist, and persons with conditions that increase the risk of becoming hypercalcemic should be cautioned about taking megadoses of vitamin D. The acceptable upper limit dose has been set at 2000 IU/day, but there have not been any observable adverse effects at levels of 10,000 IU/day. Symptoms of high serum calcium levels may be tiredness, confusion, unstable gait, constipation, decreased appetite, increased urination, and bone pain.

In summary, vitamin D is essential for bone health, and because many persons do not get enough exposure to sunlight to maintain adequate vitamin D levels, routine vitamin D supplementation has been recommended for persons at risk for osteoporosis, particularly for individuals in at-risk groups, such as residents of a nursing home. The American Academy of Pediatrics recommends 400 IU/day for all children. There have been a few reports of rickets in breastfed infants, and therefore, the media routinely highlights the recommendation that these infants receive vitamin D supplements. Further discussion regarding vitamin D supplementation and its use as a specific pharmacotherapeutic agent is discussed later in this chapter.

Vitamin E

Vitamin E is a fat-soluble antioxidant vitamin including four tocopherols (α, β, γ, δ) and four tocotrienols (α, β, γ, δ). α-tocopherol is the most abundant form in nature. Vitamin E supplements usually are in the form of α-tocopheryl acetate, but they may be synthetic or natural. Synthetic forms are only half as active as the natural form, requiring twice the dosage as the latter to obtain bioequivalence.

The antioxidant activity of vitamin E lies in the ability to prevent free radical reactions. The current RDI for vitamin E is 15 mg α-tocopherol/day (30 IU). However, intakes of 80–12,200 mg (1200–18200 IU) may have antiplatelet effects and cause bleeding; and doses of > 12,200 mg/day may result in headaches, fatigue, nausea, cramping, weakness, blurred vision, and gonad dysfunction.[29] Controlled, double-blinded studies in humans have shown that vitamin E has very low toxicity, and no consistent adverse effects were reported in doses ranging between 600 and 3200 IU/day.[30] However, there are some exceptions. For example, an individual with malabsorption syndrome or a person using anticoagulant therapy may be asymptomatic until vitamin E is taken. Thus it is advised that vitamin E not be given under those conditions. Long-term vitamin E administration should be accompanied by concomitant administration of vitamin K to maintain a balance in the clotting process.[31]

Vitamin K

Vitamin K is actually a group of different compounds. Vitamin K_1, phylloquinone, is a protein-bound version of vitamin K found in green leafy vegetables. Pancreatic enzymes and bile salts are needed to alter vitamin K_1 into a form that is absorbable.[32] Vitamin K_2, menaquinone, is converted from K_1 by intestinal bacteria and can also be found in small amounts in dairy products. Vitamin K_2 is more potent and has a wider range of action than vitamin K_1. Vitamin K is the one fat-soluble vitamin that is not stored in the body, and therefore must be supplied on a daily basis.

Vitamin K was discovered in the 1930s by Danish biochemist Henrik Dam, who was doing research on chicks. After the first clinical trials found efficacy for using vitamin K to treat persons with obstructive jaundice, it was administered to newborns who were suffering from hemorrhagic disease. This use of vitamin K lowered the mortality from the disease from 4.6% to 1.8% and led to the Nobel Prize for Henrik Dam and Edward Doisy, who later isolated vitamin K.[33] See Box 5-2.

Vitamin K plays an essential role as the cofactor for the enzyme that activates several vitamin K-dependent proteins. There are several vitamin K-dependent proteins

---

Box 5-2 Vitamins and the Nobel Prize

Vitamins were not all discovered at the same time. For several years, the Nobel Prizes in medicine, physiology, or chemistry recognized the growth of knowledge about vitamins. Among the various Nobel Prizes in medicine or physiology awarded for the discovery of vitamins were Eijkman in 1929 for vitamin B_1; Whipple, Minot, and Murphy in 1934 for vitamin B_{12}; and Dam, who was said to discover vitamin K and shared the award in 1943 with Doisy, who isolated it. Nobel Prizes in medicine or physiology also were awarded to Reinhold-Windaus (1928) for isolation of vitamin D; Szent-Gyorgyi (1937) for vitamin C, and Kuhn (1938) for vitamins B_1 and B_6. Several other Nobel laureates received awards for work in the area, such as Dorothy Crowfoot Hodgkin (1964), one of only three women to receive a Nobel Prize in chemistry, for her confirmation of the structure of vitamin B_{12} as well as the structure of penicillin. Like many other laureates, Hodgkin and Doisy made other major contributions to science. While at her home university of Oxford, the British Hodgkin also confirmed the structures of insulin, ferritin, and tobacco, among other things. The midwestern American Edward Doisy isolated estrogen and extracted it from sows' ovaries even before he conducted his work on vitamin K, all during his long tenure at St. Louis University.

in the coagulation cascade that create the fibrin mesh that traps platelets including prothrombin and coagulation factors II, VII, IX and X. Conversely, the anticoagulant pathway also has vitamin K-dependent proteins including proteins C, S, and Z. The drug warfarin (Coumadin) blocks the enzyme that converts vitamin K to its active form in the liver, and vitamin K is used therapeutically to counter the effects of warfarin when necessary.

Although the role of vitamin K in the coagulation process is the most well known, vitamin K has additional metabolic functions including bone mineralization, vascular calcification, and cell growth. Newborn hemorrhagic disease is the classic example of vitamin K deficiency. Newborns do not initially have intestinal microflora for the production of vitamin K_2 and, therefore, vitamin K injections are given prophylactically to prevent hemorrhagic disease.

Vitamin K deficiency from inadequate absorption can also occur in the setting of liver disease, celiac disease, postbariatric surgery, biliary obstruction, malabsorption syndromes, and disorders of fat malabsorption. Use of cholestyramine (Questran); the bile acid sequestrant orlistat; mineral oil; or the fat substitute olestra can result in vitamin K deficiency. Persons taking cholestyramine sometimes will be instructed to take vitamin K supplements. Finally, excessive doses of vitamin A or vitamin E can interfere with vitamin K absorption. Prolonged use of antibiotics can decrease the population of microflora that synthesize vitamin K.

Vitamin K also has other drug–vitamin interactions in addition to that associated with warfarin (Coumadin). Vitamin K can therapeutically improve the effectiveness of bisphosphonates.[32] There are no known toxicities associated with vitamin K supplementation.[34]

Water-Soluble Vitamins

Water-soluble vitamins are excreted rapidly and thus deficiency symptoms can occur within several days of low dietary intakes. Small amounts of water-soluble vitamins can be stored in the body since they are excreted in urine when in excess. The exception is vitamin B_{12}, which can be stored up to 1 year in the liver.

The B Vitamins

The eight B vitamins listed in Table 5-1 are involved in cell metabolism. Vitamin B_4 and vitamin B_8 have been declassified as vitamins because both are synthesized by the human body.

Thiamine (Vitamin B_1)

Thiamine is an essential coenzyme for several intracellular reactions that generate energy and has an independent role in nerve impulse propagation. Thiamine is plentiful in modern diets.

Thiamine (vitamin B_1) deficiency is the cause of beriberi and Wernicke-Korsakoff syndrome. Beriberi is a disease of historic note that is rarely encountered today. However, Wernicke-Korsakoff syndrome does occur in specific settings. Wernicke's encephalopathy is characterized by a classic triad of confusion, ocular abnormalities, and ataxia. This disorder can develop into Korsakoff's psychosis if untreated. Persons who abuse alcohol can develop Wernicke's encephalopathy secondary to nutritional deficits, inadequate absorption (thiamine is not absorbed in the presence of alcohol), and decreased hepatic storage.[35] In addition, pregnant women with hyperemesis, anyone with pernicious vomiting, and persons who have had bariatric surgery can develop Wernicke's encephalopathy. Regardless of the cause, treatment is 50 mg per day for several days until the individual can eat a balanced diet.

Riboflavin (Vitamin B_2)

Riboflavin is a cofactor for various oxidations/reduction reactions. Pure riboflavin deficiency is rare but can be part of a deficiency of other B vitamins. Symptoms include sore throat, cracked lips, mouth ulcers, stomatitis, and ocular irritations. Persons susceptible to riboflavin deficiency include persons with anorexia nervosa, those on a vegan diet, individuals with malabsorption syndromes, and those on anticonvulsant medications (these drugs induce hepatic enzymes that metabolize riboflavin). Riboflavin, folate, and vitamin B_{12} play complementary roles in certain metabolic transformations. Therefore riboflavin deficiency will exacerbate deficiencies of other B vitamins. This is why B vitamin supplements are often grouped together into a B-complex formulation.

Niacin (Vitamin B_3)

Niacin (nicotinic acid or vitamin B_3) is a water-soluble vitamin with various derivatives such as nicotinamide adenine dinucleotide (NAD^+) and nicotinamide adenine dinucleotide phosphate (NADP). Niacin and its derivatives have an essential role in energy metabolism in living cells and DNA repair.

Niacin is synthesized endogenously through the conversion of tryptophan, an amino acid that constitutes approximately 1% of the protein in foods. The current recommendation for niacin is 16 mg/day for men and

14 mg/day for women older than 13 years of age.[8] Findings indicate that niacin intake is adequate in adults and adolescent boys, although young girls may be at risk for low intake.[36]

Niacin deficiency results in pellagra, a disease associated with diets that lack both vegetables and protein. Pellagra is endemic today in Africa, South America, and some areas of China and Indonesia. Pellagra is most common in settings where the food staple is corn. Interestingly, the tryptophan in protein can be endogenously converted to niacin. The niacin deficiency that occurs in the United States today is deficiency secondary to prolonged use of isoniazid (INH).

The use of routine niacin supplementation in clinical practice has been limited due to adverse side effects including cutaneous flushing and hepatic toxicity. Flushing is caused by the release of prostaglandin D2 and possibly other eicosanoids from cells in skin.[37] Furthermore, less well-defined side effects of niacin include blurred vision due to macular edema, nausea and vomiting, and the aggravation of peptic ulcers.[38] Administering aspirin or other inhibitors of cyclooxygenase 30 minutes to 1 hour before niacin intake can substantially reduce the incidence of flushing.[39]

Pantothenic Acid (Vitamin B_5)

Pantothenic acid, also known as coenzyme A (CoA), is a coenzyme for fatty-acid synthesis and breakdown. *Pantos* means "everywhere" in Greek, and indeed, sources of pantothenic acid are abundant. Pantothenic acid deficiency is extremely rare; it is found primarily in severely malnourished individuals. There is no known toxicity for pantothenic acid.

Pyridoxine (Vitamin B_6)

Pyridoxine is well known to pregnant women and their providers because it has mild antinausea properties and is very safe to take in pregnancy. Like the other B vitamins, pyridoxine is a coenzyme for multiple metabolic reactions including histamine metabolism, amino acid metabolism, and synthesis of several neurotransmitters. This vitamin also has a role in providing amino acids used in gluconeogenesis. The active form of pyridoxine is pyridoxal phosphate.

Pyridoxine deficiency is rare because it is so abundant in a variety of food products. The most common symptoms are glossitis, conjunctivitis, and peripheral neuropathy. Deficiency can occur in persons who abuse alcohol or in those with malnutrition or malabsorption disorders.[40] The elderly are more prone to vitamin B deficiency because the ability to absorb some nutrients decreases with aging, and the elderly are more prone to having inadequate diets.[41] Some persons have inborn errors that affect pyridoxine metabolism. For example, X-linked sideroblastic anemia can be improved by treatment with pyridoxine.

Pyridoxine has some clinically important drug–vitamin interactions. Deficiency in the form of sideroblastic anemia can also occur in persons on long-term isoniazid (INH) and pyrazinamide (PZA) because both these antituberculosis medications are vitamin B_6 antagonists. Pyridoxine is used to treat isoniazid seizures that occur when isoniazid is overdosed.[42] It also is used to treat theophylline seizures, but the data on the efficacy of pyridoxine in treating theophylline poisoning is controversial.[42]

Toxicity can occur when megadoses of > 250 mg/day are consumed. Symptoms are peripheral neuropathy, dermatoses, photosensitivity, and nausea.

Biotin (Vitamin B_7)

Biotin also is involved in production of fatty acids and metabolism of amino acids. Biotin is necessary for the conversion of folate, which suggests deficiency symptoms would be clinically significant, but because biotin is readily made by bacteria in the intestine, deficiency is rare. Biotin also has a role in glucose metabolism, and although biotin supplementation does lower postprandial glucose levels, studies on use in clinical practice are ongoing.[43]

Folate (Vitamin B_9)

Folate (folic acid) is a water-soluble vitamin that assists in production and maintenance of cells, red blood cell production, and synthesis of DNA bases. *Folium*, the Latin word for *leaf*, hints at the food sources of folate, which include green leafy vegetables. Folic acid is the synthetic form of folate.

Folate undergoes a series of metabolic reactions once absorbed before the active form, 5-methyltetrahydrofolate, is produced, and in this form, it has multiple biologic functions. Folic acid is particularly important during growth periods such as infancy and pregnancy. It also may assist in reducing bone fractures[44] and improving cognition.[45]

Data from the NHANES III (1988–1991) found that average dietary intakes of folate were approximately 60% of the current recommendation.[46] In 1996, the FDA mandated the addition of folic acid to enriched breads, cereals, flours, corn meals, pastas, rice, and other grain products.[47]

Following such fortification, the mean total intake of folate increased by 79 mcg, although this improved intake still fails to meet current recommendations.[48]

Folic acid is easily destroyed by cooking, which may influence how well it is obtained via food sources. In dietary supplements, folic acid typically is found in its simple form, which is pteroylmonoglutamic acid. Folinic acid, another form of folate found in foods, also is available as a supplement, and can help bypass certain biochemical steps that occur once folate has been absorbed from the intestine. Although folic acid is more bioavailable from supplements when compared to food sources, the degree and significance of this difference has not been determined.[49]

Folate Deficiency   A low protein intake can cause a deficiency of folate-binding protein, which is required for optimal absorption of folate from the intestine. In addition, low protein intake results in an insufficient supply of the amino acids that directly participate in folate metabolism. Folate absorption can be impaired several ways. Excessive intake of alcohol, smoking, and heavy coffee drinking can contribute to folate deficiency.

The role of folic acid in helping build DNA bases is particularly important. Folate deficiency results in inadequate DNA in cells that turn over rapidly, and thus the classic sign of folate deficiency is pernicious anemia, which is megaloblastic anemia. This is discussed in more detail in the section on vitamin B_{12}, and additional information can be found in Chapter 16. Pregnant women who have folate deficiency have an increased risk for having a fetus with neural tube defects (discussed later in this chapter). Finally, low serum folate is a strong risk factor for high levels of homocysteine in the blood—a condition associated with cardiovascular disorders.[50] Additional information can be found in Chapter 15 regarding cardiovascular conditions and the association of folate with homocystinemia.

Signs of folate deficiency include diarrhea, loss of appetite, weight loss, headaches, heart palpitations, irritability, forgetfulness, and behavioral disorders.

A number of drugs interfere with the biosynthesis of folic acid.[51] See Table 5-3. Persons who are taking methotrexate (Rheumatrex) can take folinic acid (Leucovorin), a form of folate that can function as folic acid and reverse the effects of methotrexate.

Folate Toxicity   Folate toxicity is rare, but it may occur following folate intakes of approximately 1000–2000 mcg. The current Upper Limit for folate is 1000 mcg for men and women ≥ 19 years of age and was designed to apply

Table 5-3 Examples of Drugs That Interfere with Folate Metabolism

Drug—Generic (Brand)
Aminopterin (Alimta)
Carbamazepine (Tegretol)
Methotrexate (Trexall)
Estrogen-containing agents (e.g., combined oral contraceptives)*
Phenobarbital (Luminal)
Phenytoin (Dilantin)
Primidone (Mysoline)
Pyrimethamine (Daraprim)
Sulfasalazine (Azulfidine)
Trimethoprim (Trimpex)

* Data controversial as to whether women in early studies had preexisting low folate levels.

only to synthetic folate—the forms obtained from supplements and/or fortified foods.

Excessive folic acid supplementation can have long-term adverse health effects. Folate can ameliorate megaloblastic anemia, which can be the result of either folate deficiency or vitamin B_{12} deficiency. Thus folate supplementation can mask vitamin B_{12} deficiency.

Vitamin B_{12} (Cyanocobalamin)

Vitamin B_{12} is a structurally complex, water-soluble vitamin composed of cobalt and corrin ring molecules that must be synthesized by bacteria that inhabit the intestine. Subsequent forms of the vitamin are metabolized in the body into an active coenzyme form. The only dietary sources of vitamin B_{12} are animal foods such as meat and dairy products. Vitamin B_{12} absorption is unusual. The vitamin B_{12} that is ingested is called *extrinsic factor*, which forms a complex with a glycoprotein called *intrinsic factor* that is excreted by gastric parietal cells. This complex is then absorbed into the systemic system.

Vitamin B_{12} is involved in the metabolism of every cell of the body, including DNA synthesis and regulation, as well as fatty acid synthesis, maintenance of the myelin sheath that surrounds nerves, and energy production, particularly in the brain and nervous system.

As discussed previously, vitamin B_{12} and folate functions are intertwined and deserve special mention. Vitamin B_{12} is required for a specific demethylation step in the production of DNA bases. If this step does not occur, folic acid cannot complete the function and DNA synthesis will be impaired. Because red blood cells are made frequently, both vitamin B_{12} deficiency and folate deficiency will result in the production of large, immature red cells or megaloblastic anemia. However, large doses of folate can overpower the vitamin B_{12} steps and mask vitamin B_{12} deficiency in hematologic evaluations. Unfortunately, additional folate cannot correct other neurologic abnormalities associated with vitamin B_{12} deficiency, and there is some suggestion that large doses of folate can be associated with cognitive declines in elderly persons who might be vitamin B deficient.[4] The evaluation of iron and folate deficient anemia is discussed in more detail in Chapter 16.

Vitamin B_{12} absorption is complex and requires an acidic environment in the stomach for the orally administered vitamin B_{12} complex to be released from its bound proteins, as well as the presence of an intrinsic factor secreted by the gastric parietal cells. When there is a problem with these parietal cells and intrinsic factor is not secreted, the free vitamin B cannot be absorbed. When this occurs and an individual becomes vitamin B_{12} deficient, large amounts of vitamin B_{12} from injections are required so that sufficient amounts can be absorbed.

Anticonvulsants have been associated with decreased vitamin B_{12} absorption.[52] H_2-receptor antagonists including cimetidine (Tagamet), famotidine (Pepcid), nizatidine (Axid), and ranitidine (Zantac) cause a reduction in gastric acid that can reduce absorption of dietary sources of vitamin B_{12}. Metformin (Glucophage) inhibits vitamin B_{12} absorption and enhances the requirement of B_{12} among persons with diabetes.

No toxicity of vitamin B_{12} has been found when oral supplements do not exceed the RDI, although data are lacking about consumption of greater amounts.

Vitamin C

Vitamin C also is a water-soluble vitamin known as ascorbic acid or ascorbate. Albert Szent-Gyorgyi was awarded the Nobel Prize in 1939 for isolating ascorbic acid. This vitamin is involved in collagen synthesis, acts as an antioxidant, and aids iron absorption. Vitamin C is abundant in many fruits and vegetables.

Vitamin C intake from the 1999 to 2002 NHANES was 88 mg/day, which exceeds the RDI of 75 mg for adults aged 19 or older.[53] Smokers need higher intakes of ascorbic acid to achieve similar serum ascorbic acid concentrations to that of nonsmokers, as smokers are naturally more likely to have low ascorbic acid concentrations.[54]

The effects of vitamin C deficiency or scurvy have also been known for millennia. James Lind, a British naval surgeon, first used oranges and limes to cure scurvy. Vitamin C deficiency causes scurvy, an unusual disease in modern society, but one that was prevalent in the past and continues in some developing countries (Box 5-3).

In a review of vitamin C toxicology, it was reported that the acute, subacute, chronic, and subchronic toxicity of vitamin C is low and that high doses are well tolerated without consistent side effects because it is water soluble and is rapidly cleared by the renal system via a reabsorption mechanism in the renal tubules that maintains a predetermined plasma level very efficiently.[55] It has been suggested that intakes of up to 2000 mg (nearly 35 times the vitamin C RDI) are still well tolerated; however, intake beyond this range may be less desirable, as it may result in nausea and diarrhea.[29]

Vitamin C and the Common Cold

Linus Pauling, was an American chemist who won the Nobel Prize in chemistry for determining how to predict chemical bonds and won the Nobel Peace Prize for fighting above-ground nuclear testing. Dr. Pauling vocally advocated using megadoses of vitamin C to prevent getting colds. In a review of 21 placebo-controlled trials, a vitamin C dose of ≥ 1 g/day failed to reduce the incidence

Box 5-3 The Case of Scurvy

Scurvy is a disease of vitamin C deficiency. Historically, the scourge of scurvy was described by Hippocrates, documented during the Crusades, and recognized as an occupational hazard among naval officers and pirates alike. The eventual connection between lack of vitamin C and scurvy caused the British Royal Navy to stock vitamin-rich foods for long voyages, giving rise to the slang name *limey* for the British sailors. Although the empirical connection was made between citrus and other food, it was not until 1932 that American researcher Charles King of the University of Pittsburgh was able to establish the scientific connection between vitamin C and scurvy.

Although scurvy is rare in the United States today, one potential problem in modern society is that vitamin C is destroyed through pasteurization, so that infants who are bottle-fed with regular milk may develop scurvy if vitamin supplements are not provided. This problem is unusual in North America, because regular milk is not recommended for newborns and breast milk has sufficient vitamin C for nursing infants.

of the common cold in the general population; however, for all 21 studies, vitamin C reduced the duration of episodes and the severity of the symptoms of the common cold by approximately 23% ($P < .05$).[56] In at least one small study that combined vitamin E (400 IU) and C (500 mg), the antioxidant capacity of plasma was improved more than these treatments given singly, indicating that the combination of these two vitamins may have a synergistic effect with regard to their effect on uncomplicated viral illness.[57]

Minerals

Minerals are inorganic compounds that support many cellular processes, act as electrolytes, or have a structural function. Forty minerals exist, of which approximately 16 are essential and need to be consumed in the diet. Minerals are inorganic compounds used in biochemical processes. If the daily requirement is ≥ 100 mg, the compound is called a mineral. If the daily requirement is less, it is called a **trace element**.

Minerals are required in specific amounts to prevent deficiency. Many persons in the United States do not have adequate intakes of minerals.[10,11] The function and importance of the key minerals and how they relate to cardiovascular, cancer, and other clinical diseases are described next.

Calcium

Calcium is the most abundant mineral in the human body. More than 99% of calcium in the body is found in the bones and teeth where it plays an important structural function.[58] The remaining 1% is found in the blood, muscle, and interstitial fluid, where it mediates vascular contraction and vasodilation, muscle contraction, nerve transmission, and secretion of hormones and enzymes. Calcium is required for almost all body processes. As a result, a series of regulatory systems exist to maintain constant blood calcium levels.

Calcium is found primarily in dairy foods and to some degree in collard greens, kale, and broccoli. Several calcium-fortified foods also are available, including fruit juices, tofu, and cereals. Calcium absorption is affected by the calcium status of the body, calcium content of a meal, age, pregnancy, vitamin D status, and plant components in the diet.[58] Similar to many other vitamins or minerals, calcium absorption increases when calcium stores are low or when dietary calcium declines.[59] Calcium absorption is highest in infancy and early puberty, and is also increased during the last two trimesters of pregnancy. Calcium absorption declines gradually with age in both men and women.

Calcium absorption is enhanced by vitamin D.[60] Conversely, phytic acid and oxalic acid, both of which are found in plant foods, inhibit calcium absorption.[58,61] Foods that include oxalic acid include spinach, collard greens, sweet potatoes, rhubarb, whole grain bread, beans, seeds, nuts, grains, and soy isolates. For unknown reasons, soybeans contain large amounts of phytic acid, but calcium absorption is relatively high from this food.[62]

Calcium recommendations are listed in Table 5-4. It is essential for young women to obtain calcium as they are building peak bone mass. Calcium recommendations are higher for adults older than 50 years of age because calcium absorption declines with age. There are no changes in calcium recommendations during pregnancy and lactation because the body becomes more efficient at absorbing calcium to meet the increased needs of the mother and fetus/newborn during pregnancy and lactation.

Lactose-intolerant individuals should consume nondairy sources of calcium. Options to meet calcium needs include a calcium supplement, lactaid supplement (lactaid hydrolyzes lactose), or lactaid-treated dairy products. Some other possible foods include aged cheeses (cheddar and Swiss), which contain little lactose; yogurt that contains live active cultures, which aids in lactose digestion; or lactose-free milk.

Table 5-4 Adequate Intake for Calcium Consumption*

Life-Stage Group	Adequate Intake (mg/day)
0–6 months	210
6–12 months	270
1–3 years	500
4–8 years	800
9–18 years	1300
19–50 years	1000
> 51 years	1200
Pregnant women	
≤ 18 years	1300
19–50 years	1000
Lactating women	
≤ 18 years	1300
19–50 years	1000
Postmenopausal Women†	1200

* Upper limits are either 2500 mg/day or undetermined.
† ≥ 51 years of age.

Calcium deficiency over a long time can result in osteoporosis. Hypocalcemia due to low dietary calcium is uncommon but can result from a medical condition or treatment like renal failure, surgical removal of the stomach, or the use of loop diuretics (e.g., furosemide). Hypocalcemia can cause numbness and tingling in fingers, muscle cramps, convulsions, lethargy, poor appetite, and mental confusion, as well as abnormal heart rhythms and death.

The upper limit for calcium for anyone older than 1 year of age is 2500 mg/day.[58] Excessively high intakes can have adverse effects including impaired kidney function and impaired absorption of other minerals such as iron, zinc, magnesium, and phosphorus. Calcium toxicity from diet and supplements is rare because calcium absorption is limited by the gastrointestinal tract. Hypercalcemia can result from malignant cancer and from excess intake of vitamin D (supplement overuse at doses of 50,000 IU or higher). Symptoms of calcium toxicity include lax muscle tone, constipation, large urine volumes, nausea, and ultimately confusion, coma, and death. Although it had been theorized that kidney stones resulted from high calcium,

more recent studies have shown that a high dietary calcium intake actually decreases the risk of kidney stones.[63,64]

The two primary forms of calcium in supplements are calcium carbonate and calcium citrate. Calcium carbonate is most popular because it is inexpensive and readily available. Calcium citrate is absorbed better than calcium carbonate, especially by individuals with decreased stomach acid; however, it is more expensive and requires more pills to obtain the same amount of elemental calcium. Other forms of calcium in supplements include calcium gluconate, calcium lactate, and calcium phosphate. The amount of elemental calcium in each type of supplement and the benefits and disadvantages of each are listed in Table 5-5.[65,66]

Since calcium absorption decreases as the dose of calcium increases, calcium supplements should be taken two times per day if doses are greater than 500 mg/day. The most common side effects of calcium supplements are gas, bloating, and constipation. These conditions may be ameliorated by spreading the dose throughout the day, changing the supplement brand, and/or taking the supplement with meals.

Table 5-5 Calcium Content of Calcium Supplements

Supplement	Elemental Calcium by Weight	Clinical Considerations
Calcium carbonate	40%	Most commonly used. Less well absorbed in persons with decreased stomach acid (e.g., elderly or those on antacid medicines). Natural preparations from oyster shell or bone meal may contain contaminants such as lead. Least expensive.
Calcium citrate	21%	Better absorbed, especially by those with decreased stomach acid. May protect against kidney stones. More expensive than carbonate.
Calcium phosphate	38% or 31%	Tricalcium or dicalcium phosphate. More common in Europe. Absorption similar to calcium carbonate.
Calcium gluconate	9%	Used intravenously for severe hypocalcemia. Well absorbed orally, but low content of elemental calcium. Very expensive.
Calcium glubionate	6.5%	Available as syrup especially for pediatric use. Least amount of elemental calcium.
Calcium lactate	13%	Well absorbed, but low content elemental calcium.
Calcium-fortified water, juice, and soy milk		Several companies offer calcium-fortified water or flavored juices. Bioavailability varies greatly. Calcium can settle at the bottom of the drink. The exception is calcium-fortified mineral water, which has bioavailability equal to milk.
Calcium-fortified chocolate		Healthy Indulgence and Adora: each piece contains 500 mg calcium carbonate. Thompson Candy Co.: calcium-fortified chocolate for children.
Calcium-fortified chewable tablets		Viactiv: each caplet has 500 mg of calcium carbonate.
Calcium-fortified fiber		Metamucil plus calcium: 5 capsules contain 300 mg of calcium carbonate.

Sources: Adapted from Gregory PJ 2000[65]; Kessenich CR 2008.[66]

There are multiple drug–drug and drug–food interactions associated with calcium supplements. Table 5-6 lists common interactions that have clinical implications.

Cobalt

Cobalt, a transition metal that exists in oxidation states Co^{+2} and Co^{+3}, is an essential trace element. This mineral is an integral part of the chemical structure of vitamin B_{12}, which is essential for folate and fatty acid metabolism. Cobalt mainly is absorbed from the pulmonary and the gastrointestinal tracts; with smaller amounts absorbed through the skin.[67] High concentrations of cobalt are found in fish (0.01 mg/kg), nuts (0.09 mg/kg), green leafy vegetables (0.009 mg/kg), and fresh cereals (0.01 mg/kg), and most of the cobalt ingested is inorganic. The mean population intake of cobalt is 0.012 mg/day.[68]

No RDI has been set for cobalt. Cobalt has been recommended for treating anemia, nephritis, and infection in addition to the usual hemopoietic agents. Conversely, cobalt supplementation has been associated with risks including allergic dermatitis, rhinitis, and asthma. At very high doses, cobalt toxicity can cause death.

Copper

Copper is an essential component of numerous copper metalloenzymes that are required for normal oxidative metabolism. The total amount of copper in the body is 75–100 mg overall, with copper present in every tissue of the body. This mineral is stored primarily in the liver, with smaller amounts found in the brain, heart, kidney, and muscles. Copper is needed for synthesis of hemoglobin, proper iron metabolism, and maintenance of blood vessels. This mineral also aids in overall healthy functioning of the blood vessels, nerves, immune system, melanin, and bones. Copper is a component of lysyl oxidase, an enzyme that participates in the synthesis of collagen and elastin, two important structural proteins found in bone and connective tissue. Tyrosinase, a copper-containing enzyme, converts tyrosine to melanin, the pigment that gives hair and skin its color. Copper is involved in energy production,

Table 5-6 Selected Drug–Food Interactions with Calcium Supplements*

Drug Generic (Brand)	Clinical Implications
Drug Interactions	
Alendronate	Calcium interferes with absorption of alendronate.
Aluminum-containing antacids	Calcium increases absorption of aluminum and can cause aluminum toxicity.
Anticonvulsants: phenytoin	These drugs decrease calcium absorption by increasing the metabolism of vitamin D.
Aspirin	Calcium increases urinary pH to the level required for increased urinary elimination of salicylates.
Bile acid sequestrants	These medications decrease the absorption of calcium.
Calcium channel blockers	Calcium can interfere with effectiveness of calcium channel blockers and reverse the hypotensive effect of the calcium channel blocker.
Corticosteroids	Corticosteroids decrease calcium absorption, increase calcium excretion, and inhibit bone formation.
Digoxin	Fatal cardiac arrhythmias are possible if hypercalcemia occurs in the presence of digoxin.
H_2 blockers and proton pump inhibitors	These drugs make the gastric environment less acidic, which decreases absorption of calcium citrate.
Ketoconazole	Calcium decreases effectiveness of ketoconazole.
Levothyroxine (Synthroid)	Calcium decreases levothyroxine absorption via formation of insoluble complexes.
Loop diuretics	These diuretics increase urinary excretion of calcium.
Quinolone antibiotics	Calcium decreases antibiotic absorption via formation of insoluble complexes.
Thiazide diuretics	These diuretics decrease excretion of calcium and can cause hypercalcemia or milk alkali syndrome.
Tetracyclines	Calcium decreases tetracycline absorption via formation of insoluble complexes.
Food Interactions	
Caffeine	Caffeine increases urinary excretion of calcium.
Iron, zinc, and magnesium	Calcium decreases absorption of these minerals.
Sodium	Sodium increases urinary excretion of calcium.
Spinach and rhubarb	The oxalic acid in these foods forms an insoluble compound with calcium and decreases absorption.

* There are multiple drug interactions with calcium-containing antacids. Prescribers should ask about use of antacids and calcium supplements when prescribing any drug.

the conversion of dopamine to norepinephrine, and blood clotting. Copper also is important for the production of thyroxine and is necessary for the synthesis of phospholipids found in myelin sheaths that cover and protect nerves.

Dietary copper is absorbed through the mucosa in the jejunum and transported via the portal blood to the liver. Copper is competitive with zinc for absorption sites, so high levels of zinc can cause copper deficiency, and the reverse is also true. Much of the copper taken up by the liver is incorporated into ceruloplasmin, released into the blood, and delivered to tissues. Endogenous copper is lost via the bile, being excreted back into the gastrointestinal tract. This copper combines with small amounts of copper from pancreatic and intestinal fluids and intestinal cells and is eliminated from the body. Good dietary sources of copper are oysters and other shellfish, whole grains, beans, nuts, potatoes, organ meats (kidneys, liver), dark leafy greens, dried fruits such as prunes, cocoa, black pepper, and yeast. The average daily Western diet is adequate for copper, containing 4 to 6 mg, approximately 40% of which is absorbed with an equivalent amount returned to the gastrointestinal tract from the bile.[69]

Copper deficiency causes an extensive range of symptoms, including iron deficiency anemia, ruptured blood vessels, osteoporosis, joint problems, brain disturbances, elevated low-density lipoprotein cholesterol (LDL-C) levels, reduced high-density lipoprotein cholesterol (HDL-C) levels, increased susceptibility to infections due to poor immune function, loss of pigments in the hair and skin, weakness, fatigue, breathing difficulties, skin sores, poor thyroid function, and irregular heart beat. Persons at risk for copper deficiency include infants who are bottle-fed and persons with chronic diarrhea. Certain medications/drugs may interact with copper. Table 5-7 lists some of the most common of these.

Iodine

Iodine is a nonmetallic trace mineral required for the synthesis of thyroid hormones (triiodothyronine (T_3) and thyroxine (T_4) for normal thyroid function. Thyroid hormones regulate a number of physiologic processes, including growth, development, metabolism, and reproductive function. The pituitary gland secretes thyroid-stimulating hormone (TSH), which stimulates iodine trapping, thyroid hormone synthesis, and release of T_3 and T_4. Iodine deficiency causes hypothyroidism. TSH levels become persistently elevated, which leads to hypertrophy of the thyroid gland, often expressed as a goiter. Thyroid function has a profound impact on overall health via modulation of carbohydrate, protein,

Table 5-7 Examples of Drug Interactions with Copper

Drug/Vitamin/Mineral Generic (Brand)	Effect
Estrogen-containing agents (e.g., combined oral contraceptives)	Increase the absorption of copper.
Nonsteroidal anti-inflammatory medications, including etodolac (Lodine), ibuprofen, nabumetone (Relafen), naproxen, and oxaprozin	Copper may enhance the anti-inflammatory effects.
AZT (Azidothymidine, Zidovudine, Retrovir)	Reduces blood levels of copper.
Antisecretory antihistamines such as famotidine (Pepcid, Pepcid AD), and nizatidine (Axid, Axid AR)	Cause copper deficiency by inhibiting absorption.
Vitamin C, iron, and manganese	Inhibit copper absorption.
Calcium and phosphorous	Increase copper excretion.

and fat metabolism; vitamin utilization; the digestive process; hormone secretion; sexual and reproductive health; and many other physiologic parameters. Thyroid dysregulation may elicit a wide variety of signs and symptoms because of the sheer number of systems affected. Goiters also may be found among individuals with hypothyroidism, a condition common among older women. More discussion on thyroid conditions can be found in Chapter 19.

The amount of iodine found in most foods is typically quite small and varies depending on environmental factors such as the soil concentration of iodine and the use of fertilizers. Rich food sources often are processed foods that contain iodized salt, as well as breads that contain iodate dough conditioners. Excellent dietary sources of iodine also include sea vegetables, yogurt, cow's milk, eggs, mozzarella cheese, and strawberries.

Voluntary fortification of salt with iodine was introduced in 1924 and resulted in a virtual elimination of endemic goiter from hypothyroidism in the United States. The Institute of Medicine's RDI is 150 mcg/d of iodine for adults and adolescents, 220 mcg/day for pregnant women, 290 mcg/d for lactating women, and 90–120 mcg/d for children aged 1–11 years.[70] The adequate intake for infants is 110–130 mcg/day. A multivitamin/multimineral supplement that contains 100% of the daily value (DV) for iodine provides 150 mcg of iodine.

In the Total Diet study, an ongoing project since 1961 designed to monitor the US food supply for chemical contaminants, nutritional elements, and toxic elements, the US population dietary iodine intakes ranged from 138 to 353 mcg/day, generally an adequate level.[71] Iodine deficiency is rare in the United States, but it can be found in areas of Africa, Asia, and eastern Europe, with goiter as one of most visible signs of iodine deficiency.

Iron

Iron has a key role in many enzymes and proteins and also is involved in regulation of cell growth and cell differentiation.[70] Iron serves as the site for oxygen binding in the hemoglobin molecule, which contains almost two-thirds of the total body iron. Twenty-five percent of total body iron is stored as ferritin and hemosiderin, primarily in the liver, spleen, and bone marrow. These stores are readily mobilized to meet daily needs when iron intake or absorption is inadequate.

The RDA for iron is 18 mg/day for women age 19–50 years, 27 mg/day during pregnancy, 9 mg/day during lactation, and 8 mg/day for postmenopausal women.[70] Dietary iron comes in two forms: heme iron and nonheme iron. Heme iron consists of iron tightly bound to a porphyrin ring, such as in hemoglobin, myoglobin, and cytochromes. Heme iron is found exclusively in animal products, including meat, fish, and poultry. Nonheme iron refers to iron in all other forms and is found in plant foods such as legumes, green leafy vegetables, strawberries, and some whole grains. Nonheme iron from plant foods is the sole source of dietary iron for individuals on a vegan diet.

The three most important factors that influence iron absorption are: (1) the level of iron stores, (2) the type of iron (heme or nonheme) consumed, and (3) the effects of other foods consumed with the iron. The amount of iron stored has the greatest influence on iron absorption. Iron absorption increases when stores are low and decreases when stores are high to prevent toxicity.

Nonheme iron is less efficiently absorbed than heme iron.[72] Thus, although the total dietary iron intake in a vegetarian diet may meet recommended levels, less of it will be absorbed compared with diets that include meat. Vegetarians need to consume almost two times more iron each day than nonvegetarians.[70]

Absorption of nonheme iron is affected by other meal components. Nonheme iron absorption is inhibited by phytate (found in legumes and whole grains), polyphenols (found in tea, chocolate, grains, and red wine), tannins (found in coffee and tea), and calcium (found in dairy products).[70] Vitamin C promotes absorption of nonheme iron by reducing iron in the ferric form (+3) to the ferrous form (+2), which is better absorbed.[70] Therefore, it is recommended to include sources of vitamin C with foods containing nonheme iron (i.e., plant sources), especially when daily intake is low, when losses are high (e.g., menorrhagia), when requirements are

high (e.g., pregnancy), and for those on a vegetarian diet.[73] Foods high in vitamin C include orange juice, grapefruit juice, lemon and lime juice, green peppers, broccoli, melon, and strawberries.

Iron needs are higher for women during their reproductive years and especially during pregnancy.[70] Iron needs also are higher in women than in men because of a woman's menstrual blood losses. Data currently are insufficient to establish an RDI for iron for infants from birth through 6 months of age. The recommended intake is based on the AI, which reflects the average iron intake for healthy infants fed breast milk, which is estimated to be 0.27 mg/day.

Anemia

Approximately 80% of the world population may be iron deficient, while an estimated 30% has iron deficiency anemia.[74] Iron deficiency limits the delivery of oxygen to cells, resulting in fatigue, decreased exercise and endurance capacity, poor work performance, and an impaired immune response. Iron deficiency anemia also is associated with decreased work and school performance, slow cognitive and social development during childhood, reduced exercise and endurance capacity, impaired cognitive function, decreased immune function, and glossitis (an inflamed tongue).[75,76]

Table 5-8 lists measurements commonly used to evaluate iron status. In early iron deficiency, low iron stores only are reflected by low serum ferritin concentration, because the iron stores are used to maintain normal serum iron levels. When iron deficiency anemia occurs, iron stores as well as other serum iron measures including transferrin saturation, hemoglobin concentration, and mean cell volume are low. Hemoglobin usually increases within 2 to 3 weeks of beginning iron supplementation and continues to increase approximately 1 g/dL (10 g/L) every 2 to 3 weeks.[77] The determination of iron status is complicated during inflammatory conditions because both serum ferritin and serum iron are acute phase reactants to inflammatory cytokines. The presence of inflammation should be ruled out when diagnosing iron deficiency. Additional information about anemia and anemia in pregnancy can be found in Chapters 16 and 35.

Iron Toxicity

A significant risk of iron toxicity exists from oversupplementation because iron accumulates in body tissues and organs. Although cases of long-term iron overload are unusual, they can occur following intakes of 200 to 1200 mg/day for long

Table 5-8 Laboratory Measurements Commonly Used to Evaluate Iron Status*

	Normal Values in Women	Iron Deficiency Without Anemia	Mild Anemia	Severe Anemia
Hgb (g/dL)	12–16	12–16	9–12	6–7
MCV (fL)	80–100	80–100	< 80	< 80
Ferritin (ng/mL)	10–291	< 40	< 20	< 10
Serum iron (mcg/dL)	60–150	60–150	< 60	< 40
TIBC (mcg/dL)	300–360	300–400	350–400	> 410
Transferrin saturation (%)	20–50	30	< 15	< 10

* These value ranges may be slightly different in individual laboratories depending on the assays used to determine reference ranges.

periods of time. The tolerable upper intake level (UL) for adults is 45 mg/day of iron, a level based on the incidence of gastrointestinal distress as an adverse effect.[70]

In children, death has occurred from ingesting 200 mg of iron supplements, and, therefore, iron supplements should be tightly capped and kept away from children's reach. An estimated 30% of pediatric drug fatalities result from unintended overdoses of iron supplements. Pediatric ingestions of > 40–60 mg/kg elemental iron have been associated with serious iron toxicity. A lethal dose of elemental iron in children is 2000–10,000 mg.

Early symptoms of iron overdose include gastrointestinal (GI) disturbances (nausea, vomiting, and diarrhea) and shock, followed by acidosis, edema, liver failure, and vasomotor collapse. Iron toxicity is diagnosed by measuring serum iron concentration and can be treated with parenteral administration of deferoxamine mesylate (Desferal), a detoxifying agent that chelates and sequesters free iron as well as iron bound to ferritin and hemosiderin.

Drug–Iron Interactions

The most notable drug–drug interactions with oral preparations of iron affect drug absorption. Antacids, histamine$_2$ receptor antagonists, and proton pump inhibitors have all been shown to decrease iron absorption, while tetracycline and fluoroquinolone absorption may be inhibited if coadministered with iron. These medications should be taken at least 2 hours before or after iron administration. Vitamin C (ascorbic acid) coadministration results in an increase in both iron absorption and iron-associated side effects. Oral preparations should be administered between meals, as food can decrease iron absorption by 50%.

Iron Supplements

Oral preparations of iron include tablets and liquid formations. Iron supplements are available in ferrous and ferric forms. Carbonyl iron consists of purely aggregated elemental iron. Ferrous iron salts (ferrous fumarate, ferrous sulfate, and ferrous gluconate) are the best absorbed forms of iron supplements. Information about parenteral forms of iron can be found in Chapter 16.

The amount of elemental iron (amount available for absorption) varies depending on the type of iron supplement (Table 5-9). The amount of iron absorbed decreases with higher doses, so it is recommended that individuals take their daily iron supplements in two or three equally spaced doses throughout the day. The Centers for Disease Control and Prevention (CDC) recommends that persons take 50–60 mg of elemental iron orally twice daily for 3 months for treatment of iron deficiency anemia, which is equivalent to approximately one 300 mg tablet of ferrous sulfate taken once a day.[78]

Ferrous sulfate is the drug of choice for treating iron deficiency anemia and is the preferred prophylactic treatment for preventing iron deficiency anemia when dietary iron intake is not sufficient, including iron deficiency anemias resulting from pregnancy and chronic blood loss not associated with gastric bleeding. Extended release capsules are also available and purport to decrease GI side effects; however, they are significantly more expensive and may lead to varied iron release that may prolong the required course of treatment. A once-daily dose of 150–300 mg ferrous sulfate is recommended to avoid iron deficiency during pregnancy.

Ferrous gluconate and ferrous fumarate differ from ferrous sulfate in the percentage of elemental iron contained in each tablet. When doses are adjusted to have equal amounts of iron, all iron salts possess equal efficacy and equal likelihood to produce GI disturbances. Those not responding to ferrous sulfate will not respond to ferrous gluconate or ferrous fumarate.

One purported benefit of carbonyl iron is that it may have less risk of toxicity, and thus less risk of inadvertent poisoning in children, in comparison to ferrous sulfate.[79]

Table 5-9 Oral Iron Preparations

Generic (Brand)	Formulation and Elemental Iron Content	Dosing and Indications	Contraindications/Precautions
Iron Salts			
Ferrous sulfate (Feosol, Fer-gen-sol, Fer-Iron Drops, Fero-Grad, Mol-Iron, Slow Fe*)	65-mg elemental iron in 325-mg tablet.	3 tablets tid on an empty stomach for treatment of iron deficiency anemia in adults. Iron deficiency anemia (*drug of choice*). Prevention of iron deficiency (e.g., during pregnancy or chronic blood loss).	Use with caution in patients in GI distress. May decrease dosing to qd/bid or take with food if GI side effects become problematic. Extended-release formulations are more expensive and may have less bioavailability. Discoloration of stool (dark green/black) should not be interpreted as sign of bleeding. Fatal toxicity may occur in children from unintended overdose (lethal dose is 2–10 g in children).
Ferrous fumarate (Femiron, Feostat, Feostat Drops, Hemocyte, Ircon, Nephro-Fer, Palafer, Span-FF)	33% elemental iron available in 63-, 195-, 200-, 324-, and 325-mg tablets, chewable 100-mg tablets, controlled-release 300 mg; oral suspended 100 mg/5 mL, 45 mg/0.6 mL; 108 mg elemental iron in 325-mg tablet.	PO 200 mg tid-qid; no specific instructions available for pregnancy iron deficiency anemia. Prevention of iron deficiency (e.g., during pregnancy or chronic blood loss).	Same as ferrous sulfate.
Ferrous gluconate (Fergon, Fertinic, Novoferrogluc)	12% elemental iron available in 300-, 320-, 325-mg tablets; 86-, 325-, 435-mg capsules, 300-mg film coated, and 300 mg/5 mL elixir; 35 mg elemental iron in 325-mg tablet.	PO 300–600 mg/day in divided doses. Iron deficiency anemia. Prevention of iron deficiency (e.g., during pregnancy or chronic blood loss).	Same as ferrous sulfate.
Carbonyl iron (Feosol caplets, Feosol elixir, Icar-C, Icar C Plus SR Oral)	45-mg caplets (Feosol), 65-mg tablets, 15-mg chewable tablets (Icar-C), 15-mg/1.25 mL suspension (Icar), 0.4-mg tablets (Icar C Plus SR Oral).	Feosol-1 tablet or caplet qd, or 5 mL daily. Icar C. Icar C Plus SR Oral—0.4 mg. Iron deficiency anemia. Prevention of iron deficiency (e.g., during pregnancy or chronic blood loss). Icar C PLUS used for folic acid-deficient megaloblastic anemia and prevention of neural tube defects.	On a per-mg basis, carbonyl iron formulations contain pure (elemental) iron and thus are substantially more potent than iron salts. Hemochromatosis, hemosiderosis. Inhibits tetracycline absorption. Nausea, abdominal discomfort and pain, constipation, diarrhea, mask occult bleeding. Tooth discoloration (Feosol elixir).

* Iron is absorbed primarily in the duodenum, so expensive enteric-coated or sustained-release formulations usually have less bioavailability and are less therapeutic.

Thus, it may be preferred for parents of small children. The formulation is readily bioavailable and may result in fewer GI side effects compared to equipotent concentrations of oral iron salts.

Side Effects/Adverse Effects of Iron Supplementation

GI-associated adverse effects, including GI irritation, pain and cramping, nausea, constipation, and vomiting, are observed in 10–20% of individuals who take iron supplements. Diarrhea and pyrosis occur with less frequency. All observed GI effects most commonly diminish with continued use of iron supplements.

These side effects are frequent only when doses exceed 200 mg of iron, and lowering the dose usually reduces these effects. Most individuals do not have problems at the normal doses of approximately 39 mg of elemental iron (e.g., 125 mg of ferrous sulfate).

Several options are available to individuals who require therapy adjustments due to gastrointestinal discomfort. Tablets may be administered less frequently (e.g., 1 tablet per day) and the frequency may be increased as tolerance develops. The formulation may be switched to a different one containing a smaller concentration of elemental iron. For example, one could switch from ferrous fumarate, which has 106 mg elemental iron/tablet to ferrous sulfate, which has 65 mg. A third option is to take the oral iron preparation with food. Since all three approaches for decreasing GI distress concomitantly decrease the amount of iron absorbed into the body, the duration of therapy necessary to achieve desired Hb and red blood cell levels will subsequently increase.

The aforementioned substances that interfere with dietary iron absorption (e.g., dairy products) also can decrease absorption. Since vitamin C enhances absorption of nonheme iron by changing it into the ferrous form, this augmentation is unnecessary for supplements already in the ferrous state, such as ferrous sulfate.

Drug–Drug Interactions

Iron absorption is decreased in the presence of many foods or pharmaceuticals. These agents include antacids, cereals, dietary fiber, caffeine (tea or coffee), milk, eggs, and specific antibiotics, especially tetracyclines. In addition, the presence of iron supplements in the gastrointestinal tract can inhibit absorption of other medications, especially antibiotics such as the tetracyclines. The primary mechanism of action is that medications form iron–drug complexes, which are not absorbed into the systemic system. Iron supplements should always be taken several hours before or after taking any other medication.

Magnesium

Magnesium is involved in the production and transport of energy and is important for the contraction and relaxation of muscles. Whereas calcium stimulates the muscles, magnesium relaxes them. Magnesium assists in protein synthesis, bone and teeth formation, absorption of calcium and potassium, and blood pressure control. Magnesium assists the parathyroid gland to process vitamin D; thus, low vitamin D can cause calcium absorption problems.

In combination with vitamin B_{12}, magnesium may prevent calcium oxalate kidney stones; it also may help to prevent depression, dizziness, muscle twitching, and premenstrual syndrome. Magnesium may help prevent cardiovascular disease (CVD), osteoporosis, certain forms of cancer, and hypercholesterolemia.

The majority of dietary magnesium comes from vegetables, particularly dark green, leafy vegetables; soy products, such as soy flour and tofu; legumes and seeds; nuts (e.g., almonds and cashews); whole grains (e.g., brown rice and millet); and fruits (e.g., bananas, dried apricots, and avocados).

Magnesium deficiency is rare. Symptoms include muscle weakness, fatigue, hyperexcitability, and sleepiness. Deficiency of magnesium can occur in persons who abuse alcohol or in persons whose magnesium absorption is decreased due to surgery, burns, or malabsorption problems. Certain medications or low serum calcium levels may be associated with magnesium deficiency. Magnesium toxicity is uncommon since the body is able to eliminate excess amounts. Magnesium excess almost always occurs associated with supplements or medications containing magnesium.

Potassium

Potassium is an electrolyte that helps maintain kidney function and is involved in contractions of cardiac, skeletal, and smooth muscle cells. Balance of potassium in the body is regulated by sodium since potassium is pumped into the cell by active transport systems that concomitantly pump sodium out of the cell. Potassium is absorbed readily in the small intestine, and excess potassium is excreted through the urine. A high-sodium diet is a risk factor for hypertension, and excessive use of sodium may deplete potassium stores. Therefore, a diet high in potassium may assist in lowering blood pressure. Sources of potassium include fruits and vegetables as well as meats, fish, soy products, and milk.

Low dietary potassium intake culminating in a potassium deficiency is uncommon, as many foods contain potassium. However, even a moderate reduction in the body's potassium level can lead to salt sensitivity and high blood pressure. A deficiency of potassium can occur in individuals with certain diseases or as a result of taking diuretics for the treatment of hypertension or heart failure. Additionally, several medications such as diuretics, laxatives, and steroids can cause a loss of potassium.

In contrast to hypokalemia, hyperkalemia is an excess of potassium caused by poor renal function (especially among individuals receiving dialysis for kidney failure), abnormal breakdown of protein, and severe infection. Symptoms of hyperkalemia may include irregular heartbeat, nausea, or a slow, weak, or absent pulse. Aldosterone is a hormone that regulates the kidneys' removal of sodium and potassium. A lack of aldosterone, as found in Addison's disease, results in increased total body potassium and subsequent hyperkalemia.

Potassium supplements are available in both oral and intravenous formulations. Potassium supplements are most often prescribed for persons taking loop diuretics and thiazides. Individuals who take potassium supplements need to be careful to balance dietary sources of sodium, and sodium-free products may be recommended. More information about use of potassium supplements can be found in Chapter X.

Selenium

Selenium was discovered in 1817 but it was not recognized as an essential nutrient until the late 1950s. Selenium is an essential trace mineral that acts on antioxidant enzymes and is important for muscular function, cardiac function, and preventing free radical damage. Plant foods are the major dietary sources of selenium in most countries throughout the world. The content of selenium in food depends on the selenium content of the soil, with northern Nebraska and the Dakotas being among the highest natural deposits in the United States.[80] Dietary selenium is related to protein content in the diet since it is incorporated into proteins to make selenoproteins, important antioxidant enzymes. Fruits and vegetables have very low protein content, hence very low selenium content.

This mineral interacts with antioxidant enzymes and it may enhance T and B lymphocyte proliferation, decrease excretion of lactic acid into the bloodstream, and enhance mitochondrial energy production. Selenium's most well-recognized role is its ability to regulate the activity of glutathione peroxidase (GPx), an enzyme that may help protect DNA from oxidative damage. At low levels of selenium, GPx levels may provide a more accurate reflection of selenium status than measurement of selenium.

Nutritional doses of selenium (approximately 40–100 mcg/day in adults) maximize antioxidant selenoenzyme activity and may enhance immune system function and carcinogen metabolism. At pharmacologic doses, approximately 200–300 mcg/day in adults, the formation of selenium metabolites, especially methylated forms of selenium, also may exert anticarcinogenic effects and antiviral effects. Selenium-dependent proteins promote regulation of thyroid function, synthesize DNA, prevent oxidative damage to cells, boost immunity, and reduce inflammation.

Selenium deficiency may contribute to the development of heart disease, hypothyroidism, and a poor immune system. Selenium deficiency also may make the body more susceptible to illnesses caused by other nutritional, biochemical, or infectious stresses.[81,82]

Chronic selenium poisoning has been reported from excessive environmental exposures to selenium and evidenced by changes in hair and nails. Garlic odor on the breath is an indication of excessive selenium exposure as a result of the expiration of dimethyl selenide.[83]

Zinc

Zinc is a cofactor for the antioxidant enzyme superoxide dismutase and is involved in a number of enzymatic reactions in carbohydrate and protein metabolism. Zinc's immunologic activities include regulation of T lymphocytes, CD4, natural killer cells, and interleukin II;

as well as facilitation of wound healing, especially following burns or surgical incisions. Zinc is essential for the maturation of sperm, normal fetal development, and sensory perception (taste, smell, and vision), and it controls the release of stored vitamin A from the liver. There are no specific storage sites known for zinc, so a regular supply in the diet is required. Zinc is found in all parts of the body; 60% is found in muscle, 30% in bone, and about 5% in skin.

Data from NHANES III suggested that all groups appear to be consuming sufficient intakes, likely the result of many common foods containing zinc.[84] Pumpkin seeds provide one of the most concentrated sources of zinc (20 g in 2/3 oz). Foods with significant sources include red meat, poultry, fortified breakfast cereal, some seafood, whole grains, dry beans, lentils, yeast, and nuts.

Zinc deficiency impairs growth, and severe depletion results in growth retardation. Zinc deficiency is generally a result of a low dietary zinc intake, disease states that promote zinc losses, or physiologic states that require increased zinc. Loss of zinc caused by diarrhea is a contributing factor common in developing countries. Signs of zinc deficiency include growth restriction, hair loss, diarrhea, delayed sexual maturation and impotence, eye and skin lesions, and loss of appetite, and there is evidence that weight loss, delayed healing of wounds, taste abnormalities, and mental lethargy can occur. Low zinc status has been observed in 30–50% of persons who abuse alcohol. Individuals who have malabsorption problems, including sprue, Crohn's disease, and short bowel syndrome, are at greater risk for a zinc deficiency.[85]

Zinc deficiency causes a decrease in appetite, which could lead to anorexia nervosa. Appetite disorders, in turn, cause malnutrition and less zinc intake. Deficiency of other nutrients such as tyrosine and tryptophan (precursors of the monoamine neurotransmitters norepinephrine and serotonin, respectively), as well as vitamin B_1 (thiamine) could contribute to this phenomenon of malnutrition-induced malnutrition.[86]

Zinc toxicity may occur and result in suppression of copper and iron absorption. There is evidence of induced copper deficiency with low intakes (100–300 mg Zn/d) of zinc. The RDI is 15 mg Zn/d; lower levels may interfere with the utilization of copper and iron.[87]

Zinc may affect other medications by inhibiting absorption, producing side effects, or enhancing actions. Insulin sensitivity is increased with zinc supplementation. Conversely, iron supplements may decrease zinc absorption. Table 5-10 displays drug interactions with zinc.

Table 5-10 Selected Drug–Drug Interactions Associated with Zinc*

Drugs—Generic (Brand)	Interactions
Amiloride (Midamor)	Reduces urinary zinc excretion and increases zinc blood levels.
Caffeine	Decreases zinc concentrations.
Captopril (Capoten) and enalapril (Vasotec)	Increase urinary zinc excretion.
Carbenoxolone analog (BX24)	Zinc sulfate may interact.
Chlorthalidone (Thalitone)	Increases serum zinc levels.
Cholera vaccine	Improves the efficacy.
Cholesterol-lowering drugs	Interact with LDL, HDL lipoproteins, and triglycerides, reducing HDL.
Cholestyramine (Questran)	Decreases zinc excretion in the urine and alkalinization of urinary zinc.
Cisplatin (Platinol-AQ)	Increases the cytotoxicity of cisplatin.
Deferoxamine (Desferal)	Increases urinary zinc elimination.
Diuretics (loop and thiazide)	Depletion of zinc; may decrease zinc absorption.
Erythromycin (E-mycin)	Decreases the absorption of erythromycin.
Estrogen	Depletion of zinc; may decrease zinc absorption.
Ethanol (alcohol)	Decreases serum zinc concentrations.
Fluoroquinolone antibiotics	May decrease the effectiveness of fluoroquinolone antibiotics.
Interferon alfa-2B (Intron A)	Prevention of interferon release.
Insulin	Improves both insulin secretion and insulin sensitivity and exerts insulin-like effects.
Pancreatic enzyme replacements	May improve absorption of zinc.
Tetracycline antibiotics	Zinc decreases absorption and serum levels of demeclocycline, minocycline, and tetracycline due to zinc binding.
Thyroid-active drugs	Alter thyroid hormone metabolism.

* This table is not comprehensive as new information is being generated on a regular basis.

Drug Interactions with Minerals

Little is known about drug interactions with trace minerals in humans; however, Table 5-11 provides a list of common nutrient interactions that have been reported. Prescription and over-the-counter medications can affect the nutrients in food by enhancing or inhibiting the absorption of nutrients. Medications can decrease appetite or change the way a vitamin or mineral is absorbed, metabolized, or excreted. For example, some cholesterol-lowering medications reduce cholesterol by removing bile acids that are needed to absorb the

Table 5-11 Selected Mineral Interactions with Drugs*

Drugs—Generic (Brand)	Nature of Interaction
Chromium	
Antacids, corticosteroids, H₂ blockers, proton pump inhibitors (e.g., omeprazole [Prilosec], lansoprazole [Prevacid])	These medications alter stomach acidity and may impair chromium absorption or enhance excretion.
Beta-blockers (e.g., atenolol or propranolol), corticosteroids, insulin, nicotinic acid, nonsteroidal anti-inflammatory drugs (NSAIDs)	Effects enhanced if taken together with chromium or they may increase chromium absorption.
Prostaglandin inhibitors (e.g., ibuprofen [Advil], naproxen [Aleve], and aspirin)	Effects enhanced if taken together with chromium or they may increase chromium absorption.
Antihypertensive medications, antihyperglycemic medications, cholesterol-lowering drugs	Effects enhanced if taken together with chromium or they may increase chromium absorption.
Magnesium, zinc, vitamin C, phosphatidyl serine, amino acid chelates	May enhance chromium absorption.
Copper	
Estrogen	Increases blood levels of copper.
NSAIDs	Copper binds to NSAIDs (such as ibuprofen and naproxen) and appears to enhance their anti-inflammatory activity.
Penicillamine (Cuprimine)	Reduces copper levels.
Allopurinol (Zyloprim)	May reduce copper levels.
Cimetidine (Tagamet)	May elevate copper levels in the body leading to damage of the liver and other organs.
Antipsychotics (haloperidol [Haldol] and risperidone [Risperdal]), nifedipine (Procardia), or oral contraceptives	May alter copper levels in the body.
Boron, vitamin C, selenium, molybdenum, and manganese	May alter (decrease or increase) copper levels in the body.
Zinc	May result in decreased copper absorption in the intestines or copper deficiency possibly due to increased synthesis of the intestinal cell protein metallothionein, which binds some metals.
Zinc	
Tetracycline (Sumycin)	Decreases the absorption of orally administered tetracycline (e.g., tetracycline).
Quinolone (e.g., ciprofloxacin [Cipro] and norfloxacin [Noroxin])	Possibly decrease the anti-infective response.
Iron and copper	May decrease zinc absorption.
Iron	
Cholestyramine and colestipol	Reduce the absorption of iron.
Tetracyclines, quinolones, ACE inhibitors	Decrease the absorption of drugs.

(continues)

Table 5-11 Selected Mineral Interactions with Drugs* (continued)

Drugs—Generic (Brand)	Nature of Interaction
Carbidopa and levodopa, levothyroxine	Iron may reduce the effectiveness or blood levels of these medications.
Calcium and copper	May decrease iron absorption.
Vitamin C	Enhances absorption.
Selenium	
Antacids	Reduce the absorption of selenium.
Chemotherapy/ radiation therapy	Selenium may reduce toxic side effects associated with chemotherapy drugs.
Corticosteroids	May decrease plasma selenium levels.
Erythropoietin (EPO)	Selenium increases the effects of erythropoietin in hemodialysis patients.
HMG-CoA reductase inhibitors	Selenium could reduce the effectiveness of other HMG-CoA reductase inhibitors.
Combination oral contraceptives	Selenium levels may be decreased.
Boron	
Calcium	Boron supplementation may result in increased calcium levels in the blood, and it may add to the effects of calcium or vitamin D supplementation.
Phosphorus	Supplemental boron may decrease phosphorus levels in the blood.
Estrogen-active supplements	Boron with estrogen-active herbs or supplements may result in increased estrogen effects.
Iodine	
Antithyroid drugs (methimazole, propylthiouracil), potassium iodide in combination with lithium salts	Hypothyroid effects may occur with the use of iodine products.
Potassium iodide with potassium-sparing diuretics, selenium deficiency	Concomitant use of iodine may increase the risk of hyperkalemia (high blood potassium levels) and may exacerbate the effects of iodine deficiency.
Potassium	
Diuretic (loop, potassium depleting—e.g., furosemide)	May decrease appetite.
Laxatives	May cause imbalance of electrolytes.
Magnesium	
Thiazide diuretics	May cause increased urinary excretion of magnesium.

* This table is not comprehensive as new information is being generated on a regular basis.

fat-soluble vitamins (A, D, E, and K), potentially reducing absorption of these vitamins. Vitamins or minerals in excess amounts may interact with other nutrients or may be toxic—e.g., large amounts of zinc can interfere with copper and iron absorption. Similarly, large amounts of iron can interfere with zinc absorption.

Multivitamins and Vitamin–Mineral Interactions

Approximately half the adult population in the United States takes a multivitamin. Unfortunately, there is no standardization for the components of multivitamins and no database that summarizes the components found in the multitude of multivitamin products available.[88] Evaluation of bioavailability is complicated because it depends on factors specific to the individual as well as type of supplement, formulation, and what combinations are present in the overall vitamin pill.

Some vitamins and/or minerals interfere with the absorption or metabolism of other vitamins. For example, zinc inhibits copper absorption, vitamin E antagonizes the action of vitamin K, and iron inhibits zinc absorption.[4] Although there is no evidence of adverse effects from use of a multivitamin by healthy individuals, toxicity can occur when megadoses are ingested. The evidence for therapeutic effectiveness and possible adverse effects related to individual vitamins is presented next.

Dietary Supplements as Pharmacotherapeutics

Several studies have assessed using vitamins, minerals, or both as treatments for major clinical conditions. The use of supplements has not been universally advised for prevention of cardiovascular disease or cancer since few studies have strongly supported reductions in these events when supplements are used. Therefore, diet remains the cornerstone in clinical management when vitamins and minerals are suggested as therapies. This section reviews the evidence to date for use of vitamins and minerals as pharmacologic agents.

The majority of observational studies evaluating the health effects of vitamins and minerals found a lower risk of chronic disease among individuals with higher circulating levels or intakes of specific nutrients, vitamins, or minerals. However, these types of observational studies often do not report whether subjects were taking other supplements before and during the study, and there is little information addressing other variables that may modify the effects of supplements. In addition, there is no standardization for dietary supplements, and trials have used different products with different bioavailabilities. For example, since food fortification has become popular, intakes of certain nutrients often exceed the RDI.

Despite limitations from early epidemiologic evaluations, randomized trials have been conducted and knowledge about the use of dietary supplements as specific pharmacotherapeutic agents is growing rapidly. For the most part, randomized trials that have compared use of a single vitamin supplement to no supplementation have found no effect on the disease of interest, and on occasion they have documented an increased risk for other disorders in the group using the vitamin.[4] These findings are discussed in the following section.

Prevention of Cardiovascular Disease

Hypercholesterolemia is a major risk factor for CVD, and there has been great interest in identifying which key bioactive nutrients and phytochemicals confer a protective effect and whether or not administration through dietary supplements can be therapeutic.

Although there is controversy concerning which nutrients consistently provide effective protection, the supplements that have been studied most include the B vitamins (folic acid, vitamin B_6, vitamin B_{12}, and niacin), antioxidant vitamins (vitamin C, vitamin E, vitamin A, and β-carotene), and more recently, vitamin D.

Antioxidant Vitamins (Vitamins A, C, and E)

A meta-analysis of five cohorts evaluated antioxidant supplementation and found a very modest, nonsignificant association between supplemental vitamin E and vitamin C intakes and coronary heart disease (CHD) events. The relative risk (RR) for CHD among subjects who consumed vitamin E supplements in amounts of < 25 mg/day and among subjects who consumed vitamin C supplements at 400–699 mg/day compared to nonusers was 0.87 (95% CI, 0.78–0.97; $P < 0.02$) and 0.72 (95% CI, 0.62–0.83; $P < .001$), respectively.[89] Additional vitamin E intakes ≥ 25 mg and vitamin C intakes ≥ 700 mg did not strengthen the association, but when all dietary sources were included in the model, there was no association between vitamin E use and CHD whereas vitamin C in high doses (700 mg/d) was modestly associated with a decreased incidence of CHD.[89]

However, a recent meta-analysis of primary and secondary prevention trials evaluated the effects of antioxidant supplements (e.g., β-carotene at 1.2–50 mg, vitamin C at 60–2000 mg, vitamin E at 10–5000 IU, vitamin A at 1333–200,000 IU, and selenium at 20–200 mcg) either alone or in combination. This meta-analysis found no significant effect of antioxidant supplements on mortality (RR = 1.02; 95% CI, 0.98–1.06). In addition, in the low-bias risk trials, mortality actually was increased by the use of the following alone or in combination: β-carotene (RR = 1.07; 95% CI, 1.02–1.11), vitamin A (RR = 1.16; 95% CI, 1.1–1.24), and vitamin E (RR = 1.04; 95% CI, 1.01–1.07).[90] β-Carotene increased the incidence of lung cancer in smokers and the HOPE trial of long-term vitamin E supplementation found a higher risk of heart failure in the group that took vitamin E.[4]

None of this research addressed the possible benefit to subgroups with increased oxidative stress, who also are at risk for increased CVD. For example, these studies did not explore whether vitamin E could reduce cardiovascular events in individuals with diabetes mellitus with the haptoglobin genotype (Hp2–2). This genotype is a determinant of CVD risk in persons with diabetes mellitus and exists in a subgroup that comprises 2–3% of the general population.[91] Further studies are required to investigate the use of antioxidant vitamins, especially by subpopulations, but given the negative findings and the possible adverse effects of vitamin E, antioxidant supplementation is not recommended for prevention of coronary artery disease at this time.

Vitamin D

Low vitamin D status recently has emerged as a potential risk factor for CVD; however, further studies are needed to assess its role in reducing CVD mortality.[92] Since the major source of vitamin D comes from sunlight exposure rather than through diet, at-risk groups who have little sunlight exposure may benefit most from supplementation.

Data from the NHANES III cohort (1988–1994) were the first to support a significant association between low 25(OH)D levels (< 37 nmol/L) and CVD risk factors in a nationally representative sample.[93] The mechanism(s) by which vitamin D may affect CVD is unclear. However, vitamin D may have immunosuppressive effects, thus reducing the proliferation of lymphocytes and the production of cytokines, which appear to have an important role in atherogenesis.[94] Vitamin D receptors are present in many cells, including macrophages, dendritic cells, monocytes, natural killer cells, B cells, and T cells.

Low 25(OH)D status, which is associated with abnormal bone turnover, has been postulated to affect CVD risk by increasing arterial calcification, therefore increasing arterial resistance and inducing hypertension.[95] However, in a large randomized trial of postmenopausal women, supplementation twice daily of 500 mg of calcium in combination with 200 IU (5 mcg) vitamin D did not affect the risk for coronary or CVD during a 7-year period.[96] In addition, another study was conducted for a shorter time period (15 weeks), but with a similar supplemental dose (calcium: 1200 mg; vitamin D: 400 IU) in women who were overweight/obese, but otherwise healthy. These supplements were compared to placebo, and researchers found LDL-C decreased by 7.3 mg/dL (0.19 mmol/L, $P < .05$) but no statistically significant changes in total cholesterol or high-density lipoprotein (HDL) ($P = .08$) were found.[97]

In summary, some studies indicate that vitamin D, particularly serum 25(OH)D levels in response to supplementation, may be important for improving markers of CVD, although not all studies support this. Long-term studies need to address the use of sunlight as a means to increase serum 25(OH)D to reduce CVD risk factors. Long-term trials to assess vitamin D supplementation and CVD risk need to be conducted in all age groups to support a beneficial effect in reducing CVD risk factors.

Potassium Supplements for Treatment of Hypertension

Hypertension is a strong risk factor for CVD, especially for ischemic stroke. Electrolytes such as potassium influence blood pressure, although the effects on clinical outcomes are unclear.

Electrolyte supplements have been studied with regard to their effect on hypertension. A review of three randomized controlled trials (RCTs) among 277 mildly hypertensive subjects suggested that combinations of potassium and magnesium supplements, with or without reduction in sodium intake, might reduce the risk of hypertension.[98] When these three trials were combined, however, there was no significant reduction in either systolic blood pressure or diastolic blood pressure among participants receiving combined supplementation.[98] Similarly, another review of six RCTs, with 8–16 weeks follow-up, using only potassium supplements, found the treatment group compared to the control group experienced a large, but statistically nonsignificant reduction in systolic blood pressure (mean difference = 11.2; 95% CI, −25.2–2.7) and diastolic blood pressure (mean difference = −5.0; 95% CI, −12.5–2.4).[99]

A food-based approach that increased dietary potassium intakes and reduced sodium intakes was favorable and reduced systolic and diastolic blood pressure. However, high supplemental doses of potassium do not appear to be beneficial for reducing blood pressure either alone or in combination with magnesium. These findings indicate that a reduction in the sodium content of processed foods including staple food items (particularly bread), together with an increase in potassium intake (through increased fruit, vegetable, and whole-grain cereal intake), appears practicable and would assist in the maintenance of optimal blood pressures. Supplements do not provide a bioequivalent result.

Magnesium and Metabolic Syndrome

Metabolic syndrome is defined by a constellation of CVD risk factors, including insulin resistance, elevated blood pressure, impaired glucose tolerance, central obesity, and atherogenic dyslipidemia as well as impaired clotting, increased inflammatory burden, and oxidative stress. Emerging experimental, clinical, and epidemiological data have provided evidence that dietary magnesium intake and supplementation are inversely associated with the risk for metabolic syndrome and its components.[100]

Prospective data from the Coronary Artery Risk Development in Young Adults study were derived from following 608 participants, starting at ages 18 to 30 years, for 15 years, during which time they developed metabolic syndrome. Data analysis revealed that these individuals were more likely to be in the lowest quartile of dietary intake of magnesium, compared to the other three quartiles.[101] A meta-analysis of seven cohort studies suggested that increase in magnesium may decrease the risk of type 2 diabetes, a major risk factor for metabolic syndrome.[102] Most of the studies involved found that an increase in magnesium by dietary manipulation to 130 mg/day was needed in order to obtain a decrease of 15% in the incidence of type 2 diabetes.[102] This amount is difficult to obtain nutritionally, as it essentially is equal to four slices of whole-grain bread, four cups of cooked oatmeal, one cup of beans, one-fourth cup of nuts, four tablespoons peanut butter, one-fourth cup of cooked spinach, or three bananas per day. This additional intake of magnesium is so high that a magnesium supplement may be necessary for this group.

Blood pressure and magnesium intake were assessed in a meta-analysis of 20 randomized controlled trials that included 1220 participants, some of whom were hypertensive and others normotensive. Magnesium intake was significantly related to small decreases in systolic blood pressure. The pooled net estimates of blood pressure (BP) change were reported to be RR = 0.6 (95% CI, −2.2 to 1.0 mm Hg) for systolic blood pressure and RR = 0.8 (95% CI, −1.9 to 0.4 mm Hg) for diastolic blood pressure. There was an apparent dose-dependent effect of magnesium, with an increase in magnesium dose resulting in reductions of 4.3 mm Hg systolic BP (95% CI, .2–6.3; $P < .001$) and of 2.3 mm Hg diastolic BP (95% CI, 0–4.9; $P = .09$) for each 10 mmol/day increase in magnesium dose.[103]

Low dietary magnesium intake appears to be associated with increased risk for metabolic syndrome. Randomized controlled studies using magnesium supplements to reduce diabetes and blood pressure are required to confirm that supplements are necessary when intakes are low. The best advice for persons with a low magnesium intake remains to consume a diet rich in food sources of magnesium, including fruits, vegetables, whole grains, and legumes.

Prevention of Cancer

Antioxidants

Cancer is the second leading cause of death in the United States after CHD. Free radical damage (oxidation) to cellular components likely plays an important role in carcinogenesis.[104] Antioxidants may help prevent this oxidative damage.[105]

The Women's Health Study evaluated the effects of β-carotene supplementation in a randomized double blind placebo trial that included 39,876 women. The β-carotene portion of the trial was terminated early at 4 years because there was no difference in the incidence of cancer in the women who took β-carotene compared to the incidence in the women who took placebo (378 cases vs 369 cases, respectively; RR = 1.03; 95% CI, 0.89–1.18).[106]

Therefore, studies question the use of antioxidants for global cancer prevention and do not provide strong support for population-wide implementation of high-dose antioxidant supplementation for the prevention of cancer. However, additional research is needed for subpopulations for whom supplements may be most helpful or more harmful.

Vitamin D and Breast Cancer

There is an association between higher dietary intakes of calcium and vitamin D and a decreased risk of developing premenopausal breast cancer.[107] The mechanism by which vitamin D may assist breast cancer reduction and other cancer types may be through the binding of the vitamin D-3

receptor (VDR), a nuclear receptor that modulates gene expression when combined with its ligand $1,25(OH)D_3$, the biologically active form of vitamin D_3. The cellular effects of vitamin D-3 receptor signaling include growth arrest, differentiation and/or induction of apoptosis, which indicate that the vitamin D pathway participates in negative-growth regulation.[108] However, other studies, including RCTs exploring supplementation with vitamin D and calcium, found conflicting results for prevention of cancer in general and for colorectal cancer in particular.[59,109] Additional studies are needed to clarify if vitamin D does provide cancer protection, and further research is required to address the expression and function of vitamin D proteins and receptors in cancer tissue and the role of vitamin D in limiting cancer growth.

Selenium

Among 1312 men and women in the Nutrition Prevention of Cancer multicenter cancer prevention RCT, selenium supplementation (200 mcg supplied as 500 mg high-selenium yeast tablets) for a mean period of 7.9 years was associated with a statistically significantly reduced risk of all cancers as measured by hazard ratios (HR = 0.75; 95% CI, 0.58–0.97). Reduction, albeit nonsignificant, also was found for lung cancer (HR = 0.70; 95% CI, 0.40–1.21) and colorectal cancer (HR = 0.46; 95% CI, 0.21–1.02).[110]

CVD and Cancer Summary

In summary, the effects of dietary supplements on cardiovascular events and cancer have generated great interest by consumers, providers, scientists, and nutritionists, as well as the private sector. The B vitamins (folic acid, vitamin B_6, vitamin B_{12}) and antioxidants (vitamin E, vitamin C, β-carotene, selenium) had great promise to decrease cancer and CVD risks based on findings from observational studies, and from studies using in vitro and animal models that demonstrated a protective effect. However, randomized controlled clinical trials have not demonstrated consistent efficacy, and some even have demonstrated adverse effects. As a result, these supplements are currently not recommended for risk reduction.[111] In addition, use of supplemental vitamin D, magnesium, potassium, and selenium has not provided consistent evidence that they can be used to reduce CVD and/or cancer risk. Particularly for vitamin D, as the major source comes from sunlight exposure rather than through diet, at-risk groups who have little sunlight exposure may benefit most from supplementation.

The American Heart Association currently recommends consumption of antioxidant-rich foods such as fruits, vegetables, whole grains, and nuts, and based on the inconsistent available evidence,[111] it should be recommended that antioxidants, vitamins, and minerals be consumed through diet rather than supplements as a means of increasing intakes. Further studies are required to assess whether long-term dietary intakes of antioxidants, vitamins, and minerals, or a combination of these, are beneficial for CVD and/or cancer risk reduction, and whether excessive dietary intakes adversely affect health in the long term.

Prevention of Other Disorders

Treating Hypercholesterolemia with Niacin

Numerous randomized trials with both men and women as participants have reported that niacin in doses ranging between 1 and 3 g/day decrease total cholesterol by 8%, LDL-C by 6–21%, and triglycerides by 16–29%; and increase HDL-C by 17–30%.[112,113] Subjects with coronary artery disease who were given extended-release niacin treatment of 500 mg nicotinic acid (Niaspan ER) for 3 months had increased HDL-C by 7.5% and decreased triglycerides by 15%; but there was no effect on total cholesterol or LDL-C.[114] In a 6-month evaluation of prolonged-release nicotinic acid (maximum dose 2000 mg/day) in statin-treated individuals with CVD and/or type 2 diabetes, HDL-C levels increased by 23%, triglycerides decreased by 15%, and LDL-C decreased by 4%.[115]

Reduction of Homocystinuria by B Vitamins

The homocysteine hypothesis for atherosclerosis was introduced by McCully in 1969, following the observation of premature atherothrombosis in children with homocystinuria.[116] Homocysteine is an amino acid produced by the metabolism of methionine via one of these two vitamin-dependent pathways: (1) remethylation, requiring folic acid and vitamin B_{12}, or (2) transsulfuration requiring vitamin B_6.[117] Controversy exists about whether B vitamins reduce the CVD risk by lowering serum homocysteine (tHcy) levels or whether the effects are independent of a decrease in tHcy. Supplementation with 0.5–5.0 mg/day of folic acid significantly reduces tHcy by 25%, and the addition of 0.5 mg/day of vitamin B_{12}, further reduces tHcy by 7%.[118]

Although results from a large prospective cohort study of healthy men and women demonstrated that serum homocysteine levels were associated with total incidence of CVD, MI, and stroke over 10 years, there were no significant associations between dietary intakes of folate or B vitamins and CVD risk.[119] Similarly, in a large, 8-year prospective study of postmenopausal women, dietary folate intake was not associated with CVD risk.[120]

In a meta-analysis of subjects with preexisting cardiovascular or renal disease, folic acid supplementation (range: 0.5 mg–15 g/day) did not reduce risk of CVD or all-cause mortality.[121] Similarly, several large, multicenter, double-blind, randomized studies evaluated the impact of B vitamin supplementation (ranging between 20 mcg and 2.5 mg folate; 200 mcg and 50 mg vitamin B_6; 0.4 mg and 1 mg vitamin B_{12}) on stroke and MI. Despite all studies finding a reduction in homocysteine, there were no effects on the primary end points (i.e., stroke, CHD events, or death) over the 2–5 year follow-up periods.[122,123]

In summary, although elevated tHcy is associated with increased CVD risk in observational studies, the results from clinical trials suggest that reducing tHcy with B vitamin supplementation does not confer any benefit. This finding supports the hypothesis that elevated tHcy may be a consequence of CVD, rather than a cause. The American Heart Association does not recommend use of folic acid and B vitamin supplements to reduce the risk of CVD, but rather recommends consumption of a healthy dietary pattern, consisting of vegetables, fruits, legumes, nuts, lean meats, poultry, fatty fish, whole grains, and cereals to meet current recommendations for all nutrients.[111]

Vitamins, Minerals, and Age-Related Macular Degeneration

Age-related macular degeneration is a leading cause of irreversible vision loss and blindness in the elderly. According to the Eye Diseases Prevalence Research Group, approximately 1.22 million US residents have neovascular age-related macular degeneration.[124] Reviews have described potential relationships between nutrients provitamin A carotenoids (α- and β-carotene), vitamin A, and α-tocopherol.[125] It has been suggested that these vitamins may play a role in the exogenous and endogenous defense and repair systems that operate in response to oxidative stress and inflammation in the retina. In the Multicenter Eye Disease Case-Control study, a higher dietary intake of carotenoids was associated with a 43% lower risk for age-related macular degeneration compared with those in the lowest dietary intake quintile (OR = 0.57; 95%

CI, 0.35–0.92; *P* = .02) although no significant finding was found for use of vitamin C and vitamin E.[126] In the Age-Related Eye Disease study, supplementation with antioxidants (vitamin C, 500 mg; vitamin E, 400 IU; and β-carotene, 15 mg) and zinc (80 mg) reduced the development of advanced age-related macular degeneration (OR = 0.72; 99% CI, 0.52–0.98) compared to placebo over a 6-year period.[127] These data suggest that carotenoids and antioxidant vitamins are beneficial for reducing age-related macular degeneration.

Zinc is hypothesized to play a role in the development of age-related macular degeneration, as it is found at high concentrations in the part of the retina affected by age-related macular degeneration. In the Blue Mountains Eye Study, the RR for total zinc intake between the top decile intake and the remaining population was 0.56 (95% CI, 0.32–0.97) for any type of age-related macular degeneration and 0.54 (95% CI, 0.30–0.97) for early age-related macular degeneration.[128] Data from a large, randomized, controlled trial of daily supplementation with antioxidants (500 mg of vitamin C, 400 IU of vitamin E, and 15 mg of β-carotene) and high-dose zinc (80 mg of zinc and 2 mg of copper) found that the antioxidant combination plus high-dose zinc, and high-dose zinc alone, both significantly reduced the risk of advanced macular degeneration compared to placebo (probability of age-related macular degeneration event at year 5, combination: 0.202, zinc alone: 0.216, vs placebo: 0.278) in individuals with signs of moderate to severe macular degeneration in at least one eye.[127] These data suggest that zinc may be beneficial for reducing age-related macular degeneration; however, further studies are needed to confirm these findings.

Calcium, Vitamin D, and Bone Health

The incidence of osteoporosis increases as women age because the decrease in ovarian estrogen that occurs postmenopause accelerates bone remodeling and bone loss. Because osteoporosis significantly increases the risk for fracture and disability, treatments to prevent and ameliorate osteoporosis have received a great deal of attention. Osteoporosis is directly related to calcium intake, but the question emerges whether or not supplemental calcium and/or supplemental vitamin D prevent osteoporosis?

There have been several randomized trials of calcium supplementation, vitamin D supplementation, and both calcium and vitamin D supplementation.[129-131] A 2008 meta-analysis of randomized clinical trials of calcium supplementation with or without vitamin D (n = 53,260) found that vitamin D alone is not sufficient to prevent fractures.[131] However, vitamin D and calcium combined

reduce the risk of fracture by 25% (95% CI, 4–42) and the risk of nonverbal fractures by 23% (95% CI, 1–40) compared to vitamin D supplementation alone.[131] It is recommended today that women at risk for osteoporosis and those with osteoporosis supplement with vitamin D and calcium. More information about prevention and treatment of osteoporosis can be found in Chapter 34.

Calcium in Diet and Blood Pressure

Observational studies reported an inverse relationship between calcium intake and blood pressure.[132,133] Randomized clinical trials have supported this finding and have demonstrated a modest decrease in blood pressure with calcium supplementation. A meta-analysis of 40 randomized controlled clinical trials demonstrated that calcium supplementation reduced systolic BP by 1.86 mm Hg and reduced diastolic BP by 0.99 mm Hg. Participants with a relatively low calcium intake (≤ 800 mg per day) had a slightly greater reduction in systolic (−2.63 mm Hg) and diastolic (−1.30 mm Hg) blood pressure.[134] Calcium supplementation during pregnancy has been found to reduce the incidence of preeclampsia. Preeclampsia is discussed in more depth in Chapter 35.

Calcium obtained by diet also has been shown to lower blood pressure. The Dietary Approaches to Stop Hypertension (DASH) study was the first to show that blood pressure could be reduced by diet to the same extent as antihypertensive drugs. One DASH study compared an average American diet with a diet high in fruit and vegetables and with a diet high in fruits, vegetables, and low-fat dairy products.[135] In another DASH diet study, 412 participants were randomized to consume either a DASH diet or a typical American diet, and further randomized to consume these diets with either a high sodium intake (a target of 150 mmol per day with an energy intake of 2100 kcal, reflecting typical consumption in the United States), intermediate sodium intake (a target of 100 mmol per day, reflecting the upper limit of the current national recommendations), or a low sodium intake (a target of 50 mmol per day, reflecting a level that may produce an additional lowering of blood pressure).[136] Reducing sodium intake from the high to the intermediate level reduced systolic blood pressure by 2.1 mm Hg (*P* < .001) in the control diet and by 1.3 mm Hg (*P* = .03) in the DASH diet. Reducing sodium intake from the intermediate to the low level caused additional systolic reductions of 4.6 mm Hg in the control diet (*P* < .001) and 1.7 mm Hg in the DASH diet (*P* < .01). Reducing sodium intake to levels below the current recommendation of 100 mmol per day in combination with the DASH diet lowered blood pressure also. The research strongly supports lowering sodium intake below what is currently recommended in order to improve blood pressure readings.

In a report of the Council on Science and Public Health, it was concluded that 1265 mg/d lower lifetime intake of sodium translates into an approximately 5 mm Hg smaller rise in systolic BP in persons aged 25–55 years. This dietary amount is equivalent to approximately 1 ounce of potato chips, one slice white bread and two slices of bacon; or one meal of macaroni and cheese or one half of a cup of cream of tomato soup.[137]

Special Populations

Pregnant Women

Nutrients are important for brain development during fetal and early postnatal life. Certain nutrients have greater effects on brain development than others, such as protein, certain fats, iron, zinc, copper, iodine, selenium, vitamin A, choline, and folate. Nutrient deficiency or excess can affect brain development, depending on its timing, dose, and duration of exposure.[138]

Many women in low-income countries consume inadequate levels of micronutrients due to limited intake of animal products, fruits, vegetables, and fortified foods that can potentially lead to anemia, hypertension, complications of labor, and even death.[139] At least 50 million pregnant women in low-income countries are anemic, primarily due to iron deficiency, and approximately 100 million women of reproductive age suffer from iodine deficiency.[140,141] It has been estimated that 82% of pregnant women have inadequate intakes of zinc, and more than one-third of breastfeeding women have inadequate intakes of vitamin B$_6$ based on breast milk concentrations.[142]

Some have questioned the effectiveness of multimicronutrient supplements because of possible interactions of nutrients resulting in impaired absorption. Studies have shown that high doses of iron may impair the absorption of zinc.[143] Manganese supplementation also decreases iron absorption.[144] Calcium also has been shown to have an absorption-depressing effect on iron.[145] More evidence is required before multimicronutrient supplementation programs are implemented on a global scale. Consumers may be modifying diets and using self-prescribed supplements themselves in attempts for various health outcomes. For example, some women are changing their diets or adding vitamins and minerals in attempts to conceive or even preferentially conceive a specific gender, although evidence is currently scant in this area. More about use of vitamin and mineral use in pregnancy can be found in Chapter 35.

Folate

Pregnant women are at risk for folate deficiency because many pregnant women do not consume sufficient amounts of folate from foods. Folate is required to support the increase in red cell volume during pregnancy. Low maternal folate levels are associated with an increase in neural tube defects. In a study of 23,228 women, an additional 500 dietary folate equivalents (approximately 300 mcg) consumed per day decreased the prevalence of neural tube defects by 0.78 cases (95% CI, 0.47–1.09) per 1000 pregnancies.[146] In a group of White participants, following mandatory fortification with folic acid, there was a reduction in anencephaly by 16% (95% CI, 0.73–0.97) and spina bifida by 35% (95% CI, 0.59–0.72).[147] These studies indicate the importance of additional supplements and folate-fortified food consumption before and during pregnancy. More details about pregnancy and folate can be found in Chapter 35.

Iron

Iron needs are approximately doubled during pregnancy (RDA is 27 mg/day) due to the fetal need for iron and the large increase in maternal blood volume.[70] Iron deficiency anemia is associated with an increased risk for preterm birth and low-birth-weight infants.[1,148] Severe anemia (hemoglobin < 4 g/dL) is also associated with increased perinatal maternal mortality.[1,148] The frequency of iron deficiency anemia in the first, second, and third trimesters is 2%, 8%, and 27%, respectively, in pregnant women in low-income areas in the United States.[149] The CDC recommends daily low-dose iron supplementation (30 mg elemental iron/day) for all pregnant women beginning at their first prenatal visit.[78] However, a meta-analysis of 40 randomized, controlled trials conducted in several countries with 12,706 participants showed that neither routine iron supplements alone nor iron supplements with folic acid demonstrated any clinically significant benefits and suggested that data were insufficient to promote routine supplementation.[150] More information about this controversy can be found in Chapter 35.

Zinc

Low maternal intake of zinc has been associated with several adverse outcomes of pregnancy, including low birth weight, premature birth, overall labor and delivery complications, and congenital anomalies. A systematic review of 17 randomized, controlled trials found that zinc supplementation (20–90 mg/day) during pregnancy was associated with a 14% reduction in premature deliveries; the lower incidence of preterm births was observed mainly in low-income women (RR = 0.86; 95% CI, 0.76–0.98 in

13 RCTs; n = 6854).[151] Supplementation did not have any effect on maternal health indicators, weight gain, or intra-uterine growth restriction. Further studies are required to determine if zinc supplementation during pregnancy is warranted for all pregnant women.

Vitamin A

Increased teratogenic risk may be associated with excess vitamin A intakes > 10,000 IU/day in pregnant women.[152] Fetal exposure to isotretinoin (Accutane), a synthetic retin-oid used for the treatment of severe acne, increased the risk of a malformation 25 times.[153] It is proposed that this occurs when both natural and synthetic retinoids affect the development of cephalic neural-crest cells and their deriv-atives. This action causes interference with the closure of the neural tube.[154] Evidence indicates that the teratogenic effect of retinoids may be derived from the expression of the homeobox gene *Hoxb-1* that regulates axial patterning in the embryo.[155,156]

Iodine

Iodine deficiency is the leading preventable cause of intellec-tual impairment worldwide. The fetus depends on maternal thyroid hormones for its normal development. The main form of thyroid hormone is T4 since very low amounts of maternal T3 reach fetal tissues.[157] In a review of iodine supplementa-tion before or during pregnancy in areas of iodine deficiency, two of the three trials (n = 1551 women) found iodine supple-mentation was associated with a reduction in deaths during infancy and early childhood (RR = 0.71; 95% CI, 0.56–0.90). Supplementation was associated with decreased prevalence of endemic cretinism at 4 years old (RR = 0.27; 95% CI, 0.12–0.60) and better psychomotor development scores between 4 and 25 months of age.[158] Iodine supplementation in a population with high levels of endemic cretinism appears to be important for reducing the incidence of the condition with no apparent adverse effects.

Iodine excess does not appear to adversely affect the pregnant mother or neonate. If a pregnant woman is ingest-ing 300 mg of iodine daily, supplementation with 200 mg/day iodine during a period of approximately 15 months (pregnancy plus lactation) does not endanger the fetus and newborn, as the total amount is well below the quan-tities required to block the developing thyroid gland.[159] Currently, the American Thyroid Association recommends that during pregnancy and lactation, women receive 150 mcg iodine supplements/day, and that all prenatal vitamin/mineral preparations contain 150 mcg of iodine.[160]

Elderly

Both physiologic and lifestyle changes that affect the elderly have an impact on absorption and utilization of vitamins and minerals. For example, as we age, we absorb vitamin D less efficiently. Elderly persons who are in nursing homes do not get sufficient sunlight. This combination potenti-ates the problem to result in the well-known risk elderly persons have for falls and fractures. Chapter 34 reviews physiologic changes of aging and implications for pharma-cologic therapies in more detail.

▍Conclusion

The available data do not demonstrate benefits of vitamin, mineral, or antioxidant supplementation for decreasing risk of CVD or cancer. Vitamins and minerals should be consumed through food, rather than as a supplement, since food provides a variety of nutrients, which may act synergistically to promote health. This approach is central to current dietary guidelines that support a food-based approach for meeting nutrient needs and decreasing risk of chronic diseases.

Pregnant women may need supplements for the health benefits of the fetus. There is a wealth of information sup-porting folate supplements to prevent neural tube defects as well as iodine and iron supplementation for adequate nutrient status and a good pregnancy outcome. Although a food-based approach is strongly recommended as the forefront for increasing nutrient intakes, pregnant women should have a high nutrient intake of many nutrients, and in some cases these intakes cannot be achieved through diet alone, and prenatal vitamins and iron can be recom-mended or prescribed.

╬ References

1. Hasler CM, Bloch AS, Thomson CA, Enrione E, Manning C. Position of the American Dietetic Association: Functional foods. J Am Diet Assoc 2004;104:814–26.
2. Cao Y, Zhang J, Kris-Etheron PM. Chapter 4, Effects of nutrient supplements and nutraceuticals on risk for cardiovascular disease. In Gotto AM, Toth P. Comprehensive management of high risk cardiovascular patients. New York: Informa Health Care, 2006:p. 79–145.

3. Vora CK, Mansoor GA. Herbs and alternative therapies: relevance to hypertension and cardiovascular diseases. Curr Hypertens Rep 2005;7:275–80.

4. Lichtenstein AH, Russell RM. Essential nutrients: foods or supplements: where should the emphasis be? JAMA 2005;294:351–8.

5. Harper AE. Contributions of women scientists in the US to the development of the recommended dietary allowances. J Nutr 2003;133:3698–702.

6. Anon. How should the recommended daily allowances be revised? Washington, DC: National Academy Press, 1996.

7. Food and Nutrition Board, Institute of Medicine. Dietary reference intakes: a risk assessment model for establishing upper intake levels of nutrients. Washington, DC: National Academy Press, 1998.

8. National Academies of Sciences. Dietary reference intakes (DRIs): recommended intakes for individuals, vitamins. 2004. Available from: *http://www.iom .edu/Object.File/Master/21/372/0.pdf* [Accessed December 30, 2008].

9. Huang H, Caballero B, Chang S, Alberg A, Semba R, Schneyer C, et al. Multivitamin/mineral supplements and prevention of chronic disease. Rockville, MD: US Department of Health and Human Services, Agency for Healthcare Research and Quality, 2006.

10. Dwyer JT, Holden J, Andrews K, Roseland J, Zhao C, Schweitzer A, et al. Measuring vitamins and minerals in dietary supplements for nutrition studies in the USA. Anal Bioanal Chem 2007;389:37–46.

11. Ervin RB, Kennedy-Stephenson J. Mineral intakes of elderly adult supplement and non-supplement users in the third national health and nutrition examination survey. J Nutr 2002;132:3422–7.

12. Wintergerst ES, Mani S, Hornig DH. Contribution of selected vitamins and trace elements to immune function. Ann Nutr Metab 2007;51:301–23.

13. Rothman KJ, Moore LL, Singer MR, Nguyen US, Mannino S, Milunsky A. Teratogenicity of high vitamin A intake. N Engl J Med 1995;333:1369–73.

14. Underwood BA. Vitamin A deficiency disorders: international efforts to control a preventable "pox." J Nutr 2004;134:2315–65.

15. Leo MA, Lieber CS. Alcohol, vitamin A, and B-carotene: adverse interactions including hepatotoxicity and carcinogenicity. Am J Clin Nutrition 1999;69:1071–85.

16. Nau H. Teratogenicity of isotretinoin revisited: species variation and the role of all-trans-retinoic acid. J Am Acad Dermatol 2001;45:S183–7.

17. Bendich A, Langseth L. Safety of vitamin A. Am J Clin Nutr 1989;49:358–71.

18. Feskanich D, Singh V, Willett WC, Colditz GA. Vitamin A intake and hip fractures among postmenopausal women. JAMA 2002;287:47–54.

19. Rosa FW, Koren G. Retinoid embryopathy in humans. New York: Marcel Dekker, 1993.

20. Holick MF. Vitamin D deficiency. N Engl J Med 2007;357:266–81.

21. DeLuca HF. Overview of general physiologic features and functions of vitamin D. Am J Clin Nutr 2004;80(suppl):1689S96S.

22. Mimball S, Fuleihan GH, Vieth R. Vitamin D: a growing perspective. Crit Rev Clin Lab Sci 2008;45: 339–414.

23. Murphy P. Vitamin D and mood disorders among women: an integrative review. JMWH 2008;53:440–6.

24. Grieger JA, Nowson CA. Nutrient intake and plate waste from an Australian residential care facility. Eur J Clin Nutr 2007;61:655–63.

25. Holick MF. Vitamin D: importance in the prevention of cancers, Type 1 diabetes, heart disease, and osteoporosis. Am J Clin Nutr 2004;79:362–71.

26. Binkley N, Novotny R, Krueger D, Kawahara T, Daida YG, Lensmeyer G, et al. Low vitamin D status despite abundant sun exposure. J Clin Endocrinol Metab 2007;92:2130–5.

27. Matsuoka LY, Wortsman J, Hanifan N, Holick MF. Chronic sunscreen use decreases circulating concentrations of 25-hydroxyvitamin D: a preliminary study. Arch Dermatol 1988;124:1802–4.

28. Diamond TH, Ho KW, Rohl PG, Meerkin M. Annual intramuscular injection of a megadose of cholecalciferol for treatment of vitamin D deficiency: efficacy and safety data. Med J Aust 2005;183:10–2.

29. Ziegler EE. Present knowledge in nutrition. Washington, DC: International Life Sciences Institute, 1996.

30. Tsai AC, Kelley JJ, Peng B, Cook N. Study on the effect of megavitamin E supplementation in man. Am J Clin Nutr 1978;31:831–7.

31. Kappus H, Diplock AT. Tolerance and safety of vitamin E: a toxicological position report. Free Radic Biol Med 1992;13:55–74.

32. Pizzorno L, Pizzorno L. Vitamin K: beyond coagulation to uses in bone, vascular and anticancer metabolism. Integrative Med 2008;7:24–30.

33. Zetterstrom RH, Dam CP, Doisy EA. The discovery of antihaemorrhagic vitamin and its impact on neonatal health. Acta Paediatr 2006;95:642–4.

34. Institute of Medicine Food and Nutrition Board. Press NA. Dietary reference intakes for vitamin A, vitamin K, boron, chromium, copper, iodine, iron, manganese, molybdenum, nickel, silicon, vanadium, and zinc. Washington, DC: Institute of Medicine, 2001.

35. Donnino MW, Vega J, Miller J, Walsh M. Myths and misconceptions of Wernicke's encephalopathy: what every emergency physician should know. An Emerg Med 2007;50:715–21.

36. Donald EA, Esselbaugh NC, Hard MM. Nutritional status of selected adolescent children. V. Riboflavin and niacin nutrition assessed by serum level and subclinical symptoms in relation to dietary intake. Am J Clin Nutr 1962;10:68–78.

37. Morrow JD, Awad JA, Oates JA, Roberts LJ 2nd. Identification of skin as a major site of prostaglandin D2 release following oral administration of niacin in humans. J Invest Dermatol 1992;98:812–5.

38. Guyton JR, Bays HE. Safety considerations with niacin therapy. Am J Cardiol 2007;99:22C–31C.

39. Oberwittler H, Baccara-Dinet M. Clinical evidence for use of acetyl salicylic acid in control of flushing related to nicotinic acid treatment. Int J Clin Pract 2006;60:707–15.

40. Halstaed CH. Nutrition and alcohol liver disease. Sem Liver Disease 2004;24:289–304.

41. Ferrario CG. Geropharmacology: a primer for advanced practice acute care and critical care nurses. Part 1. AACN;2008;19:23–35.

42. Lheureux P, Penazloza A, Gris M. Pyridoxine in clinical toxicology: a review. Eur J Emerg Med 2005; 12:78–85.

43. Campbell RK. A critical review of chromium picolinate and biotin. US Pharmacist 2006;31:11v.

44. Sato Y, Honda Y, Iwamoto J, Kanoko T, Satoh K. Effect of folate and mecobalamin on hip fractures in patients with stroke: a randomized controlled trial. JAMA 2005;293:1082–8.

45. Raman G, Tatsioni A, Chung M, Rosenberg IH, Lau J, Lichtenstein AH, et al. Heterogeneity and lack of good quality studies limit association between folate, vitamins B-6 and B-12, and cognitive function. J Nutr 2007;137:1789–94.

46. Ford ES, Ballew C. Dietary folate intake in US adults: findings from the third National Health and Nutrition Examination survey. Ethn Dis 1998;8:299–305.

47. Crandall BF, Corson VL, Evans MI, Goldberg JD, Knight G, Salafsky IS. American College of Medical Genetics statement on folic acid: fortification and supplementation. Am J Med Genet 1998;78:381.

48. Dietrich M, Brown CJ, Block G. The effect of folate fortification of cereal-grain products on blood folate status, dietary folate intake, and dietary folate sources among adult non-supplement users in the United States. J Am Coll Nutr 2005;24:266–74.

49. Gregory JF III. The bioavailability of folate. In McNulty H, Pentieva K. Folate bioavailability. Proc Nutr Soc 2004;63:529–36.

50. Wierzbicki AS. Homocysteine and cardiovascular disease: a review of the evidence. Diab Vasc Dis Res 2007;4:143–50.

51. Hernandes-Diaz S, Werler MM, Walker AM, Mitchell AA. Folic acid antagonists during pregnancy and the risk of birth defects. N Engl J Med 2000;343:1608–14.

52. Aslan K, Bozdemir H, Unsal C, Guvenc B. The effect of antiepileptic drugs on vitamin B_{12} metabolism. Int J Lab Hematol 2008;30:26–35.

53. Kant AK, Graubard BI. Secular trends in the association of socio-economic position with self-reported dietary attributes and biomarkers in the US population: National Health and Nutrition Examination Survey (NHANES) 1971–1975 to NHANES 1999–2002. Public Health Nutr 2007;10:158–67.

54. Schectman G, Byrd JC, Hoffmann R. Ascorbic acid requirements for smokers: analysis of a population survey. Am J Clin Nutr 1991;53:1466–70.

55. Hanck A. Tolerance and effects of high doses of ascorbic acid. Int J Vitam Nutr Res Suppl 1982; 23:221–38.

56. Hemila H. Does vitamin C alleviate the symptoms of the common cold? A review of current evidence. Scand J Infect Dis 1994;26:1–6.

57. Lara-Padilla E, Kormanovski A, Grave PA, Olivares-Corichi IM, Santillan RM, Hicks JJ. Increased antioxidant capacity in healthy volunteers taking a mixture of oral antioxidants versus vitamin C or E supplementation. Adv Ther 2007;24:50–9.

58. Standing Committee on the Scientific Evaluation of Dietary Reference Intakes, Food and Nutrition Board, Institute of Medicine. Dietary reference intakes for calcium, phosphorus, magnesium, vitamin D, and fluoride. Washington, DC: The National Academies Press, 1997.

59. Lappe JM, Travers-Gustafson D, Davies KM, Recker RR, Heaney RP. Vitamin D and calcium supplementation reduces cancer risk: results of a randomized trial. Am J Clin Nutr 2007;85:1586–91.

60. Zafar TA, Weaver CM, Zhao Y, Martin BR, Wastney ME. Nondigestible oligosaccharides increase

calcium absorption and suppress bone resorption in ovariectomized rats. J Nutr 2004;134:399–402.

61. Basu TK, Donaldson D. Intestinal absorption in health and disease: micronutrients. Best Pract Res Clin Gastroenterol 2003;17:957–79.

62. Heaney RP, Weaver CM, Fitzsimmons ML. Soybean phytate content: effect on calcium absorption. Am J Clin Nutr 1991;53:745–7.

63. Curhan GC, Willett WC, Speizer FE, Spiegelman D, Stampfer MJ. Comparison of dietary calcium with supplemental calcium and other nutrients as factors affecting the risk for kidney stones in women. Ann Intern Med 1997;126:497–504.

64. Hall PM. Preventing kidney stones: calcium restriction not warranted. Cleve Clin J Med 2002;69:885–8.

65. Gregory PJ. Calcium salts: Prescriber's Letter, 2000: Document #160313.

66. Kessenich CR. Alternative choices for calcium supplementation. JNP 2008;4:36–40.

67. Lauwerys R, Lison D. Health risks associated with cobalt exposure—an overview. Sci Total Environ 1994;150:1–6.

68. MAFF UK. Duplicate diet study of vegetarians: dietary exposure to 12 metals and elements. Food surveillance information sheet. No. 193, 2000. Available from: http://archive.food.gov.uk/maff/archive/food/infsheet/2000/no193/193vege.htm [Accessed December 30, 2008].

69. Milne DB. Copper intake and assessment of copper status. Am J Clin Nutr 1998;67:1041S–5S.

70. Institute of Medicine, Food and Nutrition Board. Dietary reference intakes for vitamin A, vitamin K, arsenic, boron, chromium, copper, iodine, iron, manganese, molybdenum, nickel, silicon, vanadium, and zinc. Washington, DC: National Academy Press, 2001.

71. Murray CW, Egan SK, Kim H, Beru N, Bolger PM. US Food and Drug Administration's Total Diet study: dietary intake of perchlorate and iodine. J Expo Sci Environ Epidemiol 2008;18(6):571–80.

72. Miret S, Simpson RJ, McKie AT. Physiology and molecular biology of dietary iron absorption. Annu Rev Nutr 2003;23:283–301.

73. Monsen ER. Iron nutrition and absorption: dietary factors which impact iron bioavailability. J Am Diet Assoc 1988;88:786–90.

74. Stoltzfus R. Defining iron-deficiency anemia in public health terms: a time for reflection. J Nutr 2001;131:565S–7S.

75. Zimmermann MB, Hurrell RF. Nutritional iron deficiency. Lancet 2007;370:511–20.

76. Pollitt E. Iron deficiency and educational deficiency. Nutr Rev 1997;55:133–41.

77. Killip S, Bennett JM, Chambers MD. Iron deficiency anemia. Am Fam Physician 2007;75:671–8.

78. CDC Recommendations to prevent and control iron deficiency in the United States. MMWR Recomm Rep 1999;47:1–29.

79. Spiller HA, Wahlen HS, Stephens TL, Krenzelok EP, Benson B, Peterson J, et al. Multi-center retrospective evaluation of carbonyl iron ingestions. Vet Hum Toxicol 2002;44:28.

80. Combs GF Jr, Gray WP. Chemopreventive agents: selenium. Pharmacol Ther 1998;79:179–92.

81. Zimmermann MB, Kohrle J. The impact of iron and selenium deficiencies on iodine and thyroid metabolism: biochemistry and relevance to public health. Thyroid 2002;12:867–78.

82. Beck MA, Levander OA, Handy J. Selenium deficiency and viral infection. J Nutr 2003;133:1463S–7S.

83. Barceloux DG. Selenium. J Toxicol Clin Toxicol 1999;37:145–72.

84. Briefel RR, Bialostosky K, Kennedy-Stephenson J, McDowell MA, Ervin RB, Wright JD. Zinc intake of the US population: findings from the third National Health and Nutrition Examination Survey, 1988–1994. J Nutr 2000;130:1367S–73S.

85. Menzano E, Carlen PL. Zinc deficiency and corticosteroids in the pathogenesis of alcoholic brain dysfunction—a review. Alcohol Clin Exp Res 1994;18:895–901.

86. Shay NF, Mangian HF. Neurobiology of zinc-influenced eating behavior. J Nutr 2000;130:1493S–9S.

87. Fosmire GJ. Zinc toxicity. Am J Clin Nutr 1990; 51:225–7.

88. Yelty EA. Multivitamin and multimineral dietary supplements: definitions, characterization, bioavailability, and drug interactions. Am J Clin Nutr 2007;85(suppl): 269S–76S.

89. Knekt P, Ritz J, Pereira MA, O'Reilly EJ, Augustsson K, Fraser GE, et al. Antioxidant vitamins and coronary heart disease risk: a pooled analysis of 9 cohorts. Am J Clin Nutr 2004;80:1508–20.

90. Bjelakovic G, Nikolova D, Gluud LL, Simonetti RG, Gluud C. Mortality in randomized trials of antioxidant supplements for primary and secondary prevention: systematic review and meta-analysis. JAMA 2007;297:842–57.

91. Milman U, Blum S, Shapira C, Aronson D, Miller-Lotan R, Anbinder Y, et al. Vitamin E supplementation reduces cardiovascular events in a

subgroup of middle-aged individuals with both type 2 diabetes mellitus and the haptoglobin 2–2 genotype: a prospective double-blinded clinical trial. Arterioscler Thromb Vasc Biol 2008;28:341–7.

92. Zittermann A, Koefer R. Vitamin D in the prevention and treatment of coronary heart disease. Curr Opin Clin Nutr Metab Care 2008;11:752–7.

93. Martins D, Wolf M, Pan D, Zadshir A, Tareen N, Thadhani R, et al. Prevalence of cardiovascular risk factors and the serum levels of 25-hydroxyvitamin D in the United States: data from the Third National Health and Nutrition Examination survey. Arch Intern Med 2007;167:1159–65.

94. Jouni ZE, Winzerling JJ, McNamara DJ. 1, 25-Dihydroxyvitamin D3-induced HL–60 macrophages: regulation of cholesterol and LDL metabolism. Atherosclerosis 1995;117:125–38.

95. Watson KE, Abrolat ML, Malone LL, Hoeg JM, Doherty T, Detrano R, et al. Active serum vitamin D levels are inversely correlated with coronary calcification. Circulation 1997;96:1755–60.

96. Hsia J, Heiss G, Ren H, Allison M, Dolan NC, Greenland P et al. Calcium/vitamin D supplementation and cardiovascular events. Circulation 2007;115:846–54.

97. Major GC, Alarie F, Dore J, Phouttama S, Tremblay A. Supplementation with calcium + vitamin D enhances the beneficial effect of weight loss on plasma lipid and lipoprotein concentrations. Am J Clin Nutr 2007;85:54–9.

98. Beyer FR, Dickinson HO, Nicolson DJ, Ford GA, Mason J. Combined calcium, magnesium and potassium supplementation for the management of primary hypertension in adults. Cochrane Database Syst Rev 2006;3:CD004805.

99. Dickinson HO, Nicolson DJ, Campbell F, Beyer FR, Mason J. Potassium supplementation for the management of primary hypertension in adults. Cochrane Database Syst Rev 2006;3:CD004641.

100. Ford ES, Li C, McGuire LC, Mokdad AH, Liu S. Intake of dietary magnesium and the prevalence of the metabolic syndrome among US adults. Obesity (Silver Spring) 2007;15:1139–46.

101. He K, Liu K, Daviglus ML, Morris SJ, Loria CM, Van Horn L, et al. Magnesium intake and incidence of metabolic syndrome among young adults. Circulation 2006;113:1675–82.

102. Larsson SC, Wolk A. Magnesium intake and risk of Type 2 diabetes: a meta-analysis. J Intern Med 2007;262:208–14.

103. Jee SH, Miller ER 3rd, Guallar E, Singh VK, Appel LJ, Klag MJ. The effect of magnesium supplementation on blood pressure: a meta-analysis of randomized clinical trials. Am J Hypertens 2002;15:691–6.

104. Breimer LH. Molecular mechanisms of oxygen radical carcinogenesis and mutagenesis: the role of DNA base damage. Mol Carcinog 1990;3:188–97.

105. Niki E. Antioxidants in relation to lipid peroxidation. Chem Phys Lipids 1987;44:227–53.

106. Lee Im, Cook NR, Manson JE, Buring JE, Hennekens CH. Betacarotene supplementation and increase of cancer and cardiovascular risk. The Women's Health study. J Natl Cancer Inst 1999;91:2101–6.

107. Lin J, Manson JE, Lee IM, Cook NR, Buring JE, Zhang SM. Intakes of calcium and vitamin D and breast cancer risk in women. Arch Intern Med 2007;167:1050–9.

108. Welsh J, Wietzke JA, Zinser GM, Byrne B, Smith K, Narvaez CJ. Vitamin D-3 receptor as a target for breast cancer prevention. J Nutr 2003;133:2425S–33S.

109. Wactawski-Wende J, Kotchen JM, Anderson GL, Assaf AR, Brunner RL, O'Sullivan MJ, et al. Calcium plus vitamin D supplementation and the risk of colorectal cancer. N Engl J Med 2006;354:684–96.

110. Reid ME, Duffield-Lillico AJ, Garland L, Turnbull BW, Clark LC, Marshall JR. Selenium supplementation and lung cancer incidence: an update of the nutritional prevention of cancer trial. Cancer Epidemiol Biomarkers Prev 2002;11:1285–91.

111. Mosca L, Banka CL, Benjamin EJ, Berra K, Bushnell C, Dolor RJ, et al. Evidence-based guidelines for cardiovascular disease prevention in women: 2007 update. J Am Coll Cardiol 2007;49:1230–1250.

112. Goldberg A, Alagona P Jr., Capuzzi DM, Guyton J, Morgan JM, Rodgers J, et al. Multiple-dose efficacy and safety of an extended-release form of niacin in the management of hyperlipidemia. Am J Cardiol 2000;85:1100–5.

113. Knopp RH, Alagona P, Davidson M, Goldberg AC, Kafonek SD, Kashyap M, et al. Equivalent efficacy of a time-release form of niacin (Niaspan) given once-a-night versus plain niacin in the management of hyperlipidemia. Metabolism 1998;47:1097–104.

114. Kuvin JT, Dave DM, Sliney KA, Mooney P, Patel AR, Kimmelstiel CD, et al. Effects of extended-release niacin on lipoprotein particle size, distribution, and inflammatory markers in patients with coronary artery disease. Am J Cardiol 2006;98:743–5.

115. Birjmohun RS, Kastelein JJ, Poldermans D, Stroes ES, Hostalek U, Assmann G. Safety and tolerability of

prolonged-release nicotinic acid in statin-treated patients. Curr Med Res Opin 2007;23:1707–13.

116. McCully KS. Vascular pathology of homocysteinemia: implications for the pathogenesis of arteriosclerosis. Am J Pathol 1969;56:111–28.

117. Hankey GJ, Eikelboom JW. Homocysteine and vascular disease. Lancet 1999;354:407–13.

118. Anon. Lowering blood homocysteine with folic acid based supplements: meta-analysis of randomised trials: homocysteine lowering trialists' collaboration. BMJ 1998;316:894–8.

119. Zee RY, Mora S, Cheng S, Erlich HA, Lindpaintner K, Rifai N, et al. Homocysteine, 5,10-methylenetetrahydrofolate reductase 677C>T polymorphism, nutrient intake, and incident cardiovascular disease in 24,968 initially healthy women. Clin Chem 2007;53:845–51.

120. Dalmeijer GW, Olthof MR, Verhoef P, Bots ML, van der Schouw YT. Prospective study on dietary intakes of folate, betaine, and choline and cardiovascular disease risk in women. Eur J Clin Nutr 2007; 62(3):386–94.

121. Bazzano LA, Reynolds K, Holder KN, He J. Effect of folic acid supplementation on risk of cardiovascular diseases: a meta-analysis of randomized controlled trials. JAMA 2006; 296(22):2720–6.

122. Bonaa KH, Njolstad I, Ueland PM, Schirmer H, Tverdal A, Steigen T, et al. Homocysteine lowering and cardiovascular events after acute myocardial infarction. N Engl J Med 2006;354:1578–88.

123. Toole JF, Malinow MR, Chambless LE, Spence JD, Pettigrew LC, Howard VJ, et al. Lowering homocysteine in patients with ischemic stroke to prevent recurrent stroke, myocardial infarction, and death: The Vitamin Intervention for Stroke Prevention (VISP) randomized controlled trial. JAMA 2004;291:565–75.

124. Friedman DS, O'Colmain BJ, Munoz B, Tomany SC, McCarty C, de Jong PT, et al. Prevalence of age-related macular degeneration in the United States. Arch Ophthalmol 2004;122:564–72.

125. Ambati J, Ambati BK, Yoo SH, Ianchulev S, Adamis AP. Age-related macular degeneration: etiology, pathogenesis, and therapeutic strategies. Surv Ophthalmol 2003;48:257–93.

126. Seddon JM, Ajani UA, Sperduto RD, Hiller R, Blair N, Burton TC, et al. Dietary carotenoids, vitamins A, C, and E, and advanced age-related macular degeneration. Eye Disease Case-Control study group. JAMA 1994;272:1413–20.

127. Anon. A randomized, placebo-controlled, clinical trial of high-dose supplementation with vitamins C and E, beta carotene, and zinc for age-related macular degeneration and vision loss: AREDS report no. 8. Arch Ophthalmol 2001;119:1417–36.

128. Tan JS, Wang JJ, Flood V, Rochtchina E, Smith W, Mitchell P. Dietary antioxidants and the long-term incidence of age-related macular degeneration: the Blue Mountains Eye study. Ophthalmology 2008;115: 334–41.

129. Jackson RD, LaCroix A, Gass M, Wallace RB, Robbins J, Lewis CE, et al. Calcium plus vitamin D supplementation and the risk of fractures. N Engl J Med 2006;353:669–83.

130. Prince RL, Devine A, Dhaliwal SS, Dick IM. Effects of calcium supplementation on clinical fracture and bone structure. Arch Intern Med 2006;166:869–75.

131. Rizzoli R, Boonen S, Brand ML, Burlet N, Delmas P, Reginster JY. The role of calcium and vitamin D in the management of osteoporosis. Bone 2008;42(2): 246–9.

132. Jorde R, Bonaa KH. Calcium from dairy products, vitamin D intake, and blood pressure: The Tromso study. Am J Clin Nutr 2000;71:1530–5.

133. Witteman JC, Willett WC, Stampfer MJ, Colditz GA, Sacks FM, Speizer FE, et al. A prospective study of nutritional factors and hypertension among US women. Circulation 1989;80:1320–7.

134. VanMierlo LA, Arends LR, Streppel MT, Zeegers MP, Kok SJ, Grobbee DE, et al. Blood pressure response to calcium supplementation: a meta-analysis of randomized trials. J Hum Hypertens 2006;20: 571–80.

135. Appel LJ, Moore TJ, Obarzanek E, Vollmer WM, Svetkey LP, Sacks FM, et al. A clinical trial of the effects of dietary patterns on blood pressure. DASH Collaborative research group. N Engl J Med 1997;336:1117–1124.

136. Sacks FM, Svetkey LP, Vollmer WM, Appel LJ, Bray GA, Harsha D, et al. Effects on blood pressure of reduced dietary sodium and the Dietary Approaches to Stop Hypertension (DASH) diet. DASH-Sodium Collaborative research group. N Engl J Med 2001;344:3–10.

137. Dickinson BD, Havas S. Reducing the population burden of cardiovascular disease by reducing sodium intake: a report of the Council on Science and Public Health. Arch Intern Med 2007;167:1460–8.

138. Huffman SL, Baker J, Shurmann J, Zehner ER. The case for promoting multiple vitamin/mineral supplements for women of reproductive age in developing countries. Washington DC: Academy for Educational Development, 1998.

139. Ramakrishnan U, Manjrekar R, Rivera J, Gonzalez T, Martorell R. Micronutrients and pregnancy outcome. Nutr Res 1999;19:103–59.

140. Stoltzfus RJ. Iron deficiency and strategies for its control. [Report prepared for the Office of Nutrition]. Washington DC: USAID, 1993.

141. Leslie J. Women's nutrition: the key to improving family health in developing countries? Health Policy Plan 1991;6:1.

142. Caulfield LE, Zavaleta N, Shankar AH, Merialdi M. Potential contribution of maternal zinc supplementation during pregnancy to maternal and child survival. Am J Clin Nutr 1998;68:499S–508S.

143. Argiratos V, Samman S. The effect of calcium carbonate and calcium citrate on the absorption of zinc in healthy female subjects. Eur J Clin Nutr 1994;48: 198–204.

144. Sandstrom B. Micronutrient interactions: effects on absorption and bioavailability. Br J Nutr 2001;85 (Suppl)2:S181–5.

145. Rossander-Hulten L, Brune M, Sandstrom B, Lonnerdal B, Hallberg L. Competitive inhibition of iron absorption by manganese and zinc in humans. Am J Clin Nutr 1991;54:152–6.

146. Moore LL, Bradlee ML, Singer MR, Rothman KJ, Milunsky A. Folate intake and the risk of neural tube defects: an estimation of dose-response. Epidemiology 2003;14:200–5.

147. Canfield MA, Collins JS, Botto LD, Williams LJ, Mai CT, Kirby RS, et al. Changes in the birth prevalence of selected birth defects after grain fortification with folic acid in the United States: findings from a multi-state population-based study. Birth Defects Res A Clin Mol Teratol 2005;73:679–89.

148. Allen LH. Anemia and iron deficiency: effects on pregnancy outcome. Am J Clin Nutr 2000;71:1280S–4S.

149. Scholl TO. Iron status during pregnancy: setting the stage for mother and infant. Am J Clin Nutr 2005;81:1218S–22S.

150. Pena-Rosas JP, Viteri FE. Effects of routine oral iron supplementation with or without folic acid for women during pregnancy. Cochrane Database Syst Rev 2006, Issue 3. Art No: CD004736.

151. Mahomed K, Bhutta Z, Middleton P. Zinc supplementation for improving pregnancy and infant outcome. Cochrane Database Syst Rev 2007:CD000230.

152. Rothman KJ, Moore LL, Singer MR, Nguyen US, Mannino S, Milunsky A. Teratogenicity of high vitamin A intake. N Engl J Med 1995;333:1369–73.

153. Rosa FW. Teratogenicity of isotretinoin. Lancet 1983;2:513.

154. Eckhoff C, Nau H. Vitamin A supplementation increases levels of retinoic acid compounds in human plasma: possible implications for teratogenesis. Arch Toxicol 1990;64:502–3.

155. Marshall H, Studer M, Popperl H, Aparicio S, Kuroiwa A, Brenner S, et al. A conserved retinoic acid response element required for early expression of the homeobox gene Hoxb-1. Nature 1994;370:567–71.

156. Studer M, Popperl H, Marshall H, Kuroiwa A, Krumlauf R. Role of a conserved retinoic acid response element in rhombomere restriction of Hoxb-1. Science 1994;265:1728–32.

157. de Escobar GM, Obregon MJ, del Rey FE. Maternal thyroid hormones early in pregnancy and fetal brain development. Best Pract Res Clin Endocrinol Metab 2004;18:225–48.

158. Mahomed K, Gulmezoglu AM. Maternal iodine supplements in areas of deficiency. Cochrane Database Syst Rev 2000:CD000135.

159. Berbel P, Obregon MJ, Bernal J, Escobar del Rey F, Morreale de Escobar G. Iodine supplementation during pregnancy: a public health challenge. Trends Endocrinol Metab 2007;18:338–43.

160. Sullivan KM. Iodine supplementation for pregnancy and lactation: United States and Canada: recommendations of the American Thyroid Association. Thyroid 2007;17:483–4.

The classic children's board game Candy Land was created to entertain children in a San Diego hospital polio ward by a school teacher, Eleanor Abbot, who contracted polio as an adult and found herself in the same ward. Although the polio vaccine made such units a thing of the past, the game continues today.

6
Immunizations

Mary Beth Koslap-Petraco and Barbara Hackley

Chapter Glossary

Active immunity Immunity produced by a person's own immune system that is usually permanent.

Adaptive immunity The ability of the body to make specific responses to individual antigens.

Antibody Protein molecules (immunoglobulin) produced by B lymphocytes that act to help eliminate an antigen.

Antigen A live or inactivated substance capable of producing an immune response.

Cell-mediated immune response Same as cellular immunity. Immune response does not involve antibodies and does involve activated macrophages and cytotoxic T-cell lymphocytes.

Cellular immunity The immune response that involves these cellular components of the immune system: macrophages, T-cell lymphocytes, and natural killer cells.

Humoral immunity Immune response that relies on antibodies produced by B lymphocytes.

Immune globulin Preformed antibodies derived from human sera that provide passive immunization.

Immunization The provision of vaccine to an individual in order to provoke active immunity.

Inactivated vaccine Bacteria or virus that is inactivated by heat or chemicals so it cannot replicate. The components of the organism that stimulate immunity are isolated and used for the vaccine. Inactivated vaccines cannot cause disease.

Innate immunity Immune cells that respond nonspecifically to foreign material. For example, phagocytes will attack many different microbes. Innate immunity is in contrast to adaptive immunity.

Live attenuated vaccine Bacteria or viruses that are weakened so they usually do not cause disease. Very small inoculum is used to stimulate active immunity. Live attenuated vaccines could rarely cause disease in recipients with suppressed immune systems.

Passive immunity Immune protection by antibodies that are produced by an animal or human and transferred to another human, usually by injection. Passive immunity is not permanent.

Polysaccharide vaccine Inactivated vaccine that is composed of long chains of sugar molecules from the capsule of specific bacteria.

Recombinant vaccine Antigens used in vaccines that are produced by genetic engineering technology.

Toxoid Fractional vaccine made from an inactivated toxin.

Historic Review

Vaccine-preventable diseases have been a leading cause of death and disability worldwide until very recently. Hippocrates described diphtheria among other conditions in 400 BC, yet the first vaccination was not introduced until 1796 when Edward Jenner developed the first smallpox vaccine.[1] In the past, immunizations were generally perceived to be mainly for young children, but this perception has changed. The most recently approved vaccines are human papillomavirus (HPV) vaccine and herpes zostervaccine, both for age groups other than children. In fact, today the majority of cases of many vaccine-preventable diseases such as tetanus, mumps, and meningococcal disease occur in adults.[2] Therefore, the subject of immunization is of importance for healthcare providers who care for persons of any age. This chapter reviews the vaccines commonly used in primary care. Readers interested in vaccines not covered in this chapter are referred to the United States Centers for Disease Control and Prevention for information.

Public Health Impact of Immunization Programs

Reduction of Mortality Cost–Benefit Ratio

Vaccines had a significant positive impact on public health in the 20th century (Box 6-1). A 100% decrease in small-pox and diphtheria occurred because of vaccination. Other vaccine-preventable diseases such as tetanus, paralytic polio, measles, mumps, rubella, and congenital rubella have virtually been eliminated in the United States since the inception of effective immunization programs.[3] Diseases such as measles, mumps, or pertussis can be severe and can result in social and economic as well as physical costs. If immunization programs are not maintained, the incidence of many of these diseases will rise to prevaccination levels.[1]

Disparities in Vaccination Rates

Compared to immunization rates among young children, immunization rates are considerably lower for older persons. According to Behavior Risk Factor Surveillance System data from 2005, a median of only 65.5% of persons ≥ 65 years of age received the influenza vaccine in the previous 12 months, and only 65.7% ever received

pneumococcal vaccine despite universal recommendations to do so.[1] Improvements in adult immunization rates have gradually declined. According to data from the National Health Interview Survey, after a consistent increase in vaccination rates during the 1980s and early 1990s, improvements in influenza vaccination rates for adults ≥ 65 years of age have leveled off since 1997.[3] Economic and racial disparities also exist. Low-income and minority children and adults are at greater risk for underimmunization in pockets of need.[3]

Healthy People 2010 Goals

The Centers for Disease Control and Prevention (CDC) set targets for immunizations for all populations in its Healthy People 2010 goals.[4] The immunization-specific goals are: (1) Increase the proportion of young children and adolescents who receive all the vaccines recommended for universal administration; (2) adolescents will receive the universally recommended vaccines; (3) increase routine vaccination coverage levels for adolescents to at least three doses of hepatitis B vaccine, two doses of measles-mumps-rubella (MMR) vaccine, and at least one dose of varicella vaccine; and (4) increase the proportion of adults who are vaccinated annually against influenza and ever vaccinated against pneumococcal disease.[4] Providers in all settings who see persons of all ages can work to help reach these goals.

Basics of Immunity

Immunity is the ability of the human body to tolerate the presence of material indigenous to the body (self), and to

---

Box 6-1 Gone But Not Forgotten: *Haemophilus* Influenza Type B

Vaccines have saved countless lives, and great progress has been made in eliminating vaccine-preventable diseases. The World Health Organization (WHO) has spearheaded a campaign to eradicate diseases, and smallpox, which was once the scourge of the entire world, has been eliminated. The last case occurred in 1975 in India. The world was declared smallpox free in 1980, and smallpox vaccination was subsequently eliminated.

Currently the WHO is working to eradicate poliomyelitis from the world. Good progress was being made until wars and political issues greatly slowed efforts. Polio still exists in Africa, India, and Bangladesh.

Haemophilus influenza type B (Hib) disease has been virtually eliminated in the United States due to a very successful implementation of a Hib vaccination program. Hib-related meningitis and epiglottis are virtually no longer seen in the United States. At some point in the future, perhaps we will be able to remove Hib vaccine from the recommended scheduled vaccines.

eliminate foreign (nonself) material. This discriminatory ability provides protection from infectious disease, because most microbes are identified as foreign by the immune system. Immunity to a microbe is usually indicated by the presence of **antibody** to that organism. Immunity generally is specific to a single organism or group of closely related organisms.

Variations exist in individuals' ability to mount effective responses to infection. Microbes must first penetrate the physical barriers (such as the cornified epidermis of the skin or mucus produced by the respiratory tract) and chemical barriers (such as the exquisitely maintained pH of the vaginal mucosa) developed by the human body to repel microbes. If these barriers are breached, then the immune system is triggered to respond in multiple ways to isolate invading microbes, which are called **antigens**, and render them harmless.

Invading microbes first encounter the general defense mechanisms of the immune system (also known as **innate immunity**) such as circulating phagocytes, natural killer cells, nonspecific antibodies, and complement. The complement system is responsible for marking invading microbes as foreign and weakening their cell walls to allow antibodies to penetrate and kill microbes. This initial response can help contain the invading microbes until the cellular and humoral systems are activated and can respond to specific antigens.

The ability of the body to develop specific responses to specific antigens is known as **adaptive immunity** (Figure 6-1). The humoral system is comprised chiefly of B lymphocytes,

which develop and secrete antibodies against specific antigens such as bacteria or viruses. Antibodies released by B cells generally attack free-floating extracellular antigens, a process referred to as **humoral immunity**.

The cellular system is dominated by T cells, some of which help coordinate B cells and other immune responses, and others that attack infected cells directly. T cells also fight intracellular infections such as viruses and can function either offensively or defensively. The offensive T cells do not attack the virus directly, but use their chemical weapons to eliminate the cells already infected with the offending virus. Because they have been programmed by previous exposure to virus antigen, these cytotoxic T cells sense the presence of the virus in infected cells, latch onto the infected cell, and release chemicals to kill the cell and the virus inside. The defensive T cells or helper T cells defend the body by secreting chemical signals that direct the activity of other immune system components. Helper T cells assist in inactivating cytotoxic T cells and also work closely with B cells. The work done by T cells is called **cell-mediated immune response**. Any one of these pathways can be affected by the general health or genetic makeup of an individual, which can either hinder or boost the immune response.

Immunizations affect adaptive immunity, primarily by creating memory B cells that can release large numbers of antibodies directed against specific antigens once these antigens enter the human host, although some vaccines are T-cell mediated. However, because these immune mechanisms are only one part of a complex system, vaccinations

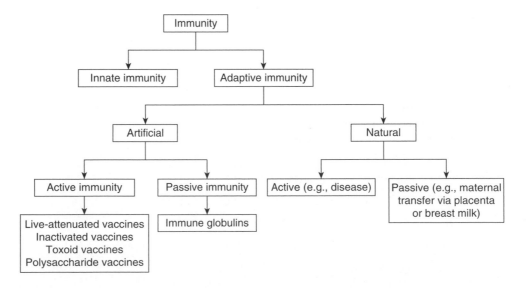

Figure 6-1 Types of immunity.

may not produce the same level or durability of protection in all individuals.

There are two basic mechanisms for developing immunity against a disease-causing pathogen: active and passive.[1,5]

Active Immunity

Active immunity is protection produced by the person's own immune system and usually is permanent. The immunity is the result of antigen stimulation of the immune system, which produces antigen-specific humoral antibody and **cellular immunity**. Vaccination therefore produces active immunity. Vaccines interact with the recipient's immune system and usually initiate an immune response similar to that stimulated by the natural infection, but vaccines do not subject the recipient to the disease and its potential complications.[3]

Passive Immunity

Passive immunity is immune protection by antibodies that are produced by an animal or human and transferred to another human, usually by injection. Passive immunity provides protection against some infections, but the protection is temporary. The most common form of passive immunity is that which an infant receives from its mother. Antibodies are transported across the placenta during the last 4 to 8 weeks of pregnancy and via breast milk to the newborn. As a result, the full-term infant generally has the same antibodies as his or her mother. Although these antibodies protect the infant more effectively from some diseases (e.g., measles, rubella, tetanus) than others (e.g., polio, pertussis), the protection tends to last for up to a year only.[3]

Vaccine Products

Immunization is the provision of the vaccine to the individual in order to provoke active immunity.[6] A vaccine is a substance that is either injected into the body or swallowed, and which mimics natural infection.[6] There are several different types of vaccines that have different pharmacologic effects and characteristics (Table 6-1), and these differences determine how the vaccine is used.

Live Attenuated Vaccines

Live attenuated vaccines are derived from wild or disease-causing viruses or bacteria. These wild viruses or bacteria are attenuated, or weakened, in a laboratory. To produce an immune response, live attenuated vaccines must replicate in a vaccinated person. A relatively small dose of the attenuated virus or bacteria is administered, which replicates in the body and creates enough of the organism to stimulate an immune response. The immune response to a live attenuated vaccine is virtually identical to that produced by a natural infection because the immune system is unable to differentiate between an infection with a weakened vaccine virus and an infection with a wild virus.[3] Table 6-2 summarizes the differences between live attenuated vaccines and inactivated vaccines.

Although live attenuated vaccines do replicate, they rarely cause the disease that occurs following exposure to the wild form of the organism. When a live attenuated vaccine does cause disease, it is usually much milder than the natural disease and is referred to as an adverse reaction.[5] There are two ways a live attenuated virus can cause severe

Table 6-1 Types of Vaccine Products

| Live Attenuated Vaccines | Inactivated Vaccines | | | | Immune Globulin |
	Other Inactivated Vaccines	Conjugated	Recombinant Vaccines	Toxoids	
Measles (M)	Acellular pertussis (given as tetanus-diphtheria-acellular pertussis, Tdap)	Pneumococcal (generally given to infants and young children)	Hepatitis B (Hep B)	Tetanus and diphtheria (Td)	VariZIG
					VZIG
Measles-mumps-rubella (MMR)	Meningococcal polysaccharide (MPSV)	Meningococcal conjugate vaccine (MCV4)			HBIG
Varicella (VAR)	Inactivated polio vaccine (IPV)				
Herpes zoster	Hepatitis A (whole cell)	*Haemophilus* influenza	Human papillomavirus (HPV)		
Rotavirus	Influenza				
Influenza (intranasal)	Pneumococcal (PPV23) polysaccharide (generally given to adults)				

VariZIG = varicella zoster immune globulin; VZIG = varicella zoster immune globulin; HBIG = hepatitis B immune globulin.

Table 6-2 Live Attenuated Vaccines and Inactivated Vaccines

Live Attenuated Vaccines	Inactivated Vaccines
Small dose of attenuated bacteria replicates and stimulates active immunity. Could rarely cause disease.	Killed bacteria or component of bacteria that stimulates active immunity. Cannot cause disease.
One dose required.	Booster doses required that stimulate B cells to make antibody that will remain in immunologic memory.
Circulating antibody can interfere with replication of the attenuated antigen and disrupt or obstruct antibody response and subsequent development of active immunity.	Circulating antibody will not affect antibody response and development of active immunity. Vaccines can be administered if antibody is present (e.g., newborn who might have transplacentally acquired antibody).
Contraindicated in pregnancy and some may be contraindicated in specific immunosuppressed states.	May be given in pregnancy.

disease. Rarely, a live attenuated vaccine may cause severe or fatal reactions as a result of uncontrolled replication (growth) of the vaccine virus. However, this phenomenon only occurs in persons with immunodeficiency (e.g., from leukemia, treatment with certain drugs such as very large doses of cortisone, or human immunodeficiency virus [HIV] infection). Secondly, a live attenuated vaccine virus could revert to its original pathogenic (disease-causing) form.[7] This has been documented to occur very rarely after use of the live oral polio vaccine (OPV).

Active immunity from a live attenuated vaccine may not develop if the antibody response in the recipient is obstructed by circulating antibody to the vaccine virus. Passively acquired antibody from any source (e.g., transplacental, transfusion) can interfere with replication of the vaccine organism and lead to poor response or no response to the vaccine, also known as vaccine failure. Currently, live attenuated viral vaccines include those for measles, mumps, rubella, vaccinia, varicella, zoster (which contains the same virus as varicella vaccine but in a much higher titer), yellow fever, rotavirus, and influenza (intranasal). Oral polio vaccine is a live viral vaccine but is no longer available in the United States. The live attenuated bacterial vaccines are bacilli Calmette-Guerin (BCG), used to immunize persons against tuberculosis and oral typhoid vaccine.[1]

Inactivated Vaccines

Inactivated vaccines are produced by growing the bacterium or virus in culture media, then inactivating it with heat and/or chemicals (usually formalin). In the case of fractional vaccines, the organism is treated further to purify only the components to be included in the vaccine (e.g., the polysaccharide capsule of pneumococcus).

Inactivated vaccines are not alive and cannot replicate. The entire dose of antigen is administered in the injection. Inactivated vaccines cannot cause disease from infection, even in an immunodeficient person. In addition, they are less affected by any preexisting circulating antibody than are live attenuated organisms. These vaccines may be administered when antibody is present in the blood (e.g., in infancy or following receipt of antibody-containing blood products).[3] Inactivated vaccines always require multiple doses. In general, the first does not produce protective immunity but primes the immune system. A protective immune response develops after the second or third dose. In contrast to live virus vaccines, in which immune response closely resembles the immune response that follows natural infection, the immune response to an inactivated vaccine primarily is humoral with little or no cellular immunity results. Antibody titers against inactivated antigens diminish over time. As a result, some inactivated vaccines may require periodic supplemental doses to increase or boost antibody titers.[3]

Currently whole-cell inactivated vaccines are limited to inactivated whole viral vaccines (polio, hepatitis A, rabies). Inactivated whole virus influenza vaccine and inactivated bacterial vaccines (pertussis, typhoid, cholera, and plague) are no longer available in the United States because alternatives have been developed or the diseases do not exist in the United States at this time. Fractional vaccines include subunits (hepatitis B, influenza, acellular pertussis, human virus) and toxoids (diphtheria, tetanus).

Toxoid Vaccines

A **toxoid** is a fractional vaccine made from a formalin-inactivated toxin.[3] Diphtheria toxoid is produced by growing toxigenic *Corynebacterium diphtheriae* in a liquid medium. The filtrate is incubated with formaldehyde to convert toxin to toxoid and is then adsorbed onto an aluminum salt. Tetanus toxoid consists of a formaldehyde-treated toxin. There are two types of toxoid available—adsorbed (aluminum salt precipitated) toxoid and fluid toxoid. Although the rates of seroconversion are about equal, the adsorbed toxoid is preferred because the antitoxin response reaches higher titers and is longer lasting than that following the fluid toxoid.[3]

Polysaccharide Vaccines

Polysaccharide vaccines are a unique type of inactivated subunit vaccine composed of long chains of sugar molecules that make up the surface capsule of certain bacteria. Pure polysaccharide vaccines are available for three diseases: pneumococcal disease, meningococcal disease, and typhoid fever.[3]

The immune response to a pure polysaccharide vaccine is typically T-cell independent, indicating that these vaccines are able to stimulate B cells to produce antibody without the assistance of helper T cells. Young children do not respond consistently to polysaccharide antigens, probably due to immaturity of the immune system.[5]

Repeat doses of polysaccharide vaccines do not cause a booster response. Antibodies induced with polysaccharide vaccines have less functional activity than those induced by protein antigens. This is because the predominant antibody produced in response to most polysaccharide vaccines is IgM, and little IgG is produced.[5]

In the late 1980s, it was discovered that these problems could be overcome through a process called conjugation, in which the polysaccharide antigen is chemically combined with a protein molecule. Conjugation changes the immune response from T-cell independent to T-cell dependent, resulting in increased immunogenicity in infants and antibody booster response to multiple doses of vaccine.[5,6] The first conjugated polysaccharide vaccine developed was for *Haemophilus* influenza (Hib). A conjugate vaccine for pneumococcal disease was licensed in 2000. A meningococcal conjugate vaccine was licensed in 2005.[3]

Recombinant Vaccines

Vaccine antigens may also be produced by genetic engineering technology. These vaccines are referred to as **recombinant vaccines**. Hepatitis B (HBV) vaccines are produced by insertion of a segment of the respective viral gene into the gene of a yeast cell. The modified yeast cell produces pure hepatitis B surface antigen or HBV capsid protein when it grows. Live typhoid vaccine (Ty21a) is *Salmonella typhi* bacteria that have been genetically modified to not cause illness. Live attenuated influenza vaccine has been engineered to replicate effectively in the mucosa of the nasopharynx but not in the lungs.[3]

Immune Globulins

Immune globulins are not vaccines but are preformed antibodies that provide passive immunization. Such preparations are considered treatment rather than prophylaxis when they are administered following exposure to the diseases they are meant to prevent. Hepatitis B immune globulin (HBIG) and varicella zoster immune globulin (VZIG) are examples of immune globulins. Table 6-3 lists the immune globulins available for treatment in the United States today.

In 2004, the only US-licensed manufacturer of VZIG (Massachusetts Public Health Biological Laboratories, Boston, Massachusetts) discontinued production. In February 2006, an investigational VZIG product, VariZIG, (Cangene Corporation, Winnipeg, Canada) became available under an investigational new drug application submitted to the FDA. This product can be requested from the sole authorized US distributor, FFF Enterprises of Temecula, California, for individuals who have been exposed to varicella and who are at increased risk for severe disease and complications.[3,8]

VariZIG

The investigational VariZIG, similar to licensed VZIG, is a purified human immune globulin preparation made from plasma containing high levels of antivaricella IgG antibodies.[8] Unlike the previous product, the investigational product is lyophilized, or freeze dried in a high vacuum. When properly reconstituted, VariZIG is approximately a 5% solution of IgG that can be administered intramuscularly. As with any product used under an investigational new drug application, persons must be informed of potential risks and benefits and must give informed consent before receiving the product.[8] Table 6-4 lists the indications for VariZIG.[9]

Hepatitis B Immune Globulin

Nonimmune individuals who are exposed to hepatitis B should be treated with hepatitis B immune globulin (HBIG) and started on the hepatitis B vaccine series as soon as possible after exposure. Exposed individuals who have completed the hepatitis B vaccine series do not require HBIG but should receive a booster dose of vaccine if they did not have postvaccination testing to confirm immunity.[9] Generic immune globulin (IG) contains low levels of anti-HBs. Because titers are relatively low, IG has no valid use in the treatment in the individuals exposed to hepatitis B virus (HBV) unless hepatitis B immune globulin is unavailable.[9]

HBIG is prepared by cold ethanol fraction of plasma from selected donors with high anti-HBs titers; it

Table 6-3 Immune Globulins* Available in the United States

Preparation	Clinical Indication
Botulinum antitoxin	Treatment of botulism. There are two antitoxins available for treatment of food-borne or wound botulism. Both are made from equine antibodies. The third antitoxin is the infant preparation (BabyBIG), which is made from human antibodies.
Cytomegalovirus immune globulin (CMV-IGIV)	Prophylaxis for organ transplant recipients. Administered intravenously.
Diphtheria toxin	Treatment of respiratory diphtheria.
Hepatitis B immune globulin (HBIG)	Prophylaxis following exposure to hepatitis B.
Immune globulin (IG)	Prophylaxis following hepatitis A or measles exposure. Used to treat rubella during first trimester of pregnancy. Also used to treat varicella if varicella zoster immune globulin is unavailable.
Immune globulin (IVIG)	Replacement for persons with antibody deficiency disorders, thrombocytopenic purpura, hypogammaglobinemia in chronic lymphocytic leukemia, neurologic disorders such as myasthenia gravis or Guillain-Barré syndrome. Administered intravenously.
Rabies immune globulin (RIG)	Treatment of rabies postexposure if unvaccinated for rabies.
Respiratory syncytial virus (RSV-IGIV or RSV-mAb)	Prevention of RSV in infants < 35 weeks' gestation or children with chronic lung disorders. RSV-IGIV is from human antibodies. RSV-mAb is from murine monoclonal antibody.
Rho(D) immune globulin (RhoGAM)	Used to prevent development of antibodies to Rh+ red cells whenever fetal cells are known or suspected of entering the maternal circulation (e.g., after spontaneous abortion or amniocentesis). Also recommended for prophylaxis at 28 weeks' gestation and following birth if the infant is Rh+.
Tetanus immune globulin	Treatment of tetanus and used postexposure for persons who are not fully vaccinated with tetanus toxoid.
Varicella zoster immune globulin	Prophylaxis for postexposure in persons who are immunocompromised or pregnant and in prenatally exposed newborns.

* Immune globulins are administered intramuscularly unless otherwise specified.

contains anti-HBs titer of at least 1:100,000, by radio immune assay. This agent is used for passive immunization to treat accidental (e.g., percutaneous, mucosal membrane) exposure, sexual contact with an individual who has hepatitis B surface antigen (HBsAg positive), perinatal exposure of a newborn, or household exposure of an infant younger than 12 months old to a primary caregiver with acute hepatitis B.

Ensuring timely completion of the postexposure vaccine series is essential in order to prevent chronic infection, particularly in the young. Of these risk groups, infants and young children exposed to hepatitis B are at highest risk of becoming chronic carriers. Neonates born to infected mothers have up to a 90% chance of becoming chronic carriers compared to 30% of exposed children less than 5 years of age and less than 5% of exposed adults.[9] Since administration of HBIG and the vaccine series is thought to be only 85% to 95% effective in preventing acute infection, prevention by immunizing susceptible individuals before exposure occurs is critical in reducing the burden of disease from hepatitis B infection.

Factors Affecting Response to Immunizations

Optimal response to a vaccine depends on multiple factors, including the nature of the vaccine and the age and immune status of the recipient. Recommendations for the age at which vaccines are administered are influenced by age-specific risks for disease, age-specific risks for

Table 6-4 Recommendations for VariZIG

Immunocompromised persons
Neonates whose mothers have signs and symptoms of varicella around the time of delivery (i.e., 5 days before to 2 days after)
Preterm infants born at 28 weeks' gestation or later who are exposed during the neonatal period and whose mothers do not have evidence of immunity
Preterm infants born earlier than 28 weeks' gestation or who weigh 1000 g or less at birth and were exposed during the neonatal period, regardless of maternal history of varicella disease or vaccination
Pregnant women

Source: Centers for Disease Control and Prevention 2006.[8]

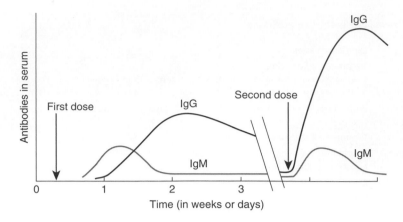

Figure 6-2 IgG and IgM following booster dose of vaccine.

complications, ability of persons of a certain age to respond to the vaccine, and potential interference with the immune response by passively transferred antibody.[10] Neonates will have received passively transferred antibodies during pregnancy and will also receive them via breast milk if the mother chooses to breastfeed.

Another factor that affects whether receipt of a vaccine will induce durable immunity is how far apart booster injections are spaced. Vaccines that require multiple boosters must not be administered earlier than recommended. Giving the booster dose too early will not increase the immune response because the immune system does not recognize the second vaccine as a separate event (Figure 6-2). Other issues that can affect a vaccine's potency and its ability to trigger durable immunity are outlined later in this chapter in the Vaccine Administration section.[11]

Vaccine Schedules

The Advisory Committee on Immunization Practices (ACIP) issues recommendations on what specific vaccines should be offered to newborns, children, adolescents, and adults. Immunization recommendations change frequently depending on the evolving epidemiology of vaccine-preventable diseases, the introduction of new vaccine products, and the supply of various agents, which can be adversely affected by production problems. Therefore, providers should regularly consult the ACIP for the most current recommended schedules. Vaccine

recommendations are released annually and are available for young children (0 to 6 years of age), older children and adolescents (ages 7 to 18 years), and adults.

Differences Between Childhood and Adolescent/ Adult Schedules

New vaccines are generally introduced first into the childhood schedule, since newborns and young children are more likely to experience complications from vaccine-preventable diseases. These vaccines are then often later recommended for use in adults because vaccine use in children pushes infection into unimmunized populations— i.e., nonimmunized adults. Consequently, adult providers must be even more vigilant than pediatric providers in screening for risk factors that could increase the likelihood that an individual could become infected with a vaccine-preventable disease and make sure to offer vaccination to these individuals (Box 6-2).

While many of the vaccines offered to adults and children are directed to the same vaccine-preventable illnesses, the specific vaccine products offered to newborns and children may need to be adapted for use in adolescents and adults. For example, tetanus, pertussis, and diphtheria vaccines have long been offered to both adults and children. Formulations offered to children include DTaP, DT, and DTP; adolescent and adult formulations include Td and Tdap.[3] While all of these products provide protection against diphtheria and tetanus, and some provide protection against pertussis, the major differences involve relative differences in dose (capitalized letter for larger doses and small letter for smaller doses) of the various components. Adult and adolescent vaccines contain reduced amounts of diphtheria toxoid but similar levels of tetanus toxoid and inactivated pertussis antigen compared with pediatric formulations[3] (Box 6-3). While dosage levels of diphtheria toxoid are higher in pediatric than adult vaccines, dosages of other vaccine products such as hepatitis B are lower.[3]

Another major difference between the various schedules is that many more products using unique combinations of vaccines are available for use in children than adults. While similar to each other, not all of them are approved for use in the exact same populations or may be used interchangeably, making the schedule very complex to administer in children. For example, there are two Tdap products available, Boostrix and Adacel. Boostrix is available for use only in individuals aged 10 to 18 years, whereas Adacel is approved for use in adolescents and adults aged 11 to 64 years.[3] To minimize potential problems, the ACIP recommends that, where possible, the same vaccine products be used for an entire series, although evidence to date suggests that using like products interchangeably does not adversely impact durable immunity.[1]

Box 6-2 A Primary Case Visit

A 60-year-old, healthy woman comes in today for a routine visit. She does not have any vaccination records and cannot remember receiving any vaccinations in years. What vaccines should you offer her?

a. Td, MMR, and varicella vaccine

b. Pneumococcal and influenza if her visit is in the fall, or if winter, Td

c. Tdap and influenza if her visit is in the fall or winter, and zoster vaccine

d. Nothing is needed since she received her complete childhood and adolescent series

Answer: c. Tdap is needed because she is overdue for her 10-year tetanus booster and because pertussis control is currently needed. ACIP recommends that Tdap replace the next Td booster dose in adults. Subsequent booster doses should be given with Td.

Influenza is recommended for all individuals older than 50 years of age since older adults are more likely to experience complications with influenza infection than younger adults. Even at younger ages, influenza vaccination can be offered to all individuals who desire to reduce their risk of becoming infected with influenza.

Zoster is recommended for the prevention of shingles and should be offered as a one-time vaccine to all individuals 60 years of age or older.

MMR and varicella are unnecessary because she is old enough to have been born at a time when these diseases were epidemic.

Pneumococcal vaccines are recommended for use starting at age 65 in healthy adults. Therefore it is too early to give this vaccine.

Box 6-3 An Annual Gynecology Visit

A 16-year-old adolescent comes to your office for a routine visit. She is taking oral contraceptives and has been in a monogamous relationship for a year. You ask to see her immunization record and it reveals the adolescent has completed her five-dose DTaP series at age 6 years, has had four doses of inactivated polio vaccine, two MMRs, two VARs, and three Hep B vaccines. What vaccines are recommended for her today?

a. Tdap

b. Meningococcal vaccine

c. HPV vaccine

d. All of the above

Answer: d. This adolescent has not had any immunizations since she was 6 years of age. A Tdap booster is indicated for all adolescents at 11 years of age with catch-up if the booster was not previously administered. Meningococcal vaccine is also indicated for all 11- to 12-year-olds with catch-up indicated. While the optimum time to give HPV vaccine is before sexual debut, it is still useful to give it to older adolescents and young women. Even if she is infected with one of the strains of HPV contained in the vaccine, the vaccine will protect her against the other strains for which it is indicated.

Adult and Adolescent Vaccines

Tetanus-Diphtheria (Td) Vaccine

Infection

The tetanus-diphtheria (Td) vaccine prevents tetanus (also referred to as lockjaw) and diphtheria. The typical clinical manifestations of tetanus are caused when tetanus toxin interferes with release of neurotransmitters blocking inhibitor impulses, which leads to unopposed muscular contraction and spasm. Seizures may occur, and the autonomic nervous system also can be affected.[3,12] The typical clinical manifestation of diphtheria is local tissue destruction and membrane formation that can involve any mucous membrane. The diphtheria toxin also is responsible for the major complication of myocarditis and neuritis and can cause thrombocytopenia and proteinuria.

Vaccine

Tetanus toxoid is combined with diphtheria toxoid to produce Td vaccine. Toxoids are formaldehyde-treated toxins. This process renders the toxin unable to cause illness, but it allows the vaccine the ability to invoke immunity.[3,12] This vaccine is indicated for persons 7 years of age and older. Booster doses are indicated every 10 years, but they may be administered earlier if the risk of tetanus is high, as might be the case after an injury.[3] Revaccination with tetanus-containing vaccine is indicated if the individual has not received a recent 10-year booster in the case of clean wounds or a booster within 5 years in the case of dirty wounds. Adults needing a booster injection who have never received a pertussis-containing vaccine should be vaccinated with Tdap. Clean minor wounds require at most receipt of Td or Tdap; however, dirty wounds may also require receipt of tetanus immunoglobulin.[13]

Local adverse reactions (e.g., erythema, induration, pain at the injection site) are common but are usually self-limiting and require no therapy. A nodule of absorbed products may be palpable at the injection site for several weeks and usually resolves without difficulty, although a rare abscess at the injection site has been reported. Fever and other systemic symptoms are not common.[3,12] See Appendices A and B for dosing schedule, contraindications, and precautions.

Exaggerated local (arthus-like) reactions are occasionally reported following receipt of a diphtheria- or tetanus-containing vaccine. An arthus-like reaction usually presents as extensive painful swelling. These reactions generally begin from 2 to 8 hours after injections and are reported most often in adults, particularly those who have received frequent doses of diphtheria or tetanus toxoid.[13] Severe systemic reactions such as generalized urticaria (hives), anaphylaxis, or neurologic complications have been reported after receipt of tetanus toxoid.[3] A few cases of peripheral neuropathy and Guillain-Barré syndrome have been reported following tetanus toxoid administration.[1] Following a recent review, the Institute of Medicine concluded that the available evidence favors a causal relationship between tetanus toxoid and both brachial neuritis and Guillain-Barré syndrome, although these reactions are very rare.[14]

Pertussis-Containing Vaccines (Tdap)

Infection

During the past two decades, pertussis is the only vaccine-preventable disease whose incidence has risen in the United States.[2] The reasons for the increase are not clear. Reported cases in adolescents have increased dramatically.[14] Adults have accounted for an increasing proportion of cases. Better recognition and diagnosis of pertussis in older age groups probably contributed to this increase of reported cases among adolescents and adults. Pertussis is characterized by bursts or paroxysms of numerous, rapid coughs, apparently due to difficulty expelling thick mucus from the tracheobronchial tree. Pertussis infection in adults and adolescents may be asymptomatic or present as illness ranging from a mild cough illness to classic pertussis with persistent cough (i.e., lasting more than 7 days). Inspiratory whoop is common but not universal in infants and young children, and not usually observed in adolescents and adults.[15] A study based on pertussis surveillance data from four states reported that the mother was the source of infection in 32% of infants for whom a source could be found.[16]

Vaccine

Because of the increased incidence of pertussis in adolescent and adult populations, a one-time booster dose of Tdap was recommended by the CDC for all adults beginning in 2006.[1] Td is currently recommended as the preferred product for use in subsequent booster doses, although if elevated levels of pertussis persist, authorities may recommend additional doses of pertussis-containing vaccines to adults.

Tdap has also replaced Td as the recommended booster dose for children ages 11–12 years. Adolescents who have not been immunized with Tdap should receive a catch-up dose. This catch-up dose of Tdap can be administered as early as 5 years after receipt of Td although repeated and early administration of tetanus-containing vaccines does seem to increase the risk of local and systemic reactions. Even earlier administration than every 5 years is acceptable when there is risk of pertussis in the community. See Appendices A and B for dosing schedule, contraindications, and precautions.

Hepatitis B Vaccine

Infection

Hepatitis B is characterized by an insidious onset of malaise, anorexia, nausea, vomiting, right upper quadrant abdominal pain, fever, headache, myalgia, skin rashes, arthralgia and arthritis, and dark urine beginning 1–2 days before the onset of jaundice. Clinical signs and symptoms occur more often in adults than in infants or children, who usually have an asymptomatic acute course. However, 50% of adults who have acute infections are asymptomatic.[3, 17]

Hepatitis B virus (HBV) is the most common known cause of chronic viremia, with more than 350 million chronically infected persons estimated worldwide.[3] HBV infection is an established cause of acute and chronic hepatitis and cirrhosis. It is the cause of up to 80% of hepatocellular carcinomas, and it is second only to tobacco among know human carcinogens.[3]

The key route of transmission of hepatitis B is via contamination of mucosal surfaces with infective serum or plasma. Fecal–oral transmission does not appear to occur. In the United States, the most important route of transmission is via sexual contact, either heterosexual or homosexual, with an infected person. Direct percutaneous inoculation of HBV by needles during injection drug use is the second most common mode of transmission. Transmission of HBV may also occur by other percutaneous exposure, including tattooing, ear piercing, and acupuncture, as well as needle sticks or other injuries from sharp instruments sustained by medical personnel. These exposures account for only a small proportion of reported cases in the United States. Breaks in the skin without overt needle puncture, such as fresh cutaneous scratches, abrasions, burns, or other lesions may also serve as routes for entry.[3]

Transmission may also occur during mouth pipetting, eye splashes, or other direct contact with mucous membranes of the eyes or mouth. Transfer of infective material to skin lesions or mucous membranes via inanimate environmental surfaces may occur by touching surfaces of various types of hospital equipment. Contamination of mucosal surfaces with infective secretions other than serum or plasma could occur with contact involving semen.[3] While most HBV infections in adults result in complete recovery, fulminant hepatitis occurs in about 1–2% of acutely infected persons.[17]

Because hepatitis B infection is common in certain subgroups in the United States and is epidemic in many parts of the world, it may be that an individual already has been infected and is not in need of vaccination. In this case, serologic testing can help distinguish whether an individual is acutely or chronically infected or is susceptible and could benefit from vaccination. Lab indices and their clinical interpretation are listed in Table 6-5.

Table 6-5 Interpretation of Hepatitis B Serologic Tests

Tests	Results	Interpretation
HBsAg	Negative	Susceptible
anti-HBc	Negative	
anti-HBs	Negative	
HBsAg	Negative	Immune due to vaccination
anti-HBc	Negative	
anti-HBs	Positive with ≥ 10 mIU/mL*	
HBsAg	Negative	Immune due to natural infection
anti-HBc	Positive	
anti-HBs	Positive	
HBsAg	Positive	Acutely infected
anti-HBc	Positive	
IgM anti-HBc	Positive	
anti-HBs	Negative	
HBsAg	Positive	Chronically infected
anti-HBc	Positive	
IgM anti-HBc	Negative	
anti-HBs	Negative	
HBsAg	Negative	Four interpretations possible†
anti-HBc	Positive	
anti-HBs	Negative	

* Postvaccination testing, when it is recommended, should be performed 1–2 months following dose No. 3.
† 1. May be recovering from acute HBV infection.
2. May be distantly immune and the test is not sensitive enough to detect a very low level of anti-HBs in serum.
3. May be susceptible with a false positive anti-HBc.
4. May be chronically infected and have an undetectable level of HBsAg present in the serum.
Source: Atkinson et al. 2007.[3]

Serologic Tests

Perinatal transmission from the mother to infant at birth is very efficient. If the mother is positive for both HBsAg (hepatitis B surface antigen) and HBeAg (antigen contained in the core of HBV and indicates high infectivity), 70–90% of infants will become infected in the absence of postexposure prophylaxis.[1,17] The risk of perinatal transmission is about 10% if the mother is positive only for HBsAg.[1,17] As many as 90% of infants who become infected will develop a chronic infection.[3] Postexposure prophylaxis requires provision of hepatitis B immunoglobulin and initiation of the three-dose vaccine series immediately after birth. Infants who weigh less than 2000 gm at birth who are born to HBsAg-positive mothers have a decreased immune response to vaccine and a high risk of exposure during birth; these infants will need an additional dose of vaccine (for a total of 4 doses) starting at 1 month of age.[18] Adherence to the recommended follow-up vaccine series is critical in preventing neonatal infection.

Because not all women are tested for hepatitis B before the birth of the infant and some women may have become acutely infected after the last test was taken, a mother's status may not be known with accuracy when she gives birth. Therefore, hepatitis B vaccination for all infants soon after birth and before hospital discharge is the preferred strategy recommended by the ACIP, even for those infants born to women who were tested and found to be HBsAg negative. Infants born to women whose status is unknown should receive hepatitis B vaccinations within 12 hours of birth and HBIG no later than 7 days after birth if the mother tests positive. Because preterm infants' immune systems respond less robustly than term infants, infants weighing less than 2000 gm who are born to women whose HBsAg status is unknown should also receive HBIG.[18]

Vaccine

Hepatitis B vaccine is produced by two manufacturers, GlaxoSmithKline (Engerix-B) and Merck (Recombivax HB). Both vaccines are available in both pediatric and adult formulations. The recommended dose of vaccine differs depending on the age of the recipient and type of vaccine. See Table 6-6 for dosing schedule. Although the antigen content of the vaccines differs, vaccines made by different manufacturers are interchangeable with one exception. Only the Merck vaccine is approved for the alternate two-dose schedule for adolescents age 11–15 years. Providers must always follow the manufacturer's dosage recommendations. Both vaccines are now available as thimerosal-free preparations.[3]

Table 6-6　Recommended Doses of Currently Approved Formulations of Hepatitis B Vaccine by Age Group and Vaccine Type

| | Single-Antigen Vaccine | | | | Combination Vaccine | | | | | |
| | Recombivax HB | | Engerix-B | | Comvax | | Pediarix | | Twinrix | |
Age Group	Dose (mcg)*	Volume (mL)	Dose (mcg)*	Volume (mL)	Dose (mcg)*	Volume (mL)	Dose (mcg)*	Volume (mL)	Dose (mcg)*	Volume (mL)
Infants (< 1 yr)	5	0.5	10	0.5	5	0.5	0	0.5	N/A**	N/A
Children (1–10 yrs)	5	0.5	10	0.5	5	0.5	10	0.5	N/A	N/A
Adolescents 11–15 yrs	10*	1.0	N/A	N/A	N/A	N/A	N/A	N/A	N/A	N/A
11–19 yrs	5	0.5	10	0.5	N/A	N/A	N/A	N/A	N/A	N/A
Adults (≥ 20 yrs)	10	1.0	20	1.0	N/A	N/A	N/A	N/A	20	1.0
Hemodialysis patients and other immunocompromised persons										
< 20 yrs§	5	0.5	10	0.5	N/A	N/A	N/A	N/A	N/A	N/A
≥ 20 yrs	40¶	1.0	40‡	2.0	N/A	N/A	N/A	N/A	N/A	N/A

* Recombinant hepatitis B surface antigen protein dose.
† Adult formulation administered on a two-dose schedule.
§ Higher doses might be more immunogenic, but no specific recommendations have been made.
¶ Dialysis formulation administered on a three-dose schedule at age 0, 1, and 6 months.
‡ Two 1.0 mL doses administered at one site, on a four-dose schedule at age 0, 1, 2, and 6 months.
** Not applicable.
Source: Atkinson et al. 2007.[3]

After three intramuscular doses of hepatitis B vaccine, more than 90% of healthy adults develop adequate antibody responses. Correct administration is also the key to durable immunity. The deltoid muscle is the recommended site for hepatitis B vaccination in adults. Immunogenicity of vaccine is lower when injections are given in the gluteus. However, there is an age-specific decline in immunogenicity. After age 40 years, approximately 90% of recipients respond to a three-dose series, and by 60 years, only 75% of persons vaccinated develop protective antibody titers.[3]

The vaccine is 80–100% effective in preventing infection or clinical hepatitis in those who receive the complete course of vaccine. Larger vaccine doses (2 to 4 times the normal adult dose) or an increased number of doses are required to induce protective antibody in a high proportion of hemodialysis patients and may also be necessary in other immunocompromised persons.[3,9]

The most common adverse reaction following hepatitis B vaccine is pain at the site of injection. Mild systemic complaints such as fatigue, headache, and irritability have been reported. Fever has been reported in 1% of adults, but serious systemic adverse reactions and allergic reactions are rarely reported following hepatitis B vaccine. No evidence has been reported that administration of hepatitis

B vaccine at or shortly after birth increases the number of febrile episodes, sepsis evaluations, or allergic or neurologic events in the newborn period.

Hepatitis B vaccine has been suggested to cause or exacerbate multiple sclerosis (MS). A 2004 retrospective study in a British population found a slight increase in risk of MS among hepatitis B vaccine recipients.[19] However, earlier large population-based studies have shown no association between receipt of hepatitis B vaccine and either the development of MS or exacerbation of the course of MS in persons already diagnosed with disease.[20,21]

Occupational Exposure to Hepatitis B

Occupational exposure to hepatitis B deserves special mention. Table 6-7 presents the recommended doses of hepatitis B vaccine for persons who are exposed to hepatitis B through occupational contact.

Hepatitis A Vaccine

Infection

Hepatitis A virus (HAV) is acquired through fecal-oral transmission and replicates in the liver. The symptoms of

---

Table 6-7 Recommended Postexposure Prophylaxis for Occupational Exposure to Hepatitis B Virus

Vaccination and Antibody Response of Exposed Workers*	Treatment		
	Source HBsAg[†] Positive	Source HBsAg[†] Negative	Source Unknown or Not Available for Testing
Unvaccinated	HBIG[‡] × 1 and initiate HB vaccine series	Initiate HB vaccine series	Initiate HB vaccine series
Previously Vaccinated			
Known responder[§]	No treatment	No treatment	No treatment
Known nonresponder[‖]	HBIG × 1 and initiate revaccination or HBIG × 2[¶]	No treatment	If known high-risk source, treat as if source were HBsAg positive
Antibody response unknown	Test exposed person for anti-HBs[#] — If adequate,[§] no treatment is necessary — If inadequate,[‖] administer HBIG × 1 and vaccine booster	No treatment	Test exposed person for anti-HBs[#] — If adequate,[§] no treatment is necessary — If inadequate,[‖] administer vaccine booster and recheck titer in 1–2 months

* Persons who have previously been infected with HBV are immune to reinfection and do not require postexposure prophylaxis.
[†] Hepatitis B surface antigen.
[‡] Hepatitis B immune globulin; dose is 0.06 mL/kg administered intramuscularly.
[§] A responder is a person with adequate levels of serum antibody to HBsAg (i.e., anti-HBs ≥ 10 mIU/mL).
[‖] A nonresponder is a person with inadequate response to vaccination (i.e., serum anti-HBs < 10 mIU/mL).
[¶] The option of giving one dose of HBIG and reinitiating the vaccine series is preferred for nonresponders who have not completed a second three-dose vaccine series. For persons who previously completed a second vaccine series but failed to respond, two doses of HBIG are preferred.
[#] Antibody to HBsAg.
Source: Centers for Disease Control and Prevention 2001[21]; Atkinson et al. 2007.[3]

acute HAV are indistinguishable from that of other types of acute viral hepatitis. The illness typically has an abrupt onset of fever, malaise, anorexia, nausea, abdominal pain, dark urine, and jaundice. Clinical illness usually does not last longer than 2 months, although 10–15% of persons have prolonged or relapsing signs and symptoms for up to 6 months. Virus may be excreted during a relapse.[3,22]

The likelihood of symptomatic illness from HAV infection is directly related to age. In children younger that 6 years of age, most (70%) infections are asymptomatic. In older children and adults, infection is usually symptomatic, with jaundice occurring in more than 70% of patients. HAV infection rarely produces fulminant hepatitis A.

Groups at increased risk for hepatitis A infection include international travelers, men who have sex with men, and persons who use illegal drugs. Food handlers are not at increased risk for hepatitis A because of their occupation, but are noteworthy because of their critical role in common-source food-borne HAV transmission.[3,22]

Children play an important role in HAV transmission. Children generally have asymptomatic or unrecognized illnesses, so they may serve as a source of infection particularly for household or other close contacts. Historically, children 2–18 years of age have had the highest rates of hepatitis A. Since 2002, rates among children have declined due to immunization, and the incidence of hepatitis A is now similar in all age groups.[23]

Vaccine

Vaccination against hepatitis A has been incorporated into the routine childhood schedule, but is generally offered only to high-risk adults. Two preparations of hepatitis A vaccine currently are licensed in the United States—Havrix, manufactured by GlaxoSmithKline, and Vaqta, manufactured by Merck. Both preparations are available in pediatric and adult formulations. A single primary dose is followed in 6 months by the booster dose. Limited data indicate that the vaccines from different manufacturers are interchangeable. For both vaccines, the booster dose given should be based on the person's age at the time of the booster dose, not the age when the first dose was given.[23] See Appendices A and B for dosing schedule, contraindications, and precautions.

The most commonly reported adverse reaction following vaccination is a local reaction at the site of injection. Injection site pain, erythema, or swelling is reported by 20–50% of recipients. These symptoms are generally mild and self-limited. Mild systemic complaints (e.g., malaise, fatigue, low-grade fever) are reported by fewer than 10% of recipients. No serious adverse reactions have been reported.[3]

Combination Hepatitis A and Hepatitis B Vaccine

Combination hepatitis A and hepatitis B vaccine (TwinRix) contains about half the adult dose of hepatitis A vaccine and the usual adult dose of hepatitis B vaccine. By giving a reduced-dose of hepatitis A vaccine, this formulation can be used in place of the three-dose single-agent hepatitis B vaccine schedule and provides good protection against both diseases. TwinRix is approved for persons 18 years of age and older.[23] Single-antigen hepatitis A vaccine may be used to complete a series begun with TwinRix and vice versa. The vaccine schedule for single TwinRix is presented in Figure 6-3.

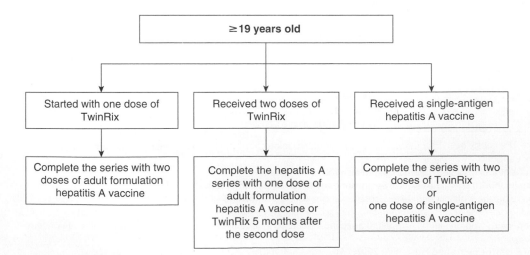

Figure 6-3 Hepatitis: A vaccine schedule using TwinRix.

Measles-Mumps-Rubella Vaccine

Infection

Measles (rubeola) is a viral illness characterized by a generalized maculopapular rash lasting 3 days or longer, with fever (101°F [38.3°C] or higher), which is accompanied by cough, coryza, and/or conjunctivitis.[24] Approximately 30% of persons with reported measles cases have one or more complications of varying severity.[24] Complications of measles are more common among children < 5 years of age and adults ≥ 20 years of age.[24] Common manifestations include diarrhea, otitis media (almost exclusively in children), and pneumonia. Acute encephalitis occurs in approximately 0.1% of cases. The risk of death is approximately 0.2% and is higher among young children and adults. Measles illness during pregnancy results in a higher risk of premature labor, spontaneous abortion, and low-birth-weight infants. For an immunocompromised person, measles may be severe and prolonged.[3, 24]

Mumps is a viral illness that is characterized by nonspecific, prodromal symptoms, which include myalgia, anorexia, malaise, headache, and low-grade fever. Parotitis is the most common manifestation and occurs in 30–40% of infected persons.[3] Symptomatic meningitis occurs in up to 15% of infected individuals and resolves without sequela. Adults are at higher risk for this complication than are children, and boys are more commonly affected than girls. Oophoritis occurs in 5% of postpubertal females.[3]

Rubella (German measles) symptoms are often mild, and up to 50% of infections are subclinical.[25] In children, rash is usually the first manifestation and a prodrome is rare. In older children and adults, there is often a 1- to 5-day prodrome with low-grade fever, malaise, lymphadenopathy, and upper respiratory symptoms preceding the rash. The maculopapular rash usually occurs initially on the face and then progresses from head to foot.[3]

Complications are not common but occur more frequently in adults compared to children. Arthralgia or arthritis occurs in 70% of the adult women who contact rubella, but it is rare in children.[3]

Prevention of congenital rubella syndrome is the main objective of rubella vaccination programs in the United States. Infection with rubella virus can be disastrous for a fetus in early gestation.[25] The virus can affect all organs and cause a variety of spontaneous defects. Infection may lead to fetal death, spontaneous abortion, or premature delivery. Of infants infected in the first trimester, 85% will be affected following birth. Deafness is the most common and is often the only manifestation. Eye defects, including cataracts, glaucoma, retinopathy, and microphthalmia may occur; cardiac defects such as patent ductus arteriosus, ventricular septal defect, pulmonic stenosis, and coarctation of the aorta are possible. Neurologic abnormalities, including microcephaly and mental retardation, and other abnormalities, such as thrombocytopenia with purpura, may occur.[25]

Vaccine

Measles vaccine, a live attenuated vaccine, is available most commonly in combination with mumps and rubella vaccines (MMR). Measles vaccine is prepared in chick embryo fibroblast tissue culture, as is the combination MMR vaccine. MMR is supplied as a lyophilized (freeze-dried) powder and is reconstituted with sterile, preservative-free water. The vaccine contains a small amount of human albumin, neomycin, sorbitol, and gelatin. Measles vaccine is available as a single antigen in limited quantities. All persons born during or after 1957 who do not have a medical contraindication should receive at least one dose of MMR vaccine unless they have documentation of vaccination with at least one dose of measles-, mumps-, and rubella-containing vaccine or other acceptable evidence of immunity such as positive titers to those three diseases. With the exception of women who might become pregnant and persons who work in medical facilities, birth before 1957 generally can be considered acceptable evidence of immunity to measles, mumps, and rubella.[26]

Adverse reactions following measles vaccine (except allergic reactions) represent replication of measles vaccine virus with subsequent mild illness. These events occur 5–12 days postvaccination and only in persons who are susceptible to infection. No evidence exists of increased risk of adverse reactions following MMR vaccination in persons who are already immune to the diseases.[26]

Fever is the most common adverse reaction following MMR vaccination. Most persons with fever following MMR vaccination are otherwise asymptomatic. MMR vaccine may cause a transient rash. Rashes, usually appearing 7–10 days after MMR or measles vaccination, have been reported in approximately 5% of cases. Rarely, MMR vaccine may cause thrombocytopenia (low platelet count) within 2 months after vaccination. The clinical course of these cases was usually transient and benign, although hemorrhage occurred rarely. Transient lymphadenopathy sometimes occurs following receipt of MMR or other rubella-containing vaccine, and parotitis has been reported rarely following receipt of MMR or other mumps-containing vaccine. Arthralgias and other joint symptoms are reported in up to 25% of susceptible adult women given MMR vaccine. This adverse reaction is associated with the rubella component. Allergic reactions are rare, and if they do occur, they generally are minor.[26]

MMR may transiently suppress the response to a tuberculin skin test in a person infected with tuberculosis. Tuberculin skin testing is not a prerequisite for vaccination with MMR vaccine. Tuberculin skin testing has no effect of the response to MMR vaccination. The tuberculin skin test and MMR vaccine can be administered at the same visit. If MMR has been administered recently, tuberculin skin testing screening should be delayed at least 4 weeks after vaccination.[3]

Contraindications

Women known to be pregnant should not receive MMR vaccine. Individuals with severe immunosuppression should also not receive the MMR vaccine. Very rarely, death from vaccine-acquired virus has been reported in severely immunocompromised recipients. Further details on immunizations in special populations can be found later in the chapter.

Inactivated Polio Vaccine (IPV)

Infection

The response to polio infection is highly variable. Up to 95% of all persons with polio infections are asymptomatic. Symptoms can vary from upper respiratory symptoms to gastrointestinal symptoms to nonparalytic aseptic meningitis. Fewer than 1% of all persons with polio infections develop flaccid paralysis. Many persons with paralytic poliomyelitis recover completely, and, in most, muscle function returns to some degree.[3]

Vaccine

Jonas Salk introduced the first inactivated polio vaccine (IPV) in 1955. Several years later Albert Sabin introduced the live attenuated oral polio vaccine (OPV). Since 1980 the only indigenous polio in the United States was vaccine acquired, with eight to nine cases occurring annually. Since the Western Hemisphere was declared polio free in 1991, this risk was no longer acceptable. In 2000, the CDC and ACIP changed the immunization schedule and opted for an IPV-only schedule, and use of the OPV was discontinued.[27] The inactivated IPV in current use in the United States is an enhanced-potency IPV that was licensed in 1987.[27]

Routine vaccination of adults (18 years of age and older) who reside in the United States is not necessary or recommended because most adults already received a complete vaccine series in childhood and are immune. In addition, wild polio has been eliminated from the United States, and so adults have a very small risk of exposure to wild poliovirus. Adults who are at risk of infection include travelers to epidemic areas (currently limited to South Asia, the eastern Mediterranean, and Africa), some laboratory workers, and healthcare personnel in close contact with individuals who may be excreting wild polioviruses. For those at risk, a three-dose series is recommended for those who have not been previously immunized.[3,27] See Appendices A and B for dosing schedule, contraindications, and precautions.

Side effects to IPV are minor local reactions (pain, redness). No serious adverse reactions to IPV have been documented.[27]

Pneumococcal Vaccines (PPV-23, PCV-7)

Infection

The major clinical syndromes of pneumococcal disease are pneumonia, bacteremia, and meningitis. Pneumococcal pneumonia is the most common clinical presentation. The overall incidence of invasive pneumococcal disease is highest among young children, especially those 2 years of age and younger. The next highest incidence is among those 65 years of age and older.[28] Infection with *Streptococcus pneumoniae* bacteria is thought to cause up to 30% of all cases of community-acquired pneumonia and 13–19% of all cases of bacterial meningitis in adults in the United States.[3] It is also a common cause of acute otitis media and pneumonia in children.

Vaccine

There are two vaccines available for use in the United States: the pneumococcal conjugate vaccine (PCV-7) and the pneumococcal polysaccharide vaccine 23-valent (PPV-23). While the PPV-23 vaccine covers more pneumococcal strains than the PCV-7 vaccine (23 compared to 7), it induces a weaker immune response in young children than in adults. Consequently, the PCV-7 vaccine is the only vaccine approved for use in children less than 2 years of age, whereas the PPV-23 vaccine is the preferred product in older children and adults because of its broader coverage and stronger immunogenicity. All adults 65 years of age, regardless of risk status, should be offered vaccination with PPV-23. Individuals aged 2 to 64 years of age with certain high-risk conditions should also be offered vaccination with PPV-23. PCV-7 has been incorporated into the routine childhood schedule and is given in a four-dose series starting at 2 months of age.[3]

The adult series consists of one dose. Revaccination after completion of the primary vaccination is generally not needed except in those at highest risk of complications from pneumococcal infection. See Appendices A and B for dosing recommendations, contraindications, and precautions.

Since the introduction of PCV-7, the incidence of pneumococcal disease in children has declined by over 80%. Rates in the elderly also have decreased. This finding may indicate that vaccination of young children has decreased transmission to elderly household contacts.

The most common adverse reactions following PPV-23 are local reactions such as pain, swelling, or erythema at the site of injection. These reactions usually persist for less than 48 hours. Local reactions are reported more frequently following a second dose of PPV-23 than following the first dose. Moderate systemic reactions such as fever and myalgia are not common. A transient increase in HIV replication has been reported following PPV-23. No clinical or immunologic deterioration has been reported in these persons.[28]

Influenza Vaccines (TIV, LAIV)

Infection

Influenza is the most common vaccine-preventable disease in the United States. The risk for complications and hospitalizations from influenza are higher among persons ≥ 65 years of age, young children, and persons of any age with certain underlying medical conditions. Classic influenza disease is characterized by the abrupt onset of fever, myalgia, sore throat, nonproductive cough, and headache.[3] The most common complication associated with influenza infection is a secondary bacterial pneumonia.

Because the influenza virus is constantly evolving, it is necessary to reformulate the vaccine each year. When there is a good match between circulating and vaccine serotypes, the influenza vaccine is estimated to be 70–90% effective in preventing infection in healthy recipients < 65 years of age. Influenza activity peaks in temperate areas between late December and early March. Vaccination is most effective when it precedes exposure. It should be offered annually, beginning in September during routine health visits. The optimal time for vaccination efforts is usually during October and November, but vaccination can be offered throughout the flu season.

Vaccines

Two types of influenza vaccine are available in the United States. These include trivalent inactivated influenza vaccine (TIV) and live attenuated influenza vaccine (LAIV). Both TIV and LAIV contain the same three influenza viruses in their makeup, which include specific strains of type A (H1N1), type A (H3N2), and type B.[29] TIV has been available since the 1940s and is administered by intramuscular route. LAIV was approved for use in the United States in 2003 and is administered by the intranasal route. Both TIV and LAIV are available in adult and pediatric formulations.[29]

LAIV is approved for healthy persons 2–49 years of age who have no underlying medical conditions. Persons in this group, including most persons in close contact with individuals in high-risk groups and those wishing to reduce their risk of influenza, now have the option of choosing either inactivated vaccine or LAIV. Viral shredding after receipt of LAIV-vaccine virus has been documented in only one case. But because of this concern, LAIV should not be given to persons who are household contacts of extremely high-risk individuals. Specific contraindications to the use of LAIV are listed in Table 6-8.[29] Until additional data are available, persons at high risk for complications from influenza should also not receive LAIV. These persons should continue to receive inactivated influenza vaccine.[29] TIV can be given to all adults, both low and high risk. See Appendices A and B for dosing schedule, contraindications, and precautions.

Table 6-8 Contraindications to Administration of Influenza Vaccine

Condition	Contraindications
Severe allergy (anaphylaxis) to egg or a prior dose of vaccine	LAIV and TIV
Moderate or severe acute illness	LAIV and TIV
Immunosuppression from any cause	LAIV
Pregnant women	LAIV
6 months of age	TIV
Children and adolescents receiving long-term aspirin therapy or other salicylates	LAIV
Children < age 2 and persons > age 50	LAIV
Chronic medical condition such as diabetes, renal dysfunction, hemoglobinopathy, or known or suspected immunosuppressed state	LAIV
History of Guillain-Barré syndrome	LAIV and TIV
Persons whose medical condition places them at high risk for complications of influenza	LAIV
Moderate or severe febrile illness	LAIV and TIV

Source: CDC 2008.[29]

Inactivated vaccines do not interfere with the immune response to live vaccines. Inactivated vaccines, such as tetanus and diphtheria toxoids, can be administered either simultaneously or at any time before or after LAIV. Other live vaccines can be administered on the same day as LAIV. Live vaccines not administered on the same day should be administered at least 4 weeks apart when possible.[3,29]

Reactions to Vaccine

Local reactions are the most common adverse reactions following vaccination with TIV. Local reactions include soreness, erythema, and indurations at the site of injection. These reactions are transient, generally lasting 1 to 2 days. Local reactions are reported in 15–20% of persons who receive the vaccine. Nonspecific systemic symptoms, including fever, chills, malaise, and myalgia, are reported in fewer than 1% of TIV recipients. These symptoms most often occur in those with no previous exposure to the viral antigen in the vaccine, develop within 6–12 hours of TIV vaccination, and last 1–2 days. Reports indicate that these symptoms are no more common than in persons given a placebo injection.

Rarely, immediate hypersensitivity, presumably allergic reactions (e.g., hives, angioedema, allergic asthma, systemic anaphylaxis) occur after vaccination with TIV. These reactions probably result from hypersensitivity to a vaccine component. The majority are most likely related to residual egg protein. Although current influenza vaccines contain only a small quantity of egg protein, this protein may induce immediate allergic reactions in persons with severe egg allergy. Persons who have developed hives, had swelling of the lips or tongue, or have experienced acute respiratory distress or collapse after eating eggs should not receive either TIV or LAIV vaccines in the primary care setting. These individuals need further evaluation by an allergist if vaccine receipt is required.[29]

Among healthy adults, a significantly increased rate of cough, runny nose, nasal congestion, sore throat, and chills was reported among LAIV vaccine recipients. These symptoms were reported in 10–40% of vaccine recipients. There was no increase in the occurrence of fever among vaccine recipients. No serious adverse reactions have been identified in LAIV recipients, either children or adults. No instances of Guillain-Barré syndrome have been reported in either children or adults. Few data are available concerning the safety of LAIV among persons at high risk for development of complications of influenza, such as immunosuppressed persons or those with chronic pulmonary or cardiac disease.

Meningococcal Vaccine

Infection

Meningitis is the most common presentation of invasive meningococcal disease. Risk factors for the development of meningococcal disease include deficiencies in the terminal common complement pathway and functional or anatomic asplenia. Persons with HIV infection are probably at increased risk for meningococcal disease. Certain genetic factors (such as polymorphisms in the genes for mannose-binding lectin and tumor necrosis factor) may also be risk factors. Family members of an infected person are at increased risk for meningococcal disease. Three to four percent of households with a case of meningitis reported a secondary case.[3] Antecedent upper respiratory tract infection and both active and passive smoking also are associated with increased risk.[30]

One of the most consistently reported risks for meningitis is overcrowding. In the United States, African Americans and persons of low socioeconomic status have been consistently at higher risk; however, race and low socioeconomic status are likely markers for differences in factors such as household crowding rather than inherent risk factors.[30] During outbreaks, bar or nightclub patronage and alcohol use have also been associated with higher risk for disease. Studies have shown that college freshmen living in dormitories are at modestly increased risk of meningococcal disease.[30] However, US college students other than freshmen living in dormitories are not at higher risk for meningococcal disease than other persons of similar age.[31]

Vaccine

There are two meningococcal vaccines currently licensed in the United States: MPSV (brand name Menomune by Sanofi Pasteur, Swiftwater, PA) and MCV4 (brand name Menactra by Sanofi Pasteur). The quadrivalent A, C, Y, W-135 meningococcal polysaccharide vaccine (MPSV; brand name Menomune) was licensed in 1978 and is administered subcutaneously. The second, MCV4 (Menactra), was first licensed in the United States in 2005 for use in individuals 11 to 55 years of age. MCV4 contains *Neisseria meningitidis* serogroups A, C, Y, and W-135 capsular polysaccharide antigens individually conjugated to diphtheria toxoid protein. MCV4 is administered intramuscularly. There is no vaccine available in the United States for serogroup B, which causes approximately one-third of all meningococcal infections.[32]

Because the polysaccharides are conjugated in the production of MCV4, it is believed that MCV4 will have a longer duration of protection than that seen after administration of MPSV. With MPSV, there is little boost in antibody titer if repeated doses are given. The antibody that is produced is relatively low-affinity IgM, and switching from IgM to IgG production is poor. Protection is estimated to last 3 to 5 years after vaccination with MPSV for adults and 1 to 3 years for children.[32] In addition, MCV4 is expected to reduce asymptomatic carriage of *N. meningitidis* and produce herd immunity, as occurs for *S. pneumoniae* and *Haemophilus influenzae* type b following administration of the respective conjugate vaccines. Pure polysaccharide vaccines have little or no effect on carriage of the vaccine organism.[30] However, studies are needed to confirm these assumptions.

Current recommendations have incorporated the MSV4 vaccine into the routine adolescent schedule. MCV4 should be administered to all children at 11–12 years of age and, as a catch-up vaccine, to all unvaccinated adolescents between 13 and 18 years of age.[3] Immunization for adults is only needed for those at risk. The ACIP has expanded its recommendations for use of MCV4 in children and now considers MCV4 to be the preferred product for individuals aged 2 to 55 years of age. In these age ranges, MPSV should be used only when meningococcal conjugate vaccine (MCV4) is unavailable. MPSV is the preferred product for use in at-risk individuals 55 years of age or older. Because MSPV vaccine is expected to be replaced by the newer meningococcal vaccine, limited supplies of MPSV are available. See Appendices A and B for dosing schedule, contraindications, and precautions.

Adverse reactions to MPSV are generally mild. The most frequent reactions are local ones, such as pain and redness at the injection site. These reactions last for 1–2 days. Systemic reactions, such as headache and malaise within 7 days of vaccination, are reported for up to 60% of recipients. Fewer than 3% of recipients reported these systemic reactions as severe.[3,30] Reported adverse reactions following MCV4 are similar to those reported after MPSV. The most frequent are local reactions, which are reported in up to 59% of recipients. Fever (100°F to 103°F) within 7 days of vaccination is reported for up to 5% of recipients. Systemic reactions, such as headache and malaise, are reported in up to 60% of recipients within 7 days of vaccination. Fewer than 3% of recipients reported these systemic reactions as severe. As of September 22, 2006, the Vaccine Adverse Event Reporting System (VAERS) received 15 confirmed case reports of Guillain-Barré syndrome in persons 11–19

years of age after receipt of MCV4 vaccine.[33] This number represents a rate of 1–2 cases per 100,000 persons immunized per year.[33] Symptom onset occurred 2–33 days after vaccination. Data are not sufficient to determine at this time if MCV4 increases the risk of Guillain-Barré syndrome in persons who receive the vaccine. Guillain-Barré syndrome is a rare illness, and the expected background population rates of Guillain-Barré syndrome are not precisely known. Because ongoing known risk for serious meningococcal disease exists, the CDC recommends continuation of current vaccination strategies. Whether receipt of MCV4 might increase the risk for recurrence of Guillain-Barré syndrome is unknown. Until this issue is clarified, persons with a history of Guillain-Barré syndrome should not receive MCV4.[33]

Revaccination may be indicated for persons previously vaccinated with MPSV who remain at increased risk for infection (e.g., persons residing in areas in which disease is epidemic). Although the need for revaccination of older children and adults after receiving MPSV has not been determined, antibody levels rapidly decline in 2–3 years, and if indications still exist for vaccination, revaccination may be considered 5 years after receipt of the first dose. MCV4 is recommended for vaccination of persons 11–55 years of age. However, use of MPSV is acceptable. More data will likely become available within the next 5 years to guide recommendations on revaccination for persons who were previously vaccinated with MCV4. At present, revaccination after receipt of MCV4 is not recommended.[33] See Appendices A and B for a list of contraindications and precautions.

Varicella Vaccine

Infection

Varicella infection may be preceded by 1 to 2 days of fever and malaise prior to rash onset, but in children the rash is often the first sign of disease. Adults may have more severe disease and a higher incidence of complications.[34] Secondary bacterial infections of skin lesions with *Staphylococcus* or *Streptococcus* are the most common causes of hospitalization and outpatient medical visits. Secondary infections with invasive group A streptococci may cause serious illness and lead to hospitalization and death. Pneumonia following varicella is usually viral but may be bacterial. Central nervous system complications range from aseptic meningitis to encephalitis.[34] Complications are more frequent in persons older than 15 years of age and infants younger than 1 year of age. Adults account for only 5% of reported cases of varicella but approximately 35% of mortality.[3] Immunocompromised persons have a high risk of disseminated disease.

The onset of maternal varicella from 5 days before to 2 days after delivery may result in overwhelming infection of the neonate and a fatality rate as high as 30%. This severe disease is believed to result from fetal exposure to varicella virus without the benefit of passive maternal antibody. Infants born to mothers with onset of maternal varicella 5 days or more prior to delivery usually have a benign course, presumably due to passive transfer of maternal antibody across the placenta.

Primary maternal varicella infection in the first 20 weeks of gestation is rarely associated with a variety of abnormalities in the newborn, including low birth weight, hypoplasia of an extremity, skin scarring, localized muscular atrophy, encephalitis, cortical atrophy, chorioretinitis, and microcephaly.[1] In a prospective study conducted in Europe between 1980 and 1993 that involved nearly 1400 mothers who had varicella during pregnancy, 2% of the infants were born with congenital varicella syndrome when maternal infection occurred during 13–20 weeks' gestation.[35]

Vaccine

Varicella vaccine (VAR; brand name Varivax by Merck) is a live attenuated viral vaccine. VAR should be administered to all adolescents and adults 13 years of age and older who do not have evidence of varicella immunity. Persons 13 years of age and older should receive two doses of varicella vaccine separated by at least 4 weeks. VAR is administered subcutaneously.[3] See Appendices A and B for dosing schedule, contraindications, and precautions.

Generally adults do not require vaccination. Those at highest risk are individuals in their 20s who were too young to have been infected when varicella was an endemic infection in the United States and too old to have been vaccinated in childhood. Therefore careful assessment of the immune status of these individuals is critical. Specific assessment efforts should be focused on adolescents and adults who are at highest risk of exposure and those most likely to transmit varicella to others.[3]

Evidence of varicella immunity includes any of the following: documentation of age-appropriate vaccination, laboratory evidence of immunity or laboratory confirmation of disease, born in the United States before 1980, a healthcare provider diagnosis or verification of varicella disease, or history of herpes zoster based on healthcare provider diagnosis.[3] For pregnant women, birth before 1980 should not be considered evidence of immunity.

The most common adverse reactions following varicella vaccine are local reactions, such as pain, soreness, erythema, and swelling. A varicella-like rash at injection site is reported by 3% of children and 1% of adolescents and adults following the second dose of VAR. A median of two lesions have been present. These lesions generally occur within 2 weeks and are most commonly maculopapular rather than vesicular. A generalized varicella-like rash is reported in 4–6% of VAR recipients with an average of five lesions. Most of these generalized rashes occur within 3 weeks and most are maculopapular. Systemic reactions are not common. The risk of varicella zoster following vaccination appears to be less than those following infections with wild-type virus. The majority of cases of zoster following vaccine have been mild and have not been associated with complications such as postherpetic neuralgia.[1] However, since zoster most commonly presents in the elderly and varicella vaccine has only been in use in children since 1995, it is too early to determine if these predictions will hold. Very rarely, secondary transmission of vaccine virus has occurred, more commonly in immunocompromised than immunocompetent recipients. Laboratory-confirmed transmission by healthy vaccine recipients to susceptible contacts has been documented in five cases.[36]

VAR does not contain egg protein or preservative; therefore, it can be administered to those who have severe allergies (anaphylaxis) to eggs. Individuals with immunosuppression due to leukemia, lymphoma, generalized malignancy, immune deficiency disease, or immunosuppressive therapy should not be vaccinated with VAR. However, treatment with low-dose (less than 2 mg/kg/day), alternate-day, topical, replacement, or aerosolized steroid preparations is not a contraindication to vaccination. Persons whose immunosuppressive therapy has been discontinued for 1 month (3 months for chemotherapy) may be vaccinated. Persons with moderate or severe cellular immunodeficiency resulting from infection from HIV, including persons diagnosed with AIDS, should not receive VAR. HIV-infected adults with a CD4 count of 200 per microliter or higher may be considered for vaccination.[3]

Herpes Zoster Vaccine

Infection

Herpes zoster, or shingles, occurs when latent varicella zoster virus reactivates and causes recurrent disease. Factors associated with recurrent disease include aging, immunosuppression, intrauterine exposure to varicella zoster virus, and having had varicella at a young age (younger than 18 months). The vesicular eruption of zoster generally occurs unilaterally in the distribution of a sensory nerve. Postherpetic neuralgia, or pain in the area of the occurrence that persists after the lesions have resolved, is a distressing complication primarily treated with pain medications.

Vaccine

Historically, when varicella infection was endemic, exposure to circulating wild virus was thought to boost the immune system and by doing so maintain immunity against varicella and help prevent zoster. Now that rates of varicella infection have fallen dramatically in the United States after the introduction of the varicella vaccine, the zoster vaccine may be critical in preventing zoster.[35] Zoster vaccine is a live viral vaccine that was approved in 2006 by the FDA for persons ≥ 60 years whether or not they report a prior episode of herpes zoster. It contains the same viral components as the varicella virus but at much higher doses.[3,36] See Appendices A and B for dosing schedule, contraindications, and precautions.

As with other vaccines, the most common reactions after receipt of zoster vaccine are local; systematic reactions such as headache are less common. In preapproval trials, varicella-like rashes were more common in vaccine than placebo recipients ($P < .05$). All but two of these rashes tested negative for Oka/Merck-strain varicella virus. To date, no evidence exists that exposure to these rashes led to transmission of vaccine-virus to susceptible contacts. Rates of serious adverse events were higher in vaccine recipients (1.9%) than in placebo recipients (1.3%), but no differences in the types or patterns of adverse events

was found between the two groups.[36] However, because zoster vaccine is new, ongoing surveillance is necessary to confirm its safety and efficacy.

Human Papillomavirus Vaccine (HPV)

Infection

Most human papillomavirus infections are asymptomatic and result in no clinical disease. Clinical manifestations of human papillomavirus infection include anogenital warts, recurrent respiratory papillomatosis, and cervical, anal, vaginal, vulvar, and penile cancers.[4] Anogenital human papillomavirus infection is believed to be one of the most common sexually transmitted infections in the United States.[37] Prevalence among adolescent girls is as high as 64%. Up to 75% of new infections occur among persons 15–14 years of age.[37] Modeling estimates suggest that more than 80% of sexually active women will have been infected by age 50.[37] The two most common types of cervical cancer worldwide, squamous cell carcinoma and adenocarcinoma, are both caused by human papillomavirus infection. Approximately 3700 women will die annually as a result of cervical cancer. Human papillomavirus is believed to be responsible for nearly all of these cases of cervical cancer, and human papillomavirus types 16 and 18 in particular are associated with 70% of these cancers[37] (Figure 6-4). In addition to cervical cancer, human papillomavirus is

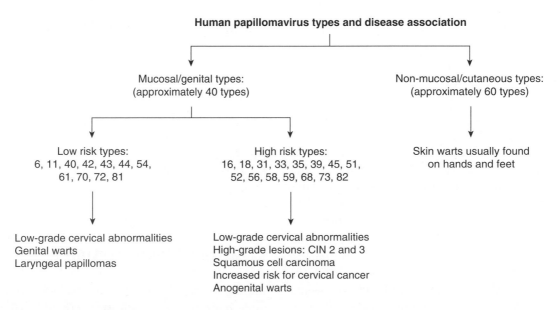

Figure 6-4 Human papillomavirus types and disease association.

responsible for 90% of anal cancers, 40% of vulvar, vaginal, or penile cancers, and 12% of oral and pharyngeal cancers.[37]

Vaccine

The currently licensed HPV (Gardasil, Merck) vaccine is a recombinant quadrivalent type with efficacy against HPV types 6, 11, 16, and 18.[38] This vaccine has been found to have high efficacy for prevention of human papillomavirus vaccine type-related persistent infection, vaccine type-related cervical intraepithelial neoplasia 2/3, and external genital lesions in women ages 16–26 years. Efficacy against cervical intraepithelial neoplasia due to HPV types 6, 11, 16, and 18 is 95%. Efficacy against HPV 6-, 11-, 16- or 18-related genital warts is 99%.[38,39]

HPV vaccine is licensed for administration to girls and women ages 9–26 years of age.[5] It is recommended for routine administration to all girls in the United States at ages 11–12 years. The vaccine can be administered to children as young as 9 years of age at the discretion of the provider. Catch-up vaccination is recommended for females 13 through 26 years of age who have not been previously vaccinated or who did not finish the three-dose series. Ideally, the vaccine should be administered before potential exposure to HPV through sexual contact. However, females who may have already been exposed to HPV still should be vaccinated. See Appendices A and B for dosing schedule, contraindications, and precautions.

Sexually active females who have not been infected with any of the HPV vaccine types will receive full benefit from vaccination. Vaccination will provide less benefit to females if they have already been infected with one or more of the four HPV vaccine types.[40] However, it is not possible for a provider to assess the extent to which sexually active females would benefit from vaccination, and the risk of HPV infections may continue as long as persons are sexually active. Pap testing or screening for HPV DNA or HPV antibody is not recommended prior to vaccination at any age. The use of HPV vaccine does not eliminate the need for Pap testing since 30% of cervical cancers are caused by HPV types not protected by the vaccine. HPV vaccine is administered via intramuscular injection in a three-dose series, and it contains no thimerosal. Interrupted series do not have to be restarted.[38]

The most common adverse reactions to HPV vaccine are pain, swelling, and erythema at the injection site. The majority of injection-site adverse experiences to HPV were mild to moderate in intensity. Serious adverse events reported in pre-licensure trials did not differ significantly between placebo and vaccine recipients.[3,38] However, because the HPV vaccine is new, ongoing surveillance is needed to confirm long-term efficacy and safety. Long-term efficacy could be undermined if immunity wanes over time or if other serotypes not covered in the HPV vaccine become more prevalent. In addition, while safety data from the prelicensure trials are reassuring, large sample sizes are needed to uncover rare events. As of 2007, 2531 adverse events, including 9 deaths, out of 7 million distributed doses have been reported to VAERS.[40] In the same time period, Health Canada reported 82 adverse events out of 162,000 distributed doses.[40] In their analysis, neither agency thought these events indicated that the vaccine was of concern.[40] A more recent analysis of VAERS data indicates increasing reports of postvaccination syncope, which in some cases caused serious injury from falling.[41]

The vaccine is not approved for use in pregnancy. Data on the safety of vaccination during pregnancy are limited. Until further information is available, initiation of the vaccine series should be delayed until after completion of the pregnancy. If a woman is found to be pregnant after initiation of the vaccine series, the remainder of the three-dose regimen should be delayed until after the completion of the pregnancy.[38] If a vaccine dose has been administered during pregnancy, no intervention is indicated. A vaccine in pregnancy registry has been established; patients and healthcare providers are urged to report any exposure to quadrivalent HPV vaccine during pregnancy. Contact information for the registry is listed in Appendix C.

Immunizations for Travelers

Travelers should check with a vaccine expert regarding what vaccines are necessary before traveling outside the United States. Vaccine recommendations vary by country and by regions within a country. Because the prevalence of vaccine-preventable diseases can change dramatically and recommendations change accordingly, international travelers could benefit from referral to a travel clinic (Appendix C).

Vaccine Administration

Improper administration of vaccine products can undermine the protection they provide against vaccine-preventable diseases. Strict adherence to vaccine handling and storage requirements and recommended techniques of administration (e.g., choice of site, deltoid vs gluteal muscle, and route, intramuscular vs subcutaneous), spacing booster doses correctly, and using proper dosages (pediatric vs adult) are essential. Failure to follow recommended guidelines can impede a complete and full immune response after vaccine receipt and can leave the recipient susceptible to infection.[10]

While failure to comply with guidelines affects all vaccines, improper handling and administration is more likely to adversely affect live viral vaccines. Anything that either damages the live organism in the vial (e.g., heat, light) or interferes with replication of the organism in the body (circulating antibody) can cause this type of vaccine to be ineffective.[5] Some vaccines seem to be more affected than others. Measles vaccine virus seems to be most sensitive to circulating antibody whereas polio and rotavirus vaccine viruses are rarely affected.

Generally, vaccines are given simultaneously at a healthcare visit. Doing so is more practical for both providers and patients and is highly recommended by the ACIP as an approach that improves the likelihood that an individual will receive all recommended immunizations on time. Simultaneous receipt of multiple vaccines, whether they are live or inactivated ones, does not impair the immune response to any agent. However, if it is determined later that another live viral vaccine is needed, vaccination will need to be delayed. Live viral vaccines need to be spaced a minimum of 4 weeks apart.[3] Giving live viral vaccines too close together negatively affects the immune response of the second vaccine. This situation is most likely to occur when providing vaccine coverage to travelers. It is highly recommended that providers consult with an expert in travel vaccines before administering any vaccines so that a determination can be made concerning which vaccines are needed, and then a plan be made to administer them in a timely, convenient fashion that does not undermine their effectiveness.

Receipt of antibody-containing products such as immunoglobulins, whole blood, or other blood products can negatively affect the immune response of live vaccines but not inactivated ones. If a live vaccine is given first, 2 or more weeks should elapse before an antibody product is given. If an antibody-containing product is given first, then 3 or more months should elapse before vaccination.[3] The recommended time interval between the two varies by product. Providers should consult vaccine package inserts or ACIP statements for guidance.

Live viral vaccines are generally also more susceptible to damage if not handled properly; inactivated vaccines are also affected but to a lesser degree. Storing the vaccine at the wrong temperature or exposing the vaccine to light can all reduce the potency of some vaccines. Resources such as the Vaccine Storage and Handling Toolkit and the Immunization Practice Toolkit listed in Appendix C are very useful for practices needing detailed information on vaccine administration issues.

Vaccines that require multiple doses also need to be spaced correctly.[10] Each dose needs to be timed so that the body recognizes it as a separate event and will reboost the immune system. Vaccine schedules list the minimum interval between doses. Individuals who are late for the next dose in the series should receive that scheduled dose and continue on in the series; those who receive vaccination later than recommended do not need to restart the series. However, if vaccines are administered earlier than recommended, even by a few days, that vaccine cannot be counted and the patient will need to return at the appropriate time for revaccination.

As more vaccines are added to the immunization schedule, questions have begun to arise regarding the ability of adolescents to sign for immunizations for themselves. Some health departments in the United States currently allow adolescents who are minors to sign for vaccines for themselves if the vaccine is part of the protocol for a visit for a sexually transmitted infection or disease. The Adolescent Working Group of the National Vaccine Advisory Committee is currently exploring this issue. Issues related to confidentiality during a visit for a sexually transmitted infection or disease are a prominent part of the discussion. How best to ensure appropriate immunization services for this population is at the heart of this discussion.

Special Populations

Vaccines considered safe in healthy adults may not be appropriate for use in all populations. Adult vaccines administered to pregnant and lactating women may be unsafe for fetuses and newborns. Individuals with chronic conditions may be more likely to experience vaccine-related adverse events. These concerns have led to close scrutiny of the safety of vaccine products in vulnerable populations, particularly pregnant women and immunosuppressed individuals.

Immunosuppression

Individuals may be immunosuppressed from a multitude of causes including cancer, chemotherapy, HIV infection, and high-dose corticosteroid use. Inactivated vaccines have been found to be well tolerated in immunosuppressed individuals.[3] However, use of live viral vaccines is problematic. Case reports have linked measles vaccine virus infection to subsequent death in at least six severely immunocompromised persons.[26] For this reason, patients who are severely immunocompromised for any reason should not receive the MMR vaccine or other live viral vaccines. Persons receiving low-dose or short-course (less than 14 days therapy), alternate-day treatment, maintenance physiologic doses, or topical, aerosol, intra-articular, bursal, or tendon injections may be vaccinated.

Healthy susceptible close contacts of severely immunocompromised persons should be vaccinated. MMR, varicella vaccines, zoster vaccine, and LAIV (but not OPV) may be given to healthy contacts living in a household with an immunosuppressed individual.[3] No special precautions need to be taken unless the vaccinated contact develops a rash after vaccination with varicella vaccine. In this case, contact should be avoided with immunosuppressed individuals until after the rash resolves.[10] Because immunosuppressed individuals are at higher risk of experiencing complications from vaccine-preventable diseases, these individuals should be vaccinated with products thought to be safe.[10] Immunosuppressed individuals should receive vaccines against influenza (use TIV vaccine), meningococcal and pneumococcal infections, HIB disease, and hepatitis B, although the response to these vaccines may be suboptimal. Adults with HIV are at risk for complications after measles infection and varicella. Therefore the ACIP recommends vaccinating asymptomatic or mildly-immunosuppressed HIV-positive individuals with MMR or varicella. Because guidelines change frequently, women's healthcare providers should consult the latest recommendations before immunizing HIV-positive individuals with live viral vaccines.

Pregnancy

Use of inactivated vaccines is considered safe in pregnancy, whereas live viral vaccines are not.[10]

Live viral vaccines have the potential to cause infection with vaccine virus and could potentially harm the fetus. Of greatest concern is rubella, since fetuses born to mothers infected with wild virus have a high risk of birth defects. While no cases of congenital rubella syndrome have been reported in infants born to women inadvertently vaccinated with rubella vaccine in pregnancy, documented cases of subclinical infection with vaccine virus have occurred.[26]

Congenital syndromes after maternal infection in pregnancy with mumps, measles, and varicella are much rarer than after infection with rubella. Consequently, adverse fetal effects from exposure to measles, mumps, and varicella vaccines are even less likely to cause birth defects than after exposure to rubella vaccine. Therefore, women who are inadvertently vaccinated with MMR or varicella vaccine in pregnancy should be reassured that fetal harm is very unlikely and only of theoretical concern. Live viral vaccine in pregnancy should not be regarded as a reason to terminate a pregnancy.[10] All pregnant women should be evaluated for immunity to rubella and varicella. Women susceptible to rubella and varicella should be vaccinated immediately after delivery and instructed to avoid pregnancy for 4 weeks. No known risk exists for the fetus from passive immunization of pregnant women with immune globulin preparations.[10]

Because of the importance of protecting women of childbearing age against rubella and varicella, reasonable practices in any vaccination program include asking women if they are pregnant or might become pregnant in the next 4 weeks, not vaccinating women who state that they are or plan to be pregnant with MMR or varicella vaccines, and counseling women who are vaccinated not to become pregnant during the 4 weeks after MMR or varicella vaccination.[10] Routine pregnancy testing of women of childbearing age before administering a live attenuated virus vaccine is not recommended.

Persons who receive MMR vaccine do not transmit the vaccine viruses to contacts. Transmission of varicella vaccine virus to contacts is extremely rare. MMR and varicella vaccines should be administered when indicated to the children and other household contacts of pregnant women.

The benefits of vaccinating pregnant women usually outweigh potential risks when the likelihood of disease exposure is high, when infection would pose a risk to the mother or fetus, and when the vaccine is unlikely to cause harm. Vaccine-preventable illnesses of concern in pregnancy include tetanus, pertussis, hepatitis B, and influenza. Pregnant women should receive Td vaccine if indicated. Compliance with the recommended vaccine schedule will protect the mother and prevent neonatal tetanus. Td is the preferred product in pregnancy.[42] In August 2006, the ACIP began recommending that pregnant and postpartum women receive Tdap in order to protect their infants less than 12 months of age from pertussis. Tdap is recommended for use in pregnancy if the risk of pertussis is high and a pregnant woman has not received a prior pertussis-containing vaccine.[42] If the risk of pertussis is low and the woman is sufficiently protected against tetanus (Table 6-9), vaccination should be deferred until after delivery. Tdap has not been evaluated for safety in pregnancy, and it is unclear if giving Tdap in pregnancy interferes with neonatal

Table 6-9 Evidence of Tetanus Immunity in Pregnancy

- < 31 years and received childhood series of 4–5 doses of pediatric DTP, DTaP, and DT
- < 31 years and received complete three-dose adult series of Td during adolescence or as an adult
- ≥ 31 years, has received childhood series of 4–5 doses of pediatric DTP, DTaP, and/or DT and ≥ two Td booster doses
- Has a protective level of serum tetanus antitoxin (≥ 0.1 IU/mL by ELISA)

Source: Centers for Disease Control and Prevention 2008.[42]

protection. It is unclear if passively transmitted antibodies from maternal Tdap will provide protection for the newborn after birth or if it interferes with the development of active immunity when the infant begins the DTaP series at 2 months of age. Women who have not received a prior pertussis vaccine and who have not been vaccinated with Td within the previous 2 years are recommended to receive Tdap after delivery prior to hospital discharge.[42]

Infection with hepatitis B in pregnancy places the exposed neonate at higher risk of chronic infection. Therefore, HBsAg status should be evaluated each pregnancy. A woman found to be HBsAg- positive should be followed carefully to ensure that the infant receives prophylactic treatment. Women found to be HBsAg negative could benefit from further evaluation to determine if they are immune. Those who may already be immune require confirmation of immunity by serologic testing or by documentation of an appropriately administered hepatitis B vaccine series. Women without prior vaccination, particularly if they have risk factors such as drug use or recent sexually transmitted infection, should be offered vaccination.

All pregnant women should be offered the TIV influenza vaccine during flu season.[11] This recommendation is for women during all trimesters of pregnancy.[3,29] The risk of hospitalization when a woman has influenza is higher during pregnancy than it is in nonpregnant individuals.[29] Excess deaths in pregnancy have only been seen in pandemics.[29] In a study of over 134,000 women that compared rates of hospitalization for pregnant women during the flu season to the rates of hospitalization for these same women a year earlier when they were not pregnant, it was found that the risk of hospitalization did not increase in healthy pregnant women who contracted influenza until the second trimester, although hospitalization rates did increase for higher risk women in the first trimester.[43] Therefore, another option would be to adhere to the earlier ACIP recommendations that low-risk pregnant women should be offered influenza vaccination in their second or third trimester, and if they have a high risk of developing

complications from influenza, the vaccination should be offered during the first trimester.[44] This would avoid vaccinating most pregnant women in the first trimester, when a fetus is the most vulnerable to insult.

While no studies to date have documented any fetal harm from influenza vaccination in the first trimester, it is impossible to design high-quality studies that can adequately address this concern. Since almost all women receive prenatal care in the second and third trimester of pregnancy, deferring vaccination for healthy women until later would not increase their risk of hospitalization from influenza or the likelihood that they would not be vaccinated.

Although it has always been assumed that vaccination during pregnancy is of benefit to the mother, recent evidence points to benefit for the fetus as well. In a randomized controlled trial of 340 pregnant women, the infants born to the women who were vaccinated with inactivated influenza vaccine had significantly fewer respiratory illnesses in the first 6 months of life when compared to the infants of the women who were not given TIV during pregnancy.[45]

Additional information about vaccines in pregnancy can be found in Chapter 35.

Lactation

Neither inactivated nor live vaccines administered to any lactating woman adversely affect the breastfeeding dyad. Breastfeeding confers to the infant passive immunity to the diseases to which the mother is immune. Breastfeeding does not adversely affect immunizations and is not a contraindication for any vaccine. Inactivated, recombinant, subunit, polysaccharide, conjugate vaccines and toxoids pose no risk for mothers who are breastfeeding or for their infants. Breast-fed infants should be vaccinated according to recommended schedules.[10]

Healthcare Workers

Healthcare workers should have evidence of immunity or evidence of vaccination to measles, mumps, rubella, and varicella. Healthcare workers who have direct contact with patients in hospitals or outpatient settings should receive a one-time dose of Tdap. It is recommended that a 2-year interval exist between this dose and the last Td. An annual influenza vaccine is also recommended.

Vaccine Safety

Vaccine safety is a prime concern for vaccine manufacturers, immunization providers, and consumers. Vaccination is among the most significant public health success stories of all time. However, like any pharmaceutical product, no vaccine is completely safe or completely effective. While almost all known vaccine adverse events are minor and self-limited, some vaccines have been associated with very rare but serious health effects.[46,47]

Today vaccine-preventable diseases are at or near record lows. By virtue of their absence, these diseases are no longer reminders of the benefits of vaccination. However, approximately 15,000 cases of adverse events following vaccination are reported in the United States each year.[46] These reactions include both true adverse reactions and events that occur coincidentally after vaccination but are not secondary to that vaccination. This number exceeds the current reported incidents of vaccine-preventable diseases.[45] As a result, parents and providers in the United States are more likely to know someone who has experienced an adverse event following immunization than a vaccine-preventable disease. Thus, the success of vaccination has led to increased public attention on health risks associated with vaccines while the benefits often are overlooked.[10,46,47]

Maintaining public confidence in immunizations is critical for preventing a decline in vaccination rates that can result in outbreaks of disease. While the majority of persons who reside in the United States believe in the benefits of immunization and have their children immunized, some have concerns about the safety of vaccines. Public concerns about the safety of whole-cell pertussis vaccine in the 1980s resulted in decreased vaccine coverage levels and the return of epidemic disease in Japan, Sweden, United Kingdom, and several other countries.[6] In the United States, similar concerns led to increases in both the number of lawsuits against the manufacturers and the price of vaccines, and to a decrease in the number of manufacturers willing to make vaccines. Close monitoring and timely assessment of suspected vaccine adverse events can help distinguish true vaccine reactions from coincidental, unrelated events and help to maintain public confidence in immunizations.[46-48] A lower risk tolerance for vaccine adverse events translates into a need to investigate the possible causes of very rare adverse events following vaccinations. Sound immunization policies and recommendations affecting the health of the nation depend upon the ongoing monitoring of the benefits and risks associated with vaccine use.[10,46-48]

Monitoring benefit is relatively easy; assessing risk is much more difficult. Even if an adverse reaction is triggered by a particular vaccine product, the exact cause of an adverse event can be difficult to determine. Vaccines are composed of substance other than the viral component, such as adjunctives and preservatives. Vaccines are often given as combination products, and several products may be given at a healthcare visit, making it difficult to discern which specific vaccine could have caused a reaction. Products could also be contaminated during their production or reconstituted with inappropriate dilutants. Vaccination could potentially trigger an adverse event only in susceptible individuals, not the general population. Vulnerability may be evident (e.g., in individuals who have experienced prior episodes of Guillain-Barré). Vulnerability can also be hidden when unrecognized genetic or physiologic differences between individuals increase the risk of adverse events. While the relationship between an adverse event and vaccination could be causal, most are thought to be coincidental. Determining which of these myriad possibilities the correct one is very challenging.

VAERS was established in order to help answer these questions. VAERS is a national vaccine safety surveillance program cosponsored by the CDC and the FDA. VAERS collects and analyzes information from reports of adverse events following immunization. Since 1980, VAERS has received over 123,000 reports, most of which describe mild side effects such as fever. Very rarely, people experience serious adverse events following immunization. By monitoring such events, VAERS can help to identify important new safety concerns.[49] While case reports submitted to VAERS cannot determine the underlying relationship between an adverse event and a vaccine, potential problems can be identified and evaluated in future research on vaccine safety. Because large sample sizes are needed to identify rare events, reporting is essential. In the case of the original rotavirus vaccine, over 1.5 million doses of vaccine were distributed before a relationship between the rotavirus vaccine and bowel obstruction was confirmed and prompted a recall of the vaccine.[50-52] Therefore, providers need to be vigilant and report minor as well as major and remote as well as recent adverse events associated with vaccine receipt. Appendix C lists the Web address where VAERS reports can be submitted.

The Vaccine Injury Compensation Program is a no-fault alternative to the traditional tort system for resolving vaccine injury claims. It was established as part of the National Childhood Vaccine Injury Act of 1986, after a rash of lawsuits against vaccine manufacturers and healthcare providers threatened to cause vaccine shortages and reduce vaccination rates. The Vaccine Injury Compensation Program covers all vaccines recommended by the CDC for routine administration to children. It is administered jointly by the US Department of Health and Human Services, the US Court of Federal Claims, and the US Department of Justice.[49,53]

Vaccine Controversies

Thimerosal

Thimerosal, a mercury-containing preservative commonly used in vaccines in the past, has been the focus of intense scrutiny by the US Congress and the news media. The concern was raised because thimerosal contains ethyl mercury. While methyl mercury is an environmental contaminant, ethyl mercury metabolizes to water (H_2O) once it enters the body. Methyl mercury remains in the tissues with the inherent danger of mercury poisoning. Attention by the news media has caused some parents and pregnant women to be concerned that thimerosal contained in vaccines might have harmed their children. However, numerous studies to date have not found any association between thimerosal and adverse outcomes.[54-56]

Removal of thimerosal from vaccines was precipitated by an amendment to the FDA Modernization Act that was signed into law on November 21, 1997.[57] The amendment gave the FDA 2 years to "compile a list of drugs and foods that contain intentionally introduced mercury compounds and . . . to provide a quantitative and qualitative analysis of the mercury compounds in the list . . . "[57] The amendment arose from a long-standing interest in lessening human exposure to mercury, a known neurotoxin and nephrotoxin.

When the FDA Modernization Act was passed, it was recommended that infants receive three different vaccines that contained thimerosal, DTP, hepatitis B, and DTP/Hib. Infants receiving all of these vaccines could have been exposed to a cumulative dose of mercury that exceeded the guidelines recommended by the US Environmental Protection Agency. The Environmental Protection Agency recommends that mercury consumption be limited to 2.05 mcg per day or 14.35 mcg per week. Trace amounts of thimerosal are established as ≥ 1 microgram of mercury per dose. Thus the FDA considers the amount of thimerosal in vaccines to be much lower than the amount needed to cause neurodevelopmental delays. Thimerosal, as a preservative, is no longer contained in any childhood vaccine, with the exception of the influenza vaccine. Most commonly used adult vaccines are also now thimerosal free. At this time, only Td (but not Tdap) and some influenza vaccine products contain thimerosal.[57]

Other Controversies

Aluminum salts are the only adjuvants currently licensed for use in the United States. Aluminum salts were initially found to enhance immune responses after immunization with diphtheria and tetanus vaccines in studies performed in the 1930s, 1940s, and 1950s. It has been used extensively in many vaccines for more than 70 years; hundreds of millions of people have been inoculated with aluminum-containing vaccines. Concern has been expressed by the lay public about the safety of aluminum in vaccines. However, exposure to aluminum from vaccination appears to

---

Box 6-4 To Treat or Not to Treat: Do Vaccines Cause Autism?

The number of children who have the diagnosis of autism has increased since the 1980s. At the same time, the number of vaccines recommended for children has increased. In 1998, Wakefield et al published an article that proposed the MMR vaccine causes autism via a series of physiologic reactions to the vaccine. The study cited the cases of 12 children with developmental delays (8 had autism) who developed the condition within 1 month of receiving an MMR vaccination.[a] Following the publication of the Wakefield article, several studies have evaluated the relationship between administration of the vaccines and subsequent development of autism.[b,c] To date, none of the many well-designed studies done have found any association between vaccines and autism or other developmental delays.

What is the relationship between autism and vaccines? The MMR is given to children at 2 years of age. This is also the time that symptoms of autism usually first appear. Thus, there is a temporal association (but no causation) between the administration of vaccine and the development of this disorder. In addition, although it appears that the number of children with autism has increased in the last several years, it is likely that the noted increase is secondary to a more inclusive case definition and improved awareness of the disorder, resulting in more reported incidents and a growth in services for autism.

a. Wakefield et al.[59]
b. Madsen, Hviid, Vestergaard, Schendel.[60]
c. DeStefano.[61]

be minimal. A recent study has found that aluminum levels postvaccination are transiently elevated above recommended levels for only a few days and then rapidly fall well below the level of concern.[58] Adverse reactions are thought only to be local and include redness or nodules at the site of injection.[58]

Numerous other potential adverse events have been linked to vaccine receipt. These include multiple sclerosis following hepatitis B vaccine, autism following vaccination with the MMR, and diabetes following influenza vaccine, among others[59-61](Box 6-4). Most of these associations have either not been found to be etiologically related or are under current investigation. While it is beyond the scope of this chapter to cover these issues in detail, further information can be found on Web sites, particularly the immunization safety review (listed in Appendix C), sponsored by the Institute of Medicine and Global Advisory Committee on Vaccine Safety, which, in turn, is sponsored by the World Health Organization.

Future of Vaccines

Imagine eating a banana or a mashed potato to become immunized against hepatitis B. Research to genetically engineer plants so they have proteins that elicit an immune response is under way. Although this research has several challenges to solve, it is a promising possibility that may in the future improve vaccine availability and lower cost.

Another future use for vaccines is in the treatment of addiction. A vaccine that would stimulate the immune system to destroy cocaine before it reaches the brain is under investigation in human trials. Vaccines against nicotine, heroin, and methamphetamines are also in development. These vaccines are made of a molecule of the drug/antigen, which is attached to a protein from a specific bacterium that is known to illicit an immune response. The bacterium protein elicits an immune response and the antibodies made are specific for the attached drug. Thus, the next time the drug is ingested, injected, or inhaled, the antibodies attach and destroy the drug before it crosses the blood–brain barrier. These vaccines are currently being developed for the purpose of treating persons with addiction. Prophylactic use for protecting against becoming addicted raises the concern that use of these vaccines is a violation of civil liberties, and thus prophylactic use is not currently being proposed.

Finally, the vaccines you are most likely to see in the future are more mucosal vaccines that, when taken orally, stimulate a local secretory IgA (SIgA) antibody response in the gut or mucosal lining that is the port of entry for an infectious organism as well as IgG antibodies. There are currently mucosal vaccines for polio, cholera, typhoid, rotavirus, and influenza. The live attenuated vaccine for polio (OPV) and typhoid live attenuated vaccine are examples of these vaccines licensed today for use internationally or in the United States. Research on development of more mucosal vaccines for other infectious agents is currently under way.

Conclusion

Immunizations are among the most cost effective measures that have been developed for health maintenance and promotion. Great strides have been made to provide vaccines that are safe and effective. Providers caring for adults who incorporate vaccines into their practice will extend the benefits of vaccination into traditionally underimmunized populations. Those who also vigilantly screen for any potential adverse events and report these to VAERS will also help ensure that the products offered to the public are the safest ones possible.

References

1. Centers for Disease Control and Prevention. Impact of vaccines universally recommended for children–United States, 1990–1998. MMWR 1999;48(12):243–8.

2. Centers for Disease Control and Prevention. Notice to readers: final 2005 reports of notifiable diseases. MMWR 2006;2006(55):32.

3. Atkinson W, Hamborsky J, McIntyre L, Wolfe S, eds. Epidemiology and prevention of vaccine-preventable diseases. 10th ed. Centers for Disease Control and Prevention. Washington DC, 2007.

4. Centers for Disease Control and Prevention. Healthy People 2010 goals. 2000. Available from: *http://healthypeople.gov/document/HTML/tracking/od14.htm#vacccoverage* [Accessed February 4, 2008].

5. Ada G. The immunology of vaccination. In: Vaccines. Plotkin S, Orenstein W, eds. Philadelphia: Saunders, 2003:31–45.

6. US Department of Health and Human Services, National Institutes of Health, National Institutes

of Allergy and Infectious Diseases. Understanding vaccines and how they work. NIH publication No. 03-4219, 2003.

7. Plotkin S. Vaccines, vaccination, and vaccinology. J Infect Dis 2003 May 1;187(9):1349–59.

8. Centers for Disease Control and Prevention. A new product (VariZIG) for postexposure prophylaxis of varicella available under an investigational new drug application expanded access protocol. MMWR 2006;55(8):209–10.

9. Centers for Disease Control and Prevention. A comprehensive immunization strategy to eliminate transmission of hepatitis B virus infection in the United States. Recommendations of the Advisory Committee on Immunization Practices (ACIP) part II: immunization of adults. MMWR 2006;55 (RR16):1–25.

10. Centers for Disease Control and Prevention. General recommendations on immunizations, recommendations of the Advisory Committee on Immunization Practices (ACIP). MMWR 2006;55(RR15):1–48.

11. Chiarella P, Massi E, De Robertis M, Fazio Vm, Signori E. Strategies for effective naked DNA vaccination against infectious diseases. Recent Pat Antiinfect Drug Discov 2008;32:93–101.

12. Wassilak S. Tetanus. In: Vaccines. 4th ed. Plotkin SA, Orenstein WA, editors. Philadelphia: Saunders, 2003: 745–81.

13. Centers for Disease Control and Prevention. Preventing tetanus, diphtheria, and pertussis among adolescents: use of tetanus toxoid, reduced diphtheria toxoid and acellular pertussis vaccines. Recommendations of the Advisory Committee on Immunization Practices (ACIP). MMWR 2006;55(RR-03):1–34.

14. Stratton K, Howe C, Johnston R, editors. Diphtheria and tetanus toxoids: adverse events associated with childhood vaccines: evidence bearing on causality. Washington, DC: National Academy Press, 1994: 67–117.

15. American Academy of Pediatrics. Pertussis (whooping cough). Summaries of infectious diseases. In: Pickering LK, Baker CJ, Long SS, McMillan JA, eds. Red Book: 2006 report of the Committee on Infectious Diseases. 27th ed. Elk Grove Village, IL: American Academy of Pediatrics, 2006.

16. Bisgard KM, Pascual FB, Ehresmann KR, Miller CA, Cianfrini C, Jennings CE, et al. Infant pertussis: who was the source? Pediatr Infect Dis J 2004 Nov; 23(11):985–9.

17. Mast E. Hepatitis B vaccine. In Plotkin SA, Orenstein WA, eds. Vaccines. 4th ed. Philadelphia: Saunders, 2003:299–337.

18. Centers for Disease Control and Prevention. A comprehensive immunization strategy to eliminate transmission of hepatitis B virus infection in the United States. Recommendations of the Advisory Committee on Immunization Practices (ACIP) part 1: immunization of infants, children and adolescents. MMWR 2005;54(RR16):1–39.

19. Hernán MA, Jick SS, Olek MJ, Jick H. Recombinant hepatitis B vaccine and the risk of multiple sclerosis: a prospective study. Neurology 2004 Sep 14; 63(5):838–42.

20. Ascherio A, Zhang S, Hernan M, Olek M, Coplan P, Brodovicz K. Hepatitis B vaccination and the risk of multiple sclerosis. N Engl J Med 2001;344:327–32.

21. Centers for Disease Control and Prevention. Updated U.S. public health service guidelines for management of occupational exposures to HBV, HCV, and HIV and recommendations for postexposure prophylaxis MMWR Recommendations and Reports June 29, 2001;50(RR11):1–42.

22. Margolis H, Atler M, Hadler M. In Evans AS, Kaslow RA, eds. Viral infections of humans. Epidemiology and control. 4th ed. New York: Plenum Medical Book Company, 1997:363–418.

23. Centers for Disease Control and Prevention. Prevention of hepatitis A through active or passive immunization. Recommendations of the Advisory Committee on Immunization Practices. MMWR 2006;55(RR-07):1–23.

24. American Academy of Pediatrics. Measles. In Pickering LK, Baker CJ, Long SS, McMillan JA, eds. Red Book: 2006 report of the Committee on Infectious Diseases. 27th ed. Elk Grove Village, IL: American Academy of Pediatrics, 2006:441–52.

25. American Academy of Pediatrics. Rubella. In Pickering LK, Baker CJ, Long SS, McMillan JA, eds. Red Book: 2006 report of the Committee on Infectious Diseases. 27th ed. Elk Grove Village, IL: American Academy of Pediatrics, 2006:574–9.

26. Centers for Disease Control and Prevention. Measles, mumps, and rubella—vaccine use and strategies for elimination of measles, rubella, and congenital rubella syndrome and control of mumps. Recommendations of the Advisory Committee on Immunization Practices (ACIP). MMWR 1998;47 (RR-8):1–57.

27. Centers for Disease Control and Prevention. Polio-myelitis prevention in the United States: updated recommendations of the Advisory Committee on Immunization Practices. (ACIP). MMWR 2000;49 (RR-05):1–22.

28. Whitney C, Shaffner W, Butler J. Rethinking recommendations for use of pneumococcal vaccines in adults. Clin Infect Dis 2001 Sep 1;33 (5):662–75.

29. Centers for Disease Control and Prevention. Prevention and control of influenza. Recommendations of the Advisory Committee on Immunization Practices (ACIP). MMWR 2008;57(RR-07):1–60.

30. Centers for Disease Control and Prevention. Prevention and control of meningococcal disease. MMWR 2005;54(RR07):1–21.

31. Granoff D, Feavers I, Borrow R. Meningococcal vaccine. In Plotkin SA, Orenstein WA, eds. Vaccines. 4th ed. Philadelphia: Saunders, 2003:959–87.

32. Gardner P. Prevention of meningococcal disease. N Eng J Med 2006;355:1466–73.

33. Centers for Disease Control and Prevention. Update: Gullain-Barré syndrome among recipients of Menactra meningococcal conjugate vaccine—United States, June 2005–September 2006. MMWR 2006;55(41): 1120–4.

34. Centers for Disease Control and Prevention. Prevention of varicella. Recommendations of the Advisory Committee on Immunization Practices (ACIP). MMWR 2007;56(RR-4):1–39.

35. Enders G, Miller E, Cradock-Watson J. Consequences of varicella and herpes zoster in pregnancy: prospective study of 1739 cases. Lancet 1994; 343:1548.

36. Centers for Disease Control and Prevention. Prevention of herpes zoster. Recommendations of the Advisory Committee on Immunization Practices (ACIP). MMWR 2008;57(RR 05):1–30.

37. Trottier H, Franco E. The epidemiology of genital human papillomavirus infection. Vaccine 2006;24 (supp11):S1–5.

38. Centers for Disease Control and Prevention. Quadrivalent human papillomavirus vaccine. Recommendations of the Advisory Committee on Immunization Practices (ACIP). MMWR 2007; 56(early release):1–24.

39. Schiller J, Lowy D. Human papillomavirus vaccines for cervical cancer prevention. In Plotkin SA, Orenstein WA, eds. Vaccines. 4th ed. Philadelphia: Saunders, 2003:1259–65.

40. Eggertson L. Adverse events reported for HPV vaccine. CMAJ 2007;177(10):1169–70.

41. Centers for Disease Control and Prevention. Syncope after vaccination—United States, January 2005–July 2007. MMWR 2008;57(17):457–60.

42. Centers for Disease Control and Prevention. Prevention of pertussis, tetanus, and diphtheria among pregnant and postpartum women and their infants. Recommendations of the Advisory Committee on Immunization Practices (ACIP). MMWR 2008;7 (04):1–51.

43. Dodds L, McNeil SA, Fell DB, Allen VM, Coombs A, Scott J, et al. Impact of influenza exposure on rates of hospital admissions and physician visits because of respiratory illness among pregnant women. CMAJ 2007;176(4):463–8.

44. Centers for Disease Control and Prevention. General recommendations on immunization. MMWR 2002; 51 (RR-02):1–36.

45. Zaman K, Roy E, Arifeen SE, Rahman M, Raqib R, Wilson E. Effectiveness of maternal immunization in mothers and infants. N Engl J Med 2008;359: 1–10

46. American Academy of Pediatrics. Vaccine safety and contraindications. In Pickering LK, Baker CJ, Long SS, McMillan JA, eds. Red Book: 2006 report of the Committee on Infectious Diseases. 27th ed. Elk Grove Village, IL: American Academy of Pediatrics, 2006: 39–50.

47. Centers for Disease Control and Prevention. Surveillance for safety after immunization. MMWR 2003;52(SS-1):1–24.

48. Centers for Disease Control and Prevention. Update: vaccine side effects, adverse reactions, contraindications, and precautions. Recommendations of the Advisory Committee on Immunization Practices (ACIP). MMWR 1996;45(RR-12):1–35.

49. Chen R, Glasser JW, Rhodes PH, Davis RL, Barlow WE, Thompson RS, et al. Vaccine Safety Datalink project: a new tool for improving vaccine safety monitoring in the United States. Pediatrics 1997;99(6):765–73.

50. Rotavirus vaccine for the prevention of rotavirus gastroenteritis among children. Recommendations of the Advisory Committee on Immunization Practices (ACIP). MMWR Recomm Rep 1999 Mar 19;48 (RR-2):1–20.

51. Centers for Disease Control and Prevention (CDC). Intussusception among recipients of rotavirus vaccine—United States, 1998–1999. MMWR 1999;48(27): 577–81.

52. Centers for Disease Control and Prevention (CDC). Withdrawal of rotavirus vaccine recommendation. MMWR 1999;48(43):1007.

53. Centers for Disease Control and Prevention (CDC). National Childhood Vaccine Injury Act: requirements for permanent vaccination records and for reporting of selected events after vaccination. MMWR 1988;37:197–200.

54. Pichichero ME, Cernichiari E, Lopreiato J, Treanor J. Mercury concentrations and metabolism in infants receiving vaccines containing thimerosal: a descriptive study. Lancet 2002;360:1737–41.

55. Heron J, Golding J, Team AS. Thimerosal exposure in infants and developmental disorders: a prospective cohort study in the United Kingdom does not show a causal association. Pediatrics 2004;114(3):577–83.

56. Hivid A, Stellfeld M, Wohlfahart J, Melbye M. Association between thimerosal-containing vaccine and autism. JAMA 2003;290:1763–6.

57. US Food and Drug Administration (FDA). Thimerosal in vaccines. 2007. Available from: *http://www.fda.gov/cber/vaccine/thimerosal.htm#pres* [Accessed October 12, 2007].

58. Keith L, Jones D, Chou C. Aluminum toxicokinetics regarding infant diet and vaccination. Vaccine 2002;20(Supplement 3):S13–7.

59. Wakefield AJ, Murch SH, Anthony A, Linnell J, Casson DM, Malik M, et al. Ileal-lymphoid-nodular hyperplasia, non-specific colitis, and pervasive developmental disorder in children. Lancet 1998;351: 637–41.

60. Madsen KM, Hviid A, Vestergaard M, Schendel J. A population-based study of measles, mumps, and rubella vaccination and autism. N Engl J Med 2002;347:1477–82.

61. DeStefano F. Vaccines and autism: evidence does not support a causal association. Clin Pharmacol Ther 2007 Dec;82(6):756–9.

Appendix A: Summary of Recommendations for Adult Immunization

Adapted from the recommendations of the Advisory Committee on Immunization Practices (ACIP)* by the Immunization Action Coalition, April 2008

Vaccine name and route	For whom vaccination is recommended	Schedule for vaccine administration (any vaccine can be given with another)	Contraindications and precautions (mild illness is not a contraindication)
Influenza Trivalent inactivated influenza vaccine (TIV) *Give IM* Live attenuated influenza vaccine (LAIV) *Give intranasally*	**Note:** LAIV may not be given to some of the persons listed below; see contraindications listed in far right column. • All persons who want to reduce the likelihood of becoming ill with influenza or of spreading it to others. • Persons age 50 yrs and older. [TIV only] • Persons with medical problems (e.g., heart disease, lung disease, diabetes, renal dysfunction, hemoglobinopathy, immunosuppression). [TIV only] • Persons with any condition that compromises respiratory function or the handling of respiratory secretions or that can increase the risk of aspiration (e.g., cognitive dysfunction, spinal cord injury, seizure disorder, or other neuromuscular disorder). [TIV only] • Persons living in chronic care facilities. [TIV only] • Persons who work or live with high-risk people. • Women who will be pregnant during the influenza season (December–spring). [If currently pregnant, TIV only] • All healthcare personnel and other persons who provide direct care to high-risk people. • Household contacts and out-of-home caregivers of children age 0–59 m. • Travelers at risk for complications of influenza who go to areas where influenza activity exists or who may be among people from areas of the world where there is current influenza activity (e.g., on organized tours). [TIV only] • Students or other persons in institutional settings (e.g., residents of dormitories or correctional facilities).	• Give 1 dose every year in the fall or winter. • Begin vaccination services as soon as vaccine is available and continue until the supply is depleted. • Continue to give vaccine to unvaccinated adults throughout the influenza season (including when influenza activity is present in the community) and at other times when the risk of influenza exists. • If 2 or more of the following live virus vaccines are to be given— LAIV, MMR, Var, and/or yellow fever vaccine—they should be given on the same day. If they are not, space them by at least 28 d.	**Contraindications** • Previous anaphylactic reaction to this vaccine, to any of its components, or to eggs. • For LAIV only, age 50 years or older, pregnancy, asthma, reactive airway disease, or other chronic disorder of the pulmonary or cardiovascular system; an underlying medical condition, including metabolic disease such as diabetes, renal dysfunction, and hemoglobinopathy; a known or suspected immune deficiency disease or current receipt of immunosuppressive therapy. **Precautions** • Moderate or severe acute illness. • For TIV only, history of Guillain-Barré syndrome (GBS) within 6 wks of previous TIV. • For LAIV only, history of GBS within 6 wks of a previous influenza vaccination.

Pneumococcal polysaccharide (PPV) *Give IM or SC*	• Persons age 65 yrs and older.
	• Persons who have chronic illness or other risk factors, including chronic cardiac or pulmonary disease, chronic liver disease, alcoholism, diabetes, CSF leak, as well as people living in special environments or social settings (including Alaska Natives and certain American Indian populations).
	• Those at highest risk of fatal pneumococcal infection, including persons who
	  - have anatomic asplenia, functional asplenia, or sickle cell disease
	  - have an immunocompromising condition, including HIV infection, leukemia, lymphoma, Hodgkin's disease, multiple myeloma, generalized malignancy, chronic renal failure, or nephrotic syndrome
	  - are receiving immunosuppressive chemotherapy (including corticosteroids)
	  - have received an organ or bone marrow transplant
	  - are candidates for or recipients of cochlear implants.
		• Give 1 dose if unvaccinated or if previous vaccination history is unknown.
		• Give a 1-time revaccination at least 5 yrs after 1st dose to persons
		  - age 65 yrs and older if the 1st dose was given prior to age 65 yrs
		  - at highest risk of fatal pneumococcal infection or rapid antibody loss (see the 3rd bullet in the box to left for listings of persons at highest risk)
			Contraindication
			Previous anaphylactic reaction to this vaccine or to any of its components.
			Precaution
			Moderate or severe acute illness.

Zoster (shingles) (Zos) *Give SC*	ACIP has voted to recommend herpes zoster (shingles) vaccine for all persons age 60 yrs and older who do not have contraindications. Provisional recommendations are online at www.cdc.gov/vaccines/recs/provisional/default.htm#acip.		

*This document was adapted from the recommendations of the Advisory Committee on Immunization Practices (ACIP). To obtain copies of these recommendations, call the CDC-INFO Contact Center at (800) 232-4636; or visit CDC's Web site at www.cdc.gov/vaccines/pubs/ACIP-list.htm; or visit the Immunization Action Coalition (IAC) website at www.immunize.org/acip. This table is revised periodically. Visit IAC's Web site at www.immunize.org/adultrules to make sure you have the most current version.

Appendix A: Summary of Recommendations for Adult Immunization (continued)

Vaccine name and route	For whom vaccination is recommended	Schedule for vaccine administration (any vaccine can be given with another)	Contraindications and precautions (mild illness is not a contraindication)
Hepatitis B (HepB) *Give IM* Brands may be used interchangeably.	• All persons through age 18 yrs. • All adults wishing to obtain immunity against hepatitis B virus infection. • High-risk persons, including household contacts and sex partners of HBsAg-positive persons; injecting drug users; sexually active persons not in a long-term, mutually monogamous relationship; men who have sex with men; persons with HIV; persons seeking evaluation or treatment for an STD; patients receiving hemodialysis and patients with renal disease that may result in dialysis; healthcare personnel and public safety workers who are exposed to blood; clients and staff of institutions for the developmentally disabled; inmates of long-term correctional facilities; and certain international travelers. • Persons with chronic liver disease. **Note:** Provide serologic screening for immigrants from endemic areas. If patient is chronically infected, assure appropriate disease management. Screen sex partners and household members; give HepB at the same visit if not already vaccinated.	• Give 3 doses on a 0, 1, 6 m schedule. • Alternative timing options for vaccination include 0, 2, 4 m and 0, 1, 4 m. • There must be at least 4 wks between doses #1 and #2, and at least 8 wks between doses #2 and #3. Overall, there must be at least 16 wks between doses #1 and #3. **Schedule for those who have fallen behind:** If the series is delayed between doses, DO NOT start the series over. Continue from where you left off. For Twinrix (hepatitis A and B combination vaccine [GSK]) for patients age 18 yrs and older only: give 3 doses on a 0, 1, 6 m schedule. An alternative schedule can also be used at 0, 7, 21–30 d, and a booster at 12 m.	**Contraindication** Previous anaphylactic reaction to this vaccine or to any of its components. **Precaution** Moderate or severe acute illness.
Hepatitis A (HepA) *Give IM* Brands may be used interchangeably.	• All persons wishing to obtain immunity to hepatitis A virus infection. • Persons who travel or work anywhere EXCEPT the U.S., Western Europe, New Zealand, Australia, Canada, and Japan. • Persons with chronic liver disease; injecting and non-injecting drug users; men who have sex with men; people who receive clotting-factor concentrates; persons who work with hepatitis A virus in experimental lab settings (not routine medical laboratories); and food handlers when health authorities or private employers determine vaccination to be appropriate. **Note:** Prevaccination testing is likely to be cost effective for persons older than age 40 yrs, as well as for younger persons in certain groups with a high prevalence of hepatitis A virus infection.	• Give 2 doses. • The minimum interval between doses #1 and #2 is 6 m. • If dose #2 is delayed, do not repeat dose #1. Just give dose #2.	**Contraindication** Previous anaphylactic reaction to this vaccine or to any of its components. **Precautions** • Moderate or severe acute illness. • Safety during pregnancy has not been determined, so benefits must be weighed against potential risk.
Td, Tdap (Tetanus, diphtheria, pertussis) *Give IM*	• All adults who lack written documentation of a primary series consisting of at least 3 doses of tetanus- and diphtheria-toxoid-containing vaccine. • A booster dose of tetanus- and diphtheria-toxoid-containing vaccine may be needed for wound management as early as 5 yrs after receiving a previous dose, so consult ACIP recommendations.* • Using tetanus toxoid (TT) instead of Td or Tdap is <u>not</u> recommended. • In pregnancy, when indicated, give Td or Tdap in 2nd or 3rd trimester. If not administered during pregnancy, give Tdap in immediate postpartum period. **For Tdap only:** • All adults younger than age 65 yrs who have not already received Tdap. • Healthcare personnel who work in hospitals or ambulatory care settings and have direct patient contact and who have not received Tdap. • Adults in contact with infants younger than age 12 m (e.g., parents, grandparents younger than age 65 yrs, childcare providers, healthcare personnel) who have not received a dose of Tdap should be prioritized for vaccination.	• For persons who are unvaccinated or behind, complete the primary series with Td (spaced at 0, 1–2 m, 6–12 m intervals). One-time dose of Tdap may be used for any dose if age 18–64 yrs. • Give Td booster every 10 yrs after the primary series has been completed. For adults age 18–64 yrs, a 1-time dose of Tdap is recommended to replace the next Td. • Intervals of 2 yrs or less between Td and Tdap may be used. **Note:** The two Tdap products are licensed for different age groups: Adacel (sanofi) for use in persons age 11–64 yrs and Boostrix (GSK) for use in persons age 10–18 yrs.	**Contraindications** • Previous anaphylactic reaction to this vaccine or to any of its components. • For Tdap only, history of encephalopathy within 7 d following DTP/DTaP. **Precautions** • Moderate or severe acute illness. • GBS within 6 wks of receiving a previous dose of tetanus-toxoid-containing vaccine. • Unstable neurologic condition. • History of arthus reaction following a previous dose of tetanus- and/or diphtheria-toxoid-containing vaccine, including MCV4. **Note:** Use of Td/Tdap is not contraindicated in pregnancy. Either vaccine may be given during trimester #2 or #3 at the provider's discretion.
Polio (IPV) *Give IM or SC*	Not routinely recommended for persons age 18 yrs and older. **Note:** Adults living in the U.S. who never received or completed a primary series of polio vaccine need not be vaccinated unless they intend to travel to areas where exposure to wild-type virus is likely (i.e., India, Pakistan, Afghanistan, and Nigeria). Previously vaccinated adults can receive one booster dose if traveling to polio endemic areas.	• Refer to ACIP recommendations* regarding unique situations, schedules, and dosing information.	**Contraindication** Previous anaphylactic or neurologic reaction to this vaccine or to any of its components. **Precautions** • Moderate or severe acute illness. • Pregnancy.

(continues)

Appendix A: Summary of Recommendations for Adult Immunization (continued)

Vaccine name and route	For whom vaccination is recommended	Schedule for vaccine administration (any vaccine can be given with another)	Contraindications and precautions (mild illness is not a contraindication)
Varicella (Var) (Chickenpox) *Give SC*	• All adults without evidence of immunity. **Note:** Evidence of immunity is defined as written documentation of 2 doses of varicella vaccine; born in the U.S. before 1980 (exceptions: healthcare personnel and pregnant women); a history of varicella disease or herpes zoster based on healthcare-provider diagnosis; laboratory evidence of immunity; and/or laboratory confirmation of disease.	• Give 2 doses. • Dose #2 is given 4–8 wks after dose #1. • If the second dose is delayed, do not repeat dose #1. Just give dose #2. • If 2 or more of the following live virus vaccines are to be given—LAIV, MMR, Var, and/or yellow fever vaccine—they should be given on the same day. If they are not, space them by at least 28 d.	**Contraindications** • Previous anaphylactic reaction to this vaccine or to any of its components. • Pregnancy or possibility of pregnancy within 4 wks. • Persons immunocompromised because of malignancy and primary or acquired cellular immunodeficiency, including HIV/AIDS (although vaccination may be considered if CD4+ T-lymphocyte counts are greater than or equal to 200 cells/mcL. See *MMWR* 2007;56,RR-4). **Precautions** • If blood, plasma, and/or immune globulin (IG or VZIG) were given in past 11 m, see ACIP statement *General Recommendations on Immunization** regarding time to wait before vaccinating. • Moderate or severe acute illness. **Note:** For those on high-dose immunosuppressive therapy, consult ACIP recommendations regarding delay time.*
Meningococcal Conjugate vaccine (MCV4) *Give IM* <u>Polysaccharide vaccine (MPSV)</u> *Give SC*	• All persons age 11 through 18 yrs. • College freshmen living in a dormitory. • Persons with anatomic or functional asplenia or with terminal complement component deficiencies. • Persons who travel to or reside in countries in which meningococcal disease is hyperendemic or epidemic (e.g., the "meningitis belt" of Sub-Saharan Africa). • Microbiologists routinely exposed to isolates of *N. meningitidis*.	• Give 1 dose. • If previous vaccine was MPSV, revaccinate after 5 yrs if risk continues. • Revaccination after MCV4 is not recommended. • MCV4 is preferred over MPSV for persons age 55 yrs and younger, although MPSV is an acceptable alternative.	**Contraindication** Previous anaphylactic or neurologic reaction to this vaccine or to any of its components, including diphtheria toxoid (for MCV4). **Precautions** • Moderate or severe acute illness. • For MCV4 only, history of Guillain-Barré syndrome (GBS).
MMR (Measles, mumps, rubella) *Give SC*	• Persons born in 1957 or later (especially those born outside the U.S.) should receive at least 1 dose of MMR if there is no serologic proof of immunity or documentation of a dose given on or after the first birthday. • Persons in high-risk groups, such as healthcare personnel, students entering college and other post–high school educational institutions, and international travelers, should receive a total of 2 doses. • Persons born before 1957 are usually considered immune, but proof of immunity (serology or vaccination) may be desirable for healthcare personnel. • Women of childbearing age who do not have acceptable evidence of rubella immunity or vaccination.	• Give 1 or 2 doses (see criteria in 1st and 2nd bullets in box to left). • If dose #2 is recommended, give it no sooner than 4 wks after dose #1. • If a pregnant woman is found to be rubella susceptible, administer MMR postpartum. • If 2 or more of the following live virus vaccines are to be given—LAIV, MMR, Var, and/or yellow fever vaccine—they should be given on the same day. If they are not, space them by at least 28 d.	**Contraindications** • Previous anaphylactic reaction to this vaccine or to any of its components. • Pregnancy or possibility of pregnancy within 4 wks. • Persons immunocompromised because of cancer, leukemia, lymphoma, immunosuppressive drug therapy, including high-dose steroids or radiation therapy. **Note:** HIV positivity is NOT a contraindication to MMR except for those who are severely immunocompromised (i.e., CD4+ T-lymphocyte counts are less than 200 cells/mcL). **Precautions** • If blood, plasma, and/or immune globulin were given in past 11 m, see ACIP statement *General Recommendations on Immunization** regarding time to wait before vaccinating. • Moderate or severe acute illness. • History of thrombocytopenia or thrombocytopenic purpura. **Note:** If PPD (tuberculosis skin test) and MMR are both needed but not given on same day, delay PPD for 4–6 wks after MMR.
Human papillomavirus (HPV) *Give IM*	All previously unvaccinated women through age 26 yrs.	• Give 3 doses on a 0, 2, 6 m schedule. • There must be at least 4 wks between doses #1 and #2 and at least 12 wks between doses #2 and #3. Overall, there must be at least 24 wks between doses #1 and #3.	**Contraindication** Previous anaphylactic reaction to this vaccine or to any of its components. **Precaution** Data on vaccination in pregnancy are limited. Vaccination should be delayed until after completion of the pregnancy.

Appendix B: Recommended Adult Immunization Schedule, United States, October 2006–September 2007

Recommended adult immunization schedule, by vaccine and age group

Age group (yrs) ▶ Vaccine ▼	19–49 years	50–64 years	≥65 years
Tetanus, diphtheria, pertussis (Td/Tdap)[1]*	1-dose Td booster every 10 yrs Substitute 1 dose of Tdap for Td		
Human papillomavirus (HPV)[2]*	3 doses (females)		
Measles, mumps, rubella (MMR)[3]*	1 or 2 doses	1 dose	
Varicella[4]*	2 doses (0, 4–8 wks)	2 doses (0, 4–8 wks)	
Influenza[5]*	1 dose annually	1 dose annually	
Pneumococcal (polysaccharide)[6,7]	1–2 doses		1 dose
Hepatitis A[8]*	2 doses (0, 6–12 mos, or 0, 6–18 mos)		
Hepatitis B[9]*	3 doses (0, 1–2, 4–6 mos)		
Meningococcal[10]	1 or more doses		

Recommended adult immunization schedule, by vaccine and medical and other indications

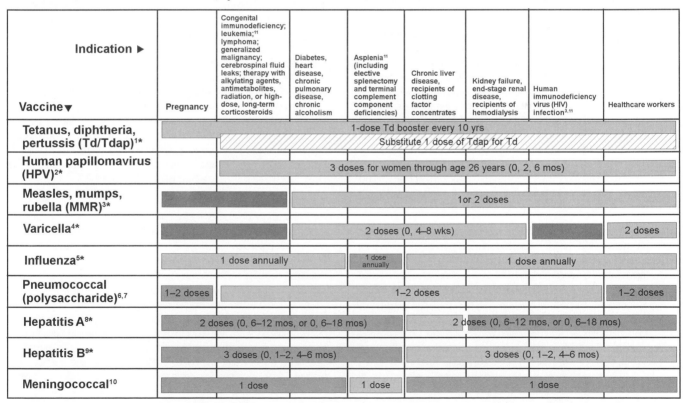

Indication ▶ Vaccine ▼	Pregnancy	Congenital immunodeficiency; leukemia;[11] lymphoma; generalized malignancy; cerebrospinal fluid leaks; therapy with alkylating agents, antimetabolites, radiation, or high-dose, long-term corticosteroids	Diabetes, heart disease, chronic pulmonary disease, chronic alcoholism	Asplenia[11] (including elective splenectomy and terminal complement component deficiencies)	Chronic liver disease, recipients of clotting factor concentrates	Kidney failure, end-stage renal disease, recipients of hemodialysis	Human immunodeficiency virus (HIV) infection[3,11]	Healthcare workers
Tetanus, diphtheria, pertussis (Td/Tdap)[1]*	1-dose Td booster every 10 yrs Substitute 1 dose of Tdap for Td							
Human papillomavirus (HPV)[2]*		3 doses for women through age 26 years (0, 2, 6 mos)						
Measles, mumps, rubella (MMR)[3]*		1 or 2 doses						
Varicella[4]*		2 doses (0, 4–8 wks)						2 doses
Influenza[5]*	1 dose annually	1 dose annually		1 dose annually				
Pneumococcal (polysaccharide)[6,7]	1–2 doses	1–2 doses						1–2 doses
Hepatitis A[8]*	2 doses (0, 6–12 mos, or 0, 6–18 mos)			2 doses (0, 6–12 mos, or 0, 6–18 mos)				
Hepatitis B[9]*	3 doses (0, 1–2, 4–6 mos)			3 doses (0, 1–2, 4–6 mos)				
Meningococcal[10]	1 dose		1 dose	1 dose				

* Covered by the Vaccine Injury Compensation Program

These recommendations must be read along with the footnotes, which can be found on the next 2 pages of this schedule.

For all persons in this category who meet the age requirements and who lack evidence of immunity (e.g., lack documentation of vaccination or have no evidence of prior infection)

Recommended if some other risk factor is present (e.g., on the basis of medical, occupational, lifestyle, or other indications)

Contraindicated

(continues)

Appendix B: Recommended Adult Immunization Schedule, United States, October 2006–September 2007 (continued)

Footnotes

1. Tetanus, diphtheria, and acellular pertussis (Td/Tdap) vaccination. Adults with uncertain histories of a complete primary vaccination series with diphtheria and tetanus toxoid–containing vaccines should begin or complete a primary vaccination series. A primary series for adults is 3 doses; administer the first 2 doses at least 4 weeks apart and the third dose 6–12 months after the second. Administer a booster dose to adults who have completed a primary series and if the last vaccination was received ≥ 10 years previously. Tdap or tetanus and diphtheria (Td) vaccine may be used; Tdap should replace a single dose of Td for adults aged < 65 years who have not previously received a dose of Tdap (either in the primary series, as a booster, or for wound management). Only one of two Tdap products (Adacel [sanofi pasteur, Swiftwater, Pennsylvania]) is licensed for use in adults. If the person is pregnant and received the last Td vaccination ≥ 10 years previously, administer Td during the second or third trimester; if the person received the last Td vaccination in < 10 years, administer Tdap during the immediate postpartum period. A one-time administration of 1-dose of Tdap with an interval as short as 2 years from a previous Td vaccination is recommended for postpartum women, close contacts of infants aged < 12 months, and all healthcare workers with direct patient contact. In certain situations, Td can be deferred during pregnancy and Tdap substituted in the immediate postpartum period, or Tdap can be given instead of Td to a pregnant woman after an informed discussion with the woman (see http://www.cdc.gov/nip/publications/acip-list.htm). Consult the ACIP statement for recommendations for administering Td as prophylaxis in wound management (http://www.cdc.gov/mmwr/preview/mmwrhtml/00041645.htm).

2. Human Papillomavirus (HPV) vaccination. HPV vaccination is recommended for all women aged ≤ 26 years who have not completed the vaccine series. Ideally, vaccine should be administered before potential exposure to HPV through sexual activity; however, women who are sexually active should still be vaccinated. Sexually active women who have not been infected with any of the HPV vaccine types receive the full benefit of the vaccination. Vaccination is less beneficial for women who have already been infected with one or more of the four HPV vaccine types. A complete series consists of 3 doses. The second dose should be administered 2 months after the first dose; the third dose should be administered 6 months after the first dose. Vaccination is not recommended during pregnancy. If a woman is found to be pregnant after initiating the vaccination series, the remainder of the 3-dose regimen should be delayed until after completion of the pregnancy.

3. Measles, Mumps, Rubella (MMR) vaccination. *Measles component:* Adults born before 1957 can be considered immune to measles. Adults born during or after 1957 should receive ≥ 1 dose of MMR unless they have a medical contraindication, documentation of ≥ 1 dose, history of measles based on health-care provider diagnosis, or laboratory evidence of immunity. A second dose of MMR is recommended for adults who (1) have been recently exposed to measles or in an outbreak setting; (2) were previously vaccinated with killed measles vaccine; (3) have been vaccinated with an unknown type of measles vaccine during 1963–1967; (4) are students in postsecondary educational institutions; (5) work in a healthcare facility, or (6) plan to travel internationally. Withhold MMR or other measles-containing vaccines from HIV-infected persons with severe immunosuppression. *Mumps component:* Adults born before 1957 can generally be considered immune to mumps. Adults born during or after 1957 should receive 1 dose of MMR unless they have a medical contraindication, history of mumps based on healthcare provider diagnosis, or laboratory evidence of immunity. A second dose of MMR is recommended for adults who (1) are in an age group that is affected during a mumps outbreak; (2) are students in postsecondary educational institutions; (3) work in a health-care facility; or (4) plan to travel internationally. For unvaccinated healthcare

workers born before 1957 who do not have other evidence of mumps immunity, consider giving 1 dose on a routine basis and strongly consider giving a second dose during an outbreak. *Rubella component:* Administer 1 dose of MMR vaccine to women whose rubella vaccination history is unreliable or who lack laboratory evidence of immunity. For women of childbearing age, regardless of birth year, routinely determine rubella immunity and counsel women regarding congenital rubella syndrome. Do not vaccinate women who are pregnant or who might become pregnant within 4 weeks of receiving vaccine. Women who do not have evidence of immunity should receive MMR vaccine upon completion or termination of pregnancy and before discharge from the health-care facility.

4. Varicella vaccination. All adults without evidence of immunity to varicella should receive 2 doses of varicella vaccine. Special consideration should be given to those who (1) have close contact with persons at high risk for severe disease (e.g., healthcare workers and family contacts of immunocompromised persons) or (2) are at high risk for exposure or transmission (e.g., teachers of young children; child care employees; residents and staff members of institutional settings, including correctional institutions; college students; military personnel; adolescents and adults living in households with children; non-pregnant women of childbearing age; and international travelers). Evidence of immunity to varicella in adults includes any of the following: (1) documentation of 2 doses of varicella vaccine at least 4 weeks apart; (2) U.S.–born before 1980 (although for healthcare workers and pregnant women, birth before 1980 should not be considered evidence of immunity); (3) history of varicella based on diagnosis or verification of varicella by a healthcare provider (for a patient reporting a history of or presenting with an atypical case, a mild case, or both, healthcare providers should seek either an epidemiologic link with a typical varicella case or evidence of laboratory confirmation, if it was performed at the time of acute disease); (4) history of herpes zoster based on healthcare provider diagnosis; or (5) laboratory evidence of immunity or laboratory confirmation of disease. Do not vaccinate women who are pregnant or might become pregnant within 4 weeks of receiving the vaccine. Assess pregnant women for evidence of varicella immunity. Women who do not have evidence of immunity should receive dose 1 of varicella vaccine upon completion or termination of pregnancy and before discharge from the healthcare facility. Dose 2 should be administered 4–8 weeks after dose 1.

5. Influenza vaccination: *Medical indications:* Chronic disorders of the cardiovascular or pulmonary systems, including asthma; chronic metabolic diseases, including diabetes mellitus, renal dysfunction, hemoglobinopathies, or immunosuppression (including immunosuppression caused by medications or HIV); any condition that compromises respiratory function or the handling of respiratory secretions or that can increase the risk of aspiration (e.g., cognitive dysfunction, spinal cord injury, or seizure disorder or other neuromuscular disorder); and pregnancy during the influenza season. No data exist on the risk for severe or complicated influenza disease among persons with asplenia; however, influenza is a risk factor for secondary bacterial infections that can cause severe disease among persons with asplenia. *Occupational indications:* Healthcare workers and employees of long-term–care and assisted living facilities. *Other indications:* Residents of nursing homes and other long-term–care and assisted living facilities; persons likely to transmit influenza to persons at high risk (i.e., in-home household contacts and caregivers of children aged 0–59 months, or persons of all ages with high-risk conditions); and anyone who would like to be vaccinated. Healthy, nonpregnant persons aged 5–49 years without high-risk medical conditions who are not contacts of severely immunocompromised persons in special care units can receive either intranasally administered influenza vaccine (FluMist®) or inactivated vaccine. Other persons should receive the inactivated vaccine.

Appendix B: Recommended Adult Immunization Schedule, United States, October 2006–September 2007 (continued)

Footnotes

6. Pneumococcal polysaccharide vaccination. *Medical indications:* Chronic disorders of the pulmonary system (excluding asthma); cardiovascular diseases; diabetes mellitus; chronic liver diseases, including liver disease as a result of alcohol abuse (e.g.,cirrhosis); chronic renal failure or nephrotic syndrome; functional or anatomic asplenia (e.g., sickle cell disease or splenectomy [if elective splenectomy is planned, vaccinate at least 2 weeks before surgery]); immunosuppressive conditions (e.g., congenital immunodeficiency, HIV infection [vaccinate as close to diagnosis as possible when CD4 cell counts are highest], leukemia, lymphoma, multiple myeloma, Hodgkin disease, generalized malignancy, organ or bone marrow transplantation); chemotherapy with alkylating agents, antimetabolites, or high-dose, long-term corticosteroids; and cochlear implants. *Other indications:* Alaska Natives and certain American Indian populations and residents of nursing homes or other long-term–care facilities.

7. Revaccination with pneumococcal polysaccharide vaccine. One-time revaccination after 5 years for persons with chronic renal failure or nephrotic syndrome; functional or anatomic asplenia (e.g., sickle cell disease or splenectomy); immunosuppressive conditions (e.g., congenital immuno-deficiency, HIV infection, leukemia, lymphoma, multiple myeloma, Hodgkin disease, generalized malignancy, or organ or bone marrow transplantation); or chemotherapy with alkylating agents, antimetabolites, or high-dose, long-term corticosteroids. For persons aged ≥ 65 years, one-time revaccination if they were vaccinated ≥ 5 years previously and were aged < 65 years at the time of primary vaccination.

8. Hepatitis A vaccination. *Medical indications:* persons with chronic liver disease and persons who receive clotting factor concentrates. *Behavioral indications:* men who have sex with men and persons who use illegal drugs. *Occupational indications:* persons working with hepatitis A virus (HAV)–infected primates or with HAV in a research laboratory setting. *Other indications:* persons traveling to or working in countries that have high or intermediate endemicity of hepatitis A (a list of countries is available at http://www.cdc.gov/travel/diseases.htm) and any person who would like to obtain immunity. Current vaccines should be administered in a 2-dose schedule at either 0 and 6–12 months, or 0 and 6–18 months. If the combined hepatitis A and hepatitis B vaccine is used, administer 3 doses at 0, 1, and 6 months .

9. Hepatitis B vaccination. *Medical indications:* Persons with end-stage renal disease, including patients receiving hemodialysis; persons seeking evaluation or treatment for a sexually transmitted disease (STD); persons with HIV infection; persons with chronic liver disease; and persons who receive clotting factor concentrates. *Occupational indications:* healthcare workers and public-safety workers who are exposed to blood or other potentially infectious body fluids. *Behavioral indications:* sexually active persons who are not in a long-term, mutually monogamous relationship (i.e., persons with > 1 sex partner during the previous 6 months); current or recent injection-drug users; and men who have sex with men. *Other indications:* household contacts and sex partners of persons with chronic hepatitis B virus (HBV) infection; clients and staff members of institutions for persons with developmental disabilities; all clients of STD clinics; international travelers to countries with high or intermediate prevalence of chronic HBV infection (a list of countries is available at http://www.cdc.gov/travel/diseases.htm); and any adult seeking protection from HBV infection. Settings where hepatitis B vaccination is recommended for all adults: STD treatment facilities; HIV testing and treatment facilities; facilities providing drug-abuse treatment and prevention services; healthcare settings providing services for injection-drug users or men who have sex with men; correctional facilities; end-stage renal disease programs and facilities for chronic hemodialysis patients; and institutions and nonresidential daycare facilities for persons with developmental disabilities. *Special formulation indications:* for adult patients receiving hemodialysis and other immunocompromised adults, 1 dose of 40 mcg/mL (Recombivax HB) or 2 doses of 20 mcg/mL (Engerix-B).

10. Meningococcal vaccination. *Medical indications:* adults with anatomic or functional asplenia, or terminal complement component deficiencies. *Other indications:* first-year college students living in dormitories; microbiologists who are routinely exposed to isolates of *Neisseria meningitidis*; military recruits; and persons who travel to or live in countries in which meningococcal disease is hyperendemic or epidemic (e.g., the "meningitis belt" of Sub-Saharan Africa during the dry season [December–June]), particularly if contact with local populations will be prolonged. Vaccination is required by the government of Saudi Arabia for all travelers to Mecca during the annual Hajj. Meningococcal conjugate vaccine is preferred for adults with any of the preceeding indications who are aged ≤ 55 years, although meningococcal polysaccharide vaccine (MPSV4) is an acceptable alternative. Revaccination after 5 years might be indicated for adults previously vaccinated with MPSV4 who remain at high risk for infection (e.g., persons residing in areas in which disease is epidemic).

11. Selected conditions for which *Haemophilus influenzae* type b (Hib) vaccination may be used. Hib conjugate vaccines are licensed for children aged 6 weeks–71 months. No efficacy data are available on which to base a recommendation concerning use of Hib vaccine for older children and adults with the chronic conditions associated with an increased risk for Hib disease. However, studies suggest good immunogenicity in patients who have sickle cell disease, leukemia, or HIV infection or have had splenectomies; administering vaccine to these patients is not contraindicated.

This schedule indicates the recommended age groups and medical indications for routine administration of currently licensed vaccines for persons aged ≥19 years, as of October 1, 2006. Licensed combination vaccines may be used whenever any components of the combination are indicated and when the vaccine's other components are not contraindicated. For detailed recommendations on all vaccines, including those used primarily for travelers or that are issued during the year, consult the manufacturers' package inserts and the complete statements from the Advisory Committee on Immunization Practices (http://www.cdc.gov/nip/publications/acip-list.htm).

Report all clinically significant postvaccination reactions to the Vaccine Adverse Event Reporting System (VAERS). Reporting forms and instructions on filing a VAERS report are available at http://www.vaers.hhs.gov or by telephone, 800-822-7967.

Information on how to file a Vaccine Injury Compensation Program claim is available at http://www.hrsa.gov/vaccinecompensation or by telephone, 800-338-2382. To file a claim for vaccine injury, contact the U.S. Court of Federal Claims, 717 Madison Place, N.W., Washington, D.C. 20005; telephone, 202-357-6400.

Additional information about the vaccines in this schedule and contraindications for vaccination is also available at http://www.cdc.gov/nip or from the CDC-INFO Contact Center at 800-CDC-INFO (800-232-4636) in English and Spanish, 24 hours a day, 7 days a week.

Approved by the Advisory Committee on Immunization Practices, the American College of Obstetricians and Gynecologists, the American Academy of Family Physicians, and the American College of Physicians

Appendix C Selected Vaccine Information Web Sites

CDC National Center for Immunizations and Respiratory Diseases Immunization Web site	*www.cdc.gov/vaccines*
Immunization Action Coalition	*www.immunize.org*
Children's Hospital of Philadelphia Vaccine Education Center	*www.vaccine.chop.edu*
National Network for Immunization Information	*www.immunizationinfo.org*
Johns Hopkins University School of Public Health, Institute for Vaccine Safety	*www.vaccinesafety.edu*
Pregnancy registries	
HPV vaccine	*www.merckpregnancyregistries.com/gardasil.html* 800-986-8999
VARIVAX	*www.merckpregnancyregistries.com/varivax.html*
National Center for Infectious Diseases Travelers' Health	*http://wwwn.cdc.gov/travel/contentVaccinations.aspx*
Vaccine Storage and Handling Toolkit	*http://www2a.cdc.gov/nip/isd/shtoolkit/splash.html*
Immunization Practice Toolkit	*http://www2.cdc.gov/nip/isd/immtoolkit/content/clinicops/improverates.htm*
Global Advisory Committee on Vaccine Safety (GACVS), WHO	*www.who.int/vaccine_safety/en/*
VAERS Submission Web page	*https://secure.vaers.org/VaersDataEntryintro.htm*
Immunization Safety Review, Institute of Medicine	*www.iom.edu/?ID=4705*
Travelers vaccine information	
Centers for Disease Control and Prevention Travelers' Health	*wwwn.cdc.gov/travel/*
TravelersVaccines.Com	*www.travelersvaccines.com/En/Index.cfm*

"You can never be too rich nor too thin."

ATTRIBUTED TO WALLIS,
DUCHESS OF WINDSOR

7
Drugs to Promote Optimum Weight

Cecilia Jevitt

Chapter Glossary

Anorexia nervosa A serious mental illness in which the individual suffering from the condition incorrectly perceives herself as overweight and engages in extreme means (such as starving and purging) to lose weight.

Binge eating disorder The most common eating disorder; the individual suffering from the condition regularly eats excessive amounts of food.

Body mass index (BMI) A relative measure of weight for height using a standard calculation.

Bulimia nervosa A condition in which an individual eats excessively (see binge eating disorder), followed by purging the food using a variety of methods (e.g., vomiting).

Diet General foods eaten by an individual. The word often is used imprecisely to connote weight reduction. However, a "diet" may be configured to gain, lose, or maintain weight.

Fen-Phen Brand name for the drug made up of a combination of fenfluramine and phentermine, used for weight loss. It is no longer available.

Obesigenic agents Pharmacologic medications whose side effects include weight gain.

Obese A person with a BMI of 30.0 or greater. This may be subdivided further into 3 classes. Class 3 obesity (a BMI of 40 or greater) may be termed morbid obesity.

Overweight An individual with a BMI between 25.0 and 29.9.

Yo-yo dieting A cycle of weight loss and weight gain.

Introduction

Maintaining an optimum weight is a health challenge. Before mechanization, hours were spent each day gathering or growing food; these are physical activities that use energy. Expenditure usually balanced intake. However, during the last half century, food intake has remained stable while activity levels have fallen. Mechanized farming, manufacturing, and information technology along with individual car ownership and hours watching broadcast entertainment minimize energy use. Few residents of postindustrial nations do daily heavy manual labor, and thus intake regularly exceeds energy expenditure. For weight loss to occur, regardless of medication use, energy expenditure must exceed intake. Medications can support planned weight loss by suppressing appetite and signaling satiety.

Unlike the excessive intake of other illness-producing substances, such as tobacco or alcohol, food cannot be avoided entirely. Some food must be consumed several times a day for health and always remains an object of potential excessive intake. Eating has been integrated into family and work patterns as three meals a day. Meals are designated rest, relaxation, and communication times. Holidays have culturally specific celebratory foods, and religions have ceremonial meals and foods. Persistent willpower is necessary to avoid overeating in societies with an abundance of resources, regular relaxation times, and frequent celebrations.

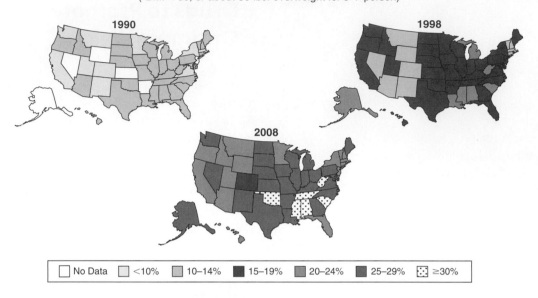

Figure 7-1 Obesity trends among US adults. *Source:* CDC Behavioral Risk Factor Surveillances System.

Thirty percent of American women are **overweight** and another 30% are **obese**.[1] Optimum weight is not defined by clothing size or physical attractiveness; rather, optimum weight is weight that does not increase risk for disease. Obesity increases women's risks for abnormal menstrual patterns, infertility, early pregnancy loss, fetal malformations, surgical birth, postpartum hemorrhage, lactation difficulties, depression, diabetes, hypertension, heart disease, sleep apnea, joint pain, and a variety of cancers.[2] Being overweight is not as strongly linked with risk for disease; however uncontrolled weight gain is the first step to obesity. The prevalence of overweight and obesity in postindustrial societies, as illustrated in Figure 7-1, mandates that clinicians of all specialties view **body mass index (BMI)** as a vital sign and be familiar with obesity prevention strategies and pharmacologic treatments.

Overweight and Obesity

BMI is a relative measure of weight for height using the formula[3] [weight (pounds)/height (inches)^2] × 703. Overweight is defined as a BMI between 26 and 29.9, and a BMI ≥ 30 indicates obesity.[3,4] BMI is an imperfect measure of adiposity because it can be inflated by large bone and muscle mass.[3,4] Table 7-1 lists the BMI categories. Each

Table 7-1 Weight Classifications by BMI and Body Fat Content

Classification	BMI	Women: Percentage of Body Fat	Men: Percentage of Body Fat
Underweight	< 18.5	23–31	13–21
Normal	18.7–24.9	31–37	21–25
Overweight	25.0–29.9	37–42	27–31
Obesity class I	30.0–34.9	> 42	> 31
Obesity class II	35–39.9		
Obesity class III	≥ 40		

Note: BMI is a relation between weight and height. It can be calculated in several ways, based on choice of measurement instruments.
BMI = weight in kilograms divided by (height in meters)^2 or
BMI = weight in pounds × 703 divided by (height in inches)^2 or
BMI = weight in pounds × 4.88 divided by (height in feet)^2
Source: Institute of Medicine 2002.[4]

BMI level represents approximately 5 pounds (2.27 kg). In general, women have a higher percentage of body fat per BMI level than men because men have more muscle mass.

Waist measurements in women (measured just above iliac crest) > 35 inches (88.8 cm) indicate excess abdominal fat and are correlated with the same health risks as obese BMIs. Abdominal fat is metabolically active. It produces hormones including leptin and inflammatory substances such as cytokines.[5,6] It has been hypothesized that chronic inflammation may be the root of many of obesity's comorbid diseases.

Women often strive for a weight they perceive as attractive instead of healthy. If, for example, a woman is 5'6" and weighs 196 pounds (168 cm, 88.9 kg), she has a BMI of 32. Losing 5% of total body weight (10 pounds [4.54 kg], BMI 30) reduces risk for hypertension, diabetes, dyslipidemia, and heart disease.[3] Another 10% loss (20 pounds [8.94 kg], BMI 27) further reduces risk and is achievable by most women with decreased intake and increased physical activity.[6] A study published in 2007 reported that for each 1 kg (2.2 pounds) lost, the risk of metabolic syndrome was reduced by 8%.[7] To attain a normal or healthy BMI of 25, a 40-pound (18 kg) weight loss would be required. Losing and sustaining a loss of more than 10% body weight is difficult,[7] yet women often strive to be unrealistic weights. For example, a loss of almost 80 pounds (36 kg) would be necessary for this woman to wear a size 8 dress.

Healthy intake reductions and exercise increases produce a 1-pound-a-week weight loss.[4] Once weight is lost, intake limitations and activity increases must continue or weight will be regained.[4] Controlling appetite and sustaining the motivation to exercise for years is a challenge that makes weight loss and control medications attractive.

▌ Physiology of Weight Gain and Loss

Weight abnormalities can be caused by alterations in appetite and energy expenditure, physical or mental disease, eating disorders, and medications.

Mechanical and Neurohormonal Control of Energy Homeostasis

The body strives to balance energy intake with expenditure through central nervous system control. Hunger is stimulated before eating by afferent visual and olfactory sensory signals that prepare the body to eat and digest food. Peripheral distention and chemoreceptors in the gut and energy conversion in the liver signal intake via the vagus nerve in the area postrema and the nucleus of the solitary tract.[8] Brain stem receptors detect circulating levels of nutrients and their metabolites.

Ingested neurotransmitter precursors alter central nervous system neuron-chemical activity, such as serotonin production, particularly in the hypothalamic nuclei and the limbic areas.[8] The serotonin, dopamine,

norepinephrine, and endocannabinoid systems all modulate feelings of hunger and satiety. Food intake and meal size are both decreased when serotonin (5-HT) or its precursors tryptophan and 5-HTP are increased. Selective serotonin receptor agonists are under investigation as appetite modulators.[9] Serotonin reuptake inhibitors, such as phenterimine (Adipex-P), fenfluramine (Pondimin), and sibutramine (Meridia) are known to reduce hunger. Noradrenaline mechanisms, rather than 5-HT, may account for the appetite-reducing action of sibutramine (Meridia). Eating causes an increase in endogenous noradrenaline.[9] Medications such as amphetamine, phenylpropanolamine, and sibutramine, which increase noradrenaline, reduce appetite and intake. Dopamine activation decreases food intake. If D_1 or D_2 receptors are stimulated by selective dopamine agonists, food consumption decreases.[9] Bupropion (Wellbutrin) is both a noradrenaline and dopamine reuptake inhibitor. Bromocriptine (Parlodel), a D_2 receptor, is under investigation as an appetite suppressant.[9] Endogenous cannabinoids interact with cannabinoid type 1 (CB_1) receptors in fat, liver, skeletal muscle, and other tissues to stimulate appetite. The exogenous cannabinoid found in cannabis sativa, or marijuana, is an example of this effect. Selective CB_1 receptor-blockers, such as rimonabant (Acomplia), decrease appetite with psychoactive effects.[10]

In addition to the effects of neurotransmitters, a variety of hormones are involved in appetite and satiety including insulin, leptin, ghrelin, neuropeptide Y, cholecystokinin, pancreatic polypeptide, peptide YY and glucagon-like peptide.[6] Many of these hormones are under investigation for use in weight control. Gut distention, adequate levels of nutrients, and neurotransmitters produce feelings of satiety.[8] Medications to optimize weight could, therefore, intervene in excessive intake through increasing and prolonging gastrointestinal distention, decreasing chemoreceptor signaling, or increasing the amount of neurotransmitters necessary for satiety.

Most body cells undergo periods of growth, programmed aging, and death (apoptosis). Adipose cells do not die but expand or contract to accommodate excess energy stored as fat. Leptin, produced in abdominal fat stores, signals hunger to increase eating and conserve fat stores. Leptin is produced even after weight loss, signaling the body to eat and regain lost weight.

Age Variations in Energy Expenditure

Body size and composition, resting metabolic rate differences that are independent of body composition, and the thermal effect of food (the ability of intake to increase energy expenditure) are influenced by genetic inheritance.[4] Studies attribute 25–50% of body composition to genetic factors.[4] The genetics of weight homeostasis are being studied.

As women age, their caloric needs change. Growth to 18 years of age uses more calories than necessary for weight maintenance. Children's linear and ponderal growth occur at different times, preventing the reliable use of BMI under age 18; instead, reference weights for children that have been established by the World Health Organization should be employed. Children who are less than the 3rd percentile of weight for age/height (length) are undernourished while, conversely, overweight children exceed the 97th percentile of weight for length.[4]

Women's thermal energy expenditures are approximately 16% lower than men's, giving them lower daily caloric requirements. For reproductive-aged women, basal metabolic rate and resting metabolic rate increase slightly during the luteal phase of the menstrual cycle. An adult woman with a BMI between 18.5 and 25 and low activity level needs approximately 2000 calories per day to maintain body weight while men in the same BMI and activity categories need 2500 calories per day. Institute of Medicine and US Department of Agriculture nutrition guidelines are based on a 2000-calorie-per-day **diet**. Measuring intake against this standard may lead some women to unwittingly overeat, as some sedentary women need only 1500 to 1700 calories per day, particularly those with heights less than 63 inches and women who are over the age of 30.[4]

The decline in resting energy expenditure with age, coupled with a loss of fat-free body mass, lowers the basal metabolic rate. In men with stable weights, basal metabolic rate drops 1–2% per decade. However, this decline accelerates for women after age 50, and resting metabolic rate and fat-free mass further decrease postmenopausally in the absence of hormone replacement therapy.[4]

Diseases Associated with Weight Alterations

Many physical diseases alter weight homeostasis. Physical causes of weight change, such as diabetes and thyroid abnormalities, must be investigated before weight maintenance therapies are initiated. Nicotine suppresses appetite. Tobacco cessation without lifestyle changes and behavioral therapy commonly is followed by weight gain. Unfortunately, some women recognize this association and do not discontinue smoking for fear of weight gain, and women who stop tobacco use for pregnancy often restart in the postpartum period in an effort to control their weight.

The hormonal disturbances associated with obesity may cause anovulation, thereby reducing fertility. Weight losses of as little as 10% of body weight have been demonstrated to restore ovulation and fertility. Many published studies have shown that metformin (Glucophage) enhances insulin sensitivity and has been used preconceptionally to enhance weight loss and restore ovulation.[11-14] However, a meta-analysis of metformin and glitazone use in polycystic ovary syndrome questions the methodology and power of these studies, thus the utility of metformin in ovulation restoration.[15]

Binge Eating Disorder

Most individuals occasionally overeat or binge, but persons with **binge eating disorder** regularly eat excessive quantities of food.[16] Binge eating disorder is the most common eating disorder.[16] It is more common among women than men, and it affects about 2% of the adult population living in the United States. Individuals with binge eating disorder are most often obese or go through cyclic bingeing and dieting (**yo-yo dieting**), alternating periods of overweight with obesity. Table 7-2 provides a list of the symptoms of binge eating disorder. Treatment plans using second-generation antidepressants such as fluvoxamine (Luvox) and fluoxetine (Prozac, Sarafem) along with weight-optimizing medications have been studied to reduce food binges.[17]

Bulimia Nervosa

Binge eating is a component of **bulimia nervosa**. Persons with bulimia nervosa eat excessively and then purge using induced vomiting, diuretics, or laxatives in an attempt to prevent weight gain. Binge eating alternates with purging, fasting, and excessive exercise.[16] Antianxiety agents along with weight-optimizing medications are being studied for treatment of this disorder.

Anorexia Nervosa

Anorexia nervosa is a serious mental illness. Individuals with this disease see themselves as overweight and starve and purge to attain abnormally low body weight (Table 7-2). Anorexia nervosa is most common in female adolescents and young women, with an estimated 0.5 to 3.7% of American women suffering with anorexia during their lives.[18] Challenges in treatment of anorexia are to overcome obsessions with eating and weight while

Table 7-2 Signs of Eating Disorders

Binge Eating Disorder	Anorexia Nervosa
Consume an unusually large quantity of food	Resistance to maintaining body weight at or above a minimally normal weight for age and height
Eat much more quickly than usual during binge episodes	
Continue eating until uncomfortably full	Intense fears of gaining weight or becoming fat, even though underweight
Consume large amounts of food even when not hungry	Disturbances in the way in which body weight or shape is experienced, undue
Eat alone because of embarrassment about the amount of food eaten	influence of body weight or shape on self-evaluation, or denial of the seriousness of the current low body weight
Feel disgusted, depressed, or guilty after overeating	Infrequent or absent menstrual periods in females who have reached
Feel eating is out of control	puberty

Source: National Institute of Mental Health.[18]

stimulating appetite and changing self-image. Anorexia nervosa generally requires individual treatment with psychotropic medications within a program of biobehavioral support. Individuals with a history of anorexia never should be prescribed weight-loss medications.

Obesigenic Medications

Several drug categories have weight gain as a possible or even common side effect. Table 7-3 lists some common drug categories whose side effects include weight gain. Prominent among these **obesigenic agents** are glucocorticoids and various psychiatric agents.

Glucocorticoids

Long-term use of glucocorticoids promotes weight gain. All glucocorticoids stimulate gluconeogenesis in the liver and inhibit peripheral glucose use. Glucocorticoids also cause protein breakdown in muscle, bone, and skin, which increases circulating amino acids. These amino acids stimulate hepatic enzyme activity, causing increased glycogen deposition and decreased glycolysis. High-dose exogenous steroid use promotes insulin resistance with resulting carbohydrate intolerance and fasting hyperglycemia. Long-term steroid use mobilizes and remodels adipose deposits resulting in characteristic fat deposits on the neck, supraclavicular area, and face.

Medications for Schizophrenia

Individuals with schizophrenia have a high prevalence of obesity and metabolic syndrome.[19] Olanzapine (Zyprexa), risperidone (Risperdal), quetiapine (Seroquel), and clozapine (Clozaril) are antipsychotic medications

Table 7-3 Drugs That May Cause Weight Gain

Drugs	Examples Generic (Brand)
Class of drugs that cause weight gain	
Antipsychotics	Olanzapine (Zyprexa), risperidone (Risperdal), quetiapine (Seroquel), clozapine (Clozaril)
Beta-blockers	Atenolol (Tenormin), labetalol (Trandate), metoprolol (Lopressor)
Corticosteroids	Methylprednisolone (Solu-Medrol), prednisone (Deltasone)
Sulfonylureas	Chlorpropamide (Diabinese), glyburide (Micronase)
Thiazolidinedione (glitazones)	Rosiglitazone (Avandia), pioglitazone (Actos)
Tricyclic antidepressants	Amitriptyline (Elavil), nortriptyline (Aventyl), imipramine (Tofranil)
Individual drugs that cause weight gain	
Insulin	
Lithium (Eskalith)	
Valproate (Depakote)	

used in the treatment of schizophrenia that cause weight gain that often progresses to obesity.[20-22] Investigations using sibutramine (Meridia), topiramate (Topamax), or metformin (Glucophage) to counter this weight gain are ongoing.[19,21,22]

Hormonal Contraceptives

Excessive weight gain is a commonly reported side effect of hormonal contraceptives such as combined oral contraceptive pills and medroxyprogesterone acetate (DMPA); however, this side effect of contraceptives is not supported by FDA premarketing research.[23] Despite this, many women continue to associate hormonal contraceptive use with weight gain. One of the newer pills on the market contains the progestin drospirenone that is chemically related to spironolactone and has antimineralcorticoid properties that produce mild diuresis. Drospirenone is used in the oral contraceptives Yasmin (3 mg drospirenone and 30 mcg ethinyl estradiol) and YAZ (3 mg drospirenone and 20 mcg ethinyl estradiol). Drospirenone is favored by some endocrinologists for use by obese women with polycystic ovarian syndrome because of its antiandrenergic properties. Early marketing of these products stressed less bloating and fluid retention. Because of the marketing and the mild diuretic effect, some consumers viewed drospiranone as a weight-loss pill, but no evidence has been found to support this claim.

Weight-Loss Guidelines

Current guidelines support antiobesity drug use only as part of a comprehensive weight optimization plan that includes dietary modification, increased physical activity, lifestyle modification, and behavioral management, because integration of these components has an additive, synergistic effect.[3,24,25] Weight management through intake reduction, increased exercise, lifestyle modifications, and behavioral therapies lack the potential physical and cognitive side effects associated with use of weight management medications alone. Therefore, non-medicinal and nonsurgical weight-loss interventions are recommended for overweight individuals (BMIs 26–29.9). A reduction of 500 to 1000 calories per day will provide for a sustainable weight loss of 1 pound per week. Total fats should be 30% or less of dietary intake.[3,24,25]

Most weight loss is accomplished by decreased calorie intake; however, increased physical activity burns calories and stabilizes blood glucose through cellular use of noninsulin glucose. A walking program incrementally increased from 10 minutes to 30 to 60 minutes a day 5 days a week can provide the physical activity necessary for weight stabilization and cardiac health.[3,25] Lifestyle modifications are accomplished through behavioral changes. Individuals need insight into their eating behaviors to change to healthier patterns. For example, through counseling, a woman might realize that she eats a quart of her favorite ice cream when she has an upsetting day at work. Substituting other stress-relieving tactics could lower consumption.

Weight-loss medications are indicated for individuals with BMIs greater than 29 or individuals whose BMIs are greater than 26 and who have comorbidities such as hypertention or type 2 diabetes. Weight regain occurs with all weight-loss medications once the medication is discontinued unless intake is kept low and physical activity is maintained.[3,25-27]

Weight-loss surgery to correct obesity includes gastric banding and gastric bypass. The potentially serious side effects of these surgeries limit their use to individuals with a BMI of ≥ 40 who have failed medical therapy, or those individuals with BMIs ≥ 35 who have comorbid conditions.[3,24,25] Following these surgeries, individuals will need vitamin and mineral supplementation for life. For example, calcium supplementation is essential to prevent postsurgical osteoporosis.

Pharmacokinetics and Pharmacodynamics of Weight Optimization Drugs

Medications to optimize weight fall into these three categories: (1) those that increase energy expenditure, (2) those that reduce appetite, and (3) those that decrease nutrient absorption (Figure 7-2). Single-drug weight-loss therapies at best produce an 8–10% loss of initial body weight.[28] Because other weight-loss treatments, such as reduction diets and exercise programs, have fewer side effects than weight-loss medications and have equal weight-loss success, the benefits and risks of weight-loss medications must be carefully considered. Weight-loss medications are most effective when they are used to control appetite and signal satiety during a program of restricted intake and increased physical activity. Weight-loss drugs may be of more value for obese individuals with mechanical arthritis or reduced cardiac function, which limits physical activity along with dietary restriction, than they would be for other obese people who could implement increased exercise programs with the dietary restrictions.

In general, weight-loss drugs should not be used by those with hepatic or renal disease. Weight loss can precipitate or exacerbate gallstone formation; therefore individuals with preexisting cholelithiasis should use weight-loss medication cautiously. Anorexia nervosa and obesity, as well as many weight-management medications, may cause menstrual irregularities and amenorrhea among reproductive-aged women. Therefore, overweight or obese women seeking treatment for metrorrhagia or oligomenorrhea should be questioned routinely about use of antiobesity medications.

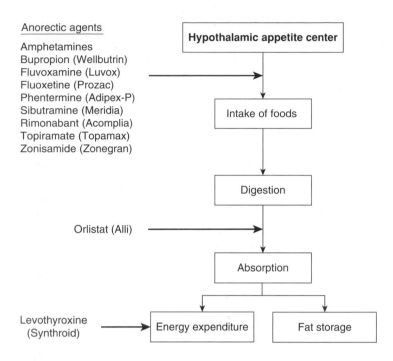

Figure 7-2 Weight loss drugs: site of action.

Drugs That Increase Energy Expenditure

Levothyroxine (T$_4$, Levo-T, Levoxyl, Synthroid, Unithroid, Thyro-Tabs, Levothroid) is the manufactured levo isomer of thyroxine. Indicated primarily for the treatment of hypothyroidism, it promotes protein and carbohydrate metabolism and increases gluconeogenesis. Levothyroxine is a cardiostimulant and decreases cholesterol concentrations in the liver and bloodstream. Physiologic doses of the drug gradually reduce overweight or obesity that is secondary to hypothyroidism.

Exogenous levothyroxine has been administered since the 1950s for weight loss. Although not FDA approved for weight loss, weight-loss clinics across the United States use high-dose levothyroxine to raise metabolism, thereby burning calories. The induced hyperthyroidism necessary for weight loss may produce serious and dangerous side effects. Withdrawal of thyroid hormone may cause hypoglycemia, and long-term, high-dose levels have been associated with osteoporosis, especially in postmenopausal females.

Levothyroxine use is contraindicated for individuals with uncontrolled adrenal insufficiency, untreated thyrotoxicosis, and myocardial infarction. It should be used cautiously by women with hypertension, angina, cardiac arrhythmias, previous myocardial infarction, and/or coronary artery disease. The cardiostimulatory effects of levothyroxine may precipitate cardiac arrhythmias and angina, and its use for individuals who are taking sympathomimetic agents for coronary artery disease treatment may result in coronary insufficiency. In addition, levothyroxine alters blood glucose levels and may alter the effectiveness of antidiabetes medications.

Drugs That Reduce Appetite

Amphetamine

Amphetamine, a schedule C-II controlled substance, is a sympathomimetic adrenergic agonist that suppresses appetite. Amphetamine was widely used in the 1950s and 1960s for weight loss. Because of its addictive properties and psychiatric effects such as insomnia, it is no longer indicated for weight loss.

Fenfluramine and Dexfenfluramine

Fenfluramine (Pondimin) and dexfenfluramine (Redux) stimulate the release of serotonin and inhibit serotonin reuptake, thereby decreasing appetite. They also increase glucose uptake by skeletal muscles. Fenfluramine was

Box 7-1 Gone But Not Forgotten: The Fen-Phen Fiasco

The Fen-Phen (fenfluramine and phentermine) regimen was introduced in 1992. Weight loss using this drug regimen was highly successful with losses of 15% of initial body weight.[28] However, associated cases of pulmonary hypertension and valvular heart disease were reported among 5–25% of women using this combination of drugs. The association was confounded by the fact that obesity alone also is associated with cardiovascular disease. However, the FDA disapproved the combination in 1996, and the manufacturers voluntarily withdrew the drugs from the American market in 1997, despite its widespread use and favorable safety record in Europe.[5]

Combined phentermine and fenfluramine is still available in Europe and over the Internet in the United States with a prescription. The severity of valvular disease decreases following the termination of Fen-Phen use; however, persons who have used Fen-Phen need to report dyspnea, decreasing exercise tolerance, syncope, angina, and edema immediately, as all of these are signs of cardiac disease.

prescribed with phentermine as the **Fen-Phen** regimen. It is no longer marketed in the United States and is not FDA approved for use, although both fenfluramine and dexfenfluramine may still be available in Europe or available via the Internet (Box 7-1).

Phentermine

Phentermine (Adipex-P, Atti-Plex-P, Fastin, Ionamin, Kraft-Obese, Pro-Fast SA, Pro-Fast SR, Tara-8), a noradrenergic drug that suppresses appetite by stimulating sympathetic activity, is chemically and pharmacologically related to the amphetamines. It is indicated for short-term (6 week) weight-loss therapy. Phentermine can be purchased over the Internet without a prescription (Table 7-4).

The most common side effects associated with phentermine include irritability, insomnia, and personality changes. Altered alertness places phentermine users at risk for accidents when driving or using heavy equipment. Phentermine use is contraindicated for persons with hypertension, heart disease, glaucoma, or depression. Because it is a sympathomimetic drug, it is also contraindicated for persons with hyperthyroidism. Long-term use of phentermine can cause dependence. Phentermine can aggravate anxiety, mania, agitation, and psychosis. Abrupt cessation of therapy is known to cause depression or extreme fatigue. Use should be gradually tapered before discontinuation. It should not be used for those with a history of anorexia nervosa, depression, or substance abuse. Phentermine interacts with monoamine oxidase (MAO) inhibitors, causing increased cardiac stimulation and hypotension. Insulin requirements and the actions of other hypoglycemic agents may be altered by phentermine use.

A phentermine-fluoxetine (phen-flu) combination is being investigated in Europe as a Fen-Phen replacement. In one study, phentermine-fluoxetine users had lower weight loss (9%) than phentermine-fenfluramine users (12.6%) but developed no cardiac valve lesions after 6 months of treatment.[28]

Sibutramine

Sibutramine (Meridia) is a serotonin and norepinephrine reuptake inhibitor that is theorized to suppress appetite by signaling early satiety. Sibutramine is indicated for weight loss for healthy individuals as part of a program of dietary management and increased physical activity. Some sources credit sibutramine with increasing resting energy expenditure. However, in a randomized trial of obese adolescents, those using sibutramine plus an energy-restricted diet and exercise had weight losses comparable to adolescents who followed the same energy-restricted diet and exercise regimen.[26] Weight-loss programs that include sibutramine have demonstrated more weight loss when compared to those using orlistat (Xenical).[27]

Sibutramine (Meridia) can be taken with or without food. In clinical trials, sibutramine has been used in the morning. The sympathetic actions of sibutramine increase blood pressure and raise pulse. Doses may be titrated to minimize these side effects. Doses as high as 20 mg per day have been studied; however significant weight loss occurs at the 10- to 15-mg dose, and side effects are markedly increased at the 20-mg dose. Some individuals demonstrate no response to sibutramine. Weight loss of 4 pounds (1.8 kg) during the first month of treatment is an indicator of successful use. At least half of individuals on the drug lose 5% of their body weight after 6–12 months of treatment. Safe use beyond 2 years has not been studied.

Table 7-4 Medications Used in Weight-Loss Therapy

Name Generic (Brand)	Formulations	Dose	Clinical Considerations
Phentermine (Adipex-P)	Tabs: 5 mg, 18.75 mg, 30 mg, 37.5 mg ER: 8 mg, 30 mg	8 mg tid PO or 17–37.5 qd PO taken 10–14 hrs before bedtime	For short-term use. Take 30 minutes before meals.
Sibutramine (Meridia)	Caps: 5 mg, 10 mg, 15 mg	15 mg qd PO. Initiate therapy with 5 mg/day and titrate up to 10–15 mg/day	For long-term use.
Topiramate (Topamax)	Tablets: 25 mg, 50 mg, 100 mg, 200 mg Available as sprinkle capsules to place over food	27–600 mg qd PO Average dose is 50 mg/day	Off-label use for binge eating disorders. Can be taken without regard to meals. Has multiple drug–drug interactions. GI side effects are common. Must be withdrawn gradually.
Zonisamide (Zonegran)	Caps: 25 mg, 50 mg, 100 mg	100 mg/day gradually increased to 400 mg/day*	Off-label use for binge eating disorders. GI side effects are common. Must be withdrawn gradually.
Fluoxetine (Prozac, Sarafem)	Caps: 10 mg, 20 mg, 40 mg Tabs: 20 mg, 40 mg	60 mg/day PO	FDA approved for binge eating disorders.
Fluvoxamine (Luvox)	Tabs: 25 mg, 50 mg, 100 mg	50 mg/day at HS May increase to maximum of 300 mg/day. If > 100 mg/day, give in divided doses	Off-label use for binge eating disorders.
Bupropion (Wellbutrin)	Tabs: 75 mg, 100 mg SR tabs: 100 mg, 150 mg, 200 mg ER tabs: 150 mg, 300 mg	150 mg q AM, increase by 100 mg/day every 3 days to a max of 350 mg/day in divided doses	Increased risk for seizures. Do not break, crush, or chew SR or ER formulations. Should allow 8 hours between doses.
Orlistat (Alli, Xenical)	Caps generic: 120 mg Caps trade: 60 mg	120 mg with each main meal containing fat. Max dose is 360 mg/day	For long-term use. Take with or up to 1 hour after a meal containing fat. Take a multivitamin containing fat-soluble vitamins at least 2 hours after taking orlistat.
Metformin (Glucophage)	Tabs: 500 mg, 850 mg, 1000 mg ER tabs: 500 mg, 750 mg	850 mg bid PO	Do not break, crush, or chew ER formulations. GI side effects are common. Contraindicated for persons with cardiac, renal, or liver disease secondary to risk for lactic acidosis.

Tabs = tablets; Caps = capsules; ER = extended release; SR = sustained release.
* Can be increased to 600 mg/day for persons who lose < 5% of body weight at the end of 12 weeks.

Sibutramine has many common side effects, including exhaustion, weakness, anxiety, insomnia, dizziness, drowsiness, sweating, and dry mouth. Gastrointestinal complaints include stomach pain, gas, nausea, vomiting, diarrhea, or constipation. Tachycardia, hypertension, chest pain, dyspnea, muscle and joint pain, and menstrual irregularities are more worrisome side effects. Sibutramine interacts with many medications including MAO inhibitors, many migraine medications including the ergotamines and the tryptans, bupropion, fentanyl, meperidine, lithium, ketoconazole, and many antidepressants and antianxiety agents. Sibutramine may interact with many over-the-counter agents, such as dextromethorphan, decongestants, and St. John's wort, to produce impaired judgement or motor skills. Medications that increase serotonin levels such as selective serotonin reuptake inhibitors (SSRIs) and triptans for migraine headaches must be avoided during sibutramine use.

Sibutramine is contraindicated for individuals with anorexia or bulimia nervosa, hypertension, heart disease, cardiac arrhythmias, seizure disorders, cholethiasis, closed-angle glaucoma, depression, hepatic disease, hypothyroidism, migraine headaches, neurologic disease, renal disease, and substance abuse. However, sibutramine use has not been associated with pulmonary hypertension or cardiac valve disease as have other serotonin-stimulating appetite suppressants.

Topiramate and Zonisamide

The ability to induce anorexia and persistent weight loss in obese individuals was discovered during clinical trials of topiramate (Topamax) and zonisamide (Zonegran), two antiepileptic drugs with similar actions and indications. Topiramate and zonisamide have multiple indications including the treatment of seizure disorders, alcoholism, bipolar disorder, diabetic neuropathy, mania, and migraine prophylaxis. The exact mechanisms of weight-loss action are unknown for topiramate and zonisamide; however, emerging research indicates that both inhibit the induction of carbonic anhydrases. Carbonic anhydrase enzymes are necessary for new lipogenesis in both the mitochondria and the cytosol of cells. Topiramate inhibits lipogenesis in adipocytes similarly to other sulfonamide carbonic anhydrase inhibitors.[29,30] Topiramate has been shown to produce significant weight loss and improve glucose homeostasis when used as an adjunct to diet and exercise therapy in persons with type 2 diabetes (Box 7-2).[31] Topiramate alone or in combination with sibutramine has been used to treat obesity associated with medications for bipolar disorder.[32,33]

Topiramate and zonisamide have multiple adverse reactions, including agitation, anorexia, depression, dizziness, drowsiness, emotional lability, euphoria, hallucinations, hypoesthesia, decreased libido, erectile dysfunction, menstrual irregularities, psychosis, tinnitus, and xerostomia. Driving and operating heavy equipment should be undertaken with caution due to the central nervous system side effects. Gastrointestinal symptoms include abdominal pain, constipation, diarrhea, gastritis, flatulence, gastroesophageal reflux, nausea, vomiting, and pancreatitis. These agents may be such effective anorexiants

---

Box 7-2   A Case of Chronic Obesity

MJ is a 37-year-old accountant who asked during her regular gynecologic visit, "Can you prescribe more of this weight-loss medication for me?" MJ revealed that her primary care provider had prescribed the phentermine a year ago but refuses to renew the prescription, partially due to concerns about her blood pressure. MJ lost 27 pounds while using phentermine, but since she discontinued it she has regained 23 pounds. MJ had four prior cycles of 25- to 30-pound (11.34–13.6 kg) weight loss and regain since age 20. Her highest weight was 212 pounds (BMI 34.2). Prior weight-loss medications included Fen-Phen, over-the-counter products with ephedra, and two cycles of phentermine.

MJ did little physical activity and disliked exercise. At this visit, her weight was 198 pounds, BMI was 32, and waist measurement was 45 inches. Her blood pressure was 146/94. Her thyroid function was normal, total cholesterol was 295 mg/dL, triglycerides were 210 mg/dL, and her HDLs were 34 mg/dL. Her fasting glucose was 112 mg/dL and her hemoglobin A1C was 6.5 mg/dL. Because of her prior Fen-Phen use, an EKG had been done; the results were normal. She is a nonsmoker.

MJ had the following four markers for metabolic syndrome: (1) obesity, (2) abdominal fat, (3) hypertension, and (4) elevated triglycerides, including elevated cholesterol and decreased high density lipoproteins. The clinician reviewed caloric needs, the effect of exercise on glycemic control and blood pressure, and metabolic syndrome. Weight optimization would be vital for preventing diabetes and heart disease. MJ would need a lifelong program of reduced intake and increased physical activity to prevent weight regain.

MJ hesitantly agreed to a referral to a local multidisciplinary weight-loss program. During program participation, she walked at lunch hour, gradually increasing her walking to 45 minutes each day. The program provided low-fat, nutritious meal cooking classes. MJ initiated sibutramine (Meridia) 5 mg per day that was increased to 15 mg per day over 6 weeks. Ten weeks after initiation of this program, she was dissatisfied with her loss and found a new provider who prescribed topiramate (Topamax) to augment weight loss. Although she lost 8 lbs during 3 weeks of topiramate use, she felt confused and stopped using the topiramate.

At 30 weeks of program participation, she had lost 25 pounds. This lowered her BMI to 27.9. Her total cholesterol was 170 mg/dL and her high density lipoproteins were 72 mg/dL. Her hemoglobin A1C was 4.8 mg/dL. Her blood pressure averaged 126/85. MJ hoped to double that loss and planned to continue sibutramine use.

that they cause hypoglycemia, anemia, osteopenia, and osteoporosis. Both topiramate and zonisamide are contraindicated for persons with biliary cirrhosis, hepatic or renal disease, chronic obstructive lung disease, emphysema, glaucoma, nephrolithiasis, and ocular disease.

Fluoxetine and Fluvoxamine

Fluoxetine (Prozac) and fluvoxamine (Luvox) are SSRIs that have been studied as components of weight-loss therapy for persons with binge eating disorder, bipolar disease-associated obesity, and obesity.[5,34] Fluoxetine (Prozac) has been approved by the FDA for the treatment of binge eating disorder in 60-mg-per-day oral doses. In studies, use of fluoxetine reduced food intake, improved insulin sensitivity, and decreased insulin requirements for individuals with type 2 diabetes.[5] Fluoxetine is not indicated for general treatment of obesity because of its frequent side effects, which include somnolence, agitation, alterations in libido and orgasmic dysfunction, diarrhea, and tremors.

Use of fluvoxamine to reduce binge eating disorders has been studied, and significant results in decreasing binge episodes and lowering BMI over 9 weeks were found. Oral doses ranged from 50–300 mg per day. The majority of participants failed to complete the study due to nausea, somnolence, and dizziness.[5] Fluvoxamine (Luvox) is currently used off label for binge eating, but it is important to note that SSRIs have recently been associated with suicidal ideation among young adults (age 18–24 years), and a black box warning currently cautions use of these drugs in persons younger than age 24 years.

Bupropion

Bupropion (Wellbutrin) is a noradrenaline and dopamine reuptake inhibitor indicated for treatment of depression. Unintentional weight loss during bupropion use suggested its utility in weight-loss therapy. This agent has also been used as adjunctive therapy for the treatment of seasonal affective disorder, nicotine dependence, bipolar disorder, and obesity. Incremental initiation reduces the risk of seizures, a potential side effect. Individuals with bulimia or anorexia nervosa who use bupropion are at increased risk for having seizures.

Bupropion may cause elevations in liver function tests. Central nervous system side effects include restlessness, agitation, anxiety, confusion, insomnia, paranoia, and hallucinations. Bupropion must be used cautiously with cardiac disease, as it may cause hypertension.

Drugs That Decrease Nutrient Absorption

Orlistat

Orlistat (Alli, Xenical) is a gastrointestinal lipase inhibitor that blocks the absorption of dietary fat by preventing gastric and pancreatic lipases from hydrolyzing dietary triglycerides into free fatty acids and monoglycerides. Numerous studies demonstrate reduced fasting insulin levels, reduced low density lipoproteins, lowered HbA1c, and improved glycemic control with orlistat use. It has minimal systemic absorption with more than 80% being excreted unchanged in feces. The brand Alli became available over the counter in the United States in 60 mg dosing in 2007, although Xenical in 120 mg capsules continues to be available by prescription only.

One orlistat capsule is administered with each main meal containing fat or within 1 hour after the meal. The dose is omitted when meals are missed or contain no fat. Orlistat has a modest effect on weight loss. One can expect to lose approximately 6 pounds more per year than can be lost with diet alone.

The most common side effects of orlistat (Alli, Xenical) are steatorrhea, flatulence, abdominal bloating, increased defecation, oily spotting, and fecal urgency and incontinence. Side effects increase with the amount of dietary fat consumed, with adverse gastrointestinal events being most common when fat exceeded 30% of intake. Poor lipid absorption decreases serum levels of β-carotene and vitamins A, D, and E, but vitamin deficiencies can be avoided by daily use of a fat-soluble vitamin-containing multivitamin that is taken at least 2 hours after orlistat use.

Rare cases of rash, urticaria, pruritis, and prolonged clotting times were reported during postmarketing surveillance. Orlistat is contraindicated in individuals with cholestasis, anorexia, or bulimia nervosa, and hyperoxaluria and clotting times must be monitored in those using anticoagulant therapy.

Other Weight-Loss Medications

Rimonabant (Acomplia) is a novel appetite suppressant that blocks the cannabinoid-1 (CB-1) receptor subtype. The use of cannabis sativa as an antiemetic and appetite stimulant in oncology established the role of endocannibinoids in appetite regulation. Rhimonabant is available in the United Kingdom and other European countries; however, the FDA denied its release in the United States in 2007,[6,35] as safety concerns centered on increased anxiety, depression, aggression, psychosis, and suicidal thoughts in rimonabant users.

The effectiveness of rimonabant is similar to that of sibutramine (Meridia) and orlistat (Xenical). Daily oral doses of 5 to 20 mg are used. Its most common side effects are nausea and diarrhea with some reports of mood disorders. Rimonabant use has been shown to improve glucose tolerance, lower blood pressure, and reduce leptin and C-reactive protein more than could be explained by weight loss alone. In a randomized, double-blind study comparing rimonabant to a placebo, a daily dose of rimonabant 20 mg was associated with significant ($P < .0001$) weight loss (-6.7 ± 0.5 kg), reduction in waist circumference (-5.8 ± 10.5 cm), increase in HDL cholesterol ($+10.0\pm1.6\%$), and a reduction in triglycerides ($-13.0\pm3.5\%$). Rimonabant may have central nervous system side effects, such as depression,[34] aggression, insomnia, psychosis, and suicidal thoughts, and it should not be prescribed for individuals with histories of psychiatric illness.[35,36] Seizures during use have been reported.

Long-term studies of rimonabant and atherosclerotic disease are under way.

Metformin

Metformin (Glucophage) is a biguanide that decreases liver glucose production while increasing insulin sensitivity in the liver and peripheral tissues. Metformin decreases intestinal glucose absorption and decreases triglycerides and low density lipoproteins while increasing high density lipoproteins. In nondiabetic individuals, metformin does not affect pancreatic β-cell function or cause hypoglycemia. Metformin induces weight loss in women with polycystic ovary disease. Metformin may be used as initial infertility treatment in anovulatory obese women with the aim of restoring ovulation following weight loss, although as aforementioned, the efficacy has been called into question (Box 7-3).[11-15] Metformin 850 mg is taken orally twice a day with meals for weight loss. This dose produces weight loss comparable to daily sibutramine doses and prescription-strength orlistat.[37]

Adverse reactions to metformin use include dizziness, headache, flushing, chills or sweating, myalgias, chest

Box 7-3 A Case of Obesity and Infertility

SH is a 24-year-old primary schoolteacher. After 3 years of marriage and 2 years of unsuccessful attempts to start a family, she has asked for fertility help during her annual gynecologic exam. She is a nonsmoker with no chronic diseases. Her menstrual cycles are approximately 70–90 day intervals with 2–3 days of painless spotting during each menses.

SH's height is 64 inches (162.6 cm), weight 207 pounds (93.9 kg), and her BMI is 35.5. Her blood pressure is 131/84, pulse 80, and respirations 18. Her physical examination was essentially normal. SH has facial acne with mild facial and abdominal hirsutism. The clinician explained the connections between excess adipose tissue, insulin resistance, excess estrogen storage, elevated androgens, and ovulatory irregularities. Her menstrual irregularities, hirsutism, and acne suggested polycystic ovary syndrome. The clinician ordered a transvaginal ultrasound to visualize ovarian mass and rule out reproductive organ anomalies, a fasting blood glucose, along with tests of her thyroid-stimulating hormone level and serum androgen level so these results would be available when SH had her appointment with the reproductive endocrinologist. SH's transvaginal ultrasound was normal, as were the serum glucose and thyroid-stimulating hormone level. Her serum androgen was near the upper limits of normal.

The reproductive endocrinologist advised SH that she most likely had polycystic ovarian syndrome and that a 5–10% loss of body weight was the easiest first treatment to restore ovulation. SH was prescribed metformin 850 mg to be taken orally twice a day with meals. She was also prescribed spironolactone (Aldactone) 50 mg orally per day to minimize androgenic action. Obesity increases the risk of fetal deformities, and SH was advised to take folic acid 400 mcg orally daily. SH joined a weight-loss program that focused on balanced, calorie-restricted nutrition, and she joined a women's gym.

(continues)

> ### Box 7-3 A Case of Obesity and Infertility (*continued*)
>
> At the end of 20 weeks, SH had lost 18 pounds (8.2 kg) and continued to take the metformin, spironolactone, and folic acid. She was losing patience with her planned meals and had stopped using the gym after 12 weeks. However, the 9% loss of body weight lowered her BMI to 32.4. Her blood pressure fell to an average of 124/70, and she had two menses that were a month apart. These successes encouraged SH to continue her planned eating and return to the gym. At the end of week 36, SH had maintained her weight at 189 pounds (85.7 kg, BMI 32) for 5 months and was pregnant.
>
> The 18-pound (8.2 kg) weight loss did not shift SH from an obese to an overweight BMI category; however, 20 pounds (9 kg) is the average annual loss associated with all weight-management therapies. Women with BMIs ≥ 30 are at increased risk for many perinatal complications, including fetal malformations, gestational diabetes, hypertension, deep vein thrombosis, macrosomia, induction of labor, cesarean birth, and shoulder dystocia. The reproductive endocrinologist advised SH to discontinue the metformin and spironolactone during pregnancy but to continue the folic acid during the first trimester. Using Institute of Medicine guidelines, SH was advised not to diet during pregnancy, but to anticipate a 15 pound weight gain.[53] A dietician reviewed carbohydrate counting and the American Diabetic Association Diet with SH, planning a 2000-calorie-per-day intake.

pressure, palpitations, and dyspnea. Metformin use may cause many gastrointestinal symptoms, including cramping, diarrhea, nausea, vomiting, flatulence, indigestion, and abnormal stools. Some individuals experience an annoying metallic taste.

Over-the-Counter Medications

A variety of herbs, vitamin and mineral supplements, and fibers are available over the counter for weight loss. Questions about over-the-counter weight diet pills or preparations should be a part of every primary care exam. Women who use these compounds are motivated to optimize weight and may be receptive to trying prescription weight-loss medications with proven efficacy.

Substances That Increase Energy Expenditure

Chromium Picolinate

An organic compound of trivalent chromium and picolinic acid, a derivative of tryptophan, is marketed as *chromium picolinate*. Chromium is an essential mineral that is an insulin cofactor. Most weight-loss compounds contain chromium picolinate in 200- to 400-mcg per day doses. One meta-analysis indicates that use over 6–14 weeks in individuals with BMIs of 28–33 provides statistically significant weight loss compared to a placebo, but clinically this amounts to approximately 2.5 pounds (1.1–1.2 kg).[38] Restricting intake by 500 calories per

day over the same time period could produce a loss of 3–7 pounds (1.4–3.2 kg). Chromium picolinate was well tolerated in the randomized controlled trials.[38]

Garcinia Cambogia

Garcinia cambogia contains hydroxy-citric acid, which suppresses de novo fatty acid synthesis and is thought to reduce intake.[38] One randomized study demonstrated significantly greater weight loss with *Garcinia cambogia* use over 12 weeks' time compared to a placebo (8.14±6.82 lb vs 5.28±6.45 lb [0.7±3.1 kg vs 2.4±2.9 kg]).[39] Another randomized study showed no significant difference in weight loss between those using *Garcinia cambogia* compared to a placebo after 12 weeks.[40]

Ephedra

An alkaloid derived from the herb *Ephedra sinica* is available as ephedra. This pharmacologic agent increases metabolism, has anorectic properties, and is a bronchodilator. Known as *ma huang* in Chinese medicine, it has been used for over 5000 years to treat asthma, hay fever, and respiratory tract infections. Ephedra was a component of many over-the-counter weight-loss pills. Ephedra has serious adverse reactions, including hypertension, dizziness, nausea, dysrythmias, heart failure, and myocardial infarction. A series of sudden heart failure deaths in ephedra users with no prior heart disease prompted the FDA to ban ephedra sales in 2004. Appeals courts upheld the ban in 2006. Ephedra is available outside the United States and is used extensively both legally and illegally by athletes for weight control. Strenuous exercise during ephedra use increases the risk of heat stroke, stroke, and sudden cardiac arrest; therefore, many sports organizations, including the International Olympics Committee, have banned its use.

Substances That Reduce Appetite

Yerba mate, an herbal product from the South American evergreen tree *Ilex paraguariensis*, contains large amounts of caffeine, which delays gastric emptying time, thereby prolonging satiety. Adverse effects have not been reported, but studies are limited. Side effects secondary to caffeine may be expected. Another evergreen tree, *Pausinystalia yohimbe*, yields yohimbine, an α-2 receptor agonist that is intended to reduce appetite. Trials of the product marketed as yohimbe have produced conflicting results.[38] Yohimbine is a purported aphrodisiac; it is contraindicated in persons with renal disease. Extracts of black, green, and mulberry teas are under investigation as weight-loss adjuvants.[41]

Other Botanical Products

Many weight-loss products contain fibers that increase the size of the intestinal food bolus, stimulating pressure receptors to signal satiety. *Amorphophallus konjac*, the konjac root, contains glucomannan, a dietary fiber comprised of a polysaccharide chain and mannose. Glucomannan is hydrophilic and creates a larger food bolus, thereby signaling early satiety. Glucomannan is used extensively in Japanese foods such as noodles and tofu. Weight loss using 2–4 grams per day has been demonstrated with few side effects.[38,42-44] In a double-blind study where the intervention subjects used 1 gram of glucomannan with 8 oz water before each of their three daily meals over 8 weeks, the glucomannan group averaged a 5.5 pound (2.5 kg) greater weight loss than control subjects with no prescribed change in intake or exercise. They also had significant reductions in serum cholesterol and LDL (21.7 and 15 mg/dL respectively) compared to placebo users.[44] Glucomannan improved lipid parameters and glycemic status in one study of individuals with diabetes but no weight loss was associated with glucomannan.[45] Guar gum, another dietary fiber, is derived from the Indian bean *Cyamopsis tetragonolobus*. It has not been shown to lower body weight. Although the water-soluble fiber psyllium is well tolerated, it has not been shown to enhance weight loss, but it can improve lipid and glucose parameters.[38,46] All fiber products have the potential to cause diarrhea, flatulence, and gastrointestinal discomfort.

Substances Intended to Decrease Nutrient Absorption

Chitosan is a polysaccharide produced from the chitin contained in the exoskeletons of marine crustaceans. Chitosan is marketed to decrease fat absorption but has not been shown to enhance weight loss. Its most frequent side effects are constipation and flatulence.[38] Over-the-counter orlistat (Alli) would be an effective substitute for chitosan.

Nonpharmacologic Weight-Loss Methods

The National Physical Activity and Weight Loss survey was a nationwide telephone survey completed in 2002 that questioned 11,211 individuals about complementary and alternative medicine (CAM) therapy use for weight loss. Of those surveyed, 3% had used a CAM therapy in the preceding 12 months for weight loss. The most popular CAM modality used was yoga, including yoga breathing (57.4%). Other methods included meditation (8.2%), massage (7.5%), acupuncture (7.7%), and Eastern martial arts (5.9%). All other CAM therapies combined accounted for 13.3% of those used.[47] A meta-analysis of acupuncture and acupressure studies revealed no convincing research that either method reduces body weight.[48] Most studies investigating the effect of hypnosis on weight loss are a decade old and do not demonstrate significant weight loss.[48]

Special Populations

Children and Adolescents

Overweight and obesity are epidemic in children in the United States; however, weight-loss medication use in children younger than 16 years old is generally not recommended. The preferred interventions are to identify children at risk for overweight, then reduce their energy intake by trading calorie-dense, nonnutritious foods, such as cookies and soda, for more nutritious foods such as fruits and complex carbohydrates, while increasing their physical activity. Play and sports participation will increase muscle mass while using stored fat for fuel. The high basal metabolic rate during children's growth augments weight loss when intake and activity are optimized.

The use of weight-loss medications has been studied in children receiving second-generation antipsychotic medications with subsequent insulin resistance, obesity, and type 2 diabetes. In one study, 10- to 17-year-olds treated with atypical antipsychotics took metformin 500 mg with their evening meal for 1 week and then added another

500-mg dose with breakfast. In week 4, metformin was increased to 850 mg twice a day. Those individuals using metformin stabilized BMI, neither gaining nor losing weight, and increased insulin sensitivity over 16 weeks. Adolescents receiving the placebo continued to gain weight.[22]

Topiramate (Topamax) was used as an anorectic in a small study of children ages 4 to 18 years with binge eating disorder or Prader-Willi syndrome. Doses were gradually increased until 7.0 mg/kg/day was achieved. Topiramate was successful in reducing obsessive food cravings. However, at this dose, 71% of children complained of memory problems and almost 30% also complained of reduced psychomotor speed and language and attention problems. These complaints disappeared after dose reductions to 3.0 mg/kg/day or cessation of topiramate.[49]

Sibutramine (Meridia) has been effective when used in combination with behavioral therapy for weight loss (−19.8±14.1 pounds, −9.0±6.4 kg) in Caucasian youth aged 14–17 years. African American adolescents in the same study did not have weight loss that differed significantly from control subjects.[50] Orlistat (Xenical, Alli) has been studied in obese adolescents and can be used safely with weight monitoring every 2–4 weeks. Forty percent of adolescents 12–16 years of age using orlistat plus mild caloric restriction, exercise, and behavioral therapy in one study had a 5–10% decrease in BMI compared to 20.2% of teens using a placebo. BMI reduction is a better measure of weight loss in adolescents because rapid adolescent height growth changes BMI. At the end of 1 year, weight had increased only 1 lb (0.53 kg) in the orlistat group while the control group gained 6.9 lb (3.14 kg).[51] Parents need to know that their offspring may purchase orlistat without a prescription and might use it during unsupervised weight-loss attempts.

Adolescents may also purchase and use laxatives for weight loss without parental knowledge. This strategy, often used for purging in eating disorders, provides a temporary 1–2 pound weight loss of fecal matter but no loss of stored fat. A study of 4,292 adolescents using the 2001 National Household Survey on Drug Abuse found that approximately 10% of adolescent females used laxatives or vomited to lose weight during the preceding year.[52] Teens of both sexes use laxatives and diuretics for small weight loss when trying to stay in a lower weight division for sports divided into weight categories, such as wrestling.

Pregnant Women

Women should not adopt dietary restrictions to lose weight during pregnancy. Recommended prenatal weight gain varies with prepregnant body mass index.[53] Physical activity can be increased to prevent excessive prenatal weight gain. Phentermine (Adipex-P) and sibutramine (Meridia) are FDA Pregnancy Category C drugs, as their safe use in pregnancy has not been determined. No data link accidental phentermine and sibutramine during pregnancy with teratogenicity. Orlistat (Xenical, Alli) is a pregnancy category B drug, with animal studies failing to demonstrate embryotoxicity or teratogenicity; however, it will limit the absorption of essential fatty acid and vitamins needed for optimal fetal development. Both topiramate (Topamax) and zonisamide (Zonegran) are contraindicated during pregnancy, as fetal effects are unknown.

Lactating Women

Milk production utilizes 500 calories a day. Lactation with calories restricted to those needed to maintain ideal body weight will cause the loss of 1 pound per week. A 500-calorie-per-day restriction augments weight loss without decreasing the quantity or quality of milk production. Lactating women should not need drug therapy for gradual weight loss. Orlistat's (Xenical, Alli) limited absorption suggests that it is not excreted in breast milk, but no research is available to support this. Both topiramate (Topamax) and zonisamide (Zonegran) are contraindicated during breastfeeding. Although not studied, potential excretion in breast milk would expose the infant to potent neuromodulators that might suppress appetite.

Elderly

Women's caloric needs drop postmenopausally. Intake must drop or activity must increase to prevent weight gain. As estrogen levels drop, adipose depots are remodeled, and fat is moved from breasts and hips to the abdomen. Waist measurements may increase without weight gain. Whether estrogen replacement therapy prevents this remodeling or not still is being studied. Women's risk for hyperlipidemia, hypertension, heart disease, and type 2 diabetes increase postmenopausally, adding importance to weight optimization. Age-related decreases in liver and renal function must be considered when prescribing weight-loss medications for postmenopausal women.

▌Conclusion

Intake and exercise adjustments can optimize body weight with few side effects or medication interactions and are the preferred method of weight loss for those who are overweight. Multiple hormonal variations make weight loss more difficult for the obese. Medications, such as antipsychotics and glucocorticoids, actually can cause obesity. Prescription weight-loss medications can augment diet, exercise, and biobehavioral therapy to initiate weight loss for the obese. Without dietary vigilance, weight will be regained once weight-loss medications are stopped. Ongoing research into neuromodulators and hormones will provide many new weight-loss therapies over the next decade.

References

1. Centers for Disease Control. 2007. National Center for Health Statistics. Obesity among adults in America. Available from: *http://www.cdc.gov/nchs/data/databriefs/db01.pdf* [Accessed January 2, 2009].

2. American College Obstetricians and Gynecologists. The role of the obstetrician-gynecologist in the assessment and management of obesity. Committee Opinion No. 319. Washington, DC: ACOG, 2005.

3. National Institutes of Health. National Heart, Lung and Blood Institute. Clinical guidelines on the identification, evaluation, and treatment of overweight and obesity in adults. 1998. Available from: *www.nhlbi.nih.gov/guidelines/obesity/ob_home.htm* [Accessed July 15, 2007].

4. Institute of Medicine. Dietary reference intakes: energy, carbohydrate, fiber, fat, fatty acids, cholesterol, protein, and amino acids. Washington, DC: The National Academies Press, 2002.

5. Palamara K, Mogul H, Peterson S, Frishman W. Obesity: new perspectives and pharmacotherapies. Cardiol Rev 2006;14(5):238–58.

6. Hofbauer K, Nicholson J, Boss O. The obesity epidemic: current and future pharmacological treatments. Annu Rev Pharmacol Toxicol 2007;47:565–92.

7. Phelan S, Wadden TA, Berkowitz RI, Sarwer DB, Womble LG, Cato RK, et al. Impact of weight loss on the metabolic syndrome. Int J Obs 2007;31:1442–8.

8. Halford J. Pharmacology of appetite suppression: implication for the treatment of obesity. Current Drug Targets 2001;2:353–79.

9. Jensen MD. Potential role of new therapies in modifying cardiovascular risk in overweight patients with metabolic risk factors. Obesity 2006;14(3):143S-9S.

10. Pacher P, Batkai S, Kunos G. The endocannabinoid system as an emerging target of pharmacotherapy. Pharmacol Rev 2006;58(3):389–462.

11. Sahin Y, Unluhizarci K, Yilmazsoy A, Yikilmaz A, Aygen E, Kelestimur F. The effects of metformin and cardiovascular risk factors in nonobese women with polycystic ovary syndrome. Clin Endocrinol 2007;67;904–08.

12. Palomba S, Orio F, Falbo A, Russo T, Tolino A, Zullo F. Clomiphene citrate versus metformin as first-line approach for the treatment of anovulation in infertile patients with polycystic ovary syndrome. J Clin Endocrin Metab 2007;92:3498–503.

13. Legro R, Zaino R, Demers L, Kenselman A, Gnatuk C, Willimas N. The effects of metformin and rosiglitazone, alone and in combination, on the ovary and endometrium in polycystic ovary syndrome. Am J Obstet Gynecol 2007;196:402.e1–402.e11.

14. Elnashar A, Fahmy M, Mansour A, Ibrahim K. N-acetyl cysteine vs metformin in treatment of clomiphene citrate-resistant polycystic ovary syndrome: a prospective randomized controlled study. Fertil Steril 2007;88:406–9.

15. Pillai A, Bang H, Green C. Metformin and glitazones: do they really help PCOS patients? J Fam Pract 2007;56(6):44–53.

16. National Institute of Diabetes, Digestive and Kidney Diseases. Binge eating disorder. US Department of Health and Human Services NIH publication 04–3589, September 2004. Available from: *http://win.niddk.nih.gov/publications/binge.htm#adread* [Accessed July 15, 2007].

17. Brownley K, Berkman N, Sedway J, Lohr K, Bulik C. Binge eating disorder treatment: a systematic review of randomized controlled trials. Int J Eating Disord 2007;40(4):337–48.

18. National Institute of Mental Health. Anorexia nervosa. Available from: *www.nimh.nih.gov/publicat/eatingdisorders.cfm* [Accessed July 15, 2007].

19. Newcomer J. Metabolic considerations in the use of antipsychotic medications: a review of the recent evidence. J Clin Psychiatry 2007;68(Suppl 1):20–7.

20. Peukens J, DeHert M, Mortimer A; SOLIANOL Study Group. Metabolic control in patients with schizophrenia treated with amisulpride or olanzapine. Int Clin Psychopharmacol 2007;22(3):145–52.

21. Henderson DC, Fan X, Copeland PM, Borba CP, Daley TB, Nguyen DD. A double blind, placebo controlled

trial of sibutramine for clozapine-associated weight gain. Acta Psychiatr Scand 2007;115:101–5.

22. Klein D, Cottingham E, Sorter M, Barton B, Morrison J. A randomized, double blind, placebo-controlled trial of metformin treatment of weight gain associated with initiation of atypical antipsychotic therapy in children and adolescents. Am J Psychiatry 2006;163: 2072–9.

23. Westhoff CL. Contraception and obesity: effectiveness. Dialogues in Contraception 2007;11(2):8,9. Available From: *http://www.usc.edu/schools/medicine/education/continuing_education/selfstudy.html* [Accessed September 3, 2007].

24. Snow V, Barry P, Fitterman N, Qaseem A, Weiss K. Pharmacologic and surgical management of obesity in primary care: a clinical practice guideline from the American College of Physicians. Ann Intern Med 2005;142:525–31.

25. Anderson D, Wadden T. Treating the obese patient: suggestions for primary care practice. Arch Fam Med 1999;8:156–67.

26. Van Mil EG, Westerterp KR, Kester AD, Delemarre-van de Waal HA, Gerver WJ, Saris WH. The effect of sibutramine on energy expenditure and body composition in obese adolescents. J Clin Endocrinol Metab 2007;92(4):1409–14.

27. Gursoy A, Erdogan MF, Cin MO, Cesur M, Baskal N. Comparison of orlistat and sibutramine in an obesity management program: efficacy, compliance, and weight regain after compliance. Eat Weight Disord 2006;11:e127–32.

28. Whigman LD, Dhurandhar NV, Rahko PS, Atkinson RL. Comparison of combinations of drugs for treatment of obesity: body weight and echocardiographic status. Int J Obesity 2007;31(5):850–7.

29. De Simone G, Supuran CT. Antiobesity carbonic anhydrase inhibitors. Curr Top Med Chem 2007;7(9): 879–84.

30. Kishore M, Gadde D, Francis D, Wagner R, Krishnan R. Zonisamide for weight loss in obese adults: a randomized controlled trial. JAMA 2003;289:1820–5.

31. Stenlof K, Rossner F, Vercruysse A, Kumar M, Fitchet M, Sjostrom L. Topiramate in the treatment of obese subjects with drug-naïve type 2 diabetes. Diabetes Obes Metab 2007;9:360–8.

32. McElroy SL, Frye MA, Altshuler LL, Suppes T, Hellemann F, Black D, et al. A 24-week, randomized, controlled trial of adjunctive sibutramine versus topiramate in the treatment of weight gain in overweight or obese patients with bipolar disorders. Bipolar Disord 2007;9(4):426–34.

33. Gabriel A. Adjunctive topiramate treatment in refractory obese bipolar patients: a descriptive open label study. Eat Weight Disord 2007;12(1):48–53.

34. Clayton AH. Extended-release bupropion: an antidepressant with a broad spectrum of therapeutic activity? Expert Opin Pharmacother 2007;8(4):457–66.

35. Padwal R, Majumdar S. Drug treatments for obesity: orlistat, sibutramine, and rimonabant. Lancet 2007; 369:71–7.

36. Depres JP, Golay A, Sjostrom L. Effects of rimonabant on metabolic risk factors in overweight patients with dyslipidemia. N Engl J Med 2005;353:2121–34.

37. Gokcel A, Gumurdulu Y, Karakose H, Melek Ertorer E, Tanaci N, BascilTutuncu N, et al. Evaluation of the safety and efficacy of sibutramine, orlistat and metformin in the treatment of obesity. Diabetes Obes Metab 2002;4(1):49–55.

38. Pittler M, Ernst E. Dietary supplements for body-weight reduction: a systematic review. Am J Clin Nutr 2004;79:529–36.

39. Heymsfield SB, Allison DB, Vasselli JR, Pietrobelli A, Greenfield D, Nunez C. *Garcinia cambogia* (hydroxy-citric acid) as a potential anti-obesity agent. JAMA 1998;280:1596–600.

40. Mattes RD, Bormann L. Effects of (-)-hydroxycitric acid on appetitive variables. Physiol Behav 2000; 71:87–94.

41. Zhong L, Furne J, Levitt M. An extract of black, green, and mulberry teas causes malabsorption of carbohydrate but not of triaglycerol in healthy volunteers. Am J Clin Nutr 2006;84:551–5.

42. Keithley J, Swanson B. Glucomannan and obesity: a critical review. Altern Ther Health Med 2005;11:30–4.

43. Birketvedt GS, Shimshi M, Erling T, Florholmen J. Experiences with three different fiber supplements in weight reduction. Med Sci Mont 2005;11:P15–8.

44. Walsh DE, Yaghoubian V, Behforooz A. Effect of glucomannan on obese patients: a clinical study. Int J Obes 1984;8(4):289–93.

45. Chen HL, Sheu WH, Tai TS, Liaw YP, Chen YC. Konjac supplement alleviated hypercholesterolemia and hyperglycemia in type 2 diabetic subjects—a randomized double-blind trial. J Am Coll Nutr February 2003;22(1):36–42.

46. Saper R, Eisenberg D, Phillips R. Common dietary supplements for weight loss. Am Fam Physician 2004;70:1731–38.

47. Sharpe P, Blanck H, Williams J, Ainsworth B, Conway J. Use of complementary and alternative medicine for weight control in the United States. J Alternative Complementary Medicine 2007;13(2):217–22.

48. Pittler MH, Ernst E. Complementary therapies for reducing body weight: a systematic review. Int J Obesity 2005;29:1030–8.

49. Aarsen F, van den Akker E, Drop S, Catsman-Berrevoets C. Effect of topiramate on cognition in obese children. Neurology 2006;67:1307–8.

50. Budd G, Hayman L, Crump E, Pollydore C, Hawley K, Cronquist J, et al. Weight loss in obese African American and Caucasian adolescents. J Cardiovasc Nurs 2007;22:288–96.

51. Chanoine JP, Hampl S, Jensen C, Boldrin M, Hauptman J. Effect of orlistat on weight and body composition in obese individuals. JAMA 2005;293:2873–83.

52. Cance J, Ashley O, Penne M. Unhealthy weight control behaviors and MDMA (Ecstasy) use among adolescent females. J Adolesc Health 2005;37:409.

53. Institute of Medicine Subcommittee on Nutritional Status and Weight Gain During Pregnancy. Nutrition during pregnancy. Institute of Medicine. Washington, DC: National Academy Press, 1990.

"Quitting smoking is easy, I've done it a thousand times."
MARK TWAIN

8
Smoking Cessation

Donna D. Caruthers and Susan A. Albrecht

Chapter Glossary

Drug discrimination Psychobiologic cues that develop with drug use (e.g., nicotine) and can prompt additional drug-using behavior (e.g., smoking another cigarette).

Lapse A momentary smoking event or slip by an abstinent tobacco user. The individual might take a puff of a cigarette or smoke a whole cigarette. This event is usually followed by an effort to become abstinent again.

Relapse When a tobacco user attempting cessation reinstitutes previous use of tobacco or more. This event often follows a lapse in smoking.

Tolerance Condition that occurs when a tobacco user's response to nicotine (a psychoactive drug) decreases and requires the individual to use large quantities or more frequent dosing of tobacco-/nicotine-containing products. Tolerance to nicotine includes psychobiologic factors.

Withdrawal symptom Symptom indicative of the decreasing level of nicotine in the body that occurs within 24 hours of abstaining from tobacco. Such symptoms include (1) depressed mood or dysphoria; (2) irritability/frustration/anger; (3) anxiety; restlessness; (4) increased appetite/hunger; (5) decreased heart rate; (6) difficulty concentrating/impaired cognitive function; (7) insomnia/sleep disturbance; (8) craving; and (9) somatic complaints of headaches, gastrointestinal disturbances, and dizziness.

Introduction

The Centers for Disease Control and Prevention (CDC) in the United States estimates that 43.5 million adults (20.8%) smoke cigarettes.[1] The prevalence of smoking is higher among men (23.9%) than women (18%), and tobacco use is the foremost cause of death in women and men in the United States today.[2] Annually, 178,000 deaths among women are attributed to cigarette smoking.[3]

The first surgeon general's report on the adverse effects of smoking specific to women was published in 1980.[4] The report identified use of cigarettes and other tobacco products with the development of cardiovascular disorders, lung cancer, pulmonary disease, and other malignancies.[5]

Lung cancer is the leading cause of cancer deaths in women and exceeds the combined total number of deaths from breast, ovarian, and uterine cancers.[6] Unfortunately most women are unaware of this information. Two-thirds of women recently surveyed about their knowledge of the leading cancer death in women incorrectly chose breast cancer.[7] As smoking prevalence in women increases or decreases, lung cancer deaths follow the direction of smoking prevalence.[8]

Efforts to reduce the morbidity and mortality secondary to tobacco use require both prevention and tobacco cessation interventions. Cessation messages, pharmacologic treatment, and cognitive behavioral therapy are most effective when combined in treating individuals with tobacco use disorder. This chapter reviews the evidence for nonpharmacologic methods used to augment treatment for smoking cessation and the pharmacologic treatment(s) for tobacco addiction in women. Because an understanding of several terms related to drug addiction is necessary, a glossary is provided at the beginning of this chapter. The definitions are specific to nicotine addiction.

Reasons Women Smoke

Most women begin smoking during adolescence. Today, girls are more likely to start smoking than are boys. Girls are also more likely to remain smokers because females develop symptoms of nicotine addiction faster than males.[9] Other reasons for smoking initiation have included perceptions of peers,[10] experimentation, and role models who smoke.[11] Adolescents may find that after they initiate tobacco use, continuing to smoke has perceived advantages with peers and elevated mood. Those suffering from negative mood and depressive symptoms may use smoking to cope with alterations in their mood. Researchers are exploring the relationship and pattern of tobacco as a gateway drug[12] and the reinforcement one obtains from combining tobacco with other substances (e.g., alcohol).[13]

Health Consequences of Tobacco Use Among Women

The continuum of the health consequences of tobacco use may begin within the womb and end with death, and the consequences are not limited to the leading fatal medical disorders, such as lung cancer and cardiovascular disease. A woman who smokes tobacco increases the probability of adversely affecting her own health and the health of those around her, including unborn children during pregnancy. Tobacco use has significant adverse effects on fertility, maternal complications in pregnancy, birth outcomes, breastfeeding, and risk for sudden infant death syndrome (SIDS). Specific maternal complications include ectopic pregnancy, preterm premature rupture of membranes (PROM), placenta previa, spontaneous abortion, hypertensive disorders, preterm birth, stillbirth, neonatal and perinatal mortality, low birth weight, and neonatal tube defects.[14] Research has also shown that women who quit smoking before or during pregnancy reduce tobacco's associated effects for adverse reproductive outcomes.

The risks of environmental tobacco smoke to the newborn child resulting from postpartum maternal smoking include lung dysfunction, acute respiratory infections, recurrent otitis media, bronchitis, pneumonia, and SIDS. The most recent published medical costs related to these illnesses are estimated to be $4.6 billion per year for direct medical expenditures and an additional $8 billion related to the cost of loss of life of 6200 children annually.[15]

Continued tobacco use contributes to early onset of menopause and the development of osteoporosis and osteoarthritis later in life.[16] According to Supervia et al., women smokers had a statistically lower level of 25 hydroxyvitamin D as compared to nonsmoking women (m = 16.8; SD = 9.9 ng/mL vs m = 31.9; SD = 15.1 ng/mL; P = .002).[16] Therefore, women smokers begin to develop a risk for osteoporosis before they reach the menopausal stage of life. Among postmenopausal women, hip fractures are 2.27 times more likely in former smokers and 3.72 in current smokers as compared to nonsmokers.[17] Heavy smokers are four to five times more likely to have facial wrinkles than nonsmokers, independent of sun exposure.[18] Sun exposure and smoking combine to have a synergistic effect in accelerating cutaneous aging.

Tobacco alters the oral mucosa and leads to the development of nonmalignant and malignant problems in the oral cavity. Smoking also increases the risk of developing periodontal disease. Due to vasoconstriction by nicotine, inhalation of carbon monoxide, and impairment of the immune system, wounds may heal slowly.

Epidemiology of Female Smokers

Cigarette smoking was rare among women in the early part of the 20th century, increased until the 1960s, and began to decline in the mid-1970s. During the 1990s, reductions in smoking prevalence among adult women were small, and teenage tobacco use increased markedly.[19] By the late 1990s, more than one in five adult women was a regular smoker, and approximately 30% of high school senior girls admitted to having smoked within the past 30 days.

Despite the overwhelming negative health effects of smoking, tobacco marketing uses positive imagery, capitalizes on issues important to women, and exploits the women's movement. Tobacco advertisers suggest women who smoke are liberated, sexually attractive, athletic, fun loving, and slim. Tobacco companies have also supported women's causes, providing funding for women's sports, women's professional organizations, and antidomestic violence programs in an attempt to align themselves with positive roles.[19]

Prevalence of smoking is highest among women aged 18 through 44 years and lowest among women aged 65 years or older. Smoking prevalence is highest among American Indian or Alaska Native women (34.5%), intermediate among White women (23.5%) and Black women (21.9%), and lowest among Hispanic women (13.8%) and Asian or

Pacific Islander women (11.2%).[19] The smoking prevalence in 2006 among women with 9–11 years of education was 31%, compared to 5% among women with higher levels of education. Smoking rates were 40% among women who obtained a general equivalency diploma. With respect to income, the highest rate of smoking (28%) occurs among women below the poverty line.[1] Thus, smoking trends have increasingly become an addiction borne by women with the least resources in society.

Smoking During Pregnancy

Reports of smoking during pregnancy range between 10.2% and 16.3% depending upon the question used to obtain the information.[20] This smoking rate is less than the average smoking rate of nonpregnant women and slightly less than the reported rate of 10.4% in 2003. Relapse at 6 months postpartum has been reported as high as 66%.[21] Researchers have examined the differences between self-reported smoking and biologic validation with cotinine. Self-reported cessation from smoking was reported to be 19.2% during the first trimester and 15.7% for the third trimester. Biologic validation studies suggest smoking rates are higher than the smoking rates from self-reports. These findings suggest that between one-third and one-half of smoking pregnant women and girls conceal the extent of their smoking from the clinician.

Natality data indicate that smoking prevalence during pregnancy differs by age and race/ethnicity. Native American women have the highest smoking rates during their pregnancy, followed by non-Hispanic White women.[22] Tobacco use during pregnancy is consistently highest among women with only some high school education and lowest for college graduates. Women who are exposed to passive smoking, have a smoking partner, or lack support from their partner to quit smoking[9] are at greater risk to continue smoking during pregnancy.[23]

▌ Facilitators and Barriers to Smoking Cessation

Research is lacking with respect to gender differences between women's and men's motivation to stop smoking. Confidence to quit smoking has been reported to be lower among women (30%) compared to men (53%).[24] Current studies suggest that multiple gender-linked biopsychologic factors might influence motivation to smoke or serve as barriers to smoking cessation that need to be taken into account when a comprehensive approach toward tobacco control among women is developed.

Premenopausal women may find quitting more difficult during the luteal phase of their menstrual cycle.[25] Depressive symptoms and irritability are nicotine withdrawal symptoms, as well as effects of the luteal phase of the menstrual cycle. Research suggests that women with severe premenstrual symptoms should consider starting to quit smoking during the follicular phase of the menstrual cycle to minimize the experience of nicotine withdrawal symptoms, particularly those that are related to negative mood in the 2 weeks before menses.[25]

▌ Physiology of Tobacco Addiction

The primary addictive substance within tobacco is nicotine, which is a water- and lipid-soluble plant alkaloid. Transportation, absorption, and metabolism of nicotine is assisted by the dual soluble nature of nicotine. The delivery of nicotine to tissues within the body can vary from absorption through the mucosa or skin or across the capillary-alveolar membranes when carried on tar droplets from cigarette smoke to the terminal airways and alveoli in the lung. Cigarette smoke is a most effective delivery method because the speed and dosing of nicotine affects the brain faster than intravenous injection due to the huge surface area of the pulmonary capillary-alveolar membrane and the subsequent acceleration provided by the arterial side of the heart that delivers blood to the brain without going through the venous system and liver.[26]

This addictive drug is an agonist that stimulates presynaptic and postsynaptic nicotinic acetylcholine receptors (nCHRs), particularly the $\alpha_4\beta_2$ subtype.[27] These receptors are located throughout the body but are found primarily in the brain. The β_2 subunit influences self-administration of nicotine, while the α_4 subunit likely influences sensitivity to nicotine.[28] The $\alpha_4\beta_2$ subunit and α_7 likely reinforce the cardiovascular effects of nicotine use. The α_7 subunit may promote rapid synaptic transmission, which could influence learning, conditioning, and sensory gating.[28] Nicotine stimulates nCHRs in the mesolimbic system, the frontal cortex, and the corpus striatum. Several different neurotransmitters are released from these nicotinic receptors (Figure 8-1).[28] In all, nicotine stimulates five different neurotransmitter classes, which include amino acids, monoamine catecholamines, monoamine indolamine, neuropeptides, and acetylcholine.

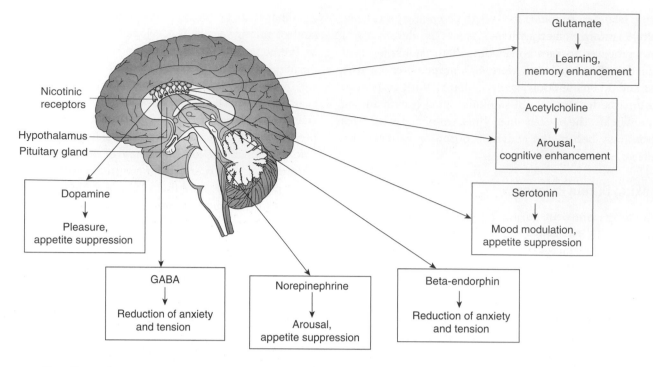

Figure 8-1 The effects of nicotine on nicotinic receptors in the brain.

Of particular importance is the dopamine release that occurs when nicotine binds to nCHRs in the ventral tegmental area located in the midbrain and the nucleus accumbens, which are part of the reward pathway.[28] This stimulation of the mesolimbic reward pathway via release of dopamine is an essential process in the development and maintenance of nicotine addiction, which is similar to other substances of abuse (e.g., heroin, alcohol, and cocaine).[28] Nicotine also stimulates the release of dopamine in the corpus striatum and frontal cortex. This pattern of spiked dopamine release in the brain is similar to the pattern of other addictive substances.

The process of addiction is a biopsychologic one. The biopsychologic conceptual framework identifies an interaction between the biologic activity at the cellular level and psychologic processes developed following sensory, mood, and environmental cues that contribute to conditioning to smoking.[28] With repeated use of nicotine, the central nervous system is remodeled through a psychopharmacologic process, which includes the development of **tolerance**, **drug discrimination**, **withdrawal symptoms**, and **relapse** potential during tobacco abstinence.[29] In addition, after some exposure to nicotine, the brain produces more acetylcholine nicotine receptors, which in turn provides more receptor sites for nicotine.[28] This part of the

remodeling becomes important in the process of smoking cessation, **lapses**, and relapse. Positive psychoactive effects of nicotine, such as improved mood, arousal, and relaxation reinforce the use of nicotine.[28] Benowitz notes that nicotine meets the US surgeon general's primary criteria for an addictive substance, since nicotine promotes compulsive self-administration, has psychoactive effects, and reinforces self-administration.[28]

There are other substances within tobacco that contribute to addiction, including nornicotine, anabasine, myosmine, nicotyrine, and anatabine.[30] In addition, an unidentified substance may contribute to addiction by decreasing monoamine oxidase (MAO) B availability. MAO B breaks down released dopamine. Nicotine has not been identified to have any interactions with MAO B. However, with the stimulated release of dopamine by nicotine and the impairment in the breakdown of dopamine, dopamine remains in higher concentrations than the body is normally subject to, which may, in turn, have an effect on the addiction process.

Nicotine and Drug Interactions

Tobacco smoking has known interactions with drugs.[31] Due to the initiation of smoking cessation, a person's drug profile may need to be reevaluated for correct dosing. For example, warfarin, theophylline (TheoDur), and insulin may require higher dosages when an individual is smoking.[31] Upon initiating smoking cessation, appropriate laboratory tests should be conducted for each drug to determine the appropriate dosage.

Nicotine Withdrawal

Nicotine addiction is marked by the development of a withdrawal process when an individual attempts to quit or has a substantial delay in smoking. Nicotine withdrawal symptoms include (1) depressed mood or dysphoria; (2) irritability/frustration/anger; (3) anxiety; restlessness; (4) increased appetite/hunger; (5) decreased heart rate; (6) difficulty concentrating/impaired cognitive function; (7) insomnia/sleep disturbance; (8) craving; and (9) somatic complaints of headaches, gastrointestinal disturbances, and dizziness.[32] Persons usually reach the peak of the physiologic withdrawal symptoms within 1–3 weeks of smoking cessation without nicotine replacement.[32]

▎ Initiating Smoking Cessation

The 1996 publication *Smoking Cessation, Clinical Practice Guideline of the Agency for Health Care Policy and Research (AHCPR)* and the 2000 US Public Health Service update recommended tobacco use be treated as a vital sign with no differential treatment guidelines by gender, except for treatment during pregnancy.[33] The 2008 update by Fiore et al. provides a practical guide to healthcare providers for this aspect of nicotine addiction treatment.[34]

The promotion and prescription of treatment for tobacco addiction starts with the healthcare provider's knowledge and commitment to providing appropriate treatment and maintaining adequate follow-up. Studies on smoking cessation suggest that lack of adherence by healthcare providers to assess, monitor, and follow up on tobacco addiction and treatment contributes to the lack of initiation to quit smoking and/or relapse from cessation.[35,36] In addition, healthcare providers may have preconceptions regarding the effectiveness of their interaction if they themselves smoke. Some surveys of healthcare providers report that they perceived a lack of adequate training in how to approach smokers regarding tobacco use, inadequate time to address the problem, and current information on the most effective strategies to promote cessation.[37,38]

Treatment for tobacco use must include screening or assessment, selecting appropriate interventions based upon the individual's willingness to quit, and identification of where the person is within the quitting process (e.g., initiation of quitting, relapse, maintenance with relapse prevention).[33] Clinical guidelines for smoking cessation intervention suggest using the "Five *A's*" to initiate and monitor smoking cessation with individuals in any medical setting.[33] The "Five *A's*" encourage the healthcare provider to ask, advise, assess, assist, and arrange follow-up. In addition, considering the assessment of smoking status, quantity, and cessation interest has been proposed as an addition to vital sign assessments.[33]

Intervention sessions of at least 10 minutes in length delivered by healthcare providers have the potential to double the cessation rate (22% versus 11%) as compared to no contact time on the topic. Although this chapter does not focus on the behavioral components of an intervention program, various resources are available to assist healthcare providers as needed.[33,39]

Pharmacologic therapy should be considered for all smokers unless those therapies are contraindicated for that particular individual (i.e., at high risk for adverse effects).[33] A dual treatment protocol is recommended, which is comprised of pharmacologic treatment and cognitive behavioral therapy following a distinct healthcare message advocating cessation.[39]

▎ Nonpharmacologic Therapies for Smoking Cessation

There is a dose–response relationship with respect to the length of behavioral intervention sessions. Intensive behavioral interventions of > 10 minutes/session are most effective with an odds ratio of 2.3 (95% CI, 2.0–2.7) and an estimated abstinence rate of 22% when compared to no provider contact time.[33] Total contact time of 90 minutes spread across more than eight sessions is recommended.[33]

Group or individual therapy and alternative intervention delivery via the Internet and telephone are also effective intervention delivery strategies. According to the latest treatment guidelines, intervention programs that combine three or more formats are more effective than a single intervention with an odds ratio of 2.5 (95% CI, 2.1–3.0) and a subsequent abstinence rate of 23%.[34] The degree of confidence in one's ability to stop smoking is predictive of relapse versus maintaining cessation.

Pharmacologic Therapies

When drug therapy is added to behavioral therapy consisting of more than eight sessions, abstinence rates can increase from 25% to 33%.[34] There are currently seven pharmaceutical agents that are FDA approved for treatment of smoking cessation. First-line therapy for tobacco dependence includes nonnicotine therapies (bupropion [Zyban]), partial nicotine receptor agonists (varenicline [Chantix]), and nicotine replacement therapies delivered via gum, patch, inhaler, spray, or lozenge. Although considered experimental in the United States, a cannabinoid receptor antagonist (rimonabant) has been developed by the Sanofi Aventis company.[39] Table 8-1 provides information about the odds ratios for effectiveness of the first-line therapies as they compare to placebo at 6 months after stopping smoking.[33,34] Costs may vary regionally. In addition, some insurance carriers are covering the prescription cessation drugs with varying requirements for the client co-pay. On average, the cost of smoking cessation products compare with the price of cigarettes, but the client purchases a 1- to 3-month supply of the drug with a higher cost up front as opposed to the weekly cost incurred with purchasing cigarettes.

Table 8-1 First-Line Smoking Cessation Medications: Odds Ratios for Abstinence 6 Months After Smoking Cessation

Medication—Generic (Brand)	Odds Ratios for Abstinence (95% Confidence Interval)
Nonnicotine Medications	
Bupropion SR (Zyban)	2.0 (1.8–2.2)
Varenicline (Chantix) 2 mg/day	3.1 (2.5–3.8)
Varenicline (Chantix) 1 mg/day	2.1 (1.5–3.0)
Nicotine Replacement Medications	
Nicotine gum (2 mg) (≥14 weeks' use)	1.5 (1.2–1.7)
Nicotine lozenge	2.05 (1.62–2.59)
Nicotine patch (6–14 weeks)	1.9 (1.7–2.2)
Nicotine patch (> 14 weeks)	1.9 (1.7–2.3)
Nicotine nasal spray	2.3 (1.7–3.0)
Nicotine inhaler	2.1 (1.5–2.9)
Combination Therapy	
Nicotine patch with prn nicotine gum or nicotine spray	3.6 (2.5–5.2)
Nicotine patch with bupropion SR	2.5 (1.9–3.4)
Nicotine patch with nortriptyline or nicotine inhaler	2.3 (1.3–4.6)
Medications That Are Not Effective	
Selective serotonin reuptake inhibitors	1.0 (0.7–1.4)
Naltrexone	0.5 (0.2–1.2)

Source: Adapted from Fiore ML 2008[34]; Nides M 2008.[41]

Nortriptyline (Aventyl) and Clonidine (Catapres)

Second-line treatment options that do not have FDA approval such as clonidine (Catapres) and nortriptyline (Aventyl) are used "off-label" in the treatment of nicotine addiction. Nortriptyline (Aventyl) requires careful monitoring by healthcare providers for adverse effects on major organs (e.g., heart, liver, and kidney), as well as adverse and side effects. Therefore, routine follow-up should include clinical (e.g., vital signs), laboratory (e.g., BUN, creatinine, liver function studies), and radiographic monitoring (e.g., chest X-ray).

Evidence of the effectiveness of nortriptyline (Aventyl) is available in the literature, but it is not consistent. Although a review of the use of nortriptyline indicates doses between 75 and 100 mg by mouth can obtain abstinence rates twice that of a placebo treatment, adverse effects of this drug are considered serious.[40,41] The 2008 treatment guideline update indicates the odds ratio for abstinence using nortriptyline (Aventyl) across studies was 1.8 (95% CI, 1.3–2.63) and estimated abstinence of 23% when compared to placebo at 6 months after smoking cessation is initiated.[33] Research on this drug using a 12-week cessation program did not find it to be significantly better than placebo.[42] The drug is not suitable for women with cardiovascular problems due to its effect on contractility changes of the heart and potential for arrhythmias.[39]

Clonidine (Catapres) lacks adequate evidence to support use as a first-line medication for the treatment of nicotine addiction.[34] In addition, side effects while taking the drug and discontinuing the drug raise concern given that other medications with established efficacy are available.[39] In the event that an individual is not able to use first-line treatment medications, these second-line treatment medications can be considered, but only under strict supervision by healthcare providers.[34]

Bupropion Sustained Release (Zyban, Wellbutrin)

Bupropion is available for smoking cessation treatment under the trade name of Zyban. The identical agent also can be found marketed as Wellbutrin, Wellbutrin SR (sustained release), and Wellbutrin XL (extended release) for treatment of depression. Zyban is the formulation that is specific for smoking cessation treatment. Zyban and Wellbutrin SR are bioidentical. Both are sustained release and both contain 150 mg of bupropion. It is important to note that Wellbutrin SR also comes as 100-mg and 200-mg tablets. Wellbutrin SR typically is taken twice a day. Differences in insurance coverage may exist for these drugs. Wellbutrin may be covered for the treatment for depression, but Zyban may not be covered for the treatment of smoking cessation. However, some health insurance companies cover both of these uses of bupropion. This issue may be important for prescribing purposes if smoking cessation drugs are not covered under a woman's insurance plan.

Initially, bupropion (Wellbutrin; Zyban) was approved for the treatment of depression. The release of bupropion for smoking cessation occurred in the mid-1990s following clinical drug trials that demonstrated efficacy for this indication. These trials were initiated after clinicians reported a decreased interest in smoking among smokers treated with bupropion. Table 8-2 provides information about nonnicotine therapies.

Mechanism of Action

Theoretically, bupropion is thought to mediate noradrenergic and dopaminergic mechanisms as well as antagonizing nicotinic receptors. Bupropion may inhibit presynaptic reuptake of the noradrenergic and dopaminergic transporters, which may mimic effects obtained from nicotine receptor stimulation and diminish nicotine withdrawal effects.[43] Bupropion is metabolized in the liver via CP450B6, which is the basis of potential drug–drug interactions reviewed later in this chapter. Approximately 87% of bupropion and

its metabolites are excreted in urine through the kidneys and another 10% via fecal elimination.[33,44,45] Dependent upon a person's comorbid disease status, laboratory values should be monitored for both liver and kidney function.

Side Effects/Adverse Reactions

The most common side effects of bupropion (Zyban) include insomnia and dry mouth. If insomnia becomes problematic, the evening dose can be moved to an earlier part of the evening with monitoring for alleviation from the insomnia. In 2009, the FDA mandated that companies producing bupropion add a black box warning to the label that warns the user of possible serous neuropsychiatric symptoms in persons who use this drug. Postmarketing surveillance studies have found a temporal relationship between bupropion and changes in behavior, hostility, agitation, suicidal ideation, and suicidal attempts. These symptoms tend to occur approximately two weeks after initiation of the drug. The actual incidence is unknown because the data comes from the FDA's Adverse Events Reporting System (AERS).

Drug–Drug Interactions

The active metabolite of bupropion, 4-hydroxybupropion, is metabolized by hepatic cytochrome P450-2B6 (CYP2B6) and possesses inhibitory effects on cytochrome

Table 8-2 Nonnicotine-Containing Medications

Drug Generic (Brand)	Preparation	Mechanism of Action	Dosing	Side Effects/Adverse Effects	Contraindications	FDA Pregnancy Category
Bupropion (Zyban)	150 mg; begin 7–14 days before scheduled quit date. By prescription	Nonsedating anxiolytic. Eliminates dysphoria by slowing metabolism of serotonin and increases firing of noradrenergic neurons. Dopamine reuptake inhibitor.	Start a week before the quit date and continue for 7–12 weeks after smoking cessation. Q day 150 mg for 3 days. Then 150 mg bid.	Insomnia, dry mouth, dizziness, nausea, constipation, runny nose, jitters, tachycardia, trouble concentrating, skin rash, agitation, change in appetite, and serious neuropsychiatric events, including suicidal ideation and suicide attempts. Rarely, bupropion can cause seizures.	History of seizures, eating disorders, uncontrolled hypertension; use of MAO inhibitor in previous 14 days; use of Wellbutrin for depression.	C
Varenicline (Chantix)	0.5 mg, 1.0 mg, 2.0 mg. By prescription	Partial nicotine receptor agonist.	First 3 days 0.5 mg Q day. Days 4–7, 0.5 mg bid. Days 8 and on, 1.0 mg bid until end of treatment.	Nausea, sleep disturbance and strange dreams, constipation, flatulence, vomiting, sensitivity to light, pancreatitis, hallucinations, and serious neuropsychiatric events, including suicidal ideation and suicide attempts.	> 18 y, alcohol and illicit drug use, use of insulin, anticoagulants, or theophylline. Use of bupropion at the same time for psychiatric disorder is not absolute contraindication but should be used with caution during pregnancy or breastfeeding.	C

NRT = nicotine replacement therapy; MAO = monoamine oxidase.

P450-2D6 (CYP2D6). Therefore, caution and observations for side effects are warranted if this medication is taken with other medications that require CYP2B6 or CYP2D6 for metabolism in the liver.[34] Table 8-3 provides

Table 8-3 Selected Drug–Drug Interactions with Bupropion*

Drug—Generic (Brand)	Clinical Effect
Alcohol	Adverse neuropsychiatric reactions.
Amantadine (Symmetrel)	Increases risk of CNS side effects.
Antiarrhythmics: flecainide (Tambocor)	Increases plasma levels of antiarrhythmic drugs.
Antipsychotics: risperidone (Risperdal)	Bupropion inhibits CYP2D6, which decreases metabolism of these drugs and potentiates their effect. Also increases risk for seizures.
Antiseizure medications: phenobarbital (Luminal), phenytoin (Dilantin), carbamazepine (Tegretol)	Hepatic metabolism of bupropion inhibited, which increases adverse effects of bupropion.
Beta-blockers	Bupropion inhibits CYP2D6, which decreases the metabolism of these drugs. Increased risk for hypotension, bradycardia, atrioventricular block.
Cimetidine (Tagamet)	Increases drug levels of bupropion.
Clopidogrel (Plavix)	Increases drug level of bupropion.
Codeines	Decreased codeine efficacy.
Cyclophosphamide (Cytoxan)	Increases drug level of bupropion.
Levodopa (Sinemet)	Increases bupropion side effects.
MAO inhibitors	Increases drug levels of bupropion. Use of bupropion within 14 days of using an MAOI is contraindicated.
Meperidine (Demerol)	Increases meperidine levels and risk of respiratory depression.
Metronidazole (Flagyl)	Increases risk of seizures.
Quinolones, all	Increase risk of seizure.
Orphenadrine (Norflex)	Increases drug level of bupropion.
Phenothiazines	Increase phenothiazine levels, prolong QT interval, and cardiac arrhythmias.
Rifampin (Rifadin)/isoniazid (INH)	Decreased efficacy of bupropion, and isoniazid increases risk of seizures.
Selective serotonin reuptake inhibitors (SSRIs)	Increase serotonin levels and increase risk for seizure (additive effect).
Steroids: oral contraceptives and hormone replacement therapy, tamoxifen	Increase drug level of bupropion. Decreases active tamoxifen metabolite levels.
Theophylline (Theo-Dur)	Lower seizure threshold and increase risk of arrhythmias (additive effect).
Tramadol (Ultram)	Increases tramadol levels.
Tricyclic antidepressants: e.g., amitriptyline (Elavil), desipramine (Norpramin)	Bupropion inhibits CYP2D6, and decreases metabolism of these drugs and potentiates their effects.
Venlafaxine (Effexor)	Increases risk of seizures.
Warfarin (Coumadin)	Increases risk of bleeding.

*This table is not comprehensive as new information is being generated on a regular basis.

an overview of the most common drug–drug interactions associated with bupropion.

Contraindications

Bupropion (Zyban, Wellbutrin) lowers the threshold for seizure activity. Contraindications for the use of bupropion include history of seizures, epilepsy, eating disorders, use of MAO inhibitors within 14 days of therapy, use of Wellbutrin for treatment of depression, bipolar condition, severe hepatic cirrhosis, active brain tumor, discontinuation of alcohol or benzodiazepines, and severe hypertension.[34,46] Although bupropion and nicotine replacement may be used in combination, ongoing assessments are necessary if there is a history of cardiovascular disease.[33] Therefore, healthcare professionals will need to monitor for side effects of both drugs. The combination of these drugs has been safely used for individuals with a diagnosis of heart failure.[47]

Prescribing Information

According to the updated treatment guidelines, bupropion is considered an FDA pregnancy class C drug.[34] Bupropion has been used among diverse populations of smokers with similar results. Clinical treatment studies have not identified gender differences in responses to bupropion for tobacco dependence. In addition, while treated with bupropion, weight gain associated with smoking cessation is attenuated in both men and women. There is a positive correlation between increasing doses from 100 mg to 300 mg and cessation rates; however, the response to therapy diminishes by 45 weeks following the end of treatment. Therefore, smokers are more likely to achieve cessation on higher doses early on in their treatment. However, this effect is not sustained and relapse occurs as with other treatments, which adds support for treatment plans that include both pharmacologic and cognitive-behavioral therapy to stop smoking and prevent relapse. There is no known difference over the life span of adults with respect to age and dosing with bupropion for tobacco dependence treatment.[33,45]

Smokers are instructed to begin taking 150 mg of bupropion SR once a day for 3 days. From day 4 until the end of treatment (12 weeks minimum suggested), the dose is increased to 150 mg twice a day. Bupropion is started approximately 7 to 14 days before a scheduled quit date from tobacco use.[33] If smoking continues beyond the 7th week of treatment, healthcare providers need to reevaluate the use of this drug. Initial assessment of kidney and liver function may be performed and should be considered for persons with comorbid conditions. Assessment is necessary for poor adherence, which may occur due to side effects. Although self-report is a typical method of assessing adherence, healthcare providers may consider reviewing medication refill rates as an additional indirect measure of adherence, if available. Requesting individuals to maintain a medication log in the first 3 months of therapy may provide information regarding adherence and side effects to medication. Furthermore, drug effectiveness may be hampered if the smoker did not adhere to a quit date. Assessing adherence with the medication may correct adherence, cessation, and/or health literacy related to the administration of the drug.

Pharmacogenomics

Sponsored genetic research is attempting to target specifics to assist in individualizing smoking cessation treatment. In a recent study, individuals with the specific variant gene of CYP2B6 were less likely to return to smoking 6 months following the initiation of smoking cessation with bupropion.[48] Genetic research regarding bupropion suggests women with a particular genetic variation may be susceptible to side effects with bupropion, which eventually leads to poor adherence to the medication and relapse to tobacco use.[49] This relationship was not found in men. These findings regarding genetic susceptibility for side effects in women suggest the need for careful monitoring by healthcare professionals. Clinical health care does not have the ability to treat smoking intervention based upon genetic makeup at this time. Although research is rapidly revealing information, clinically, we are not able to assess individuals for smoking-related genes to design treatment. Therefore, when women report difficulty with side effects to bupropion and indicate that these side effects interfere with their ability to adhere to the drug, healthcare providers should consider discontinuing the drug and offer alternative medications and strategies. Although the relay of side effects and adherence difficulties is not indicative that a woman has this genetic variation, clinicians should consider that it is a possibility and reevaluate the treatment plan with the woman. Future studies are needed to examine pharmacogenomics with all of the first-line therapies and combinations of these medications.

Varenicline (Chantix)

Varenicline (Chantix) is the most recent medication approved for tobacco dependence treatment. This drug is both a partial agonist and antagonist to neuronal nicotinic acetylcholine receptors. Quit rates in the clinical trials of the drug were reported as 44%.[50,51]

Mechanism of Action

The action of the drug is theorized to influence the reward pathway response in the mesolimbic dopamine system of the brain and decrease nicotine withdrawal symptoms. When administered, varenicline binds with $\alpha_4\beta_2$ neuronal nicotinic acetylcholine receptors and produces agonist activity at that receptor site but blocks the receptors from being stimulated by nicotine. Maximum plasma concentrations occur in 3 to 4 hours, and the half-life is approximately 24 hours. This drug is minimally metabolized by the liver with 92% of the drug excreted by the kidneys.[52]

Side Effects/Adverse Reactions

Since varenicline (Chantix) and other first-line medications (e.g., bupropion) for tobacco dependence act on nicotinic brain receptors, monitoring the response to medications should include self-reported information from the person for known side effects of each drug, changes in behavior, as well as laboratory monitoring of kidney and liver function. Changes in behavior can include agitation/anxiety, depressive symptoms or mood, suicidal ideation, and suicide.[34]

The most common side effects reported with varenicline included nausea, abnormal or vivid strange dreams, constipation, flatulence, and vomiting. The FDA issued warnings in 2007 and 2008 regarding neuropsychiatric symptoms reported with the use of varenicline (Chantix) that include agitation, depression, suicidal ideation, and completed suicide, and in 2009 these warnings were converted to a mandated black box warning that is to be placed on the label and reviewed with the person who will be taking this medication.[34] This drug was not originally tested in populations diagnosed with psychiatric illnesses. Stapleton et al. reported the use of varenicline in a sample of individuals diagnosed with mental illness (i.e., depression, bipolar disorder, or psychosis) and found that varenicline did not affect the participants' mental illness.[53] More research in this area is needed. Healthcare providers are cautioned to conduct a thorough mental/psychiatric assessment prior to prescribing this drug, and persons taking varenicline should be monitored for neuropsychiatric symptoms. In addition, prescribing this drug for individuals with known histories of drug and alcohol use and/or dependence should be done only if careful follow-up is arranged due to lack of information regarding the use of varenicline with alcohol and addictive drugs. This drug is a newly released drug with limited research in persons with various comorbid conditions or psychiatric disorders.[54]

Drug–Drug Interactions

Clinically significant pharmokinetic drug interactions have not been reported with varenicline, except with cimetidine (Tagamet). When cimetidine (Tagamet) and varenicline (Chantix) were taken together among a sample of 12 individuals, renal clearance was decreased and systemic exposure of varenicline was increased.[52] In addition, the safety of administering varenicline with bupropion SR (Zyban) has not been examined. Therefore, the use of these two drugs together is not recommended at this time. Varenicline is not recommended for combination therapy with NRT, due to the competing antagonist action of varenicline and nicotine at the same nicotinic receptor sites, as well as the partial stimulating agonist effect provided by varenicline that is similar to nicotine.[34]

Contraindications

Varenicline (Chantix) is contraindicated for persons younger than 18 years. Studies of varenicline predominantly were completed with samples of healthy subjects. Therefore, caution should be exercised when considering this drug for those with comorbid disorders. Because most of this drug is excreted unchanged by the kidneys, varenicline should not be given to individuals with renal dysfunction (creatinine clearance of less than 30 mL).[34] Furthermore, this drug is contraindicated for persons with renal insufficiency or failure. The use of alcohol and illicit drugs should be avoided due to lack of information available on the consequences of taking these agents at the same time with other drugs acting upon brain receptors. In 2009, the FDA issued a black box warning that varenicline may cause neuropsychiatric effects such as agitation, violence, suicide ideation, or suicide attempts. Persons who take this drug are given a medication guide that reviews the adverse effects and are cautioned to stop this medication if they have any of these symptoms.

Studies of varenicline (Chantix) did not find response differences by gender, a finding that is similar to studies of bupropion. Varenicline is categorized as an FDA pregnancy category C drug due to results of animal studies and reported effects on the animal offspring. These side effects included decreased birth weight and decreased fertility in the offspring of pregnant animals that were administered the drug at high doses. There are no human studies to date regarding any effects on the fetus, neonate, or during nursing, but caution is advised regarding the use of this drug in pregnant and nursing women.

Prescribing Information

Dosing of this drug is increased according to a standard regimen during the first 8 days of treatment. Administration of varenicline is reported to be unaffected by food or time of day; however, directions for administration include (1) take the varenicline after meals or food, (2) drink 8 ounces of water with each dose for renal clearance, (3) start varenicline 7 days before a selected quit day while still smoking, and (4) for support and motivation, use the Web-based GetQuit program, recommended by the manufacturer (Pfizer) during treatment.[52]

Data from clinical trials suggest there is no difference in dosing required for adults across the life span. Once individuals begin using this drug, they may report that smoking prior to their quit date is not as rewarding or satisfying as it was prior to the initiation of varenicline. Treatment is recommended for a minimum of 12 weeks, but research findings suggest that treatment may need to be continued beyond the initial 12 weeks for one additional 12-week round.

Nicotine Replacement Therapy (NRT)

NRT uses various dosing vehicles to deliver nicotine, such as gum, lozenge, patch, inhaler, and spray. Plasma levels of nicotine rarely exceed 15 ng/mL from these various dosing vehicles. An overview of the various types of NRT, availability by prescription versus over the counter, dosing, and length of therapy is provided in Table 8-4. NRT with nicotine gum was the first pharmacologic preparation designed for treatment of tobacco dependence. Each of the NRT delivery vehicles has demonstrated effectiveness in treating tobacco dependence with and without behavioral therapy; however, tobacco cessation is greatest when any of the pharmacologic therapies is coupled with a cognitive behavioral therapy.[33,34] A treatment strategy of medication and counseling can increase abstinence rates by 7% over medication alone.[34]

Mechanism of Action

Nicotine replacement products replace nicotine without the other toxic substances contained in cigarettes. It is important to remember that once nicotine-replacement medications are discontinued, abstinent individuals can experience nicotine withdrawal symptoms. Thus, these products are used to help persons withdraw from nicotine by mitigating withdrawal symptoms via exposure to less nicotine.

One cigarette contains approximately 1–2 mg of nicotine. The NRT lozenge may provide a higher plasma level of nicotine compared to nicotine gum.[55] Patch therapy has the slowest absorption rate with the lowest plasma

Table 8-4 Nicotine Replacement Therapies

Drug Generic (Brand)	Preparation	Dose	Side Effects	Contraindications	FDA Pregnancy Category
Gum (Nicorette)*	2 mg, 4 mg	< 25 cigs/day: 2 mg if smoking; > 25 cigs/day: 4 mg if smoking; 1 piece of gum q hr for 6 wks, then 1 piece q 2–4 hrs 2–4 wks, then 1 piece q 2–4 hrs for 2–4 wks, then 1 piece q 4–8 hrs.	Irritation of buccal cavity, mouth soreness, hiccups, dyspepsia, aching jaw.	Myocardial infarction, heart disease, angina pectoris, serious arrhythmias, stroke, diabetes, hypertension, hyperthyroid, stomach ulcers, liver or kidney disease, pregnancy or breastfeeding.	D
Lozenge (Commit)*	2 mg, 4 mg	Those who smoke first cig within 30 min of wakening: use 4 mg. Others use 2 mg First 6 wks, q 1–2 hrs. Wks 7–9, q 2–4 hrs. Wks 10–12, q 4–8 hrs.	Irritation of teeth, gums, and throat, dyspepsia, diarrhea, constipation, flatulence, insomnia, hiccups, headache, coughing.	Same as for gum.	D
Patch (Nicotrol, NicoDerm CQ)*	7–14 mg, light smoker; 21–22 mg, moderate smoker; 40+, heavy smoker (two 21-mg patches)	> 10 cigs/day: 21 mg/24 hr for 6–8 weeks, then ↓ to 14 mg/24 hr for 2–4 wks, then ↓ 7 mg/24 hr for 2–4 wks. ≤ 10 cigs/day: 14 mg/24 hr for 6 wks, then ↓ 7 mg/24 hr for 2–4 wks.	Skin irritation, sleep disturbance, tachycardia, dizziness, headache, nausea, vomiting, muscle aches and stiffness. Vivid dreams and nightmares. May take patch off after 16 hrs if sleep disturbances occur.	Same as for gum.	D
Inhaler (Nicotrol Inhaler) †	4-mg cartridge	6–16 cartridges/day for 12 wks, then taper dose over 12 wks.	Inflammation of mouth and throat, coughing, rhinitis, stomach irritation.	Same as for gum.	D
Spray (Nicotrol NS) †	0.5 mg per spray	1–2 spray in each nostril q hr for 3–6 mo, then taper dose over 4–6 wks.	Throat irritation, sneezing, coughing, watery eyes, runny nose.	Same as for gum.	D

*Available over the counter.
† Available via prescription only.

levels, which do not reach peak plasma levels until 8 hours following administration.

Smokers may perceive the first day on NRT to be easier than subsequent days on the same NRT dose due to residual nicotine from the previous use of tobacco products. NRT is metabolized in the liver. Cotinine is the primary active metabolite of nicotine. The half-life of nicotine is 4 hours. Excretion occurs through the kidneys into the urine, but clearance is dependent upon renal pH. Grapefruit juice inhibits the metabolism of nicotine to cotinine, and it increases renal clearance of nicotine.[56]

Side Effects/Adverse Reactions

Adverse reactions can occur with any of these products as illustrated in Table 8-4. The side effects are relative to mode of delivery. Nicotine is an irritant when it comes in contact with skin and mucosa. Side effects with nicotine gum and lozenge include irritation of the buccal cavity, mouth soreness, hiccups, dyspepsia, and an aching jaw. Initial side effect of the nicotine nasal spray may include mouth/throat irritation, sneezing, coughing, watery eyes, or runny nose. Individuals should be instructed to avoid operating motorized vehicles for 5 minutes after using the nasal spray because of the potential for coughing, watery eyes, and sneezing. In addition, coughing and rhinitis have been reported to be common side effects with inhaler use. Complaints of skin irritation have occurred in approximately half of the persons using the nicotine patch. Rotating patch sites is essential in minimizing this side effect, as well as the use of topical ointments such as over-the-counter hydrocortisone cream. With severe cases, the patch may have to be discontinued.

If individuals use NRT prior to quitting, nausea can occur due to nicotine overdosing.[57] Caution is recommended in the use of NRT within 2 weeks of a myocardial infarction, presence of serious arrhythmias, and escalating difficulty with angina pectoris, but has not been associated with increasing risk for cardiovascular events among persons with a history of such disease.[57]

Drug–Drug Information

When administering the gum, lozenge, or the inhaler, individuals should be cautioned against the ingestion of beverages such as food, coffee, juices, and soft drinks within 15 minutes of administering nicotine in these NRT forms because the absorption of the medication may be diminished.[55] Acidic beverages can interfere with the absorption of nicotine by these delivery systems.

Prescribing Information

Dosing with any of the NRT products should be individualized. The base smoking rate can assist to establish the initial dose. For example, if a person smokes a pack of cigarettes per day, a typical starting dose for the patch would be a 21- or 22-mg patch. If the individual smokes two packs per day, the 40+ mg patch may need to be prescribed (Box 8-1). Follow-up in 1- and 2-week intervals is recommended to monitor for adherence, side effects, and self-reported smoking with NRT. When daily smoking is no more than half of a pack, the 2-mg gum, 2-mg lozenge, and

---

Box 8-1 A Smoking Cessation Plan

ML is 35 years old, and although she successfully quit smoking during her pregnancy, her daughter is now 18 months old, and ML has resumed smoking one pack of cigarettes per day. During an annual visit for a PAP smear, she said she wants to stop smoking for good. Her clinician ran through the Five A's: ask, advise, assess, assist, and arrange. ML has asked for smoking cessation medication, and together, she and her clinician chose a quit date.

ML's history is significant for depression, for which she takes amitriptyline (Elavil). She has no other medical problems, and the only other medications are TriCyclen oral contraceptives and a multivitamin. She is not breastfeeding her daughter. Which of the following is the best choice for a first-line treatment for ML?

1. Bupropion SR (Wellbutrin SR)

2. Nicotine patch

3. Nicotine patch with ad lib use of other NRT products

4. Varenicline (Chantix)

Answer: ML should not take bupropion because both the antidepressant and the oral contraceptives have a potential drug–drug interaction that would increase the plasma levels of bupropion and increase the risk for seizure. Combination therapies are more efficacious than monotherapies, so the nicotine patch alone is not the best choice. Varenicline is the most effective but has an FDA black box warning that it could increase suicidal ideation. Thus, the nicotine patch with ad lib use of other NRT products is the best choice for a primary care provider who may not be able to provide the monitoring necessary for her use of varenicline.

ML's provider reviewed these options with her. The nicotine patch comes in formulations of 7 mg, 14 mg, and 21 mg (NicoDerm) designed for 24-hour use or a 15-mg (Nicotrol) formulation that is used for 16 hours. Standard practice is to give the patient the dose that corresponds to the number of cigarettes smoked per day. Thus, ML was given one 21 mg patch. Her provider gave her a prescription and education materials on how to use the patch, gum, and lozenges.

Smoking cessation is most effective if nonpharmacologic methods are combined with pharmacologic methods. ML's provider encouraged her to make an appointment with her therapist to discuss possible use of varenicline and other nonpharmacologic therapies. She was given information about a smoking cessation group as well. ML made an appointment to return 1 week after her quit date to evaluate her progress.

7- or 14-mg patch may be considered for a starting dose of NRT.

Individuals selecting to use the gum or lozenge do require instruction on proper use. The NRT gum should not be chewed like regular gum. The NRT lozenge should not be used like candy. Both the gum and lozenge require a slow alternating pace of stimulation of the product in the mouth by parking the lozenge or gum in the mouth. Stimulation of the drug, such as NRT gum with chewing, should occur with smoking urges. Individuals have complained about the effect of the gum on dental work.

The inhaler is used through the mouth. An individual selecting this method will also require administration instructions. The product looks like a cigarette. A small cartridge is placed in the device. Drug release requires activation of the device in order to inhale or puff on the device for the release of nicotine. Directions for using nicotine replacement products are listed in Table 8-5.

Most nicotine patches are applied and removed every 24 hours. The Nicotrol patch is unlike the other patches and is not used for 24 hours. Instead, this patch should only be worn for 16 hours. For women who have sleep disturbances with the use of the 24-hour patches, the 16-hour patch provides an alternative NRT. Nicotine patches have been found to be associated with sleep disturbances. Nicotine patches are similar to a sandwich. The top layer exposed to the air is not permeable. The nicotine is placed between the outer layer and a permeable layer that is placed on the skin. The nicotine is slowly released over the course of the day through the skin to the capillaries. Patches were originally all the same size and color. More recently, patches have been designed to be less obvious when worn on an area not covered by clothing (e.g., on an arm). Patch size has been scaled to reflect changes in dosage for those products that provide a stepwise reduction in nicotine dosing as part of the treatment strategy.

According to the 2008 update to the clinical guidelines, women benefit from smoking intervention medications, but perhaps not in the same way as men.[34]

Gender differences have been reported in clinical trials, but whether this evidence is clinically significant is not apparent. NRT has been more effective for men than women except with the nicotine inhaler, although differences were not always statistically significant.[58] The nicotine inhaler has been reported as an effective mode of medication delivery of NRT for women.[59] More research is needed to determine if the inhaler's delivery system with design similarities comparable to a cigarette are related to cues and triggers specific to women. Women have different cues for smoking. Research suggests these may form the basis for the improved response by women in the use of the NRT inhaler compared to other NRT products. Women are triggered by sensory cues related to smoking, such as tactile and odor cues.[25,39,60]

Combination Therapy

Within the last decade, research has investigated the efficacy of combining different types of NRT or combining NRT with bupropion to increase tobacco cessation. These trials have

Table 8-5 Directions for Using Nicotine Replacement Products

Nicotine Patch	Nicotine Gum or Lozenge	Nicotine Nasal Spray	Nicotine Inhaler
The nicotine patch provides a steady supply of nicotine that is absorbed from the skin and will continue to be absorbed several hours after the patch is removed.	Nicotine gum provides a steady supply of nicotine that is absorbed from the mucous membranes in your mouth. Any nicotine that you swallow will not have an effect.	Spray is a good form of NRT for persons who are highly addicted because the nicotine gets to the brain faster than with other products (approximately 10 min) and reduces cravings more quickly.	The inhaler comes with 42 cartridges and a mouthpiece.
• Place a new patch on your body every morning.	• Chew slowly until you notice a peppery taste.	• Each spray is approximately 0.5 mg of nicotine. Blow your nose to make it clear.	• Place the cartridge in the inhaler and then place the inhaler in your mouth.
• Place the patch on a clean, dry, nonhairy area on your upper body or arm between your neck and your waist.	• Then place the gum in the side of your mouth between your gum and your cheek.	• Slightly tilt your head back and insert bottle tip as far back as is easily done.	• Close your mouth around the inhaler.
• Use a different site every day.	• Leave each piece of gum in place for 30 minutes.	• Breathe in through your mouth and hold your breath.	• Suck on the inhaler with several short sucks to get the air saturated with nicotine into the back of your throat.
• It is safe to wear the patch in the shower, pool, or bath.	• Avoid acidic foods for 15 min before and after using this gum.	• Press the bottom of the bottle to release the spray.	• Suck or puff on each cartridge for about 20 minutes.
• If the skin becomes irritated, rub a small amount of 1% hydrocortisone cream over the irritated area once a day until healed.		• Don't sniff through your nose or swallow while spraying.	• Use at least 6 cartridges a day and no more than 16 per day.
		• Breathe out through your mouth.	
		• Apply one spray to each nostril.	
		• Use the spray at least 8 times/day but no more than 40 times/day.	

been successful. The patch provides the long-acting NRT while nicotine gum, an inhaler, or lozenge provides relief for breakthrough urges for nicotine.[61-63] Long-term use of a nicotine patch (greater than 14 weeks) with ad lib use of NRT gum or spray has had an odds ratio of effectiveness of 3.6 (95% CI, 2.5–5.2).[34] According to the latest treatment guideline update, this combination of NRT medications has an estimated abstinence rate of 36%.[34] Use of the NRT patch with bupropion had the next highest odds ratio (OR 2.5; 95% CI, 1.9–3.4) and abstinence rates (29%). Use of the patch with nortriptyline or the NRT inhaler have also demonstrated abstinence rates of 27% and 26%, respectively.[34]

Future Therapy

There are new therapies under development and testing to treat tobacco dependence. Nicotine conjugate vaccine (NicVAX) is under investigation with the potential use for treating tobacco dependence. The vaccine blocks nicotine's antibodies in the brain. Findings from Phase II trials indicate NicVAX is safe and influenced cessation efforts in 25% of smokers with smoking histories of one pack per day or more.[64,65] Furthermore, these preliminary reports suggest the nicotine vaccine has minimal to no side effects.

Alternative Therapies

Smokers have used various complementary and alternative medicine (CAM) therapies that include but are not limited to hypnosis, acupuncture, relaxation, and meditation.[66,67] A survey of 1175 tobacco users or former users found more than a quarter acknowledged using CAM to assist their tobacco cessation efforts.[67] In addition, more than two-thirds reported interest in using CAM for future attempts to treat their tobacco disorder.

Evidence is lacking for support of scheduled sessions with temporary acupuncture treatment.[68] There is no research evidence to support the use of staples in the ear for smoking cessation.

Aromatherapy may gather support as an intervention for control of tobacco cravings if future studies build upon the evidence reported by Sayette and Parrott. Malodorous and pleasant odors that did not illicit a negative-effect-related expression were most effective in minimizing urges to smoke with a 21-point drop in their reported urge to smoke as compared to the 11-point drop in reported urge

when water was sniffed ($P < .05$).[69] Research has not been reported using aromatherapy to suppress tobacco urges. Future studies may consider incorporating this suggested intervention for urge control with an array of other distraction techniques. In addition, the usefulness of this technique may be dependent upon whether individuals have limbic system sensitivity to chemical odors.[70]

A 2005 Cochrane Database systematic review indicated that one study provided evidence of support for the use of exercise to aid smoking cessation when exercise therapy is considered as a complementary intervention strategy for smoking cessation.[71] Three studies that examined using exercise as a smoking cessation intervention achieved significant differences between the exercise group and the control group at the end of the treatment phase; however, only one study demonstrated borderline effectiveness for exercise 12 months following treatment. Abstinence rates at the 3-month follow-up were 11.9% for the exercise group and 5.4% for control group.[72] Rigorous research trials are lacking in the examination of yoga as an aid in smoking cessation. Further research is needed to investigate CAM therapies for tobacco cessation.

Special Populations

Women Using Oral Contraceptives

Oral contraceptives may inhibit CP450B6 activity, which metabolizes bupropion. Thus concomitant use may increase plasma levels of bupropion SR and thereby increase the risk of seizures and bupropion side effects. This has been studied in a few small studies with inconclusive results to date. However, women on oral contraceptives may need smaller doses of bupropion when starting on this drug.[73]

Pregnancy and Lactation

The US Public Health Service guideline suggested that women may be motivated to quit during pregnancy, during which time they are likely to be susceptible to messages and reinforcement for tobacco cessation. Furthermore, healthcare providers may promote relapse prevention by emphasizing the relationship between maternal smoking and poor health outcomes for both the mother and child. Women who are able to quit smoking by 16 weeks gestation have no increased risk for low birth weight, stillbirth, or infant death compared to those who continue smoking into the second trimester.

Bupropion (FDA Pregnancy Category C) has no known teratogenic effects, but the increased risk for seizures is a concern that has limited prescriptions for use by pregnant women. NRT is classified as FDA Pregnancy Category D although there is no data on teratogenic effects in humans to date. The safety of nicotine replacement during pregnancy has been evaluated in a few clinical trials that have shown some effectiveness and no adverse effects on women or their fetuses.[74] In the absence of conclusive data, it is currently believed that the benefits of smoking cessation outweigh potential risks to the fetus from exposure to NRT products, and clinical practice guidelines in the United States recommend NRT products for pregnant women as long as the total dose of nicotine in the NRT is not larger than would have been received via the usual dose from that individual's daily smoking habit.[34]

The majority of women who quit smoking during pregnancy resume smoking within 3 months postpartum.[75] Postpartum relapse has been attributed to decreased self-efficacy, lack of effective coping strategies to resist smoking temptation, and weight concerns.[75] A systematic review of smoking interventions delivered during the postpartum period found no effect of these programs in increasing smoking cessation rates.[76] More research is needed to prevent smoking relapse in the postpartum period.

Elderly

Efforts to help women who are perimenopausal or menopausal to stop smoking deserve special mention. Smoking is significantly associated with early onset of menopause, which, in turn, increases a woman's risk for cardiovascular disorders, osteoporosis, etc. Concern about weight gain has been one reason smokers do not quit smoking. Smoking cessation drugs can be used by women who are on hormone therapy.[77] Few studies on specific NRT products used by women 65 years or older found that the nicotine patch is equally effective in this population as it is in persons in other age ranges. Because steroids inhibit CP450B6 activity, women on hormone therapy may need smaller doses of bupropion SR when starting the drug.

▌Conclusion

Pharmacologic therapy is an important treatment option for women desiring to discontinue their use of tobacco. Varenicline (Chantix) is relatively new for tobacco addiction treatment but holds promise as a new and effective therapy and as a monotherapy, and it has the highest abstinence rate compared to placebo (33.2% CI, 28.9–37.8 at 6 months).[34] Bupropion provides women with a different option that

also has the ability to attenuate weight gain with nearly a 25% abstinence rate, and is as efficacious as NRT products when used as a monotherapy.[34] For women who are highly addicted, the highest rates of abstinence occur with the combination therapy of the nicotine patch with bupropion SR followed by the combination of the nicotine patch with ad lib use of NRT gum or spray.[34] Combination therapies with varenicline have not been conducted to date.

Research supports the need to treat smokers for longer than 12 weeks, particularly in the severely addicted person.[34] Healthcare providers may need to consider menstrual cycles when initiating tobacco cessation in premenopausal women. Both the younger and older women should not be ignored due to their age when it comes to providing tobacco addiction treatment. They each can obtain great health benefits by quitting smoking.

Offering messages to promote cessation and prescribing treatment is only the beginning when assisting women to abstain from tobacco. Follow-up is vital to assist women with the support and monitoring required of their progress, use of medications, side effects, and relapse prevention. When women smoke, they have the potential of creating harm to themselves, their children, and their unborn children. When healthcare providers promote tobacco cessation and provide treatment, the promotion of health goes beyond the individual. Treatment begins with assessment and messages, which leads to the selection of the therapy plan for both pharmacologic products and cognitive behavioral therapy.

✚ References

1. Cigarette smoking among adults—United States, 2006. MMWR 2007;56(44):1157–61.
2. Mokdad AH, Marks JS, Stroup DF, Gerberding JL. Actual causes of death in the United States, 2000. JAMA2004;291(10):1238–45.
3. Annual smoking-attributable mortality, years of potential life lost, and economic costs—United States, 1995–1999. MMWR2002;51(14):300–3.
4. US Department of Health and Human Services. The health consequences of smoking for women. A report of the surgeon general. Washington, DC: US Department of Health and Human Services, Public Health Service, Office of the Assistant Secretary for Health, Office on Smoking and Health, 1980.
5. Minino AM, Heron MP, Murphy SL, Kochanek KD. Deaths: final data for 2004. Natl Vital Stat Rep 2007;55(19):1–119.

6. Henschke CI, Yip R, Miettinen OS. Women's susceptibility to tobacco carcinogens and survival after diagnosis of lung cancer. JAMA 2006;296(2):180–4.

7. Healton CG, Gritz ER, Davis KC, Homsi G, McCausland K, Haviland ML, et al. Women's knowledge of the leading causes of cancer death. Nicotine Tobacco Res 2007;9(7):761–8.

8. Edwards BK, Brown ML, Wingo PA, Howe HL, Ward E, Reis LA, Schrag D, et al. Annual report to the nation on the status of cancer, 1975–2002, featuring population-based trends in cancer treatment. J Natl Cancer Inst 2005;97(19):1407–27.

9. DiFranza JR, Savageau JA, Rigotti NA, Fletcher K, Ockene JK, McNeill AD, et al. Development of symptoms of tobacco dependence in youths: 30 month follow up data from the DANDY study. Tobacco Control 2002;11(3):228–35.

10. Albrecht SA, Caruthers D. Characteristics of inner-city pregnant smoking teenagers. J Obstet, Gynecol, Neonatal Nurs 2002;31(4):462–9.

11. Bricker JB, Peterson AV, Robyn Andersen M, Leroux BG, Bharat Rajan K, Sarason IG. Close friends', parents', and older siblings' smoking: reevaluating their influence on children's smoking. Nicotine Tobacco Res 2006;8(2):217–26.

12. Hertling I, Ramskogler K, Dvorak A, Klinger A, Saletu-Zyhlarz G, Schoberberger R, et al. Craving and other characteristics of the comorbidity of alcohol and nicotine dependence. Eur Psychiatry 2005; 20(5–6):442–50.

13. Johnson PB, Boles SM, Kleber HD. The relationship between adolescent smoking and drinking and likelihood estimates of illicit drug use. J Addic Dis 2000;19(2):75–81.

14. Werler MM. Teratogen update: smoking and reproductive outcomes. Teratology 1997;55(6):382–8.

15. Aligne CA, Stoddard JJ. Tobacco and children. An economic evaluation of the medical effects of parental smoking. Arch Pediatr Adolesc Med 1997;151(7):648–53.

16. Supervia A, Nogues X, Enjuanes A, Vila J, Mellibovsky L, Serrano S Aubia J, et al. Effect of smoking and smoking cessation on bone mass, bone remodeling, vitamin D, PTH and sex hormones. J Musculoskelet Neuronal Interact 2006;6(3):234–41.

17. Jenkins MR, Denison AV. Smoking status as a predictor of hip fracture risk in postmenopausal women of northwest Texas. Preventing Chronic Dis 2008; 5(1):A09.

18. Kadunce DP, Burr R, Gress R, Kanner R, Lyon JL, Zone JJ. Cigarette smoking: risk factor for premature facial wrinkling. Ann Intern Med 1991;114(10):840–4.

19. US Department of Health and Human Services. Women on smoking. A report of the surgeon general. Atlanta, GA: US: Department of Health and Human Services, Centers for Disease Control and Prevention, National Center for Chronic Disease Prevention and Health Promotion, Office on Smoking and Health, 2001.

20. Centers for Disease Control and Prevention. Smoking during pregnancy—United States, 1990–2002. MMWR 2004;53(39):911–5.

21. Mullen PD, Richardson MA, Quinn VP, Ershoff DH. Postpartum return to smoking: who is at risk and when. Am J Health Promotion 1997;11(5):323–30.

22. Martin JA, Hamilton BE, Sutton PD, Ventura SJ, Menacker F, Kirmeyer S. Births: final data for 2004. National Vital Statistics Report, 2006;55(1):1–102.

23. Nafstad P, Botten G, Hagen J. Partner's smoking: a major determinant for changes in women's smoking behaviour during and after pregnancy. Public Health 1996;110(6):379–85.

24. Audrain J, Gomez-Caminero A, Robertson AR, Boyd R, Orleans CT, Lerman C. Gender and ethnic differences in readiness to change smoking behavior. Women's Health 1997;3(2):139–50.

25. Perkins KA. Smoking cessation in women. Special considerations. CNS Drugs 2001;15(5):391–411.

26. Benowitz N. Nicotine pharmacology and addiction. In Benowitz N, ed. Nicotine safety and toxicity. New York: Oxford University Press, 1998:3–16.

27. Rosecrans JA, Karan LD. Neurobehavioral mechanisms of nicotine action: role in the initiation and maintenance of tobacco dependence. J Subst Abuse Treatment 1993;10(2):161–70.

28. Benowitz NL. Neurobiology of nicotine addiction: implications for smoking cessation treatment. Am J Med 2008; 121(4 Suppl 1):S3–10.

29. Henningfield J, Cohen C, Pickworth W. Psychopharmacology of nicotine. In Orleans C, Slade J, eds. Nicotine addiction: principles of management. New York: Oxford University Press, 1993:24–45.

30. Pinel J. Biopsychology, 3rd ed. Boston: Allyn and Bacon, 1997.

31. Zevin S, Benowitz NL. Drug interactions with tobacco smoking. An update. Clin Pharmacokinet 1999; 36(6):425–38.

32. Hughes JR, Gust SW, Skoog K, Keenan RM, Fenwick JW. Symptoms of tobacco withdrawal. A replication and extension. Arch Gen Psychiatry 1991;48(1):52–9.

33. Fiore MC, Bailey WC, Cohen SJ, Dorfman SF, Goldstein MG, Gritz ER, et al. Treating tobacco use and dependence. Clinical practice guidelines. Rockville, MD: US

Department of Health and Human Services, Public Health Service, 2000.

34. Fiore MC, Jaén CR, Baker TB, Bailey WC, Benowitz NL, Curry SL, et al. Treating tobacco use and dependence: 2008 update. Clinical practice guideline. Rockville, MD: US Department of Health and Human Services. Public Health Service, May 2008.

35. Segaar D, Willemsen MC, Bolman C, De Vries H. Nurse adherence to a minimal-contact smoking cessation intervention on cardiac wards. Res Nurs Health 2007;30(4):429–44.

36. Meredith LS, Yano EM, Hickey SC, Sherman SE. Primary care provider attitudes are associated with smoking cessation counseling and referral. Med Care 2005;43(9):929–34.

37. Blumenthal DS. Barriers to the provision of smoking cessation services reported by clinicians in underserved communities. J Am Board Fam Med 2007;20(3):272–9.

38. Price JH, Mohamed I, Jeffrey JD. Tobacco intervention training in American College of Nurse-Midwives accredited education programs. J Midwifery Women's Health 2008; 53(1):68–74.

39. Perkins KA, Conklin CA, Levine MD. Cognitive-behavioral therapy for smoking cessation: a practical guidebook to the most effective treatments. London: Routledge Taylor & Francis Group, 2008.

40. Hughes JR, Stead LF, Lancaster T. Antidepressants for smoking cessation. Cochrane Database Syst Rev 2007 (1):CD000031.

41. Nides M. Update on pharmacologic options for smoking cessation treatment. Am J Med 2008; 121(4 Suppl 1):S20–31.

42. Hall SM, Lightwood JM, Humfleet GL, Bostrom A, Reus VI, Munoz R. Cost-effectiveness of bupropion, nortriptyline, and psychological intervention in smoking cessation. J Behav Health Serv Res 2005;32(4):381–92.

43. Foley KF, DeSanty KP, Kast RE. Bupropion: pharmacology and therapeutic applications. Expert review of neurotherapeutics 2006;6(9):1249–65.

44. Haustein KO. Bupropion: pharmacological and clinical profile in smoking cessation. Int J Clin Pharmacol Ther 2003;41(2):56–66.

45. Boshier A, Wilton LV, Shakir SA. Evaluation of the safety of bupropion (Zyban) for smoking cessation from experience gained in general practice use in England in 2000. Eur J Clin Pharmacol 2003;59(10):767–73.

46. West R. Bupropion SR for smoking cessation. Expert Opinion Pharmacother 2003;4(4):533–40.

47. Rigotti NA, Thorndike AN, Regan S, McKool K, Patetrnak RC, Chang Y, et al. Bupropion for smokers hospitalized with acute cardiovascular disease. Am J Med 2006;119(12):1080–7.

48. Lee AM, Jepson C, Hoffmann E, Epstein L, Hawk LW, Lerman C, et al. CYP2B6 genotype alters abstinence rates in a bupropion smoking cessation trial. Biol Psychiatry 2007;62(6):635–41.

49. Swan GE, Valdes AM, Ring HZ, Khroyan TV, Jack LM, Ton CC, et al. Dopamine receptor DRD2 genotype and smoking cessation outcome following treatment with bupropion SR. Pharmacogenomics J 2005;5(1):21–9.

50. Obach RS, Reed-Hagen AE, Krueger SS, Obach BJ, O'Connell TN, Zandi KS, et al. Metabolism and disposition of varenicline, a selective alpha4beta2 acetylcholine receptor partial agonist, in vivo and in vitro. Drug Metab Dispo 2006; 34(1):121–30.

51. Gonzales D, Rennard SI, Nides M, Oncken C, Azoulay S, Billing CB. Varenicline, an alpha4beta2 nicotinic acetylcholine receptor partial agonist, vs sustained-release bupropion and placebo for smoking cessation: a randomized controlled trial. JAMA 2006;296(1):47–55.

52. Zierler-Brown SL, Kyle JA. Oral varenicline for smoking cessation. Ann Pharmacother 2007;41(1):95–9.

53. Stapleton JA, Watson L, Spirling LI, et al. Varenicline in the routine treatment of tobacco dependence: a pre-post comparison with nicotine replacement therapy and an evaluation in those with mental illness. Addiction 2008;103(1):146–54.

54. Jorenby DE, Hays JT, Rigotti NA, Azoulay S, Wastsky EJ, Williams KE, et al. Efficacy of varenicline, an alpha4beta2 nicotinic acetylcholine receptor partial agonist, vs placebo or sustained-release bupropion for smoking cessation: randomized controlled trial. JAMA 2006;296(1):56–63.

55. Choi JH, Dresler CM, Norton MR, Strahs KR. Pharmacokinetics of a nicotine polacrilex lozenge. Nicotine Tob Res 2003;5(5):635–44.

56. Hukkanen J, Jacob P III, Benowitz NL. Effect of grapefruit juice on cytochrome P450 2A6 and nicotine renal clearance. Clin Pharmacol Ther 2006;80(5):522–30.

57. Stead LF, Perera R, Bullen C, Mant D, Lancaster T. Nicotine replacement therapy for smoking cessation. Cochrane Database Syst Rev 2008 (1):CD000146.

58. Wetter DW, Fiore MC, Young TB, McClure JB, de Moor CA, Baker TB. Gender differences in response to nicotine replacement therapy: objective and subjective indexes of tobacco withdrawal. Exp Clin Psychopharmacol 1999;7(2):135–44.

59. Cepeda-Benito A, Reynoso JT, Erath S. Meta-analysis of the efficacy of nicotine replacement therapy for smoking cessation: differences between men and women. J Consult Clin Psychol 2004;72(4):712–22.

60. Perkins KA, Donny E, Caggiula AR. Sex differences in nicotine effects and self-administration: review of human and animal evidence. Nicotine Tobacco Res 1999;1(4):301–15.

61. Croghan IT, Hurt RD, Dakhil SR, Crighan GA, Sloan JA, Novotny PJ, et al. Randomized comparison of a nicotine inhaler and bupropion for smoking cessation and relapse prevention. Mayo Clin Proc 2007; 82(2):186–95.

62. Hurt RD, Krook JE, Croghan IT, Loprinzi CL, Sloan JA, Novotny PJ, et al. Nicotine patch therapy based on smoking rate followed by bupropion for prevention of relapse to smoking. J Clin Oncol 2003; 21(5):914–20.

63. Jamerson BD, Nides M, Jorenby DE, Donahue R, Garrett P, Johnston JA, et al. Late-term smoking cessation despite initial failure: an evaluation of bupropion sustained release, nicotine patch, combination therapy, and placebo. Clin Ther 2001;23(5):744–52.

64. Cerny T. Anti-nicotine vaccination: where are we? Recent Results Cancer Res 2005; 166:167–75.

65. Hatsukami DK, Rennard S, Jorenby D, Fiore M, Koopmeiners J, de Vos A, et al. Safety and immunogenicity of a nicotine conjugate vaccine in current smokers. Clin Pharmacol Ther 2005;78(5):456–67.

66. Abbot NC, Stead LF, White AR, Barnes J. Hypnotherapy for smoking cessation. Cochrane Database of Systematic Rev 1998, Issue 2. Art No: CD001008. DOI: 10.1002/14651858.CD001008.

67. Sood A, Ebbert JO, Sood R, Stevens SR. Complementary treatments for tobacco cessation: a survey. Nicotine Tobacco Res 2006;8(6):767–71.

68. White AR, Rampes H, Campbell JL. Acupuncture and related interventions for smoking cessation. Cochrane Database of Systematic Reviews 2006, Issue 1. Art. No.: CD000009. DOI: 10.1002/14651858. CD000009.pub2.

69. Sayette MA, Parrott DJ. Effects of olfactory stimuli on urge reduction in smokers. Exp Clin Psychopharmacol 1999;7(2):151–9.

70. Bell IR, Hardin EE, Baldwin CM, Schwartz GE. Increased limbic system symptomatology and sensitizability of young adults with chemical and noise sensitivities. Environ Res 1995;70(2):84–97.

71. Ussher M. Exercise interventions for smoking cessation. Cochrane Database Systematic Rev 2005 (1):CD002295.

72. Marcus BH, Albrecht AE, King TK, Parisi AF, Pinto BM, Roberts M, et al. The efficacy of exercise as an aid for smoking cessation in women: a randomized controlled trial. Arch Int Med 1999;159(11):1229–34.

73. Palovaara S, Pelkonen O, Uusitalo J, Lundgren S, Laine K. Inhibition of cytochrome P450 2B6 activity by hormone replacement therapy and oral contraceptive as measured by bupropion hydroxylation C. Clin Pharmacol Ther 2003; 74:326–33.

74. Rigotti NA, Park ER, Chang Y, Regan S. Smoking cessation medication use among pregnant and postpartum smokers. Obstet Gynecol 2008;111(2 pt 1):348–55.

75. McBride CM, Curry SJ, Lando HA, Pirie PL, Grothaus LC, Nelson JC. Prevention of relapse in women who quit smoking during pregnancy. Am J Public Health 1999;89(5):706–11.

76. Levitt C, Shaw E, Wong S, Kaczorowski J. Systematic review of the literature on postpartum care: effectiveness of interventions for smoking relapse prevention, cessation, and reduction in postpartum women. Birth 2007;34(4):341–7.

77. Allen SS, Hatsukami DK, Bade T, Center B. Transdermal nicotine use in postmenopausal women: does the treatment efficacy differ in women using and not using hormone replacement therapy? Nicotine Tobacco Res 2004 Oct;6(5):777–88.

"I can resist anything but temptation."

OSCAR WILDE

9

Drugs of Abuse

Barbara Peterson Sinclair and Shirley A. Summers

✚ Chapter Glossary

Addiction A state in which a body relies on a substance for normal functioning and develops physical dependence. Impaired control over drug use.

Craving Also called psychological dependence. An intense desire to reexperience the effects of a psychoactive substance. Craving is often the cause of relapse.

Cross tolerance The ability to tolerate one drug because of tolerance to another drug that is similar in mechanism and action, even if that other drug has not been administered or used.

Drug abuse See *substance dependence*.

Drug addiction According to the World Health Organization, "a state of periodic or chronic intoxication detrimental to the individual and society, which is characterized by an overwhelming desire to continue taking the drug and to obtain it by any means."

Drug misuse Inappropriate use of prescribed or OTC drugs. Examples include taking more prescribed or OTC drugs than indicated, for a longer period than indicated, mixing drugs to potentiate euphoria, sharing drugs with others, or discontinuing drugs early.

Gateway drug An agent whose use may lead to use of another drug. Alcohol, tobacco, and marijuana are the most commonly used first drugs.

Illicit drug Illegal drug, such as marijuana, cocaine, or LSD.

Licit drug Legal drug such as caffeine-containing agents, alcohol, or tobacco.

Narcotic The word used to refer to illegal use of opiates.

Opiate Any substance derived from opium.

Opioid All opiate-type drugs, both those manufactured synthetically and those derived naturally from opium.

Physical dependence Adverse physical symptoms that appear when a drug is withdrawn.

Psychoactive effects The result of using substances that affect the central nervous system and alter consciousness and/or perception.

Recreational drug use Use of drugs to achieve a certain mental or psychic state.

Substance abuse* Recurrent clinical adverse effects from drug use that include one or more of the following: (1) failure to fulfill major obligations, (2) use when physically hazardous, (3) recurrent legal problems, (4) recurrent social or interpersonal problems.

Substance dependence* (drug abuse) A maladaptive pattern of substance use that leads to clinically significant impairment that is manifested by at least three of the following: (1) tolerance, (2) withdrawal, (3) use of the substance in larger amounts or over a longer period of time than intended, (4) desire or unsuccessful attempts to stop use, (5) spending considerable time to acquire the substance, reducing important social, occupational, or recreational activities over a 12-month period, or (6) continued use despite adverse consequences.

Tolerance A decreased effect of a drug that develops with continued use so that larger doses are needed to elicit an effect. Dose-response curve shifts to the right.

Withdrawal syndrome A set of classic signs and symptoms that appear when a drug is discontinued in a person who has physical dependence. Also known as abstinence syndrome.

* APA DSM-IV criteria.

Sources: Adapted from Goode[64]; Hanson[65]; Cami.[3]

Introduction

During the last several decades, scientific research has shown that **drug addiction** is a true health problem similar to other physical diseases that have negative effects on normal functioning. Substance abuse was once thought to be due to a moral failing, and even today in many arenas it continues to be perceived entirely as a social problem. Although behavioral aspects have great significance, there is no question that drug addiction is a chronic disease of the brain.[1]

With advances in newer imaging techniques, neurobiologists have found that chronic drug exposure can actually enlarge or shrink certain regions of the brain. In addition, drugs can negatively influence neurotransmitter systems that link and coordinate brain cells, resulting in derangements in pathways, especially those affecting reward and pleasure. Such changes often affect abusers' cognitive and decision-making abilities as well as their perception of "feeling good" emotions.

Addiction varies among individuals depending upon biologic makeup and factors such as genetics, gender, environment, drug availability, and age at initial use. Not everyone exposed to drugs will become addicted; however, adolescents are at a greater risk than the general population. This increased risk exists because the brain continues to develop during adolescence and drugs can negatively influence some of the ongoing modifications during this developmental phase.[2] A second group at higher risk are those with psychiatric illnesses such as schizophrenia, bipolar disorder, depression, and attention deficit hyperactivity disorder. Such individuals usually have existing chemical imbalances and thus poor impulse control. They often exhibit risk-taking or novelty-seeking traits such as the use of substances, which is then perceived to make them feel better, and then they continue using substances as self-medication. In addition, persons with conditions such as schizophrenia may already have an overactive dopamine system, thus requiring much larger amounts of drug to achieve the desired feelings.[3]

Addiction to chemical substances that are deemed either legal or illicit can occur. Legal substances include alcohol, tobacco, and inhalants, or drugs with therapeutic value such as analgesics, sedatives, antihistamines, tranquilizers, and amphetamines. Illicit substances are agents whose use is against the law and commonly include marijuana, methamphetamine, cocaine, hallucinogens, and heroin.

Definition of Addiction

Although standard terminology varies, **addiction** is defined as "a primary, chronic, neurobiologic disease, with genetic, psychosocial, and environmental factors influencing its development and manifestations. It is characterized by behaviors that include one or more of the following: (1) impaired control over drug use, (2) compulsive use, (3) continued use despite harm, and craving."[4] The chapter glossary lists the definitions for common terms used in the substance abuse field as well as the American Psychological Association DSM-IV definitions of **substance abuse** and **substance dependence**.

Physiology of Brain Function and Neurotransmitters

Major brain regions with roles in addiction can be seen in Figure 9-1. The prefrontal cortex is the focal point

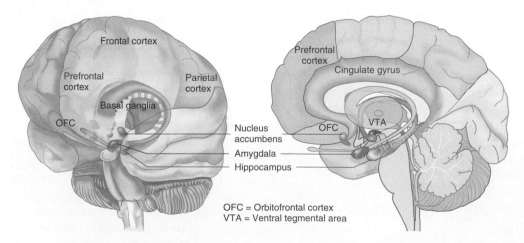

Major portions of the brain involved in addiction include the prefrontal cortex (the focus for cognition and planning) and the limbic system, which coordinates the brain's reward system and includes the ventral tegmental area, nucleus accumbens, amygdala, and hippocampus.

Figure 9-1 The brain and addiction. *Source:* ©Terese Winslow per use agreement.

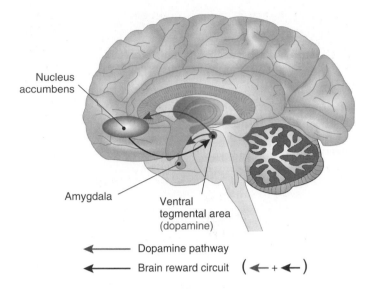

Nucleus
accumbens

Amygdala

Ventral
tegmental area
(dopamine)

⟵——— Dopamine pathway

⟵——— Brain reward circuit (⟵ + ⟵)

Increased levels of dopamine in the neuronal synapses stimulate the reward pathway, which encourages the individual
to continue taking substances that increase dopamine in the neuronal synapses.

Figure 9-2 The reward pathway.

for cognition, planning, and goal setting where rational thought can override impulsive behavior. Just below the cortex is the mesolimbic system, a group of structures that form a ring or limbus around the brain stem. The mesolimbic system structures are involved with internal homeostasis, memory, learning, motivation, and emotion. Structures in the mesolimbic system include the ventral tegmental area (VTA), nucleus accumbens (NAc), amygdala, hippocampus, and the mesolimbic pathway of neurons that connects the neuronal cell bodies in the VTA to the NAc. The mesolimbic pathway has branches that extend to the prefrontal cortex. This area of the brain is best known as the reward or pleasure system since it provides an individual with positive feelings normally associated with activities necessary for survival such as eating, biologic rhythms, and sexual behaviors (Figure 9-2).

Neurons in the brain are not physically contiguous, and in order for messages to pass from one neuron to another, the message must cross a synapse, the small space separating the cells. This movement is accomplished by receiving, processing, and sending signals down the presynaptic neuronal axon and then using chemicals called neurotransmitters that physically cross the synapse. Once in the synapse, the neurotransmitter binds to receptors on the dendrite of the postsynaptic neuron. The neurotransmitters not bound to specific receptors are either enzymatically destroyed, diffuse away, or are taken back into the presynaptic nerve via a reuptake mechanism (Figure 9-3).

The neurotransmitters most commonly altered by drugs of abuse include dopamine, a regulator of motivation and

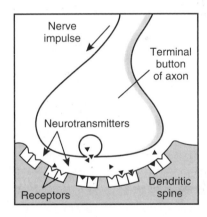

Neurotransmitters such as dopamine are released via electrical impulses from the presynaptic neuron and move through the synaptic cleft to bind with receptors on the postsynaptic neuron.

Figure 9-3 Synaptic neurotransmission.
Source: Courtesy of the National Institute of Drug Abuse.

pleasure; serotonin, which provides a sense of well-being and regulates mood; endogenous opioids, the naturally occurring pain reducers that produce euphoria; norepinephrine, which triggers alertness and arousal under stress; glutamate, a major excitatory neurotransmitter; and gamma-amino butyric acid (GABA), the major inhibitory neurotransmitter[5] (Table 9-1). Approximately 50–65% of all neurons in the brain are GABAergic—i.e., they enhance GABA activity.[6]

Dopamine is the major neurotransmitter in the mesolimbic pathway. Other neurotransmitters, such as serotonin, GABA, and the endorphins are closely linked

Table 9-1 Key Neurotransmitters

Neurotransmitter	Class	Function
Dopamine	Monoamine	Generally excitatory. Plays major role in motivation and reward. Acts as pacesetter for nerves needed to maintain desired needs and aims. Considered energizer of reward system. Stimulants and alcohol increase levels by blocking reuptake. Decreases nociception.
Endorphins	Neuropeptide	Generally inhibitory. Resembles opiates in producing analgesia and sense of well-being (euphoria). Effects are enhanced with use of actual opioids.
GABA (gamma amino-butyric acid)	Amino acid	Presynaptic inhibition. Effect augmented by alcohol and depressants that bind to receptors, causing slow reflexes and impaired motor coordination.
Glutamate	Amino acid	Excitatory. Inhibited by barbiturates and alcohol resulting in CNS depressant effects. Excessive amounts can damage cells via excitotoxicity.
Serotonin	Monoamine	Generally inhibitory. Modulates anger, aggression, mood, sleep, sexuality. Low levels may result in depressive state and schizophrenic conditions. Psychedelics mimic action and MDMA releases additional amounts.
Norepinephrine	Monoamine	Excitatory or inhibitory. Reaction to stressful events affects alertness and arousal, causing emergency responses of body. Low levels influence focus and can result in depression. Stimulants increase release and block reuptake.

Source: Cami.[3]

and can additionally impact the availability of dopamine, either by enhancing or inhibiting presynaptic release or by enhancing or inhibiting reuptake of dopamine.

Neurobiology of Addiction

On a neurobiologic level, addiction involves stimulating the pleasure or reinforcement pathway in the mesolimbic system. When drugs of abuse are used, they modulate the function of neurotransmitters in the mesolimbic system in a way that produces sensations of pleasure and positive feelings. When such drugs are used repeatedly, the mesolimbic system becomes dysregulated, and the result is a compulsion to maintain the drug use often with the need for greater amounts or more frequent dosing over time.[7]

The mesolimbic system also responds to environmental stimuli, and thus the associations that the individual makes between drugs and people, places, or objects will induce intense **cravings** in the individual when those associations are made. Such cue-induced reactions are thought to be responsible for relapse even after significant abstinence. Individuals who abuse drugs often exhibit cognitive difficulty making reasoned decisions or judging actions. This dysfunction is thought to arise from the prefrontal cortex, which is innervated by nerves from the VTA in the mesolimbic system.

The NAc is a primary target of amphetamines, opioids, cocaine, phencyclidine, ketamine, and nicotine, whereas alcohol, barbiturates, benzodiazepines, and opioids stimulate neurons in the VTA. Chronic administration of drugs such as cocaine, amphetamines, nicotine, or alcohol eventually results in a decrease in the reward/pleasure sensations, which then can lead to the compulsive drug-seeking and drug-taking behavior indicative of addiction.[8] Ultimately, addictive drugs act as both positive reinforcers via producing the feelings of pleasure and euphoria and as negative reinforcers via their ability to alleviate withdrawal symptoms.

Although drugs of abuse act on various parts of the limbic system and do so in various ways, they all enhance dopamine activity in the mesolimbic system.[9] Specific drugs of abuse affect the presence of dopamine in the synapses via different actions. For example, although dopamine is normally released at a slow, steady rate, opiates can increase the firing rate of the dopaminergic neurons. Stimulants such as cocaine and amphetamines decrease the reuptake of dopamine, thus enhancing the amount available in the synapse. Major central nervous system sedatives such as barbiturates and benzodiazepines generally augment GABA, and as a result, decrease the firing of dopaminergic neurons, which results in less dopamine in the synapse.

Continued exposure to drugs of abuse interferes with the normal communication process, especially in the prefrontal cortex, by causing synaptic remodeling to occur, resulting in a lower number of properly functioning dopamine receptors on the postsynaptic neuron. The clinical result is **tolerance**, or the need for larger or more frequent doses of the drug to obtain the same sense of pleasure. Individuals who are tolerant to one drug may also be tolerant to other drugs that have a similar mechanism of action. This is called **cross tolerance**. Addiction is a state in which the individual engages in a compulsive behavior to reinforce internal rewards, even when faced with negative outcomes.[4] A major feature of addiction is the user's loss of control in limiting intake of the substance.[4]

It remains unknown why the progression from user to abuser to addict occurs in certain individuals and not in others, but it is thought that contributing factors include individual biologic makeup and environmental/cultural/social components. Although the effect of specific drugs on the brain has been established, the degree of replication necessary for substance abuse to occur in a particular individual is simply not understood. No matter how an individual begins the process of addiction, there is a continuum or progression that moves from occasional use to compulsive use (increased frequency) to tolerance (higher doses) to dependency (creation of multiple, significant problems).

Mechanism of Action of Drugs Used by Substance Abusers

All drugs of abuse work in one of these four ways: (1) They imitate natural neurotransmitters and thereby stimulate a sense of well-being and euphoria (e.g., morphine binds to opiate receptors and stimulates the postsynaptic neuron).

(2) They stimulate the release of natural neurotransmitters (e.g., amphetamines stimulate the release of dopamine). (3) They block the release of a reuptake mechanism, thereby allowing more neurotransmitters in the synapse (e.g., cocaine blocks the reuptake of dopamine [Figure 9-4], and ecstasy blocks the reuptake of serotonin). (4) They bind to the GABA receptor and make it more effective in hyperpolarizing the postsynaptic neuron, which causes the postsynaptic neuron to be less excitable. This is the mechanism of action of alcohol, barbiturates, and benzodiazepines.

Mechanism of Action of Drugs Used to Treat Substance Abuse

Drugs used to treat substance abuse can be divided on the basis of three basic functions: (1) drugs used to treat acute intoxication or overdose, (2) drugs used to treat acute withdrawal symptoms, and (3) drugs used to sustain withdrawal from the substance that has caused addiction.

Drugs that are used to treat acute intoxication tend to be those that support basic respiratory and cardiac function. Most of the other drugs used for all three of these functions have a specific effect on the receptor for the neurotransmitter that is affected by the drug, causing

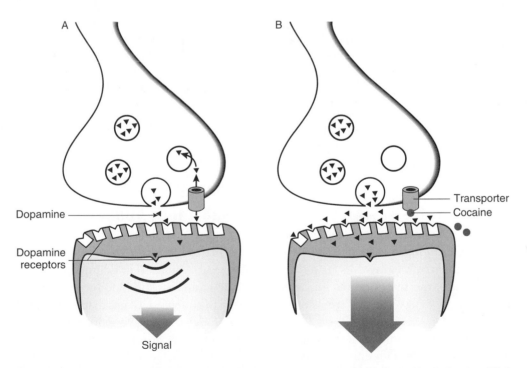

(A) Reuptake: Under normal conditions, dopamine is transported back into the presynaptic cell via the transporter. (B) Cocaine disrupts the reuptake of dopamine, causing it to accumulate in the synapse and intensify stimulation of receptors with resulting euphoria.

Figure 9-4 Effect of cocaine on dopamine reuptake. *Source:* © Terese Winslow per use agreement.

addiction. For example, naloxone (Narcan) is a competitive antagonist for the mu-opioid receptor, which is stimulated by opioids. (See Chapter 2 for a review of agonists, antagonists, and competitive antagonists.) Naloxone replaces opioids at the receptor site and blocks the action of that receptor. Methadone (Dolophine) is a full agonist for the mu-opioid receptor, but because it is also an antagonist to the glutamate receptor, the clinical result for persons taking methadone is analgesia—relief of narcotic craving— but no euphoria that stimulates the reward pathway.

Treatment of Substance Abuse and Addiction

For purposes of this chapter, substance abuse includes the nonmedical use of drugs that do or do not have medical value, whether they are illicit or legal.[10,11]

First, however, it is important to note that the healthcare delivery system in the United States is not able to provide total care to persons with drug addiction because many have limited access. In addition, the system has insufficient capacity and a lack of trained providers. To some degree, these deficits survive as a result of the social stigma that exists regarding drug use. A change in public opinion and healthcare policy could increase the availability of appropriate care needed by individuals suffering from substance abuse.[12]

The most successful approach for an individual with a substance-related disorder is comprehensive care, including both nonpharmacologic and pharmacologic therapies. Psychiatric services are often a critical component of care. Many individuals have concomitant social or behavioral problems that make their addictive disorders more difficult to treat, but even without related comorbidities, the severity of addiction ranges widely. Treatment must be tailored to fit the needs of the individual. Pharmacologic treatment as a stand-alone option is rarely sufficient to ensure long-term abstinence from alcohol or drugs. Treatment often involves urine testing for substances of abuse; the time periods for detection of the most common drugs abused are listed in Appendix 9-A.

Although an individual can become addicted to a wide variety of substances, including virtually any drug, specific ones appear to garner greater attention due to their frequent use. These will be highlighted within the classes of drugs discussed later in this chapter. (Nicotine addiction is discussed in Chapter 8.)

It should be noted that because most of the agents of abuse are used illicitly, they often have street names that are different than their formal pharmaceutical names. The most common street names are listed in the tables of this chapter; some terms vary regionally, such as cocaine, which may be termed *crack* in certain parts of the United States and *rock* in others. Regional variations also may include a polypharmacy approach wherein certain drugs are more likely to be combined with another when used in a specific area, and may even have a specific street name for the combination, such as *cheese* for a combination of acetaminophen, diphenhydramine, and heroin in the Southwest.

Nonpharmacologic Treatments for Substance Abuse

A number of scientifically based treatment options are available for individuals who are addicted to drugs and/ or alcohol. Behavioral treatments are designed to help the individual develop new coping skills, learn to identify relapse triggers, and respond appropriately to a relapse should it occur. Treatment interventions include motivational interviewing, cognitive behavioral therapy, contingency management, and skills training; however, one of the most commonly used approaches is a self-help group. Alcoholics Anonymous and Narcotics Anonymous are 12-step support groups run by former addicts who promote a lifetime of abstinence. The meetings are designed to provide mutual support to the members who do not use substances of any kind, using a one-day-at-a-time approach.

Pharmacologic Treatments for Substance Abuse

Pharmacologic properties of specific drugs affect their potential for abuse. For example, drugs that are highly lipophilic and cross the blood–brain barrier easily are more likely to be abused. Drugs that have a rapid onset and intensity of effect also have more potential for abuse. Persons who abuse the drugs discussed in this chapter often consume more than one drug or one class of drug. The specific effects of interactions between different drugs of abuse are listed in Table 9-2.

The following sections review addiction, withdrawal, and treatment for individual drugs or classes of drugs.

Table 9-2 Examples of Polypharmacy: Common Interactions of Agents and Substances of Abuse*

Drug Generic (Brand)	Combined With Generic (Brand)	Clinical Effect
Alcohol	Cocaine	This combination produces cocaethylene which has cardiotoxic properties and places the individual at increased risk for seizures. Persons using cocaine and alcohol concomitantly have a significantly increased risk for mortality.
Amphetamines	Antihypertensives	Antagonize the hypotensive effects of the antihypertensive medication.
Amphetamines	Chlorpromazine (Thorazine)	Blocks dopamine and norepinephrine receptors and can be used to treat amphetamine poisoning.
Amphetamines	Insulin	Decreased hypoglycemic effects.
Amphetamines	MAO inhibitor antidepressants	Slow metabolism of amphetamines, which increases amphetamine effect and possible hypertensive crisis, hyperthermia.
Amphetamines	Meperidine (Demerol)	Potentiates the analgesic effect of meperidine.
Amphetamines	Tricyclic antidepressants	Increased effect of the antidepressant, hypertensive crisis.
Cocaine	Insulin	Decreased hypoglycemic effect of insulin.
Diazepam (Valium)	Alcohol	Increased sedative effects.
Diazepam (Valium)	SSRI antidepressants	Increased sedative effects of the benzodiazepine (e.g., diazepam).
Heroin	Barbiturates, diazepam	Increased sedative effects.
MDMA	SSRIs	Theoretical risk for serotonin syndrome.

*Many antidepressants are based on interactions with the neurotransmitters dopamine, serotonin, and norepinephrine. Because these are the same neurotransmitters altered by the drugs discussed in this chapter, drug–drug interactions are typically additive or antagonistic. The clinical effects are secondary to too much neurotransmitter or the decreased efficacy of one drug or the other from the antagonism.

Source: Adapted from Hanson et al.[65]

It should be noted, however, that many individuals abuse more than one class of drugs and treatment is modified accordingly.

Opioids (Narcotics)

Natural opiates are derived from the opium poppy and include morphine, codeine, and thebaine. When these substances are modified, they produce semisynthetic opioids such as heroin, hydromorphone, oxycodone, and hydrocodone. Manufactured or synthetic opioids, e.g., meperidine (Demerol), propoxyphene, and fentanyl, were developed to produce anesthesia or reduce pain. Although the opioids are available by prescription only, they are among the many drugs that are abused. Terminology can be confusing. The term **opiate** refers specifically to substances derived from the opium poppy. The term **opioids** includes opiates, both the synthetic and the semisynthetic drugs that have a morphine-like effect. The term **narcotic** is frequently used when referring to opioids. However, because this term is often used in legal and common usage to refer to all **illicit drugs**, not just opioids, it is best to avoid the term narcotic.

Opioids bind to specific opiate receptors within the brain and spinal cord, resulting in decreased synaptic chemical transmission throughout the central nervous system (CNS). This, in conjunction with endogenous endorphins, inhibits the flow of pain sensations into the higher centers and the perception of pain in the higher centers (Chapter 12).

Side effects following opioid administration include drowsiness, nausea, constipation, clammy skin, and constricted pupils. Adverse effects and complications include depressed respirations and ultimately death from respiratory failure.

Concurrently, when opioids bind to mu receptors in the prefrontal cortex, they also block the release of GABA, which takes away the GABA-related tonic inhibition of dopaminergic neurons and causes more dopamine to be released into the synapse. This, in turn, overstimulates the receptor neurons, and the individual experiences euphoria.[13] With repeated use of opioids, dopamine stimulation continues unabated and the brain is never quite sated; therefore, the craving for more drugs becomes stronger. Often when street opioids are abused, since the strength and purity cannot be known, their use can result in an unintentional overdose. Table 9-3 lists the opioids that are most commonly involved in substance abuse and drug addiction.

Table 9-3 Opioids (Narcotics)

Substance Generic (Brand)	Street Name	Route of Administration	Medical Use
Schedule I			
Heroin	Big H, black tar, brown sugar, China white, junk	Inhalation, intravenous, intramuscular	None
Propoxyphene (Darvon)	None	Oral	Mild to moderate pain relief
Schedule II			
Morphine (Kadian, Avinza, MS Contin, Roxanol)	Morph, Miss Emma, M	Oral, intravenous, intramuscular, transdermal	Postsurgical pain relief, management of acute or chronic pain, breakthrough cancer pain
Hydromorphone (Dilaudid)	Drug store heroin	Oral, intravenous, intramuscular, transdermal, suppositories	Postsurgical pain relief, management of acute or chronic pain, breakthrough cancer pain
Fentanyl (Duragesic)	China girl, Fat Albert	Oral, intravenous, intramuscular, transdermal	Postsurgical pain relief, management of acute or chronic pain, breakthrough cancer pain
Oxycodone (OxyContin)	Hillbilly heroin, cotton	Oral, intravenous, intramuscular, transdermal	Postsurgical pain relief, management of acute or chronic pain, breakthrough cancer pain
Hydrocodone (Vicodin, Lortab, Lorcet)	Watson 387, vike	Oral	Moderate pain relief
Meperidine (Demerol)	Demmies	Oral, intravenous, intramuscular	Moderate to severe pain relief
Schedule III			
Codeine	Nods, lean, T-3, T-4	Oral	Pain relief, relief of cough and diarrhea

Opioid Withdrawal and Treatment

Withdrawal symptoms depend on pharmacologic characteristics of the drug involved. For instance, the short half-life of heroin results in more intense withdrawal symptoms than do opiates with longer half-lives.

Persons who have abused opioids and experience withdrawal symptoms might benefit from a medically supervised detoxification. Symptoms are similar among all classes of opioids, appearing as early as 4–6 hours after the last dose and peaking within 72 hours. Most symptoms subside after 7–10 days; however, postacute withdrawal signs may last up to a month. The larger the dose and the longer the period of use, the more severe are the withdrawal symptoms. Table 9-4 lists the stages of withdrawal

Table 9-4 Stages of Opioid Withdrawal

Stage*	Symptoms
I	Yawning, sweating, lacrimation, rhinorrhea, fear of withdrawal, anxiety, drug craving
II	Mydriasis, piloerection, muscle twitching, anorexia, diaphoresis
III	Insomnia, tachycardia, increased respiratory rate, elevated blood pressure, abdominal cramps, vomiting, diarrhea, weakness

* The time from discontinuation to onset of peak opioid-withdrawal symptoms varies and primarily depends on the half-life of the opioid involved.

symptoms.[14] Although healthcare providers suggest that symptoms are similar to the flu, most substance abusers would not support that description.

Pharmacologic treatment of opiate dependence includes medications that act as either an agonist and/or an antagonist to the opiate receptors. Methadone (Dolophine), an opioid agonist, and buprenorphine (Buprenex), a partial opioid agonist, are currently the only two medications approved by the United States FDA for treatment of withdrawal symptoms and maintenance support of opioid dependence. Naltrexone (ReVia) is an opioid antagonist approved to support abstinence after withdrawal symptoms have ceased. In addition to the medications approved by the FDA, some clinicians also have found success using clonidine (Catapres), an antihypertensive agent that is used off label for opioid withdrawal.

Withdrawal from opiate dependence can be conducted in an inpatient facility, outpatient clinic, or a private office. Methadone (Dolophine) and buprenorphine (Buprenex) are both long-acting opioids usually started in inpatient settings, but may be initiated in the outpatient setting by opioid treatment programs that are certified by the Federal Substance Abuse and Mental Health Services Administration.

The length of detoxification depends on the type of medication used, the treatment setting, the severity of the dependence and the motivation of the individual. Typically, withdrawal in an inpatient facility can last for 10–14 days. A rapid (3–10 days) and an ultrarapid (1–2 days) detoxification using an opioid antagonist such as naltrexone (Vivitrol) or naloxone (Narcan) in combination with other supportive medications like clonidine (Catapres) and/or benzodiazepines have evolved in recent years (Table 9-5). Individuals undergoing an ultrarapid detoxification are placed under anesthesia or sedated. There is the potential for adverse side effects of an ultrarapid detoxification, and patients must be well informed of any potential risk.[15] Outpatient detoxification can last 14–21 days and long-term withdrawal (often called tapering) can require up to 180 days.

Historically, outpatient treatment for opiate withdrawal was conducted exclusively in federally regulated opioid treatment programs as specified in the Narcotic Treatment Act of 1974. The law allowed only certified and registered opioid treatment programs to provide treatment services, and only methadone, a schedule II opioid medication, to be dispensed for withdrawal. Federal regulatory oversight

of these programs was transferred from the FDA to the Substance Abuse and Mental Health Services Administration (SAMHSA) in 2001. SAMHSA has developed an accreditation model for certification of opioid treatment programs in order to allow treatment providers more flexibility and greater clinical judgment in treating opiate-dependent individuals. Certain restrictions on dosage forms were eliminated so that the programs may now use solid dosage forms.[16]

The Drug Abuse Treatment Act of 2002 allowed opioid treatment programs and physicians not affiliated with a certified clinic to provide treatment services for opioid dependency by using schedule III, IV, or V medications (thus allowing for the use of buprenorphine [Buprenex]. However, the drug abuse law does not permit use of methadone for detoxification or maintenance unless the prescriber is affiliated with a certified opioid treatment program. Also,

Table 9-5 Drugs Used for Opioid Withdrawal

Drug Generic (Brand)	Category	Formulations	Dose	Clinical Considerations	FDA Pregnancy Category
Methadone (Dolophine)	mu-agonist	Solution, tablets, and injectable	Daily maintenance: 20–100 mg/day PO Detoxification: 1–5 mg daily or weekly decrease from initial dose	Restricted to inpatient settings for initiation.	C
Buprenorphine (Buprenex, Subutex)	mu-partial agonist	2- and 8-mg tablets	8 mg SL on day 1, 16 mg SL day 2, and then 16 mg SL qd for maintenance	Restricted to opioid treatment programs for dispensing. Has a ceiling effect so that increased doses do not increase the effect.	C
Buprenorphine/ Naloxone (Suboxone)	mu-partial agonist in combination with mu-antagonist	2 mg buprenorphine/ 0.5 mg naloxone or 8 mg buprenorphine/ 2 mg naloxone	16 mg SL qd for maintenance	Restricted to opioid treatment programs for dispensing. Contraindicated for persons hypersensitive to buprenorphine or naloxone. Can cause hepatotoxicity if used in higher doses. Has a ceiling effect so that increased doses do not increase the effect.	C
Clonidine (Catapres, Catapres-TTS)	Antihypertensive	0.1-, 0.2-, and 0.3-mg tablets. Transdermal patches: TTS-1 is 0.1mg/day, TTS-2 is 0.2 mg/day, TTS-3 is 0.3 mg/day	0.2 mg PO tid × 10 days for heroin withdrawal or × 14 days for methadone withdrawal	Observe for hypotension.	C
Naltrexone (ReVia)	mu-antagonist	50-mg tablets 300-mg extended-release injectable	50 mg PO daily	Used to prevent relapse. Can initiate withdrawal symptoms and should not be initiated until the individual is opioid free. SE include headache, nausea, vomiting, insomnia, dizziness, weight loss, anxiety. Can cause hepatotoxicity if used in higher doses.	C

there are certain regulations regarding the prescribing of buprenorphine, and, therefore, physicians who wish to provide buprenorphine detoxification or maintenance services must notify the Secretary of Health and Human Services and apply for certification.

Methadone (Dolophine)

Methadone (Dolophine), a long-acting, full mu-opioid agonist, is the most frequently used medication to treat opioid addiction. In essence, it takes the place of the other drugs, which results in decreased withdrawal symptoms and drug craving. Administered daily, methadone will suppress withdrawal symptoms for 24–36 hours and block the craving and effects of heroin without producing a sensation of euphoria or sedation. Methadone is used for the maintenance treatment or withdrawal of opioids.

Serious side effects of methadone include respiratory depression, hypotension, and sedation or coma. Caution should be used when medicating a person on methadone who is concurrently using alcohol or taking CNS depressants or other opioid analgesics. This is true also for an individual scheduled for general anesthesia.[16]

Methadone maintenance consists of a daily dose used as a substitute for illegal heroin with no attempt to reduce the dose. Methadone detoxification is intended to reduce the dose in a controlled manner with the goal of abstinence. Individuals can be maintained on a dose of methadone for any length of time, occasionally involving years. Critics of opioid treatment programs often claim that individuals are practicing a legal form of drug addiction. However, addiction is a chronic relapsing disease that has consequences beyond the control of the addict. Research into methadone maintenance treatment has shown reduction in the use of illicit drugs, criminal activity, needle sharing, HIV infection rates, and many other improvements in an individual's overall health and social productivity.[17] Closely related to methadone is the synthetic compound levo-alphacetylmethadol, or LAAM (ORLMM). It was approved for opioid addiction in 1993; however, recent findings regarding its cardiovascular toxicity have limited its use as a primary treatment option.

Buprenorphine (Buprenex)

Buprenorphine hydrochloride (Buprenex) is a partial mu-opioid agonist. Suboxone, a partial mu-opioid agonist/mu antagonist, is a combination of the buprenorphine hydrochloride and naloxone hydrochloride. Both drugs are approved for the treatment of opiate addiction.

Buprenorphine is a very potent drug that works at the mu-receptor site to displace morphine, methadone, and other full agonists. It reduces withdrawal symptoms, and unlike other treatment drugs, it has a lower potential for abuse and a reduced incidence of overdose or respiratory depression. Suboxone is the recommended form for maintenance treatment, as the addition of naltrexone prevents the individual from injecting the drug, thus reducing the risk of diversion.

Individuals are maintained on daily medication (usually sublingual tablets) at either an opioid treatment program or physician's office. Tablets must be placed under the tongue, allowed to fully dissolve, and must not be chewed or swallowed whole.

Neither Suboxone nor Subutex should be administered to persons who are hypersensitive to buprenorphine, and Suboxone should not be administered to those who are hypersensitive to naloxone (Narcan).[18] Drug–drug interactions are listed in Table 9-6.

Clonidine (Catapres)

Clonidine (Duraclon) is an antihypertensive medication that is used off label to treat symptoms of opiate withdrawal, primarily by suppressing restlessness, lacrimation, rhinorrhea, and sweating. Some providers and individuals prefer the use of clonidine over a traditional medication such as methadone for a variety of reasons. It is not classified under the drug schedule, therefore no special licensing is required to dispense it, it does not produce intoxication, and it does not reinforce drug-seeking behaviors. Individuals with a history of drug abuse must be monitored closely, as clonidine can cause sedation and hypotension.[19] Clonidine has additive drug–drug interactions with digitalis, calcium channel blockers, and beta-blockers that can cause bradycardia and atrioventricular (AV) block.

Naltrexone (ReVia)

Naltrexone (ReVia) is a full mu-opioid antagonist that is approved for the treatment of opioid addiction. Naltrexone blocks the effects of heroin and other opiates; therefore, it has no positive reinforcing effects. As a result, there has been little acceptance of this drug for initial treatment, as it is most effective for individuals who are already detoxified and want to prevent relapse. Treatment should not begin until the individual is opioid-free because administration of naltrexone can initiate an opioid **withdrawal syndrome** in a person who is using any type of opioid.

Table 9-6 Selected Drug–Drug Interactions Associated with Drugs Used to Treat Substance Abuse*

Drug—Generic (Brand)	Clinical Effect
Buprenorphine (Subutex) and	
Azole antifungal agents: ketoconazole	Increase effect of buprenorphine, causing opioid toxicity.
Barbiturates: phenobarbital, mephobarbital (Mebaral)	Increased CNS or respiratory depression.
Benzodiazepines: diazepam (Valium, Ativan, Xanax)	Increase effect of benzodiazepines (additive effect).
Carbamazepine (Tegretol)	Decrease effect of buprenorphine, causing possible opioid withdrawal.
Erythromycin, clarithromycin (Biaxin)	Increase effect of buprenorphine, causing opioid toxicity.
HIV protease inhibitors	Increase effect of buprenorphine, causing opioid toxicity.
Phenytoin (Dilantin)	Decrease effect of buprenorphine, causing possible opioid withdrawal.
Rifampin (Rifadin)	Decrease effect of buprenorphine, causing possible opioid withdrawal.
Clonidine (Catapres) and	
Alcohol	Potentiate CNS depressant effects (additive effects).
Barbiturates: phenobarbital, mephobarbital (Mebaral)	Potentiate CNS depressant effects (additive effects).
Beta-blockers	Cause bradycardia, AV block (additive effect).
Calcium channel blockers	Cause bradycardia, AV block (additive effect).
Digitalis	Cause bradycardia, AV block (additive effect).
Tricyclic antidepressants	The antidepressants decrease the hypotensive effect of clonidine.
Naltrexone (ReVia) and	
Disulfiram	Both naltrexone and disulfiram are hepatotoxic and should not be taken together.
Opioids	Increased dose of opioid may be necessary if given for therapeutic indication.
Benzodiazepines* and	
Anticonvulsants, opioids, barbiturates, sedatives, MAO inhibitors, phenothiazines	All drugs that cause CNS depression can cause additive effects that lead to respiratory depression.
Antacids	Lower peak concentrations of benzodiazepines secondary to slower absorption.
Cimetidine (Tagamet), ketoconazole (Nizoral), fluoxetine (Prozac), fluvoxamine (Luvox), omeprazole (Prilosec)	Increase sedative properties of benzodiazepines.
Phenytoin (Dilantin)	Metabolic clearance of phenytoin is decreased.
Theophylline or aminophylline	Reduce the sedative effects of benzodiazepines.

* Individual benzodiazepines have additional drug–drug interactions that should be assessed prior to administration.

Contraindications are abuse of any type of opioids, use of legitimately prescribed opioid analgesics, opioid withdrawal symptoms, and failure of the naloxone challenge test (a means to determine the presence of any opioids in the body).[17]

Treatment of Intoxication/Overdose

A person who has overdosed using an opioid can exhibit low blood pressure, slow respirations, pinpoint pupils, depressed sensorium, and coma. Treatment of acute overdose is to provide basic support of airway, breathing, and circulation as needed. If the patient is conscious, the stomach contents should be emptied via initiation of vomiting or gastric lavage. Persons who present with pinpoint pupils, slow respirations, and coma are presumed to be overdosed with an opioid, and naloxone (Narcan) should be administered in titrated doses every 2–3 minutes until the symptoms are reversed.

▌ Stimulants

Stimulants (Table 9-7) are a class of drugs that elevate mood, enhance physical and mental performance, increase feelings of well-being, and boost energy and alertness. Stimulants can cause irregular and abnormally fast heart rates, elevation in blood pressure, and increases in metabolism. Also, these agents may narrow blood vessels, reducing the flow of blood and oxygen to heart muscle and, in turn, to the rest of the body. Although used therapeutically for a number of purposes such as narcolepsy, weight loss, and increased concentration, the euphoria produced by stimulants often results in illicit **recreational drug use**.

Cocaine

Cocaine is made from the leaf of the *Erythroxylum coca* plant, a shrub that is native to the Andes, Mexico, West Indies, and Indonesia. Cocaine comes in the form of a white

Table 9-7 Stimulants and Depressants

Substance—Generic (Brand)	Street Name	Route of Administration	Medical Use
Stimulants—Schedule II			
Dextroamphetamine (Dexedrine, Adderall)		Oral	Obesity, narcolepsy, attention deficit hyperactivity disorder
Methylphenidate (Ritalin, Concerta)	JIF, MPH, R-ball, Skippy, smart drug, vitamin R	Oral	Attention deficit hyperactivity disorder
Cocaine/crack	Coke, snow, flake, blow, crack, rock	Oral, inhalation, intravenous, intramuscular	Topical anesthetic
Methamphetamine (Desoxyn)	Meth, speed, crystal, glass, ice, crank	Oral, inhalation, intravenous, intramuscular	None
Schedule I			
MDMA	Adam, clarity, ecstasy, Eve, lover's speed, peace, STP, X, XTC	Oral	None
Depressants—Schedule IV			
Barbiturates, mephobarbital (Mebaral), pentobarbital (Nembutal), amobarbital (Amytal), secobarbital (Seconal)	Barbs, reds, red birds, phennies, tooties, yellows, yellow jackets, blues and reds	Oral	Sedation, seizure disorder
Benzodiazepines, diazepam (Valium), chlordiazepoxide HCl (Librium), alprazolam (Xanax), clonazepam (Klonopin), triazolam (Halcion), lorazepam (Ativan)	Mother's little helper, benzos, downers, nerve pills, football, tranks	Oral	Anxiety, acute stress reaction, panic attacks, tension, sleep disorders, anesthesia (at high doses)
Flunitrazepam (Rohypnol)	Roofies, rophies, roaches	Oral	Anxiety, acute stress reaction, panic attacks, tension, sleep disorders, anesthesia (at high doses)

powder that dealers frequently mix with other substances such as sugar, talcum powder, or cornstarch and possibly with other stimulants such as amphetamines. Crack is a form of cocaine processed with ammonia or baking soda and water, heated, and then smoked in a glass pipe, which causes a crackling sound (hence its name). When cocaine or crack is combined with heroin, it is known as a speedball.

Whether snorted, smoked, injected, or rubbed onto the gums, cocaine enters the bloodstream and crosses the blood–brain barrier quickly, where it interferes with reabsorption of dopamine, causing the neurotransmitter to accumulate in the synapse. This continuous stimulation of the postsynaptic neurons is responsible for the euphoria reported by cocaine abusers[20] and is of special concern, as an inordinate degree of pleasure and the memories of that pleasure are associated with time, place, and activities. With repeated use, cocaine produces a compulsive response to similar cues, resulting in a strong desire to take the drug again.

Cocaine also inhibits reuptake of norepinephrine.[21] When norepinephrine accumulates in the synapse, some diffuses into the vascular compartment. Norepinephrine is highly vasoactive and causes vasoconstriction and hypertension, which is responsible for possible abnormalities in the heart, blood pressure, and blood vessels, as well as restlessness, agitation, erratic behavior, and occasional paranoia.[22]

Cocaine is primarily metabolized in the liver. There are several metabolites, some of which are active, which increase the potential toxicity of cocaine. In addition, when cocaine and alcohol are used concomitantly, the metabolite cocaethylene is produced, which is more toxic to liver cells than the metabolites that are produced by either drug when used alone.

Amphetamines

Amphetamines also are abused because of their action on the dopamine reward system. These agents often cause individuals to be talkative and anxious and feel exhilarated—effects similar to those of cocaine but more prolonged. Methamphetamine (Desoxyn) is usually the drug of choice, as it is potent and comes in a form that easily dissolves in water or alcohol. The smokeable form is a clear crystal of high purity that is smoked, like crack, in a glass pipe.

Short-term effects inhibit sleep, increase physical activity, and decrease appetite and may include rapid or irregular heartbeat, high blood pressure, damage to small blood vessels in the brain, shortness of breath, nausea, vomiting, diarrhea, tremors, and aggressiveness. Also, this drug can significantly increase body temperature, a situation that can be lethal if not treated rapidly. One imaging study revealed that repeated use of methamphetamine reduces the availability of dopamine transporters, and with fewer dopamine cells, individuals had inferior memory and slower motor function.[1] Long-term effects can include stroke, violent behavior, anxiety, confusion, auditory hallucinations, and delusions. Chronic heavy use may involve a paranoid psychosis that is very difficult to manage.

3, 4-Methylenedioxymethamphetamine (MDMA)

3, 4-methylenedioxymethamphetamine, also known as MDMA but better known as ecstasy, acts as both a stimulant and a psychedelic. It affects the brain by increasing three neurotransmitters, dopamine, norepinephrine, and serotonin, resulting in mood elevation, a sense of alertness, distortions in time, enhanced sensory perceptions, and decreased anxiety. MDMA can cause muscle tension, blurred vision, chills, sweating, and increases in heart rate and blood pressure. Of special concern is a possible overdose leading to hyperthermia that can result in major organ failure.[23] MDMA is currently the most popular agent at all-night dance clubs, and thus, is often referred to as a club drug. In frequent users, MDMA can cause side effects of anxiety, confusion, and insomnia that can last for days or weeks. It is not a benign drug and often is used in combination with cocaine or marijuana.

Methylphenidate

Methylphenidate (Ritalin) is a medication indicated for use by individuals with attention deficit hyperactivity disorder (ADHD), and numerous studies have shown its effectiveness when used as prescribed. However, when it is abused, methylphenidate (Ritalin) can lead to many of the same problems seen with other stimulants including appetite suppression, wakefulness, increased focus/attentiveness, and euphoria. Addiction to methylphenidate seems to occur with frequent use and high doses that produce rapid increases of synaptic dopamine in the brain.

Stimulant Withdrawal and Treatment

Stimulant withdrawal syndrome is characterized by hypersomnia, fatigue, headache, irritability, poor concentration, and restlessness—i.e., symptoms that are clinically very similar to the symptoms of depression. Persons withdrawing from stimulants should be monitored for suicide if indicated. Drug craving can be prolonged and intense. Acute toxicity can manifest as paranoia, delusions, and compulsive symptoms. These symptoms may require treatment with benzodiazepines or chlordiazepoxide (Librium).[15] Acute psychosis may also occur. No medications have been approved for treating stimulant abuse or withdrawal, and

medical complications are rare. Benzodiazepines can be provided for treatment of agitation; however, in most cases no treatment other than social support is needed for the initial phase of stimulant withdrawal.

Withdrawal symptoms may begin within 1–2 hours after the last dose of a short-acting stimulant such as cocaine and within 14 hours after last use of a long-acting stimulant such as methamphetamine. One recent study identified amphetamine withdrawal syndrome as having an acute phase characterized by craving, increased sleepiness, anxiety, dysphoria, and inactivity. The acute phase lasts for 7–10 days. The second phase or subacute phase of withdrawal continues for 2 weeks with the symptoms decreasing over time. It has been found that older individuals with higher rates of use experienced more severe withdrawal symptoms.[24] A major problem encountered after withdrawal of all substances is the risk of relapse, which continues for years after detoxification.

Currently, scientists are researching the efficacy of several medications to combat stimulant dependence and withdrawal symptoms but none yet has reached the market. Opportunities for research focus primarily on agonists that partially replace the effects of the stimulant or on antagonists that block the stimulant effects entirely. Medications involved in research that might prove promising for cocaine abuse include amantadine (Symmetrel), disulfiram (Antabuse), tiagabine (Gabitril), and baclofen (Lioresal).

Research studies also are investigating the efficacy of a cocaine vaccination. One recent study using the TA-CD vaccine found participants who were vaccinated with a series of injections made large amounts of cocaine-specific antibodies. The antibodies last for a limited period, generally less than a year. During the first 3 months when antibodies remain at a therapeutic level, users report diminished euphoric rewards if cocaine is used. To date, the TA-CD vaccine has proven safe and effective in small clinical trials.[25]

Treatment of Stimulant Overdose

All stimulants elevate endogenous catecholamine and dopamine levels. The resulting symptoms are increased arousal and hypertension (from vasoconstriction) secondary to the catecholamines, and movement disorders and hyperthermia secondary to the dopamine effects. Persons who overdose on a CNS stimulant are admitted to a hospital and treated symptomatically. Activated charcoal can be used if the agent was ingested orally. Rapid cooling of hyperthermia is a critical first step after establishing an airway. Benzodiazepines are used aggressively to treat psychomotor agitation and convulsions, and vasodilators such as nitroglycerin are used to lower blood pressure. Phenothiazines should not be given because they reduce the threshold for seizure activity and can worsen both the hyperthermia and tachycardia. Beta-blockers should be avoided because they have both alpha and beta adrenergic effects that could worsen the hypertension.

Sedatives and Hypnotics

Hundreds of substances that produce CNS depression and are used to induce sleep, relieve stress, and allay anxiety have been developed. However, the two major groups of sedatives-hypnotics that dominate both the licit and illicit market are barbiturates and benzodiazepines. Unlike most other classes of drugs frequently abused, sedative-hypnotics are rarely produced in clandestine laboratories but rather legitimate pharmaceuticals are diverted to the illicit market. A notable exception to this is a relatively recent drug, gamma hydroxybutyric acid (GHB), which is discussed later in the chapter. This class of drugs is actually a mixed group chemically, yet all are CNS depressants. Sedatives decrease CNS arousal and anxiety whereas hypnotics produce drowsiness or sleep.

Barbiturates

Barbiturates bind to GABA-sensitive ion channel receptors in the CNS, thereby allowing an influx of chloride, which hyperpolarizes the postsynaptic neuron. Barbiturates also inhibit the excitatory effects of glutamate receptors thereby depressing virtually all brain activity. Symptoms include slurred speech, loss of motor coordination, and impaired judgment.[26] Barbiturates are identified by speed and length of effects. Ultra-short-acting barbiturates, methohexital (Brevital) and thiopental (Pentothal) are highly lipophilic and produce anesthesia within approximately 1 minute after intravenous administration. Short-acting and intermediate-acting barbiturates are used primarily for insomnia and preoperative sedation with onset from 15 to 40 minutes after administration and effects lasting to 6 hours. These categories are preferred by barbiturate abusers and include products such as amobarbital (Amytal), pentobarbital (Nembutal), secobarbital (Seconal), and an amobarbital/secobarbital combination (Tuinal). Long-acting barbiturates are less lipophilic and accumulate more slowly in tissue. These agents are used primarily for insomnia, anxiety, and the treatment of seizure disorders and include phenobarbital (Luminal) and mephobarbital (Mebaral).

Barbiturate use can lead to both psychological and **physical dependence**.[3]

Benzodiazepines

Of all the drugs that affect CNS functions, benzodiazepines are among the most widely prescribed medications. They even have a song written about them. In 1967, the Rolling Stones immortalized diazepam (Valium) in their song, "Mother's Little Helper," which spoke of a housewife who used Valium to get her through the day. Therapeutically, these drugs are prescribed to produce sedation, induce sleep, relieve anxiety and muscle spasms, and prevent seizures.

Benzodiazepines have a unique mechanism of action. These drugs have a high affinity for the GABA-binding site on postsynaptic neurons in the VTA. Potentiating GABA binding results in CNS depression. Prolonged use can lead to tolerance and physical dependence even at doses recommended for medical treatment.

As a rule, benzodiazepines act as sedatives in low doses, anxiolytics in moderate doses, and hypnotics in high doses. Pharmacologic properties of the different benzodiazepines such as rapidity of onset, half-life, and activity of metabolites dictate their clinical use and are responsible for their abuse potential.[13] Short-acting preparations include flurazepam (Dalmane), temazepam (Restoril), midazolam (Versed), and triazolam (Halcion). Benzodiazepines with a longer duration of action include alprazolam (Xanax), chlordiazepoxide (Librium), diazepam (Valium), lorazepam (Ativan), oxazepam (Serax), clonazepam (Klonopin), and quazepam (Doral).

Abuse of benzodiazepines is particularly high among heroin and cocaine users, and the most frequently abused benzodiazepines are alprazolam (Xanax), diazepam (Valium), and clonazepam (Klonopin).

Flunitrazepam (Rohypnol) is a high-potency, short-acting benzodiazepine that is not manufactured or legally marketed in the United States. Flunitrazepam is also known as a date rape drug when it is placed in the drink of an unsuspecting victim in order to incapacitate that individual and prevent resistance from sexual assault. It produces anterograde amnesia, a condition in which events that occurred while under the influence of the drug are forgotten.[27]

Other Sedative-Hypnotics

A number of other sedative-hypnotics used medically are not as frequently abused as those already mentioned, most likely because the more potent drugs produce a stronger response in a shorter time or because the older agents are less available. Chloral hydrate has been given orally as a pill or syrup to induce sleep. Chloral hydrate mixed with alcohol is known as a Mickey Finn or a knockout liquid (see Box 9-1 for an explanation of the origin of the term *Mickey Finn*). Carisoprodol (Soma), a skeletal muscle relaxant, is metabolized to meprobamate, which may account for some of the properties associated with its occasional abuse.

Barbiturates and Benzodiazepines Withdrawal and Treatment

Barbiturates and benzodiazepines are drugs with moderate potential for abuse. Both substances can create physiologic and psychological dependence and require medically supervised withdrawal. Severity of the withdrawal depends on the person's history and extent of depressant use, including duration, quantity, and type (short-acting or long-acting). Withdrawal of barbiturates can be life threatening if not managed properly. Symptoms can begin within 20 hours after last use in short-acting compounds, and within 7 days for long-acting forms. Benzodiazepines generally produce a less severe withdrawal syndrome depending on dose and duration of use. Common symptoms include anxiety, insomnia, irritability, mild tremor, muscle spasms, loss of appetite, sweating, perceptual distortions, and acute awareness of stimuli. Severe symptoms can include weakness, vomiting, increased respirations, decreased blood pressure, seizures, and delirium with disorientation and hallucinations. An outpatient detoxification can last as long as 3–4 months, during which time the sedatives are

titrated at weekly intervals. Medically supervised inpatient withdrawal can last from 15 to 30 days. Generally, a long-acting medication is substituted for a short-acting one and will suppress withdrawal symptoms for a longer period of time. The rate of withdrawal will depend on the severity of the symptoms of the individual.

Treatment of Acute Overdose

Barbiturate toxicity presents as lethargy that proceeds to coma. Other symptoms include hypothermia, decreased pupillary light reflex, bradycardia, hypotension, and shock. Treatment is largely supportive, and after establishing an airway it includes intravenous hydration and use of pressor medications such as norepinephrine to correct hypotension and rewarming. Ipecac syrup is contraindicated secondary to an increased risk for aspiration from the depressed neurologic responses. Activated charcoal can be used, which is administered orally or via gastric lavage. These drugs are excreted renally, so enhanced elimination through an infusion of dextrose and sodium bicarbonate may be used.

Hallucinogens and Dissociative Anesthetics

Hallucinogens or psychedelic agents alter an individual's perception, consciousness, and mood with particular distortions associated with thought, time, and space. Hallucinogens cause their effects by disrupting the neurotransmitter serotonin, which is involved in the control of behavioral, perceptual, and regulatory systems. It can produce dreaming while the individual remains conscious. The psychedelic experience may be either pleasurable or quite terrifying. Expectations are unpredictable for each time the substance is used, and flashbacks are common. Physical effects can include elevated heart rate, increased blood pressure, tremors, dilated pupils, and hyperthermia. Table 9-8 lists the hallucinogens and other substances not in categories previously discussed that can be abused.

Lysergic Acid Diethylamide (LSD)

Lysergic acid diethylamide (LSD) is the most potent hallucinogen known to science. The effects of LSD are unpredictable. However, in the hallucinatory state, users may suffer impaired depth and time perception and disorganization in the capacity to recognize reality, think

---

Box 9-1 Gone But Not Forgotten: The Mickey Finn

According to urban legend, there once existed a Chicago bartender whose name was Mickey Finn. Mr Finn would drug unsuspecting customers while they were incapacitated and rob them. Upon his arrest, the name of Mickey Finn entered into popular culture as a synonym for the drinks he served. Slipping a Mickey to someone implied that "knockout" liquids were secretly added to the beverages. The most common drug used at the time was the sedative chloral hydrate, an agent rarely found in use today. A Mickey also can be found in many films and books during the 20th century as a plot device. However, today, a Mickey Finn may be seen as the predecessor of such date rape drugs as GHB.

Table 9-8 Other Substances of Abuse

Substance	Street Name	Symptoms	Complications
Schedule I			
Hallucinogens, phencyclidine (PCP), psilocybin	Angel dust, supergrass, boat, tic tac, zoom, Sherm	Hypothermia, nausea, perspiration, tachycardia, altered states of perception and feeling, increased body temperature and blood pressure, loss of appetite	Persisting perception disorder, acute anxiety, sleeplessness, numbness, weakness, tremors
Mescaline, peyote, mushrooms	Buttons, cactus head, shrume		
LSD	Acid, blotter acid, window pane, orange sunshine		
Ketamine	Special K		
Cannabis (marijuana)	Dope, MJ, bud grass, pot, reefer, weed, skunk weed, sinsemilla	Relaxation, euphoria, lack of motivation	Impaired memory, panic attacks, risk for cancer of the respiratory tract and lungs
GHB	Liquid ecstasy, liquid X, goop, Georgia home boy, easy lay	Vomiting, dizziness	Tremors, seizures, coma, death
Schedule II			
Anabolic steroids	Arnolds, gym candy, pumpers, roids, stackers, weight trainers, gear, juice	No intoxication, elevated blood pressure, agitation, increase in cholesterol, severe acne, fluid retention	Blood clotting and cholesterol changes; kidney cancer; premature stoppage of growth; in females, more facial and body hair, deeper voice, smaller breasts, and fewer menstrual cycles; in adolescents, may prematurely stop the lengthening of bones
Not scheduled			
Inhalants	Laughing gas, poppers, snappers, whippers	Confusion, delirium, nausea, vomiting, tremors, weakness	Asphyxiation, weight loss, disorientation, inattentiveness, irritability, depression
Dextromethorphan	CCC, triple C, skittles, robo, poor man's PCP	Confusion, dizziness, double or blurred vision, slurred speech, loss of physical coordination, abdominal pain, nausea and vomiting, rapid heart beat, drowsiness, numbness of fingers and toes, disorientation	Mild distortions of color and sound, visual hallucinations, out-of-body dissociate sensations, loss of motor control

rationally, or communicate with others; their senses are distorted. After an LSD trip, the user may suffer acute anxiety or depression, and flashbacks have been reported days or even months after taking the last dose. LSD is not considered an addictive drug; it does not produce compulsive drug-seeking behavior as do cocaine, heroin, and methamphetamine. However, LSD users may develop tolerance to the drug, meaning that they must consume progressively larger doses of the drug in order to continue to experience the hallucinogenic effects that they seek.[28]

Tryptamine and Peyote

Psilocybin and psilocin are forms of tryptamines that are obtained from certain mushrooms that grow in tropical and subtropical areas. When these substances as well as other "magic" mushrooms are dried and eaten or brewed into a liquid and imbibed, they produce hallucinogenic effects including vivid auditory and visual distortions and

emotional disequilibrium. Dimethyltryptamine (DMT) is found in a variety of plants and seeds and also can be produced synthetically with short hallucinogenic effects of less than an hour. Diethyltryptamine (DET) is an analogue of DMT with similar effects.[28]

Peyote is a small cactus containing the hallucinogen mescaline (3, 4, 5-trimethoxyphenethylamine). Mescaline also can be made synthetically, and in many instances amphetamines are added to obtain a special euphoric effect.[29]

Phencyclidine (PCP)

Phencyclidine (PCP) is classified as a dissociative anesthetic, but it has many properties of the hallucinogens. This agent affects a number of neurotransmitters, especially glutamate, and also causes an accumulation of dopamine. Low or moderate doses cause alterations in body image, distortions of space and time, feelings of invulnerability, and mental delusions. Addiction can occur, and chronic users may have memory loss, speech difficulties, and depression persisting for up to a year after the last use.[30]

Ketamine

Ketamine is currently used as an anesthetic for animals and to a limited degree with humans, primarily for emergency surgery. Its actions are similar to PCP but less potent and of shorter duration; however, some users report a frightening sensory detachment similar to a bad trip on LSD. With high or frequent doses, ketamine can produce analgesia, amnesia, and coma.[31]

Hallucinogen and Dissociative Anesthetic Withdrawal and Treatment

Chronic use of PCP can cause toxic psychosis that takes days or weeks to clear; however, PCP does not have a set of specific withdrawal symptoms. Symptoms of PCP withdrawal may include memory loss and depression. LSD and ecstasy do not produce physical dependence, although with LSD there is some evidence of hallucinogen-persisting perception disorder (HPPD), which includes flashbacks and persistent psychosis similar to those experienced following use of PCP.[29]

Treatment of Overdose

The most common adverse reaction to a large dose of a hallucinogenic agent is the bad trip. This can manifest as a psychotic state that is usually temporary. Although there are reports of permanent psychosis, it is not clear if this result was secondary to the hallucinogen or to an underlying vulnerability. The pharmacologic treatment of choice is benzodiazepines to reduce anxiety.

▌ Anabolic Steroids

Once viewed as a problem associated only with selected athletes, the abuse of anabolic steroids has increased significantly, especially among adolescents. When used in combination with exercise and a high-protein diet, anabolic steroids can promote increased size and strength of muscles, improve endurance, and decrease recovery time between workouts. Some steroids are taken orally, others are injected intramuscularly, and still others are creams or gels that are applied to the skin.

Physical effects from steroid abuse can include elevated blood pressure, fluid retention, increases in cholesterol, and severe acne. Abuse of these drugs can lead to early heart attacks, strokes, liver tumors, kidney failure, cancer, and serious psychiatric problems. In females, the steroids have a masculinizing effect, resulting in more facial and body hair, a deeper voice, smaller breasts, and fewer menstrual cycles. Several of these effects are irreversible. Abuse of steroids may interfere with the lengthening of bones.[32]

Steroid Withdrawal and Treatment

Little research has been conducted on steroid withdrawal, and there is not a recommended withdrawal protocol. Detoxification is associated with symptoms of varying degrees of intensity that appear more frequently in heavy users. Possible symptoms include craving, mood swings, reduced sex drive, fatigue, depression, restlessness, insomnia, aggression, headaches, and loss of appetite. Antidepressants can be utilized to combat depression, and analgesics can be used for body aches.[33]

▌ Cannabis

Frequently known as marijuana, cannabis is the most widely used illicit drug in the United States and is a **gateway drug**. Its ingredient, tetrahydrocannabinol (THC), is responsible for most of the **psychoactive effects** by causing the release of dopamine, which allows the user to experience a euphoric high. Stronger doses intensify reactions, whereas very high doses may result in image distortion and hallucinations. A similar but more concentrated form is called hashish, which is compressed, then broken into pieces and smoked in pipes. Physical effects of inhaling marijuana include tachycardia, relaxed and enlarged bronchial passages, and redness in the eyes. The user may become hungry and thirsty, grow cold, and feel sleepy or depressed. Effects can be greater if other drugs are taken concurrently. Regular use may result in short-term memory loss, decreased motor coordination, and cardiac or respiratory problems. Frequent users are at risk for cancer of the respiratory tract and lungs because marijuana smoke contains 50–70% more carcinogenic hydrocarbons than tobacco smoke.[34]

Although illegal nationally, a number of individual states have passed laws permitting the use of cannabis for medical purposes, such as controlling nausea and vomiting from cancer chemotherapy, stimulating appetite for individuals with AIDS, and for those with glaucoma and spasticity. The only approved THC preparation for such purposes is dronabinol (Marinol), although individuals frequently elect to obtain and use other forms of the substance. Significant studies regarding dronabinol (Marinol) are not available; however, some reports suggest that it does not give the individual the same degree of relief as marijuana. Euphoria from THC appears to decrease as women age.

Cannabis Withdrawal

Research reports vary with regard to the validity of a marijuana withdrawal syndrome, although individuals who use marijuana often report failed attempts at cessation and perceived themselves as dependent. Onset of withdrawal symptoms appears to vary among users, and medication is not generally required for marijuana withdrawal. Medical complications during the process are rare. Individuals report withdrawal symptoms can begin within 24 hours of last use and commonly include drug craving, sleep difficulty, anxiety, restlessness, irritability, and decreased appetite.[35]

Inhalants

Inhalants are volatile substances whose inhaled vapors can produce a rapid euphoria that is inexpensive and easily accessible. The chemicals involved are found in huge numbers of commercial products and are categorized as volatile solvents, aerosols, gases, and nitrites. They are available in such diverse products as model airplane glue, paint thinners, hair sprays, nail polish remover, butane lighters, nitrous oxide, video head cleaners, and whipped cream. Substances can be inhaled directly or by sniffing, bagging, huffing, or spraying. Following inhalation, there is rapid action with responses similar to the pleasurable effects of CNS depressants. The high is often followed by dizziness, uncoordinated movement, and slurred speech. Because the intoxication lasts a very short time, the tendency is to repeat inhalations. With excessive use and depending upon the type of chemical, individuals may exhibit confusion, delirium, nausea, vomiting, and tremors. Long-term effects can include weight loss, irritability, and depression. In very severe situations, damage to organs such as the liver, kidney, and brain is possible. Because inhalants may be one of the first drugs used by an individual, adolescents from 12 to 16 years of age are at particular risk.[36]

Dextromethorphan

For many years dextromethorphan (Benylin, Delsym) has been used widely as an over-the-counter antitussive available in a variety of forms, including capsules, liquids, lozenges, and tablets. At the normal dose, it is a safe and effective treatment for a cough. In 2005, the FDA issued a paper warning consumers about an increase in abuse of dextromethorphan. Recent studies have found that the agent is metabolized to an active, more potent metabolite called dextrorphan, and if genetic polymorphisms of the CYP2D6 enzyme are present, this metabolic conversion can be enhanced. Dextrorphan has mild opiate binding and also has an affinity for the PCP site of the ligand-gated channel of the N-methyl-D-aspartate (NMDA) receptor complex, suggesting an explanation for the euphoria reported with consumption of large amounts by some individuals, most likely those who are extensive metabolizers.[37] Poor metabolizers may notice sedation, but are less likely to abuse the drug. Withdrawal is described as a mild form of opiate withdrawal and usually does not require pharmacologic treatment. Overdose of the agent is associated with cardiac arrhythmias, seizures, respiratory depression, and brain injury.

Gamma Hydroxybutyric Acid (GHB)

Beginning in the mid-1990s, gamma hydroxybutyric acid (GHB) emerged as an important drug of abuse for its euphoric effects, its alleged utility as an anabolic agent for body building, sleep aid, and weapon for sexual assault (date rape). GHB is often used with alcohol by teenagers and young adults at nightclubs and rave parties. It is synthesized illegally, and overdose frequently requires emergency room care due to severe depressant effects. A significant number of GHB-related fatalities have been reported.[38]

GHB Withdrawal and Treatment

Reports of GHB withdrawal symptoms are not common among users. This may be due to the drug's rapid absorption and elimination from the body. Onset of effects begin within 10 to 15 minutes of ingestion, reaching peak levels within 45 minutes. In studies where an individual used GHB repeatedly (every 1–4 hours over 24 hours), a withdrawal syndrome has been reported. The withdrawal syndrome is characterized by anxiety, insomnia, and tremor, and in severe cases the syndrome can progress to severe delirium. Other symptoms noted during withdrawal include nausea, vomiting, confusion, and agitation. Not all individuals experience the full range of symptoms. Medications used to manage symptoms during withdrawal include lorazepam (Ativan), haloperidol (Haldol), and diazepam (Valium).[38]

Alcohol

It is estimated that approximately 7% of the overall population in the United States meets the diagnostic criteria for alcohol abuse or alcoholism.[39] Alcoholism is the third most common etiology of preventable mortality. More specifically, 5.3 million women drink alcohol in ways that have adverse health and social outcomes annually.[40] Women who are heavy drinkers have an increased risk for cardiac problems, liver damage, and both mental and physical disability when compared to men who are heavy drinkers.[40] Although the alcohol content in different drinks varies widely, one 12-ounce bottle of beer or wine cooler, one 5-ounce glass of wine or 1.5 ounces of 80-proof distilled spirits is, for clinical and research purposes, considered a standard drink.

Effects of Alcohol Consumption

Alcohol has both direct effects on brain neurotransmitters and effects that are second to intermediate products of alcohol metabolism. Alcohol affects several neurotransmitters in the brain. Increased production of GABA and decreased sensitivity to glutamate receptors lead to overall sedation; alcohol directly activates dopaminergic neurons in the VTA, which results in increased dopamine release in the NAc. The endogenous opioid circuits within the limbic system are also activated by alcohol, and as a result, more opioid receptors are upregulated.[13]

Chronic exposure causes sustained stimulation of the mesolimbic system. Over time, adaptations within the limbic system develop so withdrawal of alcohol results in hypofunction of dopamine that can last for up to 2 months following initiation of abstinence. Chronic use of alcohol is responsible for many adverse health effects including cirrhosis, cancers of the respiratory and alimentary tracts, and malnutrition.[41] Chronic alcohol use can exacerbate coexisting medical conditions such as diabetes, hypertension, and peptic ulcer disease.

Alcohol is rapidly absorbed from the gastrointestinal tract and cleared from the blood within an hour. Approximately 20% is absorbed from the stomach and 80% from the small intestine. The longer ethanol remains in the stomach, the slower it will be absorbed into the bloodstream. This is why drinking and eating appears to have a sobering effect compared to drinking the same amount of alcohol without eating at the same time. A small portion of consumed alcohol is excreted via the kidney, salivation, or exhalation (the basis of breathalyzer tests), but 98% is metabolized in the liver via several pathways. The most common pathways involve either the enzyme alcohol dehydrogenase (ADH) or aldehyde dehydrogenase (ALDH) to convert alcohol into acetaldehyde. Acetaldehyde is converted to acetate and then carbon dioxide and water.[13] The rate at which this process occurs is dependent upon the amount of enzyme available in the liver and is not dependent upon the amount of alcohol consumed. Although acetaldehyde is normally oxidized rapidly, chronic use of large amounts of alcohol can overwhelm the system and allow acetaldehyde to accumulate in concentrations that cause liver damage. The concentration of alcohol in blood and related symptoms are listed in Table 9-9.

Gender Differences in Alcohol Abuse and Addiction

It is not known why some individuals become reliant on alcohol and others do not, but a genetic predisposition plays a role for some persons.[3,42] The effects of alcohol are related to the amount imbibed and individual

Table 9-9 Concentration of Alcohol in Blood

Blood Value mg/dL	Brain Area Affected*	Impairment*	Behavior*
10–30	Frontal lobe	None	Appears normal
30–100	Frontal lobe	Incoordination, impaired judgment, increased reaction time	Euphoria, alteration in mood, loss of inhibition
100–200	Frontal and parietal lobe	Increasingly impaired judgment, slow responses, emotional instability	Slurred speech, ataxia, impaired short-term memory
200–300	Parietal lobe and occipital lobe	Blackout possible	Staggering gait, decreased sense of pain
300–400	Cerebellum, diencephalon	Decreased response to stimuli, muscular incoordination that may appear to be paralysis	Double vision, altered equilibrium, stupor
> 400	Medulla	Stupor, coma, respiratory depression, death	

* As the blood alcohol level increases, additional brain areas are affected. Impairment and behaviors noted at higher levels include those noted at lower levels.

susceptibility. Women absorb alcohol more quickly than do men and lower doses affect women when compared to the doses needed to affect men. Alcohol is more soluble in water than in fat and therefore distributes more widely in tissue containing water. Women have proportionally more fat and less water than men, and this may account for why women have higher blood-alcohol concentrations than men do after ingesting the same amount of alcohol. In addition, women become addicted faster and suffer the consequences of alcohol-related illnesses sooner than men who consume comparable amounts of alcohol.[40]

Women are at increased risk for a number of complications, including a more rapid development of cirrhosis, hypertension, anemia, and osteoporosis. Also, a woman's risk of breast cancer may rise with the amount of alcohol she consumes. In addition, women with alcoholism are at higher risk for menstrual disorders and infertility. Finally, women with alcohol abuse disorders are more likely to have eating disorders, panic disorders, depression, and posttraumatic stress disorder. Older women require less alcohol to become intoxicated, probably because they have less body fluid and slight differences in metabolism. When a woman is pregnant, she faces additional problems associated with alcohol that involve potential morphological changes and neurologic impairment in the developing fetus.

Diagnosis of Alcohol Abuse and Alcoholism

The formal definition of alcoholism used by most healthcare providers is that alcoholism is a chronic disease that includes craving, loss of control, physical dependence, and tolerance. The DSM-IV criteria states:

> Alcoholism is maladaptive alcohol use with clinically significant impairment as manifested by at least three of the following within any one-year period: 1) tolerance; 2) withdrawal; 3) taken in greater amounts or over longer time course than intended; 4) desire or unsuccessful attempts to cut down or control use; 5) great deal of time spent obtaining, using, or recovering from use; 6) social, occupational, or recreational activities given up or reduced; 7) continued use despite knowledge of physical or psychological sequelae.[43]

Alcohol Withdrawal and Treatment

Treatment for persons addicted to alcohol focuses first on treatment of withdrawal syndromes and second on treatments used to help individuals maintain abstinence.

Alcohol Withdrawal Syndrome

Alcohol withdrawal symptoms occur because alcohol is a CNS depressant, and abrupt withdrawal releases compensatory overactivity in parts of the CNS, including hyperactivity in the sympathetic autonomic system. Mild to moderate symptoms of alcohol withdrawal include restlessness, irritability, anxiety, poor concentration, emotional volatility, impaired memory and judgment, lack of appetite, insomnia, elevated heart rate, and increased blood pressure. Acute symptoms can occur when alcohol withdrawal is more severe and include hyperthermia, increased sensitivity to sound or light, tremors, agitation, paranoid or persecutory delusions, delirium tremens, known as DTs (disorientation, fluctuation in level of consciousness, auditory, visual, or tactile hallucinations), and grand mal seizures.

The primary goal of medical treatment for alcohol withdrawal syndromes is to avoid seizures and delirium tremens. Benzodiazepines including diazepam (Valium), chlordiazepoxide (Librium), lorazepam (Ativan), and oxazepam (Serax) are used to treat psychomotor agitation. Alcohol withdrawal may be best treated in an inpatient setting that provides both pharmacologic and biopsychosocial treatments.

Treatment of Acute Intoxication

An overdose of alcohol will cause stupor, delirium, and then coma. Sudden death can result if very large quantities are drunk rapidly. Medical treatment is the same as treatment for overdoses of other CNS depressants. Once an airway is established, intravenous fluids and B complex vitamins are given to counter the diuretic effect of alcohol and to protect against Wernicke's encephalopathy in case the individual is thiamin deficient secondary to chronic use of alcohol. Treatment is then supportive until the effects of intoxication wear off.

Treatment of Alcohol Dependence

Currently there are three medications approved by the FDA for the medically supervised treatment of alcohol dependence. Included are disulfiram, (Antabuse), approved in 1951; naltrexone (ReVia), approved in 1994, and naltrexone as an extended-release injectable suspension (Vivitrol), which was approved in 2006; and acamprosate (Campral), approved in 2004 (Table 9-10). Topiramate (Topamax) and several other neurotransmitter agonists and antagonists are under study but not currently used in clinical practice. All medications

Table 9-10 Pharmacologic Treatments for Maintenance of Alcohol Abstinence

Drug—Generic (Brand)	Formulations	Dose	Clinical Considerations	Side Effects/Adverse Reactions	FDA Pregnancy Categories
Disulfiram (Antabuse)	250- and 500-mg tablets	125–500 mg PO qd	Do not start until 12 hrs after last ingestion of alcohol. Disulfiram reaction can occur up to 2 weeks after discontinuing the medication. Contraindications: cirrhosis, coronary artery disease, psychoses (past or current), renal impairment.	Minor: drowsiness, headache, impotence, headache, rash, acne, fatigue, and a metal or garlic aftertaste Major: weakness, lack of energy, loss of appetite, nausea, and vomiting	C
Acamprosate (Campral)	333-mg delayed-release tablets	666 mg PO tid	Start as soon as possible after alcohol withdrawal. Do not use this drug to treat symptoms of withdrawal. Contraindicated for persons with renal impairment.	Sleep problems, headache, anxiety, depression, and weakness	C
Naltrexone (ReVia)	50-mg tablets, 380-mg injectable kit	50 mg PO qd or 380 mg ER IM q 4 weeks	Contraindicated for persons using opioids and persons with liver impairment.	Nausea, headache, dizziness, fatigue, insomnia, anxiety, and nervousness	C
Topiramate (Topamax)	25-, 50-, 100-, 200-mg tablets	Ceiling dose is 300 mg/day	Can be started prior to initiating abstinence.	Confusion and glaucoma, paresthesia, taste perversion	C

ALDH = acetaldehydase dehydrogenase.

work best when used in conjunction with behavioral therapies. Although alcoholism is a chronic disease with a high rate of relapse, all studies of alcohol treatments conducted to date have found behavioral therapies essential in all the therapeutic programs that have been studied.[44]

Disulfiram (Antabuse)

Disulfiram (Antabuse) is the most widely used medication used in the United States to treat alcohol abuse and to date, the one that appears to be most effective for persons who are highly motivated and under medical care.[45] Disulfiram blocks the complete oxidation of alcohol at the step where acetaldehyde is created. Increased levels of acetaldehyde result in the feelings of hangover, which is termed the disulfiram-alcohol reaction. Disulfiram acts as an enforcing agent for sobriety by making the individual physically ill when alcohol is consumed. The disulfiram-alcohol reaction generally lasts for 30–60 minutes, but can last for several hours based on the level of blood alcohol. To avoid such reactions, an individual should not take disulfiram for 12 hours after drinking alcohol. Contraindications to the use of disulfiram include simultaneous use of alcohol or alcohol-containing preparations and the conditions listed in Table 9-10. Individuals are encouraged to carry a safety card to notify healthcare providers or emergency personnel when they are using disulfiram.[45] See Table 9-11 for drug–drug interactions.

Acamprosate (Campral)

Acamprosate (Campral) antagonizes glutamate receptors which help return balance to the interplay between excitatory and inhibitory neurotransmission.[45] Acamprosate is prescribed for maintaining abstinence. This drug does not treat symptoms of alcohol withdrawal, nor does it affect craving that is elicited via environmental or social cues. However, unlike disulfiram (Antabuse), acamprosate (Campral) has no interaction with alcohol and is clinically well tolerated. The delayed-release tablets should be administered as soon as possible following alcohol withdrawal and should be maintained if the person relapses. The use of this drug is contraindicated for those who have previously exhibited hypersensitivity to acamprosate and for individuals with severe renal impairment. The therapeutic effect of acamprosate is modest. Mann et al. conducted a meta-analysis of 17 controlled trials that compared acamprosate to placebo and found that continuous abstinence rates at 6 months were more frequent in the cohort who got acamprosate (36.1% versus 23.4%, respectively; relative benefit 1.47; 95% CI, 1.29 to 1.69; $P < .001$).[46] Multiple trials of acamprosate conducted in Europe have substantiated these findings, but the studies done in the United States have not shown acamprosate to be efficatious.[45] The reason for this contradiction may be that the populations of alcohol-dependent persons in the studies were different in Europe when compared to the cohorts studied in the

Table 9-11 Selected Drug–Drug Interactions Associated with Drugs Used to Treat Alcoholism*

Drug—Generic (Brand)	Effect of Interaction
Disulfiram (Antabuse) and	
Alcohol intoxication	Disulfiram–alcohol reaction.
Benzodiazepines	Increase effect of benzodiazepines to cause CNS depression.
Anticoagulants	Increase prothrombin time.
Isoniazid (INH)	Unsteady gait.
Metronidazole (Flagyl)	Confusion and psychosis, mechanism unknown.
Phenytoin (Dilantin)	Phenytoin intoxication.
Products that contain alcohol: ritonavir (Norvir), sertraline (Zoloft), tipranavir (Aptivus), cough syrups	Disulfiram–alcohol reaction.
Acamprosate (Campral)	No significant drug–drug interactions.
Topiramate (Topamax) and	
Amitriptyline (Elavil)	Increase plasma levels of amitriptyline.
Antiepileptics: phenytoin (Dilantin), carbamazepine (Tegretol), valproic acid (Depakene), lamotrigine (Lamictal)	Decrease plasma levels of topiramate. Valproic acid is also associated with hyperammonemia and encephalopathy when given with topiramate.
CNS depressants	Topiramate can cause CNS depression and should be used with caution when the individual is taking other CNS depressants (additive effect).
Dichlorphenamide (Daranide) and/or acetazolamide (Diamox)	Both topiramate and dichlorphenamide are carbonic anhydrase inhibitors, which increases the risk of renal stone formation (additive effect).
Digoxin (Lanoxin)	Plasma levels of digoxin are decreased.
Hydrochlorothiazide (HCTZ)	Increase plasma levels of topiramate.
Oral contraceptives	Possible decreased efficacy of oral contraceptives and increased breakthrough bleeding.
Risperidone (Risperdal)	Decrease the plasma level of risperidone.

United States. Subanalyses of this body of work suggest acamprosate may be of most benefit for alcohol-dependent persons who have increased levels of anxiety, negative family histories of alcoholism, late age of onset, and female gender.[47] At this time, acamprosate is not used extensively in the United States.

Naltrexone (ReVia)

Oral naltrexone (ReVia) is an mu-opioid antagonist that appears to be most efficacious for persons who have a family history of alcoholism and those with strong cravings.[48] Like acamprosate, naltrexone (ReVia) has a modest effect and is more likely to facilitate abstinence if combined with behavioral therapy.[44] The COMBINE randomized trial published in 2006 is the largest study to date that compared different combinations of medical treatment, medications, and behavioral therapy.[44] Persons who received naltrexone or behavioral therapy had a higher percentage of abstinent days than did persons in the groups who received combinations of acamprosate (Campral) and therapy during the 16 weeks of treatment.[44]

Naltrexone will cause opioid withdrawal and should not be used until the individual is opioid-free for at least 7–10 days. There have been a few reports of depression and suicidal ideation following initiation of this drug, but an etiologic link between naltrexone and suicide has not been established. It is important that naltrexone not be prescribed for individuals with acute hepatitis or liver failure, and its use in those with active liver disease must be carefully considered in light of its hepatotoxic effects. Major drug interactions can occur in persons taking naltrexone who receive opioid analgesics or other medications containing opioids. Individuals taking naltrexone are encouraged to carry a health safety card to notify healthcare providers or emergency personnel of their use of naltrexone. Using opiates while taking naltrexone can create life-threatening opioid intoxication and result in respiratory arrest, coma, and circulatory collapse.

The high incidence of nausea affects compliance with this medication, and yet, compliance is important in order to assure the blood levels sufficient to have a therapeutic effect. Although the recommended dose is 50 mg/day, the COMBINE study used a dose of 100 mg/day, a factor that may account in part for the positive findings.[44]

Naltrexone is available as an extended-release injectable suspension (Vivitrol) that is administered intramuscularly at monthly intervals. This formulation was designed to allow for more stable plasma levels and a lower incidence of side effects, and it circumvents the problem of compliance, as the individual who uses this formulation does not have to remember to take tablets daily. Unfortunately, the extended-release injectable formulation does not appear to be more efficacious than oral tablets, and the adverse effects appear in the same frequency as they do if naltrexone is taken orally.[46] Of more concern, this formulation did not increase days of abstinence in women compared to placebo.[48] This lack of effectiveness in women is presumed to be secondary to a lower rate of family history of alcoholism and a higher rate of response to placebo in the women subjects.[45,48]

Topiramate (Topamax)

Topiramate (Topamax) reduces dopamine release from the presynaptic neurons and antagonized glutamate activity. It is an anticonvulsant more commonly used to treat epilepsy. However, these functions also interfere with the alcohol reward circuit and thereby decrease the desire to drink. Although topiramate (Topamax) is not FDA approved for treatment of alcoholism, it is currently the subject of research, and in a recent randomized trial, it was more effective in decreasing heavy drinking days than was a placebo (mean difference 8.44%; 95% CI, 3.07–13.8%).[49] Topiramate can be started prior to initiating abstinence. Rarely, persons taking topiramate will develop myopia, angle-closure glaucoma, or increased intraocular pressure, all of which are reversible once the drug is discontinued.[45]

Other Neurotransmitter Agonists and Antagonists

Given the effects alcohol has on the limbic system circuits' dopamine agonists, dopamine antagonists and GABA receptor agonists (e.g., baclofen) could be of clinical value. Studies of all three have been conducted. Neither the dopamine agonists nor the dopamine antagonists are effective for the treatment of alcoholism. The GABA receptor agonist baclofen (Lioresal) has been the subject of a few small studies and appears promising, but further research is needed.

Studies of selective serotonin reuptake inhibitors (SSRIs) and selective serotonin antagonists have been conducted with small numbers of participants, and to date, the results are inconclusive. SSRIs do not appear to improve days of abstinence or reduce the number of days of heavy drinking in persons without depression, although those taking serotonin antagonists such as ondansetron (Zofran) may consume fewer drinks per day. Individuals who have comorbid depression can be treated with these agents appropriately, but there is no evidence yet that they significantly improve days of abstinence.

Complementary and Alternative Medicine

Various approaches via complementary or alternative medicine (CAM) have been used to treat withdrawal of a variety of substance addictions. Among these are herbs, such as acorus, guarana seed, yohimbe, valerian root, skullcap leaf and chamomile; acupuncture, involving a number of body meridians; vitamin therapy; massage; acupressure; yoga; biofeedback; and visualization. Although many methods are mentioned in the literature or suggested by providers of CAM or extolled by believing lay populations, it is difficult to find prospective research studies that prove efficacy of such techniques. However, if individuals undergoing withdrawal find an approach that is comforting to them, it could be considered as an adjunct to the more standard treatment, assuming that there are no deleterious interactions.

Special Populations: Pregnancy and Lactation

Care of women who are abusing substances or who have a drug addiction during pregnancy can be both rewarding and challenging. Pregnancy outcomes for both the mother and neonate depend upon the type of substance abused, frequency of use, gestational age at the time of exposure, and whether multiple substances are used concurrently. It is not uncommon for substance-abusing women to minimize or avoid prenatal care because of the negative feedback from society and from healthcare providers. These women may be reluctant to seek help for fear of criminal prosecution or losing custody of their child. Although information is accessible regarding the consequences of using nicotine and alcohol during pregnancy, long-term studies that demonstrate deleterious effects and possible treatment modalities are not available for many of the drugs discussed in this chapter. Maternal and fetal/neonatal effects from common drugs of abuse are listed in Table 9-12.

Alcohol

Approximately 13% of pregnant women report having a few drinks during pregnancy, 3% report binge drinking, and 0.7% report heavy drinking.[50] Although these seem like relatively small numbers, prenatal exposure to alcohol is one of the leading causes of preventable birth defects and developmental disabilities.[51]

No amount of alcohol has been determined safe during pregnancy. The adverse effects of alcohol could be dose related, which means that there are some adverse effects at small doses and more serious effects if the fetus is exposed to larger doses. In contrast, adverse fetal effects from alcohol exposure could be a threshold effect, which means they do not occur at low doses but

Table 9-12 Substances of Abuse, Maternal Overdose, and Fetal/Neonatal Effects

Substance of Abuse	Maternal Overdose/Withdrawal	Fetal/Neonatal Effects
Alcohol	*Overdose:* Unusual behavior, depression, amnesia, hypotension *Withdrawal:* Agitation, tremors	Microcephaly, growth retardation, mental retardation, craniofacial abnormalities, abortion. Growth restriction occurs both before and after birth. Nutritional deficiencies, smoking, and polypharmacy confound data. The fetus of a woman who ingests six drinks per day is at a 40% risk of developing some features of FAS, but the threshold is still unknown.
Anticholinergics Atropine Belladonna Scopolamine	*Overdose:* Pupils dilated and fixed, increased heart rate and temperature, amnesia, vagueness *Withdrawal:* None	None noted.
Cannabis Marijuana THC Hashish	*Overdose:* Infected conjunctiva with normal pupils, decreased blood pressure when standing, increased heart rate, time and space disoriented *Withdrawal:* None	Some subtle behavioral alterations noted but no anomalies or growth delay.
CNS sedatives Barbiturates Chlordiazepoxide Diazepam Flurazepam Glutethimide Meprobamate	*Overdose:* Normal pupils, decreased, shocky blood pressure, depressed respiration, depressed tendon reflexes, coma, ataxia, slurring, convulsions *Withdrawal:* Tremulousness, insomnia, chronic blink reflex, agitation, toxic psychosis	No anomalies. Limp baby.
CNS stimulants Antiobesity Amphetamines Cocaine Methylphenidate Phenmetrazine Methaqualone	*Overdose:* Dilated and reactive pupils, shallow respirations, increased blood pressure, hyperactive reflexes, cardiac arrhythmias, dry mouth, tremors, sensorium hyperacute *Withdrawal:* muscle aches, abdominal pain, hunger, prolonged sleep, possibly suicidal	Questionable increased rate of abortion, hyperactivity in utero, depression of interactive behavior, controversy about anomalies. Cocaine has been linked with some bowel atresias and possible congenital malformations of heart, limbs, face, and GU tract as well as growth restriction. Maternal and fetal complications include sudden death and placental abruption (six-fold increase in obstetrical complications).
Hallucinogens LSD Ketamine Mescaline Dimethyltryptamine Phencyclidine (PCP)	*Overdose:* Dilated pupils, increased blood pressure, heart rate and tendon reflexes, flushed face, euphoria, anxiety, illusions, hallucinations *Withdrawal:* None	Dysmorphic face. Behavioral problems.
Opiates Codeine Heroin Hydromorphone Meperidine Morphine Opium Pentazocine Tripelennamine	*Overdose:* Constricted pupils, decreased blood pressure, heart rate and reflexes, hypoactive sensorium *Withdrawal:* Agitation, flu-like symptoms, dilated pupils, abdominal pain	Intrauterine withdrawal with increased fetal activity. Neonatal withdrawal. Depressed breathing movements. Methadone usually treatment of choice.

Source: Rayburn et al.[67]; American College of Obstetricians and Gynecologists[68]; Wang[69]; Dunbar et al.[70]

do occur if the fetus is exposed to higher doses.[52] Alcohol appears to affect the fetus both ways. There appears to be a threshold effect with regard to the effect of fetal CNS development, and binge drinking is associated with an increased risk for stillbirth.[53] There is a dose relationship that affects physical growth.[52] In addition,

polymorphisms of the alcohol dehydrogenase gene in the mother, fetus, or both may play a role in determining an individual fetus's vulnerability to the effects of alcohol. Malnutrition, comorbid medical conditions, and use of other drugs may also impact the effects of alcohol on the fetus. Thus, in the United States and Canada, abstinence from alcohol during pregnancy is recommended as the safest course. In selected European countries and Australia, an abstinence-based approach is not routinely recommended. This tactic is based on the lack of research that has delineated exact amounts of alcohol that cause problems, a concern that a recommendation of abstinence could cause undue anxiety in women with unplanned pregnancies, and in some instances, a belief that small amounts of alcohol throughout pregnancy will not cause damage.[54]

The teratogenic effects of alcohol were first noted in 1973 when researchers noted similar patterns of birth defects and developmental delays in children of mothers who were alcoholics.[55] The term fetal alcohol spectrum disorder (FASD) is used to encompass the spectrum of fetal effects that occur following maternal alcohol use. The most severe form of these effects is fetal alcohol syndrome, which is a syndrome that includes the classic craniofacial abnormalities, microcephaly, and delays in both prenatal and postnatal growth and development.[51]

FASD covers a range of effects including fetal alcohol syndrome (FAS), fetal alcohol effects (FAE), and alcohol-related neurodevelopmental disabilities (ARND).[51] Although FAS is seen most often in children born to women who chronically drink large amounts of alcohol, it is not known if the teratogenic effects of alcohol are related to amount of alcohol, frequency of use, or the gestational age of exposure. Offspring with FAE exhibit symptoms similar to those of FAS but with a lesser degree of severity. FAE usually results from drinking during the first trimester. Alcohol-related mental and behavioral problems fall within alcohol-related neurodevelopmental disabilities (ARND). These sequelae can result from drinking at any time during the pregnancy and among other problems can cause difficulties with memory, attention, judgment, language, reasoning, and recklessness.[51] Studies suggest that FAS occurs in approximately 0.2 to 2.0 infants per 1000 live births, and FASD occurs at least four times more often.[51]

A decision to suddenly stop drinking during pregnancy can result in withdrawal effects that can be dangerous to both mother and fetus; thus it is important that withdrawal be conducted under supervision. During efforts to withdraw, most programs elect to treat the woman with short-acting barbiturates (e.g., phenobarbital or secobarbital) or benzodiazepines (e.g., chlordiazepoxide or diazepam). However, because barbiturates are potentially teratogenic (FDA Pregnancy Category D), a risk-to-benefit analysis should be undertaken before they are used. Other drugs that have proven effective in decreasing alcohol intake—e.g., naltrexone and acamprosate—are FDA Pregnancy Category C, and although animal studies suggest adverse fetal effects, actual research in women has not been conducted.[56] Detailed information on the FDA pregnancy categories can be found in Chapters 1 and 35.

Marijuana

Marijuana is a widely used illicit drug that readily crosses the placenta during pregnancy and is thought to decrease the oxygen available to the fetus. The bulk of research findings have found no effect on birth outcomes following marijuana use in pregnancy.[57]

Opioids

The actual incidence of opioid use among pregnant women is unknown, but it is believed that heroin is the most commonly abused opioid. Use of opioids during pregnancy can result in complications including miscarriage, preeclampsia, intrauterine growth retardation, premature rupture of membranes, preterm delivery, and stillbirth.[57] Within 48 to 72 hours of birth, newborns of heroin users undergo withdrawal symptoms (trembling, irritability, constant high-pitched crying, fever, uncoordinated sucking, vomiting, diarrhea, and occasional seizures) and are also at higher risk for later sudden infant death syndrome.[58] The recommended treatment for maternal heroin addiction is methadone taken in divided morning and evening doses. Although the newborn may undergo withdrawal from methadone, the symptoms are not as severe and can be handled more expediently than those of heroin. Abrupt cessation of heroin should not be undertaken as it increases the risk of death in the fetus.

Other opioids used during pregnancy such as oral oxycodone, hydrocodone, and pentazocine (especially when mixed with tripelennamine) also may produce withdrawal situations in the baby. If substances are used intravenously, the baby may be at risk for growth retardation.

Cocaine

Cocaine, especially crack cocaine, is highly addictive and has been studied in depth. Adverse effects are more consistently noted in women who use cocaine during pregnancy compared to women who use other opioids during pregnancy.[57] Cocaine is a CNS stimulant that increases the levels of norepinephrine. This in turn causes vasoconstriction of arterial vessels and hypertension. Vasoconstriction of the uterine vessels is the mechanism responsible for most of the fetal effects, which include miscarriage, placental abruption, fetal growth restriction, preterm labor, low birth weight, decreased head circumference, and fetal death.[59,60]

Methamphetamine

The use of methamphetamine by a pregnant woman causes fetal growth restriction and increased risks for complications such as preterm delivery, low birth weight, and small head circumference. After delivery, some babies exhibit symptoms of withdrawal including jitteriness, lethargy, and breathing difficulties. Long-term effects are not known.[61]

Club Drugs

Very little research has been done on the gestational effects of club drugs. It is suggested that when MDMA (ecstasy) is used during pregnancy, the offspring may have risks similar to those of amphetamine users.[61] Also of concern are possible adverse effects on learning and memory. Newborns exposed to PCP may have withdrawal symptoms and could be at increased risk for learning and behavioral problems later in life. The effects of LSD on the offspring are not known; however, the disorganization and distorted senses during the trip and the anxiety and depression that can follow it may negatively affect the safety and well-being of the pregnant woman.

Managing Substance Abuse During Labor

Although drug-abusing women may be perceived as drug seekers, the pain associated with labor is real, and women should be treated accordingly. Women on maintenance programs may be taking methadone during labor, but it should be recognized that methadone is not a pain reliever. Women who are on methadone should be given their regular maintenance dose of methadone.[62] The amount of analgesia that is needed may be difficult to gauge as usual dosages likely will need to be increased. Epidurals are appropriate, as the amount of intravenous or intramuscular opioids given during labor may not fully relieve the pain.

Butorphanol (Stadol) and Nalbuphine (Nubain) are agonist-antagonists that displace methadone from opiate receptors and thereby induce opiate withdrawal

symptoms. These two drugs are the only opiates that should not be used during labor by women who are on methadone or who are abusing opiates.[62] Additionally, naloxone (Narcan) should not be administered to newborns of opioid-dependent mothers at delivery to reverse the effects of opioids, because it may cause acute withdrawal in the newborn.

▌ Substance Abuse and the Mature Woman

Historically, substance abuse treatments and programs are envisioned primarily for adolescents and young adults. However, the aging population in the United States is increasingly composed of baby boomers who may have had a different relationship with illicit substances than their elders had.

Currently, the most commonly reported issues for aging women are alcohol abuse and polypharmacy factors, usually with prescription drugs originally prescribed for their therapeutic effects.[63] By 2030, the number of individuals aged 65 or older will constitute 20% of the national population. By that time it has been suggested that the number of elderly with substance abuse problems will more than double.

Little has been studied regarding effectiveness of treatment for older Americans. Physiologic changes, including liver metabolism, have been documented for aging in general, but not applied to substance abuse. Therefore, knowledge about use of treatment drugs in particular may not be able to be extrapolated to senior citizens. The area of substance abuse and the elderly, especially women as they tend to comprise the majority of this age group, requires rigorous research in the near future.[63]

▌ Conclusion

It is vitally important that healthcare providers screen for substance abuse. **Drug misuse** can occur with illicit drugs, legal drugs used illicitly, a variety of other easy-to-obtain materials, such as nicotine, alcohol, or inhalants, and medications prescribed for individuals or their families or friends. The negative effects of substance abuse account for major health problems for the individual and for the healthcare system. Knowledge about abused substances, their symptoms, and potential negative outcomes are valuable tools for all who work in the healthcare field.

◆◆ References

1. Fowler JS, Volkow ND, Kassed CA, Chang L. Imaging the addicted human brain. Sci Pract Perspec 2007;3:2:4–16.

2. National Institute on Drug Abuse. The science of addiction. Bethesda, MD: National Institutes of Health, 2007.

3. Cami J, Farre M. Drug addiction. N Engl J Med 2003;349:975–86.

4. The American Academy of Pain Medicine, The American Pan Society and the American Society of Addiction Medicine. 2001 definitions related to the use of opioids for the treatment of pain. 2001. Available from: *www.painmed.org/pdf/definition.pdf* [Accessed March 26, 2008].

5. Howell LL, Kimmel HL. Monoamine transporters and psychostimulant addiction. Biochem Pharmacol 2008;75:196–217.

6. Schwartz RD. The GABA receptor-gated ion channel: biochemical and pharmacological studies of structure and function. Biochem Pharmacol 1988; 37:3369.

7. Ritz M. Reward systems and addictive behavior. In Niesink R, Jaspers, R Kornet, L, van Ree J, eds. Drugs of abuse and addiction: neurobehavioral toxicology. Boca Raton, FL: CRC Press, 1999:124–49.

8. Moal ME, Koob GF. Drug addiction: pathways to the disease and pathophysiological perspectives. Eur Neuropsychopharmacol 2007;17:377–93.

9. Feltenstein MS, See RE. The neurocircuitry of addiction: an overview. Br J Pharmacol 2008;1–14.

10. O'Brien PG. Addictive behaviors. In Lewis SL, Heitkemper MM, Dirksen SR, O'Brien PG, Bucher L. Medical-surgical nursing, 7th ed. St Louis, MO: Mosby Elsevier, 2007:165-91.

11. Technologies for understanding and preventing substance abuse and addiction. US Government Office of Technology Assessment Appendix C. Available from: *www.druglibrary.org/schaffer/library/studies/ota/appc.htm* [Accessed July 19, 2007].

12. Dackis C, O'Brien C. Neurobiology of addiction: treatment and public policy ramifications. Nature Neurosci 2005;8(11):1431–6.

13. Reynolds EW, Bada HS. Pharmacology of drugs of abuse. Obstet Gynecol N Amer 2003;30:501–22.

14. Kosten TR, O'Connor PG. Management of drug and alcohol withdrawal. N Engl J Med 2003;348:1786–95.

15. Fudala PJ, Woody GE. Current and experimental therapeutics for the treatment of opioid addiction. In: Davis KL, Charney D, Coyle JT, Nemeroff C, eds. Neuropsychopharmacology: the fifth generation of progress. Philadelphia: Lippincott Williams & Wilkins, 2002:1507–18.

16. National Archives and Records Administration. Opioid drugs in maintenance and detoxification treatment of opiate addiction; final rule 2001. Federal Register Part II Department of Health and Human Services 21 CFR Part 291, 42 CFR Part 8.

17. Jones ES, O'Connor PG. Diagnosis and pharmacologic management of opioid dependency. Hosp Phys 2007;43:1015–24.

18. Fudala PJ. Office-based treatment of opiate addiction with a sublingual-tablet formulation of buprenorphine and naloxone. N Engl J Med 2003;349:949–58.

19. Bigelow GE, Preston KL. Opioids. In: Bloom FE, Kupfer DJ, eds. Psychopharmacology: the fourth generation of progress. Philadelphia: Lippincott Williams & Wilkins, 1995:1731–44.

20. Nestler, EJ. The neurobiology of cocaine addiction. Sci Pct Perspec 2005;3(1):4–10.

21. Plessinger MA, Woods JR. Cocaine in pregnancy. Obstet Gyn Clin N Amer 1998;25:99–118.

22. Rampulla J. Substance abuse. In: Buttaro IM, Trybulski J, Bailey PP, Sandberg-Cook J, eds. Primary care: a collaborative practice, 3rd ed. St Louis, MO: Mosby Elsevier, 2007:1425–34.

23. Archer T. Ecstasy, toxicity and the cooling factor. Emerg Med J 2008;25:534.

24. McGregor C, Srisurapanont M, Jittiwutikarn J, Laobhripatr S, Wongtan T, White JM. The nature, time course and severity of methamphetamine withdrawal. Society for the Study of Addiction. Addiction 2005; 100:1320–9.

25. Martell BA, Mitchell E, Poling J, Gonsai K, Kosten TR. Vaccine pharmacotherapy for the treatment of cocaine dependence. Biol Psych 2005;58:158–64.

26. Katzung BG. Sedative-hypnotic drugs. In: Katzung BG, ed. Basic and clinical pharmacology, 10th ed. New York: McGraw-Hill, 2007:347–62.

27. Smith KM, Larive LL, Romanelli F. Club drugs: methylenedioxymethamphetamine, flunitrazepam, ketamine

hydrochloride, and gamma-hydroxybutyrate. Am J Health Syst Pharm 2002;59(11):1067–76.

28. Abraham HD, McCann UD, Ricaurte GA. Psychedelic drugs. In: Davis KL, Charney D, Coyle JT, Nemeroff C, eds. Neuropsychopharmacology: the fifth generation of progress. Philadelphia: Lippincott Williams & Wilkins, 2002:1545–56.

29. National Institute on Drug Abuse, Research Report. National Institutes of Health. Hallucinogens and dissociative drugs, 2006. Available from: *www.nida.nih .gov/ResearchReports/Hallucinogens.html.* [Accessed August 13, 2007].

30. Caroll ME. PCP and hallucinogens. Adv Alcohol Subst Abuse 1999;9:167–90.

31. Sinner B, Graf BM. Ketamine. Handb Exp Pharmacol 2008;182:313–33.

32. National Institute on Drug Abuse, Research Report. National Institutes of Health. Anabolic steroids, 2006. Available from: *www.drugabuse.gov/PDF/RRSteroids .pdf* [Accessed January 11, 2008].

33. National Institute on Drug Abuse, National Institutes of Health. Anabolic steroid abuse research report series, 2003. Available from: *www.drugabuse. gov/ResearchReports/Steroids/anabolicsteroids5.html #treatment* [AccessedJuly 24, 2007].

34. National Institute on Drug Abuse, National Institutes of Health. Research report: marijuana abuse, 2006. Available from: *www.nida.nih.gov/ResearchReports/ Marijuana2.html.* [Accessed August 21, 2007].

35. Smith, NT. A review of the published literature into cannabis withdrawal symptoms in human users. London: Addiction Directorate, South London and Maudsley NHS Trust, Marina House, 2001:7.

36. Eaton DK, Kann L, Kinchen S, Ross J, Hawkins J, Harris WA, et al. Youth risk behavior surveillance— United States, 2005. MMWR 2006;55(3505):1–108.

37. Shin EJ, Lee PH, Kim HJ, Nabeshima T, Kim HC. Neuropsychotoxicity of abused drugs: potential for dextromethorphan and novel neuroprotective analogs of dextromethorphan with improved safety profiles in terms of abuse and neuroprotective effects. J Pharmacol Sci 2008;106:22–7.

38. Dyer JE, Roth B, Hyma BA. Gamma-hydroxybutyrate withdrawal syndrome. Ann Emerg Med 2001, February;37:147–53.

39. US Department of Health and Human Services. 10th special report to the US Congress on alcohol and health. Bethesda, MD: National Institute on Alcohol Abuse and Alcoholism, 2000.

40. Mann K, Ackermann K, Croissant B, Mundle G, Nakovics H, Diehl A. Neuroimaging of gender differences in alcohol dependence: are women more vulnerable? Alcohol Clin Exp Res 2005;29:896–901.

41. Lieber CS. Medical disorders of alcoholism. N Engl J Med 1995;333:1057–65.

42. Kohnke MD. Approach to the genetics of alcoholism: a review based on pathophysiology. Biochem Pharm 2008;75:160–77.

43. American Psychiatric Association. Diagnostic and statistical manual of mental disorders (DSM) IV-TR. Fourth Edition, Text Revision. Washington, DC: American Psychiatric Association, 2000.

44. Anton RF, O'Malley SS, Ciraulo DA, Cisler RA, Couper D, Donovan DM, et al. Combined pharmacotherapies and behavioral interventions for alcohol dependence. The COMBINE study: a randomized controlled trial. JAMA 2006;295:2003–17.

45. Johnson BA. Update on neuropharmacological treatments for alcoholism: scientific basis and clinical findings. Biochem Pharmacol 2008;75:34–56.

46. Mann K, Lehert P, Morgan MY. The efficacy of acamprosate for alcoholism treatment: a meta analysis. Alcohol Clin Exp Res 2001;25:1335–41.

47. Verheul R, Lehert P, Geerlings PJ, Koeter MW, van den Brink W. Predictors of acamprosate efficacy: results from a pooled analysis of seven European trials including 1485 alcohol-dependent patients. Psychopharmacology 2005;178:167–73.

48. Galloway GP, Koch M, Cello R, Smith DE. Pharmacokinetics, safety, and tolerability of a depot formulation of naltrexone in alcoholics: an open-label trial. BMC Psychiatry 2005;5:18.

49. Johnson BA, Rosenthal N, Capece JA, Weingand F, Mao L, Beyers K, et al. Topiramate for treating alcohol dependence. JAMA 2007;298:1641–51.

50. Office of Applied Studies, Department of Health and Human Services. 2006 national survey on drug use and health: national findings. Available from: *http://oas .samhsa.gov/NSDUH/2k6NSDUH/2k6results.cfm#3.3* [Accessed March 25, 2008].

51. Bertrand J, Floyd RL, Weber MK. Guidelines for identifying and referring persons with fetal alcohol syndrome. Centers for Disease Control. MMWR 2005;54(RR-11):1–10.

52. Larkby C. The effects of prenatal alcohol exposure. Alcohol Health Res 1997;21:192–9.

53. Strandberg-Larson K, Nielsen NJ, Gronbak M, Anderson PK, Olsen J, Anderson AM. Binge drinking

in pregnancy and risk of fetal death. Obstet Gynecol 2008;111;602–9.

54. Marcellus L, Kerns K. Outcomes for children with prenatal exposure to drugs and alcohol: a social-determinants of health approach. In Boyd SC, Marcellus L, eds. With child substance use during pregnancy: a woman-centered approach. Winnipeg, MB, Canada: Fernwood, 2007:38–53.

55. Jones KL, Smith DW, Ulleland CN, Streissguth P. Pattern of malformation in offspring of chronic alcoholic mothers. Lancet 1973;1(7815):1267–71.

56. Lee R, An S, Kim S, Rhee G, Kwack S, Seok J. Neurotoxic effects of alcohol and acetaldehyde during embryonic development. JTEH 2005;68(23): 2147–62.

57. Kuczkowski KM. The effects of drug abuse on pregnancy. Curr Opin Obstet Gynecol 2007;6:578–85.

58. Zuckerman B, Frank D, Brown E. Overview of the effects of abuse and drugs on pregnancy and offspring. NIDA Res Monogr 1995;149:16–38.

59. Vidaeff AC, Mastrobattista JM. In utero cocaine exposure: a thorny mix of science and mythology. Am J Perinatol 2003;20:4:165–72.

60. Bauer CR, Langer JC, Shankaran S, Bada HS, Lester B, Wright LL. Acute neonatal effects of cocaine exposure during pregnancy. Arch Pediatr Adolesc Med 2005; 159:9:824–34.

61. Smith LM, LaGasse LL, Derauf C, Grant P, Shah R, Arria A. The infant development, environment, and lifestyle study: effects of prenatal methamphetamine exposure, polydrug exposure, and poverty on intra-uterine growth. Pediatrics 2006;118:3:1149–56.

62. Goff M, O'Conner M. Perinatal care of women maintained on methadone. J Midwifery Womens Health 2007;52:e236.

63. Gfroerer JC, Penne MA, Pemberton MR, Folsom RE. The aging baby boom cohort and future prevalence of substance abuse. Substance use by older adults: estimates of future impact on the treatment system. OAS Analytic Series #A-21, DHHS Publication No. (SMA) 03-3763. Rockville, MD: Substance Abuse and Mental Health Services Administration, Office of Applied Studies, 2002: Chapter 5.

64. Goode E. Drugs in American society, 5th ed. Boston: McGraw-Hill, 1999.

65. Hanson GR, Venturelli PJ, Fleckstein AE. Drugs and society, 9th ed. Sudbury, MA: Jones and Bartlett, 2006.

66. Varney H, Kriebs JM, Gegor CL. Varney's midwifery, 5th ed. Sudbury, MA: Jones and Bartlett, 2004.

67. Rayburn WF, Zuspan FP. Drug therapy in obstetrics and gynecology. St. Louis, MO: Mosby, 1992.

68. American College of Obstetricians and Gynecologists. Teratology. ACOG Educ Bull 1997;233:1–8.

69. Wang EC. Methadone treatment during pregnancy. JOGNN 1999;28(6):615–22.

70. Dunbar AE, O'Neil M, Marben L. Johns Hopkins Children's Center NICU guidebook 1999–2000. Baltimore, MD: Johns Hopkins University, 1999.

Appendix A   Detection of Substances of Abuse in Urine

Drug	Maximum length of time substance can be detected in urine
Amphetamines	30 hours for low doses and up to 120 hours for higher doses
Ethanol	< 1 day
Barbiturates	1 day for short-acting barbiturates 2–3 days for intermediate-acting barbiturates 7 days for long-acting barbiturates
Benzodiazepines	2–4 days depending on dose
Cocaine	60 hours after single dose and up to 22 days following chronic use
Methadone	3 days
Marijuana	6 days following single use and 29 days following chronic use
Opioids	
Heroin	1–4 days
Meperidine (Demerol)	4–24 hours
Morphine	84 hrs minimum

"The caution may seem useless, but it is quite surprising how many men (some women do it too), practically behave as if the scientific end were the only one in view, or as if the sick body were but a reservoir for stowing medicines into, and the surgical disease only a curious case the sufferer has made for the attendant's special information. This is really no exaggeration."

FLORENCE NIGHTINGALE

10
Complementary and Alternative Therapies

Wendell Combest, Austin J. Combest, and Juliana van Olphen Fehr

Chapter Glossary

Botanical Foods or supplements that are derived from any part of the plant, including fruits, roots, and flowers.

Botanical medicine Medicine that is derived from botanicals. Also known as phytotherapy.

Complementary and alternative medicine A group of diverse medical and healthcare systems practices and products that are not presently considered to be part of conventional medicine.

Dietary supplement Any product intended to supplement the diet that is not represented for use as a conventional food. Dietary supplements are not regulated by the FDA.

Herbal Product derived from the stem and/or stems of a plant.

Homeopathy A type of alternative treatment or alternative medicine whose main tenet is that a person with a disease or condition can be treated by minute amounts of substances that in larger doses can cause the condition or symptoms of the condition. The term homeopathy is derived from the Greek words for "similar" and "suffering."

Integrative medicine Combines conventional Western medicine with alternative and complementary treatments.

Phytoestrogen Plant-derived agent that is a nonsteroidal compound that binds to estrogen receptors.

Phytotherapy Medicine that is derived from any part of a plant, including the root, leaves, fruit, flowers, etc. Also known as botanical medicine.

Probiotic Live organism, which, when administered in adequate amounts, confers a health benefit on the host.

United States Pharmacopeia (USP) Nongovernmental, not-for-profit public health organization that serves as an official standards-setting authority for all prescription and OTC medicines, including dietary supplements sold in the United States.

USP Verified Dietary Supplement Mark This label is awarded to dietary supplements that have been approved by the USP to verify that (1) all listed ingredients are the only ingredients in the container; (2) the supplement does not contain harmful levels of contaminants; (3) the supplement will not break down and release alternate ingredients into the body; and (4) the supplement has been made using good manufacturing practices.

Introduction

Complementary and alternative medicine (CAM) is defined by the National Center for Complementary and Alternative Medicine (NCCAM) as "a group of diverse medical and health care systems practices and products that are not presently considered to be part of conventional medicine." Another widely used definition of CAM states that CAM is "a group of therapies not typically taught at US medical schools or other schools of allied health or widely available at US hospitals."[1]

The various CAM treatment modalities have been organized by NCCAM into four general domains and a fifth called whole medical systems, which combines aspects of the other four domains. The four domains are: (1) mind-body medicine (e.g., meditation, prayer, art, music, dance therapies); (2) biologically based practices (e.g., herbal medicine, vitamins); (3) manipulative and body-based practices (e.g., chiropractic, osteopathic manipulation, massage); and

(4) energy medicine involving energy fields (e.g., qi gong, Reiki, therapeutic touch) and bioelectromagnetic-based therapies (e.g., sound, magnet, and light therapies). The whole medical systems domain includes complete systems of practice and theory such as the Western practices of **homeopathy** and non-Western systems such as traditional Chinese medicine (TCM) or Indian traditional medicine, called Ayurveda.

This chapter reviews botanical therapies used by women in the United States today, which is also referred to as **botanical medicine** or **phytotherapy**. The term **herbal** refers to the herbaceous parts of a plant, such as leaves and stems. The term **botanical** refers to foods or supplements that are derived from any part of the plant, including fruits, roots, and flowers.

History of Complementary and Alternative Medicine

Many of the therapies under the mantle of CAM have been prominent components of healthcare systems in other countries, such as China and India, for centuries. Written reference to medicinal herbs can be found in the earliest records from most cultures in the world. In fact, the use of herbs for medical treatment might be the oldest form of healthcare known, and it is the field of herbalism that is the direct precursor of pharmacology as it is practiced today. Many of the drugs used today are still derived from plant sources.

Although medical use of herbs and plants is an unbroken chain that reaches back into antiquity, other CAM therapies have had a less clear path. In India and China, some of the therapies such as acupuncture and Ayurveda, which are labeled CAM in the United States, are part of mainstream medical care. In the United States, as traditional allopathic medicine became more dominant during the late 1800s and early 1900s, alternative systems of health care used in this country became less popular. CAM therapies experienced a resurgence in the late 20th century as part of the alternative health movement.

In the last few decades, CAM therapies have been subjected to scientific scrutiny with mixed results. Some therapies such as acupuncture, massage, and aromatherapy have proven benefits and are being incorporated into conventional health care. The emphasis on using both traditional biomedical techniques and CAM in a way that addresses the needs of the whole person is referred to as a new form of health care called **integrative medicine**.

In the past 10 years, an increasing number of schools of health training in the United States began including CAM in their standard curriculum, underscoring its increased popularity and acceptance. In 2002, President Bill Clinton's White House Commission on Complementary and Alternative Medicine released a report that recommended increased federal funds for CAM research in addition to many other recommendations aimed at integrating CAM into healthcare practice in the United States in a safe, efficacious, and thoughtful manner.[2] Today, many medical schools and academic institutions have centers for integrative medicine where CAM is studied and practiced.

National Center for Complementary and Alternative Medicine (NCCAM)

One of the major reasons for the rapid growth of CAM in the United States was the formation of the Office of Alternative Medicine (OAM) in 1992. In 1999, the Office of Alternative Medicine was upgraded and became one of the 27 institutes and centers of the National Institutes of Health that exists within the US Department of Health and Human Services. Its name was changed to the National Center for Complementary and Alternative Medicine (NCCAM) to adequately reflect the complementary aspects of this group of therapies.[3] The available funding budget was substantially increased (approximately $120 million per year since 2004), which has led to a marked increase in evidence-based CAM research. The mission statement of NCCAM is to "explore complementary and alternative healing practices in the context of rigorous science, train CAM researchers, and disseminate authoritative information to the public and professionals." The NCCAM has funded more than 1000 research projects by more than 200 institutions.

Office of Dietary Supplements

Another key player in the advancement of our knowledge of CAM in the United States is the Office of Dietary Supplements (ODS) at NIH, which was established in 1995 as a mandate of the Dietary Supplement Health and Education Act of 1994. Its mission is to "strengthen knowledge and understanding of dietary supplements by evaluating scientific information, stimulating and supporting research, disseminating research results, and educating the public to foster an enhanced quality of life and health for the U.S. population." The ODS has a collaborative relationship with other NIH branches, especially NCCAM, supporting research and information databases. The International Bibliographic Information on

Dietary Supplements is an extensive database provided and maintained by ODS and various NIH agencies as well as the United States Department of Agriculture and the Food and Nutrition Information Center. This database provides access to bibliographic citations and abstracts from the published research literature on dietary supplements. The ODS, along with NCCAM, funds six dietary supplement research centers that are mainly university based. These centers focus their research on the safety, efficacy, and biologic mechanisms of action of potentially useful botanical medicines.

German Commission E Monographs

Although no longer active, the German Commission E deserves mention. This commission was formed in Germany in 1978. It produced 380 monographs on the safety and efficacy of drugs before being disbanded in 1995. The monographs were imported, translated into English, and published by the American Botanical Council in 1998.[4] However, the English translations do not have citations, and the information in these monographs is not dated.

Regulation of Dietary Supplements

In the United States, botanical medicines are sold and regulated as **dietary supplements**. The Food and Drug Administration (FDA) regulates the marketing and sales of four categories of consumable products: food, food additives, drugs, and dietary supplements. The Federal Trade Commission (FTC) regulates the advertising of these products. The classification of botanical products as a dietary supplement instead of a medicine or drug has significant consequences for consumers and providers. Table 10-1 summarizes these differences.

The Dietary Supplement Health and Education Act (DSHEA) passed by the US Congress in 1994 amended the 1938 Food, Drug, and Cosmetic Act and broadened the definition of dietary supplements to include vitamins, minerals, amino acids, and botanical and animal products.[3] The DSHEA defines a dietary supplement as "any product intended to supplement the diet which is not represented for use as a conventional food." Therefore botanical as well as nonbotanical supplements can be sold in the United States provided they do not make any claims that the dietary supplement diagnoses, treats, cures, or prevents any disease. Doing so makes the product subject to regulation as a drug.

Table 10-1 Comparison of Dietary Supplements and Drugs in the United States

	Dietary Supplement	Drugs
Burden of proof of safety	Manufacturer	FDA
Label can denote use for treating disease	No	Yes
Must demonstrate safety before approval	No	Yes
Must demonstrate efficacy before approval	No	Yes
Requires Investigational Drug Application	No	Yes
Regulation of advertising	FDA	FTC

FDA = Food and Drug Administration; FTC = Federal Trade Commission.

In 1998, the FDA redefined the word *disease* to help clarify permissible claims by dietary supplement manufacturers. Under this new definition, the following type of statements concerning the claims of dietary supplements were not permissible: "reduces the pain and stiffness of arthritis," or "lowers elevated cholesterol." What is allowable is a statement that is called a structure/function claim.[5] For example, manufacturers selling cranberry products can claim that they support urinary health but they cannot claim that they prevent the occurrence of urinary tract infections. Following any allowable structure/function claim, the dietary supplement manufacturer must say on the product label, "This statement has not been evaluated by the FDA." Labels must also state, "This product is not intended to diagnose, treat, cure, or prevent any disease."

New requirements for labeling of dietary supplements were implemented in 1999. Under these guidelines, product name, quantity, serving size, and total weight of each ingredient must appear on the label. All ingredients including excipients must be listed in descending order of amount in the product. The identity of the plant parts present must be indicated as well as the name and location of the manufacturer or distributor. The product must state on the label that it is a dietary supplement.

Other quality control measures have recently been implemented in the dietary supplement industry. The **United States Pharmacopeia** (USP) is a nongovernmental, not-for-profit public health organization that serves as an official standards-setting authority for all prescription and over-the-counter (OTC) medicines, including dietary supplements, sold in the United States. The USP sets standards for the quality, strength, purity, and consistency of these products. Recently the USP has begun to help with the much-needed task of improving the quality standards of dietary supplements. In its newly created Dietary Supplement Verification program, many supplements are being tested for purity, potency, and overall quality. If a manufacturer meets USP's strict criteria, it is allowed to use the **USP Verified Dietary Supplement Mark** on the label of its product.

Safety of Botanical Medicines

Unlike food additives and drugs, dietary supplements do not require premarket approval for safety; therefore, the FDA must assume the burden of proving a product is unsafe if FDA personnel decide to investigate a particular product. Thus both safety and efficacy, the two standards applied to pharmaceutical products, are not necessarily assessed for botanical products.

The medically active compound in a plant can come from the leaf, root, stem, or flower. In addition, the compound of interest may be several compounds that work synergistically. This combination may only be active if the plant is picked a certain time of year or if it is dried or processed in a certain way. It is easy to see why the amount of active ingredient in the herbal supplements found on the shelf of the pharmacy varies widely. As an example, Draves et al. had 54 St. John's wort preparations analyzed and found very large variations in the actual amount of the two pharmacologically active ingredients in the products analyzed. The actual percentage of active ingredient ranged from 0 to 108.6% of what was claimed on the label.[6] In 2004, the FDA issued a rule banning ephedra from being included in dietary supplements but this was after receiving reports of 34 deaths and more than 800 adverse medical events that were submitted between 1993 and 1997. Another concern is purity; some botanical preparations are contaminated with heavy metals (e.g., iron in Ayurveda therapies imported from India). Products labeled as ginseng have been found to contain scopolamine.[7] Ginseng is very expensive to produce, which makes it an obvious target for replacement with noninseng substances.

Adverse Reactions to Botanical Medicines

Even when quality control issues are not a concern, adverse effects of botanical preparations that are pure can occur. Adverse reactions associated with herbs include idiosyncratic reactions, cardiotoxicity, renal toxicity, hepatotoxicity, convulsions, and drug–herb interactions.[5]

Hepatotoxicity, the adverse reaction most frequently reported in either case reports or small series, deserves

comment. The well known hepatotoxic effect of pyrrolizidine alkaloids is a good example of the problem. Pyrrolizidine alkaloids are present in many plants to varying degrees. Pyrrolizidine alkaloids are metabolized via CYP3A4 and CYP2B6 into pyrroles, which are capable of inducing hepatocellular injury. Comfrey contains pyrrolizidine alkaloids and large doses of comfrey tea have been the etiology of liver dysfunction in several of the case reports of herb-induced hepatoxicity. Table 10-2 lists the herbs that have been implicated in cases of hepatotoxicity. Because hepatotoxicity is rare, it can take large population exposures before a relationship between one herbal formulation and liver damage becomes evident. This may account for why some of the Chinese herbal medicines are on this list. In addition, many Chinese herbal medicines contain species of *Senecio*, which is one of the three families of plants that have large amounts of pyrrolizidine alkaloids.

Herb–Drug Interactions

Prescribers should be aware that 20% of persons in the United States use botanical products concomitantly with prescription drugs.[1] Herb–drug interactions are difficult to determine for several reasons. Herb–drug interactions are, in general, rare when taken in the prescribed manner for short periods of time. However, these interactions are undoubtedly underreported, so the true incidence is not

Table 10-2 Selected Herbs That Have Been Implicated in Cases of Hepatotoxicity

Black Cohosh (*Cimicifuga racemosa*)
Cascara sagrada (*Rhamnus purshiana*)*
Chaparral (*Larrea*)
Chinese herbal medicines:
Chaso
Sho (Do)-saiko-to
Jin Bu Huan (*Stephania sinica*)
Ma huang (Ephedra)†
Shou-wa-pian
Comfrey (*Symphytum*)
Germander (*Teucrium chamaedrys*)
Kava (*Piper methysticum*)
Mistletoe (*Viscum album*)
Pennyroyal (*Mentha pulegium*)
Sassafras oil (*Sassafras*)
Senecio (*Senecio aconitifolius*)
Senna (*Cassia acutifolia*)
Skullcap (*Scutellaria*)
Valerian (*Valeriana officinalis*)

* Case report of cholestatic hepatitis.

† In 2004, the FDA issued a rule banning ephedra from all dietary supplements.

known. Finally, most herbal preparations contain multiple compounds or a mixture of several different herbs; therefore when adverse effects are reported, it is not clear which compound is responsible for the reaction. The herbs that are associated with drug interactions include gingko, St. John's wort, ginseng, garlic, and kava.[8,9] Some of the well-known drug–herb interactions are listed in Table 10-3.

Efficacy of Botanical Medicines

The number of studies evaluating the efficacy of botanical medicines is only just beginning to increase. Because botanical medicines are complex compounds that are not easy to reproduce, determining the active ingredient(s) is a necessary first step that can take time and research. This is a step that must be completed before efficacy studies can be conducted. Most of the studies on medicinal use of herbs being published today are these basic chemistry studies that either determine the active compound or test the effects of the active compound. This chapter reviews the efficacy for specific botanical medicines where it is known and discusses the extent of knowledge about specific herbs that, to date, have not been proven to be efficacious.

It is important to recognize that the doses of botanical medicines used in randomized trials are not necessarily the same doses found on the shelf at the local drug store. Consumers and prescribers need to assess the value of the efficacy studies reported here with caution because until botanical medicines are standardized in this country, neither quality, purity, efficacy, nor safety are guaranteed.

▌ Use of CAM in the United States

The most comprehensive survey on CAM use in the United States was published in 2004, summarizing the 2002 National Health Interview survey that is conducted by the National Centers for Health Statistics of the Centers for Disease Control and Prevention. Barnes et al., from NCCAM, analyzed several questions about CAM. The survey (n = 31,044 civilian, noninstitutionalized adults aged 18 years or older) found that 36% of the adults were using some form of CAM in the 12 months prior to when the survey was conducted.[10] When prayer is included as a CAM therapy, mind-body medicine is the most commonly used domain (53%), and if prayer is excluded, biologic-based therapies (22%) were the most popular. CAM users are more likely to be women

Table 10-3 Selected Herb–Drug Interactions*

Drug—Generic (Brand)	Effects
Asian ginseng root and	
Phenelzine (Nardil)	Case report of mania.
Warfarin (Coumadin)	Decreased anticoagulant effect.[†]
Echinacea and	
Acetaminophen (Tylenol)	Both acetaminophen and echinacea are potentially hepatotoxic, and therefore, it is theorized that the combination could increase the risk of hepatotoxicity.
Garlic and	
Antiretroviral drugs	Toxic gastrointestinal effects.[‡]
Chlorpropamide (Diabinese)	Enhanced hypoglycemic effect.
Warfarin (Coumadin)	Increased anticoagulant effect.[†]
Gingko and	
Aspirin and other NSAIDs	Increased bleeding.
Digoxin (Lanoxin)	Increased blood levels of digoxin.
Hypoglycemic agents	Gingko decreases blood sugar and may enhance the antihyperglycemic effect of oral medications used for diabetes.
Omeprazole (Prilosec)	Increased metabolism of omeprazole and possible decreased effectiveness.
Thiazide diuretics	Increased blood pressure.
Trazodone (Desyrel)	Coma.
Warfarin (Coumadin)	Increased anticoagulant effect.[†]
Ginseng (panax) and	
Opioids	Ginseng can inhibit analgesic effect of opioids.
Warfarin (Coumadin)	Decreased serum concentrations of warfarin.
Kava and	
Alprazolam (Xanax)	Semicomatose state.
Levodopa (Sinemet)	Increased number of off periods.
Opioids	Increased sedation.
St. John's wort and	
Antiretroviral drugs	Decreased plasma levels of the antiretroviral drugs.
Amitriptyline	Decreased plasma levels of amitriptyline.
Benzodiazepines (midazolam [Versed], alprazolam [Xanax])	Decreased plasma levels of benzodiazepines.
Cyclosporin (Neoral)	Decreased plasma levels of cyclosporine.
Digoxin (Lanoxin)	Decreased plasma levels of digoxin.
Loperamide (Imodium)	Acute delirium.[†‡]
Methadone	Withdrawal syndrome.[‡]
Oral contraceptives	Decreased plasma levels of contraceptives. Can cause contraceptive failure.
Selective serotonin reuptake inhibitors	Serotonin syndrome.
Simvastatin (Zocor)	Decreased plasma levels of simvastatin.
Tacrolimus (Prototropic)	Decreased plasma levels of tacrolimus.
Theophylline (Theo-Dur)	Decreased plasma levels of theophylline.

NSAID = nonsteroidal antiinflammatory drugs.
* This table is not comprehensive, as new information is being identified on a regular basis.
[†] Causality uncertain.
[‡] Case reports only.

Table 10-4 Selected Botanical Medicines for Reproductive Health

Botanical Product	Clinical Indication	Evidence for Use
Blue cohosh	Induction of labor	Contraindicated.
Black cohosh	Dysmenorrhea	No evidence of effectiveness.
	Induction of labor	No evidence of effectiveness.*
	Menopausal symptoms	Conflicting studies; may have potential but more research needed.
Castor oil	Induction of labor	No evidence of effectiveness.*
Chasteberry	Dysmenorrhea	No evidence of effectiveness.
	Mastalgia	Effective.
	Premenstrual syndrome	Effective for short-term use.
Cramp bark	Dysmenorrhea	No evidence of effectiveness.*
Cranberry products	Prevention of urinary tract infection (UTI)	Good for prevention of UTI but no evidence that cranberry is effective in treating UTIs.
Dong quai	Dysmenorrhea	No evidence of effectiveness.*
Evening primrose	Premenstrual syndrome	No evidence of effectiveness.
	Mastalgia	No evidence of effectiveness.
	Menopausal symptoms	No evidence of effectiveness.
Flax	Mastalgia	No evidence of effectiveness.
Ginger	Nausea and vomiting in pregnancy	Effective.
Ginseng	Menopausal symptoms	No evidence of effectiveness.
Kava	Anxiety	Effective.
Probiotics	Prevention of UTI	No evidence of effectiveness.
Psidium guajava	Dysmenorrhea	One study found that rose tea was effective. More studies needed.
Red clover	Menopausal symptoms	No evidence of effectiveness.
Rose tea	Dysmenorrhea	One study found that rose tea was effective. More studies needed.
Sage	Menopausal symptoms	Preliminary evidence of effectiveness in one study only.
St. John's wort	Depression	Good evidence for mild to moderate depression for short-term therapy.
Soy products	Menopausal symptoms	Effective for vasomotor symptoms. Soy-based food products more effective than tablets or capsules.
Wild yam	Menopausal symptoms	No evidence of effectiveness.

* No randomized trials identified and/or few small studies that were methodologically poor.

younger than 65 years of age who are living in the western United States. They have, in general, a higher income than non-CAM users.

Botanical Medicine in Women's Health

Women are much more likely to use botanical medicines than are men. Upchurch et al. conducted a secondary analysis of the 2002 National Health Interview survey and found that 40% of the women (n = 17,295) reported recent use of one or more CAM modalities.[11] The category of CAM most frequently used was the biologically based products category (23.8%).[11] Musculoskeletal disorders and chronic pain were the conditions for which women most frequently used CAM therapies to ameliorate overall. Menopause was among the top 10 conditions because so many women choose herbal remedies for treating menopausal symptoms today.

The remainder of this chapter provides examples of major botanical therapies used predominately by women. Other chapters in this book include specific CAM therapies as well. The sections that follow are organized by disease state or health condition. Evidence-based research about use of herbs in the following areas are covered: depression, urinary tract infections, premenstrual syndrome (PMS) and premenstrual dysphoric disorder (PMDD), primary dysmenorrhea, mastalgia, nausea and vomiting during pregnancy, induction of labor, and menopausal symptoms (Table 10-4). Use of botanical medications for other disorders is addressed in separate chapters. For example, readers interested in echinacea for the common cold are referred to Chapter 20, whereas the efficacy of aloe vera for treating burns is addressed in Chapter 26.

Depression

St. John's Wort (*Hypericum Perforatum*)

Hypericum is a common ground cover with a pretty, five-petal yellow flower that blooms in the summer. The active agent, hypericin, contains many compounds including napthodianthrones that have several different versions of hypericin, flavonoids, hyperforin, amino acids, and tannins. The actual compound responsible for the therapeutic effects is unknown.[5] The mechanism for the apparent antidepressant effect of St. John's wort is unclear, but many studies indicate that this agent inhibits the reuptake of serotonin, dopamine, and norepinephrine in neuronal synapses in the brain.[10] Other pharmacologic studies indicate that various components in St. John's wort extracts bind to adenosine, gamma-amino butyric acid (GABA-A and B), and glutamate receptors in the central nervous system.[12]

Abundant evidence supports the benefit of this herbal supplement for treatment of mild to moderate depression. A meta-analysis of the clinical trials on St. John's wort that were published in the late 1990s found that St. John's wort is as effective as placebo in improving major depression (RR 2.47; 95% CI, 1.69–3.61; 29 trials, n = 5489) over a short period of treatment (mean was 6 weeks).[13] In many of these studies, the benefits of St. John's wort was shown to be equivalent to conventional antidepressant drugs. Fewer side effects were reported with St. John's wort than with the antidepressant medications.

In general, adverse effects following use of St. John's wort are minimal and lower in frequency than the side effects that occur after taking tricyclic antidepressants or selective serotonin reuptake inhibitors. That said, multiple side effects and a few adverse effects are associated with use of St. John's wort, including gastrointestinal distress, sexual dysfunction, dizziness, confusion, dry mouth, headache, and allergic skin reactions. Photosensitivity has been reported as well. Adverse effects include serotonin syndrome, which can occur when this herbal agent is taken concomitantly with selective serotonin reuptake inhibitors. In addition, there are case reports of cardiovascular collapse during anesthesia, delayed emergence from anesthesia, and hypertensive crisis in persons taking St. John's wort.[5]

St. John's wort is a potent inducer of several CYP450 enzymes and has clinically important interactions with numerous drugs such as anticoagulants, cyclosporine, digoxin, protease inhibitors, and oral contraceptives,[14] which are listed in Table 10-3 and are reviewed in more detail in Chapter 25. The FDA has issued black box warnings that advise against using St. John's wort if one is taking protease inhibitors.

Urinary Tract Infections

Urinary tract infections (UTI) include cystitis, urethral syndrome, and pyelonephritis. Lower UTIs involve the bladder, and upper UTIs involve the kidneys and ureters as well. Urinary tract infections are more common in women than in men. In fact, UTI is one of the most common bacterial infections in women.[15] Approximately 30% of all women will have a UTI before reaching the age of 24.[15]

Cranberry

Cranberry (*Vaccinium macrocarpon*) has been recommended for treating and preventing urinary tract infections. There is no evidence that cranberry is effective for treatment of UTIs. Cranberry lacks direct antibacterial activity but appears to work via compounds in the berries that prevent microorganisms such as *Escherichia coli* from adhering to epithelial cells lining the urinary tract.[16] Cranberry also lowers urine pH enough to retard the breakdown of urine by *E. coli*, thus reducing the pungent ammonia-like odor.

Cranberry may also be used as prophylaxis for prevention of UTIs. In a randomized, double-blind, placebo-controlled trial by Avorn et al.[17] involving 153 elderly women, consumption of 300 mL per day of a cranberry-containing beverage decreased the odds of bacteriuria to 42% of the odds found in the control group and decreased the odds of remaining bacteriuric if they were bacteriuric in the previous month to 27% of the odds in the control group. A Cochrane meta-analysis of 10 studies (n = 1049) found that cranberry products (400-mg tablet daily or 250-mL unsweetened undiluted juice three times/day) reduced the incidence of UTIs (RR 0.61; 95% CI, 0.40–0.91) over a 12-month period. The effectiveness was greater for women when compared to men, but dropout rates were high secondary to side effects such as cost, caloric load, and gastrointestinal upset.[18] It is important to remember that cranberry has flavonoids that may interact with warfarin (Coumadin) in a way that causes an enhanced anticoagulant effect, and therefore women on warfarin therapy should avoid using cranberry products in large amounts.

Probiotics

Probiotics are dietary supplements that contain "live organisms, which, when administered in adequate amounts confer a health benefit on the host."[19] The use of probiotics to treat and/or prevent UTIs has been researched extensively.[20,21] The mechanism by which *Lactobacillus* cultures may exhibit a protective effect is bacterial competition. In normal conditions, lactobacilli are the dominant bacteria in the vaginal flora. These bacteria are a known form of a biofilm that has some antimicrobial activity in vitro and in animal models. Infection or incomplete cure of a genitourinary infection shifts the flora in the vagina to a predominance of coliform uropathogens. Women who have recurrent UTIs are known to have vaginal microbacterial flora that does not have the usual amount of lactobacillus.[21] It has been theorized that lactobacillus-containing probiotic products placed in the vagina will allow the lactobacillus to compete with uropathogens, thereby preventing uropathogen colonization to the urethra and ascending infection into the bladder.

To date, none of the randomized trials that have evaluated the effectiveness of probiotics for prevention of UTIs have had adequate numbers to show a significant change in the incidence of UTI.[20] Although one randomized controlled trial did find a reduction in urinary tract infections from 6 per year to 1.6 per year following weekly intravaginal use of *L rhamnosus* and *L fermentum*, the control group that used a milk-based probiotic that stimulated indigenous lactobacilli was equally effective.[22] It appears that perhaps only certain strains of *Lactobacillus* are able to recolonize the vagina. More studies that utilize defined strains of lactobacillus and larger numbers of participants are needed before the efficacy of probiotics in preventing UTIs can be determined.

Lactobacillus-containing products marketed for intravaginal use have very few adverse effects. The incidence of infection with lactobacilli is very low but can occur in persons who are immunocompromised or debilitated. None of the studies done to date have enrolled persons with these risk factors.[20] More studies need to be completed for *Lactobacillus* therapy to be recommended at this time, although the treatment does seem promising.

Treatment of Primary Dysmenorrhea

Dysmenorrhea is a type of pelvic pain occurring during menstruation that can be classified as either primary or secondary. Primary dysmenorrhea is very common, occurring in as many as 50% of all menstruating women and usually presents within 3 years of menarche.[23] Uterine spasms are usually experienced as sharp intermittent pains that often radiate to the back of the legs or lower back. The etiology of the condition is not known but likely involves tissue ischemia and the release of prostaglandins, which mediate the pain and uterine contractions.[24] Several herbs have been widely used in treatments of dysmenorrhea, but evidence is generally weak supporting their efficacy.

Dong Quai

An extract from the root of the celery plant *Angelica sinensis*, dong quai, has been a popular remedy for dysmenorrhea in traditional Chinese medicine for centuries. The active constituent contains several different chemicals that have individually and in combination been tested in vitro and found to have weak estrogenic activity. One presumed mechanism of action is a presumed antagonistic effect on prostaglandin synthesis, which will then inhibit uterine contractions. This drug does inhibit prostaglandins and has anticoagulant properties and anti-platelet action; however, no clinical trials have been done showing its effectiveness for treatment of dysmenorrhea.

Adverse effects include bloating and loss of appetite. Because dong quai has possible antithrombotic effects and progesterone effects, persons taking warfarin (Coumadin), hormone replacement therapy, oral contraceptives, or other herbs that cause blood thinning may consider this herb contraindicated. Individuals with a history of an estrogen-dependent tumor should also use this drug with caution.

Cramp Bark (*Viburnum Opulus*) and Black Haw (*Viburnum Prunifolium*)

A hot water infusion (tea) of the bark from cramp bark (*Viburnum opulus*) has been a traditional folk remedy for relieving menstrual cramps for centuries in the United States. Although no clinical studies have been conducted, animal studies have demonstrated that extracted components of cramp bark have smooth-muscle-relaxing properties. Black haw (*Viburnum prunifolium*) has also been used, but we could find no studies that have evaluated either product in humans.

Rose Tea

Rose tea is widely used to treat dysmenorrhea in Eastern cultures. One randomized trial has attempted to determine the effectiveness of drinking rose tea to reduce pain associated with dysmenorrhea in Taiwanese adolescents (n = 130), and found that the experimental group (n = 59) perceived less pain and had higher psychological well-being over time (1, 3, and 6 months; $P > .001$) at each level based on scales used.[25] The adolescents in the experimental group drank two teacups of rose tea for 12 days each month for 6 months. Limitations of the study are the subjective reporting of the participants and the fact that these findings cannot be generalized to all populations. The study contributes to current knowledge about rose tea and its use in the treatment of primary dysmenorrhea; however, it also emphasizes the need for further research.

Psidium Guajava L.

A popular Mexican phytomedicine prescribed for the treatment of dysmenorrhea is *Psidium guajava* L. (Myrtaceae) extract.[26] The primary action of the flavonols in *Psidium guajava* L. is antispasmodic, in addition to its antioxidant and anti-inflammatory activity. One randomized trial (n = 197) found that a dose of 6 mg/day of the extract significantly reduced menstrual pain as measured on a visual analogue scale ($P > .001$) when compared with nonsteroidal anti-inflammatory drugs (NSAIDs) and placebo. However, all groups documented some reduction of pain associated with dysmenorrhea over the course of the trial.[27] A distinct advantage of using *Psidium guajava* L. to treat dysmenorrhea is it does not have the adverse gastrointestinal side effects of NSAIDs, but more research is needed before this supplement can be recommended for use.

Other Herbs for Dysmenorrhea

Roots of the false unicorn (*Chamaelirium luteum*) were widely used by Native Americans and 19th-century eclectic physicians in North America to treat a variety of women's conditions, including dysmenorrhea. Black cohosh and chasteberry have also been used to treat dysmenorrhea, but there are no studies documenting safety or efficacy of these agents.[27] These products are also reviewed in Chapter 30.

Premenstrual Syndrome and Premenstrual Dysphoric Disorder (PMDD)

It is estimated that 85–90% of women have regular premenstrual symptoms that include depression, irritability, mood swings, bloating, cyclic mastalgia (discussed separately later in this chapter), abdominal discomfort, emotional lability, headache, and constipation.[2] PMS is a disorder related to cyclical hormonal variation that causes disruption of both the emotional and physical well-being of women. PMS occurs during the luteal phase of the menstrual cycle and ceases after the start of menses. CAM therapies that show promise for treating PMS symptoms include calcium and vitamin B_6. The botanical medicines used for PMS include chasteberry and evening primrose oil.[28]

Chasteberry (*Vitex Agnus-Castus*)

The dried ripe fruit of the chasteberry tree has been a popular botanical treatment for reproductive disorders for centuries. Chasteberry fruit was used to decrease sexual desire in men in the middle ages, which is where it got its name.[7] Chasteberry (*Vitex agnus-castus*) is often referred to simply as *Vitex* by many herbalists. It is a deciduous shrub native to the Mediterranean, Europe, and Central Asia. The active ingredients in chasteberry fruit are progesterone, testosterone, flavonoids, alkaloids, and some volatile oils. The proposed mechanism of action is a decrease in prolactin, which reverses the normal luteal phase suppression of luteinizing hormone (LH) that then allows full development of the corpus luteum and production of more progesterone, so the PMS symptoms are less severe.[29] Several large, uncontrolled studies support the effectiveness and safety of chasteberry for treating PMS,[30] and clinical trials have shown chasteberry to be effective in reducing the symptoms of PMS as well.[29] The most recent study was a well-designed multicenter, randomized, double-blind, placebo-controlled trial including 178 women with PMS.[31] The women received either 20 mg of a standardized chasteberry extract (ZE 440) or placebo for three menstrual cycles. Slightly over half (52%) of the women in the chasteberry group reported more than a 50% reduction in symptoms, whereas 24% in the placebo group reported a 50% reduction in symptoms. Interestingly, bloating was not affected by chasteberry treatment.

Reported side effects include nausea, headache, and gastrointestinal disturbance. There are no reports of drug–drug interactions or serious adverse effects.[32] Side effects of chasteberry appear to be mild, with reports of gastrointestinal complaints, mild skin rash, headaches, acne, and increased menstrual flow.[32]

Chasteberry may have estrogenic activity and should be avoided or used with caution by persons with estrogen-sensitive disease. Chasteberry may also interfere with the efficacy of oral contraceptives and dopamine antagonists such as chlorpromazine (Thorazine) or prochlorperazine (Compazine).

One randomized, controlled trial investigated possible benefits of chasteberry in 41 women with premenstrual dysphoric disorder.[33] Chasteberry was compared to drug treatment with fluoxetine (Prozac) for 2 months. Both treatments resulted in significant improvements in symptoms (64% with fluoxetine and 57.9% with chasteberry).

To date, only one study has assessed the use of St. John's wort for treating depression associated with PMS or PMDD.[34] In this small pilot study including 19 women with PMS, anxiety, and depression, scores were significantly lowered after St. John's wort treatment (two tablets of 300-mg extract for 2 months). A larger randomized, controlled study is needed to confirm these preliminary observations. Ginkgo biloba, better known for its well-documented clinical benefits in dementia, has been shown in a single study to decrease fluid retention and congestion in PMS.[35]

Evening Primrose (*Oenothera Biennis*) Seeds

Evening primrose (*Oenothera biennis*) seeds are a rich source of the omega-6 fatty acid gamma-linoleic acid (GLA), which are precursors to the synthesis of the important antiinflammatory prostaglandin E1.[36] It has been shown that some women with PMS are deficient in GLA, particularly those who cannot convert the fatty acid linoleic acid to GLA.[37] Because of these properties, evening primrose oil (EPO) pressed from the seeds has become a popular remedy for PMS. However, little evidence supports use of this herb.[38]

Breast Pain (Mastalgia)

Mastalgia is a multifaceted condition whose cause is poorly understood. Anywhere from 50% to 80% of women can expect to have some level of mastalgia in their lifetime. Mastalgia is classified as either being noncyclical or cyclical associated with the menstrual cycle. Cyclical mastalgia in many women is associated with stress-induced hyperprolactinemia. In these women, an abnormal hyperresponse to stimulation of prolactin release is seen, which leads to hyperstimulation of the mammary gland, which often results in pain.

Chasteberry (*Vitex Agnus-Castus*)

Since 1999, evidence has accumulated supporting the potential efficacy of chasteberry for the treatment of mastalgia.[39] The mechanism of action is presumed to be secondary to diterpenes such as clerodadienols present in the dried fruit (berries), which are capable of binding to the D_2 dopamine receptors, causing suppression of prolactin release from the pituitary.[40] It has also been postulated that as-yet unidentified phytoestrogens in Vitex may be competitively binding to estrogen receptors in the breast, thereby exerting antiestrogen effects. Evidence demonstrates that fruit extracts have constituents that competitively bind to both the alpha and beta isoforms of the estrogen receptor.[41]

The results of a large noninterventional study in 1634 women with cyclic mastalgia indicated that a 3-month treatment with chasteberry decreased the frequency and severity of pain.[30] Chasteberry was found to be effective in reducing both intensity and duration of breast pain in a placebo-controlled trial and two randomized, clinical trials.[31,42]

Evening Primrose (*Oenothera Biennis*)

The oil from evening primrose seeds (referred to as EPO) is a rich source of the omega-6 essential fatty acid GLA. EPO is a popular treatment for mastalgia throughout Europe, especially in the United Kingdom. However, the few poorly designed clinical studies that have been conducted do not strongly support the effectiveness of EPO in the treatment of breast pain.

Flax (*Linum Usitatissimum*)

It has been hypothesized that the phytoestrogen lignins present in the seeds of the flax plant (*Linum usitatissimum*) may offer benefit in mastalgia. A single randomized, double-blind trial in 116 premenopausal women with severe breast pain showed that flaxseed (25 g formulated into a muffin) given daily for 6 months decreased pain as measured by a visual analogue scale.[43]

Nausea and Vomiting During Pregnancy

Approximately 50–90% of women experience at least some level of nausea during the first trimester of pregnancy, while a somewhat lower number (25–55%) have episodes of vomiting.[44] Several CAM therapies including acupressure and acupuncture, vitamin B_6, and ginger are used to treat nausea and/or vomiting that occur during pregnancy. Acupuncture and vitamin B_6 are discussed in more detail in Chapter 36.

Ginger (*Zingiber Officinale*)

Ginger (*Zingiber officinale*) has been used for centuries to treat many medical complaints, but particularly gastrointestinal disorders. Its effects are thought to be due to increasing tone and peristalsis in the gastrointestinal tract due to anticholinergic and antiserotonin action.[45] Ginger acts directly on the digestive tract.

A recent systematic review of the literature on ginger and hyperemesis gravidarum[46] described six double-blind, randomized, placebo-controlled trials (total of 675 women). Four of the six trials demonstrated that ginger was more effective than placebo.[47] The other two studies were equivalence studies that found that ginger was as effective as vitamin B_6 in treating nausea and vomiting.[44,48]

In the aforementioned published clinical trials, the dose of ginger (fresh or powdered) varied from 0.5 to 2 g daily with 1.0 g being the most typical dose. Ginger is available in a variety of forms, and an evaluation of products purchased in pharmacies and health food stores found a wide variation in the amount of active ingredients and suggested serving sizes.[49] Exact dosing relies on use of standardized extracts. Equivalent dosing is listed in Table 10-5.[50]

Ginger is a thromboxane synthetase inhibitor, and a frequently cited comment by Backon[51] cautions that ginger could affect testosterone receptor and sex steroid differentiation in the fetus. There is no clinical evidence to suggest that ginger has an adverse effect on fetal development. In traditional medical systems and herbalist literature, ginger is often contraindicated for use by pregnant women due to its reputation for inducing menstruation or promoting bleeding, but there is no clinical evidence that it acts as an abortifacient.[52] More research is needed to confirm the general belief that ginger is safe to use during pregnancy.

Table 10-5 Equivalent Dosing of Ginger Products

The following equal 1000 mg standardized extract:
1 tsp fresh grated rhizome.
2 droppers liquid extract (2 mL).
2 tsp syrup (10 mL).
4 cups (8 oz each) ginger tea prepackaged.
4 cups (8 oz each) ginger tea, steeping ½ tsp grated ginger for 5–10 min.
8 oz ginger ale, made with real ginger.
2 pieces crystallized ginger, each 1 inch square, ¼ inch thick.
Chewable tablets contain 67.5 mg.
Capsules come in various doses ranging from 100 mg to 1000 mg.

Source: Adapted with permission from Bryer E et al. 2005.[50]

Induction of Labor

A natural and safe form of inducing labor is often desired by both pregnant women and their caregivers. Acupuncture, castor oil, homeopathic compounds, and several herbs have all been used for this purpose. According to a national survey in which researchers mailed 500 questionnaires to nurse-midwives, about 50% used herbal preparations to stimulate labor.[53] Of the 50% who used herbal preparations, 93% reported using castor oil, 64% used blue cohosh, 45% used black cohosh, 63% used red raspberry leaf, and 60% used evening primrose oil.

Castor Oil

Castor oil is classified as a stimulant laxative. Its use in pregnant women is contraindicated because of the propensity to cause uterine contractions, and it is classified as pregnancy category X. A dose of 15–60 mL will produce laxative effects.[54] The mechanism of action for inducing labor remains unknown, but it is theorized that castor oil produces hyperemia in the gastrointestinal tract, which causes reflex stimulation of the uterus.[54] The active compound in castor oil is ricinoleic acid, constituting 90% of the fatty acid content.[54]

There has been one randomized trial that assessed the value of castor oil for induction of labor. In the trial, 102 women were randomized to either a single dose of castor oil or no treatment, and there were no differences between the two groups in any beneficial or adverse obstetric outcomes.[55]

Castor oil can cause nausea, vomiting, diarrhea, and gastrointestinal cramping. The ability of ricinoleic acid to cross the placenta seems plausible based on the small molecular weight, lipophilicity, and nonpolarity, although the effects of castor oil on the fetus are unknown. More studies should be conducted before castor oil use can be truly evidence based.

Blue Cohosh (*Caulophyllum Thalictroides*)

Blue cohosh (*Caulophyllum thalictroides*) is a woodland perennial native to North America. The medicinal compounds are derived from the root.[56] Other names for blue cohosh are papoose root and squaw root. It was used by Native American healers in a tea to relieve menstrual cramping and pains of labor. Interestingly, blue cohosh was listed in the US Pharmacopeia as a labor inducer until 1905.[56]

Homeopathic doses of blue cohosh have not been efficacious in stimulating labor, but some authors state this is because the dilutions used are such that there are few if any cohosh molecules left in the tincture.[56] The dose that is therapeutic is unknown.

Blue cohosh has several adverse pharmacologic effects in animal studies including toxicity to the myocardium in rats, teratogenic effects in rats, and uterotonic contraction and/or tetanus in excised uterine tissue of guinea pigs. In addition, there are several case reports of perinatal stroke,[57] myocardial infarction in a newborn, and hypoxic-ischemic encephalopathy following use of both blue and black cohosh to induce labor.[56] Given the potential for serious harm, blue cohosh should not be used by pregnant women.

Black Cohosh (*Cimicifuga Racemosa*)

Black cohosh (*Cimicifuga racemosa*) is a perennial member of the buttercup family that, like blue cohosh, is native to North America. This plant is also called bugbane, snakeroot, bugwort, and squawroot. Black cohosh is in a different family than blue cohosh, and the two should not be confused with each other. The roots and rhizomes contain a series of triterpene glycosides, mainly 27-deoxyactein and cimicifugoside, as well as isoflavone formononetin, a phytoestrogen that functions as weak partial agonists at the estrogen receptor. Black cohosh was extremely popular among eclectic physicians in the United States during the 1800s. It was a main ingredient in the famous Lydia Pinkham's Vegetable Compound used by many women for a variety of disorders, including menopause-associated hot flashes.

Although there are reports of black cohosh being used for induction of labor or correction of dysfunctional contractions, there are no studies of either efficacy or safety.[58]

▌ Menopause

Menopause is said to occur when a woman has cessation of ovulation and subsequent decrease in circulating estrogens. Menopause is signaled by permanent amenorrhea. The transitional phase prior to the onset of menopause is referred to as the climacteric or perimenopause. The menopausal symptoms most commonly reported are vasomotor symptoms such as hot flashes, headaches, and vaginal dryness. Because no pharmaceutical, including hormone therapy, is without some adverse effects, women frequently seek CAM remedies to ameliorate menopausal symptoms with natural therapies that may have less risk.

Some plant-derived agents bind to estrogen receptors, and these compounds, called **phytoestrogens**, interact with estrogen receptors to function as estrogen agonists, antagonists, or partial agonists. There are several types of phytoestrogens available in foods and marketed in dietary supplements. Isoflavones, which are found in soy and red clover, are a good example of the complexity of phytoestrogens. Isoflavones are a class of organic chemicals that are both phytoestrogens and antioxidants. They are found exclusively in legumes (the bean family) with soybeans having the highest concentration, followed by lentils, kidney beans, lima beans, broad beans, and chickpeas. Isoflavones have both estrogenic and antiestrogenic effects.[59] They have a stronger affinity for the estrogen-β receptor (found in kidney, brain, heart, and coronary arteries) than for the estrogen-α receptor (found in breast and uterine tissue).

Isoflavones from both soy and red clover have been promoted for treatment of several menopausal vasomotor symptoms, but the studies that have attempted to determine their efficacy have conflicting results. It is difficult to conduct meta-analyses or systematic reviews because these studies have used different populations with variability in endogenous estrogen at baseline, different phytoestrogen compounds that have varying bioavailability, and different study measures. That said, there is some evidence for the use of isoflavones as well as other botanical products for treating menopausal symptoms. Analysis of their safety is hampered by the same problems, yet some clinical recommendations can be made. Both safety and efficacy must be considered.

Soy (*Glycine Max*)

Soybeans are rich in isoflavones, primarily genistein and daidzein, and they have been studied extensively for their effect on multiple menopausal symptoms. High dietary intake of soy-based food products in Asia has been proposed as one explanation for the lower prevalence of menopausal symptoms in women from Japan, China, and Korea. Isoflavones appear to reduce menopausal vasomotor symptoms slightly and only in some women.[60] Approximately 30–50% of women metabolize daidzein into equol (these women are called *equol producers*), a metabolite that has estrogenic effects. This individual variability in bioavailability of isoflavones may partially explain why some women have a more positive response to isoflavones than do others. It also appears that isoflavones from food products are more efficacious than dietary supplements that have higher concentrations of isoflavones.[61] In addition, soy-based isoflavones have the most benefit for women who have mild symptoms and who are in the perimenopausal period or early menopause.[59] Therefore at this time, soy products are recommended only for women with mild to moderate symptoms and for short-term use.[62]

Soy isoflavones may be more beneficial in maintaining bone density via their effect in increasing synthesis of vitamin D. Although none of the randomized, controlled trials have demonstrated a benefit in preventing osteoporosis or bone fracture, increases in bone density have been documented.[63] Long-term effects are unknown.

Isoflavones have a beneficial effect inhibiting multiple physiologic pathways that result in atherosclerosis, and in 1999, the FDA approved the labeling of soy foods as protective for cardiovascular health. An average soy consumption of 47 mg/day (approximately half the daily recommended intake of protein) does reduce total cholesterol and LDL cholesterol by a modest amount.[64] Purified phytoestrogen pills are not as efficacious as food-based products. It is not clear if this is because the purification process destroys the effective compounds or if there are other active compounds in soy protein that are responsible for the beneficial effect. In 2006, the American Heart Association summarized additional studies and recommended that isoflavone supplements not be used for cardioprotection.[65]

In vitro, isoflavones can stimulate growth of estrogen-sensitive breast tumors, but they do not appear to stimulate endometrial tissue or breast tissue in human studies at the doses that have been evaluated in short-term therapies. This may be because isoflavones are more attracted to estrogen-β receptors than estrogen-α receptors. At this time, women with breast cancer or other estrogen-dependent malignancies should avoid isoflavone supplements.

Red Clover (*Trifolium Pratense*)

The flower of the red clover plant (*Trifolium pratense*) contains the isoflavones genistein and daidzein. In addition, red clover contains coumestrol, which has anticoagulant and estrogenic properties.[66] Red clover has been studied for its potential to decrease hot flashes in menopause, decrease cholesterol, and increase arterial compliance and bone mineral density. Several studies testing its benefits in relieving hot flashes have used the product Promensil TM, a red clover dietary supplement containing 40 mg of total isoflavones per dose.[67] These studies found improvements in symptoms, but they were not significantly more effective than placebo.

In summary, isoflavones have many beneficial effects physiologically, but it is not yet clear whether these effects

are secondary to the estrogenic activity of isoflavones or other compounds in food-based soy products. The maximum benefit may accrue through lifelong exposure to a diet that has a high intake of soy rather than isoflavone supplements.

Ginseng (*Panax Ginseng*)

Ginseng, a subcategory of the genus *Panax*, includes several species of a slow-growing perennial that has a long tradition in traditional Chinese medicine (TCM). The most commonly used species are Asian ginseng (*panax ginseng*) and American ginseng, both of which belong to the same genus. Siberian ginseng is sometimes promoted as an alternative but should not be used because it does not have ginsenosides, which are the active ingredients.

Ginseng is recommended as an adaptogen or tonic herb used to strengthen normal function and help the body deal with stress. Ginseng likely produces its beneficial effects via stimulation of the hypothalamus-pituitary-adrenal axis.[68] It has been promoted for improving mood and cognition in menopause as well as improvement in general menopausal symptoms. Wiklund et al. conducted a randomized, double-blind, placebo-controlled trial that included 384 postmenopausal women.[69] Ginseng was administered as 200 mg taken orally for 16 weeks. The women who took ginseng reported a slight improvement in menopausal symptoms overall that did not reach statistical significance, but they had a significant improvement in depression compared to the women in the control group. This study also recorded several physiologic parameters such as follicular-stimulating hormone (FSH) levels and endometrial thickness. There were no changes in any of these physical characteristics. The authors postulate that any beneficial effects of ginseng are not secondary to hormone replacement effects. Ginseng may have benefits for treating mood and cognition but needs further study.

Ginseng is in general a safe herb to use in usual doses. The most common side effects are headache, sleepiness, and gastrointestinal distress. Ginseng can induce hypoglycemia, so it should be used with caution by persons with diabetes. Herb–drug interactions are listed in Table 10-3.

Wild Yam (*Dioscorea Villosa*)

Because of the widespread belief that wild yam (*Dioscorea villosa*) roots contain dehydroepiandrosterone-like precursors of steroid hormones, it has been used in a variety of treatments for dysmenorrhea and menopausal symptoms. Wild yam roots (particularly the Mexican wild yam) contain the saponin diosgenin, which was historically used to synthesize a variety of steroid hormones, including estrogen and progesterone. However, the conversion of diosgenin to steroid hormone cannot occur in the body. To add further confusion, some manufacturers have adulterated wild yam preparations with synthetic steroid hormone, mainly progesterone, which can explain their observed effectiveness.[70]

Black Cohosh (*Cimicifuga Racemosa*)

The mechanism underlying the potential clinical effects of black cohosh (*Cimicifuga racemosa*) root probably involves the action of the various phytoestrogens. Therefore, it is likely that different preparations have different compounds, which may account for the conflicting results in the studies conducted to date. Much of the early scientific work on black cohosh was done in Germany on a highly characterized alcoholic extract called Remifemin TM, standardized to contain 2.5% 27-deoxyactein. These studies found that black cohosh was more effective than the conventional treatment for relieving the depression and anxiety associated with menopause.[71] Multiple additional clinical trials have been conducted since 1987. One of the recent well-designed studies was the Herbal Alternatives for Menopause trial,[72] a 1-year, randomized, double-blinded placebo-controlled trial of 351 menopausal or postmenopausal women who reported at least two occurrences of hot flashes per day. Participants were randomized to one of five therapies involving different combinations of black cohosh, blends of other herbs, conventional hormone therapy, or placebo to be taken for 1 year. None of the herbal treatments resulted in clinical improvement when measured at 3, 6, or 12 months. Thus, the results of the best study to date do not support the effectiveness of black cohosh for treating hot flashes. In contrast, another large randomized, multicenter, trial that included 304 menopausal women found black cohosh effective for treating menopausal symptoms.[71] Subjects were randomized to receive either Remifemin (2.5 mg isopropanolic root extract) or placebo two times a day. The reason these two studies had conflicting findings is unclear, but one possible explanation is that different black cohosh formulations were used. The Daiber study used Remifemin, an isopropanolic extract produced in Germany, whereas the Herbal Alternatives for Menopause study used a 70% ethanolic root extract.

Flaxseed (*Linum Usitatissimum*)

The seeds of flax (*Linum usitatissimum*) are rich in secoisolariciresinol diglycoside, which can be converted by colonic bacteria to the active phytoestrogen lignans enterodiol and enterolactone. Flaxseed contains 25% protein, 3–6% soluble fiber, and 30–45% unsaturated fatty acids. Flaxseed oil is a good source of the omega-3 fatty acid alpha-linolenic acid. Like the isoflavone phytoestrogens, the lignans interact with the estrogen receptor as partial agonists. Flaxseed has been shown to lower total and LDL cholesterol levels. Part of this effect may be due to the lignans, which inhibit the activity of cholesterol-7 alpha-hydroxylase.[73]

One study looking at the effects of flaxseed on menopausal symptoms and cholesterol levels in menopausal women has been done. A flaxseed-supplemented diet was compared to a conventional estrogen-progesterone replacement therapy for 2 months.[74] Both treatment groups had significant reductions in LDL cholesterol levels as well as menopausal symptoms.

Sage (*Salvia Officinalis*)

Sage (*Salvia officinalis*) has been used as a culinary and medicinal herb for hundreds of years in Europe. Medicinally, it is most often used to treat mouth and throat inflammation, excessive sweating, and dyspepsia.[74] A single small study in 1998 investigated its possible benefits in decreasing menopausal symptoms.[75] A group of 30 women received one tablet that contained extracts of 120 mg sage leaves and 60 mg of alfalfa daily for 3 months, and 12 women served as control subjects. Hot flashes and night sweats completely disappeared in 20 of the 30 women who took the sage/alfalfa supplements. Although this study is encouraging, it needs to be repeated with a larger number of subjects in a better designed trial with validated outcome measures of menopausal symptoms.

It should be noted that large amounts and prolonged exposure of sage leaf and sage essential oil could result in restlessness, vomiting, tachycardia, and seizures.[76] This toxicity is due to the presence of camphor and thujone. Levels of 12 drops of the essential oil of sage, or 15 grams of sage leaves, can engender toxic effects.[77,78]

Evening Primrose (*Oenothera Biennis*)

The seeds of the popular medicinal plant evening primrose (*Oenothera biennis*) are a rich source (~ 9% of the seed oil) of the essential omega-6 fatty acid GLA. Most of the pharmacologic effects are due to the high content of GLA. Evening primrose also contains linoleic acid that is found in many other vegetable oils. Although there is evidence that suggests evening primrose may be beneficial for a variety of diseases and conditions, only two clinical trials that have investigated the potential benefits for treatment of menopausal symptoms were found, and neither was able to show that evening primrose is therapeutically beneficial.[79]

Kava (*Piper Methysticum*)

Kava (*Piper methysticum*) has a long tradition of both social and medicinal use as a tea and ground extract of root among South Pacific Islanders. Several trials have been performed investigating the effects of kava on anxiety, and there is good evidence that kava is efficacious for reducing anxiety.[80-82] The mechanism of action appears to be secondary to kavalactones present in the kava roots, which bind to GABA receptors, antagonize dopamine, inhibit norepinephrine uptake, inhibit monoamine oxidase B, and decrease glutamine release.[83] Kava dietary supplements are available as tablets, capsules, or powder that is mixed into a drink. Doses range from 50–240 mg of kavalactones, but the exact dose that is therapeutic is actually unknown.

Common side effects include headache and gastrointestinal distress. Chronic administration of large amounts can cause an unusual rash, which is reversible.[84]

Kava is a potent inhibitor of CYP2E1, CYP1A2, and CYP2D6, so theoretically, it can interact with many drugs metabolized by these enzymes.[9] There have been many case reports of liver damage following kava use; the FDA has issued a warning about possible liver failure associated with kava use, and this herb should be used with caution.[85]

Conclusion

There is good evidence that St. John's wort can improve depression, kava can improve symptoms of anxiety, and black cohosh can improve menopausal vasomotor symptoms when used for short periods of time. It also appears that soy from food products may have beneficial effects in treating menopausal symptoms.

Most of the botanical compounds discussed in this chapter have been used for centuries, yet little is known about their safety or efficacy. This is particularly important today as more women choose dietary supplements and the number of products available in the marketplace rapidly increases. Because botanical medicines are classified as dietary supplements, they are largely unregulated. Large variations in the composition of ingredients make it difficult to determine therapeutic doses even when there is evidence for efficacy. Healthcare providers need to know more about the safety, efficacy, and adverse effects of these compounds. Drug–herb interactions are especially important as they can potentially cause adverse effects.

Although this chapter focused on the botanical medicines used for specific reproductive health issues, CAM therapies are used for a wide diversity of health problems. The practice of integrative medicine whereby alternative practices are used in combination with conventional medical therapies is becoming increasingly popular.

References

1. Eisenberg DM, Davis RB, Ettner SL, Appel S, Wilkey S, Van Rompay M, et al. Trends in alternative medicine use in the United States, 1990–1997. *JAMA* 1998;280:1569–75.
2. White House Commission on Complementary and Alternative Medicine Policy. Final report. 2002, March. Available from: *www.whccamp.hhs.gov/pdfs/fr2002_document.pdf* [Accessed February 5, 2009].
3. Kinsel JF, Straus SE. Complementary and alternative therapeutics: rigorous research is needed to support claims. Annu Rev Pharmacol Toxicol 2003; 43:463–84.
4. Blumenthal M, Goldberg A, Brinkmann J. Herbal medicine: expanded Commission E monographs. Austin, TX: American Botanical Council, 2000.
5. De Smit P. Herbal remedies. N Engl J Med 2002; 347:2046–56.
6. Draves AH, Walker SE. Analysis of the hypericin and pseudohypericin content of commercially available St. John's wort preparations. Can J Clin Pharmacol 2003;10:114–8.
7. Tesch BJ. Herbs commonly used by women. An evidence-based review. Am J Obstet Gynecol 2003; 188:S44–52.
8. Izzo AA, Ernst E. Interactions between herbal medicines and prescribed drugs. Drugs 2001;61:2163–75.
9. Hu Z, Ho PC, Chan SY, Heng PW, Chan E, Duan W, et al. Herb–drug interactions: a literature review. Drugs 2005;65:1239–82.
10. Barnes P, Powell-Griner E, McFann K, Nahin R. CDC advance data report No. 343. Complementary and alternative medicine use among adults: United States, 2002. 2004, May 27. Available from: *http://nccam.nih.gov/news/report.pdf* [Accessed February 5, 2009].
11. Upchurch DM, Chyu L, Greendale GA, Utts J, Bair YA, Zhang G, et al. Complementary and alternative medicine use among American women: findings from the national health interview survey 2002. J Womens Health 2007;16:102–13.

12. Butterweck V. Mechanism of action of St. John's wort in depression: what is known? CNS Drugs 2003;17:539–62.

13. Linde K, Berner MM, Kriston L. St. John's wort for major depression. Cochrane Database of Systematic Reviews 2008, Issue 4. Art No: CD000448. DOI: 10.1002/14651858.CD000448.pub3.

14. Zhou S, Chan E, Pan SQ, Haung M, Lee EJ. Pharmocokinetic interactions of drugs with St. John's wort. J Psychopharmacol 2004;18:262–76.

15. Foxman B. Epidemiology of urinary tract infections: incidence, morbidity, and economic costs. Dis Mon 2003 Feb;49(2):53–70.

16. Ofek L, Goldhar J, Zafriri D, Lis H, Adar R, Sharon N. Anti-*Escherichia* activity of blueberry and cranberry juice. New Engl J Med 1991;332:1599.

17. Avorn J, Monane M, Gurwitz JH, Glynn RS, Choodnovsky I, Lipsitz LA. Reduction of bacteriuria and pyuria after ingestion of cranberry juice. JAMA 1994;271(10):751–4.

18. Jepson RG, Mihalievic L, Craig J. Cranberries for preventing urinary tract infections. Cochrane Database Syst Rev, 2004(2):CD001321.

19. FAO/WHO. Health and nutritional properties of probiotics in food including powder milk with live lactic acid bacteria. Report of a joint FAO/WHO expert consultation on evaluation of health and nutritional properties of probiotics in food including powder milk with live lactic acid bacteria. Córdoba, Argentina: World Health Organization, 2001.

20. Barrons R, Tassone D. Use of lactobacillus probiotics for bacterial genitourinary infections in women: a review. Clin Therapeutics 2008;30(3):453–68.

21. Hatakka K, Saxelin M. Probiotics in intestinal and non-intestinal infectious diseases: clinical evidence. Cur Pharmaceutical Design 2008;14:1351–67.

22. Reid G, Bruce AW, Aylor M. Instillation of lactobacillus and stimulation of indigenous organisms to prevent recurrence of urinary tract infections. Microecol Ther 1995;23:32–45.

23. Proctor ML, Smith CA, Farquhar CM, Stones RW. Transcutaneous electrical nerve stimulation and acupuncture for primary dysmenorrhea. Cochrane Database of Systematic Reviews 2002, Issue 1. Art No: CD002123. DOI: 10.1002/14651858.

24. Sales KJ, Jabbour N. Cyclooxygenase and prostaglandins in pathology of the endometrium. Reproduction 2003;126:559–67.

25. Tseng Y, Chen C, Yang Y. Rose tea for relief of primary dysmenorrhea in adolescents: a randomized controlled trila in Taiwan. J Midwifery Women's Health [Electronic version] 2005;50(5):51–7. 10.1016/j.jmwh.2005.06.003.

26. Doubova S, Morales H, Hernandez S, Martinez-Garcia M, Ortiz M, Soto M, et al. Effect of a Psidii guajavae folium extract in the treatment of primary dysmenorrhea: a randomized clinical trial. J Ethnopharmacol 2007;110;305–10.10.1016/j.jep.2006.09.033.

27. Dennehy CE. Use of herbs and dietary supplements in gynecology: an evidence-based review. J Midwifery Womens Health 2006:51:402–9.

28. Fugh-Berman A, Kronenberg F. Complementary and alternative medicine (CAM) in reproductive-age women: a review of randomized controlled trials. Reproductive Toxicol 2003;17:137–52.

29. Wuttke W, Jarry H, Christoffel V, Psengler B, Seidlova-Wuttke D. Chaste tree (Vitex agnus-castus) pharmacology and clinical implications. Phytomedicine 2003;10:348–57.

30. Loch EG, Selle H, Boblitz N. Treatment of premenstrual syndrome with a phytopharmaceutical formulation containing Vitex agnus-castus. J Women's Health Gender Based Med 2000;9:315–20.

31. Schellenberg R. Treatment for the premenstrual syndrome with agnus castus fruit extract: prospective, randomised, placebo controlled study. BMJ 2001:322(7279);134–7.

32. Daniele C, Kuhn JT, Pittler MH, Ernst E. Vitex agnus castus: a systematic review of adverse events. Drug Safety 2005;28:319–32.

33. Atmaca M, Kumru S, Tezcan E. Fluoxetine versus Vitex agnus castus extract in the treatment of premenstrual dysphoric disorder. Hum Psychopharmacol 2003;18(3):191–5.

34. Stevinson C, Ernst E. A pilot study of *Hypericum perforatum* for the treatment of premenstrual syndrome. BJOG 2000;107:870–6.

35. Tamborini A, Taurelle R. Value of standardized Ginkgo biloba extract (EGb761) in the management of congestive symptoms of premenstrual syndrome. Rev Fr Gynecol Obstet 1993;88(7–9):447–57.

36. Horrobin DF. Nutritional and medical importance of gamma-linolenic acid. Prog Lipid Res 1992;31(2):163–94.

37. Hardy ML. Herbs of special interest to women. J Am Pharm 2000;40:234–42.

38. Budeiri D, Li Wan P, Durnan JC. Is evening primrose of value in the treatment of premenstrual syndrome? Control Clin Trials 1996;17:60–8.

39. Carmichael AR. Can Vitex agnus castus be used for the treatment of mastalgia? What is the current

evidence? Evid Based Complement Alternat Med 2008;5(3):247–50.

40. Jarry H, Leonhardt S, Gorkow C, et al. In vitro prolactin but not LH and FSH release is inhibited by compounds in extracts of Agnus castus: direct evidence for a dopaminergic principle by the dopamine receptor assay. Exp Clin Endocrinol 1994;102(6):448–54.

41. Liu J, Burdette JE, Xu H, Gu C, Van Breemen RB, Bhat KP, et al. Evaluation of estrogenic activity of plant extracts for the potential treatment of menopausal symptoms. J Agri Food Chem 2001;49(5):2472–9.

42. Halaska M, Beles P, Gorkov C, Sieder C. Treatment of cyclical mastalgia with a solution containing a Vitex agnus castus extract: results of a placebo-controlled double-blind study. Breast 1999;8:175–81.

43. Basch E, Bent S, Collins J, Dacey C, Hammerness P, Harrison M, Smith M, et al. Flax and flaxseed oil: a review by the Natural Standard Research Collaboration. Soc Integr Oncol 2007;5:92–105.

44. King TL, Murphy PA. Nausea and vomiting in pregnancy. J Midwifery Women's Health 2009;54:(in press).

45. Lien HC, Sun WM, Chen YH, Kim H, Hasler W, Owyang C. Effects of ginger on motion sickness and gastric slow-wave dysrhythmias induced by circular vection. Am J Physiol Gastrointest Liver Physiol 2003;284(3):G481–9.

46. Burrelli F, Capasso R, Aviello G, Dittler, MH, Izzo AA. Effectiveness and safety of ginger in the treatment of pregnancy-induced nausea and vomiting. Obstet Gynecol 2005;105(4):849–56.

47. Smith C, Crowther C, Willson K, Hotham N, McMillian V. A randomized controlled trial of ginger to treat nausea and vomiting in pregnancy. Obstet Gynecol 2004;103(4):639–45.

48. Sripramute M, Lekhyananda N. A randomized comparison of ginger and vitamin B_6 in the treatment of nausea and vomiting of pregnancy. J Med Assoc Thai 2003;86(9):846–53.

49. Schwertner HA, Rios DC, Pascoe JE. Variation in concentration and labeling of ginger root dietary supplements. Obstet Gynecol 2006;107(6):1337–43.

50. Bryer E. A literature review of the effectiveness of ginger in alleviating mild-to-moderate nausea and vomiting of pregnancy. J Midwifery Womens Health, 2005;50(1):e1–3.

51. Backon J. Ginger in preventing nausea and vomiting of pregnancy: a caveat due to its thromboxane synthetase activity and effect on testosterone binding. Eur J Obstet Gynecol Reprod Biol 1991;42(2):163–4.

52. Westfall RE. Use of anti-emetic herbs in pregnancy: women's choices and the question of safety and efficacy. Complement Ther Nurs Midwifery 2004;10(1):30–6.

53. McFarlin BL, Gibson MH, O'Rear J, Harman P. A national survey of herbal preparation use by nurse-midwives for labor stimulation. Review of the literature and recommendations for practice. J Nurse-Midwifery 1999 May-Jun;44(3):205–16.

54. Burdock GA, Carabin IG, Griffiths JC. Toxicology and pharmacology of sodium ricinoeate. Food Chem Toxicol 2006;44:1689–98.

55. Kelly AJ, Kavanagh J, Thomas J. Castor oil, bath and/or enema for cervical priming and induction of labour (abstract). Cochrane Database of Systematic Reviews 2001, Issue 2. Art No: CD003099. DOI: 10.1002/14651858.CD003099.

56. Dugoua JJ, Perri D, Seely D, Mills E, Koren G. Safety and efficacy of blue cohosh (*Caulophyllum thalictroides*) during pregnancy and lactation. Can J Clin Pharmacol 2008;15:e66–73.

57. Finkle RF, Zarlengo KM. Blue cohosh and perinatal stroke. New Engl J Med 2004;351:302.

58. Dugoua JJ, Seely D, Perri D, Koren G, Mills E. Safety and efficacy of black cohosh (*Cimicifuga racemosa*) during pregnancy and lactation. Can J Clin Pharmacol 2008;15:e257–61.

59. Tempfer CB, Bentz EK, Leodolter S, Tsherne G, Reuss F, Cross HS, et al. Phytoestrogens in clinical practice: a review of the literature. Fertil Sterility 2007;87:1243–9.

60. Lethaby AE, Brown J, Marjoribanks J, Kronenberg F, Roberts H, Eden J. Phytoestrogens for vasomotor menopausal symptoms. Cochrane Database of Systematic Reviews 2007, Issue 4. Art No: CD001395. DOI: 10.1002/14651858.CD001395.pub3.

61. Kronenberg F, Fugh-Berman A. Complementary and alternative medicine for menopausal symptoms: a review of randomized controlled trials. Ann Intern Med 2002;137:805–13.

62. Treatment of menopause-associated vasomotor symptoms: position statement of the North American Menopause Society. Menopause 2004;11:11–33.

63. Atmaca A, Kleerkoper M, Bayraktar M, Kucuk O. Soy isoflavones in the management of postmenopausal osteoporosis. Menopause 2008;15:748–57.

64. Anderson JW, Johnstone BM, Cook-Newell ME. Meta-analysis of the effects of soy protein intake on serum lipids. N Engl J Med 1995;333(5):276–82.

65. Sacks FM, Lichtenstein A, Van Horn L, Harris W, Kris-Etherton P, Winston M, for the American Heart Association Nutrition Committee. Soy protein, isoflavones, and cardiovascular health: an American Heart Association science advisory for professionals from the nutrition committee. Circulation 2006 Feb 21;113(7):1034–44. Epub 2006 Jan 17.

66. Low Dog T, Riley D, Carter T. An integrative approach to menopause. Alternative Ther 2001;7(4):45–55.

67. Umland EM, Weinstein LC, Buchanan EM. Menstruation-related disorders. In DiPiro JT, Talbert RL, Yee GC, Matzke GR, Wells BG, Posey LM, eds. Pharmacotherapy: a pathophysiologic approach. 7th ed. New York: McGraw-Hill Publishing Company, 2008:1547–65.

68. Kiefer D, Pantuso T. Panax ginseng. Am Fam Physician 2003;68:1539–42.

69. Wiklund IK, Mattsson LA, Lindgren R, Limoni C. Effects of a standardized ginseng extract on quality of life and physiological parameters in symptomatic postmenopausal women: a double-blind, placebo-controlled trial. Swedish Alternative Medicine Group. Int J Clin Pharmacol Res 1999;19:89–99.

70. Taylor M. Botanicals: Medicines and menopause. Clin Obstet Gynecol 2001;44:853–63.

71. Osmers R, Friede M, Liske E, Schnitker J, Freudenstein J, Heinrich H, et al. Efficacy and safety of isopropanolic black cohosh extract for climacteric symptoms. Obstet Gynecol 2005;105:1074–83.

72. Newton KM, Reed SD, LaCroix AZ, Grothaus LC, Ehrlich K, Guiltinan J. Treatment of vasomotor symptoms of menopause with black cohosh, multibotanicals, soy, hormone therapy, or placebo: a randomized trial. Ann Intern Med 2006 Dec 19;145(12):869–79. [Summary for patients in Ann Intern Med 2006 Dec 19;145(12):I25].

73. Tham DM, Gardner CD, Haskell WC. Potential health benefits of dietary phytoestrogens: a review of the clinical, epidemiological, and mechanistic evidence. J Clin Endocrinol Metab 1998;83:2223–35.

74. Lemay A, Dodin S, Kadri N, Jaques H, Forest JC. Flaxseed dietary supplement versus hormone replacement therapy in hypercholesterolemic menopausal women. Obstet Gynecol 2002;100(3):495–504.

75. Bisset NG, Wichtl M, eds. Herbal drugs and phytopharmaceuticals: a handbook for practice on a scientific basis, 2nd ed. Stuttgart, Germany: Medpharm Scientific Publishers, 2001.

76. De Leo V, Lanzetta D, Lazzavacca R, Morgante G. Tratment of neurovegetative menopausal symptoms with a phytotherapeutic agent. Minerva Ginecol 1998;50(5):207–11.

77. Burkhard PR, Burkhardt K, Haenggeli CA, Landis T. Plant-induced seizures: reappearance of an old problem. J Neurol 199;246(8):667–70.

78. Millet Y, Jouglard J, Steinmetz MD, Tognetti P, Joanny P, Arditti J. Toxicity of some essential plant oils: clinical and experimental study. Clin Toxicol 1981;18(12):1485–98.

79. Cancelo Hidalgo MJ, Castelo-Branco C, Blumel JE, Lanchares Perez JL, Alvarez De Los Heros JI. Effect of compound containing isoflavones, primrose oil and vitamin E in two different doses on climacteric symptoms. J Obstet Gynecol 2006;26(4):344–7.

80. Geller S, Studee L. Botanical and dietary supplements for mood and anxiety in menopausal women. Menopause 2007;14(3):541–9.

81. Cagnacci A, Arangino S, Renzi A, Zamni AL, Malmusi S, Volpe A. Kava-kava administration reduces anxiety in perimenopausal women. Maturitas 2003;44:103–9.

82. DeLeo V, La Marca A, Morgante G, Lanzeth D, Florio P, Petraglia F. Evaluation of combining kava extract with hormone replacement therapy in the treatment of postmenopausal anxiety. Maturitas 2001;39:185–8.

83. Assemi M. Herbs affecting the central nervous system: gingko, kava, St. John's wort and valerian. Clin Obstet Gynecol 2001;44:824–35.

84. Couatre DL. Kava kava: examining reports of toxicity. Toxicol Lett 2004 April 15;150:85.

85. Ulbricht C, Basch E, Boon H, Ernst E, Hammerness P, Sollars D, et al. Safety review of kava (*Piper methysticum*) by the Natural Standard Research Collaboration. Expert Opin Drug Safety 2005;4:779–94.

Appendix A Information Resources on Dietary Supplements

Aside from the databases provided by the ODS and NCCAM, there are several outstanding Web-based resource databases available. The Natural Standard (*www.naturalstandard.com*) database on CAM and integrative medicine was founded by research scientists and clinicians from over 100 academic institutions throughout the world to provide quality, evidence-based information necessary for safer therapeutic decision making. The CAM information is presented in well-referenced, peer-reviewed comprehensive monographs. Each monograph on a particular dietary supplement or CAM therapy provides rating scales to help evaluate the research evidence.

The Natural Medicine Comprehensive Database (*www.naturaldatabase.com*) is published by *Pharmacist's Letter*. It was first released in 1999 and is continually updated online. It is recognized by many as the gold standard in evidence-based information on natural products. More than 1000 natural products, including botanical products, are covered. This database provides current information on safety, efficacy, mechanism of action, adverse reactions, and interactions with herbs. A useful feature includes the Natural Product/Drug Interaction Checker, which provides information on potential interactions between natural products and drugs. The Disease/Medical Conditions Search covers information on which natural products may be effective for a given disease state or medical condition.

The American Botanical Council (ABC), founded in 1988 in Austin, Texas, is one of the nation's leading providers of science-based information on herbal medicine (*www.herbalgram.org*). *Herbalgram* is the official publication of this agency. ABC also offers the English translation of the Expanded German Commission E Monographs. The Commission E monographs produced by the German government in the 1970s evaluate the safety and efficacy of more than 300 herbal medicines.

Finally, the Phytochemical and Ethnobotanical databases were compiled by James Duke, PhD, with the Agricultural Research Service. These databases list chemical constituents and ethnobotanical uses of medicinal plants (*www.ars-grin.gov/duke/*).

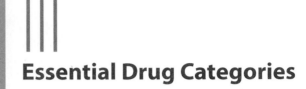

III

Essential Drug Categories

During initial organization of this book, it became apparent that many drugs were specific for the treatment of a selected condition, whereas some drug categories include medications that are used for multiple different conditions. Knowledge of the pharmacokinetics and pharmacodynamics of drugs used in many different settings enhances safe and rational prescribing. For example, understanding that a specific category of antibiotics acts by incapacitating bacterial cell wall synthesis enables the clinician not to choose that category when the bacteria in question is *Chlamydia trachomatis*, an obligate intracellular parasite without cell walls. Knowledge that selected antihistamines cause profound sedation can promote use of one for mild insomnia and avoidance of the same agent for common allergies. Since these drugs are used for many different indications, it became apparent that the same material could be repeated in a number of chapters. Therefore, the following four chapters are clustered into this section: "Anti-Infectives," "Analgesia and Anesthesia," "Antihistamines," and "Steroid Hormones."

The anti-infectives chapter includes the common antibiotics and reviews the challenges of drug resistance, especially due to overuse. Antivirals and antifungals also are included in this chapter. "Analgesia and Anesthesia" examines drugs that are often used in the primary care arena. The analgesics can be over the counter or by prescription only. Anesthesia may be used in an ambulatory setting as part of treatment for a repair of a small laceration or other procedures.

Antihistamines are an interesting drug family. Antihistamines may be employed as a treatment for such conditions as gastrointestinal diseases, allergies, or sleeping difficulties. For each of these conditions, the basic pharmacologic principles remain the same.

Steroidal hormones, specifically estrogens, progestins, and androgens, are a staple in a list of drugs used by women for multiple conditions. These drugs may be used as contraceptives, fertility drugs, menopause treatments, or as remedies for menstrual irregularities.

Although four major drug categories are addressed in this section, specific pharmacologic agents are identified by name and dose within the chapters. The chapters in following sections expand upon the information found in this section.

"I had a series of childhood illnesses; scarlet fever, pneumonia, polio. I walked with braces until I was at least nine years old. My life wasn't like the average person who grew up and decided to enter the world of sports."

WILMA RUDOLPH (1940–1994), THE FIRST AMERICAN RUNNER TO WIN 3 GOLD MEDALS AT A SINGLE OLYMPICS

11

Anti-Infectives

Tekoa L. King, Anne Marie Mitchell, Barbara J. Lannen, and Marie Daly, with acknowledgment to Lori A. Spies

Chapter Glossary

Aerobe An organism that lives and reproduces in the presence of oxygen.

Anaerobe An organism that lives and reproduces in the absence of oxygen.

Antibiotic (antibacterial) A natural or synthetic substance that destroys bacteria or inhibits their growth.

Antifungal An agent that destroys or inhibits the growth of fungi.

Anti-infective Any agent used to combat infection.

Antimicrobial Any agent that destroys or prevents the development of microorganisms.

Antiparasitic An agent that destroys parasites.

Antistaphylococcal penicillins (penicillinase-resistant penicillins) Penicillins that have a bulky side chain, which prevents the bacterial beta-lactamase enzyme from binding to the drug and making it inactive. These penicillins are useful for treating staphylococcal species and streptococci microorganisms.

Antipseudomonal penicillins Another term for the extended-spectrum penicillins, because they are primarily used to treat infections from *Pseudomonas aeruginosa.*

Antiviral A drug used to treat viral infections.

Bacteriocidal An agent that is capable of killing bacteria.

Bacteriostatic An agent that is capable of inhibiting the growth of bacteria.

Beta-lactamase An enzyme that destroys the beta-lactam ring of penicillin-like antibiotics and makes them ineffective.

Broad-spectrum Penicillin that is effective against a variety of gram-positive and gram-negative organisms.

Elimination The metabolism of the drug and how it is excreted outside the body.

Extended-spectrum A type of penicillin that has increased activity against gram-positive and gram-negative organisms.

Facultative anaerobic Bacteria that can thrive in an environment that has oxygen or in one that does not have oxygen.

Gram-negative Bacteria that lose the color of the crystal violet stain and take the color of the red counterstain in Gram's method of staining.

Gram-positive Bacteria that retain the color of the crystal violet stain in Gram's method of staining.

Half-life The time required for the serum concentration of the drug to decrease by 50%; determines the frequency of dosing.

Metabolism The process of the drug's chemical change to a compound called a metabolite.

Methicillin-resistant *staphylococcus aureus* (MRSA) *S aureus* bacteria that produce altered PBPs to which the antistaphylococcus penicillins such as methicillin are unable to bind.

Mycosis Infection caused by fungi.

Penicillin binding proteins (PBPs) Bacterial enzymes such as transpeptidases to which the penicillins and cephalosporins bind in order to act on bacterial microorganisms.

Penicillinase A bacterial enzyme that inactivates most penicillins.

Pseudomembranous colitis Colitis associated with antibiotic therapy most often caused by *Clostridium difficile*, a normal part of the intestinal flora, because of disruption

249

of the balance by broad-spectrum antibiotics. Symptoms include foul-smelling diarrhea with blood and mucus, cramps, fever, and leukocytosis. Treatment includes discontinuation of antibiotic responsible and metronidazole therapy.

Red man syndrome A reaction appearing within 4–10 minutes after the commencement or soon after the completion of an infusion, characterized by flushing and/or an erythematous rash on the face, neck, and upper torso due to nonspecific mast cell degranulation rather than an IgE-mediated allergic reaction. Hypotension and angioedema may also occur. Treated with antihistamines.

Selective toxicity The ability of an anti-infective to successfully target the cells of a microorganism without also destroying the human host cells.

Stevens-Johnson syndrome Systemic skin disease producing fever, lesions of oral, conjunctival, and vaginal mucous membrane, and cutaneous rash—often widespread and severe.

Torsades de pointes From French "twisting of the points," a rapid, polymorphic ventricular tachycardia with a characteristic twist of the QRS complex, associated with long QT intervals and hypotension; without intervention, can lead to ventricular fibrillation.

Urticaria Multiple, swollen, raised intensely itchy areas on the skin caused by vasodilation and increased permeability of capillaries of the skin as a result of mast cell release of vasoactive mediators in an immunoglobulin E-mediated reaction to allergens.

Anti-Infectives

Anti-infectives are among the most frequently prescribed pharmaceutical agents in the United States. Yet many prescriptions for anti-infectives are given for conditions that do not require anti-infective medication.[1] This chapter reviews anti-infective drugs and presents guidelines for rational prescribing.[1,2]

In simple terms, an infection is colonization of a host by a pathologic agent. An **anti-infective** is any agent that kills or inhibits the growth of microorganisms that cause infections. Arsenic and strychnine were anti-infectives used a century ago and found to be effective against the pathologic organisms, but they also tended to kill the host. The introduction of effective anti-infectives during the 20th century revolutionized health care.

The term **antimicrobial** describes all medications that are used for the treatment of infections caused by a variety of living organisms. The pathogen responsible for the infection could be a bacterium, fungus, virus, or protozoan. Antimicrobial drugs commonly are subcategorized as **antibacterials**, **antifungals**, **antivirals**, and **antiparasitics**.

Principles of Rational Antimicrobial Therapy

A systematic and rational approach to prescribing antimicrobial medications is essential, particularly in light of rapidly expanding bacterial resistance.[1] Rational prescribing requires that we maximize effectiveness, minimize risks, respect patient concerns, consider cost, and evaluate for bacterial resistance.[3] Elements central to this approach include: (1) confirmation of the presence of an infection through history and physical exam; (2) identification of the pathogen when possible; (3) confirmation of need for antimicrobial as opposed to palliative therapies and infection control measures; (4) understanding of host factors that may impact pharmacodynamics as well as the individual's concerns and resources; (5) selection of an appropriate antimicrobial agent using the dual principles of narrowest spectrum and shortest effective duration possible; (6) knowledge of the pharmacokinetics and pharmacodynamics of selected medications; (7) education of individuals and families regarding appropriate use of antimicrobials; and (8) appropriate monitoring of the therapeutic response.[1,2,4,5]

Web-based or electronic decision algorithms for antibiotic treatment of specific conditions are increasingly popular and may be found at several Web sites.[2,6,7] Decision trees such these, although not universally accepted, can be expected to decrease inappropriate antibiotic prescribing practices.[8]

Classification of Bacteria and Other Pathogens

The universe of microorganisms is quite diverse. The microbes that can be human pathogens include bacteria, fungi, protozoa, complex organism parasites, and the non-living obligate intracellular viruses. The primary mechanism of action of all antimicrobial agents is their ability to identify and target the biologic structure or function of a specific microbe that is different from normal cells in the human body, a function called **selective toxicity**.

Bacteria

Bacteria are classified and named by their shape, reaction to staining, and oxygen requirements. Bacteria are described as spherical (cocci), rod shaped (bacilli), or spiral (spirochetes). Cocci are further subdivided into (1) diplococci, e.g., those found in pairs such as *Neisseria gonorrhoeae*; (2) streptococci, which are cocci found in a chain formation; and (3) staphylococci, which are cocci that exist in clusters.

All bacteria are classified as either gram-positive or gram-negative based on the structure of the cell wall. **Gram-positive** bacteria have a phospholipid bilayer cell membrane and a cell wall that is made of peptidoglycan. Peptidoglycan is made of long sugar polymers that have peptide side chains that form strong cross-links that make the cell wall strong. In contrast, **gram-negative** bacteria have a more complex cell wall structure. The cytoplasmic membrane of gram-negative bacteria is surrounded externally by a thin peptidoglycan wall, and then the outermost layer is another phospholipid bilayer membrane (Figure 11-1). Gram-positive bacteria are so named because this outermost thick cell wall retains dye, and therefore these bacteria appear blue or violet when stained with crystal violet dye. Gram-negative bacteria do not retain the crystal violet dye and appear red or pink when stained with a counterstain.

Finally, bacteria that use oxygen are called **aerobes** (e.g., *Mycobacterium tuberculosis*), and bacteria that do not require oxygen are called **anaerobes** (e.g., *Bacteroides*). **Facultative anaerobic** bacteria can function with or without oxygen (e.g., group B streptococci).

Chlamydia is a unique category of bacteria because this organism lives in other cells. The members of this genus of bacteria are obligate intracellular pathogens that cannot replicate outside of the host cell.

Bacteria have the following three characteristics that are both essential for their survival and different from humans: (1) the unique structure of their cell wall, (2) production of bacterial proteins, and (3) replication of bacterial chromosomes. **Antibiotics** (from Latin *anti*, meaning against; and Greek βιοτικός or *biotikos*, meaning fit for life) are antimicrobial agents that interfere with the bacterial peptidoglycan cell wall, inhibit protein synthesis, or interfere with bacterial DNA synthesis.

Fungi

Fungi include molds and yeasts that consist of filaments (hyphae), which create spores. The major difference between fungi cells and human cells is that the cell membrane of fungi is made of ergosterol instead of cholesterol. Therefore, antifungal agents interfere with the production or stability of ergosterol in different ways and thereby damage fungi without damaging adjacent human cells.

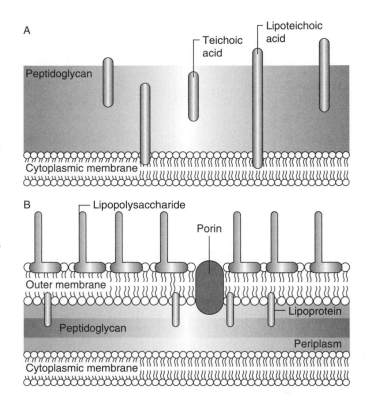

Figure 11-1 (A) Gram-positive cell wall. (B) Gram-negative cell wall. *Source:* Adapted with permission from Cabeen.[90]

Viruses

Viruses (from the Latin *virus*, meaning toxin or poison) are acellular obligate intracellular organisms made of either RNA or DNA. The viral RNA or DNA is covered by a protein coat called a capsid. The whole unit of viral genetic material and capsids is called a *virion*. Viruses cannot reproduce on their own. They have a typical life cycle that involves attachment to a host cell, release of the viral genes into the host cell, replication of viral components using host cell mechanisms, assembly of viral components, and then release of viral particles that will infect new host cells. Antiviral medications work by attacking a specific step in this life-cycle process. The best antivirals attack a viral protein that does not have a function in the human cell.

Parasites

Parasites are organisms that live on or in a host organism and can damage the host organism. Parasites that infect humans range from single-celled organisms, such as protozoa (e.g., trichomonas), to multicellular organisms, such as worms. Parasitic disease accounts for a large burden of human morbidity worldwide. Malaria in particular causes 3 to 5 million malarial episodes each year throughout the world.[9] Antiparasitic drugs are particularly difficult to develop because these multicellular organisms have many similarities with human cells.

Bacterial Resistance to Antimicrobial Drugs

The phenomenon of antibiotic resistance is one of global concern. Recognition and increased awareness of the evolving antibiotic resistance of major microbial pathogens is the first step in improving strategies to combat the rapidly growing problem.[10] Extreme care is necessary when prescribing antimicrobial therapy because overuse and inappropriate use of antimicrobial agents has contributed to the prevalence of drug resistance.

Antibiotic resistance occurs as a result of natural selection. The organism that has a point mutation that confers antibiotic resistance will survive an exposure to an antibiotic. Those organisms will pass this mutation to their offspring, and in a short time, the result is a population of microbes that are resistant to a particular antimicrobial agent. Some bacteria have an inherent or natural resistance to an antibiotic, and for others, resistance is acquired via plasmid transfer.

Antibiotic resistance can occur in one of several ways. Table 11-1 summarizes these effects and Figure 11-2 illustrates those used specifically by the beta-lactam antibiotics. Clinical implications for each type of antibiotic are discussed later.[11,12]

Antibacterial Agents

In 1929, Sir Alexander Fleming, a Scottish bacteriologist, went on vacation and incubated his agar plates of staphylococci at room temperature uncovered, thinking they would grow slower than when placed at a higher temperature and would be mature when he returned. However, when he returned, the agar plates had a mold growing on them, and he noticed that the bacteria did not grow near the mold. He named the mold *Penicillium*, and thus, the history of modern antibiotic discovery was launched.[13] Dr. Dorothy Crowfoot Hodgkin determined the molecular structure of penicillin and won the 1964 Nobel Prize in chemistry for her work. Finally, penicillin was successfully mass produced following World War II efforts by scientists in the United Kingdom and the United States. Streptomycin, chloramphenicol (Chloromycetin), and tetracycline were discovered in the 1940s through the 1950s, and new antibiotics are still being discovered today.[14]

Antibiotics are compounds that were first derived from living organisms, specifically molds and plants, although many are now produced synthetically. Antibiotics work in one of two ways—those that inhibit bacterial growth are **bacteriostatic**, and those that kill bacteria are **bacteriocidal**.

In practice, antibiotics are classified by their chemical structure and mechanism of action. Most antibiotics (1) attack the cell wall or cell membrane, (2) inhibit or alter protein synthesis, or (3) interfere with DNA replication. There are a few that have other specific mechanisms of action, as shown in Figure 11-3.

Antibiotics That Inhibit Cell Wall Synthesis: Beta-Lactams and Vancomycin

Antibiotics that inhibit cell wall synthesis are the beta-lactams (penicillins and cephalosporins) and vancomycin. Ethambutol also acts on the cell wall, but it is included

Table 11-1 Mechanisms of Antibiotic Resistance

Action of Antibiotic	Mechanism of Bacterial Resistance	Example Bacteria That Use This Mechanism of Resistance	Example Antibiotics Affected
Cell membrane alteration	Genetic alterations code for a different structure of the peptidoglycan cell wall that penicillin cannot bind to well.	Methicillin-resistant *Staphylococcus aureus*, *Neisseria gonorrhoeae*, *Streptococcus pneumonia*.	Penicillins, cephalosporins
Drug inactivation	Bacteria produce an enzyme that breaks down the antibiotic. The classic example of this is beta-lactamase, which breaks down penicillin and is produced by penicillin-resistant bacteria.	Methicillin-resistant *S aureus*, *N gonorrhoeae*, *Klebsiella*, *Bacteroides fragilis*.	Penicillins, cephalosporins
Active efflux	Some drugs develop a method to actively pump antibiotic out of the cell before it reaches its internal target.	*Escherichia coli*, *Pseudomonas aeruginosa*.	Tetracycline
Alteration of metabolic pathways	Bacteria develop alternative metabolic pathways that bypass the metabolic step with which the antibiotic interferes.	*E coli*, *Klebsiella*, *Enterobacter*, *Proteus mirabilis*, and *Proteus vulgaris*.	Sulfonamides, trimethoprim

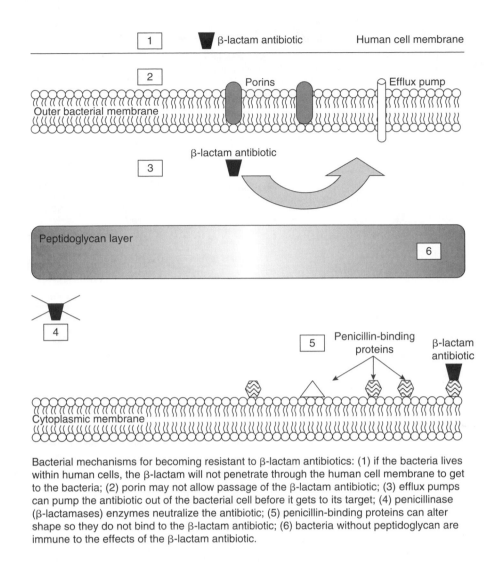

Bacterial mechanisms for becoming resistant to β-lactam antibiotics: (1) if the bacteria lives within human cells, the β-lactam will not penetrate through the human cell membrane to get to the bacteria; (2) porin may not allow passage of the β-lactam antibiotic; (3) efflux pumps can pump the antibiotic out of the bacterial cell before it gets to its target; (4) penicillinase (β-lactamases) enzymes neutralize the antibiotic; (5) penicillin-binding proteins can alter shape so they do not bind to the β-lactam antibiotic; (6) bacteria without peptidoglycan are immune to the effects of the β-lactam antibiotic.

Figure 11-2 Mechanisms of bacterial resistance to β-lactam antibiotics. *Source:* Adapted with permission from Cabeen MT et al. 2005.[90]

under the category of antimycobacterial agents. The beta-lactam family shares a basic structure that includes a thiazolidine ring attached to a beta-lactam ring that carries a secondary amino acid group. The beta-lactam ring is a critical element with respect to the antimicrobial activity of penicillin.[15] The family of beta-lactams includes the penicillins, cephalosporins, carbapenems, and monobactams.

Penicillins

Penicillins are a bacteriocidal class of antibiotics that are subdivided into one of these four categories: natural penicillins, antistaphylococcal penicillins, broad-spectrum penicillins, and extended-spectrum penicillins.

Mechanism of Action and Spectrum of Activity

Penicillins inhibit bacteria by interfering with the integrity of the cell walls of bacteria. In particular, penicillins bind to bacterial enzymes known as transpeptidases or **penicillin-binding proteins** (PBPs). When the transpeptidases and other enzymes are bound to the penicillin molecule, the construction of the bacterial cell wall is impaired, and necessary cross-links are unable to be laid, causing the cell to die. Thus penicillins are bactericidal. Penicillins are effective against gram-positive bacteria that have an exposed peptidoglycan cell wall.

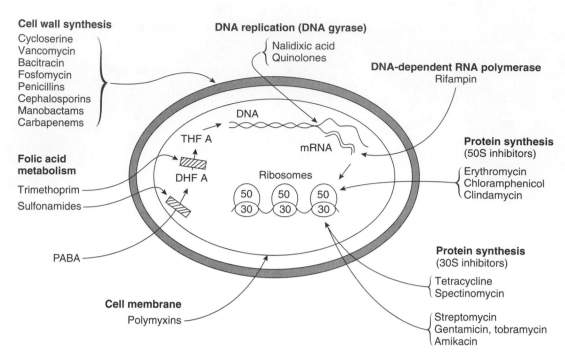

Figure 11-3 Antimicrobials: Mechanisms of action.

Resistance to Penicillins

Bacterial resistance to penicillin exists secondary to several different bacterial characteristics and/or mechanisms. First, the penicillins poorly penetrate into the intracellular space and are therefore ineffective against obligate intracellular organisms such as *Rickettsia* or *Chlamydia*. Nor are they effective against gram-negative bacteria because the peptidoglycan wall is not exposed to the antibiotic in gram-negative bacteria. Some gram-negative bacteria also have pores in the outer membrane that do not allow passage of beta-lactam antibiotics. Other bacteria have efflux pumps that remove the antibiotic from the periplasmic space. Some bacteria, such as *Mycoplasma*, do not make peptidoglycan and are therefore impervious to the mechanism of action of beta-lactam antibiotics. Bacteria that do have peptidoglycan can alter the form of peptidoglycan made so the beta-lactam antibiotics are ineffective. Finally, bacterial development of enzymes **beta-lactamase** or **penicillinase** is a common mechanism of resistance. These enzymes break open the beta-lactam ring of the penicillin molecule and render it inactive.[16]

Natural Penicillins

In the late 1920s, natural penicillins were identified, and by 1950, penicillin G was proven to be bactericidal and became available for the treatment of many gram-positive and gram-negative cocci, anaerobes, and spirochetes. Table 11-2 lists the indications, doses, and adverse reactions to the most commonly used penicillins. The two natural penicillins used today are benzylpenicillin, also known as penicillin G, which can only be given intravenously, and penicillin V, which is the oral formulation. Procaine penicillin (Bicillin CR) is penicillin G in combination with a local anesthetic (procaine), making it useful for intramuscular injection. Benzathine benzyl penicillin (Bicillin LA) is a form of penicillin G that is slowly absorbed then hydrolyzed to penicillin G internally. It is used when prolonged concentrations are required. It is important not to confuse Bicillin CR and Bicillin LA. Bicillin CR has 1.2 million units of penicillin G and 1.2 million units of procaine. Bicillin LA has 2.4 million units of penicillin G.[17]

Penicillin G remains indicated for infections caused by streptococci, meningococci, enterococci, penicillin-susceptible pneumococci, and non–beta-lactamase-producing staphylococci. This agent also is highly effective against spirochetes such as *Treponema pallidum*, *Clostridium* species, *actinomyces*, and other gram-positive rods, but it is inactive against most strains of *Staphylococcus aureus*.

Penicillin V (Veetids), also known as penicillin VK, is similar to penicillin G, except it is acid stable, and penicillin G is not. Because of its acid stability, penicillin V is the drug

Table 11-2 Penicillins

Penicillins Generic (Brand)	Indications	Doses	Route	Half-Life	Excretion	Adverse Reactions	Clinical Considerations	FDA Pregnancy Category
Natural Penicillins								
Penicillin V (Veetids, Pen-Vee K)	Minor infections—drug of choice for group A Beta hemolytic strep.	2–4 g/day in divided doses— e.g., 500 mg q 4 h.	PO	1 h	Renal	Low incidence of adverse reactions.	Stable in stomach acid, may be taken with meals. Do not give concomitantly with tetracyclines.	B
Penicillin G potassium (Pfizerpen)	Bacterial endocarditis, pneumococcal pneumonia, GBS, prophylaxis for laboring women.	8–24 million units/day in divided doses.	IV	25–50 min	Renal	Anaphylaxis, hypersensitivity reactions.	Do not give concomitantly with tetracyclines.	B
Penicillin G Benzathine with procaine (Bicillin CR)	Moderate to severe upper respiratory infections, skin, soft tissue, diphtheria.	600,000–1.2 million U/day.	IM	0.5 h	Renal	Hypersensitivity occurs in 10–15% of individuals; risk of reaction highest when combined with procaine and administered IM.	Only parenteral PCN in use in outpatient settings. Reduce dose if renal impairment and hepatic disease occur. Do not give concomitantly with tetracyclines.	B
Benzathine Penicillin G (Bicillin LA)	Syphilis, rheumatic fever, group A streptococcal pharyngitis.	600,000–1.2 million U as single dose.	IM	0.5 to 1 h	Renal	Anaphylaxis, hypersensitivity reactions.	Dose lasts 2–4 wk. Do not give IV or SQ. Do not give concomitantly with tetracyclines.	B
Penicillinase-Resistant Penicillins								
Cloxacillin (Cloxapen)	Treatment of soft-tissue infections caused by penicillinase-producing staphylococci that have demonstrated susceptibility to the drug.	250–500 mg q 6 h.	PO/ IM/IV	0.4 h	Renal/bile	High dose associated with seizures and encephalopathy. Thrombophlebitis has occurred with IV administration.	Food interferes with absorption.	B
Dicloxacillin (Dynapen)		125–500 mg q 6 h.	PO	0.8 h	Renal/bile	Anaphylaxis, hypersensitivity reactions.	Food interferes with absorption.	B
Nafcillin (Unipen)	Treatment of infections due to penicillinase-producing staphylococci.	500 mg–1 g IV q 4–6 h.	IM/IV	0.5 h	Renal/bile	Anaphylaxis, hypersensitivity reactions.	Food interferes with absorption.	B
Oxacillin (Bactocill)		250–500 mg PO q 4–6 h, 1–2 g IV q 4–6 h. Maximum of 9 g/day.	IM/IV	0.4 h		Anaphylaxis, hypersensitivity reactions.	Dose of oxacillin must be modified for persons with renal insufficiency.	B

(*continues*)

Table 11-2 Penicillins (*continued*)

Penicillins Generic (Brand)	Indications	Doses	Route	Half-Life	Excretion	Adverse Reactions	Clinical Considerations	FDA Pregnancy Category
Aminopenicillins								
Ampicillin (Principen)*	Group B *Streptococcus faecalis, Proteus mirabilis, E coli, Salmonella, Shigella, Haemophilus influenzae.*	4–12 g/day IV, 250–500 mg q 6 hr PO.	PO/IV	1.0 h	Renal/bile	Rashes, diarrhea most common; also urticaria, nausea, vomiting.	Assess for pseudomembranous colitis if diarrhea persists.	B
Amoxicillin (Amoxil, Trimox)*	Not effective against *S aureus*; used for acute otitis media, sinusitis.	250–500 mg q 8 h.	PO	1.0 h	Renal, 60%	Most common side effects are rash and diarrhea—less diarrhea than with ampicillin.	Take on an empty stomach. Amoxicillin is more acid resistant than ampicillin and blood levels are greater; therefore, it is preferred when oral therapy is indicated.	B
Extended-Spectrum Penicillins								
Ticarcillin (Ticar)	Same organisms susceptible to aminopenicillins plus *Pseudomonas aeruginosa, Enterobacter species, Proteus, Bacteroides fragilis,* and *Klebsiella.*	200–300 mg/kg/d 12–24 gm/d.	IV	1.0 h	Renal	Symptoms of sodium overload (CHF), interferes with platelet function and can promote bleeding.	Should not be mixed with aminoglycosides in same IV solution.	B
Carbenicillin indanyl (Geocillin)		1.5–3 g/d.	PO	1.0 h	Renal	Anaphylaxis, hypersensitivity reactions.	*Off market in United States.	B
Piperacillin/ tazobactam (Zosyn)		12–24 g/d.	IV	1.0 h	Renal	Diarrhea, rashes, pain at IV site, confusion, dizziness, lethargy, constipation, nausea, vomiting, urticaria.	Assess for pseudomembranous colitis (*C diff*) if diarrhea persists.	B

PCN = penicillin; GBS = group B streptococcus.

* Epstein-Barr infection, acute lymphocytic leukemia, or CMV infection increases the risk of developing ampicillin rash to approximately 60%.

of choice for oral therapy. This oral medication may be taken with meals without restriction of any particular foods.

Clinical Indications for Penicillin G and Penicillin V

Although penicillin G was once the drug of choice for treatment of gonorrhea, it has been replaced by ceftriaxone (Rocephin) or cefixime (Suprax) as the primary treatment because of the development of drug resistance of gonorrhea to penicillins over the years.[18] Penicillin G is used to treat endocarditis, meningitis (caused by *Neisseria meningitidis*), group B streptococcus sepsis, and syphilis (Chapter 23). It is used as prophylaxis for group B streptococcus sepsis in laboring women (Chapter 36). Penicillin V is also used to

treat tonsillitis, pharyngitis, and scarlet fever, as streptococcal pharyngitis has yet to demonstrate any resistance to penicillin. Penicillin V is also the first choice for prophylaxis against rheumatic fever.

Antistaphylococcal Penicillins

The second broad category of penicillins, **antistaphylococcal penicillins** or **penicillinase-resistant penicillins**, have a bulky attachment to the R-side chain that prevents the bacterial beta-lactamase enzyme from binding to them. These semisynthetic penicillins are active against most staphylococcal species and streptococci microorganisms, but are not effective against the gram-positive enterococci, anaerobic bacteria, or gram-negative cocci and rods. Therefore, antistaphylococcal penicillins have a narrow spectrum of activity. Drugs in this category include cloxacillin (Cloxapen), dicloxacillin (Dynapen), nafcillin (Unipen), and oxacillin (Bactocill). Cloxacillin and dicloxacillin are administered orally and are appropriate for the treatment of mild to moderate localized staphylococcal infections. Cloxacillin (Cloxapen) and dicloxacillin (Dynapen) should be taken 2 hours before or after a meal since food interferes with drug absorption. Individuals should be advised to always continue taking the medication until the course of therapy is completed because taking incomplete doses not only might result in a treatment failure but could also promote development of drug resistance. For systemic staphylococcal infections, nafcillin and oxacillin are indicated and should be administered intravenously. The usual dose for intravenous administration of nafcillin and oxacillin for adults is 2–12 grams in a 24-hour period given in divided doses. Ideally, a culture and sensitivity should be performed before prescribing the anti-infective of choice.

Methicillin is an antistaphylococcal penicillin that is no longer commercially available. Approximately 30% of the population in the United States is colonized with *S aureus*, and 1% are colonized with **methicillin-resistant S aureus** (MRSA),[19] a growing clinical problem. Resistance to penicillins appears to result from a production of altered PBPs to which the antistaphylococcus penicillins are unable to bind. Community-acquired MRSA infections are predominately skin infections that manifest as abscesses, boils, or pus-filled lesions. Currently, trimethoprim/sulfamethoxazole (TMP/SMX) or clindamycin (Cleocin) are recommended for treatment of dermatologic infections that are suspicious for being caused by MRSA (Box 11-1). Healthcare-associated MRSA, which is diagnosed as an invasive infection, is most often seen in persons who have been hospitalized and have some degree of immunocompromise. Vancomycin (Vanocin), alone or combined with rifampin, is the treatment of choice for infections caused by methicillin-resistant staphylococci.[18]

Clinical Indications for Antistaphylococcus Penicillins

The primary use of antistaphylococcus penicillins is for cellulitis and soft tissue infections caused by *S aureus*. Dicloxacillin (Dynapen) has been and is still the first choice for treatment of lactational mastitis.[20] That said, if any soft tissue infection has signs that suggest MRSA is the etiologic agent,

or if the individual is at risk for being infected with MRSA, then vancomycin will be the first-choice treatment.

Broad-Spectrum Penicillins

The two **broad-spectrum** penicillins available are ampicillin (Principen) and amoxicillin (Amoxil). These agents are aminopenicillins and are considered to be broad spectrum due to their ability to penetrate the gram-negative outer bacterial cell membrane. This group is generally effective against the same bacterial strains as penicillin G but have additional coverage against certain gram-negative bacteria, including *Haemophilus influenzae, Escherichia coli, Proteus mirabilis* and enterococci.

Broad-spectrum penicillins can be administered orally or intravenously. Amoxicillin is one of the most frequently prescribed antibiotics and is the preferred oral agent because it is more acid resistant, thus resulting in greater absorption and less diarrhea, and can be given three times per day rather than four times per day.

Combination aminopenicillins that consist of a beta-lactamase inhibitor with an aminopenicillin are also available. This combination allows the antimicrobial spectrum to be extended to include beta-lactamase-producing strains of bacteria. Amoxicillin in combination with clavulanic acid (Augmentin) is effective against beta-lactamase-producing *S aureus, N gonorrhoeae, H influenza, E coli, S pneumonia*, enterococci, and *Moraxella catarrhalis*.[18]

Clinical Indication for Broad-Spectrum Penicillins

Ampicillin (Principen) and amoxicillin (Amoxil) are prescribed for the treatment of upper respiratory infections, pneumonia, sinusitis, uncomplicated urinary tract infections, orthopedic infections, gastrointestinal disorders, and many genital tract infections. They are the drug of choice for meningococcal meningitis. Amoxicillin is the drug of choice for infectious or subacute bacterial endocarditis prophylaxis when indicated. Box 11-2 lists the guidelines for infectious prophylaxis from the American Heart Association.[21]

Extended-Spectrum Penicillins

The three **extended-spectrum** penicillins available in the United States are ticarcillin (Ticar), carbenicillin (Geocillin), and piperacillin (Zosyn). The drugs in this category also are classified as the **antipseudomonal penicillins** because they are used primarily for infections with *Pseudomonas aeruginosa*, a condition more commonly found among immunocompromised individuals. These infections are particularly difficult to eradicate. Extended-spectrum penicillins are limited to parenteral use only. These agents usually are used in combination with aminoglycosides such as gentamicin to eradicate the *pseudomonas.* However, these drugs should not be mixed in the same intravenous solution, as inactivation may occur under those circumstances.

Metabolism of Penicillin

Metabolism of the penicillins varies greatly depending on the route of administration, stability, and protein binding capacity. Oral dicloxacillin (Dynapen), ampicillin (Principen), and amoxicillin (Amoxil) are well absorbed by the gastrointestinal tract. Intravenous administration results in rapid absorption and wide distribution to body tissues. Intramuscular administration is clinically effective; however, pain and local irritation at the injection site are reasons to select an alternative route. Most of the penicillins are excreted as unchanged drugs through the kidneys. **Elimination** is rapid and the half-lives of penicillins are typically 30–90 minutes.

Side Effects and Adverse Reactions

Penicillins are generally nontoxic. The most common side effects of broad-spectrum penicillins are rash,

---

Box 11-1　Methicillin-Resistant *Staphylococcus Aureus* (MRSA)

Methicillin-resistant *Staphylococcus aureus* (MRSA) is a strain of *S aureus* that is resistant to all the beta-lactam antibiotics including those with beta-lactamase inhibitor combinations (e.g., Ampicillin claviculate [Augmentin]). MRSA is categorized as either healthcare-associated MRSA (HA-MRSA) or community-associated MRSA (CA-MRSA).

Historically, HA-MRSA accounted for 90% of the MRSA infections. It is associated with a recent hospitalization and is more likely to occur in the elderly, African Americans, persons with open wounds or weakened immune systems, and men. HA-MRSA has accounted for 85% of the invasive disease, which includes osteomyelitis, sepsis, and endocarditis. Vancomycin has been the standard antibiotic used for treatment of HA-MRSA.

CA-MRSA is not associated with a recent hospitalization and is unfortunately becoming more common. A recent report from the United States found that approximately 50% of the pigs and pig farmers in the United States carry MRSA. Although this is a small study, there is concern that MRSA is becoming more prevalent in the United States and that animal sources may become an important reservoir. It is theorized that the large amount of antibiotics used in pig farming (to keep the pigs healthy), may inadvertently be the right incubator for breeding bacteria that are resistant to antibiotics. MRSA is a good example of this type of bacteria.

Approximately 75% of CA-MRSA presents as soft tissue infections that present as a furuncle (boil), cellulitis, impetigo, report of spider bite, or infected wound.[19] CA-MRSA should be part of the differential diagnosis for all soft tissue infections seen in the outpatient setting. These soft tissue infections form abscesses quite often. CA-MRSA strains are more virulent than HA-MRSA strains and can spread and progress to toxic shock syndrome, sepsis, or necrotizing pneumonia.

The initial treatment is always incision, culture, and drainage. The diagnosis of CA-MRSA can be made if the culture is positive for MRSA, and if the individual does not have a medical history of MRSA infection and does not have an indwelling catheter or other medical device that passes through the skin into the body. In addition, in order to make the diagnosis, the person in question will not have any of the following within the previous year: (1) hospitalization; (2) admission to a nursing home, skilled nursing facility, or hospice; (3) dialysis; or (4) surgery.[19]

If incision and drainage is not possible or not considered sufficient treatment, the antibiotic recommendation for CA-MRSA is guided by the susceptibility of the cultured organism. If empiric therapy is started prior to knowledge of culture results, trimethoprim-sulfamethoxazole (Bactrim) 1–2 double-strength tablets every 8–12 hrs or clindamycin 300 mg by mouth four times a day for 14 days are the best first choices for women of childbearing age. Doxycycline can be used but is contraindicated for children and pregnant women. Linezolid is the big gun that will eradicate CA-MRSA, but it has potential for antibiotic resistance, is expensive, and should not be used for outpatient empiric treatment.

Box 11-2 Infectious Endocarditis Prophylaxis Guidelines

The American Heart Association no longer recommends routine prophylaxis for dental or other procedures except in the following cases:

- Presence of a prosthetic cardiac valve or prosthetic material used for cardiac valve repair
- History of previous infectious endocarditis
- Cyanotic congenital heart disease, completely repaired congenital heart disease with prosthetic material in first 6 months, or partially repaired congenital heart disease with residual defect
- Cardiac transplantation recipients developing cardiac valvulopathy

The only procedures for which subacute bacterial endocarditis (SBE) prophylaxis is recommended are:

- Invasive respiratory procedures (e.g., bronchoscopy)
- Dental procedures: Gingival or periapical region of teeth manipulated or oral mucosa perforated

When needed, the recommendation is amoxicillin 2 grams 30–60 minutes prior to procedure if given intravenously and 1 hour prior to procedure if given by mouth.

If the person receiving the drug is penicillin allergic, the alternatives are:

a. Clindamycin 600 mg by mouth 1 hour before procedure or 600 mg intravenously 30 minutes before
b. Cephalexin or cefadroxil 2 g by mouth 1 hour before
c. Cefazolin or ceftriaxone 1.0 g intramuscularly/intravenously 30 minutes before the procedure
d. Azithromycin or clarithromycin 500 mg by mouth 1 hour before

Source: From Wilson et al. 2007.[21]

---

nausea, vomiting, and diarrhea. These reactions occur more frequently with ampicillin than with any other penicillin. A nonpruritic maculopapular rash is quite common in children who take ampicillin or amoxicillin, and this is frequently assumed to be a penicillin allergy, but in fact if the rash is nonpruritic, it is not a true hypersensitivity reaction. Persons who report ampicillin rash may be able to take penicillins subsequently without experiencing real allergic reactions.[22] Prolonged anti-infective use has been implicated in the occurrence of secondary vaginal candidiasis infections due in large part to the failure to reestablish a normal lactobacilli-dominated vaginal flora following antimicrobial therapy. However, other etiologies could be responsible for the opportunistic infection and should be evaluated in instances of fungal overgrowth rather than assuming that any vaginal condition automatically is a sequela to antimicrobial therapy.

Serious adverse effects of penicillins include allergic reactions, dermatologic reactions such as photosensitivity or morbilliform rash, and more rarely, **Stevens-Johnson syndrome** or exfoliative dermatitis. Other adverse effects include encephalopathy, seizures, hepatitis, renal disorders such as interstitial nephritis, and, finally, hematologic disorders such as neutropenia or hemolytic anemia.

Ampicillin specifically has been linked to **pseudomembranous colitis**, and individuals presenting with a history of colitis or serious episodes of diarrhea associated with anti-infective therapy should be evaluated for pseudomembranous colitis, which is often called *C diff* because it is most frequently caused by an overgrowth of *Clostridium difficile*. Individuals with renal failure are vulnerable to seizures when penicillin is given in high doses, and, therefore, kidney function tests should be monitored in persons who have impaired renal function. Persons with hepatic impairment also require monitoring of liver function.

Allergic Reactions to Penicillins

Interestingly, 89–90% of persons who report a penicillin allergy are not truly allergic to penicillin.[23] Allergic reactions vary extensively. Immediate hypersensitivity reactions range from **urticaria** or angioedema to bronchospasm and anaphylaxis. Nonimmediate reactions occur 1–72 hours after administration and include blood dyscrasias such as hemolytic anemia. Late reactions usually occur more than 72 hours after administration and can range from maculopapular rash to serum sickness or drug fever[24,25] (Table 11-3). The incidence of immediate hypersensitivity

Table 11-3 Penicillin Reactions

Classification	Mechanism of Action	Time of Onset After Administration	Clinical Signs
Type I (immediate)	Penicillin-specific IgE antibodies binding to mast cells with release of histamine and inflammatory mediators.	Within minutes to 1 h.	Urticaria, erythema or pruritus, hypotension, angioedema, bronchospasm, hypotension or shock, anaphylaxis.
Type II (nonimmediate)	Cytotoxic response of IgG or IgM antibodies directed at drug–hapten-coated cells.	Variable: 1 h to 72 h.	Blood cell dyscrasias (hemolytic anemia, neutropenia, thrombocytopenia).
Type III (nonimmediate)	Immune complex reaction: tissue deposition of drug–antibody complex with complement activation and inflammation.	7–10 days.	Serum sickness, fever, rash, arthralgias, lymphadenopathy, urticaria, glomerulonephritis, vasculitis.
Type IV (delayed)	Cell-mediated response to T cells with cytokine and inflammatory mediator release.	2–21 days.	Allergic contact dermatitis, eczema, maculopapular, bullous, or pustular exanthema.

Sources: Adapted with permission from Riedl MA et al. 2003[24] and from Demoly P et al. 2005.[25]

pruritic skin rashes is approximately 4%, whereas only 1 in 5000 to 1 in 10,000 individuals will actually experience anaphylaxis as a result of receiving penicillin.[26]

Treatment of Persons Who Are Allergic to Penicillin

In persons with an established allergic response to penicillin, alternative options can often be found. However, the incidence of cross-allergenicity within the same drug class or among drugs that contain similar structural similarities, specifically first- and second-generation cephalosporins, occurs in approximately 1–20% of individuals with confirmed penicillin reactions.[18]

Approximately 90% of individuals who have experienced a severe allergic reaction to penicillin stop expressing penicillin-specific IgE over time. Skin testing with major and minor determinants of penicillin can determine which persons are currently at high risk for an allergic reaction. Major determinants are available commercially; they can identify 90–97% of currently allergic individuals, but caution must be exercised since 3–10% will still be missed without the full range of testing.[27]

When necessary, desensitization can be achieved in highly sensitive persons. The Centers for Disease Control and Prevention (CDC) has guidelines for desensitizing the individual with a history of penicillin allergy.[28] As stated earlier, for most individuals, an alternative antimicrobial can be used when penicillin allergy is present. However, there are no proven alternatives to penicillin for treating neurosyphilis, congenital syphilis, or syphilis in pregnant women. Individuals who have a positive skin test to the penicillin reagents can be desensitized through a relatively safe procedure that can be completed in 4 hours in a hospital setting. The procedure can be performed by the administration of small, gradually

increasing amounts of penicillin V, orally or intravenously. After desensitization, the individual is maintained on penicillin for the course of therapy.

Drug–Drug Interactions

In general, drug–drug interactions with penicillin are uncommon. Evidence regarding penicillin and its effect on oral contraceptives is contradictory. Oral estrogens undergo hepatic metabolism to form conjugates that gastrointestinal flora hydrolyze. This process allows for reabsorption of estrogens and maintenance of their pharmacologic effect. The alteration of gastrointestinal flora by the use of antibiotics can result in breakthrough bleeding and pregnancies. The estimated likelihood of this interaction is rare (approximately 1%), and therefore the recommendation to counsel women about the potential for oral contraceptive failure remains controversial. In addition, it is difficult to link contraceptive failure directly to penicillin use because no oral contraceptive is 100% efficacious.[29] To date, only rifampin has been positively shown to decrease the effectiveness of oral contraceptives. A number of other antibiotics, including penicillins, have been linked to unintended pregnancy anecdotally or in retrospective surveys, but prospective, randomized controlled trials have not been undertaken. A true drug interaction may occur in a small subset of women, therefore most experts agree that the conservative approach is to advise use of an additional nonhormonal contraceptive method while taking any antibiotic.

Probenecid (Benemid), an antigout pharmacologic treatment, slows tubular excretion of penicillin, thereby increasing plasma levels. Historically, probenecid was used with penicillin when treating gonorrhea to prolong blood levels of penicillin in order to augment therapy. If taken concomitantly with penicillin, tetracycline (Achromycin) or chloramphenicol (Chloromycetin) can decrease the bactericidal action of penicillin. Penicillin can increase bleeding when coadministered with an anticoagulant such as warfarin (Coumadin).[28] Penicillin can decrease clearance of methotrexate (Trexall), causing a risk for toxicity of this antifolate drug. Methotrexate, aspirin, and indomethacin can also potentially slow tubular secretion, although the clinical implication of this interaction is not clear. Cholestyramine (Questran) decreases absorption and therefore the effect of oral penicillins. Neomycin can decrease absorption of penicillin V.

Special Populations

The risk category for the most commonly used penicillins is an FDA pregnancy category B drug because there has been no risk found to fetuses in animal studies. However, human studies have been limited.[30] Penicillin in general penetrates breast milk with peak levels occurring about 6 hours after the drug is taken. Infants should be observed for any gastrointestinal upset, candidiasis, or allergic response, although major adverse effects have not been noted.

Oral penicillins generally are well tolerated. Individuals should be asked specifically about allergy to penicillin, especially because the mature woman may have difficulty remembering old allergies. Some parenteral penicillins have higher sodium content and may need to be monitored in elderly persons if they have or are at risk for cardiac and renal conditions.

Recent information suggests that infections in general may be linked to atherosclerosis and thrombosis, which are more common as we age. Assuming that phenomenon exists, it is theorized that use of antibiotics may be prophylactic. One study found that recent use of penicillin decreased stroke by 19% in elderly subjects on antihypertensive therapy (RR = 0.81; 95% CI, 0.70 to 0.94).[31]

Cephalosporins

In many respects, cephalosporins are similar to penicillins. Agents in both these categories are beta-lactam antibiotics—i.e., containing a beta-lactam ring that is primarily responsible for their antimicrobial activity. However the cephalosporins are less susceptible to cleavage by beta-lactamases than are the penicillins, and they have two sites that can be modified, which accounts for the broader number of agents available.

Cephalosporins, isolated from the fungus *Cephalosporium* shortly after penicillins were discovered, are

categorized into four generations and comprise one of the largest antibiotic classes. Their toxicity is low, and these drugs are therefore one of the most widely prescribed classes of antibiotics. First-, second-, and third-generation preparations have several alternatives. Currently, cefepime (Maxipime) is the only fourth-generation medication available (Table 11-4).

Mechanism of Action and Spectrum of Activity

The cephalosporins are bacteriocidal and inhibit cell wall synthesis of microorganisms. As with penicillins, this action involves cephalosporins binding with the PCPs, impairing construction of the bacterial cell wall. Unique properties of individual cephalosporins are determined by changes made to the structure of the nucleus of the cephalosporin formula.[18]

Cephalosporins are active against most gram-positive bacteria. The first-generation cephalosporins have the strongest activity against those gram-positive bacteria susceptible to this class of antibiotic, an important concept to remember when choosing one for specific infections. Each generation of cephalosporins has a broader spectrum of activity against aerobic gram-negative bacteria, but each generation has less activity against gram-positive bacteria. These agents have limited activity against anaerobes. In general, older first-generation formulations are less expensive but have a narrower antimicrobial spectrum of activity than the more recently developed agents.

Cephalosporins of any generation do not have appreciable activity against a number of common organisms, including penicillin-resistant *Pneumococcus*, MRSA, *Staphylococcus epidermidis, Enterococcus, Listeria, Mycoplasma, Campylobacter,* or intracellular organisms such as *Chlamydia pneumoniae* and *Chlamydia trachomatis.*

Mechanism of Resistance

Resistance to cephalosporins occurs via the same mechanisms that confer resistance to penicillins.

First-Generation Cephalosporins

First-generation cephalosporins are indicated for infections caused by gram-positive cocci, in particular, streptococci, staphylococci, and pneumococci organisms. These agents have limited activity against aerobic gram-negative organisms such as *E coli, P mirabilis,* and *Klebsiella pneumoniae.*

The primary employment of first-generation cephalosporins is to treat skin and soft tissue infections. Cefazolin

Table 11-4 Cephalosporins*

Cephalosporins Generic (Brand)	Indications	Doses	Route	Excretion	Half-Life	Adverse Reactions	Clinical Considerations	FDA Pregnancy Category
First Generation								
Cefadroxil (Duricef)		500 mg: 1 g qd–bid.	PO	Renal	1.2–1.3 h	Adverse reactions seen in all generations.*†	Most active against gram-positive organisms and the least expensive.	B
Cefazolin sodium (Ancef)	Gram-positive cocci causing skin and soft tissue infections such as *S aureus* and streptococci.	250 mg: 2 g tid.	IM/IV	Renal	1.5–2.2 h	Adverse reactions seen in all generations.*†	Cefazolin is the drug of choice for surgical prophylaxis in most surgical procedures.	B
Cephalexin (Keflex)		250–500 mg q 6 h.	PO	Renal	0.4–1 h	Adverse reactions seen in all generations.*†		B
Second Generation								
Cefotetan (Cefotan)	More active against gram-negative organisms and anaerobic organisms—used to treat serious upper and lower respiratory infections, GU infections, gonococcus *Haemophilus influenzae*, *E coli*, GABHS, staphylococci.	1–2 g q 12 h.	IV/IM	Renal	4 h	Adverse reactions seen in all generations.*† Disulfiram-like reaction if taken with alcohol.	Less effective than first generation against gram-positive organisms.	B
Cefaclor (Ceclor)		250–500 mg q 8 h.	PO	Renal	0.6–0.9 h	Adverse reactions seen in all generations.*†		B
Cefprozil (Cefzil)		250–500 mg q 12–24 h.	PO	Renal	1.3 h	Adverse reactions seen in all generations.*†		B
Cefuroxime (Ceftin)		125–500 mg q 12 h.	PO/IV	Renal	1–1.9 h	Adverse reactions seen in all generations.†‡		B
Third Generation								
Cefoperazone (Cefobid)	Serious infections resistant to first and second generations. Drugs of choice for meningitis caused by gram-negative bacilli. Nosocomial infections caused by gram-negative bacilli.	2–4 g/day divided q 12 h.	IV/IM	Biliary/ renal	2 h	Adverse reactions seen in all generations.†‡ Disulfiram-like reaction if taken with alcohol.	Good alternative to aminoglycosides due to their lack of toxicity even at high doses.	B
Ceftriaxone (Rocephin)		250 mg: 2 g qd.	IM/IV	Hepatic	5.8–8.7 h	Adverse reactions seen in all generations.†‡		B
Cefotaxime sodium (Claforan)		1–2 g bid.	IM	Renal	0.9–1.14 h	Adverse reactions seen in all generations.†‡		B
Cefdinir (Omnicef)		300 mg bid.	PO	Renal	1.7 h	Adverse reactions seen in all generations.†‡		B
Cefditoren (Spectracef)		200–400 mg bid.	PO	Renal	1.6 h	Adverse reactions seen in all generations.†‡		B
Cefixime (Suprax)		200 mg bid or 400 mg/d.	PO	Renal and hepatic	3–4 h	Adverse reactions seen in all generations.†‡		B

(continues)

Table 11-4 Cephalosporins* (*continued*)

Fourth Generation

Cefepime (Maxipime)	Very broad antibacterial spectrum.	500 mg: 1 g bid.	IM/IV	Renal	2 h	Encephalopathy, headache, bleeding, anemia.	Penetration to CSF good.	B

GABHS = Group A beta-hemolytic streptococcus; GU = genitourinary.

* This is not a complete list of the cephalosporins available in the United States today. There are several others in each of the four generations.

† Common adverse reactions and side effects for all generations of cephalosporins include diarrhea, nausea, dyspepsia, pain and inflammation at IV site, rashes, urticaria, pruritus. If diarrhea persists, assess for pseudomembranous colitis.

‡ Uncommon adverse reactions and side effects for all generations of cephalosporins include vomiting, oral or vaginal candidiasis, pseudomembranous colitis, and fever.

(Ancef and Kefzol), a first-generation parenteral antibiotic, is used often prophylactically for surgical procedures such as a planned cesarean birth. These drugs should not be used for the treatment of respiratory infections because they are not active against *H influenzae.* Cephalosporins should not be prescribed for serious systemic infections because of their limited spectrum of activity.

Second-Generation Cephalosporins

Second-generation cephalosporins are active against the organisms that are affected by first-generation drugs but interestingly, in the case of cefotetan (Cefotan) and cefoxitin (Mefoxin), less so because these two agents have an additional methoxy group that results in diminished activity against staphylococci and streptococci. Second-generation cephalosporins can be used to treat some aerobic and facultative gram-negative bacteria such as *E coli, K pneumoniae,* and *P mirabilis.* These agents are also active against beta-lactamase-producing strains of *H influenzae* and *M catarrhalis* as well as *Streptococcus pneumoniae.* Second-generation cephalosporins are indicated for the treatment of sinusitis, otitis, and lower respiratory tract infections. They also may be useful in treating peritonitis or diverticulitis.

Third-Generation Cephalosporins

Third-generation cephalosporins provide even greater gram-negative coverage in addition to being effective against the bacteria that are affected by second-generation cephalosporins, and select forms cross the blood–brain barrier, making them an effective treatment for meningitis. These agents are usually reserved for treatment of serious infections caused by organisms that are resistant to other medications, and they are the current recommended treatment for several sexually transmitted diseases (see Chapter 31). Cefixime (Suprax) is the only recommended oral antimicrobial to which *N gonorrhoeae*

has not developed resistance and is currently available as a single 400-mg dose. Ceftriaxone (Rocephin) is notable for a few special characteristics. It has a very long **half-life** and can therefore be dosed once per day. It is commonly used intramuscularly to treat endometritis, gonorrhea, and other mixed microbial infections.

A newer agent, cefepime (Maxipime), is a fourth-generation product that is highly resistant to hydrolysis by beta-lactamases. This drug has been found to be very active against penicillin-resistant strains of streptococci.

Metabolism

Cefadroxil, cephalexin, and cephradine are absorbed from the intestine. Most cephalosporins are excreted via the kidney as unchanged drugs; thus concentration in the urine remains high. Tissue concentrations are variable and tend to be lower than serum concentrations.[15] Second-generation cephalosporins have significant individual differences in activity and toxicity. Excretion of third-generation cephalosporins administered via intravenous infusion is managed through the biliary tract; thus adjustment of dosing is not necessary in instances of renal insufficiency. Cefepime (Maxipime) is able to penetrate into cerebrospinal fluid and is excreted by the kidney.

Side Effects and Adverse Reactions

Cephalosporins are generally well tolerated and the cephalosporin group is one of the safest groups of antimicrobial drugs. Serious adverse effects are rare. Serum sickness-like reactions consisting of erythema multiforme, skin rashes with polyarthritis, arthralgia, and fever have been reported in children but not in adults. Anaphylaxis is rare.

Local irritation may occur at the injection site, or thrombophlebitis may occur after intravenous administration. Maculopapular rashes and/or pruritus may also occur in approximately 1–3% of persons.[32] Gastrointestinal irritation from oral formulations may result in nausea and generalized intestinal upset. Fungal overgrowth such as vaginal candidiasis may occur with extended use.

Some cephalosporins contain an N-methylthiotetrazole group, which can cause hypothrombinemia. The mechanism is reduction of prothrombin levels through the drug's interference with vitamin K metabolism. Thus, caution is required when treating individuals with a history of bleeding disorders.[18] Another adverse reaction, pseudomembranous colitis, may occur following the administration of cephalosporins, requiring discontinuation of the drug and treatment for *C difficile*. Individuals with a history of gastrointestinal disease, especially colitis, should avoid cephalosporins.

Allergic Reactions to Cephalosporins

Hypersensitivity reactions to cephalosporins are the same as the reactions that occur after taking penicillin (see *Side Effects and Adverse Reactions* in the *Penicillins* section). Anaphylaxis and urticaria can occur immediately, but, as with penicillin, the most common reaction is a maculopapular pruritic rash.[32] However, the nucleus of cephalosporins is quite different from penicillin; therefore individuals who do not tolerate penicillin may be able to take cephalosporins without encountering an allergic response.

The story of cephalosporin cross-reactivity with penicillin allergy is interesting. The cephalosporin mold produces some penicillin-like compounds, and thus early cephalosporin antibiotics actually contained traces of penicillin. The actual mechanism responsible for cross-reactivity between cephalosporins and penicillin has not been elucidated but the incidence is approximately 8–10%.[32]

Drug–Drug Interactions

The use of alcohol when taking cefotetan (Cefotan) or cefoperazone (Cefobid) may lead to an acute disulfiram-like reaction producing headache, flushing, dizziness, nausea, vomiting, or abdominal cramps within 30 minutes of alcohol use and lasting up to 3 days. Persons taking these cephalosporins should be cautioned to not drink alcohol during the antibiotic therapy. A uricosuric such as probenecid may reduce renal excretion of some cephalosporins, allowing the drug to be maintained in the kidney or bladder for a longer therapeutic time.

Special Populations

Cephalosporins are in FDA pregnancy category B. The pharmacokinetic properties of cephalosporins change during pregnancy, resulting in shorter half-lives, lower serum levels, and increased clearance, although generally there is no necessary change in dosing.[18] Cephalosporins

are excreted in breast milk in small quantities, but no untoward effects have been found. Cefdinir has not been detected in breast milk, suggesting it might be an excellent choice when alternatives are considered.

Cephalosporins generally are safe and effective drugs for the elderly. Since renal disease is more common among aged individuals compared to younger cohorts, if an elderly individual has decreased renal function, doses may need to be decreased.

Carbapenems and Monobactams

Carbapenems and monobactams are two classes of penicillins used by hospitalists. The medications in these classes are the most broad-spectrum antibiotics in use today and thus are used to treat infections that are resistant to all other agents. Their mechanism of action is the same as the mechanism utilized by all penicillins. They interfere with the construction of the bacterial cell wall and are therefore bactericidal.

The carbapenems, imipenem (Primaxin), meropenem (Merrem IV), and ertapenem (Invanz), are all available in parenteral form only. These medications have three special characteristics. First, they are very small, which allows them to enter porins in the outer membrane of gram-negative organisms. Second, they are resistant to beta-lactamases, and third, they are able to attack a broad range of PBPs. That said, carbapenems are not effective against MRSA, which has an altered form of PBP the carbapenems cannot bind to, and they are not effective against intracellular bacteria such as *chlamydiae*.

Vancomycin

Antibiotic resistance was already becoming a problem in the 1950s, and the search was on for new agents that were active against microbes that are penicillin resistant. Vancomycin (Vanocin) was first isolated from a soil sample collected in the interior jungles of Borneo by a scientist at E. Lily.[33] This agent has traditionally been considered the drug of last resort only to be used after other antibiotics have failed to eradicate disease, and the primary use of vancomycin has been to treat infections caused by MRSA and antibiotic-induced pseudomembranous colitis.

Mechanism of Action and Spectrum of Activity

Vancomycin (Vanocin) inhibits the synthesis of the bacterial cell wall via binding with cell wall precursors, which makes it bactericidal for dividing microbes. Vancomycin is a very large molecule, which prevents it from passing through the porins in gram-negative cell membranes; thus it is only effective against gram-positive organisms and is primarily used to treat gram-positive bacteria that have resistance to penicillins and cephalosporins.

Mechanism of Resistance

The primary mechanism of resistance to vancomycin is via genetic alteration of the cell wall, so it is resistant to binding by vancomycin. Vancomycin-resistant enterococcus emerged in 1987. Vancomycin-intermediate *S aureus* (VISA), vancomycin-resistant *S aureus* (VRSA), and vancomycin-resistant *C difficile* strains were identified in the 1990s.[34,35]

Clinical Indications for Vancomycin

The CDC has guidelines that restrict the use of vancomycin to specific life-threatening, gram-positive infections.[36] This drug has several common adverse side effects such as **red man syndrome** and can rarely be the cause of nephrotoxicity and ototoxicity. It is almost exclusively used intravenously in a hospital setting. The interested reader can find more information in several recent reviews.[33,37]

Antibiotics That Inhibit or Alter Protein Synthesis

This section includes the antibiotics that work by either inhibiting or altering protein synthesis in bacteria. They include the macrolides, clindamycin (Cleocin), aminoglycosides, tetracycline, the oxazolidinone linezolid (Zyvox), and chloramphenicol (Chloromycetin).

Macrolides

Macrolides (erythromycin, clarithromycin, and azithromycin) and lincosamides (clindamycin) are a group of anti-infectives that have a high molecular weight, hence their name[38] (Table 11-5). Macrolides and lincosamides have a large macrocyclic ring containing 14–16 atoms with deoxy sugars attached to the ring. Erythromycin (E-mycin), the prototypic drug in this group, was developed in 1952 from *Streptomyces erythreus*. Clarithromycin (Biaxin) and azithromycin (Zithromax) are derivatives of erythromycin (E-mycin) and categorized as macrolides. The lincosamide clindamycin (Cleocin) is slightly different chemically from the macrolides but functions similarly and is discussed separately later in the chapter. Ketolides are a newer

generation of drugs based on macrolides that are used for resistant respiratory infections. Telithromycin (Ketek) is the only ketolide available for clinical use at this time and will not be discussed in detail here. All of these agents are considered broad spectrum.

Mechanism of Action and Spectrum of Activity

Macrolides and lincosamides bind to the P site of the 50S ribosome subunit of susceptible organisms, which inhibits RNA-dependent protein synthesis. These drugs may be bacteriostatic or bactericidal depending on the drug concentration, species of bacteria, and growth phase.

Macrolides concentrate in macrophages, polymorphonuclear cells, and other leukocytes that migrate to the site of infection. Thus, the tissue concentration is higher than the plasma concentration, and, via their leukocyte host, these drugs are the first discussed so far in this chapter that are active against intracellular microbes such as *Chlamydia*, *Legionella*, *Mycoplasma pneumonia*, and *Rickettsia* species.

Macrolides and lincosamides have an antibacterial spectrum similar to that of penicillin, but because they do not have a beta-lactam ring, they are effective against beta-lactamase-producing bacteria. Erythromycin (E-mycin) is often used to replace penicillin for persons who are allergic to penicillin, but because it is not effective against gram-negative bacteria such as *H influenzae*, it is important to remember that it is not a replacement for broad-spectrum penicillins such as ampicillin (Principen); nor is it a replacement for cephalosporins.

Succeeding generations of macrolides have a broader spectrum of activity. Clarithromycin is effective against *Bordetella pertussis*, *Campylobacter*, *Chlamydia*, *Helicobacter*, *Legionella* species, *H influenzae*, *Helicobacter pylori*, and *M tuberculosis*. Azithromycin (Zithromax) is less effective than erythromycin (E-mycin) or clarithromycin (Biaxin) against gram-positive bacteria, but is more effective against *H influenza* and *M catarrhalis*, which is why it is one of the current drugs of choice for treating community-acquired pneumonia.

Mechanism of Resistance

The primary mechanism of resistance to macrolide and/or lincosamide is via mutation or methylation of the bacterial ribosome (target-site modification) and, less often, efflux pump. Although resistance to macrolides has plateaued in the last decade, 29.5% of *S pneumoniae* in the United States is currently resistant to macrolides.[39] Because there is significant regional variation in the incidence of

Table 11-5 Macrolides and Clindamycin

Macrolides Generic (Brand)	Indications	Doses	Route	Excretion	Half-Life	Adverse Reactions	Clinical Considerations	FDA Pregnancy Category
Erythromycin (E-mycin, Ery-Tab)	Mild to moderate upper and lower respiratory tract infections, skin infections, *Bordetella pertussis*, *Corynebacterium diphtheriae*. HIV-related infections and atypical organisms—chlamydiae, rickettsiae, legionellae.	250–500 mg qid × 10 days.	PO/IV	Renal/bile	1.4 h	Ototoxicity following IV administration. Prolonged QT interval, cholestatic hepatitis can aggravate myasthenia gravis symptoms. Multiple drug–drug interactions.	Due to GI upset, compliance can be an issue; most erythromycins need to be taken with food.	B
Azithromycin (Zithromax)	Gram-negative organisms, particularly GU pathogens: *Chlamydia trachomatis*, *Neisseria gonorrhoeae*, and *Treponema palladium*.	500 mg × 1 day, then 250 mg × 4 days.	PO	Hepatic	12–68 h	Serious allergic reactions have occurred but are more common with erythromycin. Is not metabolized via CYP450 enzymes and has fewer drug–drug interactions.	Absorbed faster when taken with food, need to take loading dose to obtain effective plasma concentrations.	B
Clarithromycin (Biaxin, Biaxin XL)	*Haemophilus influenzae*, non-TB mycobacterium, and *Helicobacter pylori* (part of triple therapy for *H pylori*).	250–500 mg q 12 h × 7–14 days.	PO	Urine	3–7 h	Multiple drug–drug interactions.	Food delays the onset of action; suspension should not be refrigerated.	C
Clindamycin (Cleocin)	Serious infections caused by anaerobes or *Staphylococcus*; used in combination therapy for polymicrobial infections; bacterial vaginosis, acne vulgaris.	PO: 150–450 mg q 6 h. IM/IV: 300–600 mg q 6–8 h. Intravaginal dose as directed.	PO, IM/IV, intravaginal	Hepatic	2–3 h	Diarrhea most common; dizziness, headache, vertigo, hypotension, nausea, vomiting, rashes.	Persistence of diarrhea indicates need to assess for pseudomembranous colitis.	B

GI = gastrointestinal; GU = genitourinary.

pathogenic bacteria resistant to these agents, clinicians need to be aware of changing recommendations for treatment of common conditions such as community-acquired upper respiratory tract infections, which are often caused by *S pneumoniae* (see Chapter 20). In general, the higher the rate of resistance to penicillin, the higher the rate of resistance to macrolides and lincosamides.

Clinical Indications for Macrolides and Lincosamides

Erythromycin

Erythromycin (E-mycin) is FDA approved to treat upper and lower respiratory tract infections, especially in individuals who have a penicillin allergy. Erythromycin (E-mycin) is effective against *Streptococcus pyogenes*, *S pneumoniae*, *M pneumoniae*, and *Legionella*, with the caveat that resis-

tance to *S pyogenes* and *S pneumoniae* can be significant in some areas. This drug is the agent of choice in corynebacterial sepsis and neonatal and ocular infections. *C trachomatis*, *Helicobacter*, *Listeria*, and other mycobacteria also are susceptible to erythromycin (E-mycin), but because azithromycin (Zithromax) has a more tolerable side effect profile, it is more often recommended as first-line treatment for disorders caused by these microbes. Erythromycin (E-mycin) is still the drug of choice for individuals infected with *B pertussis*, as it eliminates *B pertussis* from the nasopharynx and lowers infectivity.[38]

Clarithromycin

Clarithromycin (Biaxin) is derived from erythromycin and is almost identical with respect to antibacterial activity. Clarithromycin has a half-life of 6 hours compared to 1.5 hours in erythromycin (E-mycin); thus less frequent dosing is possible, and it is approved for treatment of disseminated *Mycobacterium avium* infections in persons with advanced HIV infection.[40] Clarithromycin (Biaxin) also is used for the treatment of *H pylori* infection, a common cause of gastrointestinal reflux disease.

Azithromycin

Azithromycin (Zithromax) has unique properties that allow for once-a-day dosing. The slow release of the drug from tissues gives this medication a tissue half-life of 2–4 days with an elimination half-life of almost 3 days. It is rapidly absorbed, and the oral preparation is well tolerated. The benefit of prescribing azithromycin is that it has fewer gastrointestinal side effects than the other macrolides and its effect continues several days after the last dose due to the long half-life. The 15-member lactone ring results in far fewer drug–drug interactions than occur with erythromycin or clarithromycin. Azithromycin (Zithromax) is the drug of choice for treating *C trachomatis*.

Metabolism

Macrolides are weak bases, and their action is enhanced in an alkaline pH. Erythromycin base is inactivated by stomach acid and thus is manufactured as either enteric or film-coated formulations (Eryc, E-mycin).[38] Erythromycin estolate is an acid-stable salt, and erythromycin ethyl succinate (EES) is an acid-stable ester that converts to erythromycin base in vivo. Macrolides are absorbed from the GI tract, metabolized in the liver via the cytochrome P450 system, and primarily excreted in bile, with 5% excretion occurring through the urine. Erythromycin estolate and azithromycin (Zithromax) are better absorbed when taken with food, whereas erythromycin ethylsuccinate (EES) is better absorbed in the absence of food.

Side Effects and Adverse Reactions

Nausea, vomiting, diarrhea, and anorexia are the most common side effects associated with use of erythromycin and to a lesser extent clarithromycin and azithromycin. The gastrointestinal effects are frequent and significant enough that this is often the reason individuals will discontinue taking erythromycin. Although the exact mechanism of action is not clear, it is dose related. Some suggest that drinking large amounts of water with the dose of medication will minimize the gastrointestinal effects.

Erythromycin estolate has the potential to produce acute cholestatic hepatitis. Therefore, this agent is not an appropriate antibiotic for pregnant women or persons of any age who have compromised liver function.[38]

In high concentrations, erythromycin has the potential to prolong the cardiac QT interval causing the fatal dysrhythmia of **torsades de pointes**. To minimize this risk, erythromycin should be avoided in those with congenital QT prolongation.

The longer half-life associated with clarithromycin (Biaxin) and azithromycin (Zithromax) as compared to erythromycin results in reduced gastrointestinal side effects. The selection of one over the other may be determined by tolerability and cost.

Drug–Drug Interactions

Erythromycin (E-mycin) and clarithromycin (Biaxin) are cytochrome P450 inhibitors. Concomitant use of these drugs with drugs that are substrates for the CYP450 enzymes inhibited by macrolides will increase the plasma levels of the other medications.[41,42] Inhibition of CYP3A4 by erythromycin can cause fatal drug–drug interactions, and thus, knowledge of these interactions is critical when prescribing any macrolide. The most common and significant drug–drug interactions associated with use of macrolides are listed in Table 11-6. Grapefruit juice is an inhibitor of the CYP3A4 enzyme system, which is responsible for the first-pass metabolism of erythromycin (E-mycin) and clarithromycin (Biaxin). This effect causes increased bioavailability of these drugs and results in an increased serum level of the drug. Individuals should be counseled to avoid grapefruit juice during macrolide therapy.[43]

Special Populations

Erythromycin (E-mycin) is an FDA pregnancy category B drug. This drug does cross the placenta, but because plasma levels vary widely in pregnancy, it does not consistently treat the fetus for infection (e.g., syphilis) if administered to the mother.[44] Azithromycin (Zithromax), also in FDA pregnancy category B, is the drug of choice in the treatment of *C trachomatis* infections among pregnant women.

Clarithromycin (Biaxin) and dirithromycin (Dynabac) are in FDA pregnancy category C because studies in animals have revealed adverse effects on the fetus. However, no controlled studies have been conducted among women and no adverse effects have been reported as case studies. Therefore these drugs are not recommended as first-line

Table 11-6 Macrolides: Selected Drug–Drug Interactions*

Drug—Generic (Brand)	Effect if Taken with Macrolides
Erythromycin or Clarithromycin	
Amitriptyline (Elavil)	Increased concentration, risk of *torsades de pointes*.
Antiarrhythmics (Quinidine, ibutilide, sotalol, dofetilide, amiodarone, bretylium, verapamil)	Increased concentration, QT prolongation, *torsades de pointes*, death.
Antipsychotics (haloperidol, risperidone, quetiapine, clozapine)	Increased concentration, risk of *torsades de pointes*, disorientation with clozapine.
Benzodiazepines (Triazolam)†	Amnesia, psychomotor impairment, unconsciousness.
Buspirone (BuSpar)	Increased plasma levels of buspirone.
Calcium channel blockers	Increased plasma levels of calcium channel blockers causing hypotension, tachycardia, edema, dizziness.
Carbamazepine (Tegretol)	Toxic serum levels.
Clozapine (Clozaril)	Disorientation.
Corticosteroids	Increased plasma levels of corticosteroids.
Cyclosporine (Neoral)	Nephrotoxic serum levels.
Digoxin (Lanoxin)	Increased levels of digoxin, mild to moderate gastrointestinal symptoms.
Diltiazem (Cardizem, Tiazac)	Fivefold increased risk of sudden cardiac death.
Ergot alkaloids (e.g., Cafergot)	Increased risk for ergotism (peripheral vasoconstriction).
Felodipine (Plendil)	Increased plasma levels of felodipine.
Fexofenadine (Allegra)	Increased plasma levels of fexofenadine.
Fluoxetine (Prozac)	Delirium.
HMG-CoA inhibitors‡	Increased plasma levels of statins and possible rhabdomyolysis.
Itraconazole (Sporanox)	Fivefold increased risk of sudden cardiac death.
Methylprednisolone	Decreased clearance of methylprednisolone; effect unknown.
Midazolam (Versed)	Increased plasma levels of midazolam.
Pimozide (Orap)	Prolonged QT interval.
Rifabutin (Mycobutin)	Uveitis.
Sildenafil (Viagra)	Priapism.
Theophylline (Theo-Dur)	Increased plasma levels of theophylline may lead to toxicity.
Valproate (Depakote)	Increased plasma levels of valproate.
Verapamil (Calan)	Fivefold increased risk of sudden cardiac death.
Warfarin (Coumadin)	Cardiac dysrhythmias and death.
Azithromycin	
Aluminum and magnesium antacids	Decreased plasma levels of azithromycin.
Digitoxin (Crystodigin)	Increased plasma levels of digitoxin.

* This table is not comprehensive as new information is being generated on a regular basis.
† The benzodiazepines lorazepam (Ativan) and oxazepam (Alepam) are not metabolized by CYP450 enzymes and have no adverse interactions with macrolides.
‡ The HMG-CoA reductase inhibitors pravastatin (Pravachol) and lovastatin (Mevacor) are not metabolized by CYP2C9 and do not have adverse interactions with macrolides.

agents except in situations where no reasonable alternative therapy exists.[44]

Some studies have shown a correlation between erythromycin in breastfeeding mothers and infantile hypertrophic pyloric stenosis in the early newborn. Therefore, azithromycin may be a better choice during the early postpartum period.

Erythromycin is safe to use among elderly individuals who do not have severe cardiac, renal, or hepatic impairment or are not on any of several other medications that could interact with this drug.

Clindamycin

Clindamycin (Cleocin) is a synthetic derivative of lincomycin, and because it is very similar to macrolides is often classed with them. Clindamycin has broad coverage against gram-positive bacteria, many anaerobes such as *Clostridium*, and intracellular bacteria such as *Mycoplasma*. It is more active than the macrolides against several anaerobic bacteria such as *Bacteroides fragilis*. It is not effective for the treatment of disorders caused by gram-negative aerobic bacteria. The mechanism of action and mechanism of resistance to clindamycin are the same as those for the macrolides. Thus, bacteria that are resistant to erythromycin are frequently resistant to clindamycin.

Clinical Indications for Clindamycin

Clindamycin (Cleocin) primarily is used to treat serious infections caused by anaerobes or *Staphylococcus*. It is useful against polymicrobial infections such as pelvic inflammatory disease and bacterial vaginosis and is often used as part of combination therapy for polymicrobial infections. This agent is used in combination with chloroquine to treat malaria. Clindamycin is effective against acnes vulgaris, which is caused by *Propionibacterium acnes.* Although clindamycin is also effective against many gram-positive cocci, there is a high incidence of diarrhea and a risk for developing pseudomembranous colitis when clindamycin is used, which is one reason why it is not considered a first-line treatment over penicillins or cephalosporins for disorders caused by gram-positive cocci. Clindamycin can be used to treat soft-tissue infections caused by MRSA, as many strains of MRSA are still susceptible to this agent.[45]

Metabolism

Clindamycin is easily absorbed orally, and food does not affect absorption. It is also absorbed topically enough to reach therapeutic systemic levels and is formulated as a gel, cream, or lotion. It is 90% protein bound and metabolized via the liver but not via the cytochrome P450 system.

Side Effects and Adverse Reactions

Diarrhea occurs in 2–20% of persons who take clindamycin (Cleocin).[46] Pseudomembranous colitis secondary to overgrowth of *C difficile* is rare but accounts for approximately 3 million cases of diarrhea and colitis per year in the United States.[47] Hypersensitivity reactions occur in approximately 10% of persons who use clindamycin (Cleocin).

Drug–Drug Interactions

Clindamycin enhances the action of muscle relaxants such as pancuronium (Pavulon) and tubocurarine. Clindamycin should not be given concurrently with erythromycin because the two have antagonistic effects.

Special Populations

Clindamycin is an FDA pregnancy category B drug. There are no reports linking clindamycin with congenital defects. One of the more interesting uses of clindamycin is for the treatment of symptomatic bacterial vaginosis. One study found that both a 5–7-day course of clindamycin 800 mg twice daily and clindamycin 2% vaginal cream achieved cure rates similar to those for oral metronidazole, and for this reason it has been recommended by some over metronidazole in the first trimester of pregnancy.[46] Clindamycin is secreted into breast milk, but no adverse effects on nursing infants have been confirmed. It is classified as compatible with breastfeeding by the American Academy of Pediatrics.[30]

Studies have shown no clinically important differences between young and elderly subjects with normal hepatic function and normal renal function. Antibiotic-associated colitis and diarrhea occur more frequently in the elderly and may be more severe. These patients should be carefully monitored for the development of diarrhea.

Aminoglycosides

The first aminoglycoside, streptomycin, was formulated in 1943. Gentamicin was formulated in 1963 and had better coverage of gram-negative bacterial infections. Other aminoglycosides were developed, including amikacin (Amikin), netilmicin (Netromycin), and tobramycin (Nebcin). Since they are parenteral drugs used only in hospital situations, they will be only briefly discussed here. Currently there are seven aminoglycosides available for therapeutic use in the United States. The more commonly used aminoglycosides are gentamicin, tobramycin, and amikacin (Table 11-7).

Mechanism of Action and Spectrum of Activity

Aminoglycosides are potent bactericidal antibiotics that work via creating an irreversible inhibition of bacterial protein synthesis.[48] Energy is needed for the aminoglycoside uptake into the bacterial cell. Anaerobic microorganisms have less oxygen energy available for this uptake, and therefore aminoglycosides are less active against anaerobes and streptococci.[49] These agents are active against aerobic gram-negative bacteria such as *E coli, Klebsiella, P mirabilis, Enterobacter, Acinetobacter, P aeruginosa,* and some mycobacteria. Despite being active against gram-negative organisms, they are not used to treat *N gonorrhea* because there are drugs with fewer adverse reactions available for use against this organism.

Amikacin has the broadest spectrum of activity and is useful in the treatment of gentamicin- or tobramycin-resistant bacteria and in the treatment of infections caused by *Nocardia* and nontuberculous mycobacteria.

Table 11-7 Aminoglycosides

Aminoglycosides Generic (Brand)	Indications	Doses	Route	Excretion	Half-Life	Adverse Reactions	Clinical Considerations	FDA Pregnancy Category
Gentamicin (Garamycin)	Systemic infections, gram-negative bacteremia, peritonitis, meningitis, pneumonia, urosepsis *Pseudomonas aeruginosa, Escherichia coli, Klebsiella, Serratia, Proteus mirabilis.*	1.7 mg/kg q 8 h.	IV	Renal	2–3 h	Ototoxic, nephrotoxic. Hypersensitivity reactions. Hypomagnesemia common.	Inactivated by penicillin; should not be mixed in same IV fluid. Need kidney levels and electrolyte levels monitored with all aminoglycosides.	C
Amikacin (Amikin)	Bacteremia, peritonitis, meningitis.	5 mg/kg q 8 h.	IV	Renal	2–3 h		Same as gentamicin.	C
Streptomycin	Meningitis, pneumonia, urosepsis, tuberculosis, endocarditis, plague, tularemia, glanders, brucellosis.	0.5–2 g q 24 h.	IV	Renal	5–6 h	Has been associated with neurologic disorders.	First aminoglycoside discovered. Used in combinations with other drugs to treat tuberculosis.	D
Tobramycin (Nebcin, TobraDex)	Same as gentamicin. More active against *P aeruginosa* than gentamicin.	1.7 mg/kg q 8 h.	IV/IM, nebulization	Renal	2–3 h	Same as gentamicin.	Inhaled drug used for cystic fibrosis.	C
Neomycin (Neo-Fradin Cortisporin, Neosporin)	Infectious diarrhea, GI sterilization prior to surgery. Topical infections of ear, eye, and skin.	1 g × 3 doses preop, topical 1–3 × daily.	PO/topical	97% unchanged, renal 3%	2–3 h	Most ototoxic and nephrotoxic. Oral has caused intestinal malabsorption. Topical can cause dermatitis.	Not used parenterally.	PO: D Topical: C

Netilmicin has a coverage spectrum similar to that of gentamicin but is less nephrotoxic and ototoxic. Gentamicin and generic tobramycin are the drugs of choice against sensitive bacteria because of their lower cost and the extensive clinical experience with these drugs. Streptomycin is used primarily in the treatment of multidrug-resistant tuberculosis. Streptomycin is both ototoxic and nephrotoxic and is therefore not used if other efficacious drugs are available.

Metabolism

Aminoglycosides are poorly absorbed from the gastrointestinal tract and therefore are administered through the parenteral route to treat systemic infections. Excretion is rapid by glomerular filtration resulting in a half-life varying from 2 to 3 hours in a person with normal renal function.[50] Aminoglycosides have good tissue penetration but have a low concentration in cerebrospinal fluid, lungs, alveoli, and bile.

Mechanism of Resistance

Bacteria can become resistant to aminoglycosides via changes to the cell wall active transport system that facilitates entry into the intracellular compartment, via the usual alteration of the 30S ribosome to prevent binding, or via enzymatic deactivation of the drug. Many enterococci that cause urinary tract infections are resistant to aminoglycosides, and resistance to *P aeruginosa* is increasing, but otherwise, resistance to aminoglycosides is very low.[51]

Clinical Indications for Aminoglycosides

Aminoglycosides are mostly used intravenously to treat serious gram-negative infections such as *P aeruginosa*. These agents have been frequently used in combination with beta-lactam antibiotics to treat polymicrobial infections, because their effect on gram-positive and gram-negative bacteria is synergistic. The beta-lactam effect on the cell wall facilitates the uptake of the aminoglycoside into the cell cytoplasm where it can reach the ribosomes.

Readers will recognize the classic amp and gent combination that is often used in hospital settings to treat infections presumed to be caused by streptococci. That said, because aminoglycoside resistance is increasing, a fluoroquinolone is more often substituted for the aminoglycoside today. Alternatively, they are used in combination with clindamycin to extend coverage to anaerobic organisms. Gentamicin (Garamycin) in combination with tobramycin (Tobrex) and neomycin in combination with bacitracin (Neosporin ointment) are used topically to treat eye infections.

Side Effects and Adverse Reactions

Common minor side effects of aminoglycosides are nausea, vomiting, diarrhea, headache, dizziness, tinnitus, vertigo, and roaring in the ears, all of which are mild and transient. More serious adverse reactions include nephrotoxicity, ototoxicity, neuromuscular blockade, drug fever and electrolyte imbalance. A serum peak level of gentamicin and trough levels should be monitored after the second or third day of treatment and every 3 to 4 days thereafter for the duration of the therapy to ensure effectiveness and prevent toxicity.[50]

Both ototoxic and nephrotoxic effects are directly related to the length of treatment and serum levels experienced by an individual. Management during treatment should include monitoring of blood serum levels and be limited to short-term therapy. A single daily dosage of an aminoglycoside is generally safe, efficacious, and cost effective.

Drug–Drug Interactions

Drugs that are potentially nephrotoxic should not be taken concomitantly with aminoglycosides so the additive risk of nephrotoxicity is avoided. Penicillins, cephalosporins, vancomycin, and loop diuretics all have potential to increase the risk of nephrotoxicity when taken with aminoglycosides. When penicillins and aminoglycosides are present together in high concentrations, penicillins can inactivate aminoglycosides. The risk of renal damage is increased when aminoglycosides are administered with amphotericin B, cephalosporins, and vancomycin, as well as with salicylates and nonsteroidal anti-inflammatory drugs.[29]

Special Populations

The parenteral aminoglycosides are assigned to FDA pregnancy category C. Animal studies have revealed changes in size and weight among rat pups, although human teratogenic effects have not been reported. Aminoglycosides are approved for use with breastfeeding mothers by the American Academy of Pediatrics.[30] Gentamicin levels in breast milk were found to be very low and clinically irrelevant for most infants. Aminoglycosides should be used with caution among the elderly because of potential diminished renal function related to aging that may prolong the half-life of the drug and increase risk of toxicity.[50]

Tetracycline

Tetracyclines were extracted from *Streptomyces* soil microorganisms found in Missouri mud in 1948 and became the first class of antimicrobials to be labeled *broad spectrum* (Table 11-8). However, due to their widespread use in the 1950s and 1960s, there are a large number of resistant bacterial strains today, which limits their therapeutic use. Doxycycline (Vibramycin) and minocycline (Dynacin, Minocin) are the most commonly used formulations of tetracycline.

Mechanism of Action and Spectrum of Activity

Tetracyclines are primarily bacteriostatic, acting by binding to the 30S subunits of the ribosomes in susceptible microorganisms, thereby inhibiting protein synthesis.[52] These pharmaceuticals enter organisms through a combination of passive diffusion and active transport, ultimately preventing the addition of amino acids to the growing peptide.

Tetracyclines are considered broad-spectrum antibiotics effective against gram-positive aerobes and gram-negative aerobes, thereby providing a good alternative for individuals who have a penicillin allergy. However, due to increasing bacterial resistance, they are now more often prescribed for the treatment of susceptible atypical organisms such as *Mycoplasma*, *Chlamydia*, and *Rickettsia* species, *Borrelia* species (especially *Borrelia burgdorferi*, the cause of Lyme disease), and *P acnes*.[52]

This class of antibiotic should not be used for common infections unless the organism has been shown to be sensitive through a culture and sensitivity test. Tetracyclines, most specifically doxycycline (Vibramycin), are considered a first-line drug of choice for *C trachomatis*, *Ureaplasma urealyticum*, and *B burgdorferi*. This class is also used to prevent and treat malaria and may be used in different combination regimens for therapeutic treatment of duodenal ulcers caused by *H pylori*. Tetracyclines are active against *Bacillus anthracis* and *Vibrio cholerae*.

Tigecycline (Tygacil) is similar to tetracycline, although it is technically a glycylcycline. Tigecycline first became

Table 11-8 Tetracyclines

Tetracyclines Generic (Brand)	Indications	Doses	Route	Excretion	Half-Life	Adverse Reactions	Clinical Considerations	FDA Pregnancy Category
Tetracycline (Achromycin Sumycin)	Mild to moderate infections, gonorrhea, severe acne.	1-2 g/day bid–qid.	PO	Renal	6–11 h	Photosensitivity, will accumulate in kidneys, may increase BUN, can cause liver toxicities.	Not to take with products containing calcium, magnesium, zinc, or iron, antacids, and milk products. Food affects absorption.	D
Doxycycline (Vibramycin, Doxy Caps)	Mild to moderate infections, *Chlamydia trachomatis*, more severe gonorrhea, lymphogranuloma venereum, early syphilis, acne, acute exacerbation of bronchitis. Prophylaxis of rat, bat, raccoon bites, anthrax, malaria prophylaxis, *Borrelia burgdorferi* (Lyme disease).	100 mg qd–bid.	PO/IV	Hepatic	18 h	Photosensitivity, GI upset, rash, blood dyscrasias, hepatotoxicity.	Associated with less nephrotoxicity. Can be taken with food.	D
Minocycline (Dynacin, Minocin)	Urethritis, gonorrhea. Has been used to reduce symptoms of arthritis.	100 mg bid.	PO	Hepatic	16 h	Can cause damage to vestibular system, causing dizziness and vertigo and blue–black hyperpigmentation of skin and mucous membranes.	More expensive.	D
Tigecycline (Tygacil)	Broad spectrum including MRSA, vancomycin-resistant enterococci, most aerobic gram-positive and gram-negative bacteria, except *Pseudomonas aeruginosa* and *Proteus*.	100 mg IV followed by 50 mg IV q 12 h × 5–14 days.	IV	Hepatic	36 h	Diarrhea, nausea, and vomiting during first few days of therapy. Photosensitivity.	Has a structure that makes it difficult for bacteria to develop resistance.	D

MRSA = methicillin-resistant *S aureus*; BUN = blood urea nitrogen; GI = gastrointestinal.

available in the United States in 2005. It is very effective against organisms that are resistant to other forms of tetracyclines and penicillins and also is highly effective against many resistant strains of staphylococci and *S aureus*.

Mechanism of Resistance to Tetracyclines

Resistance to tetracyclines is now common among bacteria causing respiratory infections such as pneumococci, *H influenzae*, and *M catarrhalis*.[52] The primary mechanism is efflux pump of the drug out of the intracellular compartment, and to a lesser extent, genetic mutation of the ribosome, thereby preventing binding of the drug to the ribosome.

Clinical Indications for Tetracyclines

One of the most common uses of tetracyclines is for the treatment of acne vulgaris (see Chapter 26). These agents are the drugs of choice for treating infections caused by *Chlamydia*, *Rickettsia*, and spirochetal infections such as syphilis or Lyme disease. They may also be used to treat pneumonia, sinusitis, or urinary tract infections.

Metabolism

Differences among the tetracyclines include variety in absorption after oral administration and elimination from the body. Absorption occurs primarily in the upper intestinal tract and the small intestine, 60–70% for tetracycline (Sumycin), and 95–100% for doxycycline (Vibramycin) or minocycline (Dynacin, Minocin). Both doxycycline and minocycline have a longer half-life than tetracycline itself, enabling a less frequent dosing schedule to be employed. The tetracyclines are widely distributed to tissues throughout the body with the exception of cerebrospinal fluid. The shorter acting tetracyclines are eliminated unchanged without being metabolized by the liver. The longer acting tetracyclines have some metabolism by the liver and are unaffected by kidney dysfunction and therefore are safer in those individuals with renal impairment.[53]

The short-acting tetracyclines, tetracycline (Sumycin) and oxytetracycline (Terramycin), have a serum half-life of 6–8 hours. Intermediate-acting formulations, demeclocycline (Declomycin) and methacycline (Rhodomycin), have a longer serum half-life of 12 hours and are not commonly used. The longest acting agents are doxycycline (Vibramycin) and minocycline (Minocin), with a half-life of 16–18 hours, enabling a once-a-day dosing regimen.

Tigecycline has excellent tissue penetration and is excreted via the biliary tract; thus it is the preferred agent for individuals with renal compromise. Tigecycline has a very long half-life of 36 hours and is currently FDA approved for skin infections and intra-abdominal infections.

Side Effects and Adverse Reactions

Adverse effects to tetracyclines include photosensitivity, especially for individuals with fair skin. Gastrointestinal disturbances are not unusual following both oral and intravenous administration. Nausea, vomiting, and diarrhea result from direct irritation to the intestinal tract. Anorexia has also been reported. Tetracyclines, like other antibiotics, can cause the pseudomembranous colitis caused by *C difficile*, a superinfection of the bowel. In light of this potential complication, if such a diagnosis is made, tetracycline should be discontinued. Vertigo and dizziness have occurred with both doxycycline and minocycline. For individuals who have preexisting renal or liver disease, the risk for hepatotoxicity and nephrotoxicity needs to be considered.[53]

Tetracyclines are potent chelators of metal ions and can cause tooth discoloration of permanent teeth.[52] These drugs are contraindicated for pregnant women and children 8 years of age and younger.

Drug–Drug and Drug–Food Interactions

Doxycycline (Vibramycin) is the only tetracycline extensively metabolized in the liver and subject to drug–drug interactions via inhibition or induction of CYP450 enzymes. The many drug–drug interactions associated with use of tetracyclines and doxycycline in particular are listed in Table 11-9. Tetracyclines form chelate complexes with many drugs containing metal ions such as antacids, calcium, zinc, and iron, which impairs the absorption of the tetracycline. Milk products also contain ions and therefore would decrease absorption of tetracycline. The presence of food in the stomach may reduce absorption of tetracycline by 50%. However, food taken with doxycycline or minocycline only affects absorption by 20% and is not considered clinically significant.[53] Tetracyclines should not be used concomitantly with penicillins because the tetracycline diminishes the bacteriocidal activity of the penicillin.

Diuretics interact with all the tetracyclines except doxycycline by increasing the accumulation of serum urea concentration. Rifampin (Rifadin), phenobarbital (Luminal), phenytoin (Dilantin), and carbamazepine (Tegretol) stimulate liver enzymes, thereby increasing doxycycline metabolism and shortening its half-life.[52]

Special Populations

Tetracyclines are not recommended for pregnant women and are in FDA pregnancy category D. This anti-infective will deposit itself in the teeth of the unborn leading to discoloration and enamel dysplasia. It may also deposit itself in the bone of the developing fetus, causing fetal bone deformities and causing growth restrictions. Children under the age of 8 years may experience similar adverse effects.[44]

Tetracyclines are not contraindicated for breastfeeding mothers, most likely because the drug binds to milk calcium in the breast, reducing transfer to the infant and resulting in low neonatal absorption. Although the short-term exposure of infants to tetracyclines through breast milk is not contraindicated, a period greater than 3 weeks, such as the daily use of the medication for acne, has been associated with dental staining and therefore should be avoided.[27]

Reduction of kidney function is common among the elderly; thus, nephrotoxicity may ensue with the use of tetracyclines since they are not metabolized through the liver but solely eliminated through the kidneys. If a tetracycline is needed to treat an infection in an older person, the daily dose should be reduced unless doxycycline (Vibramycin) is used.[52]

Table 11-9 Tetracycline: Selected Drug–Drug Interactions*

Drug—Generic (Brand)	Effect if Taken with Tetracyclines
Drug–Drug Interactions	
Atovaquone (Mepron)	Decreased plasma levels of atovaquone by 40%. This combination is contraindicated for persons who need to take atovaquone for malarial prevention or treatment.
Barbiturates[†]	Decreased doxycycline plasma levels.
Carbamazepine (Tegretol)	Decreased plasma levels of tetracyclines.
Colestipol (Colestid)	Decreased plasma levels of tetracyclines.
Digoxin (Lanoxin)	Decreased plasma levels of tetracyclines.
Ergotamine (Cafergot)	Increased risk for ergotism. Bilateral upper limb ischemia.
Isotretinoin (Accutane)	Increased risk for idiopathic intracranial hypertension.
Lithium (Eskalith, Lithobid)	Increased lithium levels and possible toxicity.
Methotrexate (Trexall, Rheumatrex)	Increased methotrexate plasma levels and possible toxicity.
Molindone (Moban)	Decreased absorption of tetracyclines.
Oral contraceptives	Decreased plasma levels of oral contraceptives.
Phenytoin (Dilantin)	Decreased plasma levels of tetracyclines.
Quinapril (Accupril)	Decreased absorption of tetracyclines.
Quinine	Increased quinine plasma levels and possible toxicity.
Rifampin (RIF, Rifadin)[†]	Decreased doxycycline levels.
Sucralfate (Carafate)	Decreased absorption of tetracyclines.
Theophylline (Theo-Dur)	Increased theophylline levels.
Warfarin (Coumadin)	Increased plasma levels of warfarin.
Drug–OTC Preparations Interactions	
Antacids	Decreased absorption of tetracyclines.
Bismuth (Pepto-Bismol, Kaopectate)	Decreased absorption of tetracyclines.
Iron-containing vitamins	Decreased absorption of tetracyclines.
Laxatives	
Sodium bicarbonate (baking soda)	Decreased absorption of tetracyclines.
Zinc	Decreased absorption of tetracyclines.
Drug–Food Interactions	
Cheese	Decreased absorption of tetracyclines.
Ethanol[†]	Decreased doxycycline plasma levels if chronic ethanol consumption.
Iron-fortified cereals	Decreased absorption of tetracyclines.
Milk, yogurt, and dairy products	Decreased absorption of tetracyclines.

* This table is not comprehensive as new information is being generated on a regular basis.
† These interactions are specific for doxycycline as opposed to all tetracyclines.

Oxazolidinones

The first oxazolidinone was formulated in the 1970s for control of bacterial and fungal diseases of certain foliage such as tomatoes and other plants. Due to initial adverse effects they were not marketed for human use. It was not until further chemical modifications resulted in safer agents with superior properties that this class of drug became available in the United States in 2000.[54]

Mechanism of Action and Spectrum of Activity

Oxazolidinone, a monoamine oxidase (MAO) inhibitor, inhibits protein synthesis by interfering with the complex formation.[55] Because of the unique binding site of oxazolidinone, it has no known cross-resistance with other drugs. The most commonly used oxazolidinone is linezolid (Zyvox), an antimicrobial that is often bactericidal against streptococci and bacteriostatic against staphylococci and enterococci. This pharmacologic treatment is active against gram-positive anaerobic cocci and gram-positive rods as well as *Legionella, C pneumoniae,* and *H influenzae.* Linezolid (Zyvox) is also used to treat vancomycin- and methicillin-resistant infections caused by multiresistant microbes.[54,56]

Metabolism

Linezolid is rapidly and extensively absorbed after oral administration, and peak serum levels are achieved within 1–2 hours. The time to peak concentration is delayed when linezolid is administered with a high-fat meal. This drug is well distributed in the tissues and metabolized in the liver, and approximately 65% of the dose is eliminated via non-renal clearance.[57] Linezolid (Zyvox) may be administered intravenously or orally, 600 mg twice a day.

Side Effects and Adverse Reactions

Hematologic effects occur in approximately 3% of individuals who take linezolid for longer than a 2-week period of time, although the effects are reversible over time. This medication should be used cautiously among individuals on antiplatelet drugs or those with bleeding disorders. The most common reactions reported, in 2% or more of individuals receiving linezolid (Zyvox), include diarrhea, headache, nausea, vomiting, insomnia, constipation, rash, and dizziness.[57]

More serious adverse reactions include peripheral and optic neuropathy, sometimes progressing to loss of vision in individuals receiving the drug for longer than 28 days. An individual with any visual impairment occurring should have an ophthalmic evaluation performed. Seizures have been reported in individuals, and therefore those at risk should not be administered linezolid.[57]

Drug–Drug Interactions

Linezolid (Zyvox) is a weak monoamine oxidase inhibitor, and, therefore, persons taking linezolid should be counseled to avoid OTC formulations that contain sympathomimetics such as phenylpropanolamine (Dexatrim) or pseudoephedrine (Sudafed). Similarly, they should not consume foods high in tyramine to avoid the potentially serious adverse effect of a hypertensive crisis. (See Chapter 25 for a detailed description of the drug–drug interactions associated with MAO inhibitors.) A small percentage of persons (< 5%) will develop serotonin syndrome when linezolid (Zyvox) is administered concomitantly with selective serotonin reuptake inhibitors.[55]

Special Populations

Linezolid is an FDA pregnancy category C drug because of lack of studies among pregnant women. There is a paucity of data about the use of linezolid among breastfeeding women, although it is likely that it transfers through breast milk to the infant.[30] Because of potential gastrointestinal issues for the newborn, there is some suggestion that it may not be the best choice of an anti-infective agent for the breastfeeding woman.

No differences have been found in safety or efficacy when linezolid is administered to elderly individuals. However, as is true for most antibiotics, it should be used with caution by persons with severe renal and hepatic impairment regardless of age.

Chloramphenicol

Chloramphenicol (Chloromycetin) was first isolated in 1947 from *Streptomyces venezuelae,* an organism found in a soil sample in Venezuela. It is not a first-line antibiotic because of its potential for causing aplastic anemia. It is indicated only for treatment of life-threatening infections such as bacterial meningitis or rickettsial infections in individuals for whom the benefits outweigh the risks of potential toxicity.[56]

Mechanism of Action and Spectrum of Activity

Choramphenicol is a protein synthesis inhibitor and readily penetrates bacterial cells. It binds to the 50S subunit of the ribosome. It also can inhibit mitochondrial protein synthesis in mammalian cells; erythropoietic cells seem to be particularly sensitive to the drug. Chloramphenicol (Chloromycetin) has a wide range that includes activity against gram-positive, gram-negative, aerobic and anaerobic bacteria, including typhoid fever, bacterial meningitis, rickettsial diseases, and brucellosis.

Metabolism

Chloramphenicol (Chloromycetin) is well absorbed orally or intravenously; it is secreted into milk and readily traverses the placental barrier. The half-life of the active drug is 4 hours. The major route of elimination is hepatic metabolism to an inactive metabolite, which is excreted in the urine. For this reason, any renal insufficiency can result in increased plasma concentrations.

Side Effects and Adverse Reactions

Nausea, vomiting, unpleasant taste, diarrhea, and perineal irritation may occur following the oral administration of chloramphenicol. The most important adverse effect, however, is on the bone marrow, a dose-related toxicity presenting as anemia, leukopenia, or thrombocytopenia. The more rare but serious aplastic anemia is an idiosyncratic response leading in many cases to fatal pancytopenia. Hypersensitivity is uncommon and may appear as a macular or vesicular rash; fever may appear simultaneously or be the sole manifestation.[56]

Drug–Drug Interactions

Chloramphenicol (Chloromycetin) is a potent inhibitor of CYP2C619 and CYP3A4 and a weaker inhibitor of CYP2D6. Chloramphenicol prolongs the half-lives of drugs that have a narrow therapeutic window, such as cyclosporine (Neoral), chlorpropamide (Diabinese), phenytoin (Dilantin), tacrolimus (Prototropic), tolbutamide (Orinase), and warfarin (Coumadin). Drugs that induce these enzymes, such as phenobarbital (Luminal) or rifampin (Rifadin), may shorten the half-life of chloramphenicol and result in subtherapeutic concentrations.[29] Chloramphenicol in combination with cimetidine (Tagamet) has an additive effect that increases the risk for inducing bone marrow suppression and aplastic anemia. Chloramphenicol also increases the hypoglycemic effect of sulfonylurea hypoglycemic agents.

Special Populations

There are no reports linking chloramphenicol with birth defects. It crosses the placental barrier at term, however, and there have been reports of the gray baby syndrome in neonates of mothers treated at term with chloramphenicol.

For this reason, it is not recommended in pregnancy.[44] Fatal chloramphenicol (Chloromycetin) toxicity, called gray baby syndrome, may develop in neonates, especially premature babies, when they are exposed to excessive doses of chloramphenicol due to failure of the drug to be metabolized in the liver as well as inadequate renal excretion. Neonates should never be given this drug without close monitoring of serum levels.[56] Chloramphenicol is secreted in breast milk but not in high enough concentrations to produce gray baby syndrome, and no infant toxicity has been reported in the literature from use by lactating women. However, this antibiotic is not recommended for use in lactating mothers due to potential toxic effects.[44]

There are no data about increased risk in the elderly following use of chloramphenacol. Caution should be exercised, however, and when other antimicrobial drugs that are equally effective and potentially less toxic than chloramphenicol are available, they should be used.

Antibiotics That Affect DNA

There are several antibiotics that alter DNA in bacterium. Included in this section are the fluoroquinolones and antiprotozoans. Rifampin (Rifadin) and possibly isoniazid (INH) also alter bacterial DNA, but these drugs are included under the *Antimycobacterial Agents* section later in this chapter.

Fluoroquinolones

Quinolones originally were used for therapeutic treatment of gram-negative organisms found in urinary tract infections. The initial quinolone was nalidixic acid (NegGram). However, that agent is no longer used because of the prevalence of resistant organisms. The fluoroquinolones were formulated by adding a fluorine molecule to the quinolone structure, thereby increasing the drug's therapeutic use. This drug family is more commonly called fluoroquinolones today.

Like cephalosporins, fluoroquinolones are categorized by generations (Table 11-10). The second generation of fluoroquinolones includes ciprofloxacin (Cipro), enoxacin (Penetrex), lomefloxacin (Maxaquin), levofloxacin (Levaquin), ofloxacin (Floxin), and pefloxacin. Gemifloxacin (Factive) and moxifloxacin (Avelox) comprise the third generation of fluoroquinolones. The third generation has improved coverage against gram-positive organisms and a notably longer half-life. A number of broader spectrum agents have been developed (e.g., sparfloxacin, trovafloxacin) but have been withdrawn in the United States due to problems with toxicity.

Mechanism of Action and Spectrum of Activity

Fluoroquinolones block bacterial DNA synthesis by interfering with the bacterial transcription process, thus preventing replication of the bacteria or rendering it infertile. These drugs display a concentration-dependent bactericidal effect that produces a higher peak concentration, resulting in a more rapid and complete eradication of the offending microorganism.[58] Fluoroquinolones are used for various infections caused by aerobic gram-negative bacteria and other microorganisms. These drugs are also effective against *Shigella*, *Salmonella*, toxigenic *E coli*, and *Campylobacter*.

Clinical Indications

With the exception of moxifloxacin (Avelox), all fluoroquinolones may be used for the treatment of urinary tract infections caused by multidrug-resistant bacteria. Norfloxacin (Noroxin) is approved in the United States only for treatment of urinary tract infections. A 7-day course of ofloxacin (Floxin) is an alternative to doxycycline (Vibramycin) or azithromycin (Zithromax) for *C trachomatis* infections. A single oral dose of ofloxacin or ciprofloxacin (Cipro) is effective against some strains of *N gonorrhoeae* but is not first line due to increasing resistance. A 14-day course of ofloxacin (Floxin) has been effective in treatment of pelvic inflammatory disease along with an antibiotic with anaerobic activity. A 3-day course of ciprofloxacin is effective against chancroid.

Fluoroquinolones have been effective in the treatment of bone, joint, and soft tissue infections. Norfloxacin (Noroxin), ciprofloxacin (Cipro), and a 5-day course of ofloxacin (Floxin) are effective against shigellosis and traveler's diarrhea. Newer fluoroquinolones such as moxifloxacin (Avelox) and gatifloxacin (Tequin) are indicated for community-acquired pneumonia (*S pneumoniae)* and may be comparable to the beta-lactams.[58] Gemifloxacin (Factive) and moxifloxacin (Avelox) are often referred to as the *respiratory fluoroquinolones* because of their enhanced gram-positive activity against the atypical chlamydial *mycoplasma* and *Legionella* pneumonia infections. Ciprofloxacin (Cipro) or levofloxacin (Levaquin), along with azithromycin (Zithromax), are antibiotics of choice for *Legionella pneumophila*. Ciprofloxacin (Cipro) is the preferred agent for prophylaxis and treatment of anthrax.

Metabolism

Fluoroquinolones are absorbed well when taken orally, (80–95% with high bioavailability) and thus have excellent distribution to tissues and body fluids. Peak concentrations in serum are usually attained within 3 hours of administration. Food does not seem to affect the extent of quinolone absorption but may delay the time to reach peak drug concentrations in serum.[58] Serum half-life ranges from 3 to 5 hours for norfloxacin and ciprofloxacin to 20 hours for sparfloxacin. Elimination for the majority of preparations is through the renal system, and doses must be adjusted in renal failure. Pefloxacin and moxifloxacin are metabolized predominantly by the liver.[58]

Side Effects and Adverse Reactions

Fluoroquinolones are in general well tolerated. The most common effects are nausea, vomiting, and diarrhea (5–10% incidence). Various CNS effects that include headache (5% incidence), dizziness, and insomnia are the second most common side effects. Rashes overall occur in

Table 11-10 Fluoroquinolones*

Fluoroquinolone	Indications	Doses	Route	Excretion	Half-Life	Adverse Reactions[†]	Clinical Considerations	FDA Pregnancy Category
Second-Generation Quinolones								
Ciprofloxacin (Cipro)	Mild to moderate UTI, lower respiratory tract, sinusitis, GI and skin infections, prostate, typhoid fever, bone and joint infections, anthrax prevention, gonorrhea, meningococcal carrier.	250–750 mg PO qd–bid IV: 200–400 mg q 12 h.	PO/IV	Renal/biliary	3–5 h	Mild GI/CNS symptoms, blood glucose abnormalities; can cause rupture of the Achilles tendon (contraindicated for children < 18 y).	Avoid compounds with cations. Need proper hydration. Will cause precipitates to form if given in same IV line with ampicillin or aminophylline.	C
Lomefloxacin (Maxaquin)		400 mg.	PO	Renal	6–8 h	Mild GI/CNS symptoms; photosensitivity reactions can be severe; prolonged QT syndrome and tendon rupture.	Once-daily dosing. Does not elevate theophylline levels.	C
Norfloxacin (Noroxin)		400 mg bid × 3 days.	PO	Renal/biliary	3–4 h	Mild GI/CNS symptoms; risk for tendon rupture (do not use < age 18 y).		C
Ofloxacin (Floxin)		200–400 mg bid.	PO/IV	Renal/biliary	6–8 h	Dizziness, drowsiness, headache, GI symptoms, tendon rupture (do not use < age 18 y).		C
Third-Generation Quinolones								
Levofloxacin (Levaquin)	Same as ciprofloxacin plus many gram-negative bacteria.	250–500 mg qd.	PO/IV	Renal	6–8 h	Mild GI/CNS symptoms, prolonged QT syndrome, rarely peripheral neuropathy.		C
Fourth-Generation Quinolones								
Gemifloxacin (Factive)	Same as Cipro. Increased activity against S pneumoniae.	320 mg qd × 5 days.	PO	Renal	6–8 h	Mild GI/CNS symptoms prolonged QT syndrome, hypersensitivity reaction.	Used for community-acquired pneumonia and acute exacerbation of chronic bronchitis.	C
Moxifloxacin (Avelox)	Same as Cipro. Increased activity against S pneumoniae.	400 mg qd.	PO/IV	Fecal	15 h	Altered sense of taste, prolongs QT interval.		C

GI = gastrointestinal; CNS = central nervous system.

* This is not a complete list of the quinolones available in the United States today. There are several others in each of the generations.

[†] Pseudomembranous colitis may occur with all quinolones; monitor for persistence of diarrhea.

approximately 1%, but interestingly, about 14% of women younger then 40 years who take gemifloxacin (Factive) for more than 7 days develop a rash, and therefore, this drug is given for a maximum of 5 days of continuous therapy if possible. The rash is even more likely to occur if the woman is taking estrogen-containing products as well as the fluoroquinolone. Photosensitivity may occur among individuals taking lomefloxacin and pefloxacin.

There are some serious adverse effects that can occur following use of these antibiotics. In 2008, the FDA issued a black box warning noting that fluoroquinolones increase the risk for developing tendinitis and tendon rupture in persons of all ages. Levofloxacin (Maxaquin), gemifloxacin (Factive), and moxifloxacin (Avelox) are contraindicated for individuals with a known prolonged QT interval or hypokalemia, as they are known to prolong the QT interval. Fluoroquinolones occasionally can cause interstitial nephritis. The clinical presentation of an antibiotic-induced interstitial nephritis varies, and, therefore, it should be suspected in any individual on a fluoroquinolone who develops an acute renal dysfunction.[59]

Fluoroquinolone use has been associated with central nervous system effects including headaches, hallucinations, slurred speech, confusion, and even seizures in 1–2% of recipients. These symptoms usually resolve once the medication is discontinued, but the presence of a neurologic disorder might predispose to these symptoms and, therefore, needs to be assessed.[59] In addition, the development of pseudomembranous colitis secondary to overgrowth of *C difficile* is particularly associated with fluoroquinolone treatment.[60] *C difficile* is resistant to fluoroquinolones, and as use of these drugs has increased, so has the incidence of pseudomembranous colitis (Box 11-3). Finally, fluoroquinolones cause hypersensitivity reactions including anaphylaxis, albeit very rarely.

Drug–Drug Interactions

Common drug–drug interactions associated with fluoroquinolones are listed in Table 11-11. Absorption of fluoroquinolones is impaired in the presence of magnesium, calcium, aluminum, and zinc. Therefore, any form of antacid, vitamin, or dairy product containing these cations must be avoided prior to taking the medication and for several hours after administration.

When fluoroquinolones are taken with caffeine, warfarin (Coumadin), cyclosporine (Neoral), or theophylline (Theo-Dur), they cause increased serum concentrations of these drugs. There is an increased risk of seizures when ciprofloxacin is used concurrently with foscarnet (Foscavir).[30]

Special Populations

Fluoroquinolones are FDA pregnancy category C drugs due to lack of adequate studies. However, they are generally considered to be contraindicated for pregnant women and children under the age of 8 years because these drugs cause cartilage abnormalities in animals. The studies evaluating outcomes of babies born to women exposed to norfloxacin (Noroxin) or ciprofloxacin (Cipro) during the first trimester have identified no increase in teratogenic risks.[61] But because other, equally effective drugs are better studied and known to be safe in pregnancy, fluoroquinolines are contraindicated.

Current studies suggest that the amount of fluoroquinolones present in breast milk is quite low. However, if ciprofloxacin (Cipro) is used by a lactating mother, the infant needs to be observed closely for diarrhea. Ciprofloxacin was recently approved by the American Academy of Pediatrics for use in breastfeeding women.[30] Levofloxacin (Maxaquin), ofloxacin (Floxin), and norfloxacin (Noroxin) have milk plasma ratios even lower in breast milk than ciprofloxacin, and often are first-line choices for breastfeeding mothers when this class of drugs is indicated.

Antiprotozoans

There is a wide variety of protozoal parasites in humans that may be transmitted by insects, other mammals, or other humans. There are no effective vaccines, so chemotherapy is the only practical treatment, and integrity of the immune system is crucial. Protozoal infections include malaria, amebiasis, giardiasis, trichamoniasis, toxoplasmosis, giardiasis, cryptosporidiosis, and trypanosomiasis (sleeping sickness).[62] Toxoplasmosis is primarily treated with drugs discussed elsewhere, such as pyrimethamine (Daraprim), sulfadiazine, and clindamycin (Cleocin). Many of the other infective protozoans are found primarily in developing countries; this discussion will concentrate on the antiprotozoal drugs most commonly used in this country. These include the nitroimidazoles, metronidazole (Flagyl) and tinidazole (Tindamax). The drugs used to treat lice, scabies (1% permethrin [Nix]), and pinworms (mebendazole [Vermox]) are also reviewed (Table 11-12).

Metronidazole

Metronidazole (Flagyl) is a nitroimidazole drug that was introduced for the first time in 1959 for its antiprotozoal

> ### Box 11-3 Don't Forget *C Diff*
>
> You are the clinician covering triage for your practice when you get a call concerning MD, who is a 42-year-old woman who completed a course of ciprofloxacin (Cipro) for presumed Mycoplasma pneumonia 2 weeks ago. MD reported diarrhea and abdominal cramping for 4 days that had not resolved following a day of bowel rest and use of loperamide (Imodium). She was having 3–4 episodes of foul-smelling diarrhea per day and felt very ill but was afebrile.
>
> You have a suspicion that this individual may have a pseudomembranous colitis caused by *Clostridium difficile* (called *C diff*, which is pronounced "see-diff"). This gram-positive, spore-forming rod is a normal inhabitant of the intestine, but it has become resistant to fluoroquinolones, so when ciprofloxacin eradicates most of the gut flora, the *C difficile* takes off and overgrows. Infection with *C difficile* is an identified risk associated with fluoroquinolone therapy. There is some evidence that *C difficile* may also be acquired via oral ingestion of the heat-resistant spores, which then convert to the vegetative forms in the intestine.
>
> *C difficile* releases toxins that cause the symptoms of pseudomembranous colitis. If untreated, *C diff* can cause sepsis, bowel perforation, or toxic megacolon, although these complications are more common in persons at higher risk for infection—i.e., the elderly and those who were recently hospitalized with a serious medical condition or need for surgical procedure.
>
> You meet this woman in the office. The physical exam is essentially normal except for the symptoms she reported, so you determine that she does not need hospitalization. The antibiotics that effectively treat *C difficile* are metronidazole (Flagyl) 500 mg three times a day for 10–14 days or vancomycin 500 mg four times a day for 10–14 days. Metronidazole can cause a metallic taste in the mouth and nausea or occasionally vomiting. Vancomycin should be used for persons who do not tolerate metronidazole or for pregnant women. There is some evidence that probiotics are also effective in helping restore the normal gut flora in persons with *C diff*.
>
> Follow-up is very important because approximately 25% of persons with *C difficile* will become reinfected following treatment. It is not clear if these reinfections are a relapse or a true reinfection from ingesting *C difficile* spores. Treatment of reinfection is a second course of the same antibiotic used the first time, and most relapses respond to a second course if needed. MD had a resolution of symptoms 5 days after she started treatment with metronidazole (Flagyl).

activity in treating *Trichomonas vaginalis*. This drug penetrates well into the tissues and has been found to be bactericidal and effective for treatment of both anaerobic bacteria and protozoa.

Mechanism of Action and Spectrum of Activity

Metronidazole (Flagyl) is a prodrug that works in a unique way. Susceptible anaerobic organisms are able to donate electrons to the metronidazole molecule. This changes metronidazole (Flagyl) into a highly reactive nitro anion radical that kills the host organism via alteration of the DNA and perhaps other significant biologic proteins within that organism. Thus metronidazole (Flagyl) enters the cell by diffusion and is cytotoxic via the transformation into destructive free radicals.[63] Metronidazole is effective against the anaerobes *B fragilis*, *C difficile* (*C diff*), *Fusobacterium*, *Gardnerella vaginalis*, and *H pylori*. The agent is used for treatment of anaerobic intra-abdominal and pelvic infections. Because it penetrates well into the cerebrospinal fluid, it is useful for the treatment of meningitis or brain abscess caused by *B fragilis*. Metronidazole is effective against pseudomembranous colitis caused by *C difficile*. Resistance to metronidazole is being seen increasingly in all organisms that have traditionally been susceptible, so treatment failures do occur.

Clinical Indications

A single, 2-gram dose of metronidazole (Flagyl) is effective against *T vaginalis* 90% of the time[62] (Chapter 31). Metronidazole (Flagyl) is also the standard treatment for bacterial vaginosis in a 7-day course of treatment. It is the agent of choice for treatment of amebiasis and is a component of prophylaxis against postoperative mixed aerobic and anaerobic infections.

Metabolism

Metronidazole is a well-absorbed antibacterial agent that is widely distributed throughout the body tissues, and it is metabolized in the liver and excreted renally. The half-life is

Table 11-11 Fluoroquinolones: Selected Drug–Drug Interactions*

Drug—Generic (Brand)	Effect if Taken with Fluoroquinolone
All Quinolone Interactions	
Antacids	Reduced absorption of fluoroquinolone.
Antiarrhythmics: Class 1a and III (quinidine, ibutilide [Covert], Sotalol [Betapace], dofetilide [Tikosyn], amiodarone [Cordarone], verapamil [Calan])	Increased concentration of antiarrhythmic, QT prolongation, *torsades de pointes*, death.
Antipsychotics (e.g., haloperidol [Haldol], risperidone [Risperdal], clozapine [Clozaril])	Increased concentration of antipsychotic, risk of *torsades de pointes*, disorientation with clozapine.
Multivitamins containing calcium, iron, or zinc	Decreased absorption of fluoroquinolones.
Nonsteroidal anti-inflammatory drugs (NSAIDs)	CNS stimulation and convulsive seizures.
Sucralfate (Carafate)	Decreased absorption of fluoroquinolones.
Ciprofloxacin (Cipro), Enoxacin (Penetrex), Norfloxacin (Noroxin) Interactions	
Clozapine (Clozaril)	Increased levels of clozapine.
Cyclosporine (Neoral)	Increased serum concentration of cyclosporin and risk for nephrotoxicity.
Duloxetine (Cymbalta)	Increased plasma levels of duloxetine.
Foscarnet (Foscavir)	Increased risk of seizures.
Glyburide (Micronase)	Hypoglycemia requiring urgent treatment.
Nitrofurantoin (Macrobid)	Nitrofurantoin antagonizes the antibiotic effect of norfloxacin in the urinary tract.
Phenytoin (Dilantin)	Increased plasma levels of phenytoin and possible phenytoin toxicity.
Tacrine (Cognex)	Increased plasma levels of tacrine.
Theophylline (Theo-Dur)	Increased theophylline levels and potential theophylline toxicity.
Tizanidine (Zanaflex)	Increased plasma levels of tizanidine.
Warfarin (Coumadin)	Increased plasma levels of warfarin.
Drug–Food Interactions	
Caffeine	Increased plasma levels of caffeine.
Milk, yogurt, and dairy products	Decreased absorption of fluoroquinolones.

* This table is not comprehensive. New information is being identified on a regular basis.

approximately 6–9 hours. Formulations of metronidazole can be obtained in oral, parenteral, topical, and vaginal preparations.

Side Effects and Adverse Reactions

Gastrointestinal issues such as nausea, metallic taste, and diarrhea are the most commonly reported side effects. Individuals with hepatic insufficiency may have difficulty metabolizing metronidazole. More serious side effects that are rare include peripheral neuropathy, seizures, and pancreatitis. Seizures have been reported with high doses and peripheral neuropathy with prolonged use of metronidazole.[62]

Drug–Drug Interactions

Metronidazole is structurally similar to disulfiram, and if the two are taken together acute psychosis can occur. Some individuals who drink alcohol while taking metronidazole will develop a disulfiram-like (Antabuse-like) effect of pronounced GI upset, flushing, and palpitations. Therefore, individuals should be counseled to avoid alcohol while taking the agent and for at least 24 hours after the last dose. This includes alcoholic drinks, alcohol-based cough syrups, flavorings, or other products.[62] Metronidazole (Flagyl) increases the plasma levels of several drugs including cyclosporine (Neoral), carbamazepine (Tegretol), lithium (Eskalith, Lithane), phenytoin (Dilantin), tacrolimus (Prototropic), and warfarin (Coumadin). The few drugs that are CYP34A inducers, phenobarbital (Luminal), phenytoin (Dilantin), and rifampin (Rifadin), increase the metabolism of metronidazole (Flagyl), thereby decreasing the effectiveness of metronidazole.[62]

Special Populations

The use of metronidazole has been controversial in pregnancy. Early animal studies showed the drug to be mutagenic and potentially carcinogenic. Although the drug has not been shown in humans to act this way, some have advised against the use of the drug especially during the first trimester of pregnancy. However, the drug is rated as FDA pregnancy category B therapy, and most sources now advocate use during any trimester of pregnancy when the drug is needed.[30,44] No reports of untoward effects in breastfed infants with any of the dosage regimens have been published, but metronidazole is excreted into breast milk in larger than usual amounts (approximately 20%).[30] However, the American Academy of Pediatrics recommends discontinuing breastfeeding for 12–24 hours to allow excretion of the dose, or the mother can pump her breast milk and dump to not suppress lactation. Metronidazole should be used with caution in older adults who might have renal impairment or hepatic or biliary disease.

Tinidazole

Tinidazole (Tindamax) is a nitroimidazole, approved in 2004, that is similar to metronidazole in its effect against

Table 11-12 Nitromidazoles

Nitroimidazole Generic (Brand)	Indication	Doses	Route	Excretion	Half-Life	Adverse Reactions	Clinical Considerations	FDA Pregnancy Category
Metronidazole (Flagyl)	*Trichomonas vaginalis*, bacterial vaginosis, amebiasis, pseudomembranous colitis, component of treatment of polymicrobial infections.	TV: 2 g single dose. BV: 250 mg tid or 375–500 mg bid. Amebiasis: 500–750 mg tid. Pseudomembranous colitis: 250–500 mg tid–qid × 10–14 days.	PO/IV	Hepatic/ renal/ fecal	6–12 h	Dizziness, headache, abdominal pain, anorexia, nausea, vomiting, unpleasant taste, leucopenia, peripheral neuropathy, disulfiram-like reaction with alcohol.	Avoid alcohol due to pronounced GI upset, flushing, and palpitations. Caution in hepatic insufficiency.	B: some conflicting conclusions; use with caution in 1st trimester (contraindicated per manufacturer guidelines); 2nd and 3rd OK.
Tinidazole (Tindamax)	Bacterial vaginosis, *T vaginalis*, giardiasis, amebiasis.	BV: 1 g qd × 5 or 2 g qd × 2. TV, giardiasis: 2 g single dose. Amebiasis: 2 g/d × 3.	PO	Renal/ fecal	12–14 h	Dizziness, headache, constipation, dyspepsia, metallic or bitter taste, vomiting, vaginal candidiasis.	Take with food to minimize gastrointestinal discomforts. Avoid alcohol while taking.	C: very limited human studies; consider only if metronidazole is ineffective; avoid in 1st trimester.

TV = *T vaginalis*; BV = bacterial vaginosis.

amebiasis, giardiasis, and trichomoniasis, and has a better toxicity profile than metronidazole.

Mechanism of Action and Spectrum of Activity

Tinidazole (Tindamax) has a mechanism of action similar to that of metronidazole (Flagyl). Free nitro-anion radicals are generated as a result of reduction of the nitro group of tinidazole by *T vaginalis*, which is responsible for the antiprotozoal activity. The mechanism by which tinidazole acts against *Giardia* and *Entamoeba* species is unknown. Approximately 38% of *T vaginalis* isolates exhibiting reduced susceptibility to metronidazole (Flagyl) also show reduced susceptibility to tinidazole (Tindamax) in vitro, but this appears much less commonly in practice (see Chapter 31). It is recommended, in order to reduce development of resistance, that tinidazole be used only in cases where metronidazole is shown to be ineffective.

Clinical Indications

Tinidazole is indicated for the treatment of *T vaginalis* and bacterial vaginosis. It is also used in the treatment of amebiasis and for giardiasis in children older than 3 years.

Metabolism

Oral tinidazole is readily absorbed by simple diffusion. It crosses the placental and blood–brain barriers. Peak plasma concentrations are reached in 2–3 hours, and the half-life is 12–14 hours. It is excreted mainly in the urine; plasma clearance is reduced in the presence of hepatic impairment.

Side Effects and Adverse Reactions

The most common side effects include dizziness and headache, gastrointestinal effects such as constipation or diarrhea, vomiting, dyspepsia, and a metallic or bitter taste. Transient leukopenia or neutropenia may occur. It may also cause vaginal candidiasis in women.

Drug–Drug Interactions

Although studies have not been performed yet, it is assumed, due to the near relationship with metronidazole, that tinidazole will have the same drug–drug interactions. Alcohol should be avoided, as with metronidazole.

Special Populations

Tinidazole (Tindamax) is in pregnancy category C due to lack of human studies. There is some evidence of mutagenic potential, and it should be avoided in the first trimester. Current recommendations suggest interruption of breast-feeding for up to 3 days following administration of tinida-zole due to lack of safety studies. This is longer than is recommended for use of metronidazole and reflects lack of knowledge and a cautious approach by the professional organizations that issue such guidelines.

There are not enough studies of use of tinidazole (Tindamax) in the elderly to assess response. Caution should be exercised in the presence of hepatic or renal insufficiency due to decreased clearance.

Unusual Antibiotics

Antibiotics in the following sections have a mechanism of action that is different from those in the preceding sections, so they are described separately. They include the sulfonamides, trimethoprim (Trimpex, Primsol), and nitrofurantoin (Macrodantin).

Sulfonamides

Sulfonamides were the first agents formulated for the treatment of bacterial infections in the 1930s and were actually discovered in 1936 by Gerhard Domagk (1895–1965), who found that an industrial dye named Pronto-sil was able to cure infections in mice. He subsequently treated his daughter who was very ill with a streptococcal infection that failed to respond to standard treatments and won the Nobel Prize in 1938 for the discovery. Because Adolf Hitler prohibited German scientists from accepting this prize, he declined it but was given the award (without the prize money) in 1947.[64] Similar to the first-generation quinolones, sulfonamides are no longer used as single agents because of the evolution of resistant microbes. When used in combination, however, sulfonamides and trimethoprim (Primsol) both are enhanced, and the cover-age against gram-negative organisms is improved. A com-bination formulation sulfamethoxazole and trimethoprim (SMX-TMP [Bactrim, Septra]) is available (Table 11-13). Additionally, trimethoprim concentrates in vaginal fluid and prostatic fluid. This property allows the medication to have increased antibacterial activity when compared to most other formulations for infections of the vaginal and prostate tissue.

Mechanism of Action and Spectrum of Activity

Although a wide variety of chemical modifications of the sulfonamides have been synthesized, all basically share the same mechanism of action. These agents compete with para-aminobenzoic acid (PABA) for incorporation into folic acid. Once the sulfa drug is incorporated, the synthe-sis of folic acid is stopped. The sulfonamides are bacterio-static in that they inhibit bacterial growth by interfering with microbial folic acid synthesis.

Sulfisoxazole (Gantrisin) is primarily used as a pediatric preparation. These drugs are indicated for mild to mod-erate antibacterial or antiprotozoal infections. Sulfasala-zine (Azulfidine) is used for inflammatory bowel disease including ulcerative colitis and enteritis, and is discussed in Chapter 17. Acute toxoplasmosis can be treated with sulfa-diazine in combination with pyrimethamine.

Trimethoprim/Sulfamethoxazole

The combination of trimethoprim/sulfamethoxazole (TMP/SMX; Bactrim, Septra) has a unique mechanism of action whereby both drugs independently affect one part of the pathway that results in synthesis of tetrahydrofolic acid, which is essential for the production of bacterial DNA. TMP/SMX (Bactrim, Septra) has been effective against pneumonia, toxoplasmosis, and nocardiosis, as well as other bacterial infections. This combination formulation is especially therapeutic for urinary tract infections caused by *E coli*, *Klebsiella*, *Enterobacter*, *P mirabilis*, and *Proteus vulgaris* and is therefore well known to women's health-care providers. Although there is widespread resistance to both trimethoprim and sulfamethoxazole, resistance to the combination formulation is not common.[65]

Metabolism

Sulfonamides are categorized into three major groups. The first category includes the oral absorbable agents that are absorbed from the stomach and small intestine, metabolized in the liver, distributed widely throughout the body tissues, and cross the placenta barrier. Oral absorbable formulations include sulfisoxazole (Gantrisin). A second category of sulfon-amides is the oral, nonabsorbent group that includes Sulfasala-zine (Azulfidine). These drugs are relatively poorly absorbed from the gastrointestinal tract and, because of this effect, have been used in the past to suppress the susceptible bowel flora before surgery. A third category of sulfonamides includes topical preparations. For example, neomycin is available in a topical form for treatment of ophthalmic infections and skin

Table 11-13 Oral Absorbable Sulfonamides

Sulfonamides Generic (Brand)	Indications	Doses	Route	Excretion	Half-Life	Adverse Reactions	Clinical Considerations	FDA Pregnancy Category
Sulfisoxazole—generic (Gantrisin)	Antibacterial or antiprotozoal: UTI, otitis media, sinusitis, bronchitis, pneumonia, traveler's diarrhea, diverticulitis, rheumatic fever prophylaxis. Serum levels peak in 2–6 h.	1–2 g q 6 h (dose varies dependent on indication).	PO/ IM/ IV/ subQ, oral preferred.	Hepatic	5–8 h	Similar adverse reactions with all sulfonamides: nausea, rash, confusion, dizziness, diarrhea, blood dyscrasias, Stevens-Johnson syndrome, kernicterus, renal damage.	Short acting. Maximum adult daily dose is 8 g. Fluid intake should be sufficient with all sulfonamides.	C*
Sulfadiazine—generic	Same; best for prophylaxis of meningitis. When combined with pyrimethamine, is used to treat toxoplasmosis.	1 g q 4–6 h.	PO	Renal	10 h		Short acting.	C*
Trimethoprim and sulfamethoxazole TMP/SMX (Bactrim DS, Septra DS)	Same plus *Shigella flexneri*.	160/800 mg q 12 h PO, 10–20 mg/kg/day IV.	PO/IV	Hepatic/renal	6–11 h and 9–12 h	Most commonly seen are nausea, vomiting, and rash. Hyperkalemia and blood dyscrasias can occur. Many drug–drug interactions.		C*

* These drugs are not teratogenic but should not be given in the third trimester due to risk of hyperbilirubinemia, severe jaundice, hemolytic anemia, and theoretically kernicterus in the newborn.

infections and in liquid form for ear infections (Neosporin, Cortisporin). Silver sulfadiazine (Silvadene) is another topical agent with very low toxicity and is used for prevention of infection in cases of skin burns. (See Chapter 26 for more details about dermatological treatments.)

The oral absorbable sulfonamides used as antibiotics are short acting, intermediate acting, or long acting, based upon their half-lives. Sulfisoxazole (Gantrisin) is a short-acting preparation. Serum levels generally peak 2–6 hours after oral administration.

The dose of trimethoprim, when given alone, is 100 mg twice a day for acute urinary infections. When trimethoprim is given in combination with sulfamethoxazole, in a double-strength tablet, the dosing is 160 mg of trimethoprim with 800 mg of sulfamethoxazole, given every 12 hours. One-half of the regular dose may be used prophylactically to suppress recurrent urinary tract infections. This dosing regimen may safely be maintained over a period of months when prescribed for use three times a week.

Side Effects and Adverse Reactions

Sulfonamides can cause multiple side effects, including nausea, vomiting, diarrhea, rash, fever, headache, and depression.

Adverse effects such as jaundice, hepatic necrosis, drug-induced lupus, and a serum sickness-like syndrome are also well-known hypersensitivity reactions. Sulfonamides can crystalize in the renal tubules, causing an acute renal failure, and they can block secretion of creatinine. Acute pancreatitis has been associated with sulfonamides.[59] Individuals who are glucose 6-phosphate dehydrogenase-deficient (G6PD) are at risk for a sulfonamide-induced hemolytic anemia. Sulfonamides also can cause a neutropenia or agranulocytosis or induction of a thrombocytopenia.

The sulfonamides are among the most common causes of Stevens-Johnson syndrome, a rare condition that can evolve into toxic epidermal necrolysis with a mortality rate of 30%. Therefore, Stevens-Johnson syndrome should be considered if a woman presents with inflammation of the mucous membranes and a painful, blistering rash. A history of sulfonamide use will help confirm the diagnosis. Long-acting sulfonamides have been associated with fatal hypersensitivity reactions, especially in children, and this severely limits their use.[59]

Sulfa Allergy

The sulfonamide allergy is important because other frequently used classes of drugs (e.g., sulfonylureas, diuretics, celecoxib [Celebrex], dapsone, and sumatriptan [Imitrex]) have a sulfonamide moiety, and the existence of cross-reactivity has been controversial. Cutaneous rashes develop in 3–4% of persons who take drugs that have a sulfonamide component (usually 72 hours to 2 weeks after administration), and approximately 0.4% of persons who take a sulfonamide drug develop a severe hypersensitivity reaction such as anaphylaxis or Stevens-Johnson syndrome.[66] The exception is in persons who are HIV positive. Individuals who are HIV positive develop rashes to sulfonamide antibiotics 30–50% of the time for reasons that have not been fully elucidated.

The culprit responsible for these reactions is a reactive metabolite that results from the P450 cytochrome facilitated metabolism of the parent drug. Cross-reactivity of the allergic reaction between sulfonamide antibiotics and sulfonamide nonantibiotics does not occur because this reactive metabolite is not generated in the metabolism of sulfonamide nonantibiotics.[65] However, approximately 10% of persons who report a reaction to sulfonamide antibiotics will also have a reaction to sulfonamide nonantibiotics, and it is theorized at this time that these persons have an innate tendency to develop drug reactions, which in this case would be secondary to an underlying mechanism that is not related to the sulfonamide moiety.[66]

Manufacturers of sulfonamide-containing drugs vary in how the products are labeled with regard to sulfonamide allergy. Some do not mention the possibility of cross-reactivity, some warn that it might exist, and some suggest their product is contraindicated for persons who report a sulfonamide allergy. There are no clear clinical guidelines for practitioners, and therefore decisions about prescribing sulfonamide nonantibiotics to individuals who have reported a sulfa allergy following a course of a sulfonamide antibiotic must be individualized.

Drug–Drug Interactions

Sulfonamides can displace sulfonylurea hypoglycemic drugs from plasma protein-binding sites, which increases the plasma level of the sulfonylurea and results in more hypoglycemic effect and rarely bone marrow depression.[30] Sulfonamides can also potentiate the action of potassium-sparing diuretics and thiazide diuretics, causing hyperkalemia. Hyperkalemia can also occur if sulfonamides are taken in conjunction with ACE inhibitors. In addition, there are a few unusual interactions. For example, sulfonamides and amantadine (Symmetrel) taken together can cause acute mental confusion. Methenamine, which is used to prevent urinary tract infection,

can cause sulfonamides to crystalize in urine. Agents that increase the risk of sulfonamide toxicity include phenylbutazone (Butazolidin), salicylates, and probenecid (Benemid).[65] Agents that decrease the plasma levels of sulfonamides include procaine, rifampin (RIF, Rifadin), and dapsone (Aczone).

Trimethoprim is a potent inhibitor of renal tubular secretion, which can result in increased plasma levels of many drugs. Dapsone (Aczone), digoxin (Lanoxin), dofetilide (Tikosyn), methotrexate (Trexall), phenytoin (Dilantin), repaglinide (Prandin), rifampin (RIF, Rifadin), rosiglitazone (Avandia), and warfarin (Coumadin) plasma levels can be increased when administered with trimethoprim/sulfamethoxazole.

Special Populations

Sulfonamides are not teratogenic, but they should not be administered during the last month of pregnancy because they compete for bilirubin-binding sites on plasma albumin and may increase neonatal blood levels of unconjugated bilirubin, increasing the risk of kernicterus.[67] Trimethoprim has a small association with an increased risk for cardiovascular defects and oral clefts. There is the risk of megaloblastic anemia in a folate-deficient woman, more commonly seen during pregnancy, with the use of sulfonamides.

Sulfonamides should be used with caution among breastfeeding mothers with fragile newborns, premature infants, infants with G6PD deficiency or infants under the age of 2 months with hyperbilirubinemia.[44] Sulfisoxazole is considered the best choice of sulfonamides during lactation due to reduced transfer to the nursing infant.[30]

A major concern with the elderly individual is renal impairment, and, therefore, a fluid intake of 2 liters daily is advised to reduce the formation of renal crystals and stones when taking sulfonamides. With the combination of trimethoprim/sulfamethoxazole, older adults are more susceptible to the adverse effects of skin reactions and bone marrow depression. Folic acid deficiency may occur in debilitated individuals and alcoholics because of the interference of folic acid metabolism with this drug, and therefore these individuals should be advised to supplement with folic acid.

Nitrofurantoin

Nitrofurantoin (Macrodantin) is a classic urinary tract antimicrobial and is available as macrocrystals as well as a combination of monohydrate/macrocrystals (Macrobid). Nitrofurantoin is a urinary antiseptic prescribed exclusively for treatment or prophylaxis of urinary tract infections because of its pharmacologic and chemical properties.

Mechanism of Action, Spectrum of Activity, and Metabolism

The mechanism of action of nitrofurantoin is not well known; however, nitrofurantoin is involved with bacterial metabolism and may work by disrupting the bacterial cell formation.[58] Nitrofurantoin achieves high concentrations only in kidney tissue and urine where it is active against most organisms responsible for urinary tract infections. It is not effective against *Pseudomonas* and *Proteus* microbes. Nitrofurantoin (Macrodantin, Macrobid) is absorbed and metabolized efficiently, minimizing the side effects for most individuals. Excretion is through the kidneys. The drug does not obtain therapeutic levels in most body tissues and, therefore, should not be used in upper tract and complicated infections. It has minimal side effects on bowel and vaginal flora and has been used effectively in prophylaxis of urinary tract infections for more than 40 years. There is low bacterial resistance with this drug, but the cure rate of acute cystitis is approximately 80–85% when given twice daily for 7 days, which is lower than the cure rate seen following treatment with TMP/SMX (Bactrim, Septra).[65]

Side Effects and Adverse Reactions

Nitrofurantoin can cause gastrointestinal distress. This drug can cause peripheral polyneuropathy, especially in individuals with impaired renal function, anemia, diabetes, electrolyte imbalance, and vitamin B deficiency, and in those who are debilitated. This drug should be used with caution among individuals with peripheral polyneuropathy or with G6PD deficiency. A hypersensitive reaction to the drug manifests as a pulmonary reaction with an acute or chronic cough, dyspnea, and fever.

Drug–Drug Interactions

Probenecid (Benemid), an antigout agent, should be avoided because when taken simultaneously with nitrofurantoin, probenecid inhibits renal excretion of nitrofurantoin (Macrodantin, Macrobid). Concomitant magnesium or quinolones should not be administered with nitrofurantoin due to their antagonistic action with nitrofurantoin.[65]

Special Populations

Nitrofurantoin is an FDA pregnancy category B drug and often is used in pregnancy for the treatment of asymptomatic bacteruria and cystitis. Since it is not a sulfa-containing drug, there are no limitations on its use in the third trimester. No concerns have been reported among healthy breastfeeding mothers and their infants. As previously noted, nitrofurantoin should be avoided or used with caution for a lactating woman whose infant has G6PD.[30]

Nitrofurantoin is not contraindicated for a healthy, mature individual. However, the geriatric woman who has severe renal disease should avoid use of the drug because this could reduce nitrofurantoin excretion and cause a systemic toxicity.

▋ Antimycobacterial Agents

M tuberculosis is the bacterium responsible for tuberculosis infection and was first isolated in 1882 by Robert Koch, a German physician who eventually received the Nobel Prize for his discovery.[68] The mycobacterial organisms are intracellular pathogens that reside within macrophages. They are enclosed in a lipid-rich cell wall membrane and are therefore often inaccessible to pharmacologic agents. Additionally, these pathogens have the ability to develop resistance that requires combination therapies to be continued for months, or in some cases, years, to successfully eradicate the pathogen. Management of mycobacterial infections requires long-term persistence with the treatment regimen.

Thirty percent of the world's population is infected with *M tuberculosis*, making it the most common infection globally.[69] Multiple-drug-resistant tuberculosis (MDR-TB) and extensively drug-resistant tuberculosis (XDR-TB) are increasing. The World Health Organization estimates 4.6% of all cases of tuberculosis are MDR-TB, but in a widely divergent pattern geographically.[70]

Tuberculosis (TB) can affect any organ in the body, but it most often affects lung tissue. Once the infection has been acquired, it may or may not become active depending on the individual's age, immunity status, and the presence of other health factors such as HIV, renal insufficiency, body mass index (BMI) below 10% of normal, concomitant medical conditions, and other environmental conditions.

Once exposed and infected, a healthy individual will develop a cell-mediated immunity 2–12 weeks after the initial infection but remain asymptomatic because small amounts of bacteria remain in nodules that the macrophages and T cells have surrounded and isolated to prevent the spread of the infection to other body tissues. These bacteria do have the capability of becoming activated at a later point in time. Thus latent tuberculosis infection (LTBI) is an inactive form of TB that is detected through an abnormal skin test. The individual with latent TB does not yet have any lung damage, is not contagious, and is asymptomatic. However, this individual has approximately a 10% risk of developing the active form of TB and requires treatment.[70-72] The risk is higher for individuals with conditions that compromise their immunity or health.[71]

There are currently 10 drugs FDA approved for treatment of TB.[71] Table 11-14 lists the first-line drugs discussed in this chapter, and Figure 11-4 illustrates their mechanism of action. LTBI can be treated with isoniazid (INH) monotherapy. The first-line agents that form a four-drug regimen for treatment of active TB are isoniazid (INH), rifampin (RIF, Rifadin), ethambutol (EMB, Myambutol), and pyrazinamide (PZA). Streptomycin is added in situations that meet certain specifications. In addition, there are two newer forms of rifampin—rifabutin (Mycobutin) and rifapentine (Priftin)—that can be used for persons who have shown intolerance to rifampin (Rifadin).[71] Drug regimens recommended for treatment of LTBI are reviewed in Chapter 20.

Nondrug resistant TB is treated with a combination of first-line therapy. Treatment of MDR-TB requires additional drugs and regimens and is beyond the scope of this discussion. The interested reader is referred to the CDC for current guidelines.[71]

Isoniazid

Isoniazid (INH, Nydrazid, Lionized) is an antibacterial medication that has been used to both prevent and treat TB since 1952. Isoniazid should be a part of treatment for all persons with TB unless there is a compelling reason to omit it such as allergy to the pharmacologic agent.[71]

Mechanism of Action

Isoniazid is a prodrug, the exact mechanism of which remains unknown, but is theorized to have multiple mechanisms, contributing to its effectiveness. A primary mechanism of action is in the disruption of the mycolic acid, an essential component in the lipid cell wall synthesis.[73] Alternative mechanisms that have been proposed

include DNA impairment of the bacterium, decrease in cellular respiration, and lipid peroxidation of the bacterial wall.[73]

Metabolism

Isoniazid is readily absorbed by the gastrointestinal tract and diffuses well to all body tissues. The medication reaches peak plasma concentrations within 2 hours of dosing and is metabolized by the liver and excreted in the urine. The dose adjustment for individuals with hepatic insufficiency has not been specifically defined. The dose for isoniazid is 5 mg/kg/day, and a maximum dose is 300 mg daily.

Side Effects and Adverse Reactions

Isoniazid is metabolized in the liver to inactive metabolites, principally by acetylation, the rate of which is genetically determined. The rate of acetylation does not alter treatment course but does alter the half-life, and poor acetylators have an increased incidence of drug–drug interactions.[72] Side effects include, rash, fever, and neuritis, all of which occur in $\leq 2\%$ of persons taking this drug.

Isoniazid (INH) increases secretion of pyridoxine (vitamin B_6) in urine and can cause vitamin B_6 deficiency, which manifests as peripheral neuritis, although this is rare at the 5-mg/kg dose. Peripheral neuropathy is more common in pregnant women and in persons with seizure disorders, diabetes, alcoholism, malnutrition, or HIV infection. If peripheral neuropathies occur, they can be successfully treated with 25 mg/day pyridoxine with ultimate resolution without permanent disability.[71]

Isoniazid can stimulate true hypersensitivity reactions, of which hepatotoxicity is the most serious. Hepatotoxicity occurs in 5–20% of persons on a regular multidrug regimen, a wide range that reflects different vulnerabilities in different populations.[74] Adults started on isoniazid should have baseline values of liver enzymes recorded, and then monitoring during therapy is individualized.

Approximately 20% of persons taking isoniazid will develop antinuclear antibodies, but < 1% actually develop a lupus-like syndrome.[71] Rarely, persons taking isoniazid (INH) will develop seizures, mental abnormalities, or florid psychosis.

Rifampin

Rifampin (RIF, Rifadin) is a bactericidal antibiotic first introduced in the late 1960s. This agent is a semisynthetic

Table 11-14 Antimycobacterial Agents

Drug—Generic (Brand)	Indications	Doses	Route	Excretion	Half-Life	Adverse Reaction	Clinical Considerations	FDA Pregnancy Category
Isoniazid (INH, Lionized)	First-line TB. Used in pregnancy.	5 mg/kg. Max 300 mg/dose.	PO/IM	Renal	1–5 h	Peripheral neuropathies, hepatitis, nausea, vomiting, mild CNS effects.	Contraindicated in acute hepatic disease. Vitamin B_6 may prevent peripheral neuropathy and CNS effects. Drug–drug interactions: see Table 11-15.	C
Rifampin (Rifadin)	First-line TB. Used in pregnancy.	10 mg/kg. Max 600 mg/dose.	PO/IV	Renal/fecal	1.5–5 h	GI upset, hepatitis, skin rashes, blood dyscrasia, Headaches, fatigue, dizziness.	Causes orange discoloration in urine, tears, and sweat. Contraindicated in acute hepatic disease. Interferes with oral contraceptives: Use alternate method. NNRTIs and PIs contraindicated if on rifampin. Drug–drug interactions: see Table 11-16.	C
Rifabutin (Mycobutin)	For MAC prophylaxis in persons with HIV or for persons intolerant to rifampin.	300 mg/day.	PO/IV	Renal/fecal	45 h	GI upset, skin rashes, hepatotoxicity, neutropenia, thrombocytopenia, uveitis, arthralgias, and neutropenia seen with high doses.	Causes orange discoloration in urine, tears, and sweat. Has the most drug–drug interactions of the first-line TB agents. NNRTIs and PIs contraindicated if on Rifabutin. Drug–drug interactions: see Table 11-16.	C
Rifapentine (Priftin)	For MAC prophylaxis in persons with HIV or for persons intolerant to rifampin.	600 mg/wk taken as 300 mg twice wk, supplied as 150-mg tablets.	PO	Renal/fecal	14–17 h	GI upset, skin rashes, uveitis seen with high doses. Hepatotoxicity, neutropenia, thrombocytopenia rare.	Causes orange discoloration in urine, tears, and sweat. Take on an empty stomach. Drug–drug interactions: see Table 11-16.	C
Pyrazinamide (PZA)	First-line TB. Not used in pregnancy.	15–30 mg/kg. Max 2 g/dose.	PO	Renal	9–10 h	Mild elevation of serum aminotransferases and uric acid, rashes, arthralgia, GI disturbances.	Contraindicated in acute hepatic disease, acute gout. May make glucose control more difficult in persons with diabetes.	C
Ethambutol (Myambutol)	First-line TB. Used in pregnancy.	5–25 mg/kg. Max 2.5 g/dose.	PO	Renal	3–4 h	Red-green color blindness, blurred vision, GI disturbance, rash.	Extreme caution with renal failure, optic neuritis.	B

MAC mycobacterium avium complex; NNRTI = nonnucleoside reverse transcriptase inhibitors; PI = protease inhibitor.

derivative of rifamycin and one of the four drugs used in the standard regimen for treating active tuberculosis.[69,71]

Mechanism of Action and Spectrum of Activity

Rifampin inhibits DNA activity, thereby suppressing RNA synthesis. This pharmacologic agent is most active against bacteria undergoing cell division and those that are semidormant.[69,71] Rifampin is used in the treatment of gram-positive and gram-negative cocci, some enteric bacteria, mycobacteria such as TB, and *Chlamydia*. Rifampin (RIF, Rifadin) often is used in combination with isoniazid for the treatment of active TB, although it may be given alone as an alternative to isoniazid for the treatment of latent TB. Rifampin is very effective in the treatment of mycobacteria because it has the ability to penetrate phagocytic cells, killing organisms that are not well accessed by other therapeutic agents.

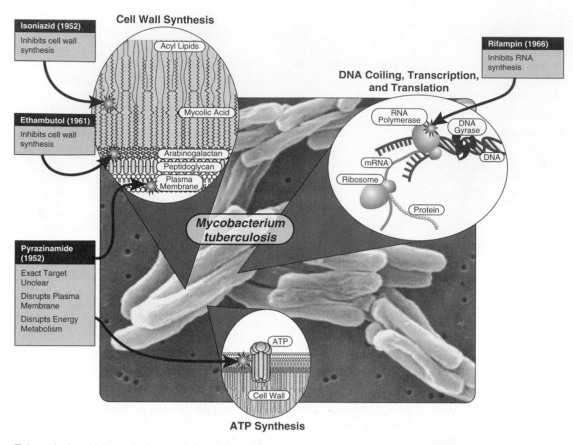

Tuberculosis, which results from an infection with *Mycobacterium tuberculosis*, can usually be cured with a combination of first-line drugs taken for several months. Shown here are the four drugs in the standard regimen of first-line drugs and their modes of action. Also shown are the dates these four drugs were discovered—all more than 40 years ago.

Figure 11-4 Mechanism of action of anti-tuberculosis drugs used in the first-line treatment protocols.

Source: National Institute of Allergy and Infectious Diseases; National Institutes of Health; Centers for Disease Control and Prevention.

Rifampin (RIF, Rifadin), in combination with a second therapeutic agent, is a good choice for the treatment of microbes that are harbored within abscesses and lung cavities. Further uses have been in the treatment of osteomyelitis, prosthetic valve endocarditis, and Hansen's disease (leprosy). Finally, rifampin has been used in the treatment of methicillin-resistant *S aureus* (MRSA) in combination with other antibiotics.

Metabolism

Rifampin (RIF, Rifadin) is well absorbed after oral administration and is metabolized and excreted by the liver through bile, primarily in the stool with a small amount being excreted in the urine. It is widely distributed to tissues.

Side Effects and Adverse Reactions

Side effects associated with rifampin may include drowsiness and dizziness. The medication stains tears, sweat, and urine orange, and all persons taking this drug will experience this effect.[70] This phenomenon does not pose any serious risk and spontaneously resolves after the medication has been discontinued. Other side effects include fever, chills, headaches, muscle aches, nausea, vomiting and gastrointestinal pain, a flu-like symptom that is rare, more likely to occur with intermittent dosing, and is not dangerous.[71] Pruritus with or without rash is also self-limited and occurs in approximately 6% of persons on rifampin.[71]

More serious adverse reactions include hepatotoxicity, which is more common when rifampin is given with isoniazid (approximately 3% incidence) than when rifampin is administered alone (1%, but this regimen is not recommended).[74] Rifampin can rarely stimulate a Type II hypersensitivity reaction that is manifest as thrombocytopenia, hemolytic anemia, acute renal failure, or thrombocytopenic purpura.

Pyrazinamide

Pyrazinamide (PZA) is a derivative of niacinamide and is active against mycobacteria and tubercle bacilli.[69,71] This agent is used in combination with isoniazid (INH) and rifampin (Rifadin) for the 6-month therapy course when treating active TB. Pyrazinamide is not used as monotherapy. The addition of pyrazinamide to the initial 2 months of treatment allows the regimen to be reduced from 9 months to 6 months.[69,71]

Mechanism of Action

Pyrazinamide (PZA) has the least well understood mechanism of action of the first-line TB drugs. Pyrazinamide, a prodrug, is metabolized to the active metabolite pyrazinoic acid. Pyrazinoic acid then inhibits fatty acid synthesis in the microbe. In addition, pyrazinoic acid lowers the pH below that which is necessary for growth of *M tuberculosis*. Pyrazinamide (PZA) is bacteriostatic and works best against dormant or semidormant mycobacterial populations. Thus when used with isoniazid (INH) and rifampin (RIF), it helps eliminate all forms of the organism faster and can allow for a shorter period of therapy.[71]

Metabolism

Pyrazinamide (PZA) is well absorbed and able to cross the blood–brain barrier when the meninges are inflamed. Pyrazinamide is metabolized in the liver, and approximately 70% of the drug is excreted in the urine.

Side Effects and Adverse Reactions

Arthralgia is the most common side effect (40%), although it rarely warrants discontinuation of the medication and can be managed with aspirin or NSAIDs.[71] Mild nausea and vomiting are also common but not severe unless higher doses are used. Transient rashes can occur, and it is important to counsel individuals that photosensitivity can occur when taking this drug. Hyperuricemia with gout has been reported, and history of gout is reason to consider avoiding pyrazinamide as the TB treatment regimen.[71] Among the four agents used for the treatment of active TB, pyrazinamide (PZA) is the most hepatotoxic. That said, the incidence is still approximately 1% at most.[71]

Ethambutol

Ethambutol (EMB, Myambutol) is bacteriostatic against actively growing *M tuberculosis* and is used in combination with isoniazid (INH), rifampin (RIF, Rifadin), and pyrazinamide (PZA), primarily to add extra coverage in case the organism is resistant to isoniazid.

Mechanism of Activity

Ethambutol (EMB) is a bacteriostatic agent that works by inhibiting the cell wall formation of the TB bacilli.[69] Ultimately, the cell wall is rendered more permeable, improving the access of the combination drugs to the microbe.

Metabolism

Ethambutol (EMB) is well absorbed from the gastrointestinal tract and widely distributed in body tissues. It is metabolized in the liver and excreted renally. Ethambutol accumulates in individuals with renal insufficiency, and the dose requires downward adjustment.

Side Effects and Adverse Reactions

Arthralgia is the most common side effect of ethambutol, but it rarely is cause for discontinuation of the medication. A decrease in the renal secretion of uric acid may result in hyperuricemia.[69,71] Adverse effects are less frequent with ethambutol than other antituberculosis agents. Loss of visual acuity may occur, and red-green color blindness may develop when the dose is continued for several months but is reversible and rare at lower doses. Cutaneous reactions and peripheral neuritis are rare adverse effects.

Drug Resistance to Antitubercular Agents

The tubercular bacilli are able to mutate into drug-resistant strains quite effectively, and thus drug resistance is an increasingly difficult problem. Drug-resistant strains to each of the primary agents used exist, but cross-resistance is not common, so combination therapies are generally effective. That said, strains that are resistant to isoniazid (INH) and rifampin (RIF), called multiple-drug resistant strains or MDR, are becoming more prevalent and require a complicated therapeutic approach best managed by specialists in this field.

Drug–Drug Interactions

Isoniazid (INH) and rifampin (RIH, Rifadin) are the two antitubercular agents that have clinically significant drug–drug interactions. Isoniazid (INH) is an inhibitor of several CYP450 enzymes, and as one would expect, it has multiple drug–drug interactions because the inhibition is permanent until new CYP450 enzyme is synthesized. Rifampin (RIF, Rifadin) is a potent inducer of several CYP450 enzymes and thus can decrease the therapeutic effects of more than 100 medications.[75] This can lead to adverse health consequences when rifampin is given to persons on some commonly used drugs such as oral contraceptives, warfarin (Coumadin), or sulfonylureas. Drug–drug interactions are among the most important considerations for persons prescribing and taking isoniazid or rifampin (RIF, Rifadin). Common drug–drug interactions of these two drugs are listed in Tables 11-15 and 11-16.[69,75]

All food can impair absorption of isoniazid and rifampin. Isoniazid is a weak MAO inhibitor, and there are case reports of a cheese reaction when isoniazid is taken with cheese or wine. (See Chapter 25 for a full description of this reaction.) Antacids inhibit oral absorption of ethambutol and should be avoided by individuals taking it.

Special Populations

Isoniazid (INH), rifampin (RIF), and pyrazinamide (PZA) are assigned to FDA pregnancy category C, whereas ethambutol (EMB) is in FDA pregnancy category B.[44] Animal studies have failed to demonstrate teratogenic effects, but few studies have been conducted among humans. All four drugs are recommended for use by pregnant women who have active TB.[71] If INH is prescribed to pregnant women, 25 mg per day of pyridoxine should be prescribed as well.[71]

All four medications are secreted in breast milk in minute quantities ranging from 0.75% to 2.3% of the maternal dose at most. Careful monitoring of the breastfeeding infant for liver toxicity and neuritis is required, but there are no contraindications to use of these drugs by lactating women and no reports of adverse effects on a nursing infant.[44]

Similarly, all four drugs are recommended for use by elderly individuals if needed. Because the elderly are more likely to have kidney or liver dysfunction, monitoring for liver toxicity is important.

▌Antifungal Agents

There has been a dramatic increase in the incidence of fungal infections over the last 20 years related to the emergence of broad-spectrum antibiotics, advances in critical care, surgery, and cancer treatment, as well as the HIV epidemic.[76] Antifungal agents have gone through revolutionary changes and have become much less toxic; however, the emergence of azole-resistant organisms as well as the increased incidence of mycotic infections have generated new challenges.

The fungi that cause infections in humans are eukaryotic organisms that grow as either multicellular filaments called hyphae (molds) or single-cell organisms (yeasts), which often branch into pseudohyphae. They usually reproduce by making spores. Fungi possess a chitinous cell wall, which is the major focus of most antifungal medications. Fungi that act as human pathogens come from the genera *Aspergillus*, *Candida*, *Cryptococcus*, *Histoplasma*, and *Pneumocystis*.

Fungal infections are called **mycoses** and are categorized as superficial (localized to skin, hair, or nails), subcutaneous (confined to the dermis or subcutaneous tissue), systemic (infection in internal organs), or opportunistic (infection secondary to immunocompromise in the host). One interesting property of these infections is that they are not transmissible. Dermatophytes are fungi that only live on dead tissue such as nails or skin.

Chemically, the five classes of antifungal agents are azoles, polyenes, allylamines and benzylamines, echinocandins, and an *other* class that contains a few antifungals with unique mechanisms of action. The antifungal agents are also categorized as (1) oral and parenteral systemic drugs, (2) oral drugs for mucocutaneous infections, and (3) topical antifungal drugs used to treat mucocutaneous infections.

Table 11-15 Isoniazid: Selected Drug Interactions*

Drug—Generic (Brand)	Effect if Taken with Isoniazid
Acetaminophen (Tylenol)	Increased plasma levels of acetaminophen and increased risk of hepatotoxicity. Risk greatest 24 h after last dose of isoniazid. Contraindicated combination.
Carbamazepine (Tegretol)	Increased plasma levels of carbamazepine and increased risk for hepatotoxicity.
Chlorzoxazone (Paraflex)	Increased plasma levels of chlorzoxazone.
Diazepam (Valium)	Increased plasma levels of diazepam.
Levodopa (Sinemet)	Hypertension, flushing, tachycardia. Isoniazid acts as an MAO inhibitor, causing excess catecholamine when given with levodopa, which is a dopamine precursor.
Phenytoin (Dilantin)	Increased plasma levels of phenytoin.
Rifampin (Rifadin)	Increased risk for hepatotoxicity.
Theophylline (Theo-Dur)	Increased plasma levels of theophylline.
Triazolam (Halcion)†	Increased plasma levels of triazolam.
Valproic acid (Depakote)	Increased plasma levels of valproic acid and increased risk of hepatotoxicity.
Warfarin (Coumadin)	Increased plasma levels of warfarin.

* This table is not comprehensive. New information is being identified on a regular basis
† This interaction is documented; there are case reports of increased plasma levels of other benzodiazepines when taken with isoniazid, but studies are needed to elucidate the relationships.

Table 11-16 Rifampin, Rifabutin, and Rifapentine: Selected Drug–Drug Interactions*

Drug—Generic (Brand)	Effect if Taken with Rifampin, Rifabutin, or Rifapentine
Antiarrhythmic	
Amiodarone (Cora)	Increased amiodarone metabolism. Avoid concomitant use.
Digoxin (Lanoxin)	Digoxin dosage may need to be increased.
Quinidine	Quinidine dosage may need to be increased.
Anticoagulant	
Warfarin (Coumadin)	Increased renal clearance of warfarin and decreased efficacy.
Antimicrobial	
Chloramphenicol (Chloromycetin)	Increased risk of aplastic anemia. Avoid concomitant use.
Doxycycline (Vibramycin)	A 50% increase in the doxycycline dosage may be necessary.
Erythromycin (E-mycin)	Erythromycin metabolism is increased and plasma levels lowered. Efficacy can be decreased.
Anticonvulsants	
Lamotrigine (Lamictal)	Increased clearance noted, monitor clinical condition; may require increase in dosage. Measurement of phenytoin and valproic acid concentrations suggested.
Phenytoin (Dilantin)	
Valproic acid (Depakote)	
Angiotensin II Receptor Blocker	
Irbesartan (Avapro)	Increased metabolism, which decreases effect of angiotensin II receptor blocker.
Losartan (Cozaar)	
Antifungal	
Fluconazole (Diflucan)	Fluconazole dosage may need to be increased.
Itraconazole (Sporanox)	Substantial reduction in plasma level noted. Concomitant use not recommended.
Ketoconazole (Nizoral)	Substantial reduction in plasma level noted. Concomitant use not recommended.
Benzodiazepines	
Buspirone (BuSpar)	Increased metabolism, which decreases effect of buspirone.
Diazepam (Valium)	Increased metabolism, which decreases effect of diazepam.
Triazolam (Halcion)	Increased metabolism, which decreases effect of triazolam.
Zolpidem (Ambien)	Increased metabolism, which decreases effect of zolpidem.
Beta-Blockers	
Carvedilol (Coreg)	Increased clearance, resulting in reduced effects. Monitor and increase dosage as necessary.
Metoprolol (Lopressor)	
Propranolol (Inderal)	

Drug—Generic (Brand)	Effect if Taken with Rifampin, Rifabutin, or Rifapentine
Calcium Channel Blockers	
Diltiazem (Cardizem)	Substantial reduction in diltiazem, verapamil, and nifedipine concentrations. Avoid concomitant use with rifampin.
Verapamil (Calan)	
Nifedipine (PO only) (Procardia)	
Glucocorticoids	
Methyl prednisolone (Medrol)	Decreased plasma levels of glucocorticoids, and dose must be adjusted.
Hormonal Therapy and Oral Contraceptives	
Contraceptives, oral	Documented clinical failures; use nonpharmacologic contraceptive agent.
Levothyroxine (Synthroid)	Decreased plasma levels of levothyroxine.
Opioids	
Methadone	Decreased plasma levels of methadone are significant and dose of methadone might need to be doubled. Morphine dose may need to be increased to have efficacy.
Morphine and codeine	
Protease Inhibitors	
Indinavir (Crixivan)	Concomitant use with protease inhibitors is contraindicated. Rifabutin should be used if a rifamycin is necessary, with appropriate manufacturer-recommended dosage adjustment.
Nelfinavir (Viracept)	
Ritonavir (Norvir)	
Saquinavir (Invirase, Fortovase)	
Psychotropic Drugs	
Haloperidol (Haldol)	Decreased plasma levels of haloperidol.
Nortriptyline (Aventyl)	Decreased plasma levels of nortriptyline.
Quetiapine (Seroquel)	Decreased plasma levels of quetiapine.
Selective Serotonin Reuptake Inhibitors	
Citalopram (Celexa)	Serotonin syndrome.
Escitalopram (Lexapro)	
Fluvoxamine (Luvox)	
Statins	
Fluvastatin (Lescol)	Increased statin metabolism and reduced efficacy. Substantially increasing dose may be necessary.
Lovastatin (Mevacor, Altocor)	
Simvastatin (Zocor)	
Sulfonylureas	
Chlorpropamide (Diabinese)	Increased hypoglycemic effect.
Glyburide (Micronase, DiaBeta)	
Tolbutamide (Orinase)	
Theophylline (Theo-Dur)	Theophylline is more extensively metabolized and plasma levels fall.

* This table is not comprehensive. New information is being identified on a regular basis.

This categorization is how they are presented in this chapter[77] (Table 11-17). We will first review the group of agents most commonly used in the clinical situation, which are the azoles, followed by agents less commonly used. Those that are parenteral only, and therefore used only in hospitalized individuals, are not reviewed in detail.

Azoles

The azoles are primarily fungistatic rather than fungicidal. Twelve drugs exist in the azole family used to treat topical fungal infections. Of these 12 drugs, 4 are also used to treat systemic mycoses, including ketoconazole (Nizoral), itraconazole (Sporanox), fluconazole (Diflucan), and voriconazole (Vfend).

Azoles are classified as imidazoles or triazoles, according to the number of nitrogen atoms they have in the azole ring.[77] The imidazoles include ketoconazole (Nizoral), miconazole (Monistat), and clotrimazole (Lotrimin). The triazoles include itraconazole (Sporanox), fluconazole (Diflucan), and voriconazole (Vfend). These agents are newer and less toxic than the imidazoles.

Mechanism of Activity and Spectrum of Activity

Both imidazoles and triazoles act by inhibiting enzyme cytochrome P450 14 α-demethylase. This enzyme is critical for the conversion of lanosterol to ergosterol, which is a requirement for fungal cell membrane synthesis. Specificity is conferred via this mechanism because human cell membranes are made with cholesterol whereas fungi cell membranes are made with ergosterol. The spectrum of action of azoles is broad and generally effective against endemic mycosis, *Cryptococcus neoformans*, the dermatophytes, and even *Aspergillus* infections.[77]

Metabolism

The azoles are rapidly absorbed in the gastrointestinal tract, but there are individual differences with regard to being affected by food intake. The azoles have good tissue penetration, are metabolized in the liver via interaction with the CYP450 enzyme system, and are eliminated by the kidneys, except fluconazole (Diflucan), which is excreted renally as unchanged drug.

Side Effects and Adverse Reactions

Over-the-counter antifungal agents have a very low toxicity. The most common adverse reactions of the oral agents are associated with gastrointestinal symptoms. The azoles are relatively nontoxic, but they have been associated with hepatotoxicity to varying degrees. Although the hepatotoxicity is usually reversible after discontinuation of the drug, a few of these drugs have FDA black box warnings about the risk of liver damage. All individuals taking azoles orally or parenterally need to be aware of signs and symptoms of hepatitis, including fatigue, anorexia, nausea, fever, and jaundice. In some situations, liver enzymes should to be monitored in those taking prescription oral antifungal agents.

Drug–Drug Interactions

Azoles are inhibitors of CYP3A4 and can therefore cause increased plasma levels of drugs metabolized by this enzyme, some of which are serious and potentially fatal. Thus they are another category of drugs wherein drug–drug interactions are a critical knowledge for the prescriber and person taking the medication. Common drug–drug interactions are listed in Table 11-18.[78-80] Ketoconazole (Nizoral) is the most potent inhibitor of CYP3A4, followed by itraconazole (Sporanox), miconazole (Monistat), and to a lesser degree, fluconazole (Diflucan).

Drug–Food Interactions

Ketoconazole (Nizoral) and itraconazole (Sporanox) require an acidic environment of absorption. Antacids, proton pump inhibitors, and H₂ antagonists should not be coadministered with these drugs. Conversely, absorption of fluconazole (Diflucan) is independent of the presence or absence of food. Grapefruit juice can delay absorption of itraconazole and, therefore, should be avoided during therapy.

Fluconazole (Diflucan)

Fluconazole (Diflucan) is the most widely used antifungal despite its high cost. It is most often used for the treatment of mucocutaneous candidiasis. Fluconazole is also active against *Tinea corporis*, *Tinea cruris*, and *Tinea pedis*. More recently, it has been used to treat mammary candidiasis in breastfeeding mothers.[81]

This agent has almost 100% bioavailability and excellent cerebrospinal fluid penetration, providing a therapeutic advantage for the treatment of cryptococcal meningitis. Fluconazole has a high degree of water solubility, and gastric absorption is not affected by pH or the presence of food. It is widely distributed in the tissues, and it is eliminated unchanged in the urine.

Table 11-17 Systemic Antifungals

Drug—Generic (Brand)	Indications	Doses	Route	Excretion	Half-Life	Adverse Reactions	Clinical Considerations	FDA Pregnancy Category
Ketoconazole (Nizoral)	Candidiasis, blastomycosis, histoplasmosis, severe tinea, onychomycosis	200–400 mg qd.	PO	Bile	2–8 h	Hepatic toxicity, headaches, dizziness, nausea.	Multiple drug–drug interactions. See Table 11-18.	C
Fluconazole (Diflucan)	Candidiasis, cryptococcal meningitis	Vaginally: 150 mg as single dose. Oral: 200 mg × 1 day, then 100 mg qd.	PO/IV	Renal, 80%	30 h	Minimal gastrointestinal side effects.	Multiple drug–drug interactions. See Table 11-18.	C
Itraconazole (Sporanox)	Candidiasis, blastomycosis, histoplasmosis, severe tinea, onychomycosis, aspergillosis	Dose varies: 100–200 mg qd.	PO	Renal	30–40 h	Cardiac dysrhythmias and bronchospasm when taken with other drugs.	Multiple drug–drug interactions. See Table 11-18.	C
Terbinafine (Lamisil)	Onychomycosis	250 mg/day × 6–12 wk.	PO/ topical	Renal	36 h	Ophthalmic changes.	Oral dose associated with some drug–drug interactions common to all azoles. Topical preparations generally considered safe.	B
Griseofulvin (Grifulvin V)	Dermatophytosis of skin, hair, and nails: tinea corporis, cruris, capitis, pedis, unguium	500 mg to 1 g daily.	PO	Renal	24 h	Headache, nausea, vomiting, diarrhea, photosensitivity, fatigue, vertigo, syncope, mental confusion.	Monitor renal, hepatic, and hematologic functions with prolonged therapy; absorbed better with fatty meal.	C
Amphotericin B (Fungizone, Amphotec, Abelcet, AmBisome)	Systemic mycoses, cutaneous candidiasis	IV: up to 5 mg/kg/day depending on product. Topical: 3% cream/ lotion. Ointment: applied 2–4 × day.	IV/ topical	Renal	Varies depending on product	Azotemia, anemia, chills, fever, myalgias, abdominal pain, weight loss and vomiting; burning, itching, erythema with topical application.	Ineffective against dermatophytic infections.	B
Flucytosine (Ancobon, 5-FC)	Cryptococcal meningitis, chromoblastomycosis	100–150 mg/kg/d. Note: Used only in combination with amphotericin B or itraconazole.	PO	Renal	3–6 h	Leukopenia, thrombocytopenia, rash, nausea, vomiting, diarrhea.	Toxicity increased in HIV; modify dose in renal impairment.	C
Echinocandins: caspofungin (Cancidas)	Aspergillosis not responsive to other drugs, invasive candidiasis	50–70 mg daily.	IV over 1 h	Renal and fecal	9–11 h	Phlebitis, histamine effect with rapid infusion.	No change with renal impairment.	C
Voriconazole (Vfend)	Aspergillosis not responsive to other drugs, invasive candidiasis	200–300 mg bid.	IV/PO	Renal	6 h	Transient visual disturbances, photophobia. Rare Stevens-Johnson syndrome.	Multiple drug–drug interactions. See Table 11-18.	D

Fluconazole (Diflucan) is the systemically used azole with the fewest side effects or adverse effects. Minor gastrointestinal upsets have been reported. The issues that limit use are that resistance in *Candida* species appears to develop quickly and drug–drug interactions must be assessed before prescribing.

Itraconazole (Sporanox)

Itraconazole (Sporanox) has largely replaced ketoconazole (Nizoral) in the treatment of systemic infections and is available in oral and intravenous formulations. Itraconazole is indicated for the treatment of dimorphic *Fungi Histoplasma, Blastomyces,* and *Sporothrix.* This agent also is active against *Aspergillus.*

The inhibiting action of itraconazole is the same as that of the other antifungal medications. The antifungal activity of itraconazole is potent but can be limited by bioavailability. Absorption is improved when taken with food but inhibited by an alkaline gastric environment. There is poor cerebrospinal fluid penetration. The half-life is 24–42 hours and itraconazole is eliminated through the hepatic system. This drug undergoes extensive hepatic metabolism and, therefore, is associated with many drug–drug interactions. Gastrointestinal disturbances as well as elevated liver enzymes may occur, and as is true of all the azoles, rarely, hepatotoxicity may occur. Itraconazole has an FDA black box warning that recommends this drug not be prescribed to persons who have ventricular dysfunction or congestive heart failure and that itraconazole is associated with hepatic toxicity. Hair loss is the other rare adverse effect associated with use of this drug.[78]

Table 11-18 Azoles: Selected Drug–Drug Interactions*

Drug—Generic (Brand)	Azole	Effect
Severe Effects: Contraindicated Combinations		
Cisapride (Propulsid)	All	Prolonged QT interval.
Cyclosporin (Neoral)	All	Nephrotoxicity.
Digoxin (Lanoxin)	Itraconazole, ketoconazole	Digoxin toxicity.
Disopyramide (Norpace)	Itraconazole	Prolonged QT interval.
Dofetilide (Tikosyn)	Itraconazole	Increased plasma levels of dofetilide and cardiac failure.
Ergotamine (Cafergot)	Itraconazole	Ergotism.
Felodipine (Plendil)	Itraconazole	Hypotension.
Lovastatin (Mevacor, Altocor)†	Itraconazole	Increased plasma levels of lovastatin and hypotension, case report of rhabdomyolysis.
Quinidine	Itraconazole	Increased plasma levels of quinidine and cardiac failure.
Pimozide (Orap)	Itraconazole	Increased plasma levels of pimozide and cardiac failure.
Moderately Severe Effects		
Carbamazepine (Tegretol)	Fluconazole	Increased carbamazepine levels.
Methyl prednisolone (Medrol)	Ketoconazole	Adrenal suppression.
Midazolam (Versed)	Fluconazole, ketoconazole, itraconazole	Increased sedation.
Phenytoin (Dilantin)	Fluconazole, miconazole	Nystagmus and ataxia.
Rifabutin (Mycobutin)	Fluconazole	Ocular toxicity (uveitis).
Rifampin (RIF, Rifadin)	Ketoconazole	Increased clearance of the azole and reduced concentrations of rifampin.
Sulfonylureas	Fluconazole, miconazole	Hypoglycemic reactions.
Tacrolimus (Prototropic)	Ketoconazole, miconazole	Decreased plasma levels of tacrolimus.
Theophylline (Theo-Dur)	All	Increased plasma levels of theophylline.
Triazolam (Halcion)	Ketonoazole, itraconazole	Increased plasma levels of triazolam and increased sedation.
Warfarin (Coumadin)	All	Increased plasma levels of warfarin.
Drugs That Alter Azole Metabolism		
Antacids	Ketoconazole, itraconazole	Decreased absorption of azole.
Barbiturates	All	Decreased plasma levels of the azole.
Carbamazepine (Tegretol)	All	Decreased plasma levels of the azole.
Cimetidine (Tagamet)	Terbinafine	Increased plasma levels of terbinafine.
H$_2$ receptor antagonists	Ketoconazole, itraconazole	Decreased absorption of the azole.
Isoniazid (INH)	Itraconazole	Decreased plasma levels of the azole.
Phenobarbital (Luminal)	Itraconazole	Decreased plasma levels of the azole.
Proton pump inhibitors	Ketoconazole, itraconazole	Decreased absorption of the azole.
Rifampin (RIF, Rifadin)	All	Decreased plasma levels of the azole.

* This table is not comprehensive. New information is being identified on a regular basis.
† This interaction is expected to occur with other statin drugs as well as lovastatin.

Ketoconazole (Nizoral)

Ketoconazole is one of the oldest azoles and most studied. It is available as a shampoo, cream, foam, or gel for treatment of superficial fungal and yeast infections. Topical agents are used to treat dermatophytosis and candidiasis, and shampoos are for treatment of seborrheic dermatitis. Once- or twice-daily applications to the affected area for 2–3 weeks should result in a resolution of a superficial fungal infection. Interestingly, the topical formulations of ketoconazole have anti-inflammatory effects that are equal to 1% hydrocortisone cream. Infections of the hair and nails may take a longer program of treatment. Ketoconazole is lipophilic and is easily stored in tissue.

Ketoconazole (Nizoral) is also available in an oral preparation for systemic use; however, it is less selective against fungal enzymes than the newer azoles that have been developed for use against systemic infections and largely replaced by itraconazole (Sporanox) because ketoconazole has more adverse effects and drug–drug interactions.

Side effects include a stinging sensation, pruritis, erythema, and general local irritation following topical use (1–2%).[78] The cream has sulfites and should not be used by persons who are allergic to sulfites. Approximately 3% of persons using this drug report nausea, vomiting, or anorexia.[78] This drug can cause mild elevations in liver enzymes or fatal hepatotoxicity. The overall rate of hepatic dysfunction is 1–2%.[78] Ketoconazole carries an FDA black box warning that addresses one warning and three contraindications: (1) ketoconazole is associated with hepatic toxicity that includes some fatalities; (2) coadministration with terfenadine (Seldane-D) is contraindicated, and subsequently, terfenadine was removed from the market in the United States; (3) coadministration with astemizole (Hismanal) is contraindicated secondary to the risk of increased plasma levels of astemizole that can cause prolonged QT syndrome; and (4) coadministration with cisapride (Propulsid), which has also been removed from the US market, is contraindicated secondary to an increased risk for cardiovascular events. Finally, more rarely, anaphylaxis, suicidal ideation, severe depression, and other hypersensitivity reactions such as hemolytic anemia have been reported.

The ability to inhibit CYP450 enzymes and cause drug–drug interactions is probably the most clinically significant aspect of ketoconazole day to day. At normal antifungal doses, this drug is a potent inhibitor of CYP34A. Interestingly, it also inhibits CYP 17 α-hydroxylase and CYP11A1, which can, at high doses of ketoconazole, block steroidogenesis. This property is used therapeutically to treat Cushing's disorder or adrenal cancer, but it is also associated with the adverse effect of adrenal insufficiency, gynecomastia, and infertility in persons with normally functioning adrenal glands.[80]

Voriconazole (Vfend)

Voriconazole (Vfend) is one of the newest azoles to be marketed in the United States and is indicated for *Candida* species infections, including those known to be resistant to other forms of therapy. This drug also is the current agent of choice for treatment of *Aspergillus* infections, fungal infections refractory to other agents, and severe corneal infections of the eye.[78] Voriconazole is used most frequently for individuals who are immunocompromised, such as those with organ transplants and hematologic cancers.

Voriconazole is metabolized by the liver and the dose should be reduced for individuals with hepatic impairment or avoided altogether. Rashes (7%) and elevated hepatic enzymes have been observed with the use of voriconazole.[78] Visual disturbances occur in 30% of individuals who are given this medication, including blurring and alterations in color vision that may resolve without intervention.

Special Populations

Ketoconazole (Nizoral), fluconazole (Diflucan), and itraconazole (Sporanox) are FDA pregnancy category C drugs due to teratogenic effects seen in animals. Breast milk, like dairy products, creates an alkaline condition and therefore inhibits transfer of the azoles to the nursing infant.[30] Voriconazole (Vfend) is in FDA pregnancy category D and should not be administered to pregnant women.

Lower dosages may be required for elderly individuals with renal impairment. Itroconazole can cause a dose-dependent inotropic effect leading to congestive heart failure in individuals with impaired ventricular function and may also cause hypokalemia with high doses, so it should be used with caution.[77]

Topical Antifungal Azoles

Topical treatment is indicated for many of the superficial fungal infections such as dermatophytosis, mucocutaneous candidiasis, *T pedis* (athlete's foot or ringworm of the foot), *T corporis* (ringworm on arms, trunk, or legs) or *Tinea capitis* (ringworm on scalp), *T cruris* (jock itch or ringworm near groin), *Tinea versicolor*, and fungal keratitis (Table 11-19). A number of agents are available for these mycoses. The preferred formulation is lotion or cream; powders are primarily

Table 11-19 Topical Azole Antifungals

Drug—Generic (Brand)	Indications	Doses	Route	Adverse Reactions	FDA Pregnancy Category
Butoconazole (Mycelex 3, Gynazole 1)	Vulvovaginal candidiasis	2% cream at HS × 3 (Mycelex 3) or × 1 (Gynazole 1).	Intravaginal	Itching, soreness, swelling, burning.	C
Clotrimazole (Gyne-Lotrimin, Lotrimin, Mycelex, Mycelex-G)	Vulvovaginal candidiasis, superficial mycoses, oropharyngeal candidiasis	Vaginal: 1% cream or 100-mg tab at HS × 7; 2% cream or 200-mg tab at HS × 3. Topical: 1% cream or solution to be applied bid × 1–4 wks.	Topical or intravaginal	Burning, itching, redness, stinging, soreness.	B
Econazole (Spectazole)	Superficial mycoses	1% cream to be applied once daily for tinea or twice daily for cutaneous candidiasis × 1–2 wks.	Topical	Burning, itching, redness, stinging.	C
Miconazole (Monistat)	Vulvovaginal or oral candidiasis, *Tinea pedis*, *T corporis*, *T capitis*, *T cruris*, and *T versicolor*	Vaginal: 2% cream or 100-mg supp at HS × 7; 4% cream or 200-mg supp at HS × 3; or 1200-mg supp × 1. Topical: 2% cream, lotion, powder, ointment, solution, spray, or tincture to be applied bid × 2–4 wks.	Topical or intravaginal	Burning, itching, redness, stinging, cramping.	C
Oxiconazole (Oxistat)	Topical dermatophytes	1% cream/lotion qd–bid × 2–4 wks.	Topical	Localized burning, redness, itching, dry skin, tenderness.	B
Sulconazole (Exelderm), sertaconazole (Ertaczo)	Topical dermatophytes	1% cream/solution qd–bid × 3–4 wks; 2% cream bid × 4 wks.	Topical	Localized burning, redness, itching, dry skin, tenderness.	C
Terconazole (Terazol)	Vaginal candidiasis	0.4% cream at HS × 7; 0.8% cream or 80-mg supp at HS × 3.	Intravaginal	Abdominal pain, irritation, itching, burning, fever, dysmenorrhea.	C
Tioconazole (Vagistat 1, Monistat-1Day)	Vaginal candidiasis	6.5% ointment: at HS × 1.	Intravaginal	Irritation, burning.	C

used for moist intertriginous areas (groin, feet). Cutaneous application is generally twice a day for 3–6 weeks. Vaginal applications are once daily for between 1 and 7 days. The most common side effect is localized burning or itching; a male sexual partner may also experience mild penile irritation when these agents are applied vaginally.[77] All of the azoles described here have extremely poor systemic absorption when applied topically.

Given the plethora of agents and formulations available in this one family, which works best? A recent Cochrane review of 67 randomized, controlled trials found that azoles overall do not work quite as well as the allylamines (discussed in the next section) for treatment of fungal infections of the skin, nails, or feet (risk ratio of treatment failure 0.63; 95% CI, 0.42–0.94 in favor of allylamines).[82] It appears azoles work better than allylamines in treating vaginal *Candida* infections, but all azole topical preparations are equally efficacious for this purpose. Resistant organisms may require additional treatments or oral fluconazole (Diflucan). Additional information about specific infections can be found in Chapters 26 and 31.

Allylamines and Benzylamines

The allylamines include naftifine hydrochloride (Naftin) and terbinafine (Lamisil), and the one benzylamine available is butenafine (Mentax). These agents work well for infections caused by dermatophytes but are not quite as effective against *Candida* infections. Naftifine hydrochloride (Naftin) is only approved for topical treatment of fungal species, and terbinafine is approved for oral and topical treatment. Topical formulations are 1% creams applied twice daily to the affected area. Butenafine is more effective than the other two in treating *Candida albicans*. Systemic oral terbinafine (250-mg tablet once daily) is effective for nail onychomycosis.

Mechanism of Action

These drugs interfere with ergosterol production but at a different point in the synthesis pathway than the conversion of sterol where azoles break the process.

Metabolism

Absorption of naftifine (Naftin) and butenafine (Mentax) is low and therefore no systemic effects have been reported.[78] Oral terbinafine undergoes some hepatic metabolism via the CYP450 enzyme system, and approximately 80% of the drug is excreted in the urine. Terbinafine accumulates in skin, nails, and fatty tissue and has a very long half-life (300 hours), which represents the slow elimination from these tissues, all of which may account for its efficacy in treating nail infections.

Side Effects and Adverse Reactions

The most common side effects that have been reported with naftifine and butenafine are burning and stinging of the affected area. Rare incidences of liver failure have occurred with the use of terbinafine along with ophthalmic changes, neutropenia, and renal adverse effects.[78] Terbinafine (Lamisil) is the final antifungal mentioned in this chapter that has an FDA black box warning applied to the oral formulation that states it is associated with hepatic toxicity.

Drug–Drug Interactions

Terbinafine is a potent inhibitor of CYP2D6 and has multiple drug–drug interactions that include increased plasma levels of tricyclic antidepressants, beta-blockers, selective serotonin reuptake inhibitors, MAO inhibitors, and caffiene.[78] Alcohol can cause increased liver damage if taken with terbinafine (Lamisil). Cimetidine (Tagamet) decreases the clearance of terbinafine and increases plasma levels. Conversely, rifampin (RIF, Rifadin) increases metabolism of terbinafine and decreases plasma levels.

Special Populations

Naftifine hydrochloride (Naftin), terbinafine (Lamisil), and butenafine (Mentax) are FDA pregnancy category B drugs. No fetal harm has been noted in animal studies, but lack of human studies does not allow a full assessment of fetal risk.[44] Terbinafine is found to be moderately safe in mothers who are breastfeeding with no untoward effects reported to the fetus.[30] Elderly individuals tend to be on more medications that may interact with these drugs. If an elderly individual has renal or hepatic impairment, the dosage of terbinafine should be reduced.

Polyenes

The polyenes include amphotericin B and nystatin (Mycostatin). From 1950 until recently, amphotericin B was the only antifungal agent available for treating systemic fungal infections. Amphotericin B is a broad-spectrum antifungal drug that is available for topical and intravenous use. Therapy with this agent is limited due to its nephrotoxicity and other adverse effects as noted later, but it does remain the drug of choice for many systemic mycoses, usually during life-threatening situations.[78] Nystatin is limited to topical use and is effective against *Candida* but not other dermatophytes. It is available as a cream, ointment, powder, liquid, suspension, and pastille that is used to treat oral candidiasis (thrush). Although it is well tolerated vaginally, other medications such as the imidazoles or triazoles are more effective for vaginal candidiasis.

Mechanism of Action and Spectrum of Activity

Amphotericin and nystatin bind to ergosterol in the fungal cell membrane resulting in leakage of the cell and reduced viability, which makes them both fungistatic and fungicidal.[79] This agent has coverage against *C albicans*, *C neoformans*, *Histoplasma capsulatum*, *Blastomyces dermatitidis*, *Coccidioides immitis*, and *Aspergillus fumigatus*. Topical amphotericin is limited to treatment of candidiasis of the skin.

Metabolism

Gastrointestinal absorption of amphotericin B is negligible, and this drug is only available parenterally. With parenteral administration, it is distributed throughout the body and excreted by the kidneys; however, there is extensive binding to tissues so that there is a terminal phase of elimination with a half-life of 15 days.[77]

Side Effects and Adverse Reactions

Nystatin has very few side effects or adverse effects.[78] Renal damage is the most significant dose-dependent adverse reaction associated with amphotericin B and can be irreversible, and newer formulations that have the drug surrounded by lipid envelopes are beginning to be used in the hope that these formulations will decrease the incidence of renal damage. Hematologic effects have occurred with administration of this medication. Individuals taking nystatin should be regularly monitored for anemia. Almost all persons receiving amphotericin intravenously experience chills, fever, myalgias, joint pain, abdominal pain, weight loss, and vomiting. Other side effects include burning, itching, and erythema from topical application.[77,78]

Drug–Drug Interactions

If amphotericin B and azole antifungals are given at the same time, the antifungal effect of amphotericin B is antagonized. Amphotericin B in combination with a long list of individual agents can cause nephrotoxicity, hypokalemia, or prolonged QT syndrome.[79]

Special Populations

Amphotericin B and nystatin are in FDA pregnancy category B. There are no reports linking these drugs with fetal congenital defects. They may be used during pregnancy if the individual would clearly benefit from them.[44] They are not absorbed through the gastrointestinal tract, and, therefore, the amount in breast milk would not be clinically significant to cause any untoward effects to the nursing infant.[30] Amphotericin B should not be administered to an elderly person who might have renal impairment.

Echinocandins

Caspofungin acetate (Cancidas), micafungin (Mycamine), and anidulafungin (Eraxis) belong to the newest class of antifungal agents, the echinocandins. In susceptible fungi, they cause lysis of the cell wall. These agents are approved for treatment of esophageal candidiasis, disseminated and mucocutaneous Candida infections, invasive aspergillosis intolerant of other drugs, and in febrile neutropenic patients in whom a fungal infection is suspected.[77,78] They are available only in intravenous form because they are not absorbed when administered orally. These agents are not metabolized via the CYP459 enzymes and thus do not have the drug–drug interactions associated with the azoles and allylamines. All are FDA pregnancy category C drugs.

Other Antifungals

Griseofulvin (Fulvicin, Grifulvin V)

Griseofulvin (Fulvicin, Grifulvin V) is an older antifungal medication that has not been as widely used due to the enhanced safety panel of some of the newer antifungal agents. Griseofulvin is used to treat superficial mycoses such as ringworm of the skin and nails and is available as a suspension or in tablets.

Mechanism of Action and Spectrum of Activity

Griseofulvin (Fulvicin, Grifulvin V) interferes with cell division of the fungal cells by inhibiting mitosis, and it also acts at the cellular level to protect new skin and nail growth from becoming infected. It is not effective against Candida species but has for years been the agent of choice for treating T capitis. Although now largely replaced by other agents, griseofulvin (Fulvicin, Grifulvin V) is more effective in treating Microsporum canis infections than is terbinafine (Lamisil), which is one of the dermatophytes that cause T capitis.

Metabolism

Griseofulvin is better absorbed when taken with a fatty meal. Elimination is by hepatic metabolism and renal excretion.[78]

Side Effects and Adverse Reactions

Gastrointestinal discomfort such as nausea, vomiting, and diarrhea may occur when an individual takes griseofulvin. Headaches have been observed in as many as 15% of individuals, and they usually disappear spontaneously with continued therapy. Additionally, some individuals experience photosensitivity, fatigue, vertigo, syncope, and mental confusion. Periodic monitoring of liver and renal function is important.[78]

Drug–Drug Interactions

Griseofulvin is an inducer of the enzymes that facilitate metabolism of oral contraceptives and warfarin (Coumadin). Thus concomitant use may interfere with oral contraceptive or warfarin effectiveness. It can also increase sensitivity to alcohol, causing a serious reaction. Griseofulvin can decrease the effects of warfarin and decrease levels of barbiturates and cyclosporine.[77,79]

Special Populations

Griseofulvin is an FDA pregnancy category C drug due to lack of studies in humans. The drug has been studied in a limited number of breastfeeding women without any adverse effects to the infant.[30] No special considerations have been noted for the use of griseofulvin among the elderly.

Flucytosine

Flucytosine is a water-soluble pyrimadine analog effective against *C neoformans*, some *Candida* species, and chromoblastomycosis. Clinical therapeutic use is limited to treatment of cryptococcal meningitis in conjunction with amphotericin B and to treatment of chromoblastomycosis in conjunction with itraconazole (Sporanox). It is well absorbed from the gastrointestinal tract and widely distributed in the body with peak plasma concentrations in 1–2 hours. About 80% of the drug is excreted unchanged in the urine. Normal half-life is 3–6 hours, but in the presence of renal impairment is much more prolonged; patients with renal failure or HIV must have plasma levels monitored frequently. Side effects include rash, nausea, vomiting, diarrhea, and enterocolitis. Flucytosine may also depress the bone marrow, causing leucopenia and thrombocytopenia.[77]

▌ Antiviral Agents

Virus is from the Latin word that means *toxin* or *poison*. Viruses consist of RNA or DNA genetic material and a protein coat that protects the genetic material, and some have a fat envelope that surrounds the protein coat. All viruses are obligatory intracellular pathogens with a unique ability to cause infections in humans via hijacking the normal functions of human cells.

Antiviral therapy was the focus of pharmacologic research in the 1950s when the effort to find a cure for cancer viruses was directed to finding compounds that could inhibit DNA synthesis. Current research is directed toward finding antiviral agents that have greater specificity with fewer toxic effects on the host cell.

The influenza virus has two proteins of import that are the antigens that current antiviral agents attack. Hemagglutinin works to allow the virus entry into the host cell. Neuraminidase is involved in the budding of new virions out of the host cell. Mutations in either of these surface proteins will allow the virus to evade antiviral medications. Mutations are both common and frequent in the influenza virus, a process that is referred to as *antigenic drift*. As more and more point mutations occur, strains of the virus that are able to evade the antibodies made by the human host during a previous infection with influenza appear.

Viral replication consists of several generic steps (Figure 11-5), which include (1) binding and fusion or attachment to the host cell, (2) penetration into the host cell, (3) reverse transcription or uncoating of the virus to reveal the genetic material, (4) integration into the cell nucleus and replication of the genetic material, (5) assembly of virus particles, and (6) lysis of the host cell to release the newly made viruses. A key point regarding viral invasion is that the replication of the virus actually peaks before the individual has any manifestations of clinical symptomatology. This situation provides the virus with a distinct advantage and poses additional challenges to the host and the clinician in providing remedial curative and finally preventative efforts.

Antiviral agents can target any one of the viral replications processes.[83] Uncoating inhibitors amantadine (Symmetrel, Symadine) and rimantadine (Flumadine) prevent the viral genetic material from being released from the protein coat once the virus is inside the host cell. Nucleic acid synthesis inhibitors are phosphorylated by the virus within the host cell into a metabolite that accumulates and inhibits replication of DNA or RNA. Acyclovir (Zovirax) is a nucleic acid synthesis inhibitor. Nucleoside reverse transcriptase inhibitors also prevent DNA or RNA replication after the drug is phosphorylated, but in this case, cellular kinases do the job instead of viral kinases. These drugs are approved for treatment of HIV. Nonnucleoside reverse transcriptase inhibitors bind to HIV reverse transcriptase and block viral reproduction; they are also part of the regimen used to treat HIV. Finally, protease inhibitors inhibit the proteolytic enzymes that are needed for production of new viruses. These drugs work synergistically with nonnucleoside reverse transcriptase inhibitors as part of the HIV regimen.[83]

There are many viruses that are pathogenic in humans. Viruses cause cold sores, cytomegalovirus (CMV), Epstein-Barr virus (EBV), hepatitis, herpes simplex virus (HSV), HIV, influenza, and varicella-zoster virus (VZV), to name just a few. There are eight herpes viruses within the family *Herpesviridae* that are pathogenic in humans. This is not a conclusive list; rather it is a selective one of the viruses most often encountered in generally healthy adults who seek treatment in primary care practice. Women's healthcare providers in the primary care setting are most often called upon to provide an antiviral therapy for herpes simplex virus (HSV), influenza, varicella-zoster virus (VZV) infection, and hepatitis. The antiretroviral drugs used to treat HIV/AIDS are listed in Table 23-16 but will not be discussed in depth. Readers interested in the pharmacologic issues surrounding antiretroviral therapy are referred to the national AIDS Web site at *www.AIDS.gov* for detailed information about treatment of persons with HIV/AIDS.

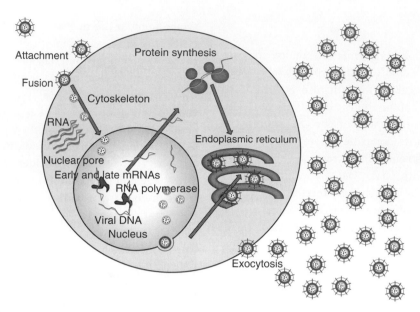

Figure 11-5 Viral life cycle.

Drugs for Herpes: Acyclovir, Famciclovir, Valacyclovir

Acyclovir (Zovirax) is the first of three nucleoside analog formulations known to be effective for the treatment of intracellular viral parasites. Famciclovir (Famvir) and valacyclovir (Valtrex) are the other systemic agents available. All three are similar in their method of action and indications. Acyclovir is the only preparation that is available for intravenous use in the United States (Table 11-20).

Mechanism of Action and Spectrum of Activity

All three of these drugs have the same mechanism of action. They require viral kinase or a trigger for initial phosphorylation. The active metabolite accumulates only in the infected host cells and then inhibits viral replication via attachment to the end of a growing DNA chain and blocking further growth. Valacyclovir (Valtrex) is a prodrug of acyclovir and is converted rapidly and completely to acyclovir after oral administration.

Acyclovir (Zovirax) is indicated for the treatment of HSV, prevention of recurrent HSV, and treatment of VZV infections. When used for the treatment of genital herpes, oral acyclovir has been found to shorten the symptoms of the infection by about 2 days and also reduces viral shedding by 7 days. Famciclovir (Famvir) and valacyclovir (Valtrex) are preferred for the treatment and prevention of HSV because both have been found to have a slight superiority in effectiveness when compared to acyclovir in that they

reduce the pain and shorten the duration of the outbreak more than does acyclovir.[83,84] The EBV, CMV, and human herpesvirus-6 (HHV-6) have been treated with acyclovir; however, the in vitro activity has been found to be weak.[85]

Metabolism

The bioavailability of acyclovir (Zovirax) is low, approximately 15–30%. It is poorly absorbed from the gastrointestinal tract. Acyclovir diffuses into most tissues and penetrates into cerebrospinal fluid. It is excreted through the renal system as an unchanged drug; the liver only metabolizes 10%, and the half-life is approximately 3 hours for individuals with normal renal function. Famciclovir (Famvir) and valacyclovir (Valtrex) are both more bioavailable than acyclovir. The bioavailability of famciclovir is 70–80% and the bioavailability of valacyclovir is approximately 50%.[83]

Side Effects and Adverse Reactions

Acyclovir (Zovirax), famciclovir (Famvir), and valacyclovir (Valtrex) are all generally tolerated with minimal discomfort. The primary complaints are headache, nausea, and diarrhea. Intravenous infusion has been associated with renal complications. Adequate hydration and avoidance of rapid infusion rates can prevent adverse effects. More serious side effects have been noted with long-term use of the drugs. Acyclovir should be used cautiously with individuals who have neurologic disorders, because approximately 1% of individuals who have received parenteral acyclovir have reported neurologic reactions.

Table 11-20 Antivirals

Drug—Generic (Brand)	Indications	Doses	Route	Excretion	Half-Life	Adverse Reactions	Clinical Considerations	FDA Pregnancy Category
Acyclovir (Zovirax)	Herpes simplex, genital, herpes zoster, varicella	Initial: 200 mg 5 ×/day × 10 days. Chronic suppressive therapy: 400 mg bid × 12 mo. Acute: 800 mg 5 ×/day × 7–10 days. 800 mg qid × 5 days.	PO/IV/ topical	Renal	2.5 h	Nausea, vomiting, headache, CNS reactions, rash, malaise. Caution in those with renal impairment for all antivirals.	Do not exceed maximum dosage. Start all antiherpes drugs as soon as symptoms begin.	PO, IV: B Topical: C
Famciclovir (Famvir)	Herpes simplex, genital	1500 mg one dose. 1000 mg bid × 1 day.	PO	Renal	2.3 h	Headache, GI side effects, numbness.	Can decrease duration of postherpetic neuralgia.	B
	Herpes zoster	500 mg tid × 7 days.						
Valacyclovir (Valtrex)	Herpes simplex, genital	2 g bid × 1 day. 500 mg bid × 3 days.	PO	Renal	2.5–3.3 h	GI side effects, dizziness, headache, abdominal pain.	Not approved for immunocompromised individuals; not affected by food.	B
	Herpes zoster	1 g tid × 7 d.						
Anti-Influenza								
Amantadine (Symmetrel)	Influenza A	200 mg qd–bid.	PO	Renal	17 h	Have caused anxiety, irritability, and confusion— can exacerbate psychological problems. Seizures or other CNS effects. Observe for renal or hepatic effects.	Exercise caution with hazardous activities.	C
Rimantadine (Flumadine)	Influenza A	100 mg bid × 7 days.	PO	Renal, 25%	25 h	Nervousness, sleep disturbances.	Fewer side effects seen than with amantadine.	C
Zanamivir (Relenza)	Influenza A and B	2 inh bid × 5 d.	PO	Renal	2.5–5 h	Can exacerbate respiratory symptoms.	Not recommended for individuals with COPD or asthma.	C
Oseltamivir (Tamiflu)	Influenza A and B	75 mg bid × 5 days.	Inhaled	Renal	6–10 h	Nausea, vomiting.	Reduce nausea by giving with food.	C
Antihepatitis								
Interferons: Alpha 2-b (Intron A) Alphacon-1 (Infergen)	Hepatitis B, C	HBV: 5 mL U qd or 10 mL U 3 ×/wk × 16 wks. HCV: 3 mL U 3 ×/wk × 16 wks; continue × 18–24 mo if normalization of ALT occurs.	SQ or IM	Renal	Alpha 2-b: 2–5 h Alphacon-1: 6–10 h	Flu-like syndrome within 6 h; with chronic therapy: depression, confusion, somnolence, fatigue, weight loss, rash, anemia, reversible hearing loss.		C
Ribavirin (Copegus, Rebetol, Virazole)	Hepatitis C	Ribavirin: 1200 mg/day in two divided doses. Rebetol: 400 mg bid.	PO	Renal	Ribavirin: 120–170 h Rebetol: 24–44 h	Anemia, fatigue, cough, rash, pruritus, nausea, insomnia, dyspnea, depression.	Should not attempt to conceive for at least 6 months following treatment.	X

Drug–Drug Interactions

Probenecid (Benemid), cimetidine (Tagamet), and theophylline (Theo-Dur) all increase plasma levels of acyclovir (Zovirax) and valacyclovir (Valtrex). Famciclovir potentiates digoxin, and, when coadministered, the levels of digoxin need to be monitored.[84,85]

Special Populations

Acyclovir (Zovirax), valacyclovir (Valtrex), and famciclovir (Famvir) are FDA pregnancy category B drugs and are actually recommended for use in the third trimester of pregnancy for the prevention of recurrent outbreaks.[86] No concerns have been reported for breastfeeding while taking acyclovir. Valacyclovir is metabolized into acyclovir, and little is transferred to the breast milk; thus it has been found to be safe. Less data are available regarding famciclovir, and therefore acyclovir would be the preferred drug in breastfeeding moms. Intravenous administration of acyclovir is the method of treatment for the newborn with neonatal HSV infection or herpes simplex encephalitis, and few adverse reactions have been noted. Because renal dysfunction is more likely among the elderly, close monitoring should be undertaken and the dose of acyclovir may need to be reduced if the individual, regardless of age, has renal impairment.

Anti-Influenza Agents

Influenza virus strains are classified by their proteins (A, B, or C), species of origin, and geographical site of isolation. Influenza A, the only known type to cause pandemics, has many known subtype bases on the surface proteins and can infect people, animal hosts, or birds. Rapid mutations have been reported within poultry flocks, specifically from a low pathogenic state to a higher pathogenic viral form. Influenza B viruses in general only infect humans. The anti-influenza drugs are used to treat and prevent influenza during an epidemic that is confirmed by viral cultures. The four agents approved for treatment of influenza are amantadine (Symmetrel), rimantadine (Flumadine), oseltamivir (Tamiflu), and zanamivir (Relenza). Amantadine (Symmetrel) and rimantadine (Flumadine) are preferred for first-line therapy due to their relative inexpense.[87]

Mechanism of Action and Spectrum of Activity

Amantadine (Symmetrel) and rimantadine (Flumadine) are used for the treatment of influenza A viruses and are not effective against influenza B. Amantadine and rimantadine act within the infected host cell to inhibit the uncoating of the viral RNA, preventing its replication. Therefore, these agents act by inhibiting the spread of the virus rather than killing the virus. Unfortunately, many of the influenza strains are resistant to amantadine.[87]

When used to prevent clinical symptoms following exposure to the virus, dosing is 100 mg twice a day or 200 mg once a day. This regimen has been found to be 70–90% effective in preventing clinical disease. When started promptly after the detections of symptoms, the duration of illness is reduced by 1–2 days.[87]

Metabolism

These drugs are well absorbed in the gastrointestinal tract. Drug distribution into the tissues is not fully understood. Rimantadine (Flumadine) has a much longer half-life than does amantadine. Both are excreted in the urine, although amantadine is excreted unchanged, and rimantadine is first extensively metabolized in the liver, which makes it a better drug for use in the elderly.

Side Effects and Adverse Reactions

The most common adverse effects of these agents are gastrointestinal, including loss of appetite and nausea. Central nervous system disturbances include insomnia, light-headedness and difficulty concentrating. Blurred vision has been reported. An individual taking amantadine (Symmetrel) or rimantadine (Flumadine) should be cautioned to avoid tasks that require acute vision or physical coordination. Serious, even fatal, neurotoxic reactions may occur in the presence of high amantadine plasma concentrations; these are more likely in persons with renal insufficiency.[87]

Drug–Drug Interactions

An individual should avoid alcohol when taking amantadine or rimantadine to prevent further CNS disturbances. These drugs may increase effects of anticholinergic or CNS active drugs, including antihistamines. The effect of amantadine is potentiated when used with trimethoprim/sulfamethoxazole (Bactrim, Septra DS) or with the diuretics hydrochlorothiazide (Maxzide, Dyazide), triamterene (Dyrenium), or amiloride (Midamor).[88]

Special Populations

Amantadine is an FDA pregnancy category C drug because birth defects have been reported in animal studies, but there is no conclusive evidence of adverse effects in humans.[30] Amantadine has been shown to suppress milk production by suppressing prolactin levels and therefore should be avoided during lactation. The dosages of amantadine and rimantadine should be reduced, and plasma concentrations should be monitored in the elderly, particularly if renal or hepatic impairment is present.[88]

Neuraminidase Inhibitors

Oseltamivir (Tamiflu) and zanamivir (Relenza) are classified as neuroaminidase inhibitors and were first introduced in 1999. These agents are indicated for the treatment of Influenza A and B viral strains; they cost more than amantadine (Symmetrel) but have a wider spectrum of activity. Replication of the virus peaks in 24–72 hours after onset of the infection and early administration is crucial to effective therapy.

Mechanism of Action and Spectrum of Activity

Oseltamivir (Tamiflu) and zanamivir (Relenza) act by interfering with the release of the influenza virus from the infected cells to new host cells. Oseltamivir is administered orally and zanamivir is administered directly to the respiratory tract through inhalation.

Metabolism

Oseltamivir (Tamiflu) is well absorbed in the gastrointestinal tract, is metabolized in the liver, peaks at about 2.5–6 hours with a half-life of 6–10 hours, and is eliminated in the urine. Zanamivir (Relenza) is inhaled into the oropharynx and throat. Up to 20% of the drug reaches the tracheobronchial tree and lungs.[87] Approximately 5–15% of the dosage is absorbed and excreted in the urine with minimal metabolism.[87]

Oseltamivir (Tamiflu) is given in a 75-mg oral dose once daily for both prevention and treatment of influenza. Zanamivir (Relenza) is given by inhalation, 10 mg once a day for prevention and 10 mg twice a day for treatment of influenza.

Side Effects and Adverse Reactions

CNS side effects have not been reported with these drugs. Gastrointestinal symptoms such as diarrhea, nausea, vomiting, and abdominal pain have been reported with oseltamivir (Tamiflu). Food may decrease gastrointestinal effects and does not interfere with absorption.[87] Zanamivir (Relenza) should be avoided among individuals with underlying airway disease or asthma since it has been reported to exacerbate bronchial spasm and cause respiratory compromise.

Drug–Drug Interactions

An individual receiving oseltamivir (Tamiflu) or zanamivir (Relenza) should not be administered the live influenza vaccine within 2 weeks prior to or 48 hours after treatment.

Special Populations

Oseltamivir (Tamiflu) is an FDA pregnancy category C drug because of lack of studies. Zanamivir (Relenza) is an FDA pregnancy category B drug, and due to the poor absorption and low plasma levels it is unlikely to cause untoward effects in the fetus.[30] Oseltamivir (Tamiflu) and zanamivir (Relenza) are rarely used for breastfeeding mothers because of the short time of efficacy with these drugs, unless they are necessary for high-risk individuals with other medical conditions.[30]

Oseltamivir (Tamiflu) and zanamivir (Relenza) are not contraindicated for the elderly. However, these agents should be used with caution in any individual with cardiac, respiratory, or hepatic impairment.

Antihepatitis Agents

Hepatitis means damage to the liver. Hepatitis can be caused by toxins or an autoimmune process, but most cases of liver damage are secondary to infection with one of the several hepatitis viruses, CMV, and more rarely EBV. The antiviral medications used to treat hepatitis cannot cure the infection but they can stop viral replication and prevent further liver damage. The antiretrovirals lamivudine (Epivir), adefovir (Hepsera), and entecavir (Baraclude), which are reviewed in Chapter 23, are the first-line treatment for hepatitis B. In the following sections, we will discuss the interferons and ribavirin, which are also used to treat hepatitis B and hepatitis C infections.

Interferons

Interferons have been investigated for many clinical applications. They are potent cytokines and possess antiviral and immunomodulating effects. There are three major classes of human interferons with antiviral properties: alpha, beta, and gamma.[87] One critical application of interferons is the suppression of hepatitis B virus (HBV) and hepatitis C virus (HCV). Among individuals with chronic HBV infection, treatment with interferon-alpha is associated with a higher incidence of hepatitis e-antigen conversion and undetectable HBV and DNA levels. Attainment of this goal in clinical trials has been correlated with a decrease in the risk of hepatocellular carcinoma and cirrhosis and a reduced need for liver transplant.

Mechanism of Action and Spectrum of Activity

Interferons are proteins that act to prohibit viral penetration, translation, transcription, maturation, and release of viral agents. Inhibition of protein synthesis is the major inhibitory effect. These agents are active against HBV, HCV, and human papillomavirus (HPV).[87] Dosing for HBV is 5 million units given either intramuscularly or subcutaneously once a day or 10 million units subcutaneously three times per week for 16 weeks. Higher doses are required for coexisting delta hepatitis. Approximately 20–30% of persons given interferon will have normalization of liver enzymes and loss of hepatitis B viral DNA.

Metabolism

Oral administration of interferons does not result in absorption, but after intramuscular or subcutaneous injection, interferon absorption exceeds 80%. The interferons are metabolized primarily in the kidney and liver and excreted in the urine.[87]

Side Effects and Adverse Reactions

Interferons have been associated with depression, confusion, somnolence, fatigue, weight loss, rash, anemia, and reversible hearing loss. Headache, fever, myalgias and malaise have been found to occur among some individuals within 6 hours of administration. Individuals with hepatic compromise, a history of cardiac arrhythmia, or autoimmune disease should not be given interferon. Caution should be exercised when giving this medication to individuals with a history of mood disorders.

Interferons can cause myelosuppression with granulocytopenia and thrombocytopenia. Elevations of hepatic enzymes, triglycerides, alopecia, proteinuria, interstitial nephritis, pneumonia, and hepatotoxicity may occur.

Drug–Drug Interactions

Interferons can significantly increase levels of drugs such as theophylline (Theo-Dur), zidovudine (Retrovir), methadone (Dolophine), and ribavirin (Rebetol). Caution is needed when administering interferons with other hepatotoxic drugs such as nucleoside reverse transcriptase inhibitors; in particular, use with didanosine (Videx) is not recommended.[87] Hematologic abnormalities may occur when interferons are coadministered with ACE inhibitors.

Special Populations

Interferons also could impair fertility and are abortifacient in primates.[87] That said, alpha-interferons are considered FDA pregnancy category C drugs due to lack of studies. No teratogenic or reproductive toxicity has been confirmed in humans, but because of antiproliferative activity, these drugs should be used only if the potential benefit to the mother justifies the possible risk to the fetus.[85] Interferons are large in molecular weight and, therefore, not easily transferred into human milk. No concerns have been reported with the administration of interferons in breastfeeding moms.[30] Caution is required with use in elderly individuals, as they might be at greater risk of adverse effects if they are on many medications or have renal or hepatic impairment.

Ribavirin

Mechanism of Action and Spectrum of Activity

Ribavirin (Rebetol) inhibits the replication of a wide range of viruses. The mechanism of action involves alteration of the cellular nucleotide pools and inhibition of viral messenger RNA synthesis but is not clearly understood. Oral ribavirin in combination with interferon is standard treatment for chronic HCV infection.[87] In aerosol form, it is approved for treatment of bronchiolitis and pneumonia in hospitalized children only.

Metabolism

Ribavirin (Rebetol) is actively taken up in the small bowel, is metabolized by the liver, and is excreted in the urine. Food increases plasma levels. Renal insufficiency can decrease clearance by threefold.[87]

Side Effects and Adverse Reactions

Dose-related anemia may occur in those taking ribavirin. Fatigue, cough, rash, pruritis, nausea, insomnia, dyspnea, and depression all have been noted and may lead to early discontinuation of treatment. The aerosol form may cause conjunctivitis, irritation, and occasional reversible decreased pulmonary function.[87]

Special Populations

Ribavirin (Rebetol) is an FDA pregnancy category X drug.[30] Animal studies indicate that ribavirin is teratogenic, embryotoxic, and oncogenic. No human studies have been done. Pregnant women should not care for individuals receiving the aerosol form of ribavirin.[44,87] No data on humans using ribavirin during lactation is available. Because decreased renal function can cause decreased ribavirin clearance, this drug should be used with caution in the elderly.

▌ Conclusion: Appropriate Prescribing Practices

A 2007 study in Canada looked at predictors of inappropriate antibiotic prescribing among primary care providers.[89] It found that inappropriate antibiotic prescribing increased with time in practice and that those providers with higher volume practice were more likely to prescribe antibiotics for viral infections. They were also more likely to prescribe second- and third-line antibiotics as first-line treatment. Using a longitudinal study design to observe provider prescribing habits over time, these authors found that the providers tend to be softer to the clients' demands for antibiotics and engage less frequently in client health education (Box 11-4). Other mechanisms such as the influence of pharmacologic marketing were also found to influence the providers prescribing unnecessary second- and third-line antibiotics versus first-line drugs for bacterial infections.[89]

The use of inappropriate antibiotic prescribing practices is a worldwide problem that is promoting antibiotic resistance. Not only is antibiotic resistance augmented, but there is the risk of adverse drug effects anytime a medication is prescribed, and there exists the increased cost to the individual and the healthcare system.

One of the central elements to rational prescribing presented earlier in this chapter is education. *Not* prescribing an antibiotic does require more time spent with the individual in teaching her about the cause of her illness, prevention, and symptomatic relief measures. This is an essential practice to follow, however, if we are to make a truly genuine attempt to decrease the trend of antibiotic resistance.

Unfortunately, the legal risks of possibly missing a diagnosis and being sued later is difficult to ignore. No one has ever been sued for contributing to antibiotic resistance. However, by educating the individual as discussed, and allowing her to make an informed decision regarding taking an antibiotic prescription, clinicians may be able to minimize such legal risks while at the same time building a more knowledgeable public. Follow-up and monitoring of response and outcome, the final element of a rational approach to prescribing presented, is also crucial in this situation as well. While some individuals will not feel comfortable leaving without a prescription, most, if educated and followed up appropriately, will be willing to utilize symptomatic relief measures and return or call as needed for further treatment.

Clinical guidelines as noted previously can be of great value to the clinician, not only in reviewing symptoms to determine a diagnosis, but also in selecting the most appropriate antibiotic when such is warranted. This will help ensure that the principle of the narrowest spectrum drug for the shortest duration is followed. The clinician's own knowledge of the pharmacodynamics of the medications he or she is prescribing is not to be neglected, nor is the thorough history and examination as well as elicitation of the individual's concerns, needs, and resources.

Anti-infectives are an essential tool in the primary health care of women. As clinicians, it is incumbent on us to use this resource wisely and well; it can be of great benefit to the women for whom we care. It can also have unintended consequences if used carelessly or without a systematic approach. The principles presented in this chapter will assist the clinician in maximizing the effectiveness of this resource.

Box 11-4 To Treat or Not to Treat? A Case of Sinusitis

AM is a 32-year-old being seen for her annual Pap smear. In the process of giving an interval history, AM tells her provider that she is glad her visit was scheduled for today because she has sinusitis and needs a prescription for antibiotics, which she says always work best when she gets the symptoms of sinusitis.

In providing her history, AM reports the onset of headaches and pain over her right eye for 2 days. These symptoms appeared as she was getting over a bad head cold that included coughing and yellow-green discharge from her nose. She has been afebrile. AM is in good health and takes no medications other than birth control pills. She does not have a maxillary toothache. AM has not used any medications to treat these symptoms.

On exam, AM is afebrile. She does not have maxillary sinus tenderness. The posterior pharynx is red but there is no discharge. The cervical lymph nodes are not enlarged or tender.

The provider makes a diagnosis of viral sinusitis that does not require antibiotic treatment at this time. To help AM resolve these symptoms, the provider explains how inflammation of the sinuses occurs following a viral illness and that it usually lasts 7–11 days but resolves spontaneously. She recommends that AM use a decongestant on a regular basis for 3 days, humidify the bedroom at night, increase fluids, and monitor for the development of more symptoms. They discuss the pros and cons of nasal sprays versus oral decongestants, and AM decides to use phenylpropanolamine (Tavist-D), which is an extended release systemic agent she can take every 8–12 hours. The provider advises AM not to use antihistamines. They discuss pain control and AM is able to take NSAIDs to treat the headache and sore throat. This provider has free prescription pads from the Centers for Disease Control and Prevention "Get Smart: Know When Antibiotics Work"[2] campaign, and she uses it to record the recommended treatment for AM. The provider tells AM that antibiotics are indicated if her symptoms do not improve by 10 days or if they get worse in 4 days despite this treatment. AM is given the voice mail phone number for the provider and they agree that she will call in 4 days to report her progress or lack thereof. AM gives the provider the name of her pharmacy.

Four days later, AM calls to say her headache is better when she takes the decongestant but it returns when the decongestant wears off, and she now has facial pain over her right eye that is worse. AM has the classic biphasic illness that is one of the signs of bacterial sinusitis. Bacterial sinusitis is usually caused by *H influenzae*, *Branhamella M catarrhalis*, or *S pneumoniae*. These bacteria are susceptible to beta-lactam antibiotics if they are not beta-lactamase producing organisms. The provider reviews AM's history to make sure she is not allergic to penicillin, and then calls her pharmacy to prescribe amoxicillin clavulanate (Augmentin) 500 mg to be taken three times per day for 10 days. This agent was chosen because the clavulanate extends coverage to include efficacy against beta-lactamase-producing bacteria.

Ten days later, AM calls and leaves a message for her provider that her symptoms started resolving 3–4 days after she started the amoxicillin clavulanate (Augmentin) and she was feeling well.

References

1. Roe V. Antibiotic resistance: a guide for effective prescribing in women's health. J Midwifery Womens Health 2008;53:216–26.
2. Centers for Disease Control and Prevention. Get smart: know when antibiotics work, materials for health care providers. Available from: *http://www.cdc.gov/drugresistance/community/healthcare-provider.htm* [Accessed August 29, 2008].
3. Waller DG. Rational prescribing: the principles of drug selection and assessment of efficacy. Clin Med 2005;1(5):26–8.
4. Gonzales R, Bartlett JG, Besser RE, Cooper RJ, Hickner JM, Hoffman JR, et al. Principles of appropriate antibiotic use for treatment of acute respiratory tract infections in adults. Ann Emerg Med 2001;37:680–7.
5. Cadieux G, Tamblyn R, Dauphinee D, Libman M. Predictors of inappropriate antibiotic prescribing among primary care physicians. Can Med Assoc J 2007;177:895–6.

6. National Guideline Clearinghouse. Available from *http://www.guideline.gov/* [Accessed August 29, 2008].

7. Infectious Diseases Society of America. Standards, practice guidelines and statements developed and/or endorsed by IDSA. Available from *http://www.idsociety.org/Content.aspx?id=9088* [Accessed September 2, 2008].

8. Niederman MS. Principles of appropriate antibiotic use. Int J Antimicrobl Agents 2005;26(Suppl 3):S170–5.

9. Guinovart C, Navia M, Tanner M, Alonso P. Malaria: burden of disease. Curr Mol Med 2006;6:137–40.

10. Rossoilini GM. Redesigning B-lactams to combat resistance: summary and conclusions. Clin Microbiol Infect 2007;13:30–3.

11. Shapiro JA. Thinking about bacterial populations as multicellular organisms. Annu Rev Microbiol 1998;52:81–104.

12. Lenski RE. The cost of antibiotic resistance from the perspective of the bacterium. Ciba Found Symp 1997;207:131–40.

13. Friedman M, Friedman GW. Alexander Fleming and antibiotics. In: Friedman M, Friedman GW, eds. Medicine's ten greatest discoveries. New Haven, CT: Yale University Press, 1998:168–91.

14. Spring M. A brief survey of the history of the antimicrobial agents. Bull N Y Acad Med 1975;51:1013–6.

15. Chambers HF. Beta-lactam antibiotics and other inhibitors of cell wall synthesis. In: Katzung BG, ed. Basic and clinical pharmacology, 10th ed. New York: McGraw-Hill, 2007:734–54.

16. Jacoby GA, Munoz-Price LS. The new beta lactamases. N Engl J Med 2005;352:380–91.

17. Centers for Disease Control and Prevention (CDC). Inadvertent use of Bicillin C-R to treat syphilis infection—Los Angeles, California, 1999–2004. MMWR Morb Mortal Wkly Rep 2005 Mar 11;54(9):217–9.

18. Petri WA Jr. Penicillins, cephalosporins, and other β-lactam antibiotics. In: Brunton LL, Lazo JS, Parker KL, eds. Goodman & Gillman's the pharmacological basis of therapeutics, 11th ed. New York: McGraw-Hill Medical, 2006:1127–54.

19. Kriebs J. Methicillin resistant *Staphylococcus aureus* infection in the obstetric settings. J Midwifery Womens Health 2008;53:247–50.

20. Betzold CM. An update on the recognition and management of lactational breast inflammation. J Midwifery Womens Health 2007;6:595–605.

21. Wilson W, Taubert KA, Gewitz M, Lockhart PB, Baddour LM, Levison M, et al. Prevention of infective endocarditis: guidelines from the American Heart Association: a guideline from the American Heart Association Rheumatic Fever, Endocarditis, and Kawasaki Disease Committee, Council on Cardiovascular Disease in the Young, and the Council on Clinical Cardiology, Council on Cardiovascular Surgery and Anesthesia, and the Quality of Care and Outcomes Research Interdisciplinary Working Group. Circulation 2007 Oct 9;116(15):1736–54.

22. Salkind AR, Cuddy PG, Foxworth JW. Is this patient really allergic to penicillin? An evidence-based analysis of the likelihood of penicillin allergy. JAMA 2001;285:2498–505.

23. Imhof M, Lipovac M, Kurz C, Barta J, Verhoeven HC, Huber JC. Propolis solution for the treatment of chronic vaginitis. Int J Gynecol Obstet 2005;89:127–32.

24. Riedl MA, Casillas AM. Adverse drug reactions: types and treatment options. Am Fam Physician 2003;68:1781–90.

25. Demoly P, Romano A. Update on beta-lactam allergy diagnosis. Curr Allergy Asthma Rep 2005;5:9–14.

26. DeShazo RD, Kemp SF. Allergic reactions to drugs and biologic agents. JAMA 1997;278:1895–906.

27. Gruchalla RS, Pirmohamed M. Antibiotic allergy. N Engl J Med 2006;354:257.

28. Centers for Disease Control and Prevention. Management of patients who have a history of penicillin allergy. Sexually transmitted diseases treatment guidelines. 2006. Available from: *http://www.cdc.gov/STD/treatment/2006/penicillin-allergy.htm* [Accessed May 10, 2008].

29. Pai MP, Momary KM, Rodvold KA. Antibiotic drug interactions. Med Clin North Am, 2006;90:25–7.

30. Weiner CP, Buhimschi C. Drugs for pregnant and lactating women. Philadelphia: Churchill Livingston, 2004.

31. Brassard P, Bourgault C, Brophy J, Kezouh A, Suissa S. Antibiotics in primary prevention of stroke in the elderly. Stroke 2003;34:163–7.

32. Kekar PS, Li JTC. Cephalosporin allergy. N Engl J Med 2001;345:804–9.

33. Levine DP. Vancomycin: understanding its past and preserving its future. South Med J 2008;101:284–91.

34. Smith TL, Pearson ML, Wilcox KR, Cruz C, Lancaster MV, Robinson-Dunn B, et al. Emergence of vancomycin resistance in *Staphylococcus aureus*. Glycopeptide-Intermediate *Staphylococcus aureus* Working Group. N Engl J Med 1999;340(7):493–501.

35. McDonald LC, Killgore GE, Thompson A, Owens RC, Kazakova SV, Sambol SP, et al. Emergence of an

epidemic, toxin gene variant strain of *Clostridium difficile* responsible for outbreaks in the United States between 2000 and 2004. N Engl J Med 2005;353:2433–41.

36. CDC. Recommendations for preventing the spread of vancomycin resistance. Recommendations of the Hospital Infection Control Practices Advisory Committee (HICPAC). MMWR 1995;44(RR12);1–13. Available from: *http://wonder.cdc.gov/wonder/prevguid/m0039349/m0039349.asp* [Accessed March 15, 2009].

37. Moellering RC Jr. Vancomycin: a 50-year reassessment. Clin Infect Dis 2006;42:S3–4.

38. Chambers HF. Chloramphenicol, tetracyclines, macrolides, clindamycin, and streptogramins. In: Katzung BG, ed. Basic and clinical pharmacology. New York: McGraw-Hill, 2007:754–64.

39. Doern GV, Richter SS, Miller A, Miller N, Rice C, Heilmann K. Antimicrobial resistance among *Streptococcus pneumoniae* in the United States: have we begun to turn the corner on resistance to certain antimicrobial classes? Clin Infect Dis 2005;41:139–48.

40. Mofenson LM, Oleske J, Serchuck L, Van Dyke R, Wilfert C, CDC, National Institutes of Health, Infectious Diseases Society of America. Treating opportunistic infections among HIV-exposed and infected children: recommendations from CDC, the National Institutes of Health, and the Infectious Diseases Society of America. MMWR Recomm Rep 2004;53(RR-14):1–112.

41. Pai MP, Graci DM, Amsden GW. Macrolide drug interactions: an update. Ann Pharmacother 2000;34:495-513.

42. Von Rosenstiel NA, Adam D. Macrolide antibacterials: drug interactions of clinical significance. Drug Saf 1995;13:105–22.

43. Kanazawa S, Ohkubo T, Sugawara K. The effects of grapefruit juice on the pharmacokinetics of erythromycin. Eur J Clin Pharmacol 2001 Jan-Feb;56(11): 799–803.

44. Briggs GG, Freeman RK, Yaffe SJ. Drugs in pregnancy and lactation, 8th ed. Philadelphia, PA: Lippincott Williams & Wilkins, 2006.

45. Daum RS. Clinical practice. Skin and soft-tissue infections caused by methicillin-resistant *Staphylococcus aureus*. N Engl J Med 2007;357(4):380–90.

46. Stevens H. Clindamycin. Prim Care Update Ob/Gyns 1997;4:251–3.

47. Freeman J, Wilcox MH. Antibiotics and *Clostridium difficile*. Microbes Infect 1999;1:377–384.

48. Bennett C. The aminoglycosides. Prim Care Update OB/Gyns 1996;3:186–189.

49. Gonzalez LS, Spencer JP. Aminoglycosides: a practical review. Am Fam Physician 1996;58:1811–20. Available from: *http://www.aafp.org/afp/981115ap/gonzalez.html*. [Accessed May 13, 2008].

50. Chambers HF. Aminoglycosides. In: Brunton LL, Lazo JS, Parker KL, eds. Goodman & Gillman's the pharmacological basis of therapeutics, 11th ed. New York: McGraw-Hill Medical, 2006:1155–71.

51. Chow JW. Aminoglycoside resistance in enterococci. Clin Infect Dis 2000;31:586–9.

52. Alestig K. Tetracyclines and chloramphenicol. In: Cohen J, Powderly WG, eds. Infectious diseases, 2nd ed. Edinburgh, Scotland: Elsevier Mosby, 2004:568–9.

53. Meyers B, Salvatore M. Tetracycline and chloramphenicol. In: Mandell GL, Bennett JE, Dolin R, eds. Principles and practice of infectious diseases, 6th ed. Philadelphia, PA: Elsevier, 2005:356–66.

54. Khardori N. Antibiotics—past, present, and future. Med Clin North Am 2006;90:1049–76.

55. Archer GL, Polk RE. Treatment and prophylaxis of bacterial infections. In: Fauci AS, Kasper DL, Longo DL, Braunwald E, Hauser SL, Jameson JL, et al., eds. Harrison's principles of internal medicine, 17th ed. New York: McGraw-Hill Medical, 2008:851–63.

56. Chambers, HF. Protein synthesis inhibitors and miscellaneous antibacterial agents. In: Brunton LL, Lazo JS, Parker KL, eds. Goodman & Gillman's the pharmacological basis of therapeutics, 11th ed. New York: McGraw-Hill Medical, 2006:1179–82.

57. Paladino JA. Linezolid: an oxazolidinone antimicrobial agent. Am J Health Syst Pharm 2002;59: 2413–25.

58. Petri WA Jr. Sulfonamides, trimethoprim-sulfamethoxazole, quinolones, and agents for urinary tract infection. In: Brunton LL, Lazo JS, Parker KL, eds. Goodman & Gillman's the pharmacological basis of therapeutics, 11th ed. New York: McGraw-Hill Medical, 2006:1119–22.

59. Granowitz EV, Brown RB. Antibiotic adverse reactions and drug interactions. Crit Care Clin 2008; 24:421–42.

60. Sunenshine RH, McDonald LC. *Clostridium difficile*-associated disease: new challenges from an established pathogen. Cleveland Clin J Med 2006;73: 187–97.

61. Hooper DC. Quinolones. In: Mandell GL, Bennett JE, Dolin R, eds. Principles and practice of infectious diseases, 6th ed. Philadelphia, PA: Elsevier, 2005:451–67.

62. Phillips MA, Stanley SL. Chemotherapy of protozoal infections. In: Brunton LL, Lazo JS, Parker KL, eds. Goodman & Gillman's the pharmacological basis of therapeutics, 11th ed. New York: McGraw-Hill Medical, 2006:1057–60.

63. Salvatore M, Meyers B. Metronidazole. In Mandell GL, Bennett JE, Dolin R, eds. Principles and practice of infectious diseases, 6th ed. Philadelphia, PA: Elsevier, 2005:388–94.

64. Raju TN. The Nobel chronicles. Lancet 1999;353:681.

65. Nicolle LE. Empirical treatment of acute cystitis in women. Int J Antimicrob Agents 2003;22:1–6.

66. Strom BL, Schinner R, Apter AJ, Margolis DJ, Lautenbach E, Hennessy S. Absence of cross-reactivity between sulfonamide antibiotics and sulfonamide nonantibiotics. N Engl J Med 2003;349:1628–35.

67. Niebyl JR. Antibiotics and other anti-infective agents in pregnancy and lactation. Am J Perinatol 2003;20:405–14.

68. Kaufmann SH, Baumann S, Nasser EA. Exploiting immunology and molecular genetics for rational vaccine design against tuberculosis. Int J Tuberc Lung Dis 2006;10:1068–79.

69. Shi R, Itagaki N, Sugawara I. Overview of anti-tuberculosis (TB) drugs and their resistance mechanisms. Mini Rev Med Chem 2007;7:1177–85.

70. WHO. Report No 4, Anti-tuberculosis drug resistance in the world. The WHO IUATLD Global Project on Anti-Tuberculosis Drug Resistance Surveillance: Geneva, Switzerland: The World Health Organization, 2008.

71. American Thoracic Society, CDC, and Infectious Diseases Society of America. Treatment of tuberculosis, MMWR 2003;52(RR-11):1-60. Available from: *http://www.cdc.gov/mmwr/preview/mmwrhtml/rr5211a1.htm* [Accessed March 15, 2009].

72. American Thoracic Society. Diagnostic standards and classification of tuberculosis in adults and children. Official statement of ATS, Centers for Disease Control and Prevention. September 1999. Am J Respir Crit Care Med 2000;161:1376–95.

73. Timmins GS, Deretic V. Mechanism of action of isoniazid. Mol Microbiol 2006;62(5):1220–7.

74. Tostmann A, Boeree MJ, Aarnoutse RE, de Lange WCM, van der Ven AJAM, Dekuijzen R. Antituberculosis drug-induced hepatotoxicity. J Gastroenterol Hepatol 2008;23:192–202.

75. Yew WW. Clinically significant interactions with drugs used in the treatment of tuberculosis. Drug Saf 2002;25:111–33.

76. Sobel JD. Practice guidelines for the treatment of fungal infections. Guidelines from the Infectious Diseases Society of America [editorial]. Clin Infect Dis 2000;30:652.

77. Bennett JE. Antimicrobial agents: antifungal agents. In: Brunton LL, Lazo JS, Parker KL, eds. Goodman & Gillman's the pharmacological basis of therapeutics, 11th ed. New York: McGraw-Hill Medical, 2006:1225–41.

78. Zhang AY, Camp WL, Elewski BE. Advances in topical and systemic antifungals. Dermatol Clin 2007; 25:165–83.

79. Albengres E, Le Louet H, Tillement JP. Systemic antifungal agents, drug interactions of clinical significance. Drug Saf 1998;18:83–97.

80. Como JA, Dismukes WE. Oral azole drugs as systemic antifungal therapy. N Engl J Med 1994;330:263–8.

81. Morrill JF, Heining MJ, Pappagianis D, Dewey KG. Risk factors for mammary candidosis among lactating women. J Obstet Neonatal Nurs 2005;34(1):37–45.

82. Crawford F, Hollis S. Topical treatments for fungal infections of the skin and nails of the foot. Cochrane Database of Systematic Reviews 2007, Issue 3. Art No: CD001434. DOI: 10.1002/14651858.CD001434.pub2.

83. Burpo RH. Common antiviral agents used in women's and children's care part 1. JOGNN 2000;29:181–90.

84. Brantley JS, Hicks L, Sra K, Tyring SK. Valacyclovir for the treatment of genital herpes. Expert Rev Anti Infect Ther 2006;4:367–76.

85. Safrin S. Antiviral agents. In: Katzung BG, ed. Basic and clinical pharmacology, 10th ed. New York: McGraw-Hill Medical, 2007:801–27.

86. Hollier LM, Wendel GD. Third trimester antiviral prophylaxis for preventing maternal genital herpes simplex virus (HSV) recurrences and neonatal infection. Cochrane Database of Systematic Reviews 2008, Issue 1. Art No: CD004946. DOI: 10.1002/14651858.CD004946.pub2.

87. Hayden FG. Antiviral agents (nonretroviral). In: Brunton LL, Lazo JS, Parker KL, eds. Goodman & Gillman's the pharmacological basis of therapeutics, 11th ed. New York: McGraw-Hill Medical, 2006:1243–71.

88. Guay DR. Amantadine and rimantadine prophylaxis of influenza A in nursing homes. A tolerability perspective. Drugs Aging 1994;5:8–19.

89. Cadieux G, Tamblyn R, Dauphinee D, Libman M. Predictors of inappropriate antibiotic prescribing among primary care physicians. Can Med Assoc J 2007;177:895–6.

90. Cabeen MT, Jacobs-Wagner C. Bacterial cell shape. Nat Rev Microbiol 2005;3:602.

12
Analgesia and Anesthesia

Tekoa L. King and Elissa Lane Miller

Chapter Glossary

Acute pain Predicted physiologic response to a noxious chemical, thermal, or mechanical stimulus, typically associated with invasive procedures, trauma, or disease.

Agonist Drug that stimulates a response or pharmacologic action when bound to a cell receptor, as opposed to antagonist, in which the action is inhibited.

Agonist-antagonist A drug that has agonist properties for one opioid receptor and antagonist properties for a different type of opioid receptor.

Analgesia* The absence of pain in response to stimulation that would normally be painful.

Anesthesia Total or partial loss of sensation.

Antagonist Drug that prevents a response when bound to a receptor.

Atypical analgesic Antiseizure, antidepressant, or other medication that is not a classic analgesic but has analgesic properties and is used as an adjunct analgesic.

Breakthrough pain Transitory flare of moderate to severe pain that occurs unexpectedly despite otherwise controlled pain.

Ceiling effect Dose beyond which no additional therapeutic effect is gained.

Chronic pain Pain that lasts longer than 3–6 months.

Equianalgesic Different doses of two analgesics that provide approximately equal analgesic effect. 30 mg of morphine is a common standard for calculating equianalgesic doses.

Hyperalgesia* An increased response to a stimulus that is normally painful; e.g., persons with neuropathy have an increased pain response to painful stimuli.

Modulation Process in which efferent nerve fibers in the CNS send impulses back down the spinal tract and, at the dorsal horn, release neurotransmitters that inhibit afferent transmission of pain impulses.

Multimodal analgesia The use of more than one medicine or class of medication or the use of more than one analgesic technique to produce analgesia through multiple mechanisms.

Neuropathic pain* Pain that is secondary to injury or malfunction in the peripheral or central nervous system.

Nociceptive pain* Pain that is secondary to local tissue damage.

Opiate Opioids that contain compounds found in opium.

Opioid Any natural or synthetic drug that has actions similar to morphine.

Pain* An unpleasant sensory and emotional experience associated with actual or potential tissue damage or described in terms of such damage.

Note: The inability to communicate verbally does not negate the possibility that an individual is experiencing pain and is in need of appropriate pain-relieving treatment. Pain is always subjective. Each individual learns the application of the word through experiences related to injury in early life.

Pain perception Perception of pain, which occurs in the cortex of the CNS.

Pain threshold* The least experience of pain that a person recognizes.

Pain tolerance The greatest intensity of painful stimulation that an individual is able to tolerate.

Partial agonist A drug molecule that elicits a partial pharmacologic response.

Patient-controlled analgesia (PCA) A method of allowing a person in pain to self-administer pain medication.

Perception Conscious awareness of pain.

Physical dependence[†] A state of adaptation that is manifested by a drug-class-specific withdrawal syndrome that can be produced by abrupt cessation, rapid dose reduction, decreasing blood level of the drug, and/or administration of an antagonist.

Preemptive analgesia Use of analgesia before the onset of noxious stimuli or a painful procedure.

Pseudo-addiction Addictive behavior (e.g., repeated requests for pain medication, pain complaints that seem excessive) that is secondary to inadequately treated pain and resolves with adequate pain relief.

Referred pain Pain experienced at a site adjacent to or at a distance from the site of injury.

Somatic pain Pain from stimulation of nociceptive receptors in the skin and superficial structures.

Tolerance[†] A state of adaptation in which exposure to a drug induces changes that result in a diminution of one or more of the drug's effects over time. Tolerance is also the term used when need for an increased dosage of a drug to produce the same level of analgesia that previously existed appears.

Transduction Process by which nerves translate painful stimuli into painful impulses.

Transmission Process by which pain impulses are transmitted to the central nervous system.

Visceral pain Pain that originates from compression, infiltration, stretching, or ischemia in internal organs.

* Definitions from the International Association for the Study of Pain available at: *www.iasp-pain.org.*

† Definitions from the American Academy of Pain Medicine, The American Pain Society, and the American Society of Addiction Medicine, 2001.

Introduction

Pain is the most common reason persons seek medical attention.[1] It is estimated that as many as 15% of all adults have chronic pain,[2] and virtually every person will have acute pain requiring pain management at some point in their lives. An estimated 20% of adults in the United States use an over-the-counter medication or prescription medication for pain relief daily.[3,4] Aspirin and nonsteroidal anti-inflammatory drugs (NSAIDs) are the most widely used analgesic in the United States today, yet they both have adverse effects that are frequently the cause of hospitalizations and significant morbidity.

The ability to accurately diagnose and treat pain is essential for all healthcare providers. Pain is a subjective experience, and no tests exist to specifically measure the qualitative or quantitative nature of a person's pain. Prescribing pain medication is largely empiric, based on the type of pain and intensity. However there is wide individual variability in the response to drugs used to treat pain.[5] Because many factors affect a person's perception, experience, and expression of pain, accurate assessment, diagnosis, and management of pain can be extremely challenging for even the most experienced practitioner. This chapter reviews the pharmacology of drugs used to treat pain and drugs used to induce anesthesia.

Definitions: Pain and Analgesia

Pain is defined by the International Association for the Study of Pain as "an unpleasant sensory and emotional experience associated with actual and potential tissue damage or described in terms of such damage."[6] But it is more complex than that. Pain is both sensory and emotional, it involves both peripheral and central mechanisms, and there is a host of receptors and substances involved in transmission of pain and modulation of pain. Because there are multiple pathways involved, several physiologic and psychologic targets need to be affected for pain relief to be adequate.[7] The **pain threshold** is the amount of stimulation required before the sensation of pain is experienced by an individual.[6] **Pain tolerance** is the greatest intensity of painful stimulation that an individual is able to tolerate.[6] **Pain perception**, or the actual experience of pain by an individual, is influenced by many factors and is widely variable among as well as within individuals.

Age and gender are among the factors that influence an individual's perception and response to pain. The elderly are more likely to have chronic pain than their younger cohorts. Research has indicated that women are more likely than men to report frequent, recurrent, or severe levels of pain and pain of longer duration.[8] Additionally, a woman's pain is more likely to be dismissed or underappreciated by healthcare providers, who may erroneously assume psychogenic origins. Finally, pain unique to women such as that associated with menstruation, pregnancy, and childbirth has been underappreciated by the medical community. Research in gender variations in pain has only recently begun to uncover the biologic basis for these differences.[9]

Types of Pain

Pain may be classified according to duration, etiology, and/or intensity. **Acute pain** is a "predicted physiological response to a noxious chemical, thermal or mechanical stimulus ... typically ... associated with invasive procedures, trauma and disease ..."[10] and is "generally time-limited."[10]

Chronic pain is differentiated from acute pain on the basis of duration. Most experts characterize pain as chronic when it lasts longer than 3–6 months.[11,12]

Referred pain occurs when an individual experiences pain at a site adjacent to or at a distance from the site of injury. One classic example of referred pain is the pain one feels in the shoulder when an ectopic pregnancy ruptures, which is referred from the bleeding that irritates the peritoneum. **Breakthrough pain** is a transitory flare of moderate to severe pain that occurs unexpectedly despite otherwise controlled pain. Breakthrough pain typically lasts 30 minutes or less; however, it may occur several times daily.[13] Each of these types of pain requires different pharmacologic techniques.

Nociceptive Pain

Pain may also be differentiated by etiology; it is either nociceptive or neuropathic. **Nociceptive pain** occurs in the presence of local tissue damage. Activation of nociceptive receptors located in the skin and other tissues activate a variety of chemical mediators such as bradykinin, prostaglandin, potassium, leukotrienes, or histamine that cause transmission of impulses via the afferent C and A delta fibers to the substantia gelatinosa located in the dorsal horn of the spinal cord. There, the nerve impulses cross the dorsal horn and are transmitted along the spinothalamic tract to the thalamus and eventually to the cerebral cortex where the perception of pain occurs (Figure 12-1).

Nociceptive pain may be further subdivided into **somatic pain** and **visceral pain**. Visceral pain originates from receptors located in the internal organs, which are activated by compression, infiltration, stretching, or ischemia. Visceral pain is often diffuse and poorly localized and may be referred to other regions of the body. Examples of visceral pain include pain associated with myocardial infarction, cholelithiasis, and appendicitis.

Somatic pain is caused by stimulation of nociceptive receptors located in the skin and other superficial structures. Somatic pain tends to be easily localized and may be described as dull or aching. Examples of somatic pain include musculoskeletal injuries, tendinitis or bursitis, and postsurgical pain. Nociceptive pain is typically well managed by drugs from the NSAID and opioid families.

Neuropathic Pain

Neuropathic pain results from an injury or malfunction in the peripheral or central nervous system. Although pain may be initially the result of an injury, neuropathic pain persists long after the original injury has resolved. The resulting compression or injury to a peripheral nerve or to the central nervous system may persist for months to years. While acute pain may be useful as a warning signal of injury, neuropathic pain serves no useful purpose and may be classified as a disease state in and of itself. Neuropathic pain is frequently described as burning, lancinating, tingling, or like an electrical shock. Typically, neuropathic pain does not respond well to opioids or NSAIDs. Complete resolution of neuropathic pain may not always be possible, but it can often be improved by use of antidepressants, anticonvulsants, or local anesthetics. Examples of neuropathic pain include postherpetic neuralgias, nerve entrapment syndromes, diabetic neuropathies, and phantom limb pain.

An individual may also experience a mixture of nociceptive and neuropathic pain that requires a combination of therapies, pharmacologic and nonpharmacologic. Cancer pain is often mixed and requires several different treatment modalities.

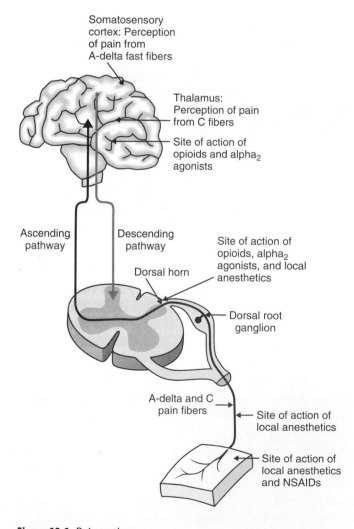

Figure 12-1 Pain pathway.

Types of Analgesia

Analgesia is the absence of pain in response to stimulation that would normally be painful.[14] The word comes from the Greek *an-* (without) and *-algesia* (to feel pain). Research on pain and methods to ameliorate pain did not begin in earnest until after Ronald Melzack and Patrick Wall published their gate control theory in 1965.[15] The neurologic pathways responsible for conducting pain from the periphery to the central nervous system (CNS) were well known but did not explain many aspects of the pain phenomenon. Melzack and Wall proposed a gating mechanism present in the spinal cord that modulated pain signals as they travel from the periphery to the CNS. This theory created a new concept that supported a subsequent body of research, which has expanded knowledge and has led to many adjunctive techniques used to ameliorate pain today.

At the other end of the scale, **anesthesia** is the condition of having pain sensation blocked. The term anesthesia was originally coined by Dr. Wendell Holmes in 1846 after he saw a demonstration of the use of ether for excision of a neck tumor at Massachusetts General Hospital.[16] From that first use of ether, the field of anesthesia has grown tremendously, and today there are several forms of anesthesia in use.

Analgesia today is not confined to treating pain via one modality with a single agent after the pain occurs. Anesthetic and analgesic drugs can be given through many different delivery systems to provide regional anesthesia, local anesthesia, or systemic analgesia. New transdermal techniques are being explored for treatment of chronic pain.

Atypical analgesics is the term used for use of drugs that can mitigate pain but are not in the opioid or nonsteroidal anti-inflammatory families. Drugs used for treating seizures, for example, have some efficacy in mitigating neuropathic pain. These agents will be discussed in further detail later in this chapter.

In addition to new techniques and new agents, older agents can be used in new ways. **Multimodal analgesia** refers to the use of more than one medicine or class of medication or the use of more than one analgesic technique to produce analgesia through multiple mechanisms.[17] Multimodal techniques use different physiologic mechanisms to block pain, which produce a synergistic or potentiating effect on pain control that allows use of lower doses of the individual agents. **Preemptive analgesia** refers to the administration of analgesic medication prior to a painful procedure or surgery for the purpose of decreasing CNS sensitization to painful stimuli, thereby decreasing postoperative pain. The theory is good, and animal studies have been promising, but to date, the clinical studies have yielded mixed results, and while promising, preemptive analgesia is not yet studied

enough to be part of clinical practice.[18] Finally, analgesic techniques can be defined by the protocols for administration. **Patient-controlled analgesia** is being used increasingly for acute and postoperative pain because when individuals are able to control the timing for administering pain medications, they have better medical outcomes, higher patient satisfaction scores, and no increase in the incidence of adverse reactions.[19] Traditionally, opioids have been administered as needed following surgery or painful medical procedures, but this frequently results in inadequate pain control and is being increasingly replaced by more explicit set dosing based on the individual situation.[20]

Pathophysiology of Pain

The perception of pain is dependent upon the cascade of physiologic events that start with detection of a noxious stimulant, followed by conduction of pain impulses to the brain, where the insult is interpreted as pain. Most pain medications affect the neurotransmitters that perpetrate the pain signal in the synapse between nerve cells at some point in the path from the site of injury to the brain (Figure 12-1). Several neurotransmitters such as endorphins, serotonin, norepinephrine, and substance P play a role as a physiologic agonist or antagonist to the pain signal. Therefore, the drugs used to treat pain interfere with one or more steps in a cascade that starts with transduction, continues with transmission, and then, in the central nervous system, concludes with perception and modulation. Although a detailed review of the pathophysiology and neurobiology of pain is beyond the scope of this chapter, the interested reader is referred to reviews by Melzack et al.[14,21-24]

In the first step of the cascade, **transduction**, a noxious stimulus releases biochemical mediators such as prostaglandins, histamine, leukotrienes, bradykinin, and/or substance P that stimulate nociceptors and initiate nerve conduction or signal transduction. Nonsteroidal antiinflammatory drugs inhibit the release of prostaglandins at the site of injury.

In **transmission**, the nerve signal travels along afferent fibers and terminates in the dorsal horn of the spinal cord. These fibers emit neurotransmitters that stimulate ascending nerve tracts, and the impulse is then carried to the thalamus or midbrain where it is interpreted as pain. Opioids bind to opioid receptors in the nerves of the spinal cord and prevent transmission to the brain.

Modulation is the process of decreasing or increasing the pain signal as it moves to the central nervous system. This occurs in the dorsal horn of the spinal cord and in the CNS. The nerve fibers that terminate in the midbrain connect to a reflex of efferent nerve fibers, which descend back down the spinal cord and release neurotransmitters that block the ascending message. Tricyclic antidepressants inhibit the reuptake of serotonin, which prolongs the effect of this neurotransmitter, thereby enhancing the reflex that blocks afferent fibers in the spinal cord.

Perception occurs in the cortex. Fibers from the thalamus send the message to several centers in the cortex that identify the type of pain, location, etc. There are several different neurotransmitter receptors in the CNS that cause a mild euphoria and decrease in pain perception when stimulated or antagonized by specific opioids.

Gender Differences in Pain Response

Gender differences in the pain response have been studied extensively in the last decade. Most studies have focused on acute rather than chronic pain. That sex differences exist regarding the response to opioid analgesia seems clear. However, the neurobiologic causes of variability in pain responses between men and women have yet to be adequately explored, especially in humans. Whether these differences are due to pharmacodynamic or pharmacokinetic differences is not yet clear.[25]

There is some evidence that estrogen reduces the efficacy of mu opioid agonists and, thus, these drugs may be less effective in the treatment of visceral pain in women than in men.[26] There is also evidence that low estrogen levels result in suppression of endogenous neurotransmissions affecting the mu receptors, resulting in higher levels of pain.[27]

▌Pain Assessment and Diagnosis

A comprehensive assessment of pain is mandated by the Joint Commission-approved pain assessment and management standards that were established in 1999. Thus a formal assessment and documentation of that assessment is now mandated for all persons cared for by institutions accredited by the Joint Commission. Pain assessment has become the fifth vital sign.

Pain assessment begins with a thorough history and physical examination. Determination of the etiology of a specific pain event is necessary so it may guide the selection of specific pain management strategies and, hopefully, methods to eliminate the cause.

Initial assessment can be guided by the PQRST (provokes, quality, radiation, severity, time) mnemonic[28] as described in Table 12-1. Several different pain scales that can be used to help the person in pain objectively measure

and quantify personal pain exist. Examples include the Short-Form McGill Pain Questionnaire[29] (Table 12-2), the Visual Analog Scale, and Faces Pain Scale. Anatomic drawings also can be used to help persons communicate the location of their pain.

Table 12-1 PQRST Mnemonic for Assessing Pain

PQRST	Additional Questions	Descriptors
Precipitating or palliative factors	What makes the pain worse? What makes the pain better? What have you already tried to treat the pain?	
Quality	Can you describe the pain?	Sharp, dull, burning, aching, shooting, stabbing, constant, throbbing
Region and radiation	Where does it hurt? Does the pain travel?	Deep versus superficial Diffuse versus localized
Severity and affect on quality of life	Ask the individual to rate pain using a pain scale. Does the pain prevent you from sleeping, eating, working? Are there associated symptoms?	Associated symptoms: dizziness, loss of balance, nausea Diaphoresis
Timing	Is pain related to any particular time? Is pain related with any particular activity?	Day, night, weekly, monthly

Table 12-2 The Short-Form McGill Pain Questionnaire

	None (0)	Mild (1)	Moderate (2)	Severe (3)
1. Throbbing				
2. Shooting				
3. Stabbing				
4. Sharp				
5. Cramping				
6. Gnawing				
7. Hot—burning				
8. Aching				
9. Heavy				
10. Tender				
11. Splitting				
12. Tiring—exhausting				
13. Sickening				
14. Fearful				
15. Punishing—cruel				
Score calculation				

Score by adding the values. Descriptors 1–11 represent the sensory component, 12–15 the affective component.
The patient's pain experience can be quantified by summing the indicated values.

Careful attention by the provider to the description of the pain can yield important clues to its origin. For instance, visceral pain often is described as diffuse, dull, or aching, while superficial pain frequently is categorized as throbbing or burning and typically can be localized.

A comprehensive pain assessment requires that supplemental information to the PQRST evaluation tool be gathered. Details of the individual's previous experience with pain, medication history, psychosocial history, and general health history can be of particular importance when caring for the person with chronic pain, but those details also can be critical in assessing acute pain. Finally, a careful physical examination for objective signs of pain is necessary to complete the pain assessment. Such findings as changes in heart or respiratory rate, blood pressure, level of consciousness, or affect may accompany pain. Localized redness, heat, edema, or alteration in function also may be present. However, absence of such findings does not mean that pain does not exist. Persons may experience significant pain without exhibiting any physical changes. Pain is a subjective experience, and the best approach to pain assessment is to believe the individual's self-description of the pain.

Approach to Therapy

In 1990, the World Health Organization (WHO) introduced the analgesic ladder for the treatment of pain.[30] Although originally intended as a standard for the management of cancer-associated pain, the analgesic ladder is a useful guideline for the management of both acute and chronic pain from any causes. The WHO ladder is a stepwise approach to pain management. Step 1 recommends treatment of mild pain with nonopioid analgesics such as acetaminophen, aspirin, or NSAIDs. Step 2 adds a

moderate opioid agonist in combination with nonopioids for moderate pain or pain of shorter duration, such as postoperative pain. Step 3 recommends use of stronger opioids on a round-the-clock rather than as-needed (prn) schedule for persistent pain. Figure 12-2 illustrates the WHO stepped approach to pain management. Adjunctive agents may be added for the treatment of severe pain as needed, especially in pain that has neural involvement. Neuropathic pain may be managed entirely with the use of adjunctive agents.

Pain management begins with the selection of the appropriate analgesic at the appropriate dosage and administration regimen. Management of chronic pain is best achieved when medications are administered on a regular, rather than as-needed, schedule.[31] Individuals and families should be taught that anticipating rather than chasing the pain results in better pain control with fewer side effects. Breakthrough pain is best managed with rapid-onset medications that have short half-lives. Alternately, pain that consistently recurs before the onset of regularly scheduled medication may indicate opioid **tolerance** or disease progression and signals the need for dose escalation and reevaluation.[32]

Nonopioid Analgesics

Nonopioid analgesics include two major classes: NSAIDs and acetaminophen. There are six classes of NSAIDs based on chemical structure. However in clinical practice, the term *NSAID* is not used to refer to salicylates (aspirin), and the other NSAIDs that are frequently used are categorized as selective or nonselective based on their mechanism of action.

Acetaminophen, aspirin, and NSAIDs are the most frequently used drugs for relief of mild to moderate acute pain. These drugs may be used in combination with opioids

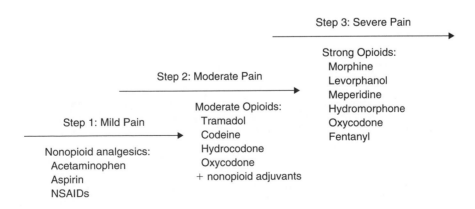

Figure 12-2 World Health Organization (WHO) analgesic scale.

for the relief of severe pain. The primary difference between nonopioid analgesics and opioid analgesics are the following: (1) NSAIDs have a **ceiling effect**, and therefore, after achieving a certain plasma level, increasing the dose will increase the side effects but not the analgesic effect; (2) NSAIDs are antipyretic and opioids do not have this effect; and (3) NSAIDs do not produce **physical dependence** or psychological dependence.[33]

Mechanism of Action of Nonopioid Analgesics: NSAIDs

All drugs in the NSAID family mitigate pain via inhibition of cyclooxygenase (COX), the enzyme responsible for synthesis of prostaglandins, prostacyclin, and thromboxane. Prostaglandins cause pain through promotion of inflammatory responses such as edema and local vasodilation, and by stimulating nociceptors (signal transduction) to transmit pain impulses.

COX converts arachidonic acid from the cell membrane into prostaglandin H_2, the precursor of a variety of different prostaglandins (Figure 12-3). Cyclooxygenase has three forms, COX-1, COX-2, and COX-3. COX-1 is constitutive and found in virtually all tissues and is involved in the production of prostaglandins that have many important "housekeeping" functions, including: (1) protection of gastric mucosa, (2) inhibition of gastric secretions,

(3) stimulation of platelet aggregation, (4) renal vasodilation, and (5) stimulation of uterine contractions. COX-2 is inducible in macrophages and at tissue injury sites. At the site of tissue injury, COX-2 forms and then converts arachidonic acid to prostaglandins that mediate local inflammatory responses and sensitize receptors to painful stimuli. COX-2 is constitutive in some tissues. In the brain, COX-2 facilitates synthesis of prostaglandins that mediate fever and pain perception, and constitutive COX-2 in the kidney facilitates production of prostaglandins that support renal function. COX-3 is a variant of COX-1 with a mutation, and therefore, some scientists prefer the term *COX-1b* or *COX-1 variant* (COX 1v). COX-3 only acts centrally within the blood–brain barrier to regulate fever and pain sensitivity. Figure 12-3 summarizes the COX pathways.

NSAIDs are generally classified according to the specific COX enzyme that is inhibited. Aspirin and other first-generation NSAIDs inhibit all three COX enzymes and are therefore called nonselective COX inhibitors. Second-generation NSAIDs inhibit both COX-2 and COX-3. Acetaminophen is hypothesized to affect only COX-3, which may explain its lack of anti-inflammatory effect.[34] Although all NSAIDs prevent production of prostaglandins via inhibition of the COX enzymes, there are clinically important differences in pharmacokinetics and pharmacodynamics, which are discussed later in this chapter.

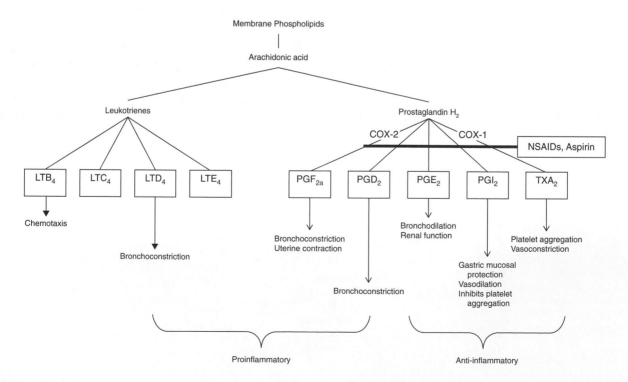

Figure 12-3 COX pathways.

Aspirin

Aspirin, or acetylsalicylic acid (ASA), is considered the prototype nonsteroidal anti-inflammatory drug. Aspirin-containing compounds have been used to treat pain since the beginning of recorded history. Medicine made from willow bark, which contains salicin, was recommended for treatment of fever, pain, and inflammation by the ancient Greeks.[35] Introduced as a patented pill by Bayer in 1899, aspirin's mechanism of action was unclear until 1971, when its COX-inhibiting abilities were demonstrated.[36] Since then, newer NSAIDs have been developed, but aspirin continues to be one of the most valuable and widely used agents and remains the standard to which all other NSAIDs are compared. Aspirin is a member of the salicylate family. Other members of this family less commonly used are listed in Table 12-3 and Table 12-4. Other salicylates produce effective analgesia with fewer gastrointestinal side effects and less impact on platelet aggregation. However, they are no more effective than most of the newer NSAIDs.[37]

Pharmacokinetics

Aspirin is a weak acid poorly absorbed in the stomach. Most is absorbed in the small intestine. Absorption following oral administration is rapid and complete. Following absorption, aspirin is rapidly converted to salicylic acid, the active metabolite. The half-life of salicylic acid varies depending on the amount present, ranging from 2 hours at low therapeutic levels to more than 20 hours when high levels are present.

Salicylic acid is distributed to all body tissues via plasma albumin, to which it is extensively bound. Once the plasma proteins are saturated, the unbound fraction increases disproportionately, which can lead to aspirin toxicity. Aspirin modifies COX-1 and COX-2 irreversibly so the duration of action is secondary to the rate at which the COX system replaces itself in the affected target organ. Excretion of salicylic acid and its metabolites occurs renally and is dependent upon urinary pH. Excretion is facilitated by alkalinization of the urine and inhibited by acidic urine. A summary of the pharmacokinetics of aspirin and NSAIDs is provided in Table 12-5.

Pharmacodynamics

Aspirin has four major therapeutic indications: (1) reduction of fever, (2) relief of mild to moderate pain, (3) reduction of inflammation, and (4) suppression of platelet aggregation. Aspirin's antipyretic effect is achieved by lowering the set point of the hypothalamus through inhibition of COX-2. By inhibiting prostaglandin synthesis in the hypothalamus, aspirin reduces fever, but does not lower normal body temperature.

The analgesic effects of aspirin are achieved both peripherally and centrally. By suppressing prostaglandin synthesis at the site of local tissue injury, local pain receptors are rendered less sensitive. Central prostaglandin inhibition results in decreased transmission of pain impulses through the spinal column. Aspirin suppresses inflammation through nonselective inhibition of the COX system, which results in an overall reduction of prostaglandins.

Aspirin is an initial drug of choice for inflammatory conditions such as rheumatoid arthritis, tendinitis, and bursitis. However, aspirin must be given in doses to produce plasma drug levels of 150 mcg/mL to 300 mcg/mL to achieve sufficient anti-inflammatory effects. Because signs of salicylate toxicity can begin at levels as low as 200 mcg/mL, becoming severe at levels above 400 mcg/mL, the usefulness of aspirin for relief of chronic inflammatory conditions can be limited by adverse effects. Aspirin and other NSAIDs have a ceiling effect; increasing the dose beyond a certain amount will not increase analgesia but will increase toxicity.[38]

Platelet aggregation occurs through the action of thromboxane A_2 (TXA_2), a prostaglandin-related compound regulated by COX-1. By irreversibly acetylating COX-1, aspirin inhibits the formation of thromboxane A_2 and thereby reduces platelet stickiness and inhibits platelet aggregation. Because platelets do not have the ability to synthesize new COX-1, platelet aggregation is inhibited for the life of the platelet, which is approximately 8–10 days.

Clinical Indications for Aspirin

Aspirin is indicated for relief of mild to moderate pain, including arthritis, fever reduction, and suppression of inflammation. Aspirin also is useful for treatment of dysmenorrhea, although it may increase menstrual bleeding when used for this purpose. Aspirin is not effective for visceral pain.

The antiplatelet aggregation effect of aspirin promotes bleeding. A daily dose of baby aspirin is recommended to inhibit platelet aggregation for persons with or at risk for ischemic stroke, transient ischemia attacks, acute myocardial infarction, and chronic stable angina. In the past, persons who took aspirin daily to prevent clotting have been counseled to stop taking the aspirin several days before having a surgical procedure. Recent studies comparing the benefits and risks of aspirin therapy have concluded that

Table 12-3 Over-the-Counter Nonopioid Analgesics for Treating Mild Pain

Medication Generic (Brand)	Formulations	Usual Adult Dose	Maximum Daily Dose	Clinical Considerations
Acetaminophen (Tylenol)	Regular strength 325 mg; extra strength 1000 mg; extended release 650 mg	650–975 mg q 4 h	4000 mg/24 h*	Acetaminophen has antipyretic and analgesic properties but is not anti-inflammatory. Should be avoided in patients with liver impairment or those who regularly consume more than three alcoholic drinks/day.
Nonsteroidal Anti-Inflammatory Drugs (NSAIDs)				
Aspirin[†]	Baby ASA 81 mg Adult tablets come as 165, 325, 500, or 650 mg	650–975 mg q 4 h	4000 mg	Aspirin is associated with Reye's syndrome in children. Antiplatelet effect is irreversible for life of platelet. Gastritis and bleeding are common with chronic use. Persons with asthma may be intolerant to ASA. Discontinue 1 week prior to elective surgery.
Ibuprofen (Motrin, Advil, Nuprin, Rufen)[†]	200 mg	400–800 mg q 4–6 h[‡]	3200 mg	Analgesic and antipyretic effects are relatively immediate. Anti-inflammatory effects require longer therapy and higher doses. Contraindicated in third trimester of pregnancy.
Naproxen (Aleve)[†]	200, 250, 375, 500 mg	200–800 mg q 4 h[§]	1500 mg	Analgesic and antipyretic effects are relatively immediate. Anti-inflammatory effects may require longer therapy.

* The recommended maximum dose per day is currently 4000 mg. Because there is a narrow margin between this dose and the risk for hepatotoxicity, some authors suggest that 2600 mg should be the maximum dose per day that is recommended for healthy individuals and that the maximum recommended dose be lower for persons at risk for hepatic injury.
† NSAIDs contraindicated during pregnancy.
‡ OTC guidelines suggest the maximum dose of ibuprofen should be 400 mg per dose and 1200 mg/day for a maximum of 10 days.
§ OTC guidelines suggest the maximum dose of naproxen should be 440 mg per dose and 660 mg/day for less than 10 days.

stopping aspirin before surgery is not always necessary and depends on the individual risk and procedure being performed.[39,40] Although regular use of high-dose aspirin has been found to decrease the risk of colorectal cancer (these cancers overexpress COX-2), the United States Preventive Services Task Force does not recommend the use of aspirin or NSAIDs for this purpose at this time because of the significant risk of gastrointestinal bleeding that is associated with the use of aspirin.[41]

Side Effects/Adverse Effects

The most common side effects of aspirin therapy are gastrointestinal. The incidence of gastrointestinal complications varies depending on specific population characteristics, use of additional medications, and differences in doses. Overall, approximately 50% of persons who take aspirin will report some gastric upset. Nausea, heartburn, and gastric distress may be seen with low or intermittent dosing secondary to suppression of the prostaglandins that facilitate production of gastric mucosa. Long-term use may result in gastric ulceration and bleeding. Aspirin-induced ulcers are often asymptomatic and perforation and hemorrhage can occur without premonitory signs. To date, there is no evidence that enteric-coated or buffered tablets decrease the risk of GI bleeding.[42]

In 2009, the FDA issued a new regulation that requires all products that contain aspirin to: (1) display the names *aspirin* and *NSAID* prominently on the principal display panel of the label, (2) add a warning about severe gastrointestinal bleeding on the outside of the container or wrapper of the package, and (3) replace an older warning about

Table 12-4 Prescription Nonopioids for Treating Mild Pain

Medication Generic (Brand)	Formulations	Usual Adult Dose	Maximum Daily Dose	Clinical Considerations
Salicylic Acid Derivatives				
Choline magnesium trisalicylate (Trilisate)	500, 750, 1000 mg	1000–2000 mg q 12–24 h	4500 mg	Does not inhibit platelet aggregation. Less effective analgesia than aspirin or ibuprofen.
Choline salicylate (Arthropan)	870 mg/ 5 mL	870 mg q 3–4 h	6 doses	Same basic side effects as aspirin.
Diflunisal (Dolobid)	250, 500 mg	1000 mg initially followed by 500 mg q 8–12 h	1500 mg	Slower onset than aspirin but 500 mg of diflunisal is superior to 650 mg of aspirin. May take up to 14 days for full therapeutic effects to be reached. Severe gastric toxicity associated with diflunisal, which may require withdrawal of the drug.
Nonsteroidal Anti-Inflammatory Drugs (NSAIDs)*				
Etodolac (Lodine)	200, 300 mg	200–800 mg bid	1200 mg	Relatively minor GI side effects in comparison with other NSAIDs. Also available in extended-release formulations for once-daily dosing.
Fenoprofen (Nalfon)	200, 300, 600 mg	200–600 mg q 6–8 h	3200 mg	Fenoprofen is the most nephrotoxic of all NSAIDs. Drug-induced nephritic syndrome has been reported.
Ketoprofen (Orudis)	12.5-, 25-, 50-, 75-mg capsules; 100-, 150-, and 200-mg ER	25–60 mg q 6–8 h	300 mg	Severe gastric toxicity associated with ketoprofen may require discontinuation. Also available in extended-release formulation for once-daily dosing.
Ketorolac tromethamine (Toradol)	10-mg tablets, 15 mg/mL, 30 mg/ mL	25–75 mg q 6–8 h	Oral: 40 mg IV: 120 mg	Therapy should be limited to 5 days. Step down to ibuprofen after 5 days.
Meclofenamate sodium (Meclomen)	50 mg, 100 mg	50–100 mg q 4–6 h	400 mg	Relatively severe gastric toxicity may require coadministration of a cytoprotective agent. May cause photosensitivity. Use sunscreen.
Mefenamic acid (Ponstel)	250 mg	500 initially, then 250 mg q 6 h	1000 mg	FDA approved for treatment of primary dysmenorrhea, but no clinical evidence that it is more effective than other NSAIDs. Treatment of mild to moderate pain should be limited to less than 7 days.
COX-2 Selective Inhibitors NSAIDs				
Celecoxib (Celebrex)	100, 200, 400 mg	100 mg bid	400 mg	COX-2 specific: Avoid in patients with sulfonamide allergy or sensitivity. Use cautiously in the elderly, and in persons with asthma, renal or hepatic disease, or on anticoagulants or antihypertensives.

* Use cautiously in the elderly and in patients with asthma, renal or hepatic disease, or on anticoagulants or antihypertensives. Contraindicated in pregnancy.

alcohol use with one that warns of severe liver damage if large doses are used or if the consumer drinks ≥ 3 glasses of alcohol per day.

Approximately 50 million persons in the United States (36% of the adult population) take aspirin daily for cardiovascular protection.[43] In the Women's Health Study, approximately 50% of the participants reported some gastric upset, whereas the incidence of any gastrointestinal bleeding was 5% and the incidence of a GI hemorrhage that required a blood transfusion was 0.6%.[44] The incidence of gastrointestinal complications appears to be dose related and increases in persons taking larger doses; however, even the lowest 81-mg dose doubles the incidence of gastrointestinal complications when compared to placebo.[43]

Factors that increase the risk of gastric ulceration include advanced age, previous history of peptic ulcer disease, infection with *Helicobacter pylori*, history of intolerance

Table 12-5 Pharmacokinetics of Aspirin, Salicylates, Acetaminophen, and NSAIDs

Drug Generic (Brand)	Time to Peak Concentration (Hours)	Half-Life (Hours)	Protein Binding	Metabolism
Acetaminophen (Tylenol)	0.7	1–4	> 50%	CYP2E1 and CYP1A2
Salicylates				
Aspirin	Variable	0.3	75–90%	Liver
Choline salicylate (Arthropan, Trilisate)	0.5	2–3	80–90%	Liver
Magnesium salicylate (Magan, Doan's caplets)	0.5	2–3	80–90%	Liver
Sodium salicylate (generic)	0.5–0.75	2–3	80–90%	Liver
Diflunisal (Dolobid)	2–3	8–12	99%	Liver
First-Generation NSAIDs (Nonselective COX Inhibitors)				
Diclofenac (Voltaren, Cataflam)	2	2	99%	CYP2C9
Etodolac (Lodine)	1.5	7.3	99%	CYP2C9
Fenoprofen (Nalfon)	2	3	99%	Liver
Flurbiprofen (Ansaid)	2.5	5.7	99%	CYP3C9
Ibuprofen (Motrin, Advil, others)	1–2	1.8–2	99%	CYP2C9 and CYP2C19
Indomethacin (Indocin)	21.5	4.5	90%	CYP2C9
Ketorolac (Toradol)	2–3	5–6	99%	CYP2C9
Ketoprofen (Orudis, Oruvail)	0.5–2	2	99%	CYP2C9
Mefenamic acid (Postel)	2–4	2	90%	CYP2C9
Meloxicam (Mobic)	4–5	20	99%	CYP2C9
Meclofenamate (generic)	0.5–2	1.3	99%	Liver
Nabumetone (Relafen)	9–12	22	99%	CYP2C9 and CYP1A2
Naproxen (Aleve, Anaprox, Naprosyn)	2–4	12–17	99%	CYP2C9
Piroxicam (Feldene)	3–5	50	99%	CYP2C9
Sulindac (Clinoril)	2–4	7.8	93%	Liver
Tolmetin (Tolectin)	0.5–1	2–7	99%	Liver
Second-Generation NSAIDs (COX-2 Inhibitors)				
Celecoxib (Celebrex)	3	11	97%	CYP2C9 and CYP3A4

of ASA or other NSAIDs, cigarette smoking, and alcohol use. Concomitant use of a proton pump inhibitor or histamine 2 antagonist to reduce gastric acid production can be useful for those on long-term aspirin therapy (Chapter 21). Misoprostol (Cytotec), a synthetic prostaglandin, promotes gastric mucus production and is the only agent proven effective for the prevention and/or treatment of clinically significant ASA-associated ulcers.[45]

Although short-term use of aspirin at low therapeutic levels rarely causes serious adverse effects, toxicity is associated with long-term use at high-dose anti-inflammatory levels. Prostaglandins promote renal vasodilation and other normal renal functions. High-dose or long-term use of ASA by persons with renal impairment can result in acute renal function impairment by inhibition of prostaglandin through the COX-1 pathway. Sodium retention, edema, decreased urine output, and increased blood urea nitrogen and serum creatinine all are signs of renal impairment that must be monitored for those individuals taking high-dose, long-term ASA therapy. Interruption of ASA therapy

typically results in a reversal of these effects. Renal papillary necrosis also may be associated with long-term ASA use.

Aspirin can also cause hepatic injury and various blood dyscrasias, although these complications are rare. Hepatotoxicity from aspirin is most likely to occur in children who have a concomitant viral illness that results in the clinical presentation called *Reye's syndrome*.[46] Reye's syndrome is not common today, secondary to the recommendation that children not be given aspirin.

Finally, daily aspirin therapy is associated with a small increased risk for hemorrhagic stroke that in all trials conducted to date is offset by a much larger reduction in myocardial infarction and stroke from clots.[44] Therefore when considering daily aspirin therapy for cardiovascular protection, the risk of gastrointestinal hemorrhage and hemorrhagic stroke must be compared to the risk for a cardiovascular event, and the recommendation for taking aspirin needs to be individualized when considering prophylactic use of aspirin. (See Chapter 15 for more detailed information on use of aspirin for cardiovascular protection.)

Aspirin Hypersensitivity

Aspirin is associated with three types of hypersensitivity reactions including aspirin-exacerbated respiratory disease (AERD), aspirin-intolerant urticaria/angioedema, and rarely anaphylaxis.[47,48] AERD has a prevalence of 0.2–0.6% in the general population. The prevalence is increased to 4.3–11% in persons with asthma, and some authors suggest it is as high as 20%.[49] However, AERD occurs in approximately 34% of persons who have asthma and nasal polyps.[48] AERD is also more common in women than in men and generally develops in adulthood.

In 1922, Widel first described the clinical syndrome of aspirin allergy, asthma, and nasal polyps, a syndrome later named Samter's triad.[48] The mechanism of action of Samter's triad is not fully elucidated, but it appears that the aspirin inhibition of the COX pathways shifts arachidonic acid metabolism to the leukotriene pathway, which results in increased production of leukotrienes that cause bronchoconstriction. There appears to be a genetic component to the disorder as well.[50] The symptoms usually appear 30–120 minutes after ingesting aspirin.

Aspirin-intolerant urticaria is the least understood and appears to occur secondary to aspirin-stimulating histamine release of cutaneous mast cells. True anaphylaxis from aspirin use is probably extremely rare.

Persons with aspirin hypersensitivity can be treated with leukotriene receptor antagonists such as zileuton (Zyflo) or montelukast (Singular). Aspirin desensitization can be performed if aspirin is necessary, but this should be done in a hospital under close supervision. Finally, avoiding aspirin and aspirin-containing products is the best way to prevent these symptoms. Approximately 20% of persons with aspirin allergy will also exhibit allergic reactions to nonselective NSAIDs because they cross-react with aspirin. Thus, nonselective NSAIDs should be avoided as well by persons with aspirin allergy. Selective COX-2 inhibiting NSAIDs and nonacetylated salicylates are recommended for treatment of pain in persons who have an aspirin hypersensitivity.

Salicylism: Aspirin Toxicity

Salicylism, or aspirin toxicity, occurs when serum plasma levels rise above 300 mcg/mL, which is just slightly higher than therapeutic levels. Signs of salicylism include tinnitus, dizziness, headache, sweating, and tachypnea. Acid–base imbalances may result in respiratory alkalosis. In most cases, salicylism is easily reversed by discontinuing the drug. Some experts suggest that tinnitus can be used as a marker for high therapeutic levels of ASA.[51] The dosage level at which tinnitus occurs is considered the individual's maximal therapeutic level. However, this method for determining maximal dosing is not safe for the elderly, who may not develop tinnitus until toxic levels are present. Many over-the-counter drugs contain aspirin, and therefore, aspirin overdose can occur unintentionally.

Drug–Drug Interactions

Aspirin can be involved in drug–drug interactions via several mechanisms. Aspirin's ability to compete for plasma protein sites can result in increased plasma levels, a well-known drug–drug interaction when valproic acid (Depakote) and aspirin are taken concomitantly. When aspirin is used in combination with other NSAIDs, the two medications have an additive effect on the risk for developing gastrointestinal side effects. More importantly, NSAIDs compete for the site where aspirin and NSAIDs block COX-1, thereby preventing aspirin from having the irreversible anticoagulation effect that is one of the desired therapeutic outcomes.[52] Significant drug interactions are summarized in Table 12-6.

Contraindications

Absolute contraindications to ASA use include previously demonstrated hypersensitivity, recent history of gastrointestinal bleeding, and bleeding disorders. Aspirin should not be used by children and adolescents suspected of having influenza or varicella because there is a reported association between use of aspirin to treat viral syndromes and the development of Reye's syndrome. The etiologic relationship is controversial but the recommendation that children not be given aspirin stands nonetheless. Aspirin should be used cautiously in patients with renal impairment, cigarette or alcohol use, *H pylori* infection, gout, mild diabetes, uncontrolled hypertension, or heart failure.

Special Populations

Pregnancy and Lactation

Aspirin is classified as a Pregnancy Category D drug. ASA suppression of COX-2 has a theoretical risk of interfering with implantation, but this has not been proven in human studies. Conversely, suppression of prostaglandins is necessary for the maintenance of pregnancy so there is a theoretical benefit to use of aspirin later in pregnancy.[53] Known risks of chronic ASA use during normal pregnancy include anemia from occult gastrointestinal blood loss. Inhibition of prostaglandin production may also suppress spontaneous uterine contractions and delay or prolong labor.[54]

Table 12-6 Selected Drug–Drug Interactions Associated with Aspirin/Salicylates and NSAIDs*

Drug Generic (Brand)	Drug–Drug Interactions if Taken Concomitantly with Aspirin or NSAIDs
Alcohol	Increases gastrointestinal bleeding.
Aminoglycosides	Nonsteroidal antiinflammatory drugs (NSAIDs) inhibit aminoglycoside renal clearance.
Antacids	Increased pH of gastric contents may affect enteric-coated acetylsalicylic acid (ASA). Aluminum hydroxide decreases naproxen absorption.
Anticoagulants	ASA and NSAIDs prolong bleeding time.
Antihypertensive agents	NSAIDs antagonize antihypertensive effects of beta-blockers, ACE inhibitors, vasodilators, and diuretics. Hyperkalemia may occur when NSAIDs are used with ACE inhibitors or potassium-sparing diuretics.
Cephalosporins	Increase bleeding risk with ASA.
Corticosteroids	Increase risk of gastrointestinal ulceration and reduction of serum salicylate levels.
Digoxin (Lanoxin)	NSAIDs inhibit renal clearance of digoxin.
Fluconazole (Diflucan)	Increases plasma concentration levels of celecoxib.
H_2 receptor antagonists	Increase potential salicylate toxicity. Reduce effectiveness of naproxen sodium.
Hypoglycemic agents	Large doses of ASA may increase the hypoglycemic effect of these drugs.
Lithium (Eskalith, Lithobid)	NSAIDs increase the steady-state concentration of lithium and can lead to lithium toxicity.
Methotrexate (Rheumatrex, Trexall)	All NSAIDs except celecoxib result in reduced clearance of methotrexate with resulting increased plasma methotrexate levels.
NSAIDs	Routine but not intermittent use of ibuprofen reduces the antiplatelet effects of ASA.
Phenobarbital (Luminal)	ASA levels may be reduced via enzyme induction.
Phenytoin (Dilantin)	ASA and ibuprofen increase serum phenytoin levels by competition for protein-binding sites.
Propranolol (Inderal)	Competition for receptors may reduce anti-inflammatory effectiveness of ASA.
Pyrazolone derivatives (phenylbutazone, oxyphenbutazone, and possibly dipyrone)	Concomitant use with ASA increases the risk of gastric ulceration.
Selective serotonin reuptake inhibitors	NSAIDs increase risk of gastrointestinal bleeding.
Spironolactone (Aldactone)	ASA may decrease sodium excretion.
Uricosuric agents (probenecid, sulfinpyrazone, and phenylbutazone)	ASA decreases effectiveness.
Urinary alkalinizers	Reduction of ASA effectiveness by increasing renal elimination of salicylic acid.
Valproate (Depakote)	ASA inhibits oxidation of valproate and reduces clearance with resulting potential increase in valproate toxicity.

* This table is not comprehensive as new information is being generated on a regular basis.

Very-low-dose aspirin has been suggested during the second and third trimesters for prevention of fetal growth retardation, premature birth, preeclampsia, and stillbirth in high-risk pregnancies.[55] Although aspirin does decrease the incidence of preeclampsia in women at risk for preeclampsia, more studies are needed, and it is not yet recommended for use in clinical practice.[56,57]

Low-dose aspirin is also sometimes recommended for women at risk for thrombotic events (e.g., antiphospholipid antibody syndrome), but again, the efficacy is unproven and the recommendation is not yet universal.

Aspirin freely crosses the placenta. There is anecdotal evidence that routine use of high-dose ASA at or near term is associated with restriction or premature closure of the ductus arteriosus in the fetus, although a causal relationship is uncertain.[58] Routine high-dose aspirin use in pregnancy has also been associated with stillbirth, renal toxicity, and intracranial hemorrhage in preterm infants.[59]

The American Academy of Pediatrics (AAP) lists ASA as a drug that has been associated with serious neonatal side effects and should be avoided during lactation.[60] Metabolic acidosis in the neonate has been reported.[61]

Elderly

The elderly are more susceptible to the adverse effects of aspirin than younger persons are. Gastrointestinal, renal, and central nervous system effects are all more frequently found among the elderly. Additionally, increased risk for drug interactions exist. Increase in serum potassium for those with chronic renal insufficiency or those on potassium-sparing antibiotics is a rare but serious adverse effect.

Other Salicylates

Nonacetylated salicylates include choline salicylate (Arthropan), magnesium salicylate (Doan's pills), sodium salicylate, and diflunisal (Dolobid). Like aspirin, these drugs inhibit both COX-1 and COX-2 and have similar indications for use, including mild to moderate pain. However, these agents do not have the same antiplatelet effect, and they are not recommended for protection against stroke or myocardial infarction. The most common side effects are gastrointestinal, although the incidence of gastric ulceration is much reduced compared to the frequency of side effects associated with use of ASA.

▌ Nonsteroidal Anti-Inflammatory Drugs (NSAIDs)

Nonselective NSAIDs: First-Generation NSAIDs

Nonselective NSAIDs were developed to achieve the benefits of aspirin with fewer side effects. In 1969, ibuprofen (e.g., Advil, Motrin), the prototype drug, was introduced to the United Kingdom market.[35] Since that time, numerous NSAIDs have been developed, and NSAIDs are today the most frequently used drugs in the United States. As the population ages, we can assume more persons will take NSAIDs, and more adverse effects will occur.[62,63] Therefore, an in-depth knowledge of the pharmacologic effects of this class of drugs is essential for all primary care providers.

Pharmacokinetics

NSAIDs are weak organic acids that are well absorbed in the stomach and have negligible first-pass metabolism.[33] They achieve peak concentrations within 1–4 hours and are clinically divided into short-acting (< 6 hours) or long-acting (> 6 hours) depending on individual half-lives. Food does not interfere with absorption. All NSAIDs are highly protein bound and undergo hepatic metabolism via the CYP450 enzymes and excretion via the kidney. Like aspirin, ibuprofen (Advil) and other first-generation NSAIDs nonselectively inhibit COX-1 and COX-2 and have antipyretic, anti-inflammatory, and analgesic properties. Unlike aspirin, NSAIDs' effect on platelet inhibition is reversible. Probably the most important clinical aspect of NSAID pharmacokinetics and pharmacodynamics is that there is considerable individual variability in response, the mechanism of which is not well known. Regardless, if one NSAID does not produce a therapeutic response, trying a different one may elicit the desired response.

Clinical Indications

Clinical indications for NSAIDs are the same as for use of aspirin with a few exceptions. Because NSAIDs do not have a permanent effect on platelet aggregation, they are not used for clotting prophylaxis or heart health.

Dosing

For those taking ibuprofen (Advil), 2400 mg/day is therapeutically equivalent to 4 g of aspirin/day. It is important to remember that lower doses can be used for treatment of pain, but higher doses are needed to treat inflammation. In addition, it takes 2–4 weeks of regular use to get the full anti-inflammatory benefit. NSAIDs are more effective than a daily 4-gram dose of acetaminophen for treatment of osteoarthritis and rheumatoid arthritis.[64] Twice as many persons with osteoarthritis prefer NSAIDs over acetaminophen.[65]

Side Effects/Adverse Effects

NSAIDs are associated with multiple adverse/side effects, which are listed in Table 12-7. One relatively recent finding is the increased incidence of hypertension in women who take NSAIDs on a regular basis. An analysis of the Nurses' Health Study found a relative risk of 1.78 (95% CI, 1.21–2.61) among older women and 1.60 (95% CI, 1.1–2.32) among younger women for developing incident hypertension if taking NSAIDs daily (for pain other than headache).[66] This may be secondary to inhibition of prostaglandins involved in maintaining normal renal and cardiovascular function.

Gastrointestinal Complications

Although most NSAIDs have minimal side effects following short-term recommended OTC use, the most common by far is gastrointestinal distress. Approximately 15–40% of persons using NSAIDs will experience gastric symptoms such as dyspepsia, heartburn, or nausea, and 10% will discontinue the drug secondary to these symptoms.[67] In addition, asymptomatic ulcers and gastrointestinal mucosal erosion will occur in 5–20% of users, and 1–2% will experience peptic ulcer, gastrointestinal hemorrhage, or perforation. The mortality of these serious gastrointestinal disorders is 10%.[67,68]

Most persons who develop a serious GI adverse event while taking a nonselective NSAID are asymptomatic prior to the event. However, five specific risk factors have been identified[69-71] (Table 12-8).

Ibuprofen (Advil) is associated with the lowest relative risk of gastrointestinal events when compared to other

Table 12-7 Adverse Effects of Nonsteroidal Anti-Inflammatory Drugs

System	Nonselective NSAIDs	COX-2 Selective NSAIDs	Adverse Effects	Clinical Considerations
Cardiovascular	Yes	Yes	COX-2 selective NSAIDs increase risk for myocardial infarction and cardiovascular events. NSAIDs may exacerbate existing heart failure and hypertension.	Contraindicated for persons recovering from coronary bypass surgery. Ibuprofen (Advil) and celecoxib (Celebrex) at high doses associated with an increased risk for myocardial infarction. Naproxen (Naprosyn) is not associated with myocardial infarction.
Central nervous system	Yes	Yes	Aseptic meningitis, psychosis, cognitive dysfunction. ASA can cause tinnitus.	Psychosis and cognitive dysfunction most prevalent in the elderly and associated most with use of indomethacin.
Gastrointestinal	Yes	Less than nonselective NSAIDs	Nonselective NSAIDs increase risk for peptic ulcer and GI hemorrhage.	Risk increases with age.
Hepatic	Yes	Yes	Hepatotoxicity is rare but increases if individual is using other medications with NSAIDs. Diclofenac (Voltaren) reported to cause hepatitis.	Acute liver injury 3.7/100,000 NSAID users. Sulindac (Clinoril) increased risk to 27/100,000 NSAID users. Some authors recommend checking liver function tests 8 wks after starting chronic therapy.
Hematologic	Yes	No	Nonselective NSAIDS have reversible effect on platelet aggregation. Chronic aspirin therapy slightly increases the risk for hemorrhagic stroke.	Concomitant use of NSAID and aspirin will negate effect of aspirin on platelet aggregation.
Renal	Yes	Yes	Nonselective and COX-2 selective NSAIDs can cause acute renal failure, but risk is higher with use of COX-2 selective. Interstitial nephritis, nephrotic syndrome more likely with nonselective NSAIDs.	Risk is highest in first 30 days of therapy. COX-2 selective NSAIDs should be avoided in persons with renal compromise.
Pulmonary	Yes	No	Bronchospasm in persons with aspirin hypersensitivity.	ASA and NSAIDs have some cross-reactivity.
Skin reactions	Yes	Yes	Stevens-Johnson syndrome and toxic epidermal necrolysis.	Rare: reported in approximately 1/100,000 persons using NSAIDs.
Allergic reaction	Yes	Yes	COX-2 selective NSAIDs have a sulfa group and should induce allergic reactions in persons who are allergic to sulfa drugs. Case reports exist but it does not appear to be common.	Use COX-2 selective NSAIDs cautiously in persons who are allergic to sulfa drugs.

NSAIDs = nonsteroidal anti-inflammatory drugs; ASA = aspirin.

nonselective NSAIDs. Aspirin and naproxen (Naprosyn) are intermediate, and ketoprofen (Orudis), although it has OTC status, has one of the highest incidences of gastrointestinal hemorrhage.[72,73] Because previous consumer education programs have not decreased the incidence of NSAID-related gastrointestinal bleeding, the 2009 FDA regulation requires all OTC products containing NSAIDs to display the product's name and the word *NSAID* prominently on the label and to carry a warning about severe gastrointestinal bleeding that includes reference to an increased risk if ≥ 3 glasses of alcohol are consumed per day.

Prevention and Treatment of Gastrointestinal Ulcers

Primary and secondary prevention and/or treatment of NSAID-induced ulcers is an important component of

therapy. Choices include use of COX-2 selective NSAIDs instead of a nonselective NSAID or the addition of medications that affect acid production in the gastrointestinal tract, which include mucosal barrier agents (e.g., sucralfate), proton pump inhibitors (PPIs) (e.g., omeprazole [Prilosec]), histamine receptor antagonists (H$_2$RAs) (famotidine [Pepcid]), and misoprostol (Cytotec). COX-2 selective NSAIDs do not induce gastrointestinal complications, but this class of drugs is associated with an increase in myocardial infarction (discussed in more detail later in this chapter) and is therefore not recommended for persons at risk for cardiovascular events.

Mucosal barrier agents and histamine receptor antagonists are not sufficiently effective and are not recommended.[70] Misoprostol is quite effective and reduces the incidence of ulcers by approximately 40%, but it must be

Table 12-8 Risk Factors for Upper Gastrointestinal Complications from NSAID Use

Known Risk Factors
Anticoagulation (warfarin)
Corticosteroid therapy

High doses of NSAIDs (≥ 2 × normal dose)
    Use of multiple NSAIDs
    Low doses of aspirin and concomitant NSAID use

Older age (≥ 60 y)
    16–44 y: 5/10,000*
    45–64 y: 15/10,000*
    65–74 y: 17/10,000*
    > 75 y: 91/10,000*

Prior clinical event (ulcer, hemorrhage)
Serious systemic disorder
Possible Risk Factors
Alcohol consumption
Cigarette smoking
Infection with *Helicobacter pylori*

* Risk for serious gastrointestinal bleeding.
Sources: From Lanzi LL 1998[69]; Wolfe MM et al. 1999[63]; and AHRQ.[71]

taken several times per day and has unpleasant side effects (diarrhea).[74] Therefore, proton pump inhibitors are the drug of choice for both primary prevention and secondary prevention in persons who have experienced a previous NSAID-induced ulcer.[70] Omeprazole (Pepcid) is more effective than ranitidine (Zantac). Proton pump inhibitors are not effective in preventing the less common lower GI events.

Various authors have slightly different recommendations concerning who should be offered PPI therapy for prophylaxis, and therefore readers are encouraged to know local recommendations and standards. In general, PPIs are preferred for persons who have additional risk factors for ulcers. Persons at high risk for gastrointestinal hemorrhage (e.g., history of previous NSAID-induced ulcer) should be offered either a COX-2 selective NSAID if they are not at risk for myocardial infarction or a nonselective NSAID and PPI. Finally, it is important to remember that when nonselective NSAIDs are taken by persons who are on daily, low-dose aspirin for cardiovascular protection, the NSAID can counter the effect of aspirin on platelet aggregation by competitively taking the COX-2 binding site aspirin would like to occupy on the platelet, thereby negating the therapeutic effect of aspirin.

Drug–Drug Interactions

Because most NSAIDs are tightly bound to plasma proteins, there is a potential for many drug interactions. Coadministration of aspirin and some NSAIDs may reduce the cardioprotective effects of aspirin because of competition for binding sites on the COX enzyme.[75,76] Significant drug interactions are summarized in Table 12-6.

Special Populations

Pregnancy and Lactation

NSAIDs are not generally recommended for use in pregnancy. Naproxen (e.g., Naprosyn, Aleve) and ibuprofen (Advil) are Pregnancy Category B but should not be used after 36 weeks of pregnancy to avoid increased blood loss during parturition and to avoid premature closure of the ductus arteriosus in the fetus.[77] There is some suggestion that NSAIDs may also decrease the amount of amniotic fluid. NSAIDs are excreted in breast milk. The American Academy of Pediatrics considers their use compatible with lactation.[60] However, some authors recommend caution when exposing NSAIDs to newborns because they competitively displace bilirubin from plasma proteins and can increase the incidence of newborn jaundice.[78]

Elderly

The elderly are more susceptible to the adverse effects of gastrointestinal bleeding, hypertension, and renal function compromise if taking NSAIDs.[71] Persons over age 65 who are considering long-term NSAID therapy should be evaluated for *H pylori* infection, and it should be treated prior to initiation of NSAIDs if it is present. In general, if NSAIDs are needed, COX-2 selective NSAIDs are recommended secondary to their decreased risk of GI complications. Because the elderly often experience persistent pain and practice polypharmacy, the potential for significant drug–drug or drug–herb interactions should be carefully evaluated when considering routine NSAID therapy for them.

COX-2 Selective NSAIDs: Second-Generation NSAIDs

Celecoxib (Celebrex) is the only selective COX-2 inhibitor currently available in the United States. Rofecoxib (Vioxx; Box 12-1) was voluntarily withdrawn from the market following research studies that demonstrated an increased risk of myocardial infarction among individuals using rofecoxib. Valdecoxib (Bextra) was also voluntarily withdrawn for similar concerns.[79,80]

Mechanism of Action

Celecoxib (Celebrex) selectively inhibits COX-2 to mediate inflammation and pain. Because it has minimal effect on COX-1, celecoxib does not have significant effects on gastric irritation, renal function, or platelet aggregation.

Pharmacokinetics

COX-2 selective NSAIDs are rapidly absorbed from the gastrointestinal tract. Taking NSAIDs with food delays absorption but does not affect peak concentration. Like the nonselective NSAIDs, COX-2 selective NSAIDs are extensively protein-bound and are metabolized in the liver and excreted through the kidneys.

Clinical Indications

Celecoxib (Celebrex) is indicated for relief of signs and symptoms of osteoarthritis, rheumatoid arthritis in adults, juvenile rheumatoid arthritis in children ≥ 2 years, and for treatment of ankylosing spondylitis, primary dysmenorrhea, or acute pain.

Adverse Effects

Adverse effects of COX-2 selective NSAIDs are listed in Table 12-7. Despite early hopes that celecoxib might have all the advantages of COX-2 inhibition without increased gastrointestinal toxicity, such promises have not been clearly demonstrated. The Celecoxib Arthritis Safety Study (CLASS) demonstrated a reduced incidence of gastric ulceration with short-term use (< 6 months).[81] However, the same study did not show any statistically significant reduction of gastric ulceration when celecoxib was compared with long-term use of traditional NSAIDs (> 12 months).[81] Subsequent studies have had mixed results.[82] In summary, at this time, the benefits of celecoxib for preventing gastrointestinal adverse effects remain unclear, especially with long-term use.

The most serious adverse effects of COX-2 inhibitors are cardiovascular. Persons taking high doses of celecoxib (400–800 mg/day) demonstrated an increased risk of both fatal and nonfatal myocardial infarctions (0.52% in persons taking a placebo versus 0.74% in persons taking rofecoxib [Vioxx] and 0.8% in persons taking celecoxib [Celebrex]).[83] Celecoxib also increases the risks of hypertension, edema, and congestive heart failure because of its adverse impact on renal function. To minimize these effects, celecoxib should be given at the lowest therapeutic dose and should be used cautiously in those with increased risks for cardiovascular or renal disease.

Box 12-1 The Story of Vioxx

The FDA approved rofecoxib (Vioxx) for relief of arthritis symptoms in 1999 based on data from trials of 3–6 months' duration. In 2000, the Vioxx Gastrointestinal Outcomes Research (VIGOR) study, which compared rofecoxib (Vioxx) with naproxen (Aleve), indicated an increased risk for myocardial infarction in individuals taking 50 mg of rofecoxib (Vioxx).[79] Merck & Co. voluntarily withdrew its arthritis medication rofecoxib (Vioxx) from the market on September 30, 2004.

This was the largest prescription drug withdrawal in history and precipitated a public outcry against the FDA's drug approval and monitoring process. Merck claimed that the data were flawed and that the increased incidence of myocardial infarction among those taking rofecoxib was due to the cardioprotective nature of naproxen (Aleve) in the group who took naproxen, although naproxen has not been shown to have a cardioprotective effect. Although the FDA reviewed the data, it chose not to act but to await further investigation.

The Adenomatous Polyp Prevention on Vioxx (APPROVe) trial was the final blow.[80] Even after excluding those individuals with a history of cardiovascular disease from the trial, the risk of MI was almost twice for those taking rofecoxib (Vioxx) as it was for those taking a placebo. The study was halted early, and at that point, Merck voluntarily withdrew rofecoxib from the market.

The proposed mechanism by which rofecoxib increases the risk of myocardial infarction is through inhibition of COX-2, which mediates prostaglandin I_2 production. Prostaglandin I_2 inhibits platelet aggregation, causes vasodilation, and prevents vascular smooth muscle cell proliferation.

Although this mechanism is thought to be a class action, celecoxib (Celebrex) is less COX-2 specific than either rofecoxib (Vioxx) or valdecoxib (Bextra) and may drive the mechanism less toward thrombosis. In April 2005, the FDA requested Pfizer to withdraw valdecoxib from the market. Currently, celecoxib is the only selective COX-2 inhibitor marketed in the United States.

Drug–Drug Interactions

Like first-generation NSAIDs, celecoxib is highly protein bound and may displace other protein-bound drugs, leading to adverse reactions. Unlike nonselective COX inhibitors, celecoxib does not interfere with the antiplatelet effect of aspirin, since mature human platelets lack COX-2. Drug–drug interactions are listed in Table 12-6.

Contraindications

Celecoxib (Celebrex) is contraindicated for those with known hypersensitivity to celecoxib. It should not be given to individuals allergic to sulfonamides or those who have had asthma or urticarial or allergic reactions to aspirin or other NSAIDS.

Special Populations

Pregnancy and Lactation

Celecoxib (Celebrex) is a Pregnancy Category C drug. Like other NSAIDs, celecoxib is contraindicated in the third trimester of pregnancy because it may promote premature closure of the ductus arteriosus. Celecoxib is transferred into human milk, but levels are so low that harm is unlikely.[84] The American Academy of Pediatrics does not make any recommendations regarding the use of celecoxib during lactation.

Elderly

Celecoxib peak plasma concentrations are approximately 40% higher in the elderly than in younger individuals. For this reason, and because of the increased incidence of underlying comorbidities, the risk of significant cardiovascular and GI events and acute renal failure are increased when celecoxib is used by persons over the age of 65.

Acetaminophen

Acetaminophen (Tylenol) is similar to aspirin and other NSAIDs in that it has both antipyretic and analgesic properties. However, acetaminophen has no clinically significant anti-inflammatory properties, nor does it suppress platelet aggregation, reduce renal blood flow, or increase gastric irritation.

Mechanism of Action

Acetaminophen (Tylenol) is a selective inhibitor of prostaglandin synthesis. Unlike aspirin and other NSAIDs that inhibit prostaglandin both in the central nervous system and the periphery, acetaminophen's effects primarily are found in the central nervous system, with only limited effects at peripheral sites.

Pharmacokinetics

Acetaminophen (Tylenol) readily is absorbed following oral dosing and is widely distributed. Metabolism takes place in the liver by two different pathways. At therapeutic doses, most acetaminophen is conjugated with glucuronic acid and other liver enzymes into nontoxic metabolites and excreted through the kidney. Small amounts are converted into toxic metabolites by a secondary pathway in the CYP450 system. Relatively small amounts of this toxic metabolite can be further converted by glutathione into nontoxic forms for excretion.

When liver function is impaired or overdose occurs, the primary metabolic pathway is overwhelmed and the drug must be metabolized via the secondary system. (For more detailed explanation of acetaminophen hepatotoxicity, see Chapter 4.) Alcohol or large amounts of acetaminophen deplete glutathione, preventing the further metabolism of the toxic metabolites, and liver damage results.

Clinical Indications

Acetaminophen is indicated for relief of mild to moderate pain and reduction of fever. It is safe for use in children and adolescents suspected of having influenza or varicella because it has never been linked to Reye's syndrome. Acetaminophen is the preferred analgesic for persons with gastric ulceration or aspirin hypersensitivity.

Side Effects/Adverse Effects

Adverse effects of acetaminophen are rare at therapeutic doses. However, overdose can cause severe and sometimes fatal liver damage. Acetaminophen is the leading cause of liver injury in the United States. It is relatively easy to overdose on acetaminophen. The minimum toxic single dose for healthy adults is between 7.5 and 10 grams, but liver toxicity can occur at normal therapeutic doses of acetaminophen in persons who consume alcohol in large amounts or regularly (Box 4-3). In 1998 the FDA issued a regulation mandating that products containing acetaminophen have an alcohol warning on the label that cautions users to check with their physician before using acetaminophen if they drink more than 3 alcoholic drinks per day. Secondly, many OTC combination products contain acetaminophen; however, the consumer may not be aware that acetaminophen is in the medication, and therefore over-dose can occur inadvertently. The FDA has recommended that OTC combination products stop using the abbreviation APAP to designate the presence of acetaminophen on the product label because most consumers do not know that APAP represents acetaminophen. To date this is a voluntary recommendation and has not been widely implemented.

In 2009, the FDA issued a regulation requiring that all OTC analgesic preparations prominently display the names of the ingredients and that acetaminophen labels carry a warning that describes the risks of liver failure.

Also in 2009, an FDA advisory committee recommended the following changes for acetaminophen preparations: (1) decrease the maximum daily dose from 4 gms to 3.250 gms; (2) decrease the maximum single dose to ≤ 650 mg (currently, OTC formulations of 500 gms allow a single dose to be 1000 gms); and (3) eliminate some combination products, such as Vicodin and TheraFlu. Although the FDA is not required to accept the recommendations of their advisory committees, these recommendations are often accepted and placed in formal regulations.

Routine use of acetaminophen at doses of ≥ 5 grams per day has been associated with an increased risk for hypertension in women.[66] A causal relationship between acetaminophen and hypertension has not been clearly established, nor is the mechanism of action whereby acetaminophen might cause elevations in blood pressure known.

Drug–Drug Interactions

Alcohol is the most significant drug interaction. Alcohol increases the risk of liver toxicity, and the FDA now requires alcohol warnings on acetaminophen products.[85] Acetaminophen should not be used by persons who consume more than three alcoholic drinks per day. See Chapter 4 for a detailed description of liver toxicity secondary to acetaminophen and alcohol use. Concurrent use of acetaminophen and drugs that induce CYP450 enzymes in the liver such as rifampin (Rimactane), barbiturates, carbamazepine (Tegretol), and sulfinpyrazone (Anturane) also increases the risk of liver toxicity and may decrease the effectiveness of acetaminophen. (See Table 4-6.)

Routine use of acetaminophen can increase the risk of bleeding in those taking warfarin (Coumadin). The mechanism of interaction is unknown, although it is speculated that acetaminophen may inhibit CYP1A2 metabolism of warfarin.[86] However, the study identifying acetaminophen–warfarin drug interaction included a large number of febrile persons who also had reduced oral intake. Both fever and dehydration independently affect warfarin metabolism.[87] Episodic use of acetaminophen has not been shown to increase the international normalized ration test of bleeding time for individuals on warfarin, and acetaminophen remains the drug of choice for analgesic and antipyretic control for these persons.

Contraindications

Acetaminophen should be avoided by persons with impaired liver function or acetaminophen hypersensitivity. Acetaminophen can theoretically cause hemolytic anemia in persons with known G6PD deficiency. Although there are case reports linking acetaminophen to hemolytic anemia in persons with G6PD deficiency, other studies suggest acetaminophen is safe in this population, and thus, at this time there is no clear contraindication to its use.

Special Populations

Pregnancy and Lactation

Acetaminophen crosses the placenta but has not been associated with birth defects. It is considered safe for short-term use in pregnant women. Acetaminophen is excreted in breast milk, but no adverse effects among nursing infants have been reported. The American Academy of Pediatrics considers acetaminophen compatible with breastfeeding.[60]

Elderly

The elderly may be at increased risk for acetaminophen toxicity because of frequently undiagnosed subclinical hepatic insufficiency. When used at low doses with increased dosing frequencies, acetaminophen is safer than other drugs typically used for persistent pain.

Opioid Analgesics

Opioid refers to any natural or synthetic drug with actions similar to morphine. **Opiate** refers only to those opioids that contain compounds found in opium. *Narcotic* is a less precise term that has been used to refer to any drug that causes central nervous system depression or has a potential for causing physical dependency, which includes nonopioid drugs and therefore tends to be used more commonly within a jurisprudence framework.

The Controlled Substances Act of 1970 created five schedule classifications for opioids, which are at least partially based on the potential for opioid dependence and addiction. The Drug Enforcement Administration and the FDA assign individual opioids to a specific schedule. The schedules are listed in Table 1-5. Prescriptive authority to prescribe opioids is regulated by the states.

Mechanism of Action of Opioids

There are three main opioid receptors: mu, kappa, and delta. All are G protein-linked receptors that are embedded in the plasma membrane of neurons. Mu receptors are located primarily in the central nervous system pain-modulating areas, the dorsal horn of the spinal cord, and the intestinal tract. Activation of mu receptors results in analgesia, euphoria, and respiratory depression. Morphine is the prototypical mu receptor agonist. Kappa receptors are concentrated in the cerebral cortex of the brain and in the substantia gelatinosa of the dorsal horn of the spinal cord and uterus. Activation of kappa receptors results in analgesia and sedation. The third primary opioid receptor, delta, is located in the limbic area of the brain and in the spinal cord. Delta receptors are thought to play a part in euphoria and may have a role in analgesia at the level of the spinal cord. In addition to the mu, delta, and kappa family, sigma and epsilon receptors are less well understood, and their functions remain unclear. The responses of opioid receptor activation are summarized in Table 12-9.

All drugs have intrinsic affinity, which is a measure of the strength of the interaction between the drug and receptor, and efficacy, which refers to the effect the drug has on the receptor. In the case of opioids, agonists have both strong affinity and efficacy, partial agonists have affinity but elicit weak efficacy, and antagonists have affinity but do

Table 12-9 Stimulation of Opioid Receptors

Drug Generic (Brand)	Mu (μ)	Kappa (κ)	Delta (δ)
Effect	Analgesia, sedation, vomiting, respiratory depression, pruritus, constipation, urinary retention, euphoria, physical dependence.	Analgesia, sedation, dyspnea, respiratory depression, euphoria, dysphoria.	Sedation, release of growth hormone.
Pure Agonists			
Codeine	Weak agonist	—	Weak agonist
Fentanyl (Duragesic, Sublimaze)	Agonist	—	—
Hydrocodone (Vicodin, Vicoprofen, Lortab, Lorcet)	Agonist	—	—
Hydromorphone (Dilaudid)	Agonist	—	—
Levorphanol (Levo-Dromoran)	Agonist	—	—
Meperidine (Demerol)	Agonist	—	Agonist
Methadone (Dolophine)	Agonist	—	—
Morphine	Agonist	Weak agonist	Weak agonist
Oxycodone (Percocet, OxyContin, Roxicodone)	Agonist	Weak agonist	Weak agonist
Oxymorphone (Opana, Numorphan)	Agonist	Weak agonist	Weak agonist
Propoxyphene (Darvocet)	Weak agonist	—	—
Sufentanil (Sufenta)	Agonist	Weak agonist	Weak agonist
Agonists-Antagonists			
Butorphanol (Stadol)	Weak antagonist	Agonist	—
Nalbuphine (Nubain)	Antagonist	Agonist	—
Partial Agonist			
Buprenorphine (Buprenex, Suboxone)	Weak agonist	Antagonist	—
Antagonists			
Nalmefene (Revex)	Antagonist	Antagonist	Weak antagonist
Naltrexone (ReVia)	Antagonist	Antagonist	Weak antagonist
Naloxone (Narcan)	Antagonist	Antagonist	Weak antagonist

not elicit any efficacy. The pharmacologic effects of opioids relate to their differing degrees of affinity and efficacy at the mu, kappa, and delta opioid receptors.

Gender Differences in Opioid Response

There is evidence that women experience more analgesia from opioid agonists and agonist-antagonists than do men.[88] This phenomenon is thought to be a result of potentiation of kappa-receptor agonists by progesterone or estrogen, but the exact cause is not fully understood.[89]

Classification of Opioids

Opioids are either hydrophilic or lipophilic and can be classified by their chemical makeup (natural, semisynthetic, or synthetic), by their potency (strong, moderate, weak), or by their action on different types of receptors (agonist, partial agonist, agonist-antagonist, pure antagonist), which is the classification used in this chapter (Table 12-10).

Opioid Agonists

Agonists elicit a pharmacologic action by activating opioid receptors. An opioid with high intrinsic ability, such as morphine, achieves maximal pharmacologic effects with relatively low receptor occupancy, whereas codeine is a weak mu agonist and as such is not a potent analgesic.

Opioid agonists produce analgesia via binding to opioid receptors in the central nervous system, spinal cord, and gastrointestinal tract. Pure mu agonists are generally preferred for the management of moderate to severe pain. Not only are they available in a variety of formulations, but pure mu opioid agonists have no analgesic ceiling. This characteristic makes them particularly useful for treatment of chronic pain, since doses may be increased indefinitely as long as adverse effects are avoided.

Pharmacokinetics of Opioid Agonists

Most opioids are easily absorbed from the gastrointestinal tract, undergoing variable, but significant hepatic first-pass effects. Thus, opioids administered orally typically require significantly larger doses than other forms for **equianalgesic** effects. Opioids are poorly protein bound. Most opioids are metabolized through the CYP2D6 and CYP34A systems and excreted through the kidney. Genetic variations and impaired hepatic or renal function all impact appropriate dosing in individuals. For example, some persons genetically have a duplication of CYP2D6, which makes

Table 12-10 Classification of Opioids

Effect on Receptor Generic (Brand)	Chemical Origin Generic (Brand)	Potency Generic (Brand)
Agonists Alfentanil (Alfenta), fentanyl (Duragesic, Sublimaze), morphine, sufentanil (Sufenta)	*Natural* Codeine, morphine	*Strong* Alfentanil (Alfenta), fentanyl (Duragesic, Sublimaze), morphine, sufentanil (Sufenta)
Partial Agonists Buprenorphine (Buprenex, Suboxone)	*Semisynthetic* Buprenorphine (Buprenex), hydromorphone (Dilaudid), hydrocodone (Vicodin), oxycodone (OxyContin, Percocet), oxymorphone (Numorphan)	*Intermediate* Butorphanol (Stadol), nalbuphine (Nubain), pentazocine (Talwin)
Antagonist-Agonist Butorphanol (Stadol), nalbuphine (Nubain), pentazocine (Talwin)	*Synthetic: Phenylpiperidines* Fentanyl (Duragesic, Sublimaze), meperidine (Demerol), sufentanil (Sufenta)	*Weak* Codeine
Antagonist Naloxone (Narcan), nalmefene (Revex), naltrexone (ReVia)	*Synthetic: Pseudopiperidines* Methadone (Dolophine), propoxyphene (Darvon)	

them ultrametabolizers of codeine. Because codeine is a prodrug and its metabolite is the active drug morphine, ultrarapid metabolism can result in plasma levels of morphine that are 50% higher than expected, causing an exaggerated analgesic and potentially toxic effect.[90] Conversely, persons who have a genetic polymorphism that results in less CYP2D6 or who are taking drugs that are CYP2D6 inhibitors (e.g., selective serotonin reuptake inhibitors, tricyclic antidepressants) often have an insufficient analgesic response to codeine secondary to decreased metabolism of the ingested prodrug.[91]

Lipid solubility varies widely among opioids and accounts for the variations in onset and duration of action among these drugs. Morphine has relatively low lipid solubility at 25–30%, which accounts for its slow onset and prolonged duration of action in relation to more lipid-soluble drugs such as fentanyl. Lipophilic opioids are more easily administered through transdermal and buccal routes. Many opioids have active metabolites that affect the pharmacodynamic response with regard to both analgesic effects and adverse effects. Table 12-11 summarizes the pharmacokinetics of commonly used opioids.

Dosing Considerations

Opioids are commonly prescribed for moderate to severe pain. These drugs may be administered in a variety of ways, including oral, rectal, parenteral, transdermal, buccal, intranasal, and epidural routes. Each route has specific advantages and disadvantages. For instance, most opioids have a high hepatic first pass, requiring larger oral doses for equianalgesic effects. Rectal routes tend to have erratic absorption. Morphine is the prototype mu opioid agonist

Table 12-11 Pharmacokinetics of Opioids

Drug Generic (Brand)	Bioavailability	Time to Peak Effect (Hours)	Onset of Action (Minutes)	Half-Life (Hours)	Duration of Action (Hours)	Clinical Considerations
Pure Agonists						
Morphine	20–40%	Oral: 1–2 IV: 0.5–1	IV: 3–5 IM: 10–20	2–3	3–6	Active metabolite morphine-6 glucuronide is more potent than parent drug.
Morphine (CR) (Kadian)	20–40%	6–8	120	2–3	8–12	Administered once or twice daily.
Morphine (SR) (MS-Contin)	20–40%	6–8	120	2–3	12–24	Administered once or twice daily.
Hydromorphone (Dilaudid)	24%	Oral: 1–2 IM/IV: 0.5–1	30–45	2–3	Oral: 3–6 IM/IV: 3–4	Preferred for individuals with renal impairment.
Oxymorphone (Numorphan)	10%	Oral: 1.5–3 IM/IV: 0.5–1	3–6	3–4	Oral: 4–6 IM/IV: 3–6	Useful for individuals subject to multiple drug interactions because it does not affect CYP2D6 or CYP34A enzymes.
Levorphanol (Levo-Dromoran)	20–40%	Oral: 1–2 IM/IV: 0.5–1	10–60	12–15	3–6	Half-life can be as long as 30 h with repeated dosing, which suggests drug accumulation occurs.
Meperidine (Demerol)	50–60%	0.5–1	10–45	3–4	2–4	Not preferred for long-term use because of increased risk of toxicity from active metabolites.
Oxycodone (various)	60–87%	1–2	15–30	2–3	3–6	Available as a single entity or in combination with acetaminophen or aspirin.
Hydrocodone (Vicodin)	Unknown	0.5–1	10–30	2–4	3–6	Available only in combination with acetylsalicylic acid or acetaminophen.
Codeine	80%	0.5–1	10–30	2–4	4–6	About 10% is metabolized to morphine. Slow metabolizers will have poor pain control.
Fentanyl (Duragesic)	NA	IV/SQ: < 10 min	7–12	3–12	1–2	Fentanyl is highly lipid soluble. Risk of delayed respiratory depression is less than that of morphine.
Fentanyl (Duragesic) transmucosal	50%	15–30 min	7–12 h	3–12	1–2	
Fentanyl (Duragesic) transdermal	92%	12–24	NA	3–12	72	
Methadone (Dolophine)	80%	1–2	30–60	12–150	4–7	May prolong QT interval. Use cautiously in patients with heart disease or those on medications that affect QT interval. Sedation lasts 24–48 h.
Propoxyphene (Darvon)	40%	2–2.5	30–60	6–12	4–6	Label has FDA black box warning about risk of overdose. Medication guide must be provided when prescription is filled. Avoid in elderly and in persons with renal insufficiency. Accumulation of toxic metabolites may cause hyperexcitability.

and is the standard by which all other opioids are compared for equianalgesic dosing, a term referred to as a *morphine equivalent dose* (Table 12-12). Parenteral routes produce a more rapid onset of action but may be problematic for long-term use. Tables 12-13 and 12-14 list doses of opioid agonists and opioid agonist-antagonists used to treat moderate to severe pain.

The opioid dose required to achieve analgesia varies widely among individuals. A person's response to prior exposure to the drug, hepatic and renal function, and route of administration should be considered when determining specific doses. Conversion to a different route or different drug requires careful consideration of the pharmacodynamics and pharmacokinetics of the preparation.

Side Effects/Adverse Effects

Gastrointestinal side effects include nausea, vomiting, and constipation. Nausea and vomiting are the most common side effects in the early stages of therapy and may require coadministration of a phenothiazine for control. Tolerance to these effects develops quickly, however, and routine use of phenothiazines to treat opioid-induced nausea is controversial. Although they are commonly used, there

Table 12-12 Equianalgesic Doses of Opioids

Drug Generic (Brand)	Intravenous (mg)	Oral (mg)
Morphine	10	30
Buprenorphine (Buprenex)	0.3	—
Butorphanol (Stadol)	2	—
Codeine	120	200*
Fentanyl (Sublimaze)	0.1	—
Hydrocodone† (Vicodin, Vicoprofen, Lortab, Lorcet)	—	20–30†
Hydromorphone (Dilaudid)	1.5	7.5
Meperidine (Demerol)	75	300‡
Methadone (Dolophine)	10	3–5
Nalbuphine (Nubain)	10	—
Oxycodone (Percocet)	—	20
Propoxyphene (Darvocet)	—	180–200
Sufentanil (Sufenta)	0.002	—

— = not available.

* Equianalgesic doses of codeine are not well defined because of the variability in codeine metabolism.

† These products contain 5, 7.5, or 10 mg of hydrocodone per tablet with either acetaminophen or aspirin. The equianalgesic doses of hydrocodone are not calculated for combination products because the analgesic efficacy is potentiated by the combination drugs.

‡ Contraindicated in persons receiving MAO inhibitors. Maximum dose is 600 mg/24 hours because toxic metabolites can accumulate and cause seizures.

Table 12-13 Opioids for Treating Moderate-Severe Acute or Chronic Pain

Drug Generic (Brand)	Usual Initial Adult Dose		Clinical Considerationns
	Oral	**IV or IM**	
Codeine	30–60 mg	130 mg	60 mg PO is equivalent to 650 mg of aspirin. Some persons have no analgesic effect from codeine.
Fentanyl (Duragesic, Sublimaze)	N/A	50–100 mcg q 1–2 h	Not recommended for acute pain except as component of regional anesthesia. Can be given transdermally q 72 h for chronic, malignant pain. Use only in opioid-tolerant individuals.
Hydrocodone (Vicodin)	5–10 mg	NA	10 mg PO equivalent to 60–80 mg of codeine. Available in combination formulations only with aspirin, ibuprofen, or acetaminophen.
Hydromorphone (Dilaudid)	2–4 mg q 3–4 h	1.5–4 mg q 3–4 h	Hydromorphone has the same efficacy as morphine, but is five times more potent in oral form. Causes less nausea, vomiting, constipation, and euphoria than morphine. Should be reserved for severe, chronic pain.
Levorphanol (Levo-Dromoran)	2–4 mg	2 mg	Long half-life and risk of accumulation and CNS depression with repeated dosing.
Meperidine (Demerol)	300 mg q 2–3 h	75–100 mg q 3 h	Not recommended for chronic use (> 48 h) or in the elderly. Accumulation of active metabolite can cause dysphoria and seizures, especially at amounts totaling > 600 mg/24 h.
Morphine	30 mg q 3–4 h*	10 mg q 3–4 h	The ability of advanced-practice nurses to prescribe these drugs is limited in many states.
Oxycodone (Percocet, OxyContin)	5 mg	NA	10 mg is equivalent to 90 mg of codeine PO or 10 mg of morphine SQ. Available in combination formulations and in sustained-release tablets. Has high potential for abuse.
Tramadol (Ultram)	50–100 mg q 4–6 h		50 mg is equivalent to 60 mg of codeine. 100 mg is equivalent to 60 mg of codeine with 650 mg of aspirin. Tramadol has both opioid and nonopioid properties. It also inhibits reuptake of serotonin and norepinephrine but does not have the anticholinergic side effects of tricyclic antidepressants. Most useful for moderate pain. Unlike other opioids, it has a limited dose of 400 mg/24 h.

Source: Adapted from Miller E 2004.[126]

Table 12-14 Opioid Agonist-Antagonists for Moderate Pain of Limited Duration*

Drug Generic (Brand)	Dose per Tablet	Usual Initial Adult Dose	Clinical Considerations
Buprenorphine (Buprenex)*	Oral formulations combined with naloxone and used to treat opiate addiction	1 mL q 6 h	Associated respiratory depression, which may not be fully reversible with naloxone.
Butorphanol (Stadol)*	2 mg/mL	0.5–2 mg q 3–4 h IV 1–4 mg q 3–4 h IM	Also available as a nasal spray.
Nalbuphine (Nubain)*	10 or 20 mg/mL	10 mg q 3–4 h IM	Dysphoria is less common than with pentazocine, but more common than with morphine.
Pentazocine (Talwin)*	30 mg/mL	50 mg PO 30 mg q 3–4 h	Confusion and dysphoria are frequent side effects, especially in the elderly. Overdose is treatable with naloxone (Narcan) but not by other narcotic antagonists.

* Unlike pure opioid agonists, agonist-antagonists do have a ceiling effect. Usefulness in patients with severe or chronic pain is limited. Use of agonist-antagonists may cause opioid withdrawal.
Source: Reprinted with permission from Miller E 2004.[126]

is a suggestion that their use may have additive sedating and dysphoric side effects without significantly increasing pain control. Tolerance for constipation does not develop, and individuals on long-term narcotic therapy should be started on a bowel regimen to minimize this effect.

Opioids produce excellent analgesia but have significant adverse effects, including respiratory depression, orthostatic hypotension, nausea, constipation, urinary retention, and dysphoria. Most of these adverse effects can be minimized by titrating slowly up to the lowest effective dose. Respiratory depression is the most serious adverse effect, but it does not frequently occur with therapeutic doses. However, the respiratory rate should be monitored for all individuals receiving intravenous opioids, and the drug should be withheld from those with respiratory rates less than 12 breaths per minute. Tolerance to respiratory depression develops with long-term use of opiates such as those with chronic pain.

Opioid overdose is characterized by the classic symptom triad of coma, respiratory depression, and pinpoint pupils. Treatment is aimed at ventilatory support and reversal of opioid toxicity by administration of opioid antagonists such as naloxone (Narcan). Since naloxone has a shorter half-life than many opioids, repeat dosing may be necessary. A newer antagonist, nalmefene (Revex), has a longer half-life and may be preferred in some settings. Table 12-15 provides a summary of adverse effects of opioids and treatment/prevention strategies.[92]

Contraindications

All pure opioid agonists should be used cautiously in patients with impaired pulmonary function such as asthma, emphysema, or other respiratory compromise. Caution should also be exercised when using them in persons with head injuries, liver impairment, inflammatory bowel disease, prostatic hypertrophy, preexisting hypotension, or reduced blood volume.

Drug–Drug Interactions

The sedation and respiratory depression caused by opioids can be intensified by any drug that causes central nervous system depression. Barbiturates, benzodiazepines, and alcohol are especially problematic, and providers should caution those for whom they prescribe opioids about the dangers of mixing any of these medications.

Morphine and other opioids may exacerbate hypotension in individuals taking antihypertensive drugs or other medications that lower blood pressure. Constipation and urinary retention may also be exacerbated by anticholinergic drugs. Monamine oxidase (MAO) inhibitors combined with meperidine may produce a syndrome of delirium, convulsions, hyperpyrexia, excitation, and respiratory depression, which can be fatal. Table 12-16 provides a summary of major drug interactions of opioids.[93]

Morphine

Morphine is primarily metabolized by demethylation and glucuronidation. Because only a very small portion is metabolized via the CYP450 enzymes, drug–drug interactions are extremely rare, and there are no genetic differences in response to this drug.[93]

Codeine

Codeine is a natural mu opioid agonist and is actually a prodrug metabolized to morphine by CYP2D6. Codeine has an analgesic potency of about 50% that of morphine.

Table 12-15 Adverse/Side Effects of Opioids

Adverse Effect	Clinical Considerations
Biliary colic	Avoid use of morphine in patients with biliary dysfunction. Substitute meperidine.
Constipation	Increase fluids, fiber, and physical activity. Routine use of stimulant laxatives and/or stool softeners is warranted.
Cough suppression	Codeine and hydrocodone are sometimes administered for this purpose. When cough suppression is undesirable, auscultate lungs for presence of rales. Instruct in deep breathing and coughing at regular intervals.
Euphoria/dysphoria	Euphoria may enhance pain relief but contributes to addiction potential. Dysphoria is most likely to occur when opioids are taken in the absence of pain.
Hormonal	Decreased estrogen and testosterone leads to decreased libido, osteoporosis, and reduced bone mineral density. Can also cause amenorrhea or hypomenorrhea.
Increased intracranial pressure (ICP)	Increased intracranial pressure corresponds to respiratory depression. At normal respiratory rate, ICP remains normal.
Miosis	Keep room lights bright during waking hours to avoid impaired vision.
Neurotoxicity	Maintain hydration and reduce dose.
Nausea and vomiting	Pretreat with antiemetic when necessary. Having the patient lie still may reduce incidence. Although opioids directly stimulate the vomiting center in the brain, some nausea and bloating may be indicative of delayed gastric emptying. Use of a prokinetic drug such as metoclopramide may be helpful.
Orthostatic hypotension	Change positions slowly. Assist with ambulation as necessary.
Pruritus	Opioids cause a histamine release.
Respiratory depression	Monitor respirations. Titrate slowly. Avoid simultaneous use of other respiratory depressants. Agonist-antagonists have less respiratory depression than pure agonists.
Sedation	Administer smaller doses more often; use drugs with shorter half-lives; administer small doses of a CNS stimulant in the morning and early afternoon.
Urinary retention	Encourage voiding every 4 hours. Palpate for bladder distention. Catheterization may be required.

Because codeine is metabolized by CYP2D6, it is subject to multiple drug–drug interactions. There are a large number of polymorphisms of the CYP2D6 enzyme. As stated previously, persons who are ultrarapid metabolizers of codeine have minimal analgesia when using codeine. The FDA recently released a public health advisory about codeine secondary to a rare unusual effect. A nursing mother who is an ultrarapid metabolizer took codeine for postpartum pain, and the high levels of morphine in her breast milk resulted in a fatal neonatal respiratory depression. Lactating women should use the lowest effective dose of codeine.[94] Codeine has an unusual emetic response. Low doses are more emetic than higher doses. The mechanism underlying this response is not clear. At doses of > 60 mg, the incidence of side effects and adverse effects increases without a concomitant increase in analgesia.

Fentanyl (Duragesic, Sublimaze)

Fentanyl is a strong synthetic mu opioid agonist approximately 80 times more potent than morphine. Fentanyl is a drug with a short duration of action and is mostly metabolized by CYP3A4 to inactive metabolites. CYP3A4 inhibitors can cause increased fentanyl levels.

Hydrocodone (Vicodin)

Hydrocodone is the most commonly used opioid. It is recommended for the treatment of moderate or moderately severe pain and is also used to treat persistent cough. Hydrocodone is also a prodrug and is metabolized via CYP2D6 to hydromorphone, which is the active metabolite. So like codeine, persons who are CYP2D6 deficient secondary to a polymorphism or those who take CYP3D6 inhibitors may have a decreased analgesic effect.

Hydromorphone (Dilaudid)

Hydromorphone is a semisynthetic potent mu opioid agonist that like morphine is minimally metabolized via the CYP450 enzyme system. The metabolites of hydromorphone are not active.

Meperidine (Demerol)

Meperidine is a semisynthetic weak mu opioid with approximately 10% of the effectiveness of morphine.[93] Meperidine has an active metabolite, normeperidine, which has a longer half-life (15–30 hours) than the parent drug (3 hours). Normeperidine has some analgesic

Table 12-16 Significant Drug–Drug Interactions of Opioids

Opioid—Generic (Brand)	Drug—Generic (Brand)	Effect
All	Antihistamines, CNS depressants (barbiturates, alcohol), chlorpromazine (Thorazine)	Potentiates sedation and respiratory depression.
All	Warfarin (Coumadin)	Increased warfarin levels.
All	Cimetidine (Tagamet)	Inhibits opioid metabolism, resulting in increased CNS toxicity.
All	MAO inhibitors	Increased risk of hypertensive crisis.
All	Erythromycin	Increased opioid effects.
Codeine	Quinidine, bupropion, celecoxib (Celebrex), cimetidine (Tagamet), MAO inhibitors	Inhibits CYP2D6, thereby inhibiting codeine conversion to morphine, decreasing analgesic effect. MAO inhibitors and codeine increase the risk for serotonin syndrome.
Fentanyl (Duragesic)	Ketoconazole (Nizoral)	Increased levels of fentanyl through inhibition of CYP3A4.
Methadone (Dolophine)	CYP3A4 inducers: carbamazepine (Tegretol), erythromycin, phenytoin (Dilantin), antiretroviral medications, rifampin (Rifadin)	Increased methadone metabolism. May induce withdrawal.
	CYP3A4 inhibitors: Fluconazole (Diflucan), SSRIs, TCAs	Increased methadone levels. Methadone can also increase TCA levels.
	CYP3A4 inhibitors: Grapefruit and ciprofloxacin (Cipro)	Prolonged QT syndrome and *torsades de pointes*.
Meperidine (Demerol)	MAO inhibitors	Hyperpyrexia
	Phenytoin (Dilantin), phenobarbital	Decreased meperidine levels.
Morphine	Antihypertensives	Increased orthostatic hypotension.
	Dexamethasone, rifampin	Induced CYP2D6, thereby increasing plasma levels of morphine.
	Tricyclic antidepressants	Inhibit morphine glucuronidation, which causes increased blood levels of morphine. Morphine also causes decreased metabolism of TCAs, which causes toxicity of TCAs.
Propoxyphene (Darvocet)	Carbamazepine (Tegretol), doxepin (Sinequan), beta-blockers	Increased plasma levels of these drugs and beta-blockers.
	Benzodiazepines	Decreases excretion of benzodiazepines, causing accumulation and overdose.
Tramadol (Ultram)	SSRIs and MAO inhibitors	Use with SSRIs causes decreased analgesic effect and increased risk for serotonin syndrome.
	CYP2D6 inhibitors such as quinidine	Tramadol is a CYP2D6 substrate. Decreased or abolished analgesic effect of tramadol.

CNS = central nervous system; TCAs = tricyclic antidepressants; SSRI = selective serotonin reuptake inhibitor; MAO = monoamine oxidase.

effect, but more importantly, it can cause CNS hyperexcitability that is exhibited as anxiety, mood changes, myoclonus, and seizures.[95] Normeperidine can cause respiratory depression in newborns whose mothers were given meperidine in labor. Although meperidine was the drug of choice for treating moderate to severe pain for much of the 20th century, the toxic effects are significant, and meperidine is no longer recommended for treatment of postsurgical pain, labor pain, or pain in the elderly.[96] Meperidine is also contraindicated for individuals who take MAO inhibitors.

Methadone

Methadone is a synthetic full mu agonist that has been used to treat heroin addicts but is also very useful for the treatment of chronic and neuropathic pain states. Methadone is metabolized by CYP3A4 and CYP2D6 and excreted via feces, so it can be used by persons with renal impairment. Methadone is associated with multiple drug–drug interactions (Table 12-16). This drug has no active metabolites, but the analgesic effect lasts approximately 4–8 hours, and the plasma half-life is 24 hours. Thus, repeated dosing can result in accumulation of the drug, which causes confusion and sedation. Changing doses must be done with caution. The pharmacokinetics of methadone are discussed in more detail in Chapter 9.

Oxycodone (OxyContin, Percocet)

Oxycodone is a semisynthetic opioid that is an agonist for the mu, kappa, and delta receptors. Oxycodone is an analgesic by itself, but the metabolite oxymorphone also has analgesic effects. Oxycodone is metabolized by CYP2D6 and is therefore subject to drug–drug interactions. Tablets must not be crushed, broken, or chewed. There are no food–drug interactions. Adverse effects and efficacy are similar to morphine.

Oxymorphone (Opana, Numorphan)

Oxymorphone is a semisynthetic mu agonist that is approximately 6–8 times more potent than morphine. Oxymorphone is slightly more toxic than morphine but less toxic than the full synthetic preparations. It is used to treat acute and chronic pain and has a safety and efficacy profile similar to morphine and oxycodone. Oxycodone is not metabolized by the CYP450 enzymes and therefore has a favorable profile with regard to drug–drug interactions.[97] An immediate and long-acting oral formulation was recently released, making oxymorphone available for outpatient treatment.

Propoxyphene (Darvocet)

Propoxyphene is a weak synthetic mu agonist that is often a component of combined formulations with aspirin or acetaminophen. Nordextropropoxyphene, the major metabolite of propoxyphene, can cause CNS and cardiac depression. In addition, propoxyphene has multiple drug–drug interactions. Some pain experts recommend that propoxyphene no longer be used because the adverse effects outweigh the modest analgesic effects, and it is contraindicated for elderly persons.[98] However, some individuals report greater analgesic efficacy with propoxyphene than with hydrocodone, and it is often used in primary care practice.

Partial Agonists

Opioids with low intrinsic ability such as buprenorphine (Buprenex) achieve relatively minimal pharmacologic effects even when drug receptor occupancy is high; these opioids are termed **partial agonists**. The pharmacologic properties of buprenorphine are discussed in more detail in Chapter 9.

Agonist-Antagonists

Agonist-antagonists, such as butorphanol (Stadol) and nalbuphine (Nubain), elicit agonist effects at one receptor while producing antagonist effects at another. Agonist-antagonists produce analgesia but typically result in less respiratory depression than pure agonists. Unlike pure agonists, agonist-antagonists do exhibit a ceiling effect.

Increasing dosage beyond the maximal dose does not increase pain relief but does increase toxicity. Concurrent use with pure agonists may cause a reduction of analgesia and/or narcotic withdrawal symptoms if the agonist-antagonist inhabits a receptor normally inhabited by the pure agonist.

Antagonists

Opioid **antagonists**, such as naloxone (Narcan), reverse or block the activity of opioids at the mu and kappa sites. Naloxone (Narcan) is a competitive antagonist for the mu opioid receptor and binds to the site heroin or morphine use. Naloxone is used to counter opiate overdose. An intravenous dose works in about 2 minutes and effects last approximately 45 minutes. Naloxone should be used with extreme caution in persons who are opioid dependent. Abrupt reversal of opioid effects can precipitate acute withdrawal symptoms.

Naltrexone (ReVia) is a competitive antagonist of the mu and kappa opioid receptors. This drug is used to treat alcohol and opioid dependence. The clinical uses of naltrexone are discussed in more detail in Chapter 9.

Miscellaneous Analgesic Agents

Tramadol

Tramadol (Ultram) is a unique opioid that does not fit in the usual classifications and is not a scheduled drug. Tramadol is a synthetic weak mu opioid agonist and an inhibitor of serotonin and norepinephrine. The mechanism of action is not completely understood. Tramadol is used for management of moderate to severe pain and can be used to treat both acute and chronic pain. This drug is metabolized by CYP2D6 and CYP3A4 and has the usual drug–drug interactions associated with these enzyme inducers and inhibitors. Tramadol can decrease the threshold for seizures when combined with serotonin reuptake inhibitors or tricyclic antidepressants or in persons with epilepsy. However, drug–drug interactions are not common when tramadol is used in therapeutic doses.

Dextromethorphan

Dextromethorphan (Benylin, Triaminic Cold and Cough, Robitussin) is a common constituent of cold and cough preparations. Dextromethorphan is an opioid derivative that relies on the opioid property of suppressing bronchospasm to elevate the threshold for coughing. Dextromethorphan is metabolized by CYP2D6, and therefore it should not be taken concomitantly with selective serotonin inhibitors, tricyclic antidepressants, or MAO inhibitors.

Although used primarily as an antitussive, dextromethorphan will enhance the analgesic properties of morphine. Interestingly, when high doses are ingested, dextromethorphan acts as a dissociative hallucinogenic drug, and many retailers have moved dextromethorphan-containing products to behind the counter to prevent theft and misuse.

Special Populations

Treatment of Persons with Chronic Pain

Treatment of nonmalignant chronic pain is an increasingly frequent problem as the population ages, and treatment with opioids is increasing as concern about addiction becomes less important than treating pain in the medical community. In general, pharmacologic treatment of chronic pain is directed at these two fronts: the underlying disease process and the treatment of pain. The NSAIDs, aspirin, acetaminophen, opioids, and adjunctive analgesics all have a role depending on the specific situation.[99] In practice, balancing pain relief and unacceptable side effects is an ongoing clinical challenge.

When increasing doses are needed to treat chronic pain, the underlying problem could be progressive disease process or a therapeutic paradox called opioid tolerance and/or opioid **hyperalgesia**. The interaction between these two phenomena reduces analgesic efficacy, and it is important that prescribers recognize these syndromes.[100] Opioid tolerance is known to occur and is increasingly being treated with a technique called opioid rotation. Development of tolerance to one opioid does not confer cross-tolerance to another, and therefore rotating opioids toward equianalgesic dosing is proposed as a mechanism for treating opioid tolerance.

Opioid hyperalgesia is a state of nociceptive sensitization caused by exposure to opioids that occurs secondary to neuroplastic changes in the CNS.[101] N-methyl-D-aspartic acid (NMDA) receptor agonism appears to play a role in the development of hyperalgesia. There are preliminary data that suggest NMDA antagonists such as ketamine can prevent or reverse opioid hyperalgesia, and research on newer agents that inhibit NMDA receptors is ongoing.[102]

Pseudo-addiction is a third behavior that affects use of opioids and is an important one to understand. Addiction is "a primary, chronic, neurobiologic disease, with genetic, psychosocial, and environmental factors influencing its development and manifestations. It is characterized by behaviors that include one or more of the following: impaired control over drug use, compulsive use, continued use despite harm, and craving."[37] Pseudo-addiction occurs when pain is not sufficiently relieved with a standard opioid dose and the individual then exhibits some of the signs of addiction, such as tolerance and frequent requests to obtain analgesic drugs.

The distinction between opioid addiction and pseudo-addiction can be difficult to make. There are no specific distinctions between the two because pseudo-addiction behaviors are somewhat dependent upon staff responses to requests. In short, undertreatment of pain causes the sufferer to adopt more exaggerated expressions of pain, which in turn causes additional miscommunication. Careful history and a willingness to treat with larger doses as needed is an important clinical strategy when caring for a person with acute or chronic pain.

Pregnancy and Lactation

All opioids cross the placental barrier and are excreted in breast milk. Use of codeine in the first trimester has been linked to respiratory malformations of the fetus.[103] Use of opioids is common for pain control during labor (Chapter 35). The healthcare provider must remember that although the mother may not experience respiratory depression, the newborn may exhibit significant respiratory depression after birth, especially when the mother has been medicated within 2 hours of delivery. The American Academy of Pediatrics considers opioids to be compatible with breastfeeding, although excessive use may result in increased sedation of the newborn.[60]

Elderly

Chronic pain of multiple etiologies is a common problem for the elderly population, and it is often undertreated. Treatment of pain for older individuals is complicated by the frequency of comorbidities such as renal or hepatic impairment and cardiovascular disease that increase the risks associated with opioid use, and polypharmacy among the elderly increases the risk of drug interactions. In addition, age-related decreases in hepatic blood flow and renal function tend to decrease metabolism and excretion of drugs, which could result in drug toxicities.

Older persons may be more sensitive to both the analgesic and adverse effects of opioids. Opioid use should be carefully monitored to achieve maximum analgesia with minimum adverse effects. Individualization of dosage, method of delivery, and careful attention to the person's response to any medication is necessary for individualized therapy to achieve maximum analgesia while minimizing adverse effects. The use of propoxyphene (Darvon) and meperidine (Demerol) should be avoided in the elderly.[104] Use of propoxyphene in elderly persons has been associated with an increased risk for hip fracture.[105] The active metabolite of meperidine, normeperidine, accumulates in the elderly because of slowed renal clearance and can result in serious CNS side effects including tremors, seizures, confusion, and hyperexcitability.[106]

Combination Analgesics

Because there are multiple pain pathways and receptors involved in the pain response, many fixed-dose formulations that combine agents with different physiologic targets are available. There are several rationales for fixed-dose combination analgesics. Combining analgesics with different mechanisms of action can potentially increase the analgesic result beyond what the individual agents are capable of via a synergistic effect. Sometimes the analgesic effect is maximized secondary to pharmacokinetic properties of the two drugs (e.g., shorter onset and longer duration). A secondary goal then is to decrease dose-related adverse

effects and improve compliance.[107] Most of the combination products on the market today include acetaminophen, aspirin, or ibuprofen in combination with an opioid, and the majority of studies on the effectiveness of pain relief supports the theory that these combination products relieve pain better than single agents.[108] Combination therapy is recommended by the World Health Organization and the American Pain Society.

When using combination products, the dose-limiting factor is the nonopioid rather than the opioid component. Individuals taking combination products should be cautioned to pay close attention to the total daily dosage of acetaminophen, ibuprofen, or aspirin from any source. Table 12-17 provides a list of the common opioids and combination products with doses that are recommended for treatment of mild, moderate, and severe pain.

Atypical Analgesics

Atypical analgesics are used alone or in combination with other analgesics to enhance the analgesic effect or reduce symptoms that exacerbate pain. Atypical agents, also called *adjunctive agents*, allow for lower doses of the primary analgesic when used in combination and are particularly

Table 12-17 Combination Opioids for Moderate Pain or Pain of Limited Duration

Medication (Brand Name)	Dose per Tablet	Usual Initial Adult Dose	Clinical Considerations
Oxycodone/acetaminophen* (Tylox)	Tylox (5/500) mg	5–10 mg oxycodone† q 3–4 h	Dose is typically prescribed by opiate strength, but maximum dosage may be limited by acetaminophen content.
	Percocet (2.5/325; 5/325; 7.5/500; 10/650)	5–10 mg oxycodone† q 3–4 h	
Oxycodone/aspirin	Percodan (5/325)	5–10 mg oxycodone q 3–4 h	Dose is typically prescribed by opiate strength, but maximum dosage may be limited by aspirin content.
Hydrocodone/ acetaminophen*	Vicodin (5/500)	5–10 mg hydrocodone q 4–6 h	Dose is typically prescribed by opiate strength, but maximum dosage may be limited by acetaminophen.
	Vicodin ES (7.5/750)	5–10 mg hydrocodone q 4–6 h	
	Lortab (2.5/500; 5/500; 7.5/500; 10/500)	5–10 mg hydrocodone q 4–6 h	
	Lorcet (10/650)	5–10 mg hydrocodone q 4–6 h	
Codeine/acetaminophen*	Tylenol No 1 (7.5/300)	30–60 mg codeine q 4–6 h	Nausea and vomiting are common side effects.
	Tylenol No 2 (15/300)	30–60 mg codeine q 4–6 h	Codeine is a weak analgesic.
	Tylenol No 3 (30/300)	30–60 mg codeine q 4–6 h	Doses above 65 mg have increased side effects without increased pain relief.

(continues)

Table 12-17 Combination Opioids for Moderate Pain or Pain of Limited Duration (*continued*)

Medication (Brand Name)	Dose per Tablet	Usual Initial Adult Dose	Clinical Considerations
Tylenol No 4 (60/300)	30–60 mg codeine q 4–6 h	Dose is typically prescribed by opiate strength, but maximum dosage may be limited by acetaminophen.	
Propoxyphene/ acetaminophen*	Darvocet N-50 (50/325)	50–100 mg q 4–6 h	Black box warning on label that warns of risk of overdose. Medication guide will be given when prescription is filled. Coma, seizures, and death have been reported. Safety is not established in pregnancy. Use cautiously.
	Darvocet N-100 (100/650)	50–100 mg q 4–6 h	Black box warning on label that warns of risk of overdose. Medication guide will be given when prescription is filled. Coma, seizures, and death have been reported. Dose is typically prescribed by opiate strength, but maximum dosage may be limited by acetaminophen.
Propoxyphene/aspirin/ caffeine	Darvon compound (65 mg/389/32.4)	Darvon comes as a single combination. Dose specification not necessary.	Black box warning on label that warns of risk of overdose. Medication guide will be given when prescription is filled. Common side effects include hypotension, dizziness, paradoxic excitement, and insomnia. Coma, seizures, and death have been reported. Use cautiously in elderly and in patients with renal impairment.

* Maximum daily dose on a particular combination product should not exceed the maximum dose of acetaminophen (4000 mg/day). Many OTC drugs used to relieve cold symptoms have acetaminophen. Thus, prescribers should review all medications a patient is taking before prescribing and determining a dosing schedule for an analgesic that contains acetaminophen.
† Oxycodone (OxyContin) is also available as a single entity for severe pain.
Source: Reprinted with permission from Miller E 2004.[126]

useful for the management of neuropathic pain (Box 12-2). Commonly used atypical analgesics include tricyclic antidepressants, antiepileptics, local anesthetics, central nervous system stimulants, antihistamines, muscle relaxers, glucocorticoids, and bisphosphonates. Table 12-18 provides examples of the use of adjunctive agents with summaries of the risks and benefits.[109]

Anesthetics

Anesthetics are drugs that produce a loss of sensitivity to stimuli. General anesthetics produce unconsciousness. Local and regional anesthetics block pain without loss of consciousness. General anesthetics may be delivered by

Box 12-2 Neuropathic Pain

Ms J is a 67-year-old White female who comes to the clinic with complaints of sharp, burning pain and increased skin sensitivity in her scapular area. She states that her skin is so sensitive that she has trouble wearing a bra. On inspection, there are no lesions, redness, or edema. Light touch with a cotton ball produces complaints of stabbing pain. A careful health history reveals that Ms J experienced an outbreak of shingles 6 weeks ago that spontaneously resolved without treatment. The healthcare provider diagnoses postherpetic neuralgia (PHN).

Post herpetic neuralgia is generally a self-limiting condition, but it can last indefinitely. PHN is defined as pain that lasts beyond 1 month after the vesicular rash subsides. Age is the greatest risk factor for PHN. At age 60 years, approximately 60% of persons with shingles develop PHN, and the incidence increases with age. Treatment is aimed at pain control while waiting for the process to subside.

(*continues*)

■ Box 12-2 Neuropathic Pain (continued)

Because the pain is neuropathic in nature, treatment rarely requires the use of opioids, although they may be indicated in some cases. A variety of treatments have proven useful in treating PHN. Although acetaminophen may be adequate to treat mild cases of PHN, more troublesome cases usually require more definitive treatment with tricyclic antidepressants (TCAs), antiepileptic drugs (AEDs), or topical analgesics.

Amitriptyline, imipramine, and nortriptyline are suitable first-line TCAs. TCAs are best tolerated when started at small doses and given at bedtime. Dosage can be titrated upward slowly every 2–4 weeks to achieve effective pain relief. TCAs may require as long as 3 months to achieve therapeutic results.

Gabapentin and carbamazepine are suitable first-line AEDs. Pregabalin (Lyrica) is a newer AED that is FDA approved for PHN, but cost may make it prohibitive to persons on fixed incomes. AEDs may have significant side effects such as memory impairment, sedation, liver toxicity, or electrolyte disturbances, which can make them problematic for some elderly persons. However, analgesic effects are typically achieved at relatively low doses, which helps to reduce the incidence of these problems.

Topical analgesics such as capsaicin have proven efficacious but must be used 5–7 times daily for effective relief. Lidocaine patches have also been effective, but pain relief typically lasts only 4–12 hours.

After reviewing treatment options, Ms J chooses to try lidocaine patches for immediate pain relief and start amitriptyline at 25 mg to be taken nightly. If pain relief is not adequate, her amitriptyline may be titrated upward by 25 mg every 2–4 weeks until adequate analgesia or a maximum dose of 150 mg per day is achieved.

Table 12-18 Atypical Analgesics

Drug Category	Beneficial Effects	Adverse Effects/Side Effects	Clinical Considerations
Tricyclic antidepressants; e.g., amitriptyline (Elavil)	Reduce neuropathic pain, elevate mood, promote sleep, enhance appetite.	Increase anticholinergic effects of opioids (dry mouth, urinary retention, constipation), nightmares, confusion, cardiotoxicity.	Inhibit serotonin and norepinephrine uptake. Effective for diabetic neuropathy and postherpetic neuralgia. Weight gain may limit usefulness. Use in elderly is controversial.
Antiepileptics; e.g., carbamazepine (Tegretol), gabapentin (Neurontin), pregabalin (Lyrica)	Reduce neuropathic pain. Pregabalin is also indicated for fibromyalgia. Carbamazepine effective for treating pain of trigeminal neuralgia.	Carbamazepine is myelosuppressive; use cautiously in patients with bone marrow suppression. Though rare, pregabalin may cause angioedema.	Gabapentin (Neurontin) is currently the first choice for neuropathic pain secondary to proven efficacy, a low side effect profile, and minimal drug–drug interactions.
Local anesthetics; e.g., lidocaine	Reduce neuropathic pain.	Minimal adverse effects if using transdermal formulations.	Available in transdermal patches and have good efficacy for postherpetic pain.
CNS stimulants; e.g., dextroamphetamine (Concerta, Ritalin)	Potentiate analgesia and reduce opioid-induced sedation.	Nausea, loss of appetite, diarrhea, constipation, nervousness, insomnia, irritability in first days of therapy, hypertension.	Can be habit forming. Contraindicated for persons with glaucoma, hypertension, cardiovascular disease, substance abuse, hyperthyroidism.
Antihistamines; e.g., hydroxyzine (Vistaril)	Enhance analgesia, reduce anxiety, promote sleep, reduce nausea.	Increased risk of respiratory depression.	Use cautiously in the elderly secondary to increased risk for tardive dyskinesia.
Corticosteroids; e.g., dexamethasone (Decadron)	Reduce edema, reduce inflammation, enhance appetite.	Long-term therapy may cause gastric ulceration, osteoporosis, hyperglycemia, immunosuppression, adrenal insufficiency, or psychosis.	Risk of adverse effects increases with increases in dose and longer duration of therapy.
Bisphosphonates; e.g., etidronate (Didronel), pamidronate (Aredia)	Reduce cancer-related bone pain.	Osteonecrosis of the jaw.	Mechanism of action not understood.

(continues)

Table 12-18 Atypical Analgesics *(continued)*

Drug Category	Beneficial Effects	Adverse Effects/Side Effects	Clinical Considerations
GABA agonists; e.g., baclofen (Lioresal)	Potentiate antineuralgia effect of carbamazepine.	Drowsiness, weakness, hypotension, confusion.	Require slow tapering to avoid possible seizures.
SNRIs; e.g., duloxetine (Cymbalta)	Duloxetine is FDA approved for treatment of pain from diabetic neuropathy but not as effective as TCAs.	No anticholinergic or antihistamine effects, but minimal analgesic effects.	The SNRIs have minimal analgesic effect, but are helpful in reducing anxiety, depression, and insomnia that accompany chronic pain. Bioavailability of duloxetine is reduced by about 1/3 in smokers, but dosage adjustment is not recommended.
Alpha agonists; e.g., clonidine (Catapres)	Reduces sympathetically mediated pain.	Anticholinergic effects (dry mouth, urinary retention, constipation), headache, nausea, allergic reaction.	Synergistic with opioids to produce antinociceptive effects.
Topical: capsaicin	Used in topical creams to relieve pain of peripheral neuropathy.	Burning at site of application.	Analgesic effect is dose dependent and can last for weeks following one dose.
NMDA antagonists; e.g., ketamine	Inhibit hyperalgesia effect from opioids and are synergistic in analgesic effect of opioids.	Hallucinations, memory impairment.	Ketamine has a narrow therapeutic window.
Cannabinoids	Decrease hyperalgesia effect from opioids and are synergistic in analgesic effect of opioids.	CNS depression.	Analgesic effect is mild, studies comparing cannabinoids to placebo reveal efficacy, but studies comparing cannabinoids to other drugs are lacking.

TCA = tricyclic antidepressants; SNRI = selective serotonin and norepinephrine reuptake inhibitors; CNS = central nervous system; GABA = gamma-aminobutyric acid; NMDA = N-methyl-D-aspartic acid.

inhalation or intravenous administration. With few exceptions, general and regional anesthetics are administered by specialists in anesthesia and are outside the scope of this discussion. One exception, nitrous oxide (Nitronox), a tasteless, odorless gas administered by inhalation, is sometimes used for anesthesia during labor or dental procedures without specialist supervision. Nitronox is a blend of 50% oxygen and 50% nitrous oxide, which is self-administered by the laboring woman through a mask or mouthpiece. Nitrous oxide's onset of effect is rapid (1 minute or less) and is equally rapidly reversed upon discontinuation, making it especially useful during the second stage of labor with few effects on the newborn.[110]

Local Anesthetics

The first local anesthetic used in clinical practice was cocaine. Sigmund Freud first noticed the anesthetic properties of cocaine, and his friend Karl Koller performed the first operation using cocaine as a topical ocular anesthetic.[111] There are two major groups of local anesthetics, esters and amides.

Esters (cocaine, procaine [Novocaine], tetracaine [Pontocaine], and benzocaine) have a shorter duration of action than amides, and their pharmacokinetics have not been studied in detail because their half-life in plasma is

< 1 minute. Hypersensitivity is more common with ester-type anesthetics. Individuals who experience an allergic response to an ester-type anesthetic should be considered allergic to all ester-type anesthetics. Allergic reactions to the amides are uncommon, but some products contain preservatives that may provoke an allergic reaction.

The amide local anesthetics are used more often in clinical practice. The amides include lidocaine (Xylocaine), mepivacaine (Carbocaine), bupivacaine (Marcaine), prilocaine (Citanest), and ropivacaine (Naropin). These agents have a low molecular weight and are highly lipophilic, which contributes to their ability to be widely distributed, especially in highly perfused organs. The amides are metabolized in the liver via the P450 enzyme system.

Mechanism of Action

Local anesthetics control pain by blocking sodium channels in the axonal membranes, which stops the conduction of sensory impulses. Local anesthetics block all action potential in all neurons to which they have access. Pain sensations, carried by small, nonmyelinated neurons, are blocked first, followed by other sensory sensations such as sensitivity to cold, heat, touch, and pressure. Motor neurons are also affected. Onset and duration of action are dependent upon molecular size, lipid solubility, and degree of ionization and vary among local anesthetics (Table 12-19).

Duration of action is also influenced by regional blood flow. For this reason, local anesthetics are often combined with a vasoconstrictive drug such as epinephrine. Epinephrine decreases local blood flow, thereby delaying systemic absorption and reducing the risk of toxicity by prolonging the achieving maximum duration of local anesthesia with less anesthetic. However, use of epinephrine may result in systemic effects such as palpitations, tachycardia, hypertension, and nervousness. In most cases, these effects are negligible and treatment is symptomatic.

Side Effects/Adverse Effects

The two major mechanisms of local anesthetic toxicity occur secondary to accidental injection into the bloodstream and subsequent systemic effects or direct toxicity from inadvertent intrathecal injection. The first symptoms of systemic toxicity are tongue numbness and a metallic taste. Dizziness, tinnitus, seizures, and then cardiac arrest can follow. Coadministration of epinephrine can reduce toxicity by reducing local blood flow and slowing systemic absorption to allow for a more even balance of drug distribution and metabolism. Direct toxicity following an intrathecal injection results in a very rapid onset of the regional block, hypotension, respiratory depression, and loss of consciousness.

Lidocaine

Lidocaine is the most common local anesthetic used in primary care. Lidocaine works by blocking sodium channels at the axonal membrane, which prevents sodium entry, resulting in a temporary halt to impulse conduction. Lidocaine is completely absorbed following parenteral administration. Peak anesthetic effect occurs within 2–5 minutes and lasts from 15 to 45 minutes. Combination with a vasoconstrictor such as epinephrine delays systemic absorption of lidocaine, thereby prolonging the anesthetic effect. Lidocaine is rapidly metabolized by the liver and excreted through the kidneys. It is available for subcutaneous injection or topical application for local anesthetic purposes. Topical use is discussed in Chapter 26.

Lidocaine suppresses myocardial excitability and conduction and may be given intravenously for its antidysrhythmic properties. Given in excess, it can cause bradycardia, heart block, and reduced myocardial contractility and cardiac arrest. Lidocaine also causes peripheral vasodilation, which can result in hypotension. Allergic reactions to lidocaine are rare but do occur. Cutaneous lesions, urticaria, edema, or anaphylactoid reactions are characteristic of lidocaine allergy.

Complementary and Alternative Medicines

Relief of pain is the most common reason for the use of complementary and alternative medicine (CAM).[112] CAM is used for a variety of reasons, including a common perception that CAM therapies are safer than prescription medications. Individuals may also choose CAM therapies because previous medically supervised treatments have been unsuccessful. CAM therapies are combined with conventional therapies. Unfortunately, many CAM therapies have been inadequately studied, and little evidence is available as to safety or efficacy or possible interaction with conventional medications. This section presents commonly used CAM therapies for pain within the context of the available scientific evidence.

Herbals

Arnica (Arnica Montana, leopard's bane) is used topically as a counterirritant, anti-inflammatory, and pain reliever.

Table 12-19 Characteristics of Local Anesthetics

Classification	Drug—Generic (Brand)	Maximum Adult Dose (Plain)	Maximum Adult Dose with Epinephrine	Onset of Action	Duration of Action
Amides	Bupivacaine (Marcaine)	175 mg	250 mg	5 min	4–8 h
	Lidocaine (Xylocaine)	300 mg*	500 mg†	2 min or less	30–120 min
Esters	Procaine (Novocain)	500 mg	600 mg	2–5 min	30–45 min
	Tetracaine (Pontocaine)	100 mg	100 mg	15 min or less	2–3 h

* 4 mg/kg, which is 30 cc of 1% lidocaine.
† 7 mg/kg, which is 50 cc of 1% lidocaine with epinephrine solution.

Studies have shown arnica to be as effective as ibuprofen for treatment of osteoarthritis of the hand,[113] as well as safe and effective for treatment of mild to moderate osteoarthritis of the knee.[114] Arnica interacts with antihypertensive drugs and is considered poisonous when taken internally.

Capsaicin (*Capsicum frutescens*, African chilies, Mexican chilies, grains of paradise) has been used topically to treat postherpetic neuralgia, diabetic neuropathy, osteoarthritis, and rheumatoid arthritis. Capsaicin works by binding to nociceptors in the skin. Initial excitation of the neurons is perceived as sensations of itching or burning and is accompanied by local vasodilation. Following this initial excitation, there is a period of reduced sensitivity, which, with repeated applications, may cause degeneration of epidermal nerve fibers resulting in persistent hypoanalgesia.[115] A systematic review of capsaicin for the treatment of chronic pain found it to have poor to moderate efficacy in the treatment of chronic musculoskeletal or neuropathic pain.[116]

Devil's claw (*Harpagophytum procumbens*) has been found to be possibly effective in controlling pain associated with osteoarthritis of the knee and hip and with nonspecific low back pain and is most efficacious when taken as an aqueous extract of 50–100 mg.[117] It has been used in the treatment of menstrual cramps, but there are no studies of its effectiveness for this use. Devil's claw interacts with warfarin, causing an increase in anticoagulation.[118] It may also have hypoglycemic effects and should be used cautiously by diabetics using hypoglycemic agents.

Ginger (*Zingiber officinale*) has been used for the treatment of inflammation associated with rheumatoid arthritis. It is believed to inhibit prostaglandin and leukotriene synthesis.[119] Randomized studies have not demonstrated any increased efficacy of ginger over placebo or ibuprofen. However, no side effects or drug interactions have been reported.[120]

Willow bark (*Salix alba*) has moderate evidence of efficacy for treatment of nonspecific low back pain. Daily doses standardized to 120 mg or 240 mg salicin, the active ingredient in willow bark, were better than placebo for short-term improvements in pain and rescue medication.[121] However, it has not been found to be effective in treatment of osteoarthritis.[122] Although there is little research on safety and drug interactions of willow bark, salicin is a salicylate, and individuals should be advised to take the same precautions as they would with aspirin.[123]

Butterbur (*Petasites hybridus*) has been found to reduce the frequency, intensity, and duration of migraine attacks in persons who have three to seven attacks per month.[124] Butterbur is in the same plant family as ragweed, marigolds, and chrysanthemums and may cause allergic reactions in some individuals. Some butterbur preparations contain pyrrolizidine alkaloids, which may cause liver toxicity.[125]

Conclusion

As knowledge of molecular mechanisms of action and technology advance, new medications and new modalities for administering pain medications are coming through the research pipeline and into clinical practice. Researchers looking for new analgesics are exploring molecular receptor targets for new drugs and genetic variability in both pain perception and response to pain medications. The role of the immune system in pain pathways is just beginning to become clear. The latest modality for delivering systemic drugs is transdermal iontophoresis, which is a process that facilitates delivery of a charged molecule across intact skin using a small electrical current. Fentanyl is being used this way in palliative hospice settings and may be superior to patient-controlled analgesia in certain settings.

Unrelieved pain causes needless suffering, and healthcare providers have an obligation to assess, believe, and document a person's report of pain and to intervene to relieve or avert pain. Because pain is a highly subjective and variable experience, treatment must be individualized, taking into account the type of pain, comorbid conditions, gender, age, and other individual characteristics.

References

1. American Pain Society. Pain assessment and treatment in the managed care environment: a position statement from the American Pain Society. Glenview, IL: American Pain Society, 2000.
2. Verhaak PF, Kerssens JJ, Deker J, Sorbi MJ, Bensing JM. Prevalence of chronic benign pain disorder among adults: a review of the literature. Pain 1998;77:231–9.
3. Paulose-Ram R, Hirsch R, Dillon C, Gu Q. Frequent monthly use of selected non-prescription and prescription non-narcotic analgesics among US adults. Pharmacoepidem Drug Safety 2005;14:257–66.
4. Hersh EV, Pinto A, Moore PA. Adverse drug reactions involving common prescription and over-the-counter analgesic agents. Cl Therapeut 2007;29:2477–97.

5. Rollason V, Samer C, Piguet V, Dayer P, Desmeules J. Pharmacogenetics of analgesics: toward the individualization of prescription. Pharmacogenomics 2008; 9: 905–33.

6. International Association for the Study of Pain. Subcommittee on Taxonomy. Classification Chronic Pain 1986;3:S1–226.

7. Barkin RL. Acetaminophen, aspirin, ibuprofen in combination analgesic products. Am J Ther 2001;8: 433–42.

8. Uruh AM. Gender variations in clinical pain experience. Pain 1996:65;123–67.

9. Craft RM. Sex differences in drug and non-drug induced analgesia. Life Sciences 2003;72:2675–88.

10. Carr DB, Goudas LC. Acute pain. Lancet. 1999; 353: 2051–58.

11. Schaible HG, Richter F. Pathophysiology of pain. Langenbecks Arch Surg 2004;389:237–43.

12. Russo CM, Brose WG. Chronic pain. Annu Rev Medicine 1998;49:123–33.

13. Portenoy RK, Bennett DS, Rauck R, Simon S, Taylor D, Brennan M, et al. Prevalence and characteristics of breakthrough pain in opioid-treated patients with chronic noncancer pain. J Pain 2006;7:583–91.

14. Merskey H, Bogduk N, eds. Part III: Pain terms: a current list with definitions and notes on usage. In Classification of chronic pain: descriptions of chronic pain syndromes and definitions of pain terms. Seattle, WA: IASP Press, 1994:209–14.

15. Melzack RW, Wall P. Pain mechanisms: a new theory. Science 1965;150:171–9.

16. Snow SJ. Anaesthesia: symbol of humanitarianism. BMJ 2007;334(suppl 1):s5.

17. Kehlet H. Multimodal approach to control postoperative pathophysiology and rehabilitation. Br J Anesth 1997;78:606–17.

18. Polomano RC, Rathmell JP, Krenzischek D, Dunwoody CJ. Emerging trends and new approaches to acute pain management. J Peri Anesthes 2008;1(suppl 1):S43–53.

19. Hudcova J, McNicol ED, Quah CS, Lau J, Carr DB. Patient controlled opioid analgesia versus conventional opioid analgesia for postoperative pain. Cochrane Database of Systematic Reviews 2006, Issue 4. Art No: CD003348. DOI: 10.1002/14651858. CD003348.pub2.

20. Gordon DR, Dahl J, Phillips P, Frandsen J, Cowley C, Foster RL, et al. The use of "as needed" range orders for opioid analgesics in the management of acute pain.

A consensus statement for the American Society of Pain Management Nursing and the American Pain Society. Pain Manage Nurs 2004;5:53–8.

21. Melzack R. Pain—an overview. Acta Anaesthesiol Scand 1999;43:880–4.

22. Melzack R. Pain and the neuromatrix in the brain. J Dent Edu 2001;65(12):1378–82.

23. Melzack R. From the gate to the neuromatrix. Pain 1999;82(S):S121–6.

24. Zimmerman M, Herdegen T. Plasticity of the nervous system at the systemic, cellular and molecular levels: a mechanism of chronic pain and hyperalgesia. Prog Brain Res 1996;110:233–59.

25. Craft RM. Sex differences in opioid analgesia: "from mouse to man." Clin J Pain 2003;19:175–86.

26. Sandner-Kiesling A, Eisenach JC. Estrogen reduces efficacy of mu but not kappa-opioid agonist inhibition in response to uterine cervical distention. Anesthesiology 2000;96:375–80.

27. Smith YR Stohler CS, Nichols TE, Bueller JA, Koeppe RA, Zubieta JK. Pronociceptive and antinociceptive effects of estradiol through endogenous opioid neurotransmission in women. J Neurosci 2006; 26:5777–85.

28. Krohn B. Using pain assessment tools. Nurs Pract 2002;27:54–6.

29. Melzack R. The short-form McGill pain questionnaire. Pain 1987;30:191–7.

30. World Health Organization. Cancer pain relief and palliative care: report of a WHO expert committee. World Health Organization Technical Report Series 804, Geneva, Switzerland: WHO, 1990.

31. Miaskowski C, Cleary J, Burney R, Coyne P, Finley R, Foster R, et al. Guideline for the management of cancer pain in adults and children. Glenview, IL: American Pain Society, 2005.

32. Fine PG, Portenoy RK. A clinical guide to opioid analgesics. Minneapolis, MN: McGraw-Hill, 2004.

33. Munir M, Enany N, Zhang JM. Nonopioid analgesics. Med Clin N Amer 2007;91:97–111.

34. Chandrasekharan NV, Hu Dal K, Roos LT, Evanson NK, Tomisk J, Elton TS, et al. COX-3, a cyclooxygenase-1 variant inhibited by acetaminophen and other analgesic/antipyretic drugs: cloning, structure, and expression. PNAS 2002;99:13926–31.

35. Brune K, Hinz B. The discovery and development of anti-inflammatory drugs. Arthritis rheum 2004;50: 2391–99.

36. Vane, JR. Inhibition of prostaglandin synthesis as a mechanism of action for aspirin-like drugs. Nature New Bio 1971;231:232–35.

37. Mas MB, Pain R, Edwards WT, Sunshine A, Inturrisi CE. Principles of analgesic use in the treatment of acute pain and cancer pain, 4th ed. Glenview, IL: American Pain Society, 1999.

38. Brown C. Effective use of nonsteroidal anti-inflammatory drugs. Female Patient 2002;27:20–30.

39. Bybee KA, Powell BD, Valeti U, Rosales AG, Kopecky SL, Mullany C, et al. Perioperative aspirin therapy is associated with improved postoperative outcomes in patients having coronary artery bypass grafting. Circulation 2005;112(suppl 9):1286–92.

40. Douketis JE, Berger PB, Dunn AS, Spyropoulos AD, Becker RC, Ansell J. The perioperative management of antithrombotic therapy: American college of chest physicians evidence-based practice guidelines, 8th ed. Chest 2008;133(suppl 6):299S–339S.

41. Dube C, Rostom A, Lewin G, Tsertsvadze A, Code C, Sampson M, et al. Use of aspirin and NSAIDs to prevent colorectal cancer. Rockville, MD: Agency for Healthcare Research Quality, 2007. Available from: www.ahrq.gov/clinic/uspstf07/aspcolo/aspcoloes.pdf [Accessed October 31, 2008].

42. Kelly JP, Kaufman DW, Jurgelon JM, Sheehan J, Koff RS, Shapiro S. Risk of aspirin-associated major upper-gastrointestinal bleeding with enteric-coated or buffered product. Lancet 1996;348:1413–6.

43. Campbell CL, Smyth S, Monalescot G, Steinhubl SR. Aspirin dose of the prevention of cardiovascular disease: a systematic review. JAMA 2007;297:2018–24.

44. Ridker PM, Cook NR, Lee IM, Gordan D, Gaziano JM, Manson JE, et al. A randomized trial of low-dose aspirin in the primary prevention of cardiovascular disease in women. N Engl J Med 2005;352:1293–304.

45. Silverstein FE, Graham DY, Senior JR, Davies HW, Struthers BJ, Bittman RM, et al. Misoprostol reduces serious gastrointestinal complications in patients with rheumatoid arthritis receiving nonsteroidal antiinflammatory drugs. A randomized, double-blind, placebo-controlled trial. Ann Intern Med 1995;123:241–9.

46. Aithal GP, Day CP. Nonsteroidal anti-inflammatory drug-induced hepatotoxicity. Clin Liver Dis 2007; 11:563–75.

47. Palikhe NS, Kim SH, Park HS. What do we know about the genetics of aspirin intolerance? J Clin Pharm Ther 2008;33:465–72.

48. Kong JS, Teuber SS, Gershwin ME. Aspirin and nonsteroidal anti-inflammatory drug hypersensitivity. Allergy Immunol 2007;32(1):97–110.

49. Babu KS, Salvi SS. Aspirin and asthma. Chest 2000;118:1470–7.

50. Palikhe NS, Kim SH, Park HS. What do we know about the genetics of aspirin intolerance? J Clin Pharm Ther 2008;33:465–72.

51. Burk A, Smyth E, FitzGerald GA. Analgesic-antipyretic agents: pharmacology of gout. In Brunton L, Lazo J, Parker K, eds. Goodman and Gillman's the pharmacologic basis of therapeutics, 11th ed. New York: McGraw-Hill, 2006:671–715.

52. Lau WC, Gurbel PA. Antiplatelet drug resistance and drug–drug interactions: role of cytochrome 450 3A4. Pharm Rev 2006;23:2691–707.

53. James AH, Braneazio LR, Price T. Aspirin and reproductive outcomes. Obsetet Gynecol Surv 2007;63:49–57.

54. Lewis RB, Schulman JD. Influence of acetylsalicylic acid, an inhibitor of prostaglandin sythesis, on the duration on human gestation and labor. Lancet 1973;2:1159–61.

55. Askie LM, Duley L, Henderson-Smart DJ, Steward LA, PARIS Collaborative Group. Antiplatelet agents for prevention of pre-eclampsia: a meta-analysis of individual patient data. Lancet 2007;369:1791–8.

56. Leitch H, Egarter C, Husslein P, Kaider A, Schemper M. A meta-analysis of low dose aspirin for the prevention of IUGR. Br J Obstet Gynecol 1997; 104:450–9.

57. James AH, Braneazio LR, Price T. Aspirin and reproductive outcomes. Obsetet Gynecol Surv 2007;63:49–57.

58. Levin DL, Fixler DE, Morriss FC, Tyson J. Morphologic analysis of the pulmonary vascular bed in infants exposed in utero to prostaglandin synthetase inhibitors. J Pediatr 1978;92:478–83.

59. Turner G, Collins E. Fetal effects of regular salicylate ingestion in pregnancy. Lancet 1975;2:338–9.

60. American Academy of Pediatrics. The transfer of drugs and other chemicals into human milk. Pediatrics 2001;108:776–89.

61. Clark JH, Wilson WG. A 16-day-old breast-fed infant with metabolic acidosis caused by salicylate. Clin Pediatr 1981;20:53–4.

62. Slone Epidemiology Center: Patterns of medication use in the United States 2005. Boston, MA: Slone

Epidemiology Center, 2005. Available from: www.bu
.edu/slone/SloneSurvey/AnnualRpt/SloneSurveyWeb
Report2005.pdf [Accessed November 2, 2008].

63. Wolfe MM, Lichtenstein DR, Singh G. Gastrointestinal
toxicity of nonsteroidal antiinflammatory drugs.
N Engl J Med 1999;340:1888–99.

64. Geba GP, Weaver AL, Polis AB, Dixon ME, Schnitzer
TJ, for the VACT Group. Efficacy of rofecoxib, celecoxib, and acetaminophen in osteoarthritis of the
knee: a randomized trial. JAMA 2002;287:64–71.

65. Pincus T, Koch G, Lei H, Mangal B, Sokka T,
Moskowitz R, et al. Patient preference for placebo,
acetaminophen (paracetamol) or celecoxib efficacy
studies (PACES): two randomised, double blind, placebo controlled, crossover clinical trials in patients
with knee or hip osteoarthritis. Ann Rheum Dis
2004;63:931–9.

66. Forman JP, Stampfer MJ, Curhan GC. Non-narcotic
analgesic dose and risk of incident hypertension in US
women. Hypertension 2005;46:500–57.

67. Vonkeman HE, van de Laar MAFJ. Nonsteroidal anti-
inflammatory drugs: adverse effects and their prevention. Semin Arthritis Rheum. In press.

68. Tramer MR, Moore RA, Reynolds DJ, McQuay HJ.
Quantitative estimation of rare adverse events which
follow a biological progression: a new model applied
to chronic NSAID use. Pain 2000;85:169–82.

69. Lanzi LL. A guideline for the treatment and prevention of NSAID-induced ulcers. Am J Gastroenterol
1998;93:2037–46.

70. García Rodríguez LA. Variability in risk of gastrointestinal complications with different nonsteroidal
anti-inflammatory drugs. Am J Med 1998 Mar 30;
104:30S–4S.

71. Agency for Health Care Research and Quality. Choosing non-opioid analgesics for osteoarthritis. Clinicians Guide. Available from: http://effectivehealthcare
.ahrq.gov/ [Accessed November 2, 2008].

72. Hersh EV, Moore PA, Ross Gl. Over-the-counter analgesics and antipyretics: a critical assessment. Clin
Ther 2000;22:500–47.

73. Henry D, Lim LL, Carcia Rodriguez LA, Perez Gut-
thann S, Carson JL, Griffin M, et al. Variability in risk
of gastrointestinal complications with individual nonsteroidal antiinflammatory drugs. Results of a collaborative meta-analysis. MBJ 1996;312:1563–6.

74. Rostom A, Dube C, Wells G, Tugwell P, Welch V,
Jolicoeur E, et al. Prevention of NSAID-induced

gastroduodenal ulcers. Cochrane Database of Systematic Reviews 2002, Issue 4. Art No: CD002296. DOI:
10.1002/14651858.CD002296.

75. MacDonald TM, Wei L. Effect of ibuprofen on cardioprotective effect of aspirin. Lancet 2003;361:573–4.

76. Kimmel SE, Berlin JA, Reilly M, Jaskowiak J, Kishel L,
Chittams J, et al. The effects of nonselective non-aspirin
non-steroidal anti-inflammatory medications on the
risk of nonfatal myocardial infarction and their interaction with aspirin. J Am Coll Cardiol 2004;43:985–90.

77. Hennessy MD, Livingston EC, Papagianos J, Killam AP.
The incidence of ductal constriction and oligohydram-
nios during tocolytic therapy with ibuprofen (abstract).
Am J Obstet Gynecol 1992;166:324.

78. Temprano KK, Brandlamudi R, Moore TL. Antirheumatic drugs in pregnancy and lactation. Semin Arthritis Rheum 2005;35:112–21.

79. Bombardier C, Laine L, Reicin A, Shapiro D,
Burgos-Vargas R, Davis B, et al. Comparison of upper
gastrointestinal toxicity of rofecoxib and naproxen
in patients with rheumatoid arthritis. VIGOR Study
Group. N Engl J Med 2000;343:1520–8.

80. Bresalier RS, Sandler RS, Quan H, Bolognese JA,
Oxenius B, Horgan K, et al. Cardiovascular events associated with rofecoxib in a colorectal adenoma chemoprevention trial. N Engl J Med 2005;352:1092–102.

81. Silverstein FE, Faich G, Goldstein JL, Simon LS,
Pincus T, Whelton A, et al. for the Celecoxib Long-
Term Arthritis Safety Study. Gastrointestinal toxicity with celecoxib vs nonsteroidal anti-inflammatory
drugs for osteoarthritis and rheumatoid arthritis. The
CLASS Study: a randomized controlled trial. JAMA
2000;284:1247–55.

82. Hippesley-Cox J, Coupland K, Logan R. Risk of
adverse gastrointestinal outcomes in patients taking
cyclo-oxygenase-2 inhibitors or conventional nonsteroidal anti-inflammatory drugs: population based
nested case-control analysis. BMJ 2005;331:1310–6.

83. Mukherjee D, Nissen SE, Topol EJ. Risk of cardiovascular events associated with selective COX-2 inhibitors. JAMA 2001;286:954–8.

84. Hale TW, McDonald R, Boger J. Transfer of celecoxib
into human milk. J Hum Lact 2004;20:397–403.

85. Food and Drug Administration. Over-the-counter
drug products containing analgesic/antipyretic active
ingredients for internal use: required alcohol warning;
final rule; compliance date. Food and Drug Administration HHS Fed Regist 1999;64:13066–7.

86. Hylek EM, Heiman H, Skates SJ, Sheehan MA, Singer DE. Acetaminophen and other risk factors for excessive warfarin anticoagulation. JAMA 1998;279:657–62.

87. Kwan D, Bartle WR, Walker SE. The effects of acetaminophen and pharmacokinetics and pharmacodynamics of warfarin. J Clin Pharm 1999;39:6845.

88. Gear RW, Miaskowski C, Gordon NC, Paul SM, Heller PH, Levine JD. Kappa-opioids produce significantly greater analgesia in women than in men. Nat Med 1996;11:1248–50.

89. Fillingim RB, Ness TJ. Sex-related hormonal influences on pain and analgesic responses. Neurosci Biobehav Rev 2000;24:485–501.

90. Kirchheiner J, Schmidt H, Tzvetkov M, Keulen J-THA, Lotsch J, Roots I, et al. Pharmacokinetics of codeine and its metabolite morphine in ultra-rapid metabolizers due to CYP2D6 duplication. Pharmacogenomics J 2006;7:1–9.

91. Sindrup SH, Brosen K. The pharmacogenetics of codeine hypnoanalgesia. Pharmacogenetics 1995;6:335–46.

92. Benyamin R, Trescot AM, Datta S, Buenaventura R, Adlaka R, Sehgal N, et al. Opioid complications and side effects. Pain Physician 2008;11:S105–20.

93. Trescott AM, Datta S, Lee M, Hansen H. Opioid pharmacology. Pain Physician 2008;11:S133–53.

94. Medwatch safety labeling change. Available from: www.fda.gov/medwatch/safety/2007/safety07.htm#Codeine [Accessed November 12, 2008].

95. Latta K, Bingsberg B, Barkin R. Meperidine: a critical review. Am J Ther 2002;9:53–68.

96. Institute for Clinical Systems Improvement (ICSI). Assessment and management of acute pain. Bloomington, MN: Institute for Clinical Systems Improvement (ICSI), March 2008: 58. Available from: www.guideline.gov/summary/summary.aspx?doc_id=12302&nbr=006371&string=pain [Accessed June 25, 2009].

97. Chamberlin KW, Cottle M, Neville R, Tan J. Oral oxymorphone for pain management Ann Pharmacother 2007;41(7):1144–52. Epub June 26, 2007.

98. Barkin RL, Barkin SJ, Barkin DS. Propoxyphene (Dextropropoxyphene): a critical review of a weak opioid analgesic that should remain in antiquity. Am J Ther 2006;13:534–42.

99. Lynch ME. The pharmacotherapy of chronic pain. Rheum Dis Clin N Am 2008;34:368–85.

100. Chang G, Chen L, Mao J. Opioid tolerance and hyperalgesia. Me Clin N Am 2007;91:199–211.

101. Chu LF, Angst MS, Clark D. Opioid-induced hyperalgesia in humans, molecular mechanisms and clinical considerations. Clin J Pain 2008;24:479–96.

102. Knotkova H, Pappagallo M. Adjunct analgesics. Med Clin N Am 2007;91:113–24.

103. Inturrisi CE. Clinical pharmacology of opioids for pain. Clin J Pain 2002;18:S3–13.

104. Heinonen OP, Slone D, Shapiro S. Birth defects and drugs in pregnancy. Littleton, MA: Publishing Sciences Group, 1977.

105. Beers MH. Explicit criteria for determining potentially inappropriate medication use by the elderly. Arch Intern Med 1997;157:1531–6.

106. Shorr RI, Griffin MR, Daugherty JR, Ray WA. Opioid analgesics and the risk of hip fracture in the elderly: codeine and propoxyphene. J Gerontol 1992;47:M111–5.

107. Chutka DS, Takahashi PY, Hoel RW. Inappropriate medications for elderly patients. Mayo Clin Proc 2004;79:122–39.

108. Barkin RL. Acetaminophen, aspirin or ibuprofen in combination analgesic products. Am J Ther 2001;8:433–42.

109. Moore A, Collins S, Carroll D, McQuay H, Edwards J. Single dose paracetamol (acetaminophen), with and without codeine, for postoperative pain. Cochrane Database of Systematic Reviews 1998, Issue 4. Art No: CD001547. DOI: 10.1002/14651858.CD001547.

110. Rosen MA. Nitrous oxide for relief of labor pain: a systematic review. Am J Obstet Gynecol 2002;186:S131–59.

111. Ruetsch YA, Boni T, Borgeat A. From cocaine to ropivacaine: the history of local anesthetic drugs. Curr Top Med Chem 2001;1:175–82.

112. Astin JA. Why patients use alternative medicine: results of a national study. JAMA 1998;279:1548–53.

113. Widrig R, Suter A, Saller R, Melzer J. Choosing between NSAID and arnica for topical treatment of hand osteoarthritis in a randomised, double-blind study. Rheumatol Int 2007;6:585–91.

114. Knuesel O, Weber M, Suter A. Arnica montana gel in osteoarthritis of the knee: an open, multicenter clinical trial. Adv Ther 2002;19:209–18.

115. Nolano M, Simone DA, Wendelschafer-Crabb G, Johnson T, Hazen E, Kennedy WR. Topical capsaicin in humans: parallel loss of epidermal nerve fibers and pain sensation. Pain 1999;81:135–45.

116. Mason L, Moore RA, Derry S, Edwards JE, McQuay HJ. Systematic review of topical capsaicin for the treatment of chronic pain. BMJ 2004;328:991–9.

117. Brien S, Lewith GT, McGregor G. Devil's claw (Harpagophytum procumbens) as a treatment for osteoarthritis: a review of efficacy and safety. J Altern Complement Med 2006;10:981–93.

118. Izzo AA, Di Carlo G, Borrelli F, Ernst E. Cardiovascular pharmacotherapy and herbal medicines: the risk of drug interaction. Int J Cardiol 2005;98:1–14.

119. Srivastava KC, Mustafa T. Ginger (Zingiber officinale) in rheumatism and musculoskeletal disorders. Med Hypotheses 1992;39:342–8.

120. Bliddal H, Rosetzsky A, Schlichting P, Weidner MS, Andersen LA, Ibfelt HH, et al. A randomized, placebo-controlled, cross-over study of ginger extracts and ibuprofen in osteoarthritis. Osteoarthritis Cartilage 2000;8:9–12.

121. Gagnier JJ, van Tulder M, Berman B, Bombardier C. Herbal medicine for low back pain. Cochrane Database Syst Rev 2006;CD004504.

122. Beigert C, Wagner I, Ludtke R, Kotter I, Lohmuller C, Gunaydin I, et al. Efficacy and safety of willow bark extract in the treatment of osteoarthritis and rheumatoid arthritis: results of 2 randomized double-blind controlled trials. J Rheumatol 2004;11:2121–30.

123. Clauson KA, Santamarina ML, Buettner CM, Cauffield JS. Evaluation of presence of aspirin-related warnings with willow bark. Ann Pharmacother 2005;39:1234–7.

124. Lipton RB, Gobel H, Einhaupl KM, Wilks K, Mauskop A. Petasites hybridus root (butterbur) is an effective preventive treatment for migraine. Neurology 2004:63:2240–4.

125. Danesch U, Rittinghausen R. Safety of a patented special butterbur root extract for migraine prevention. Headache 2003;43:76–8.

126. Miller E. The World Health Organization analgesic ladder. J Midwifery Womens Health 2004;49:542–5.

Histamine

"By your real name of alias-Ergamine
You give asthmatics wheezes,
Pollinosis patients sneezes-
You smooth muscle stimulating Histamine
Trauma, bums and inflammation.
Headache, pain and constipation
Show the finger-prints of some malicious fiend,
And the one that gets accused
Is that amine so abused-
Beta iminazol ethylamine."

CARL A. DRAGSTEDT, MD, PHD (1895–1983)

13
Antihistamines

Lillie Rizack and Lawrence Carey

Chapter Glossary

Anticholinergic Drug that blocks the effect of the neurotransmitter acetylcholine both peripherally and centrally. This inhibition results in symptoms such as dry mouth, cessation of perspiration, urinary retention, mydriasis, confusion, blurred vision, and light-headedness. Several classes of drugs have anticholinergic effects.

Antihistamine Class of drugs that blocks the effect of endogenously released histamines.

Basophil Type of white blood cell that contains granules of histamine, which are released as part of the inflammatory response.

Inflammatory response A series of cellular and vascular responses that are triggered when the body is injured or invaded by an antigen. Damaged cells release histamine and other chemicals that initiate the response.

Mast cells Cells that reside in various tissues and contain granules of histamine and heparin, which are released following injury or stimulation by members of the complement system.

Osteoclastogenesis Process by which osteoclasts are formed in the bone marrow. Osteoclasts work to remodel bone by removing bone tissue.

Paradoxical reaction When a drug has the opposite effect of the one expected. With regard to antihistamines, a paradoxical effect would be increased pruritus following administration of diphenhydramine (Benadryl).

Histamines

Histamine, as the quote above alludes to, is involved in many different physiologic and pathophysiologic processes.

Therefore, it is not surprising that **antihistamines**, which are a class of drugs that block the effects of histamine, are used to treat so many different disorders. Histamines are naturally occurring proteins that are central players in the immediate hypersensitivity reaction and the inflammatory response. In addition, they act as neurotransmitters; stimulate gastric secretions; and act on smooth muscle in the heart, vascular system, and respiratory system. Table 13-1 and Figure 13-1 provide an overview of the effects of histamine on various organ systems.

Histamine Synthesis

One of the primary functions of histamines is to mediate the body's inflammatory response. Histamines are synthesized and stored in **mast cells** and **basophils**. These cells release histamine after exposure to an antigen or trauma. Histamine in turn induces vasodilation and increases permeability of local capillaries as part of the **inflammatory response**. Pruritus, hypotension, and/or bronchoconstriction are additional histamine effects during an inflammatory response.

Histamine is also synthesized in neurons in the central nervous system where it acts as a neurotransmitter. Other sites of histamine synthesis include the enterochromaffin-like cells found in the gastric mucosa where its release increases production of gastric acid secretions.[1]

Histamine Receptors

Histamine receptors are found in numerous tissues of the body as listed in Table 13-1. Currently, four subtypes of histamine receptors have been identified and are termed H_1, H_2, H_3, or H_4. Most histamine clinical expressions

Table 13-1 Histamine's Effects on Various Organ Systems

System	Histamine Effect	Physical Manifestation	Receptor
Cardiovascular			
Cardiac	Increased heart rate Increased contractility	Not usually clinically evident	H_2
Vascular	Dilation of arterioles and capillaries Constriction of veins and vascular endothelial cells Increased permeability of endothelial cells	Erythema Edema	H_1, H_2
Nervous			
CNS	Neurotransmission	Circadian rhythms Wakefulness	H_1, H_2, H_3
Afferent	Sensitization of nerve endings due to depolarization	Pruritus Pain	H_1, H_3
Gastrointestinal	Potentiates gastrin-induced acid secretion	Increased gastric acid	H_2, H_3, H_4
Skin	Combined vascular and afferent nerve effects	Urticaria	H_1
Respiratory			
Lungs*	Bronchoconstriction Prostanoid secretions	Wheezing Inflammation	H_1, H_2, H_3
Nose	Triggers goblet cells to decrease mucus viscosity Afferent nerve effects Vascular effects	Rhinorrhea Rhinitis Congestion secondary to edema	H_1, H_2, H_3

* Individuals with asthma may have increased sensitivity to histamines.
Sources: Adapted from Sahasrabudhe A et al 2005[1]; Bielory L et al 2005[4]; Holgate ST et al 2005[55]; Taylor-Clark T et al 2005.[56]

to be involved in circadian rhythms, alertness, allergic reactions, and possibly carcinomas.[3-9] H_4 receptors have been located in immune cells, hematopoietic cells, and breast tissue and play a role in inflammation and allergic reactions.[3,6-8,10-16]

Histamine receptors are G protein coupled receptors (Figure 13-2; Chapter 2). Antihistamines traditionally are called histamine receptor antagonists or competitive antagonists. However, newer research classifies them as inverse agonists. Histamines are agonists that increase activity, and antihistamines are inverse agonists that promote inactivity or decrease activity.[10-12,14-17] Agonists will steady the active state of a receptor while inverse agonists calm the inactive state and decrease signaling from the receptor.

Traditionally, new drugs are created based on their ability to stimulate or inhibit a receptor. However, as knowledge about G protein signaling activities has emerged, new options for drugs also have presented themselves. For example, agents that target the signaling pathways or change the G protein itself rather than the receptor may provide new agents in the future. Active research is being conducted based on this expanding knowledge about histamines in order to develop new antihistamines.[18] It has been suggested that the term H_1 (or H_2) antihistamines (versus H_1 or H_2 blockers or antagonists) be used to reflect this new understanding of histamine receptors and antihistamines. This will be the terminology used in this chapter.

As more is revealed about the role of H_3 and H_4 receptors, new drugs targeting these receptors are expected to emerge. For example, studies are beginning to demonstrate that H_3 and H_4 receptors have several functions. Some of these functions include expressions that control cell proliferation, inflammation, and regulation of neurotransmitters. These findings may result in the future development of novel oncologic, neurologic, and anti-inflammatory agents.[6,19,20]

are theorized to be the result of agonist stimulation of the H_1 and H_2 receptors. H_1 receptors found in vascular, smooth muscle, and nervous tissue are primarily involved in inflammation, immediate hypersensitivity, and allergic reactions. H_1 receptors in the brain are concentrated in the cerebellum and forebrain where histaminergic neurons are thought to play a role in excitation of the neuronal circuit and arousal when stimulated.[2] Agonist stimulation of H_2 receptors, located primarily in the gastric mucosa, induces secretion of gastric acid.

Research currently is being conducted to assess location and function of H_3 and H_4 receptors. H_3 receptors appear to be found primarily in the brain and have also been located in eye, heart, and breast tissue. These receptors appear

▎ Antihistamines

Antihistamines as a class of drugs have a pharmacologic profile that allows use in a variety of clinical applications based on their histamine receptor subtype. Drugs targeting H_1 receptors generally are used to treat allergies and allergic reactions, nausea and vomiting, and motion sickness. First-generation H_1 antihistamines are subdivided into five categories based on their chemical structures: alkylamines, ethanolamines, ethylenediamines, phenothiazines, and piperazines (Table 13-2). Although these chemical classes are well delineated, there is no distinct pharmacologic quality that separates

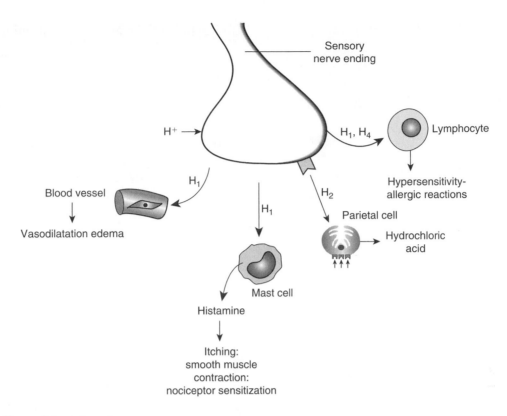

Figure 13-1 The effects of histamine release.

one from the other. Some agents, however, are used for specific therapeutic reasons; for example, piperazines such as hydroxyzine (Vistaril) are used mainly for treatment of allergic reactions and for synergistic use with opiates, while the activity of meclizine (Antivert) is limited to prevention of motion sickness and nausea and vomiting. On a clinical basis, these subgroups are rarely discussed; rather, the first-generation antihistamines are chosen based on their side effect profile and distinct indication.

Drugs that inhibit stimulation of H₂ receptors are used to treat a variety of gastrointestinal disorders, such as peptic ulcer disease, erosive esophagitis, and gastroesophageal reflux disease. They are also used to treat hypersecretory conditions such as Zollinger-Ellison syndrome, wherein increased levels of the hormone gastrin are produced.

▍H₁ Antihistamines

Clinically, H₁ antihistamines are classified into two generations (or categories). The older first-generation agents have a short duration of activity (of approximately 4–6 hours) and cause a plethora of central nervous system effects, while the second-generation H₁ antihistamines have a longer duration (up to approximately 24 hours) and have

minimal side effects. However, the second-generation drugs have more drug–drug interactions (Table 13-3). All H₁ antihistamines, regardless of type, are metabolized in the liver.[21] These drugs are usually well absorbed after oral administration. The first-generation of H₁ antihistamine medications are classified together based primarily on their side effect profiles. These drugs are used primarily for allergic reactions, sedation, motion sickness, and on occasion, treatment of nausea and vomiting, and they are highly lipophilic. They cross the blood–brain barrier where they act upon the central nervous system resulting in sedation, their best known side effect. In some cases, H₁ antihistamines are used to enhance sedation. However, tolerance to this effect appears to develop quickly, generally within 3–4 days.[22,23] Risk of tolerance explains why over-the-counter antihistamines such as diphenhydramine hydrochloride (Benadryl and Unisom SleepGels) and doxylamine succinate (Unisom SleepTabs) that are used as sleep aids are recommended for short-term, intermittent use only. Many of these medications also have **anticholinergic** side effects, which can aid in the treatment of allergy-related rhinorrhea or the prevention of nausea, but can also occasionally cause urinary retention and blurred vision. H₁ antihistamines are frequently formulated in over-the-counter combination products (Box 13-1).

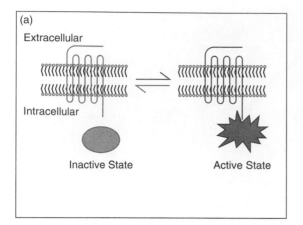

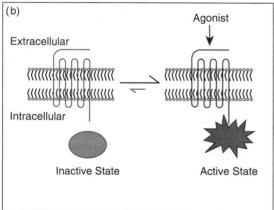

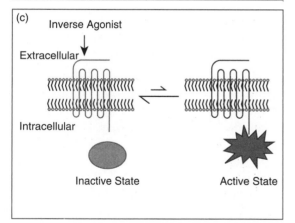

(a) Constitutive activity: Without agonist binding, this receptor initiates some agonist response.

(b) Effect of agonist: When the agonist binds to the receptor, it stimulates a classic agonist response that is stronger or more frequent than that which occurs as constitutive activity.

(c) Effect of inverse agonist: When the inverse agonist binds to the receptor, it stimulates an agonist response that is weaker or less frequent than that which occurs as constitutive activity; thus, although the inverse agonist causes an agonist response, the clinical effect is as though it is an antagonist.

Figure 13-2 Stimulation of histamine receptors.
Source: Adapted with permission from Leurs et al 2002.[17]

Clinical Indications for H₁ Antihistamines

The H₁ antihistamines have also been utilized in the treatment of tremor secondary to Parkinson's disease, although they are not considered current first-line therapy for this indication.[24,25] When used as an adjunct in the treatment of Parkinson's, antihistamines can help control some of the extrapyramidal effects of antipsychotics. Diphenhydramine (Benadryl) in particular is given intravenously for the treatment of acute dystonic reactions.[26]

Box 13-1 Beware of Brand Names

Much has been written about the confusion that sound-alike brand names can cause. However, little has been written about the variations of drugs under the *same* brand name. For example, most consumers and providers assume that the same brand name in different packaging indicates the same agent with different formulations or perhaps just marketed by different companies. Unfortunately, this assumption is proving to be increasingly false.

On occasion, a brand name is so well recognized that the manufacturer chooses to use it in an overall market strategy. For example, Tylenol is a major drug brand selling in excess of $100 million annually. The average person may think that Tylenol is synonymous with the generic drug acetaminophen, and that agent is found in its remedy for allergy symptoms, Tylenol Allergy Multi-Symptom, although in this case, acetaminophen is accompanied with the antihistamine chlorpheniramine maleate. However, Tylenol Simply Sleep, another of the company's products, has no acetaminophen and is composed solely of diphenhydramine hydrochloride, an antihistamine used as a sleep aid.

Another well recognized brand name used for sleep is Unisom. Currently, when a Unisom product is used, the active ingredient will be an antihistamine—but not necessarily the same one. Tablets (Unisom SleepTabs) are doxylamine succinate, whereas liquid/gelatin preparations (Unisom SleepGels) have diphenhydramine hydrochloride in them.

In spite of changes involved with branding, there is one constant. Reading labels continues to be a wise recommendation for all.

Contraindications to Use of H$_1$ Antihistamines

Contraindications to the H$_1$ antihistamines include any condition in which anticholinergic effects are not desired (e.g., angle-closure glaucoma, hyperthyroidism, prostatic hypertrophy, bladder neck obstructions), or those conditions where drowsiness poses a problem (e.g., driving, operating machinery, consumption of alcohol). Because antihistamines are secreted via urine, individuals with renal impairment may need reductions in the antihistamine

Table 13-2 Uses and Side Effects of Antihistamines

Antihistamine Generic (Brand)	Uses	Side Effects			
		CNS Sedation	GI	Anticholinergic	CV
H$_1$—First Generation					
Alkylamines					
Brompheniramine (Dimetane)	Allergies, pruritus, conjunctivitis	Low		Moderate	High
Ethylenediamines					
Antazoline (Clear-Eyes)	Allergic conjunctivitis	Moderate	Moderate	Low	Low
Tripelennamine (Pyribenzamine)	Allergies	Moderate	Low	Low	Low
Chlorpheniramine (Chlor-Trimeton)	Allergies, rhinitis, conjunctivitis, pruritus, urticaria	Moderate		High	Moderate
Ethanolamines					
Clemastine (Tavist)	Allergies, rhinitis, pruritus, angioedema	High	Low	High	
Dimenhydrinate (Dramamine)	Antiemetic	High		High	High
Diphenhydramine (Benadryl, Unisom SleepGels)	Insomnia, upper respiratory allergies	High	Low	High	Low*
Doxylamine (Somnil, Unisom SleepTabs)	Insomnia, nausea	High			
Piperazines					
Hydroxyzine (Atarax)	Allergies, pruritus, nausea and vomiting, insomnia	Moderate		Low	Low*
Meclizine (Antivert, Bonine)	Antiemetic	Low			
Phenothiazines					
Prochlorperazine (Compazine)	Psychotic disorders, nausea	Low		Moderate	Low
Chlorpromazine (Thorazine)	Psychotic disorders, nausea, hiccups	Moderate		Moderate	Moderate
Promethazine (Phenergan)	Allergies, nausea and vomiting	High		High	
H$_1$—Second Generation					
Cetirizine (Zyrtec)	Allergies	Low*	Low	Low	Low
Desloratadine (Clarinex)	Allergies	Low	Low	Low	Low
Fexofenadine (Allegra)	Allergies	Low*		Low	Low
Loratadine (Claritin, Alavert)	Allergies	Low*	Low	Low	Low*
H2					
Cimetidine (Tagamet)	PUD, GERD, HS		Low		
Famotidine (Pepcid)	PUD, GERD, HS, E		Low		
Nizatidine (Axid)	PUD, GERD, HS, E		Low		
Ranitidine (Zantac)	PUD, GERD, HS		Low		

CNS = central nervous system; GI = gastrointestinal system; AC = anticholinergic; CV = cardiovascular; PUD = peptic ulcer disease; GERD = gastroesophageal reflux disease; HS = hypersecretion, E = esophagitis.
* May be seen in higher doses.
Sources: Sahasrabudhe A et al. 2005[1]; Ergun T et al. 2005[2]; Leurs R et al. 2002[17]; Golightly LK et al. 2005[32]; Siepler JK et al. 2005[41]; Nagel D et al. 2005[42]; Brock TP et al. 2005.[57]

dose. **Paradoxical reactions** have occasionally been noted in this class of medications and appear with a higher occurrence in children. Paradoxical reactions can include dermal reactions and hyperactivity.[27-29]

Drug–Drug Interactions with H$_1$ Antihistamines

The primary drug–drug interactions of importance are the additive sedative effect the H$_1$ antihistamines have when taken with other medications that cause sedation such as sedatives, narcotics, antipsychotics, anxiolytics, alcohol, barbiturates, and hypnotics (Table 13-3). These sedating antihistamines also have an additive antimuscarinic action with drugs such as atropine and tricyclic antidepressants.

▌Second-Generation H$_1$ Antihistamines

Second-generation H$_1$ antihistamines are more highly selective to peripheral H$_1$ receptors than those in the central nervous system.[30] They are used in the treatment of allergic and inflammatory reactions. Generally, they are less sedating and have fewer anticholinergic side effects than the traditional H$_1$ antihistamines. However, since allergic reactions can themselves be sedating, it can be difficult to differentiate an antihistamine sedation side effect from sedation caused by the allergic condition alone.[22,23,30-32] Studies on sedative effects of antihistamines all have been conducted with healthy volunteers who are not experiencing the fatigue of an allergic response.

The longer half-life of second-generation H$_1$ antihistamines allows once-a-day dosing. This along with their favorable side effects profile often makes second-generation antihistamines preferable. Two drugs in this class, astemizole (Hismanal) and terfenadine (Seldane-D), were removed from the market secondary to the occurrence of arrhythmias, which were the result of drug–drug interactions with such agents as erythromycin and ketoconazole[33,34,26,35] (Box 13-2). Some second-generation antihistamines—azelastine (Optivar), emedastine (Emadine), epinastine hydrochloride (Elestat), and olopatadine (Patanol)—are used primarily in ophthalmic or topical solutions.[4,36]

Contraindications to Use of Second-Generation H$_1$ Antihistamines

The contraindications to use of second-generation H$_1$ antihistamines are essentially the same as the contraindica-

---

▌Box 13-2 The Terfenadine (Seldane-D) Story

Terfenadine (Seldane-D) is an antihistamine introduced for the treatment of allergies. Terfenadine is a prodrug, which is metabolized to the active drug fexofenadine by intestinal CYP3A4. However, when taken in high doses, terfenadine can cause prolonged QT interval and cardiac arrhythmias. This toxicity became apparent about 10 years after terfenadine was first introduced in clinical practice. Why did it take so long for the adverse effects of this drug to become apparent?

Most cases of terfenadine toxicity occurred in persons with preexisting cardiac disease and/or in persons who took an overdose of the drug. The active agent fexofenadine is not toxic, but when too much was taken, less was metabolized, and the toxic effects became evident. In addition, two oral antifungal agents, ketoconazole (Nizoral) and itraconazole (Sporanox), were first introduced in the 1980s. Both of these drugs block the metabolism of terfenadine.

The first report of cardiotoxicity secondary to use of terfenadine was published in 1989. In early 1997, the FDA recommended that terfenadine-containing drugs be replaced by fexofenadine. Seldane-D was removed from the US market in late 1997 after the manufacturer of Seldane-D received approval for fexofenadine (Allegra).

---

tions to use of first-generation H$_1$ antihistamines especially in conditions where anticholinergic effects would be adverse. Although the sedation effect of second-generation H$_1$ antihistamines is much less than the sedation experienced by persons who take first-generation H$_1$ antihistamines, persons who drive a car or who work with heavy machinery should take the first few doses when not operating vehicles or equipment.

Drug–Drug Interactions with Second-Generation H$_1$ Antihistamines

Few drug–drug interactions have been reported involving second-generation H$_1$ antihistamines (Table 13-3). Drug–drug interactions can theoretically occur among compounds that interact and/or affect cytochrome P450 (CYP) activity. Loratadine (Claritin) and fexofenadine

Table 13-3 Common Doses and Drug–Drug Interactions Associated with Antihistamines

Antihistamine Generic (Brand)	Usual Adult Dose	Known Drug–Drug Interactions and Adverse Effects
H₁—First Generation		
Alkylamines		
Brompheniramine (Dimetane)	4 mg PO q 4–6 h or 8–12 mg of sustained-release form bid to tid; max dose 12 mg/24 h	MAO inhibitors can prolong and intensify the effects of the antihistamines.
Chlorpheniramine (Chlor-Trimeton)	4 mg PO q 4–6 h; max dose 24 mg/day Extended-release forms: 8–12 mg bid or tid; max dose 24 mg/day	MAO inhibitors, tricyclic antidepressants, phenothiazines, and benztropine can cause additive anticholinergic effects. CNS depressants can cause additive CNS depressant effects.
Ethanolamines		
Clemastine (Tavist)	1–2 PO mg bid	MAO inhibitors, clozapine, tricyclic antidepressants, phenothiazines, and other H₁ antagonists can cause additive anticholinergic effects. Alcohol, antipsychotics, barbiturates, chloral hydrate, opiate agonists, and hypnotics can cause enhanced CNS depressant effects.
Dimenhydrinate (Dramamine)	50–100 mg PO, IV, IM q 4–6 hr Max PO dose = 400 mg/24 hr Max IM dose = 300 mg/24 hr	MAO inhibitors, clozapine, tricyclic antidepressants, phenothiazines, and other H₁ antagonists can cause additive anticholinergic effects. Alcohol, antipsychotics, barbiturates, chloral hydrate, opiate agonists, and hypnotics can cause enhanced CNS depressant effect.
Diphenhydramine (Benadryl, Unisom SleepGels)	25–50 mg PO, IM, IV q 4–6 h; max dose 300 mg/day	MAO inhibitors, tricyclic antidepressants, phenothiazines, and benztropine can cause additive anticholinergic effects. Alcohol, antipsychotics, barbiturates, chloral hydrate, opiate agonists, and hypnotics can cause enhanced CNS depressant effects.
Doxylamine (Somnil, Donormyl, Dozile, Restavit, Unisom SleepTabs)	12.5 mg PO bid (can be used in combination with pyridoxine for treating nausea)	MAO inhibitors, clozapine, tricyclic antidepressants, phenothiazines, and other H₁ antagonists can cause additive anticholinergic effects. Increased sedation if used in combination with other CNS depressant drugs. May enhance effects of epinephrine. May partially counteract the effects of heparin or warfarin.
Piperazines		
Hydroxyzine (Atarax)	25 mg tid to qid for allergies 25–100 mg tid for nausea and vomiting 50–100 mg PO before bedtime for insomnia	MAO inhibitors, tricyclic antidepressants, phenothiazines, and benztropine can cause additive anticholinergic effects. Alcohol, antipsychotics, barbiturates, chloral hydrate, opiate agonists, and hypnotics can cause enhanced CNS depressant effects.
Meclizine (Antivert, Bonine)	25–50 mg PO one h before travel, 25–50 mg PO qd	MAO inhibitors, tricyclic antidepressants, phenothiazines, and benztropine can cause additive anticholinergic effects. Alcohol, antipsychotics, barbiturates, chloral hydrate, opiate agonists, and hypnotics can cause enhanced CNS depressant effects.
Phenothiazines		
Chlorpromazine (Thorazine)	10–50 mg PO bid–qid, 25–50 mg IM which can be repeated in one h. Maximum is 2000 mg/day	Chlorpromazine is an alpha-adrenergic antagonist, so increased pulse and hypotension can occur. Use cautiously if individual has heart disease, a history of alcohol abuse, or is elderly. Can lower seizure threshold, so do not use if taking anticonvulsants. Antihistamines may lead to prolonged QT interval. Can exacerbate psychotic symptoms in persons on amphetamines, SSRIs, St. John's wort, or barbiturates.
Prochlorperazine (Compazine)	5–10 mg PO, IM, IV tid–qid, Maximum dose 40 mg/day. Sustained-release formulations available 25 mg PR q 12 h for nausea	Can cause sedation, extrapyramidal symptoms, anticholinergic effects. May be potentiated if given concomitantly with metoclopramide. MAO inhibitors, tricyclic antidepressants, phenothiazines, and benztropine can cause additive anticholinergic effects. Antacids that contain aluminum or magnesium, warfarin, or antiseizure drugs potentiate sedation of opioids and sedatives. Can reverse vasopressor effect of epinephrine.

(continues)

Table 13-3 Common Doses and Drug–Drug Interactions Associated with Antihistamines (*continued*)

Antihistamine Generic (Brand)	Usual Adult Dose	Known Drug–Drug Interactions and Adverse Effects
Promethazine (Phenergan)	12.5–25 mg PO, PR, IM, IV q 4–6 h	FDA black box warning that intra-arterial and subcutaneous administration can cause gangrene and other serious tissue injury. Sedation, extrapyramidal symptoms, and anticholinergic effects are known side effects. May be potentiated if given concomitantly with metoclopramide. MAO inhibitors, tricyclic antidepressants, phenothiazines, and benztropine can cause additive anticholinergic effects. Can reverse vasopressor effect of epinephrine.
H₁—Second Generation		
Cetirizine (Zyrtec)	5–10 mg PO qd	Alcohol,* barbiturates, tricyclic antidepressants, and opiate agonists can increase CNS depressant effects.
Desloratadine (Clarinex)		
Fexofenadine (Allegra)	60 mg PO qd	Most fruit juices, erythromycin, ketoconazole, rifampin, antacids, verapamil.
Loratadine (Claritin, Alavert)	10 mg PO qd	Macrolide antibiotics, ketoconazole, cimetidine, amiodarone, nefazodone interfere with metabolism of loratadine, resulting in increased concentrations of loratadine. Alcohol, antipsychotics, barbiturates, chloral hydrate, opiate agonists, and hypnotics can cause enhanced CNS depressant effects.
H₂		
Cimetidine (Tagamet)	800 mg PO qhs or 300 mg PO qid with meals and qhs, or 400 mg PO bid for Rx of ulcer. 400 mg PO qhs for prevention of ulcer 200 mg PO prn with max of 400 mg/day × 14 days for OTC Rx of heartburn	Decreases absorption of ketoconazole, itraconazole. Increased levels of alcohol, amiodarone, benzodiazepines, calcium channel blockers, carbamazepine, cyclosporine, diazepam, labetalol, lidocaine, loratadine, phenytoin, procainamide, propranolol, quinidine, theophylline, tricyclic antidepressants, valproic acid, verapamil, and warfarin.
Famotidine (Pepcid)	40 mg PO qhs or 20 mg PO bid for Rx of ulcer 20 mg PO qhs for maintenance 20 mg PO bid for Rx of GERD 10–20 mg PO prn for OTC Rx of heartburn	Alcohol. Decreases absorption of ketoconazole, itraconazole.
Nizatidine (Axid)	300 mg PO qhs or 150 mg PO bid for Rx of ulcer 150 mg bid for Rx of GERD 75 mg PO prn for OTC Rx of heartburn with max of 150 mg/day	Alcohol. Decreases absorption of ketoconazole, itraconazole.
Ranitidine (Zantac)	150 mg PO bid or 300 mg qhs for Rx of ulcer 150 mg PO bid for Rx of gastric ulcer or GERD 75–150 mg PO prn for OTC Rx of heartburn with max of 300 mg/day	Alcohol, warfarin. Decreases absorption of ketoconazole, itraconazole.

* Increased sedation seen primarily in women.

(Allegra) are metabolized via the liver and the CYP450 system. Other drugs that can affect CYP activity include antifungals, macrolides, and grapefruit juice; so, it is prudent to exercise caution when combining loratadine and fexofenadine with other drugs that are metabolized by one of the CYP450 enzymes.[30] Drug interactions can also be additive. For example, cetirizine hydrochloride (Zyrtec) was found in one study to cause additional sedation when taken with alcohol.[32] Additional studies did not initially replicate the finding, but upon reexamination of the first study, these effects were found to be more common among women even when controlling for weight and body mass.[32,37]

Topical antihistamines are used for the treatment of allergic rhinitis and allergic conjunctivitis, atopic dermatitis, and chronic urticaria. The onset of action is rapid with duration similar to oral administration.[32,38,39] Antihistamines have a role in the control of inflammatory responses such as the flare and wheal in skin reactions. Additionally, they are used as adjunctive therapy when attempting to control pruritus of the eyes and skin. Diphenhydramine (Benadryl) and promethazine (Phenergan) occasionally are used as local anesthetics for individuals allergic to the standard agents. These agents work in the same way as procaine and lidocaine by blocking sodium channels.[26]

H$_2$ Antihistamines

H$_2$ antihistamines are used to treat gastric disorders where hyperacidity is a factor. These drugs competitively and reversibly inhibit the action of histamine at H$_2$ receptors, without the troublesome side effects encountered when using anticholinergic drugs for similar gastrointestinal problems.[26] Several are available over the counter (Box 13-3).

H$_2$ receptors are also present in other organ tissues throughout the body; however, the therapeutic dose needed for decreasing gastric acid usually has little effect on other systems. Of the four currently available agents, cimetidine (Tagamet) is administered most frequently (up to four times daily) while the other three agents ranitidine (Zantac), famotidine (Pepcid), and nizatidine (Axid) are dosed once or twice daily. All of the H$_2$ antihistamines have a half-life that is extended in situations involving renal impairment (that may result in increased effects or toxicity due to lack of elimination) so it is wise to monitor renal function if long-term use is indicated.[40]

Contraindications

As these drugs are rather benign from a contraindication standpoint, they are generally considered safe to use except in those cases where a hypersensitivity to an individual drug has been identified.

Side Effects

Side effects with H$_2$ drugs primarily are gastrointestinal with an occasional mild central nervous system or dermatologic reaction. Table 13-4 provides a summary of the side effects seen with the different classes of antihistamines.

Box 13-3 A Case of Heartburn

LN is a 40-year-old female reporting a 3-month history of heartburn. She says it started after she was diagnosed with tension headaches, for which she takes nonsteroidal anti-inflammatory agents (NSAIDs), such as naproxen. Upon further questioning, it becomes evident that she has been taking the NSAID without food. There is a strong suspicion that she has developed a gastric complication secondary to the NSAID use, such as peptic ulcer disease.

Treatment

The first line of treatment is to switch the pain reliever to acetaminophen, which does not cause gastric ulceration. Secondly, consider starting an H$_2$ antagonist, such as ranitidine at a dose of either 150 mg administered orally twice daily, or 300 mg administered orally once a day for up to 8 weeks (in conjunction with treatment of *Helicobacter pylori* as appropriate). LN may need longer maintenance treatment of 150–300 mg taken orally each day at bedtime. Other H$_2$ antihistamines may be used; however, famotidine should not be a consideration for LN because approximately 4–5% of individuals taking that agent have headaches associated with the drug itself.

Those at higher risk for side effects include the elderly, persons taking high doses, and persons with impaired renal function.

Drug–Drug Interactions

Cimetidine also affects CYP450-mediated drug metabolism, resulting in decreased clearance of coadministered medications, especially those using the same pathway. This is most significant with medications that have a limited therapeutic range. Ranitidine is also cause for this concern but to a lesser extent (Table 13-3). All of the H$_2$ antihistamines theoretically can be involved in drug–drug interactions as a result of altered gastric pH.[1,41,42] Additional information about the H$_2$ drugs can be found in Chapter 21.

Cimetidine (Tagamet) can cause gynecomastia in men, and although this is a well-known side effect, the

Table 13-4 Examples of Side Effects Seen Within Antihistamine Classes

Side Effect	H$_1$ Antihistamines (First Generation)	H$_1$ Antihistamines (Second Generation)	H$_2$ Antihistamines
Neurologic	Drowsiness, dizziness, sedation, somnolence	Same as first generation, but with less frequency	Headache, dizziness, insomnia
Gastrointestinal	Anorexia, constipation, epigastric distress	Abdominal pain, diarrhea, vomiting (especially in children)	Diarrhea
Anticholinergic	Urinary retention, blurred vision, constipation, dry mouth, dry mucous membranes	Rare	N/A
Cardiovascular	Changes in heart rate, changes in blood pressure	Rare	Rare changes in heart rate or rhythm

Sources: From Sahasrabudhe A et al 2005[1]; Ergun T et al 2005[2]; Leurs R et al 2002[17]; Golightly LK et al 2005[32]; Siepler JK et al 2005[41]; Nagel D et al 2005[42]; Brock TP et al 2005.[57]

mechanism of action is not clear. However, cimetidine has also been implicated in causing a beneficial effect of increasing HDL and lowering LDL in both men and women. The clinical significance of this effect remains unclear.

Special Populations

Pregnancy

Antihistamines are widely used drugs both for the treatment of nausea and vomiting and for allergies. These drugs, particularly doxylamine succinate (Unisom) and most first-generation H$_1$ antihistamines, are effective for nausea and vomiting in pregnancy (See Chapter 35).[43,44] Data from studies back to the 1960s have failed to show significant fetal malformations associated with the use of any H$_1$ antihistamines for nausea and vomiting and for allergies during pregnancy.[43-47]

There is limited data on the use of H$_2$ antihistamines in pregnancy. However, two studies have confirmed the generally held belief that there are no known teratogenic associations.[48,49] All of the H$_2$ antihistamines are in FDA category B for use in pregnancy. As with any medication

use in pregnancy, it is important to consider the risk and benefits of use or nonuse with the known and potential risks.

Lactation

The use of first-generation H$_1$ antihistamines during lactation is not considered safe, because they are secreted in breast milk and can cause neonatal sedation.[2] If an antihistamine is necessary, cetirizine (Zyrtec) and loratadine (Claritin) are preferable, as they have been found in low levels in breast milk.[2] In regard to H$_2$ antihistamine use during lactation, cimetidine (Tagamet) is considered by the American Academy of Pediatrics to be most compatible with breastfeeding.[50] Growth depression has been seen in rats following administration of both famotidine (Pepcid) and nizatidine (Axid). Ranitidine (Zantac) has been shown to be excreted in breast milk, more so than with nizatidine and famotidine; it would appear that nizatidine and famotidine may be the preferred H$_2$ antihistamines for lactating women.[51,52] In addition, there is some suggestion that the sedating antihistamines may decrease milk supply due to their anticholinergic effects.[53]

Elderly

Few studies specifically have investigated the effects/use of antihistamines among the elderly. One research study noted that histamine has a role in bone metabolism. The study in question focused on postmenopausal women with pollen allergies who received no antihistamine or steroid treatment. The rate of fracture was three times greater in the untreated allergic women as compared to nonallergic postmenopausal women (34.9% versus 13.0%, respectively, $P = .003$).[54] The investigators also found a decreased incidence of fracture among postmenopausal pollen-allergic women who used antihistamines. The researchers speculated that antihistamines block histamine-induced **osteoclastogenesis**.

Conclusion

Antihistamines are a large class of drugs with several subdivisions. H$_1$ antihistamines generally are employed for the treatment of allergic reactions. These agents also are used for sedation and as antiemetics. There are two generations of H$_1$ antihistamines. The second generation generally is more specific with fewer side effects but more drug interactions. H$_2$ antihistamines are used specifically for gastrointestinal disorders related to increased gastric acid. All of the antihistamines are generally safe with caution advised with use in polypharmacy or specific conditions.

References

1. Sahasrabudhe A, Rando RR. Histamine pharmacology. In Golan D, ed. Principles of pharmacology: the pathophysiologic basis of drug therapy. Philadelphia, PA: Lippincott Williams & Wilkins, 2005:647–54.

2. Ergun T, Kus S. Adverse systemic reactions of antihistamines: highlights in sedating effects, cardiotoxicity and drug interactions. Curr Med Chem-Anti-inflammatory Anti-Allergy Agents 2005;4(5):507–15.

3. Bakker RA. Histamine H3-receptor isoforms. Inflamm Res 2004;53(10):509–16.

4. Bielory L, Ghafoor S. Histamine receptors and the conjunctiva. Curr Opin Allergy Clin Immunol 2005;5(5):437–40.

5. Levi R, Seyedi N, Schaefer U, Estephan R, Mackins CJ, Tyler E, Silver RB. Histamine H3-receptor signaling in cardiac sympathetic nerves: identification of a novel MAPK-PLA2-COX-PGE2-EP3R pathway. Biochem Pharmacol 2007;73(8):1146–56.

6. Medina V, Cricco G, Nunez M, Martin G, Mohamad N, Correa-Fiz F. Histamine-mediated signaling processes in human malignant mammary cells. Cancer Biol Ther 2006;5(11):1462–71.

7. Muller T, Myrtek D, Bayer H, Sorichter S, Schneidere K, Zissel G. Functional characterization of histamine receptor subtypes in a human bronchial epithelial cell line. Int J Mol Med 2006;18(5):925–31.

8. Sugata Y, Okano M, Fujiwara T, Matsumoto R, Hattori H, Yamoto M, et al. Histamine H4 receptor agonists have more activities than H4 agonism in antigen-specific human T-cell responses. Immunology 2007;121(2):266–75.

9. Parmentier R, Anaclet C, Guhennec C, Rousseau E, Bircout D, Giboulot T, et al. The brain H3-receptor as a novel therapeutic target for vigilance and sleep–wake disorders. Biochem Pharmacol 2007;73(8):1157–71.

10. de Esch IJ, Thurmond RL, Jongejan A, Leurs R. The histamine H4 receptor as a new therapeutic target for inflammation. Trends Pharmacol Sci 2005;26(9):462–9.

11. Dunford PJ, O'Donnell N, Riley JP, Williams KN, Karlsson L, Thurmond RL. The histamine H4 receptor mediates allergic airway inflammation by regulating the activation of CD4+ T cells. J Immunol 2006;176(11):7062–70.

12. Dunford PJ, Williams KN, Desai PJ, Karlsson L, McQueen D, Thurmond RL. Histamine H4 receptor antagonists are superior to traditional antihistamines in the attenuation of experimental pruritus. J Allergy Clin Immunol 2007;119(1):176–83.

13. Fogel WA, Lewinski A, Jochem J. Histamine in idiopathic inflammatory bowel diseases—not a standby player. Folia Med Cracov 2005;46 (3–4):107–18.

14. Fung-Leung WP, Thurmond RL, Ling P, Karlsson L. Histamine H4 receptor antagonists: the new antihistamines? Curr Opin Investig Drugs 2004;5(11):1174–83.

15. Lim HD, Smits RA, Leurs R, De Esch IJ. The emerging role of the histamine H4 receptor in anti-inflammatory therapy. Curr Top Med Chem 2006;6(13):1365–73.

16. Zhang M, Venable JD, Thurmond RL. The histamine H4 receptor in autoimmune disease. Expert Opin Investig Drugs 2006;15(11):1443–52.

17. Leurs R, Church MK, Taglialatela M. H1-antihistamines: inverse agonism, anti-inflammatory actions and cardiac effects. Clin Exp Allergy 2002;32(4):489–98.

18. Chasse SA, Dohlman HG. RGS proteins: G protein-coupled receptors meet their match. Assay Drug Dev Technol 2003;1(2):357–64.

19. Espenshare TA, Fox GB, Krueger KM, Baranowski JL, Miller TR, Kang CH, et al. Pharmacological and behavioral properties of A-349821, a selective and potent human histamine H3 receptor antagonist. Biochem Pharmacol 2004;68(5):933–45.

20. Thurmond RL, Desai PJ, Dunford PJ, Fung-Leung WP, Hofstra CL, Jiang W, et al. A potent and selective histamine H4 receptor antagonist with anti-inflammatory properties. J Pharmacol Exp Ther 2004;309(1):404–13.

21. Martens J. Histamine and antihistamines. In Minneman K, Wecker L, eds. Brody's human pharmacology: molecular to clinical, 4th ed. Philadelphia, PA: Elsevier-Mosby, 2005;701–10.

22. Richardson GS, Roehrs TA, Rosenthal L, Koshorek G, Roth T. Tolerance to daytime sedative effects of H1 antihistamines. J Clin Psychopharmacol 2002;22(5):511–5.

23. Verster JC, Volkerts ER. Antihistamines and driving ability: evidence from on-the-road driving studies during normal traffic. Ann Allergy Asthma Immunol 2004;92(3):294–303; quiz 303–5, 355.

24. Riley T, Massey E. Managing the patient with Parkinson's disease. Postgrad Med 1980;68(3):85–92.

25. Brocks D. Anticholinergic drugs used in Parkinson's disease: an overlooked class of drugs from a pharmacokinetic perspective. J Pharm Pharmaceut Sci 1999;2(2):39–46.

26. Katzung BG. Histamine, serotonin, & the ergot alkaloids. In Katzung B, ed. Basic and clinical pharmacology, 10th ed. New York: McGraw Hill, 2007;255–76.

27. Schroter S, Damveld B, Marsch WC. Urticarial intolerance reaction to cetirizine. Clin Exp Dermatol 2002;27(3):185–7.

28. Demoly P, Messaad D, Benahmed S, Sahla H, Bousquest J. Hypersensitivity to H1-antihistamines. Allergy 2000;55(7):681.

29. Chae KM, Tharp MD. Use and safety of antihistamines in children. Dermatol Ther 2000;13(4):374–83.

30. Walsh GM, Annunziato L, Frossard N, Knol K, Levander S, Nicolas JM, et al. New insights into the second generation antihistamines. Drugs 2001; 61(2):207–36.

31. Schweitzer PK, Muehlbach MJ, Walsh JK. Sleepiness and performance during three-day administration of cetirizine or diphenhydramine. J Allergy Clin Immunol 1994;94(4):716–24.

32. Golightly LK, Greos LS. Second-generation antihistamines: actions and efficacy in the management of allergic disorders. Drugs 2005;65(3):341–84.

33. Paakkari I. Cardiotoxicity of new antihistamines and cisapride. Toxicol Lett 2002;127(1–3):279–84.

34. Salmun LM. Antihistamines in late-phase clinical development for allergic disease. Expert Opin Investig Drugs 2002;11(2):259–73.

35. Greaves MW. Antihistamines in dermatology. Skin Pharmacol Physiol 2005;18(5):220–9.

36. Bielory L. Role of antihistamines in ocular allergy. Am J Med 2002;113(suppl 9A):34S–7S.

37. Vermeeren A, Ramaeker JG, O'Hanlon JF. Effects of emedastine and cetirizine, alone and with alcohol, on actual driving of males and females. J Psychopharmacol 2002;16(1):57–64.

38. Korsgren M, Andersson M, Larsson L, Alden-Raboisson M, Greiff L. Onset of action of topical antihistamine as assessed by histamine challenge-induced plasma exudation responses. Ann Allergy Asthma Immunol 2006;96(2):345–8.

39. Abelson M, Gomes P, Pasquine T, Edwards MR, Gross RD, Robertson SM. Efficacy of olopatadine ophthalmic solution 0.2% in reducing signs and symptoms of allergic conjunctivitis. Allergy Asthma Proc 2007; 28(4):427–33.

40. Bonat J, Dragon C, Arcangelo V. Gastroesophageal reflux disease and peptic ulcer disease. In Arcangelo V, Peterson A, eds. Pharmacotherapeutics for advanced practice: a practical approach, 2nd ed. Philadelphia, PA: Lippincott Williams and Wilkins, 2006;372–85.

41. Siepler JK, Smith-Scott C. Upper gastrointestinal disorders. In Koda-Kimble MA, Young LY, Kardjan WA, et al., eds. Applied therapeutics: the clinical use of drugs, 8th ed. Philadelphia, PA: Lippincott Williams & Wilkins, 2005;27-1–27-25.

42. Nagel D, Shields H. Integrative inflammation pharmacology: peptic ulcer disease. In Golan D, ed. Principles of pharmacology: the pathophysiologic basis of drug therapy. Philadelphia, PA: Lippincott Williams & Wilkins, 2005;683–94.

43. Magee LA, Mazzotta P, Koren G. Evidence-based view of safety and effectiveness of pharmacologic therapy for nausea and vomiting of pregnancy. Am J Obstet Gynecol 2002;186(5):S256–61.

44. Mazzotta P, Magee LA. A risk-benefit assessment of pharmacological treatments for nausea and vomiting of pregnancy. Drugs 2000;59(4):781–800.

45. Kallen B. Use of antihistamine drugs in early pregnancy and delivery outcomes. J Matern Fetal Neonatal Med 2002;11:146–52.

46. Werler M, McCloskey C, Edmonds L, Olney R, Honein MA, Reefhuis J. Evaluation of an association between loratadine and hypospadias—United States, 1997–2001. MMWR 2004;53(10):219–21.

47. Asker C, Norstedt Wikner B, Kallen B. Use of antiemetic drugs during pregnancy in Sweden. Eur J Clin Pharmacol 2005;61(12):899–906.

48. Garbis H, Elefant E, Diav-Citrin O, Mastriacovo P, Schaefer C, Vial T, Clementi M, et al. Pregnancy outcome after exposure to ranitidine and other H2-blockers. A collaborative study of the European Network of Teratology Information Services. Reprod Toxicol 2005;19(4):453–8.

49. Mazzotta P, Koren G. Nonsedating antihistamines in pregnancy. Can Fam Physician 1997;43:1509–11.

50. Drugs Co. The transfer of drugs and other chemicals into human milk. Pediatrics 2001;108(3):776–89.

51. Roberts CJ. Clinical pharmacokinetics of ranitidine. Clinical Pharmacokinetics 1984;9(3):211–21.

52. Hagemann TM. Gastrointestinal medications and breastfeeding. J Hum Lact 1998;14(3):259–62.

53. Hale T. Medications and mother's milk, 12th ed. Amarillo, TX: Hale Publishing, 2006.

54. Ferencz V, Meszaros S, Csupor E, Toth E, Bors K, Falus A, et al. Increased bone fracture prevalence in postmenopausal women suffering from pollen-allergy. Osteoporos Int 2006;17:484–91.

55. Holgate ST, Canonica GW, Simons FE, Taglialatela M, Tharp M, Timmerman H, et al. Consensus Group on New-Generation Antihistamines (CONGA): present status and recommendations. Clin Exp Allergy 2003;33(9):1305–24.

56. Taylor-Clark T, Sodha R, Warner B, Foreman J. Histamine receptors that influence blockage of the normal human nasal airway. Br J Pharmacol 2005;144(6):867–74.

57. Brock TP, Williams DM. Acute and chronic rhinitis. In Koda-Kimble MA, Young LL, Kardjan WA, et al., eds. Applied therapeutics: the clinical use of drugs, 8th ed. Philadelphia, PA: Lippincott Williams & Wilkins, 2005;25-1–25-32.

"The overall assumption (was) that reproductive hormones had to do with reproduction, period, until it became obvious that these hormones have global effects."

J. JOHNSON, PHYSIOLOGY PROFESSOR AT THE
UNIVERSITY OF TEXAS HEALTH SCIENCE CENTER,
SAN ANTONIO[1]

14

Steroid Hormones

Mary C. Brucker and Frances E. Likis

Chapter Glossary

Androgen One of the major sex steroids and the original anabolic steroid. The most common endogenous androgen is testosterone. Although usually attributed to males because of large production from testes (from the Greek for *men and production*), it is also a major sex steroid for women. Androgens are precursors for estrogens.

Androstane derivative Sex steroid that possesses 19 carbons. This category includes androgens.

Androstenedione An androgen that is converted along with testosterone to estrone from fat and other tissues.

Antiestrogen Agent that generally falls into one of two groups: either pure antiestrogens or compounds with both agonist and antagonistic activities. An example of antiestrogenic activity is that of tamoxifen inhibiting binding to selected estrogen receptors in the breast.

Antiprogestin Agent that blocks the action of progestogens. An example is mifepristone (RU486), a 19-nortestosterone derivative with five times the affinity for the progesterone receptors.

Aromatization A chemical reaction that produces a more stable compound. During steroidogenesis, aromatization of androgens (by addition of a benzene ring) produces estrogens.

Cholesterol The basic building block in steroidogenesis and precursor for all sex steroids.

Conjugation Chemical process, such as esterification and micronization, used for estrogens to promote absorption. The most commonly prescribed estrogen today is a conjugated equine estrogen (CEE) marketed with the brand name Premarin.

Esterification Chemical process, such as conjugation and micronization, used for estrogens to promote absorption.

Estradiol The main endogenous estrogen of the reproductive years, which is also known as E_2.

Estrane derivative Sex steroid that possesses 18 carbons. This category includes estrogens.

Estriol A weak estrogen, also known as E_3, which is produced primarily by the placenta.

Estrogen One of the major sex steroids for women. The term is derived from the Greek for *mad desire*.

Estrogen ligand The compound that binds with an estrogen receptor. It may change receptor properties, which may explain differences among estrogens such as conjugated equine estrogens, estradiol, and selective estrogen receptor modulators.

Estrogen receptor Type of cell found throughout the body that binds with estrogens through the cell membrane.

Estrone The major estrogen of the postmenopausal period. It is derived from peripheral conversion from body tissues/fat as opposed to estradiol's origins in biosynthesis from the ovary. Also known as E_1.

Micronization Chemical process, such as conjugation and esterification, used for estrogens to promote absorption.

Peripheral aromatization Extraglandular (fat tissue) conversion of androstenedione and testosterone to estrone (E_1). Of particular importance during the postmenopausal period.

Phytoestrogen Nonsteroidal botanical that possesses estrogenic activities or is metabolized into compounds with estrogen activity.

Potency Ability to interact with receptors and cause clinical manifestations. Some agents are more potent than others.

Pregnane derivative Sex steroid that possesses 21 carbons. These derivatives include progestins and corticoids.

Progesterone One of the major endogenous sex steroids for women. The term is derived from the Latin for *for pregnancy*.

Progestin The umbrella term for naturally occurring agents (progesterone) and synthetic (progestogens).

Progestogen Synthetic progesterone for exogenous use.

Relative binding affinity (RBA) A method that attempts to characterize progesterone potency by addressing binding affinity with progesterone receptors. Often mentioned in terms of animal studies but rarely used in clinical practice because of lack of clear clinical significance.

Sex hormone-binding globulin (SHBG) Globulin produced in the liver. It binds steroids in inverse proportion; e.g., the lower the SHBG, the more free circulating hormone.

Steroidogenesis Process by which steroid hormones are derived. The pathways may differ among species; however, in humans, steroidogenesis is initiated from cholesterol, and through a series of steps, estrogen, progesterone, androgens, testosterone, cortisol, corticoids, and aldosterone are produced endogenously.

Testosterone Derived from the androgen group, it is the principal major male sex steroid. Although men produce 40–60 times the amount of testosterone than women, it is necessary to women's health.

Introduction

Endogenous hormones are essential players in physiologic functions within the human body. However, it was not until the 20th century that these agents were isolated and ultimately synthesized. From the modern perspective wherein sophisticated chemical analysis is done every day, it may seem amazing that it took US chemist Edward Doisy 4 tons of sows' ovaries (approximately 8000) to obtain a mere 12 milligrams of **estradiol** in the late 1920s.[2] A few months later, the German scientist Adolf Butenandt reported that he independently isolated 20 milligrams of estradiol from the urine of more than 2000 pregnant women. Butenandt also is credited with isolating **testosterone** with an experiment in which he obtained 15 milligrams of androsterone from approximately 17,000 liters of male urine.[3] Eventually, both Doisy and Butenandt received Nobel Prizes in chemistry.

Isolation of **progesterone** followed within less than a decade but was also a major project. In 1937, Russell Marker, an American chemist, was the first to isolate pregnanediol and then convert it to progesterone. Marker had been intrigued with botanicals and imported Mexican yams, purportedly illegally, into his laboratory for study. It is reported that it took him 9–10 tons of Mexican yams to ultimately produce approximately three kilos of progesterone. At the time, these few kilos were highly valuable, with an estimated worth of approximately a quarter of a million dollars. Those kilos of progesterone provided Marker with the ability to cofound a new pharmaceutical company. Named *Syntex*, a word derived from combining *synthetic* and *Mexican*, it flourished for years, even after Marker left, primarily producing oral contraceptives and cortisol until it was acquired and subsumed by Roche Group, the pharmaceutical division of the Swiss company Hoffman-La Roche AG, in 1990.[4,5]

Today, **estrogens**, **progestins**, and **androgens** are popular pharmaceuticals; they are used for a wide variety of indications, especially in the area of women's health care. Synthetic agents are common. However, the future of hormone therapies is likely to be the development of agents that are more than simple replication of endogenous hormones. New designer hormones, such as selective estrogen receptor modulators (SERMs) and selective estrogen enzyme modulators (SEEMs), attempt to maximize therapeutic effects while minimizing adverse effects and have opened a new realm of possibilities in treatments.

The classic definition of a hormone is an agent produced in one gland that travels through the bloodstream to stimulate, via chemical action, a function in another part of the body (Greek *horman*, "to urge on"). Hormones are agents that provide paracrine communication (intercellular communication via local diffusion of regulating substances that affect nearby tissue) and autocrine communication (intracellular communication whereby a single cell produces regulating substances that act upon receptors on or within the same cell).

Based on their chemical composition, hormones are subdivided into several classes: amines, peptides, prostaglandins, and steroids. All steroid hormones are derived from **cholesterol**, yet small changes in the molecules produce the three different types of steroids: (1) mineralocorticoids, such as aldosterone, that act on salt (mineral) balance; (2) glucocorticoids, like cortisol, that act on glucose metabolism; and (3) gonadocorticoids, or sex steroids.[6] The sex steroids include estrogen, progesterone, and androgen. These agents are grouped as a family because of their mutual effect on reproductive function. This chapter provides an overview of the pharmacology of the sex steroid hormones. Pharmacotherapeutics of sex steroids are discussed in depth in Section E of this book.

Physiologic Function of Sex Steroids

Steroidogenesis

Steroidogenesis is the process by which steroids are biosynthesized or produced endogenously. All steroids are formed from cholesterol, a 27-carbon steroid. Sex steroids are formed when cholesterol is broken down further into three groups. These groups are classified by their number of carbon atoms: **pregnane derivatives** with 21 carbons, **androstane derivatives** with 19 carbons, and **estrane derivatives** with 18 carbons. These groups, the precursors of progesterone, androgens, and estrogens, respectively, are summarized in Table 14-1 and depicted in Figure 14-1.[2,7]

Estrogen and Progesterone

Estrogen and progesterone are the primary sex steroids in females. Estrogen is responsible for the majority of the development and maintenance of the female reproductive system and secondary sex characteristics. Estrogen also has roles throughout the rest of the body, including contributions to skeletal shape, urogenital tone and elasticity, and bone changes that allow for the growth spurt that occurs during puberty.[8]

Progesterone primarily acts on the reproductive tract, where it causes the endometrium to change from proliferative to secretory during the second half of the menstrual cycle and is a potent mitogen or promoter of cell division in the development of normal breast tissue.[9] Progesterone also thickens the cervical mucus. Both hormones

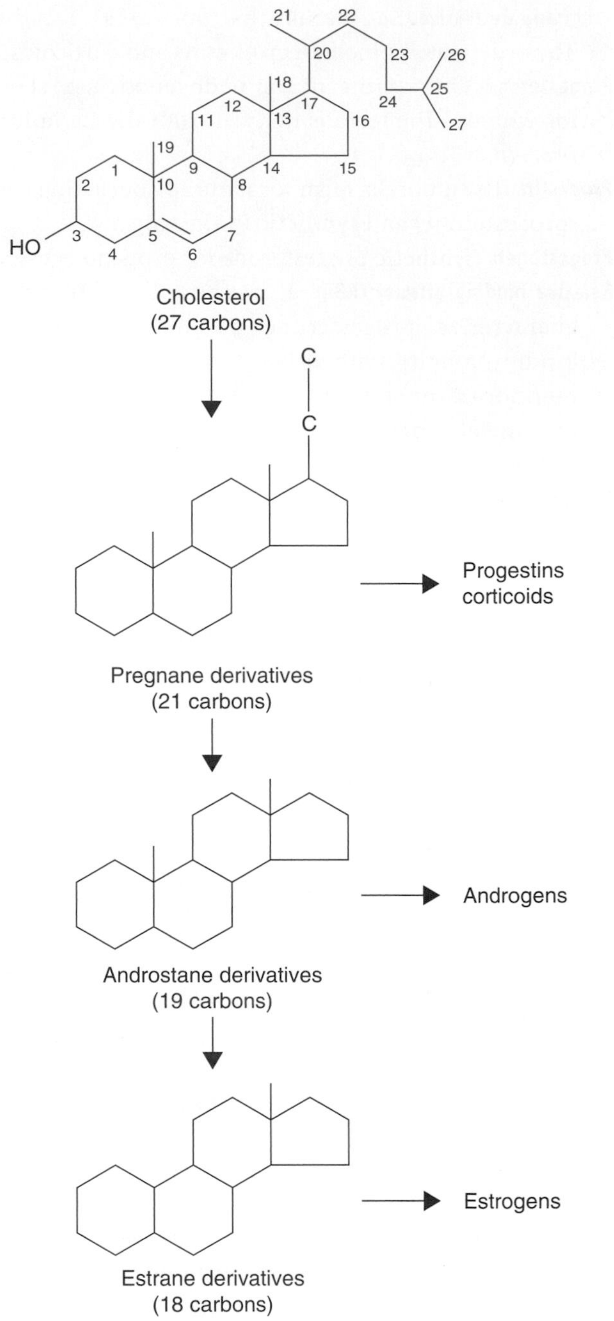

Figure 14-1 Biosynthesis of sex steroids.

have essential roles in the menstrual cycle and during pregnancy/lactation.

Overview of the Menstrual Cycle

Knowledge of menstrual physiology is needed to understand the pharmacologic applications of sex steroid hormones.

Table 14-1 Cholesterol Derivations and Products

Derivation from Cholesterol	Number of Carbons	Products
Pregnane	21	Progestogens and corticoids
Androstane	19	Androgens
Estrane	18	Estrogens

Details about the complexity involved in this natural phenomenon have continued to emerge in the last few decades as researchers have studied primates and humans. This body of research has revealed that some assumptions based on rat models have been proven false and that fluctuating levels of estrogen and progesterone are not the only necessary factors for a normal cycle. The following provides a brief overview of this sophisticated process; however, the interested reader is directed to reproductive physiology texts, such as Speroff and Fritz, for more detailed information.[2]

The menstrual cycle is the result of intricate interactions among a number of hormones in the hypothalamic-pituitary-ovarian axis as illustrated in Figure 14-2. During the first half or follicular ovarian phase of the menstrual cycle, release of gonadotropin-releasing hormone (GnRH) from the hypothalamus stimulates secretion of follicle-stimulating hormone (FSH) and luteinizing hormone (LH) from the pituitary. FSH promotes maturation of follicles in the ovaries that begin to secrete estrogen as they mature. Simultaneously, during this first half of the menstrual cycle, the endometrium proliferates under the influence of estrogen. Table 14-2 presents a summary

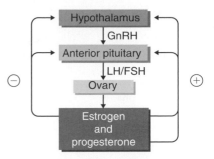

The hypothalmus–pituitary–ovarian axis operates under a negative feedback loop except during the immediate preovulatory period of days 12–14, when it becomes a positive feedback loop.

Figure 14-2 Hormonal regulation of the menstrual cycle.

of hormonal fluctuations during the normal menstrual cycle. Once critical blood levels of estrogen are attained, feedback to the pituitary signals a release of LH and more FSH. The surge of LH results in ovulation, the release of an egg from the dominant follicle.

In the second half or luteal ovarian phase of the menstrual cycle, the follicle becomes the site of the

Table 14-2 Overview of Endogenous Estrogen and Progesterone During the Menstrual Cycle

Days	Ovarian Cycle	Endometrial Cycle	Estrogen and Progesterone	Actions
1–5	Follicular	Menstrual	Low estrogen and progesterone	Inhibin falls. LH and FSH begin to slowly rise starting approximately day 27.
6–14	Follicular	Proliferative	Building estrogen and (to lesser extent) progesterone	LH initiates luteinization and progesterone production in the granulosa layer. The rise of progesterone facilitates positive feedback action of estrogen and may be necessary for the midcycle FSH peak, although complete reason for midcycle FSH peak remains unclear. Estrogen production becomes sufficient to achieve and maintain the threshold concentration of estradiol that is required in order to induce the LH surge. A midcycle increase in local and peripheral androgens occurs, derived from the thecal tissue of unsuccessful follicles. A few hours after the LH surge, changes in hormone levels release suppression of oocyte maturation.
14	Ovulation	Proliferative	High estrogen and building progesterone	High levels of estrogen induce the LH surge at midcycle, and high levels of estrogen lead to sustained, elevated LH secretion. Suppression of inhibition of oocyte maturation allows final maturation of the oocyte. LH surge occurs and is responsible for luteinization of the granulosa, and synthesis of progesterones and prostaglandins in the follicle. Progesterone and prostaglandins work together to digest, weaken, and eventually rupture the follicular wall. The midcycle FSH peak frees the oocyte from follicular attachments and ensures sufficient LH receptors to allow an adequate normal luteal phase.

(continues)

Table 14-2 Overview of Endogenous Estrogen and Progesterone During the Menstrual Cycle (*continued*)

Days	Ovarian Cycle	Endometrial Cycle	Estrogen and Progesterone	Actions
15–26	Luteal	Secretory (implantation phase)	Progesterone most dominant, but estrogen present	Progesterone from corpus luteum acts both centrally and within the ovary to suppress new follicular growth. High levels of progesterone inhibit pituitary secretion of gonadotropins by inhibiting GnRH pulses at the level of the hypothalamus. High levels of progesterone antagonize pituitary response to GnRH by interfering with estrogen action. Regression of the corpus luteum may involve luteolytic action of its own estrogen production, mediated by an alteration in local prostaglandin concentration. In early pregnancy, hCG maintains luteal function until placental steroidogenesis is established.
27–28	Luteal	Late secretory (ischemic)	Dropping estrogen and progesterone	The degeneration of corpus luteum results in low levels of estrogen, progesterone, and inhibin. The low level of inhibin removes the suppression of FSH on the pituitary. The low level of estrogen and progesterone allows an increase in GnRH pulsatile secretion and the removal of the pituitary from the negative feedback suppression. The removal of inhibin and estradiol and increased GnRH pulses allow an increase in FSH (and, to a lesser extent, LH). The increasing FSH is instrumental in the maturation of a dominant follicle.

corpus luteum, which primarily secretes large amounts of progesterone. Under the influence of progesterone, the endometrium height stabilizes while the glands become tortuous, layers of the endometrium develop, and a glycogen-rich fluid is secreted from the endometrium. These endometrial changes are in preparation for implantation should fertilization occur. If fertilization of the egg does not occur, levels of estrogen decrease due to lack of stimulation of follicles by FSH, and progesterone levels decrease secondary to the demise of the corpus luteum. The change in hormone levels results in ischemia of the endometrium and initiation of menstruation.

In addition to their association with the ovaries and endometrium, estrogen and progesterone also influence cyclic changes in other reproductive organs. As estrogen increases immediately prior to ovulation, the cervical mucus becomes clear, thin, abundant, and stretchy. During the second half of the menstrual cycle, when progesterone predominates, the cervical mucus decreases in amount and becomes opaque, thick, and viscous. Estrogen stimulates movement in the fallopian tubes to facilitate ovum transport, while progesterone reverses this effect.[2,10] Understanding the physiologic functions of estrogen and progesterone is essential for rational prescribing of the pharmacologic preparations of both hormones and their clinical applications.

Estrogen

Estrogen is the generic term for a chemically similar family of endogenous hormones and exogenous compounds with an affinity for **estrogen receptors**.[6,8] Two types of estrogen receptors (ER_α and ER_β) have been identified throughout the body in both males and females. These receptors have different tissue distributions with more ER_α receptors in the female reproductive organs and liver and more ER_β receptors in other tissues.[8] More receptor activity is likely to appear in cells with alpha receptors, although major research about ER_β is under way and may result in a deeper understanding of estrogen receptors in general.[11]

ER_α is expressed in the tissue of the uterus, ovary (theca cells), bone, breast, brain, liver, and adipose tissue. ER_β is expressed in the colon, ovary (granulosa cells), bone marrow, salivary gland, vascular endothelium, and brain.[12] The complexity of this distribution becomes important when designing new drugs. One type of drug, a SERM, is an agent that can bind to either ER_α or ER_β and can cause either agonist or antagonist properties at either receptor site.[6] SERMs are discussed later in this chapter. Receptors remain under intensive study, and there is discussion of potential cloning of receptors as well as investigation about the relationships between specific receptors and risks of cancer. Estrogen receptors also are important factors when a woman is being treated for an estrogen-sensitive cancer. Other chemotherapeutic agents that interfere with estrogens are addressed in Chapter 28 in the discussion of cancer drugs.

Estrogens are derived from androgens via **aromatization**, or development of a benzene ring, as cholesterol undergoes steroidogenesis. Three estrogens are produced naturally in the female body. They are **estrone** (E_1), estradiol (E_2), and **estriol** (E_3). The three estrogens vary in quantity and in potency, which is defined as their affinity for estrogen receptors. Among reproductive-aged women, 17β-estradiol (estradiol or E_2) is produced in the largest quantity through biosynthesis in the ovary. Following menopause, estradiol levels drop to 10% or less of premenopausal levels. More than 95% of endogenous estradiol is produced in the ovaries with the remainder produced via **peripheral aromatization** of estrone.[8] Of the three types of estrogens produced endogenously, estradiol is the most potent because it has the highest binding affinity for estrogen receptors, and it binds to both ER_α and ER_β receptors. Estrone (E_1) is a metabolite of estradiol and is less potent. Estrone primarily is produced via the conversion of **androstenedione** in adipose tissue.

Among postmenopausal women, the ovary ceases producing estradiol, but the adrenal gland continues making androstenedione, the immediate precursor to estrone; additionally, estrone continues to be produced in the tissues of the body, particularly in adiposity or fat, so the levels of estrone remain unchanged while the plasma levels of estradiol fall markedly. As a result, estrone begins to be the estrogen in largest quantity in postmenopausal women.[8]

The third endogenous estrogen, estriol (E_3), is a metabolite of estradiol and estrone in the periphery and is not secreted by the ovaries. Estriol is the principal estrogen produced by the placenta during pregnancy, although it can be found in small quantities among women who are not pregnant.[2,8]

Pharmacologic Uses of Estrogen

The clinical uses of estrogen are discussed in depth in the chapters within Section E of this textbook. In brief, exogenous estrogens primarily are used for contraception and menopausal hormone therapy. In the 1960s and 1970s, sequential contraceptives contained estrogen only for the first several weeks before progesterone was added. These contraceptives were removed from the market in the mid 1970s and all of today's estrogen-containing contraceptive methods are composed of tablets that contain both estrogen and a progestin; thus they often are known as combined contraceptives. Three major contraceptive methods contain estrogen: combined oral contraceptives, the contraceptive vaginal ring (NuvaRing), and the transdermal contraceptive patch (Ortho Evra). The estrogenic component of combined contraceptives exerts its major effect on FSH. Suppression of FSH prevents the selection and emergence of a dominant follicle. Estrogen also stabilizes the endometrium to minimize breakthrough bleeding or provide cycle control. In addition, estrogen potentiates the action of the progestational component, which allows for lower progestin doses.[6] Additional information about hormonal contraception can be found in Chapter 29.

Hormone therapy for treatment of menopausal symptoms includes the following two categories: estrogen therapy, or estrogen provided for women who have had a hysterectomy and no longer have a uterus; and estrogen plus progestin therapy, sometimes called hormone therapy. A progestin is added to estrogen for women with an intact uterus to protect from estrogen-induced endometrial cancer. More information on these therapies can be found in Chapter 34. Note that the word *replacement* (e.g., hormone replacement therapy) is no longer recommended because these formulations do not contain dosages sufficient to reach or replace premenopausal hormone levels.[13] Estrogen is prescribed for perimenopausal and postmenopausal women to alleviate menopausal symptoms that are troublesome for individual women.

Pharmacologic Properties of Estrogen

Estrogens, like all steroids, are highly lipid-soluble and, therefore, once produced, they diffuse easily through cell membranes into the circulation. When estrogen reaches one of the many different tissues that contain cells with estrogen receptors, it diffuses into the cell and through the nuclear membrane. Inside the nucleus, it attaches to an estrogen receptor via an **estrogen ligand** (a substance that binds to a receptor). Ligands may change receptor properties and, thus, this may explain some of the differences among estrogen-specific agents. The ligand-receptor complex binds to DNA and initiates gene transcription. Such transcription provides a virtual script that directs the production of specific proteins that will affect the physiologic action initiated by estrogen in the target tissue.[14]

In the bloodstream, the vast majority of estrogen (69%) is bound to a protein called **sex hormone-binding globulin** (SHBG). Another 30% of estrogen is loosely bound to albumin, which leaves only 1% of free estrogen that is available to diffuse into tissues.[2] SHBG levels are increased in hyperthyroidism and pregnancy and when exogenous estrogens are present; conversely, this globulin is decreased when androgens, progestins, insulin, and corticoids are administered or when central obesity exists.[15] Thus, the amount of circulating free estrogens is also influenced by these factors.

The effect of estrogen, whether produced endogenously or administered exogenously, is dependent upon several factors. The first consideration is the relative potency of the estrogen type. As stated previously, potency depends upon affinity for estrogen receptors, which includes how long the estrogen remains bound to the receptor and the amount of free hormone available to diffuse across cell membranes and bind to receptors. The amount of free hormone available depends upon the amount of SHBG present. SHBG is produced in the liver. Ultimately, the effect estrogen has on physiologic function depends upon the agonist or antagonist response that occurs following binding to the estrogen receptor within the target cell.[14]

Following potency and receptor agonist or antagonist properties, the metabolism of endogenous estrogen is the next important factor to be considered in evaluation of pharmacologic products. Estrogens are well absorbed from the gastrointestinal tract as well as through the skin or mucous membranes.[13] Estrogen is metabolized into biologically less active or inactive forms via these two mechanisms: (1) **conjugation** into water-soluble and nonbiologically active metabolites that can then be excreted via the kidney; and (2) conversion into estrone or estriol, which are biologically active, but approximately 10 times less potent than estradiol.[14]

Estrogens are conjugated naturally in the liver, where they are altered to become structurally similar to bile acids. Then they are excreted into the gastrointestinal tract via the bile ducts. In the intestine, normal bacterial flora unconjugate estrogen, making it once again lipid soluble. This lipid-soluble, biologically active form is reabsorbed via the entero-hepatic circulation and is thereby recycled back into the circulation as an active metabolite.[14]

Orally ingested exogenous estrogen is metabolized rapidly into estrone (E_1) in both the intestine and liver before reaching the general circulation. This first-pass effect markedly decreases the amount of estrogen available for circulation. Nonoral estrogen formulations circumvent this first-pass effect and can reach therapeutic plasma levels at lower doses than oral formulations, although often it takes a longer time to reach peak levels when nonoral formulations are used. For example, an oral contraceptive reaches peak plasma levels at 2 hours, and the estrogen patch (Ortho Evra) takes 48 hours.

Estrogen Preparations

Pharmacologic estrogen preparations can be divided into six main groups: (1) human natural estrogens, (2) nonhuman natural estrogens, (3) synthetic estrogen mixtures, (4) synthetic estrogen analogs with a steroid molecular structure, (5) synthetic estrogen analogs without a steroid skeleton, and (6) plant-based estrogens without a steroid skeleton (Table 14-3).[13] The plant-based estrogens, also known as **phytoestrogens**, are naturally occurring products that are available without a prescription and are discussed later in this chapter as well as in Chapters 10 and 34. Estrogen formulations can either be single-entity estrogens or combination products with varying amounts of chemically distinct estrogens. All formulations have a high affinity for estrogen receptors and simulate estrogen function.[14]

The only human estrogen that is available as an FDA-approved drug is 17β-estradiol, and it is used for menopausal hormone therapy. Oral estradiol is micronized to enhance absorption. It should be noted that other methods are used to promote absorption including **esterification** and conjugation, yet these are all chemical terms that have little clinical significance. Estradiol also is absorbed rapidly through the skin, and it is commonly used in nonoral formulations such as transdermal and topical estrogen products.[1,4]

The nonhuman conjugated equine estrogens (CEEs) are derived from the urine of pregnant mares and primarily used for menopausal hormone therapy. As aforementioned, conjugated formulations of estrogen are made water soluble to promote oral absorption. CEE (Premarin) contains at least 10 active estrogens—primarily sodium estrone

Table 14-3 Pharmacologic Formulations of Estrogen

Category	Available Formulations
Human estrogens, including estrone (E_1), 17β-estradiol (E_2), and estriol	17β-estradiol
Nonhuman estrogens	Conjugated equine estrogens (CEEs)
Synthetic estrogen mixtures	Synthetic conjugated estrogens Esterified estrogens
Synthetic estrogen analogs with a steroid molecular structure	Ethinyl estradiol Estropipate (formerly piperazine estrone sulfate)
Synthetic estrogen analogs without a steroid skeleton	None
Phytoestrogens	Found in a wide variety of foods and botanics, although dosing is not standardized

Source: Adapted from North American Menopause Society 2007.[13]

sul-fate (approximately 45%) and sodium equilin sulfate (approximately 25%). CEEs are not only the most frequently used estrogen product worldwide, but they are also the estrogen formulation that has been used in the majority of clinical trials to date.[13,14] There is no generic preparation for CEE (Premarin) approved in the United States at this time.

Two types of synthetic estrogen mixtures exist that are primarily used for menopausal hormone therapy: synthetic conjugated estrogens and esterified estrogens. The synthetic conjugated estrogen mixtures are derived from yam or soy plants and contain several types of estrogen. Both synthetic conjugated estrogen products available in the United States (Cenestin with 9 estrogens and Enjuvia with 10 estrogens) contain the primary estrogens in CEE, but the products are not considered equivalent to Premarin. The esterified estrogens (Menest) are derived from CEE, and their principal component is sodium estrone sulfate.[13,14]

Prior to **micronization**, estradiol could not be well absorbed by the gastrointestinal tract. Ethinyl estradiol was a breakthrough when it was realized that adding ethinyl to estradiol creates an estrogen that is active orally.[2] Ethinyl estradiol and estropipate (formerly known as piperazine estrone sulfate) are the two synthetic estrogen analogs with a steroid molecular structure. Ethinyl estradiol is the estrogen found in the contraceptive vaginal ring (Nuva Ring), the transdermal contraceptive patch (Ortho Evra), some menopausal treatments (e.g., Femhrt) and almost all combined oral contraceptives. A few older combined oral contraceptives containing mestranol instead of ethinyl remain on the market but have been virtually replaced by those with ethinyl estradiol. Estropipate (Ortho-Est) is used for postmenopausal hormone therapy and is an oral form of estrone sulfate with piperazine added for solubility and stability.[13]

Nonsteroidal synthetic estrogen analogs include diethylstilbestrol (DES), dienestrol, benzestrol, hexestrol, methestrol, methallenestril, and chlorotrianisene.[9] None of these compounds are currently available in the United States.[10,16] DES has an important role in the history of prescribing sex steroids as summarized in Box 14-1.

Routes of Administration

Routes for estrogen administration include oral, vaginal, topical, transdermal, and injection. Vaginal formulations of estrogens include creams, rings, and tablets. Transdermal and topical estrogen products include patches, gels, and emulsions. An estrogen spray for postmenopausal vasomotor symptoms is marketed as Evamist.[17]

Box 14-1 Gone But Not Forgotten: Diethylstilbestrol (DES)

Diethylstilbestrol (DES) was the first synthetic estrogen produced. This agent initially was prescribed to pregnant women in an attempt to prevent spontaneous abortion, although later studies found that it proved to be ineffective for this indication. An estimated 5–10 million persons in the United States were exposed to DES between 1938 and1971, including women who took DES during pregnancy, and their children, who now are known as DES daughters and DES sons. The Food and Drug Administration advised cessation of the prescription of DES in 1971 due to the risk of clear cell adenocarcinoma of the vagina and cervix in DES daughters. Women who took DES during pregnancy have an increased risk of breast cancer. DES daughters (women exposed to DES in utero) are at risk for reproductive tract abnormalities and cancers, pregnancy complications, and infertility, illustrating how this agent has multigenerational adverse effects.

Source: Centers for Disease Control and Prevention 2008.[16]

Estrogen Benefits

Estrogen's efficacy as a contraceptive, for treatment of vasomotor symptoms and vulvovaginal atrophy, and for prevention of osteoporosis is well established. The contraceptive methods containing estrogen and progestins are highly effective for preventing pregnancy. As women age and endogenous estrogen levels decline, perimenopausal/menopausal symptoms such as hot flashes and night sweats may occur. Exogenous estrogens are an effective treatment for these vasomotor symptoms when they are troublesome for a woman. Decreased estrogen levels can also lead to vulvar and vaginal atrophy. Estrogen improves this atrophy and associated symptoms, such as vaginal dryness and dyspareunia. Estrogens decrease bone resorption, which prevents bone loss and reduces the risk of osteoporotic fracture. Estrogen use by mature women is discussed in detail in Chapter 34.

Several other benefits of estrogen have been investigated. Toward the end of the 20th century, there was a body of observational data that suggested estrogen could be cardioprotective for mature women. However, findings regarding estrogen's ability to reduce the risk of heart disease have been conflicting. These discrepancies may be related to the time between when the study participants experienced menopause and the time when they began taking estrogen, as well of the ages of the participants and their preexisting coronary conditions. It has been theorized that premenopausal use of estrogens decrease risk of arteriosclerosis, but by the postmenopausal period, many women already have subclinical disease, and hormone therapy may cause plaque instability, resulting in cardiac events.[18] The North American Menopause Society does not recommend estrogen for protection against developing heart disease for women of any age.[12] Additional benefits of perimenopausal and postmenopausal estrogen use that have been reported in a number of studies include improved sleep, improved mood, increased sexual desire, and maintained or improved cognition, but the evidence for these effects is inconclusive to date.[12,13]

Side Effects/Adverse Effects

Like all medications, estrogen can have side effects that are not dangerous, but bothersome, as well as adverse effects that result in serious complications. The most common side effects of estrogen include nausea, breast tenderness, headache, and dizziness. Nonoral formulations can have side effects specific to the route of delivery. For example, women using estrogen patches may experience skin irritation.

Endometrial Cancer

Estrogen, when administered alone (often termed *unopposed*), increases the risk of endometrial cancer. For this reason, women who take estrogen and who have a uterus also should receive a progestin periodically for the express purpose of decreasing the risk of endometrial cancer.

Breast and Ovarian Cancer

Estrogen is theorized to be related, at least to some degree, to the development of breast cancer, although not necessarily as the single etiologic agent. Most breast tumors have estrogen receptors and some have progesterone receptors. It is believed that there is increased risk for breast cancer in persons who also have obesity, infertility, delayed pregnancy, early menarche, and late menopause, all of which are associated with times of added estrogen exposure without the protection of progesterone.[2] Progesterone's role is less clear in breast cancer, even though it is well known that progesterone plays a role in mitotic activity as

demonstrated during both the thelarche and luteal phases of the menstrual cycle.

During the Women's Health Initiative Study, it was found that women taking both estrogen and progestin had a small but significant increase in breast cancer (HR = 1.26; 95% CI, 1.00–1.59; N = 290 cases) while women taking only estrogen had no significant increase in risk at all.[19,20] A later review of women and breast cancer investigated risks for women 5 years after the initial Women's Health Initiative report. In this study, scientists found that taking combined hormone therapy for 5 years doubled the risk for breast cancer, although risks decline rapidly after discontinuation.[21] These findings underscore the importance of informed consent. Women should be told that all risks, and even benefits, are likely to be unknown at this time as part of an informed consent (or refusal) process. If they choose to use hormone therapy it should always be the lowest dose that relieves symptoms, and use should be reviewed at each visit.

Ovarian cancer appears to be less influenced by estrogen and progestins than either endometrial or breast cancer, and studies show no clear evidence of an increased risk of ovarian cancer in women who use these agents and no effect with increasing duration of use.[2] For postmenopausal hormone treatments for women with genetically linked breast and ovarian cancer, there is a 60% lifetime risk of ovarian cancer in women with the BRCA1 gene, and women with the BRCA2 have a 30% lifetime risk of developing ovarian cancer.[22]

Thromboembolic Disease

Another major risk associated with the use of estrogen is that of deep vein thrombosis (DVT) and other associated thromboembolic events such as pulmonary emboli. Early studies of oral contraceptives noted that the incidence of DVT decreased as the dosage of estrogen was lowered.[23] In 2007, it was suggested that use of transdermal contraceptive patches may incur an increased risk of DVT and other associated conditions such as stroke and myocardial infarction due to increased circulating estrogens (because transdermal patches avoid the first-pass effect), although this area of research remains under investigation.[24] The risk of DVT also appears to be associated with use of estrogen postmenopausally, although this relationship was discovered later than that with contraceptives, most likely because of the decreased potency or strength of formulations used in hormone therapy. In addition to estrogen, some progestins used in contraceptives appear to be associated with a risk for developing DVTs either independently or synergistically with estrogen.

Phytoestrogens

Phytoestrogens are weak plant-derived substances that are structurally similar to estrogens and bind to estrogen receptors.[8,25] Some scientists advocate that phytoestrogens should be termed *phytoSERMs* because these foods and supplements bind to estrogen receptors and can be viewed as SERMs, the so-called designer drugs that are discussed later in this chapter.

Phytoestrogens can be classified into three groups: isoflavones, lignans, and coumestans. The most common pharmacologic use of phytoestrogens is for the treatment of menopausal symptoms, and isoflavones are the most widely used and studied for this purpose. The isoflavones include genistein, daidzein, glycitein, biochanin A, and formononetin. Isoflavones appear to have a higher binding affinity for ER_β receptors than ER_α receptors, and these phytoestrogens can act as both estrogen agonists and antagonists.[13,14] Soy and red clover are commonly used sources of isoflavones. Soy supplementation appears to have a positive impact on serum lipids, but the clinical implication is not fully known.[26,27] Food sources of soy include soybeans, soy flour, soy protein isolate, miso soup, tempeh, tofu, and soy milk. Soy supplements are available as over-the-counter products (e.g., Health Woman, Soy Care, GeniSoy), as are supplements containing red clover (e.g., Promensil). These soy and red clover products are considered dietary supplements and as such are subject to less regulation than prescription drugs with regard to safety and efficacy.[13] In general, efficacy of most phytoestrogen supplements remains unproven, although most data suggest that dietary supplements are less useful than foods containing the agents.

Xenoestrogens (Ecoestrogens, Estrogen Look-Alikes)

Nonpharmacologic agents such as pesticides also may metabolize into estrogen components or activate estrogen receptors. These agents have been known by several names, including estrogen look-alikes, xenoestrogens (from the Greek for *stranger*), or ecoestrogens, particularly because of their association with environmental pesticides. Estrogen look-alikes were discovered several years ago when animal reproduction plummeted in areas where the water was polluted. Subsequent investigation revealed feminization of and decreased fecundity in alligators. Ecoestrogens often appear to have long half-lives. Questions have emerged concerning whether ecoestrogens are involved with the decreasing sperm counts among men in modern society, especially considering the food chain wherein animals may be exposed to xenoestrogens in their environments. Few studies have been conducted in this area. There is some suggestion that organochlorines may be associated with shortened menstrual cycles for women who ate fatty fish from polluted waters more than once a month. Thus, environmental pollutants may have negative effects via steroidal pathways and endocrine disruption.[28] Xenoestrogens theoretically may be estrogenic or antiestrogenic.

SERMs and SEEMs

Antiestrogens are medications that are estrogen antagonists. Pure antiestrogens, such as fulvestrant (Faslodex, used to treat resistant breast cancer), have no agonist effects. Most antiestrogens have both antagonist and agonist properties. Medications that have estrogenic effects on some tissues while blocking the effect of estrogen on other tissues are called *selective estrogen receptor modulators (SERMs).*

The term *SERM* may be relatively new, but such agents have existed for decades. Clomiphene citrate (Clomid) and tamoxifen citrate (Nolvadex) are mixed antagonist-agonist compounds derived from triphenylethylene. Raloxifene hydrochloride (Evista) is an estrogen antagonist-agonist derived from benzothiphene.[2] These medications differ in their indications and properties, and thus each is described separately.

Selective estrogen enzyme modulators (SEEMs) are agents that do not necessarily activate or block estrogen receptors, but rather interfere with enzymatic pathways that result in synthesis of the estrogen itself. This concept is of particular value in treatment of women with cancer, particularly breast cancer. Among pharmaceuticals that may be characterized as SEEMs are various progestins as well as tibolone (Livial) and its metabolites, since some inhibit enzymatic activities, while others can stimulate the local production of estrogen sulfates or block the aromatase action. The concept of SEEMs is more recent than SERMs and may ultimately result in another group of designer drugs.

Clomiphene Citrate

The SERM clomiphene citrate (Clomid, Serophene, Milophene) is an estrogen antagonist and agonist used as an ovulatory stimulant. This agent acts as an estrogen antagonist unless endogenous estrogen levels are extremely low, in which case it acts as an estrogen agonist. Clomiphene works by binding to estrogen receptors in the pituitary gland, thereby blocking those receptors from detecting circulating estrogen. As a result, the hypothalamus increases its secretion of gonadotropin-releasing hormone

(GnRH), which stimulates the pituitary to secrete follicle-stimulating hormone (FSH) and luteinizing hormone (LH). These hormones stimulate and initiate an ovulatory menstrual cycle. Side effects of clomiphene include hot flashes, mood swings, ovarian enlargement, and multiple gestation, as well as less frequent symptoms that include visual disturbances, breast tenderness, pelvic discomfort, and nausea. In pregnancies that occur among women taking clomiphene, 8% are multiple gestations and the vast majority of these are twins. There is no evidence that clomiphene increases the risk of congenital anomalies, nor is there evidence for a causal relationship between clomiphene and ovarian cancer.[29] Clomiphene is contraindicated for women who are pregnant (FDA Pregnancy Category X), those who have ovarian enlargement, and those who have abnormal vaginal bleeding.[29,30]

Tamoxifen Citrate

Tamoxifen citrate (Nolvadex, Soltamox) is a nonsteroidal antiestrogen used to treat breast cancer, to reduce the incidence of breast cancer recurrence, and to prolong survival in women who have been treated for breast cancer, as well as to prevent breast cancer in women who are at high risk. Tamoxifen is actually a prodrug metabolized by CYP2D6 to endoxifen, which is the active metabolite. Tamoxifen is an estrogen receptor antagonist at selected sites (e.g., breasts) and acts as an estrogen agonist at other sites (e.g., endometrium, bones, and lipids). Thus, tamoxifen has positive benefits of protection from breast cancer and promotion of bone density, but also potential serious risks such as endometrial cancer and thromboembolic events (e.g., deep vein thrombosis). The most common side effects are hot flashes, nausea, vomiting, and irregular menses (including amenorrhea and oligomenorrhea). Persons who have genetic polymorphisms that result in reduced amounts of CYP2D6 may get benefit from taking tamoxifen, and this is one of the drugs wherein genetic tests to determine the status of the CYP2D6 genes prior to prescribing the drug is being discussed. Tamoxifen contraindications include concomitant use of warfarin-type (Coumadin-type) anticoagulant therapy, history of thromboembolic event, or pregnancy (FDA Pregnancy Category D).[2,30,31] Toremifene citrate (Fareston) is a SERM that is similar in structure to tamoxifen, and it is used to treat metastatic cancer in postmenopausal women.[9]

Raloxifene

Raloxifene HCl (Evista) is a SERM that is FDA approved for the prevention and treatment of osteoporosis in post-menopausal women. Raloxifene also is as effective as tamoxifen in reducing the risk of invasive breast cancer (RR = 1.02; 95% CI, 0.82–1.28).[32] Raloxifene acts as an estrogen agonist in bone but, unlike tamoxifen, does not cause endometrial proliferation. Raloxifene is associated with thromboembolic events, but the risk is lower than that of tamoxifen. Almost 30% of women taking raloxifene report hot flashes, and approximately 10% report leg cramps. Contraindications to raloxifene use include lactation, pregnancy (FDA Pregnancy Category X), and active or past history of thromboembolic events.[32]

Tibolone

Tibolone (Livial, Tibofem), a SEEM, is a synthetic steroid that is structurally related to 19-nortestosterone commonly used in contraceptives. It has weak estrogenic, androgenic, and progestogenic properties. This drug is effective in relieving symptoms including hot flashes, in improving mood, and possibly in increasing libido and sexual response. Tibolone does not cause endometrial proliferation, thus avoiding irregular vaginal bleeding and does not require a periodic use of progestin. In clinical practice, some premenopausal women continue to experience intermittent and occasional breakthrough bleeding when taking tibolone. This clinical sign does warrant investigation to rule out endometrial abnormalities. Such bleeding is likely not from endometrial proliferation but rather polyps, fibroids, or elevated endogenous estrogen levels. Ultrasound, hysteroscopy, or serum estrogen levels might be considered. Tibolone decreases HDL, a cause for potential concern for some individuals. Tibolone also serves to prevent bone loss and may decrease fracture risk; however, its effects on breast cancer remain unknown.[33] While it is available in 90 countries, tibolone has not received FDA approval because of its association with an increased risk of stroke and the 12% incidence of uterine bleeding that results in the need for investigation.

▌ Progesterone

Progesterone is the precursor to androgens and estrogens. The primary source of endogenous progesterone production is the corpus luteum, and levels of this hormone are highest during the second half of the menstrual cycle. If pregnancy occurs, progesterone also is produced by the placenta. Small amounts of progesterone are secreted by the adrenal glands in women of all ages.

Endogenous progesterone binds to the progesterone receptor, resulting in dissociation of selected proteins, phosphorylation of the receptor itself, and activation of transcription factors. Progesterone inhibits estrogens by decreasing the number of estrogen receptors and increasing metabolism of estrogen to inactive metabolites. Progesterone induces secretory changes in the endometrium, thus decreasing risk of endometrial hyperplasia; decreases uterine contractility during pregnancy; and maintains pregnancy.

There are two forms of progesterone receptors, designated as PR-A and PR-B. The two forms are structurally identical except that PR-B contains 164 additional amino acids. The latter has yet to be associated with clinical significance.

The endogenous product is commonly known as *progesterone*. However, similar exogenous compounds have used different names, including progestins, progestational agents, progestagens, progestogens, and gestogens.[34] For clarity, the term *progestin* will include both naturally occurring progesterone and other synthetic progestational agents. The term **progestogens** is used to describe synthetic bioactive agents that are similar to progesterone.

Pharmacologic Uses of Progestins

Progestins are primarily used for contraception and for menopausal hormonal therapy to oppose estrogenic-related endometrial hypertrophy, which is known to be a precursor of endometrial cancer. Progestins can be used for contraception either alone or in combination with estrogen. Progestin-only contraceptive formulations include pills (so-called *minipills*, a misnomer because it implies low dose to some), injection (Depo-Provera MPA), implant (Implanon), the levonorgestrel-releasing intrauterine system (Mirena), and emergency contraceptive pills (Plan B). Combined contraceptive formulations that contain estrogen and progestin include combined oral contraceptives, the contraceptive vaginal ring, and the transdermal contraceptive patch. The mechanisms of action of progestins that prevent pregnancy include suppression of the LH surge that prevents ovulation and thickening of the cervical mucus that inhibits sperm penetration and transport.

Progestins usually are administered in conjunction with estrogen in the form of estrogen plus progestin therapy in women who have a uterus. Although not as effective as estrogen for vasomotor therapy, progestins also can be used to treat these symptoms of menopause.

A progesterone challenge or progesterone test continues to be used occasionally. If a woman is not pregnant and her hypothalamus/pituitary/ovarian axis is intact, vaginal bleeding should result within a few days after cessation of the progesterone agent. Bleeding indicates that the woman is producing endogenous estrogen. This progesterone withdrawal often is used to induce bleeding in women who are amenorrheic or to regulate menses when a woman is experiencing abnormal uterine bleeding. The progesterone challenge test is described in more detail in Chapter 30.

Progestins also have been advocated for use during infertility treatments, especially as vaginal suppositories administered in early pregnancy to support the endometrium for women who have experienced past spontaneous abortions, although clear evidence is lacking for this action.[35] Progesterone in the form of 17-hydroxy-progesterone also has been suggested as a method to reduce preterm labor for selected groups of women at risk, although some authorities suggest additional research is needed in order to clearly identify for whom the agent is indicated.[36,37] These pregnancy-related uses of progestins are discussed in more detail in Chapters 30 and 35.

Use of progestin for treatment of premenstrual symptomatology has had a long history. However, studies have failed to demonstrate a clear benefit for the use of this agent, and the controversy continues.[38] More discussion about progestin is found in Chapter 30.

Pharmacologic Properties of Progesterone

Half-Life

Progesterone is rapidly absorbed and has a half-life of 5 minutes.[9] Early oral progesterone products had rapid inactivation and poor bioavailability. These limitations were the impetus for the development of synthetic progestins. More recently, techniques to micronize crystals have been developed. Oral absorption is improved when oral progesterone, like oral estrogen, is micronized.[4]

Relative Binding Affinity and Progesterone Potency

In the 1970s, it was common for providers to attempt to tailor an oral contraceptive to a specific individual. Clinical symptoms such as nausea, acne, and weight gain were characterized as excessive estrogen or androgen effects and progestins were divided into different categories, such as estrogenic, in order to determine the exact combined oral contraceptive (COC) for a woman. To a large degree, these decisions were made based on studies about relative binding affinity or progesterone potency. **Relative binding**

affinity has limited clinical importance, especially because most data are derived from studies of other species. Neither is potency of clinical significance, as agents have been formulated to accommodate the dose of a specific type progestin needed for contraceptive effect. **Potency** occasionally continues to be mentioned, as some COCs are advertised with the lowest steroidal content, a marketing technique of questionable veracity. The concept of the quest for the perfect COC for an individual woman has been addressed by Speroff and Darney, who stated, "Clinical advice based on potency is an artificial exercise that has not stood the test of time."[39]

Progestin Pharmacologic Preparations

Two types of progestins exist; they are natural progesterone and synthetic progestogens. The primary distinction between the two is whether or not they are identical to endogenous progesterone.[13] Classification of the progestins is depicted in Figure 14-3.

Natural Progesterone

Natural progesterone pharmacologic agents are chemically identical to endogenous progesterone.[4] Progesterone products approved by the FDA include oral capsules (Prometrium), vaginal gels (Crinone and Prochieve), a vaginal insert (Endometrin), and an intramuscular injection (Progesterone).[10,40] These progesterones have fewer undesirable side effects than medroxyprogesterone acetate (MPA), the most commonly prescribed progestin.

Synthetic Progestogens

Synthetic progestogens are similar, but not identical, to endogenous progesterone. Most progestogens are derived from progesterone or testosterone. The one exception is drospirenone, which is derived from spironolactone.[41] Drospirenone is a novel progestin that possesses antimineralocorticoid activity with a potassium-sparing diuretic effect similar to that in spironolactone and is found in some combined oral contraceptives (Yasmin, Yaz). Drospirenone possesses antimineralocorticoid activity, and therefore potassium levels are often determined to establish baseline or continued monitoring while used. This activity is seen clinically in its effects on physiologic parameters, body weight, general well-being, and fluid-related symptoms, and it is generally not recommended for women who have hypertension. Drospirenone-containing COCs were initially characterized as a weight-loss contraceptive, but the average woman neither gains nor loses weight; however, there are some reports that users experience less breast tenderness, abdominal bloating, fatigue, and depressed mood than associated with other COCs.[42]

The progestogens that are structurally related to progesterone are divided into the pregnanes, which possess a methyl group at carbon 10, and the norpregnanes, which lack this methyl group. Pregnanes are derived from 17 α-hydroxyprogesterone, and the norpregnanes are

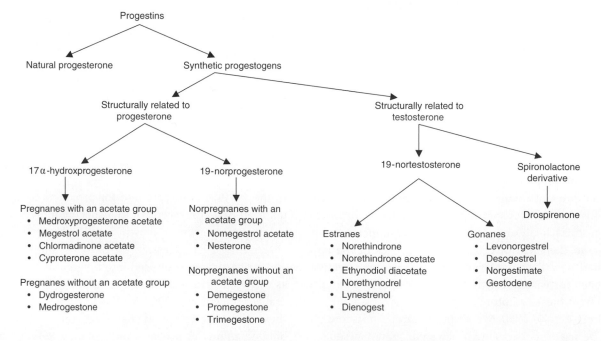

Figure 14-3 Classification of progestins. *Source:* Adapted from Simon JA 2007[41]; Stanczyk FZ 2003.[43]

derived from 19-norprogesterone. The pregnanes and norpregnanes can be further subdivided according to whether or not they contain an acetate group (Figure 14-3).[43] Pregnanes used in current clinical practice are medroxyprogesterone acetate and megestrol acetate (Megace). Medroxyprogesterone acetate, which is commonly called by its abbreviation, MPA, is available in oral and injectable formulations. The oral formulation (Provera) is primarily used as the progestin component of estrogen and progestin therapy and may be prescribed separately or combined with estrogen in one product (Premphase, Prempro). Intramuscular and subcutaneous formulations are used for contraception. The intramuscular formulation depot medroxyprogesterone acetate (DMPA) is marketed under the brand name Depo-Provera. Megestrol acetate (Megace) is used for breast and endometrial cancer treatment and is also given as an appetite stimulant for women with anorexia or cachexia.

Progestogens that are derived from testosterone are classified as estranes or gonanes. The estranes and gonanes are primarily used in oral contraceptives, although some menopausal hormone therapy formulations contain these progestins. The estranes are norethindrone and other progestins that metabolize to norethindrone, including norethindrone acetate, ethynodiol diacetate, norethynodrel, lynestrenol, and dienogest. The gonanes are levonorgestrel and related progestins, including desogestrel, norgestimate, and gestodene.[44] Some nonoral progestogen formulations contain active metabolites of these progestins. For example, the transdermal contraceptive patch (Ortho Evra) contains norelgestromin, which is the active metabolite of norgestimate. The contraceptive vaginal ring (NuvaRing) and single-rod implant (Implanon) contain etonogestrel, which is the active metabolite of desogestrel.

Routes of Administration

Routes for progesterone administration include oral, vaginal, transdermal, injection, implant, and intrauterine. Oral formulations include progestogens and micronized progesterone. A vaginal progesterone gel (Prochieve) and the contraceptive vaginal ring containing progestin (NuvaRing) are currently available. A ring for estrogen plus progestin therapy is in development. Transdermal patches with estrogen and progestin are available for contraception (Ortho Evra) and estrogen plus progestogen therapy (CombiPatch, Climara Pro). Transdermal progestin delivery via a gel and a spray are under investigation.[45,46]

Progestin Benefits

Progestins have several well-recognized benefits. Contraceptives containing progestins either exclusively or in combination with estrogen are highly effective agents. The progestin is theorized to inhibit ovulation and promote thickening of cervical mucus. Progestins have a powerful influence on the endometrium, including transformation of the endometrium to a secretory type, thus decreasing the risk of endometrial hyperplasia and ultimately endometrial cancer. These agents also can help stabilize the endometrium for treatment of abnormal uterine bleeding.

Side Effects/Adverse Effects

Side effects of progestins often include a wide variety of symptoms including abnormalities of menstruation (breakthrough bleeding, amenorrhea), weight gain or loss, breast tenderness, and somnolence, among others. The cluster of symptoms of edema, breast tenderness, mild depression, and somnolence often are described as premenstrual-like and may contribute to women self-discontinuing therapy. There are many anecdotal reports of clinicians caring for women for whom they have prescribed both estrogens and progestins for vasomotor symptoms of menopause, only to find women choosing to take estrogen only.

Certain progestins contain oils that may be allergy provoking for women. These include vaginal gels (Crinone, Prochieve) that contain palm oil; capsules (Prometrium) that contain peanut oil, and progestin injectables containing sesame oil.

Thromboembolic Events

Initially it was theorized that estrogen in combination oral contraceptives accounted for the increased risk of deep vein thrombosis and other thromboembolic events. This theory was further supported when DVT rates decreased directly with decreases in estrogen dose. However, with the advent of new COCs in the 1990s, there appeared to be a disparity in risk of DVT regardless of the same dose and type of estrogen between those using older and newer types of progestins, especially among women at inheritable risk. It has been proposed that progesterone tends to inhibit the thrombotic activity of estrogen; however, the third-generation progestins do so less efficiently, especially for women with Factor V Leiden.[47] Women taking estrogen-progestin therapy for contraception, abnormal uterine bleeding, menopausal symptoms, or other reasons should be counseled about this potential adverse effect. Reproductive-aged women should be reassured that these risks are still lower than the risk of DVT during pregnancy.

Cardiovascular Risks

Several progestins, including the gonanes, estranes, and MPA, have been reported to increase LDL levels and may slightly decrease HDL levels, although micronized progesterone has not been found to affect lipid levels to any significant degree.[34] The relationship of estrogen and progestin for the heart health of mature women and risk of subsequent cardiac events continues to be explored and is discussed in Chapter 34.

Progestins and Breast Cancer

Estrogen was first associated with breast cancer, and this association continues even today in the minds of most women. However, additional studies have called into question the role of progestins in association with the disease.[48] As with estrogen, progestins clearly are not a simple etiological agent for the disease. However, it is known that progesterone has major effects on the normal breast. As mentioned in the section discussing estrogen, the Women's Health Initiative found that women taking both estrogen and progestin experienced a small but significant increase in breast cancer. Postmenopausal mammograms have been reported to be more difficult to read for women taking progestins.[49] Therefore, the role of progestins and breast cancer continues to be an enigma, but since breast cancer is an area of intense scrutiny today, answers are hopefully coming in the near future.

Progestins and Bone

As with many other areas of progestins, controversy exists concerning the relationship between progestins and bone development. In the late 1990s, studies emerged suggesting that long-term use of the contraceptive injection medroxyprogesterone acetate in oil (Depo Provera or DMPA) by adolescents was of question based on decreased bone density. Conversely, studies of postmenopausal women using estrogen alone or estrogen and progesterone tended to demonstrate bone protection. Recent studies have indicated that progestins appear to be extensively metabolized in osteoblasts and involved with progesterone receptors in bone.[50] Until more information is available, it is generally advised that progestins not be considered for bone protection, and long-term use of depot medroxyprogesterone acetate (DMPA) be prescribed cautiously, particularly for the young woman as well as the perimenopausal woman who is about to experience the most significant loss of bone in her life once menopause occurs.

The Myth of Phytoprogesterones

Unlike phytoestrogens, there are no phytoprogesterones. Although some consumers may think that consumption of certain foods, like Mexican yams, will increase progesterone levels, that concept is a myth. This misconception may have developed based on Marker's work with yams. However, in order to isolate progesterone in food, certain laboratory manipulations are necessary, and the food itself cannot provide progesterone naturally.

Antiprogesterones and Progesterone Receptor Modulators

Mifepristone (Mifeprex, formerly RU486), a derivative of norethindrone, is a progesterone and glucocorticoid antagonist, indicating that it competes for binding to these receptors. Mifepristone usually is an **antiprogestin** but has agonist activity in some situations and is thus a progesterone receptor modulator.[34] Mifepristone currently is approved in the United States for use in conjunction with the prostaglandin analog misoprostol (Cytotec) to terminate pregnancies of gestation less than 50 days' duration. The vast majority of women will have a complete medical abortion following administration of mifepristone and misoprostol; the remainder will require surgical intervention to complete the abortion. Mifepristone also is effective as an emergency contraceptive agent. This pharmacologic agent has potential as a long-term contraceptive and as a treatment for uterine fibroids, endometriosis, steroid-receptive cancers, Cushing's disease, psychotic major depression, and Alzheimer's disease.[46] However, the politics of abortion influence funding for research and the conduct of studies in this area. Onapristone is an antiprogestin that is structurally similar to mifepristone, and there are numerous other selective progesterone receptor modulators under investigation.[46]

Androgens

Although androgens typically are viewed as male hormones, they are also important for women's health. Androgens primarily are produced in the corpus luteum and the adrenal cortex. Androstenedione and dehydroepiandrosterone are weak androgens that are the precursors to testosterone, which is a precursor for estrogen biosynthesis. For the normal woman, testosterone levels decline gradually from a high among women in their 20s, to a nadir during menopause. For women who experience a surgical menopause, levels drop dramatically. Androgens have high binding affinity, so it is estimated that almost 40% of endogenous testosterone is bound to SHBG and approximately 60% is bound to albumin, leaving 2% or less in the female circulation.[51]

Androgens are reported to affect women's sexual desire, muscle mass and strength, hair, bone mineral density, adipose tissue distribution, energy, and psychological well-being.[13] Exogenous androgenic agents are available, although they are less commonly used in clinical practice than the estrogens and progestins discussed earlier in this chapter. As with estrogens and progestins, receptor-mediated activity appears to be the major mechanism of action for androgens. Androgens penetrate cell membranes of the target cell and bind to androgen receptors located in the cytoplasm.

The primary indication for prescribing androgens is in the area of sexual well-being of the mature woman. After menopause, some women report that they not only have a lower libido, but that they are less responsive sexually. In addition, some women can experience fatigue and general lack of muscle strength in addition to lack of sex drive. The agents that are suggested for women with these symptoms include estrogen with testosterone. Several preparations exist, including Estratest, Estratest HS, and Premarin with methyltestosterone. Methylation of testosterone enables it to be orally ingested and allows it to be changed to estrogen more slowly than testosterone alone.[52,53] Use of testosterone for the mature woman is controversial and is discussed in more detail in Chapter 33.[54]

A weak androgen, danazol (Danocrine), may be used in the treatment of endometriosis. Endometriosis is a condition wherein portions of the endometrium grow outside of the uterus. These danazol implants have been found to have androgen receptors. The use of danazol (Danocrine) is discussed in Chapter 30.

Benefits of Androgens

Some studies have suggested that androgens may successfully be used to treat women with hot flashes of menopause, but strong evidence is lacking.[55] Although not FDA indicated for bone protection, estrogen and testosterone have been found to increase bone density, even when compared to estrogen alone.[56]

Side Effects/Adverse Effects

Side effects of testosterone include acne, alopecia, edema, a deepened voice, enlarged clitoris, irregular menses, and hirsutism. Serious adverse effects in some studies have included increased LDL/decreased HDL cholesterol levels. High doses of testosterone have been associated with liver cancer. The relationship between breast cancer and androgenic therapy is unknown, although most breast cancer tumors have androgen receptors. Testosterone is the prototype drug for anabolic steroids, a category of drugs of potential abuse, especially in the area of weight training and bodybuilding.

Bioidentical Compounds

Bioidentical hormones are compounds with the same chemical and structure as hormones produced in the body.[57] Although it is possible to formulate a bioidentical version of any hormone, this discussion is limited to bioidentical estrogen, progesterone, and testosterone. Advocates for bioidentical hormones believe that these products are natural, safer, and more effective than synthesized hormones, despite the lack of evidence to support this assertion.[58]

There are some FDA-approved bioidentical agents, including 17β-estradiol products (Table 14-3) and natural progesterone formulations including oral capsules (Prometrium), vaginal gels (Crinone and Prochieve), a vaginal insert (Endometrin), and an intramuscular injection (Progesterone).[18,40] However, usually when the term *bioidentical hormone* is used in relation to a sex steroid hormone agent, it most often indicates products formulated by compounding pharmacies. It is common for these products to be customized based on saliva or blood tests of endogenous hormone levels. However, evidence of efficacy for these formulations is currently lacking. Compounded bioidentical hormones are not monitored by the FDA for dosage and purity, and inconsistencies have been found for both.

The position of the Endocrine Society, which is endorsed by the North American Menopause Society, is that the public is receiving potentially misleading or false information about the benefits and risks of bioidentical hormones. They recommend that all hormones—bioidentical and synthetic—be regulated and overseen by the FDA.[57] In 2008, the FDA sent letters to seven pharmacies warning them that their claims about their bioidentical hormone products are unsupported by current evidence and considered false and misleading by the agency.[59]

■ Conclusion

Although estrogens, progesterones, and androgens first were isolated less than a century ago, their use in women's health care today is ubiquitous. Moreover, use of hormone therapy in the future will likely continue to expand as new agents are developed or designed through increased understanding of selective estrogen receptor modulators, selective estrogen enzyme modulators, and progesterone receptor modulators. These new designer drugs will promote therapeutic effects with decreasing risks associated with endogenous hormones. Simultaneously, additional studies are likely to add to knowledge about other naturally occurring hormones such as phytoestrogens and xenoestrogens.

References

1. Kreeger KY. The rhythms that bind women. Scientist 2001;15(15):20.

2. Speroff L, Fritz MA. Clinical gynecologic endocrinology and infertility, 7th ed. Philadelphia, PA: Lippincott Williams & Wilkins, 2005.

3. Sneader W. Drug discovery: a history. New York: John Wiley and Sons, 2005.

4. Lehmann PA. Early history of steroid chemistry in Mexico: the story of three remarkable men. Steroids 1992;57(8):403–8.

5. O'Dowd MJ. The history of medications for women: materia medica woman. New York: Parthenon Publisher, 2001.

6. Likis FE. Contraceptive applications of estrogen. J Midwifery Womens Health 2002;47(3):139–56.

7. Dahlman-Wright K, Cavailles V, Fuqua SA, Jordan VC, Katzenellenbogen JA, Korach KS, et al. International Union of Pharmacology. LXIV. Estrogen receptors. Pharmacol Rev 2006;58(4):773–81.

8. Food and Drug Administration, Center for Drug Evaluation and Research. FDA statement on generic Premarin. 1997. Available from: *www.fda.gov/cder/news/cepressrelease.htm* [Accessed February 16, 2008].

9. Chrousos GP. The gonadal hormones & inhibitors. In Katzung BG, ed. Basic & clinical pharmacology, 10th ed. New York: McGraw-Hill, 2007:653–82.

10. US Food and Drug Administration, Center for Drug Evaluation and Research. Electronic orange book: approved drug products with therapeutic equivalence evaluations, 2007. Available from: *www.fda.gov/cder/ob/default.htm* [Accessed August 10, 2007].

11. Morani A, Warner M, Gustafsson JA. Biological functions and clinical implications of oestrogen receptors alfa and beta in epithelial tissues. J Intern Med 2008;264(2):128–42.

12. North American Menopause Society. Estrogen and progestogen use in peri- and postmenopausal women: March 2007 position statement of the North American Menopause Society. Menopause 2007;14(2):168–82.

13. North American Menopause Society. Menopause practice: a clinician's guide, 3rd ed. Cleveland, OH: North American Menopause Society, 2007.

14. Ruggiero RJ, Likis FE. Estrogen: physiology, pharmacology, and formulations for replacement therapy. J Midwifery Womens Health 2002;47(3):130–8.

15. Schorge J, Schaffer J, Halvorson L, Hoffman B, Bradshaw K, Cunningham FG. In William's gynecology. Polycystic ovarian syndrome and hyperandrogenism. New York: McGraw Hill, 2008:383–401.

16. Centers for Disease Control and Prevention. DES update home: for consumers, health care providers, and DES update partners. 2008. Available from: *www.cdc.gov/DES/index.html* [Accessed March 1, 2008].

17. Buster JE, Koltun WD, Pascual ML, Day WW, Peterson C. Low-dose estradiol spray to treat vasomotor symptoms: a randomized controlled trial. Obstet Gynecol 2008;111(6):1343–51.

18. ESHRE Capri Workshop Group. Hormones and cardiovascular health in women. Hum Reprod Update 2006;12(5):483–97.

19. Rossouw JE, Anderson GL, Prentice RL, LaCroix AZ, Kooperberg C, Stefanick ML, et al., writing group for the Women's Health Initiative Investigators. Risks and benefits of estrogen plus progestin in healthy postmenopausal women: principal results from the Women's Health Initiative randomized controlled trial. JAMA 2002;288(3):321–33.

20. Stefanick ML, Anderson GL, Margolis KL, Hendrix SL, Rodabough RJ, Paskett ED, et al. Effects of conjugated equine estrogens on breast cancer and mammography screening in postmenopausal women with hysterectomy. JAMA 2006;295:1647–57.

21. Chlebowski RT, Kuller L, Anderson G, Mason JA, Schenken R, Rajkovic A, et al. Breast cancer after stopping estrogen plus progestin in postmenopausal women. Presented at: The Women's Health Initiative 31st Annual San Antonio Breast Cancer Symposium (SABCS); December 12, 2008. Abstract 64.

22. Neves-E-Castro M. Association of ovarian cancers with postmenopausal hormonal treatments. Clin Obstet Gynecol 2008;51(3):607–17.

23. Westhoff CL. Oral contraceptives and thrombosis. Am J Obstet Gyncol 1998;179:S38.

24. Cole JA, Norman H, Doherty M, Walker AM. Venous thromboembolism, myocardial infarction and stroke among transdermal contraceptive system users. Obstet Gynecol 2007;109:333–46.

25. Krebs EE, Ensrud KE, MacDonald R, Wilt TJ. Phytoestrogens for treatment of menopausal symptoms: a systematic review. Obstet Gynecol 2004;104(4):824–36.

26. Reynolds K, Chin A, Lees KA, Nguyen A, Bujnowski D, He J. A meta-analysis of the effect of soy protein supplementation on serum lipids. Am J Cardiol 2006;98(5):633–40.

27. Dewell A, Hollenbeck PL, Hollenbeck CB. Clinical review: a critical evaluation of the role of soy protein and isoflavone supplementation in the control of plasma cholesterol concentrations. J Clin Endocrinol Metab 2006;91(3):772–80.

28. Singleton DW, Khan SA. Xenoestrogen exposure and mechanisms of endocrine disruption. Front Biosci 2003;8:s110–8.

29. Practice Committee of the American Society for Reproductive Medicine. Use of clomiphene citrate in women. Fertil Steril November 2006;86(suppl 5): S187–93.

30. US Food and Drug Administration. Center for Drug Evaluation and Research. 2007. Available from: *www .fda.gov/cder/index.html* [Accessed August 9, 2007].

31. Thomson Healthcare. PDR.net. 2007. Available from: *http://pdr.net* [Accessed August 9, 2007].

32. Vogel VG, Costantino JP, Wickerham DL, Cronin WM, Cecchini RS, Atkins JN, et al. Effects of tamoxifen vs raloxifene on the risk of developing invasive breast cancer and other disease outcomes: the NSABP Study of Tamoxifen and Raloxifene (STAR) P-2 trial. JAMA 2006;295(23):2727–41.

33. Cummings SR, Ettinger B, Delmas PD, Kenemans P, Stathopoulos V, Verweij P, et al., LIFT trial investigators. The effects of tibolone in older postmenopausal women. N Engl J Med 2008;359(7):697–708.

34. Loose DS, Stancel GM. Estrogens and progestins. In Brunton LL, Lazo JS, Parker KL, eds. Goodman & Gilman's the pharmacological basis of therapeutics, 11th ed. New York: McGraw-Hill, 2006: 1541–72.

35. Haas DM, Ramsey PS. Progestogen for preventing miscarriage. Cochrane Database of Systematic Reviews 2008, Issue 2. Art No: CD003511. DOI: 10.1002/14651858.CD003511.pub2.

36. Meis PJ, Kebanoff M, Thom E, Dombrowski MP, Sibai B, Moawad AH, et al., for the National Institute of Child Health and Human Development Maternal–Fetal Medicine Units Network. Prevention of recurrent preterm delivery by 17 alpha-hydroxy-progesterone caproate. New Eng J Med 2003;348: 2379–85.

37. Dodd JM, Flenady V, Cincotta R, Crowther CA. Prenatal administration of progesterone for preventing preterm birth. Cochrane Database of Systematic Reviews 2006, Issue 1. Art No: CD004947. DOI: 10.1002/14651858.CD004947.pub2.

38. Ford O, Lethaby A, Mol B, Roberts H. Progesterone for premenstrual syndrome. Cochrane Database of Systematic Reviews 2006, Issue 4. Art No: CD003415. DOI: 10.1002/14651858.CD003415.pub2.

39. Speroff L, Darney PD. A clinical guide for contraception. Philadelphia, PA: Lippincott Williams & Wilkins, 2005:92.

40. North American Menopause Society. Hormone products for postmenopausal use in the United States and Canada. June 2007. Available from: *www .menopause.org/edumaterials/htcharts.pdf* [Accessed August 1, 2007].

41. Simon JA. Exogenous progestogens through the life cycle: with a focus on their role in secondary amenorrhea and menopause. Women's Health Care: Pract J Nurse Pract 2007;6(4):7–12.

42. Foidart J. Added benefits of drospirenone for compliance. Climacteric 2005;8(3):28–34.

43. Stanczyk FZ. All progestins are not created equal. Steroids 2003;68(10–13):879–90.

44. Wallach M, Grimes DA. Modern oral contraception. Totowa, NJ: Emron, 2000.

45. Sitruk-Ware R. Routes of delivery for progesterone and progestins. Maturitas 2007;57(1):77–80.

46. Chabbert-Buffet N, Meduri G, Bouchard P, Spitz IM. Selective progesterone receptor modulators and progesterone antagonists: mechanisms of action and clinical applications. Hum Reprod Update 2005;11(3): 293–307.

47. Kemmeren JM, Algra A, Meijers JC, Bouma BN, Grobbee DE. Effects of second and third generation oral contraceptives and their respective progestogens on the coagulation system in the absence or presence of the factor V Leiden mutation. Thromb Haemost 2002;87(2):199–205.

48. Lange CA, Yee D. Progesterone and breast cancer. Womens Health (London, England) 2008;4(2):151–62.

49. Warren R. Hormones and mammographic breast density. Maturitas 2004;49(1):67–78.

50. Quinkler M, Kaur K, Hewison M, Stewart PM, Cooper MS. Progesterone is extensively metabolized in osteoblasts: implications for progesterone action on bone. Horm Metab Res 2008;40(10):679–84.

51. Snyder PJ. Androgens. In Brunton LL, Lazo JS, Parker KL, eds. Goodman & Gilman's the pharmacological basis of therapeutics, 11th ed. New York: McGraw-Hill, 2006:1573–1586.

52. Shulman LP. Androgens and menopause: more fuel for the fire. Menopause 2006;13(2):168–70.

53. Penteado SR, Fonseca AM, Bagnoli VR, Abdo CH, Junior JM, Baracat EC. Effects of the addition of methyltestosterone to combined hormone therapy with estrogens and progestogens on sexual energy and on orgasm in postmenopausal women. Climacteric 2008;11(1):17–25.

54. Somboonporn W, Davis S, Seif MW, Bell R. Testosterone for peri-and postmenopausal women. Cochrane Database Syst Rev. 2005;9(4):CD004509.

55. Watts NB, Notelovitz M, Timmons MC, Addison WA, Wiita B, Downey LJ. Comparison of oral estrogens and estrogens plus androgen on bone mineral density, menopausal symptoms, and lipid-lipoprotein profiles in surgical menopause. Obstet Gynecol 1995;85:529–37.

56. Davis SR, McCloud PI, Strauss BJG, Burger HG. Testosterone enhances estradiol's effects on post-menopausal bone density and sexuality. Maturitas 1995;21:227–36.

57. The Endocrine Society. Bioidentical hormones position statement. October 2006. Available from: *www.menopause.org/bioidenticalHT_Endosoc.pdf* [Accessed August 10, 2007].

58. Cirigliano M. Bioidentical hormone therapy: a review of the evidence. J Womens Health 2007;16(5):600–31.

59. US Food and Drug Administration, Center for Drug Evaluation and Research. FDA takes action against compounded menopause hormone therapy drugs. 2008. Available from: *www.fda.gov/bbs/topics/NEWS/2008/NEW01772.html* [Accessed March 1, 2008].

IV
Pharmacotherapeutics for Common Conditions

Pharmacotherapeutics is the study of effects of drugs in clinical practice. This section on pharmacotherapeutics includes more chapters than the other sections, and here you will find the nuts and bolts of pharmacologic management for common medical conditions. This section starts with "Cardiovascular Conditions," which are the number one killer of women today. "Hematology" discusses such problems as anemia and venous thromboemboli. Multiple sclerosis, lupus, and other conditions often occur more frequently among women than among men, and these disorders are addressed in the chapter "Autoimmune Conditions." The next chapter, "Diabetes," discusses the disease of the same name, whose incidence is frequently increasing and whose pharmacologic repertoire for treatment similarly is growing.

The chapter titled "Thyroid Disorders" examines another condition that is more common among women than men, and one that requires close monitoring for appropriate treatment. "Respiratory Conditions" includes treatments of mild allergic responses to potentially severe pneumonias. "Gastrointestinal Conditions" encompasses treatments for women who experience difficulty with the alimentary tract, from heartburn to constipation. "Lower Urinary Tract Disorders" includes infections as well as incontinence. Professionals who care for women are often presented with challenges addressed in the next chapter, "Sexually Transmitted Infections."

The central nervous system plays an important role in health and disease. The chapter, "Drugs and the Central Nervous System," starts with a basic review of the anatomy and function of the central nervous system, followed by a review of pharmacologic management of epilepsy, Parkinson's disease, and Alzheimer's disease, among others. Psychotropic drugs, antianxiety drugs, and other drugs used to promote mental health are evaluated in the chapter "Mental Health."

"Dermatology" includes a discussion of the expected topical agents for acne and other skin blemishes. This chapter also includes a discussion of a new area of dermatology—cosmeceuticals. "Otic and Ophthalmic Disorders" reviews agents used for specific conditions in this highly specialized area. The last chapter in this section, "Cancer," acknowledges the importance of chemotherapeutics with an overview of chemotherapy.

Many of these chapters present an overview of drugs that are not commonly initiated by primary care providers. For example, chemotherapeutics are the purview of the oncology team. However, it is common that women continue to seek concomitant care with their trusted healthcare professional and may seek help for some of the side effects of the anticarcinogenic agents. Certainly such women will be likely to return for general care after they are deemed cancer survivors. Similarly, women with lupus may initially be diagnosed and treated by specialists, but continuing care often occurs in a primary care site. Thus, an individual scope of practice may be broader or more limited, yet basic information necessary for the primary care provider can be found in these chapters.

"Not all those who know their minds know their hearts as well."

La Rochefoucauld

15
Cardiovascular Conditions

Angela R. Mitchell and
Tekoa L. King

Chapter Glossary

α₁-Receptor antagonists Class of drugs that act as antagonists when bound to the alpha adrenergic receptors located on vascular smooth muscle. Most are competitive antagonists to norepinephrine.

Adrenergic receptors Class of G protein-coupled receptors that are the targets for catecholamines norepinephrine and epinephrine.

Adult Treatment Panel III (ATP III) Treatment guidelines for high levels of serum cholesterol from National Cholesterol Education Program Adult Treatment Panel III published in 2002.

Angiotensin I Formed by the action of renin on angiotensinogen, which is constitutively present in plasma. Angiotensin I has no biologic activity. It is the precursor of angiotensin II, which is biologically active.

Angiotensin II A peptide hormone that causes increased blood pressure via vasoconstriction, release of aldosterone, increased heart muscle contractility, and sympathetic discharge. Angiotensin II is formed from angiotensin I, which is formed from angiotensinogen.

Angiotensin II receptor blockers (ARBs) A class of pharmaceuticals used to treat hypertension. These drugs block the binding of angiotensin II to AT₁ receptors, thereby preventing the agonist effect of angiotensin II.

Angiotensin-converting enzyme inhibitors (ACE inhibitors) A class of pharmaceuticals used to treat hypertension. These drugs prevent the conversion of angiotensin I to angiotensin II.

Atherosclerosis Chronic inflammatory process that occurs in the walls of the arteries and results in atherosclerotic plaques that decrease the diameter of the blood vessel.

Baroreceptor Stretch-sensitive receptors that detect pressure of blood in the arteries. Baroreceptors communicate this detection to the CNS, which regulates peripheral resistance and cardiac output to maintain blood pressure within a narrow range.

Benzodiazepines A class of calcium channel blockers that is both a cardiac depressant and a vasodilator. Example: diltiazem (Cardizem).

Beta-adrenoreceptor antagonists (beta-blockers) A class of pharmaceuticals used to treat hypertension. These drugs bind to beta-adrenergic receptors, thereby blocking the binding of norepinephrine and epinephrine.

Calcium channel blockers A class of pharmaceuticals used to treat hypertension. These drugs prevent calcium from entering muscle cells, which results in muscle relaxation and widening of blood vessels. Also called calcium channel antagonists and calcium channel receptor antagonists.

Catecholamines Hormones derived from tyrosine. Norepinephrine, epinephrine, and dopamine are all catecholamines.

Central α₂-agonists Agents that suppress stimulation of sympathetic discharge in the central nervous system. Also called selective α₂-receptor agonists.

Chronotropic Effect of making the heart rate faster or changing the rhythm.

Dihydropyridines A class of calcium channel blocker that has a selective effect of relaxing the smooth muscle that surrounds arterial vessels. Used to treat hypertension. Example: nifedipine (Procardia).

Direct renin inhibitors A class of pharmaceuticals used to treat hypertension. These drugs inhibit the action of renin.

Diuretic Any drug that increases the amount of urine and causes a diuresis.

Epinephrine A hormone and a neurotransmitter in the sympathetic nervous system. Epinephrine plays a central role in the "flight or fight" stress response by causing increased heart rate, increased stroke volume, increased blood sugar levels, constriction of arterioles in the intestinal tract, and dilation of arterioles in the skeletal muscles. Epinephrine is a nonselective agonist for all adrenergic receptors (both beta and alpha receptors). Also referred to as adrenaline.

Fibrillation Rapid and irregular contraction of the heart muscle that is not synchronized, so the contraction is directional.

High-density lipoprotein (HDL) Lipoprotein–cholesterol complex that transports cholesterol to the liver from peripheral tissue for metabolism and excretion.

Inotropic Effect of strengthening the contraction of the heart muscle.

Low-density lipoprotein (LDL) Lipoprotein-cholesterol complex that transports cholesterol to peripheral tissue.

Negative chronotropic effect Lowering of heart rate via slowing the action potential that controls the rate of contraction in the heart. *Chrono* means time.

Negative inotropic effect Decreasing strength of contraction of the heart muscle.

Norepinephrine Like epinephrine, a hormone and neurotransmitter in initiating the physiologic actions that appear during the flight-or-fight stress response. Norepinephrine increases vascular tone via action as an alpha-adrenergic receptor agonist.

Phenylalanines The class of calcium channel blockers that predominately suppress cardiac function and are used to treat angina. Example: verapamil (Calan).

Reentry circuit An auxiliary electrical conduction circuit in the heart that travels in a circle rather than moving from one end of the heart to the other and then stopping.

Renin-angiotensin-aldosterone system (RAAS) Hormone system that functions as a negative feedback loop to control blood pressure and fluid balance.

Selective α_1-receptor antagonists Class of drugs that block the α_1-receptors peripherally causing decreased peripheral vascular resistance.

Selective α_2-receptor agonists Also called central α_2-agonists. These agents suppress stimulation of sympathetic discharge in the central nervous system.

Sodium chloride symporter An ion pump that removes sodium and chloride ions from the distal convoluted tubule of the kidney.

Statin A class of drugs that inhibit 3-hydroxy-3-methylglutaryl coenzyme A (HMG-CoA) reductase. This enzyme is part of an essential early step in the biosynthesis of cholesterol.

Sympathetic response Also called the "flight or fight" response, the set of physiologic responses to epinephrine and norepinephrine release that prepare the body for physical action. It is initiated when acute stress or danger is perceived.

Torsades de pointes A French term that means "twisting the points," which is used to describe a particular type of ventricular tachycardia that occurs when the QRS complex is altered. *Torsades de pointes* can evolve into ventricular fibrillation, which causes sudden death.

Triglycerides Major components of very-low-density lipoprotein, these are the major storage form of fatty acids, which are used for energy if glucose is not available. High levels of triglycerides in blood increase the risk for cardiovascular events.

Very-low-density lipoprotein (VLDL) Low-density lipoprotein that has given up the cholesterol.

Introduction

Cardiovascular disease (CVD) is the most common cause of death in women in the United States.[1,2] For the purposes of this chapter, the term CVD refers to several diseases including hypertension, hyperlipidemia, coronary heart disease (CHD), angina, heart failure, and peripheral arterial disease. More than 1 in 3 adults residing in the United States has CVD, and one in three persons has multiple forms of CVD.[1] The incidence of a first major cardiovascular event is 7/100 in persons ages 45–54, but it then rises to 68/100 for women older than 85.[1] The prevalence of CVD in women is equivalent to the prevalence in men during the ages of 40–59, but after the age of 60 the prevalence of CVD is greater in women than in men.[2] Treatment of persons with CVD is costly, with direct and indirect costs of CVD estimated at 431.8 billion dollars per year in the United States.[1] This chapter reviews treatments for CVD disorders. There are various degrees of illness associated with this constellation of disorders. The American Heart Association (AHA) outlines the varying levels of risk for CVD (Table 15-1).[3]

Prevention of Cardiovascular Disease

Primary prevention of CVD is an important component of healthcare services offered to women. Evidence-based

Table 15-1 Recommendations for Prevention of Cardiovascular Disease in Women

	Risk Factors	Recommendations
High Risk		

10-year Framingham global risk > 20%*	Established coronary heart disease
	Cerebrovascular disease
	Peripheral artery disease
	Abdominal aortic aneurysm
	End-stage or chronic renal disease
	Diabetes mellitus
		Smoking cessation
		Physical activity/cardiac rehabilitation
		Diet therapy
		Healthy weight
		Blood pressure control
		Cholesterol therapy
		Aspirin therapy
		Beta-blocker therapy
		ACE inhibitor or ARB therapy if ACE inhibitors are
		   contraindicated
		Glycemic control of diabetes
		Evaluate and treat for depression for class IIa
		Omega 3 fatty acid supplementation and folic
		   acid supplementation for class IIb

Intermediate Risk		

Framingham global risk > 10% and < 20%	≥ 1 major risk factor for CVD including cigarette
	   smoking, poor diet, physical inactivity
	Obesity, especially central obesity, family history of
	   premature CVD (CVD < 55 y of age in male relative
	   and < 65 y of age in a female relative)
	Hypertension, dyslipidemia
	Evidence of subclinical vascular disease
	Metabolic syndrome
	Poor exercise capacity on treadmill and/or abnormal
	   heart rate recovery after stopping exercise
		Smoking cessation
		Physical activity
		Heart-healthy diet
		Healthy weight
		Blood pressure control
		Lipid control
		Aspirin therapy for class IIa

Low Risk		
Framingham global risk < 10%	Healthy lifestyle with no risk factors	Smoking cessation Physical activity Heart-healthy diet Healthy weight Treatment of individual risk factors as indicated

* Data from the Framingham Heart Study has been used to develop a risk assessment tool that estimates one's 10-year risk for having a myocardial infarction or coronary death.
Source: Mosca L et al. 2007.[3]

strategies for primary prevention of CVD in women have not been conclusively determined secondary to the lack of research in this area, despite of the fact that more than half the deaths from CVD occur in women.[1] Until recently, most of the studies that evaluated prevention and treatment strategies for CVD included only middle- or older-aged men.[3] However, there has been a recent focus on including women and racial or ethnic minorities in primary prevention studies of CVD,[3] and in 2004, the American Heart Association published evidence-based guidelines for CVD prevention in women.[3]

The first step is to determine one's individual risk for developing CVD. This can be done by using the Framingham Point Score Calculator that estimates the 10-year CHD risk.[3] There are separate prevention strategies recommended for women who are at low risk, intermediate risk, and high risk for developing CVD (Table 15-1).

Lifestyle modification is the cornerstone of any CVD risk-reduction strategy.[4] The Nurses' Health Study demonstrated that women with the following characteristics have a low risk of having a cardiovascular event when compared to women without this exact lifestyle profile (RR = 0.17; 95% CI, 0.07–0.41)[5,6]: (1) do not smoke; (2) have a body mass index (BMI) < 25; (3) drink an average of at least half a drink of alcohol per day; (4) engage in moderate-to-vigorous physical activity for at least half an hour per day; and (5) eat a diet high in cereal fiber, omega 3 fatty acids, and folate, with a high ratio of polyunsaturated to saturated fat and low in trans fat. The study also found that 82% of the recorded coronary events experienced by study participants were attributed to women failing or unable to follow a low-risk CVD lifestyle.[7]

The AHA recommends that women who have a high risk for developing CVD add omega 3 fatty acid supplementation to their diets; however no specific amounts are recommended.[7] Individuals have a 23–32% lower incidence of cardiovascular mortality when they eat diets rich in omega 3 fatty acids such as those in fish and nuts.[8-10] Interestingly, current research does not support the use of antioxidant vitamin supplements to prevent CVD (Chapter 5). Diet changes, absorption, etc., may be a better source of antioxidants than are vitamin supplements.[7] It is also important to remember that it is difficult to attribute the decrease in mortality seen in these dietary studies solely to diet, because often when individuals make one change in their life, they make others that may not be controlled.

Obesity and physical inactivity are additional primary risk factors that are modifiable. There is a known relationship between BMI and development of CVD and other metabolic disorders.[11] When helping individuals with BMIs in the range of 27–35 design a weight loss program, cutting 300–500 calories per day will achieve a 10% weight loss in 6 months. For the person whose BMI is > 35, reducing calories by 500 to 1000 calories per day should achieve a weight loss of 1–2 pounds per week. The Dietary Approaches to Stop Hypertension (DASH) diet has been shown to result in weight loss and decreased blood pressure and cholesterol by focusing on a diet rich in fruits and vegetables, but low in fat.[11,12] More specific information about the DASH diet can be found at the National Heart, Lung and Blood Institute Web site.[13] Sodium intake should be limited to no more than 2.4 grams daily and no more than 1 ounce of alcohol consumption per day.[14]

A healthcare provider cannot address the issue of obesity and increased CVD risk without discussing physical activity. Weight reduction is possible through regular, near-daily aerobic activity of at least 30 minutes' duration. Pharmacologic treatment for weight loss may be of benefit for individuals with BMIs > 30 with no CVD risk factors, and those with BMI > 27 with CVD risk factors. Persons with a BMI > 40 with no CVD risk factor or those with a BMI > 35 with CVD risk factors who have failed medical management may be candidates for surgical treatment.[15]

Other approaches to lifestyle modification are holistic. Reductions in elevated glucose and LDL have also been found through activities such as relaxation, meditation, yoga, breathing exercises, and stress management. These activities decrease the sympathetic responses that cause elevations in glucose and cholesterol levels.

What about that daily dose of aspirin? Although currently recommended, there is controversy about the efficacy of a daily dose of aspirin for the prevention of CVD.[16] Additionally, this story is an excellent example of how gender can affect the effectiveness of specific pharmacologic treatment regimens. A total of 55,580 individuals (11,466 women) in five randomized trials received aspirin therapy and had a 32% reduction in the risk of the first myocardial infarction (MI) and a 15% reduction in the risk of all vascular events.[17] However, subsequent findings from the observational studies of the Women's Health Initiative (WHI) found that there was no risk reduction in recommending daily aspirin therapy for women who are at low risk for CVD. This was demonstrated more definitively by Ridker et al.,[2] who conducted a randomized, controlled trial (n = 39,876 women) wherein they randomized participants to daily aspirin 100 mg or placebo and then followed them for 10 years. Overall, there were 477 major cardiovascular events in the group of women who took aspirin, compared to 522 cardiovascular events in the women who were in the placebo group. A reduction of 9% in CVD was demonstrated, although it was not a statistically significant reduction (RR = 0.91; 95% CI, 0.80–1.03; P = .13).[2] This study did find that 100 mg of aspirin taken daily resulted in a significant reduction in the incidence of cardiovascular events in women who are > 65 years old.[2] However, it cannot be assumed that gender differences exist for other pharmacologic agents. Recent studies suggest that the common treatments for hypertension and hyperlipidemia may benefit men and women alike.[18]

In summary, programs that include counseling, smoking cessation, education, increased physical activity, and dietary modification are most likely to achieve successful lifestyle modification.[19] Even when successful, maintaining the new lifestyle modifications remains a challenge for most individuals. When rigorous lifestyle modifications are insufficient to achieve therapeutic goals within 3–6 months, pharmacotherapy is recommended. Drug therapy is utilized to control hypertension, dyslipidemia, and to reduce morbidity and mortality among women with CVD. When selecting therapy, all of these goals should be considered.

Hypertension

Hypertension is often known as a silent killer since it affects many women without their knowledge. The findings of the Women's Health Initiative found that the prevalence of hypertension increases with age. Twenty-seven percent of women aged 50–59 compared to 53% of women aged 70–79 are diagnosed with hypertension.[6] It was also found that the risk of hypertension increased with African American race, CVD risk factors, BMI > 27.3, inactivity, excess alcohol intake, and history of hyperlipidemia or diabetes. The Women's Health Initiative found that 38% of the women in the study had diagnosed hypertension, yet only 36% of the women with hypertension had blood pressure values in the goal range. Healthcare providers continue to do a poor job of counseling individuals about goal blood pressure levels and prescribing enough agents to obtain goal blood pressure.[1,6] The drugs used to control hypertension each affect one or more steps in several blood pressure regulatory systems. Thus a brief review of those systems is in order.

Physiology of Blood Pressure Control

Arterial blood pressure is the pressure that is exerted on the artery wall. There are two measurements: systolic and diastolic. The difference between these two measurements is referred to as the pulse pressure. Diastole represents two thirds of the cardiac cycle, which is greatly influenced by peripheral resistance, and the remaining cardiac cycle is spent in systole, which is greatly influenced by cardiac output. The mean arterial pressure is the average pressure maintained in the arteries through the entire cardiac cycle. The factors that influence mean arterial pressure include heart rate, stroke volume, and peripheral resistance. Venous blood pressure is determined by the volume present in the vessels and the degree of compliancy of the venous walls.

Several factors are involved in regulating arterial blood pressure, including the renin-angiotensin-aldosterone system (RAAS), the **sympathetic response** of the autonomic nervous system, peripheral autoregulation, and disturbances in electrolytes.

The Renin-Angiotensin-Aldosterone System

The **renin-angiotensin-aldosterone system** (RAAS) is the target of many antihypertensive agents (Figure 15-1). The juxtaglomerular cells in the kidneys produce renin in response to decreased perfusion in the juxtaglomerular system. The production of renin is controlled by several factors, including drop in blood pressure, decrease in sodium in the kidney, and β-adrenergic stimulation. Once renin is produced and is in the circulation, it converts angiotensinogen into angiotensin I. **Angiotensin I**, although active, is converted into **angiotensin II** by angiotensin-converting enzyme (ACE). Angiotensin II can bind to two receptors—AT_1 and AT_2. AT_1 receptors are located throughout the body, including the brain, kidney, myocardium, peripheral vasculature, and adrenal glands. AT_2 receptors are located in the adrenal medullary, uterus,

and brain and have no impact on blood pressure. Angiotensin II causes blood pressure elevation through potent vasoconstriction via stimulation of **catecholamines** and activation of the central sympathetic nervous system. Angiotensin-converting enzyme also stimulates the production of aldosterone, which stimulates more sodium reabsorption in the kidney. The increased sodium reabsorption leads to a decreased production of renin, which becomes the final link in the negative feedback loop that controls blood pressure in the glomerulus. Angiotensin II is converted to angiotensin III within the adrenal gland, and both angiotensin II and angiotensin III stimulate aldosterone production. This cascade of events is a sophisticated hormonal system that affects peripheral vascular resistance and blood pressure.

Arterial blood pressure is also controlled by the central and autonomic nervous systems. **Norepinephrine** and **epinephrine** are the primary neurotransmitters in the sympathetic nervous system, and receptors for these hormones, called **adrenergic receptors**, are located in most organs. Adrenergic receptor stimulation in the smooth muscle that encases arteries and veins, for example, causes vasoconstriction or vasodilation. There are two subtypes of adrenergic receptors, α and β. These receptors are further subdivided into α_1, α_2, and three β subtypes. α_1-Receptors mediate contraction of arterial and venous smooth muscle causing vasoconstriction or vasodilation. α_2-Receptors suppress release of norepinephrine presynaptically, thereby inhibiting the sympathetic response. β-Receptors are located in skeletal muscle, heart, liver, adrenal gland, blood vessels, and lungs. There are two major subtypes of β-receptors, β_1 and β_2, and a third type, β_3, that stimulates lipolysis in adipose tissue that will not be discussed here. Cardiovascular structures typically have more β- than α-receptors. The β_1-receptors are concentrated in the cardiac muscle, conduction nodes, and kidney, whereas β_2-receptors are located in the lungs, liver, pancreas, and coronary arterioles.

In general, catecholamine binding to the α-receptor results in stimulation and catecholamine binding to the β-receptor results in relaxation. Stimulation of α_1-receptors located in arterioles and venules results in vasoconstriction, whereas stimulation of β_2-receptors in the arterioles and venules causes vasodilation. Stimulation of β_1-receptors in the heart causes increased heart rate and increased contractility.

Another player in blood pressure regulation is the **baroreceptor** reflex that originates in the aortic arch. The baroreceptors are nerve endings in the wall of the artery that sense when there is a change in pressure. When the pressure drops, the baroreceptor initiates a release of norepinephrine

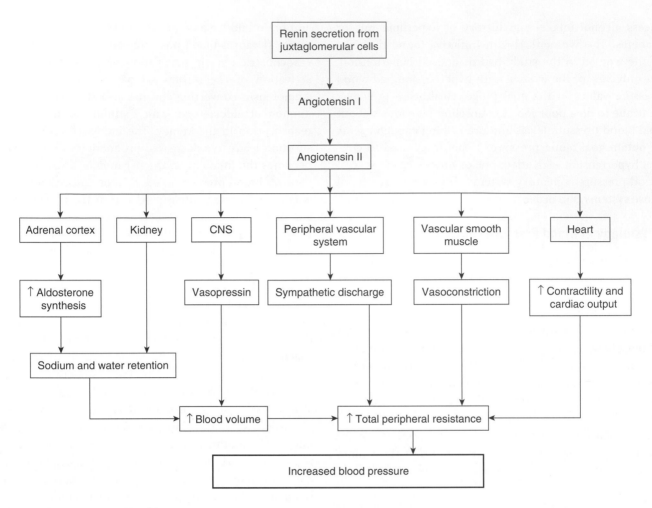

Figure 15-1 Renin-angiotensin-aldosterone system.

that then binds to β_1-receptors in the heart, which causes a subsequent rise in heart rate and contractility.

Diagnosis of Hypertension

Hypertension is diagnosed when systolic arterial blood pressure is ≥ 140 mm Hg or the diastolic blood pressure is ≥ 90 mm Hg on three separate occasions.[20] Hypertension can be described as primary or secondary. Primary hypertension is also known as essential or idiopathic, because there is no clear etiology. Secondary hypertension is caused by a primary disease of the kidney, adrenal gland, thyroid gland, coarctation of the aorta, and drugs such as combined oral contraceptives, estrogen, corticosteroids, sympathetic stimulants, appetite suppressants, antihistamines, and monoamine oxidase inhibitors. The majority of individuals with the diagnosis of hypertension have primary hypertension.

The seventh report from the Joint National Committee (JNC 7) summarizes the current guidelines for the prevention, detection, evaluation, and treatment of hypertension.[20] JNC 7 lists new staging of hypertension, including a category for prehypertension, stage 1 hypertension, and stage 2 hypertension, all of which are defined in Table 15-2. Pharmacologic treatment should be offered if blood pressure values are consistently elevated and lifestyle modification has had no impact. Lifestyle and pharmacologic treatment should be initiated immediately if a person has end organ damage secondary to elevated blood pressure.

Treatment of Hypertension

The treatment goal for persons with hypertension is to decrease the risk of cardiovascular disease.[20] The primary focus of treatment is control of systolic blood pressure. Once systolic blood pressure control is achieved, it is likely that diastolic blood pressure also will be in the normal range. A goal blood pressure of < 140/90 mm Hg is appropriate for most persons; however, individuals with comorbid

Table 15-2 Classification and Management of Blood Pressure in Adults*

Blood Pressure Classification	Systolic Blood Pressure mm Hg		Diastolic Blood Pressure mm Hg	Lifestyle Modifications	Initial Drug Therapy for Persons Without Compelling Indication	Initial Drug Therapy for Persons with Compelling Indications
Normal	< 120	and	< 80	Encourage	No antihypertensive drugs indicated.	Drugs for compelling indications.‡
Prehypertension	120–139	or	80–89	Yes	No antihypertensive drugs indicated.	
Stage 1 hypertension	140–159	or	90–99	Yes	Thiazide-type diuretics for most. May consider ACEI, ARB, BB, CCB, or combination.	Drugs for compelling indications.‡ Other hypertensive drugs such as diuretics, ACEI, ARB, BB, CCB as needed.
Stage 2 hypertension	≥ 160	or	≥ 100	Yes	Two-drug combination for most,† which is usually thiazide-type diuretic and ACEI, ARB, BB, or CCB.	

ACEI = angiotensin-converting enzyme inhibitors; ARB = angiotensin receptor blockers; BB = beta-blockers; CCB = calcium channel blockers.
* Treatment determined by highest blood pressure category.
† Initial combination therapy should be used cautiously in persons at risk for orthostatic hypotension.
‡ Treat persons with chronic kidney disease or diabetes to a blood pressure goal of ≤130/80 mm Hg.
Source: National Heart, Lung, and Blood Institute 2004.[20]

Box 15-1 Regular Follow-up Visit for Diabetes and Hypertension

SW is a 53-year-old White female presenting for routine follow-up care for her diabetes, hyperlipidemia, hypertension, coronary artery disease, and depression. SW had a myocardial infarction 2 years ago. She is able to manage her medications; however, she struggles with her diet and exercise regimens. She successfully quit smoking 6 months ago. She has been checking her glucose and blood pressure routinely and brings her log book with her to the visit. Her glucose has been controlled well as evidenced by a hemoglobin A1c of 6.8 mg/dL at her last visit, as well as her LDL of 75 mg/dL, HDL of 46 mg/dL, and triglycerides of 110 mg/dL. Her blood pressure recordings from her log book are 142/89, 138/92, 145/88, and 135/83. Over the past few visits, her blood pressure readings have been elevating. Today her vital signs are height 5′ 5″ (161.1 cm), weight 220 lbs (99.8 kg), blood pressure 140/90, heart rate 82, respirations 17, and pulse oximetry 98%. Current medications include metformin (Glucophage) 1000 mg bid, ASA 81 mg daily, exenatide (Byetta) 5 mcg SQ bid, metoprolol succinate (Toprol XL) 50 mg daily, sertraline (Zoloft) 100 mg daily, atorvastatin (Lipitor) 20 mg daily, and HCTZ (HydroDiuril) 25 mg daily. She has no problems to report. Her physical exam is unremarkable.

SW is considered a high-risk patient given her history of coronary artery disease and diabetes. She has taken some steps to reduce her risk based on quitting smoking and tight control of her diabetes and lipids. When initially diagnosed, she would have been counseled about her diet and need for exercise. Providing her with practical ideas and tips on how to start making change may be helpful. Her blood pressure goal should be less than 130/80. Previously her blood pressure was controlled well on the above agents. She has a compelling indication for metoprolol succinate (Toprol XR) because of her previous myocardial infarction. Thiazide diuretics have been shown to be beneficial in risk reduction. However, she is not at her goal and ACE inhibitors are preferred for persons with type 2 diabetes. She would benefit from the addition of an ACE inhibitor, and it can be given in combination with HCTZ. A reduction in the HCTZ may need to be done in the initialization of the ACE inhibitor because of the synergist effect of the medications. If she develops a troublesome cough that is interfering with her daily activities, a change to an ARB would be recommended.

---

conditions such as diabetes or chronic kidney disease will require a more aggressive goal of < 130/80 mm Hg. It is important to note that with every increase of 20/10 mm Hg increments, the risk for developing CVD doubles.[20] The greater the reduction in blood pressure, the greater the reductions in the subsequent incidence of CVD and renal disease[2,7] (Box 15-1).

Pharmacologic Treatments for Hypertension

The goal of antihypertensive therapy is to protect target organs such as the heart and kidney. The major categories of antihypertensive drugs include **diuretics**; **angiotensin-**

converting enzyme inhibitors (ACE inhibitors); **beta-adrenoreceptor antagonists**, also called **beta-blockers**; **angiotensin II receptor blockers** (ARBs); calcium channel antagonists, also called **calcium channel blockers** (CCBs); **direct renin inhibitors** (DRIs); vasodilators; **α₁-receptor**

antagonists; and **selective α₂-receptor agonists**, also called **central α₂-agonists**. Figure 15-2 presents JNC 7's algorithm for the treatment of hypertension.[20]

Historically, pharmacologic management of hypertension used a stepwise progression, starting with one drug

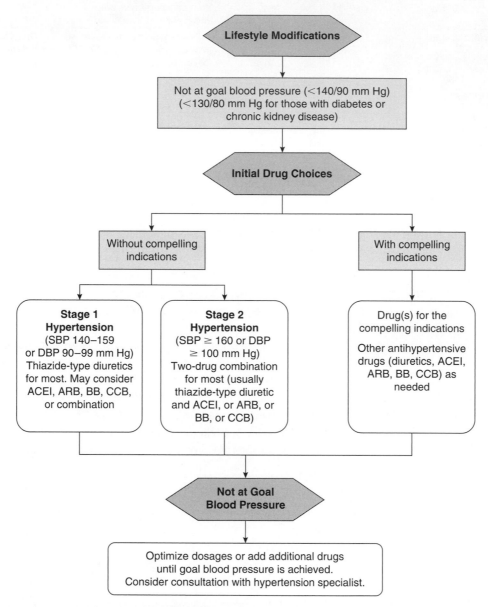

SBP = systolic blood pressure; DBP = diastolic blood pressure; ACE = angiotensin converting enzyme inhibitor; ARB = angiotensin receptor blocker; BB = beta-blocker; CCB = calcium channel blocker.

Compelling indications are comorbid conditions such as ischemic heart disease, heart failure, postmyocardial infarction, high risk for coronary artery disease, chronic kidney disease, diabetes, and history of stroke. When these conditions are present, a specific class of drugs is indicated to treat the comorbid condition, which needs to be addressed concomitantly with drugs used to treat hypertension.[21]

Figure 15-2 Joint National Committee on Prevention, Detection, Evaluation, and Treatment of High Blood Pressure (JNC 7) algorithm for hypertension treatment. *Source:* National Heart, Lung, and Blood Institute 2004.[20]

(usually beta-blockers) and then adding other agents until the blood pressure goal was reached. However, there have been many trials comparing the efficacy of these different types of drugs, and to date, there is no clear advantage of any one of them for initial therapy. That said, individual characteristics such as race, ethnicity, and age affect responses to specific classes of antihypertensives. For example, the calcium channel blockers appear to work best in persons who are African American, whereas ACE inhibitors work best for young White males. Knowledge of these different efficacy profiles will help prescribers choose the best hypertensive agent for individual patients.

Overall, thiazides are recommended as the first choice for treating persons with stage 1 hypertension because they are consistently superior or equal to all other classes of drugs in decreasing the incidence of cardiovascular complications of hypertension; they are generally well tolerated and the least expensive.[20] However, clinical trials have shown that many individuals benefit from specific combinations of antihypertensive drugs, even during initial management depending on the risk factors for CVD present at the onset of therapy.[3] Two thirds of individuals with hypertension require more than one drug to obtain a goal blood pressure.[3,21,22] When an individual has a blood pressure of > 20 mm Hg above the systolic goal or > 10 mm Hg above the diastolic goal, a second agent is indicated, which can be prescribed as an additional agent or in a fixed combination formulation.

It is important to note that individuals who have hypertension in addition to comorbid conditions require initial therapy with specific classes of drugs. Healthcare providers caring for persons who have both hypertension and comorbid medical conditions are referred to the JNC 7 guidelines for a summary of the recommended pharmacologic treatments.[20]

When initially prescribing antihypertensives, vigilance and follow-up are necessary. The most common reason for discontinuing antihypertensive therapy is the development of side effects that adversely affect quality of life. For example, beta-blockers can cause impotence; ACE inhibitors can cause a persistent, dry cough; and calcium channel blockers are associated with headaches, flushing, and edema.

Each of the classes of drugs discussed in this section has a different mechanism of action. Beta-blockers affect the adrenergic response. Thiazides stimulate the RAAS, whereas ACE inhibitors suppress it. Because the RAAS is physiologically intertwined with the actions of insulin, there is a specific concern regarding the effect of antihypertensive medications on diabetes.

Antihypertensives and New Onset Diabetes

Persons with hypertension have an increased incidence of diabetes when compared to persons who are normotensive. Observational studies and randomized, controlled trials that have compared the efficacy of different classes of antihypertensive medication have consistently noted that beta-blockers and thiazides increase the risk for developing new onset diabetes. Because diabetes incurs an independent increased risk for cardiovascular complications, there is concern that this side effect of these two types of antihypertensive agents could abrogate the benefits associated with their use. However, none of the studies conducted have found that beta-blockers and thiazides are associated with more cardiovascular complications. So, should prescribers (1) ignore this metabolic complication; (2) prescribe these two types of antihypertensives only to individuals who have a high risk for cardiovascular problems already and who therefore need the lowered blood pressure as a priority; or (3) avoid use of these two types of medication? Although the answer to these questions is not totally resolved, to date, the recommendation is that thiazides and beta-blockers continue to be employed as recommended by the JNC 7 guidelines, which means thiazides are still the recommended first-line treatment, and beta-blockers are recommended as a choice for the second agent.

Drug–Drug Interactions with Antihypertensives

There are a few drug interactions that affect all classes of antihypertensives. NSAIDs inhibit vasodilation, and they also promote salt and water retention. Thus, NSAIDs can interfere or reverse the antihypertensive effect of these drugs. Vasoconstricting agents in over-the-counter (OTC) cold remedies and nasal vasodilators also found in OTC preparations can also increase blood pressure. OTC drugs that increase blood pressure should be discussed with the individual when a prescription is given for an antihypertensive agent.

There are also some drugs given for indications other than hypertension that will increase or decrease blood pressure as an additive effect with the antihypertensive medication or as a counter to it. Tricyclic antidepressants can lower blood pressure, and when taken concomitantly with antihypertensives, nocturnal or orthostatic hypotension can occur. Table 15-3 lists some examples of drugs that have an independent effect on blood pressure.

Diuretics

All diuretics work via increasing the salt concentration in urine, which causes increased water excretion as well. The general mechanism of action is via a reduction in reabsorption of sodium ions, as these ions move through the renal tubule cells. There are three classes of diuretics categorized by where they inhibit sodium reabsorption; thiazide-type diuretics act in the distal tubule and

connecting segment, loop diuretics act in the ascending limb of the loop of Henle, and potassium-sparing diuretics affect the aldosterone-sensitive principal cells in the cortical collecting tubule (Figure 15-3).

Most diuretics are derived from sulfanilamide, which is in the family of sulfa drugs; thus individuals who are allergic to sulfonamides may be allergic to diuretics. The clinical relevance of this potential cross-reactivity is unclear and controversial. Although the Food and Drug Administration (FDA) has approved labeling that states sulfanilamide diuretics may be contraindicated for persons who are allergic to sulfa drugs, the existence of this cross-reactivity is rare. Prescribers should be aware of the issue, and individuals with a sulfa allergy should be monitored carefully if diuretics are initiated.

Thiazides

Thiazide diuretics are recommended as the first-line treatment for patients with stage 1 hypertension who do not have other compelling reasons for other agents (Table 15-4). The Antihypertensive and Lipid-Lowering Treatment to Prevent Heart Attack Trial (ALLHAT) study demonstrated that diuretics are a cost-effective treatment option for persons with mild hypertension.[3,22] Hydrochlorothiazide (HydroDIURIL) and chlorthalidone (Thalitone) are the two most commonly used in practice.

This class of diuretic inhibits the **sodium chloride symporter** in the distal convoluted tubule. Inhibition of

Table 15-3 Drugs That Affect Blood Pressure

Hypotensive Effect	Hypertensive Effect
Anesthetics	Bromocriptine (Parlodel)
Atypical antidepressants (e.g., trazodone [Desyrel])	Corticosteroids
Antipsychotics (e.g., Clozapine [Clozaril])	Cyclosporine (Sandimmune)
Benzodiazepines (e.g., lorazepam [Ativan], alprazolam [Xanax])	Estrogens (oral contraceptives)
Digoxin (Lanoxin)	Herbs: feverfew, ginseng, goldenseal, St. John's wort
Dopamine agonists (levodopa-carbidopa [Sinemet])	Immunosuppressants (e.g., cyclosporine [Sandimmune], tacrolimus [Prograf])
Nitrates (e.g., nitroglycerin [Nitrostat])	MAO inhibitors (phenelzine [Nardil])
Opiates	NSAIDs (ibuprofen [Motrin], celecoxib [Celebrex])
Tricyclic antidepressants (amitriptyline [Elavil])	Stimulants (e.g., nicotine, amphetamines)
	Sympathomimetics (pseudoephedrine [Sudafed])
	Weight loss agents (e.g., sibutramine [Meridia], phentermine [Adipex])

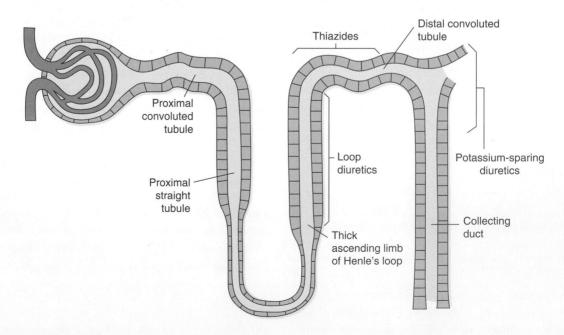

Figure 15-3 Site of action of diuretics.

Table 15-4 Thiazides Diuretics*

Drug—Generic (Brand)	Formulation	Dose per Day	Frequency per Day	Half-Life (Hours)	FDA Pregnancy Category†
Bendroflumethiazide (Naturetin)	5-mg, 10-mg tablets	2.5–10 mg	Single dose	3–3.9	C
Benzthiazide (Exna)	Tablet	25–100 mg	2 divided doses	5–15	C
Chlorothiazide (Diuril)	250-mg, 500-mg tablets	500 mg–1 g	2 divided doses	~ 1.5	C
Chlorthalidone (Hygroton)	15-mg, 25-mg, 50-mg tablets	50–100 mg	Single dose	40–60	B
Hydrochlorothiazide (e.g., Esidrix, HydroDIURIL, Microzide)	25-mg, 50-mg tablets 12.5-mg capsules	12.5–100 mg	Single dose	~ 2.5	B
Hydroflumethiazide (Diucardin, Saluron)	Tablet	25–100 mg	2 divided doses	~ 17	D
Indapamide (Lozol)	1.25-mg, 2.5-mg tablets	2.5–10 mg	Single dose	14–18	B
Methyclothiazide (Enduron)	5-mg scored tablets	2.5–10 mg	Single dose	ID	B
Metolazone (Zaroxolyn)	2.5-mg, 5-mg, 10-mg tablets	2.5–10 mg	Single dose	ID	B
Polythiazide (Renese)	2 mg	1–4 mg	Single dose	ID	D
Quinethazone (Hydromox)	Tablet	50–100 mg	Single dose	ID	C
Trichlormethiazide (Achletin, Diu-Hydrin, Triflumen)	Tablet	2–8 mg	Single dose	ID	C

ID = insufficient data.
* Use cautiously in individuals who have renal impairment, hepatic impairment, gout, diabetes, and dehydration. These drugs are used in combination with several other antihypertensive drugs.
† The thiazide diuretics are FDA Pregnancy Category D if the woman has pregnancy-induced hypertension, and they are therefore contraindicated for treatment of pregnancy-induced hypertension.

the sodium (NaCl) channel transport results in increased NaCl excretion and therefore increased water excretion. Because most of the filtered plasma is reabsorbed in the loop of Henle, thiazides are less potent than other diuretics. Overall, approximately 3–5% of the filtered sodium is inhibited from reabsorption if thiazides are used at maximal doses. Thiazides have no overall effect on renal blood flow, but they do have a synergistic relationship with other antihypertensive drugs.

The antihypertensive effect of hydrochlorothiazide (HydroDIURIL) or chlorthalidone (Thalitone) is optimal at 12.5–50 mg per day. Doses above 50 mg do not offer much benefit and result in a higher incidence of electrolyte abnormalities. Thiazides can be used as monotherapy or in combination with other medications. Chlorthalidone has an extremely long half-life and more pronounced reduction in blood pressure when compared to hydrochlorothiazide.

Side Effects/Contraindications

As a class of drugs, thiazides generally are well tolerated. Most of the side effects involve metabolic effects secondary to fluid and electrolyte imbalance such as hypokalemia, hyperuricemia, hypercalcemia, hyponatremia, impaired carbohydrate tolerance, and hyperlipidemia, the most common being hypercalcemia. These side effects can be minimized with lower doses of hydrochlorothiazide (HydroDIURIL) or chlorthalidone (Hygroton), such as 6.25–12.5 mg per day.

Few central nervous system or gastrointestinal effects are associated with thiazide use. Thiazides can also cause photosensitivity and rarely leukopenia or pancreatitis.

Drug–Drug Interactions

Cross-sensitivity is known to exist between thiazides and sulfa drugs; thus, an allergic reaction is possible if an individual has a sulfa allergy and takes a thiazide-type drug. Caution should be taken when an individual combines thiazides with nonsteroidal anti-inflammatory drugs (NSAIDs) or steroids, because the antihypertensive effect of the thiazide can be diminished while the risk of acute renal failure is increased. Thiazides can increase lithium levels and should not be administered in combination with quinidine, as a prolonged QT interval may result in polymorphic ventricular tachycardia.

Special Populations

There are conflicting thoughts about the use of diuretics during pregnancy, and the FDA pregnancy category varies for thiazide diuretics. However the most popular diuretic, hydrochlorothiazide (HydroDIURIL), is FDA Pregnancy Category B. Thiazides have been used successfully for treating chronic or gestational hypertension; however, they should not be used for the treatment of preeclampsia. Diuretics can cause decreased amniotic fluid volume and decreased placental perfusion, and there have been case reports of neonatal hypoglycemia, hypokalemia, and hyponatremia when taken close to delivery.

Providers need to be cautious in prescribing thiazides for the elderly and should start with a lower-than-recommended daily dose such as hydrochlorothiazide 6.25–12.5 mg daily. One benefit of hydrochlorothiazide is that over several years of treatment, small improvements in total body bone density have been noted.[23]

Loop Diuretics

Loop diuretics act as a membrane transporter that is made up of sodium, potassium, and chloride in the thick ascending limb of the loop of Henle by competing for the chloride binding site (Table 15-5). They are potent and will be effective even in persons with significant renal failure. Because calcium and magnesium reabsorption depends on the concentrations of sodium and chloride, these diuretics enhance urinary loss of calcium in contrast to thiazide diuretics, which promote calcium retention. This is a clinically useful effect when treating persons with hypercalcemia. These diuretics also have direct vascular effects such as increasing systemic venous capacitance, which decreases left ventricular filling pressure and subsequently lowers blood pressure. In short, the effects of decreased blood volume and vasodilation result in lowered blood pressure and decreased edema. Loop diuretics are excreted renally.

Loop diuretics are not as effective as thiazides in lowering blood pressure, but they are the most efficacious for persons who have edema secondary to congestive heart failure.

Side Effects/Contraindications

The majority of side effects of loop diuretics are related to overdiuresis leading to electrolyte disturbances such as hyponatremia, hypokalemia, hypomagnesia, and hypercal-

cemia. The same sodium/potassium/chloride membrane transporters exist in the inner ear, and therefore loop diuretics can (albeit rarely) cause ototoxicity if given in high doses intravenously. The major contraindications to starting loop diuretics include sodium depletion, volume depletion, and allergic reaction due to potential cross-sensitivity in persons with a sulfa allergy.

Drug–Drug Interactions

Loop diuretics can have many drug–drug interactions. When taken with aminoglycosides or cisplatin (Platinol), there is a synergism that can increase the risk of ototoxicity. Increased plasma levels of anticoagulants, digitalis (Digoxin), lithium (Eskalith, Lithobid), and propranolol (Inderal) occur if loop diuretics are also taken. Sulfonylureas and loop diuretics in combination can increase the risk for hyperglycemia. Conversely, there is blunted diuretic effect if NSAIDs or probenecid (Benemid) are taken with loop diuretics. There is an increased risk of hypokalemia when these drugs are taken concomitantly.

Potassium-Sparing Diuretics

Potassium-sparing diuretics act by blocking the effects of aldosterone on the collecting and late distal tubule (Table 15-6). There are two types of potassium-sparing diuretics: the ENaC channel blockers triamterene (Dyrenium) and amiloride (Midamor), and the aldosterone antagonists (e.g., spironolactone [Aldactone]). Triamterene and amiloride block sodium channels in cells in the late distal tubule. This causes a subsequent change in the transepithelial potential that drives the secretion of potassium into the lumen via potassium channels, which is why these drugs are called *potassium sparing*. The aldosterone antagonists competitively block the intracellular receptor for aldosterone. When the aldosterone receptor is bound to aldosterone, proteins are synthesized that activate sodium channels and

Table 15-5 Loop Diuretics*

Drug Generic (Brand)	Formulations	Dose per Day*	Half-Life (Hours)	FDA Pregnancy Category
Furosemide (Lasix)	20-mg, 40-mg, 80-mg scored tablets Maximum of 600 mg/day	20–80 mg usual starting dose for hypertension	~ 1.5	C
Bumetanide (Bumex)	0.5-mg, 1-mg, 2-mg scored tablets	0.5–2 mg	~ 0.8	B
Ethacrynic acid (Edecrin)†	25-mg scored tablets Maximum of 400 mg/day	50–200 mg	~ 1	B
Torsemide (Demadex)	5-mg, 10-mg, 20-mg, 100-mg scored tablets Maximum of 200 mg as single dose	2.5–20 mg	~ 3.5	B

* All of these drugs can be prescribed in a single daily dose or as a divided dose taken twice daily.
† Ototoxicity possible; rarely used.

Table 15-6 Potassium-Sparing Diuretics

Drug—Generic (Brand)	Formulations	Dose per Day	Half-Life (Hours)	FDA Pregnancy Category
Triamterene (Dyrenium)*	50-mg, 100-mg tablets	50–100 mg qd or in 2 divided doses. Maximum 300 mg per day. Combination with HCTZ 37.5 mg/25 mg.	~ 4.2	B
Amiloride (Midamor)*	5-mg tablets	5 mg qd or in 2 divided doses. Maximum 20 mg per day. Combination with HCTZ 5/50 mg.	~ 21	B
Spironolactone (Aldactone)*	25-mg, 50-mg, 100-mg tablets	25–100 mg qd or in 2 divided doses.	~ 1.6	D
Eplerenone (Inspra)†	25-mg, 50-mg tablets	Hypertension: initially 25–50 mg daily and may increase to bid. Heart failure: initially 25 mg daily and may titrate to 50 mg daily.	4–6	B

* Contraindicated for persons with renal impairment, electrolyte disturbances, or serum or potassium > 5.5 mEq/L. Concomitant use of lithium or NSAIDs should be undertaken with caution as triamterene can cause lithium toxicity and NSAIDs can increase renal toxicity. In addition, concomitant use with ACE inhibitors or other potassium-sparing agents increases the risk for hyperkalemia and is generally contraindicated.
† Dosage adjustment per serum potassium concentrations for persons with congestive heart failure. Contraindications include serum potassium > 5.5 mEq/L, creatinine clearance ≤ 30 mL/min, or concomitant use of strong CYP3A4 inhibitors such as ketoconazole (Nizoral), clarithromycin (Biaxin), and ritonavir (Norvir).

increase the synthesis of new potassium channels. The net result is more sodium is reabsorbed and more potassium is excreted into the intrastitial fluid that will become urine. Thus, the aldosterone antagonists reduce sodium reabsorption and reduce potassium secretion. Potassium-sparing diuretics are eliminated by renal excretion, with an exception of triamterene (Dyrenium), which is metabolized into an active metabolite that is then eliminated via urinary excretion.

Potassium-sparing diuretics rarely are used as first-line agents in the treatment of hypertension. Potassium-sparing diuretics do have some antihypertensive effect, although their primary function is in the treatment of heart failure. Aldosterone antagonists will be discussed later in the chapter in the section on heart failure.

Side Effects/Contraindications

The most common side effect of potassium-sparing diuretics is hyperkalemia, especially when a potassium-sparing diuretic is administered in combination with other agents that have some potassium-sparing properties, such as ACE inhibitors and ARBs. These drugs can cause rapid contraction of the extracellular space as a compensatory mechanism following the decrease in the intracellular space. This can cause an increase in plasma bicarbonate concentration, which can result in metabolic alkalosis. Potassium levels need to be determined prior to initiation of treatment and monitored if potassium-sparing diuretics are to be used in addition to other agents that increase the risk of hyperkalemia.

Drug–Drug Interactions

As is true for other diuretics, potassium-sparing diuretics should not be used concomitantly with NSAIDs or lithium. They should be used with caution if other drugs that spare potassium such as beta-blockers or ACE inhibitors are also prescribed.

Special Populations

The FDA pregnancy category for triamterene (Dyrenium) and amiloride (Midamor) is B; however, there are limited studies looking at these drugs. It is recommended that diuretics and thiazides be avoided during pregnancy secondary to the risk that use will result in decreased placental perfusion. Close monitoring is recommended for any individual who is taking a potassium-sparing diuretic and any other medication that has the potential to increase potassium levels (e.g., birth control pills that contain drospirenone).

Beta-Adrenoreceptor Antagonists (Beta-Blockers)

Drugs categorized as beta-adrenoreceptor antagonists are generally referred to as beta-blockers. These drugs are effective and generally well tolerated (Table 15-7). Prior to the introduction of new antihypertensive drugs such as ACE inhibitors and angiotensin receptor blockers (ARBs), beta-blockers and diuretics were first-line drugs used to treat hypertension. Newer clinical trials have found that ACE inhibitors and ARBs are of more benefit than are

Table 15-7 Beta-Blockers

Drug Generic (Brand)	Formulations	Dose	Cardioselective	Half-Life (Hours)	FDA Pregnancy Category
Acebutolol (Sectral)	200-, 400-mg caps	Initially 400 mg daily in 1–2 divided doses, maintenance 200–800 mg, max 1.2 g/day.	Yes	2–4	B
Atenolol (Tenormin)	25-, 50-, 100-mg tab 0.5 mg/mL parenteral Combination with chlorthalidone 50/25 mg, 100/25 mg	Initially 50 mg daily, increase after 1–2 weeks, max 100 mg daily.	Yes	5–8	D
Betaxolol (Kerlone)	10-, 20-mg tab	Initially 10 mg daily, max 20 mg daily.	Yes		C
Bisoprolol (Zebeta)	5, 10 mg Combination with HCTZ 2.5/6.25 mg, 5/6.25 mg, 10/6.25 mg	5 mg daily, max 20 mg daily.	Yes		C
Carvedilol (Coreg, Coreg CR)	3.125-, 6.25-, 12.5-, 25-mg tabs 10-, 20-, 40-, 80-mg caps	Initially 6.25 mg twice daily, increase over 1–2 week periods, max 25 mg bid. Coreg CR initially 10 mg daily increasing over 1–2 weeks to a max dose of 80 mg daily.	No		C
Labetalol (Trandate)	100-, 200-, 300-mg tab 5 mg/mL parenteral	Initially 100 mg twice daily, maintenance 200–400 mg daily, max 2.4 g daily.	No	4–6	C
Metoprolol (Lopressor, Toprol XL)	50-, 100-mg tab 50-, 100-, 200-mg tab 1 mg/mL parenteral Combination with HCTZ 50/25 mg, 100/25 mg, 100/50 mg	Metoprolol initially 100 mg in 1–2 divided doses, maintenance 100–450 mg daily. Metoprolol XL: initially 25–100 mg daily, max 400 mg daily.	Yes	3–4	C
Nadolol (Corgard)	20-, 40-, 80-, 120-, 160-mg tab Combination with bendroflumethiazide 40/5 mg, 80/5 mg	Initially 40 mg daily, maintenance 40–80 mg daily, max 320 mg daily.	No	10–20	C
Penbutolol (Levatol)	20-mg tab	20 mg daily.	No		C
Pindolol (Visken)	5-, 10-mg tab Combination with HCTZ 40/25 mg, 80/25 mg	Initially 5 mg twice daily, may increase dose after 3–4 weeks in 10-mg increments, max 60 mg.	No	3–4	B
Propranolol (Inderal, Inderal LA, InnoPran XL)	10-, 20-, 40-, 60-, 80-, 90-mg tab 4-, 8-mg/mL oral sol 80 mg/mL sol Oral sustained-release 60-, 80-, 120-, 160-mg cap	Propranolol: initially 40 mg twice daily, maintenance 120–240 mg daily, max 640 mg daily. Propranolol LA/XL initially 80 mg daily, maintenance 120–160 mg daily.	No	3–5	C
Timolol (Blocadren)	5-, 10-, 20-mg cap Combination with HCTZ 10/25 mg	Initially 10 mg twice a day. Usual maintenance 20–40 mg day with max of 60 mg/day in 2 divided doses.	No	3–5	C

beta-blockers for individuals who do not have a compelling indication for beta-blockers such as coronary artery disease.[24] Beta-blockers are the first choice for management of hypertension if the person has a history of a prior MI. In this scenario, beta-blockers have been found to reduce mortality and morbidity.

In general, all beta-blockers inhibit or block the effects of norepinephrine and epinephrine outside of the central nervous system, thereby disallowing the natural effect of these neurotransmitters. Beta-blockers are subdivided into two different categories: nonselective and selective. Drugs that are more selective for β_1-receptors in the heart versus β_2-receptors in the bronchi and peripheral blood vessels are classified as cardioselective beta-blockers. Medications such as atenolol (Tenormin), betaxolol (Kerlone), bisoprolol (Zebeta), and metoprolol (Lopressor,

Toprol XL) are cardioselective. Since these drugs are less likely to cause bronchoconstriction or vasoconstriction than nonselective beta-blockers, they generally are preferred for use by individuals who have chronic obstructive pulmonary disease or peripheral arterial disease. The cardioselective nature of these drugs is lost at higher doses; this varies from individual to individual.

Mechanism of Action

The mechanism of action of beta-blockers in relation to the effects on hypertension remains unclear. Initially the drugs were hypothesized to be vasoconstrictors, and the hypotensive side effect was unexpected. However, beta-blockers' inhibition of the beta-adrenergic receptor does not allow any activation of the receptor. Many of these receptors are in the cardiac muscle, and inhibition of those receptors results in negative **inotropic** and **chronotropic** effects, thereby decreasing cardiac conduction velocity and automaticity. Currently it is theorized that the antihypertensive mechanism primarily is related to reduction in cardiac output, reduction in renin release from the kidneys, and a central nervous system effect to reduce general sympathetic activity. Such effects should be carefully considered. For example, slowing of the atrioventricular conduction with increased P–R interval could be a desired therapeutic effect for one person, whereas it could be potentially life threatening for another. The beta-blockers are well absorbed after oral administration; peak concentrations occur in about 1–3 hours, and sustained-released formulations are available. Many beta-blockers are available in an immediate-release dose or a sustained- or extended-release formulation.

Side Effects/Contraindications

Beta-blockers with short half-lives have more negative effects following abrupt withdrawal than beta-blockers with longer half-lives. Common side effects of beta-blockers include bradycardia, hypotension, fatigue, dizziness, and dyspnea. Other side effects that need to be considered prior to use include second- or third-degree atrioventricular block, cold extremities, diarrhea, nausea, depression, and impotence.[20]

Unfortunately, as with any drug category, adverse effects can also occur. Negative effects on blood glucose levels and lipid levels can develop when beta-blockers are taken. The Glycemic Effects in Diabetes Mellitus Carvedilol-Metoprolol Comparison in Hypertensives (GEMINI) trial demonstrated that newer generations of beta-blockers do not have the same negative effect on glycemic control.[24]

A few beta-blockers, particularly carvedilol (Coreg, Coreg CR) and extended-release metoprolol (Toprol XL), are indicated for the treatment of heart failure. Abrupt withdrawal of these drugs can cause exacerbation of ischemic heart disease because of the sudden increase in sympathetic response. There is no specific method for tapering a person off of a beta-blocker; however, decreasing the dose slowly and over an extended period of time has been found to decrease the clinical negative adrenergic effects.[25]

Prolonged use, such as more than 6 months of treatment, with these drugs may lead to increases in very-low-density lipoprotein (VLDL) levels. The nonselective and newer beta-blockers have less of an effect on lipids. Beta-blockers are also associated with an increased risk for developing diabetes (RR = 1.28; 95% CI, 1.04–1.57).[26]

There are also drug–drug interactions associated with use of beta-blockers that generally fall into the category of additive effects, which cause hypotension or bradycardia or inhibition, negating the therapeutic effect of the beta-blocker. Drug–drug interactions associated with beta-blockers are listed in Table 15-8.

Special Populations

The FDA pregnancy categories for beta-blockers are listed in Table 15-7. Some of the beta-blockers are used during pregnancy to control hypertension, thyrotoxicosis, and arrhythmias. Labetalol (Trandate) is recommended as an alternative to methyldopa (Aldomet) for the management of hypertension. Atenolol (Tenormin) is associated with adverse fetal outcomes and reduced placental function and should be avoided.[27] Propranolol (Inderal), labetalol (Trandate), atenolol (Tenormin), nadolol (Corgard), and metoprolol (Lopressor) are excreted into breast milk. Since no adverse outcomes have been found among lactating dyads when beta-blockers are used, they are recommended by the American Academy of Pediatrics (AAP) for use during breastfeeding.[28]

The only considerations for the elderly are those with comorbidities such as peripheral arterial disease (PAD), chronic obstructive pulmonary disease (COPD), or asthma. Beta-blockers are not used as first-line antihypertensive agents for the elderly unless they have a compelling indication such as heart failure, postmyocardial infarction, high coronary disease risk, and diabtes.[20] Diuretics, ARBs, and CCBs are more effective for preventing cardiovascular outcomes and stroke and are associated with decreased morbidity in the elderly.[29]

Angiotensin-Converting Enzyme Inhibitors (ACE Inhibitors)

We have the Brazilian viper to thank for ACE inhibitors. The Nobel Prize–winning scientist Sir John Vane noted

Table 15-8 Drug–Drug Interactions Associated with Beta-Blockers*

Drug—Generic (Brand)	Effects
Aminophylline	Inhibits bronchodilation effect of aminophylline.
Amiodarone (Cordarone)	Bradycardia or arrhythmia.
Ampicillin (Principen)	Reduced effect of atenolol.
Antidiabetic agents	Enhanced hypoglycemia, hypertension.
Calcium channel blockers	Potentiation of bradycardia, myocardial depression, hypotension.
Chlorpromazine (Thorazine)	Potentiates the effect of propranolol (Inderal) and generally contraindicated in persons taking beta-blockers.
Cimetidine (Tagamet)	Prolongs half-life of propranolol (Inderal).
Clonidine (Catapres)	Rebound hypertension during clonidine withdrawal.
Digoxin (Lanoxin)	Increased serum levels of digoxin and possible digoxin toxicity.
Diltiazem (Cardizem)	Bradycardia.
Epinephrine	Hypertension, bradycardia.
Ergot alkaloids (e.g., Cafergot)	Excessive vasoconstriction.
Fluoxetine (Prozac)	Potentiates beta-blocker effects.
Glucagon	Inhibition of hyperglycemic effect.
Indomethacin (Indocin)	Inhibition of beta-blocker hypotensive effect.
Isoproterenol (Isuprel)	Isoproterenol and beta-blockers inhibit the effects of each other, resulting in hypertension and inhibition of bronchodilation.
Levodopa (Sinemet)	Antagonizes the hypotensive effect of levodopa.
Lidocaine	Propranolol (Inderal) increases lidocaine levels, which causes potential lidocaine toxicity.
Methyldopa (Aldomet)	Hypertension.
Nonsteroidal anti-inflammatory drugs (NSAIDs)	Attenuation of beta-blocker effect if NSAIDs are used for a prolonged period of time.
Phenothiazines	Additive hypotensive effects.
Phenytoin (Dilantin)	Additive cardiac depression.
Prazosin (Minipress)	Augmentation of first-dose syncope, hypotension.
Quinidine	Enhanced hypotensive effect.
Reserpine (Reserpaneed)	Excessive sympathetic blockade.
Rifampin (RIF, Rifadin)	Increased metabolism of beta-blockers.
Theophylline (Theo-Dur)	Attenuation of bronchodilation effect of theophylline. Can be minimized by using cardioselective beta-blockers.
Thioridazine (Mellaril)	Significant hypotensive effect, generally contraindicated.
Tricyclic antidepressants	Inhibits effect of beta-blockers.
Verapamil (Calan)	Bradycardia, heart block.

* This table is not comprehensive. New information is being identified on a regular basis.

that the toxic effects of snake venom were secondary to a profound drop in blood pressure, and he went on to determine the active substance in snake venom is a potent inhibitor of angiotensin-converting enzyme. He and other scientists at the pharmaceutical company Squibb worked with snake venom to creat a synthetic ACE inhibitor and ultimately succeeded in inventing captopril (Capoten). Today there are many angiotensin-converting enzyme inhibitors, which are commonly called ACE inhibitors. This is a widely used class of antihypertensive drugs (Table 15-9).

The ACE inhibitors are broadly effective and do not have the adverse lipid and glucose metabolic effects associated with beta-blockers and thiazides. The majority of ACE inhibitors are available in a generic formulation. Currently

11 types of ACE inhibitors are available, and they vary based in potency and pharmacokinetics. Despite the different formulations, there is no significant reason to choose one ACE inhibitor rather than another with the exception of pragmatic reasons such as local cost or coverage on a formulary. ACE inhibitors are approved for the treatment of hypertension, left ventricular systolic dysfunction, myocardial infarction, chronic kidney disease, renal protection in persons with diabetes, and for individuals who are at high risk for cardiovascular events.

Some pharmacogenomic variations appear to exist with these drugs, and there is significant individual variability in response to them. African Americans may not have the same benefit in blood pressure reduction with ACE inhibitors

Table 15-9 Angiotensin-Converting Enzyme Inhibitors

Drug Generic (Brand)	Formulations	Dose	Half-Life* (Hours)	FDA Pregnancy Category
Benazepril (Lotensin)	5-mg, 10-mg, 20-mg, 40-mg tab Combination benazepril/HCTZ: 5/6.25 mg, 10/12.5 mg, 20/12.5 mg, 20/25 mg Combination benazepril/amlodipine: 2.5/10 mg, 5/10 mg, 5/20 mg, 5/40 mg, 10/20 mg, 10/40 mg	Initially 10 mg, maintenance 20–40 mg daily, max 80 mg daily.	22	C/D‖
Captopril (Capoten)[†]	12.5-mg, 25-mg, 50-mg, 100-mg tab Combination with HCTZ: 25/15 mg, 25/25 mg, 50/15 mg, 50/25 mg	Initially 25 mg 2–3 times day, max 450 mg/daily.	2	C/D‖
Enalapril (Vasotec)	2.5-mg, 5-mg, 10-mg, 20-mg tab Combination with HCTZ: 5/12.5 mg, 10/25 mg Combination with felodipine: 5/2.5 mg, 5/5 mg	Initially 2.5 mg daily, maintenance 10–40 mg daily, max 40 mg daily.	11	C/D‖
Fosinopril (Monopril)	10-mg, 20-mg, 40-mg tab	Initially 10 mg daily, maintenance 20–40 mg daily, max 80 mg/daily.	11.5–12	C/D‖
Lisinopril (Prinivil, Zestril)	2.5-mg, 5-mg, 10-mg, 20-mg, 30-mg, 40-mg tab Combination with HCTZ: 10/12.5 mg, 20/12.5 mg, 20/25 mg	Initially 10 mg daily, maintenance 20–40 mg daily, max 40 mg daily.	12	C/D‖
Moexipril (Univasc)	7.5-mg, 15-mg tab Combination with HCTZ: 7.5/12.5 mg, 15/12.5 mg, 15/25 mg	Take 1 h before meals, initially 7.5 mg daily, maintenance 15–30 mg daily, max 30 mg daily.	2–10	C/D‖
Perindopril (Aceon)	2-mg, 4-mg, 8-mg tab	Initially 4 mg daily, maintenance 4–8 mg daily, max 16 mg daily.	25–120	C/D‖
Quinapril (Accupril)	5-mg, 10-mg, 20-mg, 40-mg Combination with HCTZ: 10/12.5 mg, 20/12.5 mg, 20/25 mg	Initially 10 mg daily, maintenance 20–80 mg daily, max 80 mg daily.	2–25	C/D‖
Ramipril (Altace)[‡]	1.25-mg, 2.5-mg, 5-mg, 10-mg	Initially 2.5 mg daily, maintenance 2.5–20 mg daily, max 20 mg daily.	13–17	C/D‖
Trandolapril (Mavik)[§]	1-mg, 2-mg, 4-mg tab Combination with verapamil 2/180 mg, 1/240 mg, 2/240 mg, 4/240 mg	Initially 1 mg daily, maintenance 2–4 mg daily, max 8 mg daily.	6–10	C/D‖

* Half-life of active metabolite.
[†] Take 1 hour before meals.
[‡] May sprinkle in applesauce or 4 oz of water if individual cannot swallow pills.
[§] Initial dose for African American individuals is 2 mg daily.
‖ FDA Pregnancy Category C for the first trimester and Category D for the second and third trimesters. These categories may change as recent studies have found an association between ACE inhibitors and birth defects. Currently the prescribing information for ACE inhibitors recommends that they be stopped as soon as possible if pregnancy occurs.

when compared to the response to calcium channel blockers or thiazide diuretics, and these drugs are therefore not recommended as the first-line treatment for this population.[30]

Mechanism of Action

Most ACE inhibitors are actually prodrugs metabolized in the liver to an active metabolite. These agents prevent the conversion of angiotensin I into angiotensin II, hence the name *ACE inhibitor*. The ACE that catalyzes the alteration of angiotensin I into angiotensin II exists primarily in endothelial tissue in the pulmonary vasculature, and angiotensin II is therefore primarily produced in the blood vessels as blood passes through the lungs. ACE, in addition to its effects on angiotensin, blocks the degradation of plasma bradykinin and stimulates the synthesis of vasodilating prostaglandins. Bradykinin is a vasodilator; thus, the

excess bradykinin levels that result following use of ACE inhibitors results in vasodilation, decreased peripheral vascular resistance, and a lowered blood pressure through this independent pathway. ACE inhibitors work well in combination with thiazides. The thiazides induce sodium depletion, which activates the RAAS and shifts blood pressure control to angiotensin, which is then blocked by the ACE inhibitor. The mechanism of action whereby the ACE inhibitor suppresses the RAAS may also be why ACE inhibitors are not associated with new onset diabetes. RAAS inhibition improves sensitivity to insulin and glycemic control.

Side Effects/Contraindications

Common side effects of ACE inhibitors include cough and angioedema related to elevated levels of bradykinin and substance P. The excess bradykinin is responsible for the dry cough that up to 20% of persons who take these drugs develop and for angioedema, which is rare. In the Antihypertensive and Lipid-Lowering Treatment to Prevent Heart Attack Trial (ALLHAT), angioedema was seen more among African Americans who took ACE inhibitors compared to other races.[30] If an ACE inhibitor cough develops, the drug should be discontinued. If the individual is taking an ACE inhibitor because of a compelling indication such as diabetes, an ARB should be substituted if possible.

The major serious risks associated with ACE inhibitors are hyperkalemia and deterioration of renal function. Prior to initiating these drugs, a baseline serum creatinine and potassium level should be obtained. These values should be checked after the first week of use in persons who are at low risk for renal impairment and after 4 days in persons who have a higher risk of developing renal compromise (e.g., peripheral vascular disease, diabetes, preexisting renal compromise). A small rise in both creatinine and potassium is expected. A > 20% rise in the serum creatinine level is considered significant and warrants further investigation and possible referral. If the potassium level rises to > 5.6–6.0 mEq/L, the ACE inhibitor should be stopped and renal function monitored carefully.

Severe hypotension can occur in persons who have hypovolemia as a result of diuretics, salt restriction, or gastrointestinal fluid loss. It is suggested that any diuretic be discontinued 2–3 days before the initial administration of an ACE inhibitor. If a goal blood pressure cannot be obtained, the diuretic could be resumed at a reduced dose. However, if the diuretic cannot be stopped prior to starting the ACE inhibitor, a lower starting dose and careful monitoring are recommended as these drugs in combination can precipitate acute renal failure. There are also case reports of ACE inhibitors leading to hypoaldosteronism. Metabolic acidosis is another adverse reaction that can occur when ACE inhibitors are used. The inhibition of angiotensin II results in lower levels of aldosterone, which causes a decreased reuptake of sodium and an excessive retention of hydrogen ions, which is the cause of metabolic acidosis.

Drug–Drug Interactions

Since ACE inhibitors can cause hyperkalemia, they should be used cautiously by individuals taking potassium supplements, potassium-sparing diuretics, or ARBs. ACE inhibitors are primarily eliminated by the kidneys; therefore, the dose may need to be altered based on renal function. The combined use of ACE inhibitors, diuretics, and NSAIDs has been referred to as the *triple whammy* secondary to

a significant risk for acute renal failure, especially in the elderly. Both ACE inhibitors and NSAIDs can cause functional renal insufficiency, and therefore this drug combination is considered potentially nephrotoxic. Drug–drug interactions associated with ACE inhibitors are listed in Table 15-10.

Special Populations

ACE inhibitors have been shown to increase the risk of birth defects in the last 6 months of pregnancy; therefore, they are FDA Pregnancy Category C in the first trimester and Category D in the second and third trimesters. These drugs should not be used by childbearing-age women who are considering pregnancy unless there is a compelling indication that outweighs the risk. ACE inhibitors do transfer in the breast milk at low levels and should only be used if no other alternatives are available.

Age is not a contraindication in the use of ACE inhibitors. There are multiple benefits of the elderly using ACE inhibitors, including reduced decline of muscle strength.[31] ACE inhibitors are known to prevent physical decline in persons with congestive heart failure (CHF). Onder et al. assessed the effects of ACE inhibitors in elderly women who did not have CHF. The participants who continuously took ACE inhibitors were found only to have muscle strength decreased by –1.0 kg compared to –3.7 kg in the control group of women taking other antihypertensives (P = .016). When the women who took ACE inhibitors were compared to elderly women who did not take any antihypertensives, the women who took ACE inhibitors had significantly less decline in their muscle strength (P = .026). The exact mechanism of action leading to reduced muscle strength decline is not known.[31]

Angiotensin Receptor Blockers

Angiotensin II receptor blockers (ARBs) are also known as angiotensin II receptor antagonists (Table 15-11). These drugs are a class of antihypertensive drugs effective for the treatment of hypertension as well as heart failure and as prophylaxis for persons who are at high risk for cardiovascular events. Although many of the ARBs are not currently available in a generic formulation, others can be found in formulations combined with other antihypertensive drugs.

Mechanism of Action

There are two types of receptors for angiotensin II—the AT_2 and AT_1 receptors. ARBs possess a high affinity to bind specifically to the AT_1 receptor, thereby blocking the

Table 15-10 Drug Interactions Associated with ACE Inhibitors and Angiotensin Receptor Blockers (ARBs)*

Drug—Generic (Brand)	Agent	Effect
Allopurinol (Zyloprim)	ACE inhibitors	Stevens-Johnson syndrome.
Alpha-blockers	ACE inhibitors	Augmentation of first-dose syncope associated with alpha-blockers.
Antidiabetic drugs	ACE inhibitors	Enhances insulin sensitivity of ACE inhibitor; increases hypoglycemic effect of antidiabetic agents.
Aspirin	ACE inhibitors and ARBs	Possible antagonism of ACE-inhibitor effects. Not usually clinically significant at low doses of aspirin.
Beta-blockers	ACE inhibitors	Rebound hypertension following withdrawal of clonidine (Catapres).
Cimetidine (Tagamet)	Losartan (Cozaar)	Increased serum levels of cimetidine.
Chlorpromazine (Thorazine)	ACE inhibitors	Increased concentrations of chlorpromazine (Thorazine).
Digoxin (Lanoxin)	Captopril (Capoten)	Increased serum levels of digoxin.
Fluconazole (Diflucan)	Losartan (Cozaar)	Reduced efficacy of losartan (Cozaar).
Grapefruit juice	Losartan (Cozaar)	Delayed absorption and lower serum levels of losartan.
Ketoconazole (Nizoral)	Losartan (Cozaar)	Inhibits CYP enzyme responsible for metabolizing losartan and thereby decreases effectiveness.
Lithium (Lithobid)	ACE inhibitors and ARBs	Lithium toxicity.
Nonsteroidal anti-inflammatory drugs (NSAIDs)	ACE inhibitors and ARBs	NSAIDs decrease efficacy of ACE inhibitors and ARBs.
Oxypurinol	Losartan (Cozaar)	Increased risk for developing renal calculi.
Phenobarbital (Luminal)	Losartan (Cozaar)	Phenobarbital induces CYP3A4 and decreases serum levels of losartan.
Potassium-sparing diuretics	ACE inhibitors and ARBs	Enhanced hyperkalemic effect.
Rifampin (Rifadin)	Losartan (Cozaar)	Induces CYP enzyme responsible for metabolizing losartan and shortens half-life.

* This table is not comprehensive. New information is being identified on a regular basis.

effects of angiotensin II on these receptors. These drugs have a slow dissociation from the AT_1 receptor that results in a long half-life, which has some clinical benefits. For example, the effects continue even if a dose is missed. It is hypothesized that these drugs are more effective in inhibiting the effects of angiotensin II than are ACE inhibitors because there is more than one physiologic pathway that creates angiotensin II other than conversion from angiotensin I. ARBs in combination with a thiazide work well, and this is a common combination when two agents are needed to meet blood pressure goals.

Side Effects/Contraindications

The rate of discontinuation of ARBs due to side effects is similar to the discontinuation rate of placebo tablets, making them a generally well tolerated category of drug.[32] Although cough can occur in persons taking ARBs, the incidence is lower (3.8%) compared to ACE inhibitors (8.8%).[33] However, hyperkalemia may occur, as well as changes in renal function. A synergistic effect occurs when ARBs are used in combination with other antihypertensive drugs. Hyperkalemia and a rise in serum creatinine are frequent concerns for persons using ARBs. If serum values of potassium or creatinine rise, the provider should review the individual's medication list, recommend the initiation of a low potassium diet, and consider a diuretic such as a loop or a thiazide to increase potassium excretion. When a person with chronic kidney disease is started on these drugs, serum potassium levels should be evaluated in 1–2 weeks. If the potassium is > 5.6 mEq/L despite diet changes and lower doses, the drug should be discontinued.

Management of individuals taking ARBs can be complex. For example, a person with a baseline serum creatinine of 1.8 mg/dL who starts taking an ACE inhibitor or ARB will have a repeat creatinine in a few weeks. The repeat creatinine may be 2.2 mg/dL. The clinician might want to discontinue the drug because the higher level is perceived to be a reflection of worsening renal function. However, angiotensin II normally effects a constriction of the efferent arterioles of the glomeruli in the kidney; thus, when the medication is used, the sudden lack of angiotensin results in vasodilation and lower intraglomerular pressure that allows an initial decrease in the glomerular filtration rate, which leads to a rise in serum creatinine levels and does not reflect actual worsening of renal function. The provider should obtain another creatinine level a few weeks after the elevation is found to determine if it

Table 15-11 Angiotensin Receptor Blockers

Drug Generic (Brand)	Formulations	Dose	Half-Life (Hours)	Clinical Considerations	FDA Pregnancy Category
Candesartan (Atacand, Atacand HCT)	4-mg, 8-mg, 16-mg, 32-mg tab Combination with HCTZ 16/12.5 mg, 32/12.5 mg	Initially 16 mg, maintenance 8–32 mg daily, max 32 mg. Daily or divided dose.	9	Drug interaction with lithium.	C/D in 2nd and 3rd trimesters
Eprosartan (Teveten, Teveten HCT)	400-mg, 600-mg tab Combination with HCTZ 600 mg/12.5 mg, 600 mg/25 mg	Initially 600 mg daily, maintenance 400–600 mg, max 800 mg daily.	5–9	Single or divided dose.	C/D in 2nd and 3rd trimesters
Irbesartan (Avapro, Avalide)	75-mg, 150-mg, 300-mg tab Combination with HCTZ 150/12.5 mg, 300/12.5 mg, 300/25 mg	Initially 150 mg daily, maintenance 300 mg, max 300 mg daily.	11–15		C/D in 2nd and 3rd trimesters
Losartan (Cozaar, Hyzaar)	25-mg, 50-mg, 100-mg Combination with HCTZ 50/12.5 mg, 100/12.5 mg, 100/25 mg	Initially 50 mg daily, maintenance 25–100 mg daily, max 100 mg daily.	6–9 active metabolite	Drug interaction with fluconazole and rifampin. Hepatic insufficiency or hypovolemia lower starting dose of 25 mg daily.	C/D in 2nd and 3rd trimesters
Olmesartan (Benicar, Benicar HCT)	5 mg, 20 mg, 40 mg tab Combination with HCTZ 20/12.5 mg, 40/12.5 mg, 40/25 mg	Initially 20 mg daily, maintenance 20–40 mg, max 40 mg daily.	13		C/D in 2nd and 3rd trimesters
Telmisartan (Micardis, Micardis HCT)	20-mg, 40-mg, 80-mg tab Combination with HCTZ	Initially 40 mg daily, maintenance 20–80 mg, max 80 mg daily.	24	Drug interaction with digoxin.	C/D in 2nd and 3rd trimesters
Valsartan (Diovan, Diovan HCT, Exforge)	40-mg, 80-mg, 160-mg, 320-mg tab Combination with HCTZ 80/12.5 mg, 160/12.5 mg, 160/25 mg, 320/12.5 mg, 320/25 mg Combination with amlodipine	Initially 160 mg daily, maintenance 80–320 mg, max 320 mg daily.	6		C/D in 2nd and 3rd trimesters

has stabilized. A 20–30% rise in creatinine is an expected outcome, and the individual should continue on the drug. If a person has a ≥ 30% rise in creatinine within a few weeks of initiating therapy, the level should be repeated, and if the level continues to rise, then the drug should be discontinued.

Drug–Drug Interactions

Interactions between ARBs and other drugs are similar to those associated with ACE inhibitors, but as a rule, drug–drug interactions with ARBs are seen less often in clinical practice than are drug–drug interactions associated with use of ACE inhibitors (Table 15-10). Angioedema can occur if ARBs are taken in combination with ACE inhibitors. Hypotension can occur in volume- or salt-depleted individuals, and therefore, these agents should be used cautiously in combination with potassium-sparing diuretics and potassium supplements. Losartan (Cozaar) is the one exception to the benign

profile enjoyed by most ARBs. Losartan is metabolized by CYP2C9 into an active metabolite that accounts for the therapeutic effect, and therefore, agents that inhibit CYP2C9 such as ketoconazole (Nizoral) decrease the effectiveness of losartan. Conversely, rifampin (Rifadin) induces CYP2C9 and shortens the half-life of losartan, again decreasing effectiveness.

Special Populations

The FDA pregnancy categories for ARBs are listed in Table 15-11. The same concerns with ACE inhibitors during pregnancy apply to ARBs. These drugs should be avoided by all women of childbearing age if possible unless there is a compelling indication that outweighs the risk. ARBs are not recommended while a woman is breastfeeding; although a small amount of the drug gets into breast milk, infants are highly susceptible to ACE inhibitors and therefore a theoretic risk to the infant exists. The elderly are found to benefit from ARBs.

Direct Renin Inhibitors

Direct renin inhibitors are agents that act on the RAAS. Aliskiren (Tekturna) is the first drug in this category approved for use by the FDA in 2007.

Mechanism of Action

Direct renin inhibitors suppress plasma renin activity thereby preventing the conversion of angiotensinogen into angiotensin I. This agent interferes with the beginning of the RAAS cycle, ultimately decreasing the amount of angiotensin II and aldosterone that is produced. The release of renin in the kidney is controlled by three major pathways. The macula densa pathway, and intrarenal baroreceptor pathway are within the kidney, and the beta-adrenergic receptor pathway is in the central nervous system. If the conversion of angiotensinogen into angiotensin I is blocked, this blockade effectively inhibits all three pathways that stimulate the RAAS reflex response, and the overall production of angiotensin I, angiotensin II, and plasma active renin are reduced. Direct renin inhibitors have a distinctly different effect from the ACE inhibitor rebound effect of angiotensin II to pretreatment levels and the ARB increases of angiotensin I and II. It is theorized that angiotensin II may play an important role in the development of cardiovascular disease by promoting endothelial dysfunction, thus direct renin inhibitors may have the additional benefit of protection against this effect.[34] Therefore, direct renin inhibitors are an appropriate agent to use in stage 1 or stage 2 hypertension.

The recommended starting dose of aliskiren is 150 mg daily; however, if the goal blood pressure is not obtained, the dose can be increased to 300 mg daily. This agent can be used in monotherapy or in combinations with all other antihypertensive agents. Aliskiren (Tekturna) added to amlodipine (Norvasc), ramipril (Altace), and hydrochlorothiazide has been found to have significantly greater reduction in blood pressure when compared to monotherapy.[34]

Pharmacokinetics

Peak plasma levels are reached in 1–3 hours following administration of aliskiren, and the half-life is approximately 24 hours. It is unknown how much of the drug that is absorbed is metabolized, although one fourth of the drug found in urine is unchanged from the parent drug.[34]

Side Effects/Contraindications

Many of the same side effects seen with use of ACE inhibitors and ARBs are seen with use of direct renin inhibitors, such as angioedema, hypotension, or hyperkalemia. There are no cited contraindications for use. Similarly, the same concerns about possible impaired renal function and hyperkalemia apply to the use of direct renin inhibitors, and the same precautions should be used in monitoring individuals who use direct renin inhibitors as are used when monitoring individuals who take ACE inhibitors or ARBs.

Special Populations

The FDA pregnancy category for aliskiren is C for the first trimester and category D for the second and third trimester for the same reasons as ACE inhibitors and ARBs. When pregnancy is detected, the medication should be discontinued as soon as possible, as there is a risk of injury such as neonatal skull hypoplasia, anuria, reversible or irreversible renal function, and fetal death.[34]

Calcium Channel Antagonists

Calcium channel antagonists are most often referred to as calcium channel blockers (CCBs). One of the key factors leading to elevated blood pressure is peripheral resistance. Calcium channel antagonists reduce peripheral resistance via dilation of the peripheral arterials (Table 15-12). These drugs are easy to identify because their generic names all end in *pine*.

Many of the calcium channel blockers are available in generic preparations and, thus, are cost effective. In addition to being useful as antihypertensives, the calcium channel blockers subcategorized as nondihydropyridines also are effective for the treatment of cardiac arrhythmias. Calcium channel blockers, however, should not be the first-line choice for management in general. For example, although persons with uncomplicated hypertension tend to respond well to calcium channel blockers, such drugs should be avoided in individuals with left ventricular hypertrophy; a history of a previous myocardial infarction, the presence of atrioventricular or sinoatrial nodal abnormalities, or overt heart failure. These drugs are effective in reducing high blood pressure not caused by elevated renin levels, which is more common among African Americans. Calcium channel blockers are also effective for treatment of hypertension in persons who also have asthma, hyperlipidemia, diabetes, or renal dysfunction.[30] Calcium channel blockers reduce mortality in the elderly with hypertension. Many other antihypertensive agents work synergistically with calcium channel blockers such as ACE inhibitors, selective beta-blockers, and diuretics. Many combination formulations of antihypertensive agents are now on the market, which helps individuals take these medications.

Table 15-12 Calcium Channel Blockers

Drug Generic (Brand)	Formulations	Dose	Half-Life (Hours)	Clinical Considerations	Side Effects*	FDA Pregnancy Category
Dihydropyridines						
Amlodipine (Norvasc)	2.5-mg, 5-mg, 10-mg tab	2.5 mg, 5 mg, 10 mg tab Initially 5 mg daily, maintenance 5–10 mg, max 10 mg daily.	30–50	Contraindicated if unstable angina, aortic stenosis, or s/p myocardial infarction.	Rare: depression, insomnia, hepatitis, Stevens-Johnson syndrome, hyperglycemia	C
Amlodipine/benazepril (Lotrel)	2.5/10-mg, 5/10-mg, 5/20-mg, 5/40-mg, 10/20-mg, 10/40-mg cap	When combination therapy is appropriate, initial dose 2.5/10 mg daily. May titrate amlodipine or benazepril appropriately.	30–50	Same contraindications as amlodipine with addition of pregnancy.	Common: headache cough Rare: anaphylaxis, angioedema, hyperkalemia	X
Amlodipine/valsartan (Exforge)	5/160-, 10/160-, 5/320-, 10/320-mg cap	When combination therapy is appropriate, initial dose 5/160 mg daily. May titrate amlodipine or valsartan appropriately.	30–50	Same contraindications as amlodipine.	Common: sensitivity to bright light	X
Felodipine (Plendil)	2.5-mg, 5-mg, 10-mg cap	Initially 5 mg daily, maintenance 2.5 mg–10 mg, max 10 mg daily.	10–16	Hypersensitivity possible. Take without food or with light meal. Do not crush or chew. Many drug–drug interactions; do not take with grapefruit juice.	Rare: severe hypotension	C
Enalapril/felodipine (Lexxel)	5/2.5-mg and 5/5-mg tab	When combination therapy is appropriate, initial dose 5/2.5 mg daily. May titrate enalapril and/or felodipine appropriately.	10–16	Hypersensitivity possible. Take without food or with light meal. Do not crush or chew. Many drug–drug interactions; do not take with grapefruit juice.	Rare: severe hypotension	X
Nicardipine (Cardene, Cardene SR)	Nicardipine: 20 mg, 30 mg Cardene SR: 30 mg, 45 mg, 60 mg	Cardene: start 20 mg PO tid, maintenance dose 20–40 mg PO tid, maximum dose 120 mg/day. Carden SR: start 30 mg PO bid, maintenance dose 30–60 mg PO bid, maximum dose 120 mg/day.	8.6	Can take without regard to meals.	Common: reflect tachycardia more common with nifedipine than with other CCBs	C
Nifedipine (Adalat CC, Procardia XL)	Adalat CC: 30-mg, 60-mg, 90-mg ER tab. Procardia XL: 30-mg, 60-mg, 90-mg ext tab	Adalat CC: initially 30 mg daily, maintenance 30–60 mg daily, max 90 mg daily. Procardia XL: initially 30–60 mg daily, max 120 mg daily.	3.7–4.3	Swallow whole on empty stomach. Titrate over 7–14 days.	Long-acting nifedipine formulations are much better tolerated than short-acting because they do not cause tachycardia, flushing, and palpitations as often as is seen with the short-acting formulations	C
Nisoldipine (Sular)	10-mg, 20-mg, 30-mg, 40-mg ER tab	Initially 20 mg daily, maintenance 20–40 mg, max 60 mg daily.	7–12	Do not crush; do not take with high-fat meal or grapefruit juice.	Well-tolerated	C

(continues)

Table 15-12 Calcium Channel Blockers (*continued*)

Drug Generic (Brand)	Formulations	Dose	Half-Life (Hours)	Clinical Considerations	Side Effects*	FDA Pregnancy Category
Nondihydropyridines						
Diltiazem (Cardizem CD, Cardizem LA, Tiazac, Dilacor XR, Dilacor XT)	Cardizem CD: 120 mg, 180 mg, 240 mg, 300 mg, 360 mg Cardizem LA: 120-mg, 180-mg, 240-mg, 300-mg, 360-mg, 420-mg ER tab Tiazac: 120-mg, 180-mg, 240-mg, 300-mg, 360-mg, 420-mg ext tab Dilacor XR Dilacor XT: 120-mg, 180-mg, 240-mg ER caps	Cardizem CD: initially 180–240 mg daily, max 480 mg daily. Cardizem LA: initially 180–240 mg daily, max 540 mg daily. Tiazac: initially 120–240 mg daily, max 540 mg daily. Dilacor XR/XL: initially 180 mg, maintenance 180–480 mg, max 540 mg daily.	4–10	Cardizem CD: titrate 2-week intervals. Cardizem LA: swallow whole, take at the same time daily. Tiazac: may sprinkle contents on food. Dilacor XR/XT: Take in am on empty stomach. Combination with digoxin and beta-blocker may lead to AV block.	Common: stuffy nose, rash, prurutis Rare: Stevens-Johnson syndrome, photosensitivity, hyperpigmentation	C
Verapamil (Calan, Calan SR, Isoptin SR, Verelan, Verelan PM)	Calan: 40-mg, 80-mg, 120-mg tab. Calan SR: 120-mg, 180-mg, 240-mg ER caps. Isoptin SR: 120-mg, 180-mg, 240-mg ER caps Verelan: 120-mg, 180-mg, 240-mg, 360-mg ER caps Verelan PM: 100-mg, 200-mg, 300-mg ER caps	Calan: initially 80 mg three times daily, max 360 mg daily. Calan SR: initially 180 mg daily, max 480 mg daily. Isoptin SR: initially 120–180 mg daily, max. Verelan: initially 120 mg daily, maintenance 120–240 mg, max 480 mg daily. Verelan PM: initially 200 mg daily, maintenance 200–400 mg, max 400 mg daily.	6–10 active metabolite	Drug–drug interaction with digoxin can cause digoxin toxicity Calan: take with food in the AM, initially 120 mg for elderly. Isoptin: take with food. Verelan: take a single dose in the AM. May sprinkle on applesauce. Verelan PM: Give at bedtime.	Common: constipation, dizziness and nausea Rare: heart failure, hypotension, AV block, gynecomastia, urinary frequency, oligomenorrhea, irregular menses	C

max = maximum; AV = atrioventricular; CCB = calcium channel blocker.

* Common side effects of all calcium channel blockers include peripheral edema, headache, flushing, dizziness, palpitations, hypotension, reflex tachycardia, gingival hypertrophy.

Mechanism of Action

Calcium channel blockers bind to L-type calcium channels located on the cell membranes of vascular smooth muscle, cardiac muscle, and cardiac nodal tissue, thereby preventing the influx of calcium into the cell. The contraction of vascular smooth muscle is extremely dependent on the influx of calcium. These drugs inhibit the influx of calcium into the arterial smooth muscle but have little effect on venous vasculature. Ultimately, calcium channel blockers cause dilation of the peripheral arterials, and a reduction in blood pressure ensues. The net effect is that the cell cannot contract as strongly with less calcium to drive the intracellular contraction mechanism. This is called a **negative inotropic effect**. The heart rate also slows because the calcium channel blocker inhibits the influx of calcium into the nerves that direct contraction so the action potential along the nerves is slowed. This is

called a **negative chronotropic effect**. The clinical effects of calcium channel blockers are peripheral vasodilation, decreased heart rate, increased cardiac contractility and decreased cardiac conduction.

There are three different classes of calcium channel blockers, each of which differs in basic chemical structure and mechanism of action. The **dihydropyridines** reduce systemic vascular resistance and arterial pressure. They are used to treat hypertension. The **phenylalanines** are selective for suppressing myocardium but have minimal vasodilation effects. They are used to treat angina. Finally, the **benzodiazepines** are an intermediate class that has both cardiac suppression and vasodilation effects.

The effect of calcium channel blockers is slightly different within the cardiac cell. The depolarization of the sinoatrial and atrioventricular nodes is controlled primarily by the recovery of the slow calcium channels. Verapamil (Calan) and diltiazem (Cardizem) depress the rate at which the sinus node fires because they slow the recovery of these channels. This phenomenon can be extremely helpful in treating a person with supraventricular tachycardia, but could be detrimental when given to someone who has a preexisting heart block.

Side Effects/Contraindications

In the mid-1990s, observational studies indicated that short-acting, immediate-release calcium channel blockers might cause an increase in myocardial infarction, gastrointestinal bleeding, and cancer, which lead to a drop-off in use. Subsequent randomized trials have shown that long-acting channel blockers decrease cardiovascular events and that there is no association between these drugs and gastrointestinal bleeding or cancer.

Most of the side effects of calcium channel blockers stem from the very mechanism that helps reduce blood pressure. As the peripheral resistance is lowered, stimulation of baroreceptor-mediated sympathetic response is initiated, which causes tachycardia and increased stroke volume. Approximately 22% of persons who take calcium channel blockers will develop peripheral edema (ankle swelling); diuretics are not helpful in alleviating this side effect. Headache, palpitations, and flushing are also common side effects. Thus, combining calcium channel blockers with beta-blockers is a useful way to treat hypertension by using two drugs that ameliorate the adverse effects of each other. Rare adverse effects include urinary retention, bradycardia, and AV node block.

Drug–Drug Interactions

Many of the calcium channel blockers inhibit CYP3A4. Thus, most of the drug–drug interactions result in increased levels of either the calcium channel blocker or the interacting drug and enhanced therapeutic responses that can become toxic effects. For example, the use of verapamil (Calan) by persons also taking digoxin will require monitoring the digoxin level on a regular basis to avoid digoxin toxicity. The combination of a calcium channel blocker and quinidine may lead to severe hypotension. Drug–drug interactions associated with calcium channel blockers are noted in Table 15-13.

Special Populations

Calcium channel blockers have been used in pregnancy when the benefit of blood pressure reduction outweighs the risk. They are all FDA Pregnancy Category C. Long-acting formulations of nifedipine (Procardia) doses of 30 to 90 mg daily have been used without major adverse

Table 15-13 Drug–Drug Interactions Associated with Calcium Channel Blockers*

Drug Generic (Brand)	Effect
Amiodarone	Additive reduction in heart rate and myocardial contractility.
Anesthetics	Additive effect of increasing hypotensive effect.
Atorvastatin (Lipitor)	Increased serum levels of atorvastatin.
Azole antifungals	Increased hypotensive effect.
Beta-blockers	Generally well tolerated and can be used therapeutically, but there is an additive effect that can cause bradycardia and heart block.
Buspirone	Increased serum levels of buspirone.
Carbamazepine (Tegretol)	Increased serum levels of carbamazepine via reduced elimination.
Cimetidine (Tagamet)	Potentiation of calcium channel blocker effects.
Cyclosporin	Increases effect of cyclosporin so dose can be reduced.
Digoxin (Lanoxin)	Increased levels of digoxin and possible digoxin toxicity. This effect is especially potent with verapamil, and combining digoxin with verapamil is contraindicated.
Erythromycin (E-Mycin)	Increases hypotensive effect, bradycardia.
Grapefruit juice	Increases serum levels of calcium channel blockers.
Lithium (Eskalith)	Increased risk of neurotoxicity.
Lovastatin (Mevacor)	Increased serum levels of lovastatin.
Opiates	Hypotension.
Nafcillin	Reduced effect of the calcium channel blocker.
Quinidine	Excessive hypotension.
Phenobarbital (Luminal)	Increases clearance of verapamil (Covera).
Phenytoin (Dilantin)	Reduced effect of calcium channel blocker.
Phenobarbital (Luminal)	Increased clearance of verapamil.
Propranolol (Inderal)	Increased serum levels and bioavailability of propranolol.
Rifampin (Rifadin)	Decreased effect of calcium channel blocker, hypertension.
Simvastatin (Zocor)	Increased serum levels of simvastatin.
Theophylline (Theo-Dur)	Decreased clearance of theophylline and increased serum levels.

* This table is not comprehensive. New information is being identified on a regular basis. In addition, individual calcium channel antagonists may have a specific drug–drug interaction that others in the same class do not have.

reactions. Nifedipine is regularly used as a tocolytic to stop preterm labor. Calcium channel blockers do cross into breast milk, but the American Academy of Pediatrics approves them in use with breastfeeding.[28]

Selective α₁-Receptor Antagonists

Selective α₁-receptor antagonists are not commonly used as first-line monotherapy, but because they are complementary to the other groups of antihypertensives, they can be added when monotherapy is not sufficient to meet blood pressure goals (Table 15-14).

Mechanism of Action

Selective α₁-receptor antagonists block the α₁-receptors in the peripheral vasculature, thereby inhibiting the effect of catecholamines, which results in vasodilation and decreased peripheral resistance. α₂-Receptor antagonists inhibit the release of norepinephrine presynaptically.

Nonselective α₁- and α₂-receptor antagonists are not used in the treatment of hypertension despite theoretical advantages. Antagonism of the α₂-receptor will stimulate insulin release. Therefore, use of nonselective alpha-receptor antagonists could be of benefit to persons with hypertension and diabetes or impaired glucose syndromes. However, the ALLHAT trial compared the effects of thiazide diuretics and α₁-receptor antagonists on cardiovascular outcomes and glucose levels in 8749 persons with diabetes and 1690 individuals newly diagnosed with impaired fasting glucose. α₁-Receptor antagonists were found to increase the risk of combined cardiovascular disease and heart failure (RR = 1.85; 95% CI, 1.56–2.19) in persons with diabetes (RR = 1.63; 95% CI, 1.05–2.55) and in those with newly diagnosed impaired fasting glucose (IFG) despite lower glucose levels in these participants.[35] Most of the α-receptor antagonists in use today are selective for the α₁-receptor.

Side Effects/Contraindications

The primary side effect of these drugs is the first-dose syncope, which is postural hypotension and tachycardia that occurs 1 to 3 hours after the initial doses of α₁-antagonists. This side effect can be reduced with a lower initial dose, the avoidance of concurrent use of diuretics, and ingestion at bedtime. Other common side effects are fatigue, nasal congestion, and headache. Women who are taking an α₁-receptor antagonist are at increased risk of floppy iris syndrome if undergoing cataract surgery.

Drug–Drug Interactions

The drug–drug interactions associated with use of α₁-receptor antagonists are primarily secondary to additive effects or inhibitory effects from concomitant use of drugs that have an independent effect on blood pressure as discussed previously.

Special Populations

These drugs are FDA Pregnancy Category C because there are no reports of use of this drug during pregnancy. There is not much information about α₁-receptor antagonists in pregnancy and lactation. It is unknown if these drugs are excreted in breast milk.[28] There are no alterations in dosing for the elderly; however, consideration for increased dizziness and syncopal episodes should be considered. In addition, because these drugs cross the blood–brain barrier, they can cause depression, vivid dreams, and lethargy, all of which can be more troublesome to the elderly.

Selective α₂-Receptor Agonists

Selective α₂-receptor agonists, which are also called central α₂-agonists, are not first-line antihypertensive drugs (Table 15-15). These drugs exert their effects primarily by stimulating the α₂-receptors within the central nervous system, which reduces the sympathetic outflow from the vasomotor center and increases vagal tone. The result is a slower heart rate and decreased cardiac output.

Table 15-14 Selective α₁-Receptor Antagonists

Drug Generic (Brand)	Formulations	Dose	Clinical Considerations	FDA Pregnancy Category
Doxazosin (Cardura)	1-mg, 2-mg, 4-mg, 8-mg tab	Initially 1 mg daily, max 16 mg daily.		C
Prazosin (Minipress)	1-mg, 2-mg, 5-mg caps	First dose at bedtime, 1 mg 2–3 times daily, maintenance 6–15 mg daily, max 20–40 mg daily.	Limit alcohol intake, hypotensive with propranolol, diuretics, false + pheochromocytoma test.	C
Terazosin (Hytrin)	1-mg, 2-mg, 5-mg, 10-mg caps	1 mg at bedtime; may increase dose slowly, maintenance 1–5 mg, max 20 mg/day. May be given in single or divided dose.		C

Table 15-15 Selective α₂-Receptor Agonists

Drug Generic (Brand)	Formulations	Dose	Half-Life (Hours)	Clinical Considerations*	FDA Pregnancy Category
Clonidine (Catapres, Catapres TTS)	0.1-, 0.2-, 0.3-mg tab 0.1-, 0.2-, 0.3-mg weekly patch	Initially 0.1 mg twice daily, maintenance 0.2–0.6 mg daily, max 2.4 mg daily.	8–12	Patch must be applied to an intact, hairless patch of skin; rotate sites. Contraindicated in persons with sinus node or AV node conduction dysfunction.	C
Guanfacine (Tenex)	1-mg, 2-mg tab	Initially 1 mg daily at bedtime, maintenance 1–3 mg daily, max 3 mg daily.	17	Contraindicated in persons with known hypersensitivity.	B
Guanabenz (Wytensin)	4-mg, 8-mg tabs	Initially 2–4 mg twice daily, max 8 mg twice daily.	4–6	Dosage adjustments for hepatic impairment.	C
Methyldopa (Aldomet)	125-mg, 250-mg, 500-mg tabs	Initially 250 mg bid to tid, maintenance 500–2000 mg daily, max 3000 mg daily.	~ 2–3	Contraindicated in persons with hepatic disease, hypersensitivity to methyldopa, pheochromocytoma, or use of MAO inhibitors. May interfere with lab tests.	B

* All of the central α₂ agonists can cause severe hypertension if abruptly withdrawn.

Side Effects/Contraindications

Side effects of centrally acting α₂-receptor agonists include sedation, dizziness, and dry mouth (which can occur in up to 50% of persons who take Clonidine [Catapres]). CNS effects also include parkinsonian symptoms and decreased libido, which can result in sexual dysfunction and impotence. The incidence of these symptoms is lower in persons who use the transdermal patch, yet this route of administration can cause contact dermatitis in approximately 15–20% of persons who use it. Abrupt discontinuation of these drugs may cause withdrawal symptoms such as headache, tachycardia, tremors, or sweating secondary to the sudden increase in sympathetic discharge. In addition, the arterial pressure can rebound and rise higher than it was previously. Rarely, a symptomatic bradycardia or sinus arrest can occur in persons with sinoatrial node dysfunction or persons who are taking other medications that affect the atrioventricular node.

Methyldopa (Aldomet) has active metabolites that have adverse effects. Methyldopa can induce a transient sedation, depression, and it has the rare potential to cause hemolytic anemia and/or liver disease. Hyperprolactinemia can become significant enough to cause gynecomastia and galactorrhea. Hepatotoxicity is a rare but serious adverse effect associated with the initiation of methyldopa. It is recommended that clinicians obtain a baseline complete blood count (CBC) and conduct liver function tests prior to starting this drug. Methyldopa is contraindicated for persons with hepatic disease, hypersensitivity to methyldopa, and those taking MAO inhibitors because the combination of methyldopa and MAO inhibitors can cause hallucinations and severe hypertension.

Both clonidine and guanfacine (Tenex) should be used with caution by persons who have had a recent myocardial infarction, cerebrovascular disease, diabetes (as it may mask signs of hypoglycemia), or renal impairment.

Drug–Drug Interactions

Selective α₂-receptor agonists are antagonized by tricyclic antidepressants, and they can potentiate the effects of CNS depressants such as alcohol, phenothiazines, and barbiturates. Methyldopa can increase the risk for lithium toxicity and the effect of levodopa. Conversely, iron tablets can decrease the extent of methyldopa absorption. The use of clonidine with beta-blockers may potentiate bradycardia and worsen rebound hypertension when the beta-blockers are discontinued.

Special Populations

The FDA pregnancy categories for this group of drugs vary. Methyldopa (Aldomet) is FDA Pregnancy Category B and has been used during pregnancy to manage moderate to severe hypertension.[36] It also crosses into breast milk at a low level, and the AAP reports that it is compatible with breastfeeding. Guanfacine (Tenex) is Category B, and no information is available about use of guanfacine during lactation. Clonidine (Catapres) is Category C and crosses the placenta, and caution should be used secondary to rebound hypertension if it is stopped abruptly. Clonidine does enter the breast milk and may concentrate. The effect of clonidine on the newborn is not clear.[27] Methyldopa can cause drug-induced immune-mediated hemolysis leading to a positive Coombs test. There are no dosing changes based on a patient's age; however, these medications should be used cautiously in the elderly because they can cause increased CNS depression.

Vasodilators

Vasodilators were among the first antihypertensive drugs available for the US market (Table 15-16). Today, hydralazine (Apresoline) and minoxidil (Loniten) are not used as single agents in the treatment of hypertension, but they are effective in combination with other agents. Hydralazine (Apresoline) is a common addition if needed after assessing the effects of the first-line drugs nifedipine (Procardia) and/or methyldopa (Aldomet).

Mechanism of Action

Vasodilators result in dilation of blood vessels (arterioles more so than veins) and by doing so, increase perfusion to the heart. These drugs stimulate the sympathetic nervous system, which results in both a faster heart rate and increased contractility.

Side Effects/Adverse Reactions

Common side effects include headache, nausea, diarrhea, palpitations, and nasal congestion. Less common side effects are blood dyscrasias, a lupus-like drug syndrome, and a positive direct Coombs test. Individuals who have mitral valve rheumatic heart disease should not take vasodilators.

Complementary Treatments for Hypertension

Many studies have been done over the past several years investigating alternative treatments for hypertension. However, the data in most of these studies are conflicting and often fail to provide a clear answer. There are no proven effective herbals for treatment of hypertension. However, there are a few that have some promise as diuretics.[37]

Hyperlipidemia

Hyperlipidemia is a major risk factor for CVD. The National Cholesterol Education Program Expert Panel's report (Adult Treatment Plan III) in 2004 and its revision in 2005 provide recommendations for screening and treatment for dyslipidemia.[38] To better understand the pharmacologic interventions for dyslipidemia, a brief review of the physiologic mechanisms of cholesterol and lipid metabolism are in order.

Cholesterol, a fat-like substance produced in the liver, is an essential element in bile salts, the precursor of steroid hormones, and a major component of cell membranes. Approximately 15% of cholesterol comes from diet, and the rest is made endogenously in the liver and intestinal cells. Cholesterol, one of the most important lipids in the body, is insoluble and therefore transported in the circulation bound in lipid protein complexes called lipoproteins (Figure 15-4).

All lipoproteins contain **triglyceride**, cholesterol, proteins, and other lipids besides cholesterol, but they vary with regard to the proportion of lipid to protein. The lipoproteins that have more lipid are less dense, and those that have a greater proportion of protein are more dense. The three most commonly discussed lipoproteins that transport cholesterol include **low-density lipoprotein** (LDL), which transports cholesterol to peripheral tissues and is absorbed by the liver when cholesterol is needed for liver function; **high-density lipoprotein** (HDL), which transports cholesterol from the tissues to the liver, where it is broken down to become bile; and **very-low-density lipoprotein** (VLDL), which transports triglycerides from the liver to peripheral tissues. Once VLDLs give up triglycerides, they convert to LDLs.

Table 15-16 Vasodilators

Drug Generic (Brand)	Dose	Half-Life	Side Effects	Contraindications	FDA Pregnancy Category
Hydralazine (Apresoline)	Usual dose 40–200 mg per day	2–4 hours but effects observed longer	Headache, anorexia, nausea, vomiting, diarrhea, palpitations, tachycardia, angina pectoris, peripheral neuritis, and systemic lupus erythematosus.	CAD and mitral valvular rheumatic heart disease.	C
Minoxidil (Loniten)	Starting dose: 5 to 10 mg per day	4.2	Headache, sweating, and hypertrichosis. Reflex sympathetic stimulation and sodium and fluid retention.	Beta-blockers: tachycardia, palpitations, angina, and edema.	C

CAD = coronary artery disease.

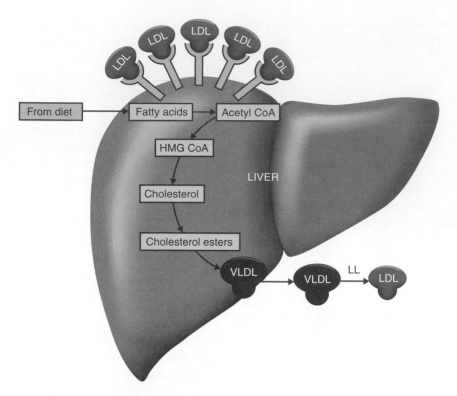

HMG CoA = 3-hydroxy-3-methyl-glutaryl-CoA reductase; LDL = low density lipoprotein;
LL = lipoprotein lipase; VLDL = very low density lipoprotein.

Figure 15-4 Cholesterol metabolism.

Low-density lipoprotein comprises 60–70% of total cholesterol and is a major atherogenic lipoprotein. Lowering LDL reduces an individual's overall risk for CVD.[38]

Atherosclerosis is a chronic inflammatory process that occurs within the walls of arteries. It is not a phenomenon that develops overnight. Atherogenesis begins with entrapment of LDLs in the blood vessel wall. The LDLs are digested by macrophages that fill with lipid and become foam cells that also get trapped in the endothelial wall. These foam cells coalesce into a fatty streak, which is a smooth, raised plaque just beneath the endothelium. The fatty streaks form early in life and can progress to become rough, calcified atherosclerotic lesions that cause arterial stenosis and/or infarctions.

Atherogenesis starts to occur at LDL levels of approximately 100–129 mg/dL, occurs at a faster rate if LDL levels are in the 130–159 mg/dL range, and is accelerated at LDL levels of 160 mg/dL or higher.[39] The atherogenesis process is influenced by the plasma levels of HDL, VLDL, LDL, and triglycerides. In measuring these values, the combination of VLDL and LDL is considered non-HDL. The non-HDL can be calculated from the total cholesterol minus the HDL. Non-HDL is considered more

of an atherogenic risk than LDL alone. Lower levels of HDL, characterized as less than 35 mg/dL, have been shown also to be an independent risk factor for CVD and are a predictor of coronary heart disease in women.[21] Conversely, elevated levels of HDL have been shown to decrease overall CVD risk. Overall, women have higher plasma levels of HDL than men; therefore, women's target values may be different than those for men. Finally it is important to remember that risk factors for CVD that are associated with elevated cholesterol include genetic predisposition, diet, obesity, physical inactivity, smoking, hypertension, and diabetes. Table 15-17 shows the target levels of LDL, HDL, and triglycerides.

Some medications used for other indications have an independent effect on lipids. For example, glucocorticoids, thiazide diuretics, cyclosporines, and tacrolimus raise the blood levels of triglycerides, LDL cholesterol, and HDL cholesterol. Estrogens increase blood levels of triglycerides and HDL cholesterol while lowering levels of LDL cholesterol. Androgens have an opposite effect of increasing triglycerides and LDL cholesterol while lowering levels of HDL cholesterol. Progestins raise blood levels of LDL cholesterol but lower levels of triglycerides and HDL cholesterol.

Table 15-17 Lipid Goals

Lipoprotein	Description	Level
Low-density lipoprotein (LDL)	Optimal	< 100 mg/dL
	Near optimal	100–129 mg/dL
	Borderline high	130–159 mg/dL
	High	160–189 mg/dL
	Very high	≥ 190
High-density lipoprotein (HDL)	Low	< 50
Triglycerides	Normal	< 150 mg/dL
	Borderline	150–199 mg/dL
	High	200–499 mg/dL
	Very high	≥ 500
Very-low-density lipoprotein (VLDL)	Normal with triglycerides less than 150	≤ 30
		≥ 30
	Normal with triglycerides greater than 150	

Source: National Cholesterol Education Program 2002.[38]

Pharmacologic Treatments for Hyperlipidemia

Decreasing the plasma levels of atherogenic lipoproteins such as LDL, non-LDL, VLDL, and triglycerides reduces the risk of developing CVD.[20] Treatment may be accomplished via several nonpharmacologic and pharmacologic treatments alone or in combination. Initial treatment should target the underlying cause of the hyperlipidemia. For many people, lifestyle modification is a necessary first step in treatment/risk reduction. However, for some individuals, this is not sufficient, and drugs are required to obtain optimal goals. Statins, bile-acid sequestering agents, nicotinic acid, fibric acid derivatives, cholesterol absorption inhibitor, and combinations of these agents are available in helping individuals reach their goals. Each has a different effect on LDLs, HDLs, and triglycerides (Table 15-18).

HMG CoA Reductase Inhibitors (Statins)

HMG CoA reductase inhibitors (**statins**) are the first-line treatment in reducing LDL (Table 15-19). These agents are the most effective class of drug available to reduce cholesterol levels. Statins have demonstrated ability to reduce a woman's risk for developing CVD. It has also been shown that an aggressive reduction of LDL in persons who have stable CAD reduces the risk of major cardiovascular events.[39]

Statins also greatly benefit women who have other CVD risk factors such as smoking, type 2 diabetes, or peripheral arterial disease. The Collaborative Atorvastatin Diabetes Study found a significant reduction in

Table 15-18 Effect of Drugs on Dyslipidemia

Drug	LDL	HDL	Triglycerides
Statins	Effective	Modest effect	Modest effect
Bile acid sequestrants	Modest effect	No effect	Minimal effect or increase
Fibrates	Minimal to no effect or increase	Modest effect	Effective
Niacin	Modest effect	Effective	Effective
Ezetimibe (Zetia)	Effective	Modest effect	No effect

LDL = low-density lipoprotein; HDL = high-density lipoprotein.

several cardiovascular events with the use of atorvastatin (Lipitor) 10 mg versus placebo in persons with diabetes. This trial was terminated 2 years early because the results were striking. The incidence of cardiovascular events was decreased by 37% ($P = .001$). When each event was evaluated separately, there was a reduction in each category: 36% in acute coronary events, 31% in coronary revascularization events, and 48% in stroke. The death rate was also reduced by 27% ($P = .059$) with atorvastatin (Lipitor).[40]

Mechanism of Action

Statins reduce cholesterol production by the liver via inhibition of 3-hydroxy-3-methyl-glutaryl-CoA reductase (HMG CoA), an enzyme involved in cholesterol production. These agents stimulate the upregulation of LDL receptors in the liver, which bind to LDL and thereby increase the extraction of LDL from the plasma pool. Some statins will cause a reduction in triglycerides and elevation of HDL, which is secondary to the primary mechanism reducing LDL. In addition to LDL reduction, statins have cardioprotective effects by improving endothelial function, improving plaque stability, and reducing endothelial inflammation.[41]

Dosing Considerations

Statins all have the same basic mechanism of action, but there are significant differences in their potency and pharmacokinetic profiles that are of clinical import (Box 15-2). Not all statins are equally aggressive in lowering LDL. Atorvastatin (Lipitor), lovastatin (Mevacor), lovastatin ER (Altoprev), and simvastatin (Zocor) are metabolized via the CYP3A4. Fluvastatin (Lescol) and fluvastatin ER (Lescol XL) are metabolized by CYP2C9. Pravastatin (Pravachol) and rosuvastatin (Crestor) are minimally metabolized. In addition, lovastatin (Mevacor) and simvastatin (Zocor) are prodrugs that have active metabolites. There is considerable individual variability in response, which may

Table 15-19 HMG CoA Reductase Inhibitors (aka Statins)

Drug Generic (Brand)	Formulations	Dose	Half-Life (Hours)	Metabolism	Effects on Lipids	Clinical Considerations	FDA Pregnancy Category
Atorvastatin (Lipitor)	10-mg, 20-mg, 40-mg, 80-mg tabs	Initially 10–20 mg daily, maintenance 10–80 mg daily, max 80 mg daily	9–32	CYP3A4	LDL ↓ 39–60%; HDL ↑ 5–9%; trig 19–37%	Do not take with food. Can be taken any time of day.	X
Amlodipine/ atorvastatin (Caduet)	2.5/20 mg, 2.5/40 mg, 5/10 mg, 5/20 mg, 5/40 mg, 5/80 mg, 10/10 mg, 10/20 mg, 10/40 mg, 10/80 mg	Combination product; see dosing for individual components	9–32	CYP3A4	LDL ↓ 39–60%; HDL ↑ 5–9%; trig 19–37%	Do not take with food. Can be taken any time of day.	X
Fluvastatin (Lescol)	20 mg, 40 mg tabs	Initially 20 mg daily, maintenance 20–80 mg, max 80 mg daily	~ 3	CYP2C9	LDL ↓ 33–38%; HDL ↑ 3–11%; trig ↓ 12–25%	Do not take with food. Take at night.	X
Fluvastatin ER (Lescol XL)	80-mg ext release tab	Initially 80 mg daily	~ 3	CYP2C9	LDL ↓ 33–38%; HDL ↑ 3–11%, trig ↓ 12–25%	Do not take with food. Take at night.	X
Lovastatin (Mevacor)	10-mg, 20-mg, 40-mg tabs	Initially 10–20 mg daily, max 80 mg daily	~ 3	CYP3A4	LDL ↓ 25%; HDL ↑ 7–11%; trig ↓ 19–25%	Take with meals. Take at night.	X
Lovastatin ER (Altoprev)	10-mg, 20-mg, 40-mg, 60-mg ext rel tab	Initially 10–60 mg daily at bedtime	10	CYP3A4	LDL ↓ 21–42%; HDL ↑ 2–10%; trig ↓ 6–27%	Take with meals. Take at night.	X
Pravastatin (Pravachol)	10-mg, 20-mg, 40-mg, 80-mg tabs	Initially 40 mg daily, max 80 mg daily	~ 3	Minimal metabolism	LDL ↓ 24–41%; HDL ↑ 9–13%; trig ↓ 10–25%	Do not take with food. Take at night.	X
Rosuvastatin (Crestor)	5-mg, 10-mg, 20-mg, 40-mg tabs	Initially 10 mg daily, maintenance 5–20 mg daily, max 40 mg daily	20	Minimal metabolism	LDL ↓ 22–37%; HDL ↑ 8–14%; trig ↓ 15–24%	Not affected by food intake. Can be taken any time of day.	X
Simvastatin (Zocor)	5-mg, 10-mg, 20-mg, 40-mg, 80-mg tabs	Initially 20–40 mg daily, maintenance 5–80 mg daily, max 80 mg daily	~ 3	CYP3A4	LDL ↓ 45–63%; HDL ↑ 8–14%; trig ↓ 10–35%	Not affected by food intake. Take at night.	X

aka = also known as; trig = triglycerides; LDL = low-density lipoprotein; HDL = high-density lipoprotein; ↑ = increased; ↓ = decreased.

▌ **Box 15-2** Case Study: Statin Failure

PC is a 56-year-old woman who is being evaluated for side effects from statin therapy. She reports that she originally started on atorvastatin (Lipitor) 20 mg daily and developed leg pain and fatigue so she discontinued use of the drug. She was then started on ezetimibe (Zetia) 10 mg daily. She denies any problems at this time. Her vital signs are height 5'8" (172.7 cm), weight 150 lbs (68 kg), blood pressure 115/72, heart rate 72, and respirations 16. She had her fasting lipid panel done and the results were total cholesterol 302 mg/dL, LDL 181 mg/dL, HDL 60 mg/dL, and triglycerides 307 mg/dL; her other fasting lab results were all within normal ranges.

PC is similar to many individuals who experience fatigue and muscle aches without a rise in the blood levels of CPK when starting statins. It is often difficult to convince a person who has no symptoms of disease of the benefit of a medication when symptoms from the treatment appear. The provider discussed diet and exercise habits with PC. She agreed to attempt another statin, rosuvastatin (Crestor) 10 mg daily at bedtime and continue on the ezetimibe (Zetia). She will be reevaluated in 6 weeks for repeat of her AST/ALT values.

The other item of concern is her hypertriglyceridemia. If she tolerates the statin, other agents such as omega 3 fatty acids and fibrates (excluding gemfibrozil) may need to be added to lower her triglycerides. It would also be reasonable to try any other statin at a low dose.

be secondary to genomic polymorphisms that direct the activity of the metabolizing enzymes, and there are differences in drug–drug interactions as well.[42]

Atorvastatin (Lipitor) is the most potent statin, followed by rosuvastatin (Crestor), then simvastatin (Zocor); lovastatin (Mevacor) is equal to pravastatin (Pravachol) with regard to potency, with fluvastatin (Lescol) being the least potent. Therefore, statins with increasing potency can be used for individuals who are unable to meet lipid value goals on less potent formulations given at their highest doses.

Lovastatin (Mevacor) needs to be taken with meals, whereas the others should be taken 2 hours before or after meals. Some individuals are intolerant to statins or cannot afford daily therapy. However there are now generic statins available that can help address the issue of cost as a barrier of treatment.

The FDA has approved label instructions that recommend evaluation of liver transaminase levels prior to initiating therapy with statins, 12 weeks after starting statin therapy, after a dose increase, and periodically thereafter. At this time, routine monitoring of liver function is not supported by research because the actual incidence of liver damage is very rare. However, until the FDA evaluates and changes its recommendations, these guidelines should be followed. An effect should be seen after 6 weeks of therapy and in general will not continue to improve beyond that time frame, so 6 weeks is a good time to reassess initially.

Individuals are encouraged to take their statin at night because HMG CoA is more active in the evening and when the individual is not eating.[43] Timing the dose this way allows for the highest plasma levels of statins when there are the highest levels of HMG CoA the statin will inhibit.

Statins confer some protection against the development of colon cancer. Although statins are not recommended for primary prevention, persons who take statins have a significantly lower risk for developing new onset colon cancer.[44]

Side Effects/Adverse Effects

The most common side effects of statins are muscle pain and soreness or muscle cramps, which occur in approximately 1–3% of individuals who start these drugs. Other side effects include abdominal pain, constipation, diarrhea, and nausea. Many patients cannot tolerate higher doses of statins secondary to myalgias. Often decreasing the dose or initially starting at the lowest possible dose and slowly titrating can overcome these problems.

There are two uncommon side effects associated with statins. First, asymptomatic elevations in aminotransferase (AST and ALT) activity can occur, which is more likely in persons with underlying liver disease. Elevations that are less than three times higher than the baseline value are considered normal and do not require intervention. The other adverse reaction is skeletal muscle abnormalities, which can range from simple myalgia to rare development of rhabdomyolysis.[41] Creatinine kinase levels should be obtained if an individual reports significant muscle pain or weakness. The statin should be discontinued if the creatinine kinase (CK) level is elevated more than 10 times the upper limit of normal and/or the individual has intolerable symptoms. Individuals taking statins should be educated about the warning signs of rhabdomyolysis (muscle weakness, muscle aching, and/or dark colored urine).

Myopathy is more likely if statins are given concomitantly with other drugs that elevate the plasma levels of statins. In August of 2001, cerivastatin (Baycol) was removed from the market because of 31 deaths worldwide associated with its use. The majority of those deaths were associated with the combined use of cerivastatin (Baycol) and gemfibrozil (Lopid), which caused rhabdomyolysis with renal failure. Since then, reports of adverse effects have fallen significantly.

Adverse effects are rare at effective doses of the statin. Statins are contraindicated for persons who are pregnant or who have active liver disease with persistent elevation of liver enzymes. However, persons with stable chronic liver disease can take these drugs if indicated.

Drug–Drug Interactions

Drug–drug interactions associated with use of statins are listed in Table 15-20. Once efficacy has been determined, an increase in the statin dose does not result in increased efficacy but there is an increase in adverse effects, especially drug–drug interactions. Lovastatin (Mevacor, extended-release Altoprev), simvastatin (Zocor) and atorvastatin (Lipitor) are CP3A4 substrates, and therefore their metabolism can be inhibited by CP3A4 inhibitors such as macrolide antibiotics, selective serotonin receptor inhibitors, cyclosporine (Neoral), ketoconazole (Nizoral), verapamil (Calan), ritonavir (Norvir), tacrolimus (Prototropic), and grapefruit juice.[45] Conversely, fluvastatin (Lescol), an inhibitor of CP450–2C9, can cause increased plasma values of diclofenac (Voltaren), warfarin (Coumadin), and phenytoin (Dilantin) if taken simultaneously.[41] Finally, statins are contraindicated for persons taking gemfibrozil (Lopid) because gemfibrozil increases plasma levels of the statins via an effect that blocks biliary excretion and is associated with a significant risk for rhabdomyolysis.[45]

Table 15-20 Drug–Drug Associations with Statins*

Drug Generic (Brand)	Agent Affected	Effect
Calcium channel blockers	All statins	Increased serum levels of statins and increased risk for myopathy and rhabdomyolysis.
Cimetidine (Tagamet)	All statins	Increased oral bioavailability of statins thereby increasing serum levels.
Cyclosporin (Neoral)	All statins but increased significantly with pravastatin (Pravachol)	Increased serum levels of statins and increased risk for myopathy and rhabdomyolysis.
Diclofenac (Voltaren)	Fluvastatin (Lescol)	Increased serum levels of diclofenac.
Digoxin (Lanoxin)	All statins	Increased serum levels of statins and increased risk for myopathy and rhabdomyolysis.
Digoxin (Lanoxin)	Atorvastatin (Lipitor) and simvastatin (Zocor)	Increased serum levels of digoxin leading to increased risk for digoxin toxicity.
Diltiazem (Cardizem)	Simvastatin (Zocor)	Rhabdomyolysis.
Fibrates	All statins	Additive increased risk for myopathy and rhabdomyolysis.
Fluconazole (Diflucan)	Fluvastatin (Lescol)	Increased anticoagulant effect of the warfarin.
Grapefruit juice†	All statins except pravastatin (Pravachol)	Increased oral bioavailability of statins, thereby increasing serum levels.
Itraconazole (Sporanox)	All statins, especially simvastatin (Zocor)	Increased serum levels of statins and increased risk for myopathy and rhabdomyolysis.
Ketoconazole (Nizoral)	All statins	Increased serum levels of statins and increased risk for myopathy and rhabdomyolysis.
Macrolide antibiotics (e.g., erythromycin [E-Mycin])	All statins	Increased serum levels of statins and increased risk for myopathy and rhabdomyolysis.
Niacin	Lovastatin (Mevacor), pravastatin (Pravachol) and simvastatin (Zocor)	Increased serum levels of statins and increased risk for myopathy and rhabdomyolysis.
Protease inhibitors	All statins	Increased serum levels of statins and increased risk for myopathy and rhabdomyolysis.
Phenytoin (Dilantin)	Atorvastatin (Lipitor) and simvastatin (Zocor)	Decreased serum levels of statin with subsequent subtherapeutic effect.
Phenytoin (Dilantin)	Fluvastatin (Lescol)	Increased serum levels of phenytoin.
Rifampin (Rifadin)	All statins	Decreased serum levels of statin with subsequent subtherapeutic effect.
Sildenafil	All statins	Increased serum levels of statins and increased risk for myopathy and rhabdomyolysis.
SSRIs	Atorvastatin (Lipitor), Lovastatin (Mevacor), and simvastatin (Zocor)	Increased serum levels of statins and increased risk for myopathy and rhabdomyolysis.
Tacrolimus (Prograf)	Atorvastatin (Lipitor), Lovastatin (Mevacor) and simvastatin (Zocor)	Increased serum levels of statins and increased risk for myopathy and rhabdomyolysis.
Verapamil (Calan)	Atorvastatin (Lipitor), Lovastatin (Mevacor), and simvastatin (Zocor)	Increased serum levels of statins and increased risk for myopathy and rhabdomyolysis.
Warfarin (Coumadin)	All statins	Increased serum levels of statins and increased risk for myopathy and rhabdomyolysis.
Warfarin (Coumadin)	Fluvastatin (Lescol)	Increased anticoagulant effect of the warfarin.

SSRIs = selective serotonin reuptake inhibitors.
* This table is not comprehensive. New information is being identified on a regular basis.
† Significant interaction only if large quantities of grapefruit juice are ingested. A single glass of grapefruit juice per day does not result in clinically significant increases in serum levels of the statin.

Special Populations

Statins are FDA Pregnancy Category X. Statins cause adverse fetal outcomes and central nervous system and limb abnormalities in animal studies. Statins enter breast milk and are contraindicated for women who are breastfeeding. Providers should be cautious prescribing women of childbearing age with statins and consider nonpharmacologic treatments if possible. There are no special considerations for the elderly.

Fibric Acid Derivatives

Fibric acid derivatives (fibrates) are drugs of choice for persons with hypertriglyceridemia and are often used in combination with statins for the treatment of dyslipidemia (Table 15-21). These drugs are not used for monotherapy.[46]

Mechanism of Action

Fibrates typically decrease serum triglycerides by approximately 30–50% and increase HDL by 5–15%. Their effect on LDL is variable. The primary mode of action is via activation of nuclear transcription factors called peroxisome proliferators activated receptors. These factors, primarily located in the liver and brown adipose tissue, affect several changes in lipid metabolism once bound to the fibrate. They reduce triglyceride production by stimulating triglyceride oxidation in the liver and increasing the activity of lipoprotein lipase, an enzyme that hydrolyzes the lipids in VLDL into free fatty acids, which then increases the clearance of triglyceride-rich VLDL. However, for those with extremely high triglyceride levels, a rise in LDL may occur when gemfibrozil (Lopid) is used.[41]

Fibrates also affect coagulation and fibrinolysis in a way that supports anticoagulation. This helps prevent thromboembolic complications of atherosclerosis.[46]

Side Effects/Contraindications

Side effects of fibric acid derivatives include skin rashes, nausea, diarrhea, myopathy, arrhythmias, hypokalemia, and elevation in liver transaminase values (AST and ALT).

Liver transaminase levels should be monitored and the drug discontinued if the AST or ALT increases more than three times the upper limit of normal. These drugs also should be discontinued in persons who develop an elevation of plasma creatinine phosphokinase (CPK). Fibrates appear to slightly increase the risk that an individual will develop pulmonary embolism and/or pancreatitis (1.1% with fibrates versus 0.7% with placebo and 0.8% with fibrates versus 0.5% with placebo, respectively).[47]

Interactions may occur with warfarin (Coumadin), and the dose of warfarin may need to be decreased. Fibrates should be avoided by persons who have hepatic or renal dysfunction, including hepatic disease and biliary cirrhosis.

Special Populations

Fibrates are FDA Pregnancy Category C. There are no studies of fibrates in pregnant women, and in animal studies these drugs have shown embryocidal and teratogenic effects. Therefore these drugs should be avoided in pregnant women. These drugs are also secreted in breast milk and in animal studies have been shown to cause tumor formation. Fibrates have a lower molecular weight that suggests they transfer into breast milk easily and should not be used by breastfeeding women secondary to the potential for newborn toxicity. There are no specific dosing considerations for the elderly.

Bile Acid Sequestrants

Bile acid sequestrants (Resins) are among the oldest treatments for hyperlipidemia and remain the only drugs approved for pediatric use (Table 15-22). These drugs can be used alone or in combination with statins. Bile

Table 15-21 Fibric Acid Derivatives

Drug Generic (Brand)	Formulations	Dose	Effect on Lipids	FDA Pregnancy Category
Fenofibrate (TriCor)	48-mg, 145-mg tabs	Initially 145 mg daily, 145 mg max daily. Renal or elderly initially 48 mg.	↓ LDL 20–30%; ↑ HDL 10–20%; ↓ trig 23–54%.	C
Fenofibrate (Triglide)	160 mg	50–160 mg per day.	↓ LDL 20–30%; ↑ HDL 10–20%; ↓ trig 23–54%.	C
Fenofibrate (Lofibra)	54-mg, 160-mg tabs	Initially maintenance 54–160 mg daily. Adjust dose for renal impairment.	↓ LDL 20–30%; ↑ HDL 10–20%; ↓ trig 23–54%. Avoid statins.	C
Fenofibrate (Antara)	43-mg, 130-mg tabs	Initially 130 mg daily, maintenance 43–130 mg daily. Renal, hepatic impairment, or elderly initially 43 mg.	↓ LDL 20–30%; ↑ HDL 10–20%; ↓ trig 23–54%. Avoid statins.	C
Gemfibrozil (Lopid)	600 mg	600 mg twice daily 30 minutes prior to meals.	↓ LDL 0–10%; ↑ HDL 10–20%; ↓ trig 20–60%. Avoid statins	C

↑ = increased; ↓ = decreased; HDL = high-density lipoprotein; LDL = low-density lipoprotein.

Table 15-22 Bile Acid Sequestrants

Drug Generic (Brand)	Formulations	Dose	Effect on Lipids	FDA Pregnancy Category
Cholestyramine (Questran)	4 g per 9-g packet	Initially 1 packet mixed with fluid 1–2 times daily, maintenance 2–4 packets daily, max 6 packets.	↓ LDL 15–30%; ↑ HDL 0–5%; ↓ trig 0–10%	C
Colesevelam (WelChol)	625-mg tab	Initially as monotherapy 3 tabs twice daily or 6 tabs daily. If used with statins, 4 to 6 tabs daily.	↓ LDL 15–18%; ↑ HDL 3–5%; ↓ trig 0–10%	C
Colestipol (Colestid)	5-g packet	5–30 g daily or divided doses.	↓ LDL 15–30%; ↑ HDL 0–5%; ↓ trig 0–10%	C
	1-g tablet	Initially 2 g daily or twice daily, maintenance 2–16 g daily, max 16 g.		

↑ = increased; ↓ = decreased; HDL = high-density lipoprotein; LDL = low-density lipoprotein.

acid sequestrants reduce the incidence of cardiovascular events.[1] Resins are useful for persons with renal or hepatic disease because these drugs are not absorbed by the intestines. Gastrointestinal side effects are the primary reason for discontinuation, and it is often difficult for an individual to reach treatment goals using these agents. A majority of persons with hyperlipidemia, just as in hypertension, need multiple drugs to get them to their treatment goals in reducing their risk of CVD. Resins are drugs that have beneficial effects when used in combination with statins.[47]

Mechanism of Action

Bile acids are metabolites of cholesterol and are normally absorbed in the intestinal lumen. Bile acid sequestrants bind to bile acids in the intestine and thereby prevent them from being reabsorbed.[48] This results in an increase in conversion of cholesterol into bile acids in the liver. When bile acid sequestrants are used to treat primary hypercholesterolemia, a reduction of 9–18% ($P = .001$) can be expected in serum cholesterol levels.[49] The mean reduction in LDL is 20% with a dose of 4.5 g per day of colesevelam.[49] Another use of these drugs is to reduce pruritus caused by the accumulation of bile acids in persons with cholestasis.

Side Effects/Contraindications

Side effects of bile acid sequestrants are bloating and dyspepsia. Severe hypertriglyceridemia is a contraindication because these drugs can increase triglycerides. Resins can interfere with the intestinal absorption of other medications such as thiazides, propranolol cardiac glycosides, coumarin anticoagulants, some vitamins, and statins. Other medications should be given 1 hour prior to taking bile acid sequestrants or 4–6 hours after. The use of these medications is contraindicated in persons with biliary and bowel obstruction.

Special Populations

Bile acid sequestrants are FDA Pregnancy Category C. These medications are not absorbed systemically but can interfere with intestinal absorption of vitamins A, D, E, and K and folic acid and iron. When used by pregnant women to treat intrahepatic cholestasis of pregnancy, the addition of a vitamin K supplement is recommended because vitamin K is not absorbed if bile salts are not present. The value of supplementing other fat-soluble vitamins is not clear. These medications are not found in appreciable amounts in breast milk, but if they are taken for long periods of time so that the mother becomes deficient in fat-soluble vitamins, this deficiency could have an adverse effect on an infant. There are no specific dosing considerations for the elderly.

Niacin (Nicotinic Acid)

Niacin (nicotinic acid) reduces LDL and effectively increases HDL (Table 15-23). It is one of the oldest drugs used to treat dyslipidemia. Niacin is also the one drug used to treat dyslipidemia that can be obtained over the counter without a prescription.

Mechanism of Action

Niacin is a water-soluble B vitamin, also named vitamin B_3, which inhibits the breakdown of fat in adipose tissue. The reduced plasma levels of free fatty acids results in a decrease in the secretion of VLDL and cholesterol from the liver, and that, in turn, leads to a reduction in LDL. When the production of LDL is decreased, the liver

Table 15-23 Nicotinic Acid

Drug Generic (Brand)	Formulations	Dose	Clinical Considerations	FDA Pregnancy Category
Niacin ER (Niaspan)*	500 mg, 750 mg, 1000 mg	Initially 500 mg once daily, maintenance 1–2 g daily, max 2 g daily.	Needs to be taken at bedtime with a low-fat snack. Take ASA or NSAID 30 min prior to the niacin.	C
Niacin/Lovastatin (Advicor)	500/20 mg, 750/20 mg, 1000/20 mg, 1000/40 mg	After a patient is on a stable dose of niacin, can add lovastatin.	Combination statin with immediate-release niacin. Dosing considerations same as those for lovastatin alone.	X
Niacin (Niacor)*	Immediate-release 500-mg tabs	Initially 500 mg daily, maintenance 1–2 g bid to tid.	Take in divided doses with food to minimize GI irritation.	C

GI = gastrointestinal.

* FDA approved for use as a lipid-altering agent. The others are approved as dietary supplements.

increases absorption of LDL from plasma. Then the overall breakdown rate of HDL in the liver decreases, and HDL plasma levels increase. Niacin also decreases the amount of circulating fibrinogen and increases tissue plasminogen, which slows the rate of atherogenesis or thrombosis. Nicotinic acid (Niacin) has slowed the progression of arteriosclerosis of the carotid arteries in studies that have been done using this agent.[50] Niacin is more effective at increasing HDL (30–40%) than are other agents such as statins (5–11%).[50] Niacin has also been found to be as effective in reducing triglycerides as are fibrates.

Dosing Considerations

Niacin can be found in both immediate-release and extended-release formulations. The immediate-release formulations are likely to cause flushing and a feeling of warmth secondary to a prostaglandin-stimulated vasodilation. The extended-release formulations do not cause flushing and can be more attractive because they do not engender uncomfortable side effects. However, these formulations are less effective than immediate-release formulations and have a rare association with hepatotoxicity when taken in doses > 2 g/day. Extended release niacin (Niaspan), one of the niacin formulations that is FDA approved for treating dyslipidemia, has a pharmacokinetic profile between the immediate-release and extended-release formulations and has minimal adverse side effects. Niacin can be used in combination with statins, but the combination increases the risk of myopathy; therefore, serum CPK levels should be monitored if this combination is prescribed.

Side Effects/Contraindications

Facial flushing is the most common side effect associated with taking niacin. The flushing and pruritus can be quite intense for 15–30 minutes and are dose dependent. However,

325 mg of aspirin taken 30 minutes prior to taking the dose of niacin or 200 mg of ibuprofen taken daily can block the flushing. Gradually titrating the dose over several days will allow the individual to develop a tolerance so that the flushing does not occur. Finally, taking niacin in combination with a low-fat snack can substantially decrease flushing.

There are three additional important side effects associated with niacin, which include: (1) hyperuricemia, (2) myopathy, and (3) impaired insulin sensitivity. The possibility of myopathy is why the combination of niacin and statins (niacin/lovastatin [Advicor]) is associated with an increased risk for rhabdomyolysis. Niacin should be used with caution by persons with diabetes and by persons with a history of gout. This drug should be avoided by individuals with peptic ulcer disease because it can cause release of histamine, which results in increased gastric motility and acid production. Liver function should be monitored secondary to the increased risk of hepatotoxicity.

Drug–Drug Interactions

The combination of statins and niacin should be closely monitored, as there is an increased risk for rhabdomyolysis when these two drugs are taken in combination. If the individual is also taking bile acid sequestrants, the dose of niacin should be taken 4–6 hours after or before the bile acid sequestrant to ensure absorption.

Special Populations

Niacin is FDA Pregnancy Category C. Although niacin is a B vitamin, which is necessary in fetal development, the doses used to lower cholesterol are high and it is not known if these higher doses used to treat hyperlipidemia have an adverse effect on the fetus. Therefore it is generally recommended that these doses not be used by pregnant women. Niacin enters breast milk but is compatible with lactation.

Cholesterol Absorption Inhibitors

Cholesterol absorption inhibitors are the newest class of drug in the treatment of hyperlipidemia. Ezetimibe (Zetia) is the only drug in this class. This drug is used alone and is also marketed in a fixed combination formulation with a simvastatin (Vytorin). The combination therapy of ezetimibe and simvastatin (Vytorin) was found to reduce LDL more than monotherapy with either drug.[51] However, the combination product did not appear to improve intima-media thickness within arteries, which was used as a surrogate marker for atherosclerosis. More research is needed before the clinical efficacy of ezetimibe (Zetia) alone or in combination products is clear.

Mechanism of Action

The mechanism of action of ezetimibe is via inhibition of intestinal absorption of cholesterol, which occurs primarily in the duodenum and proximal jejunum. The only formulation available is a 10-mg tablet. The agent has a half-life of 22 hours. The major side effects are abdominal pain and diarrhea. Ezetimibe (Zetia) should be given at least 2 hours before or 4 hours after bile acid sequestrants.

Special Populations

Ezetimibe is FDA Pregnancy Category C. No research has been conducted in pregnant women using ezetimibe, and this drug should only be used if the benefits outweigh the risks. It is unknown if the medication is excreted in breast milk, and its use during lactation should be avoided.

Combination Products

When treating dyslipidemia, the primary target is reduction of LDL. When the LDL goals are not met using monotherapy with a statin, combination therapy using an agent with a different mechanism of action is the next logical step. Statin combinations such as statin/niacin, statin/fibrates, and statin/ezetimibe are available, and studies of their efficacy are ongoing.[52]

Complementary Therapies for Hyperlipidemia

The two effective dietary supplements for the treatment of hyperlipidemia include niacin and omega 3 fatty acids. Other products such as oat bran, plant sterols, and blond psyllium have potential benefit but no solid evidence for use at this time.

Omega 3 Fatty Acids

Fish oils that are high in omega 3 fatty acids are known to have beneficial effects on the cardiovascular system.[52] Both omega 3 and omega 6 fatty acids must be obtained via diet. The normal Western diet is high in omega 6 fatty acids (e.g., nuts, cereals, eggs, poultry, most vegetable oils), which have proinflammatory and prothrombotic properties, in contrast to omega 3 fatty acids (e.g., fish, flaxseed oil), which are anti-inflammatory and antithrombotic. The AHA recommends that women who are at high risk for developing CVD take 1000 mg daily of omega 3 fatty acids if they are unable to get this amount of fatty acids in their diet.[3] Omega 3 acid ethyl ester (Lovaza) is the only FDA-approved prescription omega 3 fatty acid available on the market. Each tablet of omega 3 acid ethyl ester (Lovaza) contains 900 grams of eicosapentaenoic acid (EPA) and docosahexaenoic acid (DHA). The FDA has approved using Lovaza for the treatment of severe hypertriglyceridemia (> 500 mg/dL), and the AHA recommends use of this drug as an adjunct to other therapies by persons who have hypertriglyceridemia that has not responded to lifestyle changes for secondary prevention of myocardial infarction. There are also a wide variety of over-the-counter preparations of fish oils that might not be at the same concentration of pharmacologic-grade omega 3 fatty acids.

Mechanism of Action

The exact mechanism of action of omega 3 fatty acids is unknown at this time. It is hypothesized that omega 3 fatty acids reduce triglyceride levels via the inhibition of acyl CoA:1,2 diacylglycerol acyltransferase, increased hepatic beta-oxidation, or a reduction in the hepatic synthesis of triglycerides.

Drug–Drug Interactions

Omega 3 acid ethyl ester may increase bleeding time and therefore needs to be used cautiously by persons who are also taking anticoagulants and/or NSAIDs. Beta-blockers, thiazides, and estrogen decrease the effectiveness of omega 3 acid ethyl ester.

Side Effects/Contraindications

The most common side effect of omega 3 fatty acid is related to gastrointestinal symptoms such as taste aversion.

Special Populations

The FDA pregnancy category of omega 3 fatty acids is C. There are no well controlled studies of omega 3 fatty acid use during pregnancy, and, therefore, omega 3 acid ethyl ester should only be used if the benefit outweighs the risk.

Cerebral Vascular Disease

A cerebral vascular event is defined as a sudden neurologic deficit in the brain caused by either ischemia or hemorrhage. Ischemic stroke is the most common type of stroke, accounting for 87% of all strokes. It is estimated that 700,000 people have an ischemic or hemorrhagic stroke in the United States each year; 200,000 of these strokes occur in persons who have had a previous stroke.[53] Individuals who have had a previous stroke or transient ischemic attacks (TIAs) are at increased risk of another event.[53] The discussion in this section focuses on medications used for secondary prevention of stoke. First, however, a short review of platelet activation and aggregation is in order.

The Life Cycle of a Platelet

Technically, platelets are not cells because they do not have a nucleus. Rather, platelets are fragments of cytoplasm from a large cell called a megakaryoblast. Platelets are formed when the cell membrane of the megakaryoblast sends tendrils of membrane into the cytoplasm, which divides it into many compartments. These compartments seal off and are extruded from the megakaryocyte as a platelet. Each platelet has cytoplasm and numerous granules that contain the chemicals involved in clotting.

The platelet must be activated before it engages in clotting activity. Endothelial damage triggers this activation whereby the platelet changes from smooth and round to swollen with extruded spiky processes that are sticky. This change in shape exposes a phospholipid surface that is used by various coagulation factors. Once attached to the endothelial wall at the site of injury, the degranulation occurs, and chemicals that initiate the clotting process are released. Adenosine diphosphate (ADP) attracts more platelets to the area; thromboxane A_2 attracts more platelets and triggers more degranulation. Pharmacologic therapies for prevention of stroke are targeted at inhibiting platelet coagulation.

Pharmacologic Treatment for Cerebrovascular Disease

Several of the drugs discussed previously in this chapter have beneficial effects in supporting endothelial function to prevent platelet aggregation. Meta-analyses have found that the combination of ACE inhibitors and thiazide diuretics results in a 40–45% reduction in risk of recurrent stroke, whereas beta-blockers and ACE inhibitors alone do not reduce the incidence of recurrent stroke as effectively.[54,55]

There is a suggestion that persons who have had a stroke or transient ischemic attack suspected to be arthrosclerotic in nature need to be started on statin therapy.[53] The Angio-Scandinavian Cardiac Outcomes Trial—Lipid Lowering Arm (ASCOT-LLA) evaluated the ability of statins to prevent coronary and stroke events in 19,342 hypertensive individuals who had at least three other cardiovascular risk factors. These participants were randomly assigned to the atorvastatin (Lipitor) 10 mg or placebo group. The study was stopped at 3.3 years because atorvastatin (Lipitor) was associated with a 27% ($P = .0236$) reduction in the incidence of stroke, and no difference was found between men and women.[56]

Pharmacologic therapy that specifically targets platelet aggregation includes aspirin, aspirin/extended-release dipyridamole combination (Aggrenox), ticlopidine (Ticlid), and clopidogrel (Plavix). Evidence-based recommendations for use of these agents was released by the American Heart association and American Stroke Association in 2008.[53]

Acetylsalicylic Acid (Aspirin)

Aspirin is the most widely used drug used specifically to prevent stroke. Aspirin is recommended for primary prevention of CVD for men and women whose 10-year risk of a first CHD event is $\geq$ 6–10% percent as determined by the Framingham risk score.[3] Two studies have compared different doses of aspirin for the prevention of a second ischemic stroke (1200 mg/d versus 300 mg/d and 283 mg/d versus 30 mg/d).[57,58] The lower doses of aspirin were as effective as high-dose aspirin in risk reduction. Analysis of the different effects of antiplatelet therapy based on age and sex showed no significant difference between genders with regard to the efficacy of therapy.[58]

Mechanism of Action

Aspirin irreversibly inhibits platelet cyclooxygenase (COX) via establishment of a covalent bond at the active site of the COX enzyme inside the platelet cell (see Chapter 12 for a full description of the mechanism of action of aspirin). When aspirin is not present, the COX enzyme facilitates the conversion of arachidonic acid into thromboxane A$_2$. Thromboxane A$_2$ then diffuses across the platelet membrane and binds to a receptor on another platelet, which results in platelet aggregation. Aspirin's effect lasts for the life of the platelet, which is 5 to 7 days.[53]

Dosing Considerations

The recommended dose of aspirin for reducing the risk of a cardiovascular event is 50–325 mg daily. Multiple studies have shown that low-dose aspirin, 81 mg, is as effective and associated with fewer bleeding events than higher doses.[58] The antiplatelet effect of aspirin has an onset of less than 60 minutes, and doses of ≤ 100 mg can have an inhibitory effect on cyclooxygenase.[53]

Side Effects/Contraindications

Aspirin has multiple drug–drug interactions and side effects that are listed in Tables 12-7 and 12-8. The most concerning adverse effect is bleeding and gastrointestinal irritation that can evolve into perforated ulcers. The incidence of adverse bleeding events following use of low-dose aspirin is approximately 1% compared to 9.18% in persons who are not on antiplatelet drugs.[59] In addition, it is clear that higher doses do not enhance the anticlotting therapeutic effect, and they do increase the incidence of bleeding. Thus it is important to use the low dose for prevention of CVD.

Special Populations

Aspirin is FDA Pregnancy Category D, and it is specifically contraindicated in the third trimester of pregnancy because use of aspirin close to delivery may cause premature closure of the ductus arteriosus in the fetus. Aspirin does cross into breast milk, and the AAP recommends avoiding aspirin therapy while breastfeeding.[28] There are no specific dosing considerations for the elderly.

Aspirin and Extended-Release Dipyridamole

The fixed dose formulation of aspirin and extended-release dipyridamole (Aggrenox) was the first combination agent to show more benefit than is obtained via use of aspirin alone and is today a recommended first-line treatment for secondary prevention of stroke in addition to aspirin alone.[52]

Mechanism of Action

Dipyridamole inhibits the function of an intracellular enzyme that normally breaks down cyclic adenosine monophosphate (cAMP). cAMP remains active, increasing the reuptake of intracellular calcium into the storage tubules, and this prevents platelet activation and excretion of the granules that contain clotting factors.

Dosing Considerations

Aggrenox is a combination of dipyridamole ER and aspirin (200 mg and 25 mg respectively) that is taken twice daily. Slow titration can be done by introducing the medication at bedtime for 2 to 3 days then increasing to twice-daily dosing.

Side Effects/Contraindications

Headache is a common side effect and is more common among women than men. Because dipyridamole/aspirin (Aggrenox) contains aspirin, the side effects, adverse effects, and contraindications that exist for aspirin are also applicable to use of dipyridamole/aspirin (Aggrenox). These side effects are common and are the reason individuals stop therapy more often with Aggrenox than with low-dose acetylsalicylic acid alone.

Ticlopidine

Ticlopidine (Ticlid) is more effective than aspirin for secondary prevention of stroke and other vascular events.[53] However, ticlopidine has a significant side effect profile and has been mostly replaced by clopidogrel (Plavix) or reserved for individuals who are intolerant to aspirin.[53] Cost is a second consideration; a month of therapy of ticlopidine (Ticlid) is much more expensive than aspirin.

Mechanism of Action

Ticlopidine (Ticlid) interferes in platelet activation via blocking activation of a G protein-coupled ADP receptor on the membrane that results in the initial change in shape, which occurs once the platelet is activated. The exact mechanism is not completely understood, as ticlopidine may be a prodrug, which is converted into an active metabolite that then blocks this receptor. Ticlopidine (Ticlid) is prescribed as one 250-mg tablet taken orally twice a day.

Side Effects/Contraindications

More than 50% of persons taking ticlopidine complain of at least one side effect, with gastrointestinal upset being the most common. Up to 2% of individuals will experience neutropenia, which is reversible once the drug has been stopped. Persons who are taking this drug must be closely followed the first 3 months of therapy with twice weekly complete blood counts to rule out blood dyscrasias, including neutropenia. Ticlopidine has also been reported to increase the risk of thrombotic thrombocytopenia purpura (ITP). Other side effects include diarrhea, ulcers, and bleeding. This drug should not be prescribed for persons with a history of gastrointestinal bleeding.

Drug–Drug Interactions

Ticlopidine (Ticlid) has multiple drug–drug interactions. Ticlopidine (Ticlid) potentiates the effects of aspirin and NSAIDs on platelet aggregation, which increases the risk of bleeding. Antacids can reduce plasma levels of ticlopidine, whereas cimetidine (Tagamet) reduces clearance of ticlopidine. This drug should be used with caution by persons who are taking other drugs metabolized by the CP450 enzymes and by persons with liver disease. Ticlopidine can decrease the plasma levels of citalopram (Celexa), diazepam (Valium), methsuximide (Celontin), phenytoin (Dilantin), propranolol (Inderal), sertraline (Zoloft), amphetamines, selected beta-blockers, dextromethorphan, fluoxetine (Prozac), lidocaine, mirtazapine (Remeron), nefazodone (Serzone), paroxetine (Paxil), risperidone (Risperdal), ritonavir (Norvir), tricyclic antidepressants, and venlafaxine (Effexor). The following drugs may decrease the effect of ticlopidine (Ticlid): aminoglutethimide (Cytadren), carbamazepine (Tegretol), nafcillin, nevirapine (Viramune), phenobarbital (Luminal), phenytoin (Dilantin), and rifamycin (Rifadin).

Special Populations

Ticlopidine is FDA Pregnancy Category B, and it is unknown if this drug is excreted into breast milk. There are no specific dosing considerations for the elderly.

Clopidogrel

Clopidogrel (Plavix) is closely related to ticlopidine in mechanism of action. It, too, exerts its antiplatelet effect on the membrane G-coupled receptors that lead to platelet shape change. Clopidogrel is more effective than aspirin in reducing the combined risk of ischemic stroke, MI, or vascular death among individuals with atherosclerotic vascular disease.[60]

Mechanism of Action

The GpIIb-IIIa complex is a receptor on the platelet surface that facilitates platelet reshaping once activated. Clopidogrel irreversibly blocks ADP, therefore inhibiting activation of the platelet. Clopidogrel is a prodrug that needs to be metabolized, most likely via CYP3A4.

Dosing Considerations

The usual dose of clopidogrel is 75 mg daily; however, often a loading dose of 300 mg is given, as the onset of action is delayed by 3–7 days before antiplatelet effect is maximized.

Side Effects/Contraindications

The side effects of clopidogrel are less toxic than the side effects associated with ticlopidine. Although the incidence of gastrointestinal bleeding is less than is seen in persons taking aspirin, it is a risk associated with use of clopidogrel. Clopidogrel (Plavix) is contraindicated for individuals with active bleeding, peptic ulcer disease, and coagulation disorders. In addition, the combination of aspirin with clopidogrel is no longer recommended because in some persons there is an increased incidence of moderate bleeding associated with this combination that is not countered by a significant increase in efficacy.[53]

Drug–Drug Interactions

Clopidogrel (Plavix) should be used cautiously with other antiplatelet agents, as their effects may be potentiated.

Special Populations

Clopidogrel's FDA pregnancy category is B. There have been no teratogenic effects observed in animal studies; however, it should only be used if benefit outweighs risk. It is unknown if clopidogrel (Plavix) is excreted in breast milk; therefore, use of this drug during lactation is not recommended. There are no specific dosing considerations for the elderly.

Peripheral Arterial Occlusive Disease

Approximately 5 million people in the United States suffer from peripheral arterial occlusive disease, which is also known as peripheral vascular disease and PAD.[61] The American College of Cardiology and the American Heart Association have clinical practice guidelines for the screening, evaluation, risk reduction, and treatment of persons with peripheral arterial disease. Peripheral arterial disease is defined, for the purpose of this chapter, as a disease of noncoronary arterial circulation secondary to occlusion or dilation. Atherosclerosis is the most common pathophysiology contributing to peripheral arterial disease. Individuals with peripheral arterial disease have a 20–60% increased risk of cardiovascular events such as MI or stroke. Many women older than 65 years are asymptomatic, yet have a high risk of mortality secondary to this disorder, and it is recommended that they be treated. Those with severe ischemic peripheral arterial disease and a low ankle brachial pressure index score have a 25% annual mortality.[61]

Common symptoms of peripheral arterial disease are pain in legs at rest, intermittent claudication, and poor healing in wounds that are in the extremities. The risk factors for peripheral arterial disease are the same as the risk factors for most other CVDs. Smoking is a powerful predictor of peripheral arterial disease, with over 80% of those with PAD being current or past smokers. Diabetes, a cardiovascular risk equivalent, is also a major risk factor, and improved glycemic control can reduce the risk. Hyperlipidemia, elevated LDL, and reduced HDL also have a strong relationship with the progression of peripheral arterial disease. Hypertension has a weaker relationship with peripheral arterial disease, but use of ACE inhibitors has shown some benefit in treatment of peripheral arterial disease. Peripheral arterial disease has major implications for the development of chronic disease, decreased functional capacity, amputation, and risk of death.[61,62]

The diagnosis of peripheral artery disease is based on symptoms and physical exam that compares pulses and blood pressure readings in both arms and both legs. Doppler ultrasonography can be used to directly measure blood flow if needed.

Nonpharmacologic Treatment

The foundation of PAD treatment is lifestyle modification, which includes time-intensive interventions that can have long-reaching impact on a person's quality of life. Smoking cessation is essential in treating any person with symptoms of PAD. Increasing physical activity has been shown to have positive effects with weight reduction, blood pressure reduction, and LDL reduction.[3,52]

Pharmacologic Treatment of Peripheral Arterial Occlusive Disease

Antiplatelet therapy is a cornerstone of treatment of peripheral arterial disease, and 75–325 mg of aspirin taken daily is the recommended first-line drug. Clopidogrel (Plavix) is as effective as aspirin but is more expensive and not readily available. In addition, the American College of Cardiology and the American Heart Association recommend that persons who are at risk for or who have peripheral arterial occlusive disease be treated for risk factors that cause this disease.[61] In the **Adult Treatment Panel III** (ATP III) guidelines, peripheral arterial disease is a CVD equivalent and, therefore, the optimal LDL will be less than 70 mg/dL.[38] If a person has an elevated blood pressure, it should be treated per the current guidelines. ACE inhibitors are of benefit in the reduction of cardiovascular events for those with existing CVD such as peripheral arterial disease.[63] Individuals with concomitant peripheral arterial disease and diabetes benefit from tight glycemic control with antiglycemic agents, either oral or parenteral.

Heart Failure

Heart failure is a growing concern as our nation ages. In 2005, over 5 million adults in the United States were diagnosed with heart failure. Women account for the majority of heart failure deaths in the United States annually.[64] The two leading causes of heart failure are coronary artery disease and hypertension.

The most common clinical signs of heart failure are fluid retention, fatigue, and dyspnea. Heart failure is categorized as diastolic or systolic in nature. Diastolic heart failure occurs when the ventricle fails to properly fill, and systolic dysfunction occurs when there is reduced contractility. The incidence of diastolic heart failure increases with age and is more common in women than in men.[65] Heart failure is classified by the American College of Cardiology and the American Heart Association into four stages, which are defined in Table 15-24. The guidelines for management are listed in Figure 15-5.

Diastolic Heart Failure

Diastolic heart failure is a concept that is not as clearly defined as systolic heart failure. The exact prevalence of

Table 15-24 Stages of Heart Failure

Stage	Definition	Examples
A	Person is at high risk for developing heart failure but has no structural disorder of the heart.	Person has high blood pressure, coronary artery disease, diabetes, a history of drug or alcohol abuse, a personal history of rheumatic fever, or a family history of cardiomyopathy.
B	Person has a structural disorder of the heart but has never developed symptoms of heart failure.	Person has structural changes to the left ventricle, has heart valve disease, or has had a heart attack.
C	Person has past or current symptoms of heart failure associated with underlying structural heart disease.	Person has shortness of breath or fatigue caused by left ventricular systolic dysfunction or is without symptoms and is receiving treatment for prior symptoms of heart failure.
D	Person has end-stage disease and requires specialized treatment strategies.	Person is frequently hospitalized for heart failure or cannot be safely discharged from the hospital; person is in the hospital awaiting a heart transplant; person is at home receiving continuous intravenous support for symptom relief or being supported with a mechanical circulatory assistive device; or person is in a hospice setting for the management of heart failure.

Source: Hunt SA et al. 2005.[67]

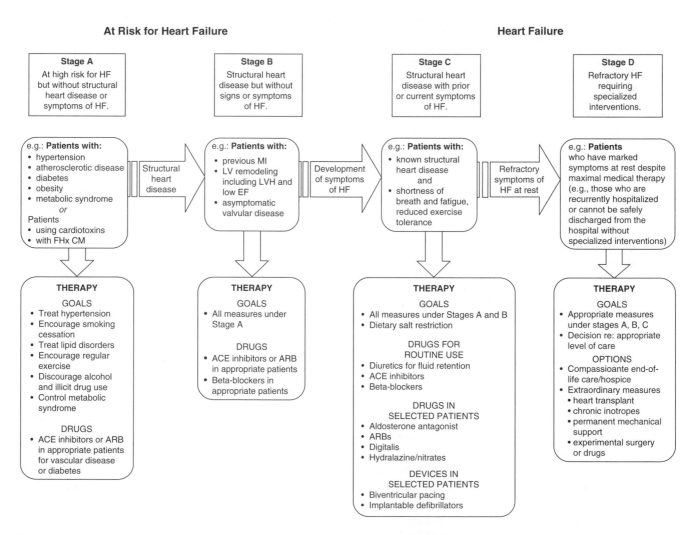

Figure 15-5 ACC/AHA heart failure staging and treatment guidelines. *Source:* Reprinted with permission from American College of Cardiology/American Heart Association Guideline Update for the diagnosis and management of chronic heart failure in the adult.[67]

diastolic dysfunction without overall heart failure is unknown. Of the individuals over the age of 70 with heart failure who present for outpatient services, 50% have diastolic heart failure. However, measuring diastolic dysfunction is limited in clinical practice because there is significant overlap between diastolic and systolic heart failure in signs and symptoms that are detected on physical exam, ECG, and radiograph studies.[66] Therefore, diagnostic criteria that are based on specific studies of systolic and diastolic function have been developed.[67]

Pathophysiology of Diastolic Heart Failure

Diastolic heart failure occurs when there is impaired or incomplete myocardial relaxation and ventricle filling, which results in the clinical symptoms of heart failure. Diastolic dysfunction is technically abnormal function of the ventricle. There are two leading causes of diastolic dysfunction: (1) cardiac ischemia and (2) left ventricular hypertrophy. In addition, there are two types of ischemia, one related to supply and one related to demand. Demand ischemia is seen when there is an increased oxygen demand as occurs when physical activity is increased. In this scenario, there is a relative insufficient supply of blood. Supply ischemia is seen when there is insufficient coronary blood flow.[67]

▎Pharmacologic Treatment of Diastolic Heart Failure

The treatment for diastolic heart failure is based on the 2005 American Heart Association and American College of Cardiology joint recommendations.[67] Many of the medications that are used for the treatment of systolic heart failure are the same medications used for the treatment of diastolic heart failure; however, they are used for different reasons. There are special considerations when selecting treatment for individuals with diastolic heart failure.

Addressing the etiology of the diastolic dysfunction is key.[68] Left ventricular hypertrophy related to hypertension is a cause of diastolic dysfunction. ARBs, calcium channel blockers, and ACE inhibitors reduce left ventricular mass somewhat better than diuretics or beta-blockers, but all can be used depending on the individual indication.[69]

Addressing other issues such as atrial fibrillation that stress the heart is vital in the management of diastolic heart failure. Medications that improve coronary ischemia need to be considered. Beta-blockers have beneficial effects in slowing the heart rate and improving ventricular filling.

Many calcium channel blockers would not be considered for use in systolic heart failure, but verapamil (Calan) is especially helpful in relaxing the myocardium, improving ventricular filling, and decreasing ischemic episodes.

Drugs that affect neurohumoral activation such as the RAAS are also effective in the treatment of diastolic heart failure. However, positive inotropic drugs such as digoxin have a limited role in diastolic heart failure because persons with diastolic heart failure already have a normal left ventricular ejection fraction.[68]

▎Systolic Heart Failure

Pathophysiology of Systolic Heart Failure

Systolic heart failure is a progressive syndrome that starts with an insult or injury to the myocardium. Over time, the accumulated injury leads to structural changes the size of heart chambers. These changes cause hemodynamic stresses to the wall of the heart that eventually result in decreasing cardiac performance such as poor filling or ejection. The poor performance continues to cause further cardiac remodeling.

When a person has poor cardiac output, the RAAS is activated secondary to reduced renal blood flow. The result of this process is production of angiotensin II, which increases peripheral vascular resistance via vasoconstriction. Angiotensin II also directly stimulates the release of catecholamines from noradrenergic receptors, which increases heart rate and contractility, and finally, it stimulates the adrenal cortex to release aldosterone, which stimulates reabsorption of sodium and water. These effects initially maintain cardiac output, but over time in the presence of a damaged myocardium, these effects become maladaptive. Drugs that block or inhibit angiotensin II have demonstrated positive effects on long-term outcomes.[68]

Ultimately, there are many neurohormonal peptides involved in the development and progression of heart failure, such as increased levels of norepinephrine, endothelin, vasopressin, and cytokines. Norepinephrine is known to increase heart rate and vasoconstriction. Individuals with heart failure who also have higher levels of norepinephrine have a poorer prognosis than those with lower norepinephrine levels because the constant activation of the sympathetic nervous system down regulates the β-receptors. Therefore, drugs that cause suppression of the sympathetic nervous system are beneficial for persons with systolic heart failure. Aldosterone increases retention of sodium.

There are new findings that aldosterone is also involved in the development of cardiac fibrosis. Significant reductions in mortality have been found with the use of drugs that reduce aldosterone levels. Angiotensin II is known to be a potent vasoconstrictor, which leads to increased vascular resistance.

Treatment of Systolic Heart Failure

Treatment for heart failure is based on the stage of the disease. Each of the four stages is based on the risk of developing worsening dysfunction[67] (Table 15-25).

Stage A Heart Failure

The purpose of identifying a person at stage A is to recognize risk factors for heart failure early and aggressively reduce those risks. If an individual does smoke, smoking cessation should be discussed and positive reinforcement should be offered to nonsmokers and especially ex-smokers.

ACE inhibitors continue to have benefit for the treatment and prevention of heart failure even beyond blood pressure reduction. ACE inhibitors reduce risk by blocking, but not completely halting the effects of the renin angiotensin aldosterone system.[70] It has also been demonstrated that ACE inhibitors improve survival and decrease mortality in women as well as in men.[71] Overall, the dose of an ACE inhibitor should be titrated to standard or maximum dose, but the benefit of an ACE inhibitor at a lower dose is superior to none at all.[72] Not all ACE inhibitors have indications for use in heart failure. The following ACE inhibitors have been approved for use in heart failure: captopril (Capoten), enalapril (Vasotec), lisinopril (Prinivil), quinapril (Accupril), ramipril (Altace), fosinopril (Monopril), and trandolapril (Mavik). The precautions for prescribing ACE inhibitors that exist when treating hypertension are the same and need to be taken into consideration when using them to manage heart failure (see the section on hypertension near the beginning of this chapter).

There are conflicting studies that indicate aspirin may negate the positive benefits of ACE inhibitors because the ACE inhibitors effect results from increased levels of kinins, which causes release of prostaglandins. Acetylsalicylic acid is a prostaglandin inhibitor that is therefore able to decrease the effectiveness of ACE inhibitors. In a meta-analysis of five trials, the researchers found that aspirin did not have significant effect on ACE inhibitors' benefits of mortality.[73] The current recommendation is to prescribe aspirin if indicated, and that 160 mg or less can be used daily.

Stage B Heart Failure

If structural changes are present but no symptoms of heart failure are found, the individual meets the criteria for stage B. The provider should continue to recommend all treatments used for persons with stage A heart failure. An individual with stage B heart failure may have a history of myocardial infarction or may have a left ventricular ejection fraction $\leq$ 40%. This person will benefit from a use of both a beta-blocker and an ACE inhibitor.[67] Beta-blockers, specifically bisoprolol (Ziac), carvedilol (Coreg, Coreg CR), and sustained-release metoprolol succinate (Toprol XL) have been shown to reduce morbidity and mortality.[74,75] Not all beta-blockers are indicated in the treatment of heart failure, and some, such as propranolol (Inderal), atenolol (Tenormin), and metoprolol (Lopressor) actually exacerbate symptoms of heart failure. Table 15-25 outlines the initial and target doses of these three drugs.[76]

Because ACE inhibitors do not block the entire RAAS pathway, other physiologic pathways to producing angiotensin II continue to function and may have negative effects on the cardiovascular system. There is some benefit to adding an ARB to ACE inhibitor therapy in order to cover ACE escape. ACE escape is the concept that ACE inhibitors do not inhibit all the major pathways of angiotensin II formation. ARBs block the effect of angiotensin II more completely than ACE inhibitors do and have been shown in multiple trials to be effective for persons with heart failure. ARBs should be considered for individuals who are unable to take ACE inhibitors. Women taking ARBs have benefited from longer survival than when they were on ACE inhibitors.[77] The two ARBs approved for use in heart failure are candesartan (Atacand) and valsartan (Diovan).

Initially there was some concern that a person taking ACE inhibitors, beta-blockers, and ARBs may have more negative outcomes. However, the Candesartan in Heart Failure: Assessment of Reduction in Mortality (CHARM)

Table 15-25 Initial and Target Doses of Beta-Blockers for the Treatment of Heart Failure

Drug Generic (Brand)	Initial Dose	Target Dose
Carvedilol (Coreg, Coreg CR)	3.125 mg bid	25 to 50 mg bid
Metoprolol CRXL (Toprol XL)	12.5 to 25 mg daily	200 mg daily
Bisoprolol (Ziac)	1.25 mg daily	5 to 10 mg daily

Source: From Chavey W, 2000.[76]

trial[78] demonstrated that combination therapy may be beneficial, although this finding was not supported in other studies, and more research is needed.[79]

Digoxin (Lanoxin) is a medication that once was extremely popular for the treatment of heart failure. However, the positive effects of digoxin are robust enough to counter the potential harms. Therefore digoxin (Lanoxin) is contraindicated for individuals with no symptoms of heart failure even if they have a low ejection fraction and a sinus rhythm.[80] Nor are calcium channel blockers recommended because they have negative inotropic effects.[67]

Stage C Heart Failure

Individuals who have symptoms of heart failure with structural changes in the myocardium have progressed to stage C heart failure. There are several medications that can be added to help with symptom management and reduce hospitalizations, morbidity, and mortality. These additional medications are ARBs, aldosterone antagonists, nitrates, hydralazine (Apresoline), and other antihypertensive agents.

When a person has fluid overload, there is also a benefit to the use of diuretics. Such individuals optimally should be titrated with a beta-blocker and ACE inhibitor or ARB if indicated. The addition of diuretics such as thiazides or loop diuretics along with salt restriction will help control fluid overload. The diuretics may be used as needed or may need to be a part of ongoing therapy. Initially, loop diuretics are recommended to manage edema. Often furosemide (Lasix) is the drug of choice; however, the pharmacokinetics of furosemide are not as predictable as other loop diuretics such as torsemide (Demadex) or bumetanide (Bumex). Failure to respond to one loop diuretic suggests that another may be tried and benefit may be gained. Individuals with normal renal function have expected benefit with normal maximum dosing. However, those with renal insufficiency may require higher doses such as 160–200 mg of furosemide (Lasix), 2–3 mg of bumetanide (Bumex), or 20–50 mg of torsemide (Demadex) to obtain a plasma concentration required to reach a desired effect.

Aldosterone Antagonists

Aldosterone antagonists have a role in heart failure management beyond their diuretic effect. Aldosterone is a key player in the development of hypertension and heart failure secondary to its role in stimulating sodium and water retention. In the Randomized Aldactone Evaluation Study (n = 1663), 386 (46%) participants in the placebo arm

died compared to 284 (35%) in the spironolactone arm (RR death 0.70; 95% CI, 0.60 to 0.82; $P < .001$).[81] This 30% reduction in risk of death was attributed to the slowing of the progression of heart failure and risk factors for sudden death. Spironolactone (Aldactone) blocks the aldosterone receptors when prescribed at 12.5 to 25 mg per day. However, hyperkalemia can develop if spironolactone is taken at doses of ≥ 50 mg per day.

Because many of the drugs (e.g., ACE inhibitors, ARBs) used to treat heart failure can cause potassium retention, electrolyte levels should be monitored carefully when these drugs are used in combination. Prior to starting an individual on spironolactone (Aldactone), the creatinine level should be less than 2 mg/dL and serum potassium less than 5.0 mEq/dL. There is also a risk of elevated levels of digoxin when used in combination with spironolactone (Aldactone). Other common side effects are gynecomastia and breast pain in men.[81] The triple therapy of ACE inhibitors, spironolactone (Aldactone), and ARBs should be avoided, as the incidence of adverse effects outweighs the benefits. Eplerenone (Inspra) is a more selective aldosterone antagonist that has fewer of the side effects seen with spironolactone.

Vasodilators

The vasodilators isosorbide dinitrate (Isordil, Sorbitrate) and hydralazine (Apresoline) also reduce mortality in persons with heart failure. These drugs cause vasodilation of both arteries and veins and can be added to a well-established therapy of ACE inhibitors, beta-blockers, and diuretics. They have been shown to reduce mortality initially when taken with diuretics and digoxin.[82] In addition, there is benefit seen among African Americans with use of these drugs and in combination with other standard treatment(s).[83] The standard dose of hydralazine (Apresoline) is 25 mg three times daily, which is commonly titrated up, a dose of 100 mg three times daily may be indicated. This standard dosing is combined with isosorbide dinitrate (Isordil, Sorbitrate) at a dose of 40 mg four times daily.

Calcium Channel Blockers

In general, calcium channel blockers are not recommended because they have an inotropic effect, which can lead to worsening of symptoms and mortality. However, amlodipine (Norvasc) and felodipine (Plendil) are the two calcium channel blockers that do not have negative effects on heart failure. Both of these agents are able to provide benefit via improved blood pressure control and decreased angina symptoms.[84] Caution needs to be taken when using these drugs, as they are associated with a high incidence of peripheral edema.

Digoxin

The benefits of digoxin were first announced in press in a treatise entitled *Account of the Foxglove and Some of Its Medical Uses with Practical Remarks on Dropsy and Other Diseases,* published by Sir William Withering in 1785. Sir Withering, the chief physician of Birmingham General Hospital, conducted an early but elegant pharmacologic inquiry. Given a gypsy remedy for dropsy, he identified the one active ingredient contained in the potion made of 20 botanical substances. That ingredient was the powdered leaf of foxglove or digitalis. Over the course of multiple observations, Sir Withering determined the dose of foxglove that would induce diuresis without inducing bradycardia.[85] Although Sir Withering's work was the first scientific analysis of foxglove, its toxic effects were known for centuries. It has been suggested that the visual symptoms of digoxin toxicity played a role in Vincent Van Gogh's use of swirling green and yellow colors in his paintings.

Digoxin (Lanoxin) is a medication that has now been used for over 200 years and, until recent years, was felt to be a mainstay of therapy for heart failure. Digoxin can be beneficial for persons with current or prior symptoms of heart failure and reduced left ventricular ejection fractions in order to decrease hospitalizations for heart failure. The use of this drug has been well established for treating arrhythmias such as atrial fibrillation. Digoxin is approved for use in combination with ACE inhibitors, beta-blockers, and diuretics with the caveat that the individual is assessed and monitored for drug interactions.

One important item to remember about use of digoxin for persons with heart failure and normal sinus rhythm is that this drug improves morbidity but does not improve mortality rates.[80] It is concerning, however, that there appears to be an increase in total mortality and secondary outcomes of death from CVD or worsening heart failure with the use of digoxin in women when compared to the outcomes in men.[80] There are several theories offered to explain this finding. Women perhaps have higher serum levels of digoxin or it is possible that hormonal therapy may interfere with the metabolism of digoxin, leading to higher levels of digoxin.[86] Women may continue to benefit from digoxin levels and should be monitored closely and maintained at a lower end of the therapeutic window.

Mechanism of Action

Digoxin (Lanoxin) has an inotropic effect on the heart, making the force of the myocardial muscle stronger during contraction. This is caused by inhibition of the sodium/potassium ATPase pump on cell membranes, which increases the intracellular calcium and results in increased contractility. The half-life of digoxin is 36 hours with an onset of action of 1.5–6 hours.

Side Effects/Adverse Effects

Digoxin has a very narrow therapeutic index, and therefore persons taking this medication must be educated about the signs and symptoms of toxicity, which include nausea, vomiting, palpitations, confusion, blurred vision, disturbances of color vision with a tendency to see yellow-green coloring, photophobia, abdominal pain, and seizures. These symptoms are not hard to miss. Digoxin toxicity usually appears at a serum level of 2 ng/mL. However, clinical symptoms of digoxin toxicity are seen in some individuals before reaching this level. When toxicity is found, the drug is withheld until the symptoms resolve or the value returns to normal levels. For those with normal renal function, 60–80% of the drug is excreted in the urine unchanged. Therefore, impaired renal function is an increased risk for toxicity.

Drug–Drug Interactions

Because digoxin (Lanoxin) has a narrow therapeutic index, there are several significant drug interactions, which are listed in Table 15-26.

Stage D Heart Failure

Stage D is the final stage of heart failure, and end-of-life care should be discussed with persons with this diagnosis. At this point, all pharmacologic options have been maximized. Often these individuals benefit from routine, continuous infusions of positive inotropic drugs for palliation. Control of fluid status is a key to providing comfort in order to decrease hospitalizations related to pulmonary edema.[87]

Cardiac Arrythmias

Abnormal electrical conduction in the heart causes irregular rate and/or rhythm. The term *cardiac arrhythmia* refers to several different conditions, some of which are

Table 15-26 Drug Interactions Associated with Digoxin*

Drugs—Generic (Brand)	Effects
Aluminum-containing antacids	Reduces the bioavailability of digoxin.
Amiodarone (Cordarone), alprazolam (Xanax), itraconazole (Sporanox), ketoconazole (Neoral), nicardipine, nifedipine (Procardia), Quinidine (Quinaglute), ritonavir (Norvir), spironolactone (Aldactone), saquinavir (Fortovase), verapamil (Calan)	Reduces clearance of digoxin, which raises serum levels and causes possible digoxin toxicity.
Beta-blockers, calcium channel blockers, methyldopa (Aldomet)	Slows heart rate leading to additive effect of hypotension.
Macrolide antibiotics, tetracycline (Sumycin)	Increases intestinal absorption of digoxin, which raises serum levels and causes potential digoxin toxicity.
Antacids, metoclopramide (Reglan), kaolin-pectin, sulfasalazine (Azulfidine), neomycin (Neo-Fradin), cholestyramine (Questran)	Interfere with intestinal absorption, which lowers serum levels and decreases therapeutic effect.
Potassium-depleting diuretics	Uncorrected potassium depletion makes the heart more sensitive to digoxin, and this combination can cause digoxin toxicity and/or arrythmias.
Rifampin (Rifadin)	Increases nonrenal clearance and decreases therapeutic effect.
Thyroid or synthetic thyroid medications	Decreased therapeutic effect.
Sympathomimetics	Cardiac arrhythmias.

* This table is not comprehensive. New information is being identified on a regular basis. Because digoxin has a very narrow therapeutic window, there are multiple drug–drug interactions possible.

asymptomatic, whereas others are life threatening. The most common symptomatic arrhythmia, atrial fibrillation, is reviewed in this chapter. Although treatment of other arrhythmias differ somewhat, the management of atrial fibrillation can be used as an example to illustrate the general principles used in the management of all arrhythmias.

Normally, electrical conduction controls the rhythm of the heartbeat. Each beat originates in the sinoatrial (SA) node in the right atrium. The electrical impulse spreads through the bundle of His in the atrioventricular node (AV) and then down the Purkinje fibers in both ventricles, which initiates ventricular contraction. The ability of the SA node to automatically stimulate a contraction is called *automaticity*. The cells in the SA node and AV node are different than other heart muscle cells in another way. These cells are dependent on calcium for the initial depolarization phase of the action potential, whereas other cells in the heart are dependent on sodium for the depolarization phase.

The atria and ventricles are electrically separate except for the anteroseptal region in the AV node the bundle of His exists. In addition to the specialized cells that generate the coordinated electrical impulses, all heart muscle cells have the capacity to contract without electrical stimulation. The cells that make up the atrioventricular node, bundle of His, and Purkinje fibers can initiate an action potential strong enough to stimulate a contraction.

Other cells can join in abnormal circuits called reentry circuits.

Usually, the sinoatrial node is faster than other cells and therefore controls the usual rate and rhythm that results in a heart rate of 60 to 100 beats per minute. However, when the heart muscle contracts secondary to stimulation by a cell other than those in the SA node, an ectopic beat occurs. Because every cell in the heart can transmit an action potential, abnormal electrical conduction circuits can develop. These abnormal circuits can cause **fibrillation** when one chamber of the heart responds to an abnormal circuit, bradycardia, tachycardias, or other types of arrhythmias, which are manifestations of **reentry circuits**. Arrhythmias are classically divided into two types—those that alter automaticity of the SA node and those that are secondary to abnormal impulse conduction.

Persons at risk for developing arrhythmias include those who have hypertension, coronary artery disease, congestive heart failure, congenital heart abnormality, hyperthyroidism, diabetes, sleep apnea, alcohol consumption, use of stimulant drugs, and advanced age. As we age, our heart muscle gets weaker and more susceptible to abnormal conduction and abnormal firing.

The risks associated with arrhythmias include fainting, falling, and fractures secondary to syncope, but more importantly, thromboembolic events that lead to stroke can occur when the blood in the heart is in stasis.

Table 15-27 Classes of Drugs Used to Treat Arrhythmias

Class I	Class II	Class III	Class IV
Class Ia	Acebutolol (Sectral)	Amiodarone (Cordarone)	Diltiazem (Cardizem)
Disopyramide (Norpace)	Atenolol (Tenormin)	Azimilide (Stedicor)	Verapamil (Calan, Covera-HS)
Procainamide (Procan, Procan)	Betaxolol (Kerlone)	Bepridil (Vascor)	
Quinidine(Cardioquin, Quinora)	Bisoprolol (Zebeta)	Dofetilide (Tikosyn)	
Class Ib	Carvedilol (Coreg)	Ibutilide (Corvert)	
Lidocaine (Xylocaine)	Esmolol (Brevibloc)		
Mexiletine (Mexitil)	Metoprolol (Toprol-XL, Lopressor)		
Class Ic	Nadolol (Corgard)		
Flecainide (Tambocor)	Propranolol (Inderal)		
Moricizine (Ethmozine)	Sotalol (Betapace)		
Propafenone (Rythmol)	Timolol (Blocadren)		

Pharmacologic Treatment of Arrythmias

The drugs used to treat arrhythmias fall into four categories (Table 15-27) based on mode of action. The class I drugs are sodium channel blockers that decrease the automaticity of the SA node and slow the heart rate. The class II drugs are the beta-blockers that inhibit the tonic sympathetic influence on the SA node, thereby slowing the heart rate so the myocardium does not have to work as hard. The class III drugs inhibit repolarization by blocking potassium channels, which both slows the heart and prevents reentry circuits. The class IV drugs are the calcium channel blockers that act on the SA and AV nodes because the cells in these nodes are more calcium dependent than sodium dependent for the depolarization phase of the action potential.

Atrial Fibrillation

Atrial fibrillation is the most common cardiac dysrhythmia in adults and affects approximately 1% of the general population in developed nations. The incidence varies with ethnicity, gender, and age. Although men are more likely to have atrial fibrillation than are women, the absolute difference in incidence and prevalence is not big. Atrial fibrillation is more common in Whites, and the incidence increases sharply after the age of 60 years.[88] Atrial fibrillation can be asymptomatic or can cause palpitations (the most common symptom), weakness, chest pain, or fatigue. The risk of having an ischemic stroke is approximately 3–8% per year. The medications used to treat atrial fibrillation are directed at the following: (1) controlling the rate, (2) preventing thrombus formation, and (3) correcting the rhythm disturbance if controlling the rate is unsuccessful. Digoxin

(Lanoxin) is used as indicated for any underlying cardiomyopathy.[88] Beta-blockers and calcium channel blockers described earlier in this chapter are the drugs used to stabilize a heart rate, and the drugs used to prevent thrombus are discussed in more detail in Chapter 16. Therefore this section will focus on a brief description of the class I and class III antiarrhythmic drugs used to correct rhythm disturbances in individuals who are hemodynamically stable, require additional medication, and who can be managed in the outpatient setting with careful monitoring and frequent supervision. Initiation and management of women who need antiarrhythmic drugs is usually outside the scope of primary care, although primary care providers may care for persons using these agents for other healthcare concerns. The interested reader is referred to the 2006 guidelines from the American College of Cardiology and American Heart Association Task Force and the European Society of Cardiology Committee for Practice for a description of currently recommended management of arrhythmias.[88]

Antiarrhythmic Drugs

Class Ia, Ic, and III antiarrhythmic drugs are used to convert atrial fibrillation into a regular rhythm if standard pharmacologic therapies or electrical conversion has been unsuccessful. The success rate of converting atrial fibrillation into a sinus rhythm is not perfect and incurs an independent increased risk for thromboembolism. Therefore, either electrical conversion or pharmacologic conversion is offered to persons already on anticoagulants.

Antiarrythmic drugs affect the electrical conduction within the heart, and therefore all have the potential to create arrhythmias and must be used with caution. The side effect of greatest concern is **torsades de pointes** or prolonged QT interval, which can evolve into ventricular fibrillation and sudden death. Quinidine (Cardioquin) has been the prototype but is used much less often today because it increases digoxin (Lanoxin) levels and has multiple drug–drug interactions.

Amiodarone (Cordarone) is the class III drug most often recommended for outpatient management. The dose of amiodarone is based on the severity of the arrhythmia. Side effects include pulmonitis, optic nerve neuropathy, hypotension, hyper- or hypothyroidism, peripheral neuropathy, headache, ataxia, and skin discoloration. This drug also has multiple drug–drug interactions. Amiodarone is contraindicated for individuals with severe SA node dysfunction, second- or third-degree AV heart block, sinus bradycardia, and hypotension.

In summary, cardiac arrhythmias are common in the elderly and a frequent comorbidity in persons with hypertension or other cardiovascular disease processes. The management of cardiac arrhythmias is complex and requires specific knowledge and training in cardiac physiology and the pharmacology of a class of drugs that have multiple adverse effects.

Conclusion

Women need to know the importance of their cardiovascular health. Primary prevention can lead to significant reduction in their lifetime risk of developing CVD. Screening and recognizing risks early is the key to reducing CVD events. Many cardiac events occur in combination and require multiple pharmacologic interventions. Often one drug is insufficient to reach clinical goals, and multiple drugs will be needed. The healthcare provider needs to be aware of the individual's risk factors and existing CVD conditions in order to provide optimal treatment. Continued monitoring of risk factors and maintenance treatment goals need to be evaluated frequently. In the area of CVD pharmacology, recommendations and guidelines frequently change as we learn more about this amazing physiologic system.

References

1. American Heart Association. Heart disease and stroke statistics—2008 update: a report from the American Heart Association statistics committee and stroke statistics subcommittee. Circulation 2007;117:e25–e146.
2. Ridker PM, Cook NR, Moin Lee I, Gordon D, Gaziano JM, Manson JE, et al. A randomized trial of low-dose aspirin in the primary prevention of cardiovascular disease in women. N Engl J Med 2005;1293–304.
3. Mosca L, Appel LJ, Benjamin EJ, Berra K, Chandra-Strobos N, Fabunmi RP, et al. Evidence-based guidelines for cardiovascular disease prevention in women: 2007 update. Circulation 2007;115:1481–501.
4. Franco OH, Kinderen AJ, Laet CD, Peeters A, Bonneux L. Primary prevention of cardiovascular disease: cost effectiveness comparison. Int J Technology Assess Health Care 2007;23:71–9.
5. Elmer PJ, PREMIER Collaborative Research Group. Effects of comprehensive lifestyle modification on diet, weight, physical fitness, and blood pressure control: 18-month results of a randomized trial. Ann Intern Med 2006;144:485–95.
6. Stampfer MJ, Hu FB, Manson JE, Rimm EB, Willett WC. Primary prevention of coronary heart disease in women through diet and lifestyle. N Engl J Med 2000; 343:16–22.
7. Kris-Etherton PM, Harris WS, Appel LJ. Fish consumption, fish oil, omega-3 fatty acids, and cardiovascular disease. Arterioscler Thromb Vascular Biol 2003;23:e20–e30.
8. Bucher HC, Hengstler P, Schindler C, Meier G. N-3 polyunsaturated fatty acids in coronary heart disease: a meta-analysis of randomized controlled trials. Am J Med 2002;112:298–304.
9. Wang C, Chung M, Lichtenstein A, Balk E, Kupelnick B, DeVine D, et al. Effects of omega-3 fatty acids on cardiovascular disease. Evid Rep Technol Assess (Summ) 2004;(94):1–8.
10. Scisney-Matlock M. Development and evaluation of DASH diet tailored messages for hypertension treatment. Appl Nurs Res 2006;19:78–87.
11. Dahlof B, Sever PS, Poulter NR, Wedel H, Beevers DG, Caulfield M, et al. Prevention of cardiovascular events with an antihypertensive regimen of amlodipine adding perindopril as required versus atenolol adding bendroflumethiazide as required, in the Anglo-Scandinavian Cardiac Outcomes Trial-Blood Pressure Lowering Arm (ASCOT-BPLA). Lancet 2005;366:895–906.
12. National Heart, Lung and Blood Institute. The DASH eating plan. Available from: *www.nhlbi.nih.gov/health/ public/heart/hbp/dash/* [Accessed November 18, 2007].
13. McNeill AN, Rosamond WD, Girman CJ, Golden SH, Schmidt MI, East HE, et al. The metabolic syndrome and 11 year risk of incident cardiovascular disease in the atherosclerosis risk in communities study. Diabetes 2005;28:385–90.

14. Weinstein AR, Sesso HD, Lee IM, Cook NR, Manson JE, Buring JE, et al. Relationship of physical activity vs. body mass index with type 2 diabetes in women. JAMA 2004;292:1188–94.

15. National Heart, Lung, and Blood Institutes of Health. Clinical guidelines on the identification, evaluation and treatment of overweight and obesity in adults. Washington, DC: National Institutes of Health, 1998.

16. Belch J, MacCuish A, Campbell I, Cobbe S, Taylor R, Prescott R, et al. for the Prevention of Progression of Arterial Disease and Diabetes Study Group; Diabetes Registry Group; Royal College of Physicians Edinburgh. The prevention of progression of arterial disease and diabetes (POPADAD) trial: factorial randomised placebo controlled trial of aspirin and antioxidants in patients with diabetes and asymptomatic peripheral arterial disease. BMJ. 2008 Oct 16; 337:a1840.

17. Eidelman RS, Hebert PR, Weisman SM, Hennekens CH. An update on aspirin in the primary prevention of cardiovascular disease. Arch Intern Med 2003;163: 2006–10.

18. Oparil S. Women and hypertension: What did we learn from the women's health initiative? Cardiology in Review 2006;14:267–75.

19. Pritchett AM, Forest JP, Mann DL. Treatment of the metabolic syndrome: the impact of lifestyle modification. Curr Artheroscler Rep 2005;7:95–102.

20. National Heart, Lung and Blood Institute. The seventh annual report of the Joint National Committee on Prevention, Detection, Evaluation, and Treatment of High Blood Pressure. Bethesda, MD: National Institutes of Health, 2004.

21. ALLHAT Officers and Coordinators for the ALLHAT Collaborative Research Group. Major outcomes in high-risk hypertensive patients randomized to angiotensin-converting enzyme inhibitor or calcium channel blocker vs diuretic: the Antihypertensive and Lipid-Lowering Treatment to Prevent Heart Attack Trial (ALLHAT). JAMA 2002;288:2981–97.

22. Appel LJ. The verdict from ALLHAT: thiazide diuretics are the preferred initial therapy for hypertension. JAMA 2002;288:3039.

23. Bolland MJ, Ames RW, Horne AM, Orr-Wa BJ, Gamble GD, Reid IR. The effect of treatment with thiazide diuretics for 4 years on bone density in normal postmenopausal women. Osteoporos Int 2007;4:479–86.

24. Bakris GL, Fonseca V, Katholi RE, McGill JB, Messerli FH, Phillips RA, et al. Metabolic effects of carvedilol vs metoprolol in patients with type 2 diabetes mellitus

and hypertension: a randomized controlled trial. JAMA 2004;292:2227–36.

25. Houston MC. Abrupt discontinuation of antihypertensive therapy. South Med J 1981;74:12–23.

26. Gress TW, Nieto FJ, Shahar E, Wofford MR, Brancati FL. Hypertension and antihypertensive therapy as risk factors for type 2 diabetes mellitus. N Engl J Med 2000;342:905–12.

27. Podymow T, August P. Hypertension in pregnancy. Adv Chronic Kidney Dis 2007;14:178–90.

28. American Academy of Pediatrics Committee on Drugs. The transfer of drugs and other chemicals into human milk. Pediatrics 2001;108:776–88.

29. Tu K, Campbell NRC, Chen Z. Use of beta blockers hypertension in the elderly: a cause of concern. J Hum Hypertens 2007:21:271–5.

30. Wright JT Jr, ALLHAT Collaborative Research Group. Outcomes in hypertensive black and nonblack patients treated with chlorthalidone, amlodipine, and lisinopril. JAMA 2005;293:1595–608.

31. Onder G, Penninx BW, Balkrishan R, Fried LP, Chaves PHM, Williamson CC, et al. Relation between use of angiotensin-converting enzyme inhibitors and muscle strength and physical function in older women: an observational study. Lancet 2002;359 926–30.

32. Burnier M, Brunner HR. Angiotensin II receptor antagonists. Lancet 2000;355(9204):637–45.

33. Goldberg AI, Dunlay MC, Sweet CS. Safety and tolerability of losartan potassium, an angiotensin II receptor antagonist, compared with hydrochlorothiazide, atenolol, felodipine ER, and angiotensin-converting enzyme inhibitors for the treatment of systemic hypertension. Am J Cardiol 1995;75:793–5.

34. Müller DN, Derer W, Dechend R. Aliskiren-mode of action and preclinical data. J Mol Med April 29, 2008. [Epub ahead of print].

35. Barzilay JI, for the ALLHAT Collaborative Research Group. Cardiovascular outcomes using doxazosin vs. chlorthalidone for the treatment of hypertension in older adults with and without glucose disorders: a report from the ALLHAT study. J Clin Hypertens 2004; 6:116–25.

36. Umans JG. Medications during pregnancy: antihypertensives and immunosuppressives. Adv Chronic Kidney Dis 2007;14:191–8.

37. Wright CI, Van-Buren L, Kroner CI, Koning MM. Herbal medicines as diuretics: a review of the scientific evidence. J Ethnopharmacol 2007;114(1):1–31.

38. National Cholesterol Education Program. Detection, evaluation, and treatment of high blood cholesterol in

adults (adult treatment panel III). Final report. Third report of the expert panel NIH Pub No 025215. Bethesda, MD: National Heart, Lung, and Blood Institute, 2002.

39. LaRosa JC, Grundy SM, Waters DD, Shear C, Barter P, Fruchart J. Intensive lipid lowering with atorvastatin in patients with stable coronary disease. N Engl J Med 2005;352:1425–35.

40. Colhoun HM, Betteridge DJ, Durrington PN, Hitman GA, Neil HAW, Livingstone SJ, et al. Primary prevention of cardiovascular disease with atorvastatin in type 2 diabetes in the Collaborative Atorvastatin Diabetes Study (CARDS): multicentre randomized placebo-controlled trial. Lancet 2004;364:685–96.

41. Bottorff MB. Statin safety and drug interactions: clinical implications. Am J Cardiol 2006;97(suppl):27C–31C.

42. Kajinami K, Akao H, Polisecki E, Schaefer EJ. Pharmacogenomics of statin responsiveness. Am J Cardiol 2005;96(9A):65K–70K[discussion 34K–35K].

43. Gotto AM. Statins: Powerful drugs for lowering cholesterol: advice for patients. Circulation 2002; 105:1514–6.

44. Poynter JN, Griuber SB, Higgins PR, Almog R, Bonner JD, Rennert HS. Statins and the risk for colorectal cancer. N Engl J Med 2005;352:2184–92.

45. Bliznakov EG. Lipid-lowering drugs (statins), cholesterol, and coenzyme Q10. The Baycol case—a modern Pandora's box. Biomed Pharmacother 2002;56:56–9.

46. Grundy SM, Vega GL, Yuan Z, Battisti WP, Brady WE, Palmisano J. Effectiveness and tolerability of simvastatin plus fenofibrate for combined hyperlipidemia: the SAFARI Trial. Am J Cardiol 2005;95:462–8.

47. Keech A, Simes RJ, Barter P, Best J, Scott R, Taskinen MR, et al. Effect of long-term fenofibrate therapy on cardiovascular events in 9795 people with type 2 diabetes mellitus (the FIELD study): randomised controlled trial. Lancet 2005;366:1849–61.

48. Jacobson TA, Armani A, McKenney JM, Guyton JR. Safety considerations with gastrointestinally active lipid-lowering drugs. Am J Cardiol 2007;99:47C–55C.

49. Insull W, Toth P, Mullican W, Hunninghake D, Burke S, Donovan JM, et al. Effectiveness of colesevelam hydrochloride in decreasing LDL cholesterol in patients with primary hypercholesterolemia: a 24-week randomized controlled trial. Mayo Clin Proc 2001;76:971–82.

50. Taylor AJ. Arterial biology for the investigation of the treatment effects of reducing cholesterol (ARBITER) 2: a double-blind, placebo-controlled study of extended-release niacin on atherosclerosis progression in secondary prevention patients treated with statins. Circulation 2004;110:3512–7.

51. Kastelein JJ, Akdim F, Stroes ESG, Zwinderman AH, Bots ML, Stalenhoef AFH, et al. Simvastatin with or without ezetimibe in familial hypercholesterolemia. N Engl J Med 2008;358;1431–43.

52. Barter P, Ginsberg HN. Effectiveness of combined statin plus omega-3 fatty acid therapy for mixed dyslipidemia. Am J Cardiol 2008;102(8):1040–5. [Epub July 31, 2008].

53. Adams RJ, Albers G, Alberts MJ, Benavente O, Furie K, Goldstein LB, et al. American Heart Association, American Stroke Association. Update to the AHA/ASA recommendations for the prevention of stroke in patients with stroke and transient ischemic attack. Stroke 2008;39(5):1647–52.

54. Rashid P, Leonardi-Bee J, Bath P. Blood pressure reduction and secondary prevention of stroke and other vascular events: a systematic review. Stroke 2003;34;2741–8.

55. Yusuf S, Sleight P, Pogue J, Bosch J, Daview R, Dagenais G. Effects of an angiotensin-converting-enzyme inhibitor, ramipril, on cardiovascular events in high-risk patients: the Heart Outcomes Prevention Evaluation Study Investigators. N Engl J Med 2000;342:145–53.

56. Sever PS, Dahlof B, Poulter NR, Wedel H, Beevers G, Caulfield M, et al. Prevention of coronary and stroke events with atorvastatin in hypertensive patients who have average or lower than average cholesterol concentrations, in the Anglo-Scandinavian cardiac outcomes trial lipid lowering arm (ASCOT-LLA): a multicentre randomized controlled trial. Lancet 2003;361:1149–58.

57. Antiplatelet Trialists' Collaboration. Collaborative overview of randomized trials of antiplatelet therapy: III. Reduction in venous thrombosis and pulmonary embolism by antiplatelet prophylaxis among surgical and medical patients. BMJ 1994;308:235–46.

58. Albers GW, Amarenco P, Easton JD, Sacco RL, Teal P. Antithrombotic and thrombolytic therapy for ischemic stroke: the seventh ACCP conference on antithrombotic and thrombolytic therapy. Chest 2004;126:483S–512S.

59. McQuaid K, Laine LD. Systematic review and meta-analysis of adverse events of low-dose aspirin and clopidogrel in randomized controlled trials. Am J Med 2006;119:624–38.

60. CAPRIE steering committee. A randomized, blinded, trial of clopidogrel versus aspirin in patients at risk of ischemic events (CAPRIE). Lancet 1996;348:1329–39.

61. Hirsch AT, Haskal ZJ, Hertzer NR, Bakal CW, Creager MA, Halperin JL, Hiratzka LF, et al. ACC/AHA Guidelines for the Management of Patients with Peripheral Arterial Disease (Lower Extremity, Renal, Mesenteric,

and Abdominal Aortic): A Collaborative Report from the American Association for Vascular Surgery/Society for Vascular Surgery, Society for Cardiovascular Angiography and Interventions, Society for Vascular Medicine and Biology, Society of Interventional Radiology, and the ACA/AHA Task Force on Practice Guidelines (Writing Committee to Develop Guidelines for the Management of Patients With Peripheral Arterial Disease). Circulation 2006;113:e436–e65.

62. Belch JJ, Topol EF, Agnelli G, Bertrand M, Califf RM, Clement DL, et al. Critical issues in peripheral arterial disease detection and management: a call to action. Arch Intern Med 2003;163:884–92.

63. Lonn E, Roccaforte R, Ji Q, Dagenais G, Sleight P, Bosch J, et al. Effect of long-term therapy with ramipril in high risk women. J Am Coll Cardiol 2002;40:693–702.

64. Keyhan G, Chen SF, Pilote L. The effectiveness of β-blockers in women with congestive heart failure. J Gen Intern Med 2007;22:955–61.

65. Masoudi FA, Havranek EP, Smith G, et al. Gender, age, and heart failure with preserved left ventricular systolic function. J Am Coll Cardiol 2003;41:217–23.

66. Zile MR, Brutsaert DL. New concepts in diastolic dysfunction and diastolic heart failure part I: Diagnosis, prognosis, and measurements of diastolic function. Circulation 2002;105:1387–93.

67. Hunt SA, Abraham WT, Chin MH, Feldman AM, Francis GS, Ganiats TG, et al. ACC/AHA 2005 guideline update for the diagnosis and management of chronic heart failure in the adult-summary article: a report of the American College of Cardiology/American Heart Association task force on practice guidelines (writing committee to update the 2001 guidelines for the evaluation and management of heart failure). Circulation 2005;112:1825–52.

68. Zile MR, Brutsaert DL. New concepts in diastolic dysfunction and diastolic heart failure part II: causal mechanism and treatment. Circulation 2002;105:1503–8.

69. Klingbeil AU, Schneider M, Martus P, Messerli FH, Schmieder RE. A meta-analysis of the effects of treatment on left ventricular mass in essential hypertension. Am J Med 2003;115(1):41–6.

70. Meurin P. The ASCOT trial: clarifying the role of ACE inhibition in the reduction of cardiovascular events in patients with hypertension. Am J Cardiovasc Drugs 2006;6:327–34.

71. Keyhan G, Chen SF, Pilote L. Angiotensin-converting enzyme inhibitors and survival in women and men with heart failure. Eur J Heart Fail 2007;9:594–601.

72. Rochon PA, Sykora K, Bronskill SE, Mamdani M, Anderson GM, Gurwitz JH, et al. Use of angiotensin-converting enzyme inhibitor therapy and dose-related outcomes in older adults with new heart failure in the community. J Gen Intern Med 2004; 19(6):676–83.

73. Flather MD, Yusuf S, Kober L, Pfeffer M, Hall A, Murray G, et al. Long-term ACE-inhibitor therapy in patients with heart failure or left-ventricular dysfunction: a systematic overview of data from individual patients. ACE-Inhibitor Myocardial Infarction Collaborative Group. Lancet 2000;355:1575.

74. Deedwania PC, Giles TD, Klibaner M, Ghali JK, Herlitz J, Hildebrandt P, et al. Efficacy, safety and tolerability of metoprolol CR/XL in patients with diabetes and chronic heart failure: experiences from MERIT-HR. Am Heart J 2005;149:159–67.

75. Packer M, Fowler MB, Roecker EB, Coats AJS, Katus HA, Krum H, et al. Effect of carvedilol on the morbidity of patients with severe chronic heart failure: results of the Carvedilol Prospective Randomized Cumulative Survival (COPERNICUS) study. Circulation 2002; 106:2194–99.

76. Chavey W. The importance of beta blockers in the treatment of heart failure. Am Fam Physician 2000;62:2453–62.

77. Hudson M. Sex differences in the effectiveness of angiotensin receptor blockers and angiotensin converting enzyme inhibitors in patients with congestive heart failure: a population study. Eur J Heart Fail 2007;9:602–9.

78. Bhakta S, Dunlap ME. Angiotensin-receptor blockers in heart failure: evidence from the CHARM trial. Cleve Clin J Med 2004;71:665–73.

79. Ramasubbu K, Mann DL, Deswal A. Anti-angiotensin therapy: new perspectives. Cardiology Clin 2007; 25:573–80.

80. The Digitalis Investigation Group. The effects of digoxin on mortality and morbidity in patients with heart failure. N Engl J Med 1997;336(8):525–33.

81. Pitt B, Zannad F, Remme WJ, Cody R, Castaigne A, Perez A, et al. The effect of spironolactone on morbidity and mortality in patients with severe heart failure. Randomized Aldactone Evaluation Study. N Engl J Med 1999;341:709–17.

82. Cohn JN, Johnson G, Ziesche S, Cobb F, Francis G, Tristani F, et al. A comparison of enalapril with hydralazine-isosorbide dinitrate in the treatment of chronic congestive heart failure. N Engl J Med 1991;325: 303–10.

83. Taylor AL, Ziesche S, Yancy C, Carson P, D'Agostino R Jr, Ferdinand K, et al. Combination of isosorbide dinitrate and hydralazine in blacks with heart failure. N Engl J Med 2004;351:2049–57.

84. O'Connor CM, Carson PE, Miller AB, Pressler ML, Belkin RN, Neuberg GW, et al. Effect of amlodipine on mode of death among patients with advanced heart failure in the PRAISE trial. Prospective randomized amlodipine survival evaluation. Am J Cardiol 1998;82:881–7.

85. Trohler U. Withering's 1785 appeal for caution when reporting on a new medicine. J Royal Soc Med 2007;100:155–6.

86. Rathore SS, Wang Y, Krumholz H. Sex based differences in the effect of digoxin for the treatment of heart failure. N Engl J Med 2002;347:1403–11.

87. Ali S, Hong M, Antezano ES, Mangat I. Evaluation and management of atrial fibrillation. Cardiovasc Hematol Disord-Drug Targets 2006;6:233–44.

88. Zipes DP, Camm AJ, Borggrefe M, Buxton AE, Chaitman B, Fromer M, et al. ACC/AHA/ESC 2006 guidelines for management of patients with ventricular arrhythmias and the prevention of sudden cardiac death: a report of the American College of Cardiology/American Heart Association task force and the European Society of Cardiology committee for practice guidelines (writing committee to develop guidelines for management of patients with ventricular arrhythmias and the prevention of sudden cardiac death); developed in collaboration with the European Heart Rhythm Association and the Heart Rhythm Society. Circulation 2006;114(10):e385–e484. [Epub August 25, 2006].

"The blood is the life!"

BRAM STOKER, *DRACULA*

16
Hematology

*Patrick J. M. Murphy, Brian Meadors,
and Tekoa L. King*

Chapter Glossary

Anticoagulant A substance that prevents coagulation.

Antiplatelet drug A class of drugs that decrease platelet aggregation.

Contact activation pathway See *intrinsic pathway*.

Embolism An object that moves from one part of the body to another distant part where it causes an occlusion of a blood vessel.

Erythrocyte Red blood cell. Erythrocytes are filled with hemoglobin, the molecule that binds to oxygen.

Erythropoiesis The development of red blood cells that undergo several divisions before becoming mature RBCs.

Erythropoietin (EPO) Glycoprotein hormone that controls erythropoiesis. Erythropoietin is produced in the endothelial cells in the kidney.

Extrinsic pathway (tissue factor pathway) The series of reactions within the coagulation process that begins when coagulation factor VII comes in contact with tissue factor expressed on the surface of cells. When FVII binds to tissue factor, the complex formed initiates a series of reactions that result in the formation of thrombin. This pathway is now referred to as the *tissue factor pathway*, and it is this pathway that initiates the coagulation process.

Ferritin A protein-iron complex that is the intracellular storage for iron.

Folate Water-soluble vitamin B_9. The name folate comes from the Latin word *folium*, which means leaf. Folate is found in large amounts in leafy, green vegetables.

Folic acid The synthetic form of folate.

Hypochromic anemia Anemia characterized by red blood cells in which the central area is enlarged and pale. It is secondary to a deficiency of hemoglobin, which contains the pigment that imparts the red color to the cell.

Intrinsic factor Glycoprotein produced by the parietal cells of the stomach. Vitamin B_{12} binds to intrinsic factor in the ileum, and the vitamin B_{12}/intrinsic factor complex is then able to enter the portal circulation.

Intrinsic pathway (contact activation pathway) Series of transformations of coagulation factors that are initiated by factors present in blood. The intrinsic cascade begins when coagulation factors present in blood come in contact with collagen from subendothelial connective tissue that is exposed when endothelial cells are injured. Also referred to as the *contact activation pathway*.

Macrocytic anemia Anemia characterized by red blood cells that are larger than usual.

Mean corpuscular volume (MCV) The measure of red blood cell volume. The MCV is a reflection of the type and amount of hemoglobin present.

Megaloblastic anemia A type of macrocytic anemia characterized by deficient DNA synthesis. Megaloblastic anemia is frequently secondary to a deficiency of vitamin B_{12} or folic acid.

Microcytic anemia Anemia characterized by red blood cells that are smaller than usual.

Pernicious anemia Anemia that is secondary to vitamin B_{12} deficiency.

Racemic mixture Mixture with equal amounts of left- and right-handed enantiomers of a molecule. These molecules have the same chemical composition, but the structure of the left-handed and right-handed versions is different.

Reticulocyte Immature red blood cell. Reticulocytes are released into the circulation and transform into mature red blood cells within 7 days. Typically, 1% of the red blood cell mass is composed of reticulocytes.

Thrombin Activated coagulation factor II$_a$. Thrombin plays a central role in propagating the coagulation process and in starting the fibrolysis process.

Thromboembolism A thrombus that breaks loose from its point of origin and blocks or obstructs a blood vessel at a point distant from where it was formed.

Thrombolytic drugs A class of drugs that dissolve blood clots via thrombolysis.

Thrombosis Disorder that occurs when a thrombus blocks the blood vessel and causes ischemia in tissues nourished by the vessel.

Thrombus (plural: thrombi) A blood clot within a blood vessel.

Tissue factor pathway See *extrinsic pathway*.

Total iron-binding capacity (TIBC) A laboratory test that measures the blood's capacity to bind iron with transferrin.

Transferrin Blood plasma protein that reversibly binds to iron and transfers iron in blood to tissues.

Virchow's triad The three factors that cause venous thrombus formation. The factors include (1) venous stasis, (2) damage to epithelium, and (3) hypercoagulation.

Introduction

Nonneoplastic hematologic disorders in women commonly include anemias and coagulopathies that can cause a thrombus or embolus. Drugs used to treat anemias and coagulopathies act by activating, inhibiting, or supplementing biomolecules normally present in the vasculature. This chapter reviews the physiologic and pathophysiologic states associated with decreased red blood cell concentrations and then addresses treatments for the most common forms of anemia. The second half of the chapter presents an overview of coagulopathies and drugs used to treat coagulation disorders.

Erythropoiesis

Erythropoiesis, which is the term for the development of red blood cells (RBCs), begins in red bone marrow with differentiation of a pluripotent stem cell and concludes in

the blood with the formation of the mature **erythrocyte**, which is commonly called an RBC. **Erythropoietin** and cytokines stimulate pluripotent stem cell differentiation into a proerythroblast, which upon subsequent cell divisions incorporates hemoglobin (Hgb) and forms an erythroblast. The erythroblast incorporates increasing amounts of hemoglobin while undergoing several rounds of cell division and gradually extrudes its nucleus, resulting in the development of a **reticulocyte**. The reticulocyte enters systemic circulation and over 7 days loses its remaining nuclear components, forming a mature RBC. RBCs constitute 40–50% of total blood volume and circulate for 120 days before being catabolized in the spleen and reticuloendothelial system.

Role of Erythropoietin, Hemoglobin, and Iron in Erythropoiesis

Erythropoietin and hemoglobin are essential for RBC maturation. Erythropoietin is a glycoprotein produced by the kidneys in response decreased oxygen levels in the blood. Once released, erythropoietin stimulates production of RBCs via interactions with growth factors involved in the transformation of RBC precursor cells. Erythropoietin also protects RBCs from apoptosis. Under normal physiologic conditions, erythropoietin maintains a constant rate of new RBC production that balances natural RBC loss. When erythropoietin production or release is impaired, such as in chronic kidney disease, RBC production decreases.

Hemoglobin is composed of an iron-porphyrin ring and four globin chains, two alpha-globin chains and two beta-globin chains. Hemoglobin reversibly binds to oxygen, which is the mechanism the body uses to transport oxygen from the lung and release it to tissues. Hemoglobin comprises > 90% of the protein content in the mature RBC and provides the characteristic red (normochromic) appearance. Hemoglobin forms in the erythroblast stage of RBC maturation—a process coordinated by iron-containing heme prosthetic groups. Approximately 75% (2.5 g) of the iron in the body is present in hemoglobin. Following destruction of RBCs by the reticuloendothelial system, iron and other cellular components are recycled for the production of future erythrocytes.

Role of Folate and Vitamin B$_{12}$ in Erythropoiesis

Vitamin B$_{12}$ (also known as cobalamin) and **folate** (also known as **folic acid**, vitamin B$_9$) are nutrients required for DNA synthesis. Blood cell lineage development and erythropoiesis specifically, is particularly sensitive to folate and vitamin B_{12} concentrations in the body due to the relatively high fraction of RBC cells undergoing cellular division at any one time. Within the cell, vitamin B_{12} demethylates the inactive dietary form of folate (5-methyl THFA) into folinic acid (THFA), which is the active metabolite. Folinic acid is an enzyme that facilitates DNA synthesis through production of thymidylate (dTMP) and the thymidylate synthase pathway.

Absorption of vitamin B_{12} occurs in the ileum and is dependent on **intrinsic factor**, a glycoprotein secreted from parietal cells of the gastric mucosa that complexes with vitamin B_{12} to facilitate robust vitamin B_{12} absorption. When superphysiologic levels of inactive folate are present within cells, an alternative pathway can facilitate the conversion of inactive folate to its active metabolite, even in the absence of vitamin B_{12}.

The Role of Iron

Orally administered iron is absorbed into mucosal cells within the duodenum and proximal jejunum. While the recommended daily iron intake is 10–30 mg, only a fraction (5–30%) of the ingested iron is absorbed, although more iron is absorbed when body stores are depleted. The charged state of the iron atom affects intestinal absorption, with ferrous (Fe^{2+}) iron being more readily absorbed by the intestine than ferric (Fe^{3+}) iron. Most iron in the body is present in hemoglobin, and the remainder is present in the muscle protein myoglobin, an iron-containing enzyme; iron storage proteins such as **ferritin**, or iron transporter proteins such as **transferrin**.

Once absorbed, iron is transported to red bone marrow by transferrin, where it is then incorporated into hemoglobin and subsequently into the developing erythroblast. Following catabolism of an RBC by the spleen, iron is recycled by the body. It is again bound to transferrin and returned to the bone marrow for a successive round of erythropoiesis. Ferritin is a globular protein that is the intracellular iron storage repository. Free iron is toxic to cells because it can catalyze the formation of free radicals; therefore, iron is bound to proteins in various ways so that it can be released for use as needed. Blood levels of ferritin reflect the total body store of iron, and thus, the ferritin level will reflect the severity of the anemia.

Daily requirements of iron are intricately linked to RBC production, and elevated iron demand corresponds to increased erythropoiesis. Increased RBC production occurs during pregnancy, infancy, early childhood, and chronic blood loss. During pregnancy and the early postpartum period (2–3 months postdelivery), the recommended daily allowance of dietary iron increases to 27 mg/day; this necessitates dietary supplementation. Over the course of an uncomplicated pregnancy, a woman requires an additional 1000 mg of iron for the expanded maternal blood volume, fetus, and placenta. Premenopausal adult women have a greater recommended dietary allowance for iron (18 mg/day elemental) than adult males, due to the need for replacing iron lost through menstruation. Following menopause, the recommended daily allowance for women and men is equivalent to 8 mg/day (Table 16-1).

Anemias

Anemias are a collection of medical conditions characterized by: (1) a loss of hemoglobin (e.g., hemorrhage or increased hemolysis of red blood cells), (2) a decrease in production of hemoglobin (e.g., aplastic anemia), (3) production of variant forms of hemoglobin (e.g., thalassemia, sickle cell anemia). Anemias occur secondary to one of

Table 16-1 Recommended Dietary Allowances for Women and Dietary Sources of Iron, Folate, and Vitamin B_{12}

	Recommended Daily Allowance for Nonpregnant Women	Recommended Daily Allowance for Women During Pregnancy and Lactation	Dietary Sources Rich in Nutrients
Elemental iron	18 mg/day	27 mg/day during pregnancy 9 mg/day during lactation	Red meat, liver, prune juice, spinach, egg yolks, fish, and fortified grains and grain products (e.g., cereals, breads, pasta, rice, and flour)
Folic acid	400 mcg/day	400 mcg/day during pregnancy 500 mcg/day during lactation	Green vegetables (e.g., lettuce, spinach, and broccoli), whole-wheat grains, fortified grains, and grain products (e.g., cereals, breads, pasta, rice, flour)
Vitamin B_{12}	2.4 mcg/day	2.6 mcg/day during pregnancy 2.8 mcg/day during lactation	Fish, meat, poultry, eggs, dairy products, and fortified cereals

several factors, including deficiency of a nutrient essential for the development and maturation of RBCs (e.g., folate or vitamin B_{12} deficiency), impaired bone marrow production of RBCs, hemolysis, chronic infection, or blood loss. Anemias may be caused by underlying physiologic states such as pregnancy or pathophysiologic states such as cancer or chronic kidney disease. Anemia can also be secondary to genetic alterations in the type of hemoglobin made, which is the underlying pathophysiology of sickle cell anemia and the thalassemias.

The most common anemias are nutritional deficiency-associated anemias that occur after a period of inadequate consumption or inadequate absorption of iron, vitamin B_{12}, and/or folic acid. Treatment in primary care is directed at replacing the absent nutrient with vitamin supplementation. Successful therapeutic intervention requires identification of the type of anemia as well as the underlying cause of the disease. The treatment goals for the individual who is anemic are to ameliorate the symptoms, rectify the underlying cause, and prevent recurrence.

Anemias are most commonly observed in adult women, occurring in 3.5 million women in the United States each year.[1] Anemia occurs less frequently in women taking estrogen-progestin oral contraceptives and at substantially higher levels in women using an intrauterine device. An estimated 10–20% of menstruating women and > 20% of pregnant women are classified as anemic based on the presence of low hemoglobin concentrations (< 11 g/dL during the first and third trimesters, < 10.5 g/dL during the second trimester). Low birth weight, preterm birth, and newborn mortality are all associated with maternal anemia during pregnancy.[2]

Anemia-Induced Morphologic Changes in Red Blood Cells

Changes in RBC development and morphology are key clues to the type of anemia that is present. Aberrant erythrocyte maturation, which may be manifested as changes in RBC size and color, plasma concentration, and/or hemoglobin content, can aid in reaching a specific diagnosis. Anemias caused by deficiencies of either folic acid or vitamin B_{12} may be identified as **macrocytic anemia** and **megaloblastic anemia**, whereas anemias caused by iron deficiencies are classically identified as **microcytic anemia** and **hypochromic anemia**. A typical mature RBC is the same diameter as the nucleus of a white blood cell. When the measured RBC diameter is greater than the nucleus of surrounding white blood cells, the RBCs are termed macrocytic. Conversely when the RBC diameter is less than the nucleus of

white blood cells, they are microcytic. Megaloblasts are oversized erythroblasts present in the bone marrow and macrocytes are oversized erythrocytes present in the circulation. Both megaloblasts and macrocytes are present in substantially increased concentrations when insufficient stores of either folic acid or vitamin B_{12} are available to the bone marrow. Microcytes are abnormally small circulating erythrocytes, and their pale (hypochromic) coloration may result from severely decreased hemoglobin content. Anemias in which RBCs have a normal RBC cell size (normocytic) and normal concentrations of hemoglobin and coloration (normochromic) may be caused by recent blood loss, which may be chronic or acute. Since anemias that are either mild or in their initial stages may not display the classical morphologic changes, it is important to carefully assess the physiologic condition and collected laboratory values for diagnosis.

Microcytic Anemia: Iron Deficiency

Iron deficiency is the most common nutritional deficiency and the most common cause of anemia, affecting 1–2% of the US population.[3] Common etiologies of iron deficiency anemias involve states where the body requires increased RBC synthesis. Examples of these conditions include maternal blood volume expansion during pregnancy, occult blood loss from a gastrointestinal ulcer or tumor, and overt blood loss from excessive menstruation or during birth. Less common etiologies of iron deficiency anemia involve decreased iron utilization occurring from dietary insufficiency or impaired intestinal absorption, which may be caused by celiac disease or other intestinal dysfunction. In contrast to men, premenopausal adult women have markedly reduced iron stores, making them more prone to developing iron deficiency anemia.

Diagnosis

Iron deficiency anemia is determined via patient history, complete blood count, and evaluation of the peripheral blood smear. Hematologic indices of anemia can be found in Table 5-8. Classic signs of iron deficiency anemia include the presence of microcytic and hypochromic RBCs that have a **mean corpuscular volume** (MCV) that is < 80 fL; however, these may not be observed in all instances. Additionally, serum iron concentrations are < 60 mcg/dL in mildly anemic individuals and < 40 mcg/dL in severely anemic individuals.

Plasma ferritin concentrations of < 20 ng/mL are particularly useful for identifying a reduction of iron stores. Aggregated ferritin stores in bone marrow are depleted or absent when iron deficiency anemia becomes clinically evident. Other indicators that may aid in confirming iron deficiency include reduced concentrations of circulating RBCs, reticulocytes, and hemoglobin. Transferrin concentration, as measured through serum **total iron-binding capacity** (TIBC) is increased (> 350 mcg/dL) while the saturation of transferrin is decreased (< 15%). In most instances, analysis of serum ferritin concentrations negates the need for bone marrow testing. During pregnancy and with oral contraceptive use, serum transferrin concentrations may be elevated in the absence of anemia.

Symptomatically, individuals suffering from significant iron deficiency anemia may display weakness, listlessness, and fatigue due to decreased oxygen carrying capacity. An initial trial dose of iron therapy given to the putatively diagnosed individual can serve to verify the diagnosis, improve symptoms, and confirm the anticipated treatment approach. If successful, an increased percentage of reticulocytes will be observed within 1 week of initiation of iron therapy and hemoglobin content will increase 2–4 g/dL within 1 month of the beginning of treatment.

Guidelines for Treating Iron Deficiency Anemia

It is important to identify the cause of iron deficiency in an individual to assure sustained and adequate treatment. In each case, treatment is intended to increase production of hemoglobin and RBCs. A test dose of oral iron may be used to empirically determine response because oral formulations of iron are inexpensive, efficacious, and generally quite safe.

Iron deficiency anemia is particularly prevalent during pregnancy, and the United States Preventive Services Task Force recommends universal routine screening during pregnancy. Women who are clinically anemic have a twofold-threefold increased risk for preterm delivery and infant mortality.[2,4]

Following the initiation of successful therapy, it is expected that the number of circulating reticulocytes will begin to increase within 4–7 days of initiated iron therapy and the hematocrit should increase after 1 week. Treatment should continue until hemoglobin levels become normal, which may take 1–2 months. Treatment may continue for 4–6 months to replace ferritin stores; however, dietary adjustments alone often suffice. For this reason, treatment is commonly discontinued once the hemoglobin concentration and anemia are corrected.

Preparations of Iron for Treating Iron Deficiency Anemia

Iron is available in both oral and parenteral preparations. Oral preparations are safer, less expensive, and equally effective as parenteral preparations, making the oral formulations overwhelmingly preferred. The three orally administered iron salts, ferrous sulfate, ferrous gluconate, and ferrous fumarate, are efficacious and well tolerated. Detailed information on oral formulations of iron can be found in Chapter 5 in Table 5-9.

The three parenteral iron preparations, iron dextran, ferric gluconate, and iron sucrose, are generally limited for use by individuals who are either unable to absorb sufficient quantities of orally administered iron or who cannot tolerate the gastrointestinal-associated side effects of oral iron therapy.

The recommended dose of oral iron for treating iron deficiency anemia in adults is 50–60 mg of elemental iron per day or in 2–4 divided doses. This is equivalent to one 300 mg tablet of ferrous sulfate taken once daily. Due to the relatively limited intestinal absorption of orally administered iron, divided dosing is required. The amount of elemental iron present in oral iron preparations varies from approximately 10% to 33% and must be factored when calculating the dose. Table 5-9 lists the amount of elemental iron and recommended dosing for each of the three iron salts that are available.

Food decreases intestinal iron absorption by 50% and iron is best absorbed in an acidic environment. Therefore, the iron tablet should be taken between meals, and many recommend taking 250 mg of ascorbic acid (vitamin C) with the iron to enhance absorption. Because iron is absorbed in the proximal portion of the small intestine, enteric-coated formulations do not supply the iron needed and should be avoided. Failure to respond to oral iron therapy may be due to malabsorption or continued blood loss, both of which are indicative of the need for further evaluation. Additional information about iron toxicity and drug–drug interactions can be found in Chapter 16.

Side Effects/Adverse Effects

The most common side effects of oral iron therapy are gastrointestinal complaints including nausea, epigastric distress, and constipation. All three of the iron salts on the market produce these gastrointestinal side effects. The reported side effects of oral iron therapy correlate to the concentration of elemental iron ingested. As such, equipotent doses of oral iron therapy should have the same degree of side effects. Patient education is important when prescribing oral iron therapy. Antacids decrease iron absorption significantly and should not be used to treat iron-related gastrointestinal symptoms.

Parenteral Preparations of Iron

The three parenteral preparations of iron are iron dextran (Dexferrum, INFeD), which has 50 mg of elemental iron/mL; ferric gluconate (Ferrlecit), which has 12.5 mg iron/mL; and iron sucrose (Venofer), which has 20 mg of iron/mL. Parenteral iron preparations are generally limited to use in individuals who are unable to absorb sufficient quantities of orally administered iron or cannot tolerate the gastrointestinal side effects of oral iron therapy (Table 16-2). For example, persons with celiac disease have limited oral iron absorption and may not obtain therapeutic levels with oral therapy. Persons being treated for peptic ulcers, inflammatory bowel disease, enteritis, or ulcerative colitis may benefit from parenteral iron therapy as it will not exacerbate their preexisting condition or cause additional gastrointestinal side effects. Parenteral therapy is commonly used for individuals undergoing cancer chemotherapy or hemodialysis. In individuals undergoing hemodialysis, intravenously administered iron is required to maximize RBC synthesis stimulated by coadministered erythropoietin (Procrit, Epogen).

Iron dextran (Dexferrum, INFeD) can be administered intramuscularly. Ferric gluconate (Ferrlecit) and iron sucrose (Venofer) are approved for intravenous use. Both ferric gluconate complex and iron sucrose have significantly less incidence of anaphylaxis and life-threatening adverse drug events than the low molecular weight dextran-containing iron formulation. For ferric gluconate, ferric sucrose, and dextran the incidence of adverse effects are 0.9, 0.6, and 3.3 per million doses, respectively.[5,6]

Iron Dextran (Dexferrum, INFeD)

Iron dextran (Dexferrum, INFeD) contains ferric hydroxide complexed to glucose polymers. Iron dextran is available in formulations containing high molecular weight dextran (Dexferrum) and low molecular weight dextran (INFeD). Iron dextran is commonly formulated in 1-mL and 2-mL single-dose vials containing 50 mg/mL elemental iron. For each administration of iron dextran, a 25-mg test dose is given over 30 seconds or 5 minutes depending on formulation and followed by an observation period of up to 60 minutes. If no allergic reaction occurs after the test dose, the remaining dose may be administered. The total dose required for restoration of hemoglobin and body stores of iron can be calculated using the equation listed in Table 16-2.

When given intramuscularly, iron dextran must be given via the Z-track method so discoloration at the injection site

Table 16-2 Parenteral Iron Formulations

Drug Generic (Brand)	Formulations	Dose	Clinical Considerations	FDA Pregnancy Category
Iron dextran (INFeD, Dexferrum)*	Injection: 50 mg elemental iron/mL (2 mL)	IM (Z-track technique) or slow IV bolus. Test dose: 25 mg over 30 seconds (INFeD) or 5 min (Dexferrum). Observe up to 60 min prior to administration of remaining dose. Dose (mL) = 0.0442 (desired Hgb − observed Hgb) × LBW + (0.26 × LBW).	Contraindications: Hypersensitivity to iron dextran; any anemia not associated with iron deficiency. IV route preferred (vs. IM) because of decreased risk of anaphylaxis. Low MW dextran shown to have fewer serious adverse drug events than high MW dextran.	C
Ferric gluconate (Ferrlecit)	Injection: 12.5 mg elemental iron/mL (5 mL)	IV: 125 mg elemental iron infused over at least 10 min. Typically 1 g of elemental iron over 8 consecutive dialysis treatments. Test dose: 25 mg elemental iron infused over 60 min.	Contraindications: Hypersensitivity to ferric gluconate; any anemia not associated with iron deficiency; iron overload. Adverse effects: Flushing/hypotension; may augment hemodialysis-induced hypotension.	B
Iron sucrose (Venofer)	Injection: 20 mg elemental iron/mL (5 mL, 10 mL)	IV: 100 mg infused over 5 min or diluted in up to 100 mL 0.9% saline and infused over 15 min. Typically 1 g of elemental iron over 10 consecutive dialysis treatments.	Contraindications: Hypersensitivity to iron sucrose; any anemia not associated with iron deficiency. Adverse effects: Hypotension has been reported frequently.	B

LBW = lean body weight in kg; MW = molecular weight.
* INFed is low molecular weight and Dexferrum is high molecular weight.

does not occur. The Z-track intramuscular injection can be quite painful. Mobilization of iron from intramuscular sites is slow.

Side Effects/Adverse Effects

Pain and localized discoloration at the injection site are the most common reported side effects. Headache, fever, and arthralgia can also occur. The most serious and potentially fatal side effect of iron dextran is anaphylaxis. Anaphylactic reactions occur in < 5% of individuals due to its polymerized glucose (dextran) component. The low molecular weight dextran formulations have demonstrated a threefold lower incidence of serious toxicity (11.3 versus 3.3 life-threatening adverse drug events per mission doses).[5] Iron dextran requires first administering a test dose to ensure no allergic reactions develop. Epinephrine and respiratory support should be available in anticipation of an adverse drug event. Following iron dextran therapy, the individual should be educated about the signs of an allergic reaction and told to contact a healthcare provider if rash, dizziness, or respiratory distress occurs.

Ferric Gluconate Complex (Ferrlecit) and Iron Sucrose (Venofer)

Ferric gluconate (Ferrlecit) and iron sucrose (Venofer) are only approved for intravenous administration for the treatment of iron deficiency for individuals undergoing chronic hemodialysis. These medications are administered in conjunction with erythropoietin to maximize RBC production. Both parenteral iron preparations lack significant risk of producing anaphylaxis.

Ferric gluconate is commonly formulated in 5-mL ampules containing 62.5 mg elemental iron per mL. The standard dose is 125 mg elemental iron infused slowly (over 10 minutes) to decrease side effects. Prior to the initial round of treatment, a 25-mg (2 mL) test dose is administered, infused over 60 minutes.

Iron sucrose (Venofer) has been used in Europe for more than 4 decades. Anaphylaxis has not been commonly observed with iron sucrose, and no test dose is required prior to the initial round of therapy. The drug is administered intravenously directly into a dialysis line at an infusion rate of 100 mg infused over 5 minutes or diluted in up to 100 mL 0.9% saline and infused over 15 minutes. The typical duration of therapy is 1 administration during each of 10 consecutive hemodialysis sessions, providing a total of 1000 mg elemental iron. The injections may cause flushing and hypotension as well as general malaise, weakness, and localized pain.

Macrocytic Anemia: Folate Deficiency

The cause of folate (folic acid) deficiency anemia primarily involves inadequate ingestion, absorption, or storage of dietary folic acid. Folate deficiency, which causes megaloblastic anemia, can be found during pregnancy, in the elderly, among individuals who are alcoholics, or as an adverse drug reaction. Anticonvulsants, phenytoin (Dilantin) and phenobarbital (Luminal) interfere with absorption and/or metabolism of folate. Additional drug–drug interactions associated with folic acid are listed in Table 5-3.

Grains in the United States are fortified with folate, and green vegetables are also a good source of the nutrient. Folate is absorbed in the small intestine and stored in the liver, where it undergoes enterohepatic recirculation. In contrast to iron, which is heavily recycled, the body requires daily replacement of folate. Folate deficiency develops within weeks if the nutrient is not replaced.

The results of folate deficiency include anemia, damage to rapidly dividing cells in the oral and gastrointestinal mucosa, and other blood cell lineages. Folate deficiency anemia is classically diagnosed via the presence of megaloblastic macrocytic anemia coupled with decreased blood levels of folate, normal vitamin B_{12} blood levels, and a normal reticulocyte count. Serum folate concentrations serve as an initial screening test; however, the recent ingestion of a dietary supplement or folate-rich meal, for example, will result in a normal serum folate concentration in an individual with folic acid deficiency. RBC folate concentration provides a time-averaged indicator of folate bioavailability, but is a more expensive test and it, too, has some problems with interpretation. Serum folate concentrations are used as a screen and when the serum folate level < 2 ng/mL are suggestive of the nutrient deficiency.

Deficiencies of either folate and/or vitamin B_{12} can result in the production of significant quantities of macrocytes (RBC mean corpuscular volume > 100 fL). Therefore, it is important to distinguish which nutrient deficit is present in order to provide the appropriate treatment approach. Excessive folic acid ingestion can correct the macrocytic anemia but does not correct the underlying pathology of vitamin B_{12} deficiency, which is described in the next section.

Folate is used prophylactically to prevent folic acid-deficient megaloblastic anemias and used therapeutically to treat folic acid deficiency and for the initial stages of treatment for severe vitamin B_{12}-deficient megaloblastic anemias. Folic acid is very well tolerated by the body and has minimal adverse effects, even if taken at supertherapeutic doses.

The most common indications for prophylactic treatment are pregnancy and lactation. In early pregnancy, folate deficiency increases the risk of neural tube defects in a developing fetus, and folic acid supplementation decreases the risk of neural tube defects by approximately 36% in women who do not have an increased risk for neural tube defects. In 1992, the Centers for Disease Control and Prevention recommended that all women of childbearing age take a folic acid supplement of 400 mcg/day via ingestion of fortified foods or supplements and that a 400 mcg/day supplement be continued during the first trimester of pregnancy.[7]

Pharmacotherapeutic doses of folic acid are most commonly administered orally and are readily absorbed (Table 16-3). For individuals with diagnosed folic acid deficiency anemia or who have impaired folate absorption, a dose of 1–2 mg/day of an oral supplement is sufficient to force absorption and stimulate erythropoiesis. Replacement therapy should continue for 4 months.

In the case of severe folic acid deficiency anemia, treatment may include intramuscular injections of both folate and vitamin B_{12}, followed by subsequent doses of oral folic acid alone (1–2 mg/day for 1–2 weeks, followed by 400 mcg/day maintenance doses). Megaloblasts will dissipate from the bone marrow after 48 hours of treatment, reticulocyte levels will increase after 2–3 days, and RBCs and hemoglobin concentrations will increase to normal levels within 2–6 weeks.

Macrocytic Anemia: Vitamin B_{12} Deficiency

Vitamin B_{12} is an essential vitamin also known as cobalamin, a name referencing its molecular structure, which is coordinated by an atom of cobalt. As with folic acid deficiency, severe vitamin B_{12} deficiency presents as megaloblastic macrocytic anemia. Vitamin B_{12} deficiency causes neuropsychiatric disorders as well as macrocytic anemia and can be caused by impaired gastrointestinal absorption of the vitamin from regional enteritis, celiac disease, decreased gastric acid secretion, aging, or a lack of intrinsic factor. There may be insufficient intrinsic factor present or the intrinsic factor-vitamin B_{12} complex cannot be absorbed. Individuals with atrophic gastritis, for example, have

Table 16-3 Folic Acid and Vitamin B_{12} Formulations

Drug Generic (Brand)	Formulations	Indication/Dose	Clinical Considerations	FDA Pregnancy Category
Folic acid (Folacin-800)	Tablet: 0.4, 0.8, 1 mg Injection: 5 mg/mL (10 mL)	Usual: 0.4 mg/day. Pregnancy/lactating: 400 mcg/day.*	Contraindications: Hypersensitivity to folic acid Not appropriate for anemias other than megaloblastic/macrocytic anemia, vitamin B_{12} deficiency, uncorrected pernicious anemia.	A
Leucovorin calcium (Wellcovorin)	Tablet: 5, 10, 15, 25 mg Injection: 50, 100, 200, 350 mg powder; 10 mg/mL (50 mL)	For folate deficient megaloblastic anemia. IM: Up to 1 mg/day.	Contraindications: Hypersensitivity to folic acid. Only for use if not responsive to folate; much more expensive than folate.	C
Cyanocobalamin (Twelve Resin-K, Nascobal, CaloMist)	Tablet/lozenge: Multiple formulations. Injection: 1000 mcg/mL. Nasal spray: 500 mcg/ actuation (Nascobal) 25 mcg/actuation (CaloMist)	*For cobalamin deficiency:* PO: 250 mcg/day. Intranasal: 500 mcg in one nostril once weekly. 25 mcg in each nostril daily to twice daily (following correction of deficiency). IM/SQ: 30 mcg/day for 5–10 days; maintenance 100–200 mcg/month. *Pernicious anemia:* PO: 1000–2000 mcg/day. IM/deep SQ: 1000 mcg/day for 1 week, then 1000 mcg/week for 4 weeks, then 1000 mcg/month. Intranasal: 500 mcg in one nostril weekly.	Contraindications: Hypersensitivity to cyanocobalamin or any component of formulation. Avoid IV administration: anaphylaxis can occur. Test dose is recommended for patients suspected of cyanocobalamin sensitivity prior to administration. IM/SQ/PO routes are used for treatment; oral and intranasal administration are used after hematologic remission and no signs of nervous system involvement. Administer nasal sprays at least 1 h before or after ingestion of hot foods/liquids.	C

* Recommended dose for women with a history of neural tube defects is 4 mg per day for 4 months prior to pregnancy and during the first 4 months of pregnancy.

decreased intrinsic factor secretion. **Pernicious anemia** is the term for anemia resulting from impaired vitamin B$_{12}$ absorption secondary to a lack of intrinsic factor. In contrast to folic acid deficiency, it can take months to years of impaired vitamin B$_{12}$ absorption before the deficiency is detected clinically because there are robust body stores of vitamin B$_{12}$.

Most vitamin B$_{12}$ is localized in the liver and the total body store of this vitamin is approximately 2–5 mg. Estimated daily requirements of the nutrient are 2.4–2.8 mcg/day for adults. Vitamin B$_{12}$ excretion is small (2–3 mcg/day) relative to normal body stores. The nutrient is only obtained from meat and dairy products, and 10–30% of adults > 50 years of age are unable to absorb sufficient quantities of vitamin B$_{12}$ through diet and require supplements of vitamin B$_{12}$-fortified foods or vitamins.[6,7]

The anemia associated with vitamin B$_{12}$ deficiency occurs because vitamin B$_{12}$ is an essential step in activating folic acid, which is required for RBC production. In addition to anemia, vitamin B$_{12}$ deficiency can lead to neurologic damage (e.g., paresthesias and cognitive impairment, possibly due to myelin synthesis). The vitamin B$_{12}$-associated neurologic effects are not observed in persons with folic acid deficiency and are unrelated to RBC production. Vitamin B$_{12}$-associated neurologic damage may take longer to correct than vitamin B$_{12}$ deficiency anemia and may be irreversible if not treated within 2–6 months of developing symptoms. High doses of folate can successfully treat the hematologic consequences of vitamin B$_{12}$ deficiency; however, folate will not resolve the neurologic effects. Plasma vitamin B$_{12}$ levels should be measured every 3–6 months following the start of replacement therapy.

Vitamin B$_{12}$ deficiency is diagnosed when the diagnostic evaluation reveals megaloblastic macrocytic anemia coupled with decreased blood levels of vitamin B$_{12}$ and normal folate levels. Serum concentrations of vitamin B$_{12}$ that are < 200 pg/mL are consistent with vitamin B$_{12}$ deficiency (normal concentration > 300 pg/mL). The classic assay for demonstrating vitamin B$_{12}$ malabsorption is the Schilling test. The individual is first given radiolabeled vitamin B$_{12}$ and an intramuscular injection of unlabeled vitamin B$_{12}$ at the same time. The unlabeled vitamin B$_{12}$ saturates the tissues and therefore the radiolabeled vitamin B$_{12}$ is excreted in the urine and measured. Interestingly, this test actually partially treats the disorder at the same time it tests for it. Although still available in some locations, use of the Schilling test has substantially dissipated in recent years and been replaced with tests measuring homocysteine and methylmalonic acid. Serum concentrations of homocysteine and methylmalonic acid are increased in individuals with vitamin B$_{12}$ deficiency (96% and 98%, respectively), whereas homocysteine levels but not methylmalonic acid levels are increased in folic acid deficiency (91% and 12%, respectively)[8] (Box 16-1).

Box 16-1 Why Is JL So Tired?

JL is a 22-year-old college student who comes into the school healthcare clinic because she is always tired and unable to keep up with her schoolwork. In taking JL's history, the clinician learns that JL has been a vegetarian for several years and is now following a vegan diet. She does not eat any dairy products. Her menses are regular and she has very light bleeding.

JL's physical examination is normal. She does not have any symptoms of viral or infectious disease. She does not have any neurologic symptoms of vitamin B$_{12}$ deficiency. The clinician suspects JL may be anemic and queries her further about her diet. JL is working and going to school simultaneously. She has relied on cooked beans/burritos and pasta because they are quick and easy to prepare, and she says she has not been hungry recently. The clinician orders a complete blood count (CBC) with differential, ferritin level, homocysteine, and methylmalonic acid level. She arranges for JL to return in a week to review the results.

JL's CBC reveals a macrocytic anemia with a normal folate level and high homocystine level, which results in a presumptive diagnosis of vitamin B$_{12}$ and/or folate deficiency. Folate is fortified in grains and would be present in pasta so the clinician suspects the source of this anemia is vitamin B$_{12}$ deficiency. The clinician reviews dietary sources of these vitamins. She tells JL how to obtain folate in green, leafy vegetables. Because vitamin B$_{12}$ is highly bioavailable in dairy products, she explores the idea of eating dairy products and JL agrees to consider it. The clinician gives JL a vitamin supplement that contains both vitamin B$_{12}$ and folate. She tells JL that it can take a few months for the anemia to resolve and arranges for a follow-up visit in 1 month.

Cyanocobalamin (Cyanoject), a crystalline form of vitamin B_{12}, is the drug of choice for treating all forms of vitamin B_{12} deficiency. Intramuscular injections are able to treat all forms of vitamin B_{12} deficiency and do not require dose adjustments for individuals who have impaired vitamin B_{12} absorption. Following the return to normal RBC and hemoglobin concentrations, monthly injections may be continued until the underlying deficiency is corrected. The injections may cause mild pain at the injection site. For pernicious anemia, cyanocobalamin is most commonly administered 1000 mcg/day intramuscularly for 1 week, followed by 1000 mcg per week for 4 weeks, followed by 1000 mcg every month for life.

Other formulations include oral tablets and an intranasal spray solution. A low-efficiency transporter system that does not rely on intrinsic factor facilitates absorption of high doses (1000–2000 mcg per day) of orally administered cyanocobalamin, even in the absence of intrinsic factor. While previous cyanocobalamin treatment regimens required substantially lower (e.g., 100 mcg) doses of the nutrient, the higher dose is well tolerated, nontoxic, and beneficial for addressing neurologic effects of vitamin B_{12} deficiency.[8] As a result, high-dose oral administration may replace intramuscular injections as the vitamin B_{12} formulation of choice.[9] Intranasal cyanocobalamin is available as a metered dose inhaler and releases 500 mcg of a cyanocobalamin per actuation. The solution should be used only after initial therapy with oral tablets or intramuscular injections fail, and the solution should not be used by an individual experiencing rhinitis or nasal blockage. The intranasal preparation has not been tested for improvement of neurologic symptoms following severe vitamin B_{12} deficiency.

While moderate vitamin B_{12} deficiency results primarily in impaired RBC production, severe vitamin B_{12} deficiency may also lead to decreases in all blood cell lineages, including leukocytes and thrombocytes, which increases the risk for infection and bleeding, respectively. Treatment of severe vitamin B_{12} deficiency includes initial intramuscular injections of both vitamin B_{12} and folic acid. Folic acid hastens the recovery of hematopoiesis; however, it does not improve the neurologic damage caused by vitamin B_{12} deficiency; therefore, it is used as an adjunct.

The hematologic response to vitamin B_{12} drug therapy is typically rapid (< 48 hrs), with reticulocyte concentrations becoming elevated 3–4 days following the start of replacement therapy and hemoglobin and RBC levels returning to normal levels in 1–2 months. Neurologic impairments may improve more gradually over 6 months for treatment.

Hemorrhagic Anemia: Hemoglobinopathies: Sickle Cell Anemia and Thalassemias

The hemoglobinopathies are a diverse set of disorders that are the result of mutations of the genes that encode for the globin chains within the hemoglobin molecule. The two categories of hemoglobinopathies are sickle cell disorders and thalassemias. Persons who are heterozygous with one gene that codes for an abnormal globin chain are usually asymptomatic and not anemic. Conversely, persons who have homozygous genes for the aberrant globin chain have profound anemia and are primarily cared for by hematology specialists. Therefore, this family of disorders is reviewed briefly.

Sickle cell disease is composed of a group of conditions that are based on mutations of the beta globin. In homozygous sickle sell anemia, both beta globins are abnormal, and the result is a type of hemoglobin called HbS. This abnormal hemoglobin forms long polymer chains when deoxygenated, which causes the red blood cell to be rigid and shaped like a sickle. The rigid elongated cells occlude the vasculature, which causes a vasoocclusive crisis typified by ischemia, pain, and ultimately organ damage. These sickle red blood cells are more easily destroyed than are regular red blood cells, which is why sickle cell disease causes a hemolytic anemia.

Historically the primary treatment for sickle cell vasoocclusive crises has been liberal use of opioids to decrease pain. As the molecular mechanisms that underlie function of sickle red blood cells become more apparent, new and novel pharmacotherapeutic treatments are being investigated. At this time, the FDA has approved use of hydroxyurea (Hydrea), which increases the production of another type of hemoglobin, fetal hemoglobin (Hbf). Fetal hemoglobin has two alpha-globin chains and two gamma-globin chains, and this type of hemoglobin does not form polymer chains.[10] Hydroxyurea significantly decreases the incidence of vasoocclusive crises and need for blood transfusions in persons with sickle cell disease.[10]

Thalassemias are conditions that result from reduced or no production of one of the globin chains. Reduction of the alpha chains causes alpha thalassemia, and reduction in the beta chains causes beta thalassemia. Persons with beta thalassemia (Cooley's anemia) are dependent on transfusions for survival. Frequent blood transfusions can result in iron overload, and then iron chelation is necessary to remove excess iron.[11]

Alpha thalassemia is usually a milder form of thalassemia. There are four genes that encode for the alphaglobin chain. No alpha globin is made in the most serious form of the disease wherein all four genes are inactive, and the resulting hemoglobin is called Bart's hemoglobin. This is a fatal condition that causes hydrops fetalis and intrauterine demise. When three of the four genes are inactive, the individual will have moderate anemia that is periodically severe and treated with transfusions. Iron overload is the expected complication and it is treated with iron chelation. Iron chelation is accomplished with desferrioxamine (Desferal). Desferrioxamine is administered intravenously or subcutaneously. The most common side effect of desferrioxamine is irritation at the site of administration, but it can rarely cause high frequency hearing loss, allergic reactions, or decreased night vision.

Aplastic Anemia

Aplastic anemia occurs when the bone marrow does not produce enough new cells to replace red blood cells in the circulation. Aplastic anemia can develop secondary to an autoimmune process, exposure to radiation or chemotherapy, or more rarely, it can be caused by drugs. Interestingly, Marie Curie died of aplastic anemia that probably developed following her exposure to radiation. A detailed discussion of aplastic anemia is beyond the scope of this chapter; however the drugs that can cause this disorder include chloramphenicol (Chloromycetin), antiepileptic drugs, nonsteroidal anti-inflammatory drugs, sulfonamides, quinine, gold, ticlopidine (Ticlid), and arsenicals.[12]

Coagulation Disorders

Coagulation disorders include disorders that predispose the individual to hemorrhage or to thrombosis and some that predispose to both hemorrhage and thrombosis.

Bleeding disorders include the hemophilias and von Willebrand disease. The most common disease that causes bleeding is von Willebrand disease. Hemophilias are a group of genetic disorders that are primarily evident in males.

Thrombophilias cause clotting. Thrombophilias can be inherited or acquired. Approximately 5–8% of the population in the United States has a genetic thrombophilia, yet most persons never have any problems with clotting until an additional risk factor is present. Several coagulation disorders are accentuated by the use of oral contraceptives and pregnancy, which is why women are more likely to experience venous thromboembolism during childbearing years than are men of comparable ages.[13] Common thrombophilias in women include deep vein thrombosis (DVT), stroke, and pulmonary embolism (pulmonary embolism). Less common etiologies include inherited disorders such as factor V Leiden, protein C deficiency or protein S deficiency, and acquired disorders such as antiphospholipid antibody syndrome. Overall, the incidence of thromboembolism increases with age and is usually considered a disease of older ages.[13]

Drugs used to treat coagulation disorders include **anticoagulants**, **antiplatelet drugs**, and **thrombolytic drugs**. Anticoagulants are indicated for acute or prophylactic treatment for thrombosis. Examples of anticoagulants include activators of antithrombin (e.g., heparin) and the oral anticoagulant warfarin (Coumadin). Antiplatelet drugs are regularly used for treating arterial thrombi. Aspirin and adenosine diphosphate (ADP) receptor antagonists such as clopidogrel (Plavix) are examples of antiplatelet medications. Thrombolytics, such as streptokinase (Streptase) and tissue plasminogen activator (tPA), are used to dissolve preexisting clots. A brief review of hemostasis is in order.

Hemostasis

Hemostasis is achieved through the formation of a platelet plug that is subsequently strengthened by the recruitment and activation of fibrin. Historically, the coagulation process was described as a cascade of events that occurred in two pathways. Coagulation initiated via the **intrinsic pathway** used coagulation factors present in blood, and coagulation initiated via the **extrinsic pathway** started after exposure to tissue factor from the cells just outside the endothelial cells that line the vasculature. These two "waterfall" cascades converge into a common pathway that results in the generation of a fibrin clot.[14] Today it is clear that the pathways are linked from the outset and rather than a focus on two cascade-type pathways, coagulation is reframed as a process with four distinct phases.[15]

First is the initiation phase, wherein two events occur. Tissue factor, a lipoprotein that is constitutively expressed on the cell membrane of cells is not usually exposed to plasma. When tissue factor is exposed to plasma via injury or damage to the endothelial cell lining of the vasculature, it binds to factor VII$_a$ (the subscript *a* means this factor is activated, and there is always a small amount of activated factor VII in plasma). Other coagulation factors are then activated and the result is the production of **thrombin**. This process is referred to as the **tissue factor pathway**. Four of the coagulation factors involved in the production of thrombin—factors VII, IX, X, and prothrombin—require vitamin K for their biosynthesis. Inhibition of vitamin K decreases serum concentration of these factors, which inhibits coagulation.

Thrombin is also the final product of the **contact activation pathway**. In this set of steps, several coagulation factors enzymatically react after coming in contact with exposed collagen from the subendothelial tissue. This process was originally characterized as the intrinsic pathway but is now referred to as the contact activation pathway. Although both pathways exist, the tissue factor pathway is the primary pathway that initiates coagulation and the formation of blood clots. The contact-activation pathway is slower than the tissue-factor pathway.

The second part of the initiation phase involves platelets. When endothelial cells are damaged, platelets aggregate in response to the presence of exposed collagen from the endothelial cells. Glycoprotein II$_b$/III$_a$ (GP II$_b$/III$_a$), a receptor on the cell membrane of the platelet, is activated. Once activated, GP II$_b$/III$_a$ undergoes a conformational change and joins with other GP II$_b$/III$_a$ receptors to form a heterodimer (Figure 16-1). This heterodimer

binds to fibrinogen, which is present in plasma and forms cross-links with other platelets in the area that have activated GP II$_b$/III$_a$ receptors on their extracellular surface. At this point, von Willebrand factor, a large glycoprotein that is constitutively produced in endothelial cells, joins the show and further strengthens the bonds by forming links between the GP II$_b$/III$_a$ receptors and collagen from the endothelial cell. The adhesion activates the platelets.[16]

There are polymorphisms in the GP II$_b$/III$_a$ receptor. It appears that estrogen may have more of a platelet aggregation effect in women with certain polymorphisms of this receptor. This might explain why hormone therapy increased the incidence of cardiovascular events in women who took nonphysiologic doses of estrogen in the recent randomized trials of estrogen therapy for postmenopausal symptoms.[17]

The second phase of coagulation is the amplification phase and formation of the loose platelet plug. Thrombin plays a central role in setting the stage for phase three by activating the platelets that are present. The activated platelets expose receptors and binding sites, and they release granules that contain ADP and thromboxane A$_2$, which signals additional platelet activation and increased clotting. This becomes a positive feedback mechanism that propagates the process. The platelets change shape to accommodate the formation of the plug. Thrombin also activates additional coagulation factors on the surface of these activated platelets, which prepares their surfaces to become the factory for stage three. Interestingly, thrombin also initiates the processes (phase four of the coagulation process) that create the chemicals that slow and stop the clot process, specifically activation of protein C and protein S.

Phase three of the coagulation process is the propagation phase in which a large burst of thrombin that alters fibrinogen into fibrin stabilizes and creates the actual blood clot.[18]

Finally, the fibrinolytic system, which thrombin originally initiated in phase two, matures, and the fourth phase of fibrinolysis can occur. There are three types of natural anticoagulants that come into play during the final phase of the coagulation process. Antithrombin inhibits the following five of the activated clotting factors: IX$_a$, X$_a$, XI$_a$, XII$_a$, and thrombin. Inhibition of factor X$_a$ and thrombin are especially important because inhibition of these two coagulation factors stops the acceleration of clotting that is initiated from either the tissue factor pathway or the contact-platelet process. The consequence of

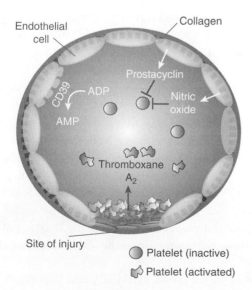

Figure 16-1 Formation of platelet plug.

antithrombin activity is that fibrinogen is prevented from being converted into fibrin, which is thus unable to extenuate clotting. Antithrombin is unable to disrupt fibrin that has already polymerized, and is thus ineffective at removing a clot that has already formed. Plasmin is an enzyme normally present in the blood in the inactive precursor form of plasminogen. Once converted from plasminogen, plasmin is able to digest fibrin polymers and dissolve fully formed blood clots once tissue repair has concluded. The third players, protein C and protein S, which inhibit two of the coagulation factors, are both dependent on vitamin K for their synthesis.

Thrombosis and Thrombocytic Structures

A **thrombus** is a pathogenic blood clot that adheres to the wall of a blood vessel or the heart and prevents blood flow. Venous **thrombosis** and arterial thrombosis differ in etiology and clinical presentation. While an arterial thrombus most commonly causes localized tissue injury at the site of formation, a venous thrombus typically causes harm at a remote location in the vasculature.

In the formation of an arterial thrombosis, an atherosclerotic plaque or other damage to the arterial wall leads to platelet recruitment and platelet adhesion at the site of injury. Platelet adhesion causes the cellular release of ADP and thromboxane A_2 into the blood and activation of additional platelets. As the number of thrombocytes increases, the size of the platelet plug expands and the blockage of the artery increases. Impaired blood transport activates the coagulation process and reinforcement of the platelet plug with a fibrin meshwork. The thrombus prevents blood flow and downstream tissue perfusion, resulting in localized tissue injury.

The classic factors to which venous thrombus formation is attributed are referred to as **Virchow's triad**, which includes venous stasis, damage to epithelium, and hypercoagulation. An arterial thrombosis most commonly develops secondary to formation of an atherosclerotic plaque or other damage to an arterial wall. A venous thrombosis originates as a result of slow moving or stagnant blood flow leading the activation of the coagulation cascade and formation of fibrin. The morphology of a venous thrombus is different from its arterial counterpart. Venous thrombi typically possess long tails of accumulated platelets and RBCs. The tail of the venous clot may detach and travel through the vasculature to a distant site, resulting in an **embolism**, which is referred to as **thromboembolism**.

Deep Vein Thrombosis, Pulmonary Embolism, and Ischemic Stroke

The two most common and life-threatening manifestations of venous thromboembolism are deep vein thrombosis (DVT) and pulmonary embolism (pulmonary embolism). DVT is a disorder in which a thrombus is localized to the iliac or femoral vein. Pulmonary embolism is an obstruction of the pulmonary artery or one of its branches, most commonly caused by a blood clot originating in a lower limb, and is fatal in 10–15% of affected individuals. An ischemic stroke results from occlusion of a vessel by a thrombus or embolus resulting in impaired perfusion to a region of the brain.

Significant risk factors for thromboembolic disorders include coronary and peripheral artery disease, major surgery, immobility, malignancy, atrial fibrillation and other cardiovascular diseases, prosthetic heart valve replacement, smoking, and advanced age.[19] Venous thromboembolism occurs in both hospitalized patients and ambulatory individuals. It is the major cause or contributing factor in > 10% of reported hospital deaths. Prophylactic therapy for pulmonary embolism has been shown to substantially improve clinical outcomes of individuals with symptomatic DVT.[20] The most commonly employed venous thrombosis prophylactic therapies include administration of a parenteral or oral anticoagulant.[21]

Venous Thromboembolism and Women's Health

Of particular note for women, long-term hormone replacement therapy, pregnancy, and oral contraceptive use are all correlated with an increased incidence of thrombosis and subsequent pathologies. The increased risk of thrombosis during pregnancy results in increased venous thromboembolism most often observed during the early postpartum period.[22] It may be attributed to impaired venous return by the uterus or the presence of the hypercoagulable state associated with pregnancy and delivery. Pregnant women who have an inherited thrombophilia (e.g., mutations in protein C signaling or heterozygosity for the factor V gene Leiden mutation) are at an even greater risk for thrombosis.[23] The risks of developing a venous thromboembolism during delivery are threefold to fivefold greater when the birth occurs via cesarean delivery when compared to vaginal birth.[24] The Royal College of Obstetricians and Gynaecologists[25] and the American College of Chest Physicians[26] have both developed expert opinion-based treatment guidelines for venous thromboembolism prophylaxis during pregnancy. Women at high risk for DVT and pulmonary embolism (e.g., inherited thrombophilia or previous idiopathic venous thromboembolism event) should be considered candidates for being treated antepartum for thromboembolism prophylaxis.

Estrogen-progestin oral contraceptives are the most common cause of thrombosis in young adult women.[27] In a 2008 study, women smokers on oral contraceptives had an 8.8 times higher risk (95% CI, 5.7–13) for venous thrombosis when compared to nonsmoking women who did not use oral contraceptives.[28] The HERS and Women's Health Initiative (WHI) trials on hormone replacement therapy (HRT) indicate a twofold increase in venous thromboembolisms[29,30] (Chapter 34).

Parenteral Anticoagulants

Parenteral anticoagulants are used for prophylaxis and acute treatment of thrombosis, particularly venous thrombosis (Table 16-4). Antithrombin inhibitors include unfractionated heparin, multiple formulations of low molecular weight heparin, and fondaparinux (Arixtra). These drugs significantly increase the activity of antithrombin by forming a drug-antithrombin protein complex. As a result of

Table 16-4 Anticoagulants

Drug Generic (Brand)	Formulations	Indication/Dose	Clinical Considerations	FDA Pregnancy Category
Unfractionated heparin	Multiple injection and solution formulations ranging from 1 unit/mL to 20,000 unit/mL	*DVT prevention:* SQ: 5000 units every 8–12 hours *DVT/PE treatment:* IV: 80 units/kg IVP followed by infusion of 18 units/kg/h to maintain antifactor X_a levels 0.3–0.7 units/mL SQ: 17,500 units or 250 units/kg then 250 units/kg q 12 h to maintain antifactor X_a levels of 0.3–0.7 units/mL	Contraindications: Hypersensitivity to heparin or any component of the formulation; thrombocytopenia; uncontrolled active bleeding except when due to DIC; suspected intracranial hemorrhage. Heparin is supplied in a wide range of strengths. Fatal medication errors related to overdose have occurred. Initial bolus is weight based followed by infusion titrated based on aPTT or antifactor X_a determinations.	C
Low molecular weight heparins: Enoxaparin (Lovenox)	30 mg/0.3 mL 40 mg/0.4 mL 60 mg/0.6 mL 80 mg/0.8 mL 100 mg/mL 120 mg/0.8 mL 150 mg/mL 300 mg/3 mL (multiple-dose vial)	*DVT prophylaxis:* SQ: Dosing ranges from 30 mg q 12 h–q 24 h to 40 mg q 24 h dependent on type of surgery. Duration is usually for approximately 10 days postsurgery or until risk of DVT has diminished or patient is anticoagulated on warfarin. *DVT treatment:* SQ: 1 mg/kg/dose q 12 h or 1.5 mg/kg/dose q 24 h	Contraindications: Hypersensitivity to heparin or any component of the formulation, hypersensitivity to pork products, thrombocytopenia, major bleeding. FDA black box warning: Persons with recent or anticipated epidural or spinal anesthesia are at risk of spinal or epidural hematoma and subsequent paralysis. Adverse effects: Bleeding/hemorrhage most common. There are multiple dosing regimens for prophylaxis and treatment for each low molecular weight heparin. They are dependent on variables such as weight, age, type of surgery, overall risk, condition (i.e., pregnancy, cancer, etc.), renal function, and others.	B
Dalteparin (Fragmin)	Injection: 2500–5000 IU/0.2 mL 7500 IU/0.3 mL 10,000 IU/mL 12,500 IU/0.5 mL 15,000 IU/0.6 mL 18,000 IU/0.72 mL	*DVT treatment:* SQ: 200 units/kg daily in one to two divided doses		B
Tinzaparin (Innohep)	Injection: 20,000 IU/mL (2 mL)	*DVT prophylaxis:* SQ: 3400 units q 24 h for 5–10 days *DVT treatment:* SQ: 175 anti-X_a IU/kg q 24 h ≥ 6 days and until adequate anticoagulation with warfarin (INR ≥ 2 for 2 consecutive days)		B

(continues)

Table 16-4 Anticoagulants (*continued*)

Drug Generic (Brand)	Formulations	Indication/Dose	Clinical Considerations	FDA Pregnancy Category
Fondaparinux (Arixtra)	Injection: 2.5 mg/0.5 mL 5 mg/0.4 mL 7.5 mg/0.6 mL 10 mg/0.8 mL	*DVT prophylaxis:* SQ: 2.5 mg q 24 h; after homeostasis established, initial dose is given 6–8 hours after surgery, usual duration 5–9 days *DVT treatment:* SQ: < 50 kg: 5 mg q 24 h; 50–100 kg: 7.5 mg q 24 h; > 100 kg: 10 mg q 24 h Usual duration 5–10 days	Contraindications: Hypersensitivity to fondaparinux, hemophilia, leukemia with bleeding, peptic ulcer disease, hemorrhagic stroke, surgery, thrombocytopenic purpura, weight < 50 kg, severe renal disease. FDA black box warning: Patients with recent or anticipated epidural or spinal anesthesia are at risk of spinal or epidural hematoma and subsequent paralysis. Adverse effects: Bleeding/hemorrhage most common.	B
Oral Anticoagulant				
Warfarin (Coumadin)	Tablet: 1, 2, 2.5, 3, 4, 5, 6, 7.5, 10 mg Injection: 5 mg powder	*Thrombosis/embolism treatment/ prevention:* PO: usual 2.5–10 mg daily dose adjusted based on INR results; wide interpatient variability with dosing IV: 2–5 mg daily (IV form rarely used)	Contraindications: Hypersensitivity, hemophilia, leukemia with bleeding, peptic ulcer disease, thrombocytopenic purpura, hepatic disease (severe), malignant hypertension, subacute bacterial endocarditis, acute nephritis, blood dyscrasias, pregnancy, eclampsia, preeclampsia, and more; see drug reference. FDA black box warning: May cause major or fatal bleeding. Adverse effects: Bleeding/hemorrhage most common. Multiple drug–drug interactions.	X

DVT = deep vein thrombosis; INR = international normalized ration; DIC = disseminated intravascular coagulation; PTT = partial thromboplastin time.

complex formation and increased antithrombin activity, factor X_a is inhibited, thus preventing coagulation signaling and fibrin production from either the tissue factor or the contact pathway. Anticoagulants must be used with extreme caution by individuals predisposed to hemorrhage. Uncontrolled bleeding is the major side effect of all these medications and should be carefully monitored.

Unfractionated Heparin

Unfractionated heparin was first isolated from an extract of liver in 1916, but it was not available for clinical use until the 1930s. The process of synthesizing a pure form of heparin suitable for use in humans was devised by Dr. Charles Best, who applied the same techniques he used in his discovery of insulin. The first formulations of clinically usable insulin and heparin were both produced by the Canadian team from the University of Toronto.

Heparin is commonly used to prevent or treat DVT, pulmonary embolism, and atrial fibrillation with embolus. The drug prevents coagulation during surgical procedures requiring extracorporeal circulation, such as heart surgery and renal dialysis, and it is also used as an adjunct to thrombolytics following an acute myocardial infarction. Heparin is the preferred anticoagulant used during pregnancy when an emergent clotting disorder develops, including treatment of pulmonary embolism, stroke, or DVT.[26]

Heparin is a polysaccharide mixture consisting of molecules with molecular weights ranging from 3 to 30 kDa. Heparin is obtained from animal sources including swine and cattle. A five-sugar (pentasaccharide) sequence that forms the site of interaction between heparin and antithrombin is intermittently dispersed along the molecule. Its multiple negatively charged sugar moieties makes heparin a large, highly polar molecule that must be administered intravenously or subcutaneously. The size and polarity of heparin substantially prevent heparin from transferring across cellular membranes, including the placenta, and heparin is not detected in breast milk.

Heparin has no effect on existing clots; rather, it prevents formation of new thrombi. Under normal conditions, the plasma protein antithrombin forms complexes with thrombin (factor II_a), factor IX, and factor X. These complexes effectively block the ability of these factors to propagate the coagulation process. Unfractionated heparin forms a complex with antithrombin that vastly accelerates the rate that these reactions take place.

Heparin is metabolized in the liver and excreted through the kidneys. The drug has a half-life of 1.5 hours in individuals with normal liver and kidney function. The duration may increase severalfold if hepatotoxicity or nephrotoxicity is present. Heparin displays extensive plasma protein binding and pharmacologic use requires ongoing monitoring. The anticoagulant response to unfractionated heparin varies among individuals. The use of activated partial thromboplastin time (aPPT) is used commonly to verify heparin concentrations are within the desired therapeutic range and to ensure proper dosing.[31] A normal aPPT is 40 seconds, and a therapeutic dose of heparin elevates the aPPT to 60–80 seconds. The therapeutically desired aPPT ratio (i.e., ratio of normal aPPT to heparin-treated aPPT) is 1.5:2.5. Another approach to monitoring heparin levels is by obtaining antifactor X_a levels with a therapeutic range from 0.3–0.7 unit/mL. A standard low dose unfractionated heparin administered for prophylaxis of venous thromboembolism is 5000 units administered subcutaneously 2 hours prior to surgery, followed by 5000 units every 8–12 hours postoperatively.

Side Effects/Adverse Effects

Heparin-associated side effects commonly relate to the drug's action and potential for initiating the immune response. The most common side effects (> 10%) of heparin therapy are excessive bleeding and thrombocytopenia. Individuals should be observed for blood loss. Heparin-induced thrombocytopenia is an immunogenic reaction observed in < 3% of individuals receiving extended (> 4 days) heparin therapy. It occurs when antibodies develop to the heparin-platelet complex. The paradoxical effect of heparin-induced thrombocytopenia results in vascular damage and activation of the clotting cascade, potentially leading to thrombosis and DVT, pulmonary embolism, and myocardial infarction. Hypersensitivity reactions to heparin may result due to the animal source of the drug. A test dose prior to fully commencing therapy can be used to verify the lack of a hypersensitivity reaction for an individual.

Protamine sulfate (Protamine) may be administered to treat a heparin overdose. Protamine sulfate is a positively charged protein that binds and sequesters the negatively charged molecules of heparin. The drug dose is calculated based on a concentration of 1–1.5 mg protamine per 100 units of unfractionated heparin. Typical administration is via a slow intravenous infusion of 50 mg at least 10 minutes.

Low Molecular Weight Heparins

Low molecular weight (LMW) heparins comprise a class of drugs that are smaller (2–9 kDa) and more uniform than unfractionated heparin. They result in fewer adverse drug events, only require once/day or twice/day dosing, and do not require aPPT monitoring, thus making them more amenable for ambulatory and in-home care settings.[32] LMW heparins are the drugs of choice for treating and preventing postoperative and established DVT. In contrast to unfractionated heparin, LMW heparins result in fewer incidents of major bleeding (0.9% versus 3.2%) and recurrent DVT (2.7% versus 7.0%).[33]

LMW heparins form a complex with antithrombin, like unfractionated heparin; however, LMW heparins are smaller, and the heparin-antithrombin complex blocks factor X_a very well but does not block the action of thrombin. Despite slightly different mechanisms of action, both types of heparin are equally efficacious for most disorders that require anticoagulation.

The pharmacokinetic properties of LMW heparins provide several advantages over unfractionated heparin. Distribution and bioavailability of LMW heparins is greater. LMW heparins display decreased nonspecific binding to plasma proteins and a half-life (3–9 hours) that is 2–6 times longer than unfractionated heparin, thus decreasing the needed frequency of administration. LMW heparins have a wider therapeutic range compared to the therapeutic range of unfractionated heparin, thus LMW heparins are administered subcutaneously on a fixed dose and do not require aPPT monitoring. A standard treatment regimen for postoperative DVT prophylaxis is 7–10 days.

There are currently three LMW heparin preparations available in the United States—enoxaparin (Lovenox), dalteparin (Fragmin), and tinzaparin (Innohep). All are suitable for both the prevention and treatment of DVT. For this reason, LMW heparins are administered following hip replacement surgery, knee replacement surgery, and abdominal surgery. Enoxaparin (Lovenox) and dalteparin (Fragmin) are also approved for the treatment of unstable angina and non-Q-wave myocardial infarction, and enoxaparin alone is approved for treating an established myocardial infarction. Tinzaparin (Innohep) is approved for treating acute DVT and can be administered in combination with the oral anticoagulant warfarin (Coumadin). While for most individuals, LMW heparin therapy will be supplemented and then replaced by warfarin (Coumadin) (an FDA Pregnancy Category X drug), women who are pregnant may receive continued, long-term LMW heparin therapy. Studies comparing tinzaparin (Innohep) and dalteparin (Fragmin) for treating DVT or pulmonary embolism found no significant difference in hemorrhagic side effects, clinical efficacy, or thromboembolism recurrence.[34] It is of note that standard dosing for enoxaparin (Lovenox) is presented in mg, whereas dosing for dalteparin (Fragmin) and tinzaparin (Innohep) is in antifactor X_a international units (IU).

Side Effects/Adverse Effects

Hemorrhage is the most common adverse effect of LMW heparins, although the associated risk is less with LMW heparins than with unfractionated heparin. Thrombocytopenia is tenfold less likely to occur with LMW heparin; however, it is still a serious concern. Protamine sulfate may be used in the treatment of LMW heparin overdose, although it is an unlabeled use. The dose of protamine sulfate varies with the specific formulation (e.g., 1 mg protamine per 1 mg enoxaparin [Lovenox]; 1 mg protamine per 100 IU of dalteparin [Fragmin] or tinzaparin [Innohep]).

Fondaparinux (Arixtra)

Fondaparinux (Arixtra) is a synthetic preparation of the active pentasaccharide present in both unfractionated heparin and LMW heparins. Like LMW heparins, fondaparinux (Arixtra) selectively interacts with antithrombin to form an inhibitory complex that prevents factor X_a from converting prothrombin to thrombin. Fondaparinux reversibly binds to antithrombin and has a higher affinity than unfractionated heparin or LMW heparin. Routine laboratory evaluation of bleeding times (e.g., aPPT) are not necessary for persons on fondaparinux (Arixtra). The drug is approved for postoperative DVT prophylaxis and for the treatment of currently formed DVT and pulmonary embolism. Similar to the LMW heparin tinzaparin (Innohep), fondaparinux is administered with warfarin (Coumadin) for treating an acute manifestation of DVT or pulmonary embolism. Most fondaparinux treatment regimens are prescribed for 5–10 days. A 2003 study comparing once-daily subcutaneously administered fondaparinux to continuous intravenous infusion of unfractionated heparin for individuals with a pulmonary embolism demonstrated similar therapeutic outcomes and similar frequency of adverse effects.[35]

Fondaparinux (Arixtra) is highly bioavailable (> 99%) and has a half-life of 20 hours, which is longer in individuals with renal impairment. This extended half-life of fondaparinux makes once-a-day dosing possible. Plasma concentrations peak 2–4 hours following administration. Fondaparinux may cause a decrease in platelet concentrations (1–3% of participants); however, the drug does not produce the allergic response or heparin-induced thrombocytopenia observed with other antithrombin activators.

A standard treatment of fondaparinux (Arixtra) includes 2.5 mg/day administered as a single daily subcutaneous injection for surgical prophylaxis of venous thromboembolism, beginning 6–8 hours postoperatively. A higher dose of fondaparinux (5–10 mg per day) is approved to be used in conjunction with warfarin to treat acute symptomatic DVT and pulmonary embolism. Although fondaparinux is classified as an FDA Pregnancy Category B drug and there have been some small studies indicating its safety during pregnancy,[36] heparins have been more extensively studied and are still preferred for use during pregnancy for women who do not have adverse effects from heparin.

Oral Anticoagulants

Warfarin (Coumadin)

Warfarin is a vitamin K antagonist that indirectly inhibits the coagulation cascade. This drug was initially produced as a pesticide for rats and mice and is still used for this purpose. As is the case for many of the drugs used today, the origins begin with observations of animal diseases. In the early 1920s, cattle in the United States and Canada began to hemorrhage following ingestion of moldy sweet clover hay. The etiology of the agent in the moldy hay that caused the cattle to become deficient in prothrombin was a mystery until the 1940s when chemists at the University of Wisconsin were able to isolate the active chemical. A few years after it was on the market as a pesticide, warfarin (Coumadin) was found to be effective in preventing thrombosis and embolism.[37]

Warfarin (Coumadin) is the only oral anticoagulant available in the United States and is used extensively for long-term prevention of thrombus formation. Warfarin (Coumadin) disrupts the biosynthesis of four vitamin K-dependent coagulation factors, which blocks activation of the tissue factor pathway, contact pathway, and common coagulation pathways. It also inhibits the synthesis of the vitamin K-dependent protein S and protein C. Warfarin is the anticoagulant of choice for prophylaxis of venous thrombosis. Long-term warfarin (Coumadin) therapy has been shown to markedly reduce recurrent DVT and the risk of pulmonary embolism.

While parenteral anticoagulants produce a therapeutic effect within minutes of intravenous administration, warfarin requires 2–4 days for peak therapeutic effects to develop. Warfarin prevents the synthesis of new vitamin K-dependent clotting factors but has no effect on the factors currently in circulation, which accounts for the delay in warfarin anticoagulant effect. Therefore, heparin is typically coadministered for the first 4–5 days of warfarin treatment.[38] Warfarin has been shown to be more efficacious than aspirin or placebo for preventing DVT in individuals recovering from hip surgery.[39]

Warfarin (Coumadin) therapy commonly follows an initial treatment with either unfractionated heparin or LMW heparin and is continued for at least 3–6 months to prevent recurrence of a thrombosis that is secondary to a nonrecurring event (e.g., surgery). Individuals who are receiving treatment for an initial DVT or pulmonary embolism and those who have an irreversible risk factor (e.g., an inherited thrombophilia) are usually prescribed warfarin (Coumadin) for 6–12 months and then evaluated for ongoing treatment. Individuals who have experienced two or more venous thromboembolisms are candidates for chronic warfarin (Coumadin) treatment. Chronic warfarin treatment may also be indicated in individuals with chronic atrial fibrillation as prophylactic therapy against ischemic stroke and other thromboembolic events.[40]

Warfarin (Coumadin) is able to pass through cell membranes with relative ease and is readily absorbed from the intestine. Once in the blood, warfarin is extensively (99%) bound to plasma albumin. The drug has a half-life of 36–48 hours and is metabolized in the liver. Anticoagulant effects will continue up to 5 days postdiscontinuation of the drug due to its long half-life.

Side Effects/Adverse Effects

The most common and significant adverse drug reaction of warfarin is bleeding, and warfarin labeling includes an FDA black box warning that the drug can cause severe bleeding. If uncontrolled bleeding develops, warfarin should be immediately discontinued. Due to the drug's long half-life, anticoagulant activity may persist for several days following cessation of drug administration.

Contraindications

Warfarin is contraindicated for individuals with impaired liver activity secondary to alcoholism because the vitamin K deficiency common in persons with impaired liver function increases the anticoagulant effect of warfarin. Other contraindications include history of hemorrhagic stroke, known hypersensitivity to warfarin, pregnancy, threatened abortion, history of blood dyscrasias, planned optic or central nervous system surgery, malignant hypertension, active bleeding, history of falls, and inability to adhere to therapy.

Clinical Management

The two most common methods for monitoring therapeutic actions of warfarin are calculation of prothrombin time (PT, normal value = 12 seconds) and international normalized ratio (INR, the desired value for treatment of venous thrombosis, pulmonary embolism, and acute myocardial infarction = 2.0–3.0). If an individual on warfarin (Coumadin) has an INR above or below the desired value, the dose of warfarin can be appropriately altered.[41] There may be a relatively long (2- to 4-day) lag time between a modification of a warfarin dose and the peak therapeutic effects as measured by subsequent INR. It is usually suggested that individuals not change brands because different formulations may have differing bioavailabilities; however, comparisons of different formulations have, to date, failed to find different pharmacokinetics, and this recommendation remains controversial. Regular monitoring of PT and INR decreases the risk of both hemorrhage from excessive warfarin administration and thrombus from insufficient drug dosing. A usual starting dose of warfarin (Coumadin) is 5 mg per day, and maintenance dose ranges from 2–10 mg per day. A starting dose of ≤ 5 mg is suggested in postmenopausal women. The maintenance dose is determined empirically and should result in an INR ranging from 2.0 to 3.0. Individuals with INRs > 3.0 are at an increased risk of hemorrhage and are not receiving any greater therapeutic drug effect.

Warfarin has a narrow therapeutic range. In addition, the activity and metabolism of this drug is highly variable from one person to another, which makes achieving a therapeutic level difficult in clinical practice.[42] The etiology of this variability in action is partially genetic. Warfarin (Coumadin) is actually a **racemic mixture** of R- and S-warfarin. S-warfarin has more anticoagulant activity than does R-warfarin, and the two are metabolized by different CYP450 enzymes within the liver. S-warfarin is metabolized by CYP2C9, and polymorphisms in CYP2C9 (specifically CYP2C9*2 and CYP2C9*3) explain much of the differences in clinical response to warfarin.[42,43] These CYP2C9 variants are found in approximately 10–20% of Caucasians and African Americans. Polymorphisms in the gene VKORC1, which encodes for vitamin K function, also affects warfarin activity, and variants of this gene also contribute to genetic variation. The frequency of the variant VKORC1 gene is approximately 80% in Asians.

In 2007, the FDA approved a label change for warfarin (Coumadin) that provides information about how warfarin pharmacokinetics are altered in persons with specific genetic polymorphisms. Healthcare providers are not required to do genetic testing prior to initiating warfarin therapy, but these tests are available and are increasingly being used to help manage persons who take this drug.

In addition to genetic polymorphisms, diet and use of other drugs affect metabolism and biologic activity of warfarin. The amount of vitamin K in the diet can impact the effect of warfarin. Individuals are counseled to stay on a regular diet without changing the proportions or types of food ingested. Foods that have large and moderate amounts of vitamin K are listed in Table 16-5. The vitamin K content of most foods can be found in charts that are available from the USDA food composition lists.

Drug–Drug Interactions Associated with Warfarin (Coumadin)

Warfarin (Coumadin) has an extensive collection of drug–drug, drug–food, and drug–herb interactions (Table 16-6). These interactions are of import for primary care providers. Approximately 17–26% of persons who are on warfarin use herbal supplements,[42,44] and in one study of 17,861 persons on warfarin, 68% were prescribed at least one agent that interacts with warfarin.[45] The PT or INR should be assayed when other drugs are added to an individual's therapeutic regimen.

Drugs may increase or decrease the anticoagulant effects of warfarin and thus increase the potential for hemorrhage or thrombosis, respectively.[44,46] Drugs can increase

Table 16-5 Vitamin K Content of Foods*

High Vitamin K Content ≥ 25 mcg per Serving Size of ½ Cup to 1 Cup	Moderate Vitamin K Content 10–24 mcg per Serving Size of ½ Cup to 1 Cup	Low Vitamin K Content 0–9 mcg per Serving Size of ½ Cup to 1 Cup
Apples, green peel	Alfalfa seeds	Alcoholic beverages
Asparagus; canned, cooked, frozen	Apple peel, red	Apple juice
Avocados, peeled	Apple pie	Apple sauce
Beans, snap, raw	Artichokes	Apple, gala, golden delicious, red delicious
Blueberries	Beans, kidney	Bacon
Broccoli	Beans, snap (raw)	Bagels
Brussels sprouts†	Blackberries	Banana
Cabbage	Bread stuffing	Barley
Cabbage, Chinese	Carrots	Beans, baked, pinto, white
Coleslaw	Cauliflower	Beef
Collard greens†	Celery	Biscuits
Cow peas	Chicken	Burritos
Cucumber skin, raw only	Grapes	Butter
Endive, raw†	Leeks	Cake
Fish, tuna in oil	Lentils	Candy
Kale†	Margarine	Cereals
Lettuce, red leaf†	Miso	Cheese
Mayonnaise	Oranges	Chicken
Nuts, pine, pistachio	Peppers, green, boiled	Cookies
Okra	Pies	Corn
Parsley†	Plums	Dairy products
Peas	Potatoes	Eggs
Prunes	Raspberries	Fish
Spinach*	Salad dressing	Fruit melons, peaches, pears
Swiss chard†	Tomatoes	Ham
Tea*		Melons
Turnip greens		Milk
		Pasta
		Potatoes
		Rice

* This list is not comprehensive. The vitamin K content of most foods, including most brands' packaged foods can be found in charts that are available from the USDA food composition lists.
† These foods have very high amounts of vitamin K (≥ 200 mcg).

Table16-6 Drug–Drug Interactions Associated with Warfarin (Coumadin)*

Drugs That Increase Anticoagulation Effect Generic (Brand)	Drugs That Decrease Anticoagulation Effect Generic (Brand)
Acetaminophen (Tylenol)	Antacids
Allopurinol (Zyloprim)	Alcohol
Androgens	Antihistamines
Aspirin	Azathioprine (Imuran)
Amiodarone (Cordarone)	Barbiturates
Cephalosporins, second and third generation	Carbamazepine (Tegretol)
Cimetidine (Tagamet)	Cholestyramine (Questran)
Ciprofloxacin (Cipro)	Clozapine (Clozaril)
Disulfiram (Antabuse)	Dicloxacillin (Dynapen)
Dong Quai	Diuretics
Erythromycin (E-Mycin)	Estrogens
Fish oil	Garlic
Fluconazole (Diflucan)	Griseofulvin (Grifulvin V)
Fluorouracil (Efudex, Fluoroplex)	Nafcillin (Unipen)
Fluoxetine (Prozac)	Oral contraceptives
Gingko	Phenobarbital (Luminal)
Ginseng	Phenytoin (Dilantin)
Glucagon	Rifampin (Rifadin)
Isoniazid (INH)	Secobarbital (Seconal)
Metronidazole (Flagyl)	Spironolactone (Aldactone)
Omeprazole (Prilosec)	Sucralfate (Carafate)
Sertraline (Zoloft)	St. John's wort
Sulfonamides	Trazodone
Tamoxifen (Nolvadex)	Vitamin C, high doses
Tetracycline	Vitamin K
Trimethoprim/sulfamethoxazole (Bactrim)	

* This table is not comprehensive as new information is being identified on a regular basis.

warfarin effects by displacing warfarin from albumin or inhibiting hepatic warfarin metabolism, while other drugs may decrease warfarin effects, reversing the inhibition of clotting factor biosynthesis or increasing hepatic warfarin metabolism. In addition, warfarin can affect the metabolism of other drugs. For example, the metabolism of hypoglycemic agents and anticonvulsants are decreased when taken with warfarin, which can lead to toxic effects.

Special Populations

Warfarin is an FDA Pregnancy Category X drug. It is able to pass across the placenta and can cause spontaneous abortion; multiple birth defects such as central nervous system abnormalities and urinary tract abnormalities; fetal growth restriction; and stillbirth. It also is detected in breast milk at high levels. Gross malformations, CNS defects, fetal bleeding, and fetal mortality have all been attributed to maternal warfarin use. Women of childbearing age should

be informed of the teratogenic effects of warfarin. Heparin is the preferred anticoagulant to administer during pregnancy.

Adverse effects other than hemorrhage, drug–drug interactions, and teratogenesis are relatively infrequent. Long-term (> 1 year) use of warfarin may increase the risk of osteoporosis and hip fracture. A small dose (2.5 mg orally) of vitamin K can compete with warfarin and reverse the warfarin-induced inhibition of clotting factor biosynthesis, thus making it a useful treatment for warfarin overdose.

Direct Thrombin Inhibitors

Direct thrombin inhibitors (DTIs) are a new class of anticoagulants that bind to thrombin.[47] There are two types of direct thrombin inhibitors that are classed on the basis of their interaction with thrombin. The bivalent DTIs bind to two sites on thrombin, and the univalent DTIs bind only to the active site on thrombin.

The first direct thrombin inhibitor used medicinally was *Hirudo medicinalis* or the European medical leech. This leech produces hirudin in saliva, which inhibits thrombin. Leeches have been used medically for centuries. They were used for bloodletting by the Greeks as a method of balancing humors to rid the body of various diseases and for treating numerous disorders throughout history. In 2004, the FDA approved the use of leeches as medical devices used to stimulate blood flow in areas where microsurgery has been performed.

Pharmacologic studies of hirudin led to the development of DTIs. Direct thrombin inhibitors are an attractive alternative to heparin for persons who need anticoagulation but who cannot use heparin. These drugs must be administered intravenously and are currently used in limited settings. However, thrombin has multiple actions within the coagulation process, and there are many possible therapeutic actions that DTIs might have as researchers continue to explore this class of drug.

Antiplatelet Drugs

Antiplatelet drugs inhibit the activation of platelets and prevent the formation of a platelet plug. The principal indication for antiplatelet drugs is the prevention of arterial thrombosis (Table 16-7). Examples of antiplatelet drugs include aspirin and ADP receptor antagonists (e.g., clopidogrel). The mechanism of action of antiplatelet drugs is shown in Figure 16-2.[48]

Aspirin

The general principles of aspirin pharmacotherapy are discussed in Chapter 12. The discussion in this chapter is limited to the role of aspirin for the prevention and treatment of arterial thrombosis. Aspirin therapy is indicated for prevention of myocardial infarction, ischemic stroke, and chronic stable and unstable angina in persons who have an increased risk for these disorders.

Aspirin prevents platelet aggregation by irreversibly inhibiting the platelet enzyme cyclooxygenase (COX). The effects of aspirin in the platelet last for 7–10 days, which is the duration of the platelet life span. Cyclooxygenase catalyzes the conversion of arachidonic acid to thromboxane A_2. In the absence of aspirin, thromboxane A_2 is produced in significant quantities and serves as an intracellular platelet signal to cause a conformational change in the GP II_b/III_a receptor, receptor activation, and fibrinogen binding. Thromboxane A_2 also is released from the platelet and serves as an extracellular signal to stimulate vascular

Table 16-7 Antiplatelet Drugs

Drug Generic (Brand)	Formulations	Indication/Dose	Clinical Considerations	FDA Pregnancy Category
Aspirin	Tablet, caplet, gum, suppository: Multiple formulations/strengths ranging from 81 to 600 mg	*MI/stroke prophylaxis:* PO: 81–325 mg/day *Acute MI/stroke:* PO: 160–325 mg/day	Contraindications: Hypersensitivity to salicylates, or any component of the formulation, GI bleeding, bleeding disorders, children < 12 y, FDA Pregnancy Category D, vitamin K deficiency, peptic ulcer, NSAIDs use. Adverse effects: Bleeding is most common; see drug reference.	C D in third trimester
Ticlopidine (Ticlid)	Tablet: 250 mg	*Stroke prevention:* PO: 250 mg bid with food	Contraindications: Hypersensitivity, severe liver disease, blood dyscrasias, active bleeding. FDA black box warning: May cause life-threatening hematologic reactions including neutropenia, agranulocytosis, thrombotic thrombocytopenia purpura, and aplastic anemia. Adverse effects: Bleeding, hemorrhage most common.	B
Clopidogrel (Plavix)	Tablet: 75, 300 mg	*Reducing the risk of stroke, MI, peripheral arterial disease in high-risk patients, acute coronary syndrome:* PO: 75 mg daily with or without food	Contraindications: Hypersensitivity, active bleeding, coagulation disorders. Adverse effects: Bleeding/hemorrhage most common.	B

MI = myocardial infarction; NSAID = nonsteroidal anti-inflammatory drugs.

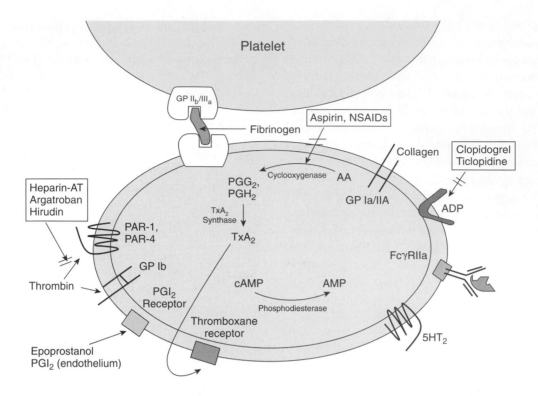

Sites of action of currently approved antiplatelet drugs. Antiplatelet drugs inhibit platelet activation by blocking cell surface receptors and inhibiting the generation of bioactive substances. These drugs inhibit platelet aggregation by blocking fibrinogen binding to glycoprotein II$_b$/III$_a$.

AA = arachidonic acid; AT = antithrombin; GP = glycoprotein; PG = prostaglandin; Tx = thromboxane.

Figure 16-2 Mechanism of action of antiplatelet drugs. *Source:* Adapted with permission from Messmore HL 2005.[48]

smooth-muscle contraction. The irreversible inhibition of platelet COX prevents both the intracellular and extracellular actions of thromboxane A$_2$, which prevents subsequent rounds of hemostasis. Aspirin may increase the risk of gastrointestinal bleeding due to its actions on COX enzymes in the stomach.

Aspirin has been shown to decrease risk of cardiovascular disease in persons with an increased risk for cardiovascular disorders.[49] However, the effects of aspirin on men and women differ. Aspirin does not reduce the risk of myocardial infarction in women but does reduce the risk of strokes approximately 17%.[49,50] In contrast, aspirin does reduce the risk for myocardial infarction in men and does not reduce the risk of stroke. In 2009, the United States Preventive Services Task Force revised previous recommendations for aspirin use. The current recommendation is that aspirin be taken by women who are between the ages of 55 and 79 years when the potential benefit of aspirin in decreasing the risk of a stroke outweighs the risks of

gastrointestinal bleeding. Aspirin is not recommended for women who are younger than age 55 years.[50]

The recommended dose of aspirin to help protect against a heart attack is the relatively low dose of 81 mg given orally once per day for long term. An initial, short-term dose for an emergent condition is 325 mg given orally once per day. While aspirin has been shown to decrease frequency of venous thrombosis following surgery (versus placebo), it is significantly less efficacious when compared to LMW heparin or warfarin and thus is not a recommended treatment approach.

ADP Receptor Antagonists

The two ADP receptor antagonists, clopidogrel (Plavix) and ticlopidine (Ticlid), irreversibly inhibit platelet ADP receptors. Blocking the receptors prevents ADP activation, which in turn prevents activation of the GP II$_b$/III$_a$ receptor and platelet activation. The drugs are useful for prevention of stroke and myocardial infarction. Similar to aspirin, the cellular machinery of the platelet is unable to resynthesize receptors to replace the ones irreversibly inhibited by these drugs. As such, the antiplatelet effects of ADP receptor antagonists last for the duration of the platelet lifespan (7–10 days). Clopidogrel (Plavix) has fewer adverse drug effects than ticlopidine (Ticlid). Both drugs are slightly more efficacious than aspirin for treating conditions, and they are substantially more expensive. Because ADP receptor antagonists do not inhibit the prostaglandin pathway in the gastric mucosa, these drugs do not cause the gastrointestinal side effects observed with aspirin therapy.

Clopidogrel (Plavix) is currently recommended for postmyocardial infarction individuals who have not responded to aspirin or cannot tolerate the aspirin side effects. It is a drug of choice for both acute and long-term treatment for individuals who have experienced a non-ST elevation myocardial infarction. Combination therapy with clopidogrel and aspirin reduces the risk of vascular events in persons with atrial fibrillation who cannot use vitamin K-antagonist drugs.[51] Its antiplatelet activity can be observed within 4 hours of initiating therapy and will plateau at days 4–6. Clopidogrel (Plavix) is administered as a prodrug that converts into an active form following absorption. It undergoes extensive first-pass metabolism

and is administered as a single 75-mg tablet administered orally once per day.

Ticlopidine (Ticlid) is approved for prevention of thrombotic stroke and is indicated for individuals who have not responded to aspirin or cannot tolerate the side effects. Like clopidogrel, ticlopidine is readily absorbed and undergoes extensive first-pass metabolism. Ticlopidine has been shown to cause severe neutropenia in a small number (2–3%) of individuals surveyed, and the condition improved following the discontinuing of the drug. The standard dose is 250 mg orally twice per day.

Thrombolytics

Thrombolytics are used to dissolve preexisting clots and are typically only administered to individuals in whom pulmonary embolism or DVT has been verified (Table 16-8). The five available drugs in this class are streptokinase (Streptase), alteplase (t-PA, Activase), tenecteplase (TNKase), reteplase (Retavase), and urokinase (Kinlytic). Of the five, streptokinase (Streptase), alteplase, and urokinase have been studied most extensively. The drugs are indicated for use in treating severe thrombosis. All five medications facilitate the conversion of plasminogen to

Table 16-8 Thrombolytic Drugs

Drug Generic (Brand)	Formulations	Indication/Dose	Clinical Considerations	FDA Pregnancy Category
Steptokinase (Streptase)	Injection: 250,000, 600,000, 750,000, 1,500,000 IU powder	*DVT, pulmonary embolism, arterial thrombosis, arterial embolism, lysis of coronary artery thrombi after MI, acute evolving transmural MI:* IV: 1.5 million IU infused over 30–60 min Intracoronary infusion: 20,000 IU bolus, 2000–4000 IU/min for 60 min	Contraindications: Active bleeding, recent cerebrovascular accident; intracranial/intraspinal surgery, intracranial neoplasm, severe uncontrolled hypertension. FDA black box warning: Neurotoxicity/ototoxicity/ nephrotoxicity have been reported. Adverse effects: Hypotension and bleeding most common. Precautions: Recent major surgery, recent serious bleed, hypertension, and more. Consult drug reference.	D
Alteplase (Activase, t-PA)	Injection: 50 mg (29 million international units/ vial), 100 mg (58 million international units/vial)	*Acute pulmonary embolism:* IV: 100 mg over 2 h *Acute ischemic stroke:* IV: 0.9 mg/kg (max 90 mg) infused over 1 h (administer 10% of total dose over 1 min initially) *Coronary artery thrombi/MI:* IV: 100 mg over 3 h	Contraindications: Hypersensitivity, active internal bleeding, recent CVA, severe uncontrolled hypertension, intracranial/ intraspinal surgery/ trauma, aneurysm. Adverse effects: Bleeding/hemorrhage most common.	C

(continues)

Table 16-8 Thrombolytic Drugs (*continued*)

Drug Generic (Brand)	Formulation	Indication/Dose	Clinical Considerations	FDA Pregnancy Category
Tenecteplase (TNKase)	Injection: 50 mg powder	*Acute MI:* IV: < 60 kg: 30 mg ≥ 60 to < 70 kg: 35 mg ≥ 70 to < 80 kg: 40 mg ≥ 80 to < 90 kg: 45 mg ≥ 90 kg: 50 mg	Contraindications: Hypersensitivity, arteriovenous malformation, aneurysm, active bleeding, intracranial, intraspinal surgery, CNS neoplasms, severe hypertension. Adverse effects: Bleeding hemorrhage most common.	C
Reteplase (Retavase)	Injection: 10.4 unit (18.1 mg reteplase) powder	*Acute MI:* IV: 10 IU bolus over 2 min followed by a second dose 30 min later	Contraindications: Hypersensitivity, active internal bleeding, history of cerebrovascular accident, recent intracranial or intraspinal surgery or trauma, intracranial neoplasm, cerebral arteriovenous malformation, aneurysm, known bleeding diathesis, a history of intracranial hemorrhage, suspected aortic dissection, recent (within 3 months) closed-head or facial trauma, or severe uncontrolled hypertension. Adverse effects: Bleeding/hemorrhage most common.	C
Urokinase (Kinlytic)	Injection: 250,000 IU powder	*Acute PE/DVT:* IV: 4400 IU/kg over 10 min; maintenance 4400 IU/kg/h × 12 h. Anticoagulation treatment recommended after completion of infusion.	Contraindications: Hypersensitivity, internal active bleeding, intraspinal surgery, neoplasms of CNS, recent trauma, arteriovenous malformation or aneurysm, uncontrolled arterial hypertension. Adverse effects: Bleeding/hemorrhage most common.	B

DVT = deep vein thrombosis; MI = myocardial infarction; CVA = cardiovascular vascular accident; PE = pulmonary embolism.

plasmin. Thrombolytics pose the risk of serious bleeding and should be used only when safer treatment approaches have been exhausted. The most serious potential consequence is an intracranial hemorrhage, which may result from the systemic dissolution of blood clots and impairment of clotting factor formation. While thrombolytics readily dissolve blood clots associated with DVT and pulmonary embolism, studies have not indicated a conclusive improvement in posttreatment mortality[52]; however, severe pulmonary embolism (e.g., pulmonary embolism presenting with persistent hypotension or severe hypoxemia) is nonetheless regarded as a suitable indication for thrombolytic drug therapy.

Streptokinase (Streptase) forms an active complex with plasminogen that then serves to convert other plasminogen proteins. It is indicated for massive occlusions, including acute myocardial infarction, DVT, and massive pulmonary embolism. Streptokinase is administered intravenously (1.5 million IU infused over 30–60 minutes) or as an intracoronary infusion (20,000 IU bolus, 2000 IU/minutes for 60 minutes). The half-life of the drug is approximately 1 hour. Streptokinase is derived from a bacterial source. In addition to the bleeding concern, streptokinase has the potential to elicit an immunologic response. Most allergic reactions are mild and can be managed with antihistamines. Although the reaction is generally rare and involves urticaria, headaches, and itching, it is advisable to switch to another fibrolytic drug if a second treatment is needed within a week of the initial therapy. Hypotension is reported in 1–10% of individuals and is not seemingly related to the bleeding or allergic reaction.

Alteplase, tenecteplase, and reteplase are produced through recombinant DNA technology. Alteplase is genetically identical to human tissue plasminogen activator and is the only therapy currently approved for treatment of acute stroke. Treatment must be initiated as soon as possible and should begin within 3 hours of symptom onset.[53] Because Alteplase can be administered at a relatively low dose, activation of plasminogen in the general circulation is minimized. Alteplase does not cause hypotension or produce an allergic reaction, as does streptokinase, and it requires the shortest intravenous infusion time. Despite these advantages, one major drawback to alteplase is its price: A single course of treatment costs in excess of $2500.

Several studies have demonstrated the efficacy and relative safety of thrombolytic agents in menstruating women.[54,55] Thrombolytics have been shown to cause only moderate increases in bleeding during the first day of menstruation; however, fibrinolytic therapy should be used with caution in women who have a history of excessive uterine bleeding.

The Role of Vitamin K

Vitamin K is essential for the formation of several clotting factors and anticoagulant proteins. Two forms of vitamin K, phylloquinone (vitamin K_1) and menaquinones (vitamin K_2), are normally absorbed in the intestine in the presence of bile salts. These precursors of vitamin K are ubiquitous in most diets (Table 16-4) and also produced by the bacteria that inhabit the intestine. Deficiency is extremely rare, except in the case of newborns, because they do not have intestinal flora at the time of birth. Chapter 39 reviews the use of vitamin K therapy for newborns. Vitamin K deficiency can also occur if the bile is obstructed, if its action is blocked by warfarin (Coumadin), other drugs that are vitamin K antagonists (e.g., anticonvulsants, antibiotics, isoniazid [INH]), parenchymal liver diseases such as cirrhosis, or malabsorption syndromes.

Vitamin K can be administered intravenously, intramuscularly, or orally. The intravenous formulation AquaMEPHYTON is used for newborns to prevent hemorrhagic disease of the newborn. The American College of Chest Physicians publishes recommendations for vitamin K therapy if persons on anticoagulant therapy have an INR that is higher than therapeutic values.[38] After one oral dose of vitamin K, the blood coagulation factors increase in approximately 6–12 hours. Oral formulations of vitamin K are recommended for pregnant women who need to take an anticonvulsant agent (e.g., phenytoin [Dilantin]) and for individuals on long-term isoniazid (INH) therapy.

Conclusion

Erythropoiesis and the coagulation cascade play a vital role in complete understanding of hematologic disorders. Accurate diagnosis through laboratory interpretation, symptom recognition, and patient presentation is one piece to the puzzle. Proper drug choice and treatment regimen depends upon knowledge of the pharmacodynamic properties of drugs used to treat these disorders, their adverse effect profiles, evidence-based guidelines, and overall condition of the patient. Treatment is adjusted based on recommended monitoring parameters and patient tolerance to the drug. Understanding the etiology and pathophysiology of anemias and coagulopathies combined with appropriate diagnosis and pharmacologic selection will together help persons with hematologic disorders achieve optimal outcomes.

References

1. Bailit JL, Doty E, Todia W. Repeated hematocrit measurements in low-risk pregnant women. J Reprod Med 2007;52:619.
2. Sifakis S, Pharmakides G. Anemia in pregnancy. Ann N Y Acad Sci 2000;900:125.
3. Looker AC, Dallman PR, Carroll MD, Gunter EW, Johnson CL. Prevalence of iron deficiency in the United States. JAMA 1997;277:973.
4. Schorr TO, Hediger ML. Anemia and iron-deficiency anemia: compilation of data on pregnancy outcome. Am J Clin Nutr 1994;59(suppl):492S–501S.
5. Chertow GM, Mason PD, Vaage-Nilsen O, Ahlmen J. Update on adverse drug events associated with parenteral iron. Nephrol Dial Transplant 2006;21:378.
6. Figlin E, Chetrit A, Shahar A, Shpilberg O, Zivelin A, Rosenberg N, et al. High prevalences of vitamin B_{12} and folic acid deficiency in elderly subjects in Israel. Br J Haematol 2003;123:696.
7. Centers for Disease Control and Prevention. Recommendations for the use of folic acid to reduce the number of cases of spina bifida and other neural tube defects. MMWR 1992;41(No. RR-14):1–7.
8. Savage DG, Lindenbaum J, Stabler SP, Allen RH. Sensitivity of serum methylmalonic acid and total homocysteine determinations for diagnosing cobalamin and folate deficiencies. Am J Med 1994; 96:239.
9. Andrès E, Dali-Youcef N, Vogel T, Serraj K, Zimmer J. Oral cobalamin (vitamin B_{12}) treatment. An update. Int J Lab Hematol 2009;31(1):1–8.
10. Madigan C, Malik M. Pathophysiology and therapy for hemoglobinopathies. Part 1: sickle cell disease. Expert Rev Mol Med 2006;8:1–23.
11. Cappellini MD, Piga A. Current status in iron chelation in hemoglobinopathies. Curr Mol Med. 2008;8(7): 663–74. Review. PubMed PMID: 18991652.
12. Vandendries ER, Drews RE. Drug-associated disease: hematologic dysfunction. Crit Care Clin 2006; 22:347–55.

13. Heit JA. The epidemiology of venous thromboembolism in the community. Arterios Thromb Vascul Biol 2008;28:370–6.

14. Macfarlane RG. An enzyme cascade in the blood clotting mechanism and its function as a biological amplifier. Nature 1964;202:498–9.

15. Riddel JP, Aouizerat BE, Miaskowski C, Lillicrap DP. Theories of blood coagulation. J Ped Oncol Nurs 2007;24:123–31.

16. Billett HH. Antiplatelet agents and arterial thrombosis. Cardiol Clin 2008;26:189–201.

17. Boudoulas KD, Montague CR, Goldschmidt-Clermont PJ, Cooke GE. Estradiol increases platelet aggregation in Pl(A1/A1) individuals. Am Heart J 2006;152(1):136–9.

18. Hoffman M, Monroe DM. Coagulation 2006; a modern view of hemostatic. Hemat Onc Clin 2007;21:1–11.

19. Vasconcelos OM, Poehm EH, McCarter RJ, Campbell WW, Quezado ZM. Potential outcome factors in subacute combined degeneration: review of observational studies. J Gen Intern Med 2006;21:1063.

20. Gerotziafas GT, Samama MM. Prophylaxis of venous thromboembolism in medical patients. Curr Opin Pulm Med 2004;10:356.

21. Geerts WH, Pineo GF, Heit JA, Bergqvist D, Lassen MR, Colwell CW, Ray JG. Prevention of venous thromboembolism: the Seventh ACCP Conference of Antithrombotic and Thrombolytic Therapy. Chest 2004;126:338S.

22. Bates SM, Greer IA, Hirsh J, Ginsberg JS. Use of antithrombotic agents during pregnancy: the Seventh ACCP Conference on Antithrombotic and Thrombolytic Therapy. Chest 2004;126:627S.

23. Kupferminc MJ. Thrombophilia and pregnancy. Reprod Biol Endocrinol 2003;1:111.

24. Lindquist P, Dahlback B, Marsal K. Thrombotic risk during pregnancy: a population study. Obstet Gynecol 1999;94:595.

25. Royal College of Obstetricians and Gynaecologists. Report of the Working Party on Prophylaxis Against Thromboembolism in Gynaecology and Obstetrics. London: RCOG, 1995.

26. Bates SM, Greer IA, Hirsh J, Ginsberg JS. Use of antithrombotic agents during pregnancy: the Seventh ACCP Conference on Antithrombotic and Thrombolytic Therapy. Chest 2004;126:627S.

27. Kujovich JL. Hormones and pregnancy: thromboembolic risks for women. Br J Haematol 2004;126:443.

28. Pomp ER, Rosendaal FR, Doggen CJ. Smoking increases the risk of venous thrombosis and acts synergistically with oral contraceptive use. Am J Hematol 2008;83:97.

29. Hulley S, Furberg C, Barrett-Connor E, Cauley J, Grady D, Haskell W, et al. Noncardiovascular disease outcomes during 6.8 years of hormone therapy: heart and estrogen/progestin replacement study follow-up (HERS II). JAMA 2002;288:58.

30. Cushman M, Kuller LH, Prentice R, Rodabough RJ, Psaty BM, Stafford RS, et al. Estrogen plus progestin and risk of venous thrombosis. JAMA 2004;292:1573.

31. Colvin BT, Barrowcliffe TW on behalf of BCSH Haemostasis and Thrombosis Task Force. The British Society for Haematology guidelines on the use and monitoring of heparin 1992: second revision. J Clin Pathol 1993;46:97.

32. Koopman MMW, Prandoni P, Piovella F, Ockelford PA, Brandjes DP, van der Meer J, et al. Treatment of venous thrombosis with intravenous unfractionated heparin administered in the hospital as compared with subcutaneous low molecular weight heparin administered at home. N Engl J Med 1996;334:682.

33. Siragusa S, Cosmi B, Piovella F, Hirsh J, Ginsberg JS. Low molecular weight heparins and unfractionated heparin in the treatment of patients with acute venous thromboembolism: results of a meta-analysis. Am J Med 1996;100:269.

34. Wells PS, Anderson DR, Rodger MA, Forgie MA, Florack P, Touchie D, et al. A randomized trial comparing two low molecular-weight heparins for the outpatient treatment of deep vein thrombosis and pulmonary embolism. Arch Intern Med 2005;165:733.

35. The Maisse Investigators. Buller HR, Davidson BL, Decousus H, Gallus A, Gent M, Piovella F, et al. Subcutaneous fondaparinux versus intravenous unfractionated heparin in the initial treatment of pulmonary embolism. N Engl J Med 2003;349:1695–702.

36. Mazzolai L, Hohlfeld P, Spertini F, Spertini F, Hayoz D, Schapira M, et al. Fondaparinux is a safe alternative in case of heparin intolerance during pregnancy. Blood 2006;108:1569.

37. Link KP. The discovery of dicumarol and its sequels. Circulation 1959;19:97–107.

38. Ansell J, Hirsh J, Hylek E, Jacobson A, Crowther M, et al. The pharmacology and management of the vitamin K antagonists: American College of Chest Physicians evidence-based clinical practice guidelines. Chest 2008;133(6)(suppl):160S–98S.

39. Powers PJ, Gent M, Jay R, Julian DH, Turbie AG, Levine M, Hirsh J. A randomized trial of less intense postoperative warfarin or aspirin therapy in the prevention of venous thromboembolism after surgery for fractured hip. Arch Intern Med 1989;149:771.

40. Sacco RL, Adams R, Albers G, Alberts MJ, Benavente O, Furie K, et al. Guidelines for prevention of stroke in patients with ischemic stroke or transient ischemic attack: a statement for healthcare professionals from the American Heart Association/American Stroke Association Council on Stroke: co-sponsored by the Council on Cardiovascular Radiology and Intervention. Stroke 2006;37:577.

41. Hull R, Hirsh J, Jay R, Carter C, England C, Gent M, Turpie AG, et al. Different intensities of oral anticoagulant therapy in the treatment of proximal-vein thrombosis. N Engl J Med 1982;307:1676.

42. Gage BF, Milligan PE. Pharmacology and pharmacogenetics of warfarin and other coumarins when used with supplements. Thromb Res 2005;117(1–2):55–9.

43. Hill CE, Duncan A. Overview of the pharmacogenetics in anticoagulation therapy. Clin Lab Med 2008; 28:513–24.

44. Daugherty N, Smith KM. Dietary supplement and selected food interactions with warfarin. Orthopedics 2006;29:309–14.

45. Snaith A, Pugh L, Simpson CR, McLay JS. The potential for interaction between warfarin and coprescribed medication: a retrospective study in primary care. Am J Cardiovasc Drugs 2008;8(3):207–12.

46. Greenblatt DJ, von Moltke LL. Interaction of warfarin with drugs, natural substances, and foods. J Clin Pharmacol 2005;45(2):127–32.

47. Di Nisio M, Middeldorp S, Buller HR. Direct thrombin inhibitors. N Engl J Med 2005;353:1028–40.

48. Messmore HL Jr, Jeske WP, Wehrmacher W, Coyne E, Mobarhan S, Cho L, et al. Antiplatelet agents: current drugs and future trends. Hematol Oncol Clin North Am 2005;19(1):87–117.

49. Berger JS, Roncaglioni MC, Avanzini F, Pangrazzi I, Tognoni G, Brown DL. Aspirin for the primary prevention of cardiovascular events in women and men: a sex-specific meta-analysis of randomized controlled trials. JAMA 2006;295:306–13.

50. US Preventive Services Task Force. Aspirin for the prevention of cardiovascular disease: U.S. Preventive Services Task Force recommendation statement. Ann Intern Med 2009;150(6):396–404.

51. The Active Investigators. Effect of clopidogrel added to aspirin in patients with atrial fibrillation. N Engl J Med 2009;360:2066–78.

52. Thabut G, Thabut D, Myers RP, Bernard-Chabert B, Marrash-Chahla M, Mal H, et al. Thrombolytic therapy of pulmonary embolism: a meta-analysis. J Am Coll Cardiol 2002;40:1660.

53. Hacke W, Donnan G, Fieschi C, Kaste M, von Kummer R, Broderick JP, et al. Association of outcome with early stroke treatment: pooled analysis of ATLANTIS, ECASS, and NINDS rt-PA stroke trials. Lancet 2004;363:768–74.

54. Karnash S, Granger CB, White HD, et al., for the GUSTO-I Investigators. Treating menstruating women with thrombolytic therapy: insights from the Global Utilization of Streptokinase and Tissue Plasminogen Activator for occluded coronary arteries (GUSTO-I) trial. J Am Coll Cardiol 1995;26:1651.

55. Wein TH, Hickenbottom SL, Morgenstern LB, Demchuk AM, Grotta JC. Safety of tissue plasminogen activator for acute stroke in menstruating women. Stroke 2002;33:2506.

17

Autoimmune Conditions

Rebekah L. Ruppe

Chapter Glossary

Aminosalicylates Salts of aminosalicylic acid that act as anti-inflammatories.

Antigen A substance that provokes B-cell production of antibodies and the immune response. Most antigens are bacteria or viruses that invade the body.

Antigen-presenting cell Any cell that digests an antigen and presents a portion of it on the cell surface. B cells can turn into antigen-presenting cells.

Anti-inflammatories Substances that suppress the body's inflammatory response.

Antimetabolite A substance that interferes with cell growth by competing with or replacing the endogenous metabolite involved in the physiologic process.

Antiphospholipid antibody syndrome (APS) Disease initiated by autoimmune production of antibodies to the phospholipids in cell membranes. The result is a disorder of coagulation that causes blood clots.

Autoimmunity A condition of abnormal immune system response in which the body produces antibodies against its own cells, tissues, or organs.

Cytokines Molecular messengers or glycoproteins that facilitate and enhance or control various steps in the immune response. Cytokines can be interferons, interleukins, or growth factors.

Glucocorticoids Adrenocortical steroid hormones with general anti-inflammatory properties.

Immunomodulatory agents Substances that modify immune system response by competing with or mimicking the action of immune cells or products involved in the immune process.

Immunosuppressive drugs Substances that diminish immune system activity by blocking or inhibiting the function of immune cells or products involved in the immune process.

Interferons (INFs) Glycoproteins produced by immune cells in response to pathogen exposure that regulate immune response.

Interleukins (ILs) Cytokines that are produced by white blood vessels, thus the name *leukin*.

Major histocompatibility complex The most gene-dense area found in most vertebrates on the mammalian genome. Major histocompatibility is integral to competent immune system and reproductive success.

Monoclonal antibodies Antibodies cloned from a single cell typically originating from mice that have been exposed to a specific antigen to induce production of the desired antibody.

Nonsteroidal anti-inflammatory drugs (NSAIDs) A group of chemically similar nonsteroidal substances that exhibit anti-inflammatory effects by inhibiting the enzyme cyclooxygenase.

Overview of Autoimmune Disorders

Immune system disorders fall into one of the following three categories: inflammatory diseases, whereby hypersensitivity reactions cause organ or cell damage; autoimmune disorders, whereby autoantibodies that cause damage are generated from an aberrant immune response; and immunologic deficiency disorders that are the result of a genetic or acquired deficiency in a component of the immune system. Autoimmune disorders are categorized as one of two types: those that cause systemic damage to many organs (e.g., systemic lupus erythematosus [SLE]) and those that cause damage to one organ (e.g., diabetes). This chapter addresses the most common systemic autoimmune disorders. Pharmacotherapy for diabetes and thyroid disorders is addressed in Chapters 18 and 19, respectively.

While the etiology of autoimmune disorders remains unknown, it is widely accepted that both genetic and environmental factors play a role. Studies of multiplex families, twin concordance, and geographic clusters suggest a variable but likely relationship between genes and environment in the pathology of autoimmune disorders.[1] There is evidence that inherited protein deficiencies or mutations in genes involved in immune response and regulation can increase a person's predisposition to autoimmune disorders. Specific susceptibility genes have been located in alleles of the **major histocompatibility complex**. Autoimmune disorders most likely require multiple susceptibility genes and environmental triggers to manifest.[2] This chapter reviews the pharmacologic treatments for the most common autoimmune disorders that affect women.

Gender plays a significant role in the development of autoimmunity. Over 75% of individuals with autoimmune disorders are women, a finding that supports the hypothesis that sex hormones play a role in disease susceptibility. The majority of autoimmune disorders have a skewed female-to-male ratio that ranges from 2 to 3:1 in the case of rheumatoid arthritis (RA) and multiple sclerosis (MS) and as high as 9:1 in persons with SLE.[3,4] Other conditions, such as type 1 diabetes and inflammatory bowel disease (IBD), occur with similar frequencies in men and women.[4] This variation suggests that sex hormones modulate rather than induce autoimmunity at least in regard to these conditions.

Pathophysiology of Autoimmune Disorders

A brief review of the components of the immune system referred to in this chapter can be found in Chapter 6. A normal functioning immune system relies on complex physiologic mechanisms that recognize and react to invading pathogens while remaining unresponsive to self-antigens.

Autoimmunity occurs when these regulatory mechanisms break down and the immune system loses tolerance to proteins or antigens that are self. Autoimmune disorders result when the self-directed immunologic reaction causes tissue injury. The underlying pathophysiology is production of autoantibodies that cause an adverse reaction and/or initiation of a hypersensitivity reaction that causes organ damage. Both of these initiating events are the result of and aberrant immune response to an endogenous protein.

Figure 17-1 presents the roles of B cells and T cells in initiating the immune response and highlights one of the theories that describe how an autoimmune disorder starts. In the figure, the B cell has attached to an **antigen**, processed that antigen, then presented a piece of it on the surface of the B cell. This attracts a mature T cell to couple with the B cell. The T cell helps the B cell work via release of **cytokines** that encourage the B cell to proliferate. This process is mutually stimulating and can continue unchecked in autoimmune disorders. The end result is an inflammatory reaction and/or production of autoantibodies. Therefore, the focus of therapy is to interrupt one of the signals that perpetrate the aberrant immune response process.

Cytokines are the molecular messengers that control many of the steps in the immune response. Cytokines are produced and released by many of the immune system cells and are broadly divided into those that are proinflammatory or anti-inflammatory (Figure 17-2). Individual cytokines are categorized as **interferons** (INFs), **interleukins** (ILs), or growth factors.

Overview of Pharmacologic Agents Used to Treat Autoimmune Disorders

Treatment(s) for autoimmune disorders focuses on providing symptomatic relief and reducing disease progression. Pharmacologic approaches to therapy consist of (1) **anti-inflammatories**, (2) **immunosuppressive drugs**, and (3) **immunomodulatory agents**. Anti-inflammatories suppress nonspecific inflammatory cells (e.g., basophils, neutrophils, macrophages), immunosuppressives inhibit the cell and humoral-mediated immune response (T-cell and B-cell activation), and immunomodulators manipulate specific interactions and responses within the immune system without necessarily suppressing overall activity.

Anti-inflammatories are generally used to manage mild disease states, with glucocorticoids reserved for acute

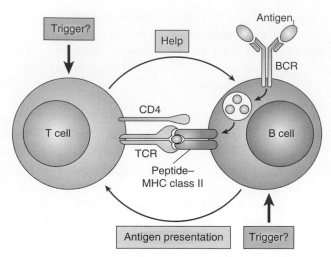

The two-way interaction between B cells and T cells provides the basis for the concept that in certain autoimmune diseases, an amplification cycle might allow persistent immunopathology to arise from a minor "trigger" factor. Such a trigger might initiate the cycle through events in either the B-cell or the T-cell compartment, including the stochastic generation of both B-cell receptors (BCR) and T-cell receptors (TCR).

Figure 17-1 B-cell and T-cell interactions in immune system response. *Source:* Reprinted with permission from Edwards JC and Cambridge G.[2]

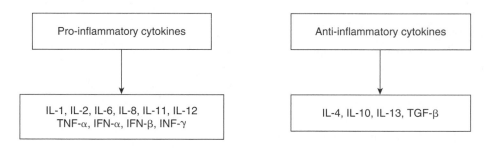

Figure 17-2 Cytokines.

flares or symptomatic episodes. Immunosuppressant and immunomodulatory therapy may be used either for acute symptomatic treatment (induction of remission) or for ongoing treatment (maintenance therapy), depending on the disorder. Some therapies modify the natural course of disease and reduce disability. These disease-modifying therapies are used for chronic disease management of some disorders even in persons who are asymptomatic.

Anti-Inflammatories

Glucocorticoids

Glucocorticoids (e.g., prednisone, methylprednisolone, budesonide) are potent anti-inflammatory agents that have direct effects on lymphoid cells (Table 17-1). These

agents reduce inflammation by inhibiting lymphocyte proliferation and suppressing cell- and humoral-mediated immune response. With large doses, antibody production is reduced.[5]

The primary therapeutic action of **nonsteroidal anti-inflammatory drugs** (NSAIDs) in treating autoimmune disorders is most likely through the inhibition of prostaglandin synthesis and the down-regulation of cytokine secretion.[6] See Chapter 12 for a thorough discussion of the pharmacotherapeutic actions of NSAIDs.

Aminosalicylates

Sulfasalazine (Azulfidine, Sulfadine) is a combination of sulfapyridine and 5-aminosalicylic acid in one molecule. 5-aminosalicylic acid is also called mesalamine in

Table 17-1 Anti-Inflammatory Drugs Commonly Used in the Treatment of Autoimmune Conditions

Drug Generic (Brand)	Uses	Adverse Effects	Precautions	Monitoring
Glucocorticoids Prednisone (Deltasone), methylprednisolone (Medrol), budesonide (Entocort)	IBD RA SLE	Hypertension, hyperglycemia, hyperlipidemia, hypokalemia, osteoporosis, avascular necrosis, cataract, weight gain, infection, fluid retention	Preexisting osteoporosis or renal insufficiency, latent or active TB, recent vaccination	BP, glucose, potassium, total cholesterol at baseline Glucose dipstick every 3–6 months Bone density in high risk
Nonsteroidal anti-inflammatories Ibuprofen (Motrin) naproxen (Aleve)	RA SLE	Gastrointestinal bleeding, hepatic toxicity, renal toxicity, hypertension	Preexisting renal insufficiency or liver disease, concomitant methotrexate use	CBC, creatinine UA, LFTs at baseline CBC, LFTs yearly
Aminosalicylates Sulfasalazine (Azulfidine, Sulfadine)	IBD RA	Nausea, diarrhea, mouth ulcers, headache, fever, rash, reversible oligospermia, hepatic impairment, myelosuppression	Preexisting hepatic or renal impairment, glucose-6-phosphate dehydrogenase deficiency (G6PHD)	CBC, LFTs, G6PHD at baseline CBC every 2–4 weeks for 3 months, then every 3 months
5-aminosalicylic acid (Asacol, Canasa, Colazal, Lialda, Pentasa, Rowasa)	IBD	Nausea, vomiting, headache, arthralgia, diarrhea, constipation, hepatic impairment Rare: leukopenia, acute nephritis	Current renal or hepatic impairment or history of renal disease	CBC, LFTs at baseline Consider creatinine monitoring for the first few weeks

RA = rheumatoid arthritis; SLE = systemic lupus erythematosus; IBD = inflammatory bowel disease; CBC = complete blood count; UA = urinalysis; LFTs = liver function tests.
Sources: Lake DF et al. 2007[5]; Imboden J et al. 2001[9]; American College of Rheumatology 2002[21]; Friedman S et al. 2005[25]; Goodin DS et al. 2002[60]; Klareskog L et al. 2006.[73]

the United States and mesalazine in European countries. Sulfasalazine (Azulfidine, Sulfadine) and other preparations of 5-aminosalicylic acid preparations (e.g., Canasa, Pentasa, Rowasa) have a direct anti-inflammatory effect on intestinal mucosa and connective tissue. The most likely mechanism of action of the **aminosalicylates** is through inhibition of nuclear factor κB (NF-κB) activation. NF-κB, which is normally in the cytoplasm of all cells, migrates to the nucleus and controls transcription of many of the genes that initiate the inflammatory process. When this factor is inactivated, multiple inflammatory pathways are affected within both cell and humoral-mediated responses and the cyclooxygenase-mediated inflammatory activity. Sulfasalazine (Azulfidine, Sulfadine) and mesalamine (Lialda) inhibit inflammation via inhibition of interleukin 1 (IL-1) and TNF-α production; inhibition of prostaglandin, leukotriene and cytokine activity; and impairment of leukocyte adhesion and function.[7]

Immunosuppressants

Antimetabolites

Antimetabolites are metabolite analogs that antagonize or inhibit the synthesis of nucleic acids. When the nucleic acids that are essential components of RNA or DNA are not made, then the proteins that the DNA and RNA are coded for cannot be made. The three most commonly used antimetabolites for autoimmune therapy are azathioprine (Azasan, Imuran), leflunomide (Arava), and methotrexate (Rheumatrex, Trexall) (Table 17-2).

Azathioprine (Azasan, Imuran) is a prodrug of mercaptopurine, which is a synthetic analog of purine and an inhibitor of purine synthesis. Purines are essential components of many biomolecules including DNA and RNA. The inhibition of purine synthesis leads to decreased production of B cells and T cells. The active metabolites of azathioprine are 6-mercaptopurine (6-MP) and 6-thioinosinic acid. Azathioprine inhibits cell- and humoral-mediated immune response and is cytotoxic to stimulated lymph cells.[5]

Leflunomide (Arava) inhibits dihydroorotate dehydrogenase, which ultimately interferes with new pyrimidine synthesis that in turn prevents proliferation of activated T cells. Its antiproliferative and anti-inflammatory effects are primarily due to suppression of cell-mediated immunity and inhibition of matrix metalloproteinase and osteoclasts.[8]

Methotrexate (Rheumatrex, Trexall) is a folic acid antagonist that inhibits the function of dihydrofolate reductase. Inhibition of dihydrofolate reductase results in functional folate deficiency. Because folate is a cofactor in DNA synthesis, cell proliferation is blocked, and cell death occurs. The mechanism of action in low-dose methotrexate therapy for autoimmune disorders is not completely

Table 17-2 Immunosuppressants Commonly Used to Treat Autoimmune Conditions

Drug Generic (Brand)	Uses	Adverse Effects	Precautions	Monitoring
Azathioprine (Azasan, Imuran)	MS SLE	Rash, fever, nausea, vomiting, diarrhea, jaundice, myelosuppression, pancytopenia, liver dysfunction, lymphoproliferative disorders	Preexisting liver disease, allopurinol (increases risk of toxicity), thiopurine methyltransferase (TMPT) deficiency (increases risk of myelotoxicity)	TMPT prior to therapy, LFTs, CBC, creatinine at baseline CBC every 1–2 weeks with change in dose, every 1–3 months with stable dose AST yearly Routine Pap smear
Cyclophosphamide (Cytoxan)	SLE	Amenorrhea, nausea, vomiting, alopecia, myelosuppression, myeloproliferative disorders, bladder carcinoma, electrolyte imbalance, hemorrhagic cystitis, secondary infertility Rare: Stevens-Johnson syndrome	Preexisting renal or liver dysfunction, leukopenia, or thrombocytopenia	CBC, UA at baseline and monthly Urine and cervical cytology annually for life
Cyclosporine (Sandimmune)	IBD MS SLE	Nausea, paresthesias, tremor, headaches, gingival hypertrophy, hair growth, anemia, liver function impairment, hyperglycemia, hyperkalemia, altered mental status, seizures Rare: hypertension, renal impairment, sepsis	Multiple drug interactions, hypomagnesemia (increases seizure risk) Antibiotic prophylaxis needed with concomitant immunosuppressant use Should not be used in hypertension, renal impairment, or severe infection	BP, LFTs, CBC, creatinine, uric acid, electrolyte panel at baseline Creatinine every 2 weeks until stable dose reached Serum drug concentration until stable dose reached then monthly Consider periodic CBC, LFTs, potassium
Hydroxychloroquine (Plaquenil)	RA SLE	Nausea, vomiting, diarrhea, abdominal pain, rash, nightmares, myopathy Rare: retinal toxicity/macular damage	Exposure ≥ 6.5 mg/kg per day or 10 years increases risk for retinal toxicity	Eye exams every 6 to 12 months
Leflunomide (Arava)	RA	Nausea, alopecia, rash, diarrhea, hypertension Rare: leukopenia, hepatitis, thrombocytopenia	Preexisting liver disease, viral hepatitis, alcoholism, severe immunodeficiency, rifampin Pregnancy (teratogenic-cholestyramine wash-out therapy prior to conception)	CBC, creatinine, LFTs every month for 6 months, then every 1–2 months Hepatitis B and C serology in at-risk persons
Methotrexate (Rheumatrex, Trexall)	IBD MS RA SLE	Nausea, mucositis, liver enzyme elevations, myelosuppression, liver and renal toxicity, hepatic fibrosis, interstitial pneumonitis	Pregnancy (teratogenic) Preexisting severe renal or liver impairment, significant lung disease, alcohol abuse	CBC, creatinine, LFTs every month for 6 months, then every 1–2 months Hepatitis B and C serology in at-risk persons
Mitoxantrone (Novantrone)	MS	Hair loss, nausea, vomiting, diarrhea, urinary tract infection, menstrual irregularities, blue-green urine and sclera (up to 24 h), acute myeloid leukemia, myelosuppression, hepatotoxicity, cardiotoxicity (risk increases with cumulative dose)	Liver impairment, significantly reduced left ventricular ejection fraction, maximum cumulative dose 140 mg/m²	CBC, LFTs, echocardiogram (baseline and routine)

RA = rheumatoid arthritis; SLE = systemic lupus erythematosus; IBD = inflammatory bowel disease; MS = multiple sclerosis; BP = blood pressure; CBC = complete blood count; VS = vital signs; LFTs = liver function tests; UA = urine analysis; TB = tuberculosis.
Sources: Lake DF et al. 2007[5]; Imboden J et al. 2001[9]; American College of Rheumatology 2002[21]; Friedman S et al. 2005[25]; Goodin DS et al. 2002[60]; Klareskog L et al. 2006.[73]

understood. Many in vivo and in vitro effects that may contribute to its potent anti-inflammatory effect have been observed. These actions include interference with adenosine-mediated inflammation, decreased cytokine and IgG production, and inhibited COX-2 activity.[8] The most likely pathway for these effects is through inhibition of aminoimidazole carboxamide ribonucleotide transformylase and thymidylate synthetase.[6] Methotrexate action in mitigating inflammatory bowel disease is not known.

Cyclophosphamide (Cytoxan) is a cytotoxic alkylating agent that induces cell death by transferring an alkyl group to the DNA of proliferating and resting lymphoid cells. Cyclosporine (Sandimmune) is a peptide antibiotic that inhibits the activation of T cells by interfering with the intracellular signaling pathway. Cyclosporine enters cells and binds to cytoplasmic cyclophilin, creating a cyclosporine-cyclophilin complex. This complex ultimately prevents translocation of nuclear factor of activated T cells in the nucleus of T cells, which prevents T-cell activation.[9] Cyclosporine selectively inhibits T-cell-mediated responses, including cytokine secretion.[10] Since cyclosporine does not block the action of already activated T cell or interaction with antigen, there is little risk of myelosuppression. Bioavailability of the drug is highly variable (20–50% of administered drug is absorbed) and due to P450 metabolism, risk of drug interaction is high.[5]

Hydroxychloroquine (Plaquenil) is an antimalarial agent. This agent has an anti-inflammatory action in rheumatic disease that may be attributed to interference with antigen presentation by antigen-presenting cells, T-cell response, antigen presentation, and deoxyribonucleotide synthesis.[6]

Mitoxantrone hydroxide (Novantrone) is a synthetic antineoplastic anthracenedione that inhibits DNA replication and repair and DNA-dependent RNA synthesis. As a result, mitoxantrone suppresses T-cell, B-cell, and macrophage proliferation and decreases secretion of proinflammatory cytokines.[11]

Immunomodulators/Biologic Agents

In recent years, genetically engineered agents that have selective immunomodulatory effects in autoimmune disorders have been developed (Table 17-3). Many of these therapies are used for only one specific disorder. However, some multiuse therapies have been studied and are indicated for more than one disorder.

Interferons (INFs) are cytokines that have antiviral, antiproliferative, and immunomodulatory activity. INF-βs are type I INFs produced by fibroblasts during the normal immune response to invading pathogens. Therapeutic action is most likely a result of reduced T-cell activation, modulated cytokine production, and inhibition of blood–brain barrier leakage.

Monoclonal antibodies are engineered antibodies that can be used to target specific areas and functions of the immune system. Monoclonal antibodies are formed by replacing non-antigen-specific components of murine monoclonal antibodies with comparable regions of human antibodies. Chimeric monoclonal antibodies have less complete replacement of the murine components than humanized monoclonal antibodies. The resulting hybrid monoclonal antibodies have less antigenicity and a longer half-life than complete murine antibodies.[5]

Natalizumab (Tysbri) is a humanized recombinant IgG4κ monoclonal antibody that binds to the surface of leukocytes, which blocks adhesion to vascular endothelium and subsequent transmigration of the leukocyte from the vasculature to the inflamed tissue.[12] Treatment with natalizumab (Tysbri) carries an increased risk of progressive multifocal leukoencephalopathy and is contraindicated for persons with history of or existing progressive multifocal leukoencephalopathy.[12] People being treated with natalizumab need to be monitored closely for signs and symptoms of progressive multifocal leukoencephalopathy.[13] Other opportunistic infections during natalizumab therapy are rare, but herpes reactivation and a case of cryptosporidial gastroenteritis have been reported.[14,15] Individuals meeting strict treatment criteria can enroll in the Tysabri Outreach: Unified Commitment to Health (TOUCH) Prescribing Program to begin natalizumab therapy. The TOUCH program was developed by Biogen Idec and Elan Pharmaceuticals to closely monitor natalizumab therapy and adverse effects. This program, created with input from the FDA, registers and monitors authorized prescribers, infusion centers, and pharmacies administering natalizumab.[16] Since the initiation of this program, there have been three cases of progressive multifocal leukoencephalopathy associated with natalizumab therapy, which correlates to one case per 10,000 patient years.[17,18] This risk is considerably lower than incidence reported in prior clinical trial data (1 in 1000; CI = 0.2–2.8 with mean treatment of 17.9 months).[19]

Rituximab (Rituxan) is a chimeric anti-CD20 monoclonal antibody that selectively depletes B cells. In vitro evidence suggests the following possible mechanisms of action: complement-mediated cytotoxicity, antibody-mediated cytotoxicity, and induction of programmed cell death. A small percentage of persons treated with rituximab develop anti-rituximab antibodies. The clinical significance of these antibodies is not well understood.[20]

Adalimumab (Humira) and infliximab (Remicade) are monoclonal antibodies that act as tumor necrosis factor-alpha (TNF-α) antagonists. TNF-α is an inflammatory cytokine involved in the pathogenesis of many chronic inflammatory diseases. Overexpression of TNF-α can cause an inflammatory response and local tissue damage. Blocking TNF-α activity results in suppression of IL-1, IL-6, and inflammatory adhesion molecules.[5]

Anti-TNF-α agents reduce inflammation through a variety of mechanisms. Infliximab (Remicade) is a chimeric monoclonal antibody that binds to TNF-α and TNF-β

Table 17-3 Immunomodulators and Biologics Commonly Used to Treat Autoimmune Disorders

Drug Generic (Brand)	Uses	Adverse Effects	Precautions	Monitoring
Abatacept (Orencia)	RA	Headache, nausea, upper respiratory infection, nasopharyngitis	Chronic obstructive pulmonary disease, use with biologics (serious infections, neoplasms)	Respiratory status
Adalimumab (Humira)	IBD	Headache, rash, nausea, infusion reactions, anemia, leukopenia, lymphoma, reactivation of infection, exacerbation of congestive heart failure	Preexisting congestive heart failure, diabetes, MS, renal failure	TB screen, infection at baseline CBC, ALT baseline and monthly until stable dose reached, then every 1–3 months
Infliximab (Remicade)	RA	Rare: new-onset demyelinating disease, exacerbation of MS, drug-induced lupus	Preexisting congestive heart failure, diabetes, MS, renal failure	TB screen, infection at baseline CBC, ALT baseline and monthly until stable dose reached, then every 1–3 months
Anakinra (Kineret)	RA	Injection site reaction, increased susceptibility to infection, headache dizziness, nausea	Asthma, chronic obstructive pulmonary disease (greater risk of pulmonary infections)	CBC monthly for 3 months, then every 3 months
Etanercept (Enbrel)	RA	Headache, rash, nausea, infusion reactions, anemia, leukopenia, lymphoma, reactivation of infection, exacerbation of congestive heart failure Rare: new-onset demyelinating disease, exacerbation of MS, drug-induced lupus	Preexisting congestive heart failure, diabetes, MS, renal failure	TB screen, infection at baseline CBC, ALT baseline and monthly until stable dose reached, then every 1–3 months
Glatiramer Acetate (Copaxone)	MS	Nausea, arthralgia, facial edema, pain at the injection site, postinjection reaction (within 30 min, benign chest pain, tachycardia, palpitations, anxiety)	Severe or prolonged postinjection reaction	Neurologic exam for MS status
Interferon β-1a (Avonex, Rebif)	MS	Injection site reaction, flulike symptoms, fever, malaise, fatigue, nausea, anorexia, dysrhythmias, seizures, depression, suicidal ideation	Preexisting cardiovascular disease, seizure disorder, or depression (may exacerbate condition)	Consider LFTs, CBC at baseline
Interferon β-1b (Betaseron)	MS	Injection site reaction, flulike symptoms, fever, malaise, fatigue, nausea, anorexia, dysrhythmias, seizures, depression, suicidal ideation Rare: injection site necrosis	Preexisting cardiovascular disease, seizure disorder, or depression (may exacerbate condition)	Consider LFTs, CBC at baseline
Natalizumab (Tysabri)	IBD MS	Skin irritation, arthralgia, headache, fatigue Serious: PML	Not for use in persons with history of or existing PML; not for concomitant use with other immunosuppressants	Signs and symptoms of PML, opportunistic infections, CBC
Rituximab (Rituxan)	RA	Moderate to severe infusion reactions, severe mucocutaneous eruption, failure to response to vaccines	Preexisting cardiac arrhythmias, SLE, hepatitis B infection	CBC, vital signs during infusion

MS = multiple sclerosis; PML = progressive multifocal leukoencephalopathy; IBD = inflammatory bowel disease; RA = rheumatoid arthritis; TB = tuberculosis; CBC = complete blood count; ALT = alanine aminotransferase; LFTs = liver function tests.
Sources: Lake DF et al. 2007[5]; Imboden J et al. 2001[9]; American College of Rheumatology 2002[21]; Friedman S et al. 2005[25]; Goodin DS et al. 2002[60]; Klareskog L et al. 2006.[73]

and reduces activity through lysis of TNF-producing cells. Adalimumab is a humanized monoclonal antibody that binds to TNF-α, preventing interaction with its receptors.

Rarely, some individuals develop anti-TNF-α antibodies and antinuclear antibodies (ANA). Antibodies to infliximab (Remicade) may decrease the clinical benefit of infliximab (Remicade) therapy. Concomitant administration of methotrexate (Rheumatrex, Trexall) reduces anti-infliximab antibody formation. Antibodies to adalimumab have been reported rarely.[8]

Other Biologic Agents

Other engineered immunomodulators used in treating autoimmune disorders stimulate or block immune response by imitating naturally occurring biomolecular activities in the immune cascade. This is currently the area of greatest research and development for treatment of autoimmune disorders.

Abatacept (Orencia) is a fusion protein composed of a human immunoglobulin component and cytotoxic T lymphocyte-associated antigen 4 (CTLA-4). Abatacept binds to the B7 receptor (CD 80/86) on **antigen-presenting cells** with high affinity and prevents binding by CD28 receptors on T cells. Through this competitive binding, abatacept blocks T-cell activation and prevents subsequent cytokine release.[5]

Anakinra (Kineret) is a recombinant human form of interleukin-1 receptor antagonist (IL-1Ra) that competitively binds to the IL-1 receptor and prevents the activation of target cells and cytokine-mediated inflammation.[5,21]

Etanercept (Enbrel) is a dimeric recombinant fusion protein of human TNF receptor bound to human IgG_1, which binds competitively to TNF-α and TNF-β receptors.[5] Etanercept acts as a TNF antagonist and has similar efficacy and side effect profiles as the anti-TNF-α monoclonal antibodies.

Glatiramer acetate (Copaxone) is a synthetic amino acid polypeptide composed of glutamine, lysine, alanine, and tyrosine. Glatiramer acetate was initially developed to mimic myelin basic protein and induce an MS-like condition in experimental animal models.[22] Instead, glatiramer acetate prevented disease development in the animals that were inoculated. Through competitively binding to major histocompatibility complex-class II molecules and inducing glatiramer acetate-reactive suppressor T-cells, glatiramer acetate inhibits myelin-reactive T cells and mediates bystander suppression in the central nervous system (CNS).[23,24]

Inflammatory Bowel Disease

Inflammatory bowel disease (IBD) includes two related but distinct gastrointestinal (GI) disorders: ulcerative colitis and Crohn's disease. The latter may affect the entire GI tract from the mouth to the anus, but those affected primarily have intestinal disease, including ileitis (30–40%), ileocolitis (40–55%), and colitis (15–25%).[25] Ulcerative colitis affects the mucosa of the large intestine and almost always involves the rectum with proximal extension that involves all or part of the colon, such as proctosigmoiditis (30–50%), left-sided colitis (30–40%), or total colitis (20%).[25]

The exact cause of inflammatory dysregulation in the intestines of persons with IBD is unknown, but a general imbalance between pro- and anti-inflammatory mediators exists. Exogenous pathogens may trigger the initial inflammatory response that goes uncontrolled, or the person's body may perceive normal intestinal flora as a pathogen. In Crohn's disease, activated T cells secrete inflammatory cytokines, induce inflammatory B cells and macrophages, and recruit lymphocytes to the intestine.[25] Interleukin-1, TNF and INF-γ production is increased. Transmural tissue damage results from the local cytokine activity and may result in mucosal inflammation and ulceration, structuring, fistulas, and abscess formation. In ulcerative colitis, T-cell activation may also play a role in the development of superficial mucosal inflammation, a characteristic of the disease.[25]

Epidemiology and Natural History

Approximately 1.4 million people in the United States suffer from IBD, with incidence rates of 7 and 11 per 100,000 for Crohn's disease and ulcerative colitis, respectively.[25,26] The highest incidences of IBD are seen in the United States, United Kingdom, and northern Europe. Incidence is lower in southern and central Europe, Africa, South America, Asia, and Australia.[25,26] In recent years, rates in low-prevalence areas have been on the rise while rates in historically high-prevalence areas have stabilized.[26] There is a slight predominance of women with Crohn's disease and men with ulcerative colitis. Disease activity typically presents during adolescence and young adulthood with a possible second peak between the sixth and eighth decades of life.[26] While associated with significant morbidity, IBD has only a modest impact on mortality. Higher mortality rate in IBD is seen in the earliest and latest years of disease, the later due to the increased risk of colon cancer.[25]

Multiple factors play a role in the development of IBD. Genetic studies of affected populations have identified several possible susceptibility genes, and three distinct polymorphisms of gene CARD15 have been associated with IBD.[27] Genetic influence is further supported by concordance and familial studies.[28,29] There is a 10% lifetime risk to a first-degree relative with IBD. Children of parents with IBD carry a 36% risk of developing the disease.[25] Likely environmental factors include appendectomy (may decrease risk of ulcerative colitis) and cigarette smoking (mixed effect). There appears to be an inverse relationship between cigarette smoking and ulcerative colitis. Current smokers are less likely than nonsmokers to have ulcerative colitis while ex-smokers have greater risk of disease. In Crohn's disease, cigarette smoking, recent or current, increases risk of disease.[26] Studies have failed to demonstrate any connection between dietary intake and risk of IBD.

Disease Classification

Disease activity in ulcerative colitis and Crohn's disease is classified based on clinical symptoms and/or response to therapy.[25,30] Ulcerative colitis and Crohn's disease have both active and quiescent disease states.

Presentation and Diagnosis

Typical presenting symptoms of IBD include diarrhea, fever, bloody stools, and abdominal pain or cramping. Additional history and physical examination data can lead to a diagnosis of either ulcerative colitis or Crohn's disease in approximately 85–90% of cases.[25] In the remaining cases it may be impossible to differentiate between ulcerative colitis and Crohn's disease, and a diagnosis of indeterminate colitis is made (Table 17-4 and Table 17-5).

Ulcerative colitis almost always involves the rectal mucosa, leading to gross blood and mucus in stools. Those affected also may report tenesmus, colicky abdominal pain, and constipation, particularly if ulcerative colitis involves only the distal portion of the colon. Abdominal pain and diarrhea increase in frequency and severity as ulcerative colitis spreads proximally. Endoscopy reveals continuous or nearly continuous mucosal involvement, and biopsy findings are negative. Hemorrhage, toxic megacolon, and intestinal perforation are rare but possible complications of severe attacks in ulcerative colitis.

Crohn's disease most frequently involves the small bowel and the proximal end of the colon. The rectum is rarely involved in Crohn's disease, but anal fissures and perianal abscesses are common. Abdominal pain is often severe, and persons affected may report symptoms of intestinal obstruction. Ten percent of women with Crohn's disease colitis will have rectovaginal fistulas resulting in significant morbidity and distress.[25] Endoscopic evaluation reveals patchy and irregular ulcers, fistulas, and lesions. Strictures,

Table 17-4 Classification of Disease Severity in Inflammatory Bowel Disease

Classification	Ulcerative Colitis
Mild	Fewer than four bowel movements a day with small amount of blood and mild anemia without fever or tachycardia
Moderate	Four to six moderately bloody stools a day with fever, tachycardia, and often anemia
Severe	More than six grossly bloody stools daily with fever, tachycardia, and anemia
Remission	Asymptomatic (spontaneous or in response to medical or surgical treatment)
Classification	**Crohn's Disease**
Mild to moderate	Ambulatory without dehydration, high fever, abdominal tenderness, mass, or obstruction and is able to tolerate oral intake
Moderate to severe	Treatment failure for mild to moderate disease or presence of prominent symptoms (fever, weight loss, abdominal pain or tenderness, nausea, vomiting, anemia)
Severe fulminant	Continued symptoms despite steroid therapy or presence of high fever, persistent vomiting, intestinal obstruction, rebound tenderness, cachexia, or abscess
Remission	Asymptomatic (spontaneous or in response to medical or surgical treatment)

Sources: Adapted from Friedman S et al. 2008[25]; Hanauer SB et al. 2001.[30]

Table 17-5 Clinical Differences Between Ulcerative Colitis and Crohn's Disease

Clinical Feature	Ulcerative Colitis (UC)	Crohn's Disease (CD)
Mucus, blood in stool	Often	Rarely
Systemic symptoms	Sometimes	Often
Rectal sparing	No	Often
Perianal involvement	Rarely	Often
Continuous bowel involvement	Yes	No
Small bowel involvement	No	Often
ANCA-positive	Often	Rarely
ASCA-positive	Rarely	Often
Depth of inflammation	Shallow into the mucosa	May be transmural and deep into tissues
Endoscopic findings	Continuous ulcers	Linear and serpiginous (snakelike) ulcers

ANCA = antineutrophil cytoplasmic antibodies; ASCA = anti-Saccharomyces cerevisiae antibodies.
Source: Adapted from Friedman S and Blumberg RS.[25]

fistulas, and abscesses are typical findings on radiographic examination, particularly in severe disease.

Serologic markers can play an important role in ulcerative colitis and Crohn's disease diagnosis and differentiation. Perinuclear antineutrophil cytoplasmic antibodies (pANCAs) and anti-*Saccharomyces cerevisiae* antibodies (ASCAs) are present among persons with IBD at greater frequencies than in the general population. Perinuclear antineutrophil cytoplasmic antibodies are more frequently found in persons with ulcerative colitis while anti-*Saccharomyces cerevisiae* antibodies are more common among individuals with Crohn's disease. Performing these tests in combination results in sensitivity, specificity, and positive predictive values of 57%, 97%, and 92.5%, respectively, for ulcerative colitis and 49%, 97%, and 96%, respectively, for Crohn's disease.[31] Other autoantibodies have been identified in sera of persons with IBD but do not play a role in diagnosis or management of the disease.

Approximately one third of all persons with IBD have at least one extraintestinal manifestation of disease. Persons with perianal Crohn's disease are more likely than persons with other types of IBD to have disease activity in other systems.[25] Systems most frequently affected are dermatologic, rheumatologic, ocular, hepatobiliary, urologic, and cardiopulmonary. Extraintestinal attacks may occur in conjunction with disease activity or during periods of remission.

Complications and Comorbidity

IBD that is unresponsive to pharmacotherapy may require surgical treatment. More than half of ulcerative colitis sufferers with extensive disease will undergo surgery within 10 years of diagnosis.[25] Surgical intervention may be through postcolectomy and ileostomy placement or through mucosal dissection and creation of an ileal pouch. The latter is effective in preserving continence. The most common complications of surgery are hemorrhage, sepsis, and neural injury. Nearly all persons with Crohn's disease will have surgery during the course of their disease; there is a 50% chance of surgery in persons who have Crohn's disease colitis and an 80% chance in persons with Crohn's disease who have small bowel involvement.[25] Surgical therapy in Crohn's disease may include small bowel resection, stricturoplasty, or postcolectomy with ileostomy depending on disease location and severity. Complications may include hemorrhage, fistula, abscess, leakage, restructure, short bowel, and recurrence.

IBD disease and therapy can impact body image and sexuality. Negative body image can result from fecal incontinence, extraintestinal manifestations of disease, or presence of a stoma or ostomy bag. Women with Crohn's disease may experience dyspareunia and sexual difficulties related to rectovaginal fistula, perianal abscess, surgical scarring, or fear of pain or embarrassment.

Pharmacologic Therapies for Inflammatory Bowel Disease

Overall, treatment of IBD includes dietary changes and medications. Counseling and support groups may be helpful for some individuals dealing with the psychosocial and emotional impact of IBD. Pharmacologic therapy is individualized and dependent upon disease location, severity, and coexisting complications. Figure 17-3 shows the various targets for pharmacologic agents. Most medications fall into one of the following categories: anti-inflammatories, immunosuppressants, and immunomodulators/biologic agents (Table 17-6).

Anti-Inflammatories

Within the category off anti-inflammatory agents, aminosalicylates are first-line therapies for the induction and maintenance of remission in mild to moderate ulcerative colitis and induction therapy in distal Crohn's disease. Choice of specific preparation depends on disease location. Glucocorticoids are generally used for active IBD, particularly if it is unresponsive to first-line aminosalicylates therapy. Other immunosuppressants and immunomodulators are reserved for refractory IBD or severe Crohn's disease.

Aminosalicylates

The mainstay of IBD therapy is 5-aminosalicylic acid, also named mesalamine (Asacol, Canasa, Pentassa, Rowasa). However, when administered orally, 5-aminosalicylic acid is rapidly absorbed in the jejunum, and therefore, effectiveness in treating distal small bowel or colonic disease is significantly limited. By changing the chemical structure of 5-aminosalicylic acid, direct delivery can be achieved. The first agent developed for bowel delivery of 5-aminosalicylic acid was sulfasalazine (Azulfidine).

Sulfasalazine (Azulfidine) is partially absorbed in the small intestine and broken down into its active sulfa and 5-aminosalicylic acid moieties in the colon. This direct delivery increases the therapeutic effects for persons with IBD. Sulfa hypersensitivity reactions and side effects, however, limit its use for many individuals.

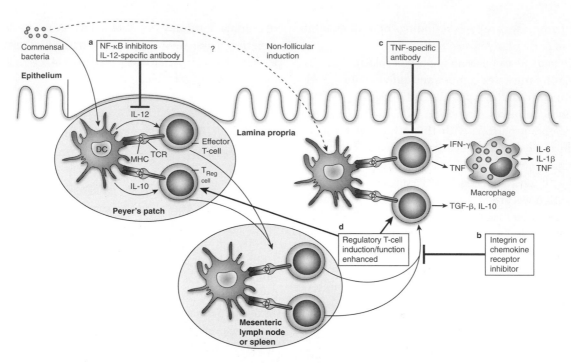

General pathogenesis of mucosal inflammation in inflammatory bowel disease and potential points of therapeutic intervention. (a) Secretion of inductive cytokines such as IL-12 or IL-13 can be inhibited with nuclear factor κB (NF-κB) inhibitors or with cytokine-specific monoclonal antibodies. This can occur in the mucosal follicle as shown or at other sites. (b) The traffic of effector cells into the lamina propria can be blocked by inhibitors or monoclonal antibodies specific for integrins or chemokine receptors involved in homing. (c) TNF expressed on the surface of effector cells can be crosslinked by antibodies specific for TNF leading to apoptosis of the effector cell. (d) Regulatory T-cell induction or function could be enhanced so as to counteract effector T-cell function. This can be achieved by the delivery of vectors that encode for regulatory cytokines.

Figure 17-3 Overview of therapeutic targets in inflammatory bowel disease. *Source:* Reprinted with permission from Bouma G et al. 2003.[135]

The newer sulfa-free 5-aminosalicylic acids (i.e., mesalamine, olsalazine, balsalazide) have similar efficacy to sulfasalazine with fewer side effects.[25] The drug is delivered to specific areas of the GI tract depending on their preparation. Azo-bonded olsalazine (Dipentum) and balsalazide (Colazal) are activated by bond-cleaving bacteria in the colon. Enteric-coated mesalamine (Asacol) disintegrates from the small bowel to the splenic fissure and is effective in treating ulcerative colitis and Crohn's disease involving the ileum or colon. Continuous-release mesalamine (Pentasa) delivers 5-aminosalicylic acid throughout the small bowel to the distal colon. Topical preparations (Canasa) and enemas (e.g., Rowasa) are effective in treating proctitis and distal colonic disease[25] and may be more effective in treating active ulcerative colitis or proctitis than oral agents or topical steroid preparations.[32] Remission rates with topical 5-aminosalicylic acid preparations range from 75% to 90% at 6 months and from 61% to 90% at 12 months.[32]

Effectiveness of aminosalicylate maintenance therapy in Crohn's disease colitis and ileocolitis is unclear. It is possible that 5-aminosalicylic acid agents will reduce postoperative recurrence of Crohn's disease. Continued therapy in ulcerative colitis may decrease future risk of colon cancer.[33]

Glucocorticoids

Glucocorticoids, such as prednisone (Deltasone), methylprednisolone (Medrol), and budesonide (Entocort) are effective in rapidly reducing disease activity and inducing remission in IBD. Their use is generally reserved for moderate to severe disease or mild to moderate Crohn's disease that has not responded to first-line therapy (salicylates).[34] Mild to moderate Crohn's disease may be treated with steroid therapy in specific instances. Ileal-release budesonide (Entocort) is indicated for ileal or right-sided colonic Crohn's disease, while topical preparations (budesonide or hydrocortisone) are preferred for distal colonic inflammation.[34] Oral preparations are sufficient for therapy in all cases except unresponsive or fulminant IBD. In this case, hospitalization and treatment with parenteral glucocorticoids are recommended. If intestinal obstruction or abscess is suspected, a CT scan should be obtained before parenteral steroid administration since intravenous steroids should be withheld in the case of abscess.

Once remission is achieved, the oral dose should be slowly tapered in accordance with disease activity.

Table 17-6 Medications Used in the Treatment of Inflammatory Bowel Disease

Drug Generic (Brand)	Dose	Indications
Balsalazide (Colazal)	2.25 to 6.75 g PO qd	Mild to moderate UC (induction and maintenance) Colonic CD (induction only)
Olsalazine (Dipentum)	1–3 g PO qd	Mild to moderate UC (induction and maintenance) Colonic CD (induction only)
Sulfasalazine (Azulfidine)	4 to 8 g PO qd, then 2 to 6 g PO qd	Mild to moderate UC (induction and maintenance) Colonic CD (induction only)
Budesonide, ileal release (Entocort EC)	9 mg PO qd for 2 to 3 months, then taper	Ileocecal CD (induction, short-term maintenance)
Mesalamine, enteric coated (Asacol)	2.4 to 4.8 g PO qd, then 1.6 to 4.8 g PO qd (continue at higher doses for CD)	Distal UC (induction and maintenance) Ileocolonic CD (induction only)
Mesalamine, topical enema (Rowasa) Suppository (Canasa)	4 g PR qd or q hs 1000 mg supp PR qd or q hs 500 mg supp PR bid–tid	Active distal UC/proctitis (induction and maintenance)
Mesalamine, sustained release (Pentasa)	2 to 4 g PO qd, then 1.4 to 4 g PO qd	Extensive UC (induction and maintenance) Active CD (induction, postoperative prophylaxis)
Methotrexate (Rheumatrex, Trexall)	15–25 mg IM q wk	Active CD steroid dependent Chronic active CD (induction and maintenance)
Prednisone (Delacort)	40 to 60 mg PO qd for 7–14 d, then taper by 2.5 to 5 mg/wk	Active IBD Active UC, 5-ASA refractory (induction only)
Methylprednisolone (Medrol)	40 to 60 mg IV qd	Active IBD, PO steroid refractory Severe IBD (induction only)
Azathioprine (Azasan, Imuran)	2 to 3 mg/kg PO qd	Severe IBD to reduce steroid dose
Cyclosporine (Sandimmune)	2–4 mg/kg IV qd	Fulminant UC, steroid refractory Fistulizing CD (induction only)
Infliximab (Remicade)	5 mg/kg IV at 0, 2, and 6 wks, then q 8 wks (slow infusion over 2 h)	Moderate to severe IBD, therapy resistant/intolerant (induction and maintenance)
Adalimumab (Humira)	160 mg SC week 1, 80 mg SC week 2, then 40 mg SC q 2 wks	Moderate to severe, active CD, therapy resistant/intolerant (induction and maintenance)
Natalizumab (Tysbri)	300 mg IV q 28 d (infused slowly over 1 h)	Moderate to severe CD, refractory (induction and maintenance)

UC = ulcerative colitis; CD = Crohn's disease; IBD = inflammatory bowel disease.
Sources: Loftus EV 2004[26]; Clark M et al. 2007.[35]

Glucocorticoids have no benefit in maintenance therapy for IBD. After induction, maintenance with salicylates or immunomodulators should be considered based on overall disease status.[34] If the agents can be tapered successfully, the daily dose can be reduced to 20 mg in 4 to 5 weeks and discontinued after several months.[25] Inability to taper is an indication for parenteral steroid therapy.

Immunosuppressants

Azathioprine (Azasan, Imuran) and 6-Mercaptopurine (Purinethol)

Azathioprine (Azasan, Imuran) and 6-mercaptopurine (Purinethol) are treatment options for individuals with refractory disease. For persons with chronic, severe IBD that is steroid resistant or tolerant, azathioprine or 6-mercaptopurine may provide relief of symptoms and allow for steroid tapering without relapse. Azathioprine and 6-mercaptopurine are effective for maintenance in Crohn's disease, but effectiveness in ulcerative colitis has not been confirmed. Azathioprine or 6-mercaptopurine therapy for persons who have Crohn's disease and are postoperative may prevent disease recurrence.[34]

Cyclosporine (Sandimmune)

Cyclosporine (Sandimmune) has a faster onset of action than azathioprine (Azasan, Imuran) or 6-mercaptopurine (Purinethol) and is effective in treating severe refractory ulcerative colitis. Intravenous administration induces remission in severe ulcerative colitis and may provide an alternative to colectomy.[25] After clinical response is achieved, cyclosporine can be orally used in short-term maintenance of ulcerative colitis, until slower acting azathioprine or 6-mercaptopurine can take effect. Intravenous cyclosporine is effective for induction in persons who have fistulizing Crohn's disease, but oral maintenance therapy is not appropriate as disease often reflares. Azathioprine or 6-mercaptopurine must be used for maintenance.[34]

Significant toxicity may result with cyclosporine (Sandimmune) therapy. Individuals should be monitored for renal dysfunction, and if creatinine levels are elevated, cyclosporine should be given at a lower dose or discontinued.[25]

Methotrexate (Rheumatrex, Trexall)

Methotrexate (Rheumatrex, Trexall) is indicated for use in chronic active Crohn's disease, but its use in ulcerative colitis is not supported.[34] For individuals who are steroid dependent, methotrexate administration allows for steroid tapering and induction and maintenance of remission. The role of liver biopsy in chronic methotrexate therapy is not clear. The American Gastroenterological Association Institute recommends either liver biopsy or discontinuing methotrexate in persons with persistently abnormal liver function tests.[34]

Immunomodulators/Biologic Agents

The primary biologic agents used in the treatment of IBD are tumor necrosis factor-alpha (TNF-α) antagonists, infliximab (Remicade), and adalimumab (Humira). These agents reduce inflammation in intestinal mucosa by blocking the proinflammatory action of TNF-α. Natalizumab (Tysbri), a selective adhesion molecule inhibitor, blocks adhesion and migration of leukocytes into the gut, thereby reducing inflammation.

Infliximab (Remicade)

Infliximab (Remicade) is extremely effective for the treatment of severe, refractory fistulizing Crohn's disease. Use is also indicated for severe active ulcerative colitis in persons who are nonresponsive or intolerant to conventional therapies.[35] Lawson et al.[36] conducted a meta-analysis of seven randomized trials that tested the efficacy of anti-TNF-blocking agents and found that in persons who have moderate to severe ulcerative colitis, infliximab (three intravenous infusions at 0, 2, and 6 weeks) was more effective than placebo in inducing clinical remission (RR = 3.22; 95% CI, 2.18–4.76).

When remission is achieved with infliximab (Remicade), steroids should be tapered and individuals should receive maintenance therapy. Scheduled therapy is more effective at maintaining remission than episodic therapy. If people receiving induction therapy fail to respond, additional treatment is not recommended.[34] Some individuals may develop antibodies to infliximab and lose response to therapy. In these situations, an increased dose may be administered and therapeutic response may be restored. Concomitant administration of azathioprine (Azasan, Imuran), 6-mercaptopurine (Purinethol), or methotrexate (Rheumatrex, Trexall) and scheduled infusion therapy may reduce antibody development.[35]

Adalimumab (Humira)

Adalimumab (Humira) is effective for induction and maintenance of remission in moderate to severe and extraintestinal Crohn's disease. Data are insufficient to support use in ulcerative colitis.[35] Subcutaneous administration of adalimumab is a potential advantage over infliximab for those who prefer self-administration. No studies have been conducted to compare the two therapies directly, but it appears that both medications have similar results in disease treatment.

Adalimumab (Humira) may be given to those individuals who have poor outcomes with infliximab (lose response, develop antibodies, or experience infusion reaction). Reported rates of anti-adalimumab antibodies are lower than with infliximab.[35] In a recent trial of adalimumab in Crohn's disease, therapy was generally well tolerated, and there were no cases of serious infection, tuberculosis, lupus-like syndrome, or lymphoma.[37] These complications, however, have been reported with adalimumab use in other diseases.

Natalizumab (Tysbri)

Natalizumab (Tysbri) may be effective for inducing and maintaining remission in some persons with moderate to severe active Crohn's disease. Use should be reserved for those who have confirmed, active Crohn's disease intolerant or refractory to other immunomodulator therapy and for whom surgery is not an option.[35]

Some people using natalizumab (Tysbri) may experience colitis or worsening Crohn's disease. One case of progressive multifocal leukoencephalopathy has been reported with concomitant azathioprine therapy.[38] Natalizumab may be particularly beneficial in individuals who have not responded to conventional therapy or infliximab (Remicade)[39]; however, potential benefits must be weighed against risk of progressive multifocal leukoencephalopathy (approximately 1 in 1000).[35] Screening for the virus may identify individuals at greater risk for progressive multifocal leukoencephalopathy.

Lifestyle Modifications

There is no evidence that IBD is caused or affected by dietary factors, and there are no dietary modifications that impact the course of disease. Individual diet changes may be indicated for the management of symptoms during exacerbations. A low-residue diet should be followed during periods of acute inflammation to decrease intestinal pain and possibly promote healing. Crohn's disease ileitis or ileocolitis is associated with indigestion and malabsorption. Supplementation or enteral nutrition should be provided to individuals with extensive small bowel involvement. Vitamin B_{12} injections may be necessary for some people with Crohn's disease ileitis. Other supplementations may be indicated for deficiencies associated with disease therapy. Adequate hydration is important, especially if significant diarrhea occurs.[40]

Complementary, Alternative, and Adjuvant Therapies

Alternative therapies investigated for treatment of IBD focus on reducing inflammation and altering the gastrointestinal environment. This approach is reasonable since disease may be triggered by an inappropriate immune response to intestinal pathogens. Studies involving antibiotics, probiotics, and prebiotics have yielded inconclusive results.[41]

Several small studies have suggested that acupuncture, *Boswellia serrata* (frankincense), traditional Chinese medicine, and digestive herbal therapies (*Aloe vera* and wheat grass juice) may improve measures of disease activity during exacerbations.[42] Safety and efficacy data for these therapies are lacking, particularly when used in conjunction with conventional therapy.

Special Populations

Pregnancy and Breastfeeding

Women with inactive IBD have normal rates of fertility. Women with active Crohn's disease have a slightly higher rate of spontaneous abortion.[43] Reproductive complications may develop secondary to fallopian tube scarring, rectovaginal fistulae, or perianal abscess found associated with inflammatory Crohn's disease.

Rates of stillbirth and neonatal death are not increased in women who have IBD; however, they do have an increased risk of preterm delivery and low-birth-weight infants.[43,44] This may be due to common underlying mechanisms or systemic effects of inflammation associated with IBD.[45] Elbaz et al.[46] found that IBD is an independent risk factor for preterm birth and reported a twofold increase in preterm birth among women with IBD when compared to non-IBD control subjects (OR = 2.0; 95% CI, 1.2–3.5; P = .012). Preterm birth is slightly more common in women who have Crohn's disease than in those with ulcerative colitis.[45,46]

Persons with Crohn's disease are more likely to smoke cigarettes than are persons with ulcerative colitis or the general population.[26] As cigarette smoking is an independent risk factor for preterm birth and low-birth-weight infants, women with Crohn's disease should be counseled about this effect.

The course of ulcerative colitis and Crohn's disease during pregnancy is related to disease activity at conception. It is best to plan pregnancy, if possible, during periods of disease quiescence.[25,43] Remission may be more difficult to induce during pregnancy. If disease is in remission prior to conception, it will likely remain inactive. Pregnancy has little effect on disease activity and progress.[43]

Medications used to treat IBD appear to be safe during pregnancy with the exception of methotrexate (Rheumatrex, Trexall), an FDA Pregnancy Category X, antifolate drug with known teratogenic and abortifacient effects. Sulfasalazine (Azulfidine) therapy is not associated with increased fetal anomalies or spontaneous abortion; however, folic acid supplementation is recommended for women using sulfasalazine in pregnancy due to its interference with folic acid absorption.[43,47] As in nonpregnant women, therapeutic selection of sulfasalazine (Azulfidine), mesalamine, and glucocorticoid preparations should be made based on disease severity and location. Due to lack of data on newer biologic agents, they are not recommended as first-line therapy during pregnancy.[43,47] There are, however, no data to support withholding biologic agents if clearly needed.

If disease is in remission with maintenance therapy, medication should be continued throughout pregnancy. Most disease flares during pregnancy are due to treatment withdrawal. Poorer obstetric outcomes seem to result from increased disease activity rather than from pharmacologic therapy.[35] Route of delivery in IBD should generally be determined on the basis of obstetric factors. Episiotomy may be performed in women with Crohn's disease if indicated for obstetric reasons, provided they do not have active perianal disease.[43] Persons with Crohn's disease who have fistulizing disease and perineal abscess may have better outcomes with cesarean section.[25]

Breastfeeding is not contraindicated for women with IBD. Sulfasalazine (Azulfidine), mesalamine, and steroids can be used during lactation. Aminosalicylates may cause watery diarrhea in breastfeeding infants, but this reaction reverses when the drug is discontinued. Slow growth has been reported in infants exposed to olsalazine (Dipentum) and should be used with caution in women who are breastfeeding. Although no adverse effects have been reported, the manufacturers of azathi-oprine (Azasan, Imuran), and 6-mercaptopurine (Purinethol) advise against use during lactation.[43] Due to concerns about impaired growth, carcinogenesis, immune suppression, and neutropenia, cyclosporine, cyclophosphamide, and methotrexate should be avoided during lactation.[48]

Effective contraception should be used by all women on methotrexate and those with active disease. Choice of contraceptive is not affected by IBD itself but by potential complications of disease or therapy. Women using long-term steroid therapy should have bone density evaluation before initiation of depot medroxyprogesterone acetate (DMPA) injection. Combined oral contraceptives are effective for women with large bowel disease but may have reduced efficacy for women with small bowel disease or malabsorption. Despite previous reports, combined oral contraceptives are not implicated in the pathogenicity of ulcerative colitis, and use is not contraindicated.[49]

Elderly

Menopause does not appear to influence or be influenced by the activity of IBD. Hormone therapy may decrease disease activity in the postmenopausal period due to the anti-inflammatory effects of estrogen. Postmenopausal osteoporosis is more prevalent in women with IBD than in the general population. This may be related to use of glucocorticoids, disease activity, and lifestyle factors. Many women with IBD are physically less active due to the symptoms of IBD flare and may suffer from malnutrition related to malabsorption or long-term avoidance of dairy products.

Postmenopausal women should have bone mineral density scans, especially if there are other risk factors for osteoporosis present.

Multiple Sclerosis

Multiple sclerosis (MS) is a chronic inflammatory, demyelinating autoimmune disorder of the central nervous system. In the early, inflammatory course of MS, autoreactive T cells cross the blood–brain barrier attacking myelin proteins leading to local inflammation and axonal demyelination. As the inflammatory process continues, macrophages and microglial cells contribute to the local autoreactive response. In the earlier phases of MS, remyelination may follow, but repeated injury results in astrocytes proliferation and gliosis forming the characteristic plaques or lesions of MS, and neurodegeneration follows[50] (Figure 17-4).

Epidemiology and Natural History

MS affects approximately 350,000 persons in the United States and over 1 million worldwide.[51] The onset of disease typically occurs between 20 and 40 years of age with nearly twice as many women affected as men. Greater prevalence of disease is seen in northern areas of North America and western Europe and is less common in Asia, the Middle East, and equatorial Africa.[1,51]

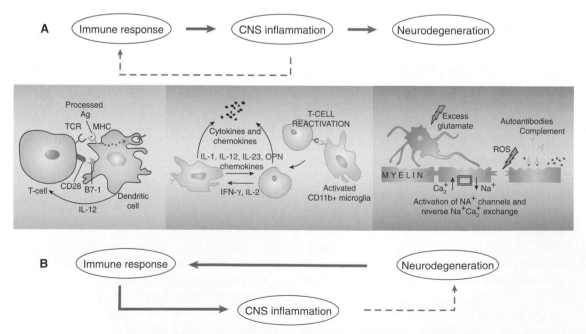

(A) The traditional neuropathological view of MS highlights CNS injury as a consequence of an autoimmune response. (B) An alternative hypothesis proposes that activation of autoimmune cells occurs as a consequence of toxic insults to CNS cells. Infections, for example, may be asymptomatic but cause cytopathic effects to target cells in the course of an antiviral response. The prolonged release of neural antigens may then induce inflammatory responses.

Figure 17-4 Models of disease pathogenesis in multiple sclerosis. *Source:* Reprinted with permission from Hauser SL et al. 2006.[50]

The disease burden of MS varies greatly. Given the variability of disease onset, severity, and progression, it is difficult to predict the overall disease course of an individual with MS. Relapsing-remitting MS has a better prognosis than progressive forms of the disease. Prognosis is relatively good when initial symptoms are visual or sensory rather than motor, relapses are infrequent, and full recovery is enjoyed between clinically active periods.[51,52] Overall, 10–20% of persons with MS may remain relatively unimpaired 20 years after diagnosis. Long-term follow-up studies have found that 30–50% of individuals will have some degree of disability within the first 10 years of disease onset while approximately 90% will have significant disability after 25 years of disease.[53]

Disease Classification

In 1996, the National Multiple Sclerosis Society developed a standardized terminology for classifying MS disease based on clinical criteria (Table 17-7).[54] Disease progression is quantified through neurologic examination and scoring with the Kurtzke Expanded Disability Status Scale.[55] Grading is based on functional status, ambulatory ability, use of assisted devices and distance walked. The nonlinear rating scale ranges from 0 (normal exam) to 10 (death due to MS).

Presentation and Diagnosis

Diagnosing MS remains a challenge due to variability in presentation and course of the disease and the lack of definitive diagnostic tests. Most individuals who are eventually diagnosed with MS, particularly relapsing-remitting multiple sclerosis (RRMS), have an initial demyelinating episode, or clinically isolated syndrome, resulting in visual or sensory deficit. An MRI of the brain and spinal column after a clinically isolated syndrome will give important prognostic and diagnostic information. A normal MRI suggests a low risk (< 20%) of developing MS, whereas an abnormal MRI (T_2-weighted lesions or gadolinium-enhancing lesions identified) suggests high risk for future MS.[51,56] Diagnosis of clinical-definite MS requires an additional clinical episode and/or evidence of disease progression (new lesions on MRI).

The International Panel on the Diagnosis of Multiple Sclerosis developed and revised guidelines for diagnosing MS incorporating MRI with other paraclinical studies and neurologic history and examination findings.[57] These criteria are 83% sensitive and specific for MS diagnosis within 36 months of a clinically isolated syndrome.[56] Clinical presentation and dissemination of lesions in space and time (increase in number of MRI lesions over time or lesions found in previously unaffected areas) continue to be the cornerstone of diagnosis. In the absence of MRI and ancillary testing, MS can still be reliably diagnosed by an experienced clinician.[57]

Therapy for Persons with Multiple Sclerosis

The goal of MS therapy is to prevent clinical relapse and postpone neurodegeneration and the subsequent accumulation of disability. Current therapies have had some success in reducing relapses, but few have been shown effective in slowing disease when in the progressive phase (primary progressive and secondary progressive). Acute MS exacerbations are generally treated with glucocorticoids while biologic agents (interferons or glatiramer acetate) are the first-line therapies for prophylactic treatment of clinically isolated syndromes and maintenance therapy in RRMS. Immunosuppressant therapy may be initiated for persons with poor response to first-line therapies or in progressive forms of MS (Table 17-8).

Anti-Inflammatories

Glucocorticoids

Glucocorticoids reduce the intensity and duration of MS relapses. There is no evidence that functional disease course is altered with short-term glucocorticoid administration for acute relapse. Routine administration of intravenous methylprednisolone (Medrol) has been shown to delay brain atrophy and decrease the volume of black hole (hypointense) lesions on T_1-weighted MRI.[58] Black hole lesions

Table 17-7 Multiple Sclerosis Disease Classification

Classification	Clinical Criteria
Relapsing-remitting (RRMS)	Clearly defined relapses followed by full recovery with or without residual deficits and no disease progression between relapses
Secondary progressive (SPMS)	Initial RR course followed by disease progression with or without relapses, remissions, and plateaus in disease activity
Primary progressive (PPMS)	Disease progresses steadily from onset with no attacks or relapses and only temporary minor improvements or plateaus
Progressive relapsing (PRMS)	Disease progresses from onset with superimposed relapses with or without recovery and continued disease progression between relapses

Source: Thrower BW et al. 2007.[56]

Table 17-8 Medications Used in the Treatment of Multiple Sclerosis

Drug Generic (Brand)	Dose	Indications
Glatiramer acetate (Copaxone)	20 mg SC qd	RRMS
Interferon-β1a, intramuscular (Avonex)	30 mcg IM q wk	CIS RRMS SPMS with relapses
Interferon-β1a, subcutaneous (Rebif)	8.8 mcg SC three times a week for 2 weeks 22 mcg SC three times a week for 2 weeks 44 mcg SC three times a week, maintenance	CIS RRMS SPMS with relapses
Interferon-β1b (Betaseron)	0.0625 mg SC every other day, increase q 1 to 2 wks by 25% up to 0.25 mg SC every other day, maintenance dose	CIS RRMS SPMS with relapses
Methylprednisolone (Medrol)	160 mg PO/IV qd for 1 week, then 64 mg PO every other day for 1 month	Acute relapse
Methotrexate (Rheumatrex, Trexall)	7.5 mg PO weekly	SPMS
Mitoxantrone (Novantrone)	12 mg/m^2 IV every 3 months	RRMS, refractory SPMS PRMS
Natalizumab (Tysbri)	300 mg IV q 28 d (infused slowly over 1 h)	RRMS
Prednisone (Deltasone)	200 mg PO qd for 1 wk, then 80 mg PO every other day for 1 month	Acute relapse

CIS = clinically isolated syndrome; RRMS = relapsing/remitting multiple sclerosis; SPMS = secondary progressive multiple sclerosis with relapses; PRMS = progressive multiple sclerosis.
Sources: Goodin DS et al. 2002[60]; Zivadinov R et al. 2001.[61]

are associated with greater disability. While this may prove to be useful in long-term management in relapsing/ remitting multiple sclerosis (RRMS), steroids are not currently recommended as first-line treatment for MS.[59,60] In a study by Zivadinov et al.,[61] persons receiving scheduled intravenous methylprednisolone pulse therapy were 32% less likely to have sustained disability worsening and had reduced expansion of black hole volume when compared to persons receiving symptomatic therapy (+1.3 mL versus +5.2 mL, *P* < .0001).

Episodic therapy may be initiated when the individual or the provider desires as long as infection has been ruled out. There is no evidence of clear benefit regarding a particular route of administration, dose, or choice of glucocorticoid for treatment of exacerbation in clinically definite MS. In persons with a first episode of optic neuritis, however, intravenous methylprednisolone (Medrol) administration decreases the risk of optic neuritis recurrence and progression to clinically definite MS within 2 years (RR = 0.34; 95% CI, 0.16–0.74 versus placebo; RR = 0.38; 95% CI, 0.17–0.83 versus oral).[62]

Immunosuppressants

Azathioprine (Azasan, Imuran)

Azathioprine (Azasan, Imuran) may reduce relapse in RRMS, but beneficial effect on disease progression has not been shown.[60] When considered in light of its side effect profile, azathioprine is most appropriate for people who have not responded to first-line drugs or other, less toxic alternatives.

Cyclosporine (Sandimmune)

Cyclosporine (Sandimmune) may provide some benefit to persons with progressive MS; however, the degree of potential improvement is likely outweighed by the risk of nephrotoxicity. The American Academy of Neurology and the MS Council for Clinical Practice Guidelines have determined the risk/benefit ratio to be unacceptable.[60]

Methotrexate (Rheumatrex, Trexall)

The use of methotrexate (Rheumatrex, Trexall) in MS has not been definitively determined. Given its potent immunosuppressive activity, it could have a role in MS therapy, but significant improvements in relapse or disease progression have not been found. Results from a single trial suggest that methotrexate may slow progression and relapse rate.[58] More studies are needed to determine if methotrexate is beneficial in MS therapy.

Mitoxantrone (Novantrone)

Mitoxantrone (Novantrone) is approved to treat both relapsing and progressive forms of MS. Persons treated with mitoxantrone should experience a reduction in clinical and MRI attack rate and may have reduced clinical disability.[11] Due to the potential cardiotoxicity of the drug, mitoxantrone therapy should be reserved for persons with progressive disease or those with RRMS who have rapidly worsening disease.[11] While the risk of cardiotoxicity increases with cumulative dose, this serious complication can occur at any time during therapy. Mitoxantrone should only be used to treat RRMS after first-line immunomodulatory therapies have been used. At dosing recommended for MS therapy, the maximum cumulative dose (140 mg/m²) is generally reached in 2 to 3 years.[11]

Immunomodulators/Biologic Agents

Interferon Beta (INF-β)

There are two subtypes of INF-β, 1a (Avonex, Rebif) and 1b (Betaseron). No evidence exists that suggests differences in clinical effectiveness between the two subtypes of INF-β.[60] In fact, their side effect profile and potential complications are quite similar.

INF-β therapy has been shown to reduce attack rate for people with clinically isolated syndrome and in RRMS or SPMS with relapses.[59,63] The effectiveness of INF-β in SPMS without relapse is not clear.[60] Some people develop persistent INF neutralizing antibodies (NAbs), which diminish the clinical and MRI benefits of therapy. NAbs may develop less frequently with INF-β1a, particularly when administered intramuscularly. There is no evidence to support serum monitoring of NAbs for clinical decision making. Therapy should be modified empirically if persons on INF therapy demonstrate reduced response.[59,60]

Glatiramer Acetate (Copaxone)

Glatiramer acetate (Copaxone) generally is better tolerated than INF-βs. MS sufferers receiving glatiramer acetate therapy may experience a reduced clinical attack rate, fewer new lesions on MRI, and less total brain atrophy. In a multicenter study by Comi et al.,[64] glatiramer acetate therapy reduced attack rate by 33% ($P = .012$) and number of enhancing lesions by 35% ($P = .001$) when compared to placebo. Filippi et al.[65] found that fewer new MRI lesions convert to black holes (15.6% glatiramer acetate versus 31.4% placebo; $P = .002$), which suggests that glatiramer acetate has a neuroprotective effect.[23,24] This clinical effect has yet to be confirmed, but if true, glatiramer acetate may be beneficial in long-term therapy protecting against axonal degeneration and disability accumulation.[60]

Natalizumab (Tysbri)

Natalizumab (Tysbri) suppresses leukocyte migration into the CNS and may reduce plaque formation by inhibiting leukocyte adhesion to endothelial cells in the vasculature and the brain. Natalizumab therapy greatly reduces relapses and appearance of new lesions on MRI.[12]

Natalizumab (Tysbri) is not recommended as first-line therapy for treatment of RRMS and should not be used in progressive forms of the disease[12] or in combination with immunosuppressive or immunomodulatory medications.[66] To initiate therapy, the individual should have recent disease activity with demonstrated poor response to first-line therapies, no treatment with immunosuppressives in the previous 3 months, and no leukopenia or other condition that compromises immunity.[12] Persons taking natalizumab (Tysbri) should be counseled to report signs of infection, depression, or neurologic changes.

Treatment of Secondary Symptoms

Neurologic deficits in MS affect physical, psychological, or social function. Apart from gait disturbances, individuals may report fatigue, sleep disturbance, spasticity, urinary and bowel dysfunction, sexual dysfunction, impaired speech, tremors, dysphagia, and cognitive impairment. There are no known therapies to reverse these secondary effects. Therapy is directed toward symptom relief. A multidisciplinary approach is preferred and may include physical therapy and psychosocial interventions in addition to medication.[52] Possible pharmacotherapy and lifestyle changes that may have a beneficial effect on secondary symptoms of MS are summarized in Table 17-9.

Complementary, Alternative, and Adjuvant Therapies

As with conventional therapy, treatment is focused on balancing the immune system and reducing inflammation. The most frequently used and recommended complemental alternative modalities are diet, essential fatty acids, vitamin/mineral supplementation, homeopathy, botanical products, and antioxidants.[67] There are no proven complementary or alternative therapies that reduce relapse rates or disease progression. Despite this fact, many MS sufferers turn to complementary and alternative therapies and perceive improvement in symptoms and quality of life as well as reduced relapse and disease progression.[67] Stress reduction and rest are recommended, particularly during acute attacks.

Special Populations

Pregnancy, Breastfeeding, and Contraception

Uncomplicated MS does not have adverse effects on fertility, pregnancy, labor, or birth. Rates of spontaneous

Table 17-9 Treatment of Secondary Symptoms for Persons with Multiple Sclerosis

Symptom	Lifestyle Modifications/Preventive Measures	Pharmacologic Treatments
Ataxia/tremor	Wrist weights	Clonazepam (Klonapin) 1.5 to 20 mg PO qd Propranolol (Inderol) 40 to 200 mg PO qd Ondansetron (Zofran) 8 to 16 mg PO qd
Spasticity	Physical therapy Exercise Stretching	Lioresal (Kemstro, Lioresal) 20 to 120 mg PO qd Diazepam (Valium) 2 to 40 mg PO qd Tizanidine (Zanaflex) 8 to 32 mg PO qd
Pain	Pain management program	Carbamazepine (Tegretol) 100 to 1000 mg PO qd Phenytoin (Dilantin) 300 to 600 mg PO qd Amitriptyline (Elavil) 25 to 150 mg PO qd Mexiletine (Mexitil) 300 to 900 mg PO qd
Bladder dysfunction	Evening fluid restriction Frequent voiding	Propantheline Br (Pro-Banthine) 10 to 15 mg PO qd Oxybutynin (Ditropan) 5 to 15 mg PO qd
Detrusor/sphincter dyssynergia	Catheterization	Phenoxybenzamine (Dibenzylene) 10 to 20 mg PO qd Terazosin HCl (Hytrin) 1 to 10 mg PO qd
Urinary tract infections	Intermittent catheterization Urine acidification	Appropriate antibiotic treatment
Constipation	High-fiber diet	Appropriate laxative treatment
Depression	Effective management of cognitive problems Effective coping strategies	Fluoxetine (Prozac) 20 to 80 mg PO qd Sertraline (Zoloft) 50 to 200 mg PO qd Amitriptyline (Elavil) 25 to 150 mg PO qd Venlafaxine (Effexor) 75 to 225 mg PO qd
Fatigue	Assistive devices Effective management of spasticity	Amantadine (Symmetrel) 200 mg PO qd Pemoline (Cylert) 37.5 to 75 mg PO qd Modafinil (Provigil) 100 to 400 mg PO qd
Cognitive problems	None known	Donepezil HCl 10 mg PO qd
Paroxysmal symptoms	None known	Acetazolamide (Diamox) 200 to 600 mg PO qd Carbamazepine (Tegretol) 50 to 400 mg PO qd Phenytoin (Dilantin) 50 to 300 mg PO qd
Heat sensitivity	Heat avoidance Cooling garments	None known
Sexual dysfunction	Personal lubricants Effective management of pain, spasticity, fatigue	None known

Source: Compston A et al. 2008.[52]

abortion, congenital anomalies, and fetal death are no higher among women with MS than in the general population.[68] There is no indication that women with MS require different care or management during the labor and birth process. Epidural, local, and general anesthesia can be administered to women with MS. However, the use of spinal anesthesia is associated with postoperative exacerbation.

If a cesarean birth is indicated, women with MS should be monitored very closely in the postoperative period. Women with respiratory or neurologic deficits may have more difficulty with hypoventilation and residual neuromuscular block.[68] Temperature elevations should be treated aggressively to prevent pseudoexacerbation. Pregnant women with MS tend to have fewer relapses during gestation with a subsequent increase in disease activity the first 3 months postpartum. Breastfeeding does not seem to have an influence on frequency or severity of exacerbations.[68]

Most medications used in MS treatment have not been shown to have adverse effects on pregnancy or the fetus. There are limited data for the first-line therapies, INF-β1a, INF-β1b, and glatiramer acetate (Copaxone). Women on these medications are generally advised to avoid pregnancy and to discontinue use when trying to conceive. Limited animal study data for INF-βs show possible abortifacient effects (at high doses), but no teratogenic effect.[69] Despite the FDA Pregnancy Category B designation for glatiramer acetate, some authorities consider it unsafe for use during pregnancy due to insufficient data.[68]

Of the alternate MS therapies, methylprednisolone, intravenous immunoglobulin administration, azathioprine (Azasan, Imuran), and cyclosporine (Neoral, Sandimmune) probably are safe to use in pregnancy.[68] Prematurity and fetal growth restriction have been reported with azathioprine (Azasan, Imuran) and cyclosporine (Neoral, Sandimmune); however, extensive use in SLE and posttransplant therapy has shown no increase in fetal anomalies. Methylprednisolone (Medrol) should be avoided in the first trimester due to anecdotal reports of fetal anomalies.

Cyclophosphamide, methotrexate, mitoxantrone (Novantrone), and natalizumab should not be used during pregnancy, and women seeking pregnancy should discontinue use of these medications. Cyclophosphamide may decrease fertility or result in significant fetal anomalies in pregnancies that occur during therapy.[70] Methotrexate is a known abortifacient and mutagen. There is insufficient evidence in human pregnancy to determine the safety of mitoxantrone or natalizumab. Mitoxantrone (Novantrone) and has been shown to cause premature delivery and low birth weight in animal studies.[68] Animal studies show increased rates of embryonic death with natalizumab.[12]

There is no evidence that any contraceptive method is contraindicated for women with MS. In many cases, using a reliable contraceptive method is strongly encouraged, as risks of current pharmacotherapy or degree of disability would make pregnancy undesirable. Combined oral contraceptives may improve symptoms for women who experience worsening symptoms during menstruation.[71]

Elderly

Multiple sclerosis and menopause has not been widely studied. Some women report exacerbation in the puerperium (a period of relative estrogen deficiency), and this may also be true for menopause. Worsening of symptoms noted during this period, however, may be related to the natural progression of MS. Relapsing-remitting MS often becomes more progressive with increasing age and duration of illness. As with other autoimmune illnesses, prior history of glucocorticoid use increases the postmenopausal risk of osteoporosis. Additionally, women with MS may have decreased physical activity related to fatigue and physical limitations. Prevention strategies for postmenopausal osteoporosis in women with MS include use of calcium and vitamin D supplementation, antiresorptive agents, and hormones. Hormone therapy for perimenopausal conditions is not contraindicated for women with MS.

Rheumatoid Arthritis

Rheumatoid arthritis (RA) is an autoimmune disorder characterized by joint inflammation and progressive disability. RA primarily affects synovial joints and tissues of the hands and feet, but any joint can be involved. The initial manifestation of RA is synovitis—an inflammation of the synovium fluid—which triggers an increase in cytokine and chemokine secretion. Local inflammation damages surrounding tissue. The cytokine TNF is the major player in this disease. TNF causes a massive inflammatory reaction in the synovium that results in diminished bone formation and secretion of protein-degrading enzymes (Figure 17-5). Over time, bone and cartilage damage accumulate, resulting in joint deformity and loss of function. With the exception of cervical vertebrae, the axial skeleton is typically spared. Multisystem extra-articular manifestations and comorbidities from the disease process and its therapy can occur.

Epidemiology and Natural History

RA affects approximately 1% of adults worldwide; it is present in nearly all geographic areas and among all ethnic groups.[72] Lower incidence is observed in sub-Saharan and Caribbean Blacks, which may be due to the low frequency of known susceptibility genes and variations in environmental exposure in these populations.[72] The disease typically presents between 30 and 50 years of age and affects twice as many women as men.

As with other autoimmune disorders, RA is likely to occur in a genetically predisposed individual when environmental exposures trigger disease onset. RA susceptibility is associated with HLA-DR4 and DR4-related alleles in the major histocompatibility complex. The only consistently linked environmental risk factor is cigarette smoking (current or past).[73] Climate and urbanization may provide additional triggers for RA in the genetically predisposed.[72]

For most persons with RA, symptoms present slowly over a period of weeks or months. Fatigue, anorexia, and weakness may precede the first arthritic event. Progression of the disease and ensuing disability is heterogeneous and unpredictable. Prognosis is poor for individuals who have high rheumatoid factor titers, significantly elevated erythrocyte sedimentation rate, more than 20 affected joints, and onset of disease at an early age.[72,74] RA is most aggressive and amenable to treatment in the early stages. Initiating antirheumatic therapy within the first 3 months after diagnosis is recommended and may have greater impact on disease progression.[8,21]

Joint deformity is a common feature of chronic RA. Typical hand deformities include Z-deformity, swan-neck deformity, and boutonniere deformity.[72] Joint deformities may also develop in the feet and ankles.

Fewer than 20% of persons with RA will have no disability 10–12 years after diagnosis, while more than 50% will have significant work disability.[72] Risk for disability

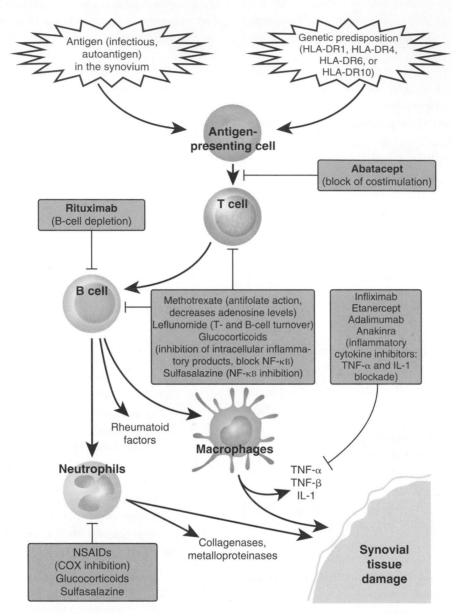

An infectious or environmental epitope in combination with a susceptible genetic background initiates the inflammatory cascade. The interaction between T and B cells often results in the production of rheumatoid factor and other autoantibodies. B cells also stimulate the activation of neutrophils and macrophages. Neutrophils secrete enzymes that directly mediate tissue damage. Macrophages are responsible for the production of inflammatory mediators (e.g., TNF-α, TNF-β, IL-1).

HLA = human leukocyte antigen; NF-κB = nuclear factor κB; TNF = tumor necrosis factor; IL = interleukin; NSAIDs = nonsteroidal anti-inflammatory drugs; COX = cyclooxygenase.

Figure 17-5 Immunopathogenesis and targeted drug therapy of rheumatoid arthritis. *Source:* Reprinted with permission from Gaffo A et al. 2006.[76]

is increased with significantly elevated rheumatoid factor (RF) titers or erythrocyte sedimentation rate (ESR), comorbid conditions, and lower socioeconomic or educational levels. Life expectancy of those with RA is decreased by approximately 3–7 years.[72] Factors associated with increased mortality include age at onset, disease duration and severity, degree of disability, glucocorticoid use, and lower socioeconomic or educational levels.

Presentation and Diagnosis

Early signs and symptoms of RA are often nonspecific and intermittent. Due to the complex and heterogeneous nature of the disease, diagnosis may not occur for months after initial onset. As the disease progresses, presentation becomes more characteristic—generally 1–2 years after actual onset.

Individuals with RA typically present with pain, swelling, and tenderness in joints; decreased mobility; and stiffness after periods of inactivity (morning stiffness). They may also report low-grade fever, anorexia, and fatigue prior to the synovial flare. Articular inflammation is generally symmetrical, involving several joints in the upper and lower extremities. In approximately 10% of cases, onset will be acute with fever, lymphadenopathy, and splenomegaly.[72]

Laboratory and radiographic findings may be helpful in the initial evaluation and diagnosis of RA. The American College of Rheumatology Subcommittee on Rheumatoid Arthritis recommends a baseline laboratory evaluation of a complete blood count (CBC), C-reactive protein (CRP), rheumatoid factor, erythrocyte sedimentation rate (ESR), and liver function tests (LFTs). The presence of rheumatoid factor, elevated CRP or ESR, increased white blood cell count (WBC), and decreased hemoglobin (Hgb) and hematocrit (Hct) are all associated with RA. Additional information gathered from liver and renal function studies can help guide choice of medication therapy.[21]

The American College of Rheumatology has developed criteria for RA classification in clinical trials, which is 91–94% sensitive and 89% specific for diagnosing RA in a population of individuals with non-RA rheumatic diseases as shown in Table 17-10.[75] Its utility is limited in a general clinical setting, particularly in early disease. The criteria may serve as a helpful guideline for differentiating RA from other possible diagnoses.[76]

Complications and Comorbidity

Persons with RA have an increased risk of osteoporosis, lymphoma, cardiovascular disease, and death due to MI.[72,77]

Table 17-10 1987 Revised Criteria for Classification of Rheumatoid Arthritis*

Criterion	Definition
1. Morning stiffness[†]	In and around joint > 1 h duration
2. Arthritis in ≥ 3 joint areas[†]	Proximal interphalangeal joint, metacarpophalangeal joint, metatarsophalangeal joint, wrist, elbow, knee, or ankle
3. Arthritis of joints in hand[†]	Wrist, MCP, or PIP
4. Symmetric arthritis[†]	Bilateral symmetric involvement of areas in No. 2
5. Rheumatoid nodules	Subcutaneous nodules (bone prominences, extensor surfaces, regions around joints)
6. Elevated rheumatoid factor (RF)	Abnormal RF
7. Radiologic changes	Evidence of bony erosions or decalcifications in or near affected joints

* At least four of the seven criteria must be met to make the diagnosis of rheumatoid arthritis.
[†] Must be present for ≥ 6 weeks.
Source: Adapted from Arnett FC et al. 1988.[75]

Long-term glucocorticoid use increases risk of osteoporosis and osteoporotic fractures while methotrexate reduces risk of cardiovascular-related death (Hazard Ratio = 0.3; 95% CI, 0.2–0.7).[78] Additional protective measures include regular exercise and dietary supplementation with vitamin D and calcium.[74] Some women are candidates for bisphosphonate therapy.

Chronic, severe RA often results in symptomatic systemic disease. Extra-articular manifestations of RA include Felty's syndrome, rheumatoid nodules, pleuropulmonary disorders, rheumatoid vasculitis, and asymptomatic pericarditis. Felty's syndrome is associated with chronic RA and consists of splenomegaly, neutropenia, and possibly anemia or thrombocytopenia. Risk of infection is increased for those with Felty's syndrome. Pleuropulmonary manifestations are more common in men and include pleural disease, interstitial fibrosis, pleuropulmonary nodules, and pneumonitis. Vasculitis may affect nearly all organ systems resulting in cutaneous ulcers, dermal necrosis, and visceral infarction. The neurologic system is generally spared, but vasculitis and inflammation may impinge nerves and result in neuropathy.[72]

Therapy for Rheumatoid Arthritis

Treatment of RA is focused on the following three factors: reducing joint inflammation, managing pain, and

Table 17-11 Medications Used in the Treatment of Rheumatoid Arthritis

Drug Generic (Brand)	Dose
Adalimumab (Humira)	40 mg SC every 2 weeks
Anakinra (Kineret)	100 to 150 mg SC qd
Azathioprine (Azasan, Imuran)	50 to 150 mg PO qd
Cyclosporine (Sandimmune)	2.5 to 5 mg/kg PO each day
Etanercept (Enbrel)	25 mg SC twice a week or 50 mg SC weekly
Hydroxychloroquine (Plaquenil)	200 to 400 mg PO qd
Infliximab (Remicade)	3 mg/kg IV at weeks 0, 2, 6, then every 8 weeks
Leflunomide (Arava)	100 mg PO qd for 3 days, then 10 to 20 mg PO qd
Methotrexate (Rheumatrex)	12 to 25 mg PO, IM or SC weekly
Rituximab (Rituxan)	1000 mg IV in 2 doses, 2 weeks apart (use with MTX)
Sulfasalazine (Azulfidine)	2 to 3 g PO qd (divided doses)

Sources: Klareskog L et al. 2006[73]; Arnett FC et al. 1988.[75]

preventing joint destruction. Initiation of an antirheumatic or biologic agent early in the disease process may limit joint damage and disability.[8,21,76] These classic medications for treatment of RA are collectively referred to as disease-modifying antirheumatic drugs (Table 17-11). In clinical practice, the classic disease-modifying antirheumatic drugs are generally used before the newer biologics.[21,72]

Nonsteroidal Anti-Inflammatory Drugs

Treatment of RA typically involves NSAIDs to control the acute inflammation and pain of synovitis. Their use is appropriate for symptomatic treatment during the initial diagnostic workup and as bridge therapy until slower-acting disease-modifying antirheumatic drugs can take effect. NSAIDs do not alter the course of RA and should not be used as monotherapy.

NSAIDs are well tolerated in short-term therapy, but toxicities may develop if they are used long term. The most common complication of long-term use is GI toxicity, including ulcers, perforation, and GI bleeding. These risks are higher for persons who are older, using steroids, or have peptic ulcer disease. Gastroprotective agents may decrease GI side effects. Chronic NSAID use is also associated with renal failure. The American College of Rheumatology recommends renal function evaluation prior to and during NSAID therapy for all persons with increased risk of renal toxicity.[79] Other associated toxicities include liver function abnormalities, cytopenia, aseptic meningitis, fluid retention, aggravation of congestive heart failure, and

angioedema. The use of COX-2 inhibitors and some other NSAIDs may increase the risk of cardiovascular events in persons with RA.[80] This risk varies from drug to drug and appears to be greater with increasing doses (RR 0.99−1.51 with lower doses versus RR 1.05−2.80 with higher doses).[80] Use should be avoided in individuals with cardiovascular risk factors.[81]

Glucocorticoids

Glucocorticoid therapy is very effective for reducing inflammation, joint tenderness, and pain in active RA. Gotzsche and Johansen[82] conducted a meta-analysis of 10 studies evaluating the efficacy of short-term glucocorticoid administration compared to NSAIDs and placebo. Glucocorticoid use was associated with significantly fewer tender joints (standard mean difference [SMD] −0.63; 95% CI, −1.16 to −0.11 versus NSAIDs; SMD −1.30; 95% CI, −1.83 to −0.78 versus placebo) and less pain (SMD −1.25; 95% CI, −2.24 to −0.26 versus NSAIDs; SMD −1.75; 95% CI, −2.64 to −0.87 versus placebo). Steroids may also improve physical function and slow the rate of joint damage; however, joint damage may increase when steroids are discontinued. Steroids are also indicated for the control of disease activity while awaiting clinical effects of newly initiated disease-modifying antirheumatic drugs therapy.

Glucocorticoids may be administered orally or through local injection. When only a few joints are involved, local injection provides rapid, but temporary symptom relief. Septic arthritis must be ruled out prior to steroid injection.[21] Despite the potential for disease modification, monotherapy with glucocorticoids is not recommended.[76] Some persons, however, will require continued low-dose steroid therapy when other treatment regimens fail.[8] Chronic use of steroids in RA should be weighed against the potential risks associated with steroid use.[21]

Methotrexate (Rheumatrex, Trexall)

Methotrexate (Rheumatrex, Trexall) is the most commonly used disease-modifying antirheumatic drug and the mainstay of RA therapy. Methotrexate is relatively inexpensive, highly effective, and has a low risk of toxicity compared to most other disease-modifying antirheumatic drugs and biologic agents. It is used as initial therapy for severe RA and has been shown to slow the progression of bone erosions.[83]

Methotrexate (Rheumatrex, Trexall) can be administered orally or by injection. Bioavailability of oral methotrexate is similar to the agent administered parenterally at low doses (0.85; 95% CI, 0.77−0.93);[84] however, at higher doses

(> 20 mg/wk), bioavailability is somewhat lower (0.64; 95% CI, 0.21−0.96).[85] Methotrexate therapy should be initiated with oral dosing, followed by parenteral administration if disease activity remains uncontrolled after increasing to high-dose oral therapy.[86]

Leflunomide (Arava)

Leflunomide (Arava) is often used for individuals who have a suboptimal or intolerant response to methotrexate.[21] Leflunomide may be used as monotherapy or in combination with methotrexate. Mechanisms of action appear to be complementary, and persons on combination therapy have somewhat better response than those on either monotherapy.[8] Liver enzyme elevations are much more common with combination therapy (60%) than with leflunomide monotherapy (5%).[21]

Hydroxychloroquine (Plaquenil)

Hydroxychloroquine (Plaquenil) is effective for symptom relief in early or mild RA. Monotherapy does not impact progression of bone erosions, but administration of hydroxychloroquine early in the disease process may improve long-term outcome.[21]

Sulfasalazine (Azulfidine)

Sulfasalazine (Azulfidine) in early or mild RA has similar effectiveness to methotrexate in providing symptom relief and slowing bone eroisions.[8] Side effects of sulfasalazine are lessened with slow and gradual titration of daily dosing. Sulfasalazine may be used as monotherapy or in combination with other disease-modifying antirheumatic drugs. If clinical response is not seen by 4 months of administration, therapy should be changed. Other antirheumatic drugs less commonly used in RA therapy include gold salts, cyclosporine (Neoral, Sandimmune), tacrolimus, and minocycline (Table 17-12).[8,21,76]

Table 17-12 Older Antirheumatics Used in the Treatment of Rheumatoid Arthritis

Drug Generic (Brand)	Dose
Gold-containing agents	
• Auranofin (Ridaura)	3 mg PO bid or 6 mg PO qd
• Gold sodium thiomalate (Myochrysine)	25 to 50 mg IM every 2 to 4 weeks
Penicillamine (Cuprimine)	250 to 750 mg PO qd
Minocycline (Minocin)	100 mg PO bid
Tacrolimus (Prograf)	1.3 to 3 mg PO qd

Source: Klareskog L et al. 2006.[73]

Immunomodulators/Biologic Agents

Biologic agents may be used as initial therapy for severe RA but more commonly are used for people with toxicity, failure, or intolerance of traditional disease-modifying antirheumatic drug therapy. The TNF-α antagonists are more effective than other biologics for the treatment of RA.[76]

Adalimumab (Humira), etanercept (Enbrel), and infliximab (Remicade) are anti-TNF-α agents that have been shown to decrease pain, improve physical function, and reduce bone erosion in individuals with RA. There is no significant difference in the effectiveness among these agents.

When used as monotherapy, each agent is as effective as methotrexate and has a more rapid onset of action.[8,76] When used in combination with methotrexate, efficacy is improved. Infliximab is approved only for use with methotrexate.[21,76] Adalimumab (Humira) and etanercept (Enbrel) may be used as monotherapy or in combination with methotrexate (Rheumatrex, Trexall) or other disease-modifying antirheumatic drugs.

Choice of anti-TNF-α therapy generally depends on cost and the person's preference for administration. If an individual does not have an adequate clinical response to a particular anti-TNF-α agent, a different anti-TNF-α inhibitor may be administered.[76] Not all individuals with RA will respond to these agents, and disease flares are common when therapy is discontinued.[21]

Abatacept (Orencia) provides symptomatic relief of RA and leads to clinical and functional improvement and a reduction in structural joint damage.[87] Abatacept can be used as monotherapy or in combination with anti-inflammatories or nonbiologic disease-modifying antirheumatic drugs in the treatment of severe, refractory RA. Use with TNF-α antagonists and anakinra is associated with increased adverse effects without significant benefit in treatment effect.

Anakinra (Kineret) improves clinical signs and symptoms of RA and reduces radiographic progression of disease. When administered with methotrexate, its effects are greater than methotrexate monotherapy.[21] Anakinra plus a TNF-α antagonist is not recommended. The combination biologic therapy is no more effective than anti-TNF-α monotherapy and may result in a higher rate of serious infections.[8,76] Anakinra is most appropriate for use by those persons who cannot tolerate TNF-α antagonist therapy.

Rituximab (Rituxan) effectively reduces rheumatoid factor titers and relieves articular signs and symptoms of RA.[20] Effectiveness in reducing progression of bone erosions has not been shown. Rituximab is currently recommended for use with methotrexate in treating severe, refractory RA that has not responded to TNF-α antagonists.[20] Retreatment is an option for some, but the optimal infusion interval has not been established. Persons receiving rituximab therapy may have slightly increased risks of infection. There have been no reports of opportunistic infections.

Combination Therapy

If monotherapy with traditional disease-modifying antirheumatic drugs fails, combination therapy may be an option for persons with RA.[21,76] Methotrexate (Rheumatrex, Trexall) plus hydroxychloroquine (Plaquenil) and methotrexate plus sulfasalazine (Azulfidine) are more effective than monotherapy. Triple combination therapy with methotrexate, hydroxychloroquine, and sulfasalazine has a greater impact than dual therapy in both early and advanced RA.[21] O'Dell et al. found a 50% improvement in RA symptoms in 40% of those treated with methotrexate and hydroxychloroquine, 29% with methotrexate and sulfasalazine and 55% with triple combination therapy.[88] Biologic agents plus methotrexate show benefit for those with suboptimal methotrexate response.[21]

Complementary, Alternative, and Adjuvant Therapies

Several nonpharmacologic therapies have been reported to improve symptoms in RA; however, studies of herbal therapies in RA treatment have inconclusive results owing in part to poor data reporting and methodologic quality of existing trials.[89] In a meta-analysis of herbal therapies, improvement in pain and stiffness was seen with gammalinoleic acid supplementation when compared to placebo (68% versus 32% and 61% versus 39%, respectively).[90] Essential fatty acid supplementation may decrease the need for anti-inflammatory medication or dose.[90] The possible benefits of *Boswellia serrata* (frankincense) and topical capsaicin need further study. Occupational therapy, spa therapy, and exercise may be of benefit.[91-93] Acupuncture and joint splinting for pain relief have yielded variable results.[94,95]

Special Populations

Pregnancy, Breastfeeding, and Contraception

Women with RA do not experience decreased fertility or poorer maternal or fetal outcomes when compared with healthy control participants. Studies have, however, reported a higher rate of nulliparity among women with RA, which most likely reflects delayed reproduction due to pain, decreased sex drive, and an impaired hypothalamic-pituitary-adrenal axis.[96] Laboratory and physical assessments should be made as in any other rheumatologic and prenatal care setting. ESR values are not a good indicator of disease activity during pregnancy.[96] Joints and range of motion should be assessed. Full rotation and mobility of the hip is important for vaginal delivery. In very rare cases, hip involvement may be so severe that vaginal birth is not possible. Apart from these cases, decisions on route of delivery should be made based on obstetric factors. Breastfeeding is not contraindicated in RA.

Disease-modifying antirheumatic drugs during pregnancy are limited to hydroxychloroquine, glucocorticoids, NSAIDs, and sulfasalazine.[97] NSAID use should be discontinued after 32 weeks' gestation to limit the risk of premature closure of the fetal ductus arteriosus.[96,97] Methotrexate (Rheumatrex, Trexall) and leflunomide (Arava) are FDA Pregnancy Category X medications and are contraindicated during pregnancy and lactation. Due to limited data regarding biologics, use during pregnancy and lactation should be avoided.[96]

RA disease activity tends to diminish during pregnancy and resume by the third postpartum month. This trend may be due to the general shift from a more anti-inflammatory cytokine profile seen in pregnancy to a proinflammatory cytokine profile in the postpartum period.[96] Some women may experience complete remission during pregnancy. Approximately 90% of women experience disease flare in the postpartum period.[96]

Any contraceptive method is appropriate for use by persons with RA provided that the woman does not have other contraindications. While some may advocate withholding intrauterine contraception (IUC) for women on immunosuppressive therapy, there are no data to substantiate this risk or determine when it is sufficient to contraindicate IUC. While the diaphragm and combined hormonal vaginal ring is not contraindicated in RA, some women with severe RA will have difficulties inserting the devices. Combined oral contraceptives have been associated with a decreased risk of developing RA but have not shown a therapeutic effect in the disease process.[98] If a woman using a combined hormonal method is anticipating surgery, it is reasonable to discontinue use prior to surgery to reduce the risk of postoperative thrombolic events.

Elderly

Women with RA have increased risk for heart disease and osteoporosis in the postmenopausal years. Women with more disease activity and greater disability may be at additional risk because of worse disease and resulting physical inactivity. The effect of menopause on RA activity is variable. Reported increases in disease activity after menopause may be related more to duration of illness than hormonal changes. Some women experience improvement in pain and joint inflammation with hormone therapy provided perimenopausally. Whether there is a clear benefit of hormone therapy on RA symptom frequency and severity is uncertain; however, hormones are not contraindicated for use in women with RA. Hormone therapy along with lifestyle changes may reduce the risk for postmenopausal heart disease and bone loss (Box 17-1).

Systemic Lupus Erythematosus

Definition

Systemic lupus erythematosus (SLE) is a chronic, inflammatory, multisystem autoimmune disorder. The primary feature of SLE is immune dysregulation of B cells that results in abnormally increased production of autoantibodies directed toward nuclear antigens (Figure 17-6). Organ and tissue damage results from deposition of immune complexes in target tissue (e.g., nephritis) or autoantibody-mediated destruction of host cells (e.g., hemolytic anemia). The deposition of immune complexes in vascular tissue increases the risk of thromboembolic events and osteonecrosis.[94]

Epidemiology and Natural History

The overall incidence of SLE in the United States is 124 per 100,000 persons. Peak onset of SLE occurs between ages 15 and 45 with a 9:1 female-to-male ratio.[99] Over 80% of cases are diagnosed in women who are in their childbearing years.[100] SLE is more common among US populations of African, Afro-Caribbean, Asian, and Hispanic descent.[101]

Interaction between susceptibility genes and environmental factors are necessary for the development of SLE. Several genes, including but not limited to those in the major histocompatibility complex region, have been associated with SLE. Environmental triggers include cigarette smoking, exposure to ultraviolet light, and infection with Epstein-Barr virus (EBV).[102]

SLE is a complex disorder characterized by periods of relative inactivity and periods of disease exacerbation (flares). Some of those affected may have relatively quiescent disease while others have chronic activity.[103] The mortality rate for persons with SLE is nearly three times

Box 17-1 Rheumatoid Arthritis and Menopause

Ms P is a 52-year-old who presents for a routine gynecologic exam. Her last menstrual period was 7 months ago. She reports frequent hot flashes, but otherwise has no significant perimenopausal symptoms. She asks her healthcare provider what menopausal therapy would be recommended for her given her history and current medications.

Ms P was diagnosed with rheumatoid arthritis (RA) 4 years ago and is currently under the care of a rheumatologist. She was initially treated with methotrexate and has received glucocorticoids for exacerbations in the past. Her course of RA has been moderately active with intermittent periods of remission. She is currently using combination therapy, methotrexate plus etanercept, and reports minimal disability with infrequent symptom flares.

Menopausal women are at greater risk for heart disease and osteoporosis. These risks are increased with RA due to chronic inflammation of the disease, physical inactivity associated with disability, and the use of glucocorticoid therapy, which decreases bone density and affects lipid metabolism. Risk-reducing strategies for these conditions include following a heart-healthy diet with moderate exercise as tolerated, limiting glucocorticoid exposure, screening for and managing dyslipidemia, screening, and prophylactic therapy for osteopenia or osteoporosis, and consideration for hormone therapy (HT). HT is not contraindicated in RA and may be beneficial in reducing risk of heart disease and osteoporosis. Some women report RA symptom reduction with HT, which is likely due to estrogen's anti-inflammatory effects. Studies have not consistently confirmed improvement in RA symptoms with HT.

Ms P's healthcare provider prescribes transdermal HT for treatment of hot flashes and for osteoporosis prevention. She also recommends 1000 mg of calcium and 800 IU of vitamin D daily and will consider adding an antiresorptive agent after reviewing the results of Ms P's bone mineral density scan ordered today.

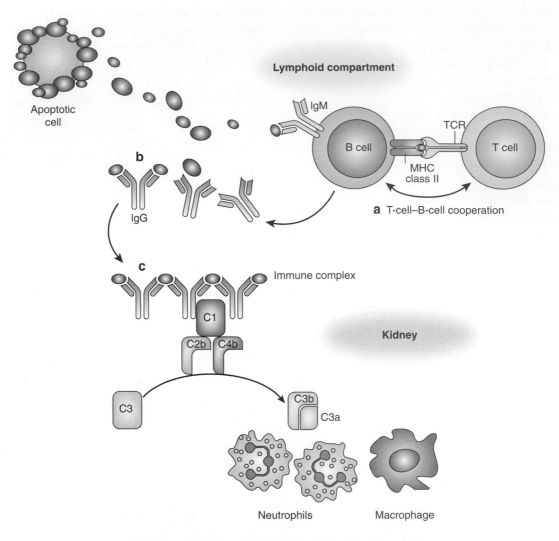

Lymphoid compartment

Apoptotic cell

b

IgG

a T-cell–B-cell cooperation

IgM

B cell

TCR

T cell

MHC class II

c

Immune complex

C1

C2b C4b

Kidney

C3

C3b

C3a

Neutrophils   Macrophage

(a) Encounter with cognate self-antigen in the presence of T-cell help induces activation.

(b) Activated B cells then form germinal centers forming both effector and memory B cells. Effector B cells release IgG autoantibodies into the circulation, where they form immune complexes in the presence of ligands (SLE antigens). Despite the normal mechanisms (such as the complement system) for the uptake and clearance of immune complexes, excess immune complexes accumulate in the small vessels of organs, such as the kidney, where they become pathogenic.

(c) Accumulated immune complexes induce inflammation through local activation of the complement system and/or the binding of Fc receptors, which leads to the degranulation of mast cells and the infiltration of neutrophils and macrophages.

C = complement component; TCR = T-cell receptor.

Figure 17-6 Autoantibody-mediated pathogenesis of systemic lupus erythematosus. *Source:* Reprinted with permission from Carroll MC 2004.[136]

that of the general population.[104] The majority of deaths in the early stages of disease are attributed to active disease (neurologic or renal) or infection. Late in the SLE disease process, women are more likely to die from atherosclerotic vascular disease, secondary complications related to organ damage, or side effects of disease treatment.[105] More than half of the persons who have SLE eventually develop permanent organ damage most commonly in the musculoskeletal, renal, and nervous systems.[106] Psychiatric manifestations—cognitive dysfunction, delirium, anxiety disorder, mood disorder, and psychosis—are common (affecting 17 to 75% of persons with SLE)[107] and are attributed to central nervous system injury, vascular pathology, and autoantibody and cytokine activity.[108]

Presentation and Diagnosis

SLE is a multisystem disorder with significant variation in presentation and course. SLE can affect all major organ systems (see Table 17-13).[105] The majority (90%) of individuals with SLE have constitutional symptoms (malaise, fatigue, anorexia, and low-grade fevers). Overall, however, the most common SLE manifestations are in the skin and musculoskeletal organs (e.g., photosensitivity, malar rash, oral ulcers, discoid rash, arthritis). There are three main categories of lupus-specific skin manifestations—acute cutaneous lupus erythematosus, subacute cutaneous lupus erythematosus, and chronic cutaneous lupus erythematosus. Acute cutaneous lupus erythematosus (ACLE) is often exacerbated by UV exposure and may be localized to the face (malar rash) or generalized; subacute cutaneous lupus erythematosus (SCLE) generally manifests as a photosensitive nonscarring maculopapular rash; and chronic cutaneous lupus erythematous (CCLE) refers to the classic scarring, discoid manifestation of lupus.[109] Pulmonary symptoms, renal involvement, CNS dysfunction, and mild hematologic abnormalities are seen in a smaller percentage of persons with SLE.[101] Other common and nonspecific symptoms include nausea, fatigue, weight loss, and alopecia.[99]

Diagnosing SLE can be challenging given the multisystem involvement and variable nature of the disease. Most individuals with SLE are diagnosed months or years after disease onset. The American College of Rheumatology has developed criteria for the classification of SLE based on clinical trials[105] (Table 17-14). These criteria demonstrate 95% sensitivity and 85% specificity for diagnosing SLE. If a person presents with fewer than 4 of the 11 criteria, a diagnosis can still be reasonably made based on the clinical scenario. SLE should be suspected if a person presents with clinical features in two or more of the systems in Table 17-14.[105]

SLE is considered mild if the disease is not life threatening and the person is clinically stable with no functional abnormalities or significant treatment toxicities. Severe manifestations of disease include nephritis, cerebritis, cardiac involvement, severe anemia or thrombocytopenia, and disease that is resistant to therapy.[105]

Complications and Comorbidity

Complications in SLE are related to disease severity, comorbidity, and the effects of long-term therapy. Close monitoring, treatment of flares, and management of comorbid conditions may be effective in reducing complications. In recent years, mortality in SLE has improved in all areas except cardiovascular deaths.

Severe active SLE can lead to serious life-threatening conditions. Lupus nephritis may lead to progressive renal failure. SLE cardiac symptoms can result in heart failure, valvular insufficiency, or pericardial tamponade. Severe SLE can also present as life-threatening anemia and thrombocytopenia.[105]

The development of **antiphospholipid antibody syndrome** (APS) and atherosclerosis increase the risk of thromboembolic events, which are a major cause of death in persons with SLE.[99,103] Cardiovascular risk reduction is recommended for all persons with SLE. Those with APS need anticoagulant therapy.[102] Long-term glucocorticoid use increases risk of infection, diabetes, obesity, osteoporosis, osteoporotic fracture, and avascular necrosis.[103] Preventive strategies to limit long-term complications include appropriate use of vaccines, suppression of recurrent

Table 17-13 Clinical Manifestations of Systemic Lupus Erythematosus

System	Symptoms	Frequency (%) At Onset	Anytime
Constitutional	Fatigue	—	90
	Fever	36	80
	Weight loss	—	40–60
Integumentary	Malar (butterfly) rash	40	30
	Photosensitivity	29	25–58
	Alopecia	—	71
	Mucosal ulcerations	11	21–30
	Raynaud's phenomenon	18–33	60
	Purpura	—	15
	Urticaria	—	9
Musculoskeletal	Arthritis	44–69	95
	Arthralgia	77	85
	Myositis	3	3
Renal	Any	16–38	50–74
	Nephrosis	5	11–18
Gastrointestinal		—	18
Pulmonary	Pleurisy	16	30–45
	Effusion	—	24
	Pneumonia	—	29
Cardiac	Pericarditis	13	23–48
	Murmurs	—	23
	ECG changes	—	34
Central nervous	Headache	12	36
	Organic	7	15–20
	Seizures	4	10–20

Source: Reprinted with permission from King TL 2004.[132]

Table 17-14 1997 Modified Criteria for Diagnosis of Systemic Lupus Erythematosus*

Feature	Definition
1. Malar rash	Fixed erythema over malar eminences, sparing nasolabial folds
2. Discoid rash	Erythematous raised patches with adherent keratotic scaling and follicular plugging; older lesions with atrophic scarring
3. Photosensitivity	Rash from sun exposure (patient or provider observation)
4. Oral ulcers	Oral or nasopharyngeal ulcers (provider observation)
5. Nonerosive arthritis	Tenderness, swelling, effusion in ≥ 2 peripheral joints
6. Pleuritis or pericarditis[†]	Pleuritis: history of pleuritic pain, rub (provider observation), or evidence of pleural effusion or Pericarditis: documented by ECG, rub, or evidence of pericardial effusion
7. Renal disorder[†]	Persistent proteinuria: > 5 g/d or > 3+ on urine dipstick or Cellular casts: RBC, Hgb, granular, tubular or mixed
8. Neurologic disorder[†]	Seizures: not drug-induced nor related to known metabolic disturbance or Psychosis: not drug induced nor related to known metabolic disturbance
9. Hematologic disorder[†]	Hemolytic anemia with reticulocytosis Leukopenia: < 4000/mm³ on ≥ two occasions Lymphopenia: < 1500/mm³ on ≥ two occasions or Thrombocytopenia: < 100,000/mm³ (not drug related)
10. Immunologic disorder[†]	Anti-dsDNA: abnormal titer of antibody to native DNA or AntiSm: antibody to Sm nuclear antigen or Positive antiphospholipid antibodies based on abnormal anticardiolipin IgG/IgM or Positive lupus anticoagulant using a standard method or False positive serologic test for syphilis for > 6 months and confirmed with *Treponema pallidum* immobilization or fluorescent treponemal antibody absorption test
11. Positive antinuclear antibody (ANA)	Abnormal ANA titer (in absence of medication use)

* The diagnosis of SLE requires 4 or more of the 11 criteria serially or simultaneously during any interval of observation.
† Diagnostic criteria require one of the listed conditions.
Source: Adapted from Hochberg MC 1997.[133]

urinary tract infections, vitamin D and calcium supplementation, and appropriate management of hypertension, dyslipidemia, hyperglycemia, and obesity. Disability in SLE is most often due to chronic renal disease, fatigue, arthritis, and pain.[102]

Drug-Induced Lupus

Drug-induced lupus is an autoimmune syndrome that shares many of the characteristic features of SLE. Common symptoms are arthralgia, myalgia, serositis, rash, and fever. Symptoms are associated with positive ANA, but rarely with anti-dsDNA. Drug-induced lupus rarely involves the central nervous or renal systems. The female predominance seen in SLE does not exist in drug-induced lupus.[110]

The cause of drug-induced lupus is not well understood. Lack of specific drug antibodies or antigen targets supports the notion that the mechanisms involved are not those of typical drug hypersensitivity reactions. Drugs implicated in drug-induced lupus may interfere with normal immune system processes, causing a disruption in tolerance to endogenous self-antigens. This may be achieved through a variety of proposed mechanisms, which include binding endogenous proteins that are then recognized as foreign, increasing proliferation of existing autoreactive lymphocytes, or disrupting processes that are involved with establishing self-tolerance.[110]

There are more than 80 drugs known to cause drug-induced lupus, including antiarrhythmics, antihypertensives, antithyroids, antipsychotics, anticonvulsants, antirheumatics, antihyperlipidemics, and antibiotics.[102]

The onset of symptoms may occur after 1 month of drug initiation or after years of therapy. Symptoms are typically mild to moderate and resolve within weeks of discontinuing the inducing drug. Severe cases, while rare, have been reported, and they generally respond to short-term glucocorticoid therapy.[110] Table 17-15 includes a list of the most common agents associated with drug-induced lupus. More information about drug-induced lupus can be found in Chapter 4.

Therapy for Systemic Lupus Erythematosus

The goal of SLE therapy is to control disease flares, suppress symptoms, and prevent organ damage. Treatment decisions are based on disease severity and organ involvement. See Table 17-16 for SLE treatments with recommended dosing and monitoring schedules.

Nonsteroidal Anti-Inflammatory Drugs

SLE arthritis and arthralgia are generally relieved by NSAID therapy. NSAIDs may also be effective in treating fever and mild serositis. Individuals with SLE are at greater risk of NSAID-induced aseptic meningitis, hypertension, edema, and renal dysfunction. Routine exams should include monitoring for these complications.[105]

Glucocorticoids

Topical, oral, and intravenous glucocorticoids are used in SLE treatment. People with mild disease typically do not need systemic therapy.[105] Systemic prednisone and methylprednisolone are generally used for treatment of severe or refractory disease. These agents are the foundation of therapy for life-threatening inflammation of major organ systems.[111] High-dose intravenous methylprednisolone may be given to treat severe, acute inflammatory manifestations followed by an oral taper to low-dose oral maintenance therapy. Some individuals continue low-dose maintenance therapy for years.[102]

Mild cutaneous lesions typically respond to topical steroids. Severe skin lesions may require treatment with intravenous steroids. If disease flares during the taper, another therapeutic agent (hydroxychloroquine, azathioprine, methotrexate) may be added to control disease activity.[102]

Immunosuppressants

Azathioprine (Imuran)

Azathioprine (Imuran) is used most often by individuals who are steroid dependent or have SLE disease activity in multiple systems.[111] Azathioprine is widely used as a steroid-sparing treatment in hematologic, pulmonary, and renal manifestations.[103] Azathioprine may be an effective treatment in lupus nephritis after cyclophosphamide induction of therapy.[99]

Table 17-15 Medications Associated with Drug-Induced Lupus

Class	Medications Strongly Associated with Drug-Induced Lupus—Generic (Brand)	Other Medications Associated with Drug-Induced Lupus—Generic (Brand)
Anti-arrhythmics	Procainamide (Pronestyl) Quinidine (Cardioquin)	Disopyramide (Norpace) Propafenone (Rythmol)
Antihyperlipidemics		Lovastatin (Altoprev, Mevacor) Simvastatin (Zocor)
Antihypertensives	Hydralazine (Apresoline)	ACE inhibitors (several) Beta-blockers (several)
Anti-infectives	Isoniazid (Nydrazid) Minocycline (Minocin)	Nitrofurantoin (Macrodantin) Terbinafine (Lamisil)
Anti-inflammatories		NSAIDs Sulfasalazine (Azulfidine)
Antipsychotics/anticonvulsants	Chlorpromazine (Thorazine) Methyldopa (Aldomet)	Carbamazepine (Tegretol) Lithium (Lithobid) Phenytoin (Dilantin)
Other		Fluorouracil (Carac, Efudex) Gold salts (Ridaura, Myochrysine) Hydrochlorothiazide (HydroDIURIL) Penicillamine (Cuprimine) Propylthiouracil (PTU)

Sources: Adapted from Hahn BH 2005[102] and Vasoo S 2006.[110]

Table 17-16 Medications Used in the Treatment of Systemic Lupus Erythematosus

Drug Generic (Brand)	Dose
Azathioprine (Azasan, Imuran)	2 to 3 mg/kg PO qd
Cyclophosphamide (Cytoxan)	0.7 to 2.5 mg/kg IV monthly for 6 months 1.5 to 3 mg/kg PO qd
Cyclosporine (Sandimmune)	2.5 to 5 mg/kg IV qd
Hydroxychloroquine (Plaquenil)	200 to 400 mg PO qd
Methylprednisolone (Medrol)	Severe: 1 g IV qd for 3 days
NSAIDs (e.g., ibuprofen [Advil])	Toward upper limits of normal ranges
Prednisone (Deltasone)	Severe: 0.5 to 1 mg/kg PO qd Mild: 0.07 to 0.3 mg/kg PO qd
Topical glucocorticoids	Low potency for face, high potency for other areas

Cyclophosphamide (Cytoxan)

Cyclophosphamide (Cytoxan) is used to treat severe renal and neuropsychiatric SLE. Cyclophosphamide is most commonly used to treat lupus nephritis in individuals who are at high risk of developing end-stage renal disease. Intravenous cyclophosphamide treatment of lupus nephritis preserves long-term renal function for the majority of sufferers.[111] After clinical response to pulse cyclophosphamide treatment of lupus nephritis is achieved, it may be followed by azathioprine to reduce adverse effects associated with cyclophosphamide therapy.[99,111]

Cyclosporine (Sandimmune, Neoral)

Cyclosporine (Sandimmune, Neoral) is generally used for those who are intolerant to other immunosuppressive therapies or who have developed myelosuppression secondary to other immunosuppressants. Cyclosporine may be particularly useful in treating severe or steroid-resistant cytopenia.[102,111] Individuals with SLE are at increased risk of accelerated atherosclerosis and should be monitored very closely for cyclosporine-induced hypertension and dyslipidemia. Cyclosporine may not be a preferred therapy for young persons with SLE because of these increased risks.[111] Cyclosporine should be discontinued gradually as rapid tapering is associated with disease flares.

Hydroxychloroquine (Plaquenil)

Hydroxychloroquine (Plaquenil) is the mainstay of therapy in serositis, arthritis, and musculoskeletal and cutaneous manifestations of SLE and should be considered for all individuals with mild SLE.[99,103,111] Topical hydroxychloroquine reduces the severity of lesions in cutaneous SLE.[102] Hydroxychloroquine has a beneficial effect on dyslipidemia and hyperglycemia as well as weak antithromboembolic effects.[99,111] Hydroxychloroquine has been shown to prevent future flares and organ damage.[103]

Methotrexate (Rheumatrex, Trexall)

Methotrexate (Rheumatrex, Trexall) is not used to treat major organ manifestations of SLE, but it may be effective in treating skin and joint disease.[102,111] For those with severe SLE arthritis, methotrexate may be an appropriate first-line therapy.[105]

Novel and Investigational Therapies

No new drugs have been approved for the treatment of SLE in the past 50 years.[103] In fact, there are no medications specifically developed for use in SLE. As many as 30% of persons with SLE have a disease that is refractory to the conventional therapies described earlier.[111] The optimal treatment strategy for major organ involvement is not known. In recent years, new therapies have been proposed for SLE, but most of these are still in trials. Emerging and experimental therapies are presented in Table 17-17.

Complementary, Alternative, and Adjuvant Therapies

Daily activity and lifestyle modifications may help reduce disease activity in SLE. Sufferers should minimize sun exposure and use sunscreen with at least an SPF of 15.[102] Moderate exercise and stress reduction may lessen fatigue without increasing the incidence of disease flares.[99]

Essential fatty acid supplementation may decrease inflammation in SLE. In animal studies of experimental SLE omega-3 fatty acids, intake is associated with increased life span, reduced frequency of SLE flares, and renal protection.[112] Dehydroepiandrosterone (DHEA) is a naturally occurring adrenocorticoid that reduces SLE flares. Chang et al.[113] found a significant reduction in flares with DHEA compared to placebo (18.3% versus 33.9%, $P = .04$). Acne and hirsutism are common among women using DHEA.[111] DHEA is not a suitable monotherapy but may be of benefit to some as an adjuvant therapy. Use of DHEA has a positive

Table 17-17 Emerging and Investigational Therapies for Systemic Lupus Erythematosus

Medication Strategies	Possible Indications
Anti-TNF-α agents	Skin and joint manifestations
Complement blockade	Antiphospholipid syndrome
Mycophenolic acid, oral	Lupus nephritis
Plasma exchange	Life-threatening thrombotic crises
Rituximab, other anti-B-cell therapies	Severe, refractory SLE
Tacrolimus (topical)	Refractory skin manifestations

impact on bone mineral density and may be steroid sparing for some people.[111]

Green tea polyphenols are potent antioxidant compounds that inhibit TNF-α–induced apoptosis and may provide epidermal protection in cutaneous manifestations of SLE.[114] There is no evidence to suggest oral consumption has an effect on SLE-related organ damage.

Special Populations

Pregnancy, Breastfeeding, and Contraception

SLE has no effect on fertility but is associated with a significant increase in morbidity and mortality during the antepartum and postpartum periods.[115-118] Among those who have SLE, there is a higher prevalence of fetal loss (spontaneous abortion and fetal demise), preeclampsia, hypertension, intrauterine growth restriction, and premature birth.[115,117,119] Dhar et al.[118] reported significantly higher rates of pregnancy-induced hypertension and preeclampsia among women with SLE when compared to control subjects (OR 4.27; 95% CI, 2.23−7.69). Newborns with antenatal exposure to anti-Ro/SSA or anti-La/SSB antibodies are at greater risk (2–20%) of developing reversible noncardiac neonatal lupus or irreversible congenital heart block.[116,117] Postpartum risks include thromboembolic events and hemorrhage (related to anticoagulant therapy). Breastfeeding is not contraindicated in SLE, and it does not seem to affect disease activity.[117] Cytotoxic medications (e.g., methotrexate, cyclophosphamide) used in the management of SLE are not recommended for women who are breastfeeding.[116,117]

If a woman with SLE is considering pregnancy, it is recommended that she postpone conception until the disease is stable or in remission. Active disease at conception and history of renal disease increase the likelihood of poor pregnancy outcome.[115,119] Women with SLE and preexisting kidney disease at conception are more likely to develop preeclampsia than women without preexisting kidney disease (66% versus 14%).[120] In 267 pregnancies observed by Clowse et al.,[115] women with increased SLE activity had fewer live births (77% versus 88%, P = .063) and fewer full-term births (26% versus 61%, P < .001) than women with lower activity SLE. There is a better pregnancy prognosis if disease is inactive for 3 to 6 months before conception.[117,119]

The effect of pregnancy on SLE activity is variable. Flares may occur in any trimester or during the postpartum period. Most flares are mild and involve arthritis or cutaneous manifestations of disease.[117,119] SLE renal flares may be difficult to differentiate from preeclampsia. Features consistent with renal flare and not preeclampsia

include SLE activity in other systems and presence of anti-dsDNA antibodies or active urinary sediments.[117]

Treatment of SLE in pregnancy is generally limited to NSAIDs, prednisone, and hydroxychloroquine (Plaquenil). Discontinuation of hydroxychloroquine therapy has been associated with a two-and-a-half-fold increase in disease activity.[121] If a woman is stable on hydroxychloroquine prior to conception, she should continue at the lowest possible therapeutic dose.[115] If a woman has antiphospholipid (aPL) antibodies, prophylactic anticoagulant therapy with low-dose aspirin is recommended. Low-dose aspirin with low-molecular-weight heparin is used in APS.[102,116] Anticoagulant therapy should be discontinued at the onset of labor and resumed postpartum for up to 3 months.[116] Azathioprine or cyclophosphamide may be indicated in severe flares of nephritis or cerebritis.[116]

Contraception recommendations for women with SLE are generally no different than those for healthy women. The method of contraception, including use of oral contraceptives, has no significant impact on SLE activity.[122,123] If a woman is aPLs positive or has APS, combination hormonal contraception should not be used.[98] While intrauterine contraception is not contraindicated for persons with SLE, appropriateness of use should be evaluated on a case-by-case basis. Women with risk factors for infection (multiple sex partners or use of aggressive immunosuppressant therapy) are generally not good candidates for intrauterine contraception.[98]

Elderly

Menopause does not appear to have an effect on SLE or SLE flares. The natural history of SLE is characterized by more significant disease activity earlier in the course of illness, so menopausal women tend to have milder disease. Disease activity in SLE has not been shown to increase menopausal symptoms or to hasten the onset of menopause. Women with SLE who receive cyclophosphamide therapy have a greater risk of premature ovarian failure. The increased risk is related to older age when treated with cyclophosphamide and higher cumulative doses. This therapy is the standard treatment for lupus nephritis and otherwise is reserved for severe flares of SLE.

Due to the systemic and inflammatory nature of SLE, women have increased risk for heart disease and osteoporosis during the postmenopausal period. Hormone therapy may increase the frequency of mild flares but does not affect the rate of severe flares. Hormone therapy is contraindicated in women with SLE who have a history of thrombosis, antiphospholipid syndrome, or positive antiphospholipid antibodies (anticardiolipin antibody or lupus anticoagulant).

Late-onset lupus, which is sometimes referred to as *elderly lupus*, presents in the early menopausal years (50 to 65 years of age). The presentation and course of late-onset lupus is generally milder than SLE that presents during the childbearing years. Women with late-onset lupus tend to have fewer skin manifestations and nephritis flares and more frequent serositis, arthritis, lung involvement, and neurologic lares. Treatment is based on symptom type and severity as with earlier onset SLE. Mortality rate and accrued organ damage is greater with late-onset lupus than with SLE.

Conclusion

A disproportionate number of persons with autoimmune disorders are women. Eighty disorders considered to have an autoimmune component affect 5–8% of the general US population, and 78% of those persons are female.[124] Classic thought regarding sex hormones and immune system function considered estrogen as an immune system stimulator and androgens as immune system suppressors.[125,126] For nonpregnant physiologic estrogen levels, this is generally true, and the increased inflammatory response explains the lower lifetime rates of infection and infection-related mortality in women as compared to men. Throughout the female reproductive life span, however, estrogen influences immune system cells in a biphasic fashion and effects in both proinflammatory and anti-inflammatory pathways. Recent research has shown that the roles of sex hormones in immune response are complex, and the sexual dimorphism of autoimmune disease is multifactorial.[4]

The effects of estrogen on autoimmunity depend in part upon the nature of the autoimmune disorder. In autoimmune disorders where B-cell activity predominates, estrogen generally stimulates at all levels. In disorders that do not have a strong B-cell involvement, there is a biphasic estrogen dose response—low levels enhance immune system activity and high levels inhibit immune response.[127] This may explain why SLE has peak onset during the childbearing years while RA may present in late reproductive and early menopausal life. In vitro studies have shown that estrogen enhances the production of autoantibodies by stimulating of B cells and inhibiting suppressor T cells.[127]

Recent trends in pharmacotherapy for autoimmune disorders focus on estrogen's immunomodulatory mechanisms of action. Estrogen stimulates tumor necrosis factor (TNF), interleukin (IL)-1β and interferon-γ. At elevated levels, as in pregnancy, estrogen stimulates IL-4, IL-10, and tumor growth factor-β (TGF-β) while inhibiting TNF, IL-1 β, IL-6, production of metalloproteinases, and natural killer cell activity.[127] The effects of estrogen on the immune system are dose dependent and are affected by the expression of estrogen receptors (ER-α and ER-β) on the target cells. Studies on animal models of MS,[128] SLE,[129] and RA[130] have shown some benefit to estrogen receptor targeted therapy. Keith et al.[130] identified a nonsteroid estrogen receptor ligand (WAY-169916) that binds to the estrogen receptor, interferes with NF-κB transcription and ultimately reduces inflammation in murine models of RA. Studies in experimental autoimmune encephalitis, the murine model of MS, has shown neuroprotective effects with estrogen receptor alpha (ER-α) agonist therapy. Treatment with ER-α agonist reduced proinflammatory cytokine secretion and decreased CNS inflammation and demelination.[128] Li et al.[129] researched the variable roles of ER-α and estrogen receptor beta (ER-β) in murine models of SLE and found that an ER-α selective agonist (propyl pyrazole triol) has an immunostimulatory effect in SLE while an ER-β selective agonist (diarylpropionitrile) has a slightly immunosuppressive effect. Current work in differentiating the specific roles of estrogen action in immune function may lead to estrogen-targeted therapies that will reduce the immunoregulatory effects of estrogen in women with autoimmune disorders.[131]

References

1. Bach JF. The effect of infections on susceptibility to autoimmune and allergic diseases. N Engl J Med 2002;347(12):911–20.
2. Edwards CW, Cambridge G. B-cell targeting in rheumatoid arthritis and other autoimmune diseases. Nature Reviews Immun 2006;6:394–403.
3. Ackerman LS. Sex hormones and the genesis of autoimmunity. Arch Dermatol 2006;142(3):371–6.
4. Gleicher N, Barad DH. Gender as risk factor for autoimmune diseases. J Autoimmunity 2007;28(1):1–6.
5. Lake DF, Briggs AD, Akporiaye ET. Immunopharmacology. In Katzung BG, ed. Basic & clinical pharmacology, 10th ed. New York, London: McGraw-Hill Medical, 2007:xiv, 931–57.
6. Furst DE, Ulrich RW. Nonsteroidal anti-inflammatory drugs, disease-modifying antirheumatic drugs, nonopioid analgesics, & drugs used in gout. In Katzung BG, ed. Basic & clinical pharmacology, 10th ed. New York, London: McGraw-Hill Medical, 2007:xiv, 576–603.

7. MacDermott RP. Progress in understanding the mechanisms of action of 5-aminosalicylic acid. Am J Gastroenterol 2000;95(12):3343–5.

8. Doan T, Massarotti E. Rheumatoid arthritis: an overview of new and emerging therapies. J Clin Pharmacol 2005;45(7):751–62.

9. Imboden J, Goodwin J, Davis J, Wofsy D. Immunosuppressive, antiinflammatory & immunomodulatory therapy. In Parslow TG, ed. Medical immunology, 10th ed. New York: Lange Medical Books/McGraw-Hill Medical Publishing Division; 2001:744–760xii, 814.

10. Griffiths B, Emery P. The treatment of lupus with cyclosporin A. Lupus 2001;10:165–70.

11. Goodin DS, Arnason BG, Coyle PK, Frohman EM, Paty DW. The use of mitoxantrone (Novantrone) for the treatment of multiple sclerosis: Report of the Therapeutics and Technology Assessment Subcommittee of the American Academy of Neurology. Neurology 2003;61(10):1332–8.

12. Ransohoff RM. Natalizumab for multiple sclerosis. N Engl J Med 2007;356(25):2622–9.

13. US Food and Drug Administration, Center for Drug Evaluation and Research. Tysabri risk minimization plan: summary of TOUCH. Available from: *www.fda.gov/cder/drug/infopage/natalizumab/RiskMAP.pdf* [Accessed August 3, 2007].

14. Polman CH, O'Connor PW, Havrdova E, Hutchinson M, Kappos L, Miller DH, et al. A randomized, placebo-controlled trial of natalizumab for relapsing multiple sclerosis. N Engl J Med 2006;354(9):899–910.

15. Rudick RA, Stuart WH, Calabresi PA, Confavreux C, Galetta SL, Radue EW, et al. Natalizumab plus interferon beta-1a for relapsing multiple sclerosis. N Engl J Med 2006;354(9):911–23.

16. Ransohoff RM. Natalizumab for multiple sclerosis. N Engl J Med 2007;356:2622–9.

17. Baldinetti F, Belcher G, Bozic C, Hyde R, Kim R, Lynn F, et al. Natalizumab utilization and safety: latest results from TOUCH and TYGRIS. Abstract SC317. Eur J Neurol 2008;15:27–8.

18. Hartung HP. New cases of progressive multifocal leukoencephalopathy after treatment with natalizumab. Lancet Neurol 2009;8(1):28–31.

19. Yousry TA, Major EO, Ryschkewitsch C, Fahle G, Fischer S, Hou J, et al. Evaluation of patients treated with natalizumab for progressive multifocal leukoencephalopathy. N Engl J Med 2006;354(9):924–33.

20. Looney RJ. B cell-targeted therapy for rheumatoid arthritis: an update on the evidence. Drugs 2006;66:625–39.

21. American College of Rheumatology. Guidelines for the management of rheumatoid arthritis: 2002 update. Arthritis Rheumatism 2002;46(2):328–46.

22. Arnon R. The development of cop 1 (Copaxone), an innovative drug for the treatment of multiple sclerosis: personal reflections. Immunol Lett 1996;50:1–15.

23. Dhib-Jalbut S. Mechanisms of action of interferons and glatiramer acetate in multiple sclerosis. Neurology 2002;58(8)(suppl 4):S3–S9.

24. Neuhaus O, Kieseier BC, Hartung HP. Pharmacokinetics and pharmacodynamics of the interferon-betas, glatiramer acetate, and mitoxantrone in multiple sclerosis. J Neurol Sci 2007;259(1–2):27–37.

25. Friedman S, Blumberg RS. Inflammatory bowel disease. In Kasper DL, Harrison TR, eds. Harrison's principles of internal medicine, 17th ed. New York: McGraw-Hill Medical Pub. Division; 2008. 1886–98.

26. Loftus EV Jr. Clinical epidemiology of inflammatory bowel disease: incidence, prevalence, and environmental influences. Gastroenterology 2004;126:1504–117.

27. Ferguson LR, Shelling AN, Browning BL, Huebner C, Petermann I. Genes, diet and inflammatory bowel disease. Mutation Res 2007;622:70–83.

28. Freeman HJ. Familial Crohn's disease in single or multiple first-degree relatives. J Clin Gastroenterol 2002;35:9–13.

29. Halme L, Turunen U, Helio T, Paavola P, Walle T, Miettinen A, et al. Familial and sporadic inflammatory bowel disease: comparison of clinical features and serological markers in a genetically homogeneous population. Scand J Gastroenterol 2002;37(6):692–8.

30. Hanauer SB, Sandborn W. Management of Crohn's disease in adults. Am J Gastroenterol 2001;96:635–43.

31. Quinton JF, Sendid B, Reumaux D, Duthilleul P, Cortot A, Grandbastien B, et al. Anti-*Saccharomyces cerevisiae* mannan antibodies combined with antineutrophil cytoplasmic autoantibodies in inflammatory bowel disease: prevalence and diagnostic role. Gut 1998;42:788–91.

32. Cohen RD, Woseth DM, Thisted RA, Hanauer SB. A meta-analysis and overview of the literature on treatment options for left-sided ulcerative colitis and ulcerative proctitis. Am J Gastroenterol 2000;95:1263–76.

33. Munkholm P, Loftus EV Jr. Reinacher-Schick A, Kornbluth A, Mittmann U, Esendal B. Prevention of colorectal cancer in inflammatory bowel disease: value of screening and 5-aminosalicylates. Digestion 2006;73:11–9.

34. Lichtenstein GR, Abreu MT, Cohen R, Tremaine W. American Gastroenterological Association Institute medical position statement on corticosteroids, immunomodulators, and infliximab in inflammatory bowel disease. Gastroenterology 2006;130:935–9.

35. Clark M, Colombel JF, Feagan BC, Fedorak RN, Hanauer SB, Kamm MA, et al. American gastroenterological association consensus development conference on the use of biologics in the treatment of inflammatory bowel disease, June 21–23, 2006. Gastroenterol 2007;133:312–39.

36. Lawson MM, Thomas AG, Akobeng AK. Tumour necrosis factor alpha blocking agents for induction of remission in ulcerative colitis. Cochrane Database Syst Rev 2006 Jul 19;3:CD005112.

37. Sandborn WJ, Hanauer SB, Rutgeerts P, Fedorak RN, Lukas M, Macintosh DG, et al. Adalimumab for maintenance treatment of Crohn's disease: results of the CLASSIC II trial. Gut 2007;56:1232–9.

38. Van Assche G, Van Ranst M, Sciot R, Dubois B, Vermeire S, Noman M, et al. Progressive multifocal leukoencephalopathy after natalizumab therapy for Crohn's disease. N Engl J Med 2005;353(4):362–8.

39. MacDonald JK, McDonald JWD. Natalizumab for induction of remission in Crohn's disease. Cochrane Database Syst Rev 2007 Jan 24; (1):CD006097.

40. Crohn's and Colitis Foundation of America. Diet & Nutrition. 2002. Available from: *www.ccfa.org/frameviewer/?url=/media/pdf/diet.pdf* [Accessed August 13, 2007].

41. Sartor RB. Therapeutic manipulation of the enteric microflora in inflammatory bowel diseases: antibiotics, probiotics, and prebiotics. Gastroenterol 2004;126:1620–33.

42. Langmead L, Rampton DS. Review article: complementary and alternative therapies for inflammatory bowel disease. Aliment Pharmacol Ther 2006;23:341–9.

43. Ferrero S, Ragni N. Inflammatory bowel disease: management issues during pregnancy. Arch Gynecol Obstet 2004;270:79–85.

44. Alstead EM, Nelson-Piercy C. Inflammatory bowel disease in pregnancy. Gut 2003;52:159–61.

45. Baird DD, Narendranathan M, Sandler RS. Increased risk of preterm birth for women with inflammatory bowel disease. Gastroenterol 1990;99:987–94.

46. Elbaz G, Fich A, Levy A, Holcberg G, Sheiner E. Inflammatory bowel disease and preterm delivery. Int J Gyaenecol Obstet 2005;90:193–7.

47. Heetun ZS, Byrnes C, Neary P, O'Morain C. Review article: reproduction in the patient with inflammatory bowel disease. Aliment Pharmacol Ther 2007;26:513–33.

48. American Academy of Pediatrics. Transfer of drugs and other chemicals into human milk. Pediatrics 2001;108:776–89.

49. Royal College of Obstetricians & Gynaecologists. Contraceptive choices for women with inflammatory bowel disease. J Fam Plann Reprod Health Care 2003;29:127–35.

50. Hauser SL, Oksenberg JR. The neurobiology of multiple sclerosis: genes, inflammation, and neurodegeneration. Neuron 2006;52:61–76.

51. Hauser SL, Goodin DS. Multiple sclerosis and other demyelinating diseases. In Kasper DL, Harrison TR, eds. Harrison's principles of internal medicine, 17th ed. New York: McGraw-Hill Medical Pub. Division; 2008. 2611–20.

52. Compston A, Coles A. Multiple sclerosis. Lancet 2008 372(9648):1502–17.53.

53. Pittock SJ, Mayr WT, McClelland RL, Jorgensen NW, Weigand SD, Noseworthy JH, et al. Change in MS-related disability in a population-based cohort: a 10-year follow-up study. Neurology 2004;62:51–9.

54. Lublin FD, Reingold SC. Defining the clinical course of multiple sclerosis: results of an international survey. National Multiple Sclerosis Society (USA) Advisory Committee on Clinical Trials of New Agents in Multiple Sclerosis. Neurology 1996;46:907–11.

55. Kurtzke JF. Rating neurologic impairment in multiple sclerosis: an expanded disability status scale (EDSS). Neurology 1983;33:1444–52.

56. Thrower BW. Clinically isolated syndromes: predicting and delaying multiple sclerosis. Neurology 2007; 68(24)(suppl 4):S12–5.

57. Polman CH, Reingold SC, Edan G, Filippi M, Hartung HP, Kappos L, et al. Diagnostic criteria for multiple sclerosis: 2005 revisions to the "McDonald Criteria." Ann Neurol 2005;58:840–6.

58. Then Bergh F, Kumpfel T, Schumann E, Held U, Schwan M, Blazevic M, et al. Monthly intravenous methylprednisolone in relapsing-remitting multiple sclerosis-reduction of enhancing lesions, T2 lesion volume and plasma prolactin concentrations. BMC Neurology 2006;6:19.

59. Kieseier BC, Hartung HP. Current disease-modifying therapies in multiple sclerosis. Sem Neurol 2003; 23:133–46.

60. Goodin DS, Frohman EM, Garmany GP Jr, Halper J, Likosky WH, Lublin FD, et al. Disease-modifying therapies in multiple sclerosis: report of the

Therapeutics and Technology Assessment Subcommittee of the American Academy of Neurology and the MS Council for Clinical Practice Guidelines. Neurology 2002;58:169–78.

61. Zivadinov R, Rudick RA, De Masi R, Nasuelli D, Ukmar M, Pozzi-Mucelli RS, et al. Effects of IV methylprednisolone on brain atrophy in relapsing-remitting MS. Neurology 2001;57:1239–47.

62. Beck RW, Cleary PA, Trobe JD, Kaufman DI, Kupersmith MJ, Paty DW, et al. The effect of corticosteroids for acute optic neuritis on the subsequent development of multiple sclerosis. The Optic Neuritis Study Group. N Engl J Med 1993;329:1764–69.

63. Johnson KP. Control of multiple sclerosis relapses with immunomodulating agents. J Neurol Sci 2007; 256(suppl 1):S23–8.

64. Comi G, Filippi M, Wolinsky JS. European/Canadian multicenter, double-blind, randomized, placebo-controlled study of the effects of glatiramer acetate on magnetic resonance imaging—measured disease activity and burden in patients with relapsing multiple sclerosis. European/Canadian Glatiramer Acetate Study Group. Ann Neurol 2001;49:290–7.

65. Filippi M, Rovaris M, Rocca MA, Sormani MP, Wolinsky JS, Comi G. Glatiramer acetate reduces the proportion of new MS lesions evolving into "black holes." Neurol 2001;57:731–3.

66. Kappos L, Bates D, Hartung HP, Havrdova E, Miller D, Polman CH, et al. Natalizumab treatment for multiple sclerosis: recommendations for patient selection and monitoring. Lancet Neurol 2007;6:431–41.

67. Shinto L, Calabrese C, Morris C, Sinsheimer S, Bourdette D. Complementary and alternative medicine in multiple sclerosis: survey of licensed naturopaths. J Altern Complement Med 2004;10:891–7.

68. Ferrero S, Pretta S, Ragni N. Multiple sclerosis: management issues during pregnancy. Eur J Obsetet Gynecol Reprod Biol 2004;115:3–9.

69. Walther EU, Hohlfeld R. Multiple sclerosis: side effects of interferon beta therapy and their management. Neurol 1999;53:1622–7.

70. Vaux KK, Kahole NC, Jones KL. Cyclophosphamide, methotrexate, and cytarabine embryopathy: is apoptosis the common pathway? Birth Defects Res Part A Clin Mol Teratol 2003;67:403–8.

71. Zorgdrager A, De Keyser J. Menstrually related worsening of symptoms in multiple sclerosis. J Neurol Sci 1997;149:95–7.

72. Lipsky PE. Rheumatoid arthritis. In Kasper DL, Harrison TR, eds. Harrison's principles of internal medicine, 17th ed. New York: McGraw-Hill Medical Pub. Division; 2008. 2083–91.

73. Klareskog L, Padyukov L, Lorentzen J, Alfredsson L. Mechanisms of disease: genetic susceptibility and environmental triggers in the development of rheumatoid arthritis. Nat Clin Pract Rheumatol 2006;2:425–33.

74. Rindfleisch JA, Muller D. Diagnosis and management of rheumatoid arthritis. Am Fam Physician 2005;72:1037–47.

75. Arnett FC, Edworthy SM, Bloch DA, McShane DJ, Fries JF, Cooper NS, et al. The American Rheumatism Association 1987 revised criteria for the classification of rheumatoid arthritis. Arthritis Rheum 1988;31:315–24.

76. Gaffo A, Saag KG, Curtis JR. Treatment of rheumatoid arthritis. Am J Health Syst Pharm 2006;63: 2451–65.

77. Maradit-Kremers H, Crowson CS, Nicola PJ, Ballman KV, Roger VL, Jacobsen SJ, et al. Increased unrecognized coronary heart disease and sudden deaths in rheumatoid arthritis: a population-based cohort study. Arthritis Rheum 2005;52:402–11.

78. Choi HK, Hernan MA, Seeger JD, Robins JM, Wolfe F. Methotrexate and mortality in patients with rheumatoid arthritis: a prospective study. Lancet 2002;359: 1173–7.

79. American College of Rheumatology. Guidelines for monitoring drug therapy in rheumatoid arthritis. Arthritis Rheum 1996;39:723–31.

80. Andersohn F, Suissa S, Garbe E. Use of first- and second-generation cyclooxygenase-2-selective nonsteroidal antiinflammatory drugs and risk of acute myocardial infarction. Circulation 2006;113:1950–7.

81. Dajani EZ, Islam K. Cardiovascular and gastrointestinal toxicity of selective cyclo-oxygenase-2 inhibitors in man. J Physiol Pharmacol 2008;59(suppl 2):117–33.

82. Gotzsche PC, Johansen HK. Short-term low-dose corticosteroids vs placebo and nonsteroidal antiinflammatory drugs in rheumatoid arthritis. Cochrane Database Syst Rev 2005;(3):CD000189.

83. Cohen S, Cannon GW, Schiff M, Weaver A, Fox R, Olsen N, et al. Two-year, blinded, randomized, controlled trial of treatment of active rheumatoid arthritis with leflunomide compared with methotrexate. Utilization of Leflunomide in the Treatment of Rheumatoid Arthritis Trial Investigator Group. Arthritis Rheum 2001;44:1984–92.

84. Jundt JW, Browne BA, Fiocco GP, Steele AD, Mock D. A comparison of low dose methotrexate

bioavailability: oral solution, oral tablet, subcutaneous and intramuscular dosing. J Rheumatol 1993;20:1845–9.

85. Hoekstra M, Haagsma C, Neef C, Proost J, Knuif A, van de Laar M. Bioavailability of higher dose methotrexate comparing oral and subcutaneous administration in patients with rheumatoid arthritis. J Rheumatol 2004;31:645–8.

86. Pavy S, Constantin A, Pham T, Gossec L, Maillefert JF, Cantagrel A, et al. Methotrexate therapy for rheumatoid arthritis: clinical practice guidelines based on published evidence and expert opinion. Joint Bone Spine 2006;73:388–95.

87. Nogid A, Pham DQ. Role of abatacept in the management of rheumatoid arthritis. Clin Therap 2006; 28:1764–78.

88. O'Dell JR, Leff R, Paulsen G, Haire C, Mallek J, Eckhoff PJ, et al. Treatment of rheumatoid arthritis with methotrexate and hydroxychloroquine, methotrexate and sulfasalazine, or a combination of the three medications: results of a two-year, randomized, double-blind, placebo-controlled trial. Arthritis Rheum 2002;46:1164–70.

89. Little CV, Parsons T. Herbal therapy for treating rheumatoid arthritis. Cochrane Database Syst Rev 2001;(1):CD002948.

90. Soeken KL, Miller SA, Ernst E. Herbal medicines for the treatment of rheumatoid arthritis: a systematic review. Rheumatol 2003;42:652–9.

91. Steultjens EEMJ, Dekker JJ, Bouter LM, Schaardenburg DD, van Kuyk MA, Van den Ende EC. Occupational therapy for rheumatoid arthritis. Cochrane Database Syst Rev 2004;(1):CD003114.

92. Van Den Ende CH, Vliet Vlieland TP, Munneke M, Hazes JM. Dynamic exercise therapy for rheumatoid arthritis. Cochrane Database Syst Rev [Online]. 2000; (2):CD000322.

93. Verhagen AP, Bierma-Zeinstra SMA, Boers M, Cardoso JR, Lambeck J, de Bie R, de Vet HCW. Balneotherapy for rheumatoid arthritis. Cochrane Database Syst Rev 2003;(4):CD000518.

94. Casimiro L, Barnsley L, Brosseau L, Milne S, Robinson VA, Tugwell P, et al. Acupuncture and electroacupuncture for the treatment of rheumatoid arthritis. Cochrane Database Syst Rev 2005 Oct 19; (4):CD003788.

95. Egan M, Brosseau L, Farmer M, Ouimet M, Rees S, Tugwell P, et al. Splints and orthosis for treating rheumatoid arthritis. Cochrane Database Syst Rev 2001;(4):CD004018.

96. Tandon VR, Sharma S, Mahajan A, Khajuria V, Kumar A. Pregnancy and rheumatoid arthritis. Indian J Med Sci 2006;60:334–44.

97. Temprano KK, Bandlamudi R, Moore TL. Antirheumatic drugs in pregnancy and lactation. Semin Arthritis Rheum 2005;35:112–21.

98. Sammaritano LR. Therapy insight: guidelines for selection of contraception in women with rheumatic diseases. Nature Clin Prac Rheumatol 2007;3:273–81.

99. D'Cruz DP. Systemic lupus erythematosus. BMJ 2006;332:890–4.

100. Mills JA. Systemic lupus erythematosus. N Engl J Med 1994;330:1871–9.

101. Gill JM, Quisel AM, Rocca PV, Walters DT. Diagnosis of systemic lupus erythematosus. Am Fam Physician 2003;68:2179–86.

102. Hahn Bevra H. Systemic lupus erythematosus. In Kasper DL, Harrison TR, eds. Harrison's principles of internal medicine, 17th ed. New York: McGraw-Hill Medical Pub. Division; 2008. 2075–82.

103. Petri M. Systemic lupus erythematosus: 2006 update. J Clin Rheumatol 2006;12:37–40.

104. Bernatsky S, Boivin JF, Joseph L, Manzi S, Ginzler E, Gladman DD, et al. Mortality in systemic lupus erythematosus. Arthritis Rheum 2006;54:2550–7.

105. American College of Rheumatology. Guidelines for referral and management of systemic lupus erythematosus in adults. American College of Rheumatology Ad Hoc Committee on Systemic Lupus Erythematosus Guidelines. Arthritis Rheum 1999;42: 1785–96.

106. Rivest C, Lew RA, Welsing PM, Sangha O, Wright EA, Roberts WN, et al. Association between clinical factors, socioeconomic status, and organ damage in recent onset systemic lupus erythematosus. J Rheumatol 2000;27:680–4.

107. Stojanovich L, Zandman-Goddard G, Pavlovich S, Sikanich N. Psychiatric manifestations in systemic lupus erythematosus. Autoimmunity Rev 2007; 6:421–6.

108. Rhiannon JJ. Systemic lupus erythematosus involving the nervous system: presentation, pathogenesis, and management. Clin Rev Allergy Immunol 2008;34:356–60.

109. Ting WW, Sontheimer RD. Local therapy for cutaneous and systemic lupus erythematosus: practical and theoretical considerations. Lupus 2001;10:171–84.

110. Vasoo S. Drug-induced lupus: an update. Lupus 2006;15:757–61.

111. Mok CC. Emerging drug therapies for systemic lupus erythematosus. Expert Opin Emerg Drugs 2006;11:597–608.

112. Ergas D, Eilat E, Mendlovic S, Sthoeger ZM. n-3 fatty acids and the immune system in autoimmunity. Isr Med Assoc J 2002;4:34–8.

113. Chang DM, Lan JL, Lin HY, Luo SF. Dehydroepiandrosterone treatment of women with mild-to-moderate systemic lupus erythematosus: a multicenter randomized, double-blind, placebo-controlled trial. Arthritis Rheum 2002;46:2924–7.

114. Hsu S, Dickinson D. A new approach to managing oral manifestations of Sjogren's syndrome and skin manifestations of lupus. J Biochem Mol Biol 2006;39:229–39.

115. Clowse ME, Magder LS, Witter F, Petri M. The impact of increased lupus activity on obstetric outcomes. Arthritis Rheum 2005;52:514–21.

116. Dhar JP, Sokol RJ. Lupus and pregnancy: complex yet manageable. Clin Med Res 2006;4:310–321.

117. Mok CC, Wong RW. Pregnancy in systemic lupus erythematosus. Postgrad Med J 2001;77:157–65.

118. Dhar JP, Essenmacher LM, Ager JW, Sokol RJ. Pregnancy outcomes before and after a diagnosis of systemic lupus erythematosus. Am J Obstet Gynecol 2005;193:1444–55.

119. Cortes-Hernandez J, Ordi-Ros J, Paredes F, Casellas M, Castillo F, Vilardell-Tarres M. Clinical predictors of fetal and maternal outcome in systemic lupus erythematosus: a prospective study of 103 pregnancies. Rheumatology 2002;41:643–50.

120. Nossent HC, Swaak TJ. Systemic lupus erythematosus. VI. Analysis of the interrelationship with pregnancy. J Rheumatol 1990;17:771–6.

121. A randomized study of the effect of withdrawing hydroxychloroquine sulfate in systemic lupus erythematosus. The Canadian Hydroxychloroquine Study Group. N Engl J Med 1991;324:150–4.

122. Sanchez-Guerrero J, Uribe AG, Jimenez-Santana L, Mestanza-Peralta M, Lara-Reyes P, Seuc AH, et al. A trial of contraceptive methods in women with systemic lupus erythematosus. N Engl J Med 2005; 353:2539–49.

123. Petri M, Kim MY, Kalunian KC, Grossman J, Hahn BH, Sammaritano LR, et al. Combined oral contraceptives in women with systemic lupus erythematosus. N Engl J Med 2005;353:2550–8.

124. U. S. Department of Health and Human Services. National Institutes of Health Autoimmune Disease Coordinating Committee Report, 2002, NIH Publication 03–05. Bethesda, MD: The Institutes, 2002.

125. Grossman CJ. Interactions between the gonadal steroids and the immune system. Science 1985;227: 257–61.

126. Olsen NJ, Kovacs WJ. Gonadal steroids and immunity. Endocr Rev 1996;17:369–84.

127. Straub RH. The complex role of estrogens in inflammation. Endocr Rev 2007;28:521–74.

128. Morales LB, Loo KK, Liu HB, Peterson C, Tiwari-Woodruff S, Voskuhl RR. Treatment with an estrogen receptor alpha ligand is neuroprotective in experimental autoimmune encephalomyelitis. J Neurosci 2006;26:6823–33.

129. Li J, McMurray RW. Effects of estrogen receptor subtype-selective agonists on autoimmune disease in lupus-prone NZB/NZW F1 mouse model. Clin Immunol 2007;123:219–26.

130. Keith JC Jr, Albert LM, Leathurby Y, Follettie M, Wang L, Borges-Marcucci L, et al. The utility of pathway selective estrogen receptor ligands that inhibit nuclear factor-kappa B transcriptional activity in models of rheumatoid arthritis. Arthritis Res Ther 2005;7:R427–38.

131. Greenstein BD. Lupus: why women? J Womens Health Gend Based Med 2001;10:233–9.

132. King TL. Systemic lupus erythematous. In Star WL, Lommel LL, Shannon ML, eds. Women's primary health care, 2nd ed. San Francisco: UCSF Nursing Press, 2004:10–27.

133. Hochberg MC. Updating the American College of Rheumatology revised criteria for the classification of systemic lupus erythematosus. Arthritis Rheum 1997;40:1725.

134. Sibilia J. Treatment of systemic lupus erythematosus in 2006. Joint Bone Spine 2006;73:591–8.

135. Bouma G, Strober W. The immunological and genetic basis of inflammatory bowel disease. Nat Rev Immunol 2003;3:521–33.

136. Carroll MC. A protective role for innate immunity in systemic lupus erythematosus. Nat Rev Immunol 2004;4:825–31.

"Diabetes is caused by melancholy."
THOMAS WILLIS, ENGLISH SCIENTIST (1621–1671)

18

Diabetes

Nancy Jo Reedy and Tekoa L. King

Chapter Glossary

Atherosclerosis Macrovascular disease of the large blood vessels.

Diabetes insipidus Increased urine production resulting from inadequate vasopressin production by the pituitary gland.

Diabetes mellitus All conditions characterized by high blood glucose levels and varying degrees of glucose intolerance.

Euglycemia Normal blood sugar—neither too high nor too low.

Gestational diabetes (GDM) Insulin resistance that occurs for the first time in pregnancy. Usually treated with diet alone or with insulin.

Glucagon Hormone secreted by pancreas in opposition to insulin.

Gluconeogenesis Manufacture of glucose by the liver.

Glycogenolysis Breakdown of fat.

Glycosuria Glucose in urine.

Glycosylation Attachment of glucose to hemoglobin, which occurs when hemoglobin is exposed to high plasma levels of glucose.

Hemoglobin A1c Measurement of glycosylated hemoglobin.

Hypoglycemia Blood glucose below normal values.

Impaired fasting glucose (IFG) Fasting plasma glucose between 100 and 125 mg/dL.

Impaired glucose tolerance (IGT) A 2-hour postglucose load plasma glucose value between 140 and 199 mg/dL.

Insulin analogs Insulin that is synthetically produced using recombinant DNA technology. Insulin analogs are slightly different from endogenously produced insulin. They are altered in ways that affect absorption, distribution, metabolism, and/or excretion. Insulin analogs bind to insulin receptors the same way endogenously produced insulin does and are able to exert all the normal metabolic functions attributed to insulin produced within the body.

Insulin resistance Condition in which normal blood levels of insulin are insufficient to produce a normal insulin response in peripheral tissues such as muscle, liver, and adipose cells.

Insulin secretagogues Medicines that stimulate the beta cells of the pancreas to secrete insulin.

Ketoacidosis Ability of glucose to chemically attach to different proteins without the stimulus of enzymatic facilitation.

Ketones Breakdown product of fat metabolism.

Latent autoimmune diabetes of adults (LADA) A form of type 1 diabetes that develops in adulthood. Persons with LADA have some insulin resistance but deficient production of insulin from the pancreas as well. These individuals usually need insulin replacement.

Lipodystrophy Loss of adipose tissue at an injection site that is usually evident as a nonpainful lump under the skin. Insulin will not be absorbed well through an area of adipose tissue that has degenerative changes. Lipodystrophy can be prevented by rotating injection sites frequently.

Lipolysis Breakdown of fat.

Metabolic syndrome A collection of risk factors that predict the occurrence of type 2 diabetes and coronary heart disease.

Polydipsia Excessive thirst.

Polyphagia Excessive hunger.

Polyuria Excessive urine production.

Prandial dose Dose of insulin given just before a meal.

Prediabetes Impaired glucose metabolism that does not meet the criteria for type 1 or type 2 diabetes. May be IGF or IGT.

Type 1 diabetes* Condition characterized by pancreatic cell destruction that is usually the result of autoimmune destruction of these cells. Persons with type 1 diabetes always need insulin replacement.

Type 2 diabetes† Condition characterized by hyperglycemia that is secondary to a combination of insulin resistance and/or insulin deficiency. May be treated with oral agents or with insulin.

* Previously called juvenile-onset diabetes and insulin-dependent diabetes.
† Previously called adult-onset diabetes and non-insulin dependent diabetes.

Introduction

Diabetes is a growth industry in the United States today. The number of persons with diagnosed diabetes tripled from 5.6 million in 1980 to 16.8 million in 2006.[1] Approximately 5.8% of the total United States population and 10% of women age 45 or older have diagnosed diabetes. In addition, 25.9% of the adults in the United States today have undiagnosed diabetes or prediabetes as ascertained by measurements of impaired fasting glucose values.[2] It is estimated that the economic cost of diabetes in both lost productivity and direct medical expenses is $132 billion per year.[3] This chapter reviews the drugs used to treat diabetes.

Definition and Classifications of Diabetes

Diabetes is derived from the Greek verb *diabainein*, which means "to stand with the legs apart" or "siphon," as in urination. The two forms of diabetes that share the one symptom of polyuria are **diabetes mellitus** and **diabetes insipidus**. Mellitus means "honey-sweet urine."[4] Diabetes insipidus comes from the Latin word that means "without taste." Diabetes insipidus is caused by a deficiency of antidiuretic hormone secondary to pituitary dysfunction. Diabetes insipidus is discussed briefly later in this chapter. Diabetes mellitus includes the diabetic conditions that are characterized by abnormally high levels of blood glucose and varying degrees of glucose intolerance.[5] Although glucose intolerance is actually a continuum, diabetes mellitus is categorized on the basis of the etiology responsible for glucose abnormalities. **Type 1 diabetes** is characterized by pancreatic cell destruction, which is usually the result of autoimmune destruction of these cells.[5] This destruction leads to absolute insulin deficiency, and thus, persons with type 1 diabetes require insulin therapy. **Latent autoimmune diabetes of adults** (LADA) is a form of type 1 diabetes that develops in adulthood. Persons with LADA have some insulin resistance but a more profound deficit of insulin production from the pancreas, and they frequently need insulin replacement soon after the initial diagnosis. The management of persons with LADA depends on the relative degrees of insulin resistance and insulin deficit present.[6] **Type 2 diabetes** is more common and is also characterized by hyperglycemia; however, in this case, the hyperglycemia is secondary to a combination of insulin resistance and/or insulin deficiency. The third type of diabetes mellitus is **gestational diabetes** (GDM), which, like type 2 diabetes, is secondary to insulin resistance that occurs for the first time during pregnancy.

In addition to the three types of diabetes mellitus, there are two types of prediabetic states that are defined on the basis of what type of plasma glucose test is obtained. Both are considered precursors to overt diabetes. Persons with **impaired fasting glucose** (IFG) have a fasting plasma glucose between 100 and 125 mg/dL. Persons with **impaired glucose tolerance** (IGT) have a 2-hour post-glucose load plasma glucose value between 140 and 199 mg/dL. Diabetes mellitus is a metabolic disorder wherein the body cannot metabolize carbohydrates, fats, and proteins secondary to insulin deficiency.

Although the definitions of the various types of diabetes are distinct, these classifications are often less clear in clinical practice. For example, a person with type 2 diabetes may over time experience destruction of pancreatic cells. Any combination of insulin resistance and insulin deficiency can be severe enough to require insulin therapy. Thus for the purpose of treating diabetes effectively, the specific diagnosis is less important than the clinical course. Nonetheless, in order to present this material in an organized fashion, each type of diabetes will be discussed separately.

Epidemiology and Complications of Diabetes

The prevalence of diabetes is higher among non-Hispanic Blacks, American Indians, Asian/Pacific Islanders, and

Hispanic/Latino American women compared to non-Hispanic Whites.[7] These populations are the racial and ethnic minorities who have the most difficulty accessing health care and the populations most likely to have some of the common complications of diabetes. The prevalence of this disease is similar in men and women, and the incidence increases sharply as we age. In 2006, 18.4% of women between the ages of 65 and 74 had diagnosed diabetes.[8] Women who have a history of gestational diabetes have a 37-fold increased risk for developing type 2 diabetes, and approximately 20% of these women will develop type 2 diabetes later in life.[9]

There are a number of adverse health outcomes associated with diabetes. In fact, the diagnosis of diabetes can be the onset of a pathophysiologic domino effect that results in both microvascular and macrovascular dysfunction.[10] These processes, in turn, lead to arteriosclerosis, hypertension, coronary artery disease, stroke, renal disease, blindness, and amputations, to name just a few[11] (Chapter 15). Although diabetes has no known cure to date, aggressive treatment can mitigate the development of complications and improve quality of life. Preventing and retarding microvascular complications is essential to effective management of diabetes. However, before discussing specific management, a review of glucose metabolism and the pathophysiology of diabetes is in order.

Physiology of Glucose Metabolism

Glucose is made available for fueling metabolism via one of the following three sources: (1) intestinal absorption of food, (2) **gluconeogenesis**, which is the manufacture of glucose by the liver, and (3) **glycogenolysis**, which is the breakdown of fat. Under normal conditions, glucose blood levels are regulated by the actions of insulin, which is produced and excreted by the beta cells of the islets of Langerhans in the pancreas. Normal insulin secretion is approximately 1 unit/kg/day in the fasting state.

There are several cast members in this play once glucose is ingested and blood levels rise. The goal is to maintain plasma glucose levels within a specific range. Gastrointestinal hormones called "incretins" stimulate the islets of Langerhans in the pancreas to release insulin as soon as food is present in the stomach and intestine. Once glucose is absorbed into the circulation, high levels of glucose also stimulate production and secretion of insulin. This initiates a series of interrelated events in which insulin is the main character (Figure 18-1).

The Role of Insulin

Insulin is in essence an anabolic hormone that acts primarily on the liver, adipose tissue, and skeletal muscle but

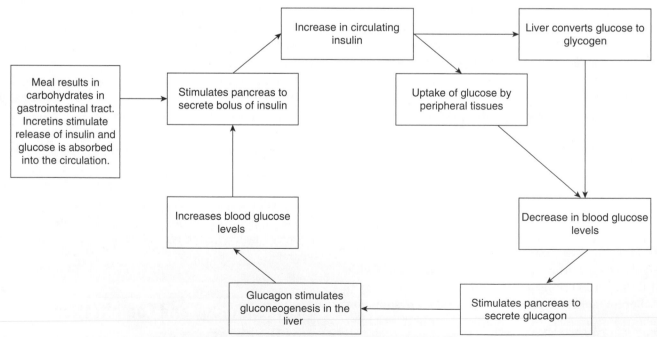

After food is ingested and blood glucose levels rise, the pancreas secretes insulin, which stimulates uptake of glucose by cells and conversion of glucose into glycogen within the liver. As blood glucose levels fall, glucagon is secreted by the pancreas. Glucagon then stimulates gluconeogenesis in the liver so blood glucose levels remain within a normal range between meals.

Figure 18-1 Regulation of glucose metabolism.

has many other functions, some of which are still being discovered. The primary function of insulin is facilitation of glucose into peripheral tissue cells. Insulin also inhibits gluconeogenesis in the liver, stimulates glycogen formation in the liver, converts fatty acids to triglyceride, discourages lipolysis, and stimulates protein synthesis. In addition, insulin encourages the production of nitrous oxide in the endothelial cells lining blood vessels throughout the vascular tree. In turn, nitrous oxide has multiple functions that protect against the formation of atherosclerosis.[12]

Most cells in the body have cell surface receptors for insulin. Once insulin binds to the insulin receptor, glucose is taken into the cell, and different enzyme-controlled reactions occur. Interestingly, there are two organs that do not have insulin receptors—the brain and the liver. However, the cells in these organs are permeable to glucose, and it passes into the cells of these two organs readily via diffusion.

Endogenous secretion of insulin has both a basal component and bolus component. The basal secretion of insulin limits **lipolysis** and gluconeogenesis in the liver while maintaining a blood level sufficient for cerebral metabolism. Nonobese, healthy adults secrete basal insulin at the rate of 0.5–1 U/hour, which maintains the plasma insulin concentration at 35–104 pmol/L. The basal insulin at normal levels results in a fasting plasma glucose of 70–110 mg/dL.[13]

Insulin secretion rises rapidly following a meal. The response to food is a fivefold to tenfold increase in insulin release as bolus insulin. This bolus of insulin inhibits gluconeogenesis in the liver and stimulates peripheral glucose utilization by muscle. The plasma concentrations of insulin rise to the peak of 417–556 pmol/L within 30–60 minutes of eating.

The release of bolus insulin occurs in a two-peak process with an initial rise immediately after the meal and a second rise that lasts up to 6.5 hours, depending on the type of food consumed. The first peak of insulin is short, limiting the circulating glucose level of the quickly absorbed carbohydrates and simple sugars in the food. The second peak is longer and is present to process the blood glucose levels that occur as carbohydrates are absorbed from the gastrointestinal tract over time. Up to 6.5 hours may be needed in the postabsorptive state—even more if the intake was high in fat.[13]

The insulin response to a meal is further affected by other factors, including the carbohydrate, fat, and protein content of the meal, transit time in the gastrointestinal system, insulin, and glucagon effect on glucose metabolism in the peripheral tissues and the liver.[14] Obese adults who are otherwise healthy show a severalfold higher rate of basal and bolus insulin response depending on the degree of obesity. Both healthy weight and obese individuals who have normal glucose metabolism will have a postprandial blood glucose level at or below 140 mg/dL. In healthy individuals, the plasma glucose level returns to basal level within 2 to 3 hours after eating.[14]

Glucagon

Playing opposite insulin is **glucagon**, a peptide hormone produced by the alpha cells within the islets of Langerhans. Glucagon is the counterregulatory hormone to insulin. It is released when blood levels of glucose are low and acts within the liver, where it stimulates gluconeogenesis, glycolysis, and ketogenesis, thereby increasing blood glucose levels. Paradoxically, once blood levels of glucose rise, this rise stimulates the release of insulin and the cycle starts over.

Pathophysiology of Glucose Metabolism: Diabetes Mellitus

Type 1 diabetes is the result of autoimmune destruction of the beta cells in the islets of Langerhans within the pancreas, which results in an absolute deficiency of insulin. Type 2 diabetes involves dysfunction in several of the steps within the glucose regulating mechanisms—insulin secretion, glucose transport, glucose production, and/or glucose utilization. However, individuals with type 2 diabetes have some degree of endogenous insulin. Over time, individuals with type 2 diabetes may lose some pancreatic function resulting in a growing deficiency of endogenous insulin requiring insulin administration.

Hyperglycemia has a multitude of adverse health consequences. Because the insulin deficiency is absolute in persons with type 1 diabetes and present but unable to transport glucose into cells in type 2 diabetes, the pathophysiology, progress of disease, and pharmacologic treatments in these two types of diabetes differ.

Type 1 Diabetes

When type 1 diabetes develops, blood concentrations of glucose are very high and the threshold for reabsorption of glucose in the proximal renal tubules is overcome. The result is **glycosuria**. Because glucose has a high osmolarity, water molecules also stay in the urine instead of being reabsorbed. This situation rapidly leads to the three classic signs of diabetes, which are **polyuria**, **polydipsia**, and

polyphagia. Secondly, the lack of basal insulin at adequate levels leads to release of hormone-sensitive lipase and free fatty acids. When the cells do not get glucose into the intracellular compartment, fatty acids are used to provide the energy for metabolic processes. Fatty acid breakdown produces **ketones**. Diabetic **ketoacidosis** can occur if this is untreated.

Type 2 Diabetes

Persons with type 2 diabetes have two primary metabolic defects: (1) resistance to insulin at the level of the cell membrane, and (2) hyperinsulinemia as more insulin is required to accomplish a specific lowering of blood glucose in persons with type 2 diabetes than in individuals without diabetes. As the disorder progresses, many individuals

with type 2 diabetes also develop a relative impairment of insulin secretion.

Because there is a degree of **insulin resistance** in the liver as well as peripheral tissue, the liver inaccurately perceives a deficit of glucose and produces excess glucose (Figure 18-2). When glucose cannot get into the cells, all the mechanisms that increase blood glucose values initiate their function, under the mistaken assumption that there is a dearth of glucose available. Thus, the gastrointestinal system reduces the production of incretin and the pancreas increases production of glucagon as well as insulin. The adipose cells respond by breaking down stored triglycerides into free fatty acids that could be used for metabolism in the absence of glucose. This results in high plasma levels of free fatty acids and an increased risk for atherosclerosis.

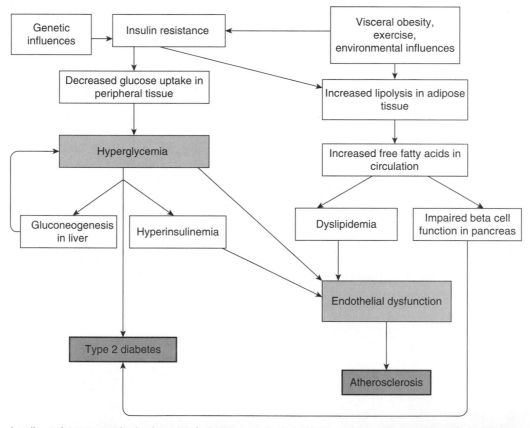

Insulin resistance results in decreased glucose uptake in peripheral tissue, gluconeogenesis in the liver, and increased lipolysis in adipose cells. The direct result of insulin resistance is hyperglycemia, which causes the pancreas to produce more insulin and stimulates gluconeogenesis in the liver. The gluconeogenesis further exacerbates the hyperglycemia. The pathophysiology of metabolic syndrome interacts with the pathophysiology of type 2 diabetes at several steps. First, the insulin resistance stimulates lipolysis, which results in increased triglycerides and dyslipidemia. Second, hyperglycemia directly contributes to endothelial cell dysfunction. Third, hyperinsulinemia directly contributes to endothelial cell dysfunction. Fourth, the increased blood level of free fatty acids impairs beta cell function within the pancreas so the hyperinsulinemia that is seen in the initial stages of type 2 diabetes, over time, results in insufficient insulin release from the pancreas.

Figure 18-2 Pathophysiology of insulin resistance and metabolic syndrome.

Once fasting plasma glucose levels are > 140 mg/dL, the beta cells in the pancreas are no longer able to increase production of insulin as compensation, and at this point, overt type 2 diabetes develops.[15] In some individuals with type 2 diabetes, the pancreas eventually shuts down completely, so glucose homeostasis requires management with exogenous insulin in addition to medications that reduce insulin resistance.

The Lipocentric Model

So far, we have described the conventional glucocentric model of diabetes. However, it is becoming clear that a lipocentric model describes the underlying pathophysiology of type 2 diabetes better and more completely.[13] Obesity is common in type 2 diabetes and is a major factor in insulin resistance. Adipocytes in the fat deposited viscerally are innately resistant to insulin, and they increase lipolysis, releasing free fatty acids into the circulation. The increase in free fatty acids that occurs when peripheral tissues perceive the presence of a hypoglycemic state further increases insulin resistance in skeletal muscle and the liver and impairs beta cell function in the pancreas. This process can be considered the tipping point, where compensation shifts to decompensation and a vicious circle of increasing hyperglycemia, causing glucose toxicity that further increases insulin resistance and pancreas suppression, which in turn further increases hyperglycemia.

Insulin Resistance and Metabolic Syndrome

Metabolic syndrome is a constellation of disorders that increases the risk for developing both type 2 diabetes and cardiovascular disease. Insulin resistance is an integral component of metabolic syndrome, which is characterized by visceral obesity, resistance to insulin, abnormalities in lipid metabolism, and hypertension. The pathophysiologic connections between metabolic syndrome, diabetes, and cardiovascular disease are important to review (briefly) because this growing field of study is challenging conventional treatment of type 2 diabetes and paving the way for new pharmacologic interventions.[16]

Three of the following five criteria must be met to acquire the diagnosis of metabolic syndrome: obesity, hypertriglyceridemia, reduced HDL cholesterol, hypertension, and impaired fasting glucose.[17] Insulin resistance is the underlying pathology that links these criteria to each other. The prevalence of insulin resistance in persons with hypertension is 58%; it is 88% in persons with dyslipidemia and almost 100% in persons with diabetes.[18] It is believed that persons with metabolic syndrome are in a state of disease evolution that includes both prediabetes and pre-atherosclerosis. Furthermore, metabolic syndrome, like diabetes, invokes an increased risk for cardiovascular disease. Treatment of the various abnormalities that comprise a diagnosis of metabolic syndrome can significantly decrease the risk for subsequent type 2 diabetes and the risk for cardiovascular disease.[5]

Complications of Diabetes

The adverse health consequences of hyperglycemia are perhaps even more debilitating than the underlying diabetes. Complications of diabetes are divided into macrovascular disorders (e.g., cerebrovascular disease, cardiovascular disease) and microvascular disorders (e.g., diabetic retinopathy, renal failure).

When the blood levels of glucose are high, the ability of glucose to chemically attach to different proteins without the stimulus of enzymatic facilitation occurs. This process is called **glycosylation**. The measurement of glycosylated hemoglobin, also referred to as **hemoglobin A1c** (HbA1c), is used to make determinations about the degree of hyperglycemia and how long it has been present. A 1% increase in HbA1c is associated with an 18% increase in the risk of having a cardiovascular event, a 12–14% increase in the risk of death, and a 37% increase in the risk of developing renal failure or retinopathy. This relationship between increasing severity of hyperglycemia and increased risk for complications is the basis for the current clinical focus on interventions that tightly regulate glucose metabolism. HbA1c levels are used to guide different steps in current clinical practice algorithms.[5,16,19]

The glycosylation of proteins produces advanced glycosylation end products (AGEs) that attach to endothelial cells that line the interior wall of all blood vessels causing them to become damaged. Endothelial cell damage is the primary initiating insult that starts the chain of adverse events that results in either macrovascular or microvascular disease.

Macrovascular disease is disease within the large vessels of the body—i.e., **atherosclerosis**. Once the endothelial cells are impaired, vasoconstrictive, proinflammatory and prothrombotic mediators are released, and over time, atherosclerotic plaque develops.[20] Coronary artery disease, cerebrovascular disease, and peripheral vascular disease are three disorders that develop in persons with atherosclerosis. All three occur more rapidly in persons with diabetes when compared to persons who do not have diabetes. Women with diabetes have a higher risk than men for developing cardiovascular complications.[21] Cardiovascular disease is responsible for 80% of the deaths that are attributed to diabetes.[22]

In addition to antihyperglycemic agents, treatment of type 2 diabetes may include use of medications that treat hypertension or dyslipidemia to lower the risk for cardiovascular disease.[5,23] A similar process occurs in the smaller vessels that cause microvascular disease. As we learn more about how the pathogenesis of diabetes takes time to develop, new pharmacologic treatments are being employed early in the hope of preventing both overt diabetes and cardiovascular disease.

Goals for Treatment of Diabetes

Treatment of type 2 diabetes is a three-pronged approach. The prongs are referred to as A, B, and C—A for lowering hemoglobin A1C levels to improve glucose control, B for lowering blood pressure, and C for managing cholesterol. The risk of developing coronary artery disease in persons with diabetes is that insulin resistance is lowered via a decrease in the plasma levels of free fatty acids.

Three organizations set standards for the diagnosis and management of diabetes. The American Association of Clinical Endocrinologists, in collaboration with the American College of Endocrinology, published medical guidelines for diagnosis and management of diabetes in 2007.[17] In 2009, the American Diabetes Association (ADA) published an updated version of its Standards of Medical Care in Diabetes.[5] The glycemic goals of both groups are listed in Table 18-1. These organizations agree that the treatment goal for all persons with diabetes is to maintain blood glucose values as close to normal as possible without **hypoglycemia**. Glycemic control is the primary key to prevention of complications. This goal is based on studies that found microvascular and neuropathic complications are reduced when normal plasma glucose values are maintained.[24] However, there is some debate about what HbA1c level is required to reduce complications and at the same time avoid hypoglycemia. A recent study[16] found that glucose control may be too tight and that individuals with type 2 diabetes who maintained their HbA1c < 6% actually had higher risks for serious cardiovascular events. At this time, the goal of < 7% or < 6.5% and not below 6% is reasonable.

Secondary goals include prevention of complications via management of hypertension, lipids, neuropathic complications, and overall prevention of microvascular

Table 18-1 Glycemic Targets for Persons with Diabetes

	American Association of Clinical Endocrinologists	American Diabetes Association*
Fasting plasma glucose	< 110 mg/dL	70–130 mg/dL
2-hour postprandial glucose	< 140 mg/dL	< 180 mg/dL*
HbA1c	≤ 6.5%	< 7%

* Goals should be individualized based on duration of diabetes, age/life expectancy, comorbid conditions, known cardiovascular disease, hypoglycemia unawareness, and individual patient considerations.
Sources: American Diabetes Association 2009[5]; American Association of Clinical Endocrinologists 2007.[19]

complications. Adjunctive management strategies that are implemented to avoid and/or minimize microvascular complications include early detection and monitoring of microvascular changes, reduction of macrovascular complications, optimal glycemic control, maintenance of normal blood pressure (< 130/85 mmHg) with angiotensin-converting enzyme (ACE) inhibitors if needed, statin drugs to maintain LDL-cholesterol at < 100 mg/dL, daily aspirin therapy to prevent emboli, elimination of smoking, and realistic exercise and weight loss of 5–10% of body weight.[5,17]

Nonpharmacologic Management of Diabetes

The primary nonpharmacologic interventions of diabetes are diet and exercise in addition to behaviors that reduce additional risk factors. The ADA has determined the most widely accepted nutrition standards with promotion of their ADA diets. For persons with diabetes, food is medicine and nutritional recommendations must be considered as part of the total medication plan for the individual. The diets are determined by individual caloric needs. Medications are added to meet the goal for glycemic control that remain after nutritional therapy is instituted. Some individuals with type 2 diabetes may be able to control blood sugar with diet alone; however, all individuals with type 1 diabetes and the overwhelming majority of individuals with type 2 diabetes will require additional medications to maintain glycemic control.

Alternative therapies such as high doses of cinnamon to assist in glycemic control have been explored.[25] None of the proposed alternative or complementary therapies has been found to be effective when subjected to rigorous study.

Prediabetes: Impaired Fasting Glucose and Impaired Glucose Tolerance

When does diabetes begin and when should interventions that affect glucose metabolism be initiated? **Prediabetes** (sometimes called borderline diabetes) has been described as impaired glucose metabolism that does not meet the criteria for type 1 or type 2 diabetes.[5] Prediabetes can be manifested as an impaired fasting glucose (IFG), which is defined as fasting plasma glucose level between 100 and 125 mg/dL, or an impaired glucose tolerance (IGT), defined as a plasma glucose level after a 2-hour post-glucose load that is between 140 and 199 mg/dL.[5] Some persons have both. It is clear that individuals with IFG and/or IGT have a fivefold to sixfold increased risk of developing type 2 diabetes.[26] According to the American College of Endocrinology,[26] 6–10% of persons with IGT progress to diabetes each year. For persons with both IFG and IGT, the cumulative risk for developing diabetes over 6 years is as high as 60%. High plasma glucose levels result in cardiovascular changes and microvascular disease before the development of type 2 diabetes. Diabetic retinopathy, hypertension, dyslipidemia, and cardiovascular disease are markedly increased in individuals with IFG and/or IGT.[26]

Strategies to prevent progression from IFG/IGT to diabetes were studied and summarized in June 2007.[19] Recommendations for interventions are focused on lifestyle changes to prevent development of diabetes and its microvascular complications. No pharmacologic interventions were recommended, and none are approved by the United States Food and Drug Administration (FDA). In 2008, the American College of Endocrinology convened a task force that addressed the issue of prediabetes and reviewed research to determine the most effective treatment. The *Consensus Statement on the Diagnosis and Management of Pre-Diabetes in the Continuum of Hyperglycemia* was issued in July of 2008.[26] The ACE statement provides guidance in the diagnosis and management of the prediabetic state, including recommendations for pharmacologic management.

Management of Prediabetes

Lifestyle changes are still the first intervention in prediabetes as in other classifications of diabetes. Nutrition to accomplish a weight reduction of 5–10% of total body weight results in lower fat mass, reduction in triglyceride and low-density lipoprotein, and lowers both blood glucose and blood pressure. Controlled sodium intake and avoidance of alcohol assist in control of blood pressure. Exercise is recommended for weight control and cardiovascular health.

Medications to reduce glucose levels are now indicated for persons with prediabetes who are at particularly high risk for diabetes. Glycemic medications should be considered for women who have prediabetes and worsening glycemia, a history of polycystic ovarian syndrome, cardiovascular disease, and/or a history of gestational diabetes. Metformin (Glucophage) and acarbose (Precose) are recommended as first-line glycemic drugs because of their safety and evidence of effectiveness in preventing progression to diabetes. Thiazolidinediones are effective in reducing progression to diabetes, but the side effects of congestive heart failure and increased incidence of fractures mitigate against their use.[26] There are no data on the effectiveness of newer glycemic agents including meglitinides, GLP-1 receptor agonists, and DPP4 inhibitors for treating prediabetes.[26] Pharmacologic management to prevent complications of diabetes in persons with prediabetes are the same as the agents recommended for individuals with type 1 or type 2 diabetes. Statin therapy is recommended to achieve the same lipid goals as desired for other diabetes conditions (LDL 100 mg/dL, non-HDL cholesterol 130 mg/dL). Niacin is not recommended for lipid control because it may adversely affect glycemic control. Ezetimibe (Zetia), bile acid sequestrants, and fibrates may be used if needed. Target blood pressure is < 130/80 mmHg. First-line antihypertensive agents in diabetes are angiotensin-converting enzyme inhibitors (ACE inhibitors) or angiotensin receptor blocking agents (ARBs) with calcium channel blockers as a second choice. As with other forms of diabetes, beta-blockers and/or thiazides should be avoided because of their potential to raise blood glucose levels. Aspirin for antiplatelet therapy is recommended unless contraindicated by hemorrhagic condition or gastrointestinal risk.

Type 1 Diabetes

Destruction of the beta cells in the islets of Langerhans within the pancreas occurs primarily in persons with a genetic predisposition who are exposed to an environmental trigger that produces autoantibodies. Once the beta cells are destroyed, an individual is unable to make sufficient insulin and thereafter must supply the body with exogenously produced insulin that is administered subcutaneously. Although the disease is not curable, insulin therapy can be quite successful in maintaining normal blood glucose levels.

Management Goals for Type 1 Diabetes

The management goal for persons with type 1 diabetes is **euglycemia** and prevention of complications associated with diabetes. Lifestyle management including intensive nutrition therapy is essential in type 1 diabetes. Exogenous insulin replacement is essential for persons with type 1 diabetes. The primary pharmacologic focus is on variations in the type of insulin, timing of administration, and routes of administration in order to maintain euglycemia without serious complications of hypoglycemia or hyperglycemia.

Insulin Therapy

The goal of insulin therapy is to simulate the normal insulin response to food, exercise, and metabolic needs of the individual. Recommendations for glycemic targets differ between the ADA and the American Association of Clinical Endocrinologists (AACE). The ADA recommends targeting therapy to a preprandial plasma glucose between 90 and 130 mg/dL, and the AACE recommends a level < 110 mg/dL. The recommended postprandial glucose measured 1–2 hours after a meal is < 180 mg/dL according to the ADA and < 140 mg/dL according to AACE.[5,19] Data support both targets, but no data are available to show a preference of one set of targets over the other. HbA1c levels indicate the effectiveness of glycemic control over the previous 30–90 days. The goal is to keep the HbA1c below 7% to minimize the complications and long-term morbidities associated with diabetes.[10]

Insulin therapy is monitored daily by checking for urinary ketones in the morning and at bedtime, fasting blood glucose levels in the morning, and then preprandial and postprandial glucoses throughout the day and once more at bedtime. Additional blood glucose readings may be needed before and after exercise and if symptoms of hypoglycemia or hyperglycemia occur. Self-monitored blood glucose levels are essential to monitor the dose and effectiveness of the insulin regimen throughout the day. According to Briscoe et al., 90% of individuals who use insulin have had at least one hypoglycemic episode.[27] Care must be taken to establish a regimen that prevents hypoglycemia. The risk of hypoglycemia is increased if the woman is ill, physiologically stressed such as during pregnancy or/labor, or undergoing surgery. Doses of insulin need to be adjusted in these situations and monitored very closely.

Insulin Delivery

Insulin is a protein that would be digested in the stomach and intestine before reaching the circulation. Insulin is therefore administered subcutaneously in multiple doses throughout the day and/or by continuous subcutaneous infusion pump. An inhaled insulin (Exubera) was approved by the FDA in 2006 but removed from the market in late 2007 due to lack of acceptance and poor sales. Transdermal delivery systems have been developed but are not yet ready for use. Several pharmaceutical companies are developing oral formulations, but none have progressed beyond the initial Phase I studies. Intravenous administration of insulin is reserved for inpatient care with intensive monitoring.

Insulin Injections

The most common method of administration of insulin is multiple injections daily. Insulin is drawn into an insulin syringe with clear markings for units of insulin. Short needles that assure injection in the subcutaneous tissue are needed. Intramuscular injection results in a very rapid absorption and metabolism of the insulin. Subcutaneous injections should be placed on the abdomen, anterior thigh, buttocks, or dorsal arm. The abdomen is the preferred site of injection in the morning because the absorption of insulin is 20–30% faster in this site than others.[27] If the woman is unwilling or unable to use the abdominal site, a consistent area (arm, thigh, or buttock) should be chosen for injections given at specific times of day. For example, morning injections would be given in the thigh and evening injections in the buttocks. Consistent use of an area will standardize the expected absorption and enable better adjustment of insulin dose.[27] Rotation within these standard sites is needed to prevent injection site reaction and lipodystrophy (Figure 18-3). An advantage of syringe injections is the ability to mix insulins; adjust administration times to accommodate changes in mealtimes, activity, and sleep/work schedules; and tailor the dose to anticipated food intake.

Insulin Pump

The insulin pump is a mechanism of providing continuous subcutaneous insulin administration. A needle is placed in the subcutaneous tissue of the abdomen and connected to a continuous pump with increasingly sophisticated computer delivery calculators to manage dose regimens. The 24-hour basal and intermittent bolus insulin can be programmed and given automatically. The pump makes it

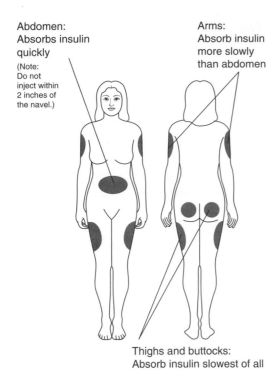

Abdomen:
Absorbs insulin
quickly

(Note:
Do not
inject within
2 inches of
the navel.)

Arms:
Absorb insulin
more slowly
than abdomen

Thighs and buttocks:
Absorb insulin slowest of all

Figure 18-3 Sites for insulin injection.

possible to deliver insulin in fractions of units if needed. Tighter control is possible. The bolus can be calculated and given for the anticipated carbohydrate intake with the upcoming meal, reduced in the situation of exercise or illness, and adjusted to various lifestyle schedules such as night employment. The disadvantage is that the pump requires careful attention because if it is kinked or empty, no insulin is given and the woman may not know it. The risk of hypoglycemia is therefore potentially increased with use of the pump. Individuals using the pump need to have backup insulin administration in the event the pump is broken. The pump is more expensive than frequent injections, and cost may be prohibitive for some women. In the future, the pumps may be able to read the glucose level in the wearer and automatically adjust the insulin dose.

Insulin Pens

Insulin pens are another method of insulin administration. Insulin pens are available with most insulins on the market today. The pen uses replaceable cartridges of insulin and disposable needles. For some insulins, a prefilled disposable pen is available. The pen is used by attaching a new needle, turning the dial on the pen for the required

units, and injecting the insulin into the desired site. The needle needs to remain in the subcutaneous tissue for 5 seconds to assure all the medicine is delivered. The pen is then removed, and the needle and cartridge discarded. The advantages of the pen are the ease of use by those who are sight or fine-motor impaired. In addition, the self-contained medication can be injected discreetly because it is already prepared. The disadvantage is that insulins cannot be mixed in a single syringe, potentially requiring more injections. The dose in the pen must be full or half—no other fractions are possible. Pens are more expensive than individual syringe injections and may be cost prohibitive for some women. As with other injections of insulins, the site must be rotated.

Insulin

Insulin was originally made from the pancreas of cattle, pigs, horses, and fish. The structure of these insulins was very close to human insulin and well tolerated, although allergic responses did occur. The allergic response was more common in persons using animal insulins because of impurities that were contained in the insulin. Better processing improved the purity of animal insulin but never could meet the purity of manufactured insulin. Only beef and pork insulin have been in common usage worldwide. Beef insulin was discontinued in the United States in 1998, and pork insulin was no longer manufactured or marketed in the United States beginning in January of 2006.[28] All insulin manufactured and marketed in the United States today is recombinant, genetically engineered human insulin or **insulin analogs**. Very few companies manufacture animal insulins, and their usage is limited to persons who have been successfully managed on animal insulin for many years. Persons in the United States who insist on animal insulin must import it for their personal use only. A mechanism exists within the FDA to accomplish the importation legally. The information is available from the FDA.

Nonanimal insulins are pure insulin with some exceptions. Neutral protamine Hagedorn insulin, which is called NPH (Humulin N, Novolin N), has the addition of the protein protamine, tiny amounts of zinc, and the buffer phosphate. Lispro (Humalog) and aspart (NovoLog) contain zinc and the buffer phosphate as well. Glulisine (Apidra) contains metacresol as a preservative—insulins may contain phenol or metacresol as preservatives. The additives are suspected to be the responsible factors when hypersensitivity and allergies-specific recombinant insulins occur.

All insulin products are measured in units. The United States has implemented this standard so all insulin is in a U-100 concentration, which is 100 units of insulin per milliliter. Regular and NPH insulin in this concentration are available over the counter without prescription. Rapid-acting and long-acting newer insulin formulations require a prescription. Higher concentrations are available by prescription for the exceptional individual on very high doses of insulin.

Side Effects/Adverse Effects

Common reactions to insulin include injection site reactions such as lipodystrophy, weight gain, pruritus, and rash. Weight gain is attributed to the anabolic effects of insulin. Peripheral edema can occur in persons on insulin therapy because insulin causes sodium retention.

Hypersensitivity Reactions

Hypersensitivity to insulin and/or any additives or buffers is possible. More serious reactions include severe hypoglycemia, hypokalemia, and rarely, anaphylaxis. In the persons who have renal or hepatic compromise, doses should be lowered and blood glucose monitored closely. Baseline creatinine clearance is recommended before initiating any insulin therapy. Decreased creatinine clearance indicates renal compromise and a decreased ability to metabolize insulin. All initial insulin doses are reduced in women with low creatinine clearance. Some insulins have specific recommendations in the amount of dose adjustment per creatinine clearance.

Skin Reaction and Lipodystrophy

Local reactions are common following insulin injection via syringe or pump. Most skin reactions resolve spontaneously when sites are changed more frequently. Careful attention to technique to prevent infection will minimize skin infections. **Lipodystrophy** is a loss of adipose tissue in injection sites. The cause of lipodystrophy is unknown. Impure animal insulin has been implicated in the development of lipodystrophy, but the complication is so rare that it is impossible to establish a cause-and-effect relationship. However, lipodystrophy is virtually unknown in individuals using insulin analogs. Treatment is individual based on the depth and extent of the area. Superficial areas may be treated with a dermatologic procedure, and others may require surgical revision.

Insulin Hypersensitivity

The incidence of insulin allergy has dropped dramatically with the transition from animal to recombinant and analog insulin. The reason for the reduction in allergy is attributed to the purer product with fewer impurities, additives, and animal proteins to stimulate allergy. Hypersensitivity still may develop in response to the minor contaminants or one of the known additives—phenol, zinc, metacresol, and phosphates. A change in the type of insulin used to remove exposure to the allergen is recommended when a hypersensitivity reaction occurs. For example, lispro insulin containing phosphates could be discontinued in favor of glulisine, which has no phosphates. If the sensitivity persists, desensitization with gradually increasing doses may be tried. Antihistamines may be used in skin reactions and hypersensitivity. Severe reactions and systemic reactions are extremely rare and may require corticosteroid therapy.

Insulin Preparations

The characteristics of insulin that are of clinical import are onset, peak time, and duration of action (Figure 18-4). Insulin preparations are categorized by duration of action—i.e., rapid-acting, short-acting, intermediate-acting, long-acting, and premixed formulations that are a combination of specific proportions of short-acting and intermediate-acting insulins. In most cases, the pharmacokinetics of insulin are dose dependent. Larger doses have earlier peak effects and a longer duration of activity. All insulin is metabolized in the liver, the kidney, and adipose tissue. Currently used insulins are summarized in Table 18-2, and an example of each type will be described.

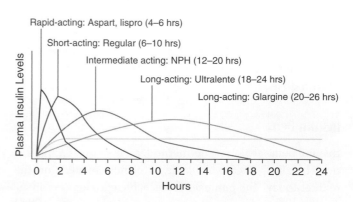

Figure 18-4 Onset, peak, and duration of action of different insulin formulations.

Table 18-2 Types of Insulin Preparations

Drug Category	Drug Generic (Brand)	Onset	Peak	Duration	Rx/OTC	Clinical Considerations	FDA Pregnancy Category	Lactation
Rapid acting	Lispro (Humalog)	< 15 min	30–90 min	5 h or less	Rx	Human	B	Probably safe
	Aspart (NovoLog)	10–20 min	1–3 h	3–5 h	Rx	Human	C	Compatible
	Glulisine (Apidra)	15–30 min	0.5–2.5 h	5 h or less	Rx	Human	C	Probably safe
Short acting	Regular (Humulin R)	30–60 min	2–3 h	4–6 h	OTC	Human	B	Compatible
	Regular (Novolin R)	30–60 min	2.5–5 h	8 h	OTC	Human	B	Compatible
Intermediate acting	NPH (Humulin N)	1.5 h	4–10 h	14–18 h	OTC	Human	B	Compatible
	NPH (Novolin N)	1.5 h	4–12 h	24 h	OTC	Human	B	Compatible
	50% NPH and 50% regular (Humulin 50/50)	30–60 min	Dual	18–24 h	OTC	Human	B	Compatible
	70% NPH and 30% regular (Humulin 70/30, Novolin 70/30)	30–60 min	Dual	24 h	OTC	Human	B	Compatible
Long acting	Glargine (Lantus)	1 hour	Constant	24 h	Rx	Insulin analog	C	Compatible
	Detemir (Levemir)	50–120 min	Constant	24 h	Rx	Insulin analog	C	Probably safe

Rx = prescription only; OTC = over the counter.

Rapid-Acting Insulins: Glulisine (Apidra)

Glulisine (Apidra) is a rapid-acting insulin analog that is similar to the other two rapid-acting insulins, aspart and lispro. Glulisine is approved for use before and *after* food intake. This postprandial property means that the glulisine dose can be adjusted on the basis of what was actually eaten at a meal. For individuals who may not eat a planned meal at a predetermined time, the postmeal regimen reduces the risk of hypoglycemia or postprandial hyperglycemia. Glulisine inhibits gluconeogenesis and stimulates peripheral glucose uptake, thereby inhibiting lipolysis and proteolysis. The result is regulation of glucose metabolism. Glulisine insulin is largely excreted by the kidney. The half-life of this rapid-acting insulin is 13 minutes when administered intravenously and 42 minutes when administered subcutaneously. Because this is such a rapid-acting and short-duration insulin, it is typically given with NPH insulin, which is one of the intermediate-acting insulins.

The dose of glulisine (Apidra) is 0.5–1 units/kg/day. Glulisine is given < 15 minutes before or < 20 minutes after meals. Glulisine can be given continuously via an insulin pump. No other medications can be mixed with glulisine in a pump, but NPH may be mixed with it in a syringe for immediate administration. Glulisine may be given intravenously in the inpatient setting under close monitoring. Doses via all routes need to be decreased if the individual has renal or hepatic compromise.

Adverse reactions that are common following use of glulisine (Apidra) include those associated with all insulins. Edema, nasopharyngitis, and respiratory infections have also been associated with glulisine. Hypertension can occur in persons using this drug. Glulisine combined in a regimen with NPH insulin increases the risk for serious cardiovascular events. Glulisine should not be given to anyone with sensitivity to metacresol, which is used as a preservative in glulisine.

Rapid-Acting Insulins: Insulin Lispro (Humalog)

Lispro (Humalog) is an insulin analog approved for use in 1996. Lispro is used in combination with a longer acting insulin for type 1 diabetes and may be used in combination with longer acting insulin as a **prandial dose** or in combination with oral medications for persons with type 2 diabetes. Lispro is metabolized in the kidney, liver, and adipose tissue. Intravenous administration is not recommended but may be used for inpatient management. Lispro is administered less than 15 minutes before meals or with continuous subcutaneous insulin pump. Lispro may be given postprandially but is not commonly used in this way. All doses need to be lowered for individuals with impaired renal or hepatic functions. Creatinine clearance evaluation is recommended before initiating lispro, and the dose should be reduced by 25% if the creatinine clearance is between 10 and 50 mL/min and the dose decreased by 50% if the creatinine clearance is less than 10 mL/min.

Short-Acting Insulin: Regular Insulin (Humulin R)

Regular insulin is a human insulin made synthetically via recombinant DNA technology. Regular insulin is a short-acting insulin that is used for type 1 diabetes and may be the primary insulin added to oral medications for persons with type 2 diabetes who need insulin therapy. The dose of regular insulin varies depending on the application and route of administration. This insulin is predominantly excreted in the urine (30–80%). The initial dose of regular insulin should be decreased by women who have renal compromise. Regular insulin is the drug of choice for treatment of both diabetic ketoacidosis and hyperkalemia because it is short acting, has a rapid onset, and can be given intravenously.

Intermediate-Acting Insulin: Insulin NPH (Humulin N)

Insulin NPH (Humulin N) is intermediate-acting insulin. Neutral protamine Hagedorn (NPH) was first created in 1936 by Hans Christian Hagedorn, who discovered that the effects of insulin could be prolonged by adding protamine.[29] It is excreted primarily in the urine (30–80%). This insulin may be mixed with other insulins, is available in premixed syringes, and has a low cost. However, NPH has a more uneven peak and duration of action than other insulins so there is a greater risk of causing hypoglycemia when using this agent. Intravenous use is not recommended for NPH insulin. NPH insulin is indicated for the management of individuals with type 1 diabetes and type 2 diabetes and may be given concomitantly with oral medications. As with all insulin, caution needs to be used in determining the dose for individuals with renal or hepatic impairment.

Long-Acting Insulins: Insulin Glargine (Lantus)

Glargine is human insulin analog. The half-life of glargine is unknown. Glargine is used as long-acting basal insulin by persons using the insulin pump. As with all basal insulin, the initial dose is calculated from 0.5 to 1 unit/kg/day depending on the individual's age and body habitus. Glargine onset of action is 1 hour with peak at 5 hours. Glargine has the unique property of maintaining that peak for 24 hours. For this reason, glargine can be given at any time in a 24-hour period and has equal effectiveness with no increase in the risk of hypoglycemia. However, the long-acting insulins are more expensive than NPH, and they cannot be mixed with other insulins in the same syringe. Exercise does not appear to affect the absorption of glargine. Glargine is absorbed equally from all injection sites, and there is no advantage to a particular site. For very lean, insulin-sensitive individuals with type 1 diabetes, absorption is improved by splitting the dose to two sites. Glargine does not mitigate the need for bolus insulin in individuals with type 1 diabetes. Glargine can be administered by pump but is usually given with a single daily injection.

Long-Acting Insulins: Insulin Detemir (Levemir)

Insulin detemir (Levemir) is a new, long-acting basal insulin analog. Detemir has a beneficial effect on weight. Individuals using this insulin have experienced a greater weight loss than those using NPH insulin.[30] As with insulin glargine, detemir has a smoother action profile compared to NPH, reducing the risks of significant hypoglycemia. The mechanism of metabolism and excretion are unknown. The onset, peak, and duration vary with route of administration.

Detemir (Levemir) can only be given subcutaneously by syringe and cannot be used intravenously or in insulin pumps. When given subcutaneously, detemir has an onset of 1 hour, no peak, and duration of 6 to 23 hours depending on the dose given. Duration is dose dependent. For persons with type 1 diabetes, detemir is given in the usual dose of 0.5–1.0 units/kg/day. If once-daily dosing is needed, the insulin is given with the evening meal or at bedtime. A short-acting insulin is also needed when detemir is used and is most effective if given prior to each meal. If insulin detemir is used by an individual with type 2 diabetes, it may be used with either oral medications or a rapid- or short-acting insulin. Detemir (Levemir) cannot be mixed in a syringe with other insulins. Individuals with impaired renal or hepatic function should use this drug in lower doses and with caution. Creatinine levels for evaluation of renal function are recommended before initiating the drug.

Premixed Insulin

Premixed formulations of insulin typically have 70% NPH or intermediate-acting insulin and 30% regular or short-acting insulin. These formulations are helpful for persons who have difficulty handling the small vials and/or persons who have poor eyesight and have difficulty measuring insulin doses.

Insulin Regimens

Historically, insulin was administered twice a day using a fixed combination of short-acting and longer acting agents. Today, many persons who use insulin either administer multiple subcutaneous injections throughout the day or use an insulin pump. Insulin regimens must be tailored to the physiologic needs and daily activity of the individual and consideration must be given to daily activity and food intake schedules. For example, if the individual exercises in the early morning or works nights, the schedule for insulin must accommodate that lifestyle. Insulin care instructions are listed in Box 18-1.

Sliding Scale Regimen

A sliding scale regimen involves using a fixed amount of long-acting insulin given at set times and then using fixed amounts of short-acting insulin prior to meals. The short-acting insulin may be adjusted based on the individual's blood glucose before each meal. The sliding scale refers to the relationship between insulin need and measured capillary glucose values. Blood glucose values are determined before mealtime, and the insulin is given 30–60 minutes before a meal. As the glucose level rises, the dose of regular insulin rises. The dose of insulin needed slides up or down based on the premeal glucose level.

Basal-Bolus Regimen

Unger[13] has outlined a step-by-step approach to prescribing a basal-bolus insulin regimen that is presented in Box 18-2. This is one example of a method to determine insulin doses for persons with type 1 diabetes. Many other algorithms are available, but the principles are the same. It is essential to consider the basal and bolus insulin and the response of the individual to the dose. The individual must

---

Box 18-1 Insulin Storage and Handling

Insulin is packaged in small, glass, multiuse vials that must be handled with care. Insulin does not work well if it is kept too long or if exposed to extreme temperatures. The following guidelines are recommended for all insulin preparations:

Storing Insulin

- Keep unopened bottles or unused pens in the refrigerator, but do not let them freeze. Insulin clumps into a precipitate when frozen.

- Before opening a new bottle, check the expiration date and do not use if it is too old.

- When you open a new bottle, write the date on it and do not use after 30 days.

- Insulin pens should not be kept at room temperature for more than 14 days.

- Insulin will stay fresh up to 30 days without refrigeration (and the shot is less painful if the insulin is not cold) as long as the temperature is less than 86°F and more than 36°F.

- Insulin that is not refrigerated should be kept away from heat and light.

- Before using, check to make sure the insulin looks like it is supposed to look.

- Very rapid-acting, rapid-acting insulin, short-acting insulin, and glargine should be clear without any cloudiness or any particles floating in the liquid.

- Intermediate-acting insulin should look uniformly cloudy.

Handling Insulin Prior to Injection

Intermediate-acting insulins and insulin pens need to be mixed before drawing the solution into a syringe or injecting it because the concentration can become unevenly distributed in the vial or pen.

- Insulin vials: Roll the vial between two hands 10 times before drawing out the solution. Do not shake vigorously.

- Insulin pens: Roll the pen 10 times back and forth and then point it up and down 10 times. The pen has a small glass bead that rolls back and forth to fully mix the layers of insulin.

Box 18-2 Establishing a Basal-Bolus Insulin Regimen

Step 1. Determine the total daily dose of insulin.

For adults, the total daily dose is calculated by taking the weight of the person in kg and multiplying it by 0.7. This calculation is adjusted for age. For example, an adolescent or adult with exceptional physical activity would need 1–2 units per kg per day. The ratio is reduced in the elderly (over 65) with 0.5–0.7 units per kg per day. For this example, consider a 32-year-old woman who does not have any comorbid conditions and who weighs 80 kg. She will require 56 units of insulin per day.

Step 2. Determine the approximate starting dose of basal insulin, which will be either glargine (Lantus) or detemir (Levemir).

The day's dose is divided into two so the morning dose will be 28 units of basal insulin and the evening dose will be 28 units of basal insulin.

Step 3. Use a simplified formula for determining baseline prandial insulin.

The baseline meal dose of insulin is calculated as 0.1 unit/kg of weight. In this case, eight units of insulin is the standard prandial dose of a rapid-acting insulin dose.

Step 4. Allow the woman to adjust the prandial dose of insulin based on the size of the meal.

The dose of rapid-acting insulin can be increased or decreased based on the planned food intake. If the meal is small, subtract 1 or 2 units. If the meal is large or heavy in calories (pizza or pasta), add 2 units.

Step 5. Establish the insulin sensitivity factor.

The insulin sensitivity factor determines how much 1 unit of rapid-acting insulin will lower the plasma glucose level. This calculation tailors the insulin dose for the individual and is very helpful for adjusting insulin to the individual lifestyle and schedule. The insulin sensitivity factor is equal to 1700 divided by the total daily basal insulin. For example, suppose a woman who weighs 80 kg uses 56 units of basal insulin a day. The insulin sensitivity factor of 1700 is divided by 56; 1700/56 = 30.3, which is rounded to 30. This means each unit of insulin is going to lower the plasma glucose by 30 mg/dL. Prior to a meal, she checks her blood glucose with her meter. If the preprandial glucose is 200, and her target is 150, she needs to lower her glucose by 50 points. For an average full meal, she will add 2 units of rapid-acting insulin to the 8 she is scheduled to take—for a total of 10 units. Additional units might be added if a large meal—or that piece of birthday cake—is anticipated.

Step 6. Allow the woman to adjust the dose of basal insulin.

One approach to adjusting basal insulin is to treat to target. The woman is advised to measure her fasting glucose in the morning and bedtime for the entire week. Every 7 days, she may adjust the basal insulin to reach the target fasting glucose of 120 agreed upon with her provider. The following chart is an example of the adjustments needed.

Average Fasting Glucose Values over 7 Days	Basal Insulin Adjustment
> 180 mg/dL	+ 8 units
140–180 mg/dL	+ 6 units
120–140 mg/dL	+ 4 units
100–120 mg/dL	+ 2 units
70–100 mg/dL	0 unit
< 70 mg/dL	− 1 unit

Source: Unger J 2007.[13]

Box 18-3 BJ Goes to College

BJ is an 18-year-old girl who has moved away from home for the first time to attend college. BJ is 5 feet, 4 inches tall, and her BMI is 23, a normal weight. She is active on the tennis team and doing well in her studies. She has had type 1 diabetes since age 3. She manages her insulin with a pump and a backup system of multiple daily injections if her pump is malfunctioning. Her insulin is glargine as a basal insulin and lispro for mealtime bolus. Her HbA1c at last evaluation when she arrived on campus was 6.8%. She takes a multiple vitamin pill every day. BJ says she is not sexually active and does not use or need contraception. She has been on campus for a semester and comes to the student health center because she has a cold. She is concerned that her pump may be malfunctioning because her postprandial glucose is consistently higher than 160 mg/dL and she usually is lower than 110 mg/dL.

On physical examination, BJ is found to have bronchitis. Upon nutritional recall, it is determined that BJ's food intake is consistent with her 1200-calorie ADA diet that she follows during the active tennis season. With further questioning about the upper respiratory infection, BJ says she has treated her symptoms with one of the over-the-counter multisymptom liquid medicines for colds, flu, and cough. She has not been able to go to tennis practice while she has been sick. Her random glucose value done on her arrival at 8 AM, approximately 1 hour after her breakfast, was 174 mg/dL.

Upon further questioning, the clinician finds that BJ does not know there is sugar in many of the over-the-counter medications marketed for treating colds. In addition, BJ is consuming her usual amount of calories for her active tennis practice but has not had that exercise while she has been ill.

The recommendation is to change to the Robitussin DM cough control for people with diabetes, or a similar formulation that does not contain glucose or sorbitol; adjust her food intake until she returns to her normal exercise regimen, and increase her lispro by a few units after meals, based on her blood glucose values. BJ checks her blood glucose levels regularly, and she should get normal values within a day or so. She is instructed to return if her blood glucose values do not return to normal, if her cold symptoms worsen, or if she develops a fever.

Table 18-3 Drugs That Cause Hypoglycemia or Hyperglycemia

Drugs That Cause Hypoglycemia Generic (Brand)	Drugs That Cause Hyperglycemia Generic (Brand)
ACE inhibitors	Atypical antipsychotics: clozapine (Clozaril), olanzapine (Zyprexa), risperidone (Risperdal)
Androgens	Beta sympathomimetics
Beta-adrenergic receptor antagonists*	Corticosteroids
Bromocriptine (Parlodel)	Clonidine (Catapres)
Ethanol	Decongestants
Indomethacin (Indocin)	Diazoxide (Proglycem)
Levofloxacin (Levaquin)	Diuretics
Lithium (Lithobid)	Epinephrine
MAO inhibitors	Estrogens
Naproxen (Aleve)	Heparin
Ofloxacin (Floxin)	HIV protease inhibitors
Oral hypoglycemic agents	Isoniazid (INH)
Pentamidine (Pentam)	Marijuana
Quinolones	Morphine
Sulfonamides	Niacin
Sulfonylureas*	Nicotine
Tetracycline (Sumycin)	Oral contraceptives
Theophylline (Theo-Dur)	Phenytoin (Dilantin)
	Thiazides
	Thyroid hormones

* Beta-adrenergic receptor antagonists and sulfonylureas are commonly prescribed medications for persons with diabetes.

be willing and able to accurately perform self-monitored blood glucose testing. The insulin dose is then adjusted to enable the individual to meet the fasting and postprandial targets (Box 18-3).

Drug–Drug Interactions

Drug–drug interactions associated with insulin are listed in Table 18-3. Many drugs can cause hypoglycemia or hyperglycemia. When one of these agents is taken by an individual who is using insulin, the action of insulin may be inhibited or potentiated. For example, beta-adrenergic receptor antagonists (beta-blockers) can potentiate hypoglycemia because they inhibit catecholamine stimulation of gluconeogenesis. In addition, beta-blockers can mask hypoglycemic symptoms (i.e., tremor or palpitations). Pentamidine (Pentam) has multiphasic effects on blood glucose and increases the risk of pentamidine-associated pancreatic beta cell toxicity.

Type 2 Diabetes

Postprandial hyperglycemia is the first blood glucose abnormality seen in persons with type 2 diabetes. The postprandial hyperglycemia is caused by loss of the first-phase insulin production of the pancreas. As this process progresses, insulin resistance increases in the liver and peripheral tissues. More insulin is required to initiate a given degree of glucose-lowering effect. Insulin resistance syndrome results in low HDL cholesterol levels and high triglycerides as well, which then contribute to an increased risk for cardiovascular events.

Management Goals for Type 2 Diabetes

The management goal for persons with type 2 diabetes is to maintain glycemic control at a level that minimizes the risk of microvascular and macrovascular complications while also minimizing the risk of hypoglycemia. Lifestyle changes and medications required to maintain normal lipid levels are an integral component of therapies for type 2 diabetes.

Pharmacologic therapy is directed at several different steps in the glucose homeostasis cycle (Figure 18-5). Sulfonylureas and meglitinides stimulate insulin secretion from the pancreas, alpha-glucosidase inhibitors decrease secretion of glucose from the intestine, and thiazolidinediones increase skeletal muscle sensitivity to insulin. If beta cell function ceases or cannot be stimulated adequately with oral medications, insulin may be required.

The American College of Endocrinology and the American Association of Clinical Endocrinologists created care maps for the management of type 2 diabetes in 2007. These road maps provide management strategies to accomplish glycemic control in persons who are newly diagnosed with type 2 diabetes (naïve to therapy) and persons receiving therapy for whom therapeutic changes are needed to

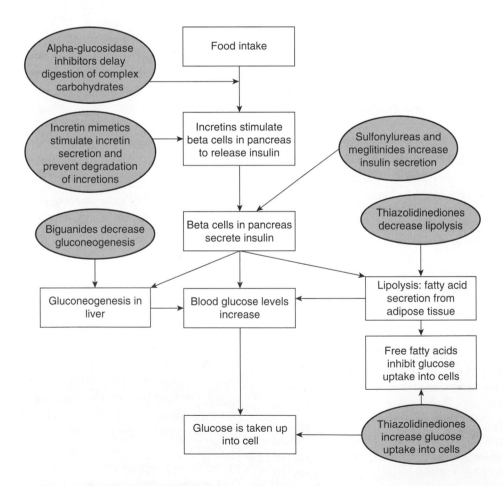

Figure 18-5 Mechanism of action of oral hypoglycemic drugs.

accomplish treatment goals. The road maps are consistent with the American Diabetes Association consensus on type 2 diabetes therapy.[31]

The choice of pharmacologic therapy first takes into consideration the contributions of fasting and postprandial hyperglycemia to the HbA1c level. Individuals newly diagnosed with type 2 diabetes who have an HbA1c < 6.5% may be managed with lifestyle modification, nutrition therapy (food is their medicine), and self-monitoring glucose. The first expression of hyperglycemia in type 2 diabetes is usually an elevated postprandial glucose level. In individuals with HbA1c < 7.3%, the postprandial glucose (usually morning) contributes 70% to the hyperglycemia with fasting levels contributing 30%. The usual medications chosen for these individuals are metformin (Glucophage), a sulfonylurea, or one of the thiazolidinediones.[19] The choice of drug balances the mechanism of action of that agent with specific characteristics of the individual (e.g., BMI, ability to take medications several times/day, risk factors for cardiovascular disease). Individuals with an HbA1c > 7.3 % and elevated fasting glucose and elevated postprandial glucose later in the day usually require combination therapy.[19,32] In

this situation, one medication is prescribed to lower the fasting glucose and an additional medication for the postprandial elevations. Fasting and postprandial hyperglycemia contributes equally when the HbA1c is between 7.3% and 8.4%. In persons with a significantly elevated HbA1c of > 10.2%, the elevated fasting glucose contributes 70% and postprandial hyperglycemia contributes 30%. Therapy to address both fasting and postprandial glucose level is needed[32] (Box 18-4).

Initial treatment and all subsequent treatment changes need to be assessed at 2- to 3-month intervals. Assessment includes review of self-monitoring glucose records and HbA1c. If the treatment goals are not met, additional pharmacologic therapy will be added and the individual assessed again in 2–3 months for effectiveness of the new regimen.

Management may need to be modified temporarily when an acute illness occurs or if a surgical procedure is needed. Individuals on oral therapy may need to be placed on insulin temporarily to enable rapid response to fluctuating glycemic status and minimize the risk of severe hyperglycemia and diabetic ketoacidosis.

Box 18-4 Initiating Treatment for Type 2 Diabetes

JP was in for her annual examination. She is 40 years old, 5 feet, 5 inches tall and weighs 205 pounds, which is a BMI of 34.1. She has three children and had gestational diabetes during her last two pregnancies. Her youngest child is 22 years. On examination today, it is noted that JP has an apple shape, indicating visceral adiposity. Her blood pressure is normal. Her laboratory findings from blood drawn a few days prior to this visit reveal an elevated lipid profile. The random blood glucose level was 190 mg/dL. The clinician suspects that JP has type 2 diabetes and schedules a fasting blood glucose and HbA1c to be obtained the next morning. Her fasting blood glucose level is 142 mg/dL and her HbA1c is 7.2%.

JP has type 2 diabetes that requires pharmacologic treatment. She should have a baseline creatinine clearance and comprehensive metabolic panel to assure that her kidney and liver are not compromised. She should be referred to an ophthalmologist for an eye examination, and she is referred to a nutritionist for diet counseling. In the past, JP would have been started on lifestyle changes and diet, and reevaluated in a few months. The current guidelines from the American College of Endocrinology (ACE) and American Association of Clinical Endocrinologists (AACE) recommend that initial treatment include lifestyle changes, diet, and metformin because the previous stepwise path frequently results in an extended period of hyperglycemia.[19] Because even slight elevations in HgA1c are associated with complications of diabetes, early aggressive treatment of hyperglycemia is recommended.[5] JP is started on metformin (Glucophage) as monotherapy and taught how to measure and record her fasting and postprandial blood glucose levels as part of a comprehensive diabetes self-management education (DSME) program. Metformin will help her lipids; it will not cause an increase in weight, and it is simple to monitor. However, because her HbA1c is > 7%, she may eventually need a sulfonylurea to become euglycemic. She will fax her blood glucose values to the office weekly and schedule another appointment for 1 month to reevaluate her regimen.

Pharmacologic Management of Type 2 Diabetes: Current and Potential Agents

Glycemic control is the mechanism for minimizing the risk of complications of diabetes. Pharmacologic management of type 2 diabetes can include both oral and injectable medications. Monotherapy with one drug may be sufficient, although multiple drug therapy will likely be required as the disease progresses over time. There are currently five classes of drugs available to lower blood glucose levels—sulfonylureas, meglitinides, biguanides, thiazolidinediones, and alpha-glucosidase inhibitors. Each class works in a different way to reduce blood glucose concentrations, but they can be subdivided into two general classes; sulfonylureas and meglitinides are hypoglycemic agents, whereas the others are antihyperglycemic agents (Table 18-4).

Table 18-4 Pharmacotherapeutic Agents for Treating Type 2 Diabetes

Drug Generic (Brand)	Dose	Maximum Daily Dose	Side Effects and Clinical Considerations	Effect on Weight
Sulfonylureas				
Glimepiride (Amaryl)	1–2 mg qd with first meal of the day	8 mg	Sulfonylureas may cause hypoglycemia. Dizziness, headaches, and sun sensitivity have been reported in approximately 2% of users. Allergic skin rashes and GI disturbances include nausea, diarrhea, and constipation. Side effects are dose dependent and disappear after lowering and/or dividing daily dose.	Weight gain
Chlorpropamide (Diabinese)*	250 mg qd	Maximum 750 mg daily		Weight gain
Glyburide (DiaBeta)	1.25–5 mg qd with first meal	20 mg in divided doses		Weight gain
Glyburide (Glynase)	0.75 mg qd	12 mg in divided doses		Weight gain
Glyburide (Micronase)	1.25–5 mg qd	20 mg a day		Weight gain
Glipizide (Glucotrol)	5 mg qd before first meal	40 mg		Weight gain
Glipizide (Glucotrol XL)	5 mg qd at first meal	20 mg		Weight gain
Meglitinides				
Repaglinide (Prandin)	0.5–2 mg before each meal	Up to 4 mg before each meal	Hypoglycemia in approximately 31% of users. Upper respiratory infections, headaches, nausea, diarrhea, sinusitis, and joint pain found in 6% or fewer.	Weight gain
Nateglinide (Starlix)	120 mg tid before meals	360 mg a day		Weight gain
Biguanides				
Metformin (Glucophage)	500 mg bid or 850 mg qd	2500–2550 mg a day	GI symptoms such as diarrhea, nausea, vomiting, abdominal bloating, and flatulence found in up to a third of people. Some need to decrease or discontinue either temporarily or permanently due to these effects. Hypoglycemia almost unknown. Rare risk for lactic acidosis that is most likely to occur in individuals with comorbid conditions.	Weight neutral
Alpha-Glucosidase Inhibitors				
Acarbose (Precose)	25 mg tid with meals	50 mg tid for women < 133 lbs and 100 mg tid for women > 133 lbs	Abdominal pain, diarrhea, flatulence, all reduced with time.	Weight neutral
Miglitol (Glyset)	25–50 mg with dinner	100 mg with every meal		Weight neutral
Thiazolidinediones				
Rosiglitazone (Avandia)	4 mg qd–bid	8 mg	Increase in LDL and HDL in clinical trials. Increased risk of hypoglycemia when taken with insulin.	Weight gain
Pioglitazone (Actos)	15 mg daily; can be taken in combination with insulin, metformin, and sulfonylureas	45 mg	No effects on lipids. Increased risk of hypoglycemia when taken with insulin.	Weight gain

(continues)

Table 18-4 Pharmacotherapeutic Agents for Treating Type 2 Diabetes (*continued*)

Name Generic (Brand)	Dose	Maximum Daily Dose	Side Effects and Clinical Considerations	Effect on Weight
DPP-4 Inhibitors				
Sitagliptin phosphate (Januvia)	100 mg qd with or without food	100 mg qd	Stuffy nose, sore throat, upper respiratory infection, and headache. Lower doses may be needed for persons with renal compromise.	Weight neutral
Incretin Mimetics				
Exenatide (Byetta)	5 mcg prefilled pen SQ bid prior to meal	5–10 mcg SQ bid prior to meal	Hypoglycemia possible if used in combination with sulfonylureas. If this occurs, dose of sulfonylurea can be decreased. Nausea, vomiting, diarrhea, headache, anorexia, and acid stomach. Side effects mostly decrease over time.	Weight neutral or weight loss

* Contraindicated for new diagnosis and initial treatment.

Insulin Secretagogues: Sulfonylureas

Insulin secretagogues are medications that stimulate the beta cells in the pancreas to secrete insulin. Sulfonylureas are beta cell stimulants. The first generation of sulfonylureas includes chlorpropamide (Diabinese), tolazamide (Tolinase), and tolbutamide (Orinase). These agents are associated with multiple drug–drug interactions and therefore are not used often today. The second-generation sulfonylureas have rare drug–drug interactions and are used in preference to the first generation. Second generation sulfonylureas include glimepiride (Amaryl), glyburide (DiaBeta, Glynase, Micronase), and glipizide (Glucotrol). These agents are the most frequently prescribed antidiabetic drugs in the United States.[33]

Mechanism of Action

Sulfonylureas counteract the insulin resistance that is characteristic of type 2 diabetes by stimulating an increase in pancreatic insulin secretion at lower glucose thresholds and increasing insulin binding to insulin receptors. These drugs close the potassium channels of the pancreatic beta cells, which opens the calcium channels enhancing the secretion of insulin. Sulfonylureas will lower HbA1c levels by 1–2% and blood glucose levels by 60–70 mg/dL.[34] Individuals must have some functional beta cells and function of liver and kidney as well for a sulfonylurea to be effective. Over time, if pancreatic beta cell function declines, this class of medications becomes ineffective. Sulfonylureas are approved for monotherapy but may be used in combination with insulin and most other oral agents. However, sulfonylureas are not used in combination with meglitinides because meglitinides have a similar mechanism of action.

Because cardiovascular disease is the most frequent complication of diabetes, the role of hypoglycemic agents in lowering or increasing the risk of cardiovascular events has been the subject of many research studies.[35] Sulfonylureas have been associated with an increased risk for cardiovascular events in some observational studies, and in 2001, the FDA added a special warning on the label of sulfonylurea agents that states there is an increased risk of cardiovascular mortality associated with the drug(s). To date, this association remains controversial, with some studies that show a relationship and others that have not found sulfonylureas associated with more cardiovascular events.[36] Sulfonylureas are also associated with an increased risk of mortality in persons who have a myocardial infarction.[36,37] The theorized mechanism for this association is the effect sulfonylureas have on ATP-dependent potassium channels in cardiac cells and cardiac vessels, which may prevent sufficient cardiac vessel dilation during a myocardial infarction.

One third of individuals placed on sulfonylureas do not reach glycemic goals with the sulfonylureas alone. The most common reasons for the drug failure include dietary intake outside recommended calorie/carbohydrate levels and/or markedly impaired beta cell function. For the approximately 66% who initially respond well to the drugs, each year 5–10% will develop secondary failure. By 10 years, half of all initial responders will have adequate control and half will have experienced secondary failure. The individual expected to have the best effect with sulfonylureas has the following profile: > 40 years of age with < 5 years with the diagnosis of type 2 diabetes, has a normal BMI, and has not used insulin in the past.

If a sulfonylurea is being added to the regimen of an individual on insulin, the individual should have normal blood glucose levels on < 40 units of insulin per day and have a fasting plasma glucose < 180 mg/dL. The optimal dose of sulfonylureas varies by the particular drug, but usually one half of the maximum dose will result in the maximum glucose-lowering effect.[19] If the desired glycemic effect is not achieved above the middle range of recommended dose, a second drug should be considered.

Side Effects/Adverse Effects

The most common side effect of sulfonylureas is hypoglycemia secondary to overproduction of insulin. The relative risk of hypoglycemia for individual drugs is listed in Table 18-5. Glipizide (Glucotrol) and glimepiride (Amaryl) do not cause hypoglycemia as often as do other drugs in this class. These agents should be used with caution by individuals who do not recognize hypoglycemia or who are unable to respond to hypoglycemia quickly.

Side effects that are common include mild hypoglycemia, nausea, headache, dizziness, and asthenia. The drugs in this category do cause some weight gain secondary to stimulation of insulin activity in adipose tissue. Therefore

they may not be the best choice for individuals who are overweight or obese. Thrombocytopenia, aplastic anemia, and pancytopenia are seen uncommonly.

Contraindications

Sulfonylureas are contraindicated for persons with a known sensitivity to any sulfonylurea or sulfonamides. Sulfonylureas are also contraindicated for use by persons taking antivirals due to an additive effect that increases the risk for hepatotoxicity. In addition, persons who use ethanol, methoxsalen (Oxsoralen), or aminolevulinic acid (Levulan) should not take sulfonylureas because these combinations also increase the risk of liver damage. These agents can be used with caution by persons who also take systemic beta-blockers. Drug–drug interactions associated with sulfonylureas are listed in Table 18-6.

▊ Insulin Secretagogues: Meglitinides

Meglitinides were first introduced in clinical practice in 1998 and are sometimes referred to as "short-acting secretagogues." Meglitinides work the same way that sulfonylureas

Table 18-5 Risk of Hypoglycemia Associated with Oral Hypoglycemic Agents

No Risk or Rare Risk Generic (Brand)	Increased Risk Generic (Brand)
Acarbose (Precose)	Insulin
Metformin (Glucophage, Glucophage XR, Glumetza, Fortamet, Riomet)	Glimepiride-containing products (Amaryl, Avandaryl, Due Fact)
Metformin/Pioglitazone (ActoPlus Met)	Glipizide-containing products (Glucotrol, Glucotrol XL, Metaglip)
Metformin/rosiglitazone (Avandamet)	Glyburide-containing products (DiaBeta Micronase, Glynase)
Miglitol (Glyset)	Nateglinide (Starlix)
Pioglitazone (Actos)	Repaglinide (Prandin)
Rosiglitazone (Avandia)	
Sitagliptin (Januvia)	

Table 18-6 Selected Drug–Drug Interactions with Oral Hypoglycemic Agents*

Drugs That Potentiate Hypoglycemic Effect Generic (Brand)	Drugs That Potentiate the Hyperglycemic Effect Generic (Brand)
ACE inhibitors	Barbiturates
Alcohol	Calcium channel blockers
Androgens	Corticosteroids
Beta-adrenergic receptor antagonists (beta-blockers)	Diuretics
Ciprofloxacin (Cipro)	Estrogen
Fluconazole (Diflucan)	Isoniazid (INH)
Gemfibrozil (Lopid)	Oral contraceptives
Insulin	Phenothiazines
Itraconazole (Sporanox)	Phenytoin (Dilantin)
MAO inhibitors	Rifampin (Rifadin)
Miconazole (Monistat, Lotrimin)	Sympathomimetics
Nonsteroidal anti-inflammatory drugs (Motrin, Aleve, Naproxen)	Thiazides
Oral hypoglycemic agents	
Salicylates	
Sulfonamide	
Trimethoprim (Primsol)	
Warfarin (Coumadin)	

* This table is not comprehensive as new information is being generated on a regular basis.

work, but they bind to a different receptor on the pancreatic beta cell. The two approved agents are Repaglinide (Prandin) and nateglinide (Starlix). The efficacy of both repaglinide (Prandin) and nateglinide (Starlix) is similar to that of the sulfonylureas in reducing HbA1c levels by 1–2% and blood glucose levels by 60–70 mg/dL.[34] Nateglinide is slightly less effective than repaglinide.[38,39]

Meglitinides are very short acting. These agents are taken before meals to increase the insulin available for the food consumed and are particularly helpful for persons who have fasting blood glucose values in the normal range but become hyperglycemic after meals and for those who have irregular meal schedules. If a meal is missed, the drug should not be taken.

Because they are short acting, less insulin is released overall compared to the effect of sulfonylureas. Therefore, meglitinides cause less hyperinsulinemia, and it is assumed they have less of an adverse effect on cardiovascular outcomes. That said, studies are lacking and the real association between meglitinides and cardiovascular events is unknown. Meglitinides have no significant effect on lipids.

Side Effects/Adverse Effects

Common side effects of meglitinides include nausea, dyspepsia, diarrhea, dizziness, upper respiratory symptoms, and hypoglycemia. Weight gain is a common side effect of these drugs. The risk of hypoglycemia associated with meglitinides is less than the risk of hypoglycemia associated with sulfonylureas. Because of the lower risk of hypoglycemia, these drugs are especially useful for persons who are unable to manage hypoglycemia well, such as the elderly and individuals with cardiac or renal disease.

Contraindications and Adverse Reactions

Contraindications to use of meglitinides are similar to those for sulfonylureas. They are contraindicated for persons with hypersensitivity to the drugs, type 1 diabetes, or diabetic ketoacidosis. These agents are metabolized via the liver and should be used with caution by persons with liver disorders. A small portion of repaglinide (Prandin) is metabolized by the kidney and should therefore be used with caution by individuals with renal impairment. Serious but rare adverse reactions associated with the use of repaglinide include anaphylaxis, severe hypoglycemia, myocardial ischemia, leukopenia and thrombocytopenia, Stevens-Johnson syndrome, pancreatitis, hepatic dysfunction, and hemolytic anemia.

▌ Biguanides: Insulin Sensitizers

The first biguanide metformin (Glucophage) was introduced into clinical practice in 1957 but was not used in the United States until 1995. Two drugs in this class, phenformin and buformin, were withdrawn due to a high risk of lactic acidosis. Metformin (Glucophage) has a much lower risk of lactic acidosis and has become the leading drug in the treatment of type 2 diabetes. It is the second most frequent drug prescribed to treat diabetes as either monotherapy or in combination with other agents.[33]

Metformin (Glucophage) reduces hepatic glucose production and increases glucose uptake in the skeletal muscles and peripheral tissue. This drug lowers fasting blood glucose levels by 50–70 mg/dL and HbA1c levels by 1–2%, which is comparable to sulfonylureas.[40] Use of metformin in combination with a sulfonylurea lowers blood glucose more than either drug does alone.[40-42]

Metformin is an oral tablet that comes in both short-acting and extended-release forms. The drug is not metabolized and passes unchanged through the body and is excreted 100% in the urine in unchanged form. The half-life in plasma is 6.2 hours and in blood 17.6 hours. A complete blood count, including red blood cell indices and a creatinine level, is recommended prior to starting metformin and then rechecked at least annually. Metformin is used by women with polycystic ovarian syndrome (Chapter 30) and has been used increasingly during pregnancy. Metformin (Glucophage) is especially helpful for persons who are overweight or obese and is the only oral agent that does not cause weight gain.

Metformin is also the only agent used to treat diabetes that improved cardiovascular outcomes (pooled OR 0.74; 95% CI, 0.62–0.89).[19,35] The drug has a positive effect on lipids with a small decrease in LDL, and a slight increase in HDL, which results in a decrease in serum triglycerides. When persons who maintained tight glycemic control with metformin were followed for 10 years, they were found to have a 21% reduction in all diabetic complications as an aggregate, a 33% reduction in the risk for myocardial infarction, and a 27% reduction in death from any cause.[43]

Side Effects/Adverse Effects

Metformin alone is less likely to cause hypoglycemia than are the sulfonylureas or meglitinides. The most common side effects are gastrointestinal complaints such as bloating, nausea, and abdominal discomfort; they are usually mild and can be mitigated if the dose is titrated up to higher doses gradually.[44] Other transient symptoms include anorexia, a metallic taste in the mouth, and rash. Extended-release formulations decrease the incidence of these side effects.

The two serious adverse reactions associated with metformin (Glucophage) are lactic acidosis and megaloblastic anemia and lactic acid.[45] Metformin interferes with absorption of folate and vitamin B_{12}, which can, over time, cause megaloblastic anemia. If the individual has other risk factors for developing megaloblastic anemia, a cyanocobalamin assessment is recommended every 2–3 years.

Lactic acidosis is a potentially life-threatening condition. The FDA has a black box warning for providers and users of metformin about the risk of lactic acidosis, which is rare but is fatal in more than half the cases when it does occur. The Cochrane Collaboration reviewed the risk of lactic acidosis with metformin and found no increased risk when the medication was used as recommended.[46]

Contraindications

Metformin is contraindicated for persons who are at risk for developing lactic acidosis. Box 18-5 lists the contraindications to use of metformin. In women over age 65, the dose of metformin should be adjusted and renal function assessed more frequently than annually. Lactic acidosis is also a risk when women on metformin undergo procedures requiring iodized contrast media. Metformin should be stopped 24 hours before the administration of iodized contrast media and restarted 48 hours later when renal function is confirmed.

Drug–Drug Interactions

Cimetidine (Tagamet) reduces renal clearance of metformin (Glucophage), which increases the blood level of metformin and increases the risk of lactic acidosis. Ethanol poses a risk with metformin because it may prolong hypoglycemia and increase the risk of lactic acidosis.

Thiazolidinediones

Thiazolidinediones (TZDs) are also known as glitazones. The three drugs in this category are troglitazone (Rezulin), rosiglitazone (Avandia), and pioglitazone (Actos). Troglitazone was withdrawn from the market in 2000 secondary to an increased risk for hepatotoxicity that was first noted in postmarketing research.

This class of drugs stimulates more effective use of glucose within cells in peripheral tissue via binding to an intracellular agent, peroxisomal proliferator-activated receptor (PPARγ) that activates genes involved in glucose and lipid metabolism. TZDs are considered insulin sensitizers because they improve insulin action in peripheral tissues and enhance glucose uptake in the cells. These agents

---

Box 18-5 Contraindications to Use of Metformin (Glucophage)

Metformin concentrates in the intestine, where it doubles the production of lactate. The lactate subsequently passes into the portal circulation and decreases the pH in the liver. This causes a further decrease in lactate metabolism. These effects combine to increase the concentration of lactate in the circulation. The contraindications to using metformin include disorders that might contribute to increased lactate concentrations. For example, hypoxia causes a shift to anaerobic metabolism, which produces lactate. The contraindications to use of metformin are the following:

1. Renal impairment (plasma creatinine level of ≥ 14 mg/dL in women)

2. Cardiac or pulmonary insufficiency that is likely to result in decreased tissue perfusion or hypoxia (e.g., congestive heart failure, chronic obstructive pulmonary disorder)

3. History of lactic acidosis

4. Profound infection that might cause impaired perfusion of peripheral tissues (e.g., sepsis)

5. Hepatic dysfunction (including alcohol-induced liver damage)

6. Alcohol abuse

Temporarily discontinue metformin at the time of or before a procedure using intravenous contrast media, withhold for 48 hours after the procedure, and restart only when renal function is assessed as normal.

decrease the HbA1c by 0.5–1.4% and reduce blood glucose values 25–50 mg/dL.[34] TZDs work synergistically with metformin and sulfonylureas.

TZDs are metabolized in the liver and excreted primarily in urine with some in feces. They have a slow onset of action with first response seen after 2 weeks of taking the drug. At least 3 months is required to see the maximal benefit of the drug in an individual. When combined with another drug such as metformin (Glucophage) or insulin, peak benefit can be seen in 4 weeks.

The primary indication for using a TZD agent is as a secondary medication for persons who have not achieved glycemic goals with insulin or metformin alone.[47] Thiazolidinediones are not used in the initial treatment of type 2 diabetes due to the risk of cardiovascular events and high cost compared to other drugs.[48] Thiazolidinediones are associated with less secondary failure than other drugs.[49] TZDs are safe for individuals with renal impairment. Blood pressured is lowered in persons who take TZDs.

Rosiglitazone (Avandia) is associated with a significant increased risk for myocardial infarction.[50] There is a second relationship between TZDs and cardiovascular compromise that is different than that of the antidiabetic drugs discussed so far. TZDs increase the risk of congestive heart failure secondary to fluid retention and edema. It is postulated that TZDs uncover latent congestive heart failure as the TZD-related fluid retention overtaxes a circulatory system that cannot accommodate the additional fluid volume. A meta-analysis conducted by Nissan et al. convinced the FDA in 2007 that these risks warrant a black box warning.[50] Rosiglitazone (Avandia) now carries an FDA-mandated black box warning that this drug is associated with a significant risk of congestive heart failure. In 2009, the final results of the Rosiglitazone Evaluated for Cardiovascular Outcomes in Oral Agent Combination Therapy for Type 2 Diabetes (RECORD) trial were released. Rosiglitazone (Avandia) did not increase the overall number of cardiovascular hospitalizations or deaths, but the risk of developing heart failure doubled in persons taking rosiglitazone compared to persons taking metformin (Glucophage) or sulfonylureas and in persons with preexisting heart failure there was a 26% increase in myocardial infarction. Rosiglitazone is also associated with an increased risk of distal fracture in older women.

Side Effects/Adverse Effects

The most common side effects of thiazolidinediones are edema and weight gain. Part of the weight gain can be attributed to fluid retention, but the majority is adiposity. Pedal edema occurs in approximately 5% of individuals who take a TZD.[44] Caution is advised if the individual has symptoms of congestive heart failure such as edema and in women with impaired liver function. Adverse symptoms including angina, pleural effusion, and pulmonary edema have all been seen with rosiglitazone.

Additional side effects include anemia and headaches. There is no risk of hypoglycemia when a thiazolidinedione is used as monotherapy; however, there is a significant risk for hypoglycemia when pioglitazone (Actos) is used in combination with other hypoglycemic agents. An increased risk for hypoglycemia also occurs when adding rosiglitazone (Avandia) to insulin or sulfonylurea therapy.

Women need to be warned that TZD can induce ovulation, and oral contraceptives may lose efficacy, so appropriate precautions need to be taken to avoid pregnancy. In addition, women on rosiglitazone have a higher incidence of bone fractures than men using the drug.

Because this class of drug is associated with an increased risk of hepatotoxicity, a baseline aminotransferase (ALT) level should be obtained, and if the value is > 2.5 times the upper limit for the reference range, the manufacturer recommends that the TZD not be prescribed. For persons who take a TZD, the ALT should be monitored every 3–6 months and more often if it is elevated.[19]

Contraindications

All TZDs are contraindicated for persons with type 1 diabetes or class III or IV congestive heart failure. The primary risk with TZDs is the risk of death from congestive heart failure and myocardial ischemia. The FDA, in July 2007, required the addition of a black box warning to packaging of rosiglitazone (Avandia), but did not remove it from the market. The warning states that the drug caused or exacerbated congestive heart failure. Contraindications to rosiglitazone (Avandia) include type 1 diabetes, hypersensitivity to the drug or class, congestive heart failure meeting New York Heart Association class III–IV requirements, congestive heart failure symptoms, and acute coronary symptoms. These contraindications may change as more information about rosiglitazone becomes available.

Drug–Drug Interactions

Thiazolidinediones are mostly metabolized in the liver via CYP3A4 and CYP2C8. Therefore, they are subject to several drug–drug interactions (Table 18-6). In particular, rifampin (Rifadin) speeds metabolism of thiazolidinediones and reduces the plasma levels, and gemfibrozil (Lopid) increases blood levels of thiazolidinediones. It is probable that the hypoglycemic effect of thiazolidinediones is decreased if other potent inducers of CYP3A4 are taken concomitantly. Drugs that are known inducers of CYP3A4 include carbamazepine (Tegretol), phenytoin (Dilantin), and St. John's wort. In contrast, these agents do not appear to alter the pharmacokinetics of other compounds.[51]

Alpha Glucosidase Inhibitors

Alpha glucosidase inhibitors prevent the digestion of carbohydrates and thus reduce the number of simple sugars absorbed through the gastrointestinal system. The agents in this class that are available in the United States are acarbose (Precose) and miglitol (Glyset). These drugs are saccharides that compete with enzymes in the brush border of the small intestine, effectively preventing the action of enzymes necessary for conversion of carbohydrate to absorbable glucose. Carbohydrates are then diges-ted in the colon.

This class of drugs is helpful particularly in controlling postprandial hyperglycemia. Alpha glucosidase inhibitors may be used as single-agent therapy or in combination with other hypoglycemic agents. The alpha glucosidase inhibitors have a short-term effect on blood glucose levels and a minimal effect on HbA1c. They decrease the HbA1c by 0.7–1.0% and the average blood glucose levels by 20–30 mg/dL.[34] The effect of alpha glucosidase inhibitors on serum lipid values and cardiovascular events is unclear. More study is recommended.[52]

The alpha glucosidase inhibitors are given orally at the start of a meal. Both are oral tablets metabolized in the gastrointestinal tract. Acarbose is excreted predominantly in feces (51%) and urine (34%). Miglitol is excreted unchanged in the urine. Because of this reliance on renal excretion, a baseline creatinine level should be obtained prior to initiating therapy with one of these agents to verify adequate renal function.

Side Effects/Adverse Effects

Side effects of alpha glucosidase inhibitors center on the gastrointestinal system with abdominal pain, cramping, flatulence, and diarrhea. Flatulence is quite common and can reduce compliance. To minimize side effects, the dose should start low and gradually increase to an effective level.

A special consideration for alpha glucosidase inhibitors is the management of hypoglycemia. If a person develops hypoglycemia while taking a drug in this class, resolution requires the intake of monosaccharides in the form of glucose tablets or gel. Carbohydrates and other sugars will be blocked by the alpha glucosidase inhibitor

and therefore only compound the hypoglycemia. Hypersensitivity is possible with drugs in this class.

In addition to the common side effects in this class of drugs, acarbose (Precose) has also been linked with serious reactions including ileus, hypersensitivity to the drug, and hepatitis. Because of the risk of hepatitis, tests of liver function are recommended in addition to the baseline creatinine test. The creatinine and alanine aminotransferase (ALT) and aspartate aminotransferase (AST) tests should be repeated every 3 months for a year. If they remain normal, they need to be rechecked at least annually.

Contraindications

Alpha glucosidase inhibitors are contraindicated for persons with gastrointestinal disease including inflammatory bowel disease or ulcers, those who are at risk for or have an intestinal obstruction, and those with malabsorption syndromes. The drugs should be avoided by individuals who use alcohol or take miglitol (Glyset), or pramlintide (Symlin) because of duplicate action and an increased risk of hypoglycemia.

Peptide Analogs

Two new approaches to glucose management are classified as incretin mimetics. As noted earlier in this chapter, incretins are a family of gastrointestinal hormones that induce insulin secretion in response to food ingestion. Glucagon-like peptide (GLP-1) and gastric inhibitory peptide (GIP) are two of the hormones in the incretion family. Dipeptidyl peptidase-4 (DPP-4) is the enzyme responsible for degrading GLP-1 and GIP.

Unfortunately, the half-life of endogenous GLP-1 is just a few minutes, and the half-life of GIP is about 7 minutes, so although direct analogs of this hormone are efficacious, they have to be continuously administered intravenously or subcutaneously, which makes their clinical utility unfeasible.[53] Therefore, the two types of incretion mimetics available attack the problem from two different angles. GLP-1 mimetics are GLP-1 receptor agonists resistant to degradation by DPP-4. These agents bind to the GLP-1 receptor and stimulate production of insulin synthesis and secretion. In contrast, DPP-4 inhibitors prevent DPP-4 from degrading endogenously produced GLP-1. These drugs are relatively new, and their effect on cardiovascular events is unknown at this time.[54-56] The interesting origin of exenatide (Byetta), the most common of these agents, is described in Box 18-6.

Box 18-6 Learning About Diabetes: From Dogs to Lizard Spit

Diabetes is a very old disease. References to the disease of sweet urine can be found in an unbroken chain of documents reaching back millennia from an Egyptian papyrus more than 3500 years ago to modern day. What may not be well known is the roles that many animals have played in the search for a cure for diabetes.

The recognition that diabetes is secondary to pancreatic dysfunction was discovered in 1899 when the European physician Minkowski removed the pancreas of a dog in his investigation of the organ. After the pancreas was removed, he noticed that the dog urinated more frequently and found the urine to be high in sugar content. This was the start of understanding diabetic pathophysiology.

The first compound used to treat diabetes was a preparation of canine pancreatic extract. Frederick Banting and Charles Best kept a diabetic dog named Alpha alive for 70 days with injections of canine pancreatic extract. This success caused the duo to consider other options as treatments. Banting had been raised on a farm so he advocated the development of concoctions made from pancreases of fetal cattle. He knew that cattle slaughtered for food would be impregnated prior to being slaughtered because pregnancy hastened their fattening. Thus, fetal calves were a source that was plentiful and easily obtained.

When Banting and Best had an extract that appeared pure enough, it was administered to Leonard Thompson, a 14-year-old boy who was dying of diabetes. After an initial hypersensitivity reaction, the extract was reformulated and a second dose resulted in a miraculous response as Leonard's blood glucose levels dropped spectacularly. When Banting, Best, and colleagues published their findings, they suggested that this product of the isles of Langerhans be called "insulin." Shortly thereafter they collaborated with the Eli Lilly company, which eventually produced an insulin made from pigs and cattle; this insulin was the predominant type for decades.

Dogs were also involved in the discovery of drugs that treat type 2 diabetes. During World War II, Marchel Janbon, a French university pharmacologist searching for a cure for malaria, noted that dogs treated with sulfonylrureas died of hypoglycemia. He quickly changed his research focus and developed sulfonylureas as a treatment for diabetes.

Since then, laboratory studies of agents that affect glucose metabolism have progressed with the sacrifice of many animals including anglerfish, catfish, salmon, laboratory rodents, transgenic mice, and most recently Gila monsters. Exenatide (Byetta), one of the newest drugs available, is a synthetic form of a hormone found in the venom of the Gila monster lizard (*Heloderma suspectum*). Studies are continuing today, and if they are successful, next up is an antidiabetic agent made from the skins of poisonous frogs.

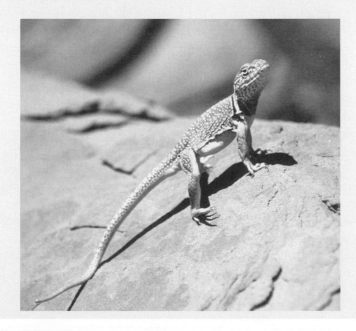

The commercially available GLP-1 mimetic is exenatide or exendin-4 (Byetta). Exenatide is an injectable medication. In the hour immediately preceding morning and evening meals, 5–10 mcg of exenatide is injected subcutaneously. Exenatide reduces the glucose impact of the food intake at that time via increasing insulin secretion, suppressing glucagon secretion, and delaying gastric emptying, which leads to decreased intake and weight loss.[57] Because the mechanism of action is in response to food intake, exenatide must only be taken prior to a meal, and if forgotten, not taken at a later time of day. A once weekly injection formulation has been developed and tested in Canada but is not available in the United States.

Exenatide is approved as adjunct therapy with oral medications such as metformin (Glucophage), biguanides, thiazolidinediones, and sulfonylureas. Exenatide provides a therapeutic advantage when paired with sulfonylureas, biguanides, and TZDs, although doses may be need to be adjusted with initiation of the combination therapy.[58] It is not currently FDA approved as monotherapy or as concurrent therapy with insulin.

Exenatide (Byetta) is metabolized in the kidney and excreted in urine. Prior to prescribing exenatide, a baseline creatinine clearance should be obtained. A creatinine clearance less than 30 indicates a degree of renal compromise that precludes use of exenatide. The half-life of exenatide is 2.4 hours. Exenatide works in response to food intake and therefore avoids some of the risks of hyperglycemia and hypoglycemia that occur with other types of medications. Exenatide also suppresses release of glucagon from the pancreas in response to food intake and hyperglycemia, thereby decreasing the postprandial plasma glucose rise in response to food intake.

Side Effects/Adverse Effects

Gastrointestinal side effects of exenatide (Byetta) include nausea, dyspepsia, vomiting, decreased appetite, and gastroesophageal reflux disease. Headaches, dizziness, and jitteriness are also reported side effects. Gastric emptying is slowed with the use of exenatide, and the sense of hunger is thus reduced. This mechanism of action has resulted in a welcome side effect of the drug—weight loss. The weight loss side effect associated with exenatide (Byetta) has made it a drug of choice for those individuals with diabetes and difficulty with weight control.

Exenatide has been associated with pancreatitis and the FDA has issued a warning that anyone on the drug who exhibits signs of pancreatitis should discontinue the drug and seek medical evaluation. The decision was controversial because pancreatitis is more common in all individuals with diabetes. Exenatide requires pancreatic function; therefore it is not for use in type 1 diabetes.

Drug–Drug Interactions

For those taking exenatide, acetaminophen and drugs that contain acetaminophen should be used with caution and monitored because absorption of exenatide will be delayed or decreased when acetaminophen is ingested concomitantly with the antidiabetic agent. Erythromycin (E-Mycin), metronidazole (Flagyl), and fosfomycin (Monurol) also delay and decreased absorption of exenatide. Women taking oral contraceptives should take the pills 1 hour before exenatide to permit maximum absorption but need to be aware that effectiveness of contraceptives may be compromised.

■ Dipeptidyl Peptidase-4 Inhibitors

Dipeptidyl peptidase-4 (DPP-4) inhibitors do just as the name describes—they inhibit the degradation of the incretin GLP-1; the result is an increase in the concentration of GLP-1 and subsequent increase in insulin release from the pancreas. The unique property of DPP-4 inhibitors is that these drugs decrease glucagon and increase insulin only in response to elevated glucose. The dose-response property reduces the risk of hypoglycemia.

There are currently two drugs in this category—vildagliptin (Galvus) and sitagliptin (Januvia). Vildagliptin is available in Europe but is not yet available in the United States. In July 2008, the FDA requested additional clinical studies to evaluate the animal results of skin lesions and renal impairment in animal studies with the use of vildagliptin. Sitagliptin (Januvia) is available in the United States.

Sitagliptin (Januvia) is an oral medication given at 100 mg daily and can be taken with or without food. The drug has a half-life of 12.4 hours. Sitagliptin is excreted predominantly in the urine (>80%) and also in feces (13%). Because the medication is excreted by the kidney, baseline creatinine clearance is recommended prior to initiation of the drug to confirm renal function.

Sitagliptin (Januvia) is recommended as a monotherapy and can be used with other oral medications, although caution is needed to avoid additive effects. Sitagliptin is often used as a second drug in combination with insulin or other oral hypoglycemic agents and has a therapeutic advantage in these combinations. Synergism is expected with sulfonylureas, metformin (Glucophage), miglitol (Glyset), nateglinide (Starlix), disopyramide (Norpace), repaglinide (Prandin), pramlintide (Symlin), rosiglitazone (Avandia), glimepiride (Amaryl), and fluoxetine (Prozac). In fact, sitagliptin has a therapeutic advantage when paired with these drugs.

Side Effects/Adverse Effects

Nasopharyngitis, headache, and upper respiratory infections are the most common side effects of sitagliptin (Januvia). Gastrointestinal discomforts include abdominal pain, diarrhea, and flatulence. Arthralgia has also been reported. Caution is recommended if renal function is impaired. Sitagliptin increases insulin release from the pancreas, so pancreatic function is required. For this reason, sitagliptin in contraindicated in type 1 diabetes. Adverse reactions that have been reported with sitagliptin include Stevens-Johnson syndrome, hypersensitivity, including anaphylaxis, and angioedema.

Drug–Drug Interactions

Combining beta-blockers with sitagliptin (Januvia) can cause an adrenergic antagonism that may alter glucose metabolism and excretion resulting in prolonged hypoglycemia. Many drugs have an antagonistic effect when used with sitagliptin, including ACE inhibitors, antihistamine/decongestant combinations, atypical antipsychotic medications, phenothiazines, isoniazid (INH), corticosteroids, estrogens, diuretics, statins, sympathomimetics, and thyroid hormones.

In addition, beta-blockers mask hypoglycemia symptoms. Caution must be used when drugs that compete for the active transport mechanism used by sitagliptin are given. These medications include adefovir (Hepsera, Preveon), cidofovir (Vistide), cimetidine (Tagamet), emtricitabine (Emtriva), and tenofovir (Viread). Androgens and MAO inhibitors have a synergistic effect that may increase the risk of hypoglycemia. Growth hormones increase insulin resistance and may increase the risk of hyperglycemia.

Amylin Analogues

Amylin analogues control glycemia by slowing gastric emptying time and suppress postprandial secretion of glucagon. Amylin is secreted by the beta cells of the pancreas along with insulin secretion. For this reason, individuals with poor beta cell secretion of insulin will also have low secretion of amylin. The only amylin analogue available in the United States is pramlintide (Symlin). Pramlintide is an injectable medication used in both type 1 and type 2 diabetes. Pramlintide is excreted in the kidney. The half-life is 48 minutes.

Pramlintide is used only by persons already taking insulin and is not a second-line drug for individuals who are using oral medications only. Pramlintide is injected subcutaneously before full meals (at least 250 calories and 30 grams of carbohydrate). The initial dose is 60 mcg before each meal. The dose is increased gradually until glycemic control is reached. The maximum dose is 120 mcg. The dose of pramlintide must be titrated with concomitant changes in insulin dose. When pramlintide is initiated, the rapid or short-acting insulin taken prior to a meal should be decreased by 50%. As pramlintide is further increased, insulin is decreased until glycemic control is achieved. Injection sites for insulin and pramlintide should be at least two inches apart to assure appropriate absorption of each drug. Blood sugar values need to be checked before and after each meal and at bedtime when using pramlintide. Hypoglycemia can occur as long as 3 hours after injection and a meal. The advantage to pramlintide is weight loss—possibly secondary to the slow gastric emptying time and the nausea experienced by some users during initiation of therapy. When the dose is increased slowly over 3–7 days, the nausea side effects are minimized.

Side Effects/Adverse Effects

Common side effects of pramlintide (Symlin) include nausea, vomiting, anorexia, arthralgia, dizziness, pharyngitis, and cough. Most side effects subside within a few weeks of initiation of the drug. The most significant adverse effect is severe hypo-glycemia, which can occur when this drug is added to an insulin regimen.

Contraindications

Contraindications for pramlintide (Symlin) include individuals with an HbA1c > 9%. This level of hyperglycemia is better managed with insulin alone because pramlintide minimally affects the HbA1c value. Individuals with gastroparesis or malabsorption syndromes may experience exacerbation with the delayed gastric emptying effect of pramlintide. Individuals with a history of severe hypoglycemia and/or hypoglycemia unawareness should not use this drug. Because of the intense monitoring required by the person taking pramlintide, persons who have difficulty managing close self-monitoring such as young teens or adults who have decreased mental capacity or motivation to consistently monitor their blood glucose should not use this medication. The risk of severe hypoglycemia is high in these populations. Pramlintide is contraindicated if the individual is also taking solid potassium salts, such as potassium phosphate, potassium citrate, potassium chloride, or potassium iodide. The administration of pramlintide slows the passage of solid potassium salts and increases the risk of ulcers/stenotic changes in the gastrointestinal tract.

Drug–Drug Interactions

Drug–drug interactions associated with pramlintide include all medications with an anticholinergic effect. Anticholinergic drugs may further delay gastric emptying and slow medication passage through the gastrointestinal tract. Drugs of concern include tricyclic antidepressants, phenothiazines, alpha glucosidase inhibitor oral hypoglycemics, antihistamines, and/or decongestants. Erythromycin given for gastrointestinal promotility is less effective when pramlintide is being used. Prokinetic activity is decreased with pramlintide and will decrease the effectiveness of cisapride (Propulsid) and metoclopramide (Reglan). The antiarrhythmic drug disopyramide (Norpace) increases the risk of serious hypoglycemia, although the mechanism is unknown.

▮ Combination Therapy with Oral Agents

When monotherapy fails to maintain euglycemia, the next step is to combine two or three medications that have different mechanisms of action. This is usually accomplished by adding a second medication. In 2008, the FDA approved the use of PrandiMet, which is a combination of repaglinide and metformin. Repaglinide is a fast-acting insulin secretagogue, and metformin is an insulin sensitizer. The drug comes in two formulations as 1/500 mg or 2/500 mg of repaglinide/metformin. One tablet is taken 2–3 times per day with meals. This drug is contraindicated for persons with renal impairment and for persons who take gemfibrozil (Lopid) or itraconazole (Sporanox). Renal function is evaluated prior to initiating therapy and assessed annually thereafter if normal at the time of initiation.

▮ Oral Agents Plus Insulin for Treating Type 2 Diabetes

When type 2 diabetes is not well controlled with lifestyle management and oral medication, insulin is indicated. Insulin may be the second agent for an individual on one oral medication. For some individuals, a second oral medication is added, and then, if needed, insulin is added as a third agent. Insulin combined with oral medications improves glycemic control, results in less weight gain than with insulin alone, and is effective with a relatively simple insulin regimen. The primary oral medication(s) is continued at its regular dose, and the insulin is added. The combination of oral medications and insulin has a synergistic effect. The therapeutic effect is achieved with lower doses of the medications when used in combination than when each is used as monotherapy. The dose of exogenous insulin is also lower than when insulin is used as a monotherapy. Insulin as a second or third agent uses fewer injections and less complicated insulin mixtures than if insulin is the single agent. The simpler regimen results in better patient acceptance because of the convenience of a less complicated dose and administration schedule when compared to insulin alone.

The basic process for initiating combination therapy including insulin is to leave the oral medication at the current dose and add regular insulin 10 units at bedtime—usually given by insulin pen. Careful attention to self-monitored blood glucose levels determines the next addition. If needed to control the fasting morning glucose level, NPH insulin may be added at bedtime. If the fasting and evening postprandial levels remain high, 70/30 insulins may be needed before the evening meal. Ultimately, basal insulin may be added. Insulin doses are increased weekly until desired blood glucose results are consistent. Insulin is increased by four units a week if the blood glucose level is ≥ 180, and increased two units a week if the blood glucose level is ≥ 140 but < 180.

▮ Pharmacotherapy for Diabetic Emergencies

Two emergency conditions can occur when treating persons with diabetes. The first emergency is hypoglycemia, and the second is hyperglycemia. Both emergencies result from potentially life-threatening blood glucose levels. Hypoglycemia (insulin shock) and hyperglycemia (sugar shock) are more common in persons with type 1 diabetes, but may occur in persons with type 2 diabetes as well.

Hypoglycemia

Hypoglycemia is defined as a plasma glucose < 70 mg/dL. Hypoglycemia may result from poor nutritional intake with regular doses of medication, too much medication (particularly insulin), illness, which increases glucose consumption by tissues, and exercise without adequate food intake. It can also be iatrogenic secondary to inaccurate insulin administration or unknown factors. Symptoms vary from a sense of feeling bad, shakiness, palpitations, tachycardia pallor clamminess, dilated pupils, nausea/vomiting, and/or headache. Typically, mental changes occur, including impaired judgment, rage and belligerence, confusion with progression to difficulty speaking, ataxia, and coma. Focal seizures may occur in severe cases. The symptoms of hypoglycemia make it difficult for affected individuals to effectively manage advanced hypoglycemia. For this reason, it is important that everyone with diabetes and everyone who lives with a person who has diabetes are taught signs, symptoms, and interventions in the first signs of hypoglycemia.

Hypoglycemic Unawareness

Hypoglycemic unawareness is a particularly serious complication of diabetes—most often seen in persons with type 1 diabetes. Individuals with recurrent hypoglycemia may develop autonomic neuropathy that prevents the release of epinephrine, which in turn signals the liver to release glucose.[59] This individual does not have the usual symptoms of tremors, jitters, or palpitations that are associated with epinephrine and that signal the onset of hypoglycemia. The same situation can occur if an individual is taking beta-blockers because they prevent the release of epinephrine and therefore the palpitations and jitter symptoms of hypoglycemia are inhibited. No symptoms of hypoglycemia are present, and the hypoglycemia can worsen until loss of consciousness occurs without the individual being aware of the hypoglycemia.

Hypoglycemia unawareness can also occur in persons with type 1 diabetes who have frequent hypoglycemic episodes that have allowed the brain to adapt to low glycemic levels so it does not signal epinephrine release. Hypoglycemic unawareness is the most dangerous form of hypoglycemia and can be life threatening if the woman is alone or does not have a responsible person nearby to provide treatment in the event of diminished mental function or loss of consciousness.

Treatment of Hypoglycemia

At the first sign of altered glucose level, a plasma glucose level should be obtained. If the glucose is < 70 mg/dL, oral glucose or carbohydrate equal to 15–20 grams of glucose should be given orally. Good choices of oral glucose are 3–4 ounces of apple, orange, or grape juice, four crackers, one slice of bread, or 5–6 ounces of regular soda. There is no advantage to more glucose—it does not absorb faster and may in fact lead to overshooting the normal glucose level desired. Fat or protein given with the glucose (peanut butter crackers) may slow the absorption of glucose. If the woman is taking acarbose (Precose) or another alpha glucosidase inhibitor, a monosaccharide sugar must be given because acarbose will prevent the breakdown of starch to sugar. Give glucose tablets, honey, or fruit juice to a woman on acarbose.

Glucagon

If a person with diabetes is unconscious, an intravenous solution with normal saline should be initiated and 2 cc of dextrose 50% should be given. An alternative is 1–2 milligrams of glucagon given intramuscularly. Glucagon is rarely used out of a hospital setting but may be used by paramedics in the field if intravenous access cannot be obtained. Care must be taken to carefully observe anyone receiving glucagon because of the danger of severe rebound hypoglycemia. For this reason, glucagon is used almost exclusively in the hospital, and if used in the field, the recipient is transferred immediately for inpatient evaluation and monitoring.

Hyperglycemia

Hyperglycemia is an elevated blood glucose level. Severe hyperglycemia is also called diabetic ketoacidosis (DKA). Diabetic ketoacidosis is defined as (1) hyperglycemia (blood glucose > 200 mg/dL) with (2) metabolic acidosis (pH < 7.3) and (3) an elevated anion gap (> 12 mmol/L) and (4) positive urinary ketones. DKA is a medical emergency. DKA may occur at blood glucose levels of < 200 mg/dL, but typically if this does occur the cause is something other than the underlying diabetes. It must be remembered that lactic acidosis presents as DKA and therefore, lactic acidosis must be considered if the individual has been taking metformin (Glucophage) or other medications that can cause lactic acidosis.

Symptoms of hyperglycemia include excessive hunger and thirst, cognitive changes, nausea, and vomiting that progress to symptoms of DKA including Kussmaul hyperventilation, stupor, ketoacidosis, and coma. Glucose is not able to enter the cells that trigger the liver to release more glucagon. Dehydration occurs due to glycosuria and osmotic diuresis in the kidney. Uncorrected, DKA is lethal.

Management requires emergency and intensive intervention by specialists in emergency, endocrine, and possibly intensive care medicine. Goals of treatment are to determine the underlying cause to assure appropriate intervention. Intravenous fluids are initiated with saline, and regular insulin is given. Plasma glucose and potassium levels are reassessed at least every 30 minutes until the patient is stable. DKA often is deep, profound, and affects multiple systems.

Hyperosmolar hyperglycemic state is a variation of DKA that does not usually exhibit the same degree of acidosis. This state is seen in lactic acidosis that may develop in persons taking metformin. Dehydration is more profound than in DKA, and more fluids are needed to correct the condition. Lower doses of insulin are often required due to increased sensitivity to insulin.

Gestational Diabetes

Gestational diabetes is diabetes that is first diagnosed during pregnancy. Diabetes appearing in pregnancy may be previously undetected type 1 diabetes, previously undetected type 2 diabetes, or gestational diabetes, which is abnormal glucose tolerance that results from the physiologic changes in the pregnancy. Data suggest that gestational diabetes mellitus (GDM) occurs in 2–5% of pregnancies but may be as high as 10% in some populations such as Native American women.[60] Gestational diabetes resolves with completion of the pregnancy.

Gestational diabetes mellitus is a disease of insulin resistance. The insulin resistance becomes significant in the early second trimester of pregnancy, and therefore screening for this condition is performed between 24 and 28 weeks of gestation. Beginning in the second trimester, insulin requirements increase to 1.5–2.5% above prepregnancy needs. This is approximately equal to the hyperinsulinemia seen in persons with type 2 diabetes. Women with GDM cannot mobilize enough insulin production in the beta cells of the pancreas to meet the increased insulin needs during pregnancy, and hyperglycemia ensues.

Risk factors for gestational diabetes are shown in Table 18-7.[61] Women who develop gestational diabetes have the same risk factors that are associated with type 2 diabetes including obesity, family history of diabetes (which suggests a genetic predisposition), age > 35, and others.

Women with GDM are at increased risk for preeclampsia, fetal macrosomia with concomitant risks for operative delivery, maternal tissue trauma, fetal injury, and infection.[61] Long term, women with GDM have a 45% risk of recurrence in subsequent pregnancies and up to 65% risk of developing type 2 diabetes in the future.[61,62]

The physiologic impact of GDM on the fetus and newborn can be profound and is the primary reason cited for aggressive management of women with GDM.[61] Glucose easily transfers from maternal circulation across the placenta into the fetal circulation via facilitated diffusion. Insulin does not cross the placenta as easily because the insulin molecule is too large, and facilitated diffusion does not occur. The result is that the fetus is exposed to hyperglycemia and responds with an increase in insulin secretion. The result of hyperglycemia, if uncorrected, is an increased incidence of macrosomia. Macrosomia places the newborn at risk for complications in the birth process and postpartum hypoglycemia when the placental infusion of elevated glucose ceases. For this reason, infants of mothers who

Table 18-7 Risk Factors for Gestational Diabetes

Maternal age over 25 years

Member of an ethnic group at increased risk for type 2 DM

    Hispanic

    African

    Native American

    South Asian or East Asian

    Pacific Islanders

Body mass index > 25

History of abnormal glucose tolerance

History of adverse outcomes associated with GDM

    Macrosomia

    Unexplained stillbirth

History of GDM in prior pregnancy

First-degree relative with diabetes

Source: Adapted from American College of Obstetricians and Gynecologists 2001.[61]

have diabetes including GDM need to be monitored with blood glucose levels in the newborn period.

Diagnosis of Gestational Diabetes

Gestational diabetes is screened for at 24–28 weeks' gestation with a screening glucose value that is obtained 1 hour after ingesting a liquid that has exactly 50 grams of glucose. The diagnosis is made with a follow-up 3-hour glucose tolerance test (GTT) if the 1-hour screen is ≥ 130 mg/dL. Some institutions use a cutoff of ≥ 140 mg/dL. Debate has persisted regarding the best threshold values for the diagnostic test, and two systems have emerged, both with excellent diagnostic credibility. No evidence exists to choose one set of criteria over the other. The criteria values for diagnosis are shown in Table 18-8.

Management of Gestational Diabetes

Several of the placental hormones contribute to insulin resistance. Because these hormones are secreted unpredictably, careful monitoring by women who have GDM is essential. Therapy may need to be changed dramatically at various times in pregnancy to accommodate the effects of maternal insulin resistance and the unpredictable hormonal secretion by the placenta.

Gestational diabetes requires careful nutritional management. Eating for two in pregnancy with diabetes means eating not *volume* for two but rather *quality and timing* to support both mother and fetus. Nutritional therapy for women with GDM is an intake of 30–36 kcal/kg per day for normal-weight women and 24 kcal/kg per day for women with body mass index > 30. Walking, swimming, and targeted exercise for women with GDM are keys to controlling blood glucose levels. Often, nutrition and exercise

alone will maintain glucose in the target range of fasting values < 105 mg/dL and the 2-hour postprandial blood glucose value of < 120 mg/dL.[61] Pharmacologic therapy is considered if nutrition and exercise fail to maintain target glucose levels.

Use of Insulin for Treating Gestational Diabetes

Insulin is the primary drug used in GDM if fasting blood glucose levels consistently exceed 95 mg/dL but postprandial levels remain < 130 mg/dL. In this scenario, a bedtime intermediate insulin such as NPH or lente may be given and correct the morning hyperglycemia. If fasting and postprandial levels are elevated, full insulin therapy is initiated.

Insulin is calculated based on the woman's weight. Total daily insulin is based on 0.5 to 0.7 units/kg of mother's weight. Combing intermediate and short-acting insulin yields the best result for most women. Two insulin doses are given daily with two thirds of the total insulin in the morning to cover energy needs of the active day and one third at night. If a woman is a night worker (RN on night shift for example), the proportions of the dose would be reversed so two thirds is given at night.

Presuming daytime is the primary time of activity, the morning dose of the insulin would cover breakfast and lunch as well as activity. The morning dose would contain one third of the total dose of the short-acting insulin and two thirds of the dose of intermediate-acting insulin. The evening dose is reversed with two thirds of short-acting insulin to cover dinner and basal needs during the night and one third of the intermediate-acting insulin to cover the activity of the evening. A standard combination for this regimen is NPH as the intermediate-acting insulin and regular insulin as the short-acting insulin.

Insulin therapy can become complex as the needs in pregnancy change. Typically, women requiring insulin or other medication during pregnancy are managed by a team of professionals with expertise in diabetes in pregnancy including maternal-fetal medicine, endocrinology, nutritionists, diabetic educators, and the primary midwife/physician.

Use of Oral Hypoglycemic Agents for Treating Gestational Diabetes

Some oral medications are safe and may be used as first-line drugs if nutrition/exercise is not adequate alone. Glyburide (DiaBeta, Micronase, Glynase) is safe for use

Table 18-8 Diagnostic Criteria for Gestational Diabetes

	Plasma Glucose Diagnostic Values*	
	American Diabetes Association (mg/dL)	National Diabetes Data Group (mg/dL)
Fasting	95	105
1 hour	180	190
2 hour	155	165
3 hour	140	145

* The 100-g test is performed on women with a positive 50-g screen. A positive 100-g test requires any two of the four values to exceed the limits noted.
Sources: American Diabetes Association 2009[5]; American College of Obstetricians and Gynecologists 2001.[61]

in pregnancy and has maternal and newborn outcomes that are similar to those seen in women who are treated with insulin.[63] Glyburide is easier to manage and is usually preferred to daily injections. For women with compromised learning or complicated lives, glyburide may be more effective because the woman is able to use it more correctly. Glyburide (DiaBeta, Micronase, Glynase) does not cross the placenta and therefore does not cause fetal/neonatal hypoglycemia.

Metformin (Glucophage) is also as effective as insulin, and although earlier studies noted a correlation between metformin use in pregnancy and an increase in the incidence of preeclampsia and stillbirth, this relationship has not been found in randomized, controlled trials.[63]

Diabetes Insipidus

Diabetes insipidus is not a disease of glucose metabolism but rather a disease of water metabolism. The common symptoms of polyuria and polydipsia resulted in the shared word *diabetes*, but the name is the only similarity between diabetes mellitus and diabetes insipidus.

Diabetes insipidus (DI) can be congenital or acquired. The disorder presents in the following four forms: neurogenic DI, gestational DI, nephrogenic DI, and dipsogenic DI. Each form has a different physiology and therefore a different method of treatment.

Neurogenic DI (also called central, hypothalamic, pituitary, or neurohypophyseal DI) is caused by a deficiency of vasopressin, the antidiuretic hormone. The deficient production may be the result of damage to the posterior pituitary secondary to trauma or disease, or it can be idiopathic. Sheehan's syndrome, a serious complication of hemorrhage that results in pituitary necrosis, is a cause of neurogenic DI. Congenital DI is a rare genetic abnormality caused by an x-linked mutation of the antidiuretic hormone V-2 receptors (80% of genetic DI). A mutation of the aquaporin 2 water channel is even more rare (10% of genetic DI).

Nephrogenic DI (also called vasopressin-resistant DI) is caused by decreased or absent sensitivity of the kidneys to the effect of vasopressin. More commonly, nephrogenic DI is caused by sickle cell disease and polycystic kidney disease that damage the kidney. The following two medications are also known causes of nephrogenic DI: lithium (Lithobid) and amphotericin B (Amphotec).

Dipsogenic DI is secondary to polydipsia caused by abnormal thirst resulting in abnormal intake of fluids including excess water. There is an abnormality in the brain perception of thirst, resulting in excess intake of water/fluids. The pituitary is unable to produce enough vasopressin to counter the excessive water intake. Dipsogenic DI is seen in some women with anorexia nervosa if the women develop hypokalemia because hypokalemia interferes with action of vasopressin.

Gestagenic or gestational DI is caused by a deficiency of vasopressin that occurs only during pregnancy. Vasopressin may be adversely affected by the enzyme vasopressinase produced in the placenta. Treatment with desmopressin acetate (DDAVP) is effective in treating this disorder. A second form of gestational DI is caused by an abnormality in the thirst mechanism. Treatment of this form of DI with desmopressin can result in water intoxication. The differential diagnosis of the two forms of gestational DI is extremely difficult and requires an endocrinologist familiar with the diseases. Both forms of gestational DI resolve spontaneously within 4–6 weeks postpartum.

Treatment of Diabetes Insipidus

Treatment of neurogenic DI management is based on the underlying pathology within the brain. If a mass or tumor of the pituitary is the cause, treatment/removal of the mass may resolve the DI. If a mass is not the cause, management includes replacement of the antidiuretic hormone (8-arginine vasopressin) desmopressin acetate (DDVAP).

Desmopressin acetate (DDVAP) is a synthetic antidiuretic hormone analogue. Desmopressin acetate is excreted in the urine and has a half-life of 1.5–2.5 hours if given orally and 3 hours if given intravenously. This drug is contraindicated in von Willebrand's disease because of drug increases in factor V2 and von Willebrand factor. It is also contraindicated for individuals with creatinine clearance < 50 mL/min because of the increased risk of hyponatremia with compromised excretion. Caution should be used in persons with hypertension, congestive heart failure, fluid/electrolyte imbalance, or polydipsia. Desmopressin acetate should not be used with polyethylene glycol and/or sodium phosphate because the combination will increase the risk of seizure from hyponatremia.

In nephrogenic DI, the kidney is the center of management. Careful attention to fluid intake and urine output is primary management. A low-sodium diet is prescribed to provide no more than 500–600 mg of sodium per day for adults. Patients should be taught to recognize the early signs of hyponatremia, which include headache and nausea followed by a disoriented or confused feeling. Failure to recognize and respond to the symptoms will lead to a worsening of the sodium level and eventual loss of consciousness progressing to seizure. Potassium-sparing diuretics such as thiazide with the possible addition of an amiloride (hydrochlorothiazide) are necessary. For some individuals, a prostaglandin inhibitor is also necessary to maintain kidney function.

Lithium-induced nephrogenic DI can usually be reversed by discontinuing the lithium. However, individuals requiring lithium for treatment of bipolar disorders typically do not manage their psychological state as well on other medications. Also, the manic phase of bipolar disease may include psychogenic polydipsia. Lithium treatment in individuals with bipolar disorder may be necessary for many years and often for life. Multiyear use of lithium may result in interstitial fibrosis of the kidney, which is irreversible. Treatment of lithium-induced DI includes a thiazide diuretic, careful monitoring of sodium intake, and use of nonsteroidal anti-inflammatory drugs (NSAIDs). It is not understood how the NSAIDS work, but they are beneficial.

Special Populations in Diabetes Insipidus

Pregnancy and Lactation

Prior to pregnancy, women with congenital DI themselves or in their family may be referred for genetic counseling to assess the risk of congenital DI in their offspring. Medications typically taken by women with DI are not contraindicated in pregnancy. Desmopressin (DDVAP) is not associated with spontaneous abortion or fetal anomalies. The dose may need to be increased in pregnancy due to the placental metabolism of vasopressin. Thiazide diuretics are not contraindicated in pregnancy

with DI. Care must be taken during common obstetric procedures to accommodate the needs of women with DI. For example, a woman with DI cannot fill her bladder for a sonogram. Hypotonic contractions may result from decreased oxytocin in women with pituitary damage. Intravenous oxytocin may be needed to induce or augment labor to accomplish a vaginal birth. Care must be taken with intravenous infusions to monitor the total fluid intake and output. An intravenous fluid bolus prior to administration of an epidural anesthetic can result in water intoxication for a woman with DI.

Women with neurogenic DI may have difficulty with milk production due to damage to the pituitary axis that resulted in the DI. Prolactin may be decreased, resulting in decreased production of breast milk. Oxytocin may be decreased, resulting in poor letdown reflex. Intranasal oxytocin (Syntocinon spray) prior to nursing may correct the letdown problem. Desmopressin is excreted in breast milk, but the amounts are very small and no adverse effects have been reported.

◼ Complementary and Alternative Treatments for Diabetes Mellitus

Dietary supplements, antioxidants, and some herbs have been recommended as effective treatments for lowering blood glucose levels. Some studies have investigated the effect of complementary therapies for preventing diabetes, and some have done so for treating type 2 diabetes. Most of the studies have been too small to generate significant results. Table 18-9 lists the most popular complementary and herbal therapies currently under investigation.

Table 18-9 Complementary and Alternative Therapies for Treating Type 2 Diabetes

Where Found	Evidence	Safety
Aloe vera[64]	Proposed mechanism: Fiber may promote glucose uptake. Dose is 1 Tb of aloe gel bid. 2 small studies: May decrease fasting blood glucose levels and triglyceride levels.	Aloe leaf contraindicated as it is a cathartic. Safety unknown.
Alpha-lipoic acid	Proposed mechanism: Antioxidant that protects against cell damage. 800 mg/day in divided doses. Some studies have found benefit but others have not. Sources: Liver, spinach, broccoli, and potatoes.	Possible hypoglycemic reaction.
Ayurvedic medicine[64,65]	Proposed mechanism: *Coccinia indica* appears to be insulin mimetic. *Coccinia indica, Gymnema sylvestre,* holy basil, fenugreek, and the herbal formulas Ayush-82 and D-44 have a glucose-lowering effect and deserve further study. Source: Ivy gourd, creeping ivy grown in India subcontinent.	Safety unknown.

(continues)

Table 18-9 Complementary and Alternative Therapies for Treating Type 2 Diabetes (*continued*)

Where Found	Evidence	Safety
Chinese herbal medicines[66]	Proposed mechanism: Unknown. Dose: Not specified. Holy basil leaves, *Xianzhen Pian, Qidan Tongmai*, traditional Chinese formulae *Huoxue Jiangtang Pingzhi*, and *Inolter* have significant hypoglycemic response. *Bushen Jiangtang Tang*, composite *Trichosanthis, Jiangtang Kang, Ketang Ling, Shenqi Jiangtang Yin, Xiaoke Tang*, and *Yishen Huoxue Tiaogan* found to be significantly better than hypoglycemic drugs.	No adverse effects reported in studies conducted.
Chromium picolinate[67]	Proposed mechanism: Insulin-sensitizing effect or direct effect on insulin receptor. Dose: 200 mcg/day capsule or tablet. Decreased HbA1c after 4 months in one study. FDA has authorized health claim that chromium picolinate may decrease insulin resistance but ADA states there is inconclusive evidence for efficacy. Source: Trace mineral found in many foods in very small amounts.	Safe in low doses. High doses can cause renal failure.
Cinnamon (*Cinnamomum cassia*)[67]	Proposed mechanism: Increases insulin sensitivity. Dose: 1–6 g/day in divided doses. Improved glucose control in one study of individuals already on sulfonylureas. Other studies have found no benefit.	Cinnamon has coumarin component. Should be taken with caution by individuals on anticoagulants.
American ginseng	Proposed mechanism: Decreases carbohydrate absorption, increases glycogen storage, and stimulates insulin secretion. Dose: 3 g before a meal. Two small clinical trials found decreases in fasting blood glucose values and HbA1c values.	Insomnia, headache, and anxiety reported side effects. Has many potential drug–drug interactions.
Nopal (*Opuntia streptacantha*)	Proposed mechanism: Decreases glucose absorption and enhances insulin delivery. Dose: 100–500 g daily of broiled stems. A few small studies in Spanish report decreases in blood glucose values following a meal with prickly pear. Additive improvement in postprandial blood glucose when added to sulfonylureas. Sources: Member of cactus family, common food in Hispanic diet. All parts of cactus can be eaten.	Diarrhea is a reported side effect.
Omega-3 fatty acids[67]	Proposed mechanism : Against cardiovascular disorders, decreases inflammation and lowers triglyceride levels. Lowers triglycerides but no effect on blood glucose levels, total cholesterol fasting blood sugars, or HbA1c. Some studies found increase in LDL cholesterol. Sources: Fish, fish oil, vegetable oils, walnuts, and wheat germ.	Safe in moderate doses. Fish oil supplements should be used with caution as mercury levels could be high. High doses interfere with warfarin (Coumadin) and some antihypertensive medications.
Polyphenols	Proposed mechanism: Laboratory studies have shown phenols may protect against cardiovascular disease and have beneficial effect on insulin and glucose control. A few small clinical trials have not found efficacy, but studies have been too small. Sources: Green tea and dark chocolate.	Safe in moderate amounts. Green tea has caffeine, which can cause insomnia or anxiety and small amounts of vitamin K, which could potentiate the effect of warfarin (Coumadin).

Sources: Adapted from Yeh GY 2003[64]; AHRQ No. 01-EO39 2001[65]; Liu JP et al. 2002[66]; Giel P et al. 2008.[67]

Special Populations

Adolescents

The incidence of diabetes is rising dramatically in adolescents. Diabetes and adolescence are an especially difficult combination. The dramatic physiologic and psychologic changes that are normal in adolescence compound the difficulty in maintaining normal glucose levels in adolescents with diabetes. The social pressures and emotional changes in adolescence have resulted in an increase in eating disorders for all teens—including those with diabetes. A new disease is *diabulemia,* for lack of a better term. Diabulemia refers to individuals, predominantly adolescents, who have type 1 diabetes and an eating disorder. Individuals with diabulemia use bulimia and/or omitting insulin to control weight. The combination of inadequate food and insufficient insulin results in significantly increased glucose levels, poor absorption of food, and resulting weight loss and hyperglycemia. Diabetic ketoacidosis is a significant risk in this population and may be the first indication that the adolescent is using the bulimia/withholding of insulin for weight control.

Pregnancy and Lactation

Preconception counseling is a key to successful pregnancy for women with diabetes. Congenital malformations pose the greatest risk to the fetus/infant of the woman with type 1 or type 2 diabetes. Women who have HbA1c levels > 1% above normal levels for nondiabetic women or HbA1c > 6% the first 6–8 weeks of pregnancy are at increased risk for fetal malformations.[5,19] To mitigate the risk, tight glycemic control with HbA1c levels in the normal range (< 6%) prior to conception significantly reduces the risk of teratogenesis. Insulin is safe in pregnancy and may be continued. Oral hypoglycemic agents such as metformin (Glucophage) and acarbose (Precose) are FDA Pregnancy Category B agents and may be continued. All other oral hypoglycemic drugs are FDA Pregnancy Category C drugs and therefore are only continued if the benefits of the drug outweigh the risks. In practical management, a woman who cannot maintain glycemic control with oral FDA Pregnancy Category B drugs will be placed on insulin during pregnancy.

The Elderly

Special considerations must be kept in mind when caring for elderly persons with diabetes. Polypharmacy and drug–drug interactions are more frequent in the elderly. In addition, exaggerated side effects to medication and drug–disease interactions are more common in the elderly than in younger populations. Elderly persons with diabetes are typically placed on oral medications for glycemic control, lipid control, hypertension and/or cardiac disease, and other comorbid conditions such as renal disease, depression, urinary incontinence, and/or cognitive impairment. It is essential to assess every medication the elder adult is taking at every visit and be certain that the medications are being taken appropriately and no adverse interactions or side effects can be anticipated.

Chlorpropamide (Diabinese) should not be used because it has a prolonged half-life that is more pronounced in older adults and leads to increased risk for hypoglycemia. Metformin (Glucophage) needs to be used with caution by older adults with impaired renal function because of the risk of lactic acidosis. The serum creatinine must be ≥ 1.4 mg/dL before metformin is initiated, and assessment of renal function should be repeated at least annually.

Conclusion

Diabetes has the unique distinction of being an ancient disease known since the beginning of recorded history, yet despite decades of research and knowledge about prevention and treatment, this is a disease that is increasingly afflicting persons in all age groups today. Primary care providers in the 21st century have to be well versed in all aspects of this disease until the epidemic of obesity is resolved.

References

1. Centers for Disease Control and Prevention, National Center for Health Statistics, Division of Health Interview Statistics. Data from the National Health Interview Survey. Data computed by the Centers for Disease Control and Prevention, National Center for Chronic Disease Prevention and Health Promotion, Division of Diabetes Translation. Available from *www.cdc.gov/diabetes/Statistics/prev/national/figpersons.htm* [Accessed June 21, 2009].

2. National diabetes information clearing house. National diabetes statistics, 2007. Prevalence of diagnosed and undiagnosed diabetes among people ages 20 years or older, United States 2007. Available from *http://www.cdc.gov/diabetes/pubs/estimates07.htm* [Accessed June 21, 2009].

3. American Diabetes Association. Economic costs of diabetes in the U.S. in 2002. Diabetes Care 2003;26: 917–32.

4. Stapley L. The history of diabetes. Trends Endocrin Metab 2001;12:277.

5. American Diabetes Association. Standards of medical care in diabetes—2009. Diabetes Care 2009;32(1): S13–61.

6. Pozzilli P, DiMario U. Autoimmune diabetes not requiring insulin at diagnosis (Latent autoimmune diabetes of the adult). Diabetes Care 2001;24:1460–7.

7. Cowie CC, Rust KF, Byrd-Holt DD, Eberhardt MS, Flegal KM, Engelgau MM, et al. Prevalence of diabetes

and impaired fasting glucose in adults in the US population: National Health and Nutrition Examination Survey 1999–2002. Diabetes Care 2006;29:1263–8.

8. Centers for Disease Control and Prevention. National diabetes fact sheet: general information and national estimates on diabetes in the United States, 2007. Atlanta, GA: US Department of Health and Human Services, Centers for Disease Control and Prevention, 2008.

9. Feig DS, Zinman B, Wang X, Hux JE. Risk of development of diabetes mellitus after diagnosis of gestational diabetes. CMAJ 2008;179:229–32.

10. The Diabetes Control and Complications Trial Research Group. The effect of intensive treatment of diabetes on the development and progression of long-term complications in insulin-dependent diabetes mellitus. N Engl J Med 1993;329:986.

11. Harris MI. Summary. In National Diabetes Data Group. Diabetes in America. National Institutes of Health National Institute of Diabetes and Digestive and Kidney Diseases NIH Publication No. 95-1468. 1995;1–13.

12. Muniyappa R, Iantorno M, Quon MJ. An integrated view of insulin resistance and endothelial dysfunction. Endocrinol Metabol Clin N Am 2008;37:685–711.

13. Unger J. Management of type I diabetes. Primary Care Clin Office Pract 2007;34:791–808.

14. Owens DR, Bolli GB. Beyond the era of NPH insulin—long-acting insulin analogs: chemistry, comparative pharmacology, and clinical application. Diabetes Technol Ther 2008:10(9):333–50.

15. DeFronzo RA. Pathogenesis of type 2 diabetes mellitus. Med Clin North Am 2004;88(4):787–835, ix.

16. The Action to Control Cardiovascular Risk in Diabetes Study Group (ACCORD). Effects of intensive glucose lowering in type 2 diabetes. N Engl J Med 2008;358:2545–59.

17. Grundy SM, Brewer B, Cleeman JL, Lenfant CL. Definition of metabolic syndrome: report of the national heart, lung, and blood institute: American Heart Association conference on scientific issues related to definition. Circulation 2004;109;433–38.

18. Ramlo-Halsted BA, Edelman SV. The natural history of type 2 diabetes: practical points to consider in developing prevention and treatment strategies. Primary Care Clin Office Pract 1999;26:771–89.

19. AACE Diabetes Mellitus Clinical Practice Guidelines Task Force. American Association of Clinical Endocrinologists medical guidelines for clinical practice for the management of diabetes mellitus. Endocrine Practice 2007;13(suppl 1):S3–67.

20. Retnakaran R, Zinman B. Type 1 diabetes, hyperglycemia and the heart. Lancet 2008;371:1790–9.

21. Vinik A, Vinik E. Prevention of complications of diabetes. Am J Managed Care 2003;9:S63–80.

22. Reasner CA. Reducing cardiovascular complications of type 2 diabetes by targeting multiple risk factors. J Cardiovasc Pharmacol 2008;52:136–40.

23. Tka'c I. Treatment of dyslipidemia in patients with type 2 diabetes: overview and meta-analysis of randomized trials. Diabetes Res Clin Pract 2007;78S:S23–8.

24. The ADVANCE Collaborative Group. Intensive blood glucose control and vascular outcomes in patients with type 2 diabetes. N Engl J Med 2008;358:2540–72.

25. Dugoua JJ, Seely D, Perri D, Cooley K, Forelli T, Mills E, et al. From type 2 diabetes to antioxidant activity: a systematic review of the safety and efficacy of common and cassia cinnamon bark. Can J Physiol Pharmacol 2007;85(9):837–47.

26. Garber AJ, Handelsman Y, Einhorn D, Bergman DA, Bloomgarden ZT, Fonseca V, et al. Diagnosis and management of prediabetes in the continuum of hyperglycemia—when do the risks of diabetes begin? A consensus statement from the American College of Endocrinology and the American Association of Clinical Endocrinologists. Endocr Pract 2006;14:934–46.

27. Briscoe VJ, Davis SN. Hypoglycemia in type 1 and type 2 diabetes. Physiology, pathophysiology, and management. Clin Diabetes 2006;24(1):115–21.

28. Davis S. Insulin, oral hypoglycemic agents, and the pharmacology of the endocrine pancreas. In Brunton LL, Lazo JS, Parker KL, eds. Goodman and Gilman, The pharmacological basis of therapeutics, 11th ed. New York: McGraw Hill, 2006:1629–1714.

29. Felig P. Landmark perspective: protamine insulin. Hagedorn's pioneering contribution to drug delivery in the management of diabetes. J Am Med Assoc 1984;51:393–6.

30. Home P, Bartley P, Russell-Jones D, Hanaire-Broutin H, Heeg JE, Abrams P, et al. Insulin detemir offers improved glycemic control compared with NPH insulin in people with type 1 diabetes: a randomized clinical trial. Diabetes Care 2004;27:1081–7.

31. Jellinger PS, Davidson JA, Blonde L, Einhorn D, Grunberger G, Handelsman Y. Road maps to achieve glycemic control in type 2 diabetes mellitus: ACE/AACE Diabetes Road Map Task Force. Endocr Pract 2007;13(3):260–8.

32. Monnier I, Collette C, Dunseath GJ, Owens DR. The loss of postprandial glycemic control precedes stepwise deterioration of fasting with worsening diabetes. Diabetes Care 2007;30:263–9.

33. Cohen FJ, Neslusan CA, Conklin JE, Song X. Recent antihyperglycemic prescribing trends for US privately insured patients with type 2 diabetes. Diabetes Care 2003;26(6):1847–51.

34. DeFronzo RA. Pharmacologic therapy for type 2 diabetes mellitus. Ann Intern Med 1999;131(4):281–303.

35. Selvin E, Bolen S, Yeh HC, Wiley C, Wilson LM, Marinopoulos SS, et al. Cardiovascular outcomes in trials of oral diabetes medications: a systematic review. Arch Intern Med 2008;168(19):2070–80.

36. Evans JM, Ogston SA, Emslie-Smith A, Morris AD. Risk of mortality and adverse cardiovascular outcomes in type 2 diabetes: a comparison of patients treated with sulfonylureas and metformin. Diabetologia 2006;49(5):930–6.

37. Simpson SH, Majumdar SR, Tsuyuki RT, Eurich DT, Johnson JA. Dose-response relation between sulfonylurea drugs and mortality in type-2 diabetes mellitus: a population based cohort study. CMAH 2006; 174:169.

38. Bolen S, Feldman L, Vassy J, Wilson L, Hsin-Chieh Y, Marinopoulos S, et al. Systematic review: comparative effectiveness and safety of oral medications for type 2 diabetes mellitus. Ann Intern Med 2007;147: 386–99.

39. Black C, Donnelly P, McIntyre L, Royle PL, Shepherd JP, Thomas S. Meglitinide analogues for type 2 diabetes mellitus. Cochrane Database Syst Rev 2007;Apr 18(2):CD004654.

40. DeFronzo RA, Goodman AM. Efficacy of metformin in patients with non-insulin dependent diabetes mellitus. The Multicenter Metformin Study Group. N. Engl J Med 1995;333:541–9.

41. Hermann LS, Schersten B, Bitzen PO, Kjellstom T, Lindgarde F, Melander A. Therapeutic comparison of metformin and sulfonylurea, alone and in various combinations. A double-blind controlled study. Diabetes Care 1994;17:1100–9.

42. Saenz A, Fernandez-Esteban I, Mataiz A, Ausejo M, Roque M, Moher D. Metformin monotherapy for type 2 diabetes mellitus. Cochrane Database Syst Rev 2005;3:CD002966.

43. Holman RR, Paul SK, Bethel MA, Mathewes DR, Neil HAW. 10-year follow-up of intensive glucose control in type 2 diabetes. N Engl J Med 2008;359:1577–89.

44. Modi P. Beyond insulin: review of new drugs for the treatment of diabetes mellitus. Cur Drug Discovery Technol 2007;4:39–47.

45. Harrington RA, Matjam MS, Beattie P. Oral agents for the treatment of type 2 diabetes: pharmacology, toxicity and treatment. Ann Emerg Med 2001;38:68–78.

46. Salpeter S, Greyber E, Pasternak G, Salpeter E. Risk of fatal and nonfatal lactic acidosis with metformin use in type 2 diabetes mellitus. Cochrane Database Syst Rev 2005;4:CD002967.

47. Fonseca V, Rosenstock J, Patwardhan R, Salzman A. Effect of metformin and rosiglitazone combination therapy in patients with type 2 diabetes mellitus: a randomized controlled trial. JAMA 2000;283: 1695–702.

48. Nathan DM. Thiazolidinediones for initial treatment of type 2 diabetes? N Engl J Med 2006;355:2477–80.

49. St. John Sutton M, Rendell M, Dandona P, Dole JF, Murphy K, Atwardhan R, et al. A comparison of the effects of rosiglitazone and glyburide on cardiovascular function and glycemic control in patients with type 2 diabetes. Diabetes Care 2002;25:2058–64.

50. Nissen SE, Wolski K. Effect of rosiglitazone on the risk of myocardial infarction and death from cardiovascular causes. N Engl J Med 2007;356:2457–71.

51. Scheen AJ. Pharmacokinetic interactions with thiazolidinediones. Clin Pharmacokinet 2007;46(1):1–12.

52. Van de Laar FA, Lucassen PL, Akkermans RP, Van de Lisdonk EH, De Grauw WJ. Alpha-glucosidase inhibitors for people with impaired glucose tolerance or impaired fasting blood glucose. Cochrane Database Syst Rev 2006;4:CD005061.

53. Knop FK, Vilsbøll T, Holst JJ. Incretin-based therapy of type 2 diabetes mellitus. Curr Protein Pept Sci 2009;10(1):46–55.

54. Conlon JM, Patterson S, Flatt PR. Major contributions of comparative endocrinology to the development and exploitation of the incretin concept. J Exp Zoolog A Comp Exp Biol 2006;305(9):781–6.

55. Patlak M. New weapons to combat an ancient disease: treating diabetes. FASEB J 2002;16(14):1853.

56. Triplitt C, Chiquette E. Exenatide: from the Gila monster to the pharmacy. J Am Pharm Assoc (2003) 2006;46(1):44–52.

57. Yoo BK, Triller DM, Yoo DJ. Exenatide: a new option for the treatment of type 2 diabetes. Ann Pharmacother 2006;40(10):1777–84.

58. Cvetković RS, Plosker GL. Exenatide: a review of its use in patients with type 2 diabetes mellitus (as an

adjunct to metformin and/or a sulfonylurea). Drugs 2007;67(6):935–54.

59. de Galan BE, Schouwenberg BJ, Tack CJ, Smits P. Pathophysiology and management of recurrent hypoglycaemia and hypoglycaemia unawareness in diabetes. Neth J Med 2006;64(8):269–79.

60. Coustan DR. Gestational diabetes. In National Institutes of Diabetes and Digestive and Kidney Diseases. Diabetes in America, 2nd ed. NIH Publication No. 95-1468. Bethesda, MD: NIH, 1995:703–17.

61. American College of Obstetricians and Gynecologists. ACOG practice bulletin. Gestational Diabetes 2001;30:1–21.

62. Kim C, Newton KM, Knopp RH. Gestational diabetes and the incidence of type 2 diabetes: a systematic review. Diabetes Care 2002;25(10):1862–8.

63. Nicholson W, Bolen S, Witkop CT, Neale D, Wilson L, Bass E. Benefits and risks of oral diabetes agents compared with insulin in women with gestational diabetes: a systematic review. Obstet Gynecol 2009; 113(1):193–205.

64. Yeh GY, Eisenberg DM, Kaptchuk TJ, Phillips RS. Systematic review of herbs and dietary supplements for glycemic control in diabetes. Diabetes Care 2003; 26(4):1277–94.

65. Ayurvedic interventions for diabetes mellitus: a systematic review. Summary, evidence report/technology assessment: number 41. AHRQ Publication No. 01-E039, June 2001. Rockville, MD: Agency for Healthcare Research and Quality. Available from: *www.ahrq .gov/clinic/epcsums/ayurvsum.htm* [Accessed June 21, 2009].

66. Liu JP, Zhang M, Wang W, Grimsgaard S. Chinese herbal medicines for type 2 diabetes mellitus. Cochrane Database Syst Rev 2002;3:CD003642.

67. Giel P, Shane-McWhorter L. Dietary supplements in the management of diabetes: potential risks and benefits. J Am Diet Assoc 2008;108:S59–65.

Shaped like a butterfly she sits within the neck
Wanting only to share her beauty throughout the body and
awakening all cells
Yet faithful to her messenger she will evolve with the
information sent
She can race forth spinning your entire being into a frenzy
Awakening you in the midst of the night saturated with
sweat and palpitating heart
Or she can lull you to sleep and make you feel so
melancholy or downright
Depressed and angry for no particular reason

ANONYMOUS

19
Thyroid Disorders

Michael W. Neville

⬦ Chapter Glossary

Diffuse goiter Type of goiter with generalized enlargement and lack of discrete nodules.

Free thyroxine index (FTI) A calculation of the amount of free T_4 available that takes into account more or less thyroid-binding hormone. The FTI is calculated by multiplying the total T_4 and the T_3 resin uptake (which indirectly measures the amount of free sites on thyroid-binding globulin) and then dividing by 100.

Goiter Enlargement of the thyroid gland; may be diffuse or nodular.

Goitrogen Any substance that interferes with thyroid function and causes goiter. The effect may be hypo- or hyperthyroidism.

Graves' disease Hyperthyroidism of unknown etiology associated with autoimmune antibodies that are developed against the TSH receptor.

Hashimoto's disease Thyroiditis secondary to chronic autoimmune disease.

Hyperthyroidism Condition secondary to excessive concentrations of T_3 and T_4. Symptoms of this disease may include goiters, palpitations, weight loss, menstrual irregularities, and exophthalmus.

Hypothyroidism Condition secondary to a deficiency of T_3 and T_4. Symptoms of this disease may include goiters, weight gain, and menstrual irregularities.

Nodular goiter Type of goiter with enlargement localized to specific areas or nodules.

Painless postpartum thyroiditis An autoimmune painless inflammation of the thyroid gland that occurs the first few weeks after giving birth. The initial phase is hyperthyroidism followed by hypothyroidism. This generally resolves spontaneously 12–18 months after the birth.

Painless sporadic thyroiditis Cause of hypothyroidism that is secondary to lymphocytic infiltration of the thyroid gland. Symptoms are mild, and approximately 50% of individuals with painless sporadic thyroiditis will have a small but detectable goiter.

Painless subacute thyroiditis Autoimmune etiology of goiter. Unlike other forms of thyroiditis, the result is usually permanent hypothyroidism.

Primary hyperparathyroidism Excessive parathyroid hormone (PTH) causing hypercalcemia, usually due to an adenoma of the parathyroid glands.

Secondary hyperparathyroidism Excessive parathyroid hormone (PTH) causing hypercalcemia, usually secondary to chronic renal failure.

Tertiary hyperparathyroidism Excessive parathyroid hormone (PTH) after prolonged period of secondary hyperparathyroidism.

Thyroglobulin Protein in which T_3 and T_4 are stored within the thyroid gland.

Thyroid-stimulating hormone (TSH) Hormone produced and released from anterior pituitary. This agent initiates production and release of T_3 and T_4. Also known as TSH.

Thyroid storm A life-threatening episode of hyperthyroidism, often called thyrotoxicosis. Symptoms of this disease may include fever, tachycardia, GI symptoms, and tremor.

Thyroiditis An inflammation of the thyroid gland, often of autoimmune origin (Hashimoto's disease) and associated with goiters.

Thyrotoxicosis Hypermetabolic clinical syndrome that results from excess thyroid hormone. Symptoms include rapid pulse; tremor; weight loss; palpitations; eyelid lag; and warm, moist skin. Hyperthyroidism is one form of thyrotoxicosis, but thyrotoxicosis can also be the result of inflammation, neoplasm, or toxic nodule.

Thyrotropin-releasing hormone (TRH) Hormone from the hypothalamus that stimulates production of thyroid-stimulating hormone (TSH). Also known as TRH.

Thyroxine (T_4) Prohormone composed of four atoms and produced exclusively in the thyroid.

Thyroxine-binding globulin (TBG) Globulin that binds to T_3 and T_4 in order to enable transfer through circulation. Also known as TBG.

Triiodothyronine (T_3) An active thyroid hormone composed of three iodine atoms that is produced in the thyroid and extrathyroidal tissue.

Wolff-Chaikoff effect A phenomenon that causes hypothyroidism when large amounts of iodine suddenly become present in plasma. This effect promotes autoregulation by inhibiting formation of the thyroid hormones inside of the thyroid follicle in response to the sudden increase in iodine. The effect lasts approximately 10–12 days. When iodine is administered to a person with hyperthyroidism, a subsequent therapeutic hypothyroid effect is explained by the Wolff-Chaikoff effect.

Introduction

Thyroid dysfunction is one of the most common endocrine disorders seen in primary care settings.[1] The recognition and treatment of thyroid disease is critical because thyroid hormones affect a myriad of body processes, including cardiovascular function, growth, and the intermediary metabolism of carbohydrates, fats, and proteins.

Physiology of Thyroid Function

The thyroid gland weighs approximately 10–20 grams in normal adults, making it one of the largest endocrine glands in the human body. The gland is located in the neck inferior to the thyroid cartilage and at approximately the same level as the cricoid cartilage (Figure 19-1).

The thyroid contains the only cells in the body that can absorb iodine. Iodine is an essential component of the thyroid hormones, and the amount of iodine available for thyroid hormone synthesis is dependent upon diet. This mineral is not stored in the body. The recommended daily allowances of iodine are 150 mcg for adolescents and adults, 220 mcg for pregnant women, and 290 mcg for lactating women.[2]

When an adequate amount of iodine is available, multiple enzyme systems and transport mechanisms work together to incorporate it into the active thyroid hormone **triiodothyronine** (T_3), which has three iodine atoms, and the prohormone **thyroxine** (T_4), which has four iodine atoms. The daily endogenous production of T_3 and T_4 is 15–30 mcg and 70–90 mcg, respectively. A majority of T_3 is produced via deionization of T_4 through the enzymatic action of 5'-deiodinase. This is why administration of usual doses of T_4 usually result in normal levels of T_3.[3] The thyroid gland produces T_3 and all the T_4 available to the body,

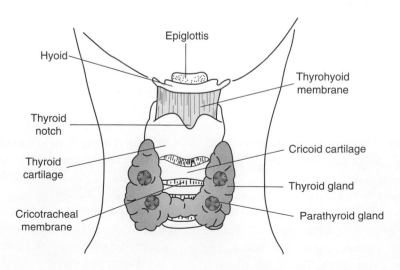

Figure 19-1 The thyroid and parathyroid glands.

whereas T_3 is also manufactured in extrathyroid tissue. Both T_3 and T_4 are stored in the thyroid gland within a protein, **thyroglobulin**, so they are readily available to meet body demands[2] (Figure 19-2).

When released into the general circulation, T_3 and T_4 are transported bound either to **thyroxine-binding globulin** (TBG), albumin, or transthyretin.[4] The plasma levels of thyroid hormone can be measured and are reported as either total T_3 or total T_4, which refers to the amount of thyroid hormone bound to a plasma protein, or it can be measured as free T_3 and free T_4, which measures the amount of hormone that is not bound to a plasma protein. The free T_3 and free T_4 are available to diffuse into tissue and initiate a metabolic response. The amount of free T_4 can also be reported as the **free thyroxine index**, which is a calculation that accounts for changes in the amount of thyroid-binding hormone present. Individuals with hypoalbuminemia can have significantly lower plasma concentrations of total T_3, total T_4, free T_3, and free T_4 and free thyroxine index unless recalculation that takes the amount of albumin into account is performed.[5]

Biosynthesis of thyroid hormones is tightly regulated in a person with a normally functioning thyroid gland (Figure 19-3). The hypothalamus, pituitary, and thyroid glands interact with one another through positive and negative feedback mechanisms to maintain plasma levels of the thyroid hormones. As the plasma level of thyroid hormones drops, the hypothalamus releases **thyrotropin-releasing hormone** (TRH). TRH concentrations increase within the hypothalamic-pituitary portal circulation and eventually stimulate the release of **thyroid-stimulating hormone** (TSH) from the anterior pituitary.[6] In response

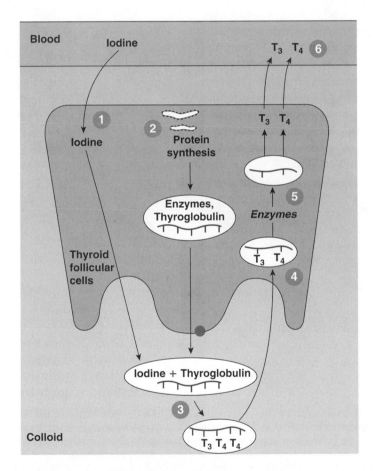

(1) Iodine is co-transported into the cell with Na^+ and transported into colloid.
(2) Follicular cell synthesizes enzymes and thyroglobulin.
(3) Enzymes add iodine to thyroglobulin to make T_3 and T_4.
(4) Thyroglobulin is taken back into the cell.
(5) Intracellular enzymes separate T_3 and T_4 from the protein.
(6) Free T_3 and T_4 enter the circulation.

Figure 19-2 Thyroid hormone synthesis and physiology.

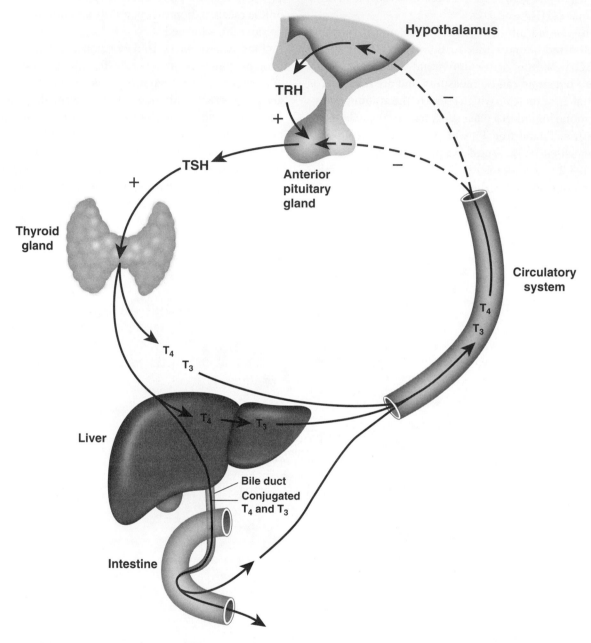

Thyrotropin-releasing hormone (TRH) increases the secretion of thyrotropin (TSH), which stimulates the synthesis and secretion of triiodothyronine (T_3) and thyroxine (T_4) by the thyroid gland. T_3 and T_4 inhibit the secretion of TSH, both directly and indirectly, by suppressing the release of TRH. T_4 is converted to T_3 in the liver and many other tissues by the action of T_4 monodeiodinases. Some T_4 and T_3 is conjugated with glucuronide and sulfate in the liver, excreted in the bile, and partially hydrolyzed in the intestine. Some T_4 and T_3 formed in the intestine may be reabsorbed. Drug interactions may occur at any of these sites.

$+$ = stimulatory pathway; $-$ = inhibitory pathway.

Figure 19-3 Regulation of thyroid hormone production and pathways of thyroid hormone metabolism.

to TSH, the thyroid gland initiates production and release of T_3 and T_4. Increasing plasma concentrations of T_3 and T_4 eventually suppress the production of TRH and TSH through a classic negative feedback mechanism.

Two important aspects of the finely tuned autoregulation of thyroid hormone production may affect pharmacologic management of persons with thyroid disorders. First is the **Wolff-Chaikoff effect**, which protects the system from responding to large variations in dietary iodine intake. Sudden large concentrations of iodine in plasma have an inhibitory effect on thyroid uptake of iodine, which decreases hormone biosynthesis, resulting in a hypothyroid effect. The sections on treatment of hypothyroidism and hyperthyroidism found later in this chapter discuss how the Wolff-Chaikoff effect is accounted for in clinical management. Secondly, the thyroid gland has a reservoir of hormone that continues to be released if there is a sudden deficit of iodine in the diet. This reservoir must also be accounted for when individuals are treated with drugs that suppress thyroid hormone production.

Alterations in thyroid function can cause changes in the normal female menstrual cycle. Increased production of TRH, often seen in women who have hypothyroidism, results in increased prolactin stimulation, and interferes with gonadotropin-releasing hormone (GnRH) production, which thereby reduces fertility.[7] Hypothyroidism is more associated with infertility than hyperthyroidism is, as thyroid hormones are critical for generation of progesterone and estrogen. Cramer et al.[7] measured serum TSH among 509 women who were receiving infertility treatment and noted that higher serum TSH concentrations were associated with decreased rates of successful in vitro fertilization of oocytes.[7]

Thyroid Disease

Thyroid dysfunction has been recognized for centuries. Chinese physicians treated goiter with the thyroid gland of sheep and pigs served either raw or powdered and diluted in wine. Several surgical and pharmacologic cures for goiter were first referred to in a book written by Rogerius Salernitanus in approximately 1180 AD. Salernitanus was a surgeon associated with the medieval Medical School of Salerno. The recommended treatment at that time was powder obtained from burnt dried marine sponges or drinking a tincture made of walnut leaves and roots, wine, and pepper. Endemic goiter was common in much of Europe; there are many paintings and wood cuts from the Renaissance that show persons with a goiter. Perhaps one of the most famous

is the Creator within the painting *Separation of Light from Darkness* that Michelangelo painted on the ceiling of the Sistine Chapel in Rome. In this painting, the neck is extended and the multi-nodular goiter is quite prominent.

Specific disorders of thyroid regulation usually result in states of either **hypothyroidism**, also known as Gull's disease after his description in 1874, or **hyperthyroidism**, which was first described by Parry in 1786 but later recognized by Graves and Basedow in 1835 and 1840.[3] Diagnosed thyroid disorders occur more frequently among women than men. The incidence of hypothyroidism is approximately 4.1/1000 women versus 0.6/1000 for men.[8] The incidence of hyperthyroidism is 0.8/1000 in women and negligible in men. The reason for the gender disparity is not well understood, but may be likely associated with the higher endogenous levels of estrogen and progesterone. Increasing age is a risk factor for hypothyroidism, but not for hyperthyroidism.[8]

Although thyroid disease often is overt, it may be asymptomatic or subclinical. Hypothyroid states are more prevalent than hyperthyroid conditions. Signs and symptoms may alert a provider to the possibility of a thyroid disease, but laboratory assessment of thyroid function is relied upon for both diagnosis and monitoring. Table 19-1 lists normal ranges for thyroid function tests.

Table 19-1 Thyroid Function Test Reference Ranges

	Normal Range: Nonpregnant	Normal Range: Pregnant*
Total T_3	95–195 ng/dL	125–275 ng/dL (usually normal or high)
Free T_4	0.8–2.0 ng/dL	0.26–1.92 ng/dL first trimester 0.59–1.56 ng/dL second trimester 0.65–1.25 ng/dL third trimester 0.8–2.0 ng/dL (normal)
FTI	4.5–12	4.5–12 (normal)
TSH*	0.45–4.5 mIU/L[†]	0.24–2.99 mIU/L first trimester 0.46–2.95 mIU/L second trimester 0.43–2.78 mIU/L third trimester

FTI = free thyroxine index; TSH = thyroid stimulating hormone; T_3 = triiodothyronine; T_4 = thyroxine.
* Normal ranges of thyroid function tests in pregnancy vary by trimester. Free T_4 values are sensitive to the amount of thyroid-binding globulin and the type of test used. Therefore the TSH and FTI are used in determining the need for replacement therapy.
[†] Both the upper and lower ranges of normal for TSH are controversial. Approximately 95% of persons who are euthyroid will have a TSH ≤ 2.5 mUI/L, and therefore, some experts argue that 2.5 mIU/L should be the upper limit of normal. Conversely, some recommend that 0.3 mIU/L should be the lowest cutoff for low TSH values. In addition, TSH values change during the course of pregnancy. They are often slightly lower in the first trimester because human chorionic gonadotropin (hCG) suppresses TSH.

Goiter is the term used when the thyroid gland is enlarged. A **diffuse goiter** indicates that the gland is uniformly enlarged. A **nodular goiter** occurs when one or more nodules develop within the otherwise normal gland. A goiter indicates that a thyroid condition exists but does not determine which type of thyroid dysfunction is present. Goiters may be associated with hypothyroidism, euthyroid state, hyperthyroidism, **thyroiditis**, or an inflammation of the thyroid gland, and rarely with thyroid cancer. Risk factors for developing a goiter include iodine deficiency, smoking, and pregnancy in areas of iodine deficiency. Conversely, alcohol use and oral contraceptives are associated with a decreased risk for developing goiter.

Any substance that alters thyroid function and causes goiter is called a **goitrogen**. Interestingly, there are several foods that have been implicated in causing goiters in areas where goiter has become endemic. For example, thiocyanate, which is present in cassava, can cause hypothyroidism and resultant goiter. Other foods that are potential goitrogens include brussels sprouts, soy products, rutabaga, turnips, radishes, cauliflower, cabbage, kale, and millet. Some suggest that these foods are not goitrogens when cooked because cooking destroys the goitrogenic compound.

Hypothyroidism

Hypothyroidism is characterized by a deficiency of T_3 and T_4 hormones. The disease may have primary or secondary causes. Although chronic autoimmune thyroiditis, which is also called **Hashimoto's disease**, is the most common cause of primary hypothyroidism in the United States,[9] other autoimmune causes include **painless postpartum thyroiditis**, **painless sporadic thyroiditis**, and **painless subacute thyroiditis**. In addition, surgical thyroid removal, radioiodine thyroid gland ablation, and thyroid hormone deficiency from iodine deficiency or drug-induced interference with thyroid function can cause primary hypothyroidism. Secondary hypothyroidism occurs as a result of pituitary disease (deficiency of TRH) or hypothalamic disease (deficiency of TSH) and is not a focus of this chapter.

The hallmark clinical features of hypothyroidism include such symptoms as fatigue, weight gain, hoarseness, hyperlipidemia, constipation, and bradycardia. Hypothyroidism is commonly a comorbid condition in individuals who have other disorders. Most notably, (1) approximately 10% of individuals with type 1 diabetes are at risk for developing chronic thyroiditis, and up to 25% of women with diabetes will develop postpartum thyroiditis (monitoring

for goiter development and TSH screening is indicated for these women); (2) women with irregular menstrual cycles and those with infertility may have underlying thyroid dysfunction, and appropriate treatment may normalize cycles and ultimately increase fertility; and (3) it is recommended that persons diagnosed with depression should be screened for hypothyroid states and monitoring for elevated TSH levels as well as for the development of positive thyroid autoantibodies.[9]

Though many theories exist regarding best methods for screening for hypothyroidism, the 2002 guidelines issued by the American Association of Clinical Endocrinologists (AACE) recommend screening by measuring TSH as a cost-efficient and effective method of detecting primary disease.[9]

Pharmacologic Treatment of Hypothyroidism

The goal of medication therapy used to treat hypothyroidism is to ameliorate symptoms and to restore a euthyroid state. This state is evidenced by normal TSH levels and a decrease in the size of goiter, if present.[1]

Thyroid Hormones

Levothyroxine (T_4) was first isolated in crystalline form in 1915; its structural formula was discovered in 1926; and it was first synthesized in 1927.[3] Triiodothyronine (T_3) was discovered around 1950.[3] T_4 and T_3 were originally manufactured from animal extracts or desiccated thyroid. Thyroid hormones obtained through animal sources varied widely with respect to their bioequivalence and included at least a small risk of allergy.[1] Consequently, synthetic preparations are used exclusively today.

Levothyroxine (T_4)

Levothyroxine (Synthroid, Levothroid, Levoxyl, Unithroid) is the preparation most commonly used to supplement or replace thyroid hormone for individuals with hypothyroidism. This agent also is used to suppress TSH in persons with thyroid cancer or in those with nodular thyroid disease.[10] The advantage of levothyroxine is that it replaces the prohormone T_4, which allows the individual to convert to the active hormone T_3 via physiologic mechanisms and thus, plasma levels of T_3 remain stable if adequate doses of levothyroxine are given.

Dosing Considerations

Levothyroxine is recognized by the Food and Drug Administration (FDA) to be a medication that has a narrow therapeutic range. Levothyroxine is available in 12 different tablet strengths, which range from 25 mcg to 300 mcg per tablet.[11] The different dose formulations are color coded. The daily dose for most persons ranges from 50 to 200 mcg per day (Table 19-2). There are several brand name and generic formulations of levothyroxine, with different bioequivalence. Persons who have a good response using one formulation—brand name or generic—should continue to use that formulation.

Levothyroxine may also be administered intravenously for persons unable to obtain it orally. Doses (available in 200 mcg and 500 mcg per vial) are reconstituted with 0.9% sodium chloride (NaCl) and administered via intravenous push at a rate of 100 mcg over 1 minute.[11]

Individuals should be instructed to avoid taking levothyroxine with other medications or with food.[11,12] The bioavailability of this drug is normally approximately 80% of the orally administered dose and it can be diminished substantially by concomitant administration of foods and/or other medications.[12] Absorption of levothyroxine occurs primarily within the jejunum and ileum. Absorption is diminished among individuals 70 years of age and older, among persons on high-fiber diets, when taken with food, and among those with lactose intolerance. Vitamins that contain iron and calcium supplements also decrease absorption of levothyroxine.

The plasma half-life of levothyroxine is approximately 7 days. Therefore, approximately 6 weeks is required to obtain a therapeutic response once therapy is initiated. Persons started on levothyroxine should have TSH and free T_4 checked 3–6 weeks after initiation of the drug, and doses should not be adjusted until steady-state values are obtained. Levothyroxine is metabolized in the liver, kidney, and other peripheral tissues and is primarily eliminated via the kidney with a small portion passing through the intestine unchanged to be eliminated via feces.

Adverse Effects

Levothyroxine is a well-established agent, in use for almost a half century (Box 19-1); adverse effects are uncommon. The most common problem is excessive dosing, which causes hyperthyroidism. The primary symptom of thyroid excess is atrial fibrillation, which is seen more often in the elderly. Subclinical hyperthyroidism can also accelerate bone loss in persons on chronic replacement over time. In instances of excessive dosing, individuals may note heart palpitations, heat intolerance, diarrhea, weight loss, nervousness, tremors, and angina.[12] Administration of levothyroxine to persons with a nontoxic or nodular goiter can cause **thyrotoxicosis**. Interestingly, tartrazine, a synthetic lemon yellow azo dye used as a food coloring that is derived from coal tar, can be found in some thyroid replacement formulations and may increase the risk of allergic reactions.[13]

When levothyroxine replacement regimens appear ineffective or individuals have conditions that seem resistant to therapy, clinicians should suspect nonadherence to the medication regimen, also known as pseudomalabsorption, as a most likely etiology.[12,14,15] In other cases, true malabsorption phenomena may be in operation and require further investigation and treatment.

Instances of true malabsorption occur in persons with gastrointestinal disease (e.g., celiac disease, lactose intolerance, vitamin B_{12} deficiency, *Giardia* infection), liver disease (e.g., cirrhosis, obstructive liver disease), pancreatic

Table 19-2 Thyroid Replacement Formulations

Drug	Brand Names	Initial Dose*	Usual Dose
Levothyroxine T_4	Levo-T Levothroid Levoxyl Synthroid	50 mcg daily	100–125 mcg per day
Triiodothyronine T_3	Cytomel Triostat	25 mcg daily	25–75 mg per day
Liotrix T_4 and T_3	Thyrolar	30 mg daily	50–100 mg per day

* Lower doses should be considered for the elderly and in those with long-standing myxedema or cardiovascular impairment.
Source: Adapted from Slagle MA 2002.[13]

Box 19-1 Gone But Not Forgotten: Thyroid Medications for Weight Loss

In years past, some providers would prescribe levothyroxine sodium for weight loss, under the assumption that the individual had hypothyroidism without confirmatory laboratory findings. However, among euthyroid individuals, there is no evidence that normal doses of levothyroxine leads to weight loss. Larger doses may be associated with weight reduction, but these doses also are associated with toxicity of the drug and should not be employed as weight loss agents.

insufficiency, gastrointestinal surgery (e.g., jejunostomy, short bowel syndrome, jejunoileal bypass), congestive heart failure, pregnancy, dietary interference (e.g., soybeans, prunes, herbs, walnuts), and ingestion of multiple medications.[12]

Drug–Drug Interactions

The drug–drug interactions associated with thyroid formulations are among the most important considerations in pharmacologic management of thyroid disorders. Table 19-3 lists the most common drug–drug interactions that are common considerations in clinical practice.

T_3 and T_4 Combinations

Liotrix (a 4:1 combination of T_4 and T_3) is not widely used in clinical practice today.[16] The AACE thyroid task force reports that there is insufficient evidence to know which

individual, if any, would have better outcomes from using combination products versus a formulation of T_4 alone.[9] In some instances, however, simply replacing T_4 to achieve normal TSH levels may be insufficient for persons treated with levothyroxine who continue to have low serum concentrations of T_3. Treatment with T_4 monotherapy can achieve a biochemical euthyroidism, culminating in some individuals continuing to be symptomatic.[16]

Triiodothyronine (T_3)

To treat persons with unremitting hypothyroid symptoms who are unresponsive to T_4 monotherapy, endocrinologists often consider the empirical addition of triiodothyronine (Cytomel, Triostat).[16] T_3 has limited use in clinical practice and is not recommended for the treatment of hypothyroidism in general.[16] The T_3 plasma half-life is 24 hours, much shorter than T_4, and causes T_3 values to vary widely.

Table 19-3 Selected Drug–Drug Interactions Associated with Levothyroxine*

Drug Generic (Brand)	Effect
Aluminum hydroxide (Amphojel)	Decreased absorption of levothyroxine.
Amiodarone (Cordarone)	Prevents conversion of T_4 to T_3.
Antidiabetic agents	Levothyroxine exacerbates diabetes, and therefore antidiabetic agents may require higher doses.
Calcium carbonate (Calci-Chew, Titralac, Tums)	Decreased absorption of levothyroxine.
Carbamazepine (Tegretol)	Carbamazepine displaces T_3 and T_4 from protein-binding sites and induces their metabolism.
Cholestyramine (Questran)	Decreased absorption of levothyroxine.
Ciprofloxacin (Cipro)	Decreased absorption of levothyroxine.
Didanosine (Videx)	Decreased absorption of levothyroxine.
Digoxin (Lanoxin)	Decreased effect of digoxin, probably secondary to increased metabolism.
Estrogens	Increased requirement for levothyroxine probably secondary to estrogen's effect in increasing thyroxine-binding globulin serum concentrations.
Ferrous sulfate (Feratab, Fer-Iron, Slow-FE)	Decreased absorption of levothyroxine.
Insulin	Hyperglycemia because levothyroxine increases severity of diabetes.
Omeprazole (Prilosec)	Decreased absorption of levothyroxine.
Phenobarbitol (Luminal)	Decreased effect of levothyroxine secondary to increased metabolism of T_3 and T_4 via stimulation of hepatic enzymes.
Phenytoin (Dilantin)	Decreased serum concentrations for levothyroxine.
Raloxifene (Evista)	Decreased absorption of levothyroxine.
Rifampin (Rifadin)	Decreased effect of levothyroxine secondary to increased metabolism of T_3 and T_4 via stimulation of hepatic enzymes.
Sertraline (Zoloft)	Decreased serum concentration of levothyroxine.
Sucralfate (Carafate)	Decreased absorption of levothyroxine.
Tetracycline (TheoDur)	Decreased theophylline effect.
Tricyclic antidepressents	Increased therapeutic and possible toxic effects of both agents including cardiac arrhythmias and CNS stimulation.
Warfarin (Coumadin)	Increased anticoagulant effect. Levothyroxine increases the catabolism of vitamin K-dependent clotting factors.

* This table is not a comprehensive list as new information is being identified on a regular basis.
Source: Adapted from England RA et al. 2006.[21]

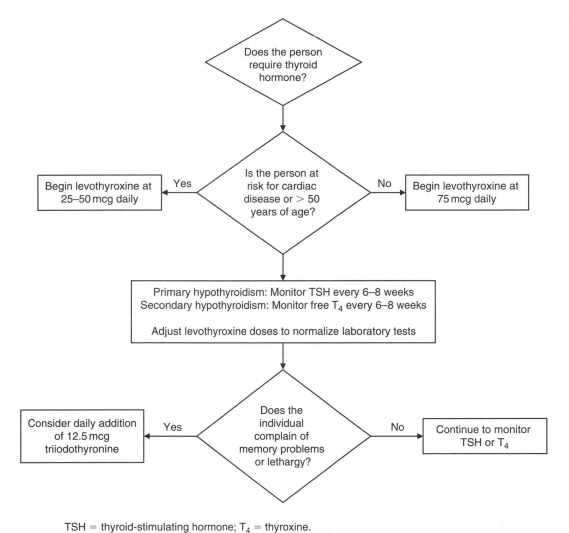

TSH = thyroid-stimulating hormone; T$_4$ = thyroxine.

Figure 19-4 Treatment of hypothyroidism. *Source:* Adapted from Klein I 2005.[1]

In addition, T$_3$ is approximately 10 times more potent than T$_4$, and because of this potency, T$_3$ can trigger hyperthyroid episodes.[16]

Figure 19-4 presents a clinical algorithm for clinicians caring for persons with hypothyroidism.

▌ Subclinical Hypothyroidism

Subclinical hypothyroidism, which may or may not cause symptoms, exists when laboratory evaluations reveal mildly elevated TSH and normal T$_3$ and T$_4$ values.[9] As many as 15% of individuals ≥ 65 years of age have a normal free T$_4$ and an elevated TSH without symptoms of hypothyroidism.[10] The causes of subclinical hypothyroidism are the same as the causes of hypothyroidism. The most common cause is autoimmune thyroiditis or Hashimoto's disease, prior radio-ablative therapy for hyperthyroidism, or suboptimal treatment of hypothyroidism.

Controversy exists regarding the best methods to treat subclinical disease. Singer et al. noted that levothyroxine supplementation is advisable, especially when thyroid autoantibodies are present, as overt disease is likely on the horizon.[10] The AACE advises clinicians to treat persons with TSH levels > 10 µIU/mL or those with TSH levels between 5 and 10 µIU/mL who also have positive thyroid antibodies, goiter, or both.[9]

Hyperthyroidism

Hyperthyroidism generally results from excess concentrations of T_3 and T_4. Etiologies vary with the most common being **Graves' disease**. Other causes include toxic adenoma, toxic multinodular goiter, excessive thyroid hormone ingestion, drug-induced (e.g., amiodarone) disease, and excessive pituitary secretion of TSH.[9]

Graves' disease is caused by autoimmune antibodies that for an unknown reason develop against the TSH receptor. When these antibodies bind to the TSH receptor, that receptor becomes chronically stimulated and excessive thyroid hormone is produced. The signs and symptoms of hyperthyroidism include but are not limited to palpitations, weight loss, menstrual irregularities, and ophthalmopathy.

Treatment of Graves' disease is two pronged. First, beta-blockers are commonly used to reduce symptoms of tachycardia, tremulousness, heat intolerance, and anxiety. Second, measures that decrease thyroid hormone synthesis, such as radioactive iodine ablation, pharmacologic doses of iodide, one of the thionamide drugs, or surgery may be employed.

Pharmacologic Treatment of Hyperthyroidism

The three primary treatments for hyperthyroidism are radioactive iodine, medication therapy with thionamides, and surgery.[11] The risk of relapse following a course of either of the two thionamides—methimazole (Tapazole) or propylthiouracil (PTU)—is approximately 37%, higher than the relapse rate following use of radioactive iodine (RAI) or surgery, making RAI the more common first-line approach. However, thionamides often are used as pretreatment prior to RAI for persons who are highly symptomatic or who may not tolerate RAI well. Table 19-4 provides a review of the results and adverse effects of the three types of treatments used for hyperthyroidism. Ablation therapy with radioactive iodine and surgical treatment result in permanent remission when successful. In most situations, an experienced clinician such as an endocrinologist or surgeon will manage the care of a woman with hyperthyroidism.

Beta-Adrenergic Antagonists for Symptomatic Relief

Beta-adrenergic antagonists or beta-blockers are not specific treatments for thyroid disorders, but rather symptomatic treatment. Beta-blockers relieve the symptoms such as palpitations and tachycardia, which are secondary to increased adrenergic tone. Atenolol (Tenormin) can be prescribed as a once-per-day dose of 25–50 mg for persons who do not have contraindications to the use of these medications. Further discussion of beta-blockers can be found in Chapter 15.

Radioactive Iodine (RAI, I_{131})

Radioactive iodine (RAI) has traditionally been offered as a treatment modality for persons diagnosed with symptoms of hyperthyroidism, Graves' disease, thyroid cancers, and those with toxic nodular goiters.[17] RAI has been considered a first-line therapy for hyperthyroid conditions since 1940, though there is a paucity of data regarding its use in children or young adults.[18] RAI destroys the thyroid gland tissue, thereby decreasing the synthesis of thyroid hormone.

Recommended RAI doses vary considerably in the literature. Fixed doses have been administered with wide variation in cure rates.[19] Cure rates appear to be related to both dose of RAI and weight of thyroid gland. Low-dose therapy is more commonly associated with treatment failure.[19]

Most individuals who receive RAI eventually will develop hypothyroidism (the goal of therapy) and will require lifelong thyroid hormone supplementation, although this is slightly more likely in men than in women. The incidence of hypothyroid states among those with Graves' disease after receiving RAI is 24%, 59%, and 82% at 1, 10, and 25 years, respectively.[17] RAI is contraindicated during pregnancy and lactation.

Dosing Considerations

RAI is administered as a one-time dose as a capsule or oral solution. It is rapidly absorbed from the GI tract and concentrates in the thyroid, whereby ablation occurs over 6–18 weeks. Occasionally an individual will require a second dose.

No consensus exists regarding the use of adjunctive oral thionamides (e.g., propylthiouracil [PTU] or methimazole [Tapazole]) with RAI or the method for calculating the RAI dose.[20] The failure of one dose of RAI to achieve therapeutic goals does not preclude the administration of subsequent doses.

Side Effects/Adverse Effects

This colorless, tasteless solution has few direct adverse effects.[21] The most common side effect of RAI is thyroid tenderness and dysphagia. Persons taking RAI should avoid being in close, prolonged contact with young children or

Table 19-4 Treatment Modalities for Hyperthyroidism

Therapy: Action and Result	Indications	Adverse Effects/Contraindications
Beta adrenergic antagonists		
Mitigates the cardiovascular and other peripheral tissue effects of thyroid hormone.	Adjunctive therapy for persons with Graves' disease or thyroid storm. May be only therapy for self-limiting thyroiditis.	Contraindicated in persons who have congestive heart failure, some forms of valvular heart disease, bradyarrhythmias, heart block, asthma, or chronic pulmonary obstructive disease.
Thionamides		
Inhibits thyroid hormone synthesis and may have immunosuppressive effects. Propylthiouracil also inhibits peripheral conversion of T_4 to T_3. Chance of permanent remission, avoids risk of permanent hypothyroidism, low cost.	First-line therapy for Graves' disease and may be used a short-term therapy prior to RAI or surgery.	**Minor:** Fever, pruritus or rash (4–6%), arthralgia (1–5%), gastrointestinal effects (1–5%), abnormal sense of taste or smell (rare).* **Major:** Polyarthritis (1–2%), thrombocytopenia, agranulocytosis (0.1%), immunoallergic hepatitis,† vasculitis (drug-induced lupus syndrome), hypoglycemia (rare).
Radioiodine (RAI)		
Radioactive iodine destroys the thyroxine-producing cells in the thyroid gland. Results in permanent resolution of hyperthyroidism and may cause permanent hypothyroidism.	Second-line therapy for Graves' disease.	**Minor:** Transient thyroid pain. Contraindicated in pregnancy, lactation.
Thyroidectomy		
Rapid permanent cure that always results in permanent hypothyroidism if thyroid completely removed.		**Major:** Recurrent laryngeal nerve injury, superior laryngeal nerve injury, postoperative hypoparathyroidism, temporary hypocalcemia.
Complications can reach 13%, but are related to surgeon's experience and surgical process.		**Major:** Vocal cord paralysis, permanent hypocalcemia, postoperative hemorrhage, wound infection.
Iodide-containing compounds		
Inhibits release of thyroid hormone from stores in thyroid gland.	Used prior to surgery and for treatment of thyroid storm.	**Minor:** Can cause skin rash, flare-up of acne, or dermatitis. **Major:** Multiple drug–drug interactions. Contraindicated in pregnancy and in persons with known sensitivity to iodides, iodine-induced goiter, or dermatitis herpetiformis. Use with caution in persons with Addison's disease, acute bronchitis, lactation.

* Occurs with methimazole (Tapazole) only.
† Occurs with propylthiouracil (PTU) only.
Source: Adapted from England RJA et al. 2006.[21]

pregnant women. A distance of one arm's length between the person being treated and others who spend more than 2 hours per every 24 hours in the presence of the person being treated is a good rule of thumb. Thus, sleeping together and other activities that require close contact for more than a brief time should be avoided. This precaution should be followed for approximately 11 days after treatment. In addition, the person being treated should be counseled to avoid sharing food or utensils. The best way to clear the RAI from the system is to drink large amounts of water and void frequently.

Adverse effects of RAI include hepatitis, arthritis, and agranulocytosis. It is estimated that fewer than 1% of women being treated for hyperthyroidism experience agranulocytosis, a condition that is more likely among women taking higher doses of antithyroid medications. No method of routine monitoring has been agreed upon, although some clinicians who monitored white blood cell counts every 2–4 weeks reported earlier detection of agranulocytosis. Regardless of the timing of diagnosis, most cases of agranulocytosis have been found to be reversible. Agranulocytosis also can be an adverse effect with use of the thionamides (see the following section on thionamides).

Pharmacologic Doses of Iodide

Persons with Graves' disease are more sensitive to the Wolff-Chaikoff effect than persons without thyroid dysfunction. Consequently, pharmacologic doses of iodide are used to rapidly induce a euthyroid state as short-term therapy for individuals with Graves' disease or thyroid storm. Five drops of saturated solution of potassium iodide (SSKI, 35 mg iodide/drop) or Lugol's solution (7 mg iodide/drop) is administered three times per day.

Thionamides: Methimazole (Tapazole) and Propylthiouracil (PTU)

Methimazole (Tapazole) and propylthiouracil (PTU) are the two commercially available oral preparations used in the United States for the treatment of hyperthyroid conditions. Thionamides actively concentrate in the thyroid gland where they inhibit thyroid hormone synthesis. These drugs also have important immunosuppressive functions. They suppress antithyrotropin receptor antibodies and may induce apoptosis of intrathyroid lymphocytes. Additionally, propylthiouracil (PTU) blocks the conversion of T_4 to T_3 in the thyroid gland and in peripheral tissue.

The goal of treatment when using thionamides is to obtain a euthyroid state within 3–6 weeks. Persons started on therapy should have thyroid function tested every 4–6 weeks until a stable euthyroid state is achieved. These agents may be administered to individuals as a primary treatment option for 6 months to 2 years in most situations and occasionally even longer.

Approximately 20–30% of individuals taking thionamides will achieve a permanent remission after therapy is discontinued. It may sound counterintuitive, but prescribers often opt to administer thyroid hormone with thionamide therapy to avoid frequent thionamide dosing adjustments.

Although these agents have been used more than half a century, no consensus exists about which is the preferred first-line agent for most individuals, nor is there consensus about optimum initial dosing[22] (Table 19-5).

Both drugs are readily absorbed from the gastrointestinal tract and peak in serum within 1–2 hours.

Methimazole (Tapazole) is essentially free in serum, whereas propylthiouracil (PTU) is 80–90% bound to protein in the serum. Methimazole acts more quickly than propylthiouracil (PTU) and has a more favorable side effect profile, but it cannot be used by pregnant women because it can have teratogenic effects. Daily doses of methimazole (Tapazole) and propylthiouracil (PTU) range from 10–40 mg and 100–600 mg, respectively.[11]

Side Effects/Adverse Effects

The most common side effects are urticaria, macular rashes, gastrointestinal upset, and arthralgias, which occur among approximately 5% of persons taking either of these two medications. Skin reactions usually resolve following treatment with antihistamines. Persons who develop arthralgias should discontinue the drug because it may signal the development of polyarthritis, which is a rare adverse effect associated with a lupus-like syndrome. Side effects are dose dependent in persons taking methimazole (Tapazole). The relationship to dose is less clear for propylthiouracil (PTU). In general, the side effect profile favors methimazole.

Adverse effects of thionamides are listed in Table 19-4. One of the most serious adverse effects reported, agranulocytosis, occurs among fewer than 0.3% of recipients.[11] Agranulocytosis is autoimmune mediated and most frequently occurs in the first 3 months of therapy, although it can occur at any time. A baseline white cell blood count should be obtained on all persons prior to initiating therapy with thionamides. Routine screening during therapy is not indicated because the onset of agranulocytosis is acute and abrupt. Individuals are counseled to stop the medication and contact their provider immediately if they develop a fever and sore throat, the two most common presenting symptoms associated with agranulocytosis.[23]

Hepatic abnormalities are medication specific. Propylthiouracil (PTU) can cause an immunoallergic hepatitis that can appear in the first several months of therapy. Because asymptomatic transient increases in liver function tests can occur in persons taking propylthiouracil (PTU), routine monitoring of liver function tests is not recommended. Methimazole (Tapazole) can rarely cause cholestasis. In either case, the medication should be stopped. Because the hepatic abnormalities have a different etiology depending on the thionamide drug involved, switching to the other drug can be recommended, albeit with caution.

The third rare, but adverse, effect of these drugs is vasculitis, which appears to be a drug-induced lupus syndrome

Table 19-5 Thionamide Dosing

Medication Generic (Brand)	Formulations	Initial Dose	Usual Dose
Propylthiouracil (PTU)	50-mg tablets	**Adult:** 300 mg per day in three equally divided doses	**Adult:** 100–150 mg per day in divided doses, up to 400–900 mg daily in divided doses.
Methimazole (Tapazole)	Trade: 5-mg, 10-mg tablets Generic: 15-mg, 20-mg tablets	**Adult:** 15 mg per day	**Adult:** 5–15 mg per day, up to 30–60 mg daily.

(Chapter 4). Symptoms include renal dysfunction, arthritis, skin ulcerations, vasculitis rash, sinusitis, and sometimes hemoptysis[24,25] (Table 19-4).

Drug–Drug Interactions

There are few known drug–drug interactions associated with thionamides. These agents can increase the anticoagulant effect of warfarin (Coumadin). Some drugs may need altered doses once an individual on a thionamide becomes euthyroid. Beta-adrenergic blockers, theophylline (Theo-Dur), and digoxin (Lanoxin) may need a dose reduction.

There are a few drug–food interactions. Thionamides should not be taken with calcium supplements or calcium-fortified orange juice because the calcium inhibits absorption of the drug.

Methimazole (Tapazole)

Methimazole (Tapazole) has an oral bioavailability of about 93%. Its half-life of 4–6 hours is longer than that of propylthiouracil (PTU), which is why it can be given once per day. It is excreted via gastrointestinal, renal, and hepatic routes.[11] Compounded formulations of methimazole (Tapazole) have been reported in the literature, but rarely used clinically except in relatively rare situations.[26] These formulations may be considered for individuals with emergent gastrointestinal surgery, bowel ileus or obstruction, or severe vomiting. In the rare situation in which this may be needed, 500 milligrams of methimazole powder USP is reconstituted with 0.9% NaCl to a final volume of 50 mL using an aseptic technique. The mixture is subsequently strained through a microfilter prior to administration. Doses are administered intravenously over 2 minutes and followed with a NaCl flush.

Propylthiouracil (PTU)

Propylthiouracil (PTU) has a short half-life of 1–2 hours and must be administered multiple times a day for optimal therapy. The oral bioavailability of this agent is approximately 73%. Propylthiouracil (PTU) is excreted via renal, hepatic, and gastrointestinal routes.[11]

Concurrent Thionamide and RAI

Individuals with severe hyperthyroidism, advanced age, or cardiac complications are frequently prescribed thionamides prior to RAI[27] (Table 19-4). It has been thought that thionamides would deplete thyroid hormones stores and reduce the chance of RAI-induced thyroid storm. Additionally, a surge in TSH antibodies may occur in the weeks following RAI, and this surge has been associated with thyroid storm development. However, thionamide pretreatment may offer radioprotection for the thyroid gland and decrease the desired ablative effects of RAI.[28] Bartalena et al. noted that this effect is likely more pronounced in those who receive propylthiouracil (PTU). They further stated that when pretreatment is desired, 2–3 months of methimazole pretreatment is preferred for individuals with Graves'-related orbitopathy, the elderly, and those with nonthyroidal illness. Alternatively, these authors encouraged the consideration of lithium therapy, initiated 2 days prior to RAI and continued for 2 weeks post-RAI to attenuate the rises in thyroid hormone levels that frequently follow RAI. More rapid reductions in goiter size have also been observed when lithium is used.[28]

Vijayakumar et al. retrospectively examined 122 subjects who were given RAI and a beta-blocker without thionamide pretreatment. No instances of thyroid storm resulted for any of the participants.[29]

Surgery

England et al. suggested that surgery should be offered as an option with RAI and thionamide therapy for the management of thyrotoxicosis.[21] These authors noted that this possible approach to treatment currently is reserved for pregnant women who cannot or do not regularly take oral thionamide therapy, children, adolescents, those with eye disease, or those with large goiters. However, they felt that persons should be provided with all options in order to support the individual in making a more informed decision.

▋ Thyrotoxicosis (Thyroid Storm)

Thyroid storm is an acute, life-threatening exacerbation of hyperthyroidism. Fever, tachycardia, nausea, vomiting, diarrhea, and tremor are the classic symptoms that can progress to dehydration and coma if not treated. Cardiomyopathy and heart failure secondary to excessive T_4 also occurs. There are four goals in treating thyroid storm, which is managed in an acute inpatient setting by experienced clinicians. These goals are: (1) decrease thyroid hormone production, (2) decrease the effect of circulating thyroid hormone, (3) provide supportive therapy, and (4) treat the underlying cause (Table 19-6). Large doses of propylthiouracil (PTU)

Table 19-6 Treatment of Thyrotoxicosis (Thyroid Storm)

Treatment Generic (Brand)	Indication
Propylthiouracil (PTU) Iodine preparations Lithium carbonate (Lithobid)	Inhibit thyroid hormone production and release from thyroid gland
Propylthiouracil (PTU) Propranolol (Inderal) Corticosteroids	Inhibit peripheral conversion of T_4 to T_3
Cholestyramine (Questran)	Increase thyroid hormone clearance
Beta-adrenergic antagonists Corticosteroids	Mitigate the hormone effect
Antipyretics Correction of electrolyte imbalances Cooling blankets and ice packs	Supportive therapy

and iodide are given together to invoke the Wolff-Chaikoff effect and inhibit release of thyroid hormone stores from the thyroid gland. In addition, cholestyramine may be administered as it decreases thyroid hormone resorption from the small intestine. Supportive therapies include corticosteroids, which inhibit peripheral conversion of T_4 to T_3, beta-adrenergic antagonists, antipyretics, and correction of electrolyte imbalances.

Special Populations

Pregnancy

Pregnancy induces multiple physiologic changes in the thyroid gland and thyroid hormone function. These changes include (1) modest thyroid gland hyperplasia, (2) modified peripheral metabolism of maternal thyroid hormones, (3) estrogen-mediated increase in production of thyroxine-binding globulin (TBG), (4) increased dietary iodine requirements coupled with increased iodine loss via the kidney and to the fetus, and (5) transient human chorionic gonadotropin (hCG)-induced stimulation of the maternal thyroid gland.[30] The result of these changes is a suppressed TSH in the first trimester and elevated T_4, yet the ratio of T_4 to T_3 remains stable and a euthyroid state persists. The fetal thyroid does not start synthesizing thyroid hormone until after 12 weeks of gestation, so all of the fetus's thyroid needs are supplied by the mother prior to this time (Box 19-2).

Some have argued that based on these physiologic changes, women should be screened during each trimester to detect subclinical hypothyroidism.[11] Proponents

of routine screening further contend that studies have identified a link between subclinical hypothyroidism and impaired brain development in children as well as preterm delivery. However, there is no evidence that treatment of subclinical hypothyroidism in pregnancy improves neonatal outcomes. Also, thionamides cross the placenta and can adversely affect the fetus. Therefore, routine screening of pregnant women to detect thyroid disease is not recommended by the United States Preventive Services Task Force or by the American College of Obstetrics and Gynecology at this time.[31] Additional information on this controversy can be found in Chapter 35.

In a clinical trial of 1560 pregnant women, investigators found that 90%, 3%, and 7% had normal, high, and low TSH levels, respectively.[32] The following conclusions were drawn: (1) most women with abnormal TSH levels early in pregnancy had no risk factors for thyroid disease; (2) there are no gestational age-specific reference ranges for TSH that can be used to guide treatment decisions; and (3) given the uncertainties of screening, recommending increased iodine intake is more logical than screening.

However, significant untreated overt maternal hypothyroidism is associated with mental retardation in the offspring, preeclampsia, placental abruption, postpartum hemorrhage, cardiac dysfunction, and stillbirth.[33] Conversely, pregnant women who have hyperthyroidism are at increased risk for spontaneous abortion, congestive heart failure, thyroid storm, preterm birth, preeclampsia, and fetal growth restriction. Overtreatment with propylthiouracil (PTU) can result in fetal hypothyroidism and fetal goiter.

Gestational transient thyrotoxicosis occurs in women with hyperemesis. This asymptomatic hyperthyroid state is the result of high levels of human chorionic gonadotropin (hCG) and overstimulation of the thyroid gland. Treatment is not warranted, and the condition resolves spontaneously as the hyperemesis is treated (Chapter 35).

Transient postpartum thyroiditis occurs in up to 10% of women in the first year postpartum, most frequently between 1 and 4 months after birth. Postpartum thyroiditis can have both a hyperthyroid phase and a hypothyroid phase. There is no standard clinical picture as some women will have both hyper- and hypothyroid phases; whereas others will only exhibit hyperthyroidism or hypothyroidism. The most common symptoms—anxiety, fatigue, insomnia, palpitations, weight loss, and irritability—are often attributed to the normal postpartum state or postpartum depression. Therefore, the thyroid dysfunction goes undetected. Treatment depends upon detection and the severity of symptoms.

Box 19-2 Hypothyroidism in Pregnancy

SL, a 28-year-old woman, comes to an ambulatory facility for a routine gynecology appointment. She reports fatigue, nausea, and constipation; she thinks she has the flu. The provider examines her and orders a complete blood count (CBC) with differential, serum chemistry, and a pregnancy test. SL's laboratory measures are normal except that she has a positive pregnancy test and an elevated TSH (7.2 mLU/L). How should the provider proceed?

The elevated TSH, accompanying clinical presentation, and diagnosis of pregnancy increase the probability of symptomatic hypothyroidism for SL. Human chorionic gonadotropin (hCG), the primary pregnancy hormone in the first trimester, has a thyroid stimulatory effect that results in a transient chemical hyperthyroidism. Therefore we expect pregnant women to have a TSH level that is on the low side, and SL's values are high.

Additional laboratory indices determined that she was pregnant. SL planned to continue the pregnancy but was worried about taking levothyroxine and wanted to know what effect this drug would have on her baby. Her provider explained that levothyroxine (Synthroid) is identical to the thyroid hormone her body makes and is not only safe but important to ensure normal development of her fetus. The fetus must get thyroid hormone from the mother because fetal production of thyroid hormone does not start until the second trimester, and even then, the majority of thyroid used by the fetus during the last months of pregnancy is supplied by the mother. SL was also told that congenital hypothyroidism is associated with abnormal brain development (Cretinism), low birth weight, and other neurologic deficits. Congenital hypothyroidism is a test included in the panel of standard newborn screening exams.

Pharmacologic treatment of postpartum hypothyroidism is not usually necessary because the symptoms are usually mild. If levothyroxine (Synthroid) is initiated, it should be continued for 6–12 months and then tapered, since 80% of women with postpartum hypothyroidism will regain normal thyroid function.

Thyroid storm can occur in the first months postpartum. Women with thyrotoxicosis may be treated with beta-adrenergic antagonists for symptomatic relief and should be monitored closely because the thyroid toxic phase is transient. Antithyroid medications are not used to treat postpartum thyroid storm as the disease is self-limiting.

Medications in Pregnancy and Lactation

Levothyroxine

Hormone replacement with levothyroxine is considered safe for pregnant women.[34] In order to maintain desirable TSH concentrations, doses of levothyroxine during pregnancy may need to be increased as much as 45%; doses should then be reduced to prepregnancy levels in the postpartum period.[33]

The American Academy of Pediatrics states that levothyroxine is safe to use during lactation.[35] Hale considers levothyroxine an L1 category drug (safest in lactation).[34] Mothers who are hypothyroid should receive levothyroxine in the postpartum period to achieve a euthyroid state that is equivalent to a normal breastfeeding female.

Thionamides

Many clinicians question when the use of thionamides in pregnancy should be considered and which agent should be selected. The agents are equally effective and therapy should be initiated when the woman becomes symptomatic and free T_4 levels exceed 2.5 ng/dL (the upper limit is 2.0 ng/dL).[32] Free T_4 concentrations should be maintained at the upper end of normal and the lowest thionamide doses should be used to avoid abnormal fetal brain development, hypothyroidism, and development of a fetal goiter.[11]

Although the FDA has categorized propylthiouracil (PTU) and methimazole as FDA Pregnancy Category D agents, thionamide preparations are used worldwide during pregnancy. The risk of the medications is more from the possibility of medication-induced fetal hypothyroidism than from a direct teratogenic effect.[11] However, they are not risk-free agents. Methimazole (Tapazole) has been associated with esophageal and choanal atresia in the fetus.[30] Clinicians in the United States usually choose propylthiouracil (PTU) over methimazole because propylthiouracil (PTU) is predominately protein bound and therefore less able to cross the placenta in significant amounts. Thus, its perceived teratogenic risk is lower. In one retrospective study of pregnant women, 99 received propylthiouracil

(PTU) and 36 received methimazole (Tapazole). The incidence of major congenital abnormalities associated with methimazole and propylthiouracil (PTU) was 3.0% and 2.7%, respectively.[36] Methimazole and propylthiouracil (PTU) also are considered compatible with lactation by the American Academy of Pediatrics.[35]

RAI

RAI is contraindicated for pregnant women. Women desiring pregnancy should use contraception for 6–12 months following RAI administration to avoid fetal thyroid ablation and the possibility of gonadal chromosomal damage secondary to the radiation effect on the ovaries.[21] RAI should also be avoided in breastfeeding women.[11]

Elderly

The elderly often are more sensitive to any treatment modality secondary to the increased incidence of comorbidities and use of other medications that can cause drug–drug interactions. When treating the elderly with hyperthyroidism, thionamide therapy should be initiated prior to RAI especially for those who are at risk for cardiovascular complications, and those with severe hyperthyroidism.[16] Clinicians who are treating the elderly with hypothyroidism should prescribe levothyroxine doses at less than 1 mcg/kg/day for those 50 years of age and older.

Thionamides are as effective in older individuals as they are in their younger counterparts. However, factors such as inability to take the medication properly, increased monitoring requirements, and a potential for adverse side effects may offset their benefit.[10]

▍ Drug–Drug Interactions Associated with Thyroid Medications

Five categories of pharmaceutical interactions are important to consider prior to prescribing thyroid replacement formulations or thionamides. They include (1) those that can induce hypothyroidism or hyperthyroidism, (2) those that interfere with thyroid laboratory results, (3) medications that when taken concomitantly with thyroid formulations can interfere with expected thyroid function effect, (4) significant drug–food interactions, and finally (5) medications that contain significant amounts of iodine.

Before instituting pharmacotherapy for the treatment of thyroid disease, the provider should perform a comprehensive medication history to rule out medication-related causes of thyroid disease.[11] A review of the most commonly prescribed drugs and their effect on either thyroid hormone laboratory test results or the development of thyroid dysfunctions can be seen in Tables 19-7, 19-8, and 19-9.

Iodine-Containing Medications

Iodine-containing medications (Table 19-10) can have a paradoxical effect depending upon the underlying thyroid disorder and dietary exposure to iodine. Individuals who are euthyroid and live in iodine-sufficient areas and those with nodular goiters with normally functioning thyroid tissue will become hyperthyroid when exposed to excess iodine. The iodine will be absorbed into the thyroid gland

Table 19-7 Medications That Cause Hypothyroidism—Generic (Brand)

Destructive Thyroiditis	Inhibition of Thyroid Hormone Synthesis and/or Release
Sunitinib (Sutent)	Aminoglutethimide (Cytadren)
Suppression of TSH Secretion	Amiodarone (Cordarone)
Bexarotene (Targretin)	Denileukin diftitox (Ontak)
Dobutamine (Dobutrex) (high dose)	Interferon-alfa (Intron-A, Roferon-A)
Dopamine (Intropin) (> 1 µg/kg/min)*	Interleukin-2 (Proleukin)
Glucocorticoids (e.g., prednisone > 20 mg/d)*	Iodine (SSKI, ThyroShield)
	Lithium (Eskalith, Lithane, Lithizine, Lithonate)
Octreotide (Sandostatin) (> 100 µg/d)*	Methimazole (Tapazole)
Phenytoin (Dilantin)	Perchloric acid salt/Perchlorate
Decreased T₄ Absorption	Propylthiouracil (PTU)
Antacids	Sulfonamide drug category (e.g., sulfa drugs)
Cholestyramine (Questran)	Sunitinib (Sutent)
Calcium supplements	Tolbutamide (Orinase)
Ferrous sulfate	
	Increase Hepatic Metabolism
	Carbamazepine (Tegretol)
	Phenytoin (Dilantin)
	Phenobarbitol (Luminal)
	Rifampin (Rifadin)

* Use of these drugs may cause a transient reduction in TSH secretion, but it is not sustained and clinical hypothyroidism does not usually occur.

Table 19-8 Medications That Can Cause Hyperthyroidism— Generic (Brand)

Stimulation of Thyroid Hormone Synthesis and/or Secretion	Immune Dysregulation
Amiodarone (Cordarone)	Interferon-alfa (Intron-A, Roferon-A)
Iodine (SSKI, ThyroShield)	Interleukin-2 (Proleukin)
Lithium (Eskalith, Lithane, Lithizine, Lithonate)	

Table 19-9 Medications That Can Alter Thyroid Laboratory Results—Generic (Brand)

Decreased TSH	Increased TSH (Usually > 10 U/L)	Increased Free T$_4$	Decreased Free T$_4$	Displaced TBG Binding
Dopamine (Intropin)	Metoclopramide[†] (Reglan)	IV furosemide[‡] (Lasix)	Phenytoin (Dilantin)	Furosemide (Lasix)
Levodopa (Sinemet)	Amiodarone (Cordarone)	NSAIDs (e.g., ibuprofen)	Carbamazepine (Tegretol)	Heparin
Bromocriptine (Parlodel)	Iodinated contrast	IV heparin		Hydantoins (e.g., phenytoin,
Glucocorticoids*	Drug interactions that	Amiodarone (Cordarone)		GABA analogues
Octreotide (Sandostatin)	decrease absorption of	Iodinated contrast		NSAIDs (e.g., ibuprofen)
Amphetamines (Adderal,	levothyroxine or increase			Salicylates (≥ 2 g per day)
Dexedrine)	thyroxine clearance			Mefenamic acid (Ponstel)
	(Table 19-3)			Phenylbutazone (Butazolidin)

TSH = thyroid-stimulating hormone; TBG = thyroid-binding globulin; NSAIDs = nonsteroidal anti-inflammatory drugs.

* > 0.5 mg/day dexamethasone or 100 mg/day hydrocortisone.

[†] doses > 1 mg/kg.

[‡] > 80 mg/day.

Source: Adapted from Dong BJ 2000.[37]

Table 19-10 Medications That Contain Iodine

Class	Drug Generic (Brand When Available)	Iodine Dose
Expectorants	Iophen	25 mg/mL
	Iodinated glycerol	15 mg/tablet
	Anhydrous calcium iodide (Calcidrine)	152 mg/5 mL
Antiasthmatic drugs	Theophylline elixir (Elixophyllin)	6.6 mg/mL
Antiarrhythmic drugs	Amiodarone (Cordarone)	75 mg/tablet
Antiamebic drugs	Iodoquinol (Yodoxin)	134 mg/tablet
Anticellulite therapy	Cellasene is the brand name for combination of gingko, grape seed, clover, evening primrose, and other ingredients	720 mcg/serving
Iodide-containing solutions	Lugol's solution	6.3 mg/drop
	Potassium iodide (Quadrinal)	145 mg/tablet
	SSKI*	38 mg/drop
Miscellaneous agents	Kelp	0.15 mg/tablet
Ophthalmic solutions	Echothiophate iodide (Phospholine iodide)	5–41 mcg/drop
	Idoxuridine solution (Herplex)	18 mcg/drop
Radiology contrast agents	Iopanoic acid	333 mg/tablet
	Intravenous preparations	140–380 mg/mL
Topical antiseptic agents	Clioquinol cream (Albaform HC)	12 mg/g
		6 mg/g
	Iodoquinol cream (Yodoxin)	40 mg/mL
	Iodine tincture	4.8 mg/100 mg gauze
	Iodoform gauze	
	Povidone-iodine (Betadine)	10 mg/mL
Vitamins	Iodine-containing vitamins	0.15 mg/tablet

* Saturated solution of potassium iodide.

and used for biosynthesis of thyroid hormone. In contrast, individuals who have autoimmune thyroid disorders such as Hashimoto's thyroiditis and subclinical hypothyroidism and persons who are euthyroid but live in iodine-deficient areas will experience the opposite effect. In these populations, increased iodine in medications and/or food will inhibit the thyroid from absorbing more iodine or experiencing a Wolff-Chaikoff effect. Subsequent production of thyroid hormone falls, and the end result is an exacerbation of hypothyroidism.

Amiodarone

Amiodarone (Cordarone) and iodine-containing contrast media (e.g., tyropanoate, iopanoic acid, and ipodate) contain very high amounts of iodine and may cause the Wolff-Chaikoff effect. Amiodarone is widely used for a wide variety of cardiac conditions. The incidence of hypothyroidism in persons taking amiodarone ranges from 2% to 24% of those who receive this drug.[37] Amiodarone can also induce hyperthyroidism, an effect that is of special concern in the elderly, who are more prone to have both cardiac disorders and thyroid nodular disease.

Amiodarone (Cordarone) can induce thyrotoxicosis via one of two mechanisms. First, amiodarone provides additional iodine that facilitates the synthesis and release of excess thyroid hormone. The second form of thyrotoxicosis is a destructive thyroiditis wherein thyroid damage occurs, causing release of excess thyroid hormone from the reservoir in the thyroid gland. In addition, amiodarone can inhibit the peripheral conversion of T$_4$ to T$_3$ in both the pituitary gland and in the peripheral circulation, which can confound the results of a thyroid function test.[37]

Corticosteroids and Beta-Blockers

Large doses of corticosteroids (e.g., 4 mg of dexamethasone) and beta-adrenergic antagonists (e.g., propranolol [Inderal]) can inhibit the peripheral conversion of T_4 to T_3 but have minimal effects on thyroid function tests. As a result, these agents often are employed in the management of severe hyperthyroidism or thyroid storm to treat symptoms of tachycardia.[11]

Lithium (Lithobid)

Lithium (Lithobid) concentrates in the thyroid gland, interferes with thyroid hormone synthesis, and may induce subclinical hypothyroidism in up to 50% of individuals. The risk appears greatest in those who receive lithium for more than 2 years.[37]

Interferon Alpha

Interferon alpha has been implicated as a transient cause of hypothyroidism for 40–50% of users and hyperthyroidism for 10–30% of recipients. However, interferon beta is rarely associated with disturbances in thyroid function.[37]

Parathyroid Disease

Parathyroid hormone is the most important factor involved in the regulation of serum calcium levels (normal range 8.8–10.5 mg/dL or 2.25–2.75 mmol/L).[4] Parathyroid hormone increases bone resorption of calcium, increases gastrointestinal calcium absorption, and decreases renal excretion of calcium. This hormone is secreted to correct hypocalcemia. Calcitonin hormone, which decreases bone resorption of calcium, decreases gastrointestinal calcium absorption, and increases renal excretion of calcium, is secreted to correct hypercalcemia. Additionally, other electrolyte abnormalities with phosphorus (normal range 2.5–5.0 mg/L or 0.5–1.25 mmol/L) and magnesium (normal range 1.8–3.0 mg/dL or 1.25–1.75 mmol/L) commonly are intertwined with altered calcium homeostasis.

Hyperparathyroidism

Hyperparathyroidism occurs in approximately 100,000 individuals each year. Women, especially those ≥ 60 years, are at the greatest risk for developing the condition.[38] Hyperparathyroid conditions may occur as a result of primary, secondary, or tertiary disease. **Primary hyperparathyroidism** is the result of excessive secretion of parathyroid hormone and usually is caused by a parathyroid tumor. **Secondary hyperparathyroidism** also is the result of excessive amounts of parathyroid hormone, usually in response to hypocalcemia. This condition is the one most likely to be amenable to pharmacologic treatments. **Tertiary hyperparathyroidism** is a condition that occurs after a long period of secondary disease.

Hyperparathyroidism was first described in 1925. This disorder is usually asymptomatic and diagnosed as a serendipitous finding of hypercalcemia. It is classically referred to as "moans, groans, stones, and bones with psychic overtones." Symptoms, when they are present, include bone disorders, kidney stones, gastrointestinal discomfort, neuromuscular dysfunction, weakness, fatigue, anxiety, and cognitive difficulties.[39] Individuals with primary and tertiary disease often develop hypercalcemia and hypophosphatemia. Chronic renal failure is the most frequent cause of secondary disease and results in an accompanying hypocalcemia and hyperphosphatemia.[40]

Treatment of hyperparathyroidism differs according to underlying disorder. Primary disease and tertiary disease are usually managed surgically while secondary disease is managed medically. As hyperphosphatemia and hypocalcemia are the hallmarks of secondary disease, phosphate-binding agents, low phosphate diets, calcium supplementation, vitamin D, and calcimimetics are used as treatments.[40]

Treatment of Secondary Hyperparathyroidism

Phosphate Binders

A variety of medications are used to bind phosphorus. These agents are generally taken 10–15 minutes before or during a meal to increase effectiveness.[41] Some include calcium (carbonate, acetate, citrate), magnesium (carbonate), and aluminum (hydroxide and carbonate). The National Kidney Foundation recommends that aluminum-based binders be considered short-term treatment and used for no longer than 4 weeks if the individual has a serum phosphorus > 7.0 mg/dL (2.26 mmol/L) to avoid the potential for aluminum toxicity.[41]

Sevelamer (Renagel) is newest among the phosphate binders and was approved in 2000[40,41] (Table 19-11). Sevelamer is indicated for the control serum phosphorus in patients with chronic renal failure who are also on dialysis.[40] The most commonly reported adverse effects seen in persons taking sevelamer are constipation, diarrhea,

Table 19-11 Pharmacologic Management of Secondary Hyperparathyroidism

Medication Generic (Brand)	Indications	Advantages	Side Effects
Calcium carbonate (Tums, OsCal)	Serum levels within target range to reduce risk of extraskeletal calcification	Inexpensive Wide variety of products	Hypercalcemia Extraskeletal calcification Constipation
Calcium acetate (PhosLo)	Same as above	Less calcium absorption than carbonate Phosphate binding similar to aluminum hydroxide	Hypercalcemia Extraskeletal calcification GI side effects
Calcium citrate (Citracal)	Not recommended	N/A	Increases aluminum absorption
Magnesium carbonate (MagneBind)	Must monitor serum magnesium	Can minimize calcium load	Hypermagnesemia Lack of long-term safety and efficacy studies
Aluminum hydroxide (AlternaGEL, Alu-Cap)	Time- and dose-limited use for hyperphosphatemia unresponsive to other binders	Effective phosphate binding	Constipation Fecal impaction Bone mineral defects Aluminum toxicity Chalky taste
Aluminum carbonate (Basaljel)	Same as aluminum hydroxide above	Same as aluminum hydroxide above	Same as aluminum hydroxide above
Sevelamer (Renagel)	Eliminates binder-related calcium load	Noncalcium Nonaluminum	GI side effects

nausea, vomiting, abdominal pain, and dyspepsia. The starting dose is one or two 800-mg or two to four 400-mg tablets by mouth three times daily with meals. Doses may be adjusted up by one tablet per meal every 2 weeks to the desired phosphorus range.[40] Sevelamer is an FDA Pregnancy Category C drug because of the lack of studies.[34]

Calcimimetics

Cinacalcet (Sensipar), a calcimimetic, was approved by the FDA in 2004 and is available in 30-mg, 60-mg, and 90-mg tablets. Its FDA Pregnancy Category is C because of lack of research, and similarly, few studies have been done regarding use during breastfeeding. This agent exerts its pharmacologic effects by altering the sensitivity of the calcium-sensing receptor on the surface of the parathyroid gland, which results in improved parathyroid hormone and extracellular calcium sensitivity.[41] Cinacalcet may be used in combination with other customary therapies (e.g., phosphate binders, calcitriol) prescribed for those with chronic renal failure. Some of the most common adverse effects seen in those who have received cinacalcet include nausea, vomiting, diarrhea, myalgia, and dizziness.[11] The starting dose is 30 mg once daily, which may be titrated up to 180 mg once daily. Providers should monitor calcium and phosphorus within the first week of initiation of therapy and intact parathyroid levels within the first 4 weeks to maintain a recommended level of 150–300 pg/mL.[11]

Hypoparathyroidism

Hypoparathyroidism is a rare disorder resulting from inadequate parathyroid hormone production. This disorder may be genetically inherited or transient, but is most often acquired secondary to damage to the parathyroid gland during thyroid surgery.[4] An elevated serum phosphorus level and low serum calcium in the absence of intestinal disorders, nutritional deficiencies, or renal failure is diagnostic of hypoparathyroidism.[4]

Therapeutic management of hypoparathyroidism primarily includes calcium replacement and vitamin D supplementation to normalize serum calcium. Intravenous calcium gluconate administered in either a bolus or continuous infusion fashion should be considered for severe hypocalcemia. Oral calcium may be given in doses of 100 mg of elemental calcium/kg/day divided in four doses per day until serum calcium levels reach 8–9 mg/dL; doses can then be reduced and adjusted as needed.[11]

Special Populations

Pregnancy

The frequency of primary hyperparathyroidism in pregnancy is rare.[42] The first reported case was documented in 1931. By 2001, 145 cases had been reported.[42] Primary hyperparathyroidism results in a pregnancy complication rate of approximately 80% in fetuses (death was noted as the complication in 27–31% of cases) and 65% in mothers. Transient cases of hypoparathyroidism have been reported to cause low birth weight and premature birth. Maternal hypercalcemia or hyperparathyroidism may also suppress parathyroid secretion in the neonate.[42]

Elderly

The aging process brings physiologic changes such as a total body water decline of about 10–15%, relative loss of lean body mass, and an increased extracellular to intracellular water ratio.[43] Although younger individuals can more easily adapt to wide fluctuations in phosphate and calcium, the elderly are much more limited in this capacity. Diseases, medications, and other factors increase this vulnerability, although exact prevalence rates are unclear.[43]

Conclusion

Women across the life span with thyroid or parathyroid dysfunction are susceptible to a wide variety of complications as these glands and their respective hormones are critical for the normal operation of many body processes. Healthcare providers have multiple pharmacologic options available to manage the derangements that may occur in these systems as a result of disease. Carefully obtained histories, physical examinations, and laboratory evaluations will help the healthcare provider provide optimal care for women with thyroid and parathyroid disorders.

References

1. Klein I. T3 and T4: are we missing half the picture? Clin Cornerstone 2005;7(suppl 2):S5–S8.
2. Food and Nutrition Board of US Academy of Sciences. Dietary reference intakes: the essential guide to nutrient requirements. Washington, DC: National Academy of Sciences, 2006.
3. Farwell AP, Braverman LE. Thyroid and antithyroid drugs. In Brunton L, Lazo J, Parker K, eds. Goodman and Gilman's the pharmacological basis of therapeutics, 11th ed. New York: McGraw Hill, 2005.
4. McCance KL, Huether SE. Pathophysiology: the biologic basis for disease in adults and children, 5th ed. St. Louis, MO: Elsevier Mosby, 2006.
5. Kassayan R, Nakhjavani M, Eghtesad M, Gouhari Hosseini L. Thyroid function tests in nonthyroidal illness: correction by mathematical method. Int J Endocrinol Metab 2003;1:6–13.
6. Katz MD. Thyroid disorders. In Chisholm-Burns MA, Wells BG, Schwinghammer TL, Malone PM, Kolesar JM, Rotschafer JC, et al. Pharmacotherapy: principles and practice. New York: McGraw Hill, 2008: 667–84.
7. Cramer DW, Sluss PM, Powers RD, McShane P, Ginsburg ES, Hornstein MD, et al. Serum prolactin and TSH in an in vitro fertilization population: is there a link between fertilization and thyroid function? J Assist Reprod Genet 2003;20(6):210–5.
8. Vanderpump MP, Turnbridge WM, French JM, Appleton D, Bates D, Clark F, et al. The incidence of thyroid disorders in the community: a twenty-year follow-up of the Whickham Survey. Clin Endocrinol 1995;43:55–68.
9. Baskin HJ, Cobin RH, Duick DS, Gharib H, Guttler RB, Kaplan MM, et al. American Association of Clinical Endocrinologists medical guidelines for clinical practice for the evaluation and treatment of hyperthyroidism and hypothyroidism. Endocr Pract 2002;8(6): 457–69.
10. Mazokopakis EE. Counseling patients receiving levothyroxine (L-T4) and calcium carbonate [3]. Mil Med 2006;171(11):vii, 1094.
11. Greenspan FS, Dong BJ. Thyroid and antithyroid drugs. In Katzung BG, ed. Basic and clinical pharmacology, 10th ed. New York, NY: McGraw-Hill, 2007: 618–34.
12. Singh N, Hershman JM. Interference with the absorption of levothyroxine. Cur Opin Endocrin Diab 2003; 10(5):347–52.
13. Slagle MA. Medication update. Thyroid supplements. Antithyroid medications. South Med J 2002;95(5): 520–1.
14. Munoz-Torres M, Varsavsky M, Alonso G. Lactose intolerance revealed by severe resistance to treatment with levothyroxine. Thyroid 2006;16(11):1171–3.
15. Lips DJ, van Reisen MT, Voight V, Venekamp W. Diagnosis and treatment of levothyroxine malabsorption. Netherlands J Med 2004;62(4):114–8.
16. Singer AJ. Combination therapy in a hypothyroid patient intolerant of elevated thyroxine. Clin Cornerstone 2005;7(suppl 2):S20–1.
17. Rosenthal MS. Patient misconceptions and ethical challenges in radioactive iodine scanning and therapy. J Nucl Med Technol 2006;34(3):143–50.

18. Metso S, Jaatinen P, Huhtala H, Auvinen A, Oksala H, Salmi J. Increased cardiovascular and cancer mortality after radioiodine treatment for hyperthyroidism. J Clin Endocrinol Metab 2007;92(6):2190–6.

19. Fitzgerald P. Endocrine disorders. In McPhee SJ, Papdakis MA, Tierney LM. Current medical diagnosis & treatment, 47th ed. New York: Lange McGraw-Hill, 2008:1123–218.

20. Bonnema SJ, Bennedbaek FN, Veje A, Marving J, Hegedus L. Continuous methimazole therapy and its effect on the cure rate of hyperthyroidism using radioactive iodine: an evaluation by a randomized trial. J Clin Endocrinol Metab 2006;91(8):2946–51.

21. England RJA, Kamath MB, Jabreel A, Dunne G, Atkin SL. How we do it: surgery should be considered equally with I131 and thionamide treatment as first-line therapy for thyrotoxicosis. Clin Otolaryngol 2006;31(2): 160–2.

22. Nakamura H, Noh JY, Itoh K, Fukata S, Miyauchi A, Hamada N. Comparison of methimazole and propylthiouracil in patients with hyperthyroidism caused by Graves' disease. J Clin Endocrinol Metab 2007; 92(6):2157–62.

23. Cooper DS. Antithyroid drugs. N Engl J Med 2005;352: 905–17.

24. Koller E, Svoboda JD, Jones F, Moore G. Atypical antineutrophil-cytoplasmic antibodies and vasculitis-like syndrome with aphthous ulcer and violaceous pinnae after retreatment with propylthiouracil for Graves disease. Endocrinologist 2006;16(1):36–40.

25. Pillinger MH, Staud R. Propylthiouracil and antineutrophil cytoplasmic antibody associated vasculitis: the detective finds a clue. Sem Arthritis Rheumat 2006;36(1):1–3.

26. Hodak SP, Huang C, Clarke D, Burman KD, Jonklaas J, Janicic-Kharic N. Intravenous methimazole in the treatment of refractory hyperthyroidism. Thyroid 2006;16(7):691–5.

27. Kubota S, Ohye H, Yano G, Nishihara E, Kudo T, Ito M, et al. Two-day thionamide withdrawal prior to radioiodine uptake sufficiently increases uptake and does not exacerbate hyperthyroidism compared to 7-day withdrawal in Graves' disease. Endocrine J 2006;53(5): 603–7.

28. Bartalena L, Bogazzi F, Pinchera A, Martino E. Treatment with thionamides before radioiodine therapy for hyperthyroidism: yes or no? J Clin Endocrinol Metab 2005;90(2):1256; author reply 1256–7.

29. Vijayakumar V, Nusynowitz ML, Ali S. Is it safe to treat hyperthyroid patients with I-131 without fear of thyroid storm? Ann Nucl Med 2006;20(6):383–5.

30. Karlsson FA, Akexsson O, Melhus H. Severe embryopathy and exposure to methimazole in early pregnancy. J Clin Endocrinol Metab 2002;87:947–9.

31. Wier FA, Farley CL. Clinical controversies in screening women for thyroid disorders during pregnancy. J Midwifery Womens Health. 2006;5:152–8.

32. Clark SM, Saade GR, Snodgrass WR, Hankins GDV. Pharmacokinetics and pharmacotherapy of thionamides in pregnancy. Ther Drug Monit 2006;28(4): 477–83.

33. Casey BM, Leveno KJ. Thyroid disease in pregnancy. Obstet Gynecol 2006;108(5):1283–92.

34. Hale TW. Medications and mother's milk, 10th ed. Amarillo, TX: Pharmasoft Publishing, 2002.

35. Academy of Pediatrics. Transfer of drugs and other chemicals into human milk. Pediatrics 2001;108(3): 776–89.

36. Wing DA, Millar LK, Koonings PP, Montoro MD, Mestman JH. A comparison of propylthiouracil versus methimazole in the treatment of hyperthyroidism in pregnancy. Am J Obstet Gynecol 1994;170:90–5.

37. Dong BJ. How medications affect thyroid function. Western J Medicine 2000;172(2):102–6.

38. Younes NA, Shagoj Y, Khatib F, Ababneh M. Laboratory screening for hyperparathyroidism. Clinic Chimica Acta 2005;353:1–12.

39. Thompson NW. The history of hyperparathyroidism. Acta Chir Scand 1990;156:5–21.

40. Ketteler M, Rix M, Fan S, Pritchard N, Oestergaard O, Chasan-Taber S, et al. Efficacy and tolerability of sevelamer carbonate in hyperphosphatemic patients who have chronic kidney disease and are not on dialysis. Clin J Am Soc Nephrol 2008 May 1;4:1125–30.

41. DeFrancisco AL. New strategies for the treatment of hyperparathyroidism incorporating calcimimetics. Expert Opin Pharmacother 2008;9(5):795–811.

42. Schnatz PF, Thaxton S. Parathyroidectomy in the third trimester of pregnancy. Obstet Gynecol Surv 2005; 60(10):672–82.

43. Allison SP, Lobo DN. Fluid and electrolytes in the elderly. Clin Nutri Metabol Care 2004;71(1):27–33.

Respiratory Conditions

Barbara W. Graves

 ## Chapter Glossary

Acute bacterial rhinosinusitis Inflammation of the sinus cavities caused by bacteria; it may or may not be preceded by a cold or allergic reaction. This condition generally lasts less than 4 weeks; if longer, it is not considered acute.

Alveolar ventilation Volume of air expired from the alveoli.

Antigenic drift Slow changes experienced by viruses by random mutations.

Antigenic shift Rapid changes experienced when two different viruses combine to produce a new subtype. These changes are usually associated with pandemics. Antigenic shifts result from recombination of the genomes of two viral strains.

Antitussive Cough suppressive or inhibitor of cough reflex.

Asthma From Greek for *pant* or *breathe with an open mouth*, a chronic respiratory condition characterized by airway constriction, inflammation, and obstruction.

Bronchitis An inflammation of the mucous membranes of the bronchial tubes, causing a persistent productive cough.

Community-acquired pneumonia Pneumonia that occurs among individuals who have not been recently hospitalized.

Decongestants Drug category of agents that reduce swelling of the mucous membranes in the nasal passages and decrease nasal congestion.

Expectorant Mucolytic or agent that dissolves or thins mucus in order to promote expulsion of sputum from the respiratory tract.

Histamine Amine released by the mast cell and responsible for such symptoms as nasal congestion, respiratory difficulty, and rhinitis.

Latent tuberculosis infection (LTBI) An infection with *Mycobacterium tuberculosis* without active tuberculosis disease or contagion.

Leukotrienes Potent endogenous inflammatory mediators that induce bronchoconstriction and airway hyper-responsiveness.

Multidrug resistant tuberculosis Tuberculosis that is resistant to at least two drugs, isoniazid (INH) and rifampin (Rifadin).

Pulmonary ventilation Mechanical movement of air in and out of the lungs.

Rhinitis medicamentosa Rebound congestion associated with discontinuation or decrease in use of topical decongestants.

Rhinorrhea Runny nose or significant increase in the amount of nasal secretions.

Rhinosinusitis Inflammation of the paranasal sinuses. This term is becoming preferred to use of *sinusitis* since it is theorized that inflammation of the sinuses cannot occur without some nasal inflammation.

Tuberculosis (TB) An infection with *Mycobacterium tuberculosis* that primarily but not exclusively affects the lungs.

Introduction

The range of diseases affecting the respiratory system is immense, and the variety of medications used to treat these illnesses is equally broad. Respiratory illness can be as mild as slight allergic rhinitis or as severe as life-threatening anaphylactic shock or adult respiratory distress syndrome. Primary care providers are usually the first contact for individuals suffering with respiratory illness. People often come for care with strongly held preconceptions of what care they should receive, but, unfortunately, these preconceptions usually are not based on any evidence. This chapter reviews the pharmacologic therapy of respiratory disorders that are frequently encountered during the delivery of primary care of women.

Respiratory Anatomy and Physiology

The function of the respiratory system is gas exchange—to allow the transfer of oxygen from the alveoli to the vascular system and subsequent delivery to tissues and removal of carbon dioxide from the vascular system. To accomplish this function, there must be inflow and outflow of air, gas exchange across the alveoli, and capillary circulation around the alveoli to carry the oxygen and carbon dioxide to and from the tissues. **Pulmonary ventilation** refers to the mechanical movement of air in and out of the lungs. Much of the volume of air in the lungs is in the dead space areas such as the trachea and bronchi that are not involved in gas exchange. **Alveolar ventilation** is the volume of air expired from the alveoli themselves.[1,2]

The trachea and main bronchi are surrounded by cartilage rings that maintain patency of the upper airways (Figure 20-1). As the bronchi further divide, there is progressively less cartilage, which disappears completely by the level of the bronchioles. The diameter of these terminal airways is about 1–1.5 mm. The walls of the bronchioles consist of smooth muscle controlled by the autonomic nervous system. These airway passages are at risk for occlusion due to their small lumen.

Autonomic Nervous System Control of the Respiratory System

The sympathetic and parasympathetic nervous systems are comprised of preganglionic neurons, ganglion, and postganglionic neurons that stimulate end target organs.[3] The respiratory tract is responsive to both sympathetic and parasympathetic stimulation. The adrenal medulla functions as part of the sympathetic nervous system via the release of the neurotransmitters epinephrine and norepinephrine.

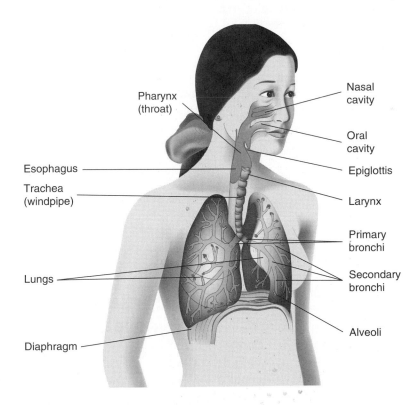

Pharynx (throat)

Nasal cavity

Oral cavity

Esophagus

Epiglottis

Trachea (windpipe)

Larynx

Primary bronchi

Secondary bronchi

Lungs

Alveoli

Diaphragm

Figure 20-1 Anatomy of the respiratory tract. *Source:* Clark RK 2005.[143]

The end organ responses to autonomic innervation are determined by both the neurotransmitter released by the postganglionic neurons and the receptor subtype displayed on the surfaces of the end organ cells. The target organs of the parasympathetic nervous system, in addition to the sweat glands, all have the muscarinic receptors that are stimulated by acetylcholine. There are two types of acetylcholine receptors: muscarinic and nicotinic. Thus, drugs that stimulate acetylcholine receptors in an agonist fashion are referred to as cholinergic drugs, and those that block muscarinic or nicotinic receptors are referred to as anticholinergic drugs. Parasympathetic innervation and stimulation in the lungs causes bronchial constriction and promotion of secretions.[3]

The sympathetic postganglionic neurons (with the exception of those innervating the sweat glands) release norepinephrine. There are more adrenergic (as in adrenaline) receptor subtypes than cholinergic, and the response of the target organ differs significantly depending on the receptor subtype present in that organ. Activation of alpha receptors, minimally constricts the pulmonary blood vessels. Beta$_1$ receptors are not present in the respiratory tract. Activation of beta$_2$ receptors in the respiratory tract causes some vasodilation of the pulmonary arterioles and a more significant effect of bronchodilation. Activation of beta$_2$ receptors has a vasoconstrictive effect on the nasal mucosa. Coincidentally, this is the same subtype of receptors that causes uterine relaxation. Finally, the adrenal medulla also releases epinephrine, which activates alpha$_1$ and alpha$_2$ receptors and beta$_1$ and beta$_2$ receptors, while norepinephrine does not activate beta$_2$ receptors.

Allergic Response of the Respiratory Tract

Mast cells are found in tissues that come in contact with the external environment, including the airway mucosa. When exposed to any of a multitude of stimuli such as antigens, anti-IgE, or anaphylotoxins, mast cells release several inflammatory mediators that include **histamine**, leukotrienes, cytokines, and prostaglandins[2] (Figure 20-2). These substances cause a cascade of responses in the respiratory tract, including bronchoconstriction and vascular permeability.[4] For example, **leukotrienes** are potent inflammatory mediators that induce bronchoconstriction and airway hyperresponsiveness. This, in turn, stimulates smooth muscle hypertrophy and mucus secretion. Continual stimulation of mast cells results in chronic inflammation characterized by edema, mucus plugging, and bronchial hyperreactivity.

The respiratory tract can be assaulted by pathogens, irritants, and allergens with subsequent responses medi-

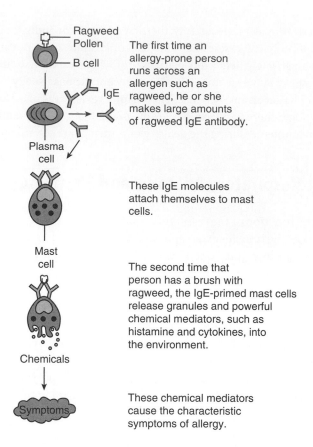

The first time an allergy-prone person runs across an allergen such as ragweed, he or she makes large amounts of ragweed IgE antibody.

These IgE molecules attach themselves to mast cells.

The second time that person has a brush with ragweed, the IgE-primed mast cells release granules and powerful chemical mediators, such as histamine and cytokines, into the environment.

These chemical mediators cause the characteristic symptoms of allergy.

Figure 20-2 The role of mast cells in the development of allergy. *Source:* From National Institutes of Health 2003.[144]

ated by many pathways. Medications used to treat respiratory disease can be effective by treating a bacterial infection, blocking mast cell stimulation, blocking the effects of histamines or leukotrienes, or enhancing activation of beta$_2$ receptors. Anti-inflammatory medications are nonspecific agents that are used to decrease the inflammation caused by chronic stimulation beta$_2$ receptors and mast cells. Many other nonspecific medications that have little or no effect on the underlying respiratory disease often are used to counter the symptoms of the illness.

Upper Respiratory Infection/ Common Cold

The common cold/upper respiratory infection (URI) can be caused by more than 200 different viruses, including rhinoviruses, parainfluenza, coronaviruses, and, less often, adenoviruses or respiratory syncytial virus (RSV). The common cold is a leading cause of healthcare visits and missed days from work and school.[5] On average, toddlers will develop 5 to 7 URIs each year, with the incidence declining to 2 to 3 per year among otherwise healthy adults.[6] Viruses responsible for the common cold are transmitted easily from one individual to another. Direct contact, especially hand to hand, is the most efficient mode of transmission, with significantly less virus found in aerosols subsequent to coughing or sneezing. Virus is rarely detectable in saliva.[7]

Prevention

Hand-to-hand direct transmission can be decreased by the use of virucidal compounds applied to the hands. While hand treatment with 2% aqueous iodine has been shown to decrease transmission, use of this compound is unlikely to be adopted due to the staining and drying effects of iodine.[8] Hand cleansers with ethanol alone have not been shown to be effective. However, hand cleansers show promising results. More than 90% of viruses remain when hands are treated with alcohol, but only 15% remain after treatment with 3.5% salicylic acid and 0% in hands treated with 1% salicylic acid plus 3.5% pyroglutamic acid.[8] To date there are no commercially available hand cleansers incorporating these compounds.

Vitamin C

Vitamin C has been recommended for both the prevention and treatment of the common cold. Findings from studies assessing the efficacy of vitamin C have been inconsistent. A Cochrane meta-analysis of trials evaluating the efficacy of vitamin C concluded that while there was little prophylactic benefit in the general public (relative risk [RR] = 96; 95% confidence interval [CI], 0.92–1.00), a greater benefit was demonstrated among athletes such as marathon runners, soldiers on sub-Arctic exercises, and skiers (RR = 0.50; 95% CI, 0.38–0.66).[9] No mechanism was proposed that explained these findings.

Echinacea

Results from studies on the effects of echinacea are even more conflicting. Echinacea refers to a collection of at least nine different species of American wildflowers commonly known as coneflowers. Echinacea is proposed to act as an immune stimulant, causing the release of tissue necrosis factor.[10] Potential side effects include allergic reactions, especially in individuals with allergies to plants such as ragweed, chrysanthemums, marigolds, and daisies. These allergic reactions may be worse than the original upper respiratory disease. The study of echinacea is complicated by the variety of species included in supplements and the inconsistent amount of active ingredient found in different

products. One study found that 10% of commercially available preparations contained no measurable echinacea.[11] The National Center for Complementary and Alternative Medicine of the National Institutes of Health has concluded that echinacea neither prevents nor ameliorates colds.[10] A 2006 Cochrane review concluded that echinacea might offer some benefit in early treatment of a cold but was not effective in preventing colds.[12] Yet another meta-analysis, which included many of the same studies as the Cochrane review and some that were excluded from the Cochrane review, concluded that the evidence supports the benefit of echinacea in both the prevention and treatment of the common cold.[13] With these contradictory findings, it is prudent to consider both the monetary cost and potential allergic reactions prior to using echinacea for either the prevention or treatment of colds.

Chicken Soup

Among the various treatments for upper respiratory infections has been a home remedy of chicken soup. Interestingly, Rennard et al. found some antiviral effects with the ingestion of chicken soup.[14] However, there are no data supporting clinical use of this gastronomic intervention.

While the common cold, with its bothersome symptoms of nasal obstruction, rhinorrhea, sneezing, scratchy throat, coughing, and headache, usually resolves spontaneously after 3–7 days, complications can include airway hyperreactivity/asthma that can persist for up to 4 weeks and acute bronchitis. In addition, approximately 25% of sufferers continue to report symptoms of cough and postnasal drip for longer than 14 days.[15] In summary, the common cold is generally a self-limited illness associated with only minimal morbidity (Box 20-1).

Pharmacologic Treatment of Upper Respiratory Infections

At this time, there is no cure for the common cold. It is inappropriate to treat a cold with antibiotics. Not only are antibiotics ineffective for decreasing symptoms or shortening the duration of a cold, their use can increase the general antibiotic-resistance of bacteria. However, without the availability of a cure, persons with colds look to medications to make them feel better. Common medications marketed to cold sufferers include antihistamines, topical and intranasal decongestants, intranasal steroids, cough suppressants, expectorants, and mucolytics. There have been several meta-analyses of

Box 20-1   Upper Respiratory Infections: To Treat or Not to Treat

Any modern pharmacy has a large amount of dedicated space for various treatments for an upper respiratory infection (URI) or the common cold. Yet research indicates that most agents are palliative at best. Antibiotics not only are ineffective but are associated with increased drug resistance and expense. Since little histamine is released with a URI, antihistamines are not indicated. Decongestants may provide mild comfort for some individuals through either topical or systemic use but are associated with unpleasant side effects. Most combination therapies include decongestants and antihistamines. It has been said that treatment of a URI risks some of the attributes of the seven dwarfs: namely Sneezy, Sleepy, Dopey, and Grumpy. Opting not to treat a URI with a pharmaceutical is a sane choice.

symptomatic treatments published in the Cochrane Database of Systematic Reviews.

Antihistamines

Although a large meta-analysis concluded that antihistamines do not provide symptomatic relief from a cold,[16] other studies have reported a decrease of sneezing, rhinorrhea, and sometimes cough, with first-generation, but not second-generation, nonsedating antihistamines.[17] Naclerio et al.[18] demonstrated that histamine is not increased in persons with experimentally induced rhinovirus and therefore probably contributes little to nasal symptoms. Sutter[16] theorized that the sedating and anticholinergic effects of the first-generation antihistamines, which are not present in the second-generation, nonsedating antihistamines, might alleviate some of the symptoms of the cold. The combination of a first-generation antihistamine with a decongestant has been shown to decrease coughing by 20–30%.[19] Chapter 13 presents a thorough discussion of antihistamines.

Decongestants

Decongestants are sympathomimetic agents that activate alpha$_1$-adrenergic receptors on the nasal blood vessels, leading to vasoconstriction, decreased swelling of the mucous membranes, and improved nasal drainage.[3] They do not, as is commonly believed, decrease nasal secretions.[20] Decongestants are available in either systemic or topical forms, and a single dose of either topical or systemic decongestant will cause some diminution of symptoms (Table 20-1). Use of a decongestant for 3–5 days often offers a significant degree of relief.

Phenylephrine (Sudafed PE) and pseudoephedrine (Sudafed) both are currently available as nonprescriptive oral decongestants. As pseudoephedrine is a key ingredient in the manufacture of methamphetamines, the Combat

Methamphetamine Epidemic Act of 2005 ruled that pseudoephedrine should be available only from pharmacists, and in limited quantities; thus it often is called a "behind the counter" drug.[21,22] Pseudoephedrine (Sudafed) is contraindicated for individuals who have severe hypertension, ischemic heart disease, or are using MAO inhibitors (e.g., selegiline). Severe, and possibly life-threatening hypertensive crises can occur if an individual taking MAO inhibitors is exposed to phenylephrine or pseudophedrine.[23] A third nonprescriptive decongestant, phenylpropanolamine, has been removed from the market due to its association with an increased risk of hemorrhagic stroke in women.[24]

Combination Therapy

The majority of cold preparations are marketed as a combination of medications. In using these preparations, one may inadvertently consume significantly higher than recommended doses of a specific medication or conversely, ingest subtherapeutic amounts.[25] In addition, combination preparations often contain medications that have no benefit for the person's symptoms. For example, guaifenesin is a common expectorant in cough preparations, but it has been shown to be of no benefit for usual cold symptoms.[26] Table 20-2 lists the ingredients in some of the common combination preparations. Note that brand names do not necessarily indicate the specific ingredients, and reformulations are common. Therefore, professionals and consumers alike should read the labels carefully.

Intranasal Ipratropium (Atrovent)

Intranasal ipratropium (Atrovent) is an anticholinergic agent that is effective in decreasing the symptoms of cough.[27] This drug is not commonly used by healthy women with minor conditions such as coughs associated with colds and allergies, but rather as adjunctive therapy for women with chronic allergies, asthma, or chronic obstructive pulmonary disease (COPD). The actions of this agent include inhibition of secretions from the nasal mucosa. Only 2–3% is absorbed systemically, and the drug quickly is metabolized into inactive metabolites. Ipratropium is categorized as an FDA Pregnancy Category B drug, with no teratogenic effects reported in rats or rabbits at doses 50 to 120 times the maximum recommended adult dose. Due to the minimal systemic absorption, it is unlikely that a clinically significant amount of the drug would cross into breast milk. Adverse reactions are rare, primarily consisting of nasal dryness or epistaxis, and lead to discontinuation of the product in fewer than 0.3% of users.[28]

Table 20-1 Medications for the Management of Allergic Rhinitis

Drug Generic (Brand)	Formulation	Dose (Sprays per Nostril for Topical Medications)
Antihistamines: Oral		
Cetirizine (Zyrtec)	5- and 10-mg tablets	5–10 mg PO qd
Chlorpheniramine (Chlor-Trimeton)	4-mg tablet (12 mg ER)	1 PO bid
Diphenhydramine (Benadryl)	25- and 50-mg tablet	1 PO tid to qid
Desloratadine (Clarinex)	5-mg tablet	1 PO qd
Fexofenadine (Allegra)	30-, 60-, 180-mg tablets	60 mg PO bid
Hydroxyzine (Atarax, Vistaril)	10-, 25-, 50-, 100-mg tablets	25–100 mg PO per day in divided doses
Loratadine (Claritin)	10-mg tablets	1 PO qd
Antihistamines: Topical		
Azelastine (Astelin)	137 mcg	1–2 bid
Decongestants		
Oxymetazoline 0.05% (Afrin 12 h, Neo-Synephrine 12 h)	Spray	2–3 sprays q 10–12 h
Phenylephrine 0.25%–1% (Neo-Synephrine Sudafed PE, and others)	Drops	2–3 drops q 4 h prn
	Spray	2–3 sprays q 4 h
	Oral	10–20 mg q 4 h
Pseudoephedrine (Sudafed and others)	30-, 60-mg tablets	60 mg q 4–6 h
	120 mg ER	120 mg q 12 h
Tetrahydrozoline 0.1% (Tyzine)	Drops	2–4 drops q 3 h
Nasal Corticosteroids		
Beclomethasone (Beconase AQ)	42 mcg/spray	1–2 bid
Budesonide (Rhinocort Aqua)	32 mcg/spray	1 daily
Flunisolide (Nasarel)	25 mcg/spray	2 bid
Fluticasone (Flonase)	50 mcg/spray	2 daily
Mometasone (Nasonex)	50 mcg/spray	1 bid
Triamcinolone (Nasacort AQ)	55 mcg/spray	2 daily
Triamcinolone (Nasacort HFA)	55 mcg/spray	2 daily
Montelukast (Singulair)	10 mg	
Anticholinergic Nasal Spray		
Ipratropium (Atrovent)	0.06%	2 tid–qid
Combination Formulations		
Fexofenadine 60 mg/pseudoephedrine 120 mg (Allegra-D) (antihistamine and a decongestant)		1 tablet bid
Loratadine 10 mg/pseudoephedrine 240 mg (Claritin D) (antihistamine and a decongestant)		1 tablet bid
Mast Cell Stabilizer		
Cromolyn sodium (NasalCrom)	5.2 mg/spray	1 tid–qid

ER = extended release; AQ = aqueous; HFA = hydrofluoroalkane (not containing chlorofluorocarbon).
Sources: Meltzer EO 2005[101]; Prenner BM et al. 2006[102]; Brunton SA et al. 2007.[103]

Table 20-2 Common Brands of Cold, Allergy, and Cough Remedies

Common Brand Names	Antihistamine	Decongestant	Cough Remedy	Analgesic
Alka-Seltzer Plus\Cold & Cough Medicine Liqui-Gels		PS	DM	AC
Alka-Seltzer Plus Cold Medicine Liqui-Gels	CH	PS		AC
Alka-Seltzer Plus Nighttime Cold Medicine Liqui-Gels	DO	PS	DM	AC
Alka-Seltzer PM Pain Reliever Sleep Aid	DI			ASA
Alka-Seltzer Plus Flu Medicine Liqui-Gels		PS	DM	AC
Chlor-Trimeton 12 Hour Allergy; Chlor-Trimeton 4 Hour Allergy; Chlor-Trimeton 8 Hour Allergy; Chlor-Trimeton Allergy Syrup	CH			
Comtrex Allergy-Sinus Maximum Strength Tablets	CH	PS		AC
Comtrex Cold & Cough Multi-Symptom Relief Maximum Strength Caplets; Comtrex Cold & Cough Multi-Symptom Relief Maximum Strength Tablets; Comtrex Cough & Cold Day-Night Maximum Strength Caplets	CH	PS	DM	AC
Comtrex Deep Chest Cold Multi-Symptom Softgels		PS	DM, GU	AC
Comtrex Non-Drowsy Maximum Strength Caplets		PS	DM	AC
Contac Day & Night Cold/Flu Caplets		PS		
Contac Severe Cold Flu Maximum Strength Caplets	CH	PS	DM	AC
Contac Severe Cold Flu Non-Drowsy Caplets		PS	DM	AC
Coricidin HBP Cold & Flu	CH			AC
Coricidin HBP Flu Maximum Strength	CH		DM	AC
Coricidin HBP Cough & Cold			DM	
Diabetic Tussin DM; Diabetic Tussin DM Maximum Strength Cough Suppressant/Expectorant			DM, GU	
Diabetic Tussin EX			GU	
Dimetapp Cold & Congestion Caplets		PS	DM, GU	
Dimetapp Cold & Fever	BR	PS		AC
Dimetapp DM Cold & Cough Elixir	BR	PS	DM	
Dimetapp Elixir	BR	PS		
Excedrin PM Caplets; Excedrin PM Geltabs; Excedrin PM Tablets	DI			
Excedrin Sinus Headache		PE		AC
Nytol QuickCaps Caplets; Nytol Quick gels Maximum Strength D	DI			
Robitussin			GU	
Robitussin Allergy & Cough	BR	PS	DM	
Robitussin Cold & Congestion Caplets; Robitussin Cold & Congestion Softgels		PS	DM, GU	
Robitussin Cold Multi-Symptom Cold & Flu Softgels		PS	DM, GU	AC
Robitussin Cold Severe Congestion Liqui-Gels		PS	GU	
Robitussin Cough & Cold Maximum Strength		PS	DM	
Robitussin Cough Gels; Robitussin Honey Cough Suppressant; Robitussin Maximum Strength Cough Suppressant			DM	
Robitussin Flu	CH	PS	DM	
Robitussin Multi-Symptom Cold & Flu Caplets; Robitussin Cold & Congestion Caplets		PS	DM, GU	AC
Robitussin Multi-Symptom Honey Flu		PS	DM	AC
Robitussin Nighttime Honey Flu	CH	PS	DM	AC
Robitussin PM Cough & Cold	CH	PS	DM	
Robitussin Sugar Free Cough; Robitussin-DM			DM, GU	
Robitussin-CF		PS	DM, GU	
Robitussin-PE		PS	GU	
Sine-Off Nighttime Relief Sinus Cold & Flu Medicine Gel Caplets	DI	PS		AC
Sine-Off Sinus Medicine Caplets		PS		AC
Sinutab Non-Drowsy Non-Drying Sinus Liquid Caps		PS	GU	

(continues)

Table 20-2 Common Brands of Cold, Allergy, and Cough Remedies (*continued*)

Common Brand Names	Antihistamine	Decongestant	Cough Remedy	Analgesic
Sinutab Sinus Allergy Maximum Strength Caplets; Sinutab Sinus Allergy Maximum Strength Tablets	CH	PS		AC
Sudafed Cold & Allergy	CH	PS		
Sudafed Cold & Cough Liquid Caps		PS	DM, GU	AC
Sudafed Nasal Decongestant		PS		
Sudafed Non-Drying Sinus Liquid Caps		PS	GU	
Sudafed PE		PE		
Sudafed PE Cold & Cough		PE	DM, GU	
Sudafed PE Multi-Symptom Severe Cold; Sudafed PE Nighttime	DI	PE		AC
Sudafed PE Nighttime Nasal Decongestant	DI	PE		
Sudafed PE Non-Drying Sinus		PE	GU	
Sudafed PE Sinus & Allergy	CH	PE		
Sudafed PE Sinus Headache		PE		AC
Sudafed Severe Cold Caplets; Sudafed Severe Cold Tablets		PS	DM	AC
Sudafed Sinus Nighttime Plus Pain Relief Caplets	DI	PS		AC
Sudafed 12 Hour Caplets, Sudafed 24 Hour		PS		
TheraFlu Cold & Cough		PE	DM	
TheraFlu Cold & Cough Nighttime Hot Liquid Regular Strength	CH	PS		
TheraFlu Cold & Sore Throat	PH	PE		AC
TheraFlu Daytime Severe Cold		PE	DM	AC
TheraFlu Daytime Severe Cold packets		PE		AC
TheraFlu Daytime Warming Relief Syrup		PE	DM	AC
TheraFlu Flu & Congestion Maximum Strength Non-Drowsy Hot Liquid		PS	DM	AC
TheraFlu Flu & Sore Throat	PH	PE		AC
TheraFlu Flu & Sore Throat Relief Syrup	DI	PE		AC
TheraFlu Flu Cold Medicine		PS		AC
TheraFlu Flu Cold Medicine for Sore Throat Maximum Strength		PS		AC
TheraFlu Nighttime Flu & Cough Maximum Strength Hot Liquid; TheraFlu Nighttime Severe Cold & Congestion Nighttime Maximum Strength Caplets	CH	PS	DM	AC
TheraFlu Nighttime Severe Cold	CH	PE	DM	
TheraFlu Nighttime Severe Cold Packet	PH	PE		AC
TheraFlu Nighttime Warming Relief Syrup	DI	PE		AC
TheraFlu Severe Cold & Congestion Maximum Strength Hot Liquid	CH	PS	DM	AC
TheraFlu Severe Cold & Congestion Non-Drowsy Maximum Strength Caplets		PS	DM	AC
TheraFlu Severe Cold & Congestion, Non-Drowsy Maximum Strength Hot Liquid		PS	DM, GU	AC
TheraFlu Thin Strips Daytime Cold & Cough	PH	PE	DM	
TheraFlu Thin Strips Nighttime Cold & Cough	DI	PE		
Triaminic AM Decongestant Syrup		PS		
Triaminic Chest		PS	GU	
Triaminic Chest & Nasal Congestion		PE	GU	
Triaminic Cold & Allergy	CH	PE		
Triaminic Cold & Allergy Softchews	CH	PS		
Triaminic Cold & Cough; Triaminic Cold & Cough Softchews; Triaminic Cold & Nighttime Cough	CH	PS	DM	
Triaminic Cough & Congestion Formula DM		PS	DM	
Triaminic Cough & Sore Throat Softchews DM, AC		PS	DM	AC
Triaminic Cough		PS	DM	
Triaminic Cough Sore Throat		PS	DM	AC
Triaminic Cough Softchews			DM	
Triaminic Day Time Cold & Cough		PE	DM	

(*continues*)

Table 20-2 Common Brands of Cold, Allergy, and Cough Remedies (*continued*)

Common Brand Names	Antihistamine	Decongestant	Cough Remedy	Analgesic
Triaminic Flu, Cough & Fever	CH	PS	DM	AC
Triaminic Nighttime Cough & Cold	DI	PE		
Triaminic Thin Strips Cold		PE		
Tylenol Allergy Multi-Symptom; Tylenol Allergy Multi-Symptom Cool Burst Caplets	CH	PE		AC
Tylenol Allergy Multi-Symptom Nighttime Cool Burst	DI	PE		AC
Tylenol Allergy Sinus Maximum Strength Caplets; Tylenol Allergy Sinus Maximum Strength Gelcaps; Tylenol Allergy Sinus Maximum Strength Geltabs	CH	PS		AC
Tylenol Allergy Sinus Nighttime Maximum Strength Caplets	DI	PS		AC
Tylenol Cold Day Non-Drowsy Multi-Symptom Caplets; Tylenol Cold Day Non-Drowsy Multi-Symptom Gelcaps		PS	DM	AC
Tylenol Cold Head Congestion Daytime Cool Burst Caplets		PE	DM	AC
Tylenol Cold Head Congestion Nighttime Cool Burst Caplets	CH	PE	DM	AC
Tylenol Cold Head Congestion Severe Cool Burst; Tylenol Cold Multi-Symptom Citrus Burst Liquid		PE	DM, GU	AC
Tylenol Cold Multi-Symptom Daytime; Tylenol Cold Multi-Symptom Daytime Citrus Burst Liquid; Tylenol Cold Multi-Symptom Daytime Cool Burst Caplets		PE	DM	AC
Tylenol Cold Multi-Symptom Nighttime Cool Burst Caplets	CH	PE	DM	AC
Tylenol Cold Multi-Symptom Severe Congestion Non-Drowsy Caplets		PS	DM, GU	AC
Tylenol Cold Multi-Symptom Severe Cool Burst		PE	DM, GU	AC
Tylenol Cold Nighttime Multi-Symptom Complete Formula Caplets	GH	PS	DM	AC
Tylenol Cough Medication with Decongestant Multi-Symptom; Tylenol Flu Day Non-Drowsy Maximum Strength Gelcaps		PS	DM	AC
Tylenol Flu Nighttime Maximum Strength	DO	PS	DM	AC
Tylenol Flu Nighttime Maximum Strength Gelcaps	DI	PS	AC	
Tylenol PM Extra Strength Caplets; Tylenol PM Extra Strength Gelcaps; Tylenol PM Extra Strength Geltabs; Tylenol Severe Allergy Caplets	DI			AC
Tylenol Sinus Congestion & Pain Daytime		PE		AC
Tylenol Sinus Congestion & Pain Nighttime	CH	PE		AC
Tylenol Sinus Congestion & Pain Severe		PE	GU	AC
Vicks 44 Cough Relief			DM	
Vicks 44D Cough & Head Congestion Relief		PS	DM	
Vicks 44E Cough & Chest Congestion Relief			DM, GU	
Vicks 44M Cough Cold & Flu Relief	CH	PS	DM	AC
Vicks DayQuil Cold/Flu		PE	DM	AC
Vicks DayQuil Multi-Symptom Cold/Flu Relief; Vicks DayQuil Multi-Symptom Cold/Flu Relief LiquiCaps		PS	DM	AC
Vicks DayQuil Sinus		PE		AC
Vicks NyQuil Cold & Flu Relief; Vicks NyQuil Cold & Flu Symptom Relief Plus Vitamin C	DO		DM	AC
Vicks NyQuil Cough; Vicks NyQuil Cough	DO		DM	
Vicks NyQuil D; Vicks NyQuil Multi-Symptom Cold/Flu Relief; Vicks NyQuil Multi-Symptom Cold/Flu Relief LiquiCaps	DO	PS	DM	AC
Vicks NyQuil Sinus	DO	PE		AC

Antihistamines: CI = clemastine; CH = chlorpheniramine; DI = diphenhydramine; DO = doxylamine; PH = pheniramine maleate; BR = dexbrompheniramine.
Decongestants: PE = phenylephrine; PS = pseudoephedrine.
Cough Preparations: DM = dextromethorphan; GU = guaifenesin.
Analgesics: AC = acetaminophen.
Sources: Adapted from Hansen WF et al. 2002[25]; US National Library and National Institute of Medicine 2009.[142]

Rebound Rhinitis (Rhinitis Medicamentosa)

Rebound congestion, also termed **rhinitis medicamentosa**, is an important side effect that can occur following prolonged use of topical decongestants.[20] As the profound local vasoconstrictive effect of the topical decongestant wears off, rebound swelling of the nasal mucosa and congestion develop. This phenomenon leads to continued, and at times increasing, use of the spray or drops in an attempt by the individual to relieve the congestion. When the longer-acting decongestants, imidazoline derivatives such as oxymetazoline (Afrin) were introduced in the 1960s, the risk of developing rebound rhinitis was believed to be small.[29] Further studies showed this was not the case.[30]

Research later found that healthy individuals who used the modern vasoconstrictors oxymetazoline or xylometazoline (e.g., Novorin, Sinutab nasal spray) for 7–21 days did not develop rebound rhinitis, while those with preexisting vasomotor rhinitis did.[31] Graf et al. pursued the relative contributions of the benzalkonium chloride, which is an ingredient that is common in decongestant preparations versus the decongestant itself. They found that both can induce rebound congestion, but benzalkonium chloride aggravates the severity and can induce rebound rhinitis after use of only a few days.[31]

Prolonged use of more than 30 days can lead to irreversible changes in the nasal mucosa.[32] Once an individual has developed a dependence on nasal decongestants, it can be a challenge to discontinue them. Research has shown that treatment with nasal corticosteroids at the time of decongestant withdrawal can ameliorate these symptoms.[33] Ipratropium bromide (Atrovent), on the other hand, reduces **rhinorrhea** but not congestion.[34] Individuals who are starting use of nasal corticosteroids when they already have significant congestion also may benefit from the short-term use of imidazoline decongestants.

Despite the risks associated with overuse of the long-acting decongestants, they do play a role in symptomatic rhinitis, whether from an upper respiratory infection or allergic rhinitis. With the common cold, short-term use to decrease congestion, especially at night, may allow for improved sleep.[31]

Cough Medicine, Expectorants, and Mucolytics

Postnasal drip is the most common etiology of the cough that accompanies the common cold. Cough medicines often are used to decrease the frequency of the cough, or as a cough suppressant or **antitussive**. Other preparations, **expectorants** or mucolytics, are used to assist in clearing the lungs of mucus. The benefit in use of these agents in decreasing the symptoms of the common cold is controversial. There is a paucity of evidence supporting any benefit of cough medicines for ameliorating symptoms of the common cold; therefore, their use is not recommended.[27,35] Conversely, a combination of a first-generation antihistamine and decongestant will lessen the cough associated with the common cold.

Naproxen (Naprosyn)

Naproxen (Naprosyn), a nonsteroidal anti-inflammatory drug (NSAID), is effective in decreasing cough, perhaps through inhibiting the inflammatory process associated with cold symptoms.[35] No studies were found investigating whether other NSAIDs might also provide this benefit.

Complementary/Alternative Regimens

Zinc lozenges and nasal spray have gained popularity over the last several years, since Mossad et al. reported their results of a study that demonstrated that the use of zinc gluconate lozenges (13.3 mg zinc) every 2 hours when awake significantly reduced the duration of cold symptoms from 7.6 days to 4.4 days ($P < .001$).[36] The theoretical mechanism for the observed beneficial effects is the belief that zinc competes for intercellular adhesion molecule (ICAM-1) receptor sites in the nasal mucosa, thereby preventing rhinoviruses from binding[37] and theoretical immunomodulation.[38]

Zinc has some potential side effects and adverse effects. The lozenges have a significant side effect profile, including foul taste and interference with the absorption of antibiotics.[39] Intranasal zinc administration has a significant risk of causing irreversible anosmia; i.e., loss of the sense of smell.[40] In 2009, the FDA banned nasal preparations of zinc because the risk of anosmia is unacceptably high. Based on a review of published research, the American College of Chest Physicians concluded that zinc preparations are not recommended in the treatment of common cold.[27]

Many over-the-counter cough lozenges contain menthol. Morice et al.[41] studied the effectiveness of menthol inhalation prior to inducing a cough challenge and found those subjects had reduced coughing when compared to a control group whose members inhaled either pine oil or air.

Saline irrigation has been shown to promote mucociliary clearance and removal of crusted mucus. Although saline sprays are often used to reduce congestion, there have not been any studies that confirmed any benefit.[42]

Special Populations: Pregnancy and Lactation

The nasal and respiratory tract mucosa become edematous as a response to the hormones present during pregnancy. Thus, nasal congestion is common during pregnancy and is more frequent as the pregnancy progresses.[43] With this physiologic change, the nasal symptoms of allergic rhinitis or upper respiratory infections are likely to be exacerbated.

Two major surveys have studied the extent of medication use during pregnancy. The National Birth Defect Prevention Study[44] is a population-based, case-control study of birth defects, conducted by performing standardized interviews of mothers of case subjects with major structural birth defects and control subjects with no major birth defects between 1997 and 2001. Mothers are asked specific questions about medications taken during pregnancy. The Boston University Slone Epidemiology Center Birth Defects Study conducts similar interviews and has presented its findings for women interviewed between 1998 and 2004.[45] In both of these studies, approximately 70–75% of pregnant women took an analgesic during pregnancy, 16–27% used a decongestant, 8–14% took an antihistamine, and 9–13% used some form of cough medicine. Surprisingly, these rates of medication use during pregnancy are higher than the reported rates during the 3 months prior to conception.[45]

None of the commonly used medications has been shown to be teratogenic, but without further research, it is impossible to state with confidence that they have no adverse effect on the fetus. In the absence of such studies, providers should caution pregnant women to avoid casual use of over-the-counter medications and offer suggestions for nonpharmacologic comfort measures instead.

Common Cold Among the Elderly

Pharmacologic therapy poses more risks in the elderly than in younger persons. The presence of comorbidities and other medications may preclude decongestant use. Confusion and altered mental status may be more common effects of cough preparations or antihistamines. Prior to recommending over-the-counter cold preparations, a complete medical history and documentation of medications used is essential. As with pregnant women,

it is prudent to offer suggestions for nonpharmacologic comfort measures rather than medications.

Acute Bronchitis

Bronchitis is an infection of the bronchi. An acute bronchitis usually is a secondary infection caused by a virus or bacteria and can last for several days or weeks in comparison to chronic bronchitis, which is prolonged irritation of the bronchial epithelium. More than 90% of cases of acute bronchitis are caused by viruses, with the rest being caused by *Chlamydia pneumoniae*, *Mycoplasma pneumoniae*, or *Bordetella pertussis*. *Streptococcus pneumoniae*, *Haemophilus influenzae*, and *Moraxella catarrhalis* are much less common causes, but they may be the etiology in individuals who have chronic lung conditions.

Acute bronchitis is a frequent reason for visits to the healthcare provider, and one of the most common causes of inappropriate prescribing of antibiotics.[46] Unlike the common cold, which rarely presents with systemic symptoms, acute bronchitis often causes such symptoms as fatigue and headaches, in addition to respiratory symptoms such as rhinorrhea, postnasal drip, dyspnea, and productive cough. The diagnosis of acute bronchitis should be considered for those whose cough persists longer than 5 days.[47] The cough of acute bronchitis often is accompanied by bronchial hyperreactivity and wheezing. Individuals with acute bronchitis rarely have accompanying fever, malaise, aches and pains, tachypnea, or rales. Individuals who present with a temperature > 100.4°F (38°C), pulse > 100 beats per minute, respiratory rate > 24 breaths per minute, or crackles on inspiration should be evaluated with a chest X-ray for pneumonia,[48] and those with a paroxysmal cough, especially one followed with emesis, should be evaluated for *B pertussis*.[49] Acute bronchitis usually resolves spontaneously within 3 weeks. Historically, treatment of acute bronchitis has fallen into one of the following three categories: antibiotics, cough suppression/expectorant, and bronchodilators.

Antibiotics

Smucny et al.[50] performed a meta-analysis of studies comparing antibiotic use with placebo for the treatment of acute bronchitis and found that antibiotics made no difference in improving night cough, frequency of productive cough, or duration of limitations on activities of daily living. Slight, albeit statistically significant decreases in the duration of cough (weighted mean difference [WMD] = 0.58 days; 95% CI, 0.01–1.16 days); duration of productive cough (WMD = 0.52 days; 95% CI, 0.01–1.03 days) and a general feeling of illness (WMD = 0.58 days; 95% CI, 0.00–1.16 days) were found, although the clinical significance of the finding is questionable.

Other reviews have failed to find any benefits from antibiotic use.[31-33] Assuming that, at best, there is a modest benefit of antibiotics and that there is the concern about developing antibiotic resistance, the routine use of antibiotics is not recommended for individuals with acute bronchitis who are otherwise healthy. Further research is necessary to provide guidance in the use of antibiotic use in various subsets of the population, such as smokers, those with asthma, or those with symptoms on the more severe end of the spectrum.

Cough Suppressants, Expectorants, and Mucolytics

Unlike their lack of efficacy in treating the common cold, cough medications may be effective in treating symptoms of bronchitis by acting on one of several pathways involved in the etiology of cough (Table 20-3). For example, a medication could alter the mucoid component, either by decreasing production, decreasing the viscosity, or improving ciliary function. Guaifenesin, which is a component of many cough medicine formulations, is a mucociliary drug and is theorized to increase volume and reduce viscosity of secretions in the trachea and bronchi. Originally derived from the guaiac tree and used by Native Americans, this agent was reported to be helpful in more study participants who used it compared to individuals who used a placebo in one study (75% versus 31%; $P < .01$),[51] but was no different than placebo in a second study ($P = .20$).[26] Interestingly, guaifenesin is also used by women to facilitate conception via thinning and increasing the amount of cervical mucus. There are no studies that have evaluated the effectiveness of this treatment.

Cough medications also may block the perception of the stimulus to cough, i.e., the afferent limb of the reflex. Two drugs, levodropropizine and moguisteine, have been found to be effective peripheral cough suppressants, but, unfortunately, are not available in the United States.[27] A third mechanism, which is probably the most common, is to suppress the cough reflex in the central nervous system. Codeine and dextromethorphan hydrobromide (Robitussin) are centrally acting cough suppressants. Both of these drugs have dissociative effects and therefore have the potential for abuse. Abuse of dextromethorphan is more prevalent than abuse of heroin, crack cocaine, methamphetamines, or anabolic steroids.[52] Coingestion of dextromethorphan and either MAO inhibitors or selective serotonin reuptake inhibitors (SSRIs) can result in serotonin syndrome,[53] which is characterized by delirium, agitation, tachycardia, diaphoresis, and hyperreflexia.[54] Recent research has found that most individuals do not have any risk of abuse to dextromethorphan; however, individuals with a CYP2D6 phenotype may be the persons at the highest risk. More information about this potential drug of abuse can be found in Chapter 9.

While there is consistent evidence to support the effectiveness of cough suppressants in the treatment of chronic bronchitis, they have not been shown to be effective in the treatment of acute bronchitis or the common cold. Despite the absence of adequate evidence of their

Table 20-3 Medications to Treat Cough

Drug Generic (Brand)	Dose	Level of Evidence*	Grade of Recommendation†	FDA Pregnancy Category
Mucociliary				
Guaifenesin (Mucinex)	200–600 mg PO qid	Good	D	C
Ipratropium	40–80 mcg inhaled qid	Fair	A	B
First-generation antihistamines	Refer to Chapter 13	Fair	A	B
Central Suppressants				
Codeine	10–20 mg PO tid–qid	Fair	B	C
Dextromethorphan polistirex (Delsym)	30 mg PO bid	Fair	C	C
Unclassified				
Benzonatate (Tessalon Perles)	100–200 mg PO tid	N/A	N/A	C
Zinc	Variable	Fair	D	N/A

* Good = evidence from randomized trials; Fair = evidence from controlled trials without randomization, cohort or case-control analytic studies, or comparisons between times or places.

† A = good evidence to recommend the action; B = fair evidence to recommend the action; C = existing evidence inconclusive and does not allow making a recommendation for or against the action; D = fair evidence to recommend against the action.

Source: Bolser DC 2006.[27]

use in acute bronchitis, the American College of Chest Physicians concluded that it is reasonable to employ them to reduce severe coughing.[55] Dextromethorphan hydrobromide is only available in the United States in combination with other drugs such as promethazine (Phenergan), pseudoephedrine, or brompheniramine, but another preparation, dextromethorphan polistirex (Delsym), is available over the counter packaged alone.[56] Benzonatate (Tessalon Perles) is a local anesthetic that can decrease cough. It is used for the treatment of opioid-resistant cough associated with lung cancer.[57] However, no evidence was found to support its use in treatment of an acute cough.

Beta₂ Agonists

The use of beta$_2$ agonists has been suggested to treat the bronchial reactivity and subsequent decreased airflow and wheezing associated with acute bronchitis. Beta$_2$ agonists activate the beta$_2$-adrenergic receptors, which increases cyclic adenosine monophosphate (cAMP), promoting bronchodilation, reducing bronchospasm, and suppressing histamine release.[3] A Cochrane review found that while there was little evidence to support the routine use of beta$_2$ agonists in the treatment of acute bronchitis, they may be effective for reducing coughing for those with evidence of airflow obstruction.[58]

Complementary and Alternative Treatments

Observational research has supported the benefit from a liquid herbal drug preparation of *Pelargonium sidoides* (EPs 7630) purported to have antibacterial and antiviral capabilities.[59] Further well controlled RCTs are needed before conclusions can be made about its efficacy.

Chinese medicinal herbs are also employed to treat the symptoms of bronchitis. Various herbs are compounded depending on the specific array of symptoms for any given individual. Some of the herbs that have been studied include yu xing cao, radix Scutellaria, radix glycyrrhizae, and Shi Wei Long Dan Hua Ke Li. While a review of the literature demonstrated some benefit, the methodologic quality of included studies was poor. There was no standardization of the purity of the herbs, nor of their dosing, nor of which herbs were included. None of the studies were blinded, and the outcomes were poorly defined. There was little information on any adverse effects of the herbs. This area is another category of herbal/pharmacologic treatment that warrants further study.[59]

Influenza

When compared to the viruses responsible for the common cold or acute bronchitis, influenza viruses cause significantly more morbidity and mortality. The onset of symptoms tend to be more acute and severe, including sore throat, cough and rhinitis, high fever, headaches, muscle aches, and extreme fatigue. In the United States, more than 200,000 persons are hospitalized from complications of influenza each year, and about 36,000 die.[60] Complications are more common among children younger than 5 years of age and adults older than 65 years of age. Mortality from complications such as pneumonia and exacerbations of chronic diseases are more common in adults over the age of 65.[60]

Two major types of influenza virus exist—influenza A and influenza B.[60] Both viruses are spread primarily by respiratory droplet transmission. Influenza A is more prone to **antigenic shifts** than influenza B is, which is why influenza A is associated with pandemics. Influenza B viruses undergo less dramatic and slower antigenic changes, known as **antigenic drift**. While these distinctions are critical for epidemiologic surveillance and vaccine development, they cannot be differentiated on the basis of clinical presentation. Moreover, antibodies against one strain of influenza virus do not confer immunity to other strains.

Following an incubation period of 1–4 days, symptoms (fever, headaches, muscle aches sore throat, cough, rhinitis, and fatigue) develop abruptly. While most of the symptoms resolve after 3–7 days in the majority of persons, the cough and malaise may continue for more than 2 weeks. Because of the overlapping symptoms with other illnesses, it is difficult to make a firm diagnosis of influenza based on clinical presentation.[60] Young children are likely to have atypical presentations, while in the elderly, the presence of fever and cough is less specific for influenza than in the general population.[60] Rapid diagnostic tests are available with sensitivities of around 70–70% and specificities of 90–95%, but they are not currently used in clinical practice. The likelihood of false positives is higher in times of low prevalence, such as toward the beginning and end of the flu season rather than the peak; therefore, influenza is usually treated empirically.[60] Influenza can lead to complications such as viral pneumonia, secondary bacterial pneumonia, or sinusitis, and it can exacerbate comorbidities.

Annual vaccination against influenza is the primary weapon against the infection and subsequent complications and is discussed in Chapter 6. A major challenge to influenza control is the low vaccination coverage in populations for whom vaccination is recommended.[60]

Antiviral Medications

Antiviral medications play a role in both chemoprophylaxis and treatment for influenza. Oseltamivir (Tamiflu) and zanamivir (Relenza) are neuraminidase inhibitors, effective against both influenza A and B. Amantadine (Symmetrel, Symadine) and rimantadine (Flumadine) are antivirals approved for the treatment of influenza, but they should no longer be used because influenza A has high levels of resistance to these medications. When used for treatment, both oseltamivir and zanamivir should be initiated within 2 days of the onset of symptoms. Such use has been associated with a 0.8-day decrease in duration of symptoms in healthy adults (95% CI, 0.3–1.3),[61] and approximately 50% reduction in hospitalizations.[62] Initiation of treatment later than 2 days after the development of symptoms has no effect on the duration of uncomplicated influenza, and there are no data available concerning any potential benefit on decreasing complications. Concern has been expressed that the majority of influenza that occurred during the 2009 flu season may be resistant to oseltamivir, illustrating one of the challenges of prescribing today.[63]

Chemoprophylaxis with Antivirals

Oseltamivir (Tamiflu) and zanamivir (Relenza) also can be used for chemoprophylaxis by individuals who have contraindications to vaccination or those at high risk for developing complications (e.g., individuals who are immunosuppressed). In this case, either antiviral should be taken daily throughout the community flu season. Chemoprophylaxis may also be appropriate for individuals who have an increased risk for complications and who are vaccinated after the flu season has begun but have not yet developed antibodies (approximately 2 weeks in adults). Chemoprophylaxis may also be appropriate in the event of an influenza outbreak with a strain not included in the vaccine; or in a residential setting such as a nursing home despite adequate vaccination. The recommended doses for oseltamivir and zanamivir are listed in Table 20-4.

Mechanism of Action

Oseltamivir (Tamiflu) and zanamivir (Relenza) both inhibit neuraminidase, an enzyme required for viral replication. Oseltamivir is well absorbed after oral administration. The drug is metabolized by the liver to oseltamivir carboxylate, the active neuraminidase inhibitor. Oseltamivir carboxylate has a half-life of 6–10 hours and is excreted in the urine by glomerular filtration and tubular secretion.

Zanamivir (Relenza) is administered as inhaled powder; with 70–87% being deposited in the oropharynx and approximately 7–21% of the orally inhaled zanamivir dose reaching the lungs. A small amount of the total amount of orally inhaled zanamivir is systemically absorbed. Systemically absorbed zanamivir has a half-life of 2.5–5.1 hours and is excreted unchanged in the urine. Unabsorbed drug is excreted in the feces.[64]

Side Effects/Adverse Effects

Nausea and vomiting occur in approximately 10% of adults taking oseltamivir compared to 4–6% of those taking placebo.[63,65] Thus, individuals taking the agent should be aware of these reactions and be closely monitored for signs of unusual behavior while taking oseltamivir.

Zanamivir (Relenza) is approved only for individuals without underlying respiratory or cardiac disease.[64] For persons with uncomplicated influenza, the frequency of adverse

Table 20-4 Recommended Daily Dose of Influenza Antiviral Medications for Treatment and Chemoprophylaxis—United States

Drug (Generic) Brand	Indication	Age Group (Years)	
		13–64	≥ 65
Zanamivir (Relenza)*	Treatment, influenza A and B	10 mg (2 inhalations) bid	10 mg (2 inhalations) bid
	Chemoprophylaxis, influenza A and B	10 mg (2 inhalations) bid	10 mg (2 inhalations) bid
Oseltamivir (Tamiflu)†	Treatment, influenza A and B	75 mg bid	75 mg bid
	Chemoprophylaxis, influenza A and B	75 mg/day	75 mg/day

* Zanamivir is manufactured by GlaxoSmithKline (Relenza—inhaled powder). Zanamivir is approved for treatment of persons aged 7 years and older and approved for chemoprophylaxis of persons aged 5 years and older. Zanamivir is administrated through oral inhalation by using a plastic device included in the medication package. Individuals will benefit from instruction and demonstration of the correct use of the device. Zanamivir is not recommended for those persons with underlying airway disease.
† Oseltamivir is manufactured by Roche Pharmaceuticals (Tamiflu—tablet). Oseltamivir is approved for treatment or chemoprophylaxis of persons aged 1 year and older. No antiviral medications are approved for treatment or chemoprophylaxis of influenza among children < 1 year of age. This information is based on data published by the Food and Drug Administration (FDA).
Source: Adapted from Fiore AE et al. 2007.[60]

effect was no different for individuals inhaling zanamivir compared to the inhaled lactose vehicle alone.[66] No specific drug interactions have been reported.[60]

Special Populations

Pregnancy and Lactation

Pregnant women are at a higher risk for complications including pneumonia from influenza than the general population.[60] It is recommended that all women who are or plan to be pregnant during flu season be vaccinated against influenza. As no clinical studies have evaluated the use of oseltamivir and zanamivir in pregnancy, they are categorized as FDA Pregnancy Category C medications. It is recommended that lactating women who were not immunized during pregnancy receive either the inactivated or live attenuated influenza vaccine in the postpartum period.[61]

The Elderly

Individuals who reside in any residential setting, such as assisted care facilities or nursing homes, should all be vaccinated at the same time before the onset of the influenza season. No reduction in the dose of oseltamivir or zanamivir is needed on the basis of age.[60]

Community-Acquired Pneumonia

Community-acquired pneumonia is an infection of the pulmonary parenchyma that is acquired in the community, as opposed to the hospital or other healthcare facilities.[67] It is the sixth leading cause and most common infectious cause of death in the United States, and a significant cause of morbidity.[67] Between 31% and 49% of low-risk individuals who access the emergency room with community-acquired pneumonia are admitted to the hospital.[68] As with influenza, prevention is an important component in the control of pneumonia. The Advisory Committee on Immunization Practices of the CDC advises that in addition to receiving influenza vaccination, individuals ≥ 65 years of age or with high-risk conditions, including chronic cardiovascular, respiratory, renal or liver disease, diabetes mellitus, alcoholism, or immunosuppression; residents of long-term care facilities; and Native Americans and Alaskan natives receive the pneumococcal polysaccharide vaccine.[69]

The pathophysiology of pneumonia involves a failure of the usual defense systems to protect the lower airways from colonization with pathogens. Microorganisms can gain access and take hold due to ineffective ciliary action,

---

> ## Box 20-2 Risk Factors for Community-Acquired Pneumonia
>
> Previous episode of pneumonia or chronic bronchitis
>
> Age > 65 years
>
> Alterations in level of consciousness
>
> Smoking
>
> Chronic obstructive pulmonary disease
>
> Bronchiectasis
>
> Use of H_2 blockers, proton pump inhibiters, or antacids
>
> Immotile cilia syndrome
>
> Alcohol consumption
>
> Cystic fibrosis
>
> Immunosuppression
>
> *Source:* Adapted from Mandell LA et al. 2007.[68]

---

decreased mucus velocity, interference with IgA, or an innate virulence of the pathogen. The most common route of exposure is by microaspiration. Any underlying condition that compromises an individual's defenses can increase the risk of pneumonia. Box 20-2 lists common risk factors.

The use of proton pump inhibitors may be associated with an increased risk of community-acquired pneumonia.[70] Implementation of guidelines for the management of community-acquired pneumonia has been associated with decreases in important clinical outcomes such as mortality and rate of hospitalization.[68] The decision regarding the appropriate site of care for individuals with community-acquired pneumonia is critical, and validated guidelines for determining who needs hospitalization versus who can be managed on an outpatient basis are available (Box 20-3). The Pneumonia Severity Index[71,72] and the British Thoracic Society Criteria[73,74] are two sets of validated criteria that the clinician can use to guide management.[76,77]

Once the diagnosis of community-acquired pneumonia has been made on the basis of clinical presentation confirmed by chest X-ray and the decision made that the individual is appropriate for outpatient therapy, further diagnostic tests are optional. Most will respond well to empiric antibiotic therapy. The most common

---

Box 20-3 A Case of a Cough

DS, a 54-year-old nurse, reports having a productive cough and fatigue for 2 weeks. She has mild intermittent asthma but has been using salmeterol (Advair) for the last week, thinking her cough was related to her asthma. She was treated for rhinosinusitis 4 weeks ago with amoxicillin (Amoxil) 500 mg three times a day for 10 days with fair relief of her symptoms.

Further questioning reveals that this cough was not preceded by any upper respiratory symptoms. While she feels generally under the weather, she denies any headache, muscle aches, or pains, except pain associated with her cough. Her physical exam is significant for a temperature of 100.8°F and respiratory rate 28; no wheezing is auscultated, but she does have crackles on inspiration in her right lower lobe.

The differential diagnosis for DS includes bronchitis, influenza, pneumonia, and tuberculosis. When questioned about possible exposure to tuberculosis, DS reports her tuberculin skin test was negative 3 months ago, and she doesn't believe she has been exposed to anyone with tuberculosis. Because her major symptom is cough unrelated to systemic symptoms such as headache or malaise, she is unlikely to have influenza. Bronchitis is usually preceded by an upper respiratory infection and is rarely associated with fever or tachypnea. As she has a low-grade fever and is tachypneic, the most likely diagnosis in community-acquired pneumonia. Following the Infectious Diseases Society of America/American Thoracic Society consensus guidelines, a chest X-ray is taken, and it confirms the diagnosis.

DS's condition is compatible with outpatient therapy. Because she has recently received antibiotic treatment, she is at risk for drug-resistant *S. pneumoniae*. Therefore, the best treatment is moxifloxacin (Avelox) 400 mg by mouth daily for 5 days. If she is still febrile after 3 days, the treatment should be extended to 7 days.

---

causative organisms in ambulatory, immunocompetent adults include *Streptococcus pneumoniae*, *Mycoplasma pneumoniae*, *Haemophilus influenzae*, and *Chlamydia pneumoniae*.[75] Respiratory viruses, including influenza, adenovirus, respiratory syncytial virus, and parainfluenza, are responsible for about as many cases as each of the above bacteria.[75]

Treatment of Community-Acquired Pneumonia

One concern about empiric treatment is the increasing drug resistance of *S pneumoniae*. Worldwide resistance of *S pneumoniae* to penicillins has been noted to be from 18.2% to 22.1%.[76] From 1987 through 2005, macrolide resistance with *S pneumoniae* has increased from 0.2% to 29.6% but appears to have leveled off since 2000.[77] Of the three macrolides, erythromycin, clarithromycin, and azithromycin, azithromycin is the least effective against *S pneumoniae* and has been most responsible for macrolide resistance, especially when used at subtherapeutic levels.[77] The ketolide telithromycin (Ketek), while similar in structure to the macrolides, has alterations that prevent

resistance in *S pneumoniae* by the two common mechanisms of macrolide resistance. Telithromycin is unique in having two binding sites, and to date, resistance is uncommon.[77] Due to several severe adverse effects, including hepatic toxicity, telithromycin is FDA approved for treatment of community-acquired pneumonia only and has an FDA black box warning on the label that notes the risk of hepatic toxicity.

In addition to macrolide resistance, *S pneumoniae* has developed significant beta-lactam resistance. Resistance to the fluoroquinolones, ciprofloxacin (Cipro) and levofloxacin (Levaquin), has also been noted. However, community-acquired pneumonia usually responds to appropriate regimens of amoxicillin (Amoxil), ceftriaxone (Rocephin), or cefotaxime (Claforan). Risk factors for drug-resistant *S pneumoniae*, include recent or repeated treatment with macrolides, fluoroquinolones, or beta-lactams, age ≥ 65, residence in a long-term care facility, and day care attendance should be considered when choosing the most appropriate antibiotic regimen.[76] The consensus guidelines of the Infectious Diseases Society of America and the American Thoracic Society for recommended antibiotic treatment of community-acquired pneumonia are presented in Table 20-5.

Table 20-5 Antibiotics Recommended for Outpatient Treatment of Community-Acquired Pneumonia

Otherwise healthy and no risk factors for drug-resistant *S pneumoniae*:

    A. Macrolide (erythromycin [EES], clarithromycin [Biaxin], azithromycin [Zithromax]) (strong recommendation; level I evidence*)

    B. Doxycycline (Vibramycin) is weak recommendation; level III evidence.*

Presence of comorbidities; alcoholism; malignancy; immunosuppression; use of antibiotics within the previous 3 months (a different class of drugs should be selected); other risks for drug-resistant *S pneumoniae*; or in regions with high prevalence of high-level macrolide-resistant *S pneumoniae*:

    A. Moxifloxacin (Avelox), gemifloxacin (Factive), or 750 mg of levofloxacin (Levaquin). Strong recommendation, level I evidence.*

    B. A beta-lactam (high-dose amoxicillin, e.g., 1 g tid) *plus* a macrolide or 2 g bid of amoxicillin-clavulanate (Augmentin). Strong recommendation, level I evidence.* Alternatives include ceftriaxone (Rocephin), cefpodoxime (Vantin), and 500 mg bid of cefuroxime (Ceftin); doxycycline (Vibramycin) is then the alternative to the macrolide. Level II evidence.*

* Level 1 evidence = evidence from well-conducted randomized controlled trials; level II evidence = evidence from well-designed trials without randomization, cohort or case-control studies, or large case series; level III evidence = evidence from case studies and expert opinion. *Source:* Adapted from Mandell LA et al. 2007.[68]

Duration of Treatment

Treatment durations of more than 5 days or regimens that use low-dose antibiotics have been associated with an increased risk of nasal colonization with penicillin-resistant *S pneumoniae*.[78] Community-acquired pneumonia has traditionally been treated for 7–10 days, although this duration was not evaluated by well-controlled studies. Several studies have demonstrated comparable efficacy with shorter durations of therapy, including use of beta-lactams in inpatients,[79] levofloxacin (Levaquin) 750 mg for 5 days versus 500 mg for 10 days,[80] 320 mg gemifloxacin (Factive) for 5 days versus 7 days,[81] and azithromycin (Zithromax) 500 mg for 3 days versus clarithromycin (Biaxin) 250 mg bid for 10 days.[82] Shorter duration of therapy can improve adherence to the regimen and reduce the emergence of resistance organisms.[83] The Infectious Diseases Society of America/American Thoracic Society Consensus Guidelines recommend that before discontinuing therapy, individuals with community-acquired pneumonia be treated for at least 5 days, be afebrile for 48–72 hours, and be clinically stable.[67]

Special Populations

Pregnancy

The incidence of pneumonia in pregnant women is similar to the incidence in the nonpregnant population of women, but with the physiologic changes in the respiratory system during pregnancy, the risk of complications, including need for mechanical ventilation, bacteremia, and empyema, is higher.[84] Asthma and use of corticosteroids for fetal lung maturation have been associated with an increased risk of pneumonia in pregnancy.[85,86] The standard management of pneumonia in pregnancy includes admission to the hospital, although a retrospective study assessing the application of either the Pneumonia Severity Index or the CURB-65 criteria to pregnant women suggests that the criteria for site of treatment may be equally applicable in pregnancy, and that hospital admission could be avoided in 25% of cases.[87] Empiric treatment with beta-lactam and macrolide antibiotics is safe and effective in pregnant women.

The Elderly

Elderly individuals are at increased risk for the development of pneumonia, may present with fewer signs or symptoms than younger individuals, and are less likely to be febrile. Tachypnea may be the most sensitive sign of pneumonia in the elderly.[67] Recommended antibiotics for the elderly are the same as for younger populations after an evaluation of other medications used and possible drug–drug interactions has been conducted.

Rhinosinusitis

Rhinosinusitis is the infection of one of the paranasal sinuses, usually following an upper respiratory infection, that leads to inflammation of the sinuses; it is somewhat arbitrarily classified as acute, subacute, chronic, or recurrent (Table 20-6).

Since this disorder is accompanied by inflammation of the nasal mucosa, rhinosinusitis has replaced sinusitis as the preferred term.[88] In the vast majority of persons afflicted, the viral URI and resultant inflammation resolve spontaneously within 10 days with no complications; however,

Table 20-6 Classification of Rhinosinusitis

Classification	Description
Acute	Symptoms last 7–10 days but less than 4 weeks, which may include purulent discharge, nasal congestion, postnasal drainage, facial pain, headache, fever, cough
Subacute	Unresolved acute rhinosinusitis, with symptoms lasting 4–8 weeks
Chronic	Symptoms lasting at least 8 weeks
Recurrent	Three or more episodes of acute rhinosinusitis per year

Source: Adapted from Slavin RG et al. 2005.[95]

the inflammation from the preceding viral URI prevents drainage of the sinuses, which sets the stage for bacterial infection in the sinuses. In the small number who do not recover spontaneously from the initial viral infection, a secondary acute aerobic bacterial infection (acute bacterial rhinosinusitis) develops, usually secondary to *S. pneumoniae*, *H. influenzae*, or *M. catarrhalis*. Over time, if the acute bacterial infection persists, the ongoing edema, compromised blood supply, and oxygen consumption by the aerobes, anaerobic bacteria, and coagulase-negative begin to take hold.[89] Antibiotics should not be prescribed earlier than 7–10 days after onset of symptoms in the absence of severe face pain, fever, or periorbital edema.

Acute Bacterial Rhinosinusitis

It is difficult to distinguish clinically between viral respiratory infections affecting the sinuses and **acute bacterial rhinosinusitis**. Unfortunately, there are no cost-effective, accurate, readily available office-based diagnostic tests. While the gold standard for diagnosis is the growth of at least 10^5 organisms from aspiration of secretions via sinus puncture, this is an invasive procedure and not indicated in uncomplicated cases.[89]

The Agency for Healthcare Research and Quality performed a meta-analysis to compare the efficacies of antibiotics and placebo in the treatment of acute bacterial rhinosinusitis.[90] Thirty-nine studies were included, with a total of 15,739 subjects, conducted from 1997 to 2004. Approximately two thirds of the persons recovered without receiving antibiotics, supporting the premise that antibiotics are often overused. Antibiotics did, however, decrease the likelihood of no improvement within 7–14 days by 25–30% ($P < .01$). In the short term, amoxicillin-clavulanate (Augmentin) was more effective than cephalosporins. The Sinus and Allergy Health Partnership promulgated guidelines for the treatment of acute bacterial rhinosinusitis in 2004.[91] These guidelines recommend treating individuals whose symptoms have not improved over the course of 10 days or have worsened after 5–7 days. They further classify individuals into two groups for initial therapy: (1) those with mild symptoms and no antibiotic use in the past 4–6 weeks, and (2) those with moderate symptoms or who have used antibiotics within 6 weeks. Depending on local patterns of antibiotic resistance, amoxicillin (Amoxil) or amoxicillin-clavulanate (Augmentin) is a reasonable first-choice antibiotic based on efficacy, cost, and side-effect profile (Table 20-7).

If there is no improvement within 72 hours of antibiotic therapy, the individual should be reevaluated, and changing the antibiotic should be considered.[53] There are limited data available regarding the optimal duration of therapy. A cure rate of 80–90% with a 10- to 14-day

Table 20-7 Antibiotics Used for Treatment of Acute Bacterial Rhinosinusitis

Drug Generic (Brand)	Route	Dose	FDA Pregnancy Category
Mild Disease with No Recent Antibiotic Use (Past 4–6 Weeks)			
Amoxicillin*	PO	1.5 g–4 g/day	B
Amoxicillin/clavulanate (Augmentin)*	PO	1.75 g–4 g/250 mg/day	B
Cefpodoxime proxetil (Vantin)*	PO	200–800 mg/day	B
Cefuroxime axetil (Ceftin)*	PO	500–1000 mg/day	B
Cefdinir (Omnicef)	PO	600 mg/day	B
If Beta-Lactam Allergic			
TMP/SMX DS (Bactrim DS)	PO	320 mg/1.6 g/day	C
Doxycycline (Vibramycin)	PO	200 mg/day	D
Azithromycin (Zithromax)*	PO	500 mg day 1, then 250 mg/day	B
Clarithromycin (Biaxin)*	PO	1 g/day	C
Mild Disease with Previous Antibiotic Use or Moderate Disease			
High-dose amoxicillin/clavulanate (Augmentin)*	PO	4 g/250 mg/day	B
Respiratory Fluoroquinolones			
Levofloxacin (Levaquin)	PO, IV	500–750 mg/day	C
Moxifloxacin (Avelox)	PO, IV	400 mg/day	C
Ceftriaxone (Rocephin)*	IM, IV	1–2 g/day	B

* Generic available.
Sources: Jackson LL et al. 2005[97]; Scheid DC et al. 2004.[92]

treatment can be expected.[92] One study found a 5-day course of azithromycin also to be effective.

Persons who present with severe unilateral maxillary pain, swelling, and fever should be treated regardless of the duration of symptoms. With the exception of these severely ill individuals, watchful waiting for 7–10 days should not increase the incidence of complications and will avoid many unnecessary courses of antibiotics.

Adjunctive Therapy

Inhaled nasal corticosteroids are potent anti-inflammatory agents and can be important adjuncts to antibiotic use in the treatment of both acute and chronic sinusitis, offering faster resolution of symptoms.[94] Steroids decrease vascular permeability, inhibit release and/or formation of histamine and leukotrienes, and prevent infiltration of inflammatory cells.[95]

There is little evidence as to the benefit or lack thereof of oral decongestants, whose vasoconstrictive properties may provide relief of symptoms. Common side effects of decongestants include increased blood pressure, central nervous system stimulation, and urinary retention.[95] Caution should be used when considering the use of oral decongestants for persons with coronary artery disease or hypertension. While over-the-counter nasal decongestants are often used to decrease congestion and have evidence supporting their short-term use with colds,[20] the FDA has ruled that any indication of use for sinusitis be removed from labeling.[96] If oral decongestants are used, their use should be limited to 3 days to avoid rebound congestion (rhinitis medicamentosa).

The use of antihistamines in the treatment of acute rhinosinusitis has no supporting evidence. The only theoretical benefit might be for individuals with a significant component of allergic rhinitis as well as acute bacterial rhinosinusitis.

Subacute Rhinosinusitis

Subacute rhinosinusitis is usually secondary to partial or inadequate treatment of acute rhinosinusitis. Treatment includes changing antibiotics and reinforcing completion of a 14- to 21-day course.

Chronic Rhinosinusitis

Individuals with rhinosinusitis symptoms that persist at least 8 weeks will benefit from referral to an otolaryngologist or allergist for further evaluation. Research supports the use of inhaled nasal steroids and saline irrigation, as well as treatment for any comorbidity.[97] High doses of guaifenesin (1200 mg bid), which is an expectorant found in many products such as Robitussin and sold as a single drug under the brand names Mucinex and Organidin NR, has been used based on its efficacy in the treatment of chronic bronchitis.

Allergic Rhinitis

Increasingly, the similarities between allergic rhinitis and asthma are leading to the concept of one airway, one disease.[98] The mucosa and submucosa are similar, with a pseudostratified epithelium, vessels, mucous glands, and nerves. While the nasal mucosa is more highly vascularized, the bronchi are characterized by smooth muscle. Both the nasal mucosa and the bronchi have similar inflammatory responses. Comorbidity is common; 80–90% of persons with asthma report nasal symptoms.[99] In addition, observational studies have demonstrated that the incidence of asthma complications is decreased by adequate treatment of allergic rhinitis.[100] Despite this interrelationship and the importance of concomitant treatment, the medications employed for these two entities are presented separately for the sake of clarity.

Allergic rhinitis, which may be either seasonal or perennial, is characterized by nasal congestion, sneezing, rhinorrhea, itchy or watery eyes, and headache. The pathology involves early-phase and late-phase symptoms. Early-phase symptoms such as rhinorrhea, nasal obstruction, sneezing, and pruritus are probably mediated through immunoglobulin E activation of mast cell and basophil release of histamine and leukotrienes. The late-phase reaction includes not only the symptoms of the early phase, but also increased nasal obstruction and inflammation from the recruitment of eosinophils, monocytes, and basophils.[100]

The treatment of allergic rhinitis is based on the severity and frequency of symptoms and personal preferences.[102] Management options for allergic rhinitis include oral and topical antihistamines (also known as H_1-receptor antagonists), oral and nasal decongestants, intranasal corticosteroids, intranasal cromolyns, and leukotriene receptor antagonists, intranasal anticholinergics, and immunotherapy[101] (Table 20-1). Omalizumab (Xolair), an antibody that binds IgE, may be available for the treatment of allergic rhinitis in the near future.

Antihistamines

Because of their proven safety and efficacy, second-generation antihistamines are recommended for the treatment of mild to moderate allergic rhinitis. First-generation antihistamines are associated with an unfavorable risk-benefit profile due to effects such as sedation, dry mouth, constipation, urinary hesitancy, and tachycardia. The second-generation antihistamines are safer, have more specific H_1-receptor selectivity, faster onset, and longer duration, and they have fewer side effects than first-generation antihistamines. Thus, they have replaced the first-generation agents as the first line of treatment.[100] Azelastine (Astelin) is a topical second-generation antihistamine that is administered as an intranasal spray twice daily. The efficacy of this agent is comparable to the oral second-generation antihistamines, and its only commonly reported side effect is a bitter taste.[101] Chapter 13 presents a thorough discussion of antihistamines.

Intranasal Corticosteroids

Intranasal corticosteroids are the mainstay of pharmacologic therapy for persons with moderate to severe symptoms or those in whom symptoms persist despite use of second-generation antihistamines.[103] All the formulations available in the United States contain either an aqueous or powder vehicle.[3] These agents have potent, long-acting, anti-inflammatory effects, reducing eosinophil infiltration, suppressing the expression of cytokines, and reducing the release of histamine and leukotrienes.[103] Although systemic corticosteroid use is associated with significant adverse effects, the minimal systemic absorption and rapid first-pass metabolism by the liver avoid such side effects with intranasal corticosteroid administration.[103] Intranasal corticosteroids have been found to be more efficacious in the relief of the nasal symptoms of allergic rhinitis than topical antihistamines,[104] oral antihistamines, nasal cromolyn, or leukotriene receptor antagonisits.[104] With its effect of decreasing nasal secretions, nasal ipratropium (Atrovent) may be considered as adjunctive therapy for individuals with profuse rhinorrhea.

Intranasal Cromolyns

Cromolyn sodium (NasalCrom) is a mast cell stabilizer that prevents the release of histamine and other mediators of inflammation. Minimal amounts are absorbed systemically and the drug is excreted unchanged. Cromolyn sodium is less effective than intranasal corticosteroids. One disadvantage of cromolyn is that it should be administered 4–6 times per day. On the other hand, it can block symptoms even when used shortly before exposure to allergens, such as cat dander. Intranasal cromolyn is an FDA Pregnancy Category B drug, and it has minimal side effects.

Leukotriene Receptor Antagonists

Leukotrienes cause nasal congestion by increasing vascular permeability and vasodilation. Medications that block the leukotriene receptor are able to decrease nasal congestion. Leukotriene receptor antagonists have no effect on sneezing or itching.[104] When used as monotherapy, they are not as effective as second-generation antihistamines or nasal steroids.[104] The combination of leukotriene receptor antagonists and second-generation antihistamines was more effective than either alone, but not better than inhaled nasal corticosteroids.[104]

The leukotriene receptor antagonist montelukast (Singulair) was approved for the treatment of allergic rhinitis in December 2002. This drug is absorbed rapidly after oral administration, and has a half-life of 2.7–5.5 hours. Leukotriene receptor antagonists are metabolized by the liver and excreted in the bile. Unique among the leukotriene receptor antagonists, montelukast does not have any significant drug interactions. These agents are in FDA Pregnancy Category B. However, postmarketing research identified a small but significant association between montelukast (Singulair), zafirlukast (Accolate), and zileuton (Zyflo and Zyflo CR) and the development of neuropsychiatric symptoms. Symptoms include agitation, aggression, anxiousness, dream abnormalities and hallucinations, depression, insomnia, irritability, restlessness, suicidal thinking and behavior (including suicide), and tremor. These medications must now have an FDA black box warning on their labels that states there is an increased risk of depression and suicide in persons who use these agents.

Immunotherapy

Immunotherapy is effective for improving symptoms of allergic rhinitis[105] and subsequent development of asthma and atopic dermatitis. The benefits from immunotherapy persist long after the treatment is finished. In the United States, only subcutaneous injections of increasing doses of allergen are available. A 2006 review of the literature on sublingual immunotherapy by the joint task force of the American College of Allergy, Asthma and Immunology and the American Academy of Allergy, Asthma and Immunology concluded that there is clear evidence supporting the benefits of sublingual therapy, but its adoption in the United States is compromised by lack of standard doses, treatment schedules, or duration of treatment. There is no sublingual allergy extract approved for use in the United States.[106]

Special Populations

Pregnancy

Twenty to forty percent of women have allergies, and as many as 30% experience worsening symptoms during pregnancy.[107] In addition, under the influence of the hormones of pregnancy, many women experience a physiologic nasal congestion, referred to as "rhinitis of pregnancy." This mucosal change can make it challenging to discriminate between rhinitis of pregnancy and other causes of rhinitis, while at the same time it can amplify the symptoms associated with comorbid conditions such as an upper respiratory infection, sinusitis, or allergic rhinitis. A detailed history will help to make the correct diagnosis.

Chlorpheniramine (Chlor-Trimeton), loratadine (Claritin), and cetirizine (Zyrtec) are FDA Pregnancy Category B drugs and believed to be safe if used at recommended doses. For those whose symptoms are not relieved by oral antihistamines, inhaled corticosteroids provide an apparently safe option. Very little of the corticosteroid is absorbed systemically. Only budesonide (Rhinocort) is an FDA Pregnancy Category B drug, so perhaps it should be the first choice for initiating inhaled steroid therapy during pregnancy. None of the other nasal corticosteroids has systemic effects at therapeutic doses, so there is no need to change medications if the woman has been using a different nasal corticosteroid prior to the pregnancy.[107]

▌ Asthma

Asthma is a significant contributor to morbidity in the United States. Approximately 22 million individuals suffer from asthma.[108] Asthma affects 7.2% of the adult population and accounts for 13.6 million office visits and 1.8 million emergency department visits each year. Asthma affects proportionally more children than adults and is more common in African Americans and among those with lower incomes.[109]

Asthma is a chronic disorder of the airways that is characterized by bronchial hyperresponsiveness, inflammation, and airway obstruction. Acute symptoms usually are due to bronchospasm, but it is the inflammation

---

Box 20-4 Nonpharmacologic Treatment of Asthma: Gone But Not Forgotten

In the mid-1500s, the physician of the archbishop of Saint Andrews removed pillows and a feather bed, and thereafter, the clergyman noticed immediate relief from his asthma. This event has been heralded as one of the earliest cases of manipulating environmental controls to treat allergic symptoms, an approach that remains integral to therapy today.

Nonpharmaceutical agents remain important in the overall treatment plan for individuals with respiratory conditions. Foremost is the reduction of exposure to allergens. Common allergens include dust mites, dander from animals, tobacco smoke, pollen, and molds.

---

that causes impaired airflow and hyperresponsiveness. Research suggests that the inflammatory process of asthma can lead to airway remodeling, which may not be prevented or treated with use of current therapies.[108]

Airborne allergens and viral respiratory infections during infancy are major environmental risk factors for asthma (Box 20-4). Exposure to house dust mites and cockroaches is an important cause of allergic sensitization. Tobacco smoke, air pollution, and diets low in antioxidants and omega-3 fatty acids are also associated with asthma.[108]

Genetics play a complex role in asthma. There are many genes involved in the clinical development of asthma, and polymorphisms can affect individual responses to treatment with both beta$_2$ agonists and corticosteroids. Further study of the differing phenotypes may lead to improved targeted treatments. There is an increasing body of evidence suggesting that polymorphisms of the gene encoding the site of action of beta$_2$ agonists have an association with the clinical response to beta$_2$ agonist therapy.[110]

While a complete discussion of the management of asthma is beyond the scope of this chapter, it is worthwhile to present a broad overview. Readers are referred to Expert Panel Report 3: *Guidelines for the Diagnosis and Management of Asthma* (2007)[108] for a comprehensive presentation of the diagnosis and management of asthma.

Exercise-Induced Bronchospasm

In some individuals, exercise is the only precipitant of asthma symptoms. Pretreatment with either short-acting beta$_2$ agonists or long-acting beta$_2$ agonists prior to exercising will prevent exercise-induced bronchospasm in the majority of such individuals. Daily pretreatment with long-acting beta$_2$ agonists has been shown to shorten the duration of that protection.

Categorization of Asthma Severity

The severity categories were previously classified as mild intermittent, mild persistent, moderate persistent, and severe persistent, but as of 2007, it has been recognized that intermittent asthma, which occurs episodically, interspersed with symptom-free periods, may present with moderate or severe symptoms. The newer category, therefore, is labeled "intermittent," and this category has no severity qualifier. Table 20-8 describes the initial classifications recommended as the basis for initiation of therapy, and Table 20-9 describes the characteristics of well-controlled, not well-controlled, and poorly controlled asthma. These terms become guides for adjusting therapy.

Certain comorbid conditions can aggravate an individual's asthma symptoms, and conversely, treatment of

those conditions can help improve asthma management. Gastroesophageal reflux disease (GERD), rhinosinusitis, obesity, obstructive sleep apnea, and allergic bronchopulmonary aspergillosis all compromise asthma control. Chronic stress or depression may also play a role, but the evidence is not as clear for a relationship between asthma and depression. Stress or depression may affect asthma severity directly, via increased production of proinflammatory mediators, or indirectly via poorer adherence to treatment regimens. Certain medications, such as aspirin and beta-blockers, are recognized precipitants of asthma, as are the sulfites found in shrimp, dried fruit, beer, and wine.

Nonpharmacologic Treatment of Asthma

While pharmacologic therapy is essential for the control of asthma, it is not sufficient in and of itself. Avoidance of environmental immunotherapy (allergy desensitization shots) factors and treatment of comorbid conditions is also critical. Clinicians should evaluate the role that allergens,

Table 20-8 Classifying Asthma Severity and Initiating Treatment Among Adolescents and Adults

| Components of Severity | Classification of Asthma Severity > 12 Years of Age | | | |
| | Intermittent | Persistent | | |
		Mild	Moderate	Severe
Symptoms	≤ 2 days/wk	≥ 2 days/wk, but not daily	Daily	Throughout the day
Nighttime awakenings	≤ 2 days/month	3–4 × /month	> 1/wk but not nightly	Often nightly
Short-acting beta agonist use for symptom control	≤ 2 days/wk	≥ 2 days/wk, but not daily, and not more than 1 × per day	Daily	Several times/day
Interference with ADL	None	Minor limitation	Some limitation	Extremely limited
Lung function	-Normal between exacerbations -FEV$_1$ > 80% predicted -FEV$_1$/FVC normal	-FEV$_1$ > 80% predicted -FEV$_1$/FVC normal	FEV$_1$ > 60% < 80% predicted -FEV$_1$/FVC reduced 5%	FEV$_1$ < 60% predicted FEV$_1$/FVC reduced > 5%
Exacerbations requiring oral systemic corticosteroids	0–1/year	≥ 2/year		
	Consider severity and interval since last exacerbation. Frequency and severity may change over time for persons in any category. Relative annual risk of exacerbations may be related to FEV$_1$.			
Recommended step for initiating treatment	Step 1	Step 2	Step 3	Step 4 or 5
			and consider short course of oral systemic corticosteroids	
	In 2–6 weeks, evaluate level of asthma control and adjust therapy accordingly.			

ADL = activities of daily living, FEV$_1$ = forced expiratory volume in 1 sec; FVC = forced vital capacity.

- Level of severity is determined considering both impairment and risk. Assess impairment by recall of prior 2–4 weeks and spirometry. Classify severity by most severe category of any feature.
- The stepwise approach is intended to assist, not replace, clinical decision making.
- In general, more frequent exacerbations indicate greater underlying disease severity. Those who require oral corticosteroids for exacerbations ≥ twice in a year may be considered as having persistent asthma.

Sources: Third Expert Panel on the Management of Asthma 2007[108]; Centers for Disease Control and Prevention 2005.[109]

Table 20-9 Assessing Asthma Control and Adjusting Therapy

Components of Control	Classification of Asthma Control for Persons > 12 Years of Age		
	Well Controlled	Not Well Controlled	Very Poorly Controlled
Symptoms	≤ 2 days/wk	≥ 2 days/wk	Throughout the day
Nighttime awakenings	≤ 2 days/mo	1–3 × /wk	Often nightly
Short-acting beta-agonist use for symptom control	≤ 2 days/wk	> 2 days/wk	Several times/day
Interference with ADL	None	Some limitation	Extremely limited
Lung function	FEV_1 > 80% predicted/personal best	FEV_1 > 60 < 80% predicted/personal best	FEV_1 < 60% predicted/personal best
Risk: Exacerbations requiring oral systemic corticosteroids	0–1/year	≥ 2/year	
	Consider severity and interval since last exacerbation.		
Risk: Progressive loss of lung function	Evaluation requires long-term follow-up care.		
Risk: Treatment-related adverse effects	Medication side effects can vary widely. The degree of intensity does not correlate to level of control, but should be considered in overall assessment of risk.		
Recommended treatment	Maintain current treatment. Regular follow-up every 3–6 months. Consider step down if well controlled for at least 6 months.	Step up one step and reevaluate in 2–4 wks. For side effects, consider alternative treatment options.	Consider short course of oral systemic corticosteroids. Step up 1–2 steps and reevaluate in 2 wks. For side effects, consider alternative treatment options.

ADL = activities of daily living; FEV_1 = forced expiratory volume in 1 sec; FVC = forced vital capacity.

- Level of severity is determined considering both impairment and risk. Assess impairment by recall of prior 2–4 weeks and spirometry. Classify severity by most severe category of any feature. Symptom assessment for longer periods reflect global assessment, such as asking if the individual's asthma is better or worse since the last visit.
- The stepwise approach is intended to assist, not replace, clinical decision making.
- In general, more frequent exacerbations indicate greater underlying disease severity. Those who require oral corticosteroids for exacerbations ≥ twice in a year may be considered as having not-well-controlled asthma.
- Before step-up therapy, review adherence to medication, inhaler technique, environmental control, and comorbid conditions. If an alternate treatment option was used in a step, discontinue and use the preferred treatment for that step.

Sources: Third Expert Panel on the Management of Asthma 2007[108]; Centers for Disease Control and Prevention 2005.[109]

both indoor and outdoor, may contribute to asthma symptoms and work with the individual to identify strategies to avoid exposure to such allergens. Skin testing may be beneficial. Immunotherapy offers the additional benefit of improving allergic rhinitis and atopy.

Pharmacologic Treatment of Asthma

Pharmacologic treatment is the key to asthma control. Appropriate therapy is based on the severity of the symptoms. Pharmacologic therapy for asthma includes short-term quick-relief medications and medications that provide long-term relief of bronchospasm. The short-term or quick-acting drugs are either beta$_2$ agonists, anticholinergics, corticosteroids, or a mixed formulation of beta$_2$ agonists and corticosteroids. The long-term control medications are inhaled corticosteroids (ICS), long-acting beta$_2$ agonists, combination formulations of

inhaled corticosteroids and long-acting beta$_2$ agonists, leukotriene modifiers, and cromolyn, which does not belong to any other class. Individuals with persistent asthma usually require both types of medications.

Many asthma medications are delivered directly to the lungs via metered-dose inhalers (MDIs), dry-powder inhalers (DPIs), or nebulizers. MDIs should be actuated during a slow, deep inspiration, followed by breath holding for 10 seconds. DPIs are actuated by the initiation of a rapid, deep inhalation. The delivery of the medication is flow dependent and is lost if the individual exhales after actuating the device but before inhaling.[108]

In the past, MDIs employed chlorofluorocarbons as propellants, and those that do so have the abbreviation *CFC* following the drug name. However, because chlorofluorocarbons contribute to reducing the earth's ozone layer, the FDA mandated that albuterol CFC be discontinued as of December 31, 2008 (Box 20-5). Most manufacturers have incorporated an alternative propellant, hydrofluoroalkane

Box 20-5 Metered-Dose Inhalers in Transition

Several types of the most commonly used metered-dose inhalers (MDIs) are being discontinued within the next few years. MDIs available for over-the-counter self-treatment, including one that is frequently prescribed for quick relief and two prescription inhalers used for long-term treatment are all being pulled from the market. What is happening here?

Metered-dose inhalers that contain chlorofluorocarbons (CFCs) are being discontinued because the CFCs that are used as propellants in these inhalers decrease the protective ozone layer above the earth. In 1987, the United States signed an international agreement called the Montreal Protocol on Substances That Deplete the Ozone Layer, and all signers agreed to discontinue sale of all products that decrease the ozone layer over a set period of time. In January of 2006, the FDA mandated that manufacture of these medications be phased out. Epinephrine CFC (Primatene Mist) will be discontinued as of December 31, 2011. Albuterol CFC ceased being sold December 31, 2008.

There has been significant controversy over this change. Persons with intermittent asthma or bronchospasm frequently self-treat their bronchospasm with over-the-counter preparations of epinephrine such as Primatene Mist. Some experts feel over-the-counter access to bronchodilators saves lives, decreases emergency room visits, and provides a safe stopgap for individuals who do not have a prescription bronchodilator available. The over-the-counter preparations are much less expensive than those obtained by prescription. However, there are no other over-the-counter bronchodilators available on the market at this time.

Albuterol CFC (ProAir, Proventil, Ventolin) has been the most frequently prescribed MDI worldwide.[123] In this case, manufacturers are changing from CFCs to hydrofluoroalkane (HFA) propellants, which act somewhat differently. These differences are important because they affect how the drug is administered. HFA inhalers taste different than the CFC formulations, and the force of the spray is softer, but more importantly, they must be cleaned and primed or the medication will not be dispersed when the MDI is used. Instructions for cleaning and priming are in the package instructions and should be reviewed with individuals when a prescription is furnished.

Finally, two of the drugs used for long-term control of asthma may no longer be recommended for treatment of asthma. Formoterol (Foradil) and salmeterol (Serevent) can cause worsening asthma symptoms and are associated with increased asthma-related morbidity and mortality. The FDA is currently reviewing studies of these two drugs to evaluate the recommendation that they no longer be indicated for treating asthma.

(HFA), which does not appear to have an effect on the ozone layer. HFA MDIs have the additional benefit of producing smaller droplets, which allow greater delivery to the lungs.[3] Unlike the MDIs that use CFCs as a propellant, the HFA MDIs require priming and periodic cleaning. Each formulation has a slightly different requirement, which necessitates detailed reading of the instructions that come with the inhaler.

Isoproterenol (Isuprel) has been discontinued as an inhaler; the metaproterenol inhaler (Alupent Aerosol) remains available by prescription. An FDA committee voted in January 2006 to take epinephrine (Primatene Mist) and Albuterol CFC (ProAir, Proventil, Ventolin) off the market due to ozone-damaging chlorofluorocarbons, and these products are disappearing from pharmacy shelves. The Expert Panel does not recommend the use of any of these medications for the treatment of asthma.[108]

Quick-Relief Medications for Treating Asthma

Short-Acting Beta$_2$ Agonists

Inhaled, short-acting beta$_2$ agonists are the most effective medications available for the relief of bronchoconstriction and prevention of exercise-induced bronchospasm[108] (Tables 20-10 and 20-11). Short-acting beta$_2$ agonists reverse bronchoconstriction and improve airflow within 3–5 minutes of use. The peak effect occurs in 30 minutes and the duration of action is 4 hours. These medications are inhaled via use of an MDI. A significant amount of inhaled medication does not reach the lungs, being deposited in the oropharynx. The use of a spacer or valved holding chamber enhances delivery to the lungs (Figure 20-3).

Table 20-10 Quick-Relief Medications for Treatment of Asthma

Drug Generic (Brand)	Formulation	Indications/Mechanisms	Potential Adverse Effects	Clinical Considerations
Short-Acting Beta₂ Agonists				
Albuterol sulfate (ProAir HFA, Proventil HFA, Ventolin HFA) Levalbuterol tartrate (Xopenex HFA) Pirbuterol (Maxair)	Oral MDI Nebulizer	Relief of acute symptoms; quick-relief medication. Preventive treatment for EIB prior to exercise. Causes bronchodilation. Binds to beta₂-adrenergic receptor, producing smooth-muscle relaxation.	Tachycardia, skeletal muscle tremor, hypokalemia, increased lactic acid, headache, hyperglycemia. Inhaled route, in general, causes few systemic adverse effects. Persons with preexisting cardiovascular disease, especially the elderly, may have adverse cardiovascular reactions with inhaled therapy.	Drugs of choice for acute bronchospasm. Inhaled route has faster onset, fewer adverse effects, and is more effective than systemic routes. For individuals who have intermittent asthma, regularly scheduled daily use neither harms nor benefits asthma control. Regular use > 2 days/week for symptom control, increasing use, or lack of expected effect indicates inadequate asthma control.
Anticholinergics				
Ipratropium bromide (Atrovent)	MDI Nebulizer	Relief of acute bronchospasm. Causes bronchodilation via competitive inhibition of muscarinic cholinergic receptors. Reduces intrinsic vagal tone of the airways. May block reflex bronchoconstriction secondary to irritants. May decrease mucus.	Drying of mouth and respiratory secretions, increased wheezing in some individuals, blurred vision if sprayed in eyes.	Reverses only cholinergically mediated bronchospasm; does not modify reaction to antigen. Does not block EIB. Multiple doses of ipratropium provide additive effects to SABA. May be alternative for those who do not tolerate SABA. Treatment of choice for bronchospasm due to beta-blocker medication.
Systemic Corticosteroids				
Methylprednisolone Prednisolone Prednisone	Oral	For short-term (3–10 days) burst: to gain prompt control of inadequately controlled persistent asthma.	Short-term use: reversible abnormalities in glucose metabolism, increased appetite, fluid retention, weight gain, mood alteration, hypertension, peptic ulcer, and rarely aseptic necrosis. Long-term use: adrenal axis suppression, growth suppression, dermal thinning, hypertension, diabetes, Cushing's syndrome, cataracts, muscle weakness, and—in rare instances—impaired immune function.	Use at lowest effective dose. For long-term use, alternate-day AM dosing produces the least toxicity. If daily doses are required, one study found improved efficacy with no increase in adrenal suppression when administered at 3 PM rather than in the morning. Consideration should be given to coexisting conditions that could be worsened by systemic corticosteroids.

MDI = metered-dose inhaler; EIB = exercise-induced bronchospasm; SABA = short-acting beta agonist.
Sources: Third Expert Panel on the Management of Asthma 2007[108]; Centers for Disease Control and Prevention 2005.[109]

Albuterol (Pro-Air HFA, Proventil HFA, Ventolin HFA) has been the drug most frequently used to treat bronchospasm, with approximately 52 million prescriptions filled per year in the United States. Albuterol consists of (R)-enantiomers and (S)-enantiomers, of which only the (R)-enantiomer is therapeutically active. In vitro studies suggest that the (S)-enantiomer actually might decrease smooth-muscle responsiveness. These findings prompted the development of levalbuterol (Xopenex), which contains only the active enantiomer. The majority of clinical trials have not demonstrated any clinical advantage of levalbuterol over albuterol.[108]

Table 20-11 Usual Doses of Quick-Relief Medications for Treatment of Asthma*

Drug Generic (Brand)	Dose per Activation	Adult Dose	Clinical Considerations
Inhaled Short-Acting Beta₂ Agonists MDI			
Albuterol HFA (ProAir HFA, Proventil HFA, Ventolin HFA)	MDI 90 mcg/puff, 200 puffs/ canister DPI 200 mcg/capsule	2 puffs every 4–6 hours as needed 1–2 capsules q 4–6 hours as needed	An increasing use or lack of expected effect indicates diminished control of asthma.
Levalbuterol tartrate (Xopenex HFA)	MDI 45 mg/actuation	2 puffs every 4–6 hours as needed	Not recommended for long-term daily treatment. Regular use exceeding 2 days/week for symptom control (not prevention of EIB) indicates the need to step up therapy. Differences in potency exist, but all products are essentially comparable per puff. May double usual dose for mild exacerbations. Should prime the inhaler by releasing 4 actuations prior to use. Periodically clean HFA activator, as drug may block/plug orifice.
Pirbuterol (Maxair)	MDI 200 mcg/puff	2 puffs every 4–6 hrs as needed	Only breath-actuated MDI available.
Inhaled Short-Acting Beta₂ Agonists Nebulizer Solutions			
Albuterol nebulizer solution	0.63 mg/3 mL 1.25 mg/3 mL 2.5 mg/3 mL 5 mg/mL (0.5%)	1.25–5 mg in 3 cc of saline q 4–8 hours as needed	May mix with budesonide inhalant suspension, cromolyn, or ipratropium nebulizer solutions. May double dose for severe exacerbations.
Levalbuterol (R-albuterol) nebulizer solution (Xopenex)	0.31 mg/3 mL 0.63 mg/3 mL 1.25 mg/0.5 mL 1.25 mg/3 mL	0.63 mg–1.25 mg q 8 hours as needed	Compatible with budesonide inhalant suspension. The product is a sterile-filled, preservative-free, unit dose vial.
Anticholinergics			
Ipratropium HFA MDI (Atrovent HFA) MDI	17 mcg/puff, 200 puffs/canister	2–3 puffs q 6 hours	Evidence is lacking that anticholinergics produce added benefit to beta₂ agonists in long-term control of asthma therapy.
Ipratropium HFA nebulizer	0.25 mg/mL (0.025%)	0.25 mg q 6 hours	
Combination Anticholinergic and Short-Acting Beta₂ Agonists			
Ipratropium with albuterol MDI (Combivent)	MDI 18 mcg/puff of ipratropium bromide and 90 mcg/puff of albuterol, 200 puffs/canister	2–3 puffs q 6 hours	Contains EDTA to prevent discoloration of the solution. This additive does not induce bronchospasm. Ipratoprium is not recommended for quick relief and is not FDA approved for this indication.
Ipratropium with albuterol nebulizer (DuoNeb)	0.5 mg/3 mL ipratropium bromide and 2.5 mg/3 mL albuterol	3 mL q 4–6 hours	

MDI = metered-dose inhaler; CFC = chlorofluorocarbon-containing; HFA = hydrofluoroalkane; EDTA = ethylenediaminetetraacetic acid; EIB = excercise-induced bronchospasm; DPI = dry-powder inhaler.
* Formulations that contain chlorofluorocarbons are being phased out and will no longer be available as soon as current supplies are exhausted.
Sources: Third Expert Panel on the Management of Asthma 2007[108]; Centers for Disease Control and Prevention 2005.[109]

The recommended treatment of intermittent asthma is short-acting beta agonists as needed, but if the need exceeds use twice a week (unless for the prevention of exercise-induced bronchospasm), initiating anti-inflammatory therapy, i.e., inhaled corticosteroid, is indicated. There is no evidence that regular use of short-acting beta agonists, when compared to as-needed use, offers any benefit, and, in fact, can lead to decreased lung function and control in some individuals.[108] There is an increasing body of evidence suggesting persons with the genotype Arg/Arg experience decreased lung function when treated with as-needed albuterol (Pro-Air HFA, Proventil HFA, Ventolin HFA).[111]

Adverse effects of current short-acting beta agonists are rare due to the selectivity of their beta₂-adrenergic agonist activity. This is not the case for older, nonselective agents such as isoproterenol (Isuprel) or metaproterenol (Alupent). These short-acting beta₂ agonists may cause excessive cardiac stimulation, especially if used in excessively high doses, and therefore these medications are not regularly used for outpatient treatment.

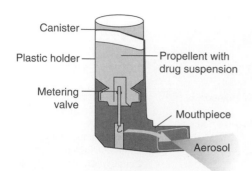

- Hold the inhaler upright and shake several times.
- Hold the mouthpiece in any of the following 2 correct positions.
    1) Seal your mouth around the mouthpiece.
    2) Hold the mouthpiece 1 to 2 inches away from your lips (a spacer may also be used).
- Do not block the inhaler opening with your tongue.
- Press down on the inhaler as you start to breathe in.
- Breathe in slowly and steadily over 3 to 5 seconds.
- Remove the inhaler from your mouth.
- Hold your breath for 10 seconds.
- Breathe out slowly.
- Rinse your mouth if using an inhaler containing corticosteroids.
- Store in dry place.

Figure 20-3 How to use a metered-dose inhaler. *Source:* Adapted from Hackley B 2007.[141]

Anticholinergics

Anticholinergics are selective antagonists of muscarinic receptors, and therefore they only reverse bronchospasm that is secondary to cholinergic input. There is a highly variable response to these agents, which is probably secondary to individual variation in parasympathetic tone and the degree of cholinergic involvement in the bronchospasm. It appears that individuals who have psychogenic exacerbations of asthma respond well to anticholinergics.

The anticholinergic used today is ipratropium bromide (Atrovent). Following administration of this agent, bronchodilation develops slowly and lasts up to 6 hours. Formulations that combine ipratropium bromide and short-acting beta$_2$ agonists generally induce better and longer lasting bronchodilation than either agent used alone.

Systemic Corticosteroids

Systemic corticosteroids are also considered quick-relief medications. These agents decrease inflammation and mucus production in the airways. Although they do not act quickly, they are used in conjunction with short-acting beta agonists for moderate and severe exacerbations and should be avoided for long-term control. One should administer systemic steroids in short courses for exacerbations in order to minimize adverse effects, which are related to both dose and duration of systemic corticosteroids.[108]

Long-Term Therapy for Treating Asthma

Inhaled corticosteroids are the mainstay for the long-term treatment of asthma. These agents are the most effective long-term therapy available for persistent asthma and are associated with few side effects. Other medications for the long-term control of asthma include long-acting beta$_2$ agonists, leukotriene receptor antagonists, immunomodulators, methylxanthines, and cromolyn sodium (NasalCrom) or nedocromil (Tilade). While none of these is as effective as inhaled corticosteroids, there may be roles for them, either when added to treatment with inhaled corticosteroids (combination therapy)[108] or as stand-alone therapy.

Inhaled Corticosteroids

Inhaled corticosteroids are potent anti-inflammatory agents that have several physiologic effects. Steroids inhibit the production and/or release of inflammatory mediators such as cytokines and leukotrienes, decrease the infiltration of eosinophils, and reduce airway edema by decreasing vascular permeability.[3] Inhaled corticosteroids improve every measurable aspect of asthma, including pulmonary function, quality of life, prevention of exacerbations, and reductions of hospitalizations, emergency visits, and deaths.[108]

Doses for inhaled corticosteroids vary significantly, depending on the preparation and delivery system. Table 20-12 displays the usual low, medium, and high doses for the currently available inhaled corticosteroids. Table 20-13 lists the medications used for long-term control. For individuals with mild or moderate asthma, increasing the dose of the inhaled corticosteroids leads to modest, at best, improvement in asthma control. Individuals with mild to moderate asthma who are started on low doses of inhaled corticosteroids show just as much improvement as those started on higher doses. In addition, many individuals with mild to moderate asthma are controlled with once-daily dosing. The Expert Panel Report notes that individuals whose asthma has been well controlled for 2 months with high-dose inhaled corticosteroids tolerate a 50% decrease in the dose without loss of control. A dose–response relationship remains in those with asthma.[108] Some individuals, such as smokers and African American children with poor

Table 20-12 Estimated Comparative Daily Doses for Inhaled Corticosteroids

Drug Generic (Brand)	Formulations	Low Daily Dose	Medium Daily Dose	High Daily Dose*
Beclomethasone HFA (QVAR)	MDI 42 or 84 mcg/actuation[†]	169–504 mcg 2–6 puffs of 84 mcg	> 504–840 mcg 6–10 puffs of 84 mcg	> 840 mcg > 10 puffs of 84 mcg
Budesonide (Pulmicort)	DPI 90, 180, or 200 mcg/actuation[‡]	200–400 mcg 1–2 inhalations	> 400–600 mcg 2–3 inhalations	> 600 mcg > 3 inhalations
Flunisolide (Flovent)	DPI 50, 100, or 250 mcg/actuation	500–1000 mcg 2–4 puffs	> 1000–2000 mcg 4–8 puffs	> 2000 mcg > 8 puffs
Flunisolide HFA (Flovent HFA)	MDI 44, 110, or 220 mcg/actuation	88–264 mcg 2–6 puffs of 44 mcg	> 264–660 mcg 2–6 puffs of 110 mcg	> 660 mcg > 6 puffs of 110 mcg
Mometasone (Asmanex)	DPI 220 mcg/actuation	220 mcg 1 puff	660–880 mcg 2–3 puffs	> 880 mcg > 4 puffs
Triamcinolone acetonide (Azmacort)	MDI 100 mcg/actuation	400–1000 mcg 4–10 puffs	1000–2000 mcg 10–20 puffs	> 2000 mcg > 20 puffs

DPI = dry-powder inhaler; HFA = hydrofluoroalkane; MDI = metered-dose inhaler.

The most important determinant of appropriate dosing is the clinician's judgment of the individual's response to therapy. The clinician must monitor the person's response on several clinical parameters and adjust the dose accordingly. The stepwise approach to therapy emphasizes that once control of asthma is achieved, the dose of medication should be carefully titrated to the minimum dose required to maintain control, thus reducing the potential for adverse effect.

* Some doses may be outside package labeling, especially in the high-dose range.

[†] MDI doses are expressed as the actuator dose (the amount of the drug leaving the actuator and delivered to the individual), which is the labeling required in the United States. This is different from the dose expressed as the valve dose (the amount of drug leaving the valve, not all of which is available to the person), which is used in many European countries and in some scientific literature.

[‡] DPI doses are expressed as the amount of drug in the inhaler following activation.

Notes: Comparative doses are based on published comparative clinical trials. The rationale for some key comparisons is summarized as follows: The high dose is the dose that appears likely to be the threshold beyond which significant hypothalamic-pituitary adrenal (HPA) axis suppression is produced, and, by extrapolation, the risk is increased for other clinically significant systemic effects if used for prolonged periods of time.

The low and medium doses reflect findings from dose-ranging studies in which incremental efficacy within the low- to medium-dose ranges was established without increased systemic effect as measured by overnight cortisol excretion. The studies demonstrated a relatively flat dose-response curve for efficacy at the medium-dose range; that is, increasing the dose of high-dose range did not significantly increase efficacy but did increase systemic effect.

Sources: Third Expert Panel on the Management of Asthma 2007[108]; Centers for Disease Control and Prevention 2005.[109]

control, have a relative insensitivity to inhaled corticosteroids therapy and present more challenges for therapy.[108]

The bioavailability of inhaled corticosteroids is significantly lower than the bioavailability of oral systemic corticosteroids; therefore there is less risk of serious side effects associated with inhaled corticosteroids compared to the risks associated with oral agents. Potential systemic effects of inhaled corticosteroids include a reduction in growth velocity in children's bone mineral density, immunosuppression, ocular effects, hypothalamic-pituitary-adrenal axis function, and glucose metabolism.[108] There appears to be a small, dose-related decrease in bone mineral density in adults,[112] but no increase in fractures was found in an observational study of older adults of 65 years of age or more who used less than 2000 mcg/day of inhaled corticosteroids.[113] Long-term inhaled corticosteroid use by adults, especially in high doses, has been associated with cataracts[114] and elevated intraocular pressure in adults,

although only in those with a family history of glaucoma.[115] There is no evidence that low- or medium-dose inhaled corticosteroid use leads to immunosuppression or altered hypothalamic-pituitary-adrenal axis function.[108]

Local adverse effects of inhaled corticosteroids include oral candidiasis, dysphonia (hoarseness), and reflex cough and bronchospasm. While most persons with asthma who use inhaled corticosteroids frequently will have positive throat cultures for candida, clinical thrush is much less common, especially at low doses.[116] Use of a spacer with non–breath-activated MDIs and rinsing the mouth after inhalation may help to prevent thrush, and topical or oral antifungals should be used to treat clinical infections.

Long-Acting Beta$_2$ Agonists

The long-acting beta$_2$ agonists salmeterol (Serevent) and formoterol (Foradil) are selective beta$_2$ agonists with increased

Table 20-13 Asthma Medications for Long-Term Control

Drug Generic (Brand)	Formulation	Indications/Mechanisms	Adverse Effects	Clinical Considerations
Corticosteroids: Inhaled				
Beclomethasone dipropionate (Qvar)	MDI	Long-term prevention of symptoms. Suppression, control, and reversal of inflammation. Reduce need for oral corticosteroid.	Cough, dysphonia, oral thrush (candidiasis). In high doses, systemic effects may occur, although studies are not conclusive, and clinical significance of these effects has not been established. In low to medium doses, suppression of growth velocity has been observed in children, but this effect may be transient, and the clinical significance has not been established.	Spacer/holding chamber devices with nonbreath-activated MDIs and mouth washing after inhalation decrease local side effects. Preparations are not absolutely interchangeable. The risks of uncontrolled asthma should be weighed against the limited risks of ICS therapy. Adjustable-dose approach to treatment may enable reduction in cumulative dose of ICS treatment over time without sacrificing maintenance of asthma control.
Budesonide (Pulmicort)	DPI			
Flunisolide (AeroBid)	MDI			
Fluticasone propionate (Flovent Diskus, Flovent HFA)	DPI MDI			
Mometasone furoate (Asmanex Twisthaler)	DPI			
Triamcinolone Acetonide (Azmacort)	MDI			
Immunomodulators				
Omalizumab (Xolair) Anti-IgE	SQ	Long-term control and prevention of symptoms in adults (≥ 12 years old) who have moderate or severe persistent allergic asthma inadequately controlled with ICS.	Pain and bruising of injection sites has been reported in 5–20% of asthmatics. Anaphylaxis has been reported in 0.2% of treated individuals. Malignant neoplasms were reported in 0.5% compared to 0.2% receiving placebo; relationship to drug is unclear.	Monitor individuals following injection. Be prepared and equipped to identify and treat anaphylaxis that may occur. The dose is administered either every 2 or 4 weeks and is dependent on the person's body weight and IgE level before therapy. A maximum of 150 mg can be administered in one injection. Needs to be stored under refrigeration at 2–8°C. Whether persons will develop significant antibody titers to the drug with long-term administration is unknown.
Leukotriene Receptor Antagonists (LTRAs)				
Montelukast tablets and granules (Singulair)	Oral	Long-term control and prevention of symptoms in mild persistent asthma for those ≥ 1 year of age. May also be used with ICS as combination therapy in moderate persistent asthma.	No specific adverse effects have been identified. Rare cases of Churg-Strauss have occurred, but the association is unclear.	May attenuate EIB for some individuals but less effective than ICS therapy. Do not use LTRA + LABA as a substitute for ICS + LABA. Administration with meals decreases bioavailability; take at least 1 hour before or 2 hours after meals.

(continues)

Table 20-13 Asthma Medications for Long-Term Control *(continued)*

Drug Generic (Brand)	Formulation	Indications/Mechanisms	Adverse Effects	Clinical Considerations
Leukotriene Receptor Antagonists (LTRAs)				
Zafirlukast tablets (Accolate)			Postmarketing surveillance has reported cases of reversible hepatitis and, rarely, irreversible hepatic failure resulting in death and liver transplantation.	Zafirlukast is a microsomal P450 enzyme inhibitor that can inhibit the metabolism of warfarin. INRs should be monitored during coadministration. Discontinue use if signs and symptoms of liver dysfunction occur. Hepatic enzymes (ALT/AST) should be monitored.
5-Lipoxygenase Inhibitor				
Zileuton tablets (Zyflo)	Oral	Long-term control and prevention of symptoms in mild, persistent asthma for those ≥ 12 years of age. May be used with ICS as combination therapy in moderate persistent asthma for those ≥ 12 years of age.	Elevation of liver enzymes has been reported. Limited case reports of reversible hepatitis and hyperbilirubinemia.	Zileuton is a microsomal P450 enzyme inhibitor that can inhibit the metabolism of warfarin and theophylline. Doses of these drugs should be monitored accordingly. Monitor hepatic enzymes (ALT/AST).
Long-Acting Beta$_2$ Agonists (LABA)				
Formoterol (Foradil)*	DPI	Long-term prevention of symptoms, added to ICS. Prevention of EIB. Compared to SABA, salmeterol has slower onset of action (15–30 minutes). Both salmeterol and formoterol have longer duration (> 12 hours) compared to SABA.	Tachycardia, skeletal muscle tremor, hypokalemia, prolongation of QT interval in overdose. Diminished bronchoprotective effect may occur within 1 week of chronic therapy. Clinical significance has not been established. Potential risk of uncommon, severe, life-threatening, or fatal exacerbation of asthma.	Not to be used to treat acute symptoms or exacerbations. Should not be used as monotherapy for long-term control of asthma or as anti-inflammatory therapy. May provide more effective symptom control when added to standard doses of ICS compared to increasing the ICS dose. Clinical significance of potentially developing tolerance is uncertain, because studies show symptom control and bronchodilation are maintained. Decreased duration of protection against EIB may occur with regular use.
Salmeterol (Serevent)*	DPI			
Combination Corticosteroid and Long-Acting Beta$_2$ Agonists				
Fluticasone/ salmeterol (Advair)	MDI Diskus DPI	Long-term control of chronic asthma.	Same as for LABAs. Corticosteroids associated with oral candidiasis, adrenal suppression. Vary rare anaphylactic reaction in persons with milk protein allergy.	Same as for LABAs. CYP3A4 inhibitors such as ketoconazole increase concentrations of fluticasone and/or budesonide, which can result in adverse effects of the corticosteroid such as adrenal suppression.
Budesonide/ formoterol (Symbicort)	MDI			
Methylxanthines				
Theophylline, sustained-release tablets and capsules	Oral	Long-term control and prevention of symptoms in mild, persistent asthma or as adjunctive with ICS, in moderate or persistent asthma.	Dose-related acute toxicities include tachycardia, nausea and vomiting, tachyarrhythmias, central nervous system stimulation, headache, seizures, hematemesis, hyperglycemia, and hypokalemia. Adverse effects at usual therapeutic doses include insomnia, gastric upset, aggravation of ulcer, or reflux.	Maintain steady-state serum concentrations between 5 and 15 mcg/mL. Routine serum concentration monitoring is essential due to significant toxicities, narrow therapeutic range, and individual differences in metabolic clearance. Multiple drug–drug interactions. Not recommended for exacerbations. There is minimal evidence for added benefit to optimal doses of SABA.

(continues)

Table 20-13 Asthma Medications for Long-Term Control *(continued)*

Drug Generic (Brand)	Formulation	Indications/Mechanisms	Adverse Effects	Clinical Considerations
Mast Cell Mediators				
Cromolyn sodium (Intal) and nedocromil (Tilade)	MDI	Long-term prevention of symptoms in mild, persistent asthma. Preventive treatment prior to exposure to exercise or known allergen.	Cough and irritation. 15–20% of persons complain of an unpleasant taste from nedocromil.	Therapeutic response to cromolyn and nedocromil often occurs within 2 weeks, but a 4- to 6-week trial may be needed to determine maximum benefit. Dose of cromolyn by MDI (1 mg/puff) may be inadequate to affect airway hyperresponsiveness. Nebulizer delivery (20 mg/ampule) may be preferred for some individuals. Safety is the primary advantage of these agents.

MDI = metered-dose inhaler; DPI = dry-powder inhaler; ICS = inhaled corticosteroids; EIB = exercise-induced bronchospasm; LABA = long-acting beta$_2$ agonist; LTRA = leukotriene receptor antagonists; INR = international normalized ratio; ALT = alanine aminotransferase; AST = aspartate aminotransferase; SABA = inhaled short-acting beta$_2$ agonist.

* In December of 2008, an expert panel of the FDA recommended that salmeterol and formoterol no longer be approved for treatment of asthma secondary to an increased risk of airway responsiveness to histamine and worsening asthma morbidity that is associated with regular use of these agents.

Sources: Third Expert Panel on the Management of Asthma 2007[108]; Centers for Disease Control and Prevention 2005.[109]

lipophilicity, which prolongs retention in the lung tissue. Due to this retention, a single dose maintains its bronchodilation action for at least 12 hours.[117] At 4–5 times the recommended dose, tachycardia, hypokalemia, and prolonged QT interval can develop.[118] In 1993, a large, randomized, controlled study of over 25,000 subjects in the United Kingdom studied inhaled salmeterol administered twice daily compared to albuterol (Pro-Air HFA, Proventil HFA, Ventolin HFA) provided four times daily. An excess death rate of 0.07% in the salmeterol group compared to 0.02% in the albuterol group resulted.[119] Although the finding was not statistically significant, it raised a concern regarding the safety of long-acting beta$_2$ agonists. A subsequent large, randomized, placebo-controlled 28-week trial of salmeterol versus placebo added to usual care in adults.[120] This study was terminated early following a planned interim analysis that showed an increased risk of asthma-related deaths and combined asthma-related deaths or life-threatening events (13 deaths out of 13,176 with salmeterol versus 3 out of 13,176 receiving placebo). The majority of the imbalance was in African Americans, raising the question of whether physiologic treatment effect, genetic factors, or personal behaviors led to the increased risk.[121] A review of this and other studies[41] prompted the FDA to issue a public health advisory stating that long-acting beta$_2$ agonists should not be the first-line treatment of asthma. Rather, they should be added only if the asthma is not controlled with low- or medium-dose corticosteroids.

There is significant support for the addition of long-acting beta$_2$ agonists for asthma that is not well controlled by inhaled corticosteroids. A Cochrane review found a reduction in severe asthma exacerbations associated with long-acting beta$_2$ agonists.[122] Further meta-analyses demonstrated that combinations of inhaled beta$_2$ agonists and inhaled corticosteroids are preferred over monotherapy with escalating doses of beta$_2$ agonists to reduce exacerbations[123] and improve symptom control. The use of both inhaled corticosteroid and long-acting beta$_2$ agonists is the preferred management regimen for moderate and severe asthma.[108]

Two combined, inhaled corticosteroid and long-acting beta$_2$ agonist inhalers are currently available—fluticasone/salmeterol (Advair) by GlaxoSmithKline and budesonide/formoterol (Symbicort) by AstraZeneca. Advair is available with three strengths of fluticasone, and Symbicort is available with two strengths of budesonide. Each has the same set dose of long-acting beta$_2$ agonist, which is 50 mcg salmeterol in the Advair and 4.5 mcg formoterol in the Symbicort. Combined inhalers offer the advantage of only having to use one inhaler rather than two. When compared to increasing the dose of inhaled corticosteroids alone, the combination products have been found to improve lung function and reduce the rate of asthma exacerbations.[112] There is some evidence that the combined inhalers are more effective than the same doses of inhaled corticosteroid and long-acting beta$_2$ agonist administered separately.[123] One study demonstrated that Advair was more effective in delivering both the fluticasone and salmeterol to the airways than separate inhalers.[123] Advair canisters have an integrated dose counter, which can help users keep track of when they need to refill their medication; the formulation and recommended dosing may improve both compliance and satisfaction.[124] Of the two long-acting beta$_2$ agonists, formoterol has a faster onset of bronchodilation, similar to that of albuterol.[117] While the Third Expert Panel currently does not recommend the use of long-acting beta$_2$ agonists for the treatment of acute symptoms, researchers are studying the use of budesonide/formoterol (Symbicort) for both relief of acute symptoms[125] and variable dosing depending on the level of symptom control.[126] If ongoing research proves such use to be both safe and efficacious, it would allow only one inhaler to be used for both maintenance and rescue.

Leukotriene Receptor Antagonists

Inhaled corticosteroids do not appear to suppress leukotriene biosynthesis, and leukotrienes incite release of inflammatory mediators, causing the inflammation component of asthma.[127] There are currently two classes of leukotriene modifiers available: the leukotriene receptor antagonists, which include montelukast (Singulair) and zafirlukast (Accolate), and the 5-lipoxygenase pathway inhibitors, which include zileuton (Zyflo). Leukotriene receptor antagonists provide some improvement in lung function when compared to placebo, but consistently less than inhaled corticosteroids.[108] They may offer benefit by decreasing exercise-induced bronchospasm. They may also be used as an alternative, but not preferred, treatment for mild, persistent asthma.

Zileuton has been associated with liver toxicity and inhibits the metabolism of theophylline and warfarin (Coumadin). For these reasons, it is a less desirable option than montelukast or zafirlukast.[108] Zafirlukast also can increase the half-life of warfarin and lead to hepatic dysfunction, so INRs must be monitored closely for individuals receiving both medications, and hepatic enzymes should be monitored if symptoms of hepatitis develop.[108] The association between leukotriene receptor antagonists and depression or suicide was noted in postmarketing research; these medications now include an FDA black box warning on their labels stating that there is an increased risk of depression and suicide in persons who use them.

Cromolyn Sodium (NasalCrom) and Nedocromil (Tilade)

Cromolyn sodium (Intal) and nedocromil (Tilade) are different medications, but both modulate release of mast cell mediators and eosinophil recruitment. Both are effective as preventive treatment for exercise-induced bronchospasm or known allergen exposure.[108] Cromolyn and nedocromil offer better symptom relief than placebo and decrease emergency visits and hospitalizations due to asthma exacerbations.[128] These agents have been found to have few if any adverse effects. Inhaled corticosteroids are more effective than nedocromil in improving outcome measures. The Expert Panel states that they may be considered as an alternative to steroids for mild, persistent asthma.[108]

Immunomodulators

Omalizumab (Xolair) is a recombinant monoclonal antibody that inhibits the binding of IgE to mast cells and basophils, thereby decreasing the release of mediators in response to an allergen.[108] Administration is accomplished by subcutaneous injection every 2–4 weeks, depending on an individual's body weight and serum IgE. While it has not been compared to other adjunctive therapies such as leukotriene modifiers, long-acting beta$_2$ agonists or theophylline (Theo-Dur), it is the only adjunctive therapy available for improving symptoms in individuals with severe persistent allergic asthma who are not well controlled with high-dose inhaled corticosteroids plus long-acting beta$_2$ agonists.

A review of postmarketing case reports demonstrated an incidence of anaphylaxis of 0.2% in persons using omalizumab, which prompted the FDA to issue an alert. As postmarketing case reports are made voluntarily, a higher incidence of anaphylaxis may exist. Anaphylaxis was noted to occur as early as with the first dose to beyond a year of receiving treatment. The majority of cases of anaphylaxis occurred within 1 hour of administration, but a small percentage developed from 1 to 4 days after administration. Because of these risks, omalizumab should be administered only in a setting that is prepared to treat anaphylaxis, and recipients should be informed of the signs and symptoms of anaphylaxis.

Methylxanthines

Theophylline (Theo-Dur) is the most commonly used methylxanthine for the treatment of asthma. Prior to the development of cromolyn sodium and inhaled corticosteroids, theophylline was one of the first-line drugs for long-term control of persistent asthma. In addition to bronchodilation, mediated by phosphodiesterase inhibition and increased cAMP, it shares many of the properties of caffeine.[3] Common side effects of theophylline

Table 20-14 Factors Affecting Serum Theophylline Levels

Factor	Decreases Theophylline Concentrations	Increases Theophylline Concentrations	Recommended Actions
Food	↓ or delays absorption of some sustained-release preparations	Fatty foods ↑ rate of absorption	Choose theophylline preparation not affected by food.
Diet	High protein ↑ metabolism	High carbohydrate ↓ metabolism	Educate; not recommended to make major dietary changes while taking theophylline.
Febrile illness		↓ metabolism	Monitor levels and adjust accordingly.
Hypoxia, heart failure		↓ metabolism	Monitor levels and adjust accordingly.
Age	↑ metabolism (1–9 years)	↓ < 6 months, elderly	Monitor levels and adjust accordingly.
Phenobarbital (Luminal), phenytoin (Dilantin), carbamazepine (Tegretol)	↑ metabolism		Monitor levels and adjust accordingly.
Cimetidine (Tagamet)		↓ metabolism	Use alternative.
Macrolides: erythromycin (E-mycin), clarithromycin (Biaxin)		↓ metabolism	Use azithromycin or alternate antibiotic.
Ciprofloxacin (Cipro)		↓ metabolism	Use alternate antibiotic or use ofloxacin if quinolone therapy is required.
Rifampin (Rifadin)	↑ metabolism		Monitor levels and increase dose accordingly.
Smoking	↑ metabolism		Advise to stop smoking; monitor levels and increase dose accordingly.

↓ = decreases.
↑ = increases.
Source: Adapted from Second Expert Panel on the Management of Asthma 1997.[129]

(Theo-Dur) include central nervous system excitation, tachycardia, CNS vasoconstriction and peripheral vasodilation, and diuresis.

Methylxanthines are administered intravenously and by mouth. Rates of metabolism are affected by many variables, such as age, comorbidity, and other medications. A list of these factors that affect metabolism and serum concentrations is presented in Table 20-14.[129] Theophylline has several clinically significant drug–drug and drug–food interactions and has a narrow therapeutic window; therefore, it is essential to monitor serum concentrations. Starting doses are 10 mg/kg/day and are increased to achieve a serum concentration of 5–15 mcg/kg after at least 48 hours on the same dose to 300 mg/kg/day. The usual maximum daily dose is 800 mg/day.[108]

Selecting theophylline as the primary long-term control medication may be considered for an individual who cannot or will not use inhaled medication or in those unable to afford long-acting beta$_2$ agonists.

Anticholinergics

Ipratropium bromide (Atrovent HFA), when used in conjunction with short-acting beta$_2$ agonists, appears to improve bronchoconstriction associated with moderate or severe asthma exacerbations.[130]

Stepwise Approach for Managing Asthma

Combining the information about the classifications of asthma severity and the medications available to treat asthma, the Expert Panel has developed stepwise guidelines for the overall management of individuals with asthma. These guidelines are presented in Figure 20-4. Drug therapy should be targeted to an individual's disease process at a given time. Neither suboptimal nor overly aggressive medication regimens are desirable, and both can lead to worsening of the asthma. Exacerbations indicate a need to step up the pharmacotherapy. Conversely, stepping down the treatment can be considered after 3 months of good control.

As with any chronic illness, drug therapy is only part of the treatment plan. Education of both the asthmatic and of providers, avoidance of allergens, and regular follow-up also are key components of the management.

Special Populations

Pregnancy

In 2007, the Expert Panel reiterated its position from the 2004 Working Group Report on managing asthma during pregnancy by stating that use of asthma medications is much safer for both the mother and fetus than having poorly controlled asthma and exacerbations.[109] Albuterol (Pro-Air HFA, Proventil HFA, Ventolin HFA)

and budesonide (Rhinocort) are the medications that have been studied the most, and, for this reason, albuterol is the short-acting beta agonist of choice. Although there are no data suggesting that other inhaled corticosteroids are unsafe,[108] budesonide is the ICS of choice when initiating therapy.[131] No evidence of fetal harm from any of the medications commonly used to treat asthma has been reported, with the possible exception of systemic corticosteroids. In that case, it is difficult to distinguish the effects of the oral corticosteroids from the effects of severe asthma.[131]

Smokers

Exposure to tobacco smoke is associated with increased symptoms and disease severity. Asthma can be more difficult to treat in smokers, who are less responsive to inhaled corticosteroids.[132] Smoking cessation results in improvement in lung function within 6 weeks; changes in response to inhaled corticosteroids may lag for some time longer.[133]

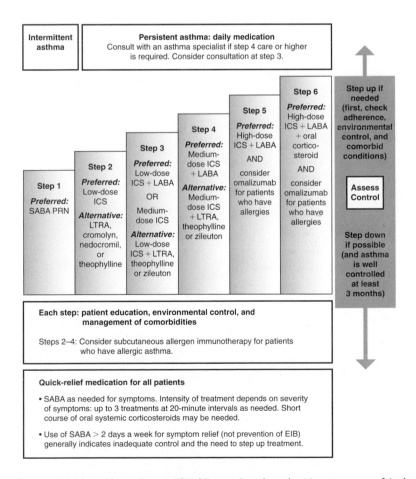

Figure 20-4 Stepwise approach to managing asthma. *Source:* Third Expert Panel on the Management of Asthma 2007.[108]

The Elderly

Irreversible airway obstruction from emphysema or chronic bronchitis is more likely to complicate the reversible airway obstruction of asthma in the elderly than in the younger individual. The elderly are also more at risk for adverse medication effects, such as tremor or tachycardia from inhaled beta$_2$ agonists, and elevated theophylline levels due to reduced clearance, and increased bone loss. Management of comorbid conditions frequently entails a long list of medications, some of which, like NSAIDs and beta-blockers, may aggravate asthma. Due to the number of comorbid conditions from which elders may suffer, they may well be under the care of numerous specialists. The primary care provider plays an important role in their management by overseeing and coordinating care. Careful attention to the diagnosis and assessment of asthma symptoms in view of all the disease processes and medications will help to decrease the risks.[108]

Tuberculosis

Mycobacterium tuberculosis is the bacteria responsible for **tuberculosis** (TB). The bacteria are transmitted by respiratory droplets spread by singing, coughing, sneezing, or talking.[134] Worldwide, one third of the population is infected with TB, and 2 million persons die from TB every year.[135] While TB is much less common in the United States, it is still a significant public health problem. Immigrants have approximately nine times the rate of TB than US-born persons have, with 21.8 cases per 100,000 persons. Racial and ethnic minorities suffer disproportionately from TB infection, as described in Table 20-15. Although the incidence of and mortality from TB is dramatically lower in the United States than in developing countries, a major concern is the rise in multidrug resistant TB. **Multidrug resistant tuberculosis** is rare among US-born individuals but occurs in 80% of cases in foreign-born persons.[136] The initial treatment of active TB infection is beyond the scope of this chapter. However, primary care clinicians commonly encounter persons for whom screening for TB and the treatment of latent TB infection is indicated, and therefore these topics are presented in this section.

Latent Tuberculosis Infection

Latent tuberculosis infection (LTBI) refers to infection in individuals who have been exposed to and harbor potentially disease-causing *M. tuberculosis* whose healthy immune systems effectively control the infection.[134] Between 5% and 10% of individuals with LTBI will progress to active disease, with the greatest risk in the first 2 years following exposure.[134] A basic principle of the control of TB in the United States is the identification and treatment of individuals who are at high risk for developing active TB (Box 20-6). A second principle is the prompt diagnosis and treatment of those with active disease as well as their close contacts.

Table 20-15 Rate of TB Infection by Race/Ethnicity, 2005

Racial/Ethnic Population	Rate of TB Infection/100,000 persons
Asian	25.8
Native Hawaiians/Pacific Islanders	13.8
Blacks	10.9
Hispanics or Latinos	9.5
American Indians/Alaskan Natives	6.9
Whites	1.3

Source: Adapted from Centers for Disease Control and Prevention 2005.[136]

Box 20-6 High-Risk Populations That Should Be Tested for Latent Tuberculosis Infections

Close contacts of persons with infectious pulmonary TB

Persons working in or served by clinics or community health organizations providing care to HIV-infected persons

Prisoners

Legal immigrants and refugees with the following:

  Chest X-ray compatible with active TB but sputum acid-fast bacillus (AFB) negative

  Chest X-ray compatible with inactive TB (no sputum specimens required)

Recently arrived refugees

Other well-defined groups in congregate living facilities

Persons enrolled in substance abuse treatment programs

Healthcare workers

Source: Adapted from Centers for Disease Control and Prevention 2000.[137]

Targeted Testing for LTBI

Tuberculin skin testing and subsequent treatment of individuals with positive tests have long been an essential component of the control of TB in the United States and other countries with a low incidence of TB. There has been a shift from widespread population-based tuberculin skin testing to targeted testing aimed at identifying individuals at high risk who would benefit from the treatment of latent TB infection. With this approach, screening of low-risk individuals is discouraged, with the exception of testing low-risk individuals whose future employment places them in healthcare settings or involves them in other activities that increase their risk for exposure.[137] State and local flexibility when defining high-risk groups is recommended; Box 20-6 lists groups who are commonly accepted as being at high risk of developing TB.

The preferred method of testing is intradermal administration of 0.1 mL of five tuberculin units of purified protein derivative (PPD) into the dorsal surface of the forearm. Tests should be read 48–72 hours after placement by measuring the diameter of induration in millimeters. Three cut-off levels for defining a positive tuberculin test have been recommended based on the sensitivity and specificity of the test, prevalence of TB in specific groups, and the risk of developing active TB (Table 20-16). Active tuberculosis should be ruled out by means of a chest X-ray and evaluation of symptoms in individuals with a positive skin test. Individuals whose X-ray is suggestive of active disease and/or those with respiratory symptoms should have three consecutive sputum samples submitted for acid-fast bacillus spear (AFB) smear and culture. Following the targeted tuberculin testing strategy, those who have a positive test but do not have active disease should be treated for LTBI.[137]

Isoniazid (INH)

In the past, pharmacotherapy for the treatment was referred to as "preventive therapy" or "chemoprophylaxis." Today, the more accurate term is *treatment of LTBI*. Adoption of this terminology emphasizes the critical nature of this component of TB control.[137] Isoniazid (INH) was found to be effective for the treatment of TB in the middle of the 20th century and was recommended for general use in 1965.[138] At that time, it was believed that the use of such a low-cost, effective treatment without identified side effects would be effective in causing a dramatic reduction in TB. By 1970, a significant association between isoniazid and hepatitis was recognized. Since that time, isoniazid toxicity, the development of alternative agents, the recognition of nonadherence, and the occurrence of

Table 20-16 Classification of the Tuberculin Skin Test Reaction

An Induration of 5 or More Millimeters Is Considered Positive In:	An Induration of 10 or More Millimeters Is Considered Positive In:	An Induration of 15 or More Millimeters Is Considered Positive in Any Person, Including:
HIV-infected persons A recent contact of a person with TB Persons with fibrotic changes on chest radiograph consistent with prior TB Persons with organ transplants Persons who are immunosuppressed for other reasons (e.g., taking the equivalent of > 15 mg/day of prednisone for 1 month or longer, taking TNF-a antagonists)	Recent immigrants (< 5 years) from high-prevalence countries Injection drug users Residents and employees of high-risk congregate settings, including prisons and jails, nursing homes and other long-term facilities for the elderly, hospitals and other healthcare facilities, residential facilities for individuals with acquired immunodeficiency syndrome (AIDS), and homeless shelters Mycobacteriology laboratory personnel Persons with clinical conditions that place them at high risk, i.e., silicosis, diabetes mellitus, chronic renal failure, some hematologic disorders (e.g., leukemias and lymphomas), other specific malignancies (e.g., carcinoma of the head or neck and lung), weight loss of > 10% of ideal body weight, gastrectomy, and jejunoileal bypass Children < 4 years of age Infants, children, and adolescents exposed to adults in high-risk categories	Persons with no known risk factors for tuberculosis

TB = tuberculosis.
Source: Adapted from Centers for Disease Control and Prevention 2000.[137]

Table 20-17 Recommended Drug Treatment Regimens for Treatment of Latent Tuberculosis Infection (LTBI) in Adults

Drug Generic (Brand)	Interval and Duration	Clinical Considerations	Rating* (Evidence)[†] HIV−	HIV+
Isoniazid (INH)	Daily for 9 months[‡]	In persons infected with human immunodeficiency virus (HIV), isoniazid may be administered concurrently with nucleoside reverse transcriptase inhibitors (NRTIs), protease inhibitors, or nonnucleoside reverse transcriptase inhibitors (NNRTIs). Directly observed therapy (DOT) must be used with twice-weekly dosing.	A (II)	A (II)
	Twice weekly for 9 months[‡]		B (II)	B (II)
	Daily for 6 months[‡]	Not indicated for HIV-infected persons, those with fibrotic lesions on chest radiographs, or children. DOT must be used with twice-weekly dosing.	B (I)	C (I)
	Twice weekly for 6 months[‡]		B (II)	C (I)
Rifampin plus pyrazinamide (RZ) [§]	Daily for 2 months	May also be offered to persons who are contacts of pyrazinamide persons with isoniazid-resistant, rifampin-susceptible TB. In HIV-infected persons, protease inhibitors or NNRTIs should generally not be administered concurrently with rifampin; rifabutin can be used as an alternative for individuals treated with indinavir, nelfinavir, amprenavir, ritonavir, or efavirenz, and possibly with nevirapine or soft-gel saquinavir. DOT must be used with twice-weekly dosing.	B (II)	A (I)
	Twice weekly for 2–3 months		C (II)	C (I)
Rifampin (Rifadin)	Daily for 4 months	For persons who cannot tolerate pyrazinamide or for persons who are contacts of persons with isoniazid-resistant, rifampin-susceptible TB who cannot tolerate pyrazinamide.	B (II)	B (III)

NNRTIs = non-nucleoside reverse transcriptase inhibitors; DOT = directly observed therapy.

* Strength of recommendation: A = preferred; B = acceptable alternative; C = offer when A and B cannot be given.

[†] Quality of evidence: I = randomized clinical trial data; II = data from clinical trials that are not randomized or were conducted in other populations; III = expert opinion.

[‡] Recommended regimens for pregnant women. Some experts would use rifampin and pyrazinamide for 2 months as an alternative regimen in HIV-infected pregnant women, although pyrazinamide should be avoided during the first trimester. Rifampin should not be used with hard-gel saquinavir or delavirdine. When used with other protease inhibitors or NNRTIs, dose adjustment may be required.

[§] The combination of rifampin and pyrazinamide has been found to cause hepatic damage and is no longer recommended for treatment of LTBI for most persons. Absolute contraindications include persons with liver disease, history of alcoholism, or INH-associated liver injury. In addition, no more than a 2-week supply should be dispensed at one time. Liver function should be tested at 2, 4, and 6 weeks of treatment.

Source: Adapted from Centers for Disease Control and Prevention 2000.[137]

the HIV epidemic has provoked researchers to evaluate the efficacy of various treatment regimens. Table 20-17 presents the 2000 recommendations of the CDC and the American Thoracic Society.[137]

Isoniazid (INH) remains the mainstay for the treatment of LTBI. It is a bactericidal antiinfective, is relatively inexpensive, and is nontoxic for most individuals. Isoniazid is well absorbed from the gastrointestinal tract and penetrates into all body fluids.

Side Effects/Adverse Effects

Severe side effects of isoniazid (INH) include hepatitis and peripheral neuropathy. Baseline testing of liver function and bilirubin should be obtained in individuals at risk for hepatic dysfunction, such as those with chronic hepatic disease or individuals who routinely consume ethanol. These tests are also indicated for persons with HIV infection, women who are pregnant, or mothers who have given birth within the prior 3 months. Routine follow-up testing is indicated if the baseline tests are abnormal or symptoms of hepatic dysfunction arise.

Peripheral neuropathy occurs because isoniazid interferes with the metabolism of pyridoxine. Peripheral neuropathy is more common in persons with underlying conditions associated with neuropathy. Supplemental pyridoxine (vitamin B$_6$) should be given to those individuals, as well as to pregnant women and individuals with seizure disorders who are taking anti-epileptic medications. Concurrent administration of isoniazid and phenytoin (Dilantin) increases serum concentrations of each drug.

Rifampin (Rifadin)

Rifampin (Rifadin), a derivative of rifamycin, also is a bactericidal anti-infective indicated for treatment of TB. Rifampin is rapidly absorbed from the gastrointestinal tract. Despite 75% of the drug being protein bound, it penetrates well into tissues and through inflamed meninges.

Side Effects/Adverse Effects

Side effects include gastrointestinal upset, skin reactions. Individuals taking rifampin should be informed that the drug causes discoloration of body fluids, including sweat, urine, and tears; permanent discoloration of contact lenses may result from tear discoloration. Rare adverse effects include hepatitis and thrombocytopenia.

Drug–Drug Interactions

Rifampin induces hepatic microsomal enzymes and may increase absorption of medications metabolized by the liver. Table 20-18 lists specific medications that may be affected. Rifampin also increases the metabolism of estrogen, potentially decreasing the effectiveness of combined hormonal contraceptives.

Special Populations

Previous Bacillus Calmette-Guérin (BCG) Vaccination

Bacillus Calmette-Guérin (BCG) vaccination can cause tuberculin reactivity of various degrees. While the reactivity tends to decrease over time, periodic skin testing can again increase reactivity.[137] Previous vaccination with BCG is not a contraindication to tuberculin skin testing. Individuals who have received BCG should be tested according to the described guidelines and treated if the tuberculin skin test result is ≥ 10 mm.[137, 138]

Table 20-18 Medications to Treat Latent Tuberculosis Infection: Doses, Toxicities, and Monitoring Requirements

Drug Generic (Brand)	Dose mg/kg (maximum oral dose in milligrams)*		Adverse Reactions	Monitoring	Clinical Considerations
	Daily	Twice Weekly			
Isoniazid (INH)	5 (300)	20–40 (900)	Rash, hepatic enzyme elevation, hepatitis, peripheral neuropathy, mild central nervous system effects. Drug interactions resulting in increased phenytoin (Dilantin) or Disulfiram (Antabuse) levels	Clinical monitoring monthly. Liver function tests† at baseline in selected cases‡ and repeat measurements if baseline results are abnormal or woman is pregnant, in the immediate postpartum period, or at high risk for adverse reactions, or if person has symptoms of adverse reactions.	Hepatitis risk increases with age and alcohol consumption. Pyridoxine (vitamin B$_6$, 10–25 mg/d) might prevent peripheral neuropathy and central nervous system effects.
Rifampin (Rifadin)	10 (600)	10 (600) in conjunction with INH	Rash, hepatitis, fever, thrombocytopenia, flu-like symptoms, orange-colored body fluids (secretions, urine, tears)	Clinical monitoring at weeks 2, 4, and 8 when pyrazinamide given. Complete blood count, platelets, and liver function tests† at baseline in selected cases‡ and repeat measurements if baseline results are abnormal or person has symptoms of adverse reactions.	Rifampin is contraindicated or should be used with caution among those infected with HIV and taking protease inhibitors (PIs) or nonnucleoside reverse transcriptase inhibitors (NNRTIs). Decreases levels of many drugs (e.g., methadone, warfarin, glucocorticoids, hormonal contraceptives, estrogens, oral hypoglycemic agents, digitalis, anticonvulsants, dapsone, ketoconazole, and cyclosporin). Might permanently discolor soft contact lenses.

(continues)

Table 20-18 Medications to Treat Latent Tuberculosis Infection: Doses, Toxicities, and Monitoring Requirements *(continued)*

Drug Generic (Brand)	Dose mg/kg (maximum oral dose in milligrams)* Daily	Twice Weekly	Adverse Reactions	Monitoring	Clinical Considerations
Rifabutin (Mycobutin)	5 (300)	5 (300)§	Rash, hepatitis, fever, thrombocytopenia, orange-colored body fluids (secretions, urine, tears) With increased levels of rifabutin, severe arthralgias, uveitis, leukopenia	Clinical monitoring at weeks 2, 4, and 8 when pyrazinamide given. Complete blood count, platelets, and liver function tests† at baseline in selected cases,‡ and repeat measurements if baseline results are abnormal, patient has symptoms of adverse reactions. Use adjusted daily dose of rifabutin and monitor for decreased antiretroviral activity and for rifabutin toxicity if rifabutin taken concurrently with PIs or NNRTIs.§	Rifabutin is contraindicated for HIV-infected patients taking hard-gel saquinavir or delavirdine; caution is also advised if rifabutin is administered with soft-gel saquinavir. Reduces levels of many drugs (e.g., PIs, NNTRIs, methadone, dapsone, ketoconazole, Coumadin derivatives, hormonal contraceptive, digitalis, sulfonylureas, diazepam, β-blockers, anticonvulsants, and theophylline). Might permanently discolor contact lenses.
Pyrazinamide (PZA)	15–20 (2.0 g)	50 (4.0 g)	Gastrointestinal upset, hepatitis, rash, arthralgias, gout (rare)	Clinical monitoring at weeks 2, 4, and 8. Liver function tests† at baseline in selected cases‡ and repeat measurements if baseline results are abnormal, patient has symptoms of adverse reactions.	Treat hyperuricemia only if patient has symptoms. Might make glucose control more difficult in persons with diabetes. Should be avoided in pregnancy, but can be given after first trimester.

* All intermittent dosing should be administered by directly observed therapy.

† AST or ALT and serum bilirubin.

‡ HIV infection, history of liver disease, alcoholism, and pregnancy.

§ If nelfinavir, indinavir, amprenavir, or ritonavir is administered with rifabutin, blood concentrations of these protease inhibitors decrease. Thus, the dose of rifabutin is reduced from 300 mg to 150 mg/d when used with nelfinavir, indinavir, or amprenavir; and to 150 mg (two or three times a week) when used with ritonavir. If efavirenz is administered with rifabutin, blood concentrations of rifabutin decrease. Thus, when rifabutin is used concurrently with efavirenz, the daily dose of rifabutin should be increased from 300 mg to 450 mg or 600 mg. Pharmacokinetic studies suggest that rifabutin might be given at usual doses with nevirapine. It is not currently known whether dose adjustment of rifabutin is required when used concurrently with soft-gel saquinavir.

Source: Adapted from Centers for Disease Control and Prevention 2000.[137]

Pregnancy and Lactation

Pregnant women with active TB during pregnancy should be treated for the disease without waiting until they give birth. Treatment of LTBI is more controversial. While some prefer to delay treatment until after delivery, many recommend that treatment be initiated at diagnosis, with close monitoring for hepatitis. Isoniazid has been shown to be safe in pregnancy and is the preferred regimen. Rifampin has also been used extensively and is probably also safe. Individuals treated for LTBI during pregnancy should also receive supplemental pyridoxine (Vitamin B$_6$).

There have been no reports of toxic effects of tuberculosis medications in breast milk, and breastfeeding is not contraindicated for those receiving treatment for TB. Serum levels in breastfed infants is < 20% of therapeutic levels and therefore inadequate for treatment of the infant.[137]

▌ Conclusion

Respiratory illness is a frequent cause of healthcare visits. Colds, bronchitis, and influenza in otherwise healthy individuals account for a significant number of visits and may be managed with self-care counseling and perhaps recommendations for symptomatic relief such as decongestants. Primary care providers do their clients a favor by educating them about the absence of proven benefit from many of the over-the-counter medications marketed to provide relief from cold symptoms. By doing so, the provider will help his or her clients save money and avoid unwanted side effects caused by nonefficacious medications.

Not every respiratory illness is benign and self-limited. Asthma, pneumonia, and tuberculosis have serious sequelae, including mortality. It is the healthcare provider's responsibility to gather a complete history and perform a thorough physical examination to assess whether an individual is suffering from an illness associated with significant morbidity and plan for appropriate care that will minimize adverse outcomes.

References

1. Glenny RW. Teaching ventilation/perfusion relationships in the lung. Adv Physiol Educ 2008;32(3):192–5.

2. Guyton AC, Hall JE. Textbook of medical physiology, 11th ed. Philadelphia, PA: Elsevier Saunders, 2006.

3. Lehne RA. Pharmacology for nursing care, 6th ed. St. Louis, MO: Saunders Elsevier, 2007.

4. Castells M. Mast cell mediators in allergic inflammation and mastocytosis. Immunol Allergy Clin North Am 2006;26(3):465–85.

5. National Institute of Allergy and Infectious Disease (NIAID). Common cold. 2006.

6. Turner RB. Epidemiology, pathogenesis, and treatment of the common cold. Ann Allergy Asthma Immunol 1997;78(6):531–9, quiz 9–40.

7. Kirkpatrick GL. The common cold. Prim Care 1996; 23(4):657–75.

8. Turner RB, Hendley JO. Virucidal hand treatments for prevention of rhinovirus infection. J Antimicrob Chemother 2005;56(5):805–7.

9. Douglas RM, Hemila H, D'Souza R, Chalker EB, Treacy B. Vitamin C for preventing and treating the common cold. Cochrane Database Syst Rev 2004; (4):CD000980.

10. Hwang SA, Dasgupta A, Actor JK. Cytokine production by non-adherent mouse splenocyte cultures to echinacea extracts. Clin Chim Acta 2004;343(1–2): 161–6.

11. Gilroy CM, Steiner JF, Byers T, Shapiro H, Georgian W. Echinacea and truth in labeling. Arch Intern Med 2003;163(6):699–704.

12. Linde K, Barrett B, Wolkart K, Bauer R, Melchart D. Echinacea for preventing and treating the common cold. Cochrane Database Syst Rev 2006(1):CD000530.

13. Shah SA, Sander S, White CM, Rinaldi M, Coleman CI. Evaluation of echinacea for the prevention and treatment of the common cold: a meta-analysis. Lancet Infect Dis 2007;7(7):473–80.

14. Rennard BO, Ertl RF, Grossman GL, Robbins RA, Rennard SI. Chicken soup inhibits neutrophil chemotaxis in vitro. Chest 2000;118:1150–7.

15. Pratter MR. Cough and the common cold: ACCP evidence-based clinical practice guidelines. Chest 2006;129(1 suppl):72S–4S.

16. Sutter AI, Lemiengre M, Campbell H, Mackinnon HF. Antihistamines for the common cold. Cochrane Database Syst Rev 2003(3):CD001267.

17. Muether PS, Gwaltney JM Jr. Variant effect of first- and second-generation antihistamines as clues to their mechanism of action on the sneeze reflex in the common cold. Clin Infect Dis 2001;33(9):1483–8.

18. Naclerio RM, Proud D, Kagey-Sobotka A, Lichtenstein LM, Hendley JO, Gwaltney JM Jr. Is histamine responsible for the symptoms of rhinovirus colds? A look at the inflammatory mediators following infection. Pediatr Infect Dis J 1988;7(3):218–22.

19. Curley FJ, Irwin RS, Pratter MR, Stivers DH, Doern GV, Vernaglia PA, et al. Cough and the common cold. Am Rev Respir Dis 1988;138(2):305–11.

20. Taverner D, Latte J. Nasal decongestants for the common cold. Cochrane Database Syst Rev 2007(1): CD001953.

21. FDA Center for Drug Evaluation and Research. Legal requirements for the sale and purchase of drug products containing pseudoephedrine, ephedrine, and phenylpropanolamine. 2006.

22. Eccles R. Substitution of phenylephrine for pseudoephedrine as a nasal decongeststant: an illogical way to control methamphetamine abuse. Br J Clin Pharmacol 2007;63(1):10–4.

23. MediTEXT Medical Managements. Monoamine oxidase inhibitors. Thomson Healthcare Series, 2007.

24. FDA Center for Drug Evaluation and Research. Phenypropanolamine (PPA) information page, 2005.

25. Hansen WF, Peacock AE, Yankowitz J. Safe prescribing practices in pregnancy and lactation. J Midwifery Womens Health 2002;47(6):409–21.

26. Kuhn JJ, Hendley JO, Adams KF, Clarh JW, Gwaltney JM Jr. Antitussive effect of guaifenesin in young adults with natural colds. Chest 1982;82:713–8.

27. Bolser DC. Cough suppressant and pharmacologic protussive therapy: ACCP evidence-based clinical practice guidelines. Chest 2006;129(1 suppl):238S–49S.

28. Boehringer Ingelheim. Atrovent (ipratropium bromide) nasal spray 0.03% prescribing information. Ridgefield, CT: Boehringer Ingelheim, 2002.

29. Kuhn A. Evaluation of a new nasal decongestant. J Indiana State Med Assoc 1966;59:1295–6.

30. Graf P, Juto JE. Decongestion effect and rebound swelling of the nasal mucosa during 4-week use of oxymetazoline. ORL J Otorhinolaryngol Relat Spec 1994;56(3):157–60.

31. Graf PM. Rhinitis medicamentosa. Clin Allergy Immunol 2007;19:295–304.

32. Passali D, Salerni L, Passali GC, Passali FM, Bellussi L. Nasal decongestants in the treatment of chronic nasal obstruction: efficacy and safety of use. Expert Opin Drug Saf 2006;5(6):783–90.

33. Ferguson BJ, Paramaesvaran S, Rubinstein E. A study of the effect of nasal steroid sprays in perennial allergic rhinitis patients with rhinitis medicamentosa. Otolaryngol Head Neck Surg 2001;125(3):253–60.

34. Graf P. Rhinitis medicamentosa: a review of causes and treatment. Treat Respir Med 2005;4(1):21–9.

35. Sperber SJ, Hendley JO, Hayden FG, Riker DK, Sorrentino JV, Gwaltney JM Jr. Effects of naproxen on experimental rhinovirus colds. A randomized, double-blind, controlled trial. Ann Intern Med 1992; 117(1):37–41.

36. Mossad SB, Macknin ML, Medendorp SV, Mason P. Zinc gluconate lozenges for treating the common cold: a randomized, double-blind, placebo-controlled study. Ann Intern Med 1996;125(2):81–8.

37. Novick SG, Godfrey JC, Godfrey NJ, Wilder HR. How does zinc modify the common cold? Clinical observations and implications regarding mechanisms of action. Med Hypotheses 1996;46(3):295–302.

38. Fraker PJ, King LE, Laakko T, Vollmer TL. The dynamic link between the integrity of the immune system and zinc status. J Nutr 2000;130(5S suppl):1399S–406S.

39. MICROMEDEX Healthcare series. ZINC. 2004.

40. Cohen DA. The efficacy of zinc lozenges and zinc nasal sprays in the treatment of the common cold. Top Clin Nutr 2006;21(4):355–61.

41. Morice AH, Marshall AE, Higgins KS, Grattan TJ. Effect of inhaled menthol on citric acid induced cough in normal subjects. Thorax 1994;49(10):1024–6.

42. Papsin B, McTavish A. Saline nasal irrigation: its role as an adjunct treatment. Can Fam Physician 2003;49: 168–73.

43. Philpott CM, Conboy P, Al-Azzawi F, Murty G. Nasal physiological changes during pregnancy. Clin Otolaryngol Allied Sci 2004;29(4):343–51.

44. Yoon PW, Rasmussen SA, Lynberg MC, Moore CA, Anderka M, Carmichael SL, et al. The National Birth Defects Prevention Study. Public Health Rep 2001; 116(suppl 1):32–40.

45. Werler MM, Mitchell AA, Hernandez-Diaz S, Honein MA. Use of over-the-counter medications during pregnancy. Am J Obstet Gynecol 2005;193(3, pt 1):771–7.

46. Gonzales R, Steiner JF, Sande MA. Antibiotic prescribing for adults with colds, upper respiratory tract infections, and bronchitis by ambulatory care physicians. JAMA 1997;278(11):901–4.

47. Wenzel RP, Fowler AA 3rd. Clinical practice: acute bronchitis. N Engl J Med 2006;355(20):2125–30.

48. Martinez FJ. Acute bronchitis: state of the art diagnosis and therapy. Compr Ther 2004;30(1):55–69.

49. Centers for Disease Control and Prevention. Epidemiology and prevention of vaccine-preventable diseases, 10th ed. Washington, DC: Public Health Foundation, 2007.

50. Smucny J, Fahey T, Becker L, Glazier R. Antibiotics for acute bronchitis. Cochrane Database Syst Rev 2004(4):CD000245.

51. Robinson RE, Cummings WB, Deffenbaugh ER. Effectiveness of guaifenesin as an expectorant: a cooperative double blind study. Curr Ther Res Clin Exp 1977;22:284–96.

52. Levine DA. "Pharming": the abuse of prescription and over-the-counter drugs in teens. Curr Opin Pediatr 2007;19(3):270–4.

53. Chyka PA, Erdman AR, Manoguerra AS, Christianson G, Booze LL, Nelson LS, et al. Dextromethorphan poisoning: an evidence-based consensus guideline for out-of-hospital management. Clin Toxicol (Phila) 2007;45(6):662–77.

54. Moore DP, Jefferson JW. Handbook of medical psychiatry, 2nd ed. Philadelphia, PA: Mosby, 2004.

55. Braman SS. Chronic cough due to acute bronchitis: ACCP evidence-based clinical practice guidelines. Chest 2006;129(1 suppl):95S–103S.

56. FDA Center for Drug Evaluation and Research. Search results for dextromethorphan, 2007; Available from: *www.accessdata.fda.gov/scripts/cder/drugsatfda/index .cfm* [Accessed August 16, 2007].

57. Doona M, Walsh D. Benzonatate for opioid-resistant cough in advanced cancer. Palliat Med 1998;12(1):55–8.

58. Smucny J, Becker L, Glazier R. Beta2-agonists for acute bronchitis. Cochrane Database Syst Rev 2006(4): CD001726.

59. Wu T, Chen X, Duan X, Juan N, Liu G, Qiao J, et al. Chinese medicinal herbs for acute bronchitis. Cochrane Database Syst Rev 2005(3):CD004560.

60. Fiore AE, Shay DK, Haber P, Iskander JK, Uyeki TM, Mootrey G, et al. Prevention and control of influenza. Recommendations of the Advisory Committee on Immunization Practices (ACIP), 2007. MMWR Recomm Rep 2007;56(RR-6):1–54.

61. Cooper NJ, Sutton AJ, Abrams KR, Wailoo A, Turner D, Nicholson KG. Effectiveness of neuraminidase inhibitors in treatment and prevention of influenza A and B: systematic review and meta-analyses of randomised controlled trials. BMJ 2003;326(7401):1235.

62. Kaiser L, Wat C, Mills T, Mahoney P, Ward P, Hayden F. Impact of oseltamivir treatment on influenza-related lower respiratory tract complications and hospitalizations. Arch Intern Med 2003;163(14):1667–72.

63. Gooskens J, Jonges M, Claas EC, Meijer A, van den Broek PJ, Kroes AM. Morbidity and mortality associated with nosocomial transmission of oseltamivir-resistant influenza A(H1N1) virus. JAMA 2009;301 (10):1042–6.

64. Colman PM. Zanamivir: an influenza virus neuraminidase inhibitor. Expert Rev Anti Infect Ther 2005 Apr;3(2):191–9.

65. FDA Center for Drug Evaluation and Research. Tamiflu information page. 2007.

66. Gravenstein S, Johnston SL, Loeschel E, Webster A. Zanamivir: a review of clinical safety in individuals at high risk of developing influenza-related complications. Drug Safety 2001;24(15):1113–25.

67. Talwar A, Lee H, Fein A. Community-acquired pneumonia: what is relevant and what is not? Curr Opin Pulm Med 2007;13(3):177–85.

68. Mandell LA, Wunderink RG, Anzueto A, Bartlett JG, Campbell GD, Dean NC, et al. Infectious Diseases Society of America/American Thoracic Society consensus guidelines on the management of community-acquired pneumonia in adults. Clin Infect Dis 2007 March1;44(suppl 2):S27–S72.

69. Advisory Committee on Immunization Practices. Recommended adult immunization schedule: United States, 2009. Ann Intern Med 2009;150(1):40–4.

70. Gulmez SE, Holm A, Frederiksen H, Jensen TG, Pedersen C, Hallas J. Use of proton pump inhibitors and the risk of community-acquired pneumonia: a population-based case-control study. Arch Intern Med 2007;167(9):950–5.

71. Lim WS, van der Eerden MM, Laing R, Boersma WG, Karalus N, Town GI, et al. Defining community acquired pneumonia severity on presentation to hospital: an international derivation and validation study. Thorax 2003;58(5):377–82.

72. Aujesky D, Auble TE, Yealy DM, et al. Prospective comparison of three validated prediction rules for prognosis in community-acquired pneumonia. Am J Med 2005;118(4):384–92.

73. Fine MJ, Auble TE, Yealy DM, Hanusa BH, Weissfeld LA, Singer DE, Coley CM, Marrie TJ, Kapoor WN. A prediction rule to identify low-risk patients with community-acquired pneumonia. N Engl J Med 1997 Jan 23;336(4):243–50.

74. Bauer TT, Ewig S, Marre R, Suttorp N, Welte T. The Capnetz Study Group. CRB-65 predicts death from community-acquired pneumonia. J Intern Med 2006; 260(1):93–101.

75. Felmingham D. Evolving resistance patterns in community-acquired respiratory tract pathogens: first results from the PROTEKT global surveillance study. Prospective resistant organism tracking and epidemiology for the ketolide telithromycin. J Infect 2002; 44(suppl A):3–10.

76. File TM. Community-acquired pneumonia. Lancet 2003 Dec 13;362(9400):1991–2001.

77. Doern GV. Macrolide and ketolide resistance with Streptococcus pneumoniae. Med Clin North Am 2006 Nov;90(6):1109–24.

78. el Moussaoui R, de Borgie CA, van den Broek P, Hustinx WN, Bresser P, van den Berk GE, et al. Effectiveness of discontinuing antibiotic treatment after three days versus eight days in mild to moderate-severe community acquired pneumonia: randomised, double blind study. BMJ 2006;332(7554):1355.

79. File TM, Mandell LA, Tillotson G. Gemifloxacin once daily for 5 days versus 7 days for the treatment of community-acquired pneumonia: a randomized, multicentre, double-blind study [authors' response]. J Antimicrob Chemother 2007;60(4):903.

80. Dunbar LM, Wunderink RG, Habib MP, Smith LG, Tennenberg AM, Khashab MM, et al. High-dose, short-course levofloxacin for community-acquired pneumonia: a new treatment paradigm. Clin Infect Dis 2003 Sep 15;37(6):752–60.

81. File TM, Mandell LA, Tillotson G. Gemifloxacin once daily for 5 days versus 7 days for the treatment of community-acquired pneumonia: a randomized, multicentre, double-blind study authors' response. J Antimicrob Chemother 2007 Oct;60(4):903.

82. O'Doherty B, Muller O. Randomized, multicentre study of the efficacy and tolerance of azithromycin versus clarithromycin in the treatment of adults with mild to moderate community-acquired pneumonia. Azithromycin Study Group. Eur J Clin Microbiol Infect Dis 1998;17(12):828–33.

83. Scalera NM, File TM Jr. How long should we treat community-acquired pneumonia? Curr Opin Infect Dis 2007;20(2):177–81.

84. Goodnight WH, Soper DE. Pneumonia in pregnancy. Crit Care Med 2005;33(10 suppl):S390–7.

85. Munn MB, Groome LJ, Atterbury JL, Baker SL, Hoff C. Pneumonia as a complication of pregnancy. J Matern Fetal Med 1999;8(4):151–4.

86. Lim WS, Macfarlane JT, Colthorpe CL. Treatment of community-acquired lower respiratory tract infections during pregnancy. Am J Respir Med 2003;2(3): 221–33.

87. Yost NP, Bloom SL, Richey SD, Ramin SM, Cunningham FG. An appraisal of treatment guidelines for antepartum community-acquired pneumonia. Am J Obstet Gynecol 2000;183(1):131–5.

88. Hickner JM, Bartlett JG, Besser RE, Gonzales R, Hoffman JR, Sande MA. Principles of appropriate antibiotic use for acute rhinosinusitis in adults: background. Ann Intern Med 2001;134(6):498–505.

89. Spector SL, Bernstein IL, Li JT, Berger WE, Kaliner MA, Schuller DE, et al. Parameters for the diagnosis and management of sinusitis. J Allergy Clin Immunol 1998;102 (6, pt 2):S107–44.

90. Ip S, Fu L, Balk E, Chew P, DeVine D, Lau J. Update on bacterial rhinosinusitis: summary, evidence report/ technology assessment No. 124. Rockville, MD: Agency for Healthcare Research and Quality, 2005.

91. Anon JB, Jacobs MR, Poole MD, et al. For the Sinus and Allergy Health Partnership. Antimicrobial treatment guidelines for acute bacterial rhinosinusitis. Otolaryngology Head Neck Surg 2004;130(suppl):1–45.

92. Scheid DC, Hamm RM. Acute bacterial rhinosinusitis in adults: part II. Treatment. Am Fam Physician 2004;70(9):1697–704.

93. Klapan I, Culig J, Oreskovic K, Matrapazovski M, Radosevic S. Azithromycin versus amoxicillin/clavulanate in the treatment of acute sinusitis. Am J Otolaryngol 1999 Jan-Feb;20(1):7–11.

94. Zalmanovici A, Yaphe J. Steroids for acute sinusitis. Cochrane Database Syst Rev 2007(2):CD005149.

95. Slavin RG, Spector SL, Bernstein IL, Kaliner MA, Kennedy DW, Virant FS, et al. The diagnosis and management of sinusitis: a practice parameter update. J Allergy Clin Immunol 2005 Dec;116(6 suppl):S13–47.

96. Food and Drug Administration H. Cold, cough, allergy, bronchodilator, and antiasthmatic drug products for over-the-counter human use; amendment of the final monograph for over-the-counter nasal decongestant drug products. Final rule. Federal Register 2005;70(195):58974–7.

97. Jackson LL, Kountakis SE. Classification and management of rhinosinusitis and its complications. Otolaryngol Clin North Am 2005;38(6):1143–53.

98. Bachert C, Vignola AM, Gevaert P, Leynaert B, Van Cauwenberge P, Bousquet J. Allergic rhinitis, rhinosinusitis, and asthma: one airway disease. Immunol Allergy Clin North Am 2004 Feb;24(1):19–43.

99. Leynaert B, Neukirch F, Demoly P, Bousquet J. Epidemiologic evidence for asthma and rhinitis comorbidity. J Allergy Clin Immunol 2000 Nov;106 (5 suppl):S201–5.

100. Corren J. The connection between allergic rhinitis and bronchial asthma. Curr Opin Pulm Med 2007;13(1):13–8.

101. Meltzer EO. Evaluation of the optimal oral antihistamine for patients with allergic rhinitis. Mayo Clin Proc 2005;80(9):1170–6.

102. Prenner BM, Schenkel E. Allergic rhinitis: treatment based on patient profiles. Am J Med 2006;119(3):230–7.

103. Brunton SA, Fromer LM. Treatment options for the management of perennial allergic rhinitis, with a focus on intranasal corticosteroids. South Med J 2007;100(7):701–8.

104. Wilson AM, O'Byrne PM, Parameswaran K. Leukotriene receptor antagonists for allergic rhinitis: a systematic review and meta-analysis. Am J Med 2004 Mar 1;116(5):338–44.

105. Calderon MA, Alves B, Jacobson M, Hurwitz B, Sheikh A, Durham S. Allergen injection immunotherapy for seasonal allergic rhinitis. Cochrane Database Syst Rev 2007(1):CD001936.

106. Nelson HS. Advances in upper airway diseases and allergen immunotherapy. J Allergy Clin Immunol 2007 Apr;119(4):872–80.

107. Incaudo GA, Takach P. The diagnosis and treatment of allergic rhinitis during pregnancy and lactation. Immunol Allergy Clin North Am 2006;26(1): 137–54.

108. Third Expert Panel on the Management of Asthma. Expert panel report 3: guidelines for the diagnosis and management of asthma. NIH publication No. 07-4051. Bethesda, MD: US Department of Health and Human Services; National Institutes of Health; National Heart, Lung, and Blood Institute; National Asthma Education and Prevention Program, 2007.

109. Centers for Disease Control and Prevention. National Center for Health Statistics. FastStats A to Z: Asthma. 2005. Available from: *http://www.cdc.gov/nchs/fastats/ asthma.htm* [Accessed October 14, 2009].

110. Wechsler ME, Israel E. How pharmacogenomics will play a role in the management of asthma. Am J Respir Crit Care Med 2005;172(1):12–8.

111. Israel E, Chinchilli VM, Ford JG, Boushey HA, Cherniack R, Craig TJ, et al. Use of regularly scheduled albuterol treatment in asthma: genotype-stratified, randomised, placebo-controlled cross-over trial. Lancet 2004 Oct 23–29;364(9444):1505–12.

112. Dahl R, Chuchalin A, Gor D, Yoxall S, Sharma R. A randomised trial comparing salmeterol/fluticasone propionate and formoterol/budesonide combinations in adults with persistent asthma. Respir Med 2006; 100(7):1152–62.

113. Suissa S, Baltzan M, Kremer R, Ernst P. Inhaled and nasal corticosteroid use and the risk of fracture. Am J Respir Crit Care Med 2004;169(1):83–8.

114. Ni Chroinin M, Greenstone IR, Danish A, Magdolinos H, Masse V, Zhang X, et al. Long-acting beta2-agonists versus placebo in addition to inhaled corticosteroids in children and adults with chronic asthma. Cochrane Database Syst Rev 2005(4):CD005535.

115. Mitchell P, Cumming RG, Mackey DA. Inhaled corticosteroids, family history, and risk of glaucoma. Ophthalmology 1999 Dec;106(12):2301–6.

116. Rinehart JJ, Sagone AL, Balcerzak SP, Ackerman GA, LoBuglio AF. Effects of corticosteroid therapy on human monocyte function. N Engl J Med 1975 Jan 30;292(5):236–41.

117. Kips JC, Pauwels RA. Long-acting inhaled beta(2)-agonist therapy in asthma. Am J Respir Crit Care Med 2001;164(6):923–32.

118. Lanes SF, Lanza LL, Wentworth CE, 3rd. Risk of emergency care, hospitalization, and ICU stays for acute asthma among recipients of salmeterol. Am J Respir Crit Care Med 1998 Sep;158(3):857–61.

119. Mann RD, Kubota K, Pearce G, Wilton L. Salmeterol: a study by prescription-event monitoring in a UK cohort of 15,407 patients. J Clin Epidemiol 1996 Feb;49(2):247–50.

120. Nelson HS, Weiss ST, Bleecker ER, Yancey SW, Dorinsky PM. The Salmeterol Multicenter Asthma Research Trial: a comparison of usual pharmacotherapy for asthma or usual pharmacotherapy plus salmeterol. Chest 2006;129(1):15–26.

121. Mann M, Chowdhury B, Sullivan E, Nicklas R, Anthracite R, Meyer RJ. Serious asthma exacerbations in asthmatics treated with high-dose formoterol. Chest 2003;124(1):70–4.

122. Walters EH, Walters JA, Gibson MD. Inhaled long acting beta agonists for stable chronic asthma. Cochrane Database Syst Rev 2003(4):CD001385.

123. Theophilus A, Moore A, Prime D, Rossomanno S, Whitcher B, Chrystyn H. Co-deposition of salmeterol and fluticasone propionate by a combination inhaler. Int J Pharm 2006;313(1–2):14–22.

124. Sheth K, Wasserman RL, Lincourt WR, Locantore NW, Carranza-Rosenzweig J, Crim C. Fluticasone propionate/salmeterol hydrofluoroalkane via metered-dose inhaler with integrated dose counter: performance and patient satisfaction. Int J Clin Pract 2006;60(10): 1218–24.

125. Buhl R, Vogelmeier C. Budesonide/formoterol maintenance and reliever therapy: a new treatment approach for adult patients with asthma. Curr Med Res Opin 2007;23(8):1867–78.

126. Lotvall J. Combination therapy in asthma—fixed or variable dosing in different patients? Curr Med Res Opin 2004;20(11):1711–27.

127. Gyllfors P, Dahlen SE, Kumlin M, Larsson K, Dahlen B. Bronchial responsiveness to leukotriene D4 is resistant to inhaled fluticasone propionate. J Allergy Clin Immunol 2006;118(1):78–83.

128. Adams RJ, Fuhlbrigge A, Finkelstein JA, Lozano P, Livingston JM, Weiss KB, et al. Impact of inhaled anti-inflammatory therapy on hospitalization and emergency department visits for children with asthma. Pediatrics 2001;107(4):706–11.

129. Second Expert Panel on the Management of Asthma. Expert panel report 2 guidelines for the diagnosis and management of asthma. NIH publication No. 97-4091. Bethesda, MD: US Department of Health and Human Services; National Institutes of Health; National Heart, Lung, and Blood Institute; National Asthma Education and Prevention Program, 1997.

130. Rodrigo GJ, Castro-Rodriguez JA. Anticholinergics in the treatment of children and adults with acute asthma: a systematic review with meta-analysis. Thorax 2005;60(9):740–6.

131. National Asthma Education and Prevention Program Asthma and Pregnancy Working Group. Working group report on managing asthma during pregnancy: recommendations for pharmacologic treatment—update 2004. NIH publication No. 05-5236. Bethesda, MD: National Asthma Education and Prevention Program, NHLBI, National Institutes of Health, US Department of Health and Human Services, 2004.

132. Chalmers GW, Macleod KJ, Little SA, Thomson LJ, McSharry CP, Thomson NC. Influence of cigarette smoking on inhaled corticosteroid treatment in mild asthma. Thorax 2002;57(3):226–30.

133. Chaudhuri R, Livingston E, McMahon AD, Lafferty J, Fraser I, Spears M, et al. Effects of smoking cessation on lung function and airway inflammation in smokers with asthma. Am J Respir Crit Care Med 2006;174(2):127–33.

134. Centers for Disease Control and Prevention. Controlling tuberculosis in the United States: recommendations

from the American Thoracic Society, CDC, and the Infectious Diseases Society of America. MMWR 2005; 54(RR-12).

135. Centers for Disease Control and Prevention. A global perspective on tuberculosis. 2007. Available from: *www.cdc.gov/tb/WorldTBDay/resources_global.htm* [Accessed September 25, 2007].

136. Centers for Disease Control and Prevention. Trends in tuberculosis, 2005—United States. 2007. Available from:*www.cdc.gov/tb/WorldTBDay/resources_global .htm* [Accessed September 25, 2007].

137. Centers for Disease Control and Prevention. Targeted tuberculin testing and treatment of latent tuberculosis infection. American Thoracic Society. MMWR Recomm Rep 2000;49(RR-6)1–51.

138. Dinnes J, Deeks J, Kunst H, Gibson A, Cummins E, Waugh N, et al. A systematic review of rapid diagnostic tests for the detection of tuberculosis infection. Health Technol Assess 2007;11(3):1–196.

139. Share with women: tuberculosis and pregnancy. J Midwifery Womens Health 2007;52(4):415–6.

140. Understanding the immune system: how it works. National Institute of Allergy and Infectious Disease. NIH publication No. 03-5423. 2003 Available from: *www.niaid.nih.gov/publications/immune/the _immune_system.pdf* [Accessed April 2, 2009].

141. Hackley B. Asthma and allergy. Hackley B, Kriebs JM, Rousseau ME, eds. Primary care of women. Sudbury, MA: Jones and Bartlett, 2007.

142. US National Library and National Institute of Medicine Medline Plus. Drugs, supplements, and herbal information. 2009. Available from: *www.nlm.nih .gov/medlineplus/druginformation.html* [Accessed March 30, 2009].

143. Clark RK. Anatomy and physiology: understanding the human body. Sudbury, MA: Jones and Bartlett, 2005.

144. National Institute of Allergy and Infectious Disease. Understanding the immune system: how it works. [Internet] NIH Publication No. 03-5423. 2003. Available from: *http://www.niaid.nih.gov/publications/immune/ the_immune_system.pdf* [Accessed April 2, 2009].

Gut Feeling

Synonym: Intuition Origin: A term that is likely derived from the fact that many people experience emotions and intuitive feelings as being centered on, or having a strong effect on, the stomach area, which is also called the gut. It is of note that after the brain, the second largest network of closely interconnected neurons is located in this enteric nervous system.

21

Gastrointestinal Conditions

Nancy Botehlo, Cathy L. Emeis, and Mary C. Brucker, with acknowledgment to Steven Deville

Chapter Glossary

Antacid Category of drugs used to reduce gastric acidity for the treatment of peptic ulcer disease, gastroesophageal reflux disease, and simple pyrosis (heartburn).

Anticholinergic An agent that blocks the acetylcholine receptor, such as the one found in the stomach that enhances production of hydrochloric acid.

Antiemetic A drug taken to prevent or relieve nausea and vomiting. Antiemetics describe a function, not a chemical category. Antiemetics include antihistamines, benzodiazepines, and some medications in other chemical classes.

Chyme-acid The term used to describe the semi-liquid mass of digested food that passes from the stomach into the lower digestive tract.

Dyspepsia Group of symptoms arising from the upper digestive tract, unrelated to colonic function.

Dyssynergia Paradoxical contraction of anus at the same time defecation is attempted secondary to failure of the pelvic muscles to relax during defecation.

Emetic A drug used to induce vomiting, especially in the case of poisoning.

Extrapyramidal symptoms (EPS) Unintentional movements that begin during the early phases of treatment with a neuroleptic drug. Early onset symptoms tend to resolve quickly and completely when the drug is discontinued. The word refers to symptoms originating in a specific part of the brain that refines and modulates movement.

Functional disorder A condition for which no physiologic or anatomic cause can be identified.

Gastric acid Secretion produced by parietal cells in the stomach. Gastric acid consists primarily of hydrochloric acid (HCl), potassium chloride (KCl), and sodium chloride (NaCl). The pH of gastric acid is 1–2.

Gastrin Hormone that stimulates release of gastric acid.

Gastroesophageal reflux disease (GERD) A condition characterized by heartburn (pyrosis), a sensation of substernal burning pain, and regurgitation of swallowed food caused by the abnormal reflux of chyme from the stomach into the esophagus.

Gastroparesis Delay in gastric emptying, often associated with diabetes.

Histamine$_2$-receptor antagonists (H$_2$-receptor antagonists) Group of drugs that inhibit acid secretion by gastric parietal cells by blockage of histamine at H$_2$ receptors (also known as H$_2$ blockers).

Helicobacter pylori A gram-negative bacterium associated with peptic ulcer disease and gastric cancer that inhabits various areas of the stomach and duodenum.

Laxative abuse Use of laxatives to lose weight.

Laxative dependency Overuse of laxatives resulting in need for laxative to have normal bowel movement.

Milk-alkali syndrome Syndrome characterized by hypercalcemia ("remember bones, stones, groans, and psychiatric overtones") that causes fractures, kidney stones, constipation, and altered mental status. Can lead to renal failure if untreated.

Pepsin A proteolytic enzyme that breaks proteins down into peptides.

Peptic ulcer disease (PUD) Condition in which ulceration in the stomach or duodenum results from an imbalance between mucosal-protective factors and various mucosal-damaging mechanisms.

Proton pump inhibitor Class of antisecretory drugs used to treat gastric conditions associated with hyperacidity by affecting proton pumps in the stomach.

Pyrosis Heartburn.

Tardive dyskinesia Involuntary repetitive movements which are a side effect of any medication that is a dopamine antagonist. Dyskinesia refers to involuntary movement and tardive indicates that the movements may continue or appear after the drug is discontinued.

Zollinger-Ellison syndrome Unusual condition in which gastrin is increased, causing increased hydrochloric acid in the stomach, usually as a result of a tumor of the pancreas or duodenum producing the hormone gastrin.

Introduction

Gastrointestinal diseases cause significant morbidity, mortality, and healthcare expenditures in the United States. It is estimated that persons in the United States spend over $10 billion per year alone on proton pump inhibitors for the treatment of gastroesophageal reflux, and 23 of the 200 most frequently prescribed drugs in the United States are for the treatment of gastrointestinal diseases.[1] This chapter reviews the pharmacologic treatments used for gastrointestinal disorders that commonly cause women to seek primary healthcare services.

Physiology of the Gastrointestinal Tract

The upper gastrointestinal tract includes the mouth, pharynx, esophagus, and stomach, and it functions primarily to ingest food and begin the digestive process through mechanical and enzymatic breakdown of the food bolus into smaller particles (Figure 21-1). The inner surface of the stomach has multiple small folds called rugae that are flattened out when the stomach is full. There are four types of cells found in the epithelial lining of the stomach: (1) chief cells that secrete **pepsin**, (2) G cells that secrete the hormone **gastrin**, (3) mucous cells that secrete an alkaline mucus that protects the stomach lining from acid and shear stress, and (4) parietal cells that secrete **gastric acid** and intrinsic factor, which is required for vitamin B_{12} absorption.

The parietal cells have receptors for histamine, acetylcholine, and gastrin (Figure 21-2). When any one of these receptors is bound to the agonist neurotransmitter, the parietal cell responds by making and secreting gastric acid. When all three receptors are bound to agonists, the amount of gastric acid secreted is voluminous.

There are several chemical, mechanical, and neural triggers that initiate secretion of gastric acid. The vagus nerve triggers release of pepsin and gastric acid when the stomach is full via release of acetylcholine, which binds to the parietal cell. Partially digested proteins increase the pH in the stomach, and this rise in pH signals the G cells to produce gastrin, which in turn stimulates release of gastric acid. The gastric acid causes the proteins to denature (unfold) and expose the peptide bonds that can then be broken. As the proteins are digested, the pH falls and gastrin production ceases. Finally, histamine is synthesized and secreted by enterochromaffin-like cells that lie underneath the gastric epithelium. The enterochromaffin-like cells are stimulated by gastrin.

After being synthesized in the parietal cell, gastric acid has to be pumped out of the cell and into the acidic environment of the stomach. This process takes energy because the gastric acid is being secreted against a pH gradient. The process is powered by a *proton pump*, which is the term used to describe the hydrogen/potassium adenosine triphosphatase enzyme system that secretes gastric acid into the stomach cavity.

Contents in the stomach mix and are ultimately moved into the lower intestinal tract via peristalsis. Distention of the stomach wall by food stimulates stretch receptors and gastrin-secreting cells that, in turn, increase the intensity

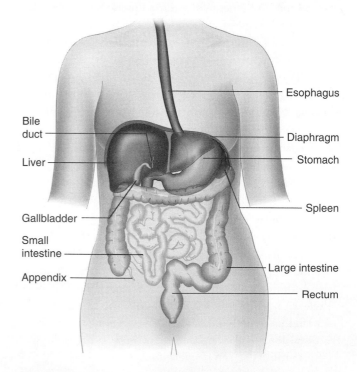

Figure 21-1 Anatomy of the gastrointestinal system.
Source: Modified from DeMatteo RP et al. 2006.[70]

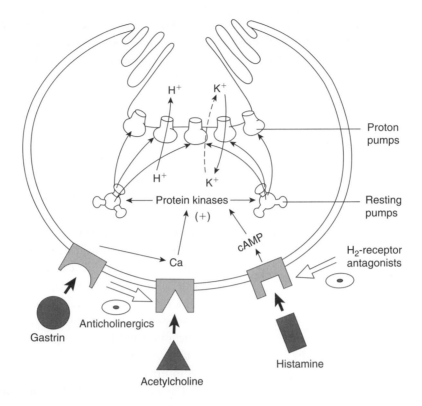

Figure 21-2 Parietal cell: stimulation of gastric acid production and secretion.

of the peristalsis. Another stimulus that activates the peristalsis reflex is serotonin (5-HT), which is synthesized by the enterochromaffin cells.

The lower gastrointestinal tract includes the small and large intestines and anus. In the small intestine, proteins, carbohydrates, and fats are further digested into constituent peptides, disaccharides/monosaccharides, and triglycerides. These nutrients are then absorbed through a variety of transport mechanisms by specialized enterocytes that line the numerous villi of the small intestine. Water, fat-soluble vitamins, and minerals also are absorbed in the small intestine.

Approximately 2 liters of **chyme-acid** and pepsin pass from the small bowel into the colon each day. The colon extracts a majority of the water from this chyme, which becomes feces and stores this waste until it can be eliminated.

Accessory organs including the liver, gallbladder, and pancreas aid in the process of digestion (Figure 21-1). Bile secreted by the liver and stored in the gallbladder plays an important role in fat absorption, and enzymes secreted by the pancreas facilitate the breakdown of proteins, fats, and carbohydrates. This complex organ system has numerous defense mechanisms that prevent infection and mucosal damage from acid or digestive enzymes. Despite these defenses and an intricate system of hormonal and neural regulation, various infectious, inflammatory, motility, malabsorptive, and structural disorders may occur.

Gastrointestinal Health

A healthy diet usually is the first choice for both prophylaxis and treatment of most gastrointestinal disorders. Although there is no single dietary pattern, the stereotypical diet in the United States—rich in meat, fat, salt, additives, and sweets; while low in natural vegetables and fruits—is characterized as unhealthy. Necessary vitamins and minerals in the average US diet range from being abnormally low to unnecessarily high. Dietary vitamins, minerals, and food supplements are discussed in detail in Chapter 5.

Dietary fiber has been touted as an important component of a healthy diet. It is recommended that individuals obtain 25–30 mg of soluble and insoluble fiber from a daily diet, even though most studies find that the Western diet falls short in this regard.[2] It is theorized that dietary fiber inhibits secretion of pancreatic enzymes, increases stool bulk, slows gastrointestinal transit, and stimulates growth of normal intestinal flora.

Two other potentially important dietary compounds include *prebiotics* and *probiotics*. Prebiotics are nondigested food ingredients such as oligosaccharides that act within the large intestine. Probiotics, from the Latin *for life*, are functional foods that improve microbiologic gastrointestinal balance. The most widely used probiotic bacteria are strains of *Lactobacillus* (e.g., *Lactobacillus acidophilus)* and *Bifidobacterium*. Controversies exist about the usefulness of prebiotics and probiotics as therapies for gastrointestinal conditions, although a number of studies now are suggesting that there may be roles for these agents. Emerging data regarding use of probiotics, especially among individuals with irritable bowel syndrome, provide hope that these agents are effective. The advantages of prebiotics and probiotics include their accessibility, lack of major adverse effects, and general low cost.

Gastrointestinal Tract Disorders

In this chapter, pharmacotherapies for the most common gastrointestinal conditions seen in primary care settings are reviewed. These conditions are clustered by the primary site of the disorder. For example, the stomach is the major area for dyspepsia, gastroesophageal reflux disease, peptic ulcers, nausea, vomiting, bleeding, and **gastroparesis**. Because many of the drugs that are used to treat these conditions are the same, pharmacologic agents are presented separately according to their major therapeutic action. Irritable bowel syndrome (IBS) is reviewed here, and inflammatory bowel disease is referred to but is reviewed in more detail in Chapter 17. Major gastrointestinal disorders such as hepatitis, pancreatitis, and colon cancer are beyond the scope of this chapter and are not addressed.

Conditions in the Upper Gastrointestinal Tract: Dyspepsia

Dyspepsia is the term used for a group of symptoms arising from the upper digestive tract, unrelated to colonic function. The estimated prevalence of dyspepsia in the United States is 25%, excluding persons with typical symptoms of **gastroesophageal reflux disease** (GERD).[3] Dyspepsia is a common reason for a visit to a healthcare provider.

Symptoms include pain in the upper abdomen that can be accompanied by bloating, early satiety, postprandial fullness, nausea, anorexia, heartburn, and burping or belching.[3] A variety of diverse factors are associated with dyspepsia including foods, medications, systemic disorders, and disorders of the gastrointestinal tract. The drugs that most commonly cause dyspepsia are nonsteroidal anti-inflammatory drugs (NSAIDs), antibiotics, and estrogens.[4] Dyspepsia may be a symptom of GERD, although it does not always occur with GERD, nor is it pathognomonic for the disorder.

When no cause can be found for dyspepsia, the condition is referred to as a **functional disorder**. Functional dyspepsia, or nonulcerative dyspepsia, the most common type of dyspepsia,[4] is defined as persistent or recurrent pain in the upper abdomen in absence of organic disease. Risk factors for functional dyspepsia include female gender and underlying psychologic disturbances.[5] The hormonal fluctuations of estrogen and progesterone associated with the menstrual cycle will often make functional symptoms worse.

Environmental and lifestyle habits such as poor socioeconomic status, smoking, increased caffeine intake, and ingestion of nonsteroidal anti-inflammatory drugs (NSAIDs) appear to be more likely to cause ulcerative dyspepsia.[5]

The first-line treatments for dyspepsia include over-the-counter antacids, **histamine$_2$-receptor antagonists** (also known as H$_2$ blockers, H$_2$ antihistamines, H$_2$-receptor antagonists, or antisecretory antihistamines), and **proton pump inhibitors**. Antibiotic therapy is indicated to treat *Helicobacter pylori* (*H pylori*) infection.

Nonpharmacologic Treatments

Alternative and complementary treatments also are a consideration for treating dyspepsia. Peppermint oil and traditional Chinese medicines have been used for centuries. A combination of enteric-coated peppermint oil and caraway has been shown in several trials to reduce symptoms of nonulcer dyspepsia.[6] The peppermint oil relaxes the lower esophageal sphincter, which alleviates the symptoms of dyspepsia. A meta-analysis of three trials of a preparation containing peppermint and caraway oils plus another herbal extract called STW5 (Iberogast) found this combination formulation to be more effective than placebo in reducing the severity of the most bothersome gastrointestinal symptoms (OR = 0.22; 95% CI, 0.11–0.47), although not all trials support these findings when compared to other agents. A fourth trial did not find any difference between the effect of STW5 and cisapride (Propulsid).[7]

Consumer-oriented Web sites tend to promote various food products such as papaya and coconut, especially in the form of macaroon cookies, as digestive remedies. Some sites also suggest hazelnuts (filberts), while others caution against their use. In summary, research about the effectiveness of these foods as a remedy for heartburn is lacking.

Peptic Ulcer Disease

Peptic ulcer disease (PUD) is an ulceration in the stomach or duodenum that occurs secondary to an imbalance between mucosal-protective factors and various mucosal-damaging mechanisms. The damage may be caused by medications such as NSAIDs or corticosteroids. Nonpharmacologic risk factors include smoking, drinking alcohol, reflux of bile acids, increased acid production, age over 40 years, male gender, drug-induced inhibition of prostaglandin synthesis, and *H pylori* infection.

In the early 1900s, B. W. Sippy advocated a dietary change as an "efficient removal of gastric juice" in the case of gastric or duodenal ulcers.[8] Milk and cream were combined with alkaline powders and administered every half hour to the individual with the ulcer. The underlying theory was that the dairy products and powders would alkalinize the stomach and promote ulcer healing. In the last half of the century, it became clear that milk products tend to increase gastric secretions as opposed to decreasing them. Eventually, clinical practice demonstrated that the so-called Sippy diet was ineffective and it is no longer advocated.

Today, the first-line medications for persons with peptic ulcer disease are H_2-receptor antagonists and proton pump inhibitors, which have demonstrated efficacy in healing ulcers. Protective agents such as sucralfate (Carafate) or antacids are used as an adjunct. These agents help relieve symptoms and have some effect on healing, but their efficacy is less than the efficacy of H_2-receptor agonists and proton pump inhibitors. Misoprostol (Cytotec) is effective for preventing NSAID-induced ulcers but has no effect on healing ulcers. Other treatments include antibiotics used to eradicate *H pylori*.

H pylori Infection

H pylori, a gram-negative bacillus, has been associated with both duodenal and gastric ulcers. The bacilli burrow into the mucosa and weaken the protective mucous coating of the stomach and duodenum, which allows acid to get through to the sensitive lining beneath. The acid and the bacteria irritate the lining of the stomach or duodenum and cause ulcers. Approximately 30–40% of the US population is infected with *H pylori* in situ, and the microorganism is said to be the most common bacillus in the world.[9] Discovery of *H pylori* took decades because the bacteria does not grow easily in cultures. In the early 1980s *H pylori* was isolated in Australia, although it took many more years to convince clinicians that ulcers were due to bacteria rather than the long-established theory of stress and spicy food. In 2005, the Australian researchers Warren and Marshall received the Nobel Prize for the discovery of the microorganism.

Many people who harbor *H pylori* never experience gastritis or ulcers. For example, it is estimated that fewer than 20% of individuals who are chronically infected with *H pylori* ever develop a peptic ulcer.[4] However, the majority of the clinical cases of gastritis and peptic ulcer disease (PUD) are caused by *H pylori*. Chronic *H pylori* infection is considered to be a carcinogen, since it is an etiologic factor in the development of gastric cancers and gastric lymphomas. Eradication of the *H pylori* organism enables the peptic ulcer to heal and decreases the recurrence rate of gastric or duodenal ulcers.[4]

H pylori is treated with two antibiotics in combination with a proton pump inhibitor. The proton pump inhibitor is given to raise the pH within the stomach, which increases the effectiveness of ampicillin (Amoxil) and erythromycin (E-Mycin). This bacterium is difficult to eradicate. *H pylori* is inherently resistant to sulfonamides, trimethoprim (Trimpex), and vancomycin. It develops resistance easily to metronidazole (Flagyl) and clarithromycin (Biaxin), but clarithromycin has the single best efficacy against *H pylori* if resistance is not present. There are currently several FDA-approved treatments for *H pylori* that have eradication rates of 61–94%, depending on the regimen used (Table 21-1). In addition, several other combinations have been used successfully.

Pylera is the brand name for a combination therapy for treatment of *H pylori* that has recently been introduced. It consists of biskalcitrate potassium 140 mg, metronidazole 125 mg, and tetracycline hydrochloride 125 mg in capsule form. A proton pump inhibitor twice daily should accompany the administration of Pylera. The recommended duration of therapy is 10 days. During pregnancy and lactation, the treatment for *H pylori* generally is deferred.[9]

Table 21-1 Treatment Regimens for *H pylori**

Regimen	Eradication Rate	Clinical Considerations
Proton pump inhibitor[†] + clarithromycin (Biaxin) 500 mg bid + amoxicillin (Amoxil) 1 g bid × 10–14 days*	77–85%	First-line treatment recommended by FDA
Proton pump inhibitor + clarithromycin (Biaxin) 500 mg bid + metronidazole (Flagyl) 500 mg bid × 10–14 days	70–85%	First-line treatment for PCN allergy
Bismuth subsalicylate (Pepto Bismol) 525 mg qid + metronidazole (Flagyl) 250 mg qid + tetracycline 500 mg qid* × 14 days + ranitidine [Zantac] 300 mg/day (or famotidine [Pepcid] 40 mg/day, or nizatidine [Axid] 300 mg/day in place of rantidine); then give H$_2$ antagonist alone for additional 14 days; avoid cimetidine (Tagamet)*	75–90%	First-line therapy; may use for PCN allergy, often used for retreatment when necessary; high pill burden; bismuth subsalicylate may turn the tongue or stools green or black—this is harmless
Lansoprazole (Prevacid) 30 mg tid + amoxicillin (Amoxil) 1 g tid × 2 wks*[‡]	77%	Lower eradication rates, useful for patients who are intolerant to clarithromycin or metronidazole
Lansoprazole (Prevacid) 30 mg bid + amoxicillin (Amoxil) 1 g bid + clarithromycin (Biaxin) 500 mg bid × 10–14 days*	85–92%	Lower eradication rates, useful for patients who are intolerant to clarithromycin or metronidazole
Omeprazole (Prilosec) 20 mg bid + amoxicillin (Amoxil) 1 g bid + clarithromycin (Biaxin) 500 mg bid × 10 days*	77–78%	Give additional 18 days of omeprazole 20 mg per day for active duodenal ulcer and 40 mg per day for up to 12 weeks for active gastric ulcer

* FDA-approved regimen.

[†] Proton pump inhibitors: omeprazole (Prilosec) 20 mg PO bid × 10 d; esomeprazole (Nexium) 40 mg PO once daily × 10 d; lansoprazole (Prevacid) 30 mg PO bid × 10 d; pantoprazole (Protonix) 40 mg PO once daily × 10 d; rabeprazole (Aciphex) 20 mg PO bid × 7 d.

[‡] Indicated for persons who are allergic or intolerant to clarithromycin or for infections that are known or suspected to be resistant to clarithromycin.

Gastroesophageal Reflux Disease

Gastroesophageal reflux disease (GERD) is characterized by heartburn (**pyrosis**), a sensation of substernal burning pain, and regurgitation of swallowed food caused by the abnormal reflux of chyme from the stomach into the esophagus. Individuals may also experience excessive salivation and the sensation of a foreign body sensation in the posterior pharynx. Other symptoms include a chronic cough, wheezing, hoarseness, sinusitis, and dental caries. These symptoms usually occur postprandially.

The resting tone of the lower esophageal sphincter (LES) normally maintains a high-pressure zone that prevents GERD. For individuals who develop reflux esophagitis, this pressure tends to be lower. Vomiting, coughing, lifting, or bending can contribute to the development of reflux esophagitis. If the chyme is highly acidic or contains bile salts and pancreatic enzymes, the refluxed chyme can be erosive. The refluxed chyme remains in the esophagus longer than normal in individuals with weak peristalsis. Delayed gastric emptying also can contribute to reflux esophagitis. Disorders that delay emptying include gastric or duodenal ulcers—which can cause pyloric edema or pyloric strictures, and hiatal hernias that weaken the lower esophageal sphincter.

Nonpharmacologic Treatment of GERD

Nonpharmacologic treatment of GERD includes lifestyle modifications that decrease the amount of reflux or decrease the damage to the lining of the esophagus from refluxed materials. Although there is a paucity of evidence on this subject, persons with GERD are often counseled to avoid foods and beverages that can decrease the LES pressure. These include chocolate, peppermint, fried or fatty foods, caffeine, and alcoholic beverages. Acidic food and beverages that can further damage the esophageal lining include tomato products and peppers. Decreasing the size of portions at mealtimes and eating at least 2–3 hours before bedtime may help to control the symptoms. The elimination of cigarettes and losing weight may also help with symptoms of GERD. Cigarette smoking prolongs clearance of acid from the stomach and relaxes the baseline LES pressure.[4] Weight gain increases intra-abdominal pressure that displaces the lower esophageal sphincter and increases the gastroesophageal gradient.[4] There is evidence that losing weight and elevating the head of the bed are effective treatments, but there is no evidence that smoking cessation or dietary modifications really improve GERD symptoms.

Finally, women should avoid medications that promote gastroesophageal reflux by reducing pressure of the lower esophageal sphincter and esophageal clearance if it is possible and clinically safe to do so. Prominent among these medications are progesterone, anticholinergics, sedatives, opiates, tranquilizers, theophylline (Theo-Dur), beta-adrenergic agonists, nitrates, and calcium channel blockers.

Pharmacologic Treatment of GERD

Antacids decrease the acidity of refluxed material and may be effective in treating mild or infrequent reflux symptoms. H_2-receptor antagonists are frequently used in the treatment of mild to moderate GERD but are less effective than are proton pump inhibitors, which are recommended for frequent or severe GERD symptoms and for persons who do not respond to H_2-receptor antagonist therapy. Proton pump inhibitors and H_2-receptor antagonists actually promote the healing of the esophagus.

The preferred empirical approach is step-up therapy; namely treat initially with an H_2-receptor antagonist for 8 weeks, and if symptoms do not improve, it is recommended to discontinue the antisecretory antihistamine and employ a proton pump inhibitor.[9]

Drugs That Reduce Gastric Acid

The common gastrointestinal conditions discussed thus far usually are treated with the medications from the same drug categories. Dyspepsia, peptic ulcer disease, and GERD all require treatment with medications that decrease secretion of gastric acid or neutralize it once it is in the stomach. No single agent has been found to be superior to others in all cases. The choice of which agent to use varies based on the individual and clinical situation.

Antacids

Antacids are one of the most frequently used classes of medications due to their safety profile, decreased cost, rapid onset, and accessibility. Antacids are the primary treatment for minor gastric symptoms or to relieve heartburn (Box 21-1). They are used as adjunct therapy for the relief of discomfort from peptic ulcers and to promote healing of peptic ulcers; for relief of stomach upset associated with hyperacidity; in prevention of stress ulcer bleeding; in treatment of duodenal ulcer; and in treatment of gastroesophageal reflux disease. Antacids contain various combinations

Box 21-1 A Case of Heartburn

JB is a 38-year-old woman who reports that she works as a nurse on the 10-hour night shift four nights a week. She reports being aroused from sleep several times a week by heartburn and mild regurgitation. She has used bismuth subsalicylate (Pepto-Bismol) as self-treatment with little success. She voices a concern that she may have an ulcer. JB is married and has two grade-school-aged children at home. Aside from bismuth subsalicylate (Pepto-Bismol), her only regular medication is Ortho Novum 777, which she takes daily for contraception. Her physical examination is unremarkable except for a BMI of 34.

Additional information is needed from JB regarding her sleep and dietary habits. Individuals who work night shifts have various sleeping patterns. Upon further discussion, she reveals that after shift she usually goes to breakfast with coworkers and shortly after arriving home, she goes to bed.

The first-line of therapy for this woman is dietary manipulation. Because of her weight and routine of sleeping shortly after eating, she is at risk for nocturnal pyrosis and regurgitation, or gastroesophageal reflux disease. Health education about weight loss and light meals before sleep may be of more value than any medication if she is able to implement these changes. However, if a medication is desired, bismuth subsalicylate (Pepto Bismol) is not the best first choice. The salicylate in this product is contraindicated for nursing mothers and for persons recovering from influenza or chicken pox because salicylate increases the risk of Reyes syndrome in these settings. Bismuth subsalicylate may be of great value for treating an ulcer, but it is unlikely from this information that she has peptic ulcer disease. Instead, an inexpensive antacid such as a combination aluminum/magnesium agent (e.g., Maalox, Mylanta) would be a reasonable first choice—but *not* taken proximate to her combined oral contraception or she may find herself with heartburn associated with pregnancy. Antacids can interfere with absorption of orally ingested hormonal contraceptives.

Table 21-2 Antacids*

Drug Generic (Brand)	Dose Range	Contraindications	Side Effects/Adverse Effects
Calcium carbonate (TUMS)	1–2 tablets (500–750 mg each) every 2 hours as needed. Maximum = 7000 mg per 24-hours.[†]	Hypercalcemia, renal calculi, hypophosphatemia, persons with suspected digoxin toxicity.	Constipation, anorexia, dry mouth, frequent urination, muscle twitching Hypercalcemia, hypophosphatemia
Aluminum hydroxide (Amphojel)	600–1200 mg between meals and at bedtime.	Hypersensitivity to aluminum salts.	Constipation, abdominal cramps, nausea, and vomiting
Magnesium hydroxide (Milk of Magnesia)	5–15 mL four times daily prn for antacid 30–60 mL prn for laxative.	Serious renal impairment; myocardial damage; heart block; colostomy or ileostomy; intestinal obstruction; impaction, or perforation; appendicitis; abdominal pain.	Hypermagnesemia, abdominal cramps, diarrhea
Magnesium/aluminum combinations (Mylanta, Maalox, Gelusil)	Variable; Maalox 2–4 teaspoons four times daily PO.	Hypersensitivity to aluminum salts. Serious renal impairment; myocardial damage; heart block; colostomy or ileostomy; intestinal obstruction; impaction, or perforation; appendicitis; abdominal pain.	Hypermagnesemia, aluminum intoxication, constipation, diarrhea, osteomalacia
Simethicone (Mylicon)	40–120 mg four times daily PO.	Hypersensitivity to simethicone or other components of the formulation.	No significant side effects
Sodium bicarbonate[‡]	Effervescent powder: 1–2 tsp in glass of water after meals (4–8 g/dose). Powder: ½ tsp in a glass of water up to every 2 h. Tablets: 325 mg–2 g qd to qid.	Persons on salt-restricted diet; pregnancy.	Excess sodium can cause alkalosis, hypertension, congestive heart failure, edema, milk-alkali syndrome possible if person has high intake of calcium
Adjunct Medications			
Oxethazaine (Mucaine)	5–10 mL four times daily PO, 15 minutes before meals and at bedtime.	Avoid if taking tetracycline, or if the individual has hypophosphatemia or renal impairment.	Dizziness, faintness, or drowsiness in doses exceeding 60 mL/day
Alginic acid (Gaviscon-2)	Chew 2–4 tablets four times daily.	Hypocalcemia, hyponatremia, vomiting, concurrent use of citrate salts, renal impairment.	Constipation, diarrhea, nausea, hyporeflexia, vomiting, muscle weakness

* Brand names of antacids can be confusing. For example, there are several formulations of Alka-Seltzer some of which include aspirin. Some antacids contain a combination of aluminum salts, magnesium salts, sodium salts, and calcium salts. Prescribers should know the constituents of specific brand names before recommending them.
[†] Milk-alkali syndrome has been reported in case studies in persons who took a maximum dose of ≥ 4 g/day.
[‡] Sodium bicarbonate is a component of several different brand names.

of metallic cations such as sodium bicarbonate, aluminum, calcium, or magnesium salts (Table 21-2).

Mechanism of Action of Antacids

All antacids neutralize gastric acid in the stomach and increase the gastric pH. Contrary to popular belief, antacids do not coat the stomach mucosal lining. Sodium bicarbonate dissociates to provide bicarbonate ions that neutralize hydrogen ion concentration, which consequently raises blood and urinary pH. The other antacids similarly dissociate to provide a base ion and neutralize gastric hydrochloric acid. When the intragastric pH is maintained above 4, the activation of pepsinogen to pepsin is decreased. Also, neutralization of gastric fluids leads to an increased lower esophageal sphincter pressure. Antacids act rapidly and empty from the stomach quickly, with a resulting reaccumulation of acid or acid rebound. The best time to take an antacid is 1 hour after a meal or as soon as symptoms appear. Liquid formulations of antacids have greater acid neutralizing capacity than do tablets, but tablets can be easier to use. Antacids are available over the counter and no randomized trials comparing antacids head to head are available. If an antacid is chosen, the side-effect profile and drug interactions should be considered prior to use.

Side Effects/Adverse Effects

Side effects of antacids are generally mild and include constipation following ingestion of aluminum antacids and calcium-containing antacids and diarrhea following use of magnesium antacids. Some antacids have a chalky taste, and sodium bicarbonate may be contraindicated for individuals with sodium restriction.

Antacids are considered relatively safe from major adverse effects. Calcium-containing antacids can cause **milk-alkali syndrome** if more than the recommended maximum dose is taken.

Drug–Drug Interactions

Many drug–drug interactions occur with antacids. A list of selected agents can be found in Table 21-3. As a general rule of thumb, individuals should refrain from using antacids with any other medications, but when necessary, they should allow at least 1 hour before and after administration of another medication.

Sodium Bicarbonate (Baking Soda, Alka Seltzer Heartburn Relief)

Sodium bicarbonate (e.g., Alka Seltzer Heartburn Relief), or baking soda, is used to treat heartburn secondary to hyperacidity. This over-the-counter agent is a component of many antacid formulations and is the only compound in baking soda. Sodium bicarbonate is well absorbed and has a rapid action, which occurs within 15 minutes. While neutralizing the acid, baking soda releases carbon dioxide, and belching is common. Like the other antacids, sodium bicarbonate is a short-term solution to indigestion.

Table 21-3 Selected Drug–Drug Interactions Associated with Use of Antacids*

Drug Generic (Brand)	Effects of These Drugs Increased by These Antacids Generic (Brand)	Effects of These Drugs Decreased by These Antacids Generic (Brand)
Sodium bicarbonate (Alka Seltzer)	Amphetamines Ephedrine Flecainide (Tambocor) Pseudoephedrine (Sudafed) Quinidine (Cardioquin, Quinaglute, Quinidex Extentabs) Quinine (Quinerva, Quinate)	Chlorpropamide (Diabinese) Iron Lithium (Lithobid) Salicylates; e.g., aspirin
Calcium carbonate (TUMS)	Digoxin (Lanoxin) toxicity	Alendronate (Fosamax) Atenolol Calcium channel blockers Iron Levothyroxine (Synthroid) Quinolone antibiotics; e.g., ofloxacin (Floxin) Sodium fluoride and tetracycline (Vibramycin) Zinc absorption
Aluminum hydroxide (Amphojel)		Allopurinol (Zyloprim) Antibiotics—tetracyclines, quinolones, some cephalosporins Bisphosphonate derivatives; e.g., alendronate (Fosamax) Corticosteroids Cyclosporine (Sandimmune) Delavirdine (Rescriptor) Imidazole antifungals Iron salts Isoniazid (INH) Mycophenolate (CellCept) Penicillamine (Cuprimine, Depen) Phenothiazines; e.g., chlorpromazine (Thorazine) Phenytoin (Dilantin) Phosphate supplements Trientine (Syprine)
Magnesium hydroxide (Milk of Magnesia)		Digoxin (Lanoxin) Indomethacin (Indocin) Iron salts Tetracyclines (Vibramycin)

(continues)

Table 21-3 Selected Drug–Drug Interactions Associated with Use of Antacids* *(continued)*

Drug Generic (Brand)	Effects of These Drugs Increased by These Antacids Generic (Brand)	Effects of These Drugs Decreased by These Antacids Generic (Brand)
Cimetidine (Tagamet)	Alfentanil (Alfenta) Amiodarone (Cordarone) Benzodiazepines; e.g., diazepam (Valium) Beta-blockers Calcium channel blockers Carbamazepine (Tegretol) Carmustine (Guadal) Clozapine (Clozaril) Cyclosporine (Sandimmune) Flecainide (Flexane) Lidocaine (Xylocaine) Metformin (Glucophage) Phenytoin (Dilantin) Procainamide (Pronestyl) Quinolones; e.g., ofloxacin (Floxin) Selective serotonin reuptake inhibitors Sulfonylureas Theophylline Thioridazine (Mellaril) Tricyclic antidepressants Warfarin (Coumadin)	Atazanavir (Reyataz) Cefpodoxime (Vantin) Cefuroxime (Ceftin) Fluconazole (Diflucan) Itraconazole (Sporanox) Ketoconazole (Nizoral)
Ranitidine (Zantac)	Warfarin (Coumadin)	Atazanavir (Reyataz) Cefpodoxime (Vantin) Cefuroxime (Ceftin) Itraconazole (Sporanox) Ketoconazole (Nizoral) Warfarin (Coumadin)
Famotidine (Pepcid AC)	Cyclosporine (Sandimmune)	Azole antifungals; e.g., miconazole (Monistat) Cefpodoxime (Vantin) Cefuroxime (Ceftin) Delavirdine (Rescriptor)
Nizatidine (Axid)		Itraconazole (Sporanox) Ketoconazole (Nizoral)
Omeprazole (Prilosec)	Carbamazepine (Tegretol) Diazepam (Valium) Phenytoin (Dilantin) Warfarin (Coumadin)	Itraconazole (Sporanox) Ketoconazole (Nizoral) Protease inhibitors

* This table is not comprehensive. New information is being generated on a regular basis.

Because of the potential for systemic alkalosis, it is not recommended for the treatment of peptic ulcer disease.

Calcium Carbonate (TUMS)

Calcium carbonate (Tums) rapidly neutralizes gastric acidity. The agent should be taken with a full glass of water 1–3 hours after a meal and remote from taking other medications including ingestion of iron supplements. Constipation occurs frequently when taking this medication, and, although rare, elevated calcium levels from calcium carbonate can lead to kidney failure. Calcium carbonate has substantial acid-neutralizing capacity; it therefore causes **gastrin** release, which stimulates gastric acid secretion and profound acid rebound.[4] Because calcium carbonate has

this contradictory side effect, it usually is not the choice for first-line therapy.

Aluminum Hydroxide (Amphojel)

Like most antacids, aluminum-containing medicines such as aluminum hydroxide (Amphojel) react chemically to neutralize or buffer gastric acid but have no direct effect on its production. These agents are indicated for the treatment of acid indigestion, heartburn, hyperacidity, dyspepsia, gastritis, reflux esophagitis, and peptic ulcerations. Aluminum binds with phosphate and decreases its absorption in the gut, which inhibits phosphate and calcium metabolism. As with calcium carbonate, the most common side effect of aluminum antacids is constipation. If large amounts of aluminum are consumed, especially over a long period of time, the person consuming them may be at risk for calcium loss, even culminating in osteoporosis.[11] Increased plasma concentration of aluminum and aluminum neurotoxicity are potential concerns for individuals who have chronic renal failure.[4] Long-term use of aluminum antacids can also increase the risk of kidney stones.[4]

Magnesium Antacids (Milk of Magnesia)

Magnesium antacids are more effective than aluminum antacids, but less effective than sodium bicarbonate.[4] Magnesium antacids also need to be used with caution by persons with renal insufficiency, as long-term use can result in magnesium toxicity. High serum magnesium can cause cardiac, central nervous system, and kidney problems. Milk of Magnesia is an example of a magnesium-containing antacid, and it can be used as an antacid or a laxative, depending upon dose.

Magnesium/Aluminum Combinations (Mylanta, Maalox, Gelusil)

Magnesium/aluminum combination antacids neutralize or reduce the acidity in the stomach. These antacids also are used for the treatment of acid indigestion, heartburn, hyperacidity, dyspepsia, gastritis, reflux esophagitis, and peptic ulcerations. The magnesium component dissociates to neutralize gastric acid while the aluminum component dissolves slowly in the stomach and provides more prolonged relief. The magnesium also has a laxative effect to counter the constipation commonly caused by aluminum. The aluminum component can impair phosphorus absorption and deplete calcium and phosphorus, resulting in bone density loss especially with prolonged use.[4]

Other Adjunctive Agents with Antacids: Oxethazaine (Mucaine)

Oxethazaine (Mucaine) is a mucosal anesthetic that also produces antispasmodic action on smooth muscles. Mucaine does not have antacid properties, but it is used in combination with an aluminum/magnesium antacid. Mucaine comes in a suspension containing oxethazaine aluminum hydroxide and magnesium hydroxide that is used for dyspepsia and also for symptom relief of hyperacidity associated with peptic ulceration, gastritis, esophageal reflux with heartburn, and gastric hyperacidity. The same side effect profile of aluminum and magnesium

antacids applies to this medication.[10] Some individuals experience dizziness, fainting, and/or drowsiness at doses greater than 60 mL per day. The rate and absorption of many drugs may be increased or decreased when taking oxethazaine. Therefore, the following medications should not be taken within 1–2 hours of oxethazaine (Mucaine): benzodiazepines (e.g., diazepam), ethambutol (Myambutol), fluoride, indomethacin (Indocin), iron salts, isoniazid (INH), nitrofurantoin (Macrobid), phenothiazines (e.g., chlorpromazine), phenytoin (Dilantin), ranitidine (Zantac), any tetracycline, or vitamin A.

Alginic Acid (Gaviscon-2)

Alginic acid (Gaviscon-2) protects the stomach mucosa and mechanically impairs reflux by forming a viscous layer on the surface of the gastric contents. Alginic acid is used for relief of mild to moderate gastroesophageal reflux symptoms and dyspepsia. Evidence for clinical effectiveness is lacking.

Special Populations: Pregnancy, Lactation, and the Elderly

Pyrosis occurs frequently during pregnancy due to the decrease in lower esophageal pressure caused by steroidal hormones, especially progesterone. Heartburn is estimated to occur in 30–50% of pregnant women, with the incidence approaching 80% in some populations.[12,13] Most antacids are considered low risk in pregnancy because they are minimally absorbed, and therefore they have no FDA pregnancy category.[14,15] Antacids that contain calcium and magnesium (Mylanta Gelcaps, Marblen, Mi-Acid Gelcaps) are recommended as the first choice because the calcium is often needed and the magnesium may reduce the incidence of preeclampsia.[15]

Alginic acid and simethicone are FDA Pregnancy Category C drugs because of lack of studies, although they, like the other antacids, are commonly used in pregnancy and are generally considered compatible with breastfeeding.[15,16] It is unknown if simethicone crosses the placenta, but it is commonly used during pregnancy. Use of simethicone is safe for breastfeeding mothers.[15,16]

However, antacids containing sodium bicarbonate should be used with caution during pregnancy because they can cause maternal or fetal metabolic alkalosis and fluid overload. Sodium bicarbonate should not be the antacid of choice for the elderly or for individuals on sodium restricted diets (e.g., people with hypertension and/or heart disease) because the increase in sodium can result in metabolic alkalosis.

H₂-Receptor Antagonists

H₂-receptor antagonists (alternately known as H₂ blockers, H₂ antihistamines, or H₂ antisecretory antihistamines) are considered second-line therapy for GERD if use of antacids does not resolve symptoms. These drugs act by blocking the stimulating effect of histamine on the gastric parietal cells (Figure 21-2). These drugs have an antagonist effect at the H₂ receptors of the parietal cells, which results in a decrease of 50–80% in basal, postprandial, and vagally stimulated acid production.[17] These medications are used for acid suppressive therapy for GERD and may be used in conjunction with non-steroidal analgesics in an effort to reduce dyspeptic symptoms and prevent NSAID-induced ulcers. For individuals with nocturnal GERD symptoms, administration of an H₂-receptor antagonist at bedtime suppresses vagally mediated, nocturnal gastric-acid secretion. All H₂-receptor antagonists originally were available by prescription only, but currently all are sold over the counter. These drugs include famotidine (Pepcid AC), cimetidine (Tagamet), ranitidine (Zantac), and nizatidine (Axid).

A combination drug composed of an H₂ blocker and an antacid now is available. This product includes famotidine, calcium carbonate, and magnesium hydroxide and is sold under the brand name Pepcid Complete. Initially there were concerns that the antacids would interfere with the pharmacokinetics of famotidine, since the agents often demonstrate drug–drug interactions. However, studies have failed to find any significant interactions, and the antacid provides rapid relief, while the H₂ blocker provides longer lasting effects.[18]

For persons with mild GERD, first-line therapy may be an antacid, particularly due to the low-risk profiles of the agents, easy availability, and low cost compared to H₂ blockers. However, over-the-counter H₂-receptor antagonists are widely advertised and are increasing in popularity (Box 21-2). The standard dose for a person with nonerosive disease is an H₂-receptor antagonist twice daily.

When erosive gastritis occurs, higher-dose H₂-receptor antagonists provide better acid control than antacids, especially if they are administered after meals. H₂-receptor antagonists and proton pump inhibitors (PPIs) are effective in the treatment of GERD, but PPI therapy is clearly superior in the treatment of severe disease and in healing of erosive esophagitis.[17,19]

The H₂-receptor antagonists are well tolerated by the majority of people who use them. These drugs impede

---

Box 21-2 To Treat or Not to Treat: Diet Versus Drugs

Several years ago, when H₂-receptor antagonists were first introduced to the over-the-counter market, there was a series of television advertisements advocating their use. These medications were promoted in one commercial by a person about to overindulge in a buffet; in another ad, a person was less than happy to go to dinner at the in-laws'; and in a third, a person was about to eat greasy pepperoni pizza. In all three situations, the individuals voiced a history of experiencing significant heartburn under similar circumstances. However, in none of the commercials did the advertisers entertain the possibility that simply changing an eating habit would avoid the need for prophylactic or therapeutic use of drugs—although the vignette with the in-laws may illustrate a valid exception to this rule.

---

gastric acid production for 6–24 hours and are useful for individuals who need persistent acid suppression. It usually takes 30–90 minutes before they are effective.

Cimetidine (Tagamet) was the first H₂-receptor antagonist approved by the Food and Drug Administration (FDA) in 1999. Many factors need to be considered for persons taking this medication. Among men, gynecomastia and impotence have been theorized to be a dose-related antiandrogen effect of cimetidine (Tagamet).[4] Because of the aforementioned effects for men, and the number of drug–drug interactions due to CYP450 metabolism, cimetidine generally is not considered a first-line H₂-receptor antagonist. However, specifically among women, this agent does appear to have an advantage of increasing HDL cholesterol.

Famotidine (Pepcid AC) is more potent than cimetidine (Tagamet), nizatidine (Axid), or ranitidine (Zantac). The most common side effect of famotidine and ranitidine is headache, which occurs in 4–5% of individuals who use famotidine and 3% of individuals who take ranitidine. Famotidine is excreted primarily via the kidney, and when used by individuals with kidney compromise, it can induce central nervous system changes such as depression, insomnia, and mental disturbances. The FDA has issued a warning that the dose of famotidine should be decreased when it is prescribed for persons who have some renal compromise.

Drug–Drug Interactions

Cimetidine (Tagamet) is associated with many clinically significant drug–drug interactions because it has the dual action of inhibiting several CYP450 enzymes and decreasing renal clearance of several drugs. Caffeine levels may increase if taken with cimetidine, whereas St. John's wort (*Hypericum perforatum*) can decrease cimetidine levels. Antacids can reduce the effect of cimetidine, and should be taken 1–2 hours before or after cimetidine is ingested. Drug–drug interactions associated with cimetidine were first noted when 300 mg were given four times per day. At current recommended over-the-counter doses (400 mg twice per day), drug–drug interactions are unlikely. The other three H_2-receptor antagonists are not CYP450 enzyme inhibitors to such a degree and are not associated with drug–drug interactions; therefore, providers recommend them more frequently.

Special Populations: Women, Pregnancy, Lactation, and the Elderly

All H_2-receptor antagonists are categorized as FDA Pregnancy Category B drugs. Of the four available currently, ranitidine (Zantac) may be preferred during pregnancy because a number of studies have documented safety, including those that assessed the effect of taking this medication in the first trimester.[17] All H_2-receptor antagonists are compatible with breastfeeding.[16]

Due to the increased risk of chronic liver and kidney disease found among the elderly, H_2-receptor antagonists should be used with caution in this population. It is recommended that individuals with moderate to severe renal/hepatic impairment receive a reduced dose of H_2-receptor antagonists.

Proton Pump Inhibitors

Proton pump inhibitors (PPIs) are the most potent and long-lasting inhibitors of gastric acid production. PPIs are indicated for treatment of peptic ulcer disease, erosive gastritis, gastric ulcer prophylaxis, NSAID-associated gastropathy, GERD, heartburn, and **Zollinger-Ellison syndrome**. These drugs suppress gastric acid secretion by directly inhibiting the parietal cell H^+/K^+ ATP pump.[4] A single dose of a PPI reduces 24-hour acid production by more than 90% and effectively stops food-stimulated acid production when taken before a major meal.[17] Proton pump inhibitors irreversibly block the hydrogen/potassium adenosine triphosphatase enzyme. The effect lasts 2–3 days, until new copies of the enzymes are produced and PPIs effectively inhibit 99% of the acid normally secreted by the parietal cells. The cost of these medications has decreased since omeprazole (Prilosec) became available in a generic formulation.

PPIs include omeprazole (Prilosec), esomeprazole (Nexium), lansoprazole (Prevacid), pantoprazole (Protonix), and rabeprazole (AcipHex). Zegerid is a new, immediate-release preparation that combines omeprazole and sodium bicarbonate. The sodium bicarbonate raises gastric pH and, thus, protects omeprazole from acid degradation.

These drugs are generally well tolerated, and their major side effects include headaches and diarrhea when used for short periods of time. Long-term use of PPIs increases the risk for hip fracture (adjusted odds ratio 1.22; 95% CI, 1.15–1.30 at 1 year and adjusted odds ratio 1.59; 95% CI, 1.39–1.80 at 4 years).[20] The increased risk for hip fracture is presumed to be secondary to malabsorption of calcium, but it may also be because proton pump inhibitors inhibit osteoclastic vacuolar proton pumps thereby inhibiting bone resorption.

Proton pump inhibitors should be ingested 1 hour before the morning meal, and peak effects occur approximately 1–2 hours after administration. The usual dose is one 20–40 mg tablet daily. PPIs are the drug of choice for achieving the goals of medical therapy in GERD, which include symptom relief, improvement in quality of life, and healing and prevention of mucosal injury.[5] For individuals with erosive gastritis, a PPI is the initial treatment of choice.[4] The PPIs may be ingested with NSAIDs as prophylaxis against ulcer formation caused by the latter.

Drug–Drug Interactions

PPIs are metabolized through the CP450 system and may alter metabolism of certain drugs (Table 21-4). Omeprazole (Prilosec) appears to have the greatest potential for drug interactions and delays the clearance of warfarin (Coumadin), diazepam (Valium), and phenytoin (Dilantin).[4]

Special Populations: Pregnancy, Lactation, and the Elderly

Omeprazole (Prilosec) was the first PPI available and is classified as an FDA Pregnancy Category C drug because at doses similar to those used in humans, it was shown to produce embryonic and fetal mortality in pregnant rats and rabbits. However, there are no reports of teratogenic effects in humans if taken during the first trimester of pregnancy.[21] Lansoprazole (Prevacid), rabeprazole (AcipHex), esomeprazole (Nexium), and pantoprazole (Protonix) are

Table 21-4 Selected Drug–Drug Interactions Associated with Use of Proton Pump Inhibitors (PPIs)*

Drug Generic (Brand)	Interacting Drugs	Implications
Esomeprazole (Nexium)	Benzodiazepines; e.g., diazepam (Valium) Clarithromycin (Biaxin)	Increased concentrations of both drugs; dose adjustment of benzodiazepines may be necessary.
Rabeprazole (AcipHex)	Clarithromycin (Biaxin)	Increased concentration of clarithromycin.
Lansoprazole (Prevacid)	Theophylline (Theolair)	Increased theophylline clearance; may need dose adjustment of theophylline.
Omeprazole (Prilosec)	Benzodiazepines; e.g., diazepam (Valium) Clarithromycin (Biaxin) Sulfonylureas; e.g., glyburide (DiaBeta) Phenytoin (Dilantin)	Increased plasma levels of clarithromycin, increase in diazepam half-life, reduction in clearance of phenytoin, hypoglycemic effects with concurrent use of sulfonylureas.
All PPIs	Warfarin (Coumadin)	Prolonged elimination and decrease in INR.
All PPIs	Digoxin (Lanoxin)	Increased serum digoxin levels.
All PPIs	Azole antifungals; e.g., miconazole (Monistat)	Decreased bioavailability of azoles.
All PPIs	Enteric-coated salicylates (Ecotrin)	Enteric coating may dissolve at increased rate and potentially cause gastric disturbance.

* This table is not comprehensive. New information is being generated on a regular basis.

FDA Pregnancy Category B drugs. Currently, the PPIs are not recommended in breastfeeding women because excretion in breast milk is unknown and studies are lacking.

Anticholinergic Agents

Anticholinergic therapy can suppress the parasympathetic muscarinic activity that triggers gastric acid secretion, especially the nocturnal surge.[19] The anticholinergic drugs affect the parietal cells by inhibiting basal and meal-stimulated gastric acid secretion via suppression of vagal-mediated activity. Anticholinergics include atropine, scopolamine (Scopace), hyoscyamine (Levsin, Levbid), glycopyrrolate (Robinul), and propantheline bromide (Pro-Banthine) and pirenzepine (Gastrozepin). All of these agents have the classic anticholinergic systemic side effects such as dry mouth, blurred vision, and urinary retention. H_2-receptor antagonists and PPIs are much more effective and have fewer side effects. These agents have limited efficacy and generally have no role in the treatment of peptic ulcer disease.

Propantheline (Gastrozepin) and hyoscyamine (Levsin, Levbid) are the exceptions. These drugs are used to treat ulcers as an adjunct to other medications because they decrease the motion of the muscles in the stomach, intestines, and bladder.

Special Populations: Pregnancy, Lactation, and the Elderly

Although anticholinergics have been used therapeutically for years, safety in pregnancy and breastfeeding of these drugs remains unclear. Both hyoscyamine (Levsin) and propantheline (Levbid) are FDA Pregnancy Category C drugs because of lack of information. Hyoscyamine is considered compatible during breastfeeding. Anticholinergics should be used with caution by the elderly because they can cause dizziness and sedation. In addition, they are contraindicated for persons with glaucoma or difficulty urinating.

Drugs to Promote Ulcer Healing: Cytoprotective Agents

Cytoprotective agents are a category of drugs specifically targeted to heal peptic ulcerations. Peptic ulceration often results as a consequence of medical therapy such as NSAIDs, which has been associated with damage to the gastric mucosa. Sucralfate (Carafate), misoprostol (Cytotec), and bismuth subsalicylate are considered to be cytoprotective or healing agents.

Sucralfate (Carafate)

Sucralfate (Carafate) is an agent indicated for short-term management of duodenal ulcers. Sucralfate is a complex salt of sucrose sulfate and aluminum hydroxide that binds with positively charged proteins in exudates and breaks down into an aluminum salt and sucrose sulfate, which forms a viscous, paste-like, adhesive substance when combined with gastric acid. This gel-like substance adheres to damaged mucosa and selectively forms a cytoprotective coating that protects the stomach lining against peptic acid, pepsin, and bile salts. This drug prevents mucosal injury, reduces inflammation, and aids healing of existing ulcers. Sucralfate should be administered before meals because it works best when the stomach is relatively empty. Antacids should not be taken within 30 minutes of ingestion.

Side effects of sucralfate include constipation, dry mouth, nausea, and abdominal pain, and it should be used in caution for those with renal dysfunction, because they may accumulate aluminum.

Drug–Drug Interactions

Sucralfate (Carafate) decreases the absorption and bioavailability of several drugs, including aminophylline, amitriptyline (Elavil), ciprofloxacin (Cipro), digoxin (Lanoxin), phenytoin (Dilantin), and theophylline (Theo-Dur). Sucralfate should not be used if fluoroquinolones are prescribed.[10]

Misoprostol (Cytotec)

Misoprostol (Cytotec) is a prostaglandin E1 analogue that binds to prostaglandin receptors, which stimulates increased production of mucus, production of bicarbonate, increased mucosal blood flow, and probably most importantly, suppression of basal and postprandial gastric acid secretion.[10] Misoprostol is indicated as a prophylactic agent to prevent ulcers in individuals who take NSAIDs. Misoprostol is in essence, a synthetic prostaglandin used to counter the effect NSAIDs have of inhibiting prostaglandin production. Misoprostol is taken with food four times per day after meals and at bedtime.

Side effects of misoprostol are largely gastrointestinal in nature and primarily include diarrhea, gastric upset, gas, vomiting, constipation, and indigestion. Diarrhea occurs in approximately 30% of persons who use this drug. Headaches have also been reported with misoprostol use.

Bismuth Subsalicylate

Bismuth subsalicylate is used for the treatment of diarrhea and dyspeptic symptoms including heartburn, although evidence for its efficacy in treating heartburn is questionable.[22] The bismuth commercially available in the United States is bismuth subsalicylate (Pepto-Bismol). The salicylate provides an antisecretory effect, while the bismuth subsalicylate exhibits an antimicrobial effect directly against bacterial and viral pathogens.[3] Bismuth subsalicylate reduces the risk of duodenal ulcer recurrence caused by *H pylori* because of the drug's cytoprotective properties. Furthermore, the agent combines with mucus to form a complex that appears to coat ulcer craters, affording protection from acid-peptic attack.[4] Bismuth subsalicylate can discolor the tongue and darken stools because it combines with trace amounts of sulfur in saliva and the gastrointestinal tract to form bismuth sulfide. This side effect is harmless and reversible once the drug is discontinued. Tinnitus could be an indication of toxicity. The usual dose

of bismuth subsalicylate is 524 mg four times/day as part of an *H pylori* eradication regimen. Bismuth subsalicylate may decrease the effect of tetracyclines and uricosurics and cause increased toxicity for persons taking it with aspirin, warfarin (Coumadin), or oral hypoglycemics.

Special Populations: Pregnancy, Lactation, and the Elderly

Sucralfate is an FDA Pregnancy Category B drug. The drug is not absorbed, so it exhibits a local rather than systemic effect. Animal studies have shown no teratogenic effects with doses up to 50 times those used in humans. Since its excretion in breast milk is minimal, sucralfate is compatible with breastfeeding. However, both misoprostol and bismuth subsalicylate are agents that should be avoided during pregnancy.

Misoprostol (Cytotec) is an FDA Pregnancy Category X drug. It is a known teratogen that can cause facial paralysis (Möbius' syndrome).[19] It is contraindicated in pregnancy and in women who wish to be pregnant because it increases uterine contractility and is associated with spontaneous abortions and premature labor. Misoprostol may induce vaginal bleeding in postmenopausal women.

Bismuth subsalicylate is an FDA Pregnancy Category C/D drug in the third trimester of pregnancy and should not be used due to the salicylate. Fetotoxicity has been reported in animals, and exposure during late pregnancy may increase the risk of constriction of the fetal ductus arteriosus with resultant pulmonary hypertension.[14] Bismuth subsalicylate should be avoided during breastfeeding or used with caution because of the potential risk of salicylate absorption.

Among the elderly, sucralfate may increase plasma and urine concentration of aluminum, most likely via increased gastric absorption of the mineral contained within the agent, although the clinical significance of this phenomenon remains unclear.[23] The pharmacokinetics of misoprostol are not changed to any major degree among the elderly.[24] There is a potential for bismuth subsalicylate neurotoxicity if bismuth is given for long periods of time, especially for persons in renal failure. Bismuth subsalicylate should also be used with caution for the elderly and individuals with salicylate sensitivity or bleeding disorders.

Drugs to Reduce Flatulence and Gas

Simethicone (Gas-X, Mylanta Gas, Maalox Advanced)

Simethicone is a gastric defoaming agent that is marketed as a single agent such as Gas-X, but more often is found as an adjunctive agent with many popular antacids. This drug is a mixture of polydimethylsiloxane and silica gel, which acts by decreasing the surface tension of gas bubbles, causing them to combine more readily into larger bubbles that should facilitate elimination. Contrary to popular belief, simethicone does not necessarily reduce the quantity of gas in the gastrointestinal tract. There is no systemic absorption with this medication, and adverse reactions are rare. Reports of its use for the relief of flatulence and postcesarean section abdominal discomfort exist, although evidence of its clinical effectiveness is sparse. There are no documented drug–drug interactions.

Alpha Galactosidase (Beano)

A nutritional supplement known by the brand name of Beano is widely advertised as a digestive aid to reduce gas. Beano contains alpha-galactosidase, an enzyme that breaks down complex sugars such as oligosaccharides found in legumes and cruciferous vegetables into simple sugars, enhancing their ability to be digested and reducing flatulence. A few small randomized, controlled trials (RCTs) have reported positive results among those who ingest alpha galactosidase.[25,26] Although larger studies are needed, the relative safety and cost of this dietary supplement suggest that it could be a reasonable agent to use for individuals who report disagreeable symptoms of gas and flatulence, especially when they are likely to be predictable.

Nausea and Vomiting

Nausea and vomiting can be a manifestation of a wide variety of conditions, including pregnancy, motion sickness, drug toxicity, radiation sickness, gastrointestinal obstruction, hepatitis, myocardial infarction, renal failure, increased intracranial pressure, asthma, Zollinger-Ellison syndrome, diabetes mellitus, thyrotoxicosis, and epilepsy.[4] Nausea and vomiting also are commonly experienced subsequent to chemotherapy and anesthesia.

Vomiting is triggered by afferent impulses to the vomiting center, which is a nucleus of cells in the medulla. The vomiting center can be stimulated by vestibular fibers, visceral afferents from the pharynx and gastrointestinal tract, and input from the chemoreceptor trigger zone (CTZ).[3] There are several neurotransmitter receptors located in the vomiting center, CTZ, and gastrointestinal tract. These receptors include serotonin (also called 5-HT$_3$), dopamine (D$_2$), and muscarinic (M$_1$) receptors. These neurotransmitter receptors are the primary targets of **antiemetic** drugs (Figure 21-3).

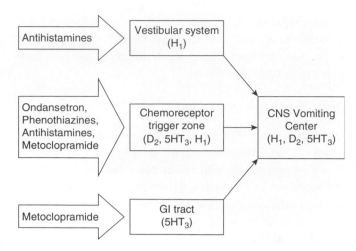

H$_1$ = Histamine-1; D$_2$ = dopamine-2; 5HT$_3$ = serotonin.

Figure 21-3 Chemoreceptor trigger zone and mechanism of action of antiemetics. *Source:* Reprinted with permission from King TL et al.[69]

Nonpharmacologic Therapies for Nausea and Vomiting

Many studies have been conducted regarding nausea and vomiting during pregnancy. Among the most common interventions have been ginger, pyridoxine (vitamin B$_6$), acupuncture, and acupressure. Additional information can be found in Chapter 35.

Fewer studies are found regarding nausea and vomiting among nonpregnant women. However, one small study of 60 women who underwent major gynecologic surgery reported that use of ginger was superior to placebo ($P < .05$) in treatment of postoperative nausea and vomiting.[27] Another study of 120 women undergoing laparoscopic gynecologic day surgery found that ginger was equal to metoclopramide (Reglan) for treating postoperative nausea and vomiting.[28]

A systematic review of P6 acupuncture at the pericardium point P6 used to treat postoperative nausea found that when compared to sham acupuncture, P6 acupoint stimulation reduced nausea (RR = 0.71; 95% CI, 0.61–0.83), vomiting (RR = 0.70; 95% CI, 0.59–0.83), and need for rescue antiemetics (RR = 0.69; 95% CI, 0.57–0.83).[29] When compared to antiemetic drugs, there was no statistically significant difference.[29] A similar meta-analysis of acupuncture studies for chemotherapy nausea and vomiting also found reduction of acute vomiting (RR = 0.82; 95% CI, 0.69–0.99), but not acute or delayed nausea compared to placebo. The researchers did not find studies comparing acupuncture to currently used antiemetics.[30]

Cannabinoids

Cannabinoids are effective antiemetic agents. Dronabinol (THC) is the major psychoactive substance in marijuana. There are limited legal uses of this medication. The only current indication for cannabinoids is the treatment of nausea and vomiting associated with chemotherapy, and it is only legal in some states. Pharmacologic effects on opiate receptors and the cortical and vomiting centers of the brain may explain the beneficial effects of cannabinoids.[4] The side effects include mood changes, anxiety, memory loss, fear, motor incoordination, hallucinations, euphoria, relaxation, and hunger. Sedation is another concern and occurs in approximately one third of users.

Pharmacologic Treatments: Antiemetics

Antiemetic drugs act by blocking the muscarinic, dopamine, histamine, serotonin, and substance P receptors within the gastrointestinal tract and those within the central nervous system. These agents are used for a wide variety of conditions, including motion sickness, ulcers, gastritis, nausea and vomiting during pregnancy, acute gastroenteritis, postoperative nausea and vomiting, vestibular neuritis, chemotherapy-induced nausea and vomiting, and other chronic disorders. Usual doses and prescribing considerations are listed in Table 21-5.

The first-line pharmacologic treatments for nausea and vomiting include antihistamines, anticholinergics, phenothiazines, serotonin receptor antagonists, prokinetic agents, and gastric acid suppression via use of H_2-receptor antagonists. Intravenous formulations and suppositories can be used by persons with persistent vomiting. The second-line treatments include corticosteroids and the all the medications used for first-line treatment plus acid suppression via proton pump inhibitors.

A systemic review of studies of eight specific drugs compared to placebo for treatment of postoperative nausea (droperidol [Inapsine], metoclopramide [Reglan], ondansetron [Zofran], tropisetron [Navoban], dolasetron [Anzemet], dexamethasone [Decadron], cyclizine [Marezine], and granisetron [Kytril]) found that none could be considered more effective than another.[31] There is individual variability in what drug is most effective for treating nausea. Because several different neurotransmitters stimulate the CTZ, adding a drug that has a different mechanism of action can be more effective than increasing the dose of an individual drug.

Antihistamines

Antihistamine is the term that describes any histamine antagonist, but in practice, this term is used to refer to H_1-receptor antagonists. Antihistamines inhibit the histamine receptors in the CTZ and limit stimulation of the vomiting center by vestibular fibers. They are particularly useful for treating nausea and vomiting associated with vestibular disturbances. Meclizine (Antivert, Dramamine Less Drossy) acts on the vestibular system and the CTZ. This drug has a slow onset of action and needs at least 1 hour before becoming effective. Other antihistamines commonly used to treat nausea and vomiting include diphenhydramine (Benadryl), dimenhydrinate (Dramamine), and doxylamine (Unisom).

Antihistamines are well absorbed following oral administration. They are metabolized in the liver by the hepatic microsomal mixed-function oxygenase system. Half-lives are variable as some antihistamines have active metabolites and many can be administered once or twice a day at most.

Although antihistamines are specific for H_1-receptors, they can also activate muscarinic cholinergic and serotonin receptors. These additional effects are the etiology of the most common side effects. The side effect most often seen is sedation followed by dizziness and anticholinergic effects. Other side effects not seen as often include confusion, tinnitus, insomnia, anxiety, dry mouth, palpitations, and headache, and rarely, hallucination or psychosis. Antihistamines have anticholinergic effects and can therefore exacerbate narrow-angle glaucoma.

Anticholinergics: Scopolamine

Scopolamine, an anticholinergic, is one of the most effective medications to treat and prevent motion sickness because it inhibits vestibular input to the central nervous system. The transdermal scopolamine patch (Transderm-Scop) has a more prolonged effect than the antihistamines. The scopolamine patch is applied behind the ear several hours before a trip, and the effects can last up to 3 days. The side effects, which are much milder among those using the patch versus those with oral administration, include the classic anticholinergic effects: constipation, dry mouth, drowsiness, blurred vision, urinary retention, and tachycardia.

Benzodiazepines

Benzodiazepines generally have weak antiemetic properties. These drugs help prevent central cortical-induced vomiting. Lorazepam (Ativan) and alprazolam (Xanax) are the drugs commonly used for chemotherapy-induced nausea and vomiting. The main side effect of benzodiazepines is sedation.

Table 21-5 Antiemetics

Drug Generic (Brand)	Dose	Major Side Effects/Contraindications	FDA Pregnancy Category
Anticholinergics			
Scopolamine (Transderm-Scop)	Apply one patch 1 hour before surgery	Side effects: dry mouth, blurred vision, dizziness, confusion, constipation.	C
Antihistamines (H₁-Receptor Antagonists)			
Meclizine (Antivert)	25–50 mg four times daily PO	Side effects: drowsiness, dry mouth, blurred vision.	B
Diphenhydramine (Benadryl)	50–100 mg q 4–6 h PO/IM/IV	Side effects: may cause drowsiness. Can be used to offset anxiety caused by metoclopramide or phenothiazines.	B
Dimenhydrinate (Dramamine)	50–100 mg q 4–6 h PO 50 mg (in 50 mL of saline over 20 min) q 4–6 h IV Maximum of 400 mg/day if single agent or 200 mg/day if taken with doxycycline	Side effects: may cause drowsiness. Can be used to offset anxiety caused by metoclopramide or phenothiazines.	B
Doxylamine (Unisom)	12.5 mg twice daily PO or 12.5 mg in morning and 25 mg at night PO	Side effects: drowsiness.	A
Benzodiazepines			
Lorazepam (Ativan)	1–4 mg PO/IM/IV every 4–6 hours	Side effects: drowsiness, sedation, amnesia. Contraindicated during pregnancy.	D
Alprazolam (Xanax)	0.25–0.5 mg PO three times daily up to 4 mg/day	Side effects: drowsiness, sedation, confusion. Contraindicated during pregnancy.	D
Phenothiazines (Central D₂-Receptor Antagonists)			
Prochlorperazine (Compazine)	5–10 mg q 4–6 h PO/IM/IV 25 mg rectal suppository twice daily Maximum dose is 40 mg/day	Side effects: sedation; anticholinergic effects; mouth, extrapyramidal side effects. Hypotension if given IV too quickly.	C
Promethazine (Phenergan)	12.5–2.5 mg q 4–6 h PO/IM/IV/per rectum Hypotension if given IV too quickly	Side effects: sedation; anticholinergic effects; mouth, extrapyramidal side effects.	C
Thiethylperazine (Torecan)	10 mg, 1–3 times per day PO/IM/per rectum	Side effects: drowsiness, dizziness, headache. Contraindicated during pregnancy.	X
Nonphenothiazine Antiemetic			
Trimethobenzamide (Tigan)	250 mg PO/PR three times daily	Side effects: pseudo-Parkinsonism, diarrhea, hypotension.	C
Benzamides (Central and Peripheral D₂-Receptor Antagonists)			
Metoclopramide (Reglan)	10 mg PO four times daily 1–2 mg/kg IV Continuous SQ dose regimens available	Side effects: extrapyramidal side effects, agitation, anxiety, acute dystonic reactions. Give 50 mg diphenhydramine before dose to prevent extrapyramidal side effects.	B
Serotonin (5-HT₃) Receptor Antagonists			
Ondansetron (Zofran)	4–8 mg PO three times daily to four times daily 4–8 mg over 15 min IV q 12 h May be given 1 mg/h continuously for 24 h	Side effects: headache.	B
Dolasetron (Anzemet)	0.35 mg/kg up to 12.5 mg approximately 15 minutes before a procedure, or 1.2 mg/kg PO up to 100 mg as tabs or injection 2 hours before surgery	Side effects: headache, drowsiness, diarrhea.	B
Butyrophenones			
Droperidol	0.625–2.5 mg IV over 15 min then 1.25 mg prn or 2.5 mg IM can be given IV continuously at 1–1.25 mg/h	Side effects: extrapyramidal side effects, prolonged QY syndrome. Give 50 mg diphenhydramine before dose to prevent extrapyramidal symptoms. Reserve for persons who have failed other regimens.	C

Dopamine Receptor Antagonists

Metoclopramide (Reglan) is the most common dopamine receptor antagonist used to treat nausea and vomiting. Metoclopramide blocks dopamine receptors and when given in higher doses, also blocks serotonin receptors in the CTZ of the central nervous system. Metoclopramide also enhances the response to acetylcholine in the gastrointestinal tract, causing enhanced motility and accelerated gastric emptying without stimulating gastric, biliary, or pancreatic secretions. It also increases lower esophageal sphincter tone. In addition to its usefulness for nausea, this agent is used to treat gastroparesis, reverse the gastric stasis induced by narcotics, and combat nausea and vomiting associated with cancer treatment medications.

Unfortunately, metoclopramide has an adverse side effect profile. This drug can induce **extrapyramidal symptoms** (also called dystonic reactions). When dopamine receptors are blocked, dopamine is unable to initiate usual physiologic functions, and the resulting effects are similar to those seen in persons with Parkinson's disease. Symptoms include restlessness, akinesia, akathisia, **tardive dyskinesia**, dystonia (involuntary spasmodic muscle movements), oculogyric crisis, and facial grimacing.[32] Although frightening, these symptoms are rarely life-threatening and they are easily reversed by administering 50 mg of diphenhydramine (Benadryl) intravenously. Metoclopramide has an FDA-mandated black box warning that reviews the risk of tardive dyskinesia. Because the risk of tardive dyskinesia increases over time, chronic use of metoclopramide is not recommended. Metoclopramide can also cause galactorrhea and has been used therapeutically for this effect when lactating women need to increase their supply of breast milk. Metoclopramide (Reglan) can also cause menstrual irregularities and occasionally amenorrhea.

Serotonin (5-HT$_3$) Receptor Antagonists

The serotonin receptor antagonists are the newest and most effective class of antiemetics. They are well tolerated and have a beneficial side effect profile, and therefore have largely replaced dopamine antagonists for treating nausea and vomiting. The four most commonly used are ondansetron (Zofran), granisetron (Kytril), dolasetron (Anzemet), and palonosetron (Aloxi). These drugs block the serotonin receptors located on the visceral afferent nerves in the gastrointestinal tract, in the solitary tract nucleus, and in the CTZ. Cisapride (Propulsid) is a serotonin receptor agonist that stimulates cholinergic nerves in the stomach.[32]

This drug was used for gastroparesis, functional dyspepsia, GERD, and intestinal pseudoobstruction. Cisapride was removed from the market in 2004 and is no longer available in the United States because it was found to cause prolonged QT syndrome.[33]

The most common side effects of serotonin antagonists are headache, diarrhea, and fatigue, although side effects are generally rare. Self-limiting asymptomatic prolongation of the QT interval and widening of the QRS complex have been noted with several serotonin antagonists.[33] Hypersensitivity reactions occur but are rare. These drugs should be used with caution by individuals who have an underlying long QT syndrome.

Phenothiazines

Phenothiazines act by antagonizing D$_2$-dopamine receptors in the postrema of the brain and have an M$_1$ muscarine and H$_1$ histamine blocker effect. The main side effects of phenothiazines are extrapyramidal side effects or reactions such as tardive dyskinesia. These medications have a sedative effect and can also cause orthostatic hypotension. Prochlorperazine (Compazine) is the most commonly used drug in this class of medications. Promethazine (Phenergan) antagonizes central and peripheral H$_1$ receptors and is also classified as a nonselective antihistamine.

Corticosteroids

Corticosteroids are effective and well-tolerated antiemetics for persons undergoing chemotherapy. These drugs enter target cells and bind to cytoplasmic receptors. The side effects include insomnia, increased energy, and mood changes. Corticosteroids have been used prophylactically for mild to moderate emetogenic chemotherapy. Corticosteroids, in addition to serotonin receptor antagonists, have been used for moderate cases of chemo-induced emesis.

Butyrophenones

Butyrophenones are tranquilizers that potentiate the action of opiates and have an antiemetic effect when used alone. Haloperidol (Haldol) and droperidol (Inapsine) block the stimulation of CTZ. Droperidol is a short-acting medication commonly used off-label to treat postoperative nausea and vomiting. Droperidol has a black box warning that warns users about possible prolonged QT interval and ventricular arrhythmias (torsades de pointes). Haloperidol has a longer half-life, so its use is more limited. The major side effects of these drugs are extrapyramidal symptoms.

Special Populations: Pregnancy, Lactation, and the Elderly

The safety of antiemetics during pregnancy is of particular importance because of gestational nausea and vomiting. Antihistamines have been used for decades, and no harm has been reported with the exception of early reports on diphenhydramine, which were unable to replicated. All the serotonin receptor antagonists are FDA Pregnancy Category C drugs, and they are commonly recommended for women who are pregnant. Scopolamine also is an FDA Pregnancy Category C drug due to lack of information, although some fetal tachycardia in labor has been reported. Corticosteroids also are FDA Pregnancy Category C drugs. In animal studies, haloperidol (Haldol) was associated with increased abortions, neonatal death, and cleft palates. Since these outcomes have not been repeated among humans, the FDA Pregnancy Category remains C.

Lorazepam (Ativan) is an FDA Pregnancy Category D drug due to potential neonatal neurodevelopment problems, cardiac or facial congenital anomalies, as well as floppy infant syndrome, also called benzodiazepine withdrawal syndrome in the neonate. Lorazepam also may inhibit fetal liver bilirubin glucuronidation, causing neonatal jaundice.

Hyperemesis gravidarum is a condition of severe nausea and vomiting during pregnancy leading to dehydration, nutritional deficiency, weight loss, and increased fetal morbidity and mortality.[34] Pharmacologic therapy includes antiemetics and antireflux medications in addition to intravenous therapy during hospitalizations. Detailed information about the treatment of nausea and vomiting during pregnancy is presented in Chapter 35.

Although much is written about gestational nausea and vomiting, there is a paucity of information about nausea associated with breastfeeding. This situation appears relatively rare, but Web chat rooms have an increasing number of discussions specifically devoted to nausea while nursing. For most women, dietary manipulation of increasing fluids and vitamin B$_6$ appear anecdotally to help. However, in the rare case that pharmacologic agents are required for nausea and vomiting while a woman breastfeeds, the aforementioned antihistamines, scopolamine, and serotonin receptor antagonists are compatible with breastfeeding.

Any of the antiemetics that can have sedative effects such as antihistamines and benzodiazepines in particular, can promote problems with balance and have been found to increase the risk of falls and fractures in the elderly.[35] Lorazepam (Ativan) has been reported to cause cognitive deficits, especially in the elderly, although discontinuation resolves the phenomenon. Since elderly have an increased risk of development of cancer, with subsequent emetic-associated chemotherapy, agents may be used prophylactically or posttreatment while cancer treatment is in process.

Gastroparesis

Gastroparesis is a condition of abnormal gastric motility characterized by delayed gastric emptying. Gastroparesis is a common cause of nausea and vomiting. The most common forms of gastroparesis are associated with diabetes, occur postoperatively, or are idiopathic. Symptoms of gastroparesis include postprandial fullness, bloating, and abdominal distention. Idiopathic gastroparesis is a term used to describe individuals (almost exclusively women) who experience intractable functional symptoms and are found to delay gastric emptying.[4]

Gastroparesis has been managed with dietary and behavioral modifications, prokinetic drugs, and surgical interventions. New advances in treatment include botulinum toxin injection (Botox), and gastric stimulation techniques have been proposed as hope to those with refractory gastroparesis.[32,33] However, the first published RCT comparing botulinum toxin A to placebo for delayed gastric emptying failed to find a statistically significant difference.[36] Further studies are needed on the different treatments used for gastroparesis.[37] More traditional pharmacologic treatment includes use of cholinergic agonists and dopamine antagonists that are prokinetic and promote gastric emptying.

Drugs to Promote Gastric Emptying

Cholinergic Agonists

Cholinergic agonists are synthetic versions of acetylcholine and therefore act as agonists at the muscarinic M$_2$ type receptors on the smooth muscle cell. Bethanechol (Urecholine) is an older cholinergic agent that is not used as often today, but is still indicated for persons with reflux and gastroparesis. This drug increases lower esophageal pressure and improves esophageal clearance. Cholinergic agonists in combination with metoclopramide (Reglan) appear to enhance the gastric emptying effects of the metoclopramide alone. The dose of bethanechol for chronic GERD is 25 mg orally four times daily given on an empty stomach or 1 hour before meals or 2 hours after meals. Adverse effects include bronchospasms, hypotension, tachycardia, and seizures.

Dopamine Antagonists

Metoclopramide (Reglan) has effects on both central and peripheral dopamine receptors, while domperidone (Motilium) operates primarily through peripheral receptors.

Metoclopramide (Reglan)

The pharmacologic treatment of gastroparesis usually begins with metoclopramide (Reglan). This drug is used orally in the treatment of diabetic gastric stasis and gastroesophageal reflux. Parenteral treatment with metoclopramide is indicated for diabetic gastric stasis, postpyloric placement of enteral feeding tubes, and prevention and/or treatment of nausea and vomiting associated with chemotherapy or postsurgery.

The usual starting dose is 5 mg given 30 minutes before meals and at bedtime. If there is an inadequate response, the dose may be increased to 10 mg. Intravenous dosing is the same. The onset of action is 0.5–1 hour when given orally but is more rapid when given parenterally (intravenously 1–3 minutes and intramuscularly 10–15 minutes).

Domperidone (Motilium)

Domperidone (Motilium) does not cross the blood–brain barrier, and thus is not associated with Parkinson and/or extrapyramidal side effects or tardive dyskinesia. Domperidone increases esophageal peristalsis, lower esophageal sphincter pressure, gastric motility, and peristalsis, and enhances gastroduodenal coordination, thereby facilitating gastric emptying and decreasing small bowel transit time.[4] This agent is indicated for symptomatic management of upper gastrointestinal motility disorders associated with chronic and subacute gastritis and diabetic gastroparesis. However, life-threatening arrhythmias and cardiac arrest have been reported with the use of domperidone, and it is not currently approved for us in the United States (Box 21-3).

In 2004, the FDA issued a letter warning that the drug had unknown risks to parents and infants, and that domestic sales were illegal even if the drug was imported from other countries.[33]

Domperidone is included in this chapter because it continues to be used as an off-label agent by many clinicians who obtain it through various means to treat individuals with gastroparesis and gastrointestinal motility disorders

---

Box 21-3 Gone But Not Forgotten: Drugs Are Safe Until Many People Use Them

Cisapride (Propulsid) was an agent that increased acetylcholine release and, thereby, increased tone of the lower esophageal sphincter among individuals with gastroesophageal reflux disease. Persons with diabetes who experienced gastroparesis also used the agent because it increased gastric emptying and had a laxative effect. Cisapride was marketed in the United States under the brand name Propulsid. However, cisapride had a major adverse effect. This drug was found to cause long QT syndrome, which is associated with cardiac arrhythmias. In 2000, the manufacturer voluntarily removed cisapride from the US market. The drug remains available for veterinary use, and commonly is used to treat feline hair balls.

Prolongation of the QT syndrome continues to be an issue among other drugs used for persons with gastrointestinal conditions. Cherbit et al.[68] have noted that this potential adverse effect continues to be possible with ondansetron (Zofran). This drug continues to be used, although with caution, especially among women with a history of cardiac abnormalities.

---

who do not respond to metoclopramide. It is available in Canada through the investigational new drug process. The usual oral dose is 10 mg 3–4 times per day, given 15–30 minutes before meals. In severe or resistant cases, this may be increased to 20 mg 3–4 times per day. Peak concentration occurs in 7 hours.

Erythromycin (E-Mycin)

Erythromycin (E-Mycin) is a macrolide anti-infective that also is a motilin agonist that is useful in treating acute gastroparesis.[38] Dhir and Richter used a gastric emptying scan to diagnose persons with dyspepsia and gastroparesis. The participants were treated with low bulk diet and low-dose oral erythromycin suspension, 50–100 mg three times per day and at bedtime. These researchers found treatment of gastroparesis with low dose erythromycin and a low bulk diet resulted in a dramatic short-term improvement in the majority of participants. In short-term follow-up, 83% experienced dramatic improvement and 17% experienced worsening symptoms or no change in symptoms ($P = .005$).

Further studies are needed to determine the effectiveness of erythromycin for gastroparesis.[39]

Erythromycin (E-Mycin) is also a CYP3A4 inhibitor and has multiple clinically important drug–drug interactions. It is contraindicated for persons also using dofetilide (Tikosyn), eletriptan (Relpax), ergotamine/caffeine (Ergomar), phenothiazines, pimozide (Orap), or ranolazine (Ranexa), and many other drugs. Side effects include stomach discomfort, cramping, headaches, urticaria, and ventricular arrhythmias.

Special Populations: Pregnancy, Lactation, and the Elderly

There are few controlled studies on the use of these agents in pregnancy. Erythromycin (E-mycin) is commonly used in pregnancy as a macrolide anti-infective and is an FDA Pregnancy Category B drug. Bethanechol (Urecholine), metoclopramide (Reglan), and domperidone (Motilium) are FDA Pregnancy Category C drugs.

Erythromycin is compatible with breastfeeding. Bethanechol (Urecholine) has been used to treat postpartum urinary retention in the first 24–48 hours postpartum. Use by lactating women is not contraindicated, but at least one case of abdominal pain and diarrhea in a newborn who was breastfed by a woman who was taking bethanechol has been reported, and use of this agent has fallen out of favor in many hospitals today.[23] Although metoclopramide and domperidone enter breastmilk, they are considered compatible with lactation, and even may be used as potential galactagogues. Additional information about galactagogues can be found Chapter 38.

Treatment of gastroparesis is particularly problematic for the elderly. Metoclopramide (Reglan) crosses the blood–brain barrier and therefore has an increased risk of drowsiness, extrapyramidal side effects, and irritability. Bethanechol (Urecholine) has been found to have significant interpersonal variability, resulting in a wide response to the agent. Erythromycin, although commonly used, is associated with drug–drug interactions. The latter is of concern with the elderly because of the increased risk of polypharmacy use.

Emetics

Emetics are substances that produce vomiting. The emetic most often used is syrup of ipecac, which is made from the dried root of a plant called ipecacuanha, which is grown in Brazil. Ipecac originally was used as an expectorant in cough syrups a century ago. However, it gained popularity as an emetic for cases of accidental poisoning. At one time, every family with children was recommended to have ipecac available in a home first aid kit.[40] However, vomiting alone does not always remove poisons from the stomach. There are no studies that show that use of ipecac changes clinical outcomes, and the risk of ipecac overdosing tends to confound diagnosis of the poison, complicating or delaying administration of effective methods such as whole bowel irrigation. The American Academy of Pediatrics recommends that parents do not use ipecac in cases of suspected poisoning. Chapter 4 has more information in use of emetics.

Conditions in the Lower Gastrointestinal Tract: Diarrhea

Diarrhea generally is defined as the passage of abnormally liquid or unformed stools with increased frequency. Chronic diarrhea is defined as the production of loose stools with or without increased stool frequency for more than 4 weeks. Pseudo-diarrhea, or the frequent passage of small volumes of stool, is often associated with rectal urgency and accompanies irritable bowel syndrome (IBS) or anorectal disorders such as proctitis.[41]

Diarrhea usually is self-limiting. Ninety percent of the cases are associated with infectious agents and are accompanied by vomiting, fever, and abdominal pain. When the viral or bacterial infection resolves, the diarrhea resolves. The remaining 10% are caused by medication, toxic ingestion, ischemia, or other conditions.[41] Most infectious diarrheas are acquired by fecal–oral transmission via direct personal contact or ingestion of food or water contaminated with pathogens from humans or animals.

Although diarrhea is most often infectious or drug related, one must be suspicious of parasites and absorption defects such as celiac disease, lactase disorders, or pancreatic insufficiency. Cancer, alcoholism, hyperthyroidism, and diabetes also should be entertained in the differential diagnosis. A temporal association between use and symptom onset may suggest etiology.

Some of the medications that cause diarrhea include antibiotics, cardiac antidysrhythmics, antihypertensives, chemotherapeutic agents, NSAIDs, antidepressants, bronchodilators, antacids, and laxatives. Since acute diarrhea is a symptom, pharmaceuticals are considered palliative rather than curative, and often it is treated with hydration and simple tincture of time.

Opiates

Opioids have significant constipating effects. They increase colonic phasic segmenting activity through inhibition of presynaptic cholinergic nerves in the submucosal and myenteric plexuses. This causes increased transit time and increased fecal water absorption. Opioids also decrease mass colonic movements and the gastrocolic reflex. Although all opioids have antidiarrheal effects, central nervous system effects and the potential for addiction limit the usefulness of opioids for treating diarrhea.

Paregoric

Paregoric, also known as camphorated tincture of opium, increases smooth muscle tone in the gastrointestinal tract, which will decrease motility and peristalsis. The usual dose is 5–10 mL orally 1–4 times per day. Until 1973, paregoric was available over the counter on a signature basis and categorized as a Schedule V drug. At that time, it was reclassified as a Schedule III narcotic and now is available only by prescription. Paregoric often is difficult to find and generally has been replaced by more accessible nonopiates.

Antiperistaltics

Antiperistaltics are synthetic opioids with a lower potential for abuse than codeine or tincture of opium.[42] Antiperistaltics control diarrhea by reducing gastrointestinal motility, inhibiting watery secretions, and increasing anal sphincter tone. Diphenoxylate (Lomotil), a synthetic opiate analogue with atropine directly affects the nerve endings and/or intramural ganglia of the intestinal wall. The usual dose is two tablets or 10 mL four times daily until diarrhea is controlled. The maintenance dose is two tablets or 10 mL daily. If there is no response within 48 hours, the medication should be discontinued. The side effects of the medication include nausea, rash, sedation, and pancreatitis. Diphenoxylate is contraindicated for people concurrently taking MAO inhibitors as it may precipitate a hypertensive crisis.

Loperamide (Imodium) may be preferred for chronic use because of its longer duration of action and fewer side effects than diphenoxylate. Loperamide is the over-the-counter treatment of choice for traveler's diarrhea (usually in combination with antimicrobial therapy).[43] Also, it crosses the blood–brain barrier poorly and is less likely to cause addiction. The ultimate goal of treatment is the gradual withdrawal of medication with the substitution of a high-fiber diet.[28]

Loperamide (Imodium) usually has a recommended dose of 4 mg by mouth initially, then 2 mg by mouth after each loose stool up to a maximum of 16 mg in a day. The side effects include dry mouth, abdominal pain, distention, constipation, drowsiness, and fatigue. Serious reactions include toxic megacolon, paralytic ileus, angioedema, and urinary retention.

Bulk-Forming Agents

Polycarbophil (FiberCon) is a bulk-forming calcium salt that acts as an absorbent. Polycarbophil is safe, effective, inert, and nontoxic. This agent may be used as a laxative as well as to increase bulk in an attempt to normalize stools. The dose is one 625-mg tablet 1–4 times per day or 1 teaspoon in 4–6 ounces of water or juice followed by another 8-ounce glass of water 1–4 times per day. Other bulk-forming laxatives are discussed in the section addressing constipation and may be used similarly.

Bismuth Subsalicylate (Pepto-Bismol)

Bismuth subsalicylate (Pepto-Bismol, Kaopectate) has a recommended dose of two tablets or caplets or 30 mL every 30–60 minutes if needed up to a maximum of eight doses per day. However, it is controversial in terms of efficacy. The side effects include blackened stools, blackened tongue, constipation, and tinnitus, and it should be used with caution by persons with coagulation disorders, diabetes, gout, or renal insufficiency. Bismuth subsalicylate may interfere with absorption of oral anticoagulants and tetracycline. Conversely, bismuth subsalicylate can enhance the effect of hypoglycemic agents. This agent should not be used by persons who are allergic to aspirin. Bismuth subsalicylate (Pepto-Bismol) has been the standard treatment of ulcers for years and is FDA approved for the treatment of indigestion, nausea, and diarrhea.

Absorbents

Charcoal, aluminum hydroxide, attapulgite, bismuth subsalts, kaolin, magnesium trisilicate, and pectin all lack clinical evidence to establish effectiveness.

Kaolin and Pectin (Kapectolin)

Kapectolin is a combination of kaolin and pectin. Although it often is purchased by individuals, there is no evidence that it is effective.

Octreotide (Sandostatin)

Somatostatin, also known as growth hormone inhibiting hormone or somatotropin release-inhibiting hormone, is a peptide hormone that interacts with G-protein coupled somatostatin receptors to inhibit release of a number of secondary hormones including gastrointestinal hormones. This causes the rate of gastric emptying to decrease, reducing smooth muscle contractions and blood flow in the intestines. Octreotide (Sandostatin) is similar to endogenous somatostatin, and it decreases blood levels of many substances including insulin, glucagon, growth hormone, and additional chemicals that affect digestion. Octreotide (Sandostatin) suppresses or inhibits the severe diarrhea associated with cancerous tumors and vasoactive intestinal peptide-secreting tumors. Octreotide (Sandostatin) reduces splanchnic blood flow and inhibits gastric acid secretions and may be employed as adjunct therapy to help control gastrointestinal bleeding when endoscopic therapy is unsuccessful or unavailable.

Special Populations: Pregnancy, Lactation, and the Elderly

Pregnant women, like any other woman, may experience diarrhea. If a medication is necessary, it is advisable to choose an agent with known effectiveness. Loperamide (Imodium) is an FDA Pregnancy Category B drug and first-line therapy. Diphenoxylate (Lomotil) is FDA Pregnancy Category C, and bismuth subsalicylate is not recommended in pregnancy because of its salicylate component and controversial effectiveness. Paregoric still is used regionally, but most often as an off-labeled treatment for a woman with prodromal labor rather than diarrhea. Octreotide (Sandostatin), an FDA Pregnancy Category B

drug, although rarely used, is compatible with breastfeeding. For the breastfeeding woman, loperamide (Imodium) remains the antiperistaltic drug of choice when one is needed, followed by diphenoxylate (Lomotil). Paregoric should be avoided because it can cause sedation in the infant.

Diarrhea is a major cause of mortality and morbidity among the elderly. Loperamide (Lomotil) generally is the preferred antiperistaltic because the usual formulation of diphenoxylate includes atropine, an anticholinergic that is unnecessary and may cause adverse effects with the elderly. Treatment of infectious diarrhea and traveler's diarrhea, for example, are the same for individuals regardless of age.

Traveler's Diarrhea

Traveler's diarrhea is a common illness that occurs when people travel from resource-rich to resource-poor regions of the world. The treatment includes fluid replacement, antibiotic therapy, and antimotility agents. For individuals who cannot tolerate dehydration, prophylactic ciprofloxacin (Cipro) or norfloxacin (Noroxin) may be prescribed, which can reduce the incidence of traveler's diarrhea by 90%. However, the CDC does not recommend antimicrobial drugs for the prevention of traveler's diarrhea.

The treatment of traveler's diarrhea includes antibiotics for 3–5 days.[44] The antibiotics are listed in Table 21-6.

Table 21-6 Medications for Treatment of Traveler's Diarrhea

Drug Generic (Brand)	Treatment Dose	Prophylaxis Dose	Clinical Considerations	FDA Pregnancy Category
Antibiotics				
Azithromycin (Zithromax)	1000 mg as a single dose	None	Fluoroquinolones are the antibiotics of choice for traveler's diarrhea	B
Ciprofloxacin (Cipro)	500 mg bid × 3 days	500 mg qd	Resistant forms of *Campylobacter* have occurred in southeast Asia and the Indian subcontinent	C
Levofloxacin (Levaquin)	500 mg qd × 3 days	None		C
Norfloxacin (Noroxin)	400 mg bid	400 mg qd	Azithromycin is active against fluoroquinolone-resistant species	C
Ofloxacin (Floxin)	200 mg bid	None		C
Rifaximin (Xifaxan)	200 mg tid × 3 days	200 mg bid or qd	Alternative to fluoroquinolones for persons who do not have bloody diarrhea or fever Not approved for use against *Salmonella, Shigella,* or *Campylobacter*	C
Antidiarrheal Drugs				
Bismuth subsalicylate (Pepto-Bismol, Kaopectate)	524 mg q 30 min for up to 8 doses in 24 h	524 mg tablet qd or 1048 mg liquid qd	May cause black tongue and black stools Contraindicated for persons with allergy to aspirin, renal insufficiency, or gout Contraindicated for persons taking anticoagulants Best for mild diarrhea	B
Loperamide (Imodium)	4 mg then 2 mg after each stool up to 16 mg per day	None	Not recommended for persons with bloody stool or fever Use for moderate or severe diarrhea	B

Trimethoprim-sulfamethoxazole (Bactrim, Septra) and doxycycline (Vibramycin) are not used because of high resistance of microbes to these medications.

Constipation

There is no one definition of constipation. Clinicians often assume constipation means infrequent bowel movements, but persons with constipation describe several symptoms, including the need to strain, incomplete emptying, hard stools, infrequent stools (fewer than three stools per week), and abdominal fullness or bloating. The Bristol Stool Form Scale, which describes seven different shapes and consistencies of stool, can be used to help individuals fully describe symptoms.[45] In addition, gut transit can be estimated by using the Bristol Stool Form Scale.[45]

Constipation occurs in approximately 30% of the population depending on demographic factors, affects all ages, and is most common in women and non-Whites.[42] Some conditions associated with constipation include pregnancy, pelvic floor dysfunction, drug interactions (calcium channel blockers and antidepressants), metabolic disorders, psychologic disorders (depression, eating disorders), endocrine disorders (hypothyroidism and hypercalcemia), and dietary variations. Severe, intractable constipation may be due to inertia or anorectal dyssynergia. Dietary fiber deficiency is a contributor to constipation. The average US citizen obtains 5–20 grams of dietary fiber a day, yet an estimated 20–50 grams of fiber per day is needed for normal bowel function.

Primary idiopathic constipation generally falls into one of three categories: (1) normal transit time, (2) slow transit time, and (3) defecatory disorders such as **dyssynergia**. Secondary constipation is a symptom of an underlying disorder such as cancer, or it can be a side effect of medication or drug–drug interactions. Drugs that can cause constipation are listed in Table 21-7.

Laxatives

Laxatives work via a variety of different mechanisms (Figure 21-4). Bulk-forming laxatives are hydrophilic cellulose derivatives that stimulate peristalsis by increasing the size of stool and modifying the consistency. Emollients are surfactant agents that facilitate mixtures of aqueous and fatty materials. This effect pulls water into the stool and softens it. Emollients are not effective for

Table 21-7 Selected List of Drugs That Can Cause Constipation

Drug Generic (Brand)	Drug Generic (Brand)
Amitriptyline (Elavil)	Diuretics
Antacids that contain calcium or aluminum	Imipramine (Tofranil)
Anticholinergic drugs	Ipratropium (Atrovent)
Anticonvulsants: e.g., carbamazepine (Tegretol), phenytoin (Dilantin)	Iron supplements
Antidepressants: e.g., nortriptyline (Aventyl), SSRIs	MAO inhibitors
Antidiarrhea drugs	NSAIDs
Antihistamines that have anticholinergic properties: e.g., all OTC antihistamines	Opioids
Anti-Parkinson's drugs: e.g., selegiline (Eldepryl)	Oxybutynin (Ditropan)
Antipsychotics: e.g., clozapine (Clozaril)	Phenothiazines
Atropine	Pseudoephedrine (Sudafed)
Benztropine (Cogentin)	Ranitidine (Zantac)
Beta blockers	Sucralfate (Carafate)
Calcium channel blockers: e.g., diltiazem (Cardizem), nifedipine (Procardia)	Terbutaline (Brethine)
Cimetidine (Tagamet)	Trazodone (Desyrel)
Clonidine (Catapres)	Tricyclic antidepressants

SSRI = selective serotonin reuptake inhibitors; MAO = monoamine oxidase; NSAID = nonsteroidal anti-inflammatory drug.

treating constipation but are a useful adjunct to prevent straining. Lubricants coat the stool and allow easier passage. Mineral oil is the only lubricant in general use. Saline cathartics retain water in the small intestine, thereby increasing the water content of stool and producing a watery stool. Magnesium stimulates peristalsis. These agents produce a watery stool. Stimulants are obtained from the bark, seeds, and roots of different plants (cascara, senna, rhubarb, and aloe). These drugs are absorbed and stimulate peristalsis. Nonabsorbable sugars have an osmotic effect in the colon, and also lower the pH in the colon, which increases peristalsis.

Drugs used to treat constipation can be divided into categories based on the amount of time it takes to produce a stool (Table 21-8). Agents that cause feces to be soft within 1–3 days include bulk-forming agents, emollients, lactulose, sorbitol, and mineral oil. Drugs that will produce a stool in 6–12 hours include bisacodyl (Carters Little Pills, Correctol), cascara sagrada, senna (Agoral), sennosides (Senokot), and magnesium sulfate (Epsom salt) in a low dose. Drugs that produce a watery stool in 1–6 hours include magnesium citrate (Citro-Mag), magnesium hydroxide (Milk of Magnesia), magnesium sulfate

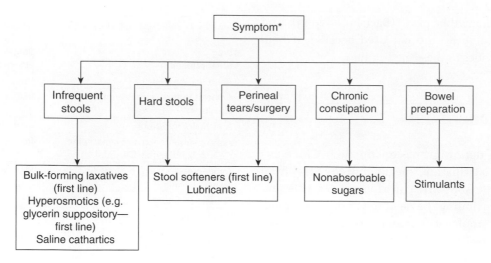

*Whenever a drug is recommended, it should be accompanied by discussion and health education about diet and bowel habits.

Figure 21-4 Mechanism of action of laxatives.

Table 21-8 Drugs Used to Treat Constipation

Drug Generic (Brand)	Dose	Clinical Considerations
Bulk-Forming Laxatives		
Calcium polycarbophil (FiberCon)	Tablets: 500, 650 mg 1–2 tablets PO qd–qid	Has effect in 1–3 days. Take each dose at the same time of day for no more than 7 days.
	Caplets 122 mg/caplet: 2 tablets PO qd–bid	Chewable tablets must be chewed thoroughly and not swallowed whole. Calcium polycarbophil can interfere with absorption of other drugs.* Calcium polycarbophil releases calcium in the GI tract and should be avoided by persons who need to restrict calcium intake.
Calcium polycarbophil (Mitrolan)	Chewable tablets: 500 mg or 625 mg/tablet 2 tablets PO qd to qid	
Carboxymethylcellulose (Citrucel)	2 caplets PO 1 to 6 ×/day	Has effect in 1–3 days. Take with 8 oz of fluid.
	1 tablespoon powder PO qd to tid	
Psyllium (Metamucil)	1–3 tsp PO qd to qid	Has effect in 1–3 days. Bulk-forming laxatives must be taken with at least 8 oz of water or they can cause a bowel obstruction.
Emollients		
Docusate sodium (Colace)	50 or 100 mg capsules taken qd to bid	Has effect in 1–3 days. Do not crush or chew the capsule. Take with 6–8 oz milk or juice. Do not take Colace within 2 hours of other medications. Contraindicated if nausea and vomiting or acute abdominal pain. Do not take Colace and mineral oil concurrently.
Docusate sodium (Peri-Colace)	50 mg docusate sodium/8.6 mg senna 1–2 tablets PO qd–bid	Has effect in 6–12 h. Combination of docusate sodium and senna, which is a laxative.
Lubricants		
Mineral oil	15–45 mL PO qd to bid	Has effect in 1–3 days. Can cause pneumonia if aspirated.

(continues)

Table 21-8 Drugs Used to Treat Constipation (*continued*)

Drug Generic (Brand)	Dose	Clinical Considerations
Saline Cathartics		
Magnesium (Milk of Magnesia)	Tablet, capsule, and liquid forms 15–30 mL PO qd to bid	Has effect in 1–6 h. Persons with renal failure should use with caution as frequent use can cause hypermagnesemia. Can cause diarrhea.
Magnesium citrate (Citroma)	1.745 g/30 mL 150–300 mL/day PO qd or as divided dose bid	Has effect in 1–6 h. Maximum dose is 300 mL/day, which equals 2.8 g elemental magnesium.
Magnesium sulfate (Epsom salts)	10–30 g/day PO Low dose is < 10 g/day High dose is 10–30 g/day	High dose has effect in 1–6 h. Low dose has effect in 6–12 h. Persons with renal failure should use with caution. Can cause hypermagnesemia
Stimulants		
Bisacodyl (Dulcolax)	5 mg/tablet or 10-mg suppositories 1–3 tablets PO qd 1 suppository per rectum up to three times per week	Has effect in 6–12 h. Stimulates mucosal nerve plexus in the colon. Do not crush, chew, or cut tablets. Avoid use within 1 hour of taking an antacid or milk.
Cascara sagrada	0.5–1.5 mL of fluid extract PO qhs	
Ricinoleic acid (castor oil)	15–60 mg PO qd	Has effect in 1–6 h. Can cause nausea, abdominal pain, diarrhea, electrolyte disorders.
Senna (Senokot, Ex-Lax)	8.6 mg/tablet or 8.8 mg/5 mL; 15 mg/5-mL granules 2 tablets qid or 4 tablets bid 10 mL syrup or 10 mL of granules (30 mg) PO qd to bid	Has effect in 6–12 h. Can cause diarrhea, nausea, abdominal bloating, flatulence, or urine discoloration. Brand X-Prep has 50 g glucose per bottle and should be used with caution by persons with diabetes.
Nonabsorbable Sugars		
Lactulose (Chronulac, Kristalose)	10 or 20 g powder/packet 10–20 g qd	Has effect in 1–3 days. Maximum dose is 40 mg/day. Can take 24–48 hours to have effect. Can cause severe diarrhea, electrolyte disorders, or metabolic acidosis if excessive doses are used. Common side effects include flatulence, diarrhea, nausea, vomiting, and abdominal bloating.
Sorbitol	15–30 mL qd–bid	Has effect in 1–3 days. Can cause abdominal cramps, flatulence, bloating.
Anticholinergic		
Loperamide (Imodium)	4 mg then 2 mg each stool not to exceed 8 mg/day if OTC or 16 mg/day if prescription	Give with clear liquids to prevent dehydration.
Absorbants		
Bismuth subsalicylate[†] (Pepto-Bismol)	30 mL or 2 tablets chewed or dissolved every 30–60 min up to 8 doses in 24 h	Has salicylate so should be avoided by persons who have allergy to aspirin, gout, or renal compromise. Contraindicated if taking anticoagulants, probenecid, or methotrexate. Possible salicylate toxicity (tinnitus).
Miscellaneous		
Polyethylene glycol electrolyte solution	240 mL of solution q 10 min up to 4 liters until fecal discharge is clear	Fast for 2–3 h before administering polyethylene glycol electrolyte solution.
Glycerin suppository	3-g suppository	Has an osmotic action in rectum, very safe, works within 30 min.

* Drug–drug interactions associated with calcium polycarbophil include decreased absorption and decreased efficacy of quinolone antibiotics, tetracyclines, digoxin, and ciprofloxacin. Can cause increased effect of glyburide.

† Suspension has 130 mg of salicylate; tablets have 102 mg of salicylate; cherry-flavored tablets and caplets have 99 mg of salicylate.

(Epsom salt) in a high dose, sodium phosphates (Fleet-Phospho-Soda), bisacodyl suppositories (Bisa-Lax), and polyethylene glycol-electrolyte (Pro-Lax) preparations.

Increased fluid intake and exercise are proven measures that help resolve constipation. Individuals with constipation should be advised to consume at least eight glasses (64 ounces) of noncaffeinated beverages and 25–50 grams of fiber per day. Many individuals report improvements in bowel function with walking 20 minutes per day. Alternative treatments such as acupuncture and Chinese herbal medication may be helpful in reducing constipation, although additional research is needed. Ideally, a laxative should be nonirritating, nontoxic, and act only on the descending sigmoid colon to produce a normally formed stool in a few hours, after which its action would cease. This ideal laxative does not exist. All laxatives can result in bowel dependency, so they should not be used for more than 1–2 weeks without consulting a healthcare provider. Women who develop **laxative dependency** or **laxative abuse** need to stop using laxatives gradually (Box 21-4). Although laxatives have not been found to be effective weight loss agents, they are frequently abused for that reason. Most of these agents are available over the counter. Laxatives and anticonstipation agents should not be used concurrently and should always be taken with at least 8 oz of water or juice. Both laxatives and stool softeners can be used to treat constipation. Laxatives cause increased frequency, whereas stool softeners do not necessarily influence the number of bowel movements, but instead change the fecal consistency. It is important to verify what the needs of the woman are prior to recommendation of the drug category.

Bulk-Forming Laxatives

Bulk-forming laxatives are indigestible, hydrophilic colloids that absorb water and form a bulky emollient gel that distends the colon and promotes peristalsis—most closely representing normal physiologic mechanisms. Common preparations include natural plant products (psyllium hydrophilic and methylcellulose) and synthetic fibers (polycarbophil). Bacterial digestion of plant fibers within the colon may lead to increased bloating and flatus.[44] Allergies to these agents rarely exist.

Psyllium hydrophilic mucilloid (Metamucil), carboxymethylcellulose (Citrucel), and calcium polycarbophil (FiberCon) are used to increase stool bulk. These agents need to be taken with 8 oz of liquid to avoid decreased efficacy or even obstruction. Consumption of the agent should be separated by at least 2 hours from other medications because they can interfere with absorption of other drugs (Table 21-7). The most common

---

Box 21-4　Laxative Dependency and Laxative Abuse

Despite their over-the-counter status and relative safety, laxatives can be overused. Laxatives are often misused in two different ways:

Laxative dependency occurs when an individual uses a laxative to treat constipation and defecate daily. The belief that defecation should occur daily can spur inappropriate use of laxatives. When laxatives are overused, the colon becomes dependent on the laxative for function and the person becomes dependent on the laxative to have a normal bowel movement. Ultimately the muscles of the colon can become damaged. Dehydration and electrolyte imbalance are also potential risks, especially in the elderly. Laxative dependency can be resolved via slowly titrating off the laxative and increasing fluids, bulk foods, and exercise.

Laxative abuse is different. Women with eating disorders sometimes use purgative laxatives to lose weight. Laxative abuse can result in laxative dependency, dehydration, and eventually can cause irritable bowel syndrome, or in rare cases, liver damage.

---

formulation of psyllium hydrophilic mucilloid (Metamucil) is contraindicated for individuals with diabetes, although sugar-free options are available. This agent also is contraindicated for individuals with phenylketonuria because it contains phenylalanine.

Emollients and Stool Softeners

Stool softeners work by permitting water and lipids to penetrate the stool material. These agents may be administered orally or rectally and are indicated for short-term therapy only. There rarely are side effects associated with the use of stool softeners. Docusate sodium (Colace) is the most common agent in this category.

Docusate sodium (Colace) facilitates the mixture of stool fat and water. When used concurrently with mineral oil, docusate sodium facilitates the absorption of mineral oil. Docusate sodium is contraindicated with the use of enemas or other laxatives, and in women with megacolon or signs and symptoms of appendicitis.

Lubricants

Mineral oil and olive oil are clear, viscous oils that lubricate fecal material and retard water absorption from stool. Lubricants are used to prevent and treat fecal impaction in young children and debilitated adults. Neither mineral oil nor olive oil is palatable, but may be mixed with juices. Care should be exercised when drinking a lubricant because aspiration can result in severe lipid pneumonitis. Long-term use can impair absorption of fat-soluble vitamins A, D, E, and K.

Saline Cathartics

The colon can neither concentrate nor dilute fecal fluid because fecal water is isotonic throughout the colon. Osmotic laxatives are soluble but nonabsorbable compounds result in increased stool liquidity due to an obligate increase in fecal fluid.[46] Magnesium oxide (Milk of Magnesia) is used in the treatment of acute or chronic constipation and is a commonly used osmotic laxative preoperatively. However, it should not be used for prolonged periods of time or by individuals with renal insufficiency due to a risk of hypermagnesemia.[47]

Hyperosmotics

Magnesium citrate, sodium phosphate (Glauber's salt), and magnesium sulfate (Epsom salt) are commonly used purgatives. High doses of osmotically active agents produce prompt bowel evacuation (purgation) within 3 hours. The rapid movement of water into the distal small bowel and colon leads to a high volume of liquid stool followed by rapid relief of constipation. Hyperosmolar agents may lead to intravascular volume depletion and electrolyte fluctuations, and thus should not be used for those who are frail, elderly, have renal insufficiency, or have significant cardiac disease.

Glycerin suppositories are safe and effective hyperosmotics. The mechanism of action is due to a combination of glycerin's osmotic effect with the local irritation of sodium stearate. Glycerin suppositories are indicated for rapid relief and usually respond within 30 minutes. Because such suppositories are local rather than systemic, few nontherapeutic effects have been attributed to them. Due to low cost, few side effects, and rapid action, glycerin suppositories are the laxative most like the ideal.

Stimulants: Anthraquinone

Anthraquinone is a laxative substance that occurs naturally in some plants including Aloe, senna, and cascara. Aloe is the harshest anthraquinone derivative, and senna is the mildest. Anthraquinone derivatives are poorly absorbed and after hydrolysis in the colon, produce a bowel movement in 6–12 hours when given orally and within 2 hours when given rectally. These drugs should not be used for more than 1 week because chronic use can lead to brown pigmentation of the colon known as melanosis coli.[47]

There is controversy about the mechanism of action of anthraquinone derivatives. The first theory is that they increase the propulsive peristaltic activity of the intestine by local irritation of the mucosa or by a more selective action on the intramural nerve plexus of intestinal smooth muscle. A competing theory is that there is no action on peristalsis; rather action is restricted to the distal ileum and colon where fluid and electrolyte secretion and absorption are altered. Long-term use of cathartics can lead to dependency and destruction of the myenteric plexus, resulting in colonic atony and dilation.

Sennosides (Ex-Lax) are a derivative of anthraquinone found in plants of the genus *Senna*. Sennosides work by increasing peristalsis. Electrolyte levels should be monitored if sennosides (Ex-Lax) are used long-term. The common side effects include nausea, bloating, cramps, flatulence, and diarrhea.

Bisacodyl, another derivative of anthraquinone can be found in such over-the-counter agents as Correctol, Dulcolax, and Carter's Little Pills. This agent is a stimulant and rarely needed for a healthy individual. Bisacodyl (Dulcolax) should not be taken within 1 hour of antacids or milk and should not be used for more than 1 week. Bisacodyl increases peristalsis by stimulating the submucosal neural plexus.

Ricinoleic acid (castor oil) increases peristalsis because it is a local irritant that stimulates intestinal motility in the small intestine. This agent is most effective when administered on an empty stomach, and due to its rapid onset (2–4 hours), it should not be taken at bedtime. Ricinoleic acid is excreted in the feces. The common side effects include dizziness, abdominal pain, nausea, diarrhea, and electrolyte disturbances. It is rarely used because of these side effects.

Nonabsorbable Sugars

Lactulose (Kristalose) and sorbitol are nonabsorbable sugars that can be used to prevent or treat chronic constipation. These sugars are metabolized by colonic bacteria that break them down into organic acids, which increase the osmotic pressure in the colon and slightly acidify the colonic contents, resulting in an increase in stool water content. The common side effects are severe flatus and abdominal cramps. Lactulose is an FDA Pregnancy Category B medication, and its safety in lactation is not known.

Lactulose (Kristalose) is contraindicated for use by individuals with galactosemia, diabetes mellitus, and colorectal electrocautery procedures. The nonabsorbable antacids may decrease the effect of lactulose (Kristalose). Common side effects include flatulence and intestinal cramps. Electrolyte levels should be monitored when therapy exceeds 6 months' duration.

Polyethylene glycol (GoLYTELY) is a solution that is lavaged for complete colonic cleansing prior to gastrointestinal endoscopic procedures. This balanced, isotonic solution contains an inert, nonabsorbable, osmotically active sugar (polyethylene glycol) with sodium sulfate, sodium chloride, sodium bicarbonate, and potassium chloride. The solution is designed so that no significant intravascular fluid shift or electrolyte shift occurs. Therefore, it is safe for all populations. The solution should be ingested rapidly (4 L over 2 hours) to promote bowel cleansing. For the treatment or prevention of chronic constipation, smaller doses of polyethylene glycol powder may be mixed with water or juices (17 g/8 oz) and ingested daily. In contrast to sorbitol or lactulose, polyethylene glycol does not produce significant cramps or flatus.[44]

Special Populations: Pregnancy, Lactation, and the Elderly

Nutritional guidance is the best intervention for pregnant women who are experiencing the common symptom of constipation. Of all the pharmacologic options, a glycerin suppository is the safest for pregnant or nursing women and is accompanied by advantages of low cost and rapid relief. However, many women today are accustomed to other routes. Bulk-forming laxatives have little systemic absorption and can be used as a first-line therapy. All other laxatives are not recommended for use in pregnancy. Ricinoleic acid (castor oil) is an FDA Pregnancy Category X drug because of its association with induction of labor.

Emollient stool softeners often are prescribed for postpartum women with perineal tears and are compatible with breastfeeding. When a laxative is needed, glycerin suppositories and bulk-forming laxatives should be among the first recommended because of their lack of systemic absorption.

It is estimated that 20–30% of individuals over the age of 65 years are dependent on laxatives. Hyperosmolar agents may lead to intravascular volume depletion and electrolyte fluctuations and thus should not be used for those who are frail, elderly, have renal insufficiency, or have significant cardiac disease.[47] When the elderly use lactulose (Kristalose), electrolyte levels should be monitored in individuals older than 60 years or if treatment lasts longer than 6 months. Elderly or chronically ill women may have difficulty defecating due to weak abdominal muscles; therefore, elevating the feet on a step or stool while on the commode may help with evacuation. Ricinoleic acid (Castor oil) is excreted in the feces and should be used with caution in the elderly.

Hemorrhoids

Hemorrhoids are dilated vascular channels located in the anal canal in three fairly constant locations: left lateral, right posterior, and right anterior. Internal hemorrhoids are located above the dentate line, while external hemorrhoids are located closer to the anal verge.[4] Hemorrhoids can cause bleeding, pain, and itching, but other anorectal diseases should be considered when individuals seek care for these symptoms. The exact pathogenesis is not clear; however, it is speculated that the internal hemorrhoids become symptomatic when their supporting structure becomes disrupted and the vascular anal cushions prolapse.[4]

One of the major causes of hemorrhoids is constipation. It is unclear how many individuals have hemorrhoidal disease, but 10–20% of the adult population is thought to be affected.[3] During pregnancy, hemorrhoids worsen because of constipation and increased venous pressure below the uterus.[4] Hemorrhoids are classified by their point of origin: internal, external, and internal-external and also are graded one to four.

Nonpharmacologic Treatment of Hemorrhoids

The initial treatment for hemorrhoids consists of a high-fiber diet (25 to 30 g daily), stool softener, and six to eight glasses of water daily. Sitz baths once or twice a day for 20–30 minutes can be soothing. Witch hazel compresses (Tucks) are commonly recommended to reduce the discomfort from hemorrhoids. The majority of research has been conducted in the area of perineal pain and hemorrhoids postchildbirth, and no strong evidence has been found as to effectiveness of any of the aforementioned treatments.[48]

In a small pilot study by Al-Waili et al., a mixture of honey, olive oil, and beeswax was found to be safe, and individuals reported a decrease in pain when the compound was used for the treatment of hemorrhoids and anal fissures.[49] Additional studies are needed to identify if this combination is effective when compared to placebo or other protectants.

Other nonpharmacologic treatment options of hemorrhoids include injection therapy with sclerosing agents, rubber banding, cryotherapy, infrared photocoagulation, electrocoagulation and heater probes, and surgery.

The agents that are used to treat hemorrhoidal symptoms include anesthetics, vasoconstrictors, protectants, counterirritants, astringents, wound-healing agents, antiseptics, and keratolytics. Each of the following categories of agents has a different mechanism of action.[4]

Pharmacologic Treatments: Anesthetics

Many over-the-counter medications are available for the treatment of hemorrhoids (Figure 21-5). Several of them contain topical anesthetics, such as benzocaine or pramaxine.[4] These drugs do not affect the underlying pathologic changes in the anal cushions. Benzocaine produces temporary pain relief, but it is quite sensitizing; the resulting allergic response may worsen the symptoms. Pramoxine is found in Anusol and Tronolane creams. It is less sensitizing than benzocaine, acts in 3–5 minutes, and lasts for several hours. The side effects of pramoxine include burning and itching, which may aggravate the inflamed tissue. Preparation H is a common over-the-counter remedy for hemorrhoids and contains shark liver oil, live yeast-cell derivatives, and phenyl mercuric nitrate. None of these agents heal hemorrhoids but they can improve symptoms.[50,51] The use of fiber-based laxatives has been demonstrated to be an effective relief measure and to decrease bleeding (decrease in symptoms RR = 0.47; 95% CI, 0.32–0.68 and bleeding RR = 0.50; 95% CI, 0.28–0.89).[52]

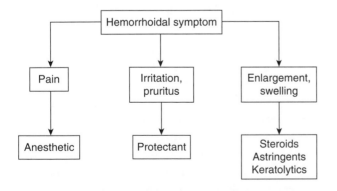

Avoid combination agents as they often contain subtherapeutic agents. Instead target treatment for major symptom.

Figure 21-5 Pharmacologic therapies for hemorrhoidal symptoms.

Vasoconstrictors

Vasoconstrictors stimulate the alpha-adrenergic receptors in the vasculature and promote constriction of the blood vessels. The vasoconstrictors relieve itching, discomfort, and irritation due to a slight anesthetic effect. These drugs include ephedrine sulfate (Levophed), epinephrine (Adrenalin), and phenylephrine HCL (Preparation H) and should not be used by persons with hypertension, diabetes, or difficulty urinating, or by those who are taking antidepressant medications.

Protectants

The protectants form a physical barrier over the skin and mucous membranes to help with itching that occurs with hemorrhoids and include aluminum hydroxide gel, calamine, cocoa butter, cod liver oil, glycerin, shark liver oil, white petrolatum, hard fat, kaolin, lanolin, mineral oil, and topical starch. In order for the protectant to be effective, it should have at least 50% of the active ingredient.

Astringents

Astringents coagulate the proteins in surface skin cells, which results in decreased cellular volume while leaving a thin layer protecting the underlying tissue. Astringents also decrease mucous and other secretions in order to decrease inflammation and irritation of the area.[4] The astringents provide relief of burning and itching, but not pain. Calamine and zinc oxide (Balmex, Desitin) in concentrations of 5–25% can be used internally and externally up to six times a day. Witch hazel or hamamelis water (Tucks) liquid or pads can be used externally in concentrations of 10–50%.

Keratolytics

Keratolytics cause desquamation and sloughing of the epidermal surface of cells in the perianal area.[51] Keratolytics are useful for reducing itching and discomfort and should only be used on external hemorrhoids. A 2-gram application of aluminum chlorhydroxy allantoinate (Alcloxa) can be used up to six times per day.

Hydrocortisone

Hydrocortisone has anti-inflammatory, lysosomal membrane stabilization, antimitotic, and vasoconstrictive properties that may be beneficial in relieving hemorrhoids. Topical hydrocortisone creams are safe and effective agents for relief of anorectal itching and swelling.

Special Populations: Pregnancy, Lactation, and the Elderly

A pregnant woman is at risk for hemorrhoids for several reasons: the hormonal milieu encourages development of varicosities due to relaxation of vessels; constipation is a common problem; and increased weight of the uterus results in more pressure on the vessels. Ice packs, warm packs, and positional changes are all suggested for treatment. Of the aforementioned pharmacologic therapies, none are contraindicated, and all are widely used during pregnancy and lactation.

As individuals age, issues of sedentary lifestyle and increased weight also may encourage the development of hemorrhoids. The pharmacologic treatments above are all indicated for use among the elderly, although dietary changes, lifestyle changes, and weight loss also may be of value.

Inflammatory Bowel Disease

Inflammatory bowel disease (IBD) is characterized by a tendency for chronic or relapsing immune activation and inflammation within the gastrointestinal tract.[53] A person with IBD often will experience cramping, abdominal pain, diarrhea, and weight loss. These symptoms are similar to those caused by other conditions. For example, irritable bowel syndrome (IBS) is frequently confused with IBD. IBS is a functional disorder that alters the motility of the small and large intestine and causes similar symptoms.

IBD includes both Crohn's disease and ulcerative colitis. Crohn's disease is an inflammatory illness that can involve any portion or portions of the digestive tract. Increased suppressor T-cell activity, alterations in immunologic A (IgA) production, and macrophage activity are associated with Crohn's disease. Crohn's disease is characterized by cycles of remissions and exacerbations of diarrhea, rectal bleeding, abdominal pain, weight loss, malnutrition, and weakness.[53] Ulcerative colitis is an inflammatory disease of the mucosa of the rectum and colon. Most commonly, it affects the most distal portions of the colon. Symptoms include rectal bleeding, diarrhea, and tenesmus, or the constant feeling of the need to empty the bowel.[53] Most authorities categorize inflammatory bowel disease as an autoimmune disease. Therefore more details about the condition and treatment of women who experience it can be found in Chapter 17.

Irritable Bowel Syndrome

Irritable bowel syndrome (IBS) is a gastrointestinal disorder characterized by altered bowel habits and abdominal pain in the absence of detectable structural abnormalities, infection, or metabolic changes on routine testing.[54] The definition of the disease is based on the clinical presentation because no clear diagnostic markers exist for IBS.[54] This syndrome is one of the most common conditions encountered in clinical practice but one of the least understood.

The burden of IBS on society is substantial. As many as 28% of referrals for gastroenterology consultations are for IBS. Absenteeism rates from school and work are significantly higher among persons with IBS than healthy individuals.[54] IBS is generally a disorder of the young, with most individuals presenting before age 45. Women are diagnosed with IBS two to three times as often as men and comprise 80% of the population with severe IBS.[46]

Individuals with IBS fall into two broad clinical groups. Most commonly, sufferers present with abdominal pain associated with diarrhea, constipation, or both. Individuals in the second group have painless diarrhea.[46,55]

The causes of IBS remain obscure.[56] Factors associated with the onset of IBS include genetic predisposition or previous history of physical, sexual, or emotional abuse, including chronic stressors such as bereavement, traumatic separation, or unemployment.[54] Autonomic signaling also differs by gender.[57] IBS may be maintained and perpetuated by psychologic factors such as general anxiety, depression, panic disorders, somatization disorder, gastrointestinal symptoms, a maladaptive coping style, or poor social support.

The pathophysiology of IBS has not been fully elucidated. Research has focused on the bidirectional signaling pathways and information processing centers between the gastrointestinal system and the central nervous system, known as the brain-gut axis. Abdominal pain and/or altered motility and bowel habits can derive from impaired activity in one or more of the stations along the brain-gut axis from the periphery (the intestinal lumen, the intestinal mucosa, the enteric nervous system) to the spinal cord and through to the higher, integrative brain centers.[58] A major factor is abnormal central processing of peripheral afferent visceral signals, leading to a lowered threshold for pain (hypersensitivity) and increased selective attention to gut-related stimuli (hypervigilance).[58]

Persons with IBS frequently report abdominal pain and constipation. For some individuals, chronic constipation is punctuated by brief episodes of diarrhea. A minority of persons experience only diarrhea.[42] These persons' stools are usually hard with narrowed caliber, possibly reflecting excessive dehydration caused by prolonged colonic retention and spasm. Most persons experience a sense of incomplete evacuation, leading to repeated attempts at defecation in a short time span.[42] Symptoms usually have been present for months to years, and it is common for those with IBS to have consulted several providers about their symptoms and to have undergone one or more gastrointestinal evaluations.[59] Persons with IBS also may have abdominal distention and increased belching or flatulence. Studies have shown these individuals have a normal amount of gas in their intestines but have an impaired transit and tolerance of intestinal gas loads. These persons also have symptoms of dyspepsia, heartburn, nausea, and vomiting. This suggests that there are other areas of the gut apart from the colon that may be involved.[30]

Bowel movements may be clustered in the morning or may occur throughout the day, but rarely is the individual awakened at night. Stools may be accompanied by an excessive amount of mucus, but blood is absent except in the presence of hemorrhoids.[59]

Women with IBS report worsening symptoms during the premenstrual and menstrual phases.[46] Several studies have reported an increased prevalence of sexual dysfunction among those with IBS, including reduced sexual drive, increased dyspareunia, and more severe IBS symptoms following intercourse. Women with IBS report a higher rate of intercourse avoidance[57] and the most common sexual dysfunction may be decreased libido. Sexual dysfunction was positively correlated with gastrointestinal symptom severity but not with psychologic symptom severity.[57] An increased incidence of chronic pelvic pain was noted among women with IBS. The prevalence of chronic pelvic pain in women with IBS was reported to be 14%. The rate of IBS in women with chronic pelvic pain ranges from 29% to 79%.[58] Because IBS affects the entire digestive tract, belching and symptoms of gastroesophageal reflux and dyspepsia are common among persons with IBS.[59] Anorexia, weight loss, fever, rectal bleeding, and nocturnal diarrhea all suggest a cause other than IBS.

Nonpharmacologic Treatment of IBS

Counseling and therapy have been advocated for individuals with IBS. Recent studies indicate that therapy may be effective in two thirds of IBS sufferers who do not respond to standard treatment.[59] Therapy can be particularly suited to persons with multiple, unexplained symptoms and comorbid functional disorders. However, a systematic

review of behavioral therapy and psychologic interventions demonstrated positive results, but the studies were small, evidence lacking for long-term effects, and in some cases the research was deemed suboptimal.[60] Hypnotherapy has been suggested as a treatment for IBS.[38] But of the four RCTs published, none were of a quality that allowed such a conclusion to be drawn.[61] A systematic review of acupuncture as a nonpharmacologic treatment for IBS also failed to find any effectiveness.[62]

Diet and Fiber Therapy

A common sense approach to diet therapy is the most appropriate. There is no need for bland foods or highly restrictive diets in the treatment of IBS. Persons should avoid foods they feel are aggravating. Substances such as coffee, disaccharides, legumes, and cabbage can be especially aggravating.[42] If lactose-containing foods produce cramps and diarrhea, they should be eliminated from the diet. The role of fiber in the treatment of IBS has been controversial. There is little objective support for its use. Several studies have found fiber supplements to be no more effective than placebos. Nevertheless, clinical experience suggests that a high-fiber diet or fiber supplements provide symptomatic relief for some.[50] High-fiber diets and bulking agents, such as bran or hydrophilic colloid, are frequently used in treating IBS. The water-holding action of fiber may contribute to increased stool bulk because of the ability of fiber to increase fecal output of bacteria.[42] Persons with cramplike abdominal pain seem most likely to benefit, although some with watery diarrhea experience a firming of their stools after the fiber content of their diet has been increased.[50]

Drugs Used to Treat Irritable Bowel Syndrome (IBS)

Irritable bowel syndrome is a chronic condition; therefore the focus of treatment is relief of symptoms. Drug therapy for IBS (Table 21-9) is tailored to the person's primary symptoms. In a systematic review of the evidence surrounding pharmacologic treatment of irritable bowel syndrome, antispasmodics, antidiarrheals, and serotonin receptor antagonists were found to be helpful, while there was inconclusive evidence for psychotropic agents.[63] Women may use various agents within categories, and individuals report relief with some drugs for which there is no evidence of efficacy. Much remains to be discovered about effective treatment of IBS.

Table 21-9 Medications with Evidence of Effectiveness for Treatment of Individuals with Irritable Bowel Syndrome

Medication Generic (Brand)	Target Dose	Clinical Considerations	FDA Approval for Symptoms or IBS
Constipation			
Laxatives: Lactulose*	15–30 mL	Strong evidence for effectiveness SE: Diarrhea, bloating, cramping	N/A[†]
Prokinetics: Tegaserod (Zelnorm)	6 mg twice daily	Strong evidence for effectiveness SE: Initial diarrhea, abdominal pain Rare AE: Cardiovascular ischemia	Both
Bloating			
Antibiotics: Rifaximin (Salix)	400 mg tid	No evidence of effectiveness SE: Abdominal pain, diarrhea, bad taste	Neither
Probiotics: Bifidobacterium infantis 35624	1 capsule daily	Some evidence for effectiveness in one RCT SE: None reported	Neither
Diarrhea			
Alosetron (Lotronex)	Initially 0.5 mg bid Up to 1 mg bid	Strong evidence for effectiveness SE: Constipation Rare AE: Ischemic colitis	Only for IBS
Loperamide (Imodium)	2–8 mg/day	Strong evidence for effectiveness SE: Constipation	
Pain			
Tricyclic antidepressants: Amitriptyline (Elavil) Desipramine (Norpramin)	Initially 10 mg qhs Up to 10–75 mg qhs	Moderate evidence for effectiveness in several RCTs SE: Dry mouth, dizziness, weight gain	Neither
SSRIs: Paroxetine (Paxil)	10–60 mg daily	Some evidence for effectiveness for IBS from one RCT SE: Sexual dysfunction, headache, nausea, sedation, insomnia, sweating, withdrawal syndromes	Neither
Citalopram (Lexapro)	5–20 mg daily	Some evidence for effectiveness for IBS and symptoms from one RCT SE: Sexual dysfunction, headache, nausea, sedation, insomnia, sweating, withdrawal syndromes	Neither

SE = side effect; AE = adverse effect; RCT = randomized controlled trial; SSRIs = selective serotonin reuptake inhibitors.
* Many over-the-counter osmotic, irritant, or fiber laxatives are available. Studies have used lactulose (Kristalose), lubiprostone (Amitiza), and polyethylene glycol (Miralax).
[†] Not evaluated as these products are over-the-counter.
Source: Adapted from Mayer E 2008.[56]

Herbals and Botanicals

Plantago seed and husk (psyllium or plantain) and chamomile tea have been suggested as herbal remedies for IBS. Chinese herbal medicines were found to be potentially effective for global symptoms such as abdominal pain, constipation, and diarrhea, but the studies tended to have methodological problems that precluded a strong recommendation of effectiveness.[64]

Nonsteroidal Anti-inflammatory Drugs (NSAIDs)

NSAIDs have anti-inflammatory effects, are available without prescription, and are absorbed well in the gastrointestinal tract. NSAIDs are suggested for treatment of some of the pain involved with IBS. However, with chronic use, gastric irritation is a common side effect. Gastric irritation is most severe with aspirin, which may cause erosion of the gastric mucosa, and because aspirin irreversibly acetylates platelets, gastrointestinal bleeding is a risk.[44]

Antispasmodics

Persons with constipation or abdominal pain may benefit from antispasmodics even though little evidence exists. These drugs are anticholinergic in their mode of action, but whether they actually relieve spasms is conjectural. A reasonable choice is dicyclomine (Bentyl) because it is less likely than others to cause unpleasant nongastrointestinal anticholinergic side effects. Persons should be cautioned about the possibility of the development of dry mouth, visual and urinary bladder disturbances, and constipation.[59]

Another antispasmodic is hyoscyamine (Levsin). Hyoscyamine is contraindicated in those with glaucoma, unstable cardiovascular status, gastrointestinal or genital-urinary obstruction, toxic megacolon, ulcerative colitis, and myasthenia gravis; and should be used cautiously in those with diarrhea, hyperthyroidism, and hiatal hernia with reflux esophagitis.

Laxatives and Prokinetics

Laxatives are not generally advised for treating IBS-related constipation. Many persons with constipation become dependent on the chronic use of laxatives and need to be withdrawn from these agents; chronic use of stimulants may ultimately cause nerve damage, and laxatives only address one symptom of IBS.[59] Increased fiber in the diet may be advised as a general good health habit.

When constipation is of concern, there is some indication that prokinetics may be of greater value to enhance gastric emptying.[65] Tegaserod (Zelnorm) was temporarily removed from the market in early 2007 because of rare cardiovascular side effects. It was returned under a restricted-access program for women who have IBS, especially constipation dominant, and no history of cardiovascular disease.[56]

Tranquilizers and Antidepressants

Tranquilizers and antidepressants are used in selected situations for the short-term management of situational anxiety and depression. Because of the potential for dependence, they have no place in long-term treatment of IBS.[59] In diarrhea-predominant IBS, the tricyclic antidepressant (TCA), imipramine (Tofranil), slows jejunal migrating motor complex transit propagation and delays orocecal and whole-gut transit time. TCAs may also alter visceral afferent neural function.

The efficacy of other classes of antidepressant agents in the management of IBS is less well evaluated. The selective serotonin reuptake inhibitor (SSRI) paroxetine (Paxil) accelerates orocecal transit, raising the possibility that this drug class may be useful in constipation-predominant individuals.[42] SSRIs are often prescribed to older persons because of their low potential for side effects and also are used to treat women with associated emotional symptoms such as anxiety, panic, obsessive disorders, and constipation in IBS.[59]

According to the American Gastroenterological Association, low doses of TCAs have more benefit than do SSRIs.[59] Low doses of TCAs treat pain and sleep disorders associated with IBS, are inexpensive, have a low potential for cardiovascular side effects, and have a rapid onset of action.

Amitriptyline (Elavil)

Amitriptyline (Elavil) is indicated for chronic pain. Side effects include orthostatic hypotension, tachycardia, elec-

trocardiogram changes, insomnia, fatigue, seizures, urinary retention, weight gain, and constipation. Amitriptyline has an FDA black box warning due to the potential increased risk of suicidal thoughts. Concomitant consumption of ethanol and grapefruit should be avoided by persons using amitriptyline because of potential drug–drug interactions.

Antiflatulence

The management of excessive gas is seldom satisfactory, except in obvious aerophagia or disaccharidase deficiency. Persons should be advised to eat slowly and avoid chewing gum; drinking carbonated beverages; and consuming artificial sweeteners, legumes, and foods in the cabbage family. Simethicone, antacids, and activated charcoal have all been tried, usually with disappointing results.[42]

Special Populations: Pregnancy, Lactation, and the Elderly

Irritable bowel syndrome has been reported in pregnancy although little has been reported other than the challenge it presents.[66] Tegaserod is an FDA Pregnancy Category B drug. However, it should be used with caution by women who are breastfeeding because it is found in breast milk. Among the antispasmodics used to treat IBS, dicyclomine (Bentyl) is an FDA Pregnancy Category B drug but is not recommended for breastfeeding women because of isolated reports of neonatal apnea of the nursing infant. Hyoscyamine (Levsin) is an FDA Pregnancy Category C drug due to lack of information, but no reports of harm have been reported for breastfeeding women.

For years it has been suggested that the elderly were less likely to suffer from IBS than younger adults. However, it now is estimated that the condition is equally distributed among all adults.[67] None of the agents are contraindicated for the elderly, but all should be used with caution because of increased risks among the elderly in regard to polypharmacy and chronic diseases such as renal and liver disease.

▋ Conclusion

Many gastrointestinal conditions disproportionately affect women. These illnesses can have a significant impact on the individual's quality of life. Yet challenges exist on many levels. Several drugs are frequently used, but with limited evidence as to effectiveness or even evidence to the contrary. Some of the most common purchases by a consumer may be for drugs that would be unnecessary if the woman is made aware of lifestyle changes that would be beneficial. Drugs such as laxatives that are considered innocuous by consumers may result in drug dependence. Systemic conditions such as irritable bowel syndrome remain unclear.

Pharmacotherapeutics for gastrointestinal conditions encompass a wide range of remedies, both nonpharmacologic and pharmacologic. This area is ripe for more research in areas of pathophysiology, diagnosis, and treatment. Until new, focused treatments emerge, clinicians will need to customize treatments based on known effectiveness, cost, availability, safety, and women's preferences. Providers, however, must be alert to the possibility of new information and would be wise to remember the words of the 20th-century author and social critic A. J. Nock, who wrote, "The mind is like the stomach. It is not how much you put into it that counts, but how much it digests."

References

1. Shaheen NJ, Hanson RA, Moragan DR. The burden of gastrointestinal and liver diseases. Gastroenterology 2006;101(9):2128–38.

2. Park J, Floch MH. Prebiotics, probiotics, and dietary fiber in gastrointestinal disease. Gastroenterol Clin North Am 2007;36(1):47–63.

3. Talley N, Vakin N. Guidelines for the management of dyspepsia. Am J Gastroenterol 2005;100:2324–37.

4. Feldman M, Friedman LS, Sleisenger MH. Gastrointestinal and liver disease: pathophysiology/diagnosis/management, 7th ed. Philadelphia, PA: W.B. Saunders, 2002:102–16, 119–26, 599–615, 747–72.

5. Mahadeva S, Goh K. Epidemiology of functional dyspepsia: a global perspective. World J Gastroenterol 2006;17:2661–6.

6. Holtmann G, Haag S, Adam B, Funk P, Wieland V, Heydenreich CJ. Effects of a fixed combination of peppermint oil and caraway oil on symptoms and quality of life in patients suffering from functional dyspepsia. Phytomedicine 2003;10(4):56–7.

7. Meltzer J, Posch W, Reichling, J, Brignoli R, Saller R. Meta-analysis: phytotherapy of functional dyspepsia with the herbal drug preparation STW 5. Aliment Pharmacol Ther 2004;20:1279–87.

8. Sippy BW. Gastric and duodenal ulcer: medical cure by an efficient removal of gastric juice corrosion. JAMA 1915;64:1625–30.

9. Chey WD, Wong CY. American College of Gastroenterology guidelines on the management of *Helicobacter pylori* infection. Am J Gastroenterol 2007;102:1808–25.

10. Kaltenbach T, Crockett S, Gerson LB. Are lifestyle measures effective in patients with gastroesophageal reflux disease? Arch Intern Med 2006;166:965–71.

11. Maher ER, Brown EA, Curtis JR, Phillips ME, Sampson B. Accumulation of aluminum in chronic renal failure due to administration of albumin replacement solutions. BMJ (Clin Res Ed) 1986;292:306.

12. Richter JE. Gastroesophageal reflux disease during pregnancy. Gastroenterol Clin North Am 2003;32:235–61.

13. Dowswell T, Neilson JP. Interventions for heartburn in pregnancy. Cochrane Database Syst Rev 2008(4):CD007065.

14. American Gastroenterology Association Institute. Technical review on the use of gastrointestinal medications in pregnancy. Gastroenterology 2006;131:283–311.

15. Richter JE. The management of heartburn in pregnancy. Aliment Pharmacol Ther 2005;22:749–57.

16. American Academy of Pediatrics Committee on Drugs. Transfer of drugs and other chemicals into human milk. Pediatrics 2001;108(3):776–89.

17. Lowe R, Wolfe M. The pharmacological management of gastroesophageal reflux disease. Minerva Gastroenterol Dietol 2004;50:227–37.

18. Zhai Q, Fu J, Huang X, Xu B, Yuan YZ, Jiang T, et al. Clinical study on the influence of a fixed-dose combination of famotidine with calcium carbonate and magnesium hydroxide on the bioavailability of famotidine. Arzneimittelforschung 2008;58(11):581–4.

19. Kahrilas P. Gastroesophageal reflux disease. N Engl J Med 2008;359:1700–7.

20. Yang YX, Lewis JD, Epstein S, Metz DC. Long-term proton pump inhibitor therapy and risk of hip fracture. JAMA 2006;296:2947–53.

21. Kallen BAJ. Use of omeprazole during pregnancy—no hazard demonstrated in 955 infants exposed during pregnancy. Eur Obstet Gynecol Reprod Biol 2001;96(1):63–8.

22. Moayyedi P, Soo S, Deeks J, Delaney B, Innes M, Forman D. Pharmacological interventions for nonulcer dyspepsia. Cochrane Database Syst Rev 2006;(4):CD001960.

23. Moore JG, Coburn JW, Saunders MC, McSorley DJ, Sirgo MA. Effects of sucralfate and ranitidine on aluminum concentrations in elderly volunteers. Pharmacotherapy 1995;15(6):742–6.

24. Nicholson PA, Karim A, Smith A. Phramacokinetics of misoprostol in the elderly, in patients with renal failure and when coadministered with NSAID or antipyrine, propranolol or diazepam. J Rheumatol Suppl 1990;20:33–7.

25. Ganiats TG, Norcross WA, Halverson AL, Burford PA, Palinkas LA. Does Beano prevent gas? A double-blind crossover study of oral alpha-galactosidase to treat dietary oligosaccharide intolerance. J-Fam-Pract 1994;39(5):441–5.

26. Di Stefano M, Miceli E, Gotti S, Missanelli A, Mazzocchi S, Corazza GR. The effect of oral alpha-galactosidase on intestinal gas production and gas related symptoms. Dig Dis Sci 2007;52(1):78–83.

27. Bone ME, Wilkinson DJ, Young JR, McNeil J, Charlton S. Ginger root—a new antiemetic. The effect of ginger root on postoperative nausea and vomiting after major gynaecological surgery. Anaesthesia 1990;45(8):669–71.

28. Phillips S, Ruggier R, Hutchinson SE. Zingiber officinale (ginger)—an antiemetic for day case surgery. Anaesthesia 1993;48(8):715–17.

29. Lee A, Done ML. Stimulation of the wrist acupuncture point P6 for preventing postoperative nausea and vomiting. Cochrane Database Syst Rev 2004;(3): CD003281.

30. Richardson MA, Vickers A, Allen C, Dibble S, Issell BF, Lao L, et al. Acupuncture-point stimulation for chemotherapy-induced nausea or vomiting. Cochrane Database Syst Rev 2006;(2): CD002285.

31. Carlisle J, Stevenson CA. Drugs for preventing postoperative nausea and vomiting. Cochrane Database Syst Rev 2006;(3):CD004125.

32. Park M, Camilleri M. Gastroparesis: clinical update. Am J Gastroenterol 2006;101(5):1129–39.

33. Kovac AL. Benefits and risks of newer treatments for chemotherapy-induced and postoperative nausea and vomiting. Drug Saf 2003;26(4):227–59.

34. Verberg N, Gillott D, Al-Fardan N., Grudzinskas JG. Hyperemesis gravidarum, a literature review. Human Reprod Update 2005;11:527–39.

35. Trewin VF, Lawrence CJ, Veitch GB. An investigation of the association of benzodiazepines and other hypnotics with the incidence of falls in the elderly. J Clin Pharm Ther 1992;17(2):129–33.

36. Fridenberg FK, Palit A, Parkman HP, Hanlon A, Nelson DB. Botilinum toxin A for the treatment of delayed gastric emptying. Am J Gastroenterol 2008;103(2):416–23.

37. van der Voort IR, Becker JC, Dietl KH, Konturek JW, Domschke W, Pohle T. Gastric electrical stimulation results in improved metabolic control in diabetic patients suffering from gastroparesis. Exp Clin Endocrinol Diabetes 2005;113(1):38–42.

38. Kendall BJ, Chakravarti A, Kendall E, Soykan I, McCallum RW. The effect of intravenous erythromycin on solid meal gastric emptying in patients with chronic symptomatic post-vagotomy-antrectomy gastroparesis. Alimentary Pharmacology Therapeutics 1997;11(2):381–5.

39. Dhir R, Richter J. Erythromycin in the short- and long-term control of dyspepsia symptoms in patients with gastroparesis. J Clin Gastroenterol 2004;38(3): 237–242.

40. Krassner L. TIPP usage. Pediatrics. 1984;74(5, pt 2): 976–80.

41. Fine KD, Schiller LR. AGA technical review on the evaluation and management of chronic diarrhea. Gastroenterol 1999;116:1464–86.

42. Longstreth G, Thompson W, Chey W, Houghton L, Mearin F, Spiller RC. Functional bowel disorder. Gastroenterology 2006;130:1480–8.

43. DuPont HL. Systematic review: the epidemiology and clinical features of travellers' diarrhoea. Aliment Pharmacol Ther. 2009 Aug;30(3):187–96.

44. Spies LA. Traveler's diarrhea: an update on prevention and treatment. J Midwifery Womens Health 2008;53(3):251–4.

45. Lewis SJ, Heaton KW. Stool form scale as a useful guide to intestinal transit time. Scand J Gastroenterol 1997;32(9):920–4.

46. Pohl D, Tutuian R, Fried M. Pharmacologic treatment of constipation: what is new? Curr Opin Pharmacol 2008 Dec;8(6):724–8.

47. Wigle P, Kim K, King A, Jones S, Schaeffer K. OTC medications for GI disorders in pregnancy. US Pharmacist 2006;31:9. Retrieved October 2, 2008, from the Medline database.

48. East CE, Begg L, Henshall NE, Marchant P, Wallace K. Local cooling for relieving pain from perineal trauma sustained during childbirth. Cochrane Database Syst Rev 2007;(4):CD006304.

49. Al-Waile N, Saloom K, Al-Waili Tk, Al-Waili AN. The safety and efficacy of a mixture of honey, olive oil, and beeswax for the management of hemorrhoids and anal fissure: a pilot study. Scientific World J 2006;6:1998–2005.

50. Clincial Practice Committee, American Gastroenterological Association. American Gastroenterological

Association medical position statement: diagnosis and treatment of hemorrhoids. Gastroenterology 2004;126:1461–2.

51. Acheson AG, Sholefield JH. Management of haemorrhoids. BMJ 2008;336:380–8.

52. Alonso-Coello P, Guyatt G, Heels-Ansdell D, Johanson JF, Lopez-Yarto M, Milles E, et al. Laxatives for the treatment of hemorrhoids. Cochrane Database Syst Rev 2005;(4):CD004649.

53. Thoreson R, Cullen J. Pathophysiology of inflammatory bowel disease: an overview. Surg Clin North Am 2007;87:1–8.

54. Sperber AD. The irritable bowel syndrome and its association with unexplained medical symptoms and other functional disorders. JCOM Case-Based Rev 2007;1(4):3–12.

55. Manabe N, Tanaka T, Hata J, Kusunoki H, Haruma K. Pathophysiology underlying irritable bowel syndrome—from the viewpoint of dysfunction of autonomic nervous system activity. J Smooth Muscle Res 2009;45(1):15–23.

56. Mayer E. Irritable bowel syndrome. N Engl J Med 2008;358:1692–9.

57. Manabe N, Tanaka T, Hata J, Kusunoki H, Haruma K. Pathophysiology underlying irritable bowel syndrome—from the viewpoint of dysfunction of autonomic nervous system activity. J Smooth Muscle Res 2009;45(1):15–23.

58. Manabe N, Tanaka T, Hata J, Kusunoki H, Haruma K. Pathophysiology underlying irritable bowel syndrome—from the viewpoint of dysfunction of autonomic nervous system activity. Smooth Muscle Res 2009 Feb;45(1):15–23.

59. Drossman DA, Camilleri M, Mayer EA, Whitehead WE. AGA technical review on irritable bowel syndrome. Gastroenterology 2002;123:2108–31.

60. Zijdenbos IL, de Wit NJ, van der Heijden GJ, Rubin G, Quartero AO. Psychological treatments for the management of irritable bowel syndrome. Cochrane Database Syst Rev 2009(1):CD006442.

61. Webb AN, Kukuruzovic R, Catto-Smith AG, Sawyer SM. Hypnotherapy for treatment of irritable bowel syndrome. Cochrane Database Syst Rev 2007(4):CD005110.

62. Lim B, Manheimer E, Lao L, Ziea E, Wisniewski J, Liu J, et al. Acupuncture for treatment of irritable bowel syndrome. Cochrane Database Syst Rev 2006(4):CD005111.

63. Jailwala J, Imperiale T, Kroenke K. Pharmacologic treatment of the irritable bowel syndrome: a systematic review of randomized, controlled trials. Ann Intern Med 2000;133(2):136–47.

64. Liu J, Yang M, Liu Y, Wei M, Grimsgaard S. Herbal medicines for treatment of irritable bowel syndrome. Cochrane Database Syst Rev 2006(1):CD004116.

65. Brenner DM, Moeller MJ, Chey WD, Schoenfeld PS. The utility of probiotics in the treatment of irritable bowel syndrome: a systematic review. Am J Gastroenterol 2009;104(4):1033–49.

66. Thukral C, Wolf JL. Therapy insight: drugs for gastrointestinal disorders in pregnant women. Nat Clin Pract Gastroenterol Hepatol 2006;3(5):256–66.

67. Ehrenpreis E. Irritable bowel syndrome: 10% to 20% of older adults have symptoms consistent with diagnosis. Geriatrics 2005;60(1):25–8.

68. Charbit B, Alvarez JC, Dasque E, Abe E, Demolis JL, Funck-Bretano C. Droperidol and ondansetron-induced QT interval prolongation. Anesthesiology 2008;109:206–12.

69. King TL, Murphy PA. Evidence-based approaches to treating nausea and vomiting in early pregnancy. J Midwifery Womens Health. In press.

70. DeMatteo RP, Symcox M, Demetri GD. 100 questions and answers about gastrointestinal stromal tumor (GIST). Sudbury, MA: Jones and Bartlett Publishers, 2006.

"In the past, the rich yellow color of urine was thought to be secondary to the presence of gold. Alchemists spent decades trying to extract gold from urine."

22

Lower Urinary Tract Disorders

Katharine K. O'Dell and Emily E. Weber LeBrun

✦ Chapter Glossary

Acute cystitis Acute onset of dysuria and frequency with or without hematuria caused by adherence of pathogenic microorganisms to the bladder wall.

Detrusor muscle Muscle of the bladder whose fibers essentially cover the inferior surface of the organ and constrict to maintain continence and relax to allow the bladder to fill.

Detrusor overactivity (DOA) Condition during which the detrusor contracts unexpectedly during bladder filling. Urodynamics are used to diagnose DOA.

Frequency Urinating too often. May be due to increased bladder sensation or contractions or to decreased bladder capacity.

Functional incontinence Inability to get to the bathroom before voiding, without undue feelings of urgency, and with normal bladder and urethral function. Associated with cognitive, psychological, or physical impairments that impede toileting.

Incompetent urethral closure mechanism Also called intrinsic sphincter deficiency. Urine loss almost continuously with minimal activity or urge to void. The urethra itself is unable to maintain a water-tight seal. It is needed to rule out vesicovaginal fistula in cases of continuous urine loss.

Interstitial cystitis Chronic bladder pain, dysuria, frequency without hematuria; increased bladder sensation. Disruption of the protective barrier of the urothelium (bladder lining).

Mixed urinary incontinence Involuntary leakage of urine associated with both urgency and exertion, effort, sneezing, or coughing. A combination of the factors associated with stress urinary incontinence and urge urinary incontinence.

Nocturia Voiding frequently during the night interfering with sleep. Associated with insomnia, increased supine urine excretion, or increased sensation and/or DOA.

Nocturnal enuresis Loss of urine while asleep. Associated factors can include DOA, sleep apnea, or medications.

Overactive bladder dry Urgency and frequency that occur without urge urinary incontinence.

Overactive bladder wet Urgency and frequency that occur with urge urinary incontinence.

Overflow incontinence Inability to empty the bladder, slow or intermittent urine stream, dribbling. Involuntary loss of urine associated with overdistention of the bladder. In women, this is most likely due to neurologic disease, obstruction due to genital prolapse or fibroids, or postpartum or postoperative edema.

Painful bladder syndrome See *interstitial cystitis*.

Stress urinary incontinence (SUI) Involuntary leakage of urine with effort, exertion, sneezing, or coughing. Bladder pressure is greater than urethral pressure due to inadequate urethral support.

Urge urinary incontinence (UUI) Involuntary loss of urine accompanied by or preceded by urgency. *DOA incontinence* is the term used to describe urine loss due to involuntary bladder contraction demonstrated on urodynamic examination.

Urgency Sudden, compelling desire to pass urine, which is difficult to defer. Result of involuntary detrusor contraction or hypersensitivity of sensory nerves.

Source: Adapted from Abrams P et al. 2003.[1]

The lower urinary tract controls the complex process of storing and eliminating urine. This process normally is painless, predictable, leak proof, and consistently under cognitive control beginning in early childhood. Reliable continence requires intact functioning of the entire urinary system, including the end organs (bladder and urethra), the communication tract (the spinal cord and peripheral and autonomic nerves), and the central control and coordination centers (the cortex and brain stem). This chapter reviews pharmacotherapeutics used to treat disorders of the urinary tract. The urinary tract is complex, and misdiagnosis or inappropriate treatment may have adverse results. Underlying anatomic, infectious, or neurologic pathology must be identified using appropriate history, physical examination, and laboratory testing before pharmacologic treatment is initiated. Additionally, it is important to remember that some lower urinary tract symptoms may be the unwanted side effects of medications prescribed for other indications (Table 22-1). Once a thorough evaluation is completed, modifiable risks are addressed, and the woman is informed of her treatment options; many lower urinary tract symptoms can be successfully treated using pharmacotherapy.

Table 22-1 Common Medications and Substances with Side Effects That Can Result in Lower Urinary Tract Symptoms

Common Medications Generic (Brand)	Mechanism of Action	Effect or Side Effect	Urinary Symptoms
ACE inhibitors	Antihypertensives	Cough	Increased SUI
Antidepressants: imipramine (Tofranil), amitriptyline (Elavil), bupropion (Wellbutrin), paroxetine (Paxil), trazodone (Desyrel)	Anticholinergics (nonmuscarinic), CNS stimulant or depressant	Impaired detrusor contractility, sedation, dizziness	Retention, overflow incontinence, constipation
Antihistamines/decongestants: diphenhydramine (Benadryl), hydroxyzine (Vistaril), pseudoephedrine (Sudafed)	Alpha-agonist	Increased outlet resistance	Voiding difficulties, dyssynergia, retention
Antiparkinson medications: amantadine (Symmetrel), bromocriptine (Parlodel), levodopa (Sinemet)	Parkinson's disease	Decreased bladder contractility	Retention
Alcohol	Diuretic, irritation of bladder lining, CNS depressant	Increased urine volume, sensory nerve stimulation, sedation	Frequency, urgency, incontinence
Alpha-adrenergic antagonists: prazosin (Minipress), terazosin (Hytrin), doxazosin (Cardura)	Antihypertensives	Urethral smooth muscle relaxant	Stress urinary incontinence
Beta-blockers	Antihypertensives	Smooth muscle relaxation; decrease urethral closure	Stress urinary incontinence
Caffeine	Diuretic, bladder lining irritant, smooth muscle stimulant	Increased urine volume, sensory nerve stimulant	Frequency, urgency, incontinence
Calcium channel blockers: verapamil (Isoptin), nifedipine (Procardia), diltiazem (Cardizem)	Antihypertensives	Reduced smooth muscle contractility	Retention
Cholinesterase inhibitors: donepezil (Aricept)	Cognitive decline; Alzheimer's disease	Slowed breakdown of acetylcholine; smooth muscle contraction	Precipitate UUI
Diuretics: furosemide (Lasix), hydrochlorothiazide (HydroDIURIL)	Diuretic	Increased output	Frequency, urgency, incontinence
Narcotics/analgesics: opioids, NSAIDs	Analgesia	Sedation, smooth muscle relaxation, delirium	Retention, overflow, constipation
Psychotropics: lithium (Lithobid)	Bipolar disorder	Mood stabilizer; mechanism of action not clear	UUI, polyuria
Sedatives: lorazepam (Ativan), diazepam (Valium)	CNS depressant	Sedation, confusion, muscle relaxation	Functional incontinence
Skeletal muscle relaxants: baclofen (Lioresal), cyclobenzaprine (Flexeril)	Spasticity	Central nervous system depressant	Urinary urgency, enuresis, and retention, overflow

SUI = stress urinary incontinence; CNS = central nervous system; UUI = urge urinary incontinence.

Physiology of the Lower Urinary Tract in Women

Anatomic components of the urinary system as they relate to pharmacologic treatments are reviewed in Figure 22-1. Four components that facilitate continence within the bladder and urethra include: (1) an intact mucoid lining that protects underlying tissue from irritants in the urine; (2) smooth muscle able to respond in a coordinated fashion to opposing parasympathetic and sympathetic nerve stimuli; (3) connective tissue support to maintain functional alignment; and (4) intact skeletal muscles with the sensory and motor innervation needed to affect voluntary control. Disease, infection, injury, or atrophy at any level in the system can produce problems in the storage or elimination of urine, resulting in the lower urinary tract symptoms common among women seeking healthcare services.

Overactive Bladder

Symptoms of painless urinary **urgency** and **frequency** are often accompanied by **nocturia** and **urge urinary incontinence** (UUI) (Box 22-1). Standardized terms to describe these symptoms include **overactive bladder dry** when urgency and frequency occur without UUI, and **overactive bladder wet** when UUI occurs.[1] Because the dome, or body of the bladder, is comprised of an elastic smooth

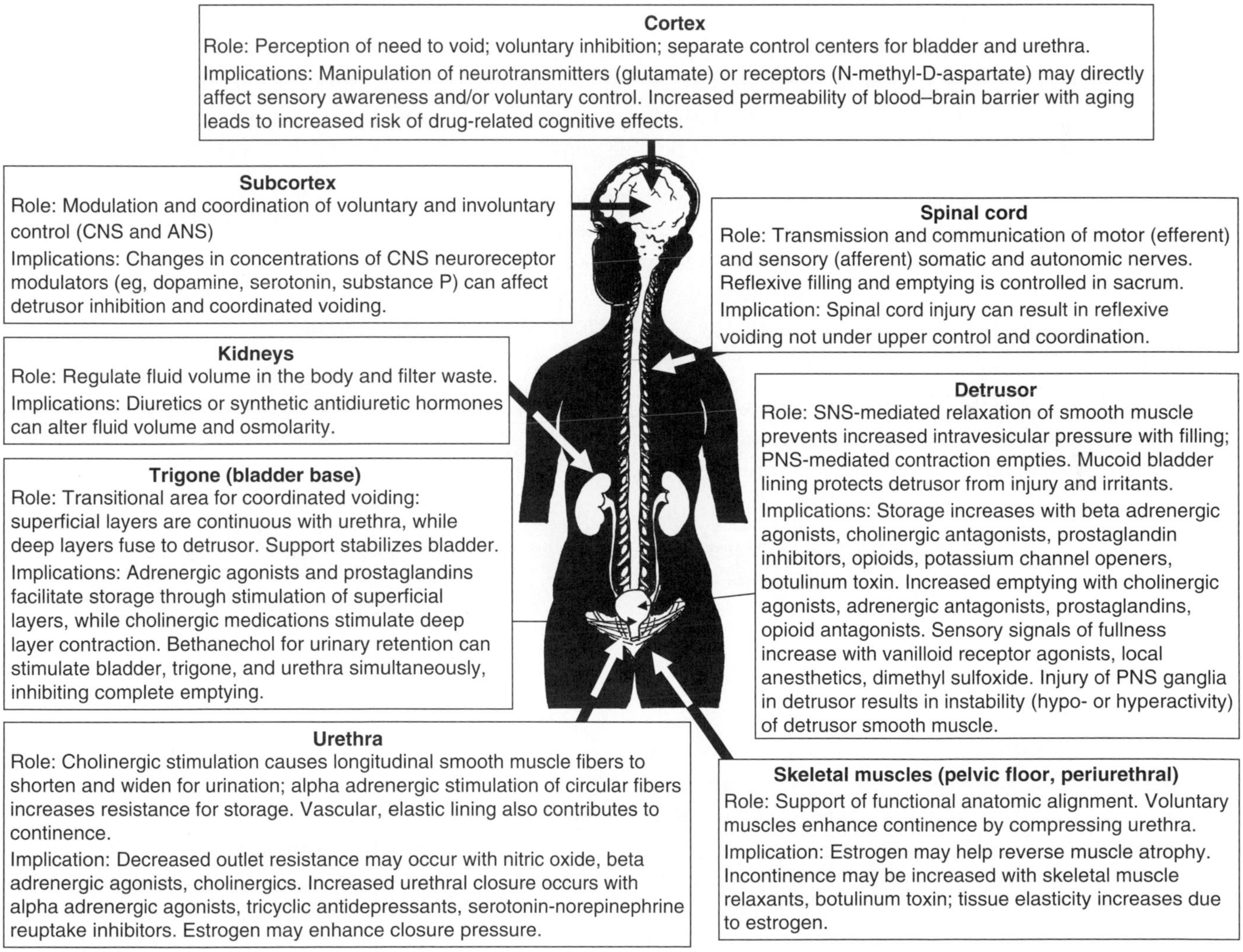

Cortex
Role: Perception of need to void; voluntary inhibition; separate control centers for bladder and urethra.
Implications: Manipulation of neurotransmitters (glutamate) or receptors (N-methyl-D-aspartate) may directly affect sensory awareness and/or voluntary control. Increased permeability of blood–brain barrier with aging leads to increased risk of drug-related cognitive effects.

Subcortex
Role: Modulation and coordination of voluntary and involuntary control (CNS and ANS)
Implications: Changes in concentrations of CNS neuroreceptor modulators (eg, dopamine, serotonin, substance P) can affect detrusor inhibition and coordinated voiding.

Spinal cord
Role: Transmission and communication of motor (efferent) and sensory (afferent) somatic and autonomic nerves. Reflexive filling and emptying is controlled in sacrum.
Implication: Spinal cord injury can result in reflexive voiding not under upper control and coordination.

Kidneys
Role: Regulate fluid volume in the body and filter waste.
Implications: Diuretics or synthetic antidiuretic hormones can alter fluid volume and osmolarity.

Detrusor
Role: SNS-mediated relaxation of smooth muscle prevents increased intravesicular pressure with filling; PNS-mediated contraction empties. Mucoid bladder lining protects detrusor from injury and irritants.
Implications: Storage increases with beta adrenergic agonists, cholinergic antagonists, prostaglandin inhibitors, opioids, potassium channel openers, botulinum toxin. Increased emptying with cholinergic agonists, adrenergic antagonists, prostaglandins, opioid antagonists. Sensory signals of fullness increase with vanilloid receptor agonists, local anesthetics, dimethyl sulfoxide. Injury of PNS ganglia in detrusor results in instability (hypo- or hyperactivity) of detrusor smooth muscle.

Trigone (bladder base)
Role: Transitional area for coordinated voiding: superficial layers are continuous with urethra, while deep layers fuse to detrusor. Support stabilizes bladder.
Implications: Adrenergic agonists and prostaglandins facilitate storage through stimulation of superficial layers, while cholinergic medications stimulate deep layer contraction. Bethanechol for urinary retention can stimulate bladder, trigone, and urethra simultaneously, inhibiting complete emptying.

Urethra
Role: Cholinergic stimulation causes longitudinal smooth muscle fibers to shorten and widen for urination; alpha adrenergic stimulation of circular fibers increases resistance for storage. Vascular, elastic lining also contributes to continence.
Implication: Decreased outlet resistance may occur with nitric oxide, beta adrenergic agonists, cholinergics. Increased urethral closure occurs with alpha adrenergic agonists, tricyclic antidepressants, serotonin-norepinephrine reuptake inhibitors. Estrogen may enhance closure pressure.

Skeletal muscles (pelvic floor, periurethral)
Role: Support of functional anatomic alignment. Voluntary muscles enhance continence by compressing urethra.
Implication: Estrogen may help reverse muscle atrophy. Incontinence may be increased with skeletal muscle relaxants, botulinum toxin; tissue elasticity increases due to estrogen.

CNS = central nervous system; ANS = autonomic nervous system; SNS = sympathetic nervous system.

Figure 22-1 Anatomy and physiology of the urinary tract system.

Box 22-1   A Case of Urinary Urgency and Incontinence

MK is a 48-year-old woman with two children. She began having irregular menses over 2 years, along with a gradual onset of increasing problems with urinary incontinence related to urgency. She has a lifelong history of frequent voiding (10–14 voids per day), including enuresis to age 8, and nocturia, typically two to three times per night. Until recently, she was able to manage her urgency by voiding frequently and modifying fluid intake. However, MK has begun experiencing increasingly intense, painless urgency. Several times a week, she leaks urine before she can reach a restroom. She now wears pads continuously. Her life is beginning to center around finding a bathroom everywhere she goes. MK rarely loses any urine with cough, sneeze, or exercise, is a nonsmoker, has not had urinary tract infections (UTIs), and has never noticed hematuria. She has no neurologic symptoms, such as incoordination, numbness, or tremor. She currently takes no prescription or over-the-counter medications. She has no other pelvic floor problems such as dyspareunia, constipation, or fecal incontinence.

MK's physical exam is normal. Her body-mass index is 24. On pelvic exam she displays moderate pelvic floor muscle strength and no evidence of prolapse. She has minimal genital atrophy. Her urinalysis and culture are negative.

Primary Care Treatment

As an initial treatment, MK was instructed to try eliminating, or decreasing, bladder irritants such as caffeine, spices, artificial sweeteners, and alcohol. MK also used other behavioral strategies, including regular, measured voiding, monitoring her fluid intake, strengthening her pelvic muscles, and using her muscles to control urgency. Though her symptoms improved, she continued to have unpredictable urine loss. Her bladder is still the focus of her daily life.

MK wants to try a medication. The review of her history indicates that she does not have contraindications to use of antimuscarinic agents or potential for drug–drug interactions. Her prescription drug plan has a tiered formulary of preferred medications. She is prescribed an inexpensive antimuscarinic agent in an extended-release formulation at the lowest recommended dose. Because MK says her biggest problem currently is restriction of her social activities due to daytime urgency, she starts taking the medication immediately on arising, anticipating peak effect in 4–6 hours.

If MK does not notice satisfactory relief within the next 2 weeks of regular use, her symptoms should guide variations in her medication use. She might choose to increase the dose within the recommended range, change agents, or add a second low-dose agent at bedtime if nighttime voiding problems increase. She was encouraged to continue using the behavioral strategies she has learned.

If medication variations do not produce satisfactory symptom relief within the next 2 months, she will be referred to a urogynecology or urology practice for further evaluation.

---

muscle called the **detrusor muscle**, symptoms associated with involuntary detrusor contraction during objective bladder testing (urodynamically) are referred to as **detrusor overactivity**.[1]

The incidence of overactive bladder is obscured by the subjective nature of the symptoms, underreporting, and variations in definition. The National Overactive Bladder Evaluation included phone interviews with 5204 adults in the United States and determined that overactive bladder increased with age from approximately 5% in those < age 25 years to approximately 30% in those > age 75 years.[2] Both men and women reported similar prevalence of overactive bladder, but women were more likely to experience overactive bladder wet, in part because of anatomically shorter urethras. In addition, continence may be impaired by external factors, including connective tissue or neuromuscular injury experienced during childbirth. In the United States, the direct and indirect costs of overactive bladder have been estimated to exceed $18 billion yearly.[2]

Pathophysiology of Overactive Bladder

Muscle and nerve changes can both play a role in the development of overactive bladder and are potential targets for pharmacologic treatment.[3] Smooth muscle changes related to overactive bladder include spontaneous or discoordinated muscle fiber firing or an increased or decreased response to normal stimuli. Skeletal muscle weakness can contribute to overactive bladder wet due to loss of voluntary urethral support. Voluntary control can also be undermined by central or somatic nervous system degeneration. For example, future therapies may have a dual purpose in maintaining the cerebral cortex, where degeneration simultaneously affects both urinary control centers and aged-related dementia.

The main target of pharmacologic treatment for overactive bladder is the autonomic neurons that control the coordinated homeostatic functioning of the bladder and urethra. Figure 22-2 displays the autonomic pathways relating to bladder function. Sympathetic motor pathways are predominantly mediated by the neurotransmitter norepinephrine.[3] Low-level release of norepinephrine stimulates beta-adrenergic receptors in smooth muscle of the bladder dome (detrusor), resulting in relaxation, while higher concentrations of norepinephrine stimulate alpha-adrenergic receptors in the urethral walls and bladder base (trigone), resulting in contraction of their smooth muscle. This synergistic activity promotes urine storage by allowing urine to fill the bladder without increasing pressure on the bladder walls.

Parasympathetic innervation is mediated by at least two neurotransmitters, acetylcholine and noncholinergic nonadrenergic transmitters. Stimulation of muscarinic cholinergic receptors in the bladder dome results in detrusor contraction and urine elimination.[3] There are five types of muscarinic acetylcholine receptors in the human body (M1–M5). Of these five, M2 and M3 receptors predominate in the detrusor, with M3 more directly affecting detrusor contraction. The primary mechanism of action of first-line medications for overactive bladder is control of detrusor instability via inhibition of cholinergic activity.

Pharmacologic Therapy with Antimuscarinic Anticholinergics

Optimal treatment of overactive bladder symptoms begins with an individualized program of behavioral management strategies, including voiding diaries, fluid management, timed voiding,[4] weight management,[5] smoking cessation, and pelvic muscle strengthening and coordination exercises.[6]

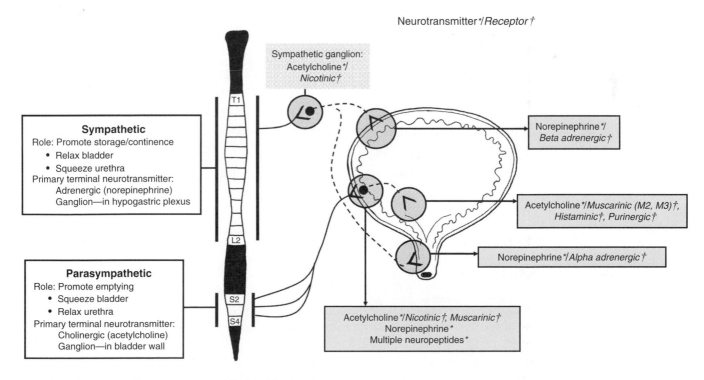

Figure 22-2 Autonomic nervous system of the bladder.

When behavioral strategies do not produce satisfactory symptom control for overactive bladder, antimuscarinic anticholinergic medications are the first-line treatment. Efficacy of antimuscarinic agents has been reported in clinical trials that followed adults for up to 24 weeks[7] and children up to 5 years.[8] Table 22-2 provides a review of current medications approved by the US Food and Drug Administration (FDA) for the treatment of overactive bladder symptoms. Meta-analysis of trials comparing antimuscarinic medications with placebo found that treatment significantly improves leakage episodes per 24 hours (RR = −0.54; 95% CI, −0.67 to 0.41), number of voids per day (RR = −0.69; 95% CI, −0.84 to −0.54), and some quality-of-life domains, including travel, social life, and emotional health.[9] Rates of discontinuation were similar in both treatment and placebo groups.

Table 22-2 Antimuscarinic Anticholinergics with FDA Approval for the Treatment of Overactive Bladder

Drug* Generic (Brand)	Action/Pharmacokinetics	Dose†/Clinical Considerations
Darifenacin (Enablex ER)	Targets M3 receptors in bladder. Metabolized in liver. Half-life 12 hours. Unlikely to cross blood–brain barrier.	7.5–15 mg PO daily with food. Clinical implications of M3-specificity are understudied but may decrease risk of side effects in women with heart disease.
Oxybutynin (Ditropan IR)	Targets M1, M3. Mild antispasmodic and anesthetic effects. Metabolized in liver. Crosses blood–brain barrier. Peak action: 1 hour. Duration: 6–10 hours.	2.5 mg or 5 mg PO daily, up to 5 mg four times daily. Available in liquid formula (5 mg/5 mL). Oxybutynin can be ground for use in intravesicular installation.
Oxybutynin (Ditropan XL)	Targets M1–M3. Mild antispasmodic. Peak action: 4–6 hours. Duration: > 24 hours.	5, 10, 15 mg PO daily, up to 30 mg daily. Cannot be chewed or crushed due to internal dispensing mechanism.
Oxybutynin transdermal (Oxytrol patch)	Targets M1–M3. Mild antispasmodic and anesthetic effects. Steady dose over 3–4 days. Avoids liver first-pass and active metabolite production, which may decrease side effects such as dry mouth. Skin irritation is a potential side effect (18%).	3.9 mg daily via patch changed twice weekly.
Solifenacin (VESIcare ER)	Targets M1, M3. Antispasmodic. Metabolized in liver. Long half-life (50 hours). Unlikely to cross blood–brain barrier.	5–10 mg daily. Can be taken with food. Clinical implications of long half-life are not known.
Tolterodine IR (Detrol)	Nonspecific antimuscarinic with low affinity for other neurotransmitter receptors. GI absorption/liver metabolism. Unlikely to cross blood–brain barrier, though CNS effects are occasionally reported. Peak: 1–3 hours. Half-life 2–6 hours.	2 mg PO daily. (1-mg and 2-mg tablets).
Tolterodine (Detrol LA)	Nonspecific antimuscarinic with low affinity for other neurotransmitter receptors. GI absorption/liver metabolism. Peak: 2–6 hours. Half-life 6–8 hours.	2–4 mg PO daily. (2-mg and 4-mg tablets)
Trospium (Sanctura IR)	Quaternary amine, nonselective peripheral effect. Minimal liver metabolism with decreased drug–drug interaction possible. Water soluble, larger molecule. Unlikely to cross blood–brain barrier and majority of drug excreted as active agent in the urine, increasing potential local anticholinergic effect. Peak effect 4–6 hours. Half-life longer than 18 hours.	20 mg PO twice daily (daily in elderly to start). Take on empty stomach as fatty foods decrease activity.

IR = Immediate release; LA, ER, and XL = long acting or extended release; M, M1, M2, M3 refer to parasympathetic muscarinic receptors.

* FDA assigned risk factors for pregnancy and lactation vary for these medications.

† For women over age 65, start with lowest possible dose.

In clinical practice, some manipulation of antimuscarinic doses and schedules may be of benefit for a woman's symptomatology (Table 22-3).

Contraindications

Table 22-4 presents a summary of contraindications to antimuscarinic drugs and precautions for their use. Contraindications and precautions for using these drugs relate in part to their metabolism and excretion. Individuals with underlying hepatic or renal disease should start therapy with the lowest potentially effective dose. In addition, the effect of antimuscarinic agents on neurotransmission to smooth muscle at other sites in the body can be a concern. Because related smooth muscle is present in the brain, orbit of the eye, heart, gastrointestinal tract, and urinary bladder; pathologies in

Table 22-3 Variations in Patterns of Antimuscarinic Use That May Improve Symptom Control Among Individual Women*

Symptom/Problem	Suggestions
Urinary incontinence is only a problem occasionally (e.g., at social gatherings or during travel).	Immediate-release agents generally work within 1 hour and may be timed for intermittent effect.
Difficulty remembering a daily medication, or prefers not to take pills/capsules/tablets.	Extended-release or transdermal agents may be easier to use.
Side effects like dry mouth are intolerable.	Extended-release and transdermal agents result in lower rates of dry mouth. Gum, sugarless candy, or sips of water can be used, but increased fluid intake to > 64 oz per day may exacerbate symptoms. Side effect profiles vary between individuals, and trial of a different agent may eliminate the symptom. Low-dose combinations of drugs may be better tolerated than a single agent at a high dose.
Nocturia is the primary problem.	Time medication use to address the symptom profile; try immediate-release agents at bedtime and extended-release formulas 2 to 4 h prior to bedtime.
Expense of medications is prohibitive.	Immediate-release agents tend to be less expensive; oxybutynin extended-release is available in generic form; pharmaceutical companies may offer programs to provide medications to the indigent.
Treatment helps somewhat, but symptoms persist.	A trial of an additional low-dose antimuscarinic may augment symptom control without exacerbating side effects.

* Recommendations based on clinical observations.

Table 22-4 General Contraindications and Precautions for Use of Antimuscarinic Agents

Contraindications	Clinical Considerations
Hypersensitivity to the agent.	Avoid use.
Narrow-angle glaucoma, uncontrolled.	Avoid use until problem is controlled; consult eye specialist prior to starting agent.
Gastric retention (gastroparesis).	Avoid use until problem is resolved.
Precautions	**Clinical Considerations**
Urinary retention.	May be used cautiously as part of a treatment plan in some cases.
Concomitant use of other anticholinergic drugs; especially in the elderly.	Use with caution.
Gastrointestinal disturbance (obstruction, atony, ulcerative colitis, severe constipation, ileostomy, colostomy).	Use with caution observing for decreasing function.
Esophageal disease (reflux, esophagitis, use of medications associated with esophageal irritation such as alendronate).	Discontinue if symptoms are exacerbated.
Hepatic or renal impairment.	Dose adjustment advised.
Myasthenia gravis.	Use with caution.
Extreme environmental heat.	Decreased sweating may lead to heat prostration in susceptible women.
Cardiac disease (arrhythmias, congestive heart failure, coronary heart disease, tachycardia, QT prolongation).	Use with caution.
Hypertension.	Monitor for increases in blood pressure.
Concurrent use of ketoconazole (Nizoral) or other potent CYP3A4 inhibitors.	Dose adjustment required.
Autonomic neuropathy.	Monitor symptoms.
Xerostomia or associated conditions (e.g., Sjögren's syndrome).	Encourage oral hygiene and monitor status.

these organs can be exacerbated by antimuscarinic use. In older adults with cognitive decline or confusion, the potential antimuscarinic side effects of dizziness and somnolence are special concerns, especially because of the potential cumulative effects related to polypharmacy.[10]

Choosing an Agent

Adherence to antimuscarinic treatments for overactive bladder has been shown to be low. In a study of 2496 California Medicaid recipients, 36.9% filled their prescription only once, and only 4% refilled at least 80% of their prescriptions over a 6-month period.[11] Although there is limited evidence to compare efficacy and tolerability of various antimuscarinic preparations, the few comparative studies that have been completed suggest extended-release and transdermal formulas result in lower rates of the most common side effect, dry mouth.[12,13] Reduction of potentially bothersome side effects may be a factor in the increased adherence found with extended-release formulas.[11] When extended-release tolterodine (Detrol) and oxybutynin (Ditropan) were compared, there was no difference in perceived improvement, leakage episodes, voids per 24 hours, or discontinuation rates, although dry mouth appeared to be more common with oxybutynin.[12] Lower doses offer similar positive effects and fewer side effects. Currently there is insufficient evidence to compare quality of life, costs, or long-term outcome of any agents.[12] Placebo-controlled trials of these drugs have been conducted; however, no research studies exist that have compared the newer agents, darifenacin (Enablex), solifenacin (Vesicare), and trospium (Sanctura), to each other. The cost to the individual may be one of the most important considerations when choosing an initial pharmacologic agent.

Side Effect Profile of Antimuscarinic Agents

All the muscarinic receptors (M1–M5) appear in smooth muscle in end-organs throughout the body. Symptoms resulting from this distribution may contribute to the adverse effects reported by approximately one third of individuals who use antimuscarinic agents.[7] The M3 receptors that predominate in the bladder are found to some extent in the exocrine glands, ocular orbits, heart, brain, and digestive tract. The most common side effects from blockade of the M3 receptor are headache, blurred vision, dry mouth, and constipation. Because of the wide distribution of receptors, even the most M3-specific antimuscarinic agents have general side effects, which also include dental caries; other gastrointestinal symptoms such as

reflux and nausea; tachycardia; sleep disturbances; confusion; and urinary retention.[10] Women taking antimuscarinic agents and living in hot climates can suffer from heatstroke if sweating is impaired. Transdermal agents may produce skin reactions and irritation.

Reasons for Treatment Failure

Pharmacologic treatment can fail for a variety of reasons.[14] First, from the individual's perspective and improved objective measures, decreased urine loss per leak or increased bladder capacity may not equate to a subjective feeling of improvement. In addition, missed diagnosis or omission of behavioral strategies can be factors. Pharmacologic explanations include inadequate dosing, inability to tolerate effective dosing due to side effects, or unusual resistance to the medication due to pharmacogenetics. Some women have symptoms that are unresponsive to antimuscarinic agents because they have atypical bladder contractions not mediated by M3 receptors, or contractions that originate in the smooth muscle itself. All of these factors are the subjects of ongoing research.[14]

Health Education

Overactive bladder can be a chronic condition. Treatment is not associated with immediate improvement but may instead take several weeks. Complete success with medication alone is unlikely, and improvement may be maintained more effectively in the context of behavioral change. Recurrence is common, making return appointments necessary. In addition, the duration of use of antimuscarinic treatment may vary. Some women, using behavioral management strategies, may be able to discontinue antimuscarinic agents after a few months of use. Others may choose to remain on medication long term. However, long-term use of antimuscarinic agents has not been well studied.[7] Unsatisfactory results with pharmacologic treatment should not be ignored. Referral to a specialist may offer additional treatment options.

Other Pharmacologic Treatment Options

Other medications are used to treat lower urinary tract symptoms, but their lack of specificity and consequent increased side effect profile result in less common use.[15] Some of these medications have FDA approval for other indications, and their use to treat overactive bladder symptoms is an off-label approach. Common medications in this category are presented in Table 22-5.

Table 22-5 Examples of Pharmacologic Agents Used Off-Label to Treat Urgency, Frequency, and Related Symptoms*

Drug Generic (Brand)	Mechanism of Action	Approved Indication	Dose	Clinical Considerations
Desmopressin/ synthetic vasopressin (DDAVP)	Antidiuretic; decreases urine production for 6 h.	Diabetes insipidus; primary nocturnal enuresis	20–40 mcg at bedtime intranasal spray. PO: 0.2–0.6 mg at bedtime.	Benefits may not outweigh risks, especially among older adults. Side effects: flushing, nausea, headache. Hypertension/hypotension, palpitations, tachyarrhythmia, hyponatremia, water intoxication syndrome, thrombotic disorder, anaphylaxis, seizures.
Dicyclomine (Bentyl)	Antispasmodic, anticholinergic	Irritable bowel syndrome	20 mg PO four times daily, up to 40 mg four times daily.	Side effect profile similar to antimuscarinic agents.
Hyoscyamine (Levsin)	Nonselective antimuscarinic	Hypermotility of the urinary tract, bladder spasm; biliary and renal colic	Extended release, 0.375–0.75 mg PO twice daily.	Side effect profile similar to other antimuscarinic agents. Also used for irritable bowel syndrome.
Imipramine (Tofranil)	Anticholinergic, antihistaminic, local anesthetic. Increases urethral resistance by blocking noradrenaline reuptake.	Tricyclic antidepressant	25 mg PO daily to three times daily.	Narrow safety profile; high risk in elderly related to dizziness, orthostatic hypotension, tremor, fatigue.
Propiverine hydrochloride (Detrunorm)	Calcium channel blocker and antimuscarinic, antispasmolytic	No FDA-approved indication	15 mg twice daily to four times daily.	Used in Europe. Side effect profile similar to other antimuscarinic agents.

* Some of these medications have US Food and Drug Administration approval for indications other than lower urinary tract symptoms.
Source: Kleeman SD et al. 2007.[15]

Estrogen Therapy

The role of estrogen in the treatment of lower urinary tract symptoms is controversial. Oral conjugated equine estrogen (Premarin) alone or with medroxyprogesterone acetate (Provera) appears to have no role in the treatment of urinary incontinence and has been found to increase incontinence in some women.[16] However, assessment of the role of vaginally inserted estrogen is ongoing. Lower urinary tract symptoms that are associated with genital atrophy are an FDA-approved indication for postmenopausal use of vaginal estrogen. Recent Cochrane reviews have concluded that topical estrogen is a safe and effective treatment for symptoms of genital atrophy.[17] Estrogen alone appears to improve symptoms of urge and stress incontinence (RR = 1.61; 95% CI, 1.04–2.49), but estrogen plus progestin therapy increased the risk of urge and stress incontinence (RR = 0.85; 95% CI, 0.76–0.95).[18] Urinary urgency, frequency, and nocturia without incontinence were not found to be significantly altered by use of vaginal estrogen in these studies.

If a trial of vaginal estrogen for genital atrophy is desired, three modes of topical estrogen replacement are available—vaginal creams, rings, and tablets. Endometrial stimulation and breast tenderness are more common with use of estrogen cream.[17,18] No studies of use longer than 1 year have been identified. In addition, a recommendation regarding concomitant progesterone use has not been rendered due to limited evidence. The North American Menopause Society, in a separate review, concluded that cyclic progesterone and routine endometrial biopsy are not necessary during use of low-dose vaginal estrogen because there is a minimal risk of endometrial hyperplasia.[19] However, women with a history of estrogen-sensitive breast cancer were cautioned to include their oncologist in their decision making about use of vaginal estrogen.

Intravesical Installation

Severe overactive bladder also is treated by direct installation of medication into the bladder via urinary catheter.[20] Intravesical installation usually takes place in a specialty-care setting. Oxybutynin (Ditropan) is used in intravesical installation to block acetylcholine in motor nerve pathways. Sensory nerves and pain perception are targeted by installation of local anesthetics and vanilloid receptor agonists (capsaicin and resiniferatoxin). The latter are plant derivatives that have a high-potency analgesic effect on the sensory neurons in the bladder.

Botulism Toxin (Botox)

Injection with botulinum toxin (Botox), which also blocks motor nerve pathways, is another promising modality currently in clinical trials.[20] This agent inhibits acetylcholine release, which causes selective, reversible muscle weakness lasting up to several months. Injection is performed transurethrally or transperitoneally. Ongoing randomized trials are being conducted to identify standard treatment and clarify expected outcomes.

Nonpharmacologic Treatments for Overactive Bladder

Nerve Stimulation

Nerve stimulation, including intravaginal, intrarectal, or perianal functional electrical stimulation (FES), and surgically implanted sacral nerve stimulation may improve symptoms of overactive bladder.[21,22]

One sacral nerve stimulation device (Interstim by Medtronic, Minneapolis, Minnesota) has received FDA approval and is marketed as a treatment for refractory overactive bladder-related symptoms. The exact mechanism behind its effectiveness is unclear, but the device has been found to significantly decrease symptoms and voiding abnormalities for up to 5 years in severely affected women.[23,24]

Complementary Therapies

Acupuncture

Acupuncture holds a theoretical place in treatment of overactive bladder-related symptoms, perhaps through decrease of symptom perception via increased endorphin levels and through neuromodulation.[25] Study of acupuncture is complicated by the difficulty in ascertaining placebo effect. One literature review concluded that efficacy of acupuncture for overactive bladder is not well established, and cost and access may be a deterrent for some women.[25] However, the low associated risk and relative speed of efficacy (when it appears to be effective, relief has typically been reported within 6 weeks), makes acupuncture a reasonable option for some women. Further research is under way in several countries.

Meditation/Mind–Body Medicine

The theoretical relationship between emotional stress and imbalances in autonomic neurotransmitter action supports recommendations of structured calming and relaxation as part of a behavioral approach to overactive bladder symptoms.[26,27] While there is little research to support meditation as a treatment, risk of relaxation techniques is low.

Herbs and Botanicals

Herbs also are understudied as a treatment for overactive bladder symptoms, making safety a concern. The German Commission E Monographs suggest that Scopolia rhizome (Scopolia root) has anticholinergic effects and likely affects the M3 receptor, because it contains hyoscyamine and scopolamine.[28] Because research evaluating efficacy, dosing, and safety is limited, general contraindications to anticholinergics should be applied.

▌ Stress Incontinence

There are several different types of incontinence. **Overflow incontinence** is the inability to empty the bladder, ultimately resulting in incontinence; **functional incontinence** is a general term designating the inability to get to a bathroom when the urge is present; and **mixed urinary incontinence** is the term used when both stress urinary incontinence and urge incontinence are present. The inability to store urine during physical activity, referred to as **stress urinary incontinence** (SUI), affects quality of life and can be a major barrier to health-promoting exercise for many women.[29] SUI is seen in nulliparous women, but prevalence appears to increase with parity, after both surgical and vaginal birth (n = 15,307; 10.1%, 15.9%, and 21.0% respectively)[30] (Box 22-2).

Pathophysiology

Urine storage is primarily controlled by the sympathetic nervous system. Stimulation of beta-adrenergic receptors that predominate in the detrusor results in relaxation, while simultaneous stimulation of alpha-adrenergic receptors in the urethra and bladder neck results in contraction and closure. Urethral closure is further enhanced by connective tissue support of the bladder neck, reflexive and voluntary contraction of skeletal muscles, and the mucovascular seal of the urethral lumen.[31]

Stress urinary incontinence (SUI) results whenever bladder pressure exceeds urethral closure pressure. Even normal urethral resistance can be overcome by extreme bladder pressure, which can occur with obesity, paroxysmal cough, strenuous activity, pregnancy, or an overly full

▌Box 22-2 A Case of Residual Urine

GB is 75 years old. Over the past 2 years she has been experiencing gradually increasing problems with urination, including urgency, frequency, nocturia, dribbling, lower abdominal discomfort, and small volume voids. Sometimes she feels like she has to urinate but is unable to do so. Other times she loses urine on the way to the bathroom. She loses urine both with urgency and with physical exertion. She often has to strain to get urine out and then feels her bladder is not really empty. She has no bowel or pelvic pain complaints, or recent urinary tract infections.

GB underwent hysterectomy at age 47 for dysfunctional uterine bleeding and fibroids. Her current medications include trazodone (Desyrel) for sleep, fentanyl transdermal patches for osteoporotic back pain, and over-the-counter diphenhydramine hydrochloride (Benadryl), which she uses for seasonal allergies.

During her examination, her postvoid residual is found to be elevated at 300 cc, but her urine sample is negative on office dipstick for blood, protein, nitrites, and leukocytes. She has atrophic genital changes, a normal-appearing urethra, and a cystocele, or anterior vaginal wall prolapse, advancing to 1 cm past her introitus in the standing position while bearing down.

Primary Care Treatment

Because GB has multiple discomforts and may have had an increased residual for several years, her provider confirms there is no kidney damage by ordering a blood test to measure urea, nitrogen, and creatinine, and she orders a renal ultrasound. A urine clean-catch dipstick for protein, blood, nitrites, and leukocytes is negative. GB does not have kidney damage or a urinary tract infection; therefore, the decision to treat her prolapse and retention are based on her symptom bother. She is currently taking several medications that can cause urinary retention (Table 22-1). These medications can be modified to help improve the contractile ability of her bladder, specifically diphenhydramine hydrochloride (Benadryl) and trazodone (Desyrel). Then she may choose to self-catheterize regularly. For example, she may self-catheterize in the morning after her first void and again at bedtime to see if intermittent complete emptying will reduce her urgency and frequency symptoms. Another primary care option is a trial of a vaginal pessary. If her bladder can be supported in an anatomic position, it may be able to function acceptably. If these approaches are not successful, she should be referred to a specialist to evaluate and treat her voiding problems. Oral medication is not indicated to treat her retention as it is due to urethral obstruction due to vaginal prolapse.

bladder. However, urethral resistance is usually sufficient to maintain continence, unless one or both of two changes occur. The first involves change in the urethra itself, including loss of elasticity and/or thinning and nonadherence of the mucovascular lining, which can result in a urethra that is structurally difficult to close. This is referred to as an **incompetent urethral closure mechanism** or intrinsic sphincter deficiency.[1] These urethral changes can occur for a variety of reasons, including surgery, radiation, childbirth, and age-related atrophy.[31] Urethral resistance can also be undermined by weakened connective tissue and/or muscle support that becomes unable to adequately stabilize and press the urethra closed. Several nonpharmacologic treatments may improve or cure SUI, including pelvic floor muscle strengthening and coordination exercises,[32] vaginal pessaries,[33] and surgical treatments,[31] and often are used in conjunction with pharmacologic interventions.

▌Pharmacologic Interventions for Stress Urinary Incontinence

Theoretically, several categories of medications can play a role in the treatment of SUI also, either by directly or indirectly enhancing closure resistance of the urethra and bladder neck or by decreasing bladder contractility. However, no oral medications have currently achieved FDA approval for SUI treatment. In part, this is due to concerns that include lack of specificity, conflicting efficacy data, or unsatisfactory risk profiles and side effects.[31] Further development and refinement eventually may increase pharmacologic specificity and effectiveness. Examples of medications that have been investigated for treatment of SUI are summarized in Table 22-6.

Table 22-6 Comparison of Pharmacologic Agents Used to Treat Mild Stress Urinary Incontinence

Class	Drug Generic (Brand)	Approved Indication	Risk/Side Effects
Alpha-adrenergic agonists*	Pseudoephedrine (Sudafed)	Decongestant	Hypertension, anxiety, cardiac arrhythmias, palpitations, tremor, weakness, insomnia, headache.
Serotonin and norepinephrine reuptake inhibitors*	Duloxetine (Cymbalta)	Antidepressant; pain of diabetic neuropathy	Increased suicide risk, nausea, fatigue, insomnia. Liver damage in susceptible women.
Tricyclic antidepressants*	Imipramine (Tofranil), Sinequan (Doxepin)	Depression	Dry mouth, blurred vision, urinary retention, constipation, orthostatic hypotension, sedation, fatigue, disorientation, cardiac arrhythmias, and decreased stroke volume.

* None of these medications currently has US FDA approval as a treatment for stress urinary incontinence, due in part to their lack of specificity and side effect or risk profiles.
Sources: Nygaard IE et al. 2004[31]; Rovner ES et al. 2004.[34]

Adrenergic Agonists

Both alpha- and beta-adrenergic agonists have a potential role in SUI treatment. The treatment effect of alpha-adrenergic agents clearly occurs because they stimulate contraction of the alpha receptors that predominate in the urethra and bladder neck. However, because beta-adrenergic receptors predominate in the detrusor itself, the apparent effect of beta-adrenergic agonists is paradoxical and not completely understood.[34]

A Cochrane systematic review reported increased efficacy of a variety of adrenergic agonists when compared to placebo, including phenylpropanolamine (Dexatrim), midodrine (ProAmatine), norepinephrine, clenbuterol, and terbutaline (Brethine).[35] However, in these studies, doses varied and improvement was modest and statistically significant only for midodrine and clenbuterol (RR = 1.55; 95% CI, 1.02–2.35 and RR = 1.96; 95% CI, 1.26–3.05, respectively). Though these adrenergic agents affect receptors outside the bladder and urethra, only 4% of women stopped treatment due to side effects (e.g., insomnia and restlessness).

Phenylpropanolamine (Dexatrim), included in the Cochrane report, has been marketed in the United States as an appetite suppressant but was withdrawn from the market in 2000 due to an increased risk of hemorrhagic stroke, especially among women. Midodrine (ProAmatine) has received an FDA black box warning related to increased risk of severe supine hypertension.[10] Other side effects of adrenergic agonists can include anxiety, insomnia, headache, tremor, weakness, palpitations, and respiratory difficulties.[34] Ephedrine and pseudoephedrine (Sudafed) are over-the-counter alpha agonists that have improved SUI symptoms anecdotally, but placebo controlled trials are lacking[34] and animal trials suggest symptom improvement is minimal.[36]

Serotonin and Norepinephrine Agonists

Serotonin and norepinephrine agonists promote continence by suppressing activity of parasympathetic receptors and enhancing both sympathetic and somatic activity.[37] A systematic review of SUI treatment with the serotonin and norepinephrine agonist duloxetine (Cymbalta) reported overall subjective cure rates over 3–36 weeks of follow-up favoring duloxetine (10.8% vs. 7.7%; RR = 1.42; 95% CI, 1.02–1.98; P = .04).[38] Side effects, predominantly nausea, were common (71% vs. 59% in placebo groups), but only resulted in one in eight stopping duloxetine treatment (17% vs. 4%). Although duloxetine (Cymbalta) has FDA approval for treatment of depression and diabetic neuropathy, application for the indication of SUI treatment was withdrawn in 2005 due to concerns about increased risk of suicide.[39] However, further study of this class of medication may change the risk-to-benefit analysis.

Tricyclic Antidepressants

Imipramine hydrochloride (Tofranil) is a tricyclic antidepressant used to promote urine storage because it both decreases bladder contractility and increases outlet resistance.[34] Although its precise mechanism of action is unknown, it appears to act by blocking norepinephrine and serotonin reuptake, affecting central and peripheral anticholinergic receptors, and producing a sedative effect presumably through antihistaminic properties at the level of the central nervous system.[10,34] FDA-approved indications are limited to treatment of depression in adults and **nocturnal enuresis** in children. However, in uncontrolled, observational studies, improvement has been reported in general continence, maximum urethral closure pressure, and quantity of urine lost.[34] While the antidepressant dose for adult outpatients ranges from 75 mg to 200 mg per day, the suggested dose for urinary incontinence (UI) in adults is 10–25 mg for up to three times a day.

The medication should be used with caution at the lowest possible effective dose when treating elderly persons and those with liver disorders. As with all antidepressants, imipramine (Tofranil) carries a black box warning regarding the potential for increased suicidality and the same general contraindications found with other anticholinergic prescriptions (Table 22-4). Serious potential side effects include cardiovascular effects such as arrhythmias, heart block, hypertension, orthostatic hypotension, palpitations, and syncope. (More information about these agents can be found in Chapter 25.) Use in pregnancy has not been evaluated. Related tricyclic medications, such as amitriptyline (Elavil), desipramine (Norpramin), doxepin (Sinequan), and nortriptyline (Pamelor, Aventyl) may have similar effects on urinary symptoms. Level I evidence of the effectiveness of tricyclic antidepressant agents in the treatment of SUI is needed.

Estrogen Therapy

Estrogen has a theoretical role in improving SUI. Because estrogen receptors are present throughout the urogenital system, estrogen therapy may increase alpha-adrenergic sensitivity in the urethral smooth muscle and the vascularity needed for coaptation of the urethral mucosa.[34] However, SUI symptoms appear to increase, not decrease, when oral estrogen is used, regardless of whether progesterone is added.[16] This phenomenon may be related to increases in the elasticity of estrogenized tissue, which in turn results in decreased urethral support. In addition to the Cochrane review that suggested an increase in stress incontinence,[18] other authors state that estrogen has no role in the treatment of the isolated complaint of SUI among postmenopausal women.[31] Future research may identify a role for estrogen in enhancing the effectiveness in dual therapies (e.g., use in tandem with alpha-adrenergic agents), but at this time, there is no evidence recommending use of estrogen either for SUI prevention or treatment.[34]

Injectable Bulking Agents

Bulking agents injected into the area around the proximal urethra are used by specialists to increase resistance and closure at the bladder neck.[40] The procedure is temporary and is repeated intermittently. Among the agents used are bovine and porcine collagen, synthetic polymers, cartilage or bone extracts, silicone, and zirconium beads. Autologous tissue injections have a potential future role.[41]

Health Education

Adherence to pelvic floor muscle strengthening and coordination exercises remains a cornerstone of SUI therapy for women who retain voluntary control of their skeletal muscles.[32] However, pelvic exercise tends to be most effective for decreasing symptoms in women who have initial weak muscle strength.[42]

Urinary Retention

Pathophysiology

In a healthy adult, a normally functioning bladder typically retains no more than 50 cc of urine after urination.[3] Emptying occurs under parasympathetic influence when acetylcholine stimulates smooth muscle contraction of the bladder dome, and norepinephrine is inhibited at both the beta receptors in the bladder dome and the alpha receptors in the bladder neck and urethra. As aging occurs, bladder coordination and contractility frequently decreases, and residual volumes up to 200 cc can be found among asymptomatic elderly individuals. Acute retention is typically managed by mechanical emptying of the bladder with a catheter, and/or removal of the obstruction. An indwelling catheter may be used temporarily to provide bladder rest and reassert contractility.

Chronic retention can also result from obstruction or from either a hyperactive or hypoactive bladder.[43] Although women with acute retention are usually uncomfortably aware of the problem, chronic retention may be asymptomatic. Hyperactivity can result from any insult to the mechanisms that inhibit bladder contraction, such as cortical lesions resulting from stroke, tumors, trauma, aging, or the neurologic deterioration seen with multiple sclerosis. On the other hand, a hypoactive or flaccid bladder can result from spinal cord injuries or lesions, or degeneration of the brain stem and subsequent sensory loss (lack of an awareness of bladder filling) and inability to initiate voiding. Peripheral nerve damage (e.g., from progressive diabetes, injury, or surgery) can also cause either sensory loss or motor nerve injury. Ultimately, chronic retention can cause upper urinary tract damage. Awareness of the complexity of evaluation and treatment planning for women with chronic retention underscores the importance of referral or consultation with a specialist.

Treatment of Chronic Retention

The mainstay of treatment for chronic retention continues to be clean intermittent self-catheterization.[3] For women who are unable to self-catheterize, an indwelling suprapubic catheter may be an appropriate treatment. Long-term indwelling urethral catheters are occasionally used as a last resort secondary to the risk of infection. Sacral nerve modulation has also been effective in selected cases.[23]

Pharmacologic Treatment of Urinary Retention

Bethanechol chloride (Urecholine), a selective cholinergic that predominantly stimulates the bladder and bowel, has been used as a treatment for chronic retention.[3] However, bethanechol often stimulates discoordinated contraction of the bladder, bladder neck, and urethra simultaneously, which decreases its clinical application. Side effects are infrequent but can include bronchial stenosis; bradycardia and orthostatic hypotension with syncope; increased sweating, salivation, and gastric acid secretion; and diarrhea and stomach cramps.

Pharmacologic agents with increased specificity and efficacy may be identified in the future. For example, although empirical evidence is lacking, there are theoretical roles for monotherapy or combined use with prostaglandins to enhance smooth muscle contraction in the bladder, as well as with cholinesterase agents, dopamine receptor antagonists (e.g., metoclopramide [Reglan]), and alpha-adrenergic antagonists to relax outlet resistance.[3] Botulinum toxin (Botox), because of its ability to block smooth and skeletal muscle contractility, has been injected transurethrally and transperineally to inhibit outlet obstruction that results from discoordinated voiding due to multiple sclerosis or spinal cord injury.[44] Research to identify optimum regimens is ongoing.

Complementary Therapies

Caffeine, provided as a cup of hot tea or coffee within 30–60 minutes of the attempt to void, has been used as a bladder stimulant in cases of urinary retention.[43] Several herbal therapies are also described in the German Commission E Monographs as treatments for urine retention, but they predominantly function as diuretics and have no direct affect on bladder function.[28] Suggested herbs include *Phaseoli fructus sine semine* (kidney bean pods without seeds),

Levistici radix (lovage root), and *Orthosiphonis folium* (java tea). *Urticae herba/folium* (stinging nettle herb and leaf) works as a diuretic and is also said to act as a weak antispasmodic in women with nephrolithiasis. *Petroselini herba/radix* (parsley herb and root) also has a reported diuretic effect, but is specifically contraindicated in pregnancy, suggesting the need for caution when using any diuretic herb in pregnancy. Because the doses in marketed formulations differ widely, it has been difficult to conduct studies with standard doses. Therefore, clinical use of these herbs and botanicals is limited to date.

Urinary Tract Infection

Adherent microorganisms in any part of the urinary tract, including the urethra, bladder, and kidneys, can result in urinary tract infection (UTI). In primary care settings, UTIs are both common and costly. A woman's lifetime risk of UTI is estimated to be 60.4% (95% CI, 55.1–65.8).[45] Treatment of UTIs accounts for over 6 million primary care visits, with overall treatment costs exceeding $2.4 billion, and outpatient prescription costs exceeding $218 million in the United States annually. The high UTI incidence in women, and the tendency for recurrence in some women, is most likely related to a combination of anatomy, genetic factors, hormonal effects, and behavioral patterns[46] (Box 22-3).

Pathophysiology of Urinary Tract Infections

The most common infective agents in the urinary tract include gram-negative bacilli, such as *Escherichia coli, Klebsiella, Enterobacter, Serratia, Proteus,* and *Pseudomonas.*[47] *Staphylococcus,* including *saprophyticus, epidermidis,* and *aureus,* are important, but less common pathologic organisms in the bladder. The gram-positive organisms *Streptococcus agalactiae* and *Enterococcus faecalis* are also found as urinary pathogens. For infection to occur, virulent strains of colonizing bacteria must adhere to the bladder wall. Asymptomatic bacterial colonization is common in adults, and treatment for asymptomatic bacterial colonization is not indicated in nonpregnant women.[47] Fungal and viral infections of the bladder are uncommon, but occasionally found among immunocompromised women. Infection ascending to the kidneys, pyelonephritis, usually manifests as sudden or gradual onset of systemic symptoms, including fever, chills, malaise, nausea, and vomiting, with or without dysuria.

Box 22-3 A Case of Acute Dysuria

BL is a 24-year-old with acute onset of dysuria, urgency, and frequency without urine loss. The pain began 2 days ago and is most intense when she begins voiding and for a few seconds postvoiding. She has tried increasing fluids and drinking cranberry juice with no relief. She denies fever, back pain, or gastrointestinal symptoms, as well as any history of UTIs. She is worried something is seriously wrong, because today she has noticed hematuria. She has a new sexual partner, and she is concerned about sexually transmitted infections. She had a normal menses about 3 weeks before and uses combined oral contraceptives regularly.

On physical examination, BL is afebrile, in no acute distress, and has no abdominal or flank tenderness. Her pelvic exam is normal, except for mild suprapubic tenderness. Gonorrhea and chlamydia tests are obtained. A urine dipstick is positive for nitrites, leukocytes, and red blood cells, and a urine pregnancy test is negative.

Primary Care Treatment

The presumptive diagnosis for BL is uncomplicated acute cystitis. Because she has no drug allergies, BL is a good candidate for any of a variety of anti-infectives. Based on cost and regional use, she is prescribed a 3-day course of trimethoprim-sulfamethoxazole (Bactrim, Septra) double-strength 160/800 mg twice a day; she is also prescribed a urinary analgesic three times a day for the first day, such as phenazopyridine (Pyridium), and is asked to increase fluid intake to avoid symptomatic irritation due to concentrated urine. A urine culture and sensitivity at the initial assessment are not necessary. Instead, treatment is empirical and BL should be instructed to take all six antibiotic doses as directed and call if her symptoms are not resolved after 48 hours. At that time, a culture could be obtained. BL is encouraged to prevent sexually transmitted infections (STIs) by using condoms until she is in a committed, long-term monogamous relationship, and is offered other appropriate STI testing.

Pharmacologic Treatment of Urinary Tract Infections

UTIs are classified as uncomplicated or complicated to aid planning the choice of agent, length of treatment, and need for hospitalization.[48] Complicating factors include evidence of pyelonephritis, recurrence, diabetes mellitus, immunocompromise, pregnancy, urinary tract obstruction (e.g., strictures, neurogenic bladder), use of an indwelling catheter, advanced age with significant comorbidity, and the presence of unusual or resistant pathogens.[48] Urine culture and longer dose therapy (7–14 days) are typically reserved for women with complicated cases and treatment failures. Although empirical treatment without culture in uncomplicated cystitis is recommended, a disadvantage of this strategy is increased difficulty in confirming a diagnosis and tracking antibacterial resistance patterns.

Figure 22-3 presents a treatment algorithm compiled from current literature. Decision to treat is based on clinical expertise. While traditional guidelines suggest antibiotic treatment be reserved for women with bacterial colony counts ≥ 100,000 colonies, many women with lower colony counts have symptomatic relief with treatment.[48] Improper handling of the specimen should be considered when colony counts are high in asymptomatic women.

Choosing an Antibacterial Agent

Because microbial resistance has increased dramatically due to overuse and misuse of antibiotics, appropriate prescription of antibacterial treatment of UTIs has become increasingly important.[49] While hospital antibiograms provide some data regarding regional antimicrobial resistance patterns, surveillance of women with uncomplicated cases of UTI is rarely performed and reports frequently overestimate actual resistance patterns found in ambulatory centers.[48] Antibiotic resistance is more likely to be found among women who have had recent or recurrent antibiotic exposures or hospitalizations or have diabetes mellitus. In addition, use of exogenous estrogen either in oral contraceptives or as estrogen replacement may increase the risk of drug resistance, although the mechanism for this is not known.[48]

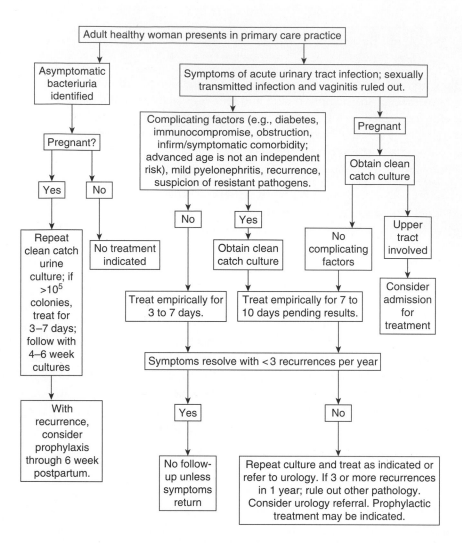

Figure 22-3 Algorithm for treatment of urinary tract infection. *Sources:* Adapted from Warren JW et al. 1999[50]; Scottish Intercollegiate Guidelines Network.[51]

When determining which antibacterial agent to use, clinicians should consider the likelihood of resistance, the site of infection (e.g., pyelonephritis or cystitis), timing (e.g., intermittent acute, postcoital, or recurrent), and severity of infection (e.g., uncomplicated vs. complicated). An optimal initial antibiotic choice should be inexpensive, have broad-spectrum coverage, and be predominately concentrated and excreted in urine. Table 22-7 reviews common antibiotic agents that meet the criteria for treatment of UTIs. Evidence-based protocols suggest that nonallergic women living in low-resistance locales with uncomplicated UTIs should be started initially on a 3-day regimen of a combination of trimethoprim and sulfamethoxazole, which is commonly termed TMP-SMX (Bactrim, Septra).[50,51] Sulfas generally are well tolerated, although there is a rare risk of Stevens-Johnson syndrome

(Chapter 11). Fluoroquinolones are recommended as the initial agent in regions where resistance to TMP-SMX has reached or surpassed 20% and among women allergic to sulfa.[48] Fluoroquinolones cost up to six times the cost of TMP-SMX. Current trends toward widespread use of fluoroquinolones is not evidence based and is likely driven by marketing efforts.[46]

A suggested algorithm for UTI treatment is presented in Figure 22-3. For uncomplicated UTIs, short-course oral treatment with confirmation of cure via resolution of clinical symptoms is appropriate.[50] Lack of resolution of symptoms requires consideration of resistant infection, structural or functional abnormalities, or sexually transmitted infections. Recurrent UTI management may be guided by culture verification prior to and after treatment.

Table 22-7 Antimicrobials Commonly Used to Treat Urinary Tract Infections*

Drug Generic (Brand)	Best Coverage of Common Microbes	Dose for Acute Episode	Prophylactic or Continuous Dose	Clinical Considerations
Trimethoprim-sulfamethoxazole (Bactrim, Septra)	*Escherichia coli, Klebsiella, Proteus, Enterobacter*	Single strength: 80 mg/400 mg PO take two bid. Double-strength: 160/800 mg one PO bid, or oral suspension: (5 mL = 40 mg/200 mg) PO bid for 3–14 days; always check label, as sometimes special suspensions compounded.	80/400 mg.	First-choice agent if resistance in area is < 20%. Allergic reactions are common; serious skin reactions and blood dyscrasias may occur. Oral suspension available.
Ciprofloxacin (Cipro)†	Broad spectrum except for anaerobes	Immediate release: 250–500 mg PO bid for 3–14 days.	125 mg PO. Extended release (XR): 500–1000 mg daily for 3–14 days.	Avoid in pregnancy and in women with epilepsy due to seizure risk. Tendon damage/rupture have been reported; elderly and steroid users at higher risk. Side effects can include nausea, vomiting, diarrhea, hypoglycemia, abdominal pain, headache, rash, arrhythmias, angina, convulsions, gastrointestinal bleeding, nephritis, joint damage. Immediate- and extended-release formulas offer similar cure rates; cost and adherence concerns can guide treatment.
Levofloxacin (Levaquin)†	Broad spectrum except for anaerobes	250 mg PO qd 3–14 days.		
Norfloxacin (Noroxin)†	*E coli, Klebsiella, Proteus, Enterobacter, Enterococcus, Staphylococcus, Serratia*	400 mg PO bid.	200 mg PO bid.	Norfloxacin not used for first-line treatment.
Amoxacillin (Amoxil), Ampicillin (Principen)	*E coli, Proteus, Enterococcus, Staphylococcus*	250–500 mg PO qid.		Beta-lactams may be less effective than other agents due to high rates of resistance. Risks include allergies, candidal overgrowth, and pseudomembranous colitis (more so with ampicillin).
Cephalexin (Keflex)	*E coli, Klebsiella, Proteus, Staphylococcus*	250–500 mg qid.	250 mg qd PO.	Not active against enterococci. Beta-lactams may be less effective than other agents. A second-generation cephalosporin may be more effective in complicated cases. Risks include allergies, hepatic dysfunction.

(continues)

Table 22-7　Antimicrobials Commonly Used to Treat Urinary Tract Infections* (continued)

Drug Generic (Brand)	Best Coverage of Common Microbes	Dose for Acute Episode	Prophylactic or Continuous Dose	Clinical Considerations
Nitrofurantoin (Macrodantin, Furadantin)	E coli	100 mg qid; macrocrystals, 100 mg PO bid.	50–100 mg PO qid.	Not active against Proteus, Pseudomonas. Resistance unlikely, but bactericidal in urine only; poor penetration into tissues. In uncomplicated UTI, a routine 7-day course is advisable. Do not use for pyelonephritis or complicated UTIs. Avoid using with alkalizing agents such as potassium citrate and in women with renal failure where dose reaching bladder will be ineffective. Side effects can include GI upset (> with macrocrystals), peripheral neuropathy, pneumonitis.
Tetracycline/doxycycline (Vibramycin, Doryx)	Gram-negative, and some gram-positive coverage; Enterococcus, Chlamydia, Mycoplasma hominis	Tetracycline: 250–500 mg every 6 hours. Doxycycline: 100 mg bid.		Less commonly used. Side effects include GI upset, skin rash, candidal overgrowth, hepatic dysfunction, nephrotoxicity. Avoid in women with renal failure and in pregnant women. Doxycycline is less likely to affect gut flora than other tetracyclines.
Fosfomycin (Monurol)	E coli, Enterococcus	Single 3-gram dose PO		Not reliable for Staphylococcus saprophyticus. Less frequently used in United States. Lower efficacy than 3 days of other agents, but resistance is rare in United States and may be option for women with multiple allergies.

* Suggested duration for uncomplicated acute cystitis (3-day course), complicated acute cystitis (7–14 day course), and uncomplicated pyelonephritis (10- to 14-day course). Most cases are associated with Escherichia coli and other gram-negative bacteria common in the gastrointestinal tract. Gram-positive bacteria, such as staphylococci, are less common. Microbial resistance varies between geographic areas.
† Ciprofloxacin is a second-generation and levofloxacin is a third-generation fluoroquinolone. Difference between generations primarily based on expanded antimicrobial activity. However, both generations of fluoroquinolones are becoming first-choice treatment where high sulfa resistance is encountered.
Sources: Miller LG et al. 2004[48]; Hooton TM et al. 2004.[49]

Complicated UTIs, including mild pyelonephritis, should be treated with 10- to 14-day regimens in women who tolerate oral medications, or, if intravenous antibiotics are needed, women with pyelonephritis may require hospitalization. If a fluoroquinolone is indicated for a non-pregnant woman, equal efficacy can be expected from all agents within the fluoroquinolone family.[52] However, ciprofloxacin (Cipro) and levofloxacin (Levaquin) appear to have the lowest potential for the associated side effects of photosensitivity, skin reactions, and insomnia.[52] Fluoroquinolones generally are avoided during pregnancy because of lack of information regarding safety, and these agents have been linked to neonatal toxicity for the breastfed infant. Referral is indicated for women who have frequent recurrence, persistent hematuria, severe pyelonephritis, evidence of kidney damage, or identification of underlying structural or functional abnormalities.

Duration of Treatment

Three-day treatment is adequate for women who have an uncomplicated UTI.[53] Higher failure rates have been demonstrated when treatment is limited to a single day. Longer regimens of 7–10 days demonstrate symptomatic cure rates similar to 3-day treatment, and, although bacteriologic cure rates are higher, increases in cost and side effects support short-course treatment. In postmenopausal women with uncomplicated UTIs, a 3-day treatment also appears to be adequate.[54]

Prevention of Recurrent Cystitis

Recurrent UTI is defined as three or more incidents of **acute cystitis** in a 12-month period. Once underlying pathology has been ruled out, there are three effective options for recurrence prevention. These include (1) self-treatment at the first sign of infection; (2) continuous, daily, low-dose therapy; and (3) postcoital therapy. In a study of healthy adult women symptomatically self-diagnosing early onset of recurrent cystitis (n = 172), infection was present in 84% of suspected cases, while an additional 11% had sterile pyuria.[55] Of the women who had confirmed infection, 92% resolved microscopically with a 3-day course of a fluoroquinolone. In women randomized to placebo or prophylactic antibiotics (continuous or postcoital), treated women had 0 to 0.9 recurrences per person per year compared to 0.8 to 3.6 for women using placebo (RR = 0.21; 95% CI, 0.13–0.34).[56] Potential side effects from treatment include vaginal and oral candidiasis and gastrointestinal symptoms.

There is little evidence comparing prophylactic agents.[57] Continuous antibiotic regimens are typically prescribed for 6–12 months, although infection may recur after discontinuation.[56] Postcoital treatments are generally taken within 2 hours after intercourse. Adverse effects have included gastrointestinal symptoms, rash, and monilial infections. Antimicrobial profiles are listed in Table 22-7.[57]

Other Pharmacologic Interventions for Urinary Tract Infections

Methenamine (Hiprex) acts as a urinary antiseptic and may have a role in preventing recurrent or chronic UTI.[51,58] The drug is converted to formaldehyde in the urine. This conversion occurs approximately 3 hours postingestion. Methenamine has been studied for prevention of recurrent UTI in continuous use up to 2 years, but study quality precludes certainty regarding its effectiveness.[58] It appears to be less effective than prophylactic treatment with nitrofurantoin (Macrodantin, Furadantin) or TMP-SMX (Bactrim or Septra) and is not effective in women with indwelling catheters. Side effects are infrequent, but include stomatitis, nausea, vomiting, and diarrhea with accompanying abdominal pain, exacerbation of preexisting liver disease, and dysuria due to crystalluria. The typical oral dose of methenamine hippurate (Hiprex) is 1 gram bid, and of methenamine mandelate (Uroqid Acid No. 2), 1 gram qid. These agents are available as tablets, granules, and liquid suspension. Tablets can be crushed for ease of ingestion. Methenamine is an FDA Pregnancy Category C drug, although specific related birth defects in humans and animals have not been identified.

Phenazopyridine (Pyridium, Uristat, Azo-Septic) acts as a urinary anesthetic and is available over the counter. The mechanism of action on the bladder mucosa is not known. The usual dose is 200 mg three times daily, taken with food, typically for the initial 2 days of antibiotic therapy. Because use of phenazopyridine can mask underlying serious disease, women should be clearly instructed to avoid using phenazopyridine as a single treatment or for extended periods of time (not to be used for more than 3 days).

Although the main indication for use of phenazopyridine is dysuria related to UTI, its side effect of turning urine bright red-orange also makes it useful as a marker for evaluation of urinary dysfunctions such as urinary incontinence or fistula. Other side effects are uncommon and mild and include headaches, vertigo, and gastrointestinal disturbances. The drug should not be used long term, to treat UTIs as a single agent, or by women with renal insufficiency. This agent is categorized as FDA Pregnancy Category B, although pregnant women with a UTI should seek medical help because of the increased risk of pyelonephritis. Nonpregnant women should be instructed to notify a provider if UTI-related dysuria persists after 2 days of treatment.

It is not clear whether treatment with estrogen plays a role in preventing recurrent UTI in postmenopausal women. One expert evidence review concluded there is no role.[51] A Cochrane review of vaginal estrogen use in UTI prevention was limited to only two randomized trials, making results questionable, although it did provide some suggestion that women using estrogen had fewer UTIs. While one study reported that postmenopausal women with a history of recurrent UTI were less likely to experience acute cystitis using a vaginal estrogen ring (Estring) versus a placebo (45% versus 20%, $P = .008$),[59] another found nitrofurantoin (Macrobid) suppression more efficacious than vaginal estrogen (48 UTIs versus 124 UTIs, $P = .0003$).[60] In the latter study (n = 171), the women using 0.5 mg estriol vaginal suppositories twice weekly did not demonstrate a change in vaginal pH or lactobacillus colonization, two hypothesized actions that were expected to inhibit pathogen colonization.

Complementary Therapies

Acupuncture

Limited evidence suggests there may be a role for acupuncture in prevention of recurrent UTI. In one study evaluating incidents of UTI and postvoid residuals, women with a history of recurrent UTI were assigned to receive either a variety of acupuncture treatments or no treatment over a period of 6 months (n = 98).[61] Women treated at acupuncture point kidney yang/qi xu demonstrated the lowest number of cystitis incidents ($P \leq .001$; incident relative rate 0.15; 95% CI, 0.05–0.42), and postvoid residuals (36.4 mL versus 12.9 mL; $P \leq .05$).

Cranberry Products

Cranberries and other berries in the genus *Vaccinium* contain proanthocyanidins, which prevent uropathogens from adhering to urinary epithelium in vitro.[48] Although there is insufficient evidence to suggest a role for treatment of acute infection, a Cochrane review concluded that two good quality trials support the use of either cranberry juice or capsules for preventing recurrent UTIs over a 12-month period (RR = 0.61; 95% CI, 0.40–0.91).[62] One of the trials used 7.5 g of cranberry concentrate in 50 mL of water daily, and the other used a 1:30 dilution of concentrate in 250 mL juice or in tablet form. Dropout rates were reportedly high. In some women with overactive bladder, cranberry-related product aggravates their symptoms. In addition, because of the potential unpredictable effect of the flavonoids in cranberry on warfarin (Coumadin) metabolism, women using warfarin as an anticoagulant are encouraged to avoid taking cranberry products in large amounts unless the health benefits outweigh risks.[50]

Other Nutritional and Botanic Supplements

Dietary changes may decrease UTI risk, but their effectiveness is understudied. At-risk women are encouraged to avoid known food allergens. Suggested dietary recommendations include increases in fresh juices, especially berry juice; fermented milk products with probiotics; onion and garlic, because of their potential antimicrobial activity; and vitamin C supplementation during acute infection (2000 mg every 2 hours for 2 days, then 2000 mg tid for 7 days) as means of acidifying the urine.[63] *Echinacea purpura herba* (purple cone flower) may have a role in supporting the immune system generally, although a specific role in UTI prevention has not been well studied. Other herbs with antimicrobial and/or diuretic properties that have been suggested for use during UTI treatment or prevention include *Hydrastis canadensis* (Golden seal), *Arctostaphylos uva-ursi* (bearberry), and *Zea mays* (corn silk). Although little research has been done to support these recommendations, risk of their use is likely to be low if active infection is also treated with prescription antibiotics.[63]

Health Education

The importance of completing the antibiotic prescription and of reporting symptoms that continue or escalate with treatment should be emphasized. Increased hydration may help remove uropathogens by encouraging bladder emptying, but overhydration also may lower levels of antibiotic in the urine.[48]

There is minimal evidence to support common recommendations for UTI prevention, including increasing fluid intake, urinating after intercourse, avoiding douching, and wiping from front to back after toileting. Evidence does support a preventive role for treatment of urine retention and genital atrophy, avoidance of indwelling catheter use, and limiting use of spermicides.[48]

Painful Bladder Syndrome and Interstitial Cystitis

In 2002, the International Continence Society defined **painful bladder syndrome** (PBS) as a complaint of suprapubic pain related to bladder filling, accompanied by other symptoms such as increased daytime and nighttime frequency, in the absence of proven urinary infection or other obvious pathology.[1] The most studied form of PBS is **interstitial cystitis** (IC). Because definitions are evolving, the incidence is difficult to determine. It is known that women experience IC/PBS more often than men, with a prevalence rate of 1.3/100,000, and an estimated outpatient visit cost of $37 million annually in the United States.[64] Although many women with IC/PBS have the symptoms described in the ICS definition, some also have retropubic pain and/or pain that does not change with voiding[50] (Box 22-4).

Pathophysiology

The pathophysiology behind the extreme, often life-changing bladder pain associated with IC/PBS is not well understood. Onset of symptoms may be related to an identifiable infection, injury, radiation, or atrophy, but often no trigger is apparent. Whatever the etiology, IC/PBS symptoms appear to occur because of disruption of the urothelium, the inner mucoid lining of the bladder. This lining acts as a barrier to bacterial and crystal adherence and prevents urinary solutes from penetrating the bladder wall.[65] The bladder lining, also called the glycosaminoglycan (GAG) or mucin layer, is predominantly composed of proteoglycans and glycoproteins.[65] In response to any injury, nerves within the detrusor appear to be susceptible to neuroplastic change.[3] Mature myelinated alpha sensory nerves, which are typical in the adult bladder, can again become the highly sensitive nonmyelinated C nerve fibers that predominate at birth. Increased permeability of the lining of the bladder appears to be one trigger to this type of change. Mast cells release characteristic granules and various hormonal mediators related to inflammation of the smooth muscle. Up-regulation of nerve growth factor, neuroplastic transformation, and chronic overstimulation of sensory nerves may play roles in perception of severe pain in the absence of obvious pathology that is typical of IC/PBS. Treatments continue to emerge as understanding of the pathophysiology evolves.

Box 22-4 A Case of Painful Bladder Syndrome

AW, a 46-year-old nullipara, reports having an isolated acute UTI 2 years ago that involved sudden onset of dysuria, urgency, frequency, and hematuria. She completed a 3-day course of antibiotics, and the hematuria resolved. Despite subsequent negative urine cultures, however, she continues to experience chronic pelvic pain with dysuria, dyspareunia, frequency, and severe nocturia. The symptoms lessen to some extent immediately after voiding and also seem to improve spontaneously for short periods of time, but they always recur. She has no other positive history, is not currently sexually active, and has no systemic symptoms. Her life now centers on the pain in her bladder area. She smokes 1 pack of cigarettes a day and drinks 5–6 glasses of wine per week. Her physical exam demonstrates tenderness only in the suprapubic region. Her neurologic exam and postvoid residual are normal. She has no anatomic abnormalities and her sexually transmitted infection testing, urinalysis, urine cytology, and culture are negative.

Treatment

At her age, bladder cancer is unlikely in the absence of hematuria. Her presumptive diagnosis is interstitial cystitis/painful bladder syndrome. She is told that her symptoms are likely to result from several related changes, including increased permeability of her bladder lining, increased sensitivity of the nerves in the walls of her bladder, and an overresponse of her immune system. These changes may have been triggered by her acute infection. However, antibiotics are not an appropriate treatment at this point. A combination of therapies is most likely to be effective.

AW starts with dietary changes to avoid acidic and high-potassium foods. She discontinues smoking and alcohol. She measures urine volumes for 24 hours and continues this occasionally, working to rebuild her bladder capacity. She tries relaxation techniques. She begins taking a trial of an antimuscarinic, antispasmodic agent, and an analgesic. If these changes are not successful in decreasing her symptoms, she will be referred for a possible cystoscopic evaluation and treatment. If a specialist starts her on a treatment plan for her painful bladder, she may choose to return to her primary care office for maintenance care.

Treatment of Interstitial Cystitis/Painful Bladder Syndrome

Nonpharmacologic Treatments

Successful management of this chronic condition requires a combination of approaches. Many of the treatments that are effective for overactive bladder symptoms also improve symptoms of IC/PBS. Suggestions for potential behavioral approaches are readily available from the Interstitial Cystitis Association. Surgical treatment options include sacral neuromodulation[23,66] or, for severe, intractable symptoms, urinary diversion and augmentation cystoplasty. A treatment specific to IC/PBS, hydrodistention, involves cystoscopically administered fluid used to stretch the bladder under anesthesia.

Pharmacologic Therapy of Interstitial Cystitis/Painful Bladder Syndrome

Several medications are used to treat IC/PBS, in combinations directed by symptom response. A universally successful treatment has not been identified. Current treatments focus on pain relief, decreasing the perception of urgency, controlling mast cell activity, and rebuilding the bladder lining using exogenous GAG replacement therapy.[50,67] Future treatment effectiveness may benefit from identification of molecular defects in IC/PBS and gene therapy.[50] Medications currently used to treat symptoms of IC/PBS are presented in Table 22-8

and also include the anticholinergics in Table 22-2, low dose tricyclic antidepressants and selective serotonin reuptake inhibitors (SSRIs), opioids for general pain management, the antiseizure medication gabapentin (Neurontin) for pain associated with sensory hyperstimulation, antihistamines, and other immunogenic agents, botulinum toxin, and the vanilloid receptor agonist resiniferatoxin.[68] These latter treatments are also discussed under treatment options for overactive bladder.

The oral medication that has FDA approval for IC/PBS treatment is pentosan polysulfate (Elmiron). It is a synthetic sulfated polysaccharide, which is theorized to work by stabilizing permeability of the mucosal lining of the bladder.[69] Rare side effects include alopecia, diarrhea, nausea, and headache. Because it promotes change in the bladder lining, the medication must be taken for several months before change in symptoms is noted. However, in a National Institutes of Health (NIH) funded pilot study (n = 121), pentosan polysulfate produced no statistically significant decrease in IC/PBS symptoms in participants when compared with placebo (34% versus 18%; P = .064).[69] Because of the low rate of effectiveness, further NIH funding for pentosan trials was deferred. Current funding is directed toward development of more efficacious treatments, such as intravesical GAG replacement.[67] Direct installation of intravesical therapy may provide pain relief for individuals with severe symptoms, usually through weekly installations performed in specialty ambulatory settings.[68]

Complementary Therapies

Complementary and alternative treatments that offer anecdotal relief for some women with IC/PBS have been used,

Table 22-8 Medications Used to Treat Interstitial Cystitis/Painful Bladder Syndrome (IC/PBS)*

Drug Generic (Brand)	Dose	FDA Approval for IC/PBS	Clinical Considerations
Pentosan polysulfate (Elmiron)	100 mg PO tid	Yes	May take up to 6 months of use to show improvement related to stabilizing permeability of the bladder lining. Symptom effect has been demonstrated in < 50% of women; may not be significantly greater than placebo.
Hydroxyzine hydrochloride (Atarax, Vistaril)	25–75 mg PO qd	No	May be useful in patients with allergy history related to decreasing mast cell activity. Also may help with sleep; drowsiness is a side effect.
Amitriptyline (Elavil) or Nortriptyline (Aventyl)	10–25 mg PO at hs	No	Nortriptyline is a metabolic by-product of the tricyclic antidepressant amitriptyline and may have lower side effects. Drug–drug interactions related to cytochrome P450 apply.
Dimethyl sulfoxide	Weekly bladder installation	Yes	This solvent has an anti-inflammatory and muscle relaxant effect and acts as a carrier to aid penetration of bladder epithelium by other therapeutic agents. Symptoms may become worse with treatment before they become better.

* Antimuscarinic agents to treat symptoms as outlined in Table 22-3 may also help some women with IC/PBS.

but have not been well studied.[70] These include stress reduction therapies such as meditation, hypnotherapy, acupuncture, trigger point injection or massage, support groups, sexual therapy, dietary supplements, and the acid neutralizer calcium glycerophosphate (Prelief).

The dietary modifications used to treat overactive bladder, such as decreasing acidity and increasing dilution of urine, may be helpful for some women. IC/PBS-specific options include a trial elimination of arylalkylamines-containing foods (bananas, beer, wine, cheese, mayonnaise, aspartame, nuts, onions, raisins, sour cream, and yogurt).[70] Women who report irritation from certain foods usually notice symptoms within 2 to 4 hours of ingestion of the irritant.[70]

Nutritional supplements that have been studied in small samples of women include L-arginine, natural mucopolysaccharides such as hyaluronic acid, chondroitin sulfate, aloe vera, and the bioflavonoid quercetin, which may inhibit histamine release.[70] One naturopathic regimen suggests 3 to 6 months of supplementation with a combination of glucosamine sulfate 500 mg tid (as a GAG replacement), L-arginine 500 mg tid (to increase nitric acid synthesis), bioflavonoids 1000 mg bid (as anti-inflammatories), buffered vitamin C 1000–2000 mg bid and mixed carotenes 50,000 IU bid (as immune support), *Zea mays* (corn silk) 2 capsules (225 mg/capsule) tid (as a demulcent to protect the mucosa), and kava kava extract 1 capsule (45–70 mg) tid (for pain relief).[71] However, research related to outcomes using this regimen was not reported.

Special Populations

Pregnancy

Transient urinary incontinence during pregnancy is common. In a study of both nulliparous and parous women at 30 weeks' gestation, almost 60% of both groups reported some episodes of urinary continence, a number more than double the prevalence in nonpregnant women.[72] Mild stress urinary incontinence is the most common type of incontinence during pregnancy, with increased risk related to parity, age, and body mass. Symptoms of urinary incontinence usually improve without intervention in the postpartum period, typically within the first 3 months. Although cesarean section appears to decrease the prevalence of urinary incontinence in the postpartum period somewhat, the prevalence of urinary incontinence in older women is similar regardless of route of birth.[73] Behavioral and exercise therapies carry lower risk than pharmacologic

interventions and are the treatment of first choice during pregnancy and lactation.

Because of the increased risk of ascending infection during pregnancy, current evidence supports use of an initial clean-catch, midstream urine culture at the first prenatal visit to identify asymptomatic bacteriuria.[47] Antibiotic treatment should be initiated when consistent presence of the same bacterial strain ≥ 100,000 colonies per milliliter is found.[47] Considerations for choice of antibiotics used to treat cystitis during pregnancy are reviewed in Table 22-9. A 3- to 7-day course of treatment is recommended.

Following treatment, regular repeat cultures should be continued throughout the pregnancy, although the optimal interval has not been determined.[47,51] Options range from repeat culture every month to every trimester for the duration of the pregnancy. Repeat surveillance is also indicated in other women at increased risk for UTI in pregnancy, including those with a prepregnancy history of UTI, sickle cell trait, or maternal comorbidities such as diabetes or structural abnormalities.

In women at risk for recurrent UTI, continuous prophylaxis for the remainder of the pregnancy and up to 6 weeks postpartum should be considered. Treatments can be administered either postcoitally or continuously with nitrofurantoin (Macrodantin) or cephalexin (Keflex). If a pregnant woman develops symptoms consistent with pyelonephritis, typical treatment involves initiation of intravenous antibiotics until the mother is afebrile, a follow-up course of oral antibiotics, and assessment of fetal well-being and preterm labor risk. Because of the risk of neonatal infection, Group B streptococcus (GBS) bacteriuria, when it is identified, should be treated with penicillin G, cephalexin (Keflex), or clindamycin (Cleocin) for women who have a true allergy to penicillin.[74] Additional screening for vaginal or rectal GBS is not needed in pregnancy as the woman with GBS bacteriuria automatically should receive intrapartum antibiotic treatment.

Women Over Age 65

Although the health of older women varies markedly, postmenopausal women are at higher risk for lower urinary tract problems.

Urinary Incontinence

The prevalence of UI increases with age, from 2% in young adults to 64% in nursing home residents.[75] Urinary incontinence among postmenopausal women is more likely to result from potentially modifiable factors, such

Table 22-9 Antibiotic Treatment and Prevention of Acute, Uncomplicated Lower Urinary Tract Infections in Pregnancy

Drug Generic (Brand)	Dose for Acute Cystitis (3- to 7-Day Regimen)	Prophylactic Dose	Clinical Considerations in Pregnancy
Clindamycin (Cleocin)	Not advised.	Not advised.	FDA Pregnancy Category B. Used as an alternative to penicillin for treatment of vaginal colonization with Group B streptococcus, but limited excretion into the bladder makes it ineffective for treatment of cystitis or asymptomatic bacteriuria secondary to Group B streptococcus. In addition, Group B streptococcus is exhibiting increasing resistance to clindamycin.
Nitrofurantoin (Macrodantin, Furadantin)	50 mg PO qid. Macrocrystals: 100 mg PO bid.	100 mg PO hs. Macrocrystals: 50 mg postcoitally 100 mg.	FDA Pregnancy Category B. Concentrates in urine only. Do not use for suspected upper tract involvement. Avoid use in last month of pregnancy due to risk of hemolytic anemia in mothers with G-6-PD deficiency, and in newborns. Small risk of maternal pulmonary reaction.
Fosfomycin (Monurol)	3 grams PO as a single dose.	Not advised.	FDA Pregnancy Category B. An aminoglycoside; infrequently used in pregnancy, resulting in limited safety and use information. Effective against uncomplicated cystitis.
Penicillin, ampicillin/amoxicillin, cephalosporins	Amoxicillin (Amoxil): 500 mg PO tid. Amoxicillin-clavulanate (Augmentin): 500 mg PO bid. Cephalexin (Keflex): 500 mg PO qid.	Cephalexin 250 mg PO qd.	FDA Pregnancy Category B. Common allergens. Use may facilitate occurrence of monilial vaginitis. High rates of bacterial resistance require culture. Penicillin or cephalexin is first choice for Group B streptococcus. Ampicillin and cephalosporins are both cleared rapidly in pregnancy, requiring higher dose options. Amoxicillin excretion is not increased.
Fluoroquinolones	Not advised.	Not advised.	FDA Pregnancy Category C. Potential for nonreversible arthropathy (joint disease) in the newborn due to impairment of cartilage development. No evidence of teratogenicity.
Sulfonamides, sulfisoxazole	Sulfasoxazole: 500 mg PO tid for 3–7 days.	Not advised.	FDA Pregnancy Category C; D near term due to increased risk of neonatal hyperbilirubinemia. Common allergen. Increasing rates of resistance limit role as first-choice agent in many localities. Hemolytic anemia a risk in women with glucose-6-phosphate dehydrogenase deficiency (G6PD). Hyperbilirubinemia of the newborn a risk due to use in late pregnancy.
Trimethoprim (Proloprim, Monotrim, or Triprim)	100 mg q 12 hours or 200 mg (two 100-mg tablets) q 24 hours.	Not advised.	FDA Pregnancy Category C. Inhibits folate metabolism. Increasing resistance limits use. Due to reports of congenital cardiovascular and palate malformations and theoretical risk of neural tube defects in exposed newborns, use in first trimester should be avoided or accompanied by ingestion of folic acid 1 mg/daily.
Tetracyclines	Not advised.	Not advised.	FDA Pregnancy Category D. Not recommended due to potential risk of minor congenital malformations, and discoloration of fetal teeth and bones if used after 5 months' gestation. High doses have been related to acute fatty liver degeneration.

Sources: Scottish Intercollegiate Guidelines Network 2006[51]; Macejko AM 2007.[74]

as delirium, depression, infections, genital atrophy, prescription medications, endocrine abnormalities such as thyroid disorders, and stool impaction. Older women are also at greater risk of anatomic abnormalities like prolapse, urine retention with overflow, or carcinoma of the bladder, and must be carefully evaluated when rapid onset of lower urinary tract symptoms occur. Serious problems secondary to UI in this age group include skin breakdown, falls, fractures, social isolation, and the financial burden of costs of supplies and care.

Nocturia

Nocturia is experienced by approximately 72% of women over age 80,[76] often due to increased nighttime urine output related to a declining glomerular filtration rate in the vertical position.[77] Although nocturia is common, related conditions, such as diabetes insipidus, obstructive sleep apnea, urinary tract infection, renal or cardiac disease, and early dementia must be ruled out. Contributors such as evening fluid intake or diuretic use, mild sleep disturbances and insomnia, decreased bladder volume, limited physical activity with frequent daytime napping, and daytime fluid retention with supine diuresis can be managed with behavioral therapy.

Many pharmacologic treatments used for lower urinary tract symptoms must be used with special caution in older women. Factors that affect treatment choice include age-related changes in drug absorption, distribution, metabolism, and excretion; comorbidities; polypharmacy; and increased incidence of typical contraindications to anticholinergics, such as gastrointestinal or urinary retention and reflux, uncontrolled narrow-angle glaucoma, unstable cardiovascular status and arrhythmias, hepatic or renal disease, and central nervous system compromise. Although anticholinergic medications are generally discouraged in older adults because of these increased risks, many older women may already be using multiple medications with potent anticholinergic effects (Table 22-2).[75]

Pharmacologic therapies used for treatment of nocturia include morning use of diuretics, topical estrogen therapy, and bedtime dosing of imipramine (Tofranil) or desmopressin (DDVAP), but any of these options should be used with caution in older women and persons with comorbidities.[15] Finally, there is little evidence comparing clinical outcomes obtained when older women use the various antimuscarinic agents. For example, darifenacin (Enablex) is M3-specific, which theoretically reduces the risk of tachycardia by sparing cholinergic receptors in cardiac muscle in women with cardiac disease. Trospium (Sanctura) is the only FDA-approved overactive bladder agent not metabolized through the cytochrome P450 pathway, and this may be an important consideration for women with liver disease or for those on multiple medications. However, no clinical significance of these variations has been identified.[78]

Urinary Tract Infection

Infection risk is also a concern in this age group; older women are more likely to have asymptomatic bacteriuria, cystitis, and urosepsis. With aging, urine becomes alkaline and contains fewer antibacterial proteins, an environment that promotes bacterial colonization. However, treating all women who have asymptomatic colonization would increase the risk of resistant organisms. On the other hand, decreases in immune response and thermoregulation often mask infection; UTI may only manifest as subtle changes in voiding patterns, behavior, or urine appearance and odor. Providers must be judicious in prescribing antimicrobials for lower urinary tract symptoms in older adults, observing for cues that may indicate a transition from colonization, which should not be treated, to infection, which should.[75]

▌ Conclusion

Lower urinary tract disorders are common problems for women and are commonly seen in primary care practice. Many of these conditions significantly affect quality of life in an adverse way. Pharmacologic treatments for urinary incontinence have significant side effects and adverse effects that require careful consideration and frequent follow-up. Because these conditions can be chronic, health education and nonpharmacologic treatments are primary interventions for amelioration of distressing symptoms. Conversely, uncomplicated UTIs are rarely associated with complications, and if the bacteria are not resistant, there are several antibiotic choices that are efficacious and safe. Women can often self-diagnose an uncomplicated UTI, and antibiotics can be prescribed without an office visit.

References

1. Abrams P, Cardozo L, Fall M, Griffiths D, Rosier P, Ulmsten U, et al. The standardization of terminology in lower urinary tract function: report from the standardization sub-committee of the International Continence Society. Urology 2003;61:37–49.

2. Stewart WF, Van Rooyen JB, Cundiff GW. Prevalence and burden of overactive bladder in the United States. World J Urol 2003;20(6):327.

3. Benson JT, Walters MD. Neurophysiology and pharmacology of the lower urinary tract. In Walters MD, Karram MM, eds. Urogynecology and reconstructive pelvic surgery, 3rd ed. Philadelphia, PA: Mosby Elsevier, 2007:31–43.

4. Eustice S, Roe B, Paterson J. Prompted voiding for the management of urinary incontinence in adults. Cochrane Database Syst Rev 2000;(2):CD002113.

5. Subak LL, Whitcomb E, Shen H, Saxton J, Vittinghoff E. Weight loss: a novel and effective treatment for urinary incontinence. J Urol 2005;174:190–5.

6. Roe B, Williams K, Palmer M. Bladder training for urinary incontinence in adults. Cochrane Database Syst Rev 2000(2):CD001308.

7. Alhasso AA, McKinlay J, Patrick K, Stewart L. Anticholinergic drugs versus non-drug active therapies for overactive bladder syndrome in adults. Cochrane Database Syst Rev 2006(4):CD003193.

8. Christoph F, Moschkowitsch A, Kempkensteffen C, Schostak M, Miller K, Schrader M. Long-term efficacy of tolterodine and patient compliance in pediatric patients with neurogenic detrusor overactivity. Urol Int 2007;79(1):55–9.

9. Nabi G, Cody JD, Ellis G, Herbison P, Hay-Smith J. Anticholinergic drugs versus placebo for overactive bladder syndrome in adults. Cochrane Database Syst Rev 2006(4):CD003781.

10. Staskin DR. Overactive bladder in the elderly: a guide to pharmacologic management. Drugs Aging 2005; 25:1013–28.

11. Yu Y, Nichol MB, Yu AP, Ahn J. Persistence and adherence of medications for chronic overactive bladder/urinary incontinence in the California Medicaid Program. Value Health 2005;8(4):495–505.

12. Hay-Smith J, Herbison P, Ellis G, Morris A. Which anticholinergic drug for overactive bladder symptoms in adults. Cochrane Database Syst Rev 2005(3): CD005429.

13. Diokno AC, Appell RA, Sand PK, Dmochowski RR, Gburek BM, Klimberg IW, et al. Prospective, randomized, double-blind study of the efficacy and tolerability of the extended-release formulations of oxybutynin and tolterodine for overactive bladder: results of the OPERA trial. Mayo Clinic Proceedings 2003;78: 687–95.

14. Wein AJ. Diagnosis and treatment of overactive bladder. Urology 2003;62(suppl B):20–7.

15. Kleeman SD, Karram MM. Overactive bladder syndrome and nocturia. In Walters MD, Karram MM, eds. Urogynecology and reconstructive pelvic surgery, 3rd ed. Philadelphia, PA: Mosby Elsevier, 2007:353–76.

16. Wein AJ. Effects of estrogen with and without progestin on urinary incontinence. J Urol 2005;174(4, pt 1): 1350–1.

17. Suckling J, Lethaby A, Kennedy R. Local oestrogen for vaginal atrophy in postmenopausal women. Cochrane Database Syst Rev 2006(4):CD001500.

18. Moehrer B, Hextall A, Jackson S. Oestrogens for urinary incontinence in women. Cochrane Database Syst Rev 2003(2):CD001405.

19. North American Menopause Society (NAMS). NAMS continuing medical education activity: the role of local vaginal estrogen for treatment of vaginal atrophy: 2007 position statement of the North American Menopause Society. Menopause 2007;14(3):355–6.

20. Reitz A, Schurch B. Intravesical therapy options for neurogenic detrusor overactivity. Spinal Cord 2004;42(5):267–72.

21. Holroyd-Leduc, Jayna M, Straus, Sharon E. Management of urinary incontinence in women: scientific review. JAMA 2004;291(8):986–95.

22. Indrekvam S, Sandvik H, Hunskaar S. A Norwegian national cohort of 3198 women treated with home-managed electrical stimulation for urinary incontinence—effectiveness and treatment results. Scand J Urol Nephrol 2001;35(1):32–9.

23. Van Kerrebroeck PE, van Voskuilen AC, Heesakkers JP, Lycklama A, Nijholt AA, Siegel S, et al. Results of sacral neuromodulation therapy for urinary voiding dysfunction: outcomes of a prospective, worldwide clinical study. J Urol 2007;178(5):2029–34.

24. Comiter C. Sacral neuromodulation for the symptomatic treatment of refractory interstitial cystitis: a prospective study. J Urol 2003;169:1369.

25. O'Dell KK, McGee S. Acupuncture for urge urinary incontinence in older women: what is the evidence? Urol Nurs 2005;26:23–9.

26. Lindmark S, Lonn L, Wiklund U, Tufvesson M, Olsson T, Eriksson JW. Dysregulation of the autonomic nervous system can be a link between visceral adiposity and insulin resistance. Obesity Research 2005;13:722–28.

27. Hulme J. Beyond Kegels: fabulous four exercises & more to prevent & treat incontinence, 2nd ed. Missoula, MT: Phoenix Publishing Co., 2002.

28. Blumenthal M, Busse WR, eds. Bundesinstitut fur Arsneimittel und Medizinprodukte. The complete German Commission E monographs: therapeutic guide to herbal medicines. Hufford CD, trans. Austin TX: American Botanical Council, 1998.

29. Nygaard IE, Girts T, Fultz NH, Kinchen K, Pohl G, Sternfeld B. Is urinary incontinence a barrier to exercise in women? Obstet Gynecol 2005;106(2):307–14.

30. Rortveit G, Daltveit AK, Hannestad YS, Hunskaar S. Urinary incontinence after vaginal delivery or cesarian section. N Engl J Med 2003;348(10):900–7.

31. Nygaard IE, Heit M. Stress urinary incontinence. Obstet Gynecol 2004;104(3):607–20.

32. Hay-Smith EJ, Dumoulin C. Pelvic floor muscle training versus no treatment, of inactive control treatments, for urinary incontinence in women. Cochrane Database Syst Rev 2006(1):CD005654.

33. Donnelly MJ, Powell-Morgan S, Olsen AL, Nygaard IE. Vaginal pessaries for the management of stress and mixed urinary incontinence. Int Urogynecol J Pelvic Floor Dysfunct 2004;15(5):302–7.

34. Rovner ES, Wein AJ. Treatment options for stress urinary incontinence. Rev Urol 2004;6(suppl 3):S29–47.

35. Alhasso AA, Glazener CMA, Pickard R, N'Dow JMO. Adrenergic drugs for urinary incontinence in adults. Cochrane Database Syst Rev 2005 Jul 20;(3): CD001842.

36. Byron JK, March PA, Chew DJ, DiBartola SP. Effect of phenylpropanolamine and pseudoephedrine on the urethral pressure profile and continence scores of incontinent female dogs. J Vet Int Med 2007;21(1): 47–53.

37. Thor KB. Targeting serotonin and norepinephrine receptors in stress urinary incontinence. Int J Gynaecol Obstet 2004;86(suppl):S38.

38. Mariappan P, Alhasso A, Ballantyne Z, Grant A, N'Dow J. Duloxetine, a serotonin and noradrenaline reuptake inhibitor (SNRI) for the treatment of stress urinary incontinence: a systematic review. Eur Urol 2007;51(1):67–74.

39. Eli Lilly and Company, Boehringer Ingelheim Pharmaceuticals, Inc. Lilly and Boehringer Ingelheim jointly announce the recision of US FDA application for duloxetine for treatment of stress urinary incontinence. Available from: *www.prnewswire.com/cgi-bin/micro _stories.pl?ACCT=916306&TICK=LLY&STORY=/www/ story/01-28-2005/0002913293&EDATE=Jan+28,+2005* [Accessed April 3, 2009].

40. Chapple CR, Wein AJ, Brubaker L, Dmochowski R, Pons ME, Habb F, et al. Stress incontinence injection therapy: what is best for our patients? Eur Urol 2005;48:552–65.

41. Bent AE. Urethral injections of bulking agents for intrinsic sphincter deficiency. In Walters MD, Karram MM, eds. Urogynecology and reconstructive pelvic surgery, 3rd ed. Philadelphia, PA: Mosby Elsevier, 2007:227–33.

42. Theofrastous JP, Wyman JF, Bump RC, McClish DK, Elser DM, Bland DR, et al. Effects of pelvic floor muscle training on strength and predictors of response in the treatment of urinary incontinence. Neurourol Urodynamics 2002;21:486–90.

43. Gray, M. Urinary retention: management in the acute care setting, part 2. Am J Nurs 2000;100(8): 36–44.

44. Schurch B. Botulinum toxin for the management of bladder dysfunction. Drugs 2006;66:1301–18.

45. Foxman B, Barlow R, D'Arcy H, Gillespie B, Sobel JD. Urinary tract infection: self-reported incidence and associated costs. Ann Epidemiol 2000;10:509.

46. Griebling TL. Urologic Diseases in America Project: trends in resource use for urinary tract infections in women. J Urol 2005;173:1281–7.

47. Nicholle LE, Bradley S, Colgan R, Rice JC, Schaeffer A, Hooton TM. Infectious Disease Society of America guidelines for the diagnosis and treatment of asymptomatic bacteriuria in adults. Clin Infect Dis 2005;40: 643–54.

48. Miller LG, Tang AW. Treatment of uncomplicated urinary tract infections in an era of increasing antimicrobial resistance. May Clin Proc 2004;79:1048–53.

49. Hooton TM, Besser R, Foxman B, Fritsche TR, Nicolle LE. Acute uncomplicated cystitis in an era of increasing antibiotic resistance: a proposed approach to empirical therapy. Clin Infect Dis 2004;39:75–80.

50. Warren JW, Abrutyn E, Hebel JR, Johnson JR, Schaeffer AJ, Stamm WE. Guidelines for antimicrobial treatment of uncomplicated acute bacterial cystitis and acute pyelonephritis in women. Infectious Diseases Society of America (ADSA). Clin Infect Dis 1999;29: 745–58.

51. Scottish Intercollegiate Guidelines Network (SIGN). Management of suspected bacterial urinary tract infection in adults. A national clinical guideline. Edinburgh, Scotland: Scottish Intercollegiate Guidelines Network (SIGN); 2006 Available from: *http://www.sign .ac.uk/pdf/sign88.pdf* [Accessed July 9, 2009].

52. Rafalsky VV, Andreeva IV, Rjabkova EL. Quinolones for uncomplicated acute cystitis in women. Cochrane Database Syst Rev 2006 Jul 19;3:CD003597.

53. Milo G, Katchman E, Paul M, Christiaens T, Baerheim A, Leibovici L. Duration of antibacterial treatment for uncomplicated urinary tract infection in women. Cochrane Database Syst Rev 2005 Apr 18;(2): CD004682.

54. Lutters M, Vogt-Ferrier NB. Antibiotic duration for treating uncomplicated, symptomatic lower urinary tract infections in elderly women. Cochrane Database Syst Rev 2008 Jul 16;(3):CD001535.

55. Gupta K, Hooton TM, Roberts PL, Stamm WE. Patient-initiated treatment of uncomplicated recurrent urinary tract infections in young women. Ann Intern Med 2001;135:9–16.

56. Albert X, Huertas I, Pereiro I, Sanfelix J, Gosalbes V, Perrota C. Antibiotics for preventing recurrent urinary tract infection in non-pregnant women. Cochrane Database Syst Rev 2004;(3):CD001209.

57. Chew LD, Fihn SD. Recurrent cystitis in non-pregnant women. West J Med 1999;170(5):274–7.

58. Lee B, Bhuta T, Craig J, Simpson J. Methenamine hippurate for preventing urinary tract infections. Cochrane Database Syst Rev 2002(1):CD003265.

59. Eriksen B. A randomized, open, parallel-group study on the preventative effect of an oestradiol-releasing vaginal ring (Estring) on recurrent urinary tract infections in postmenopausal women. Am J Obstet Gynecol 1999;180:10729.

60. Raz R, Colodner R, Rohana Y, Battino S, Rottenstrerich E, Wasser I, et al. Effectiveness of estriol-containing vaginal pessaries and nitrofurantoin macrocrystal therapy in the prevention of recurrent urinary tract infection in postmenopausal women. Clin Infect Dis 2003;36(11):1362–8.

61. Alraek T, Baerheim A. The effect of prophylactic acupuncture treatments in women with recurrent cystitis: kidney patients fare better. J Altern Complement Med 2003;9(6):979.

62. Jepson RG, Mihalievic L, Craig J. Cranberries for preventing urinary tract infections. Cochrane Database Syst Rev 2004;(2):CD001321.

63. Hudson T. Treatment and prevention of bladder infections. Altern Complementary Ther 2006;12(6): 297–302.

64. Payne CK, Joyce GF, Wise M, Clemens JQ. Urologic Diseases in America Project. Interstitial cystitis and painful bladder syndrome. J Urol 2007;177(6):2042–9.

65. Hurst RE, Moldwin RM, Grant Mulholland S. Bladder defense molecules, urothelial differentiation, urinary biomarkers, and interstitial cystitis. Urology 2007; 69(4): S1:S22–3.

66. Peters KM, Carey JM, Konstandt DB. Sacral neuro-modulation reduces narcotic requirements for the treatment of refractory interstitial cystitis: outcomes based technique. Int Urogynecol J 2003;14:223–8.

67. Kyker KD, Coffman J, Hurst RE. Exogenous glycosaminoglycans coat damaged bladder surfaces in experimentally damaged mouse bladder. BMC Urol 2005;5:4–8.

68. Phatak S, Foster HE. The management of interstitial cystitis: an update. Nat Clin Pract Urol 2006;3:45–53.

69. Sant GR, Propert KJ, Hanno PM. A pilot clinical trail of oral pentosan polysulpfate and oral hydroxyzine in patients with interstitial cystitis. J Urol 2003;170: 810–15.

70. Whitmore KE. Complementary and alternative therapies as treatment approaches for interstitial cystitis. Urology 2002;4(suppl 1):S28–35.

71. Hudson T. Treating interstitial cystitis: a natural medicine approach. Altern Complementary Ther 2001; 7(2):88–90.

72. Wesnes SL, Rortveit G, Bo K, Kunskaar S. Urinary incontinence during pregnancy. Obstet Gynecol 2007; 109:922–8.

73. Nygaard IE. Urinary incontinence: is cesarean delivery protective? Semin Perinatol 2006;30(5):267–71.

74. Macejko AM, Schaeffer AJ. Asymptomatic bacteriuria and symptomatic urinary tract infections during pregnancy. Urolog Clin N Am 2007;34(1):35–42.

75. Hazzard W, Blass JP, Halter JB, Ouslander JG, Tinetti ME. Principles of geriatric medicine & gerontology, 5th ed. New York: McGraw-Hill, 2003.

76. Middelkoop HA, Smilde-van-den Doel DA, Neven AK, Kamphuisen HA, Springer CP. Subjective sleep characteristics of 1,485 males and females aged 50–93: effects of sex and age, and factors related to self-evaluated quality of sleep. J Gerontol A Biol Sci Med Sci 1996;51(3):M108–15.

77. Van kerrebroeck P, Abrams P, Chaikin D, Donovan J, Fonda D, Jackson S, et al. The standardization of terminology in nocturia: report from the Standardization Sub-committee of the International Continence Society. Neurourol Urodyn 2002;21:179–83.

78. Chancellor MB, de Miguel F. Treatment of overactive bladder: selective use of anticholinergic agents with low drug–drug interaction potential. Geriatrics 2007;62(5):15–24.

"Virtue consisted in avoiding scandal and venereal disease."
Robert Cecil, First Viscount Cecil of Chelwood
(1864–1958)

23
Sexually Transmitted Infections

Hayley Mark, Jason Farley, and Ashley Hanahan

Chapter Glossary

Acquired immune deficiency syndrome (AIDS) Sexually transmitted infection caused by the human immunodeficiency virus (HIV) and resulting in derangements of the human immune system.

Acute retroviral syndrome Cluster of symptoms such as low-grade fever, fatigue, and lymph node enlargement that occurs after exposure to HIV and shortly before seroconversion. It is estimated that compared to men, women are more likely to manifest an acute retroviral syndrome.

Antiretroviral therapy (ART) Medications used to treat retroviruses, primarily HIV. When more than one drug is used, the term antiretroviral therapy (ART) is commonly used.

Bubo An enlarged lymph node, usually in inguinal or axillary regions. The plural is *buboes*. The word is derived from the Greek for "swollen groin."

Chlamydia trachomatis Most commonly reported bacterial sexually transmitted infection, with potential long-term effects of pelvic inflammatory disease, infertility, and pneumonia. Chlamydia is caused by *Chlamydia trachomatis* (CT).

Cluster of differentiation 4 (CD4) A type of protein molecule in human blood that is present on the surface of the majority of cells in the immune system and is the major site of destruction after infection by HIV.

Disseminated gonococcal infection (DGI) Condition that occurs subsequent to gonorrhea septicemia. The most common sign of DGI is arthritis. This condition is more common among women than men.

Enthesitis Pain and swelling of the tendon and ligaments at the sites of insertion to the bone.

Fitz-Hugh-Curtis syndrome Condition that consists of right upper quadrant pain resulting from ascending pelvic infection and inflammation of the liver capsule (perihepatitis) or diaphragm. Fitz-Hugh-Curtis is typically associated with acute salpingitis.

Gonorrhea (GC) One of the classic sexually transmitted infections. Gonorrhea is caused by *Neisseria gonorrhoeae.*

Highly active antiretroviral therapy (HAART) Several effective antiretroviral drugs that have different mechanisms of action and are used in combination in the treatment of HIV infection. ART is termed HAART when more than 4 drugs are used in a regimen for treating HIV.

Human immunodeficiency virus (HIV) Causative agent for acquired immune deficiency disease syndrome (AIDS).

Lymphogranuloma venereum (LGV) A rare sexually transmitted infection caused by invasive serovars *Chlamydia trachomatis* and characterized by buboes.

Neisseria gonorrhoeae (GC) Organism that causes the sexually transmitted infection gonorrhea.

Nucleic acid amplification testing (NAAT) Tests such as polymerase chain reaction (PCR) and other methods for amplifying DNA and RNA that facilitate rapid detection of microorganisms and have become the common test to diagnose chlamydia and/or gonorrhea.

Pelvic inflammatory disease (PID) Ascending infection of the upper genital tract and includes salpingitis. This infection is associated with infertility, ectopic pregnancies, and chronic pelvic pain.

Post-exposure prophylaxis (PEP) Short-term course of antiretroviral drugs administered after exposure to HIV to decrease the likelihood that the individual will develop the disease.

Prevention of mother-to-child transmission (PMTCT) Worldwide programs that are focused on preventing vertical (e.g., ascending) transmission of HIV from mother to child during pregnancy, labor, birth, or breastfeeding. The abbreviation PMTCT has become the shorthand expression for these programs and is so common, it is often part of the official title in individual programs.

Reactive arthritis Member of the spondylarthritis family of disorders; refers to an arthritis that appears after a bacterial infection that is associated either with urethritis or enteric illness.

Reiter syndrome An autoimmune arthritic condition whose older name was *venereal arthritis*. This syndrome is more common among men than women.

Serovars Also known as a *serotype*, subgroupings of microorganisms or viruses that are categorized on the basis of surface antigens and are used for subspecies level of classification.

Sexually transmitted disease (STD) A replacement for the term *venereal disease* (*VD*) in order to avoid the stigma attached to that term. *STD* gained popularity toward the end of the 20th century when it also became apparent that there was an increasing number of conditions that could have a sexual transmission component, such as HIV or chlamydia.

Sexually transmitted infections (STI) The current term most frequently used to identify conditions that are transmitted sexually. *STI* also is more precise than previously used terms and reflects the possibility of subclinical or latent infections.

Test of cure Repeat testing after treatment. A scheduled test of cure usually is necessary if there is a strong likelihood of treatment failure.

Venereal disease An older term used to designate contagious conditions spread primarily by sexual contact. Syphilis and gonorrhea were the major venereal diseases.

Introduction

Sexually transmitted infections have been known since ancient times. Skeletal evidence from Hippocrates's time has been said to provide evidence of syphilis. Major epidemics of syphilis, or the pox, were reported periodically during the Middle Ages, and there is a hypothesis that the sailors with Columbus were infected with the same disease during their historical exploration of the New World. Important world figures from history such as Ivan the Terrible, Lenin, Tolstoy, King Henry VIII, Lord Randolph Churchill, as well as the American Al Capone all have been known or strongly suspected of having syphilis.

Gonorrhea and syphilis were recognized as separate disorders in the Middle Ages. These conditions came to be known as **venereal diseases**. However, diagnosis preceded any effective treatment. Without therapy, the major worldwide public health approach was to stress abstinence and monogamy, often painting individuals who had a venereal disease as immoral. For example, during World War II, the U.S. military were cautioned about exposure to women who were characterized as loose or labeled as prostitutes. In some areas, such as Florida, female prostitutes were placed in quarantine in an attempt to teach them morality under the assumption that it would decrease transmission of disease.

After the war, antimicrobials became available and cure of the classic venereal diseases became possible. However, just as effective treatments for gonorrhea and syphilis emerged, more infections were found to have a sexual transmission component. In addition, effective contraceptive methods and changing mores in the 1960s accompanied an increase in the incidence of venereal diseases. By the 1990s, the term *venereal disease* began to fall into disuse, replaced by **sexually transmitted diseases** (STDs), ostensibly in an attempt to recognize the larger number of conditions as well as decrease some of the associated stigma with the original term. Within a decade, another term became popular, namely **sexually transmitted infections** (STIs). Substituting the word *infection* for *disease* enabled the use of a more precise term and allowed the acknowledgement of the number of conditions that are subclinical but still infectious. In this chapter, STI will be the term of choice, unless an alternative term is used within an historical context or for a publication.

Sexually Transmitted Infections

The United States has the highest rates of STIs of any country in the industrialized world. Approximately 19 million new infections occur each year, and more than half of all persons will be infected with an STI at some point in their lifetime.[1] Newly diagnosed STIs are most common among young persons; half of the new infections occur in persons ages 15–24 years.[2] STIs are more easily passed from men to women than vice versa, and women disproportionately bear the long-term consequences of these infections. For example, if inadequately treated, 20–40% of women infected with chlamydia or gonorrhea will develop pelvic inflammatory disease, which predisposes them to subsequent ectopic pregnancy and tubal infertility if contraception is not used. Approximately 70% of chlamydial infections and 50% of gonococcal infections in women are asymptomatic, resulting in later and less frequent treatment. Pregnant women with STIs are at greater risk of miscarriage and premature delivery than those without STIs. Some diseases can also be transmitted to the fetus or newborn. Gonorrhea and chlamydia can cause neonatal ophthalmia or neonatal pneumonia, and herpes simplex virus can cause potentially fatal neonatal viral sepsis. The prevalence and morbidity associated with STIs makes this a critical topic for healthcare providers.

The purpose of this chapter is to provide an overview of the major STIs that affect populations in the United States. One of the more minor STIs, vaginal trichomoniasis, is discussed in depth in Chapter 31. The Centers for Disease Control and Prevention (CDC) periodically publishes the *STD Treatment Guidelines* that are highly regarded and used frequently by experts in the field. These guidelines were developed after systematically reviewing evidence concerning each of the major STIs and consulting with public and private sector professionals knowledgeable in the treatment of persons with STIs. These guidelines form the basis of the pharmacologic treatments addressed in this chapter. Since most of these drugs are antimicrobials in common usage, information about using them during pregnancy or lactation or by the elderly can be found in more detail in other chapters, especially Chapter 11.

Chlamydia Trachomatis

Introduction

Chlamydia trachomatis (*C trachomatis*) is common in industrialized and developing countries and is a major cause of genital tract and ocular infections worldwide. It is estimated that there were 89 million new cases of genital chlamydia worldwide in 1997,[1] and total costs related to chlamydia morbidity in the United States exceed $2 billion per year.[2] In 2006, 1,030,911 chlamydial infections were reported to the CDC, which was nearly three times greater than the number of gonorrhea cases.[3]

Due to the often asymptomatic or nonspecific nature of the disease and the limited availability of testing, chlamydia can be undiagnosed or improperly treated. Chlamydia has become one of the leading causes of pelvic inflammatory disease (PID) and related infertility or ectopic pregnancy. It

is estimated that 20% of women with untreated chlamydia will develop PID.[4] Maternal antibodies to the organism provide limited, if any, protection for the newborn. Based upon positive cultures for *C trachomatis* in symptomatic infants, the risk for neonatal acquired conjunctivitis varies from 20% to 50% and for pneumonia from 5% to 30%.[5]

Chlamydia infections became reportable diseases in the United States in 1986, and the reported incidence has gradually increased since that time. Chlamydia is currently the most commonly reported notifiable disease in the United States.[6] The high frequency largely is due to increased screening efforts in women and improved testing methodologies that can detect active infection. The prevalence of chlamydia among adolescents and adults is estimated to be between 2.3% and 4.2%.[3] Rates of documented infection among women in the United States are three times as high as the rates among men. Additionally, substantial racial/ethnic and age disparities are present in the prevalence of both chlamydial and gonococcal infections, with non-Hispanic Black persons < 25 years of age having the greatest burden of disease.[3,4] It is important to note that there is a high rate of coinfection with gonorrhea and chlamydia; thus, these conditions should be suspected to coexist in any given woman, and dual treatment is recommended.[3,7] Chlamydial infection also appears to increase the risk of transmission of HIV.[8]

Pathogenesis, Microbiology, and Taxonomy

C trachomatis is a small gram-negative bacterium with unique biologic properties that distinguish it from all other living organisms. There are three chlamydial organisms known to cause disease in humans. The family Chlamydiaceae is divided into two genera: *Chlamydia*, which includes *C trachomatis*, and *Chlamydophila*, which includes *C pneumoniae* (a cause of atypical pneumonia) and *C psittaci* (the cause of parrot fever, for which humans are an incidental host).[9,10] All chlamydiae have a biphasic life cycle that depends upon intracellular growth. As an obligate intracellular organism, chlamydia can be found within urethral, cervical, and rectal epithelial cells but not in exudate or pus. The first phase of its life cycle occurs within 6–8 hours, and the second within 2–3 days. The long growth cycle explains the need for prolonged courses of treatment. Another critical feature of these organisms is that immunity to infection is not long lived, and as a result, persistent infection or reinfection and associated inflammatory responses are common. In ocular and genital infections, persistent inflammation may lead to scarring, resulting in blindness or infertility.[11]

C trachomatis is characterized by various **serovars** or subgroupings, based on classification related to their cell surface antigens. This is of particular importance when studying or tracking epidemiologic phenomenon relating to infectious disease. The majority of chlamydial infections of the genital tract are caused by serovars D, E, F, G, H, I, J, and K.[6] Eventually, serovars may be important in regard to treatment choices. However, although serum tests for chlamydia exist, their utility is currently limited by lack of availability of such tests.[12]

Screening

The CDC and the U.S. Preventive Services Task Force (USPSTF) have recommended that all screening protocols be guided by variations in local prevalence or geographic variation of disease, and that specific risk-based protocols be tested locally.[13] Both agencies recommend routinely screening all sexually active women ≤ 24 years of age for *C trachomatis* infection, whether or not they are pregnant. Screening of sexually active women aged > 24 years for *C trachomatis* should be considered whenever they report increased risk of infection. Risk factors for chlamydia are being ≤ 24 years of age, having multiple partners or a new sex partner during the last 3 months, inconsistent use of barrier protection, history of an STI, exchanging money for sex or drugs, and clinical evidence of mucopurulent cervicitis.[14] Because of variations in patterns of risk behaviors in individuals, specific recommendations for upper age limits for screening and for intervals between screenings have not been set. A summary of recent USPSTF chlamydial screening recommendations is listed in Table 23-1.

Transmission and Clinical Manifestations

Chlamydia is transmitted via direct, genital–genital (including anal), or oral–genital contact or perinatally to the new-born via vertical transmission from the vagina during labor and birth.

Among women, chlamydia may manifest as urethritis, Bartholin gland infection, cervicitis, salpingitis, endometritis, conjunctivitis, pharyngitis, perihepatitis (**Fitz-Hugh-Curtis syndrome**), proctitis, reactive arthritis (**Reiter syndrome**), or overt **pelvic inflammatory disease** (PID).[6] Clinical suspicion for chlamydial infection should be raised for all women < 25 years of age; any women who report multiple or new sex partners during the last 3 months; those with inconsistent use of barrier protection; and among women who have clinical evidence of mucopurulent cervicitis and cervical ectopy.[14] Since asymptomatic infection is common among both men and women, routine screening of all high-risk individuals is imperative (Table 23-1).

Among women, cervical infection is the most common chlamydial syndrome. Chlamydial cervicitis may present with mucopurulent cervical discharge, edema, ulcers, and ectopy, or the exam may be unremarkable.[15] However, no specific signs or symptoms correlate reliably with the presence of chlamydial infection, and laboratory confirmation of infection is recommended.[6] The other common sites of infection include chlamydial pharyngitis, which is generally asymptomatic, and anorectal infections, which may present with rectal burning, discharge, and painful bowel movements.[15] Urethritis may accompany cervicitis and result in symptoms often associated with urinary tract infection, including poorly differentiated lower abdominal pain, frequency, and dysuria.[6,15] Urinalysis will often reveal pyuria (i.e., the presence of 10 or more neutrophils per high-power field of unspun, voided midstream urine) without an infecting organism identified on Gram stain or traditional urine culture.[15] The differential diagnosis includes low-colony count urinary tract infection (UTI) (e.g., infection caused by *Staphylococcus saprophyticus*), or urethritis due to other STI organisms, such as *Neisseria gonorrhoeae* or Herpes simplex.[14]

Table 23-1 USPSTF Recommendations for Chlamydia Screening

Population	Recommendation for Screening for Chlamydia	Grade of Recommendation[†]
Nonpregnant women age ≤ 24 years of age who are sexually active and persons who are at increased risk*	Annual screening recommended. Benefits of screening substantially outweigh harms.	A
All pregnant women ≤ 24 years and pregnant women who are ≥ 24 years of age who are at increased risk*	Screening recommended at first prenatal visit and again in third trimester for women at continued risk or those who develop a new risk factor during pregnancy. Benefits of screening substantially outweigh harms.	B

* Increased risk = All sexually active women ≤ 24 years of age including adolescents, a history of chlamydial or other sexually transmitted infection, new or multiple sexual partners, inconsistent condom use, exchanging sex for money or drugs, clinical evidence of mucopurulent cervicitis. Risk factors for pregnant women are the same as for nonpregnant women.
[†] Grade A = good evidence that this recommendation improves important health outcomes and that the benefits substantially outweigh the harms; grade B = fair evidence that this recommendation improves important health outcomes and that the benefits outweigh the harms.
Source: United States Preventive Services Task Force 2008.[32]

Diagnosis

The obligate intracellular growth nature of chlamydia precludes its identification in samples that are exclusively purulent discharge or polymorphonuclear neutrophils (PMNs). Therefore, careful collection of columnar epithelial cells from the cervix or urethra is necessary.[6] Chlamydia cannot be cultured on artificial media, and traditionally tissue culture has been required to establish a diagnosis.[11,13] Additionally, there now are several nonculture diagnostic tests available for clinical use.

The US Food Drug Administration (FDA) approval varies by test methodology and depends on the anatomic site of specimen collection. **Nucleic acid amplification testing** (NAAT) performed on an endocervical swab specimen provides the highest sensitivity. Although less sensitive than NAATs, unamplified nucleic acid hybridization tests, enzyme immunoassays (EIAs), and direct fluorescent antibody (DFA) performed on an endocervical swab specimen also are acceptable for screening. The sensitivity of non-NAATs with urine or vaginal swab specimens is suboptimal. In the case of EIAs, specificity with vaginal swab and urine specimens is also lower than with endocervical swab specimens, and thus is not recommended. The specimen collection techniques are listed in Table 23-2.[12] Individuals who are diagnosed with chlamydia should be tested for the presence of other STIs.

Treatment

Treating women with STIs prevents transmission to sex partners, progression of disease, and transmission to infants during birth. Coinfection with *C trachomatis* frequently occurs among persons who have gonococcal infection; therefore, when treating an individual for chlamydia, presumptive treatment for gonorrhea is recommended if gonorrhea rates are high in the patient population being treated.

The CDC-recommended treatment regimens are presented in Table 23-3. The choice of a regimen should be based on ability to adhere to the regimen, cost, and side effects. Since the organism is an obligate parasite within a cell, antimicrobials that act by breaking down the cell wall will kill the otherwise healthy host, but not necessarily the microorganism. Azithromycin (Zithromax) is relatively expensive but requires only one dose so intake can be directly observed in an ambulatory facility. In general, however, macrolides such as azithromycin have distressing gastrointestinal side effects. Doxycycline (Vibramycin) is a less expensive alternative to azithromycin but requires 7 days of treatment, suggesting increased potential for missed doses. Levofloxacin (Levaquin) and ofloxacin (Floxin) are acceptable alternatives, but are more expensive and have no appreciable additional benefits.

To minimize transmission, persons treated for chlamydia should be instructed to abstain from sexual intercourse or other sexual contact for 7 days after single-dose therapy or until completion of a 7-day regimen.[4] Individuals should be encouraged to use barrier method contraception and practice safe sex to aid in prevention of repeated transmission.

To minimize the risk for reinfection, persons also should be instructed to abstain from sexual intercourse until all of their sex partners are treated.[4] Sex partners should also be treated according to standard adult

---

Table 23-2 Specimen Collection Techniques for *C Trachomatis* or *N Gonorrhoeae*

Endocervical Specimens

Nonculture specimens should be obtained as directed by the test manufacturer in the package insert, using the supplied swab or as specified.

Before obtaining a specimen, a sponge or large swab should be used to remove all secretions and discharge from the cervical os.

Insert the appropriate swab or endocervical brush 1–2 cm into the endocervical canal (i.e., past the squamocolumnar junction), rotating it against the wall of the endocervical canal > 2 times or for the period of time recommended by the manufacturer. The swab should be withdrawn without touching any vaginal surfaces and placed in the appropriate transport medium.

Urethral Specimens

Follow test manufacturer instructions in the package insert, using the swab supplied or specified by the manufacturer.

If possible, obtaining specimens should be delayed until > 1 hour after the individual has voided.

Specimens should be obtained for *C trachomatis* tests after obtaining specimens for a Gram-stained smear or *N gonorrhoeae* culture.

For nonculture tests, the urogenital swab should be inserted gently into the urethra (females, 1–2 cm; males, 2–4 cm). The swab should be rotated in one direction for > 1 revolution and withdrawn. For males or females with urethral discharge, exudate collected from the urethral meatus is sufficient for *N gonorrhoeae* culture.

An intraurethral specimen is required for *C trachomatis* testing, regardless of the presence of exudate at the meatus.

Urine Specimens

Specimens should be obtained as directed by the test manufacturer in the package insert.

If possible, specimen collection should be delayed until > 1 hour after the individual has voided.

First-catch urine (e.g., the first 10–30 cc voided after initiating the stream) should be used.

Source: Centers for Disease Control and Prevention 2007.[36]

Table 23-3 CDC Recommended Treatment Regimens for *C Trachomatis**

Nonpregnant		Pregnant	
Recommended Regimen	**Alternative Regimen**	**Recommended Regimen**	**Alternative Regimen**
Azithromycin 1 g PO in a single dose	Erythromycin base 500 mg PO qid for 7 days	Erythromycin base 500 mg PO qid for 7 days	Erythromycin base 250 mg PO qid for 14 days
Or	**Or**	**Or**	**Or**
Doxycycline 100 mg PO bid for 7 days	Erythromycin ethylsuccinate 800 mg PO qid for 7 days	Amoxicillin 500 mg PO tid for 7 days	Erythromycin ethylsuccinate 800 mg PO qid for 7 days
	Or		**Or**
	Ofloxacin 300 mg PO bid for 7 days		Erythromycin ethylsuccinate[†] 400 mg PO qid for 14 days
	Or		**Or**
	Levofloxacin 500 mg PO qd for 7 days		Azithromycin 1 g PO single dose

* Individuals who have chlamydial infection and also are infected with HIV should receive the same treatment regimen as those who are HIV negative.
[†] Erythromycin estolate is contraindicated during pregnancy because of drug-related hepatotoxicity.
Source: Centers for Disease Control and Prevention 2006.[4]

regimens, and women with *Chlamydia* infection should be encouraged to inform sex partners.

Follow-Up

Except for pregnant women, **test of cure** or repeat testing a few weeks after completing therapy is not recommended for persons treated with the recommended or alterative regimens, unless therapeutic compliance is in question, symptoms persist, or reinfection is suspected. Repeat or persistent infection occurs in 10–15% of women who are treated for *C trachomatis* infections, but antimicrobial resistance in these situations is unproven.[16] Nonculture tests that are performed less than 3 weeks after completion of antimicrobial therapy might be falsely positive because of the presence of nonviable organisms; this applies in particular to NAATs. Conversely, false-negative results might occur because of persistent infections involving limited numbers of chlamydial organisms. Thus, if a test of cure is performed, it should be performed at least 3 weeks after therapy is completed. The CDC recommends rescreening for women with *C trachomatis* infection 3–4 months after treatment is completed. This rescreening is to rule out reinfection rather than a test of cure.

Complications of Chlamydial Disease

Pelvic Inflammatory Disease

Pelvic inflammatory disease comprises a spectrum of inflammatory disorders of the upper female genital tract, including endometritis, salpingitis, tubo-ovarian abscess,

and pelvic peritonitis.[12] Women with mild to moderate PID often have vague, nonspecific symptoms (e.g., abnormal bleeding, dyspareunia, and vaginal discharge) making diagnosis difficult, and cases can go unrecognized. *Neisseria gonorrhoeae* and *C trachomatis* are implicated in many cases, but microorganisms commonly found in the vaginal flora (e.g., anaerobes, *Gardnerella vaginalis*, *Haemophilus influenzae*, enteric gram-negative rods, and *Streptococcus agalactiae*) also have been associated with PID. In addition, cytomegalovirus (CMV), *Mycoplasma hominis*, *Ureaplasma urealyticum*, and *Mycoplasma genitalium* may be associated with some cases of PID. All women who are diagnosed with acute PID should be tested for *N gonorrhoeae* and *C trachomatis* and screened for HIV infection.[12]

Diagnosis of PID is typically made on the basis of clinical findings described in Table 23-4. If the cervical discharge appears normal and there are no white blood cells on the microscopic examination of vaginal fluid, the diagnosis of PID is unlikely, and alternative causes of pain should be investigated.[12] Because of the difficulty of diagnosis and the potential for infertility from even mild or subclincial PID, healthcare providers should maintain a low threshold for the diagnosis.[12] The CDC recommends that in-hospital treatment for PID be considered under the following circumstances: when surgical emergencies cannot be excluded (e.g., appendicitis); in pregnancy; if no clinical response is apparent; for individuals who are unable to follow or tolerate outpatient oral regimens; when the presence of severe illness, nausea, vomiting, or high fever; or when tubo-ovarian abscess is suspected.[12]

Table 23-4 Criteria For Diagnosis of Pelvic Inflammatory Disease (PID)

Minimum	Additional	Most Specific
General symptoms and signs of lower genital tract, and: Cervical motion tenderness **Or** Uterine tenderness **Or** Adnexal tenderness	Oral temperature > 101°F (> 38.3°C), abnormal cervical or vaginal mucopurulent discharge Presence of abundant numbers of WBC on saline microscopy of vaginal secretions Elevated erythrocyte sedimentation rate Elevated C-reactive protein, and laboratory documentation of cervical infection with *N gonorrhoeae* or *C trachomatis*	Endometrial biopsy with histopathologic evidence of endometritis Transvaginal sonography or magnetic resonance imaging techniques showing thickened, fluid-filled tubes with or without free pelvic fluid or tubo-ovarian complex, or Doppler studies suggesting pelvic infection (e.g., tubal hyperemia) Laparoscopic abnormalities consistent with PID

Source: Centers for Disease Control and Prevention 2007.[12]

Empiric treatment of PID is recommended for sexually active young women and other women at risk for STIs who present with pelvic or lower abdominal pain and either cervical motion tenderness, adnexal tenderness, or uterine tenderness, when no other cause for the illness can be identified. Women who are treated for PID should be given an antibiotic that is effective against both *C. trachomatis* and *N. gonorrhea*. Most cases of mild to moderate PID can be treated on an outpatient basis with the use of broad-spectrum antibiotics, and there is evidence to suggest that oral therapy fares well in comparison to parenteral therapy in these cases. The optimal treatment regimen and long-term outcome of early treatment of women with asymptomatic or subclinical PID have not been extensively studied. Women who do not respond to oral therapy within 72 hours should be reevaluated to confirm the diagnosis and should be administered parenteral therapy on either an outpatient or in-hospital basis.[12] CDC recommendations for the oral and parenteral treatment for PID (Table 23-5) have recently been updated to reflect the increasing prevalence of fluoroquinolone-resistant gonorrhea in the United States.[17]

Perihepatitis

Fitz-Hugh-Curtis syndrome (perihepatitis) is an inflammation of the liver capsule; it typically occurs when women with PID develop associated peritonitis. Liver function tests usually are within normal limits. The condition is treated conservatively with anti-inflammatories while the woman is receiving treatment for the primary infection of PID.[15]

Reactive Arthritis

Reactive arthritis, a member of the spondylarthritis family of disorders, refers to an arthritis that appears after a urethritis or a diarrheal (enteric) illness.[18] *C trachomatis* and enteric pathogens are classic causative organisms. It is important to note that reactive arthritis refers to an

Table 23-5 Recommended Treatment Regimens for Pelvic Inflammatory Disease (PID)

Recommended Regimen*	Recommended Parenteral Regimen A
Ceftriaxone 250 mg IM in a single dose **Plus** Doxycycline 100 mg orally twice a day for 14 days **With or Without** Metronidazole 500 mg orally twice a day for 14 days **Or**	Cefotetan 2 g IV every 12 hours **Or** Cefoxitin 2 g IV every 6 hours **Plus** Doxycycline 100 mg orally or IV every 12 hours
Cefoxitin 2 g IM in a single dose and probenecid 1 g orally administered concurrently in a single dose **Plus** Doxycycline 100 mg orally twice a day for 14 days **With or Without** Metronidazole 500 mg orally twice a day for 14 days **Or**	**Recommended Parenteral Regimen B** Clindamycin 900 mg IV every 8 hours **Plus** Gentamicin loading dose IV or IM (2 mg/kg of body weight), followed by a maintenance dose (1.5 mg/kg) every 8 hours. Single daily dosing may be substituted
Other parenteral third-generation cephalosporin (e.g., ceftizoxime or cefotaxime) **Plus** Doxycycline 100 mg orally twice a day for 14 days **With or Without** Metronidazole 500 mg orally twice a day for 14 days	**Alternative Parenteral Regimens** Ampicillin/sulbactam 3 g IV every 6 hours **Plus** Doxycycline 100 mg orally or IV every 12 hours

* The addition of metronidazole should be considered, as anaerobic organisms are suspected in the etiology of the majority of PID cases. Metronidazole will also treat bacterial vaginosis (BV) if present.
Source: Centers for Disease Control and Prevention 2007.[17]

arthritis in which the organism cannot be extracted from the affected joint(s), differentiating it from septic arthritis. The pathogenesis of this reaction is not well understood, but it appears most commonly to affect young adults.[19] Reactive arthritis is also used to refer to the triad of postinfectious arthritis, urethritis, and conjunctivitis once called

Reiter syndrome.[19] There are no specific diagnostic criteria for reactive arthritis; however, a consensus opinion in 1999 yielded parameters that can help to guide diagnosis, and the interested reader is referred to the opinion statement.[20]

Reactive arthritis is characterized by two clinical features, arthritis and enthesitis.[15,18] **Enthesitis** refers to pain and swelling of the enthesis, which is the name for the location where the tendon and ligaments insert at the bone. This typically occurs at the heels and fingers, causing sausage digits. The classic pattern is asymmetric oligoarthritis (defined as four or fewer joints), often affecting the lower extremities or other small joints. Persons may have extraarticular signs and symptoms, including genitourinary tract symptoms, conjunctivitis, oral ulcers, nail pitting, and rashes or genital lesions and balanitis.[18] Diagnosis is dependent upon obtaining a thorough history and evaluating for overall signs and symptoms. Nonspecific tests such as C-reactive protein, sedimentation rate, and complete blood count are not of any real utility.[18]

Unfortunately, by the time reactive arthritis occurs, the original causative organism may be not readily identifiable.[21,22] However, because *C trachomatis* often is asymptomatic, it would be worthwhile to evaluate for underlying infection, particularly in persons who are at risk for chlamydia. A history of a *C trachomatis* infection preceding the symptoms increases the probability of the diagnosis.[23]

The prognosis of reactive arthritis varies. Most individuals experience remission within 6 months following initiation of treatment, although chronic persistent arthritis can occur.[24] The mainstay of therapy for reactive arthritis includes maximum-dose, around-the-clock nonsteroidal anti-inflammatories (NSAIDs).[22] A course of at least 2 weeks of anti-inflammatory doses of an NSAID is recommended before resorting to other pharmacologic interventions. Other treatments include joint injections with glucocorticoids, disease-modifying antirheumatic drugs and biologic agents (anti-TNF agents).[22] These agents are likely best used in consultation with a rheumatologist. Antibiotics are not used to treat the arthritis specifically, although they may be indicated if there is evidence of ongoing genitourinary infection or carriage of potentially pathogenic organisms. There is no evidence to suggest that long-term antibiotic therapy is of any benefit.[25]

Lymphogranuloma Venereum

Lymphogranuloma venereum (LGV) is a genital ulcer disease caused by *C. trachomatis* (serovars L1, L2, and L3). LGV is common in tropical and subtropical areas of the world, including East and West Africa, India, parts of Southeast Asia, and the Caribbean, where it is endemic.[26] LGV is predominantly a disease of lymphatic tissue as opposed to mucosal chlamydial infections. LGV predominately causes infiltration of the initial site of infection.[27] The condition is generally characterized as one that begins with ulcer formation, followed several weeks later by painful inguinal lymphadenopathy with formation and rupture of **buboes** (unilateral painful inguinal lymph nodes). An anorectal syndrome can also occur and results in an inflammatory mass present in the rectum and retroperitoneum[27] with associated rectal discharge, anal pain, fever, constipation, and/or tenesmus (inability to completely defecate or difficulty with defecation).[4] The majority of individuals with LGV proctitis in the United States have been HIV-infected homosexual males. Since men have been predominately affected by this relatively uncommon condition in the United States, a provider who suspects an individual has LGV is advised to follow the CDC recommendation to contact local or state health departments for specific, current management guidance.

Neisseria Gonorrhoeae

Neisseria gonorrhoeae was first noted by Albert Neisser in stained smears of urethral, vaginal, and conjunctival exudate in 1879.[28] The estimated global incidence of gonorrhea is 62 million infected persons annually,[1] and it is the second most commonly reported infectious disease in the United States.[3] There was an overall marked decline of gonorrhea incidence from 1975 through 1997; however, since 1997, the gonorrhea infection rate is increasing.[3] Like other sexually transmitted diseases, gonorrhea likely is substantially underdiagnosed and underreported, and approximately twice as many new infections are estimated to occur each year as are reported.[29] In medical parlance, gonorrhea is referred to as GC, an abbreviation for gonococcus, which is the abbreviation that is used in this chapter.

Geographical differences in the incidence of gonorrhea have been noted in the United States, with the southern region having the highest rates of infection.[3] Gonorrhea is estimated to be the causative organism in 40% of cases of PID.[30]

Complications of the disease include pelvic inflammatory disease (PID) in women, with subsequent risk of spontaneous abortion, preterm labor and birth, infertility, and ectopic pregnancy.[1] In approximately 1% of cases, the gonococcus becomes invasive, leading to disseminated gonococcal infection (DGI), endocarditis, and meningitis.[1] In addition, studies suggest that presence of gonorrhea infection makes an individual three to five times more likely to acquire HIV if concurrently exposed to both STIs.[30]

Substantial racial, ethnic, and age disparities are present in the prevalence of both chlamydial and gonococcal infections, with non-Hispanic Black persons under the age of 25 years having the greatest burden of disease prevalence.[7] Coinfection with GC and chlamydia is common, and both should be treated if one is identified or suspected.[7,31]

Pathogenesis, Microbiology, and Taxonomy

The genus *Neisseria* contains a number of species that are normal flora in humans and animals.[3] However, *N gonorrhoeae*, the causative organism of gonorrhea, is always considered to be pathogenic.[3] *N gonorrhoeae* is a gram-negative intracellular diplococcus that exclusively affects humans. This microorganism primarily infects the mucocutaneous surfaces of the genitourinary tract, pharynx, conjunctiva, and anus, with infections often asymptomatic.

A serological typing method for *N gonorrhoeae* was developed with monoclonal antibodies in 1984.[3] Infections with *N gonorrhoeae* are caused by a large number of different strains, and discrimination of these help with tracking epidemiologic phenomena relating to this infectious disease. Unfortunately, while there are serum tests available for gonorrhea, their utility is rather limited as serovar differentiation testing is not widely available.

Antimicrobial resistance remains an important consideration in the treatment of gonorrhea, and in 1986, the Gonococcal Isolate Surveillance Project, a national sentinel surveillance system, was established to monitor trends in antimicrobial susceptibilities of strains of *N gonorrhoeae* in the United States.[3] Recent evidence from this ongoing surveillance project has yielded important information about antibiotic susceptibility.

Prevention and Screening

The CDC and the U.S. Preventive Services Task Force (USPSTF) have recommended that all screening strategies be guided by the local prevalence of disease.[32] Because GC infections among women may be asymptomatic, an essential component of gonorrhea control in the United States continues to be the screening of those who are at high risk for STIs. Women who are younger than 25 years of age generally are at highest risk for gonorrhea infection. Other risk factors for gonorrhea include a previous gonorrhea infection, infection with other STIs, new or multiple sex partners, inconsistent condom use, commercial sex work, and drug use. Screening of low-risk populations is not recommended by the USPSTF. All pregnant women at risk for gonorrhea or living in an area in which the prevalence of *N gonorrhoeae* is high should be tested preconceptionally or at the first prenatal visit, and testing should be repeated during the third trimester for those at continued risk. A summary of recent USPSTF gonorrhea screening recommendations is shown in Table 23-6.

Transmission and Clinical Manifestations

There is considerable overlap between the signs and symptoms of gonorrhea and chlamydia infection. When symptoms occur, vaginal discharge and poorly differentiated

---

Table 23-6 USPSTF Recommendations for Gonorrhea Screening

Population	Recommendation for Screening for *Gonorrhea*	Grade of Recommendation*
Nonpregnant sexually active women who are ≤ 25 years of age	Benefits of screening substantially outweigh harms.	B
Pregnant women at increased risk[†]	Screening recommended at first prenatal visit and again in third trimester for women at continued risk or those who develop a new risk factor during pregnancy. Benefits of screening substantially outweigh harms.	B
Nonpregnant women not at increased risk	No clear certainty that benefits of screening outweigh harms.	D
Pregnant women not at increased risk	Insufficient evidence to recommend for or against routine screening.	I

* Grade B = fair evidence that this recommendation improves important health outcomes and that the benefits outweigh the harms; grade D = fair evidence that this recommendation is ineffective and that the harms outweigh benefits; grade I = evidence that this recommendation is effective is lacking, of poor quality, or conflicting, thus the balance of benefits and harms cannot be determined.
[†] Increased risk factors include a history of previous sexually transmitted infection, new or multiple sexual partners, inconsistent condom use, sex work, and drug use. In communities with a high prevalence of gonorrhea, broader screening of sexually active young people may be warranted.
Source: United States Preventive Services Task Force 2008.[32]

abdominal pain or lower abdominal pain are the most frequently reported. Pain is atypical in the absence of upper tract infection.[33-35] Gonococcal urethritis should be suspected in young, sexually active women with urinary symptoms such as frequency, dysuria, and pyuria.[34]

Diagnosis

Diagnosis of infection with *N gonorrhoeae* may be achieved by testing endocervical, vaginal, male urethral, or urine specimens.[36] Depending upon the site of collection, the CDC has outlined a guide to proper specimen collection as noted in Table 23-2.[36,37]

The gold standard for the diagnosis of gonorrhea is culture using a modified Thayer-Martin medium developed in the 1960s.[3] Cultures from endocervical specimens range in sensitivity from 80% to 100% in symptomatic women. Culture is considered to have a high specificity of ≥ 99%.[11,37]

An EIA was developed to detect gonococcal antigens from cervical swab or urine specimens, but it is not widely used because its positive predictive value is acceptable only in populations with a high prevalence of infection.[33]

DNA probes are approved by the Food and Drug Administration (FDA) for diagnosis of gonorrhea from endocervical swabs.[36] In most studies, culture and DNA probe assays have shown similar accuracy for detection of *N gonorrhoeae*.

Reporting Requirements

Because of the serious consequences of misdiagnosing gonorrhea or misidentifying strains of *N gonorrhoeae*, the CDC has recommended criteria for reporting diagnoses of gonorrhea.[3] Three levels of diagnosis are defined on the basis of clinical findings or the results of laboratory diagnostic tests (Table 23-7).

Treatment

Ongoing data from the CDC's Gonococcal Isolate Surveillance Project demonstrate that fluoroquinolone-resistant gonorrhea is now widespread in the United States and continues to increase. As a consequence, this class of antibiotics is no longer recommended for the treatment of gonorrhea in the United States (Table 23-8).

Follow-Up

Except for pregnant women with concurrent chlamydial infections, a test of cure is not recommended for persons

Table 23-7 CDC Recommendations for Three Levels of Diagnosis for *N Gonorrhoeae*

Diagnostic Category	Definition
Suggestive diagnosis	Requires *both* of the following: 1. A mucopurulent endocervical or urethral exudate on physical examination. 2. Sexual exposure to a person infected with *N gonorrhoeae*.
Presumptive diagnosis	Made on the basis of *one of the following three criteria*: 1. Typical gram-negative intracellular diplococci on microscopic examination of a smear of urethral exudate from men or endocervical secretions from women.* 2. Growth of a gram-negative, oxidase-positive diplococcus, from the urethra (men) or endocervix (women) on a selective culture medium, and demonstration of typical colonial morphology, positive oxidase reaction, and typical gram-negative morphology. 3. Detection of *N gonorrhoeae* by a nonculture laboratory test (e.g., antigen detection test such as Gonozyme [Abbott]), direct specimen nucleic acid probe test (e.g., Pace II [Gen-Probe]), nucleic acid amplification test (e.g., LCR [Abbott]).
Definitive diagnosis	Requires *both* of the following: 1. Isolation of *N gonorrhoeae* from sites of exposure (e.g., urethra, endocervix, throat, rectum) by culture (usually a selective medium) and demonstrating typical colonial morphology, positive oxidase reaction, and typical gram-negative morphology. 2. Confirmation of isolates by biochemical, enzymatic, serologic, or nucleic acid testing, e.g., carbohydrate utilization, rapid enzyme substrate tests, serologic methods such as coagglutination, or fluorescent antibody tests supplemented with additional tests that will ensure accurate identification of isolates, or a DNA probe culture confirmation technique.

* The observation of gram-negative, intracellular diplococci on microscopic examination of endocervical secretions from women must be supported by a positive result from a test from either No. 2 or No. 3.
Source: Centers for Disease Control and Prevention 2006.[4]

treated with the recommended or alternative regimens unless therapeutic compliance is in question, symptoms persist, or reinfection is suspected. If a test for cure is performed, it should be performed at least 3 weeks after therapy is completed. Health departments are encouraged to inform the CDC of *N gonorrhoeae* treatment failures and, if possible, arrange for *N gonorrhoeae* culture and testing

Table 23-8 Recommended Treatment Regimens for Gonococcal Infections

Uncomplicated Gonococcal Infections of the Cervix, Urethra, and Rectum*		Uncomplicated Gonococcal Infections of the Pharynx*
Recommended Regimens	**Alternative Regimens**	**Recommended Regimens**
Ceftriaxone 125 mg IM in a single dose	Spectinomycin 2 g in a single IM dose†	Ceftriaxone 125 mg IM in a single dose
Or	**Or**	**Plus**
Cefixime 400 mg orally in a single dose or 400 mg by suspension (200 mg/5 mL)	Single-dose cephalosporin regimens such as ceftizoxime 500 mg IM; or cefoxitin 2 g IM, administered with probenecid 1 g orally; or cefotaxime 500 mg IM‡	Treatment for chlamydia if chlamydial infection is not ruled out
Plus		
Treatment for chlamydia if chlamydial infection is not ruled out		

* These regimens are recommended for all adults and adolescents regardless of travel history or sexual behavior.
† Spectinomycin is currently not available in the United States.
‡ Some evidence indicates that cefpodoxime 400 mg and cefuroxime axetil 1 g might be oral alternatives.
Source: Centers for Disease Control and Prevention 2007.[36]

Table 23-9 Overview of Viral Hepatitis

Characteristics	HAV	HBV	HCV	HDV*	HEV*
Viral structure	RNA	DNA	RNA	RNA	RNA
Mode of Transmission					
Sex	Rare	Yes	Rare	Yes	No
Fecal–oral/food	Yes	Rare	No	No	Yes
Blood	Rare	Yes	Yes	Yes	No
Chronic infection possible	No	Yes	Yes	Yes	No
Incubation period (time between exposure and development of first symptoms)	2–10 weeks	6–20 weeks	4–10 weeks	Shortened if HBV coinfected	2–10 weeks

* Uncommon in the United States.
Source: Centers for Disease Control and Prevention, 2007.[40]

of any isolate for susceptibility to CDC-recommended regimens used for treatment.[36]

Disseminated Gonococcal Infection

A rare complication that is associated with *N gonorrhoeae* infection is **disseminated gonococcal infection** (DGI).[37] This infection is more common in women than men, a finding that is likely related to a higher incidence of asymptomatic gonococcal infection in women.[38] Other risk factors for women include recent menstruation, pregnancy or early postpartum, congenital or acquired complement deficiencies, and systemic lupus erythematosus. DGI frequently results in petechial or pustular skin lesions of limbs, asymmetrical arthralgia, tenosynovitis, or septic arthritis and, although rare, may be complicated by perihepatitis, endocarditis, or meningitis.[4] Hospitalization is recommended for initial therapy and is beyond the scope of this chapter. Individuals treated for DGI should be treated presumptively for concurrent *C trachomatis* infection, unless excluded by specific testing.[11]

▋ Viral Hepatitis

Many forms of viral hepatitis exist. Five such viral entities (i.e., hepatitis A–E) occur within the United States. The common feature of all hepatitis viruses is their ability to cause inflammatory changes in the liver. This inflammatory process can range in severity from acute elevations in liver function tests to outright liver failure. Table 23-9 summarizes key differences among these five infections.[39]

Epidemiology

The CDC collects data and reports findings about hepatitis A, B, and C infections. For all of these three causes of viral hepatitis, men are more likely to become infected than are women. This gender difference is theorized to reflect risk behaviors that currently are more common among men.[39]

As noted in Table 23-9, hepatitis A virus (HAV) is transmitted through fecal–oral transmission routes including household contacts with persons infected with HAV, ingestion of raw or contaminated foods, and international travel among both sexes. Anal sex is also a risk factor, and men who have sex with men are at greater risk of HAV infection than other groups.[39] The two most common risk factors for HBV transmission in the United States are sexual exposure followed by intravenous drug use.[39]

Hepatitis C virus (HCV) infection remains the leading cause of liver transplantation in the United States. The predominate mode of HCV transmission in the United States is intravenous drug use. While sexual transmission is possible, research on transmission has failed to be definitive.[39]

Prevention of Hepatitis

Vaccination remains the mainstay of HAV and HBV prevention. Current vaccination recommendations for these vaccines are provided in Table 23-10 and in Chapter 6.[40-42]

For the nonvaccinated person who is exposed to HAV, vaccination with hepatitis A vaccine should be initiated as soon as possible.[40] It is also recommended that individuals exposed to HAV receive an injection of immune globulin (Gamimune) that should be repeated every 3–5 months if exposure to HAV continues. Immune globulin consists of antibodies that protect against HAV and is 85% effective if given within the first 2 weeks following exposure.

Immune globulin is recommended for household contacts and sexual contacts of persons diagnosed with HAV, travelers to countries where sanitation is a problem or where HAV is prevalent, staff in institutions where an outbreak of HAV occurs, infants < 1 year of age who need protection, and persons who are exposed to HAV but who are allergic to the vaccination.

Side effects of immune globulin include soreness at the site of injection and occasionally a low-grade fever. Rarely, a life-threatening allergic reaction can occur, which is more likely if the agent is injected into an artery or vein.

For the nonvaccinated person who is exposed to HBV, clinical guidelines recommend the initiation of hepatitis B immune globulin (HBIG) 0.06 mL/kg by intramuscular injection as soon as possible after exposure (i.e., within 24 hours of needlestick or ocular or mucosal exposure or within 14 days of sexual exposure). The typical dose is 3–5 mL. In addition, the individual should begin the HBV vaccination series. HBIG is repeated at 28–30 days after exposure in nonresponders to HBV or for those who decline vaccination.[41,42]

Diagnosis

The diagnosis of HCV and HAV infections is relatively simple. HAV is diagnosed by testing for antibody (IgM)

Table 23-10 Recommendations for Hepatitis A and B Vaccination

Hepatitis A	Hepatitis B
All children at age 1 year	All newborns
Household contacts of persons with HAV	Household and sexual contacts of persons with HBV
All sexually active persons who are not in a long-term mutually monogamous relationship	All sexually active persons who are not in a long-term mutually monogamous relationship
HCV infection	HCV infection
Occupational exposure	Occupational exposure
Users of injection and noninjection illicit drugs	Current or recent injection drug users
Men having sex with men	Men having sex with men
Commercial sex workers	Commercial sex workers
Those traveling or working in countries that have endemic hepatitis A at high/intermediate levels	Those traveling or working in countries that are in HBV endemic regions
Persons with clotting factor disorders	Inmates in long-term correctional settings
Persons with chronic liver disease	Persons with chronic liver disease
Any person desiring protection from HAV infection	Any person desiring protection from HBV infection
	Residents or staff of facilities for developmentally disabled persons
	Persons with end-stage renal disease, including predialysis, hemodialysis, peritoneal dialysis, and individuals on home dialysis
	Household contacts of adoptees from HBV-endemic countries
	Immigrants and children of immigrants from areas with elevated rates of HBV
	Persons who are HIV positive
	Persons seeking evaluation or treatment for a sexually transmitted disease

Sources: Centers for Disease Control and Prevention 2001[40]; Mast EE, et al. 2005.[42]

to HAV (anti-HAV) along with either clinical signs/symptoms or liver function test elevations suggestive of acute disease.[39] Similarly, HCV disease is diagnosed by antibody to HCV infection (anti-HCV), but fewer cases result in frank signs/symptoms of infection, making serology and liver function analysis the mainstay of diagnosis. In addition to anti-HCV serology, the clinician may also obtain an HCV quantitative RNA level (i.e., viral load), which is generally detectable within 2 months of infection.[39,43] The serology for HBV infection is far more complex and is presented in Table 23-11[44] and Figure 23-1.

Table 23-11 Hepatitis B Serology

Serology	Indication of Infection
Hepatitis B surface antigen (HBsAg)	Present during acute or chronic infection and is indicative of infectious HBV infection.
Hepatitis B surface antibody (anti-HBs)	Evidence of immunization or recovery from previous infection.
Hepatitis B core total antibody (anti-HBc)	Present for life if HBV viral infection has occurred. Will not be present if immunity is secondary to vaccination.
IgM antibody to hepatitis B core antigen (IgM anti-HBc)	Demonstrates acute or recent HBV infection and will disappear within 6 months of acute disease.
Hepatitis B e antigen (HBeAg)	Individual is highly infectious.

Source: Adapted from Lok AS, McMahon BJ 2007.[44]

Treatments

The treatment of hepatitis infection is complex and is best managed by experienced clinicians, often specializing in gastroenterology or infectious diseases. Providers of women's primary care should be cognizant of the roles of various therapies and the management considerations for females. In general, the goal of treating hepatitis B and C is to reduce the viral load to undetectable limits, thereby preventing the consequences associated with chronic liver disease such as hepatocellular carcinoma.

Treatment of Hepatitis A

There is no specific treatment for hepatitis A. Administration of immune globulin and initiation of the hepatitis A vaccine is the first step following exposure. Individuals who contract HAV are treated symptomatically. The goal is to avoid liver damage. If the disease is mild and treatment is on an outpatient basis, the person is counseled to avoid alcohol and acetaminophen (Tylenol). Other prescription medications that have a risk of liver compromise may be discontinued temporarily. Persons with fulminant hepatitis will require hospitalization.

Treatment of Hepatitis B

The treatment of chronic HBV is centered on interrupting the HBV viral life cycle in a similar manner to treatment

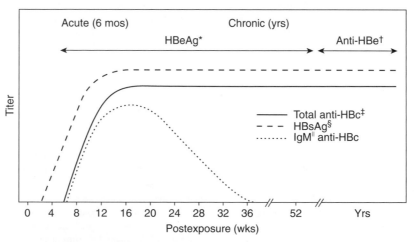

* Hepatitis B e-antigen.
† Antibody to HBeAg.
‡ Antibody to hepatitis B core antigen.
§ Hepatitis B surface antigen.
‖ Immunoglobulin M anti-HBc.

Figure 23-1 Typical serological course of acute hepatitis B virus (HBV) infection with progression to chronic HBV infection. *Source:* Centers for Disease Control and Prevention 2008.[91]

of HIV. In fact, some drugs used in the treatment of persons with HIV infection also are used to treat HBV. For this reason, persons coinfected with HIV and HBV have special treatment considerations aimed at treating both viral infections concomitantly.

Increased viral load measurements of HBV RNA are associated with a higher prevalence of hepatocellular carcinoma, hepatic failure, and cirrhosis.[45,46] Therefore, reduction in HBV DNA and prevention of complications associated with infection are considered the gold standard for monitoring success of HBV treatment. Biochemical monitoring of HBV treatment includes every-3-months-evaluation of alanine transaminase (ALT) levels, alpha-fetal protein levels (AFP), HBV RNA, and for seroconversion of hepatitis B e antigen (HBeAg) to a negative status. In addition, yearly ultrasound of the liver should be considered for high-risk individuals.[44]

Six agents have been approved for treatment of chronic HBV infection in the United States. The standard of care for treatment of the individual who has HBV but not HIV is presented in Table 23-12.

Treatment of Hepatitis C

The treatment of HCV infection is based on stimulating an appropriate antiviral immunologic response. Two FDA-approved medications for the management of HCV disease are the ones most commonly employed. The current standard of care for HCV therapy includes pegylated interferon alpha 1.5 mcg/kg/week in a subcutaneous injection. This agent requires reconstitution from powder form and usually is self-administered in combination with ribavirin, in which the dose is weight-based and usually ranging from 800 mg to 1200 mg/day.[47] The goal of HCV therapy

Table 23-12 FDA-Approved Drugs for the Treatment of Hepatitis B Infection

Drug Generic (Brand)	Class of Agent	Clinical Considerations
Pegylated interferon-alfa (Pegasys)	Synthetic interferon	Influenza-like symptoms may be severe. Avoid use during pregnancy and counsel on the use of two reliable contraceptive methods.
Lamivudine (Epivir)	Nucleoside reverse transcriptase inhibitor (NRTI)	Must be on fully suppressive ART regimen if coinfected with HIV due to cross-resistance with single-drug therapy. Abrupt discontinuation may result in severe acute HBV exacerbation. Monitor ALT for several months after stopping therapy. Lactic acidosis, a class side effect of NRTI therapy, appears to occur with greater frequency in women. Obesity and prolonged NRTI exposure may be risk factors.
Tenofovir (Viread)	Nucleoside reverse transcriptase inhibitor (NRTI)	Must be on fully suppressive ART regimen if coinfected with HIV due to cross-resistance with single-drug therapy. Abrupt discontinuation may result in severe acute HBV exacerbation. Monitor ALT for several months after stopping therapy. Lactic acidosis, a class side effect of NRTI therapy, appears to occur with greater frequency in women. Obesity and prolonged NRTI exposure may be risk factors.
Adefovir (Hepsera)	Nucleoside reverse transcriptase inhibitor (NRTI)	Must be on fully suppressive ART regimen if coinfected with HIV due to cross-resistance with single-drug therapy. Abrupt discontinuation may result in severe acute HBV exacerbation. Monitor ALT for several months after stopping therapy. Lactic acidosis, a class side effect of NRTI therapy, appears to occur with greater frequency in women. Obesity and prolonged NRTI exposure may be risk factors.
Entecavir (Baraclude)	Nucleoside reverse transcriptase inhibitor (NRTI)	Must be on fully suppressive ART regimen if coinfected with HIV due to cross-resistance with single-drug therapy. Abrupt discontinuation may result in severe acute HBV exacerbation. Monitor ALT for several months after stopping therapy. Lactic acidosis, a class side effect of NRTI therapy, appears to occur with greater frequency in women. Obesity and prolonged NRTI exposure may be risk factors.
Telbivudine (Tyzeka)	Nucleoside reverse transcriptase inhibitor (NRTI)	Abrupt discontinuation may result in severe acute HBV exacerbation. Monitor ALT for several months after stopping therapy. No HIV-associated activity.

Source: Lok AS et al. 2007.[44]

is to achieve a sustained viral response (i.e., an undetectable viral load) after completion of therapy. Individuals who have failed to achieve an undetectable viral load by 12 weeks on therapy are considered to have treatment failure and therapy is withdrawn.

Combination therapy for HCV has numerous side effects, primarily influenza-like symptoms. In addition to fevers, chills, and night sweats, combination therapy may result in significant reductions in hemoglobin and hematocrit levels that may necessitate initiation of an erythropoietin-stimulating agent. Irritability and mood swings are commonly reported among individuals undergoing HCV treatment; therefore, family-based counseling that prepares significant others for such personality changes may benefit both the individual and any personal relationships.[48]

Due to lack of available clinical trial data, combination therapy for HCV infection is contraindicated in pregnancy and women should be counseled to avoid pregnancy for 6 months posttreatment. Use of combination therapy in children less than 3 years of age currently is contraindicated.[49] Women of childbearing potential and their sexual partners should be counseled on the importance of barrier protection methods in addition to the use of a reliable and effective method of contraception during combination therapy. Everyone with HCV infection should be vaccinated against HAV and HBV infection.[49]

Human Immunodeficiency Virus

The virus that causes **acquired immune deficiency syndrome** (AIDS) was first identified in 1984, which was 3 years after the epidemic was first reported in the United States among homosexual men.[50] What came to be known as **human immunodeficiency virus** (HIV) mobilized the gay community in ways never before seen and resulted in the allocation of federal resources for pharmaceutical development. In 1987, clinical trials with the first antiretroviral drug, zidovudine (AZT, ZDV), were prematurely terminated to obtain accelerated approval by the FDA due to marked improvement in the clinical condition among recipients. Unfortunately, these improvements were soon found to be associated with worsening symptoms and the return of opportunistic infection due to the emergence of drug resistance. Zidovudine was not a cure for AIDS, but it began the reframing of HIV/AIDS as a chronic, manageable—albeit life-altering—disease.

Since the implementation of zidovudine (AZT), the list of antiretroviral medications has grown extensively and rapidly. Recently, two novel classes (e.g., entry inhibitors and integrase inhibitors) have been FDA approved, notably for treatment of drug-resistant forms of HIV. Prescribers initiating **antiretroviral therapy** (ART) for the treatment of drug-naïve women now consider pill burden and limitation of treatment-related side effects the essential aspects of regimen selection. Improvements not only in quantity, but also in quality of life are allowing more HIV-infected individuals to consider family planning options, influencing the ART regimen of choice. A thorough understanding of the key issues affecting women with HIV/AIDS will assist the provider of primary and specialty women's health services to adequately address these issues.

Epidemiology

Throughout the 1980s, the American public and scientific community tended to ignore the signs of heterosexual HIV transmission in developing countries due to the perceived and epidemiologically identified risk groups early in the US epidemic. As early as 1983, the first reports from Haiti and Africa noted heterosexual transmission with cases described in these reports from the late 1970s.[50,51] Phylogenetic testing has now tracked the origins of HIV to a primate host with the first documented human case from Africa in 1959.[52]

Unfortunately, women in the United States were not identified as targets for research or prevention efforts during the early years of the epidemic.[53] Further, stigma associated with the disease prevented open discussions about high-risk sexual practices; therefore, most early prevention campaigns failed to discuss heterosexual transmission. At the time, women represented approximately 1% of known cases in the United States,[54] making this prevention effort appear epidemiologically relatively unimportant.

However, over the years research has shown that in heterosexual relationships, women are more likely to acquire HIV infection than men. The increased risk of acquiring HIV infection in women has been attributed to a number of anatomic and biologic factors including: (1) greater exposed surface area in the female genital area; (2) higher levels of HIV in semen and pre-ejaculate; (3) more semen than vaginal fluid is exchanged during sexual acts; and (4) untreated sexually transmitted infections are more common in women.[55,56]

Statistics from 2005 reveal that women accounted for 26% of the 33,163 newly diagnosed HIV cases among adults and adolescents in the United States, and women of color were disproportionately affected. This population accounts for more than 79% of AIDS cases in women.[57]

HIV-infected women have also been documented to experience disparities in access to HIV care and prescriptions for antiretroviral therapy. Data on vertical transmission demonstrate that **prevention of mother-to-child transmission** (PMTCT) efforts have been successful. Current data indicate that fewer than 2% of infants born to HIV-positive mothers are infected. This low transmission rate is a result of several interventions including maternal treatment with ART during the antepartum and intrapartum periods, infant ART prophylaxis for 6 weeks after birth, planned cesarean section for mothers with viral loads greater than 1000 copies/mL, and avoidance of breastfeeding.[58] Providers of women's health are uniquely positioned to address the issues involving disparities in the care and treatment of HIV-infected women because they can actively provide HIV counseling, promotion of prevention, and early diagnosis of infection.[59]

The CDC currently recommends offering yearly testing for HIV infection as part of routine screening for everyone between the ages of 13 and 64. In addition, the agency recommends including HIV testing as part of pregnancy screening programs as well as HIV testing for persons presenting for treatment of other STIs at each visit.[59]

Testing Choices for Screening and Diagnosis

Women presenting with signs/symptoms consistent with acute retroviral syndrome (see *Clinical Progression of HIV to AIDS* later in this chapter) should be tested using rapid oral enzyme-linked immunosorbent assay (ELISA), if available. If positive or if rapid diagnostics are not available, a serum ELISA and western blot should be obtained. If acute seroconversion is expected, the clinician should obtain a viral load (e.g., RNA PCR), which can detect viral replication during seroconversion when the HIV antibody test is negative or indeterminate. If an individual presents for routine screening purposes, a rapid oral ELISA should be obtained, if available. If positive or if rapid diagnostics are not available, a serum ELISA and western blot should be ordered.[60]

Pathophysiology of HIV Infection

HIV Life Cycle and Corresponding Targets of Antiretroviral Therapy

After infection, the HIV viral life cycle follows a series of predictable steps. The basic steps in this process are summarized here in the order of occurrence and illustrated in Figure 23-2. Specific antiviral agents work by interfering with different steps in the life cycle.

Attachment and entry: The HIV virus requires specific receptors for attachment and cannot infect every cell of the

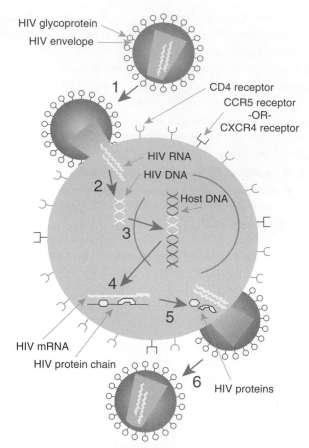

(1) Free virus. (2) Binding, fusion, and infection: Virus binds to a CD4 molecule and fuses with the cell. (3) Reverse transcription: Single strands of viral RNA are converted into double-stranded DNA by the reverse transcriptase enzyme. (4) Transcription: When infected cell divides, viral DNA is read and long HIV protein chains are made. (6) Budding and maturation: Immature virus buds out of the cell, taking some of infected cell's membranes with it; breaks free and matures into new HIV virus.

Figure 23-2 Life cycle of HIV infection. *Source:* AIDSinfo 2005.[92]

body. The **cluster of differentiation 4** (CD4) protein has a special HIV coreceptor known as gp120. Viral surface receptors (i.e., CXCR4 and CCR5) attract the CD4 proteins to the virus as well as coreceptor binding for attachment and entry.

Reverse transcription: HIV is a retrovirus, i.e., a ribonucleic acid (RNA) virus that must convert itself into deoxyribonucleic acid (DNA) before it can effectively communicate with a host CD4 cell. This conversion process is catalyzed by the enzyme reverse transcriptase, which copies the single-stranded RNA into double-stranded DNA. Reverse transcriptase inhibitors block this conversion process.

Integration: Once HIV RNA is copied into proviral DNA, the enzyme integrase forces HIV's genetic blueprint into the DNA of the CD4 protein. Production of HIV proteins is then permanently occurring whenever the CD4 protein is stimulated. Integrase inhibitors block this step and prevent proviral integration within the CD4 genome.

Transcription and translation: The CD4 cell produces the key proteins for formation of a new HIV virion or viral particle in the form of messenger RNA. Once back in the cytoplasm, the messenger RNA undergoes translation by proteins into strains of long protein sequences.

Assembly: Long protein sequences assemble near the cell surface where the HIV enzyme protease cleaves them into functional HIV proteins. Protease inhibitors block this step, resulting in a nonviable virion.

Budding and maturation: Once assembled and cut, the budding process begins through the cell wall. Maturation occurs when the viral particle has separated from the cell wall and the viral envelope is complete.

Immunologic Effects of HIV Infection

Viral infection produces a robust immunologic response. As HIV viral load increases during acute infection, millions of anti-HIV antibodies are produced. These antibodies, along with cytotoxic T cells, gradually reduce viral replication, and a viral set point for the HIV viral load of the individual is established. In general, the lower this set point, the slower the progression of HIV to AIDS. Over time and without treatment, HIV gradually depletes absolute CD4 numbers, increasing the probability of opportunistic infection.

Clinical Progression of HIV to AIDS

Shortly after infection, and generally during the process of seroconversion, a person infected with HIV may develop signs and symptoms collectively known as an **acute retroviral syndrome**. Recognition of the signs and symptoms of acute HIV infection by providers varies considerably within the literature[61,62] and has been attributed, in part, to the widely varied descriptions of symptoms associated with this syndrome (ranging from no apparent illness to severely debilitating disease).[62] When symptoms do occur, they are often similar to a mononucleosis-like illness with fever, pharyngitis, myalgias, headache, adenopathy, and rash the most commonly reported.

After seroconversion, the progression from HIV to AIDS depends on a variety of factors including the viral set point, the viral load, and access to interventions to improve and maintain general health. Gender differences in some aspects of HIV infection do exist. For example, women infected with HIV have viral load levels that are lower across the spectrum of the disease compared to infected men with similar CD4 counts.[63] This does not translate, however, into a decline in progression from HIV to AIDS for women, even when women have similar access to HIV care and treatment.[64]

Management Considerations for the Woman Infected with HIV

The management of HIV is a subspecialty practice and is the purview of clinicians with appropriate clinical training and experience in this area. However, providers in women's health care should be knowledgeable about the primary care and prevention aspects of HIV management, although initiation of ART should be undertaken with consultation with an HIV specialty provider. The best practice is to refer the individual to an HIV specialist to establish a relationship for long-term care whenever possible.

Recent Changes to the Management of HIV/AIDS

Clinical guidelines for HIV/AIDS management are routinely updated to reflect changes in practice. The most recent US Department of Health and Human Services guidelines recommend **highly active antiretroviral therapy** (HAART) for any person with an AIDS-defining illness *or* with a history of a CD4 count less than 350 cells/mm³. This change reflects recent data regarding improvements in HAART toxicity as well as clinical data demonstrating better clinical outcomes when HAART is initiated at higher CD4 counts.[65] Pregnant women, individuals with HIV-associated nephropathy, and persons with HBV should be started on HAART regardless of CD4 count.

Initiation of HAART therapy early in the clinical course of disease indicates the need for early referral to HIV care. Box 23-1 provides a brief list of primary care responsibilities of the primary care provider while awaiting HIV specialty care as noted across various treatment guidelines.[59,60,65]

General Principles of HAART

The initiation of HAART is not an emergency. The person who requires HAART also requires counseling and preparation in order to understand possible side effects as well as adherence strategies. Guidelines for the management of HIV/AIDS identify the following four factors as the primary goals of HAART: (1) maximal and durable suppression of HIV viral load; (2) restoration or preservation of immunologic function; (3) improvement in quality of life; and (4) a reduction of HIV-related morbidity and mortality.[65]

In addition to these factors, the clinician should also seek to limit the side effects of HAART. In general,

Box 23-1   HIV Primary Care Considerations for the Women's Health Provider

Refer the individual to an HIV care provider if she is currently not receiving HIV care.

Counsel regarding the need for HAART, if CD4 count and opportunistic infection history warrant.

If available, offer HIV testing to sexual and drug partners or provide counseling on the need for disclosure and follow-up testing of these persons. Offer testing of children if appropriate.

Discuss thoughts and desires regarding pregnancy. Recommendations on preconception counseling are clearly outlined in the November 2, 2007, CDC guidelines.

Give routine vaccinations (for persons with CD4 counts greater than 100 cells/ mm^3):

Influenza (yearly)

Pneumococcal vaccination (every 5 years)

Hepatitis A and B (complete series as directed)

Tetanus/diphtheria (every 10 years)

Perform yearly cervical Pap smear and gynecologic evaluation including yearly screening for gonorrhea, chlamydia, and syphilis if she is sexually active.

In addition, Women with CD4 count ≤ 200 cells/mm^3 should receive:

Cervical Pap smear every 6 months

Prophylaxis for *Pneumocystis jiroveci* pneumonia (i.e., PCP) and toxoplasmosis after a review of allergy and treatment history. Options include:

One trimethoprim-sulfamethoxazole double-strength or single-strength pill daily

Double strength if toxoplasmosis IgG is positive or unknown

Single strength if toxoplasmosis IgG is negative

One dapsone 100-mg pill daily

Aerosolized pentamidine 300 mg every 4 weeks via nebulizer

Sources: Centers for Disease Control and Prevention 2006[59]; Cooper DA et al. 1985[60]; Pham PA et al. 2005.[65]

---

antiretroviral classes of medication may have the same type of side effects across the entire class of agents due to similar mechanisms of action and pharmacologic properties.

HAART for Women of Childbearing Age

The pharmacologic properties of HAART may differ during pregnancy compared to when women are not pregnant. Additionally, there are potential drug–drug interactions between HAART medications and contraceptives (Box 23-2). The reader is referred to the *Recommendations for Use of Antiretroviral Drugs in Pregnant HIV-Infected Women for Maternal Health and Interventions to Reduce Perinatal HIV Transmission in the United States*[58] to assess specific medications and the implications of HIV treatment during pregnancy. Table 23-13 provides an overview of the potential major side effects and adverse events of each class of medication along with special considerations for women who are HIV positive.

Postexposure Prophylaxis

Professionals who provide care to women should be knowledgeable of **postexposure prophylaxis** (PEP) guidelines for healthcare workers who may experience occupational exposure as well as knowledge of PEP for persons who

Box 23-2 When HIV Is Just Another Chronic Disease

A 42-year-old nonsmoking woman has been living with HIV for more than a decade and regularly obtains health care from a specialist in infectious medicine. However, she is seeking primary care for contraception as she was widowed 3 years ago and now is entering a new relationship.

Women in their forties may have a decreased fecundity when compared to cohorts in their 20s; however, that does not mean they are infertile. Identification of the best contraception can only be made by the woman herself. However, the clinician can suggest to this woman a wide range of options. Condoms should be promoted because of the sexually transmitted nature of HIV.

In regard to the options available, some potential concerns exist about theoretical risks of drug interaction between HAART and combined oral contraceptives. In addition, many of the HAART drugs have side effects regarding insulin sensitivity and other metabolic dysregulation, an area of concern with systemic hormonal contraception.[89] The method with the most advantages is likely to be the levonorgestrel intrauterine system (Mirena) that has been found to decrease menstrual flow among women with HIV while providing contraception with minimal side effects.[90] Ultimately the most effective method is the one that the woman will use successfully.

During her primary care visit, issues such as open communication with the new partner, importance of regular Pap testing, keeping vaccinations current, and general care such as routine mammograms should be discussed.

Table 23-13 Overview of Major Side Effects and Adverse Events of HIV Medications

Drug Category	Mechanism of Action/Comments	Drug Generic (Brand)	Clinical Considerations
Nucleoside reverse transcriptase inhibitors (NRTIs)	NRTIs are faulty versions of building blocks that HIV needs to make more copies of itself. When HIV uses an NRTI instead of a normal building block, reproduction of the virus is stalled. Lactic acidosis, a class side effect of NRTI therapy, appears to occur with greater frequency in women. Obesity has been associated with prolonged NRTI exposure.	Zidovudine or AZT (Retrovir)*	Anemia may be more pronounced in menstruating women. Side effects include headaches, mania, depression, myositis, and insomnia.
		Lamivudine or 3TC (Epivir)*	
		Emtricitabine or FTC (Emtriva)†	
		Abacavir or ABC (Ziagen)†	Pharmacokinetic studies have failed to find differences between men and women.
		Tenofovir or TDF (Viread)‡	No interactions found with ethinyl estradiol/hormonal contraceptives. Avoid during pregnancy because of potential fetal bone effects. Decreases in bone mineral density may occur, necessitating monitoring, especially of perimenopausal/postmenopausal women.
		Stavudine or D4T (Zerit)‡	Side effects include peripheral neuropathy.
		Didanosine or DDI (Videx or Videx EC)†	Side effects include peripheral neuropathy.
Nonnucleoside reverse transcriptase inhibitors (NNRTIs)	NNRTIs bind to and disable reverse transcriptase, a protein that HIV needs to make more copies of itself.	Efavirenz or EFV (Sustiva)‡	Known teratogen during first trimester, although use after first trimester may be considered. Advocate reliable contraceptive method for sexually active reproductive-aged women. Induces CYP3A4 and inhibits CYP3A4, 2C9, 2C19, and 2B6. May increase concentrations of ethinyl estradiol, but clinical significance is questionable. Side effects include hallucinations and disorientation.
		Nevirapine or NVP (Viramune)	Cannot be used in women with CD4 count *greater* than 250 cells/mm³ due to risk of severe hepatotoxicity in women with high CD4 counts. Several studies have noted an increase in NVP-associated rash among women.

(continues)

Table 23-13 Overview of Major Side Effects and Adverse Events of HIV Medications (*continued*)

Drug Category	Mechanism of Action/Comments	Drug Generic (Brand)	Clinical Considerations
			Use in pregnant women with CD4 count > 250 only if benefits clearly outweigh risk. In pharmacokinetic studies, women had a 13.8% lower clearance of nevirapine. CYP3A4 > 2B6 substrate induces CYP3A4 and 2B6. May decrease efficacy of estrogen-containing contraceptives.
		Delavirdine or DLV (Rescriptor)[‡]	Data from pharmacokinetic studies suggest that plasma concentrations of delavirdine are higher in females. This difference is not considered clinically significant. May increase concentrations of ethinyl estradiol, but clinical significance is unlikely.
		Tenofovir or TDF or PMPA (Viread)	
Protease inhibitors (PIs)	PIs disable protease, a protein that HIV needs to make more copies of itself. Protease inhibitors have been associated with changes in glucose intolerance. However no study to date has verified an increase in gestational diabetes. All PI drugs influence liver metabolism through cytochrome P pathways (CYP) and thus are involved in multiple drug–drug–herb interactions, including *Hypericum perforatum* or St. John's wort—an agent that decreases efficacy of the PI. Some studies have suggested that dietary supplements of garlic, vitamin C, milk thistle, and echinacea (coneflower) also may decrease PI efficacy, but clinical significance has not been demonstrated.	Lopinavir-ritonavir or LPV (Kaletra)[‡]	Unclear pharmacokinetic data regarding dosing (2 pills bid versus 3 pills bid). Pharmacokinetic data from studies conducted in pregnant women revealed lower levels of LPV during the third trimester. Pregnant women using LPV require dose adjustments during the third trimester. Inhibits CYP3A4 > 2D6 and possibly induces CYP1A2, 2C19, 2C9, and 2B6. May decrease efficacy of estrogen-containing contraceptives.
		Indinavir or IDV (Crixivan)[†]	Inhibits CYP3A4 and may increase efficacy of estrogen-containing contraceptives.
		Fosamprenavir or FOS (Lexiva)[†]	Inhibits CYP3A4 and induces CYP3A4 and may decrease efficacy of PI when administered with estrogen-containing contraceptives.
		Atazanavir or ATV (Reyataz)[†]	Inhibits CYP3A4 and may increase efficacy of estrogen-containing contraceptives. Needs dose adjustment and ritonavir boosting when used with tenofovir.
		Darunavir or DRV (Prezista)[†]	CYP3A4 substrate and may decrease efficacy of estrogen-containing contraceptives.
		Saquinavir or SQV (Fortovase)[†]	Weak inhibitor of CYP3A4 and usually used with ritonavir, resulting in possible reduction of efficacy of estrogen-containing contraceptives.
		Nelfinavir or NFV (Viracept)[†]	Inhibits CYP3A4, 2B6 and may decrease efficacy of estrogen-containing contraceptives.
		Ritonavir or RTV (Norvir)[†]	Currently used only in lower doses to boost the effects of other PIs. Inhibits CYP3A4 > 2D6 > 2C9 > 2C19 > 2A6 > 2E1, and 2B6. Induces GT, CYP1A2, and possible 2C9, 2C19, and 2B6 and may decrease efficacy of estrogen-containing contraceptives.
Integrase inhibitors	Integrase inhibitors disable integrase, a protein that HIV uses to insert its viral genetic material into the genetic material of an infected cell.	Raltegravir (Isentress)[†]	Pharmacokinetic studies have failed to find differences between men and women.
Entry inhibitors	Entry/fusion inhibitors work by blocking HIV entry into cells.	Enfuvirtide or T-20 (Fuzeon)[†]	
		Maraviroc (Selzentry)[†]	

(*continues*)

Table 23-13 Overview of Major Side Effects and Adverse Events of HIV Medications (*continued*)

Drug Category	Mechanism of Action/Comments	Drug Generic (Brand)	Clinical Considerations
Combination drugs	Fixed-dose combination tablets contain two or more anti-HIV medications that can be from 1 or more drug classes.	Combination AZT/3TC (Combivir)*	See previous Clinical Considerations for individual agents.
		Combination TDF/FTC (Truvada)[†]	See previous Clinical Considerations for individual agents.
		Combination ABC/3TC (Epzicom)[†]	See previous Clinical Considerations for individual agents.
		Combination EFV/TDF/FTC (Atripla)[‡]	See previous Clinical Considerations for individual agents.
		Combination AZT/3TC/ABC (Trizivir)[†]	See previous Clinical Considerations for individual agents.

* Recommended for use during pregnancy for preventing mother to child transmission.
[†] Not recommended as first-line agent in pregnancy.
[‡] Avoid during pregnancy.
The use of DDI in combination with D4T is not recommended due to an increased risk for mitochondrial toxicity and peripheral neuropathy.

experience a high-risk sexual or blood exposure. The CDC has developed clear risk-based algorithms for occupational and nonoccupational exposures. In general, therapy should be initiated less than 72 hours after exposure. Before beginning any guideline-based PEP, the clinician should evaluate the pharmacologic principles of the drug, drug–drug interactions, dosing, and side effects in addition to appropriately weighing the risks and potential benefit of such treatment.[66]

Additionally, it is important to monitor for HAART-related side effects especially since individuals continue the use of these medications for several years. There is a particular need to monitor the effects of HAART when used during pregnancy to determine any patterns of adverse outcomes that might be associated with a drug or combination of drugs. The Antiretroviral Pregnancy Registry is a voluntary, prospective, observational study that collects data and analyzes it for any evidence of teratogenic events that might be associated with HAART use during pregnancy and postnatally. Persons can be registered online or via fax at the Antiretroviral Pregnancy Registry (*www.apregistry.com*). Importantly, in order to maintain confidentiality, no personal identifying information is collected. Another Web site of note for professionals is the National HIV/AIDS Clinician's Consultation Center that offers a large number of resources (*www.nccc.ucsf.edu*).

Genital Human Papillomaviruses

Introduction

Human papillomavirus (HPV) is a double-stranded DNA virus that includes more than 100 genotypes and can infect cutaneous or mucosal epithelial tissue. Thirty to 40 of the HPV virus genotypes infect the genital area. Genital HPV is the most common STI in the United States with approximately 20 million persons currently infected, and at least 50% of sexually active men and women will acquire it at some point in their lives. Approximately 50% of the individuals who become infected with HPV are sexually active adolescents and young adults between 15 and 24 years of age.[67] As with many other STIs, the majority of new HPV infections are subclinical and asymptomatic.[68]

Genital HPV types are divided into high and low risk based on their association with the development of cervical cancer Table 23-14. The two low-risk types, HPV 6 and HPV 11, cause 90% of ano-genital warts,[67] whereas HPV 16 and 18 are detected in a high percentage of cancers of the genital tract and anus. HPV types 16, 18, 31, 33, 45, 52, and 58 account for 95% of cervical cancers.[67,70] Between 5% and 30% of individuals are infected with multiple types of HPV. About 10% of women infected with HPV develop persistent HPV infections.

Persistent cervical infection with selected types of HPV is the single most important risk factor for cervical cancer.

Table 23-14 HPV Serotype Risk Classification

	High risk	Probable High risk	Low risk	Undetermined Risk
HPV Serotype	16*, 18*, 31, 33, 35, 39, 45, 51, 52, 56, 58, 59, 68, 73, 82	26, 53, 66	6[†], 11[†], 40, 42, 43, 44, 54, 61, 70, 72, 81, CP6108	34, 57, 83

* Cause of 70% of cervical cancers and 50% of precancerous cervical lesions.
[†] Etiology of anogenital warts and recurrent respiratory papillomatosis.
Sources: Adapted from Zonofrio NJ et al. 2008[73]; Kahn JA 2009.[67]

Cervical cancer is the second most common cancer in women and the third most common cause of cancer-related mortality worldwide. The incidence of invasive cervical cancer varies dramatically across populations based on the availability of screening and treatment for cervical cancer and its precursor lesions as well as the immune status of each woman.[71]

Most infections are transient and are probably self-cured by the body's immune system. A study of college students found that among 91% of women with new HPV infections, HPV became undetectable within 2 years.[69] The median duration of infections is typically 8 months. The point prevalence of cervical HPV has ranged from 14% to 35% depending on the population and sensitivity of the detection method.[69]

Pathogenesis, Microbiology, and Taxonomy

Human papillomaviruses are theorized to enter the body after slight trauma to the epithelium. The virus needs terminally differentiated epithelial cells for replication (Figure 23-3). All HPV types replicate only within the cell's nucleus, but the mechanism by which HPV types transform cells is unclear. All HPV types infect the mucous membranes of the skin; however, the various forms establish themselves in specific cell types.

Screening and Prevention

Consistent and correct use of condoms has been demonstrated to reduce transmission of HPV up to 70%.[72] In 2006, a new quadrivalent vaccine that protects against HPV types 6, 11, 16, and 18 was approved by the FDA.[67,73] The vaccine is recommended for all females ages 11–26 years old and is given through a series of three shots over a 6-month period.[67] The CDC guidelines also state that the vaccine may be given to girls at age 9 or older.

Side effects include soreness at the site of injection and bruising. As of December 2008, no adverse effects that appear directly linked to the vaccine have been reported through the postmarketing Vaccine Adverse Event Reporting System.[67] The vaccine is not recommended for pregnant women or persons who are immunocompromised because there has been limited research on these populations.[67]

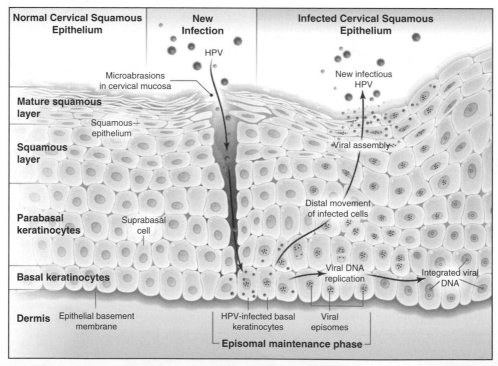

The HPV infects basal keratinocytes through microabrasions in the skin or mucosa; with viral DNA replication, the copy number of the virus is amplified to approximately 50 to 100 copies per cell. The initial genome amplification is followed by an episomal maintenance phase. Infected basal cells then enter the suprabasal compartment, where abundant expression of early and late genes and productive genome amplification to high copy numbers is triggered in the terminally differentiating compartments. Viral assembly occurs in the upper layer of the squamous epithelium, and virions are then released and may infect adjacent tissue. Because of the mechanism by which HPV infects and replicates in the host's epithelial cells, the virus is able to largely evade the host's immune system. Thus, the innate and adaptive immune responses to natural infection are limited, and although most infections are controlled, eventually antibody concentrations tend to be low or undetectable.

Figure 23-3 Human papillomavirus life cycle in the squamous epithelium. *Source:* Reproduced from Kahn JA 2009.[67] Copyright © 2009 Massachusetts Medical Society. All rights reserved.

The vaccine is relatively new and the duration of immunogenicity has not been determined.

Approximately 30% of cancers will not be prevented by the vaccine, which is why it is important for women to continue obtaining regular Pap tests.[67] Additional information about vaccination against HPV can be found in Chapter 6.

Clinical Manifestations

Genital HPV is transmitted by skin-to-skin and genital contact including vaginal, anal, and oral sex. Infection can be diagnosed clinically (genital warts), cytologically (Pap test), or virologically (DNA detection). Genital warts are typically the only visible sign of HPV infection, and they may not appear for months or years after infection. Women are more likely than men to develop warts, and they can grow on the lips of the vulva, around the clitoris, inside the vagina, around the urethra and the cervix, and in the perianal region. In immune-suppressed women (e.g., women with advanced HIV disease), progression of HPV to precancerous or cancerous lesions can be more rapid.

Treatment

In the absence of genital warts or cervical squamous intracellular lesions, treatment is not recommended for subclinical genital HPV infection. Genital warts can be removed surgically, with chemical treatment or with electrical current. The primary goal of treating visible genital warts is the removal of the warts. Genital warts have been shown to resolve spontaneously in 20–30% of women within a 3-month period. Conversely, development of new lesions or recurrence at previously treated sites is common. CDC treatment regimens are presented in Table 23-15. It is unknown whether treatment reduces transmission. Treatment can be self- or provider administered. Most women require a course of therapy rather than a single treatment, and the treatment modality should be changed when the warts have not improved substantially following the CDC treatment guidelines. Multiple treatments without improvement also suggest reconsideration of the original diagnosis, as it may suggest that the lesion is not caused by HPV.

Special Populations

Pregnancy

No link has been found between HPV and spontaneous abortion, premature delivery, or other pregnancy complications. Hormone changes during pregnancy can cause warts to multiply or enlarge. Imiquimod (Aldara), podophyllin, and podofilox (Condylox 0.5%) are contraindicated

Table 23-15 Treatment Regimens for Genital Warts

External genital warts; treatment applied by woman	Podofilox 0.5% solution or gel (Condylox 0.5%). Women should apply podofilox solution with a cotton swab, or podofilox gel with a finger, to visible genital warts twice a day for 3 days, followed by 4 days of no therapy. This cycle may be repeated, as necessary, for up to four cycles. The total wart area treated should not exceed 10 cm², and the total volume of podofilox should be limited to 0.5 mL per day. If possible, the healthcare provider should apply the initial treatment to demonstrate the proper application technique and identify which warts should be treated. The safety of podofilox during pregnancy has not been established. **Or** Imiquimod 5% cream (Aldara). Women should apply imiquimod cream once daily at bedtime, three times a week for up to 16 weeks. The treatment area should be washed with soap and water 6–10 hours after the application. The safety of imiquimod during pregnancy has not been established.
External genital warts; treatment provider-administered*	Cryotherapy with liquid nitrogen or cryoprobe. Repeat applications every 1–2 weeks. **Or** Podophyllin resin 10%–25% in a compound tincture of benzoin. A small amount should be applied to each wart and allowed to air dry. The treatment can be repeated weekly, if necessary. To avoid the possibility of complications associated with systemic absorption and toxicity, two important guidelines should be followed: (1) application should be limited to < 0.5 mL of podophyllin or an area of < 10 cm² of warts per session; and (2) no open lesions or wounds should exist in the area to which treatment is administered. Some specialists suggest that the preparation should be thoroughly washed off 1–4 hours after application to reduce local irritation. The safety of podophyllin during pregnancy has not been established. **Or** Trichloroacetic acid (TCA) or bichloracetic acid (BCA) 80%–90%. A small amount should be applied only to the warts and allowed to dry, at which time a white frosting develops. If an excess amount of acid is applied, the treated area should be powdered with talc, sodium bicarbonate (i.e., baking soda), or liquid soap preparations to remove.

(continues)

Table 23-15 Treatment Regimens for Genital Warts (*continued*)

Vaginal warts	Cryotherapy with liquid nitrogen. The use of a cryo-probe in the vagina is not recommended because of the risk for vaginal perforation and fistula formation.
	Or
	TCA or BCA 80%–90% applied to warts. A small amount should be applied only to warts and allowed to dry, at which time a white frosting develops. If an excess amount of acid is applied, the treated area should be powdered with talc, sodium bicarbonate, or liquid soap preparations to remove unreacted acid. This treatment can be repeated weekly, if necessary.
Urethral meatal warts	Cryotherapy with liquid nitrogen.
	Or
	Podophyllin 10–25% in compound tincture of benzoin. The treatment area must be dry before contact with normal mucosa. This treatment can be repeated weekly, if necessary. The safety of podophyllin during pregnancy has not been established.

* Alternative regimens include intralesional interferon OR laser surgery.
Recommended regimens for cervical warts: For women who have exophytic cervical warts, high-grade squamous intraepithelial lesions (SIL) must be excluded before treatment is initiated. Management of exophytic cervical warts should include consultation with a specialist.
Source: Centers for Disease Control and Prevention 2006.[4]

in pregnancy, and treatment is often postponed until after pregnancy if possible. In rare cases, HPV types 6 and 11 can cause respiratory papillomatosis in infants and children, which may require laser surgery. There is no evidence to support cesarean section to prevent this rare complication in the newborn.[69]

Genital Herpes Simplex Virus

Infections caused by the herpes simplex virus types 1 (HSV-1) and 2 (HSV-2) are highly prevalent.[74] These infections are associated with substantial morbidity, and can be a cofactor in the transmission and acquisition of the human immunodeficiency virus (HIV).[75] Approximately 17% of adults in the United States have antibodies to HSV-2, and 58% have antibodies to HSV-1.[74] Over two thirds of infected adults are unaware of their infections; consequently the majority of infections are transmitted by these individuals.[76] Classically, HSV-1 tends to be associated with oral herpes and HSV-2 associated with genital herpes. However, HSV-1 is now linked to increasing proportions of newly diagnosed genital herpes.[77-80] Genital herpes is more common among women than men, and is reported more frequently among African Americans than Whites. The cumulative lifetime incidence of HSV-2 is approximately 25% in White women, 20% in White men, 80% in African American women, and 60% in African American men.[74]

HSV-2 is transmitted sexually (genital to genital, oral to genital, or genital to oral) and perinatally (mother to child). The majority of genital herpes infections are transmitted by persons unaware that they have the infection and/or who have subclinical symptoms when transmission occurs.[76] Longitudinal studies of serologically discordant couples indicate a transmission rate from 3% to 12% per year. The frequency of transmission is influenced by gender and frequency of sexual activity. Women have higher rates of acquisition than men, probably due to anatomic differences that lead to greater mucosal surface area exposed in the genital area of women compared with men. Soap and water cleansing and drying readily inactivate HSV; therefore, fomite transmission is unlikely.[81]

Pathogenesis

Infection with HSV-2 occurs via inoculation of virus onto susceptible mucosal surfaces (e.g., the oropharynx, cervix, conjunctivae) or through abrasions on the skin. The initial cellular response is predominantly polymorphonuclear, followed by lymphocytic response. Concomitant with the initial infection, HSV ascends peripheral sensory nerves and establishes latency in sensory or autonomic nerve root ganglia. Latency can be established after both symptomatic and asymptomatic initial infection. Infection persists despite the host immune response, often resulting in recurrent disease. Available evidence suggests that most, if not all, HSV-2 seropositive persons have intermittent reactivations associated with HSV viral shedding on mucosal surfaces.[81] Reactivations may be symptomatic or asymptomatic. Thus, symptoms are not an accurate way to determine transmissibility or activation. Individuals who are immunocompromised have both more frequent and more severe reactivations.

Clinical Manifestations

The clinical manifestations of genital herpes differ significantly between the primary, nonprimary, and subsequent episodes. A true primary infection is the first infection with either HSV-1 or HSV-2. When symptomatic, these episodes are associated with systemic symptoms and more severe disease than nonprimary or recurrent episodes. Twenty-five percent of individuals with first clinical episode of HSV-2 have had a prior asymptomatic primary infection. Primary genital HSV-2 episodes are characterized by frequent and prolonged systemic and local symptoms including fever, headache, malaise, and myalgias. Systemic symptoms appear early in the course of the disease, usually peak within the 3–4 days of the onset of lesions, and gradually recede over the subsequent 3–4 days. Pain, itching, dysuria, vaginal or urethral discharge, and tender inguinal adenopathy are the predominant local symptoms of disease. Inguinal adenopathy peaks in weeks 2–3 after initial onset and is often the last finding to resolve. Dysuria, both external and internal, appears more frequently in women (83%) than in men (44%). The urethral discharge is usually clear and mucoid, and the severity of the dysuria is often out of proportion to the amount of urethral discharge elicited on genital exams. In both men and women with primary genital HSV infection, vesicopustular or ulcerative lesions on the external genitalia are the most frequent presenting sign. The number, size, and shape of the ulcerative lesions vary greatly between persons.[81]

Nonprimary HSV is newly acquired infection with HSV-1 or HSV-2 in an individual previously seropositive to the other virus. Manifestations tend to be milder than with primary infection. Type-specific antibody will be present, and the severity of the episode is comparable to a recurrence.

In contrast to primary or nonprimary infection, symptoms manifested during recurrent HSV-2 infections are usually localized to the genital region. As with other HSV infections, symptoms tend to be more severe in women than in men. Considerable variability exists in the severity and duration of recurrent disease both among individuals and in a single person between episodes. Recurrences may last from 2 to 16 days; be associated with significant or minimal pain, itching, and dysuria; and involve few or many lesions.

HSV Cervicitis

Approximately 70–90% of women with first-episode HSV-2 infection also have HSV cervicitis. Primary genital HSV cervicitis may be symptomatic or asymptomatic. Areas of diffuse or focal redness and bleeding, extensive ulcerative lesions of the exocervix, or severe necrotic cervicitis may be seen.

Complications: Aseptic Meningitis

Central nervous system involvement such as aseptic meningitis is not uncommon with primary HSV-2 infections. In one series of persons with primary HSV-2, such an adverse effect was reported in 36% of women and 13% of men.[81] Fever, headache, vomiting, photophobias, and nuchal rigidity are the predominant symptoms of HSV aseptic meningitis. While it appears to be a benign disease in immunocompetent persons, aseptic meningitis occasionally may require hospitalization or parenteral opiates for pain management.

Diagnosis

The clinical diagnosis of genital herpes is insensitive and nonspecific. In a prospective study of persons at risk for HSV-2 infection, only 39% of those with newly acquired HSV-2 were diagnosed on clinical grounds. In addition, 20% of those who were given a clinical diagnosis of genital herpes were not infected, suggesting that false-positive diagnosis based on clinical symptoms occurs frequently.[82] Clinical diagnosis of genital herpes should be confirmed by laboratory testing. HSV DNA polymerase chain reaction (PCR) has emerged as the best test to use when evaluating an individual who presents with genital herpes ulcers. The PCR is up to four times more sensitive than viral culture. While serologic assays for HSV-2 should be available for persons who request them, screening for HSV-1 or HSV-2 infection in the general population is not recommended.

Treatment

HSV systemic antiviral chemotherapy offers clinical benefits to the majority of individuals who are symptomatic and includes three oral medications: (1) acyclovir (Zovirax), (2) valacyclovir (Valtrex), and (3) famciclovir (Famvir). The CDC recommended treatment guidelines for the first clinical episode and suppressive and episodic therapy of genital herpes are presented in Table 23-16.

Table 23-16 Recommended Regimens for Treatment of Herpes

Treatment of First Clinical Episode of Genital Herpes*	Suppressive Therapy for Recurrent Genital Herpes	Episodic Therapy for Recurrent Genital Herpes
Acyclovir (Zovirax) 400 mg orally three times a day for 7–10 days	Acyclovir (Zovirax) 400 mg orally twice a day	Acyclovir (Zovirax) 400 mg orally three times a day for 5 days
Or	Or	Or
Acyclovir (Zovirax) 200 mg orally five times a day for 7–10 days	Famciclovir (Famvir) 250 mg orally twice a day	Acyclovir (Zovirax) 800 mg orally twice a day for 5 days
Or	Or	Or
Famciclovir (Famvir) 250 mg orally three times a day for 7–10 days	Valacyclovir (Valtrex) 500 mg orally once a day	Acyclovir (Zovirax) 800 mg orally three times a day for 2 days
Or	Or	Or
Valacyclovir (Valtrex) 1 g orally twice a day for 7–10 days	Valacyclovir (Valtrex) 1.0 g orally once a day	Famciclovir (Famvir) 125 mg orally twice daily for 5 days
		Or
		Famciclovir (Famvir) 1000 mg orally twice daily for 1 day
		Or
		Valacyclovir (Valtrex) 500 mg orally twice a day for 3 days
		Or
		Valacyclovir (Valtrex) 1.0 g orally once a day for 5 days

* Treatment might be extended if healing is incomplete after 10 days of therapy.
Source: Centers for Disease Control and Prevention, 2006.[4]

Acyclovir is an acyclic nucleoside analog that is a substrate for HSV-specified thymidine kinase (TK). Through a series of cellular enzymatic actions, acyclovir is incorporated into viral DNA where it then prevents DNA replication. Acyclovir has in vitro activity against both HSV-1 and HSV-2. Treatment with acyclovir reduces the duration of symptoms, viral shedding, and promotes lesion healing.

A major limitation of acyclovir (Zovirax) has been poor oral availability, as only a small fraction of the dose is absorbed. Valacyclovir (Valtrex), an ester of acyclovir, increases the bioavailability of acyclovir to 54%. Oral famciclovir (Famvir) is 77% bioavailable and the drug appears to be well tolerated. Acyclovir, famciclovir, and valacyclovir have all been shown to be beneficial when taken orally in reducing the duration of recurrent genital herpes.[81] Studies comparing valacyclovir to acyclovir in genital HSV infection have shown the drugs to be comparable in the immunocompetent host. Valacyclovir offers potential convenience through reduced dosing frequency.

Side effects during therapy with any of these three drugs are rare. Rare adverse effects include neutropenia, Stevens-Johnson syndrome, and hepatitis. More information on the pharmacokinetics and drug–drug interactions associated with these antiviral medications can be found in Chapter 11.

The clinical effect of acyclovir on first-episode infection is considerable, reducing fever and constitutional symptoms within 48 hours of initiating therapy and rapidly relieving symptoms. Therapy should be initiated for all women with presumptive first-episode genital HSV who present with active lesions. While treatment of first-episode infection markedly shortens the course of first-episode, it has no discernible effect on the long-term natural history of recurrences.

Suppressive Antiviral Therapy

Recurrence rates in individuals infected with HSV-2 vary. On average, individuals who report symptomatic genital HSV have five to eight recurrences in the first year after the initial outbreak. Several studies have shown that daily acyclovir therapy is effective in preventing clinical recurrences for 65–85% of those infected as long as the therapy is continued. Because frequently recurring genital herpes can affect some persons for years, many individuals choose to take oral acyclovir for prolonged periods, although few individuals use it for longer than 2 years. Suppressive therapy most often is recommended when, according to the woman, recurrences are unacceptably high, severe, painful, or associated with depression or anxiety. Suppressive therapy also may be used when a woman is undergoing a particularly stressful period or has another illness that is triggering the recurrence. No clinical or laboratory toxicities have been reported, although long-term therapy has been in clinical use for more than a decade. In addition to preventing clinical recurrences, suppressive therapy with acyclovir has been shown to reduce viral shedding, which is highest within the first year of acquisition. Thus, early suppressive therapy may prevent transmission.[81]

Episodic Therapy for HSV

Episodic therapy for some individuals with genital HSV is an option; however, the symptom control is likely to be significantly less than for those on suppressive therapy. Effective episodic treatment for recurrent herpes requires initiation of therapy within 1 day of lesion onset or during the prodrome period. The woman should be provided with the drug so she can begin therapy at the onset of symptoms. Studies indicate that it takes between 5 and 7 days for the clinical effect of episodic therapy to be apparent.[81]

Syphilis

Introduction

Syphilis is a human bacterial infection caused by the spirochete *Treponema pallidum*. Global estimated incidence of syphilis is 12 million new cases annually in 1999, with more than 90% occurring in developing countries.[1,83] In the United States, the CDC established the Syphilis Elimination Effort with an operational goal to reduce syphilis incidence to less than 1000 cases of primary and secondary syphilis reported per year.[84] Since the beginning of this initiative by the CDC in 1999, rates of congenital syphilis have declined by 39%, rates among women overall have decreased by 60%, and rates among Blacks have decreased by 37%.[84] However, data from more recent years indicate overall rates of primary and secondary syphilis have gradually been on the rise since 2001, presenting challenges and new opportunities for reframing prevention efforts.

Syphilis is usually transmitted by sexual contact or from mother to infant, although endemic syphilis is transmitted by nonsexual contact in communities living under poor hygiene conditions.[85] *Treponema pallidum* can also be transmitted by blood transfusion, and it is able to survive in the human host for several decades. It is capable of infecting all tissues and is relatively painless. It is a slowly evolving disease marked by long asymptomatic periods and short symptomatic periods during which the organism is multiplying rapidly.

Pathogenesis, Microbiology, and Taxonomy

Historically, the understanding of *T pallidum* pathophysiology has been limited by the inability to grow the organism in culture. *T pallidum* is a delicate, corkscrew-shaped organism with tightly wound spirals that can be viewed with dark-field microscopy. Syphilis is characterized by different phases that have varying signs and symptoms, depending upon the length of infection. These phases are referred to as primary, secondary, and tertiary (or late) syphilis. In pregnant women, syphilis can lead to stillbirth or congenital infection of the neonate, resulting in neonatal death or late sequelae.

Transmission and Clinical Manifestations

Syphilis is transmitted via direct, genital–genital (including anal) or oral–genital contact, and in utero through the placenta or at the time of birth. Syphilis is believed to be transmissible during early disease (primary and secondary syphilis).[4] The first stage of the disease, primary syphilis, occurs 10–90 days after infection and is characterized by a chancre—a painless ulceration—usually found on the genitals. The sore is infectious and appears at the site of inoculation. A painless chancre may aid the clinician in distinguishing it from herpes simplex virus (HSV) infection and *Haemophilus ducreyi* (chancroid), although the presence or absence of pain is not always a reliable clinical clue.[85] This entity resolves spontaneously.

Manifestations of secondary infection, appearing weeks to a few months later, include signs such as skin rash (notably on palms of hands and soles of feet), mucocutaneous lesions, and lymphadenopathy. Condylomata lata, raised, flat, papular lesions in moist areas, may occur anywhere on the genitalia, and they can be differentiated from HPV condylomata acuminata by their moist, smooth, flat appearance.[86] Meningitis is associated with syphilis and most often occurs within the first year after infection, although it can occur years later, resulting in symptoms characteristic of bacterial meningitis including headache, confusion, nausea, vomiting, and stiff neck.[87] A woman with meningitis may have visual complaints or auditory complaints. Meningitis may cause hydrocephalus as well as arteritis of small-, medium-, or large-sized vessels, leading to ischemia or infarction of brain or spinal cord, perhaps presenting as an ischemic stroke in a young person.[87] Similar to primary disease, the acute manifestations of secondary syphilis typically resolve spontaneously, even in the absence of therapy.

Tertiary or late infection occurs as a result of late syphilis, and this stage may appear at any time from 1 to 30 years after primary infection and involve a wide variety of different tissues. The most concerning manifestations of late tertiary syphilis are neurosyphilis (tabes dorsalis), a slow nerve degeneration, and cardiovascular syphilis.[85] Tabes dorsalis can result in paralysis, dementia, and blindness, and unfortunately, existing nerve damage cannot be reversed. Neurosyphilis rarely develops in persons after treatment with the penicillin regimens recommended for primary and secondary syphilis.

Latent infections (i.e., those lacking clinical manifestations) are detected by serologic testing. Latent syphilis acquired within the preceding year is referred to as early latent syphilis; all other cases of latent syphilis are either late latent syphilis or latent syphilis of unknown duration. The USPSTF recommends a longer duration of therapy for individuals with late latent syphilis due to the knowledge that the condition has a slower metabolism and a more prolonged dividing time. Clinicians having concerns about prolonged syphilis infections and complications should consult with a specialist prior to initiating a treatment regimen.

Testing

The diagnosis of syphilis is most commonly made by nontreponemal serologic tests (VDRL or RPR) that detect the presence of nonspecific antibodies that react to cardiolipin. False-positives can occur in persons with other conditions that generate these antibodies, such as pregnancy, autoimmune disorders, or a recent viral infection. False-negatives are also possible in both the primary and late stages of the disease. When titers of these tests are obtained, they will fall as treatment progresses. Therefore, the nontreponemal tests are useful for initial screening and for monitoring treatment. Treponemal-specific tests detect antibody specific to *T pallidum*. They are expensive and used only for confirming diagnosis. Culturing is not an effective method for testing.[88]

Treatment

The only known treatment for syphilis is penicillin G (Box 23-3). Penicillin G is administered parenterally for treating all stages of syphilis and is the only therapy with documented efficacy for syphilis during pregnancy[4] (Box 23-4). However, no comparative trials have been adequately conducted to guide the selection of an optimal penicillin regimen (i.e., the dose, duration, and preparation). Only the long-acting benzathine preparation (Bicillin LA) should be used for treatment of early syphilis since low and continuous levels of penicillin are necessary for the elimination of treponemes[4] (Table 23-17). Long-acting benzathine penicillin should only be given via the intramuscular route; intravenous administration has been associated with cardiopulmonary arrest and death. The preparation(s) used (i.e., benzathine, aqueous procaine, or aqueous crystalline), the dose, and the length of treatment depend on the stage and clinical manifestations of the disease. However, neither the combination of

---

Box 23-3 Gone But Not Forgotten: Syphilis

Syphilis is likely the oldest known sexually transmitted infection. In the years before antimicrobial cures and due to the stigma associated with the infection, afflicted individuals often sought to hide the telltale cutaneous signs of the disease (e.g., chancre, alopecia, rashes). Alopecia of the head was remedied by toupees; alopecia of pubic hair was disguised by merkins, or pubic wigs; and heavy makeup was used by men and women to hide blemishes. When fields of specialized medical study emerged in the 18th century, one of the areas was dermatology and venereology, a title still in use today within some medical centers and in several other countries like Singapore and China.

Attempts to deny the disease by disguising the dermatologic signs did not treat syphilis. For unknown reasons, heavy metals were used as a therapy for syphilis, dating as early as the 11th century. Shakespeare's play, *Measure for Measure*, includes a phrase about hollow bones, referring to decreased bone mineral density associated with mercury, by then a common treatment. Other interventions included drastic means, including induction of fevers by infecting the individual with malaria under the supposition that the fever might kill the disease.

By the early 20th century, an arsenic compound containing synthetic antimicrobial named salvarsan was developed in the lab of Paul Ehrlich, later immortalized in the 1940 Edward G. Robinson Academy Award–nominated film, *Dr. Erlich's Magic Bullet*. The last two words comprise the term that Ehrlich coined in his attempt to have an agent that effectively destroyed the organism without harming the host. Although the phrase *magic bullet* entered common language, Erhlich's treatment was not extremely effective, and the cure for syphilis remained elusive until the mid-20th century when penicillins became available.

■ Box 23-4 Syphilis During Pregnancy

A woman at 14 weeks' gestation has secondary syphilis. Her nontreponemal serologic test (RPR) and the treponemal test (FTA-ABS) are positive. Her nontreponemal titers (VDRL) titers are 1:256. Her past history is uneventful except she has a penicillin allergy confirmed by skin testing.

Treatment of this woman is complicated by her allergy. Syphilis has profound implications for the health of the woman and her fetus. A major cause of congenital syphilis in modern society is inappropriate therapy. The only effective method of treatment of the unborn child is through maternal penicillin therapy. If a woman reports a penicillin allergy and skin testing is negative, penicillin can be administered. However, this woman's positive skin test indicates the need for desensitization. Protocols for desensitization have been published by the CDC, and the process should be conducted in a hospital setting because of the risk of an IgE-mediated allergic reaction. The entire desensitization usually is completed within 4 hours.

After successful desensitization, this woman was treated with benzathine penicillin G 2.4 million units intramuscularly. Four weeks later, her laboratory results included VDRL 1:128. No labs were found for RPR or FTA-ABS.

Follow-up laboratory testing often does not include an RPR or a treponemal test since they often remain positive at least for a period of time. VDRL titers are used to verify treatment success through a fourfold decrease. This woman had a twofold decrease in titers. This finding can be a normal variation from the original 1:256 and does not confirm success of the therapy. Four weeks later (or at 22 weeks' gestation), this woman's VDRL was 1:16, indicating that the treatment was successful.

Health education is an important concern for persons with sexually transmitted infections. Any sexual partner should be screened and treated. A woman with syphilis also should be assessed for other STIs, including bloodborne diseases such as hepatitis and HIV as well as gonorrhea and chlamydia. This woman should know that certain laboratory levels such as treponemal-specific tests are likely to remain positive for years, if not for life. Eventually the VDRL titers may become nondetectable, although they may be reported as weakly reactive or remain sero fast for years as a 1:1 or 1:2 titer.

benzathine penicillin and procaine penicillin (Bicillin CR) nor oral penicillin preparations are considered appropriate for the treatment of syphilis. Prescribers should be aware of the similar names of these two products and avoid use of the inappropriate combination therapy agent for treating syphilis.[84]

For persons with penicillin allergy, alternative regimens include doxycycline (Dynapen), tetracycline (Sumycin), and azithromycin (Zithromax).[4] The use of these agents is not well studied in those with HIV infection, and there is some emerging evidence of azithromycin resistance; thus, close follow-up is particularly indicated for those individuals receiving alternate therapies to penicillin.[4]

For women in whom prolonged syphilitic infection (i.e., tertiary/late) or latent syphilitic infection (i.e., syphilis characterized by seroreactivity without other evidence of disease) is suspected, it is advised that consultation be made with a specialist to optimize selection of the best treatment regimen. The CDC 2006 treatment guidelines provide an overview of treatment of these uncommon conditions.[4]

Penicillin Allergy and Jarisch-Herxheimer Reaction

Penicillin allergy can be problematic as no proven alternatives to penicillin are available for treating neurosyphilis, congenital syphilis, or syphilis in pregnant women. Pregnant women with syphilis in any stage who report penicillin allergy should be desensitized and treated with penicillin.[4] Skin testing for penicillin allergy might be useful in pregnant women and others. The Jarisch-Herxheimer reaction is an acute febrile reaction frequently accompanied by headache, myalgia, and other symptoms that usually occur within the first 24 hours after any therapy for syphilis.[4] This reaction occurs most frequently among women who have early syphilis. Although it may induce early labor or cause fetal distress, therapy should still be initiated as the risk is clearly outweighed by the benefits.[4] Antipyretics may be used, but they have not been proven to prevent this reaction.

Management of Sex Partners

Persons exposed sexually to a partner who has syphilis in any stage should be evaluated clinically and serologically

Table 23-17 CDC Recommended Treatment for Syphilis in Adults

Syphilis Stage	Recommended Treatment

Primary, secondary, early latent syphilis	Benzathine penicillin G (Bicillin LA) 2.4 million units IM × 1*
	Alternative regimen:
	    Penicillin allergic, nonpregnant: (limited data to support)
	        Doxycycline (Dynapen) 100 mg PO bid × 14 days
	                    Or
	        Tetracycline (Sumycin) 500 mg PO qid × 14 days
	    Possible alternatives: (limited data to support)
	        Ceftriaxone (Rocephin) 1 g IM or IV × 8–10 days
	                    Or
	        Azithromycin (Zithormax) 2 g PO × 1 (reports of resistance)

Late latent or unknown duration, tertiary syphilis without neurologic involvement	Benzathine penicillin G (Bicillin CR) 7.2 million units IM total dose, administered as three doses of
	  2.4 million units IM each at 1-week intervals*
	Alternative regimen:
	    Penicillin allergic, nonpregnant: (limited data to support)
	        Doxycycline (Dynapen) 100 mg PO bid × 28 days,
	                    Or
	        Tetracycline (Sumycin) 500 mg PO qid × 28 days

Neurosyphilis (signs, symptoms, and/or neurologic findings), syphilitic eye disease	Aqueous crystalline penicillin G (Pfizerpen) 18–24 million units per day, administered as 3–4 million
	  units IV every 4 hours or continuous infusion for 10–14 days
	Alternative regimen: (if compliance can be ensured)
	    Procaine penicillin (Bicillin LA) 2.4 million units IM once daily for 14 days
	                    Plus
	Probenecid 500 mg PO qid for 10–14 days

* Standard benzathine penicillin, i.e., Bicillin LA, not to be confused with combination benzathine-procaine penicillin, i.e., Bicillin CR, which is not appropriate for treatment of syphilis.
Source: Centers for Disease Control and Prevention 2006.[4]

Box 23-5 CDC Guidelines for Managing the Care of Sex Partners of Persons Infected With Syphilis

Persons who were exposed within the 90 days preceding the diagnosis of primary, secondary, or early latent syphilis in a sex partner might be infected even if seronegative; therefore, such persons should be treated presumptively.

Persons who were exposed > 90 days before the diagnosis of primary, secondary, or early latent syphilis in a sex partner should be treated presumptively if serologic test results are not available immediately and the opportunity for follow-up is uncertain.

For purposes of partner notification and presumptive treatment of exposed sex partners, patients with syphilis of unknown duration who have high nontreponemal serologic test titers (i.e., > 1:32) can be assumed to have early syphilis. However, serologic titers should not be used to differentiate early from late latent syphilis for the purpose of determining treatment.

Long-term sex partners of individuals who have latent syphilis should be evaluated clinically and serologically for syphilis and treated on the basis of the evaluation findings.

For identification of at-risk sexual partners, the periods before treatment are: (1) 3 months plus duration of symptoms for primary syphilis, (2) 6 months plus duration of symptoms for secondary syphilis, and (3) 1 year for early latent syphilis.

Source: Centers for Disease Control and Prevention 2006.[4]

and treated with a recommended regimen, depending on various factors. The CDC guidelines for managing sex partners of persons infected with syphilis are presented in Box 23-5.

All individuals who have syphilis should be tested for other STIs, including HIV. In geographic areas in which the prevalence of HIV is high, individuals who have primary syphilis should be retested for HIV after 3 months if the first HIV test result was negative.[4]

Follow-Up

All individuals who have syphilis should be tested for other STIs, including HIV.[4] Clinical trial data have demonstrated that 15% of individuals with early syphilis treated with the recommended therapy will not achieve a two-dilution decline in nontreponemal titer used to define response at 1 year after treatment.

Because it is often difficult to distinguish treatment failure from reinfection with *T pallidum*, experts in infectious medicine usually are consulted or the woman is provided a referral.

Screening

The USPSTF recommends that clinicians screen for syphilis in persons at increased risk, including commercial sex workers, persons who exchange sex for drugs, and adults in correctional facilities. In addition, all pregnant women should be tested at their first prenatal visit. The USPSTF recommends against routine screening of asymptomatic persons who are not at increased risk for syphilis infection.[89]

Conclusion

Primary care clinicians have a major role in preventing, identifying, and providing services for STIs for women. STIs are extremely common and women are more frequently and severely affected by STIs than are men. Prompt diagnosis and treatment of STIs can interrupt transmission and prevent complications. The pharmacologic management of these infections is affected by resistance, compliance, and many complicated social and cultural factors. There have been several recent, important developments in therapy for STIs including global emergence of fluoroquinolone resistance in gonorrhea, new antiretroviral drugs for HIV treatment, and an understanding of the value of HSV-2 suppression for decreasing transmission to uninfected partners. Familiarity with the basic epidemiology, transmission, clinical manifestations, diagnosis, and treatment of STIs is crucial for women's health practitioners.

References

1. Weinstock H, Berman S, Cates W Jr. Sexually transmitted diseases among American youth: incidence and prevalence estimates, 2000. Perspect Sex Reprod Health 2004;36(1):6–10.
2. Cates W. Estimates of the incidence and prevalence of sexually transmitted diseases in the United States. Sex Transm Dis 1999;26(suppl.):S2–S7.
3. Centers for Disease Control and Prevention. Sexually transmitted disease surveillance, 2007. Atlanta, GA: United States Department of Health and Human Services, December 2008.
4. Centers for Disease Control and Prevention. Sexually transmitted disease treatment guidelines, 2006. MMWR Recomm Rep 2006;55(RR-11):1–95.
5. American Academy of Pediatrics. *Chlamydiatrachomatis*. In Pickering LK, ed. Red book: 2009 report of the Committee on Infectious Diseases, 28th ed. Elk Grove Village, IL: American Academy of Pediatrics:255–9.
6. Stamm WE. *Chlamydia trachomatis* infections of the adult. In Holmes K, Sparling P, Stamm W, Piot P, Wasserheit J, Corey L, et al., eds. Sexually transmitted diseases, 4th ed. China: McGraw-Hill, 2008:575–92.
7. Miller WC, Ford CA, Morris M, Handcock MS, Schmitz JL, Hobbs MM, et al. Prevalence of chlamydial and gonococcal infections among young adults in the United States. JAMA 2004;291(18):2229–36.
8. Laga M, Manoka A, Kivuvu M, Malele B, Tuliza M, Nzila N, et al. Non-ulcerative sexually transmitted diseases as risk factors for HIV-1 transmission in women: results from a cohort study. AIDS 1993;7(1):95–102.
9. Everett KD, Bush RM, Andersen AA. Emended description of the order *Chlamydiales*, proposal of *Parachlamydiaceae* fam. nov. and *Simkaniaceae* fam. nov., each containing one monotypic genus, revised taxonomy of the family *Chlamydiaceae*, including a new genus and five new species, and standards for the identification of organisms. Int J Syst Evol Microbiol 1999;49:415–40.
10. Bush RM, Everett KD. Molecular evolution of the chlamydiaeae. Int J Syst Evol Microbiol 2001;51:203–20.
11. Morrison RP, Manning DS, Caldwell HD. Immunology of *Chlamydia trachomatis* infections. In Quinn TC, ed.

Advances in host defense mechanisms. New York: Raven, 1992:57.

12. Centers for Disease Control and Prevention. Screening tests to detect *Chlamydia trachomatis* and *Neisseria gonorrhoeae* infections, 2002. MMWR 2002;51 (No. RR-15):1–27.

13. Meyers DS, Halvorson H, Luckhaupt S. Screening for chlamydial infection: an evidence update for the U.S. Preventive Services Task Force. Ann Intern Med 2007;147:135.

14. Hollblad-Fadiman K, Goldman SM. American College of Preventive Medicine practice policy statement. Screening for *Chlamydia trachomatis*. Am J Prev Med 2003;24(3):287–92.

15. Bailey PP, Green MB. Infectious processes: urinary tract infections and sexually transmitted diseases. In Buttaro TM, Trybulski J, Bailey PP, Sandberg-Cook J, eds. Primary care: A collaborative practice. St. Louis, MO: Mosby Inc, 1999:576–90.

16. Wang SA, Papp JR, Stamm WE, Peeling RW, Martin DH, Holmes KK. Evaluation of antimicrobial resistance and treatment failures for *Chlamydia trachomatis*: a meeting report. J Infect Dis 2005;191:917–23.

17. Centers for Disease Control and Prevention. Updated recommended treatment regimens for gonococcal infections and associated conditions—United States, April 2007. Available from: *www.cdc.gov/std/treatment/2006/updated-regimens.htm* [Accessed February 1, 2008].

18. Leirisalo-Repo M, Sieper J. Reactive arthritis: epidemiology, clinical features, and treatment. In Weisman MH, van der Heijde D, Reveille JD, eds. Ankylosing spondylitis and the spondyloarthropathies. St. Louis MO Mosby Elsevier, 2006:53–64.

19. Panush RS, Wallace DJ, Dorff RE, Engleman EP. Retraction of the suggestion to use the term "Reiter's syndrome" sixty-five years later: the legacy of Reiter, a war criminal, should not be eponymic honor but rather condemnation. Arthritis Rheum 2007;56:693.

20. Braun J, Kingsley G, van der Heijde D, Sieper J. On the difficulties of establishing a consensus on the definition of and diagnostic investigations for reactive arthritis. Results and discussion of a questionnaire prepared for the 4th International Workshop on Reactive Arthritis, Berlin, Germany, July 3–6, 1999. J Rheumatol 2000;27:2185–92.

21. Fendler C, Laitko S, Sörensen H, Gripenberg-Lerche C, Groh A, Uksila J, et al. Frequency of triggering bacteria in patients with reactive arthritis and undifferentiated oligoarthritis and the relative importance of the tests used for diagnosis. Ann Rheum Dis 2001;60:337–43.

22. Barth WF, Segal K. Reactive arthritis (Reiter's syndrome). Am Fam Physician 1999;60(2):499–503.

23. Sieper J, Rudwaleit M, Braun J, van der Heijde D. Diagnosing reactive arthritis: role of clinical setting in the value of serologic and microbiologic assays. Arthritis Rheum 2002;46:319.

24. Putschky N, Pott HG, Kuipers JG, Zeidler H, Hammer M, Wollenhaupt J. Comparing 10-day and 4-month doxycycline courses for treatment of *Chlamydia trachomatis*-reactive arthritis: a prospective, double-blind trial. Annals of Rheum Dis 2006;65:1521.

25. Laasila K, Laasonen L, Leirisalo-Repo M. Antibiotic treatment and long term prognosis of reactive arthritis. Ann Rheum Dis 2003;62:655.

26. Scieux C, Barnes R, Bianchi A, Casin I, Morel P, Perol Y. Lymphogranuloma venereum: 27 cases in Paris. J Infect Dis 1989;160:662.

27. Mabey D, Peeling RW. Lymphogranuloma venereum. Sex Transm Infect 2002;78:90.

28. Kampmeier RH. Identification of the gonococcus by Albert Neisser. Sex Transm Dis 1983;5:71–9.

29. Weinstock H. Sexually transmitted diseases among American youth: incidence and prevalence estimates, 2000. Perspect Sex Reprod Health 2004;36(1):6–10.

30. Fleming DT, Wasserheit JN. From epidemiological synergy to public health policy and practice: the contribution of other sexually transmitted diseases to sexual transmission of HIV infection. Sex Transm Infect 1999;75:3–17.

31. Datta D, Sternberg M, Johnson RE, Berman S, Papp JR, McQuillan G, et al. Gonorrhea and *Chlamydia* in the United States among persons 14 to 39 years of age, 1999 to 2002. Ann Intern Med 2007;147(2):89–96.

32. The U.S. Preventive Services Task Force (USPSTF). The guide to clinical preventive services, 2008: recommendations of the U.S. Preventive Service Task Force. Available from: *http://www.ahrq.gov/Clinic/pocketgd 08/index.html#Contents* [Accessed July 18, 2009].

33. Miller KE. Diagnosis and treatment of *Neisseria gonorrhoeae* infections. Am Fam Physician 2006;73(10): 1779–84.

34. Hook EW, Handsfield HH. Gonoccocal infections of the adult. In King H, Sparling PF, Stamm WE, Piot P, Wasserheit J, Corey L, et al., eds. Sexually transmitted diseases, 4th ed. New York, NY: McGraw-Hill, 2008:627–47.

35. Centers for Disease Control and Prevention. Sexually transmitted diseases treatment guidelines 2002. MMWR Recomm Rep 2002;51:1.

36. Centers for Disease Control and Prevention. Updated recommended treatment regimens for gonococcal infections and associated conditions—United States, April 2007. Available from: *www.cdc.gov/std/treatment/2006/updated-regimens.htm* [Accessed April 1, 2008].

37. Cook, RL, Hutchison, SL, Ostergaard, L, Braithwaite, RS, Ness RB. Systemic review: noninvasive testing for Chlamydia trachomatis and Neisseria gonorrhoeae. Ann Intern Med 2005;142(11):914–25.

38. O'Brien, JP, Goldenberg, DL, Rice PA. Disseminated gonococcal infection: a prospective analysis of 49 patients and a review of pathophysiology and immune mechanisms. Medicine 1983;62:395–6.

39. Centers for Disease Control and Prevention. Surveillance for acute viral hepatitis United States, 2005. *MMWR Surveill Summ* 2007;56;SS-3. Available from: *http://www.cdc.gov/ncidod/diseases/hepatitis/resource/PDFs/SS5603%20eBook.pdf* [Accessed February 8, 2008].

40. Centers for Disease Control and Prevention. Prevention of hepatitis A through active or passive immunization. Recommendations of the Advisory Committee on Immunization Practices (ACIP). *MMWR Recomm Rep* 2006;55(RR07);1–23. Available from: *http://www.cdc.gov/mmwr/preview/mmwrhtml/rr5507a1.htm* [Accessed February 8, 2008].

41. Centers for Disease Control and Prevention. Updated U.S. Public Health Service Guidelines for the Management of Occupational Exposures to HBV, HCV, and HIV and Recommendations for Postexposure Prophylaxis; Morbidity and Mortality Weekly Report, 2001;50; RR-11. Retrieved February 11, 2008 at: *http://www.aidsinfo.nih.gov/guidelines/GuidelineDetail.aspx?MenuItem=Guidelines&Search=Off&GuidelineID=10&ClassID=3*

42. Mast EE, Weinbaum CM, Fiore AE, Alter MJ, Bell BP, Finelli L, et al. Advisory Committee on Immunization Practices (ACIP) Centers for Disease Control and Prevention (CDC). A comprehensive immunization strategy to eliminate transmission of hepatitis B virus infection in the United States: Recommendations of the Advisory Committee on Immunization Practices (ACIP) Part I: Immunization of infants, children, and adolescents. MMWR 2005;54:1.

43. Farci P, Alter HJ, Wong D, Miller RH, Shih JW, Jett B, et al. A long-term study of hepatitis C virus replication in non-A, non-B hepatitis. N Engl J Med 1991;325; 98–104.

44. Lok AS, McMahon BJ. Practice Guidelines Committee, American Association for the Study of Liver Diseases (AASLD). Chronic hepatitis B: Update of recommendations. Hepatology 2007;45(2):507–539. Available from: *https://www.aasld.org/eweb/docs/chronichep_B.pdf* [Accessed February 12, 2008].

45. Chen CJ, Yang HI, Su J, Jen CL, You SL, Lu SN, et al. REVEAL-HBV Study Group. Risk of hepatocellular carcinoma across a biological gradient of serum hepatitis B virus DNA level. JAMA 2006;295:65–73.

46. Iloeje UH, Yang HI, Su J, Jen CL, You SL, Chen CJ. Predicting cirrhosis risk based on the level of circulating hepatitis B viral load. Gastroenterology 2006; 130:678–86.

47. Hoofnagle JH, Seeff LB. Peginterferon and ribavirin for chronic hepatitis C. N Engl J Med 2006;355:2444.

48. Farley JE, Dial DJ, Kearney M. Management of hematologic and neuropsychiatric side effects in persons undergoing treatment for chronic HCV infection. J Nurse Pract 2006;2(1);38–45.

49. Strader DB, Wright T, Thomas DL, Seeff LB. Practice Guidelines Committee, American Association for the Study of Liver Diseases (AASLD). Diagnosis, management, and treatment of hepatitis C. Hepatology 2004;39(4):1147–71.

50. Pitchenik AE, Fischl MA, Dickinson GM, Becker DM, Fournier AM, O'Connell MT, et al. Opportunistic infections and Kaposi's sarcoma among Haitians: evidence of a new acquired immunodeficiency state. Ann Intern Med 1983;98(3):277–84.

51. Clumeck N, Sonnet J, Taelman H, Mascart-Lemone F, De Bruyere M, Vandeperre P, et al. Acquired immunodeficiency syndrome in African patients. N Engl J Med 1984;310(8):492–7.

52. Zhu T, Korber BT, Nahmias AJ, Hooper E, Sharp PM, Ho DD. An African HIV-1 sequence from 1959 and implication for the origins of the epidemic. Nature 1998;391:594–7.

53. Centers for Disease Control (CDC). Prevention of acquired immune deficiency syndrome (AIDS): report of inter-agency recommendations. MMWR 1983; 32(8):101–3.

54. Peterman TA, Drotman DP, Curran JW. Epidemiology of the acquired immunodeficiency syndrome (AIDS). Epidemiol Rev 1985;7:1–21.

55. Padian N, Marquis L, Francis DP, Anderson RE, Rutherford GW, O'Malley PM, et al. Male-to-female

transmission of human immunodeficiency virus. JAMA 1987;258;788–90.

56. Gray RH, Wawer MJ, Brookmeyer R, Sewankambo NK, Serwadda D, Wabwire-Mangen F, et al. Rakai Project Team. Per coital act in monogamous, heterosexual, HIV-1 discordant couples in Rakai, Uganda. Lancet 2001;357:1149–53.

57. Centers for Disease Control and Prevention (CDC). Cases of HIV infection and AIDS in the United States and dependent areas, 2005; HIV/AIDS Surveillance Rep 2007 June;17(revised ed.). Available from: *www.cdc.gov/hiv/topics/surveillance/resources/ reports/2005report/default.htm* [Accessed January 21, 2008].

58. Perinatal HIV Guidelines Working Group. Public Health Service Task Force recommendations for use of antiretroviral drugs in pregnant HIV-infected women for maternal health and interventions to reduce perinatal HIV transmission in the United States. November 2, 2007, pp. 1–96. Available from: *http://aidsinfo.nih.gov/ ContentFiles/PerinatalGL.pdf* [Accessed January 24, 2008].

59. Centers for Disease Control and Prevention (CDC). Revised recommendations for HIV testing of adults, adolescents, and pregnant women in health-care settings. MMWR 2006;55(RR14);1–17.

60. Cooper DA, Gold J, Maclean P, Donovan B, Finlayson R, Barnes TG, et al. Acute AIDS retrovirus infection. Lancet 1985;1:537–40.

61. Vanhems P, Allard R, Cooper DA, Perrin L, Vizzard J, Hirschel B, et al. Acute human immunodeficiency virus type 1 disease as a mononucleosis-like illness: is the diagnosis too restrictive? Clin Infect Dis 1997;24:965–70.

62. Lavreys L, Thompson ML, Martin HL Jr, Mandaliya K, Ndinya-Achola JO, Bwayo JJ, et al. Primary immunodeficiency virus type-1 infection: clinical manifestations among women in Mombasa, Kenya. Clin Infect Dis 2000;30:486–90.

63. Lee LM, Karon JM, Selik R, Neal JJ, Fleming PL. Survival after AIDS diagnosis in adolescents and adults during the treatment era, United States, 1984–1997. JAMA 2001;285:1308–15.

64. Panel on Antiretroviral Guidelines for Adult and Adolescents. Guidelines for the use of antiretroviral agents in HIV-infected adults and adolescents. Washington, DC: Department of Health and Human Services. December 1, 2007; pp. 1–136. Available from: *http:// aidsinfo.nih.gov/* [Accessed July 22, 2009].

65. Pham PA, Flexner CW. Antiretroviral drug interactions: a practical approach. Baltimore, MD: Johns Hopkins University Press, 2005.

66. Centers for Disease Control and Prevention (CDC). Updated U.S. Public Health Service guidelines for the management of occupational exposures to HIV and recommendations for postexposure prophylaxis-September 30, 2005. [Internet] Available from: *www.cdc.gov/mmwr/preview/mmwrhtml/rr5409a1.htm* [Accessed July 20, 2009].

67. Kahn JA. HPV vaccination for the prevention of cervical intraepithelial neoplasia. N Engl J Med 2009; 361:271–8.

68. Ho GY, Bierman R, Beardsley L, Chang CJ, Burk RD. Natural history of cervicovaginal papillomavirus infection as measured by repeated DNA testing in adolescent and young women. N Engl J Med 1998;338(7): 423–8.

69. ACOG. Human papillomavirus. ACOG practice bulletin No. 61. American College of Obstetricians and Gynecologists. Obstet Gynecol 2005;105:905–18.

70. Bosch FX, Lorincz A, Munoz N, Meiher CJ, Shah KV. The causal relation between human papillomavirus and cervical cancer. J Clin Path 2002;55:244–65.

71. Corey L, Wald A. Genital herpes. In King H, Sparling PF, Stamm WE, Piot P, Wasserheit J, Corey L, et al., eds. Sexually transmitted diseases, 4th ed. New York, NY: McGraw-Hill, 2008:399–439.

72. Winer RL, Hughes JP, Feng Q, O'Reilly S, Kiviat NB, Holmes KK, et al. Condom use and the risk of genital human papillomavirus infection in young women. N Engl J Med 2006;354(25):2645–54.

73. Zonfrillo NJ, Hackley B. The quadrivalent human papillomavirus vaccine potential factors in effectiveness. J Midwifery Womens Health 2008;188–94.

74. Xu F, Sternberg MR, Kottiri BJ, McQuillan GM, Lee FK, Nahmias AJ, et al. Trends in herpes simplex virus type 1 and type 2 seroprevalence in the United States. JAMA 2006;296:964–73.

75. Freeman EE, Weiss HA, Glynn JR, Cross PL, Whitworth JA, Hayes RJ. Herpes simplex virus 2 infection increases HIV acquisition in men and women: systemic review and meta-analysis of longitudinal studies. AIDS 2006;20:73–83.

76. Brugha R, Keersmaekers K, Renton A, Meheus A. Genital herpes infection: a review. Int J Epidemiol 1997;26:698–709.

77. Schillinger JA, Xu F, Sternberg MR, Armstrong GL, Lee FK, Nahmias AJ, et al. National seroprevalence

and trends in herpes simplex virus type 1 in the United States, 1976–1994. Sex Transm Dis 2004; 31(12):753–60.

78. Coyle PV, O'Neill HJ, Wyatt DE, McCaughey C, Quah S, McBride MO. Emergence of herpes simplex type 1 as the main cause of recurrent genital ulcerative disease in women in Northern Ireland. J Clin Virol 2003;27(1):22–9.

79. Nieuwenhuis RF, van Doornum GJ, Mulder PG, Neumann HA, van der Meijden WI. Importance of herpes simplex virus type-1 (HSV-1) in primary genital herpes. Acta Derm Venereol 2006;86(2):129–34.

80. Roberts CM, Pfister JR, Spear SJ. Increasing proportion of herpes simplex virus type 1 as a cause of genital herpes infection in college students. Sex Transm Dis 2003;30(10):797–800.

81. Corey L, Wald A. Genital herpes. In King H, Sparling PF, Stamm WE, Piot P, Wasserheit J, Corey L, et al., eds. Sexually transmitted diseases, 4th ed. New York, NY: McGraw-Hill, 2008:399–439.

82. Langenberg A, Corey L, Ashley R, Leong W, Strauss S. A prospective study of new infections with herpes simplex virus type 1 and type 2. N Engl J Med 1999; 341:1432–8.

83. World Health Organization. Global prevalence and incidence of selected sexually transmitted diseases. Geneva, Switzerland: World Health Organization, 2002.

84. Centers for Disease Control and Prevention (CDC). The national plan to eliminate syphilis from the United States, 2006. Available from: *http://www.cdc.gov/StopSyphilis/plan.htm* [Accessed July 19, 2009].

85. Brown DL, Frank JE. Diagnosis and management of syphilis. Am Fam Physician 2003. Available from: *www.aafp.org/afp/20030715/283.html* [Accessed February 1, 2008].

86. Musher DM. Biology of *Treponema pallidum*. In Holmes KK, Mardh PA, Sparling PF, Stamm W, Piot P, Wasserheit J, Corey L, et al., eds. Sexually transmitted disease. New York: McGraw-Hill, 2008:205.

87. Clark EG, Danbolt N. The Oslo study of the natural course of untreated syphilis. Med Clin North Am 1964;48:613–21.

88. USPFTF. Screening for syphilis infection: recommendation statement. Ann Fam Med 2004;2:362–5.

89. Womack J, Richman S, Tien PC, Grey M, Williams A. Hormonal contraception and HIV-positive women: metabolic concerns and management strategies. J Midwifery Womens Health 2008;53:362–75.

90. Lehtovirta P, Paavonen J, Heikinheimo O. Experience with the levonorgestrel-releasing intrauterine system among HIV infected women. Contraception 2007; 75(1):37–9.

91. Centers for Disease Control and Prevention. Recommendations for identification and public health management of persons with chronic hepatitis B virus infection. MMWR 2008;57(No. RR-8):1–28.

92. AIDSinfo. The HIV life cycle. 2005. Available from: *http://www.aidsinfo.nih.gov/contentfiles/HIVLifeCycle_FS_en.pdf* [Accessed October 2, 2009].

"To think is to practice brain chemistry."

DEEPAK CHOPRA

24

Drugs and the Central Nervous System

William P. Fehder and Tekoa L. King, with acknowledgment to Jennifer Hensley

---

⚕ Chapter Glossary

Absence seizures Brief periods of unconsciousness that may or may not be accompanied by involuntary movement.

Akinesia Motor hypoactivity or muscular paralysis.

Bradykinesia Slowness of movements.

Catamenial seizure pattern Seizure exacerbation in relation to the menstrual cycle.

Convulsions Abnormal motor phenomena.

Corticospinal tract A collection of axons that travel between the cerebral cortex of the brain and the spinal cord. Also called *pyramidal tract.*

Dyskinesia Impaired ability to execute voluntary muscle movement. Also called *extrapyramidal symptoms.*

Epilepsy Disorders wherein excessive excitability of CNS neurons produce seizure activity. Seizure symptoms vary widely and include brief periods of unconsciousness, strange sensations, unusual involuntary movements, and jerking muscle movements called convulsions.

Extrapyramidal symptoms Disorders of movement associated with the removal of modifications from the extrapyramidal neurons on the pyramidal tract. These movement disorders are also called *dyskinesias.*

Gamma-amino butyric acid (GABA) Neurotransmitter in the central nervous system. GABA is the chief inhibitory neurotransmitter and is also involved in regulation of muscle tone.

Generalized seizure Seizure that involves both hemispheres of the cerebral cortex.

Glutamate The primary excitatory neurotransmitter in the central nervous system.

Inhibitory interneuron Multipolar neuron that becomes the connection between afferent neurons and efferent neurons. The cell body of the inhibitory interneuron is always in the central nervous system.

Migraine A type of neurologic disorder resulting from dysfunction of the trigeminovascular system. The disorder manifests as recurring attacks usually lasting 4–72 hours. The headaches usually involve nausea, vomiting, and photophobia.

Muscarinic One of the two types of acetylcholine receptors; the other is nicotinic.

Mydriasis Excessive dilation of the pupil.

Neocortex The outermost layer of the cerebral hemispheres. It is approximately 2–4 mm thick and is the center for higher mental functions. The neocortex is the gray matter composed of neuronal cell bodies that surrounds the deeper white matter of the cerebrum. The neocortex is composed of six horizontal layers.

Nonlinear kinetics Small increases in dose of a drug (e.g., phenytoin) that result in a much larger increase in plasma concentrations. For example, if the dose of phenytoin is increased 50% from 300 mg/day to 450 mg/day, the increase in steady state plasma concentration is 10-fold. When the pharmacokinetics of a drug are linear, increases in dose result in a proportional increase in plasma concentrations.

Partial seizures Seizures that are contained within a focal site in the cerebral cortex.

Pyramidal neuron A type of neuron in the central nervous system that has a triangular-shaped cell body and very long axon that extends through the layers of the cerebral cortex to form the corticospinal tract. The pyramidal neurons are excitatory and control motor function.

Pyramidal tract The collection of pyramidal neuron axons that extend from the cortex to the spinal cord. Also known as *corticospinal tract.*

Seizure Transient abnormal excessive neuronal activity that presents as altered mental state, tonic or clonic uncontrolled movements, or other abnormal sensations.

Transformed migraine Migraine headaches that become chronic rather than episodic.

Introduction

Health practitioners have used both naturally occurring and synthetic substances to alter processes within the central nervous system (CNS) for many years. This chapter reviews the disorders that originate in the central nervous system that are likely to be encountered by primary care providers. The pathophysiology and pharmacologic treatments for epilepsy, Parkinson's disease, Alzheimer's disease, attention deficit disorder, restless legs syndrome, and migraine headaches are reviewed with special emphasis on how these disorders affect women. Psychiatric disorders and pharmacotherapeutics are discussed in Chapter 25. This may appear to be a diverse collection of disorders, yet they have commonalities with regard to the neurotransmitter systems affected in the central nervous system, and there is significant overlap among these disorders in the drugs used to treat them. In addition, there are some interesting connections between epilepsy, migraine headaches, and witchcraft.

Seizures and Epilepsy

Epilepsy refers to a group of disorders that involve an excessive excitability of neurons of the CNS that produces symptoms ranging from brief periods of unconsciousness to jerking muscle movements termed **convulsions**. Epilepsy is an ancient disease, recognized in the earliest medical texts written as a disorder that is associated with women. Hippocrates wrote "when the uterus is near the liver and the hypochondrium and produces suffocation, the woman turns up the whites of her eyes, becomes cold, some become even livid, gnashes her teeth, saliva flows into her mouth . . ."[1] Historically, seizures were often thought of as an expression of supernatural possession or witchcraft and sometimes as a sign of genius[2] (Box 24-1).

Box 24-1 The "Sacred Disease"

Epilepsy has appeared in myths, legends, and religious writings since the beginning of recorded history. The name epilepsy was derived from the Greek word επιληψία/*epili'* and *lepsis*, which means "to attack or seize." One of the earliest suggested etiologies was a curse from the gods that explained seizures as the manifestation of an attack by demons or an evil spirit. Although an epileptic seizure might be caused by an evil supernatural being, individuals with epilepsy were also thought to have mystic powers and visions from god.

Hippocrates attempted to refute these beliefs in his text "The Sacred Disease" in which he described the characteristics of gran mal seizures and attributed it to a brain disorder as opposed to evidence of the divine. Despite Hippocrates's stature, cultural beliefs about epilepsy did not change.

Epilepsy was a particularly dangerous disease for women when the handbook on witch hunting, *Malleus Maleficarum*, was written by two Dominican friars in 1494. *Malleus Malificarum* stated that seizures were a characteristic of witches. This text became the guidebook for the Inquisition and was responsible for the deaths of more than 200,000 women who were thought to be witches.

Even today, epilepsy is misconceived and even thought to be contagious by some. It was only in the 1980s that Missouri changed its law in order to legally allow people with epilepsy to marry and South Carolina repealed its law allowing forced sterilization of women with the condition. Yet some persons who have epilepsy report having a religious experience during the postictal stage of the seizure, a phenomenon of great interest to students of neurophysiology.

In many nondeveloped cultures, persons with epilepsy continue to be stigmatized and mistreated or cared for as shamans. The book *The Spirit Catches You and You Fall Down*, written by Ann Fadiman in 1997, is a beautiful story about a Hmong child with severe epilepsy and the discord between views of her Hmong family and the western doctors who were providing medical care to her. Epilepsy is complex and the pharmacologic treatment is only one small aspect of a fascinating physiologic circumstance.

Estrogen and progesterone alter neuronal excitability. Estrogen has been shown to increase the excitatory transmitters in brain regions that are responsible for certain types of seizures.[3] Conversely, progesterone and its metabolites decrease brain excitability.[4]

Conversely, both epilepsy and the drugs used to treat epilepsy have effects on reproductive health in women. Women with epilepsy have more menstrual disturbances, higher rates of infertility, and an increased incidence of polycystic ovarian syndrome than do women who do not have epilepsy.[5] These disturbances in gonadal hormones may be due to the neuroendocrine effects of epilepsy, the effects of antiepileptic drugs (AEDs) on reproductive hormones, or both. AEDs cause women with epilepsy to have higher rates of sexual dysfunction such as anorgasmia and decreased libido.[6] Some AEDs decrease the effectiveness of oral contraceptives, and these same drugs can have teratogenic effects if used during pregnancy.[7]

Definition of Terms

In epilepsy, the normal pattern of neuronal activity becomes disturbed, causing strange sensations, emotions, behavior, and sometimes frank convulsions with loss of consciousness and muscle spasms. **Seizure** refers to transient alterations in behavior, of varying degrees, due to uncontrolled synchronous and rhythmic firing of various ensembles of neurons, usually originating in the cerebral cortex. When seizures occur in a periodic and unpredictable way, the condition is referred to as epilepsy. Individuals experiencing single seizures are not given the diagnosis of epilepsy, but they have an increased risk of developing epilepsy.

Seizure is a general term referring to all types of epileptic events, whereas the term convulsions only apply to abnormal motor phenomena. Thus, all convulsions are forms of seizures, but not all seizures are associated with convulsive events. For example, **absence seizures** are characterized by brief periods of unconsciousness but may not be accompanied by involuntary movement. Some knowledge of the anatomy and physiology of the CNS is helpful in understanding the phenomena associated with seizure disorders and the methodologies employed in the treatment of epileptic seizures.

▌Anatomy and Physiology of the Cerebral Cortex

The human cerebral cortex, which is the outermost portion of the brain, is divided into the hippocampus; the paleocortex, which is associated with the olfactory system; and the **neocortex**, which, in the evolution of the brain, developed most recently. The neocortex contains billions of neuronal cell bodies and unmyelinated fibers that are arranged horizontally in six layers. The two primary types of cells in the neocortex are **pyramidal neurons** and **inhibitory interneurons**. The pyramidal neurons have a triangular shape cell body, which is where they get their name. These neurons have a very long apical dendrite (axon) that extends vertically down through the six layers of the cortex to the white matter (Figure 24-1).

The pyramidal neurons are excitatory.[8] Their axons release the neurotransmitter **glutamate**. The inhibitory neurons connect afferent neurons and efferent neurons in neural pathways. They interrupt or restrict activity paths. The axons of the inhibitory interneuron release the neurotransmitter **gamma-amino butyric acid** (GABA). Thus, the cerebral cortex and much of the brain is organized both vertically in columns and tracts, permitting precise control of sensory and motor function as well as horizontally in association areas, which permits higher levels of processing.

Localized, discrete areas of the cerebral cortex on the surface of the brain have been extensively mapped (somatotopic maps) to establish the anatomy of motor and sensory pathways to and from the peripheral nervous system. Functional areas such as speech and memory centers (Brodmann areas) have also been identified in the cerebral cortex. The motor pathways from the cerebral cortex to the peripheral nervous system consist of large pyramidal neurons with long axons extending to the spinal cord, known as the **pyramidal tract** and also as the **corticospinal tract**.

The cerebral white matter located beneath the cerebral cortex contains myelinated nerve fibers bundled into tracts that transmit nerve impulses to and from the cerebral cortex in three directions—between hemispheres (commissural tracts), between functional areas (association tracts), and in communication with lower areas of the central and peripheral nervous system (projection tracts). Thus, between the axon collaterals of the pyramidal neurons and the white matter, there is a great deal of interconnection and coordination.

The regulation of neuronal activity in the CNS is based on a balance between excitatory neurons that use glutamate as their primary neurotransmitter and inhibitory neurons that use gamma-aminobutyric acid (GABA) as their primary neurotransmitter. The summation of excitatory and inhibitory neuronal influences on postsynaptic neurons determines whether an electric threshold is reached and an impulse in the form of an action potential is generated.

(a)

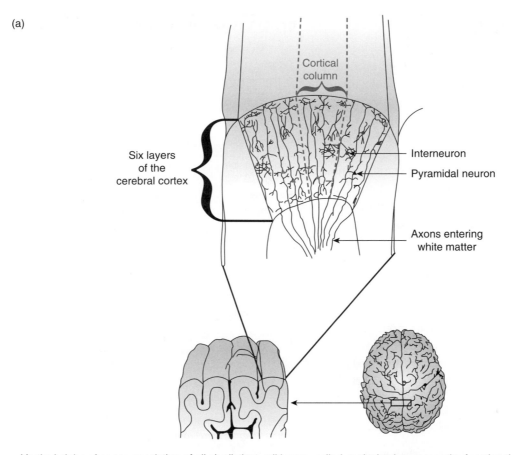

Vertical slabs of cortex consisting of all six distinct cell layers, called cortical columns, are the functional units of the cerebal cortex. Some of the cells like the large pyramidal cells have dendrites that extend through almost all layers and axons that exit the gray matter to become part of the white matter tracts, carrying information to other parts of the brain and body. There are also innumerable interneurons connecting the cells within each layer and between layers.

(b)

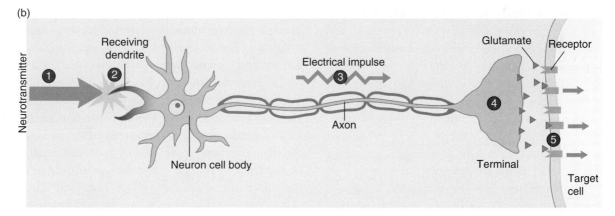

(1) Neurotransmitter agonist at receiving cell dendrite initiates an electrical impulse. (2) Neuron activated. (3) Electrical impulse travels axon. (4) Glutamate is released. (5) The neurotransmitter traverses the synapse and binds with receptor sites on the target cell.

Figure 24-1 Extrapyramidal tracts of cerebral cortex (a) and the anatomy of the pyramidal neuron (b). *Source:* Figure a is reprinted with permission from McCrossin S 2000.[8]

Seizures: An Overview

When a dysregulation of the balance between excitatory and inhibitory neuronal influences occurs, pathologic conditions such as epilepsy, Parkinson's disease, or Alzheimer's disease may arise. Behavioral manifestations of a seizure are determined by the site in the cortex at which the seizure arises. Although several types of neurons exist within the cerebral cortex, the long pyramid-shaped neurons appear to play a significant role in many types of epilepsy. The axons of pyramidal cells have collateral branches that make local connections between association areas of the cerebral cortex. Many of these axon connections are excitatory in nature, and this arrangement can result in an abnormal synchronous discharge of large numbers of neurons during an epileptic seizure. A small focus of excitatory neural activity can spread horizontally and vertically through the brain by synchronous discharge of increasing numbers of neurons producing one of several types of seizure activity depending on the extent and areas of the brain recruited. Seizure activity can be partial or generalized seizures.[9]

Types of Seizures

Nonepileptic seizures, such as those provoked by abnormal metabolic conditions or drugs, must be differentiated from epileptic seizures. Abnormal physical and metabolic conditions can cause seizures that are referred to as provoked seizures. Electrolyte imbalances, such as hypocalcemia, water intoxication, uremia, hypoglycemia, hypoxia, and alkalosis can all cause a seizure. The rapid withdrawal of sedative-hypnotic drugs such as alcohol, barbiturates, benzodiazepines, and antiepileptic drugs may precipitate seizure activity. Head trauma or other CNS insult such as cerebral bleeding, edema, or infections such as meningitis results in seizure activity for 5–10% of individuals experiencing such insults. Finally, toxemia of pregnancy (eclampsia) can result in seizure activity.

Provoked seizures can also be produced by drugs. Abuse of certain drugs such as heroin, cocaine, methadone, amphetamine, or methylenedioxymethamphetamine (MDMA or ecstasy) may come to mind first, but other drugs and drug combinations can also precipitate seizures, especially among persons with epilepsy[10] (Table 24-1). Correction or withdrawal of the factor that has provoked the seizure usually reduces the risk of recurrence of a provoked seizure. Antiseizure medications may be beneficial during the acute treatment of provoked seizures.[11]

Table 24-1 Drugs That May Lower Seizure Threshold

Category	Drugs Generic (Brand)
Antiasthmatics	Aminophylline, theophylline (Theo-Dur), albuterol
Antibiotics	Isoniazid (INH), lindane (Kwell, Kwellada lotion 1%), metronidazole (Flagyl), nalidixic acid (NegGram) penicillins, fluconazole (Diflucan)
Antidepressants	Tricyclics, serotonin-specific agents, bupropion (Wellbutrin)
Hormones	Insulin, prednisone, estrogen
Immunosuppressants	Chlorambucil (Leukeran), cyclosporine (Sandimmune)
Local anesthetics	Lidocaine, bupivacaine, procaine
Opioids	Fentanyl (Sublimaze), meperidine (Demerol), pentazocine (Talwin), propoxyphene (Darvocet), tramadol (Ultram)
Psychostimulants	Amphetamines, cocaine, methylphenidate (Ritalin), phenylpropanolamine, heroin
Neuroleptics	Clozapine, phenothiazines, butyrophenones
Other	Anticholinergics, anticholinesterases, antihistamines, baclofen (Lioresal, Kemstro), heavy metals, hyperbaric oxygen, lithium (Lithobid), mefenamic acid, oral hypoglycemics, oxytocin

Source: Adapted from Bromfield EB 1997.[10]

Epilepsy: Classification and Diagnosis

The specific type of medication that is useful for the treatment of epileptic seizures depends on the nature of the seizure and its underlying pathophysiology. For this reason, a great deal of effort has been made to differentiate seizures so clinicians can make a specific seizure diagnosis and prescribe appropriate therapy. Attempts to classify seizure disorders were first proposed in 1970 by Gastaut. The classifications were redefined in 1981 and finally in 1989 by the Commission on Classification and Terminology of the International League Against Epilepsy.[12] This classification system is based primarily on the clinical symptoms of seizures and their electroencephalogram features. The classification has been accepted worldwide and is referred to as the International Classification (Table 24-2).

In 2001, the International League Against Epilepsy proposed a classification system based on five different axes, which include seizure description (axis 1), seizure type (axis 2), epilepsy syndrome (axis 3), etiology (axis 4), and impairment (axis 5). This scheme permits modification of

Table 24-2 Classifications of Epileptic Seizures

Class	Feature	Description	AEDs Frequently Used for These Conditions	
			Conventional Antiepileptic Drugs	Newer Antiepileptic Drugs
I. Partial Seizures	Seizures with focal or localized onset.	Originate in a localized area of the cortex.		
A. Simple partial	Key feature is no loss of consciousness.	Diverse behavioral changes dependent on region of the cerebral cortex activated. Motor, autonomic, or psychic symptoms.	Carbamazepine, phenytoin, valproate	Gabapentin, lamotrigine, levetiracetam, tiagabine, topiramate, zonisamide
B. Complex partial	May occur with impairment of consciousness at onset or initially as a simple partial seizure followed by impairment of consciousness.	Impaired consciousness for 0.5 to 2 minutes often with purposeless movements such as lip smacking or hand wringing.	Carbamazepine, phenytoin, valproate	Gabapentin, lamotrigine, levetiracetam, tiagabine, topiramate, zonisamide
C. Partial evolving to generalized tonic-clonic	Simple or complex partial seizure evolving into tonic-clonic seizure.	Loss of consciousness with sustained muscle contractions (tonic) alternating with periods of relaxation (clonic). Usually lasts 1 to 2 minutes.	Carbamazepine, phenobarbital, phenytoin, primidone, valproate	Gabapentin, lamotrigine, levetiracetam, tiagabine, topiramate, zonisamide
II. Generalized Seizures	Seizures appear to begin bilaterally or may evolve from a partial seizure.	Involve diffuse regions of the brain.		
A. Absence	Abrupt onset of impaired consciousness without loss of postural control.	Formerly called *petit mal* seizures. Associated with staring and cessation of ongoing activities. Usually lasts less than 0.5 minutes.	Ethosuximide, valproate	Lamotrigine
B. Myoclonic	Brief contraction of muscles of about 1 second in duration.	Contraction similar to an electric shock. May be bilateral and generalized or restricted to the face or a single extremity.	Valproate, ethosuximide	Lamotrigine, topiramate, clonazepam, primidone, levetiracetam
C. Clonic	Rhythmic jerking or twitching movements of the extremities recurring at regular intervals of 1 to 2 seconds.	Movements may be unilateral or bilateral. Not usually followed by a period of tiredness after the seizure.	Valproate, methsuximide	
D. Tonic	Stiffening of the face, body, or extremities in a sustained contraction.	Sudden stiffening movements usually of 20 seconds' duration. Sometimes occurs during sleep.	Valproate, methsuximide	
E. Tonic-clonic	Most common major motor seizure. Alternating muscle stiffening (tonic contraction) followed by rhythmic jerking movements (clonic jerking).	Formerly called *grand mal* seizures. Period of seizure usually followed by a period of tiredness following the seizure (postictal cerebral metabolic and behavioral suppression).	Phenytoin, carbamazepine, valproate, phenobarbital, primidone	Lamotrigine, topiramate, felbamate, levetiracetam
F. Atonic	Sudden, split-second loss of muscle tone.	Also called akinetic seizures or drop attacks. Lack of muscle tone may result in dropping of jaw, drooping of a limb, or falling to the ground.	Valproate	Lamotrigine, clonazepam, felbamate

each axis because additional information is acquired and because the epilepsy evolves within an individual.[13]

Epileptic seizures can also be classified into specific epileptic syndromes of which more than 40 have been identified. These epileptic syndromes refer to clusters of symptoms that frequently occur together, such as age of onset and etiology, but they are also divided into partial or generalized epilepsies; thus both classification systems are often used together.

Seizures that begin in a focal site of the cerebral cortex are classified as **partial seizures**, whereas seizures that involve both hemispheres widely from the outset are termed **generalized seizures**. Partial seizures are subdivided into a simple type that is associated with preservation of consciousness or a complex type that is associated with impairment of consciousness.

The hormonal changes associated with menstruation produce **catamenial seizure patterns** in approximately one third of women with epilepsy. Catamenial is derived from the Greek word for monthly, *katamenios*. It has been defined as increased seizure frequency that begins either immediately before or during menses.[14] Women with this type of epilepsy may experience exacerbations of their seizures during ovulation or around the time of menstruation.

Initiating Drug Therapy

The decision to start antiepileptic medication is complex because it must balance the risks of recurrent epileptic seizures, including the rare risk of death from a seizure against the risks of medications that often have significant side effects.[15] These drugs should not be administered until a diagnosis of epilepsy has been confirmed.

Many studies indicate that between 60 and 70% of persons with a new diagnosis of epilepsy are able to become seizure free on an appropriate medication used as monotherapy. Furthermore, most individuals who achieve complete seizure control can successfully discontinue medication.[16]

The goal of drug treatment in epilepsy is to identify a single medication that is effective in eliminating or reducing the symptoms, avoiding the side effects of multiple drug therapy or becoming involved in a sequence of ineffective single medications. Ideally, an effective antiseizure agent would suppress all seizures without any side effects. Unfortunately, this drug does not exist.[17]

Antiepileptic Drugs

The term *antiepileptic drug* (AED) is used interchangeably with anticonvulsant. These drugs are increasingly being used for other conditions such as bipolar disorder, depression, chronic pain, and migraine headaches, all of which affect women more often than men.[18] The newer AEDs are also used to treat menopausal hot flashes and pelvic pain. Thus a basic understanding of how these drugs work is of import for clinicians who care for women of all ages.

Most AEDs prevent seizure activity by altering the balance of excitation and inhibition of neurons via one of three basic mechanisms: (1) modulation of voltage-gated calcium and sodium channels that perpetrate conduction of the impulse along the axon, (2) enhancement of

the neurotransmitter gamma-aminobutyric acid (GABA) that inhibits stimulation of the postsynaptic neuron, or (3) attenuation of brain excitation via inhibition of glutamate, which is the most abundant excitatory neurotransmitter in the brain (Figure 24-2).

There are no pharmacologic agents available at this time that protect against the development of epilepsy or cure it.[19] In addition, there is no effective AED for individuals with refractory epilepsy.[19] Thus, there remains a role for novel nonpharmacologic approaches, such as neurosurgery and vagus nerve stimulators for individuals who have intractable epilepsy as well as for persons who are unable to tolerate AEDs.

Classification of AEDs

The majority of the AEDs are classified into five chemical groups: hydantoins, barbiturates, succinimides, oxazolidinediones, and acetylureas (Table 24-3). The sixth "miscellaneous" classification of AEDs consists of drugs from many different chemical families.

Because eight new drugs for epilepsy were introduced in the 1990s, the drugs used to treat epilepsy are commonly

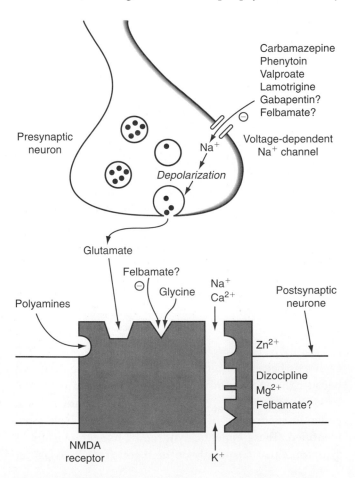

Figure 24-2 Mechanism of action of common antiepileptic drugs.

classified into the older, traditional AEDs and the newer AEDs. The traditional AEDs include carbamazepine (Tegretol), phenytoin (Dilantin), valproate (Depacon, Depakene, Depakote), and phenobarbital (Luminal). The newer agents include felbamate (Felbatol), gabapentin (Neurontin), lamotrigine (Lamictal), levetiracetam (Keppra), oxcarbazepine (Trileptal), tiagabine (Gabitril), topiramate (Topamax), and zonisamide (Zonegran). The newer AEDs were initially approved as add-on therapy for individuals who had refractory seizures despite treatment with one of the older AEDs[20] (Box 24-2).

The use of the newer AEDs, as replacements for older ones is a subject of debate in that there is no evidence of greater effectiveness and they are more expensive.[20] Some evidence-based guidelines advocate for the use of the newer AEDs because they have fewer side effects and fewer drug–drug interactions.[21]

Table 24-3 Chemical Classifications of Antiepileptic Drugs

Drug—Generic (Brand)	
Acetylureas	**Succinimides**
Acetazolamide (Diamox)	Ethosuximide (Zarontin)
Zonisamide (Zonegran)	Methsuximide (Celontin)
Barbiturates	Phensuximide (Milontin)
Mephobarbital (Mebaral)	**Miscellaneous**
Pentobarbital (Nembutal)	Carbamazepine (Carbatrol, Equetro, Tegretol)
Phenobarbital (Luminal)	Felbamate (Felbatol)
Primidone (Mysoline)	Gabapentin (Neurontin)
Benzodiazepines	Lamotrigine (Lamictal)
Clonazepam (Klonopin)	Levetiracetam (Keppra)
Diazepam (Valium)	Oxcarbazepine (Trileptal)
Lorazepam (Ativan)	Pregabalin (Lyrica)
Hydantoins	Tiagabine (Gabitril)
Fosphenytoin (Cerebyx)	Topiramate (Topamax)
Phenytoin (Dilantin)	Valproate (Depacon)
Mephenytoin (Mesantoin)	Valproic acid (Depakene)
Ethotoin (Peganone)	

Mechanisms of Action of AEDs

Some AEDs are theorized to work, at least in part, by reducing the ability of the sodium channels in the axonal membrane to recover from inactivation after an action potential, thereby prolonging the refractory period. This is the proposed mechanism of action by which carbamazepine (Tegretol), lamotrigine (Lamictal), phenytoin (Dilantin), topiramate (Topamax), valproic acid (Depakene), and zonisamide (Zonegran) inhibit the high-frequency neuronal firing characteristic of partial seizures.

Benzodiazepines and barbiturates are agonists for the $GABA_A$ receptor binding site on the postsynaptic neuron.

Box 24-2 How Are New Drugs Evaluated for Efficacy?

When a new drug is developed for treating a serious medical condition, it cannot be tested for efficacy in a randomized controlled trial that includes a placebo group because it is unethical to withhold treatment from persons with serious medical disorders. The story of how the new AEDs were evaluated is a good illustration of some of the problems involved in testing new drugs.

Eight "new AEDs" were tested in randomized controlled trials that each had two groups. The first group was treated with a traditional AED only. The second group was treated with a traditional AED and one of the newer AEDs added. Persons in both groups were followed for 8–12 weeks and if the group that took the new AED had 50% fewer seizures from their baseline rate of seizure activity, the new AED was determined to be effective. Although this design may sound reasonable, several methodological issues emerged.

Because this study design was only able to evaluate the new AED in the role of adjunct medication, the FDA only approved these drugs as adjunct medications. Moreover, this study design is likely to underestimate efficacy and overestimate toxicity. The individuals who were enrolled in the study had more seizures than most persons with epilepsy and responder rates are often less than 50%. Therefore, the new AEDs that were effective in combination with traditional AEDs were not fully evaluated for efficacy in a standard clinical population. Also, upon close reading of the studies, these drugs were titrated down much more rapidly than is currently recommended, and the sudden decreases in plasma levels were responsible for many of the toxicities that were noted in the studies.

What is a clinician to do? Monotherapy has several important advantages. Monotherapy is safer and has fewer drug–drug interactions. In addition, monotherapy is less expensive and compliance is higher. Therefore, many of the newer AEDs are used off-label as monotherapy, and as would be expected, they appear to be both efficacious and safe.

Binding to this receptor promotes the influx of chloride ions, which hyperpolarizes the neuron and raises the seizure threshold. Tiagabine (Gabitril) inhibits the reuptake of GABA by the presynaptic neuron and thus the postsynaptic neuron remains hyperpolarized and less likely to fire and cause a seizure. Similarly, vigabatrin (Sabril) interferes with the enzyme that degrades GABA, thereby promoting its duration of action.

Other AEDs inhibit the voltage-gated calcium channels that are located primarily in the presynaptic terminal membrane. Ordinarily, upon arrival of a nerve impulse, these calcium channels open and permit the passage of calcium ions into the presynaptic nerve, triggering a release of neurotransmitter in proportion to the number of calcium ions entering the terminal. Inhibition of the influx of calcium ions results in a decrease in neurotransmitter release that, in turn, reduces the likelihood that the postsynaptic neuron will fire. This mechanism is how ethosuximide (Zarontin) and valproate (Depacon, Depakene, Depakote) are thought to inhibit absence seizures.

Although gabapentin (Neurontin) and pregabalin (Lyrica) are analogs of GABA, they produce their effects by inhibiting the voltage-gated calcium presynaptic channels, thereby decreasing the release of glutamate—the primary excitatory neurotransmitter in the CNS.[19,21]

All of the older AEDs and to a lesser extent, some of the newer AEDs, interfere with folate metabolism via a mechanism that has not been fully elucidated. Folate supplementation is recommended for all women of childbearing age who are taking any AED.

Adverse Effects of Antiepileptic Drugs

All of the antiepileptic drugs have clinically significant side effects and adverse effects. In 2008, the FDA issued an alert mandating that a black box warning be placed on the label of several AEDs that are associated with a risk of suicidal ideation. Box 24-3 lists the drugs associated with an increased risk of suicidality and describes the precautions healthcare providers and persons taking these medications should take. These drugs are increasingly being used to treat conditions other than seizures, and therefore healthcare providers need a heightened awareness of this potentially fatal adverse effect.

Some persons have a genetic disposition to develop a painful and debilitating condition called porphyria that can be triggered by several AEDs. Porphyria is a metabolic disorder characterized by a deficiency of porphobilinogen deaminase. This enzyme is involved in an intermediary step of heme production. The deficiency of porphobilinogen deaminase is triggered by the presence of an AED (or other drugs, dietary changes, or hormones). The symptoms are secondary to a build-up of porphobilinogen and symptoms include abdominal pain, constipation, and muscle weakness. Barbiturates, primidone (Mysoline), phenytoin (Dilantin), mephenytoin (Mephenytoin), ethotoin (Peganone), ethosuximide (Zarontin), methsuximide (Celontin), and phensuximide (Milontin) can cause porphyria.

Anticonvulsant hypersensitivity syndrome is a condition that typically begins within 2 to 8 weeks of initiation of therapy with AEDs.[22] This syndrome usually begins with a fever developing into a rash, swollen lymph nodes, and sometimes pharyngitis. The most serious reactions involve hepatic, hematologic, renal, or pulmonary impairment. Anticonvulsant hypersensitivity syndrome is associated with the aromatic AEDs—phenytoin (Dilantin), phenobarbital (Luminal), primidone (Mysoline), carbamazepine (Tegretol), and lamotrigine (Lamictal).[25] The cross-reactivity between these different AEDs is as high as 80%. Valproate sodium (Depacon) is considered a safe alternative for treatment for persons with anticonvulsant hypersensitivity syndrome.

Drug–Drug Interactions of Antiepileptic Drugs

The AEDs are inducers, inhibitors, and substrates for various CYP450 enzymes. The older AEDs in particular have multiple drug–drug interactions that are clinically important considerations when caring for a person who is taking an AED (Table 24-4). The ability of phenytoin (Dilantin), carbamazepine (Tegretol), and other AEDs to induce CYP450 enzymes is particularly significant for women taking oral contraceptives because metabolism of the contraceptive is enhanced, which lowers plasma levels and can lead to an unplanned pregnancy.[23] The AEDs that are CYP450 inhibitors will cause a decrease in metabolism of other drugs and higher plasma levels of those drugs.

▌ Traditional Antiepileptic Drugs

Phenobarbital (Luminal) was first used to treat epilepsy in 1912, and phenytoin was first used in 1932. Both of these drugs continue to be used today. The other three traditional antiepileptic drugs have been used for several

decades. All five of the older antiepileptic drugs are efficacious and inexpensive, but uncomfortable side effects and
multiple drug–drug interactions have been the impetus for
developing newer drugs. Doses, indications, side effects,
and important clinical considerations are presented in
Table 24-5.

Box 24-3 Antiepileptic Drugs and Risk of Suicide

What is the connection between AED drugs and suicide? One of the pathogenic mechanisms that predispose a person to seizures also predisposes an individual to mood disorders, anxiety, and suicide. A decreased level of serotonin in the central nervous system is the culprit, but the exact mechanism of how AEDs increase these risks is not well elucidated.

Although persons who take AEDs have an increased risk for suicidality (which includes suicide ideation, suicide attempt, and completed suicide), this risk is actually low in absolute numbers. The FDA analyzed the pooled results of several studies of 11 AEDs and found that the risk of suicide was 4.3/1000 persons who took AEDs versus 2.2/1000 in persons who took a placebo.

Healthcare providers who prescribe these drugs need to balance the risk of suicidality with the clinical need for the drug. In addition, providers are encouraged to monitor for unusual changes in behavior and notify patients and their families of this risk.

Information given to persons who take these agents states that they should not change the medication regimen without having input from their healthcare provider and that they monitor for symptoms of suicide, which include:

  Talking or thinking about wanting to hurt yourself or end your life

  Withdrawing from friends and family

  Becoming depressed or having your depression get worse

  Becoming preoccupied with death and dying

  Giving away prized possessions

Persons using AEDs are encouraged to contact their healthcare provider if any of these behaviors occur.

The AEDs that are associated with an increased risk of suicidality are:

  Carbamazepine (Carbatrol, Equetro, Tegretol, Tegretol XR)

  Felbamate (Felbatol)

  Gabapentin (Neurontin)

  Lamotrigine (Lamictal)

  Levetiracetam (Keppra)

  Oxcarbazepine (Trileptal)

  Pregabalin (Lyrica)

  Tiagabine (Gabitril)

  Topiramate (Topamax)

  Valproate (Depakote, Depakote ER, Depakene, Depacon)

  Zonisamide (Zonegran)

Table 24-4 Selected Drug–Drug Interactions of Commonly Used Antiepileptic Drugs*

Drug Generic (Brand)	Antiepileptic Drug Generic (Brand)	Effect of Interaction
Amiodarone	Phenytoin (Dilantin)	Increased level of AED and possible toxicity.
Antacids	Phenytoin (Dilantin), carbamazepine (Tegretol), gabapentin (Neurontin), phenobarbital (Luminal)	Reduced absorption of AED leading to decreased effectiveness.
Benzodiazepines	Carbamazepine (Carbatrol, Tegretol), phenytoin (Dilantin), phenobarbital (Luminal)	Decreased plasma levels of benzodiazepines.
Carbamazepine (Tegretol)	Phenytoin (Dilantin)	Decreased plasma levels of phenytoin and increased seizure risk.
	Valproate (Depacon, Depakene, Depakote)	Increased plasma levels of active metabolite of carbamazepine. Can reach toxic levels. Valproate should not be used concomitantly with carbamazepine.
Beta-blockers; e.g., propranolol (Inderal)	Enzyme-inducing AEDs†	Decreased plasma levels of beta-blockers. These AEDs can be contraindicated for persons needing antihypertensive medications.
Chloramphenicol (Chloromycetin)	Phenobarbital (Luminal)	Increased metabolism of chloramphenicol.
	Phenytoin (Dilantin), phenobarbital (Luminal)	Increased plasma levels of AEDs, possible toxic effect.
Cimetidine (Tagamet)	Phenytoin (Dilantin), gabapentin (Neurontin)	Increased plasma levels of AED.
Clarithromycin (Biaxin)	Phenytoin (Dilantin)	Increased plasma levels of phenytoin.
Erythromycin (E-Mycin)	Carbamazepine (Carbatrol, Tegretol)	Increased plasma level of carbamazepine.
Diazepam (Valium)		
Digoxin (Lanoxin)	Phenytoin (Dilantin)	Decreased plasma levels of digoxin.
Fluconazole (Diflucan)	Phenytoin (Dilantin), valproate (Depacon, Depakene, Depakote)	Increased plasma levels of phenytoin.
Fluoxetine (Prozac)	Carbamazepine (Carbatrol, Tegretol)	Increased level of AED.
Folate	Phenytoin (Dilantin)	Bidirectional interaction. Decreased plasma levels of phenytoin and decreased plasma levels of folate.
Isoniazid (INH)	Phenytoin (Dilantin), carbamazepine (Carbatrol, Tegretol), ethosuximide (Zarontin), valproate (Depacon, Depakene, Depakote)	Increased plasma levels of AED and possible toxicity.
Ketoconazole (Nizoral)	Carbamazepine (Carbatrol, Tegretol)	Increased plasma level of carbamazepine and potential toxicity.
Lipid-lowering drugs	Phenytoin (Dilantin)	Decreased plasma levels of lipid-lowering agents.
Metronidazole (Flagyl)	Enzyme-inducing AEDs†	Decreased effectiveness of metronidazole.
	Carbamazepine (Carbatrol, Tegretol)	Increased plasma level of carbamazepine.
Oral contraceptives	Carbamazepine (Carbatrol, Tegretol), felbamate (Felbatol),‡ lamotrigine (Lamictal),‡ oxcarbazepine (Trileptal), phenobarbital (Luminal), phenytoin (Dilantin), primidone (Mysoline), topiramate (Topamax)	Enhanced metabolism of oral contraceptive, decreasing effectiveness of the contraceptive.
	Phenytoin (Dilantin)	Decreased effectiveness of oral contraceptives.
Phenobarbital (Luminal)	Phenytoin (Dilantin)	Decreased plasma levels of phenytoin and increased seizure risk.
Rifampin (Rifadin)	Phenytoin (Dilantin)	Decreased plasma levels of phenytoin and increased seizure risk.
St. John's wort	Carbamazepine (Carbatrol, Tegretol), phenytoin (Dilantin)	Decreased plasma levels of phenytoin and carbamazepine.
Sulfonamides	Phenytoin (Dilantin)	Increased plasma levels of phenytoin.

(continues)

Table 24-4 Selected Drug–Drug Interactions of Commonly Used Antiepileptic Drugs* (*continued*)

Drug Generic (Brand)	Antiepileptic Drug Generic (Brand)	Effect of Interaction
Tricyclic antidepressants	Enzyme-inducing AEDs†	Bidirectional interaction. Tricyclic antidepressant plasma levels decrease and AED plasma levels increase.
Valproate (Depakene, Depakote, Depacon)	Phenytoin (Dilantin)	Valproate displaces phenytoin on plasma protein binding sites, which causes increased plasma levels of active phenytoin.
	Oral contraceptives	Enhanced metabolism of valproate.
Warfarin (Coumadin)	Phenytoin (Dilantin)	Decreased plasma levels of warfarin.

* This list is not comprehensive as new information is being identified on a regular basis.
† Enzyme-inducing AEDs include carbamazepine (Carbatrol, Tegretol), felbamate (Felbatol), oxcarbazepine (Trileptal), phenobarbital (Luminal), phenytoin (Dilantin), primidone (Mysoline), and topiramate (Topamax).
‡ Felbamate appears to induce metabolism of progesterone component of COCs only, and clinical effect on contraceptive efficacy is unclear. There is also preliminary evidence that lamotrigine induces metabolism of progestin.

Table 24-5 First-Generation Antiepileptic Drugs*

Drug Generic (Brand)	Formulations	Therapeutic Indication	Dose	Clinical Considerations	FDA Pregnancy Category
Carbamazepine (Carbatrol, Tegretol)	Oral: 200 mg tablets, 100-mg chewable tablets; oral suspension 100 mg/5 mL; Extended-release (12 hour) capsules: Carbatrol or Tegretol XR 100-, 200-, 300-, and 400-mg capsules.	Partial and generalized tonic-clonic seizures First-line treatment for focal-onset seizures Off-label use: Chronic pain syndromes Bipolar disorder (under brand name Equetro)	Initial therapy 100–200 mg/day increasing weekly in 100- to 200-mg increments to target dose of 600–800 mg/day (may require doses as high as 1600–2400 mg/day.	Recent food intake slows absorption but may make larger doses more tolerable, so it is recommended that carbamazepine be taken with food. Extended-release capsules permit 12-hour dosing, but missed doses are more likely to result in breakthrough seizures. FDA black box warning to monitor for depression, behavior change, and signs of suicide ideation. Decreases efficacy of oral contraceptive agents. SE: Diplopia, blurred vision, vertigo, and ataxia. AE: Anticonvulsant hypersensitivity syndrome, aplastic anemia; Stevens-Johnson syndrome in susceptible individuals (most likely in Asians); increased risk of osteoporosis with long-term use.	D
Ethosuximide (Zarontin)	250-mg capsules. 250-mg/5-mL elixir.	Absence seizures	250 mg bid	Increase in 250-mg increments until seizures are controlled. Usual maintenance dose is 20 mg/kg/day. Does not decrease efficacy of oral contraceptives. Blood dyscrasias possible; periodic blood count should be evaluated. FDA black box warning to monitor for depression, behavior change, and signs of suicide ideation.	C
Phenytoin (Dilantin)	Parenteral: 50 mg/mL for IV administration. Oral: capsules 30 mg, 100 mg;	Generalized tonic-clonic seizures, partial seizures	For status epilepticus start at 10–20 mg/kg IV as a loading dose.	Large oral doses can be taken with meals to avoid gastric discomfort. Extended-release capsules are most appropriate for large single daily doses.	D

(continues)

Table 24-5 First-Generation Antiepileptic Drugs* (continued)

Drug Generic (Brand)	Formulations	Therapeutic Indication	Dose	Clinical Considerations	FDA Pregnancy Category
	chewable tablets 50 mg; oral suspension 125 mg/5 mL. Extended-release capsules phenytoin (Phenytek) 200 mg or 300 mg.	Off-label use: Neuropathic pain, motion sickness, cardiac arrhythmias	For nonacute situations, 150 mg bid increasing to 300 to 400 mg qd as tolerated.	Brands differ in rates of absorption; changing brands or formulations may result in underdosage or overdosage symptoms. Decreases efficacy of oral contraceptive agents. SE: gingivitis, nystagmus, double vision, rash, sedation AE: osteomalacia, osteoporosis with long-term use, Stevens-Johnson syndrome	
Phenobarbital (Luminal)	Tablets: 15, 30, 60, 100 mg; Oral solution: 15, 20 mg/5 mL. Parenteral solution: 20 mg/5 mL for IM or IV.	Generalized tonic-clonic seizures, partial seizures	Adult dose: 1–3 mg/kg/day in divided doses. The usual dose is 50–100 mg bid to tid.	Titration to full dose not necessary due to slow accumulation of 2–3 weeks to reach steady-state level. Decreases efficacy of oral contraceptive agents. SE: Initial sedation for first few days, but those taking it rapidly develop tolerance. Dividing doses may avoid sedation effect. OD: Symptoms of excessive dosing include nystagmus and ataxia. AE: Increased risk of osteoporosis with long-term use.	D
Primidone (Mysoline)	Tablets: 50, 250 mg.	Generalized tonic-clonic seizures, partial seizures; more effective than phenobarbital	Usual dose: 750–1500 mg/day in divided doses tid to qid with maximum of 2 g/day.	Decreases efficacy of oral contraceptive agents. CNS toxic effects more pronounced at lower doses than seen with phenobarbital; therefore requires gradual increment increases. SE: Symptoms include drowsiness, dizziness, ataxia, nausea, and vomiting. AE: Increased risk of osteoporosis with long-term use.	D
Valproate sodium (Depacon), valproic acid (Depakene), divalproex (Depakote, Depakote ER)	Valproate sodium IV solution. Valproic acid capsules 250 mg; syrup 250 mg/5 mL. Divalproex 125-, 250-, 500-mg enteric-coated tablets. Divalproex ER 250, 500 mg.	Generalized tonic-clonic seizures, partial seizures, absence seizures Off-label use: Neuropathic pain	10–20 mg/kg/day in adults.	Initial dose 5–15 mg/kg/day increasing to maintenance levels. Enteric-coated tablets (Depakote) avoid gastric upset. Individuals taking enzyme-inducing drugs such as phenobarbital may require higher doses. Does not decrease efficacy of oral contraceptives. SE: Nausea and vomiting, heartburn, weight gain, irregular menses. AE: hepatotoxicity, pancreatitis. FDA black box warning to monitor for depression, behavior change, and signs of suicide ideation.	D

SE = side effects; AE = adverse effects; OD = overdose.
* Except absent seizures.

Phenytoin (Dilantin)

Phenytoin (Dilantin) is the oldest nonsedative antiseizure drug (Table 24-5). Although it was first synthesized in 1908, its antiseizure properties were not discovered until 1938, when numerous drugs were systematically investigated for antiseizure properties.

Mechanism of Action

The major mechanism of action of phenytoin (Dilantin) is due to binding to the postsynaptic sodium channel, thereby prolonging the inactivated state of the sodium channel and stabilizing neuronal membranes. Phenytoin has some pre-synaptic actions that inhibit the release of the excitatory neurotransmitter glutamate and promote the release of the inhibitory neurotransmitter GABA.[24] These effects may explain some of the toxic symptoms associated with high levels of phenytoin. The effects of phenytoin on calcium conductance may also explain some of its usefulness as an antiarrhythmic agent.

Pharmacokinetic Properties

Phenytoin (Dilantin) is available in two different oral formulations—rapid-release tablets and extended-release capsules. The absorption varies between preparations made by different manufacturers, and therefore, the plasma phenytoin levels may vary when converting from one manufacturer to another or one formulation to another. The time to peak absorption can vary from 3 to 12 hours. Therefore, individuals should be treated with the same drug from a single manufacturer, although changes can be made if the person is monitored for seizure control or onset of toxicities. A soluble phosphate prodrug fosphenytoin (Cerebyx) is well absorbed after intramuscular injection. Fosphenytoin is converted in the body to phenytoin and is available for both intramuscular and intravenous use (Box 24-4).

Phenytoin (Dilantin) is metabolized by liver enzymes to inactive metabolites that are then excreted by the kidneys. The half-life of phenytoin ranges from 12 hours to more than 36 hours due to the variations in metabolism. At blood levels within a therapeutic range, the liver enzymes responsible for metabolizing phenytoin become saturated so small additional doses may produce large increases in phenytoin blood levels and a longer half-life. These unusual **nonlinear kinetics** result in a small and unpredictable therapeutic index. Although the average half-life at midtherapeutic range is about

24 hours, much longer half-lives occur at the higher concentration ranges.

Phenytoin (Dilantin) is extensively bound to protein (87–93%) in the plasma—primarily albumin. Only the unbound fraction is pharmacologically active because the protein-bound fraction cannot cross the blood–brain barrier. Approximately 90% of phenytoin is in the bound form if there is an adequate albumin concentration and no other drugs competing for albumin binding sites.

Side Effects/Adverse Effects

Twenty percent of persons on chronic phenytoin therapy develop gingival hyperplasia that includes swollen, tender, and bleeding gums. The overgrowth involves altered collagen metabolism and can be minimized with good oral hygiene such as flossing and gum massage.

Sedation and other CNS effects are mild within the therapeutic range. At excessively high doses, phenytoin (Dilantin) can lose its selectivity for seizure suppression and begin to elicit more diverse CNS symptoms. As plasma levels approach the upper range of therapeutic effect (20 mcg/mL),CNS effects become more common. Nystagmus (involuntary eye movements) is common, and other symptoms may include excessive sedation, cognitive impairment, diplopia (double vision), ataxia (staggering), and behavioral changes. These effects usually resolve after adjusting the phenytoin dose. Other drugs that have CNS depressive effects such as alcohol, barbiturates, benzodiazepines, and opioids will add to the CNS depressive effects of phenytoin.

Endocrine effects include inhibition of antidiuretic hormone (ADH) release, inhibition of insulin secretion resulting in hyperglycemia, and glycosuria. Softening of bones or osteomalacia occurs because phenytoin (Dilantin) interferes

---

Box 24-4 High-Risk Sound-Alikes

The most common brand name for fosphenytoin, an antiepileptic drug, is *Cerebyx*. Cerebyx is an example of a drug that is considered to be a high-risk sound-alike due to its similarity to other frequently prescribed agents. Other pharmaceuticals that are similar to Cerebyx include Celebrex, a common brand of celecoxib, a nonsteroidal anti-inflammatory often used as a treatment for arthritis; Celexa (citalopram hydrobromide), an SSRI; and a botanic, huperzine A, now marketed under the brand name of Cerebra and suggested for treatment/prevention of Alzheimer's disease, although data are lacking on effectiveness.

Since these names are so similar, extra caution must be taken when caring for individuals who report taking these agents, as they, too, can become confused about which drug is being used. The FDA has a program within its organization, the Office of Surveillance and Epidemiology, formerly Office of Drug Safety, which periodically conducts meetings and publishes findings to promote clearer and unique naming options in an attempt to decrease accidental medication errors.

with vitamin D metabolism, resulting in decreased calcium absorption. Phenytoin also increases vitamin K metabolism, which can result in increased bleeding tendencies in neonates of mothers who take phenytoin during pregnancy. Lower vitamin K levels can interfere with the production of proteins important for calcium metabolism in bone, resulting in vitamin D-resistant osteomalacia.

Between 2% and 5% of individuals taking phenytoin (Dilantin) develop a hypersensitive morbilliform (measles-like) rash that can progress to more serious skin reactions such as exfoliative dermatitis or Stevens-Johnson syndrome. Phenytoin should be discontinued if rash develops. Other adverse reactions include blood disorders such as neutropenia, leucopenia, red-cell aplasia, agranulocytosis, and thrombocytopenia.

Drug–Drug Interactions

Phenytoin (Dilantin) is an inducer of CYP1A2, CYP2C19, and CYP3A4 and has numerous drug–drug interactions (Table 24-4). Drugs that are metabolized by the same CYP450 enzymes that metabolize phenytoin (Dilantin) compete for that enzyme, which can result in decreased metabolism of phenytoin and a subsequent increased risk of toxic blood levels. Conversely, drugs that induce the CYP450 enzymes that metabolize phenytoin can decrease blood levels of phenytoin and cause a seizure. Prominent among these drugs are carbamazepine (Tegretol) and phenobarbital (Luminal). Toxic blood levels of phenytoin can also occur as the result of competition for albumin binding. Valproic acid (Depakene) competes for binding sites in this manner and is well known to increase plasma phenytoin concentrations.

Carbamazepine (Tegretol)

Carbamazepine (Carbatrol, Tegretol) is closely related chemically to the tricyclic antidepressants. Introduced in 1960 as a drug for the treatment of trigeminal neuralgia, it was approved as an antiseizure drug in 1974.

Pharmacokinetic Properties

Carbamazepine (Carbatrol, Tegretol) is only available as an oral medication and has a widely variable rate of absorption ranging from 4 to 8 hours after ingestion. The rate of absorption is slowed by recent food intake. This property may be used intentionally to slow absorption of large doses of the drug in order to make them more tolerable. Extended-release forms of the drug permit twice-daily dosing for many persons and help to avoid adverse effects.

Carbamazepine (Carbatrol, Tegretol) has an active metabolite that may contribute to its efficacy as an AED.

Side Effects/Adverse Effects

Carbamazepine (Carbatrol, Tegretol) is not sedating within the usual dose range. However, acute alcohol intoxication can have an additive effect in persons who take carbamazepine and the combination can cause CNS and respiratory depression or, conversely, hyperirritability and convulsions. More commonly, diplopia, blurred vision, vertigo, and ataxia are adverse effects related to dose, and these side effects can often be alleviated by rearranging the dosing schedule and giving a larger dose at bedtime. Gradual increases of the dose of carbamazepine over time may permit individuals to develop tolerance to the drug, alleviating CNS symptoms.

Persons who initiate therapy using carbamazepine (Carbatrol, Tegretol) should be monitored for depression, behavior changes, and suicidal ideation.[25] Carbamazepine can cause bone marrow suppression resulting in a transient leukopenia in about 10% of persons that usually resolves in the first 4 months of therapy initiation. Occasionally, transient thrombocytopenia will also occur. Irreversible aplastic anemia develops rarely, in approximately 1 in 200,000 individuals who are treated with carbamazepine, although aplastic anemia may be associated with administration of multiple drugs or prior hematologic disorders. Individuals known to have a history of a hematologic disorder or current hematologic compromise should not receive carbamazepine. Approximately 10% of persons treated with carbamazepine develop rash. Severe skin reactions such as erythema multiforme and Stevens-Johnson syndrome occur rarely and require withdrawal of the drug.

Several endocrine-related adverse effects are associated with carbamazepine. Antidiuretic hormone secretion is promoted by carbamazepine, occasionally resulting in hyponatremia from water retention promoting seizures.[26] Carbamazepine may also interfere with vitamin D metabolism, causing disordered calcium metabolism that may be associated with decreased bone mineral density.

Drug–Drug Interactions

This drug is a potent inducer of several CYP450 enzymes. Interestingly, during the initial phase of treatment, the half-life of carbamazepine is approximately 40 hours. With continued treatment, the half-life decreases to about 15 hours because this drug induces the CYP450 enzymes that metabolize it, so metabolism speeds up and doses sometimes have to be increased to compensate for this effect.

Carbamazepine (Carbatrol, Tegretol) is an inducer of CYP450 enzymes that increase the rate at which this drug and other drugs are inactivated. Other AEDs such as phenytoin (Dilantin) and phenobarbital (Luminal) are also potent hepatic enzyme inducers, so if these drugs are taken with carbamazepine as combination therapy for persons whose seizures were not controlled on monotherapy, further acceleration of the metabolism of carbamazepine can occur.

Phenobarbital (Luminal)

Phenobarbital (Luminal) is the oldest available AED and is considered one of the safest antiseizure drugs. Phenobarbital belongs to the barbiturate class of drugs, all of which have antiseizure properties. The advantage of phenobarbital over other drugs in this class is that it has a maximal antiseizure effect at a dose lower than that required for hypnosis. Other barbiturates will control seizures at doses that will make most individuals somnolent. Nevertheless, just like all barbiturates, phenobarbital can produce sedation and sleep when given in high doses. In general, however, phenobarbital is inexpensive, has a relatively low toxicity, and is very effective.

Mechanism of Action

Phenobarbital potentiates synaptic inhibition by acting on the GABA receptor in the postsynaptic neuron and decreasing excitatory transmission. When the GABA receptor is activated, it causes the opening of chloride channels that hyperpolarize the neuron, which makes it more difficult to reach threshold to create an action potential. Phenobarbital also blocks the excitatory responses elicited by glutamate.[18] Both of these actions tend to suppress the rapid firing of abnormal cortical foci inhibiting the spread of stimulation necessary for seizures to occur.

Pharmacokinetic Properties

Absorption of orally administered phenobarbital is slow. Peak plasma concentrations take several hours after a single dose of the drug. The half-life of phenobarbital is approximately 4 days, resulting in a slow time to plateau plasma concentration of 2 to 3 weeks if a loading dose is not given. This drug is actually effective for most seizure types, but it is frequently being replaced by some of the newer AEDs because the sedative properties of phenobarbital are difficult for individuals to tolerate.

Side Effects/Adverse Effects

Sedation is the most common and most troubling side effect of phenobarbital (Luminal). Phenobarbital intensifies the CNS depression caused by other drugs such as alcohol, benzodiazepines, opioids, and antihistamines. This drug interaction can result in severe respiratory depression and coma; therefore, persons on phenobarbital therapy should be warned to avoid other CNS depressants. The elderly may experience confusion and agitation with phenobarbital therapy and are especially prone to adverse drug–drug interactions. Therefore, this drug is avoided whenever possible in this population.[27]

Phenobarbital (Luminal), like all barbiturates, can cause physical dependence and should not be abruptly withdrawn as sudden withdrawal of the drug can precipitate status epilepticus.

Drug–Drug Interactions

Like the other older AEDs, phenobarbital is metabolized by CYP450 enzymes and is a potent inducer of those enzymes as well. Therefore, drugs that are metabolized by CYP450 enzymes are degraded more rapidly when administered with phenobarbital. Most notable among these drugs are the hormonal contraceptives, oral anticoagulants, and some other AEDs, especially carbamazepine (Tegretol). Conversely, valproic acid (Depakene) is known to compete with phenobarbital for hepatic degradation, increasing the plasma level of phenobarbital by as much as 100%, which necessitates a reduction in dose when the two are concomitantly administered.

Primidone (Mysoline)

Primidone (Mysoline) or 2-desoxyphenobarbital is metabolized into two compounds: phenobarbital and phenylethylmalonamide (PEMA). All three compounds are active AEDs. Primidone has more CNS toxic effects at lower doses than phenobarbital and therefore should be administered in gradual increments. Some individuals experience transient side effects such as drowsiness, dizziness, ataxia, nausea, and vomiting to such a debilitating degree that they are unwilling to take another dose. Initial dosing at bedtime often minimizes the side effects until tolerance develops. One clinical manipulation consists of taking advantage of the cross-tolerance between phenobarbital and primidone. Initial dosing with phenobarbital will allow the individual to develop a tolerance with milder side effects, and then primidone can be substituted.

Ethosuximide (Zarontin)

First introduced in 1958, ethosuximide (Zarontin) remains the drug of choice for absence seizures due to its safety and efficacy. Phensuximide (Milontin) and methsuximide (Celontin) are two other members of the succinimide family of AEDs that are not extensively used due to their toxicity profile. Ethosuximide (Zarontin) prevents synchronized firing of thalamocortical neurons that produce the large-amplitude T-current spikes associated with absence seizures.

Pharmacokinetic Properties

Ethosuximide (Zarontin) is well absorbed after oral administration, reaching a peak concentration in the plasma after about 3 hours. Ethosuximide distributes evenly throughout most of the tissues of the body except for adipose tissue.

Side Effects/Adverse Effects

Gastrointestinal complaints are common dose-related side effects that include nausea, vomiting, and anorexia. CNS effects include drowsiness, lethargy, euphoria, dizziness, headache, ataxia, and hiccups. In a manner similar to many other AEDs, some tolerance to these effects usually develops over time. Behavioral changes such as aggression, hyperactivity, and irritability also occur occasionally. Psychotic episodes including anxiety, depression, and hallucinations occur mostly in persons with a history of prior mental illness. Rare adverse effects include Stevens-Johnson syndrome, aplastic anemia, and agranulocytosis.

Drug–Drug Interactions

Although ethosuximide is metabolized by CYP450 enzymes, principally CYP3A, it does not induce its own metabolism, nor does it induce or inhibit the metabolism of other drugs by these enzymes. However, other drugs known to be CYP3A inducers, such as rifampin (Rifadin), do speed up ethosuximide metabolism, resulting in lower serum levels of this drug. Conversely, isoniazid (INH) acts as a potent inhibitor of CYP isoenzymes, and if taken concomitantly with ethosuximide, the result will be in increased serum levels of ethosuximide.

Valproate Sodium (Depacon), Valproic Acid (Depakene)

Valproic acid (Depakene) and valproate sodium (Depacon) can be used singly or in a derivative combination formulation called divalproex sodium (Depakote, Depakote ER). The active ingredient in all three formulations is Valproate ion, which is effective against myoclonic seizures, tonic-clonic seizures, and partial seizures. Valproate sodium (Depacon) is one of the major AEDs used today. The mechanism of action of valproate is not known. Hypotheses include potentiation of GABA function, inhibition of glutamate receptors, and inhibition of voltage-gated sodium channels.

Pharmacokinetic Properties

Numerous preparations of valproate are available. Oral forms of valproic acid (Depakene) and divalproex (Depakote) include capsules, tablets, and syrup for immediate release. Enteric-coated tablets consisting of different salts and formulations are provided to avoid gastrointestinal upset. Valproate sodium (Depacon) is an intravenous formulation.

Valproate is readily absorbed after oral administration, widely distributed throughout the body, and metabolized in the liver by the action of cytochrome P450 enzymes. Valproate has two active metabolites, each having its own antiseizure activity.

Side Effects/Adverse Effects

Most commonly, valproate sodium (Depacon) causes nausea, vomiting, abdominal pain, and heartburn. These effects are dose related, occur in about 16% of individuals, and may be due to direct gastric irritation by valproate sodium.[17,28] Taking valproate sodium in an enteric-coated formulation or with meals may decrease these GI effects, which are usually transient. Excessive weight gain occurs in some persons, which is hypothesized to be secondary to disordered fat metabolism rather than increased appetite.[17]

Although drowsiness, lethargy, and confusion are rarely associated with taking valproate sodium, these side effects may occur especially among those taking high doses. There is some evidence that cognitive impairment can occur in individuals receiving valproate sodium.[29] Occasionally, persons receiving valproate sodium along with another AED will develop acute mental changes, progressing to stupor or coma that is usually reversible within 2–3 days of discontinuation of either drug.

Valproate sodium has an FDA black box warning that it has caused fatal hepatotoxicity. Retrospective studies have identified the major risk factors associated with this rare, fatal condition. These factors include adults receiving valproate sodium and another AED concomitantly and persons who have developmental delays.[30] Monitoring liver enzymes might not be helpful in identifying persons developing this adverse effect because it is not preceded by progressive rise in liver enzymes, and benign enzyme elevation is common during valproate sodium therapy.[30]

Diagnosis depends on recognition of clinical features that include nausea, vomiting, anorexia, lethargy, loss of seizure control, jaundice, and edema.

Drug–Drug Interactions

Although valproate does not itself induce liver enzymes, it is sensitive to the action of other enzyme-modifying drugs. Drugs that are enzyme inducers, such as many other AEDs, when taken with valproate, will increase its metabolism, resulting in lower serum concentrations and a greater likelihood of seizures occurring.

Second-Generation Antiepileptic Drugs

The newer antiepileptic drugs are generally better than the first-generation AEDs in controlling seizures and have fewer drug–drug interactions, but these drugs also have potential adverse effects that require careful monitoring. Doses, indications, side effects and clinical considerations are presented in Table 24-6.

Lamotrigine (Lamictal)

Lamotrigine (Lamictal) appears to act on neuronal sodium and calcium channels in postsynaptic neurons, which blocks the repetitive neuronal activation characteristic of seizure disorders. Lamotrigine also blocks the release of the excitatory neurotransmitter glutamate twice as much as it blocks the inhibitory neurotransmitter GABA; thus it has a net neuroinhibitory effect. Approximately 7% of persons who take lamotrigine report having significant sedation, which is low compared to 28% of the persons who take phenytoin (Dilantin) and 25% of the persons who take carbamazepine (Tegretol).[31,32]

Pharmacokinetic Properties

Lamotrigine is well absorbed, and absorption is not affected by food or antacids. It is approximately 55% protein bound and therefore not vulnerable to drug–drug interactions that occur when drugs compete for plasma proteins. Lamotrigine is metabolized via glucuronic acid conjugation in the liver and excreted via the kidneys.

Side Effects/Adverse Effects

The most common side effects of lamotrigine are dizziness, blurred vision, insomnia, and headaches. Lamotrigine

(Lamictal) is most often used as adjunctive therapy with other antiseizure medications. Therefore, maintenance doses are tailored to the type of interaction possible with various AEDs. In addition, the FDA has specified schedules for initiation of therapy in an attempt to minimize the major adverse reaction of skin rashes. The FDA studies attribute the rashes, which can lead to hospitalization and life-threatening Stevens-Johnson syndrome, to over-rapid titration of initial therapy.[33]

Topiramate (Topamax)

Topiramate (Topamax) has recently been approved by the FDA as a monotherapeutic agent for generalized tonic-clonic seizures.[34] This drug blocks some postsynaptic neuron glutamate receptors and voltage-gated sodium channels, which limits sustained repetitive firing. Topiramate reduces high-voltage calcium currents in the postsynaptic neuron.

Side Effects/Adverse Effects

Dose-related adverse effects of topiramate usually occur within the first 4 weeks of therapy and can include fatigue, somnolence, dizziness, slowed cognition, paresthesias, nervousness, and confusion. The cognitive effects, which are most common, present as memory difficulty, word-finding difficulty, and slowed cognition. Weight loss has been observed among individuals receiving topiramate for seizure disorders as well as for conditions other than epilepsy. Those who lost weight had improved lipid profiles, glycemic control, and blood pressure. Topiramate can cause metabolic acidosis, renal calculi, and a rare ocular condition characterized by acute myopia and glaucoma that requires withdrawal from the drug.

Drug–Drug Interactions

Although the level of liver enzyme induction is less with topiramate than with the potent enzyme inducers such as carbamazepine (Tegretol), topiramate does speed the metabolism of the estrogen component of combination oral contraceptives. Therefore, women taking such oral contraceptives should receive high-dose estrogen-containing agents or use other forms of birth control. Topiramate also decreases plasma concentrations of digoxin.

Gabapentin (Neurontin) and Pregabalin (Lyrica)

Gabapentin (Neurontin) is a GABA molecule bound to a cyclohexane ring. It is highly lipid soluble and therefore

Table 24-6 Second-Generation Antiepileptic Drugs

Drug Generic (Brand)	Formulations	Therapeutic Indication	Dose	Clinical Considerations	FDA Pregnancy Category
Felbamate (Felbatol)	400- and 600-mg tablets. 600 mg/5 mL suspension.	Adjunct for refractory seizures	Average dose is 3600 mg per day.	Dose increased by 15 mg/dose in 1- to 2-week intervals. Decreases efficacy of oral contraceptives. AE: Aplastic anemia, hepatotoxicity. FDA black box warning to monitor for depression, behavior change, and signs of suicide ideation.	C
Gabapentin (Neurontin)	100-, 300-, 400-, 600-, and 800-mg tablets. 100-, 300-, and 400-mg capsules. 250 mg/5 mL solution.	Adjunct against generalized tonic-clonic seizures and partial seizures Off label use: Chronic pain, peripheral neuropathy, postherpetic neuralgia	900–1800 mg/day in three divided doses.	Dosage started with 300 mg per day and then advanced 300 mg per day until effective dose is reached. Does not decrease efficacy of oral contraceptives. SE: Drowsiness, fatigue. AE: None reported. FDA black box warning to monitor for depression, behavior change, and signs of suicide ideation.	C
Pregabalin (Lyrica)	25-, 50-, 75-, 100-, 150-, 200-, 225-, and 300-mg capsules.		150–600 mg/day in two to three divided doses.	Dosage started with 50 mg tid or 75 mg bid. Maximum dose is 600 mg per day. To discontinue drug, taper dose over 7 days. Does not decrease efficacy of oral contraceptives. FDA black box warning to monitor for depression, behavior change, and signs of suicide ideation.	C
Lamotrigine (Lamictal)*	25-, 100-, 150-, and 200-mg tablets. 2-, 5-, and 25-mg chewable tablets.	Partial seizures	300–500 mg/day PO in two divided doses.	Dose increased gradually to minimize risk of rash. Does not decrease efficacy of oral contraceptives. SE: dizziness, blurred vision, insomnia, headaches. AE: Stevens-Johnson syndrome. FDA black box warning to monitor for depression, behavior change, and signs of suicide ideation.	C
Lamotrigine (Lamictal) added to valproate			100–200 mg/day PO in two divided doses.	25 mg q other day × 2 weeks then 25 mg/day × 2 weeks, then the dose is increased by 25 to 50 mg/day every 1 to 2 weeks. Does not decrease efficacy of oral contraceptives. FDA black box warning to monitor for depression, behavior change, and signs of suicide ideation.	C
Levetiracetam (Keppra)	250-, 500-, 750-, 1000-mg tablets.	Adjunct for refractory seizures	500 mg/day. Maximum dose is 3000 mg/day.	SE: Ataxia, abnormal gait, agitation, hostility, anxiety, depression. AE: Leukopenia, psychosis, withdrawal seizures. FDA black box warning to monitor for depression, behavior change, and signs of suicide ideation.	C
Oxcarbazepine (Trileptal)	Tablets: 150, 300, and 600 mg. Oral suspension: 300 mg/5 mL.		Start at 300 mg bid increasing by max of 600 mg/ week up to a max of 2400 mg/day.	Often used as adjunctive therapy; therefore provider should monitor changes in levels of other AEDs as oxcarbazepine is added to regimen. Decreases efficacy of oral contraceptive agents.	C

(continues)

Table 24-6 Second-Generation Antiepileptic Drugs (*continued*)

Drug Generic (Brand)	Formulations	Therapeutic Indication	Dose	Clinical Considerations	FDA Pregnancy Category
				FDA black box warning to monitor for depression, behavior change, and signs of suicide ideation.	
Tiagabine (Gabitril)	2-, 4-, 12-, and 16-mg tablets.	Adjunct for refractory seizures	32–56 mg/day in two to four divided doses.	Start with 4 mg per day in 2–4 divided doses increasing 4 mg/day after 1 week, increasing 4–8 mg/day each week. Maximum dose 56 mg/day. Give with food to minimize gastric upset. Does not decrease efficacy of oral contraceptives. SE: nausea, vomiting abdominal pain, impaired concentration. AE: Status epilepticus, CNS depression. FDA black box warning to monitor for depression, behavior change, and signs of suicide ideation.	C
Topiramate (Topamax)	25-, 50-, 100-, and 200-mg tablets. 15- and 25-mg sprinkles.	Generalized tonic-clonic seizures[†], adjunct for partial seizures, atonic myotonic and atypical absence seizures, migraine headaches Off label use: Impulse control disorders, movement disorders	200–600 mg/day.	50 mg per day increasing slowly to avoid adverse effects. Decreases efficacy of oral contraceptive agents in dose of > 200 mg/day. SE: Dizziness, slowed cognition, nervousness, confusion, memory difficulty. AE: Metabolic acidosis, nephrolithiasis, glaucoma. FDA black box warning to monitor for depression, behavior change, and signs of suicide ideation.	C
Zonisamide (Zonegran)	25-, 50-, and 100-mg capsules.	Adjunct for refractory seizures	100–600 mg divided once to twice a day.	Start at 100 mg and increase every 2 weeks to max dose of 600 mg/day. Does not decrease efficacy of oral contraceptives. SE: Fatigue, nervousness, dizziness, confusion, anorexia. AE: Heat stroke, Stevens-Johnson syndrome, agranulocytosis. Contraindicated for persons allergic to sulfa. FDA black box warning to monitor for depression, behavior change, and signs of suicidal ideation.	C

SE = side effects; AE = adverse effects.
* Lamotrigine is used as an adjunct added to other AEDs.
[†] FDA approved for monotherapy.

readily crosses the blood–brain barrier. Pregabalin is also a GABA analog and closely related to gabapentin. Both drugs have been approved in the United States for treatment of seizure disorders as well as for analgesia in chronic pain conditions.

Mechanism of Action

Although they are closely related to GABA structurally, gabapentin and pregabalin do not act directly on the GABA receptors. Both drugs bind to subunits of voltage-gated calcium channels in the presynaptic neuron, which reduces entry of calcium, and this subsequently inhibits the release of glutamate. Gabapentin and pregabalin are not metabolized in the body and do not induce hepatic enzymes. Both drugs are excreted unchanged in the urine. Since they do not induce hepatic enzymes, and they are not bound to plasma proteins, the drugs have virtually no known drug–drug interactions.

Gabapentin has also been used for monotherapy for persons newly diagnosed with epilepsy and appears to be similar to carbamazepine (Tegretol) in effectiveness.[35]

Side Effects/Adverse Effects

Adverse effects of gabapentin and pregabalin include somnolence, dizziness, ataxia, and fatigue that usually resolve within 2 weeks of beginning treatment. Behavioral changes such as aggression, anger, and oppositional behavior have occurred in developmentally delayed persons and in those with attention deficit disorder. Adverse reactions are not dose related, and some individuals do not tolerate even small doses of gabapentin.

Felbamate (Felbatol), Levetiracetam (Keppra), Tiagabine (Gabitril), and Zonisamide (Zonegran)

Felbamate (Felbatol), levetiracetam (Keppra), tiagabine (Gabitril), and zonisamide (Zonegran) are used as adjunct medications when monotherapy is not effective.

Felbamate (Felbatol) can cause fatal aplastic anemia, usually within the first year of therapy. Cases of severe liver failure have also been associated with the drug.[36] Therefore, it is reserved for use as a third medication for those who have severe epilepsy that is unresponsive to several previous drugs and those who have problems with the sedative effects of other agents.

Adverse effects of levetiracetam (Keppra) mostly occur during the first 4 weeks of therapy and include ataxia, abnormal gait, and incoordination. Reported behavioral symptoms include agitation, hostility, anxiety, apathy, emotional lability, depersonalization, and depression. Reduction of the dose usually improves the behavioral problems.

Tiagabine (Gabitril) has an interesting mechanism of action in that it blocks reuptake of GABA into the glial cells and neurons. Tiagabine is extensively oxidized via the cytochrome P450 enzyme system in the liver. When coadministered with enzyme-inducing AEDs, the half-life of tiagabine is reduced from 5–8 hours to 2–3 hours due to increased clearance of the drug. Tiagabine itself neither induces nor inhibits CYP450 enzymes and is given in low enough doses that it does not displace other drugs from protein-binding sites. At low doses of 8 mg per day, tiagabine does not affect the metabolism of hormonal contraceptives, although it is not known if higher doses would produce such an effect.

Zonisamide does not induce or inhibit CYP450 enzymes, and therefore does not cause any significant alteration in the metabolism of other drugs. Adverse effects include abnormal thinking, nervousness, dizziness, anorexia, confusion ataxia, and fatigue. However, individuals who take zonisamide also take other AEDs, and the adverse effects between medications overlap, so it is difficult to assess the exact cause of a particular side effect.

Benzodiazepines for Treating Seizures

The benzodiazepines act as inhibitory neurotransmitters by binding to a specific binding site on the GABA receptor. Benzodiazepines have no action at the GABA receptor in the absence of GABA itself. Rather the benzodiazepines enhance the action of GABA at its binding site. The GABA receptor permits a greater influx of chloride ions at lower GABA concentrations when the benzodiazepine site is occupied. Thus the benzodiazepines promote the neuroinhibition produced by GABA. The potency of a specific benzodiazepine correlates with its binding affinity at the benzodiazepine sites on neuronal GABA receptors.[18]

Although benzodiazepines are effective against almost every type of seizure, the individual drugs vary in their efficacy in different types of epilepsy (Table 24-7). Long-term benzodiazepine treatment results in the phenomenon

Table 24-7 Benzodiazepines Used to Treat Seizures

Drug Generic (Brand)	Formulations	Dose	Clinical Considerations	FDA Pregnancy Category
Diazepam (Valium)	Oral: 2-, 5-, and 10-mg tablets; oral solution 5 mg/5 mL; parenteral solution 5 mg/5 mL and 5 mg/mL; rectal gel (Diastat): 2.5, 5, 10, and 20 mg.	Initial dose for status epilepticus 10–20 mg IV, 5–10 mg every few hours. Or 10 mg PR, may repeat once if necessary.	Rapid redistribution from brain to muscle tissue results in short half-life. Diazepam can be followed by longer-acting AED such as phenytoin.	D
Lorazepam (Ativan)	Oral: 0.5-, 1-, 2-mg tablets. Parenteral solution 2 mg/mL or 4 mg/mL for IV or IM.	Initial dose for status epilepticus 0.1 mg/kg up to 4 mg IV at 2 mg/min. Repeat after 10–15 min if necessary.	Longer duration of action and greater potency makes it the agent of choice in adults with status epilepticus.	D
Clonazepam (Klonopin)	Oral: 0.5-, 1-, 2-mg tablets; 0.125-, 0.25-, 0.5-, 2-mg dispersible tablets placed on tongue for absorption.	Up to 8 mg/day in 2–3 divided doses.	Not available in parenteral form in the United States.	D

of tolerance for which increasing doses of the drug are required to induce the same effect. Tolerance also increases the risk of rebound seizures upon withdrawal of the drug. Thus, the major role for benzodiazepines as AEDs is as a first-line therapy for status epilepticus and seizure clusters because these drugs have a rapid onset and proven efficacy. Status epilepticus is a life-threatening condition in which the brain is in a state of persistent seizure that manifests as one continuous seizure of ≥ 30 minutes[37] (Box 24-5).

Diazepam (Valium), Lorazepam (Ativan), Clonazepam (Klonopin)

Diazepam was the first benzodiazepine used as an AED and has become the standard drug for therapy of status epilepticus. It is available in oral, parenteral, and rectal (Diastat) forms. Diazepam rapidly enters the brain, but then its concentration decreases due to redistribution to other tissues of the body so that the initial half-life is only 1 hour resulting in a short duration of action in the brain.

Lorazepam (Ativan) has a greater potency and longer duration of action than diazepam and has become the agent of choice for initial treatment of status epilepticus in adults.[38]

Clonazepam (Klonopin) is a benzodiazepine that is often used to treat anxiety and can also be used as an AED.

Box 24-5 Emergency Treatment of Seizures

Status epilepticus is defined as either more than 30 minutes of continuous seizure activity or two or more sequential seizures without full recovery of consciousness between seizures. Status epilepticus is regarded as a medical emergency, with overall mortality rates of 30%.[37] Diazepam (Valium) has been used to treat status epilepticus due to its relative effectiveness and low likelihood of inducing respiratory depression. However, the anticonvulsant effect of a single intravenous dose of diazepam is approximately 20 minutes. A dose of 10 to 20 mg administered intravenously is followed by a continuous intravenous infusion at a rate of 20 mg per hour. Lorazepam (Ativan) has a slightly increased risk of respiratory depression when compared to diazepam. The duration of anticonvulsant effect of a single dose of lorazepam is more than 6 hours; therefore, it is becoming the favored treatment for status epilepticus. An initial dose of 4 mg is given intravenously, and it is repeated once after 10-15 minutes if needed.

It is useful for treating both acute seizures and chronic epilepsy. Clonazepam is only available in an oral formulation in the United States; therefore, it is not used in this country to treat status epilepticus. The dose of clonazepam for treating chronic epilepsy in adults is as high as 8 mg per day in two or three divided doses.

Approximately 50% of adults experience lethargy and drowsiness as an adverse effect of clonazepam, but tolerance to the drug over time decreases this effect. In children, the rate of drowsiness is as high as 85%. Other adverse effects include nystagmus, which is fairly common. Due to the high rates of adverse effects seen with clonazepam, it is usually reserved for the most difficult epileptic conditions. Furthermore, tolerance to the antiseizure effects of clonazepam usually develops after 1–6 months of administration, after which some persons do not respond to clonazepam at any dose.[39]

Alternative Therapies for Epilepsy: The Ketogenic Diet

The ketogenic diet has been used for over 80 years to provide symptomatic nonpharmacologic control of seizures associated with epilepsy. The classic ketogenic diet is composed of 80–90% fat that is meant to mimic the biochemical changes associated with periods of starvation or limited food availability.[40] In this diet, energy is derived from the utilization of dietary and body stores of fat. The traditional ketogenic diet that is based on long-chain fatty acids was originally developed by Wilder in 1921.[41] Rubenstein et al. found similar results in a retrospective study of individuals who commenced a ketogenic diet primarily due to fear of side effects they experienced with AEDs.[42] Sinha speculates about neurophysiologic mechanisms in his article on the ketogenic diet, but no definitive mechanisms have been determined for its effects in reducing seizures.[43]

Special Considerations for Women Taking Antiepileptic Drugs

Nadkarni[21] summarized recent findings of catamenial seizure variation thusly: 20–35% have an increase, 3–25% experience a decrease, while 60–85% experience no change in seizure frequency with changing hormonal levels. The following three distinct patterns have been described: perimenstrual, periovulatory, and luteal. The changes that occur may be due to hormonal fluctuations, altered protein binding that affects AED plasma levels, and perhaps other unexplained effects. Progesterone therapy may be helpful for some women with catamenial seizures as well as other forms of epilepsy.[44] Some AEDs cause metabolic changes that result in weight gain. Lamotrigine (Lamictal) may be a desirable AED for women because it does not increase weight and it does not disrupt the menstrual cycle. Topiramate lowers body weight.

Several AEDs (e.g., phenytoin) alter vitamin D metabolism and can indirectly cause osteomalacia (decreased mineralization of the bone). Supplementation with 400 IU of vitamin D has also been recommended for all women of childbearing years who are taking AEDs. Folate and multivitamin supplementation should be started prior to conception.

Antiepileptic Drugs and Contraception

Many of the antiseizure medications induce the liver enzymes that are responsible for metabolizing combined oral contraceptive (COC) agents. These result in a rapid degradation of the contraceptive agent, decreased contraceptive effectiveness, and an increased likelihood of unplanned pregnancy.[45] Tables 24-5 and 24-6 list which of the older and newer AEDs decrease the efficacy of COCs. Women using COCs who take AEDs that are metabolized via the CYP450 enzyme system have a 6% chance of contraceptive failure per year.[46] Levonorgestrel implants are contraindicated for women using these AEDs. If the woman is relying on medroxyprogesterone (DPMA) injections for contraception, the injections should be given every 10 weeks instead of every 12 weeks.[47] The most common combined oral contraceptives used today contain ≤ 35 mcg of estrogen, which makes them vulnerable to the enzyme induction effects of several AEDs. COCs with higher estrogen levels may be protected from this effect. Some authorities suggest that women with epilepsy start with a contraceptive pill that has 50 mcg of estrogen and if breakthrough bleeding occurs, consider alternative contraceptive methods.[48] However, availability of these higher estrogen dose pills is limited. Therefore, progestin-only contraceptives (POPs), injectable agents, or implantable drugs are the preferred methods.

Lamotrigine (Lamictal) has a unique dual interaction with combined oral contraceptives; while it only moderately increases their clearance, lamotrigine itself is metabolized to a greater extent during the 21-day cycle of contraceptive intake with a possible loss of antiepileptic efficacy. There is a prominent rebound of serum levels of lamotrigine during the 7-day period when no COC is taken.[49] Therefore, lamotrigine dose adjustment may be necessary during the monthly dose changes associated with the administration of combined oral contraceptives.

Antiepileptic Drugs and Osteoporosis

Carbamazepine (Tegretol), phenytoin (Dilantin), and valproate (Depacon, Depakene, Depakote) are associated with lower levels of calcium and an increased risk for fracture.[50] Therefore, all women taking these drugs should also ensure a daily intake of 1200 mg of calcium and 600 IU of vitamin D. Women who take AEDs for more than 5 years should have a bone density scan.[50]

AEDs During Pregnancy

Studies show that the older AEDs taken during the first trimester of pregnancy are associated with a twofold to threefold increase in the risk for major congenital malformations (6% in women with epilepsy versus 0.2% in the general population).[51-53] This risk also increases when multiple AEDs are administered together and may be dose related. It was originally unclear if the increase in teratogenic effects is secondary to epilepsy or secondary to AEDs, but recent research has made it clear that AEDs are the culprit. Valproate (Depacon, Depakene, Depakote) increases the risk for major congenital malformations when used as either monotherapy or part of a polytherapy regimen (6–10.2% incidence of major congenital malformations).[51,52] Additionally, there is some evidence that carbamazepine (Tegretol) increases the risk for posterior cleft palate and lamotrigine (Lamictal) in high doses is associated with an increased risk for congenital malformations. However, clinicians should not recommend discontinuing any AED for women who present for initial prenatal care and who are taking an AED. Rather, these women should be referred to a specialist for counseling and possible medication changes.

Clusters of congenital malformations were identified as early as 1963 in the offspring of women taking phenytoin (Dilantin) and its related drug, mephenytoin, for epilepsy. These malformations, which received worldwide attention, included such anomalies as craniofacial malformation, microcephalus, mental retardation, and hypoplasia of the distal phalanges and were called "fetal hydantoin syndrome."[52] The true incidence of congenital anomalies associated with the older AEDs is not conclusively known. Most studies have been too small to determine differences between the older drugs in the rate of malformations.[54] Several large, prospective pregnancy registries have been established to determine the true risk rates associated with individual agents, and specific risks are now known[55-58] (Table 24-8).

AEDs that act as folic acid antagonists such as phenytoin (Dilantin), carbamazepine (Tegretol), valproic acid (Depakene), and barbiturates increase the risk of neural tube defects.[59] Although it is not clear if folic acid supplementation will decrease the incidence of neural tube defects in women taking these AEDs, it is currently recommended that all women on AEDs take folic acid 0.4–5 mg per day from preconception until the end of the first trimester.[60]

AEDs During Lactation

The majority of AEDs are lipophilic and likely to concentrate in breast milk. Milk/plasma ratios and concentrations of many of the AEDs in breast milk are known; it is unclear what the effect is on the newborn.[61] Women with epilepsy

Table 24-8 Rates of Congenital Malformations in Women Using Antiepileptic Drugs During Pregnancy

Drug Generic (Brand)	Teratogenic Effect
Carbamazepine (Tegretol)	2.5–4% risk of major malformations (specifically posterior cleft palate, neural tube defects).*
Diazepam (Valium)	Small increased risk of pyloric stenosis and alimentary tract atresia.
Lamotrigine (Lamictal)	1.4–2.7% risk of major malformations, primarily oral clefts. Risk is not dose dependent.
Phenobarbital	6.5% incidence of major malformations. Increased incidence of cardiac malformations. Exposure during third trimester may lower IQ score of offspring by 0.5 SD.
Phenytoin (Dilantin)	Fetal hydantoin syndrome. Neural tube defects. Slight decrease in IQ scores in offspring.
Valproate, valproic acid (Depacon, Depakene)	10.73–13% risk of major malformations (including neural tube defects, facial cleft palate, and possibly hypospadias). Risk may be dose dependent. Risk increases at doses > 800–1000 mg/day. Lower IQ scores in offspring (9–10 points). Polypharmacy associated with an increased risk over monotherapy.

* Major malformation is an abnormality of an essential anatomic structure present at birth that interferes significantly with function and/or requires major intervention. Most common major malformations associated with AEDs include heart defects, cleft palate, urogenital defects, and neural tube defects.
Sources: Meador KJ et al. 2008[55]; Pennell PB 2008[61]; Meador KJ 2009.[57]

who take AEDs risk seizures and possible harm to their infants if they stop their medication while nursing. However, simply identifying the amount of the drug in breast milk is not sufficient as the drug may or may not be harmful to the newborn. As an example, ethosuximide (Zarontin) is excreted in breast milk, and the serum concentration of breastfeeding infants is relatively high at 30–50% of maternal serum concentration, but this exposure is not associated with adverse outcomes in the neonate, and the American Academy of Pediatrics considers ethosuximide compatible with breastfeeding.[53] Lamotrigine (Lamictal) reaches serum concentrations in the newborn that are potentially therapeutic and is categorized as a drug for which the effect on the newborn is unknown but may be of concern.[52,53] Benzodiazepines are in this same category. The barbiturates are associated with sedation in the newborn and should be used with caution by nursing mothers.[53] Carbamazepine (Tegretol), phenytoin (Dilantin), and valproic acid (Depakene) are considered compatible with breastfeeding.[53]

The Mature Woman

Women frequently experience an increase in seizures during the perimenopausal period and a decrease when they are postmenopausal.[62] This effect is especially common in women with the catamenial epilepsy pattern. Hormone therapy is also associated with an increase in seizure activity,[62] and the risk of fracture in this age group is especially high. Clinicians caring for women during the postmenopausal years who take AEDs will focus on interventions that decrease fracture risks and may consult with neurologists to find the best treatments for menopausal symptoms.

Restless Legs Syndrome

Restless legs syndrome (RLS) is a sensorimotor disorder that affects up to 10% of the general population and is more prevalent in women and the elderly. Although remissions occur, RLS is considered a chronic and progressive disorder. *Restless limbs syndrome* may better describe the disorder, as the legs, abdomen, and face can be affected, unilaterally or bilaterally. Women diagnosed with RLS should be reassured the disorder is not a precursor to Parkinson's disease.

Etiology of Restless Legs Syndrome

Although not clearly understood, the etiology appears to be, in part, a dopaminergic dysfunction in the substantia nigra of the basal ganglia. Anemia can contribute to this dysfunction by limiting brain iron metabolism of coenzymes and enzymes ultimately necessary for the production of dopamine. This is called the "iron-dopamine connection."

Diagnosis of Restless Legs Syndrome

Restless legs syndrome is a clinical diagnosis when all four of the following criteria are met: (1) there is an urge to move the legs accompanied by dyskinesias; (2) the dyskinesias worsen when the person is at rest, especially when sitting or lying down; (3) the dyskinesias are partially or totally relieved by movement; and (4) there is a circadian pattern with symptoms being worse in the evening and into the night, and better during the morning hours.[63] Supporting criteria for the diagnosis of RLS include a positive family history, periodic limb movements during the night as witnessed by the bed partner, and a positive response to dopaminergic therapies.[63]

Restless legs syndrome is categorized as primary (or idiopathic) or secondary. Primary RLS is subdivided into early onset (< 45 years of age), which is characterized by a slow progression of the disorder and thought to be familial, and late onset (> 45 years of age), which has a more aggressive progression. Secondary RLS may occur in persons with medical conditions that are associated with anemia, such as pregnancy, iron deficiency, and end-stage renal disease. Symptoms for primary and secondary RLS are the same; therefore, a medical workup to rule out the causes of secondary RLS is recommended.

Treatment of Restless Legs Syndrome

An algorithm for the treatment of RLS symptoms, whether primary or secondary, was devised by the Medical Advisory Board of the Restless Legs Syndrome Foundation in 2004.[64] Definitions for treatment include (1) intermittent RLS, which requires treatment as necessary; (2) daily RLS, which requires daily treatment; and (3) refractory RLS, which requires treatment adjustment or adjunct.

Dopaminergic Agents

The first line of pharmacologic treatment for primary RLS is a dopamine agonist such as ropinirole (Requip) or pramipexole (Mirapex). Both are nonergoline dopamine agonists that are believed to stimulate dopamine (D_2) receptors; the former is metabolized in the liver, the latter excreted by the kidneys. The first line of treatment for secondary RLS is to diagnose and treat the causative medical disorder, e.g., iron therapy for anemia. Pharmacologic treatments are listed in Table 24-9.[65,66]

In addition to ropinirole and pramipexole, opioids, sedative-hypnotics, and anticonvulsants have been used as

Table 24-9 Pharmacotherapy for Restless Legs Syndrome

Drug Generic (Brand)	Dose	Advantages	Clinical Considerations	FDA Pregnancy Category
Dopamine Precursors				
Carbidopa/levodopa (Sinemet)	½ or 1 tablet of 25/100 (mg carbidopa/mg levodopa) 1 h before symptom onset; not to exceed a dose of 50/200.	Can be used on a one-time basis or prn. Useful for persons with intermittent RLS as dopamine receptor agonists take longer to have an effect.	May develop augmentation, a worsening of symptoms prior to the next expected dose. Therapeutic value reduced if taken with high-protein food. Can cause insomnia, sleepiness, gastrointestinal distress.	C
Dopamine Receptor Agonists				
Pramipexole (Mirapex)	Initial dose 0.125 mg; mean effective dose is 0.375 mg; max dose is 0.75 mg.	Decreases periodic limb movements and mitigates consequences of RLS symptoms.	Can cause nausea, orthostatic hypotension, and augmentation. Associated with impulse-control disorders.	C
Ropinirole (Requip)	Initial dose 0.25 mg; average dose is 1.0 to 2.5 mg/day; max dose is 4 mg/day.			C

(continues)

Table 24-9 Pharmacologic Therapy for Restless Legs Syndrome (*continued*)

Drug Generic (Brand)	Dose	Advantages	Clinical Considerations	FDA Pregnancy Category
Opioids				
Codeine	15–30 mg; max 120 mg/day.	Opioids offer an effective alternative for persons whose RLS is not effectively treated with or cannot be treated by dopaminergic agents. Can be used on an intermittent basis or can be used successfully for QD therapy. Wide range of potencies.	Can cause constipation, urinary retention, sleepiness, or cognitive changes. Tolerance and dependence possible with higher doses of stronger agents, especially those with a shorter half-life.	C; D if prolonged use
Propoxyphene (Darvon)	65 to 130 mg/day; max 260 to 390 mg/day.			C; D if prolonged use
Hydrocodone (Vicodin)	5–10 mg/day; max 20–30 mg/day.			C; D if prolonged use
Oxycodone (Percocet, Roxicodone, OxyContin)	5–10 mg/day; max 15–20 mg/day; XR 10 mg/day; max 20–30 mg/day.			C; D if prolonged use
Tramadol (Ultram)	50–100 mg/day; max 300–400 mg/day.			C
Methadone	5–10 mg/day; max 20–40 mg/day.			B
Anticonvulsants				
Gabapentin (Neurontin)	100–300 mg/day; max 2400 mg/day.	Anticonvulsants offer an effective alternative for those whose RLS is not effectively treated with dopaminergic agents.	Disadvantages vary depending on agent but include nausea, sedation, dizziness, dermatologic conditions, hepatic disorders, and bone marrow suppression. Increases risk for suicidality.	C
Benzodiazepines				
Clonazepam (Klonopin)	0.25 mg/day; max 2 mg/day.	Sleeping aids are most effective for improving sleep quality if RLS symptoms occur at night. May be used alone if intolerant of dopaminergic drugs.	Can cause daytime sleepiness and cognitive impairment.	D
Oxazepam (Serax)	10 mg/day; max 40 mg/day.			D; first and third trimester
Temazepam (Restoril)	7.5–30 mg at bedtime; max for 1 month.			X
Zolpidem (Ambien)	5 mg/day; max 20 mg/day.			C
Triazolam (Halcion)	0.125 mg/day; max 0.25 mg/day.			X

Source: Reprinted with permission from Hensley JG 2009.[65]

adjunctive therapies for RLS. Opioids are an effective alternative for persons with RLS that is not treated effectively with dopaminergic agents and can be used intermittently. Sedative-hypnotics can improve sleep quality for persons who have symptoms at night. Gabapentin (Neurontin) is the most studied anticonvulsant and appears to be as efficacious as dopaminergic agents for controlling symptoms and has fewer drug–drug interactions. Gabapentin (Neurontin) has mild sedative properties and can be used to facilitate sleep in persons with RLS who have concomitant sleep disturbances.

Side Effects/Adverse Effects

Although nausea and other gastrointestinal upsets are the most commonly reported side effects of ropinirole (Requip) and pramipexole (Mirapex), increased somnolence can occur during daily activities such as driving.

Hallucinations, syncope, orthostatic hypotension, lack of impulse control, and increased compulsive behavior related to such events as gambling, sexual urges, and eating are rare adverse effects. These are all reasons to decrease dosing or discontinue medication. Should the medications need to be discontinued for nonemergent reasons, weaning off is recommended to avoid theoretic neuroleptic malignant syndrome.

Dopaminergic agents, especially levodopa, are associated with something called "augmentation," whereby symptoms are worsened secondary to use of the dopaminergic agent. Augmentation occurs as a paradoxical response to the medication such that the individual experiences worsening symptoms when the dose is increased. A second form of augmentation is exhibited by a shorter latency from rest to symptom onset, spread to previously unaffected body parts, increased intensity of symptoms, or shorter duration of relief following treatment. Augmentation in either form is generally treated by switching to a different agent or trying combination agents.[67]

Special Populations

Although both ropinirole (Requip) and pramipexole (Mirapex) are FDA Pregnancy Category C drugs, dopaminergic agents are generally not recommended during pregnancy due to possible teratogenic effects in animals. These medications should not be used by breastfeeding mothers as the amount of the drug secreted in the milk and its effect on the newborn is unknown. Dopamine is also known as prolactin-inhibiting factor, which could impair lactogenesis.

Migraine Headaches

Headache is a common condition, and causes of headache vary widely, ranging from stress and fatigue to more serious etiologies such as brain lesions. Although women may suffer from any form of headache, the incidence of migraine headaches has a 3:1 female to male ratio. The prevalence of migraine headaches in the United States is 18.2% in women and 6.5% in men.[68]

Migraines are a neurologic disorder characterized by recurring attacks that are most frequently severe headaches accompanied by altered body perceptions that usually include nausea, vomiting, and photophobia. Migraines have varied presentations; some persons do not have the classic aura, while others have the altered sensation but no headache. Onset typically begins in adolescence or young adulthood before the age of 30 years. Onset after the age of 50 years is rare. Migraine headaches are debilitating and represent a significant cost in terms of healthcare dollars spent, absence from work, and pain and suffering.[68]

The results of large population surveys suggest migraine headaches are undertreated.[68]

Migraines can be episodic or chronic. When migraines become chronic and occur daily, they are referred to as **transformed migraine**. It usually takes several years for episodic migraines to transform into chronic daily headaches. The diagnosis of chronic daily headache is made when the individual has a migraine without aura on ≥ 15 days per month lasting less than 4 hours, for 4 months or more. On 8 days the headache must meet criteria for migraine without aura or respond to migraine-specific treatment.[69,70]

Migraines are affected by reproductive hormones in a pattern that is similar to the changes experienced by women with epilepsy. Sixty percent of women who have migraines will have a subcategory called menstrually associated migraine. These women cyclically develop a migraine headache from 1–3 days before their menses to 3 days after the menses starts[71] (Box 24-6). They usually experience a remission during pregnancy and after menopause but often have more frequent headaches in the perimenopausal period.

One more unusual form of headache is of concern when caring for persons who have migraines. A rebound headache is one that occurs when a person uses medication frequently. A typical rebound headache occurs approximately 3–4 hours after stopping a medication. Over-the-counter analgesics and ergots are the most common types of migraine drugs that can cause rebound headaches.

Etiology of Migraine Headaches

Migraine pain results from a neural event within the brain, which causes dilation of blood vessels, resulting in pain. The neurotransmitter serotonin is the primary player involved in the migraine process. Of particular importance are the serotonin receptor ($5\text{-}HT_1$) subtypes $5\text{-}HT_{1B}$, $5\text{-}HT_{1D}$, and $5\text{-}HT_{1F}$, which influence cerebral vasodilation and trigeminal nerve stimulation.

Migraine headaches generally have four stages. The prodrome stage starts up to 24 hours before the headache occurs and is characterized by increased or decreased perception, irritability, food cravings, fluid retention, and a variety of additional nondescript symptoms. The second stage is the development of an aura, which precedes the headache by an hour and may continue as the headache begins. Auras are characterized by flashing lights, numbness, or tingling and occur in 15–20% of persons who have migraines. The third stage is the period of disability secondary to the severe headache that can last 4–72 hours. The final prodrome stage is a period of fatigue, muscle

Box 24-6 A Case of Acute Pain

MS, a 25-year-old, presents to the urgent care center complaining of a headache. She describes the headache as unilateral and throbbing in quality. She characterizes the pain as an 8 on a 10-point scale. She states that this headache has been present for about 6 hours and has been unrelieved by acetaminophen. She denies any visual disturbances but states that bright lights and noise make the pain worse. She says that she typically gets a headache with the onset of her menses and that the headache lasts anywhere from 5 to 48 hours. The pain is intense enough that she is unable to work or perform other activities of daily living and she usually misses at least 1 day of work every month because of headaches. She has tried Midrin (a combination formulation of acetaminophen 325 mg, dichloralphenazone 100 mg, and isometheptene 65 mg) to treat the pain in the past, without success.

After conducting a physical examination, the healthcare provider diagnosed a menstrually associated migraine. Several options are available to MS. Conventional abortive therapies such as NSAIDs, triptans, or ergotamines may be helpful. Abortive therapy with a long-acting triptan such as naratriptan (Amerge) or frovatriptan (Frova) can also be used as prophylaxis.

When used prophylactically, these drugs are usually started 2 days before the onset of menses and continued for 5 to 6 days. If menstrual cycles are not regular, this method of prophylaxis is not practical. NSAIDs have also been used prophylactically, starting 7 days prior to menses and continuing for 13–14 days. However, this dosing schedule may contribute to rebound headaches in some women.

Estrogen supplementation may be useful when estrogen withdrawal triggers migraine. Estrogen supplementation may be achieved by 100-mcg estrogen patches, started 2 days prior to menses and continued for 7 days. Combination monophasic oral contraceptives (COCs) such as (Mircette), which has 10 mcg of estrogen during the last 5 days of the placebo week, help prevent estrogen withdrawal migraines. Continuous-dose COCs such as (Seasonale) or (Seasonique) may also be useful in reducing the number of headaches. Women who have migraines with auras should not use COCs.

After reviewing treatment options, MS chooses to use naratriptan, 2.5 mg, to be repeated in 4 hours if there is no relief. She also plans to change her current contraception to a continuous 3-month option to reduce the number of menstrual cycles and use naratriptan prophylactically when she anticipates menses.

weakness, food intolerance, and another round of nondescript symptoms that are highly individualized.

Diagnosis of Migraine Headaches

Diagnosis of migraines is based on specific criteria (Table 24-10), and it is necessary that other etiologies of headache first be eliminated.[72] Signs that warrant further investigation include sudden onset of new, severe headache, progressively worsening headache, onset of headaches after age 50, or onset of headache after exertion or strenuous activity.

Treatment for Migraine Headaches

Traditional treatment of migraines follows a classic series of steps wherein the potency of the medication is increased as less potent regimens prove to be ineffective.

In step care, everyone starts with the same medications when the migraine starts. This approach can delay effective treatment. In contrast, the stratified care approach starts with a medication that is based on individual characteristics and level of disability. Stratified care has been definitively proven to be more efficacious in reducing the disability time and headache response 2 hours after initiating therapy.[73] The one potential disadvantage of stratified care is that more side effects of medication occur with this regimen. Concerning adverse effects do not occur more frequently.[73]

Treatment of migraine headaches includes both abortive therapy that treats the headaches when they occur and prophylactic therapy that is used continuously to prevent headaches. Abortive therapy should be combined with prophylactic therapy for persons who experience more than two or three headaches per month.

Table 24-10 Diagnostic Criteria for Migraine Headache

Migraine Without Aura*	Migraine With Aura†
A. At least five attacks fulfilling criteria B, C, and D.	A. At least two attacks fulfilling criterion B.
B. Headache attacks lasting 4–72 hours (untreated or unsuccessfully treated).	B. At least three of the following four characteristics:
C. Headache with at least two of the following characteristics:	1. One or more fully reversible aura symptoms indicating focal cerebral cortical and/or brain stem dysfunction.
Unilateral location	2. At least one aura symptom developing gradually over more than 4 minutes, or two or more symptoms occurring in succession.
Pulsating quality	3. No aura symptom lasting more than 60 minutes; if more than one aura symptom is present, accepted duration is proportionally increased.
Moderate or severe intensity (inhibits or prohibits daily activities)	4. Headache following aura with a free interval of less than 60 minutes. (It may also begin before or simultaneously with the aura.)
Aggravation by walking stairs or performing similar routine physical activity	C. At least one of the following:
D. During headache, at least one of the following events:	1. History and physical and neurologic examinations do not suggest one of the following disorders:
Nausea and/or vomiting	Headache associated with head trauma
Photophobia and phonophobia	Headache associated with vascular disorders
E. At least one of the following scenarios:	Headache associated with nonvascular intracranial disorder
History and physical and neurologic examination do not suggest one of the disorders causing secondary headaches.	Headache associated with substances or their withdrawal
History and/or physical and/or neurologic examinations suggest such a disorder, but it is ruled out by appropriate investigations.	Headache associated with noncephalic disorder
One of such disorders is present, but migraine attacks do not occur for the first time in close temporal relation to the disorder.	Headache associated with metabolic disorder
	Headache or facial pain associated with disorders of the cranium; neck; or ear, nose, and throat
	Cranial neuralgias
	2. History and/or physical and/or neurologic examinations suggest such a disorder, but it is ruled out by appropriate investigations.
	3. Such a disorder is present, but migraine attacks do not occur for the first time in close temporal relation to the disorder.

* For migraine without aura, headaches must meet criterion A; those five attacks must fulfill criteria B through D *and* must fulfill at least one of the criteria under E.

† For migraine with aura, headaches must meet criterion A; those two attacks must fulfill criteria B *and* at least one of those listed under C.

Source: Adapted from International Headache Society 2004.[72]

Abortive Treatment of Migraine Headaches

Abortive therapy for migraine headaches is aimed at achieving pain relief as rapidly as possible after onset of symptoms. Control of associated symptoms such as nausea and vomiting may also be needed. Abortive therapy alone may be sufficient for individuals who experience fewer than four attacks per month.

Abortive Agents

Mild to moderate migraine headaches may be successfully treated by acetaminophen, aspirin, or NSAIDs alone or in combination with caffeine. Occasionally, opioids may also be necessary for treatment of more severe migraines. However, because of the unique nature of migraine pain, drugs specifically designed to treat the underlying cause of pain are commonly used. These include triptans, isometheptene, and ergotamine derivatives. Detailed information on management of acute migraines is available in several published guidelines.[74,75]

Serotonin Agonists: Triptans

Triptans are the typical first-line abortive therapy for migraines. They have fewer adverse effects than other agents, but their use may be limited by their expense. Triptans are serotonin (5-HT$_1$) receptor agonists. Triptans activate serotonin receptors located in the extracerebral and intracranial blood vessels to reverse cranial vessel constriction. Although all triptans have similar chemical structures, they vary with regard to onset and duration of action, the incidence of recurrent headache, and affinity for specific receptor agonists. Therefore, failure of one agent does not preclude successful use of an alternate triptan. Variations among triptans are detailed in Table 24-11.

Side Effects/Adverse Effects

Common side effects to triptans include vertigo, fatigue, transient chest pain, pruritus, dry mouth, and paresthesias. Transient erythema may occur with injection. Intranasal formulations leave a bad taste.

Hypersensitivity to triptans is rare, but anaphylactic reactions have occurred. Other serious adverse effects

Table 24-11 Medications Used to Treat Migraine Headaches

Triptan Generic (Brand)	Dose	Maximum per 24 hrs	Time to Peak Effect	Onset of Action (Minutes)	Duration of Effect	Clinical Considerations	FDA Pregnancy Category
Almotriptan (Axert)	6.5-, 12.5-mg tablets 1 tablet q 2 h	25 mg	1–3 h	30–120		Not contraindicated with MAO inhibitors. Better tolerated than sumatriptan.	C
Eletriptan (Relpax)	20-, 40-mg tablets 1 tablet q 2 h	80 mg	1.5 h	< 120	24 h	Metabolized by CYP3A4. Do not use within 72 hours of CYP3A4 inhibitor. Bioavailability is increased by high-fat meal.	C
Frovatriptan (Frova)	2.5 mg, may repeat in 2 h	7.5 mg	2–3 h	120–180		Can be safely combined with MAO inhibitors.	C
Naratriptan (Amerge)	1- and 2.5-mg tablets 2.5 mg q 4 h	5 mg	2 h	60–180		Can be safely combined with MAO inhibitors. Fewer headache recurrences than with sumatriptan.	C
Rizatriptan (Maxalt)	5-, 10-mg tablets 1 tablet q 2 h	30 mg	1 h	30–120		Orally disintegrating tablet available.	C
Sumatriptan (Imitrex) oral	25-, 50-,100-mg tablets, 1 tablet q 2 h, may repeat in 2 h	200 mg	4 h	20–60	2.5 h	Incidence of recurrent headache within 24 hours is 40%.	C
Sumatriptan (Imitrex) intranasal	5 mg per spray 1 spray in both nostrils q 2 h	40 mg	2 h	30–60	1–1.5 h	Faster onset than with tablet forms.	C
Sumatriptan (Imitrex) SQ	6 mg, may repeat in 1 h	12 mg	2 h	15	1.5–2 h	Most rapid onset of action.	C
Zolmitriptan (Zomig) oral	2.5- and 5-mg tablets, 1 tablet q 2 h	10 mg	2–4 h	45		Orally disintegrating tablet available. Nasal spray available. Food has no significant effect on absorption.	C
Isometheptene/ acetaminophen/ dichloralphenazone (Midrin)	2 caps at onset, can use 1 caplet/h	5 caplets per attack	1–3 h	< 1 hr	3–4 h	Drowsiness, dizziness, and nausea common side effects.	X
Ergotamine tartrate (Ergomar)*	2-mg tablets, use 1 q 30 minutes	6 mg	2 h	Variable depending on duration of headache prior to administration	Variable	All ergotomine formulations are contraindicated during pregnancy and for persons with peripheral artery disease, coronary heart disease, hypertension, or impaired renal or hepatic function. Nausea and vomiting common (10% of users). Numbness and tingling in toes. Risk of rebound headache.	X
Ergotamine/ caffeine (Cafergot)*	1 mg ergotamine/ 100-mg caffeine 2 tablets at onset, 1 tablet q 30 min	6 tablets per attack	2 h	Variable depending on duration of headache prior to administration, but faster than ergotamine tartrate than with addition of caffeine	Variable		X
Ergotamine/ caffeine suppository*	2 mg ergotrate/ 100-mg caffeine rectal suppository	2	1 h	See ergotamine/ caffeine (Cafergot)	Variable		X
Dihydroergotamine mesylate (Migranal)*	Nasal spray 0.5 mg/ spray	4 sprays in each nostril per 24 h 8–16 sprays per week	15–45 min	15–30 min	8 h		X

* Ergotism possible if taken concurrently with macrolide antibiotics or other CY3A4 inhibitors. Contraindicated during pregnancy and for persons with peripheral artery disease, coronary heart disease, hypertension, or impaired renal or hepatic function. Do not take with other peripheral vasoconstricting drugs such as triptans or beta-blockers.

include coronary artery spasms, myocardial infarction or ischemia, hypertension, ventricular tachycardia and/or fibrillation, seizures, and transient ischemia attacks.

Contraindications

All triptans are contraindicated during pregnancy, as well as for individuals with uncontrolled hypertension, coronary artery disease, peripheral vascular disease, hepatic dysfunction, or those with any history of ischemic conditions. Individuals with renal impairment should use rizatriptan and sumatriptan with caution.

Drug–Drug Interactions

Triptans should not be used concurrently with ergotamine derivatives. Dosing of triptans and ergotamines should be separated by at least 24 hours to avoid the possibility of a prolonged vasospastic reaction. Different triptans should not be used in combination with each other because of the risk of vasospastic reactions. Additional drug interactions are summarized in Table 24-12.

Isometheptene

Isometheptene is a sympathomimetic agent that causes vasoconstriction of the cerebral and cranial arterioles.

Table 24-12 Selected Drug–Drug Interactions Associated with Triptans*

Drug Generic (Brand)	Effect
All Triptans	
Ergotrate derivatives	Increased incidence of vasospastic reactions.
Almotriptan (Axert)	
MAO inhibitors	Decreased clearance of almotriptan.
Potent CYP3A4 inhibitors—ketoconazole, macrolides, protease inhibitors	Increased plasma concentrations of almotriptan.
Eletriptan (Relpax)	
Potent CYP3A4 inhibitors—ketoconazole, macrolides, protease inhibitors	Increased plasma concentrations of eletriptan. Do not take within 72 hours of these drugs.
Frovatriptan (Frova)	
Oral contraceptives	Increased plasma concentrations of frovatriptan.
Propranolol	Increased plasma concentrations of frovatriptan.
Naratriptan (Amerge)	
Oral contraceptives	Increased plasma concentration of naratriptan.
Sibutramine (Meridia)	Increased plasma concentration of naratriptan.
SSRIs, SNRIs	Increased levels of SSRIs and subsequent risk of serotonin syndrome.
Rizatriptan (Maxalt)	
Propranolol	Increased plasma concentrations of rizatriptan.
MAO inhibitors	Increased plasma concentrations of rizatriptan.
Sibutramine (Meridia)	Increased plasma concentrations of rizatriptan.
Sumatriptan (Imitrex)	
SSRIs, SNRIs	Increased risk of serotonin syndrome.
MAO inhibitors	Increased plasma concentrations of sumatriptan.
Zolmitriptan (Zomig)	
MAO inhibitors, propranolol	Increased plasma concentrations of zolmitriptan.
Cimetidine (Tagamet)	Doubled half-life of zolmitriptan.
Acetaminophen (Tylenol)	Delayed maximum concentration of acetaminophen.
Oral contraceptives	Increased plasma concentration but delayed time to maximum concentration of zolmitriptan.
Isometheptene/Acetaminophen/Dichloralphenazone (Midrin)	
MAO inhibitors	Increased plasma concentrations of isometheptene.
All Ergotrate Derivatives	
Triptans	Increases incidence of vasospastic reactions.
Dihydroergotamine (Migranal)	
Azoles	Increased cerebral and peripheral ischemia through induction of CYP3A4.
Macrolide antibiotics	Increased cerebral and peripheral ischemia through induction of CYP3A4.
Protease inhibitors	Increased cerebral and peripheral ischemia through induction of CYP3A4.

SSRI = selective serotonin reuptake inhibitor; SNRI = serotonin-norepinephrine reuptake inhibitor.
* This table is not comprehensive as new information is being identified on a regular basis.

It is available in combination with acetaminophen and dichloralphenazone (Midrin). It is contraindicated for individuals with glaucoma, severe renal or hepatic disease, coronary artery or other vascular diseases, or hypertension and for persons taking monoamine oxidase (MAO) inhibitors.

Ergotamine Derivatives

Ergotamine was the etiology of an epidemic in the Middle Ages that caused countless deaths, a story that became the subject of many famous pieces of artwork from that time period. Persons who ate bread made of rye, wheat, and barley that was infected with the *Claviceps purpurea* fungus developed ergotism, which is also known as St. Anthony's fire.[76] This fungus contained ergot, which has remarkable vasoconstrictor effects and convulsive symptoms. The convulsive symptoms include nausea, vomiting, spasms, and hallucinations similar to those produced by lysergic acid diethylamide (LSD), a derivative of ergot. The vasoconstrictor effects caused gangrene.

Ergotamine derivatives include ergotamine tartrate (Cafergot) and dihydroergotamine (Migranal). Ergotamines have lost favor as first-line treatment of migraines in recent years because of adverse effects. However, they are effective if administered at the earliest sign of migraine. Their chief advantage is low cost.

Mechanism of Action

The exact mechanism by which ergotamine derivatives abort migraine attacks is unknown. Ergotamines act directly on cranial arteries to promote vasoconstriction. Recent evidence also suggests that ergotamines exert an agonist effect at the 5-HT_{IB} and 5-HT_{ID} receptor and may also block inflammation of the trigeminal vascular system.[77]

Ergotamine tartrate is the prototype ergotamine, and it is available in oral, sublingual, rectal, and inhaled preparations. Bioavailability is increased via the inhaled or rectal routes. The half-life of ergotamine tartrate is approximately 2 hours, although effects of the drug may persist for 24 hours. Dihydroergotamine is available in parenteral or inhaled forms only because of extensive hepatic first-pass effects.

Side Effects/Adverse Effects

Adverse effects of ergotamine are uncommon but include an increase in nausea and vomiting, which may be reduced by concomitant administration of a prokinetic drug such as metoclopramide (Reglan). Weakness, myalgias, numbness or tingling of fingers and toes, angina-like pain, tachycardia, and bradycardia have also been reported. Dihydroergotamine is less likely to cause nausea and vomiting but does cause diarrhea.

In overdose or chronic use, ergotamines can cause serious ischemia. Constriction of peripheral arteries results in muscle pain; intermittent claudication; pale, cold extremities; and numbness. This phenomenon is known as ergotism, and gangrene of extremities can develop if the condition is not recognized and treated. Individuals should be instructed to immediately discontinue any ergot and seek immediate medical attention should such signs or symptoms occur.

Contraindications

Ergotamines are contraindicated in pregnancy and for those with coronary artery disease, peripheral vascular disease, sepsis, uncontrolled hypertension, and renal or hepatic impairment.

Drug–Drug Interactions

Ergotamines should never be used in combination with triptans. Dosing of triptans and ergotamines should be separated by at least 24 hours to avoid the possibility of a prolonged vasospastic reaction. Dihydroergotamine is metabolized by CYP3A4 and is subject to significant drug interactions when used with drugs that inhibit CYP3A4.

Prophylactic Treatment of Migraine Headaches

The goal of preventative migraine therapy is to reduce attack frequency, duration, and severity; improve responsiveness to treatment of acute attacks; and improve function and reduce disability.[75] Preventative therapy should be considered for individuals who experience more than two migraines per month, whose disability lasts 3 or more days per month, or who do not respond to or have contraindications to abortive therapy.

Many agents are useful for migraine prevention. Table 24-13 provides a summary of the first-line agents used for migraine prophylaxis. Published practice guidelines from the United States Headache Consortium are available to help clinicians individualize preventative treatment appropriately.[75,78,79]

Triptans may also be used as short-term preventative agents for women with menstrually associated migraines. Therapy is most effective when started 2–3 days before menses and continued until 3 days after the onset. Triptans with longer half-lives, such as naratriptan (Amerge) and frovatriptan (Frova) twice daily, have demonstrated effectiveness for short-term prophylaxis.

Table 24-13 Drugs Used as Prevention Therapy for Persons with Migraine Headaches

Drug Generic (Brand)	Dose and Administration	Advantages	Side Effects/Adverse Effects	Contraindications
Tricyclic Antidepressants				
Amitriptyline (Elavil)	10–150 mg/day.	Very effective; mild to moderate side effects. Most effective in patients with mixed migraine and tension headaches. Useful in patients with comorbid depression or insomnia.	Drowsiness, weight gain, anticholinergic symptoms. Lowered seizure threshold may cause dysrhythmias in excessive doses.	Avoid in patients with acute angle glaucoma, seizures.
Antiepileptics				
Divalproex (Depakote)	250–500 mg bid. Clinical efficacy at 500–1500 mg/day.	Very effective; mild to moderate side effects. Reduces incidence of migraines by 50%.	Fatigue, weight gain, tremor, hair loss, liver toxicity, pancreatitis memory impairment, cognitive dysfunction. Teratogenic. Increases risk for suicidality for all four of these AEDs.	Avoid in pregnancy and in patients with liver impairment.
Gabapentin (Neurontin)	300–2400 mg/day. Clinical efficacy at 900–2400 mg/day.	Lower efficacy; mild to moderate side effects.		
Topiramate (Topamax)	50 mg bid.	Very effective; mild to moderate side effects.		
Valproate	Clinical efficacy at 800–1500 mg/day.	Very effective; mild to moderate side effects.		
Beta-Blockers				
Propranolol (Inderal)	80–240 mg/day.	Very effective; mild to moderate side effects. Inexpensive, useful in patients with coexisting cardiovascular disease.	Fatigue, exercise intolerance, depression, insomnia.	Avoid in patients with asthma, uncontrolled diabetes, hypotension, and heart block.
Timolol (Blocadren)	10–15 mg bid.	Very effective; mild to moderate side effects.		
Calcium Channel Blockers				
Verapamil (Calan)	240–300 mg/day.	Lower efficacy; mild to moderate side effects.	Weak evidence for migraine prophylaxis. Negative inotropic effects in heart. Increased peripheral edema, constipation, orthostatic hypotension.	Avoid in patients with bradycardia, second- or third-degree heart block, or congestive heart failure.
Estrogen				
Estrogen gel (EstroGel)	1.5 mg/day.	Useful for menstrual-associated migraines.	Headaches, breast pain, irregular vaginal bleeding or vaginal irritation, nausea and vomiting.	Known, suspected or history of breast cancer, undiagnosed abnormal vaginal bleeding, deep vein thrombosis or history of DVT, history of stroke, liver dysfunction or disease, known or suspected pregnancy.
Patch (Climara, Vivelle, Estraderm)	100 mg/day. Begin dosing 2 days before expected attack.	Useful for menstrual-associated migraines.		
ACE Inhibitors				
Lisinopril (Zestril)	20 mg/day.	Inexpensive; generally well tolerated and effective.	Increased incidence of cough. Teratogenic.	Avoid in pregnancy.
Angiotensin Receptor Blockers				
Candesartan (Atacand)	16 mg/day.	Reduces need for rescue therapy.	Teratogenic.	Avoid in pregnancy.

AED = antiepileptic drug.

Complementary and Alternative Treatments for Migraine

There are several complementary and alternative treatments for both prophylaxis and treatment of migraines that have varied efficacy. Avoiding triggers that cause migraine is an initial first step. There is consistent evidence that acupuncture, biofeedback, and relaxation training all appear to be efficacious. Dietary supplements and herbs such as feverfew, *Petasites hybridus* (butterbur), magnesium, and riboflavin have all been evaluated in small trials and appear to be worth further investigation. Additional alternative treatments for pain are reviewed in Chapter 12.

Special Populations

Pregnancy and Lactation

Triptans are FDA Pregnancy Category C drugs. Although there is no evidence of harm to human fetuses, there is evidence of teratogenesis in animal studies, and therefore, triptans are generally avoided during pregnancy. Although not FDA approved for use in pregnancy, several studies suggest no increased birth defects with sumatriptan, and it is used off-label to treat women who develop migraines during pregnancy.[80] Ergotamines are FDA Pregnancy Category X drugs because their ability to cause uterine contractions can result in fetal harm or abortion. Ergotamine tartrate has been linked to vomiting, diarrhea, and convulsions in the neonate when used in lactating women at levels required to suppress migraines.[53] Triptans may be excreted in breast milk, although adverse effects on the infant have not been well studied. Sumatriptan is approved by the American Academy of Pediatrics for use with breastfeeding.[53]

Elderly

Migraines are rare after menopause, and evidence is limited on the use of triptans in this age group. Triptans should be used cautiously because of the increased risk of comorbidities such as coronary artery disease, hypertension, or other cardiovascular conditions that may be exacerbated by triptans. Ergotamines should be used cautiously by postmenopausal women because there is an increased risk of comorbidities such as coronary artery disease, hypertension, or other cardiovascular conditions that may be worsened by ergotamines.

Adult Attention-Deficit Hyperactivity Disorder

Attention-deficit/hyperactivity disorder (ADHD) is a syndrome that is often first observed in childhood characterized by difficulty in sustaining attention, excessive motor activity, and impulsiveness. ADHD is also often associated with underachievement in school and may continue into adulthood in a modified form. In the United States, the estimated prevalence of ADHD is 8–10% among children, and approximately 40–70% of children with ADHD

will have symptoms that persist into adolescence and adulthood.[81]

The pathophysiology of ADHD has been associated with abnormalities of certain brain structures. Although ADHD most commonly is characterized as a childhood affliction, today there is a growing awareness that this condition, treated or untreated, may persist through a person's lifetime. Prevalence of adult attention-deficit/hyperactivity disorder (AADHD) is difficult to determine as many affected individuals develop coping skills that allow them to be functional members of society. Conversely, others may meet the same criteria that are used to diagnose children. Controversy exists about diagnosis, especially since hyperactivity is less common among adults than children, leading some professionals to conclude that AADHD should have a separate diagnosis. AADHD is recognized as a neuropsychiatric disability that must be accommodated under the Americans with Disabilities Act. Current research is primarily focused on variations in adult cognitive functioning.[82]

Treatment for AADHD includes medication and some form of stress management such as biofeedback or meditation. Medications help retain focus and attention but they are not effective as monotherapy in helping individuals with AADHD manage daily activities, thus the cognitive and behavioral interventions are an essential element in the overall treatment regimen for AADHD.

Drugs Used to Control AADHD

Stimulants and antidepressants are the two categories of drug used to treat AADHD. In addition, several atypical antidepressants have been used with some success.

Amphetamines

Amphetamines, which are also called sympathomimetic drugs, act as agonists at adrenergic receptors in the autonomic nervous system and are the first-line of treatment for AADHD. Approximately 75% of individuals with AADHD have improved symptoms when given sympathomimetic drugs. In addition to methylphenidate (Ritalin, Ritalin-SR), dextroamphetamine (Dexedrine) and amphetamine/dextroamphetamine (Adderall) are considered to be preferred medications for AADHD. Although the exact mechanism of action of these agents is not known, they are thought to block the reuptake of norepinephrine and increase the release of norepinephrine and dopamine, thereby inducing sympathetic nervous system activation. Table 24-14

Table 24-14 Medications Used to Treat Adult Attention-Deficit/Hyperactivity Disorder

Drug Generic (Brand)	Formulations	Dose	Side Effects/Adverse Effects	FDA Pregnancy Category
Amphetamine/ dextroamphetamine (Adderall, Adderall XR)	5-, 10-, 20-, 30-mg tablets, extended-release capsules 5, 10, 15, 20, 25, 30 mg	5–40 mg in the morning or twice a day. Extended-release capsules 20–60 mg/day. Maximum dose of 60 mg per day at a rate of 10 mg per week.	Increased heart rate, blood pressure, decreased appetite, weight loss, disturbed sleep. Hypertension is not a contraindication, but blood pressure should be monitored carefully	C
Atomoxetine (Strattera)	10-, 18-, 25-, 40-, 60-, 80-, and 100-mg capsules	80 mg in the morning. Maximum dose 100 mg per day. Larger doses may be divided twice a day.	Does not have the stimulant properties of amphetamines. Well tolerated. Rare adverse effect of hepatotoxicity, suicidal ideation.	C
Bupropion (Budeprion SR, Budeprion XL, Wellbutrin)	75-, 100-mg tablets; 100-, 150-, 200-, 300-mg extended-release tablets	100 mg three times a day. Extended release 200 mg in the morning and 100 mg in the evening.	Contraindicated in persons with a history of seizures.	C
Dextroamphetamine (Dexedrine)	5-mg tablets; 5-, 10-, 15-mg extended-release capsules	5–60 mg per day in one to three divided doses. Maximum dose of 60 mg per day if needed.	C-II controlled substance; prescription cannot be refilled, and written copy is required. Increased heart rate, blood pressure, decreased appetite, weight loss, disturbed sleep. Hypertension is not a contraindication but blood pressure should be monitored carefully.	C
Dexmethylphenidate (Focalin)	2.5-, 5-, 10-mg tablets; 5-, 10-, 15-, 20-mg extended-release capsules	2.5–10 mg twice a day; extended release 10–20 mg each morning. Maximum dose 20 mg per day.	Increased heart rate, blood pressure, decreased appetite, weight loss, disturbed sleep. Hypertension is not a contraindication, but blood pressure should be monitored carefully.	C
Imipramine (Tofranil)	10-, 25-, 50-mg tablets	10–25 mg/day to start; then increase to 100–150 mg/day.	Rare prolonged QT syndrome. ECG should be obtained before initiating therapy. Drowsiness, sexual dysfunction, weight gain, postural hypotension, and anticholinergic effects are common.	D
Methylphenidate (Concerta, Metadate, Methylin, Ritalin) Methylphenidate transdermal (Daytrana)	5-, 10-, 20-mg tablets; 18-, 27-, 36-, 54-mg controlled-release tablets Transdermal 10-, 15-, 20-, 30-mg per 9 hour patches.	5–15 mg twice or three times a day. Controlled release 18–72 mg per day. Transdermal 10- to 30-mg/9-h patch each day. Maximum dose 30 mg/9-h patch per day.	C-II controlled substance, prescription cannot be refilled, and written copy is required. Last dose should be given before 6 PM. Increased heart rate, blood pressure; decreased appetite; weight loss; disturbed sleep. Hypertension is not a contraindication, but blood pressure should be monitored carefully.	C
Nortriptyline (Norpramin)	10-, 25-, 50-, 75-mg capsules	10–25 mg/day to start; then increase to 100–150 mg/day.	Rare prolonged QT syndrome. ECG should be obtained before initiating therapy. Drowsiness, sexual dysfunction, weight gain, postural hypotension, and anticholinergic effects are common.	C

reviews the doses, side effects, and dosing considerations for the drugs used to treat AADHD.

Antidepressants

Tricyclic antidepressants inhibit the uptake of norepinephrine and serotonin. Nortriptyline (Pamelor) and desipramine (Norpramin) are preferred because they have greater effects on norepinephrine. Bupropion (Wellbutrin) is an atypical antidepressant that also appears to work well.

ADHD and Pregnancy and Lactation

In light of the high incidence of adolescent pregnancy as well as the increased recognition of ADHD, it is of note that little has been published regarding ADHD during pregnancy. Several studies have explored intrauterine factors that may contribute to the development of ADHD of the offspring, including a probable link between pediatric ADHD and maternal smoking during pregnancy.[83] However, care of the pregnant woman with ADHD has been ignored in the literature. One brief report cautioned that use of the common medications presented unknown risks although no teratogenic effects had been reported.[84] A study of transfer of dexamphetamine into breast milk revealed less than 10% maternal concentration in the milk, suggesting safety. However, only four women participated in the study, indicating that more research is needed in this area.[85]

Parkinson's Disease

There are several nervous system degenerative disorders that are characterized by an irreversible, progressive destruction of neurons from specific regions of the brain, including Parkinon's disease, Alzheimer's disease, and myasthenia gravis. In the case of Parkinson's disease the pathologic change is progressive destruction of dopamine-secreting neurons in the substantia nigra, which is located in the basal ganglia of the brain. Parkinson's disease affects men and women equally, and each of us has a 2% lifetime risk for onset of Parkinson's disease.

Women and Parkinson's Disease

There is some evidence that estrogen promotes the development and differentiation of dopaminergic neurons.[86] Premenopausal women with Parkinson's disease occasionally report increased symptoms during menstruation when there are lower levels of circulating estrogen. One study found that postmenopausal women receiving conjugated estrogen had better symptom control on the same dose of antiparkinson drugs than when they were not taking the hormone.[87] Although there is sparse evidence, this is clearly an area that deserves further research.

Pathophysiology of Parkinson's Disease

The basal ganglia are groups of neurons located deep within the cerebrum and midbrain that serve as an accessory motor system communicating bidirectionally with the cerebral cortex and the corticospinal motor system (pyramidal tract). The basal ganglia act as a modulator that regulates the flow of signals down from the motor cortex to the motor neurons of the spinal cord. Functionally, the basal ganglia modify movements controlled by the motor cortex in several ways: integrating complex patterns of motor activity such as writing, executing learned patterns of movement that are often subconscious, scaling, and timing of motions to make them appropriate to cognitive input. Disorders of movement that are secondary to basal ganglia impairment

are termed **extrapyramidal symptoms** because although the pyramidal tract remains intact and functional, it lacks adequate modification from the extrapyramidal system.

Dopamine and acetylcholine are the two neurotransmitters within this area of the brain. Dopamine is the inhibitory neurotransmitter and acetylcholine is the excitatory neurotransmitter. A deficiency of dopamine in the substantia nigra causes an imbalance in the dopamine and acetylcholine levels, which results in decreased excitation in the motor cortex.

There are four major dopamine pathways in the brain: nigrostriatal, mesolimbic, mesocortical, and tuberoinfundibular. Decreased dopamine in the nigrostriatal tract causes the altered movement symptoms of Parkinson's disease, and dopamine deficiencies in the other three tracts is the probable etiology of neuropsychiatric pathology seen in persons with Parkinson's disease.

The movement disorders or **dyskinesias** associated with Parkinson's disease have four characteristic features: (1) **bradykinesia** (slowness and poverty of movement), (2) muscular rigidity, (3) tremor while at rest that decreases with voluntary movement, and (4) impaired posture and balance that result in gait disturbance and falling.[88,89] These symptoms only appear when 65% to 80% of the dopamine is depleted.

Drugs That Cause Dyskinesias

Parkinson's disease must be distinguished from other causes of dyskinesias, which can be an adverse reaction to medications. Drugs commonly used that cause dyskinesias include antipsychotics such as chlorpromazine (Thorazine) and haloperidol (Haldol), tricyclic antidepressants, and antiemetics such as promethazine (Phenergan), prochlorperazine (Compazine), and metoclopramide (Reglan). The common mechanism of action is antagonism of dopamine, thereby inhibiting postsynaptic impulses.

Dopamine Metabolism

Since Parkinson's disease is caused by a relative lack of dopamine, the pharmacologic treatments are aimed at altering different phases of dopamine metabolism and physiology.

Dopamine is synthesized by dopaminergic neurons in a series of steps starting with the amino acid tyrosine, which is acted upon by tyrosine hydroxylase to produce L-dihydroxyphenylalanine (L-dopa), then finally dopamine that is subsequently stored in vesicles and released into a synapse when the presynaptic neuron is depolarized by entry of calcium ions. Dopamine binds to one of two important receptors to produce an effector response in the postsynaptic neuron—the D_1 or the D_2 receptor. The action of dopamine is terminated either by reuptake into the presynaptic or postsynaptic nerve terminal, or broken down by the sequential action of two enzymes, catechol-O-methyltransferase (COMT) and monoamine oxidase (MAO). Drugs used to treat Parkinson's disease work in one of the following three ways: (1) replace dopamine in the brain, (2) decrease the amount of acetylcholine, and (3) provide neuroprotection.

Medications for the Treatment of Parkinson's Disease

Dopaminergic Therapy: Levodopa (Sinemet)

Levodopa (Sinemet), also called L-dopa, is the metabolic precursor of dopamine and is the most effective treatment presently available for the treatment of Parkinson's disease. Dopamine itself does not cross the blood–brain barrier and, therefore, cannot be administered peripherally. More than 90% of individuals with Parkinson's disease respond favorably to the administration of levodopa. Orally administered L-dopa is absorbed from the small intestine and crosses the blood–brain barrier by means of special transport mechanisms for aromatic amino acids. In the brain, L-dopa is converted to dopamine by decarboxylation in the presynaptic terminals of dopaminergic neurons of the striatum. It is the dopamine itself that is responsible for the therapeutic action of the drug in Parkinson's disease therapy, as L-dopa has no effect on its own.

Levodopa also is decarboxylated by enzymes in the intestines and liver into dopamine that enters the peripheral circulation. This peripheral conversion of L-dopa results in a low availability of the drug entering the brain since dopamine itself does not cross the blood–brain barrier. Dopamine in the peripheral circulation causes undesirable effects such as nausea, orthostatic hypotension, and cardiac arrhythmias. Therefore, levodopa is usually administered with a peripherally acting decarboxylase inhibitor such as carbidopa. This combination of levodopa and carbidopa prevents much of the peripheral conversion of levodopa, resulting in increased drug availability in the brain while also avoiding the undesirable peripheral effects of dopamine. For these reasons, L-dopa is most commonly prescribed in combined form containing 25 mg of carbidopa and 100 mg of levodopa (Sinemet 25/100) (Table 24-15).

Side Effects/Adverse Effects

Levodopa therapy often has dramatic effects on the signs and symptoms of early Parkinson's disease with almost complete improvement of tremor, rigidity, and bradykinesia and long-lasting benefits possibly due to storage and release of the exogenous dopamine. At later stages of the disease, there is a loss of this buffering effect, and dramatic changes in motor ability occur secondary to each dose of levodopa, termed the *on-off phenomenon*. When this phenomenon occurs, each dose of levodopa may improve symptoms for only 1–2 hours, after which rigidity and akinesia rapidly return. Increasing the dose and frequency of dosing is limited by the possibility that a hyperdopaminergic state will induce dyskinesias. The use of sustained-release formulations or changing the dosing schedule from every 4 to 6 hours to every 2 hours, while providing the same total daily dose, sometimes helps with the on-off symptoms.

Rapid initial titration of levodopa or high doses of the pharmaceutical may result in dyskinesias. Excessive and abnormal involuntary movements such as head bobbing, tics, and grimacing develop in up to 80% of individuals treated with the drug during the first year of therapy. Reduction of the dose can decrease dyskinesias but may lead to increased symptoms of Parkinson's disease. The elderly with preexisting cognitive problems are susceptible to confusion and hallucinations requiring dose reduction, which can make treatment ineffective. Levodopa-induced psychosis can be effectively treated with atypical antipsychotic agents such as clozapine (Clozaril) that do not tend to worsen Parkinson's disease symptoms as might occur with phenothiazine antipsychotics.

Drug Interactions

Individuals taking nonspecific MAO inhibitors for depression such as phenelzine (Nardil) and tranylcypromine (Parnate) can experience a life-threatening hypertensive crisis and hyperpyrexia if they receive catecholamines such as dopamine. These drugs should be stopped at least 2 weeks before starting L-dopa administration.

Abrupt withdrawal of dopaminergic agents such as levodopa can precipitate neuroleptic malignant syndrome. Taking a dose of levodopa on a full stomach may delay absorption due to competition with other amino acids for the transport mechanism in the small intestine. Pyridoxine (vitamin B_6) enhances decarboxylase activity that may increase peripheral transformation of levodopa into dopamine, thereby decreasing its availability in the brain. Phenothiazine antipsychotic drugs decrease the therapeutic

Table 24-15 Medications Used to Treat Parkinson's Disease

Drug Generic (Brand)	Formulations	Dose	Clinical Considerations	Pregnancy FDA Category
Amantadine (Symmetrel)	100-mg tablets; 50-mg/5-mL syrup	100 mg bid.	Maximum dose 400 mg/day. SE: Confusion, nausea. AE: Hallucinations, neuroleptic malignant syndrome.	C
Benztropine (Cogentin)	0.5-, 1-, 2-mg tablets	1–2 mg bid.	Maximum dose 6 mg/day (4 mg in elderly). SE: Confusion, dry mouth, nausea.	C
Bromocriptine (Parlodel)	2.5-mg tablet, 5-mg capsule	1.25–30 mg bid to tid.	The initial dose for bromocriptine is 1.25 bid increasing 2.5 mg/day every 2–4 weeks. Maximum dose 100 mg/day.	B
Carbidopa/levodopa (Sinemet 25/100)	10/100-, 25/100-, 25/250-mg tablets and 50/200-mg controlled-release tablets	Normal dosage range for levodopa (in combination with carbidopa) is 200–1200 mg/day in two to three divided doses.	Dosage is initiated with either 10 mg carbidopa/100 mg levodopa three to four times a day; or 25 mg carbidopa/100 mg levodopa tid and increased by 1 tablet per day every 24–48 hours.	C
Entacapone (Comtan)	200-mg tablets	200 mg per dose.	Used as adjunctive treatment with each dose of carbidopa/levodopa. Maximum dose 1600 mg/day.	C
Diphenhydramine (Benadryl)	25-, 50-mg capsules; 12.5-mg/5-mL solution	25–50 mg tid to qid.	Maximum single dose 100 mg or 400 mg/day.	B
Pramipexole (Mirapex)	0.125-, 0.25-, 0.5-, 0.75-, 1-, 1.5-mg tablets	0.5–1.5 mg tid.	Given initially as 0.125 mg tid up to a dosage range of 1.5 to 4.5 mg per day.	C
Ropinirole (Requip)	0.25-, 0.5-, 1-, 2-, 3-, 4-, 5-mg tablets	3 mg tid.	The dosage for ropinirole initially is 0.25 mg tid up to a daily dosage range of 1.5 to 24 mg per day.	C
Selegiline (Eldepryl, Zelapar)	5-mg capsules, 1.25-mg dispersible tablets (Zelapar)	5 mg bid.	Maximum dose 10 mg/day.	C
Tolcapone (Tasmar)	100-, 200-mg tablets	100 mg tid.	Used as adjunctive treatment with carbidopa/levodopa. Maximum dose 200 mg tid.	C
Trihexyphenidyl (Artane)	2-, 5-mg tablets; 2-mg/5-mL elixir	6–10 mg/day in three divided doses.	Maximum dose 15 mg/day. SE: Confusion, dry mouth, nausea.	C

SE = side effects; AE = adverse effects.

effects of levodopa and are also capable of inducing Parkinsonian symptoms on their own.

Dopaminergic Therapy: Amantadine (Symmetrel)

Amantadine (Symmetrel) is used in the initial therapy of mild Parkinson's disease and may also be helpful as an adjunct for individuals receiving levodopa who have symptom fluctuations or dyskinesias. Amantadine is thought to enhance dopamine release from the presynaptic storage vesicles and is used as an early treatment to delay starting levodopa therapy.[90]

Dopamine Receptor Agonists

Bromocriptine (Parlodel)

Bromocriptine (Parlodel) is an older dopamine receptor agonist derived from ergot. Bromocriptine acts as an agonist at the D_2 receptor and is the drug used when amantadine is no longer useful. Initial treatment with bromocriptine (Parlodel) can cause profound hypotension and should be started at a low dose. Bromocriptine can induce transient nausea and fatigue as well so it can sometimes require weeks to months to slowly adjust the dose up to necessary levels. Bromocriptine is most often prescribed for persons who are already receiving levodopa to reduce motor fluctuations such as those associated with on-off symptoms or to decrease the dose of levodopa to avoid dyskinesias.

Ropinirole (Requip) and Pramipexole (Mirapex)

The newer agents, ropinirole (Requip) and pramipexole (Mirapex), are more selective for the D_2 receptor sites, better tolerated, and more quickly titrated. The two newer drugs also are less apt to cause nausea and fatigue. These selective dopamine agonists are being increasingly used as initial monotherapy for Parkinson's disease. They have the advantage of better tolerance and less likelihood of on-off phenomena due to their longer half-lives when compared to levodopa.

Acetylcholine Muscarinic Receptor Antagonists

Several acetylcholine **muscarinic** receptor antagonists, also called anticholinergic drugs, are currently used to treat early Parkinson's disease or as adjunctive therapy to dopamine agonists. These drugs include benztropine (Cogentin), diphenhydramine (Benadryl), and trihexyphenidyl (Artane). Their ability to cause smooth muscle relaxation makes them particularly useful for treating muscle rigidity and **akinesia**.

Side Effects/Adverse Effects

The side effects result from their anticholinergic properties and include sedation, mental confusion, constipation, urinary retention, and blurred vision. Anticholinergic drugs can have an additive effect with any drug or agent that causes sedation. Adverse effects include confusion, hallucinations, **mydriasis**, and photophobia. These drugs are contraindicated for persons who have narrow angle glaucoma or a history of urinary retention.

Neuroprotection: Catechol-O-Methyltransferase (COMT) Inhibitors

Catechol-O-methyltransferase (COMT) is one of the two enzymes responsible for the catabolism of levodopa and dopamine, and its inhibition prolongs the half-life of levodopa, permitting more of the drug to reach the brain, and prolongs the effect of dopamine in the synapse within the brain. Entacapone (Comtan), a COMT inhibitor, is available as a single pill combined with levodopa/carbidopa in several fixed-dose combinations. Tolcapone (Tasmar) is a potent COMP inhibitor that carries a FDA black box warning about an increased risk for hepatotoxicity and acute liver failure. Both of the COMT inhibitors are used as adjunctive treatment with levodopa/carbidopa and have similar side effects as levodopa/carbidopa, including nausea, orthostatic hypotension, vivid dreams, confusion, and hallucinations.

Selective MAO-B Inhibitors

There are two isoenzymes of MAO that are responsible for metabolism of catecholamines. These include MAO-A and MAO-B, both of which are present in periphery, but only MAO-B is predominant in the striatum and responsible for most of the metabolism of dopamine in the brain. Selegiline (Eldepryl) is an irreversible selective MAO-B inhibitor. Unlike nonspecific MAO inhibitors, selegiline does not inhibit peripheral catecholamine metabolism and does not potentiate catecholamines or tyramine as long as daily doses do not exceed 10 mg. Selegiline has a modest effect in relieving Parkinson's disease symptoms presumably by retarding the breakdown of dopamine in the striatum. Selegiline appears to have a neuroprotective effect and if started early in the course of the disease can delay progression. Metabolites of selegiline include amphetamine and methamphetamine that may cause insomnia, anxiety, and other adverse symptoms.

Special Populations

Few cases of Parkinson's are diagnosed before the age of 50 years; therefore there are not a lot of data regarding the use of these drugs during pregnancy and lactation. Anecdotal reports have been published indicating worsening of Parkinson's symptoms in women who were untreated during pregnancy.[91] Among the medications used to treat Parkinson's, only amantadine was associated with increased risk of complications during pregnancy and fetal osseous abnormalities, although animal studies would urge caution in the use of selegiline.[92] The data regarding breastfeeding while taking Parkinson's drugs are even more sparse. The potential risks of these drugs must be weighed by the mothers against the known benefits of breast milk.

Alzheimer's Disease

Alzheimer's disease is a neurodegenerative condition that results from a progressive destruction of neurons in the cerebral cortex associated with memory and abstract reasoning (i.e., the hippocampus and the association areas of the cortex). Degenerating neuronal processes and neurofibrillary tangles lead to accumulation of senile plaques consisting of the protein β-amyloid. Neuronal loss results in a reduction of neurotransmitters in the areas of the brain that have the most destruction—especially acetylcholine. Thus treatments for Alzheimer's disease focus on increasing the availability of acetylcholine in the brain. Attempts to increase the concentration of acetylcholine by administration of its synthetic pathway precursors such as choline and phosphatidyl choline (lecithin) have not been consistently successful. Clearly, much work remains to be done in the evaluation of all agents, including nutritional supplements as an aid to memory among the elderly. Pharmacologic interventions at present concentrate on drugs that inhibit the intrasynaptic enzyme (acetylcholinesterase) that breaks down acetylcholine. Acetylcholinesterase inhibitors have proven to be moderately successful in treating early symptoms of Alzheimer's disease and have also been used in combination with nutritional supplements such as choline with modest results.[93]

Drugs Used for Alzheimer's Disease

The FDA has approved four anticholinesterase-inhibiting drugs for use in the treatment of Alzheimer's disease. Tacrine (Cognex) is associated with significant side effects such as abdominal cramping, nausea, diarrhea, and anorexia, all of which are dose related. Approximately 30% of individuals taking this drug at therapeutic levels experience these symptoms. Furthermore, the risk of hepatotoxicity is greater with tacrine and has led to reduction in clinical use.[94] The three other drugs in this class, donepezil (Aricept), rivastigmine (Exelon), and galantamine (Razadyne), have less effect on peripheral tissues and are associated with fewer of the above side effects that are most pronounced with tacrine.[95]

Other pharmacologic approaches to altering brain neurotransmitters in the treatment of Alzheimer's disease are in the development stage at present. However, one new drug, memantine (Namenda), has been approved and is currently in use. Memantine is an N-methyl-D-aspartic acid (NMDA) glutamate receptor antagonist that appears to reduce neurologic excitotoxicity and might reduce the rate of clinical deterioration by that mechanism.[73] Memantine has mild and reversible side effects that include headache and dizziness and is useful for those with moderate to severe Alzheimer's disease. The dose considerations for all of the drugs used to treatment of Alzheimer's disease are summarized in Table 24-16.

▌ Myasthenia Gravis

Myasthenia gravis is a progressive incurable disorder characterized by the loss of acetylcholine receptors. The name comes from the Latin word *gravis* which means serious and the Greek words μύς, which means muscle, and σθένεια, which means weakness. The result is skeletal weakness and fatigue that is worse with exertion and milder when the individual is resting. Myasthenia gravis is an autoimmune disorder whereby circulating autoantibodies block acetylcholine receptors at the postsynaptic neuromuscular junction. The most serious complication of myasthenia gravis is weakness of the respiratory muscles, which sets the stage for pneumonia. Myasthenia gravis tends to occur more often in women when it is diagnosed during early adulthood (ages 20–30 years) and more often in men when diagnosed in persons older than 50 years.

Anticholinesterase inhibitors are the mainstay of medical treatment for myasthenia gravis. These drugs prevent cholinesterase from inactivating acetylcholine.

Table 24-16 Medications Used to Treat Alzheimer's Disease

Drug Generic (Brand)	Formulations	Dose	Clinical Considerations	FDA Pregnancy Category
Tacrine (Cognex)	10-, 20-, 30-, 40-mg capsules	20–40 mg qid	Initial dose 10 mg qid for 4 weeks, then may increase 10 mg qid every 4 weeks until desired dose reached. Maximum dose 40 mg qid. Monitor liver function.	C
Donepezil (Aricept)	5-, 10-mg tablets 5-mg dispersible tablets	5–10 mg at bedtime	Initial dose is 5 mg at bedtime for 4–6 weeks. May increase to 10 mg at bedtime if needed.	C
Rivastigmine (Exelon)	1.5-, 3-, 4.5-, 6-mg capsules 2-mg/mL liquid 4.6-, 9.5-mg/24 h transdermal patch	3–6 mg bid	Initial dose 1.5 mg bid increasing 1.5 mg per dose every 2 weeks as tolerated. Maximum dose 12 mg/day. Initial dose for transdermal patch 4.6 mg/24 h after 4 weeks, may increase to 9.5 mg/24 h.	B
Galantamine (Razadyne)	4-, 8-, 12-mg tablets 4-mg/mL liquid 8-, 16-, 24-mg extended-release capsules	8–12 mg bid	Initial dose 4 mg bid increasing 4 mg bid every 4 weeks to maximum dose of 24 mg per day. Solution should be diluted in 100 mL of nonalcoholic beverage. Extended-release capsules 8 mg in the morning initially. May increase 8 mg/day every 4 weeks for a maximum dose of 24 mg/day.	B
Memantine (Namenda)	5-, 10-mg tablets 2-mg/mL solution	10 mg bid	Initial dose 5 mg once a day. May increase 5 mg per week changing to a bid schedule. Maximum dose 20 mg/day.	B

Corticosteroids and immunosuppressants may be used to suppress the abnormal immune response. Because the thymus is frequently involved in producing the destructive antibodies, surgical removal of the thymus gland is also a common treatment.

Neostigmine (Prostigmin) and pyridostigmine (Mestinon) are two common examples of the anticholinesterase drugs. Side effects include nausea, vomiting, diarrhea, urinary frequency, and increased bronchial secretions. These agents should be used with caution by persons with bronchial asthma, or anyone on a cardiac glycoside. They are all FDA Pregnancy Category C secondary to documented fetal harm in animal studies, but no studies have been done on humans.

▌ Conclusion

Diseases that affect the central nervous system are of particular import for women. The reproductive hormones estrogen and progesterone affect the function of most neurotransmitters that are involved in this collection of disorders. Pharmacologic treatment of nervous system disorders at the present time is aimed at regulating neuronal transmission imbalances primarily at the synaptic level. The drugs available are not always able to be targeted to the specific imbalance, and thus, they may produce global effects on many body systems resulting in numerous side effects. Newer drugs have fewer side effects due to greater specificity.

The most productive area of new research most likely will be in the area of neuroprotection or the prevention of neuronal damage. Combinations of neuroprotective drugs and dietary supplements may hold the greatest hope for the future.

✚ References

1. Zanchin G. Considerations on "the sacred disease" by Hippocrates. J Hist Neurosci 1992;1:91–5.
2. Vanzan Paladin A. Women and epilepsy in the Mediterranean cultures. Ital J Neurol Sci 1997;18(4):221–3.
3. Reddy DS. Pharmacology of catamenial epilepsy. Methods Find Exp Clin Pharmacol 2004;26(7):547–61.
4. Hamed SA. Neuroendocrine hormonal conditions in epilepsy: relationship to reproductive and sexual functions. Neurologist 2008;14(3):157–69.
5. Herzog AG. Menstrual disorders in women with epilepsy. Neurology 2006;66(6)(suppl 3):S23–8.
6. Harden CL. Sexuality in women with epilepsy. Epilepsy Behav 2005;7(suppl 2):S2–6.
7. Pack AM, Morrell MJ. Treatment of women with epilepsy. Semin Neurol 2002;22(3):289–98.
8. McCrossin S. LEAP for the assessment and correction of specific learning difficulties. Positive Health 2000;50. Available from: *http://www.crossinology.com/pdf/www.positivehealthKinesiology.pdf* [Accessed October 14, 2009].
9. Fried I, Katz A, McCarthy G, Sas KJ, Williamson B, Spencer SS, et al. Functional organization of human supplementary motor cortex studied by electrical stimulation. J Neurosci 1991;11(11):3656–66.
10. Bromfield EB. Epilepsy and the elderly. In Schachter SC, Schomer DL, eds. The comprehensive evaluation and treatment of epilepsy. San Diego, CA: Academic Press, 1997:233–54.
11. Schierhout G, Roberts I. Anti-epileptic drugs for preventing seizures following acute traumatic brain injury. Cochrane Database Syst Reviews 2000(4): CD000173.
12. Terminology CoCa. Proposal for revised classification of epilepsies and epileptic syndromes. Commission on Classification and Terminology of the International League against Epilepsy. Epilepsia 1989;30(4):389–99.
13. Engel J Jr. A proposed diagnostic scheme for people with epileptic seizures and with epilepsy: report of the ILAE Task Force on Classification and Terminology. Epilepsia 2001;42(6):796–803.
14. Foldvary-Schaefer N, Falcone T. Catamenial epilepsy: pathophysiology, diagnosis, and management. Neurology 2003;61(6)(suppl 2):S2–15.
15. Hitiris N, Suratman S, Kelly K, Stephen LJ, Sills GJ, Brodie MJ. Sudden unexpected death in epilepsy: a search for risk factors. Epilepsy Behav 2007;10(1): 138–41.
16. Shorvon S, Luciano AL. Prognosis of chronic and newly diagnosed epilepsy: revisiting temporal aspects. Curr Opin Neurol 2007;20(2):208–12.
17. Perucca E, Meador KJ. Adverse effects of antiepileptic drugs. Acta Neurologica Scandinavica 2005; 181:30–5.
18. Ettinger AB, Argoff CE. Use of antiepileptic drugs for nonepileptic conditions: psychiatric disorders and chronic pain. Neurotherapeutics 2007;4(1):75–83.
19. Hitiris N, Brodie MJ. Modern antiepileptic drugs: guidelines and beyond. Curr Opin Neurol 2006; 19(2):175–80.
20. LaRoche SM, Helmers SL. The new antiepileptic drugs. JAMA 2004;291:605–14.

21. Nadkarni S, LaJoie J, Devinsky O. Current treatments of epilepsy. Neurology 2005;64(12)(suppl 3):S2–11.

22. Schlienger RG, Shear NH. Antiepileptic drug hypersensitivity syndrome. Epilepsia 1998;39(suppl 7):S3–7.

23. Perucca E. Clinically relevant drug interactions with antiepileptic drugs. Br J Clin Pharmacol 2006; 61(3):246–55.

24. Czapinski P, Blaszczyk B, Czuczwar SJ. Mechanisms of action of antiepileptic drugs. Curr Top Med Chem 2005;5(1):3–14.

25. Bialer M. Extended-release formulations for the treatment of epilepsy. CNS Drugs 2007;21(9):765–74.

26. Van Amelsvoort T, Bakshi R, Devaux CB, Schwabe S. Hyponatremia associated with carbamazepine and oxcarbazepine therapy: a review. Epilepsia 1994;35(1): 181–8.

27. Pugh MJV, Van Cott AC, Cramer JA, Amuan ME, Tabares J, Ramsay RE, et al. Trends in antiepileptic drug prescribing for older patients with new-onset epilepsy: 2000–2004. Neurology 2008;70:2171–8.

28. Guerrini R. Valproate as a mainstay of therapy for pediatric epilepsy. Paediatric drugs 2006;8(2):113–29.

29. Gallassi R, Morreale A, Lorusso S, Procaccianti G, Lugaresi E, Baruzzi A. Cognitive effects of valproate. Epilepsy Res 1990;5(2):160–4.

30. Bryant AE 3rd, Dreifuss FE. Valproic acid hepatic fatalities. III. U.S. experience since 1986. Neurology 1996;46(2):465–9.

31. Steiner TJ, Dellaportas CI, Findley LJ, Gross M, Gibberd FB, Perkin GD, et al. Lamotrigine monotherapy in newly diagnosed untreated epilepsy: a double-blind comparison with phenytoin. Epilepsia 1999;40(5):601–7.

32. Brodie MJ, Richens A, Yuen AW. Double-blind comparison of lamotrigine and carbamazepine in newly diagnosed epilepsy. UK Lamotrigine/Carbamazepine Monotherapy Trial Group. Lancet 1995; 345(8948):476–9.

33. Gilliam FG, Gidal BE. Lamotrigine. In Wyllie E, ed. The treatment of epilepsy, 4th ed. Philadelphia, PA: Lippincott Williams & Wilkins, 2006:869–75.

34. Bergey GK. Evidence-based treatment of idiopathic generalized epilepsies with new antiepileptic drugs. Epilepsia 2005;46(suppl 9):161–8.

35. Glauser T, Ben-Menachem E, Bourgeois B, Bourgeois B, Cnaan A, Chadwick D, et al. ILAE treatment guidelines: evidence-based analysis of antiepileptic drug efficacy and effectiveness as initial monotherapy for epileptic seizures and syndromes. Epilepsia 2006;47: 1094–120.

36. Dieckhaus CM, Thompson CD, Roller SG, Macdonald TL. Mechanisms of idiosyncratic drug reactions: the case of felbamate. Chem Biol Interact 2002; 142(1–2):99–117.

37. Prasad K, Krishnan PR, Al-Roomi K, Sequeira R. Anticonvulsant therapy for status epilepticus. Br J Clin Pharmacol 2007;63:640–7.

38. Lowenstein DH, Alldredge BK. Status epilepticus. N Engl J Med 1998;338:970–6.

39. Farrell K. Benzodiazepines in the treatment of children with epilepsy. Epilepsia 1986;27(suppl 1):S45–52.

40. Kossoff EH. More fat and fewer seizures: dietary therapies for epilepsy. Lancet Neurol 2004;3(7):415–20.

41. Gasior M, Rogawski MA, Hartman AL. Neuroprotective and disease-modifying effects of the ketogenic diet. Behav Pharmacol 2006;17(5–6):431–9.

42. Rubenstein JE, Kossoff EH, Pyzik PL, Vining EP, McGrogan JR, Freeman JM. Experience in the use of the ketogenic diet as early therapy. J Child Neurol 2005;20(1):31–4.

43. Sinha SR, Kossoff EH. The ketogenic diet. Neurologist 2005;11(3):161–70.

44. Pennell PB. 2005 AES annual course: evidence used to treat women with epilepsy. Epilepsia 2006;47(suppl 1): 46–53.

45. Harden CL, Leppik I. Optimizing therapy of seizures in women who use oral contraceptives. Neurology 2006;67(12)(suppl 4):S56–8.

46. Morrell MJ, Cramer JA, Darne PD, Naftolin F. Use of oral contraceptives by women with epilepsy. JAMA 1986;246:238–40.

47. Crawford P. Interactions between antiepileptic drugs and hormonal contraception. CNS Drugs 2002;16: 263–72.

48. O'Brien MD, Gilmour-White SK. Management of epilepsy in women. Postgrad Med J 2005;81(955): 278–85.

49. Sidhu J, Job S, Singh S, Philipson R. The pharmacokinetic and pharmacodynamic consequences of the co-administration of lamotrigine and a combined oral contraceptive in healthy female subjects. Br J Clin Pharmacol 2006;61:191–9.

50. Pack AM, Walczak TS. Bone health in women with epilepsy: clinical features and potential mechanisms. Int Rev Neurobiol 2008;83:305–28.

51. Tomson T, Battino D. Teratogenicity of antiepileptic drugs: state of the art. Curr Opin Neurol 2005; 18:135–40.

52. Harden CL, Meador KJ, Pennell PB, Hauser WA, Gronseth GS, French JA, et al. Management issues

for women with epilepsy—focus on pregnancy (an evidence-based review): II. Teratogenesis and perinatal outcomes. Epilepsia 2009;50:1237–46.

53. American Academy of Pediatrics. Transfer of drugs and other chemicals into human milk. Pediatrics 2001; 108:776–89.

54. Tomson T, Perucca E, Battino D. Navigating toward fetal and maternal health: the challenge of treating epilepsy in pregnancy. Epilepsia 2004;45:1171–5.

55. Meador KJ. Effects of in utero antiepileptic drug exposure. Cur Rev Clin Science 2008;8:143–7.

56. Harden CL. Antiepileptic drug teratogenesis: what are the risks for congenital malformations and adverse cognitive outcomes? Int Rev Neurobiol 2008; 83:205–13.

57. Meador KJ, Bake GA, Browning N, Clayton-Smith J, Combs-Cantrell DT, Cohen M, et al. Cognitive function at 3 years of age after fetal exposure to antiepileptic drugs. N Engl J Med 2009;360:1597–605.

58. Harden CL, Hopp J, Ting TY, Pennell PB, French JA, Hauser WA, et al. Practice parameter update: management issues for women with epilepsy—focus on pregnancy (an evidence-based review): Obstetrical complications and change in seizure frequency. Report of the Quality Standards Subcommittee and Therapeutics and Technology Assessment Subcommittee of the American Academy of Neurology and American Epilepsy Society. Neurology. 2009 April 27. Available from: *www.neurology.org/cgi/rapidpdf/WNL .0b013e3181a6b2f8v1.pdf* [Accessed August 4, 2009].

59. Tettenborn B. Management of epilepsy in women of childbearing age: practical recommendations. CNS Drugs 2006;20:373–87.

60. Yerby MS. Management issues for women with epilepsy: neural tube defects and folic acid supplementation. Neurology 2003;61(6)(suppl 2):S23–6.

61. Pennell PB. Antiepileptic drugs during pregnancy: what is known and which AEDs seem to be safest? [Review]. Epilepsia 2008;49(suppl 9):43–55.

62. Harden CL. Issues for mature women with epilepsy. Int Rev Neurobiol 2008; 83:385–95.

63. Allen R, Picchiette D, Hening W, Trenkwalder C, Walters A, Montplaisi J. Restless legs syndrome: diagnostic criteria, special considerations, and epidemiology. A report from the restless legs syndrome diagnosis and epidemiologic workshop at the National Institutes of Health. Sleep Med 2003;4:101–9.

64. Sibler MH, Ehrenber BL, Allen RP, Buchfuhrer MJ, Earley CJ, Hening WA, et al. An algorithm for the management of restless legs syndrome. Mayo Clinic Proc 2004;79(7):916–22.

65. Hensley JG. Leg cramps and restless legs syndrome during pregnancy. J Midwifery Womens Health 2009; 54:211–8.

66. Allen RP. Controversies and challenges in defining the etiology and pathophysiology of restless legs syndrome. Am J Med 2007;120(1A):S13–21.

67. Carcia-Borreguero D, Allen RP, Kohnen R, Hogel B, Trenkwalder C, Oertel W, et al. Diagnostic standards for dopaminergic augmentation of restless leg syndrome: report from a world association of sleep medicine-international restless leg syndrome study group consensus conference at the max plan institute. Sleep Med 2007;8:520–30.

68. Lipton RB, Walter F, Diamond S, Diamond M, Reed M. Prevalence and burden of migraine in the United States. Headache 2001;41:646–57.

69. Cady RK, Scheriber CP, Farmer KU. Understanding the patient with migraine: the evolution from episodic headache to chronic neurologic disease. A proposed classification for patients with headaches. Headache 2004;44:426–35.

70. Silberstein SD, Diener HC, Lipton RB, Goadsby P, Dodick D, Bussone G, et al. Epidemiology, risk factors, and treatment of chronic migraine: a focus on topiramate. Headache 2008;48:1087–95.

71. Martin VT. Menstrual migraine: a review of prophylactic therapies. Curr Pain Headache Rep 2004;8: 229–37.

72. Headache classification subcommittee of the International Headache Society. The international classification of headache disorders, 2nd ed. Cephalalgia 2004;24(suppl 1):9–160.

73. Lipton RB, Steward WF, Stone AM, Lainez MJ, Sawyer JPC. Stratified care vs step care strategies for migraine. The disability in strategies of care (DISC) study: a randomized trial. JAMA 2000;284:2599–605.

74. Matcher DB, Young WB, Rosenberg JH, Pietrzak MP. Evidence based guidelines for migraine headache in primary care setting: pharmacological management of acute attacks. April 2000. Available from: *www.aan .com/professionals/practice/pdfs/gl0087.pdf* [Accessed May 4, 2009].

75. Silberstein SD. Practice parameter: evidence-based guidelines for migraine headache (an evidence-based review): report of the quality standards subcommittee of the American Academy of Neurology. Neurology 2000;55:754–62.

76. Tfelt-Hansen P, Saxena PR, Dahlos C, Pascual J, Lainez M, Henry P, et al. Ergotamine in the acute treatment of migraine: a review and European consensus. Brain 2000;123:9–18.

77. Silbertein SD, McCrory DC. Ergotamine and dihydroergotamine: history, pharmacology, and efficacy. Headache 2003;43:144–66.

78. Kaniecki R, Lucas S. Treatment of primary headache: preventive treatment of migraine. In Standards of care for headache diagnosis and treatment. Chicago: National Headache Foundation, 2004:40–52.

79. Ramadan NM, Silberstein SD, Freitag FG, Gilbert TT. Evidence-based guidelines for migraine headache in the primary care setting: pharmacological management for the prevention of migraine. April 2000. Available from: *http://www.aan.com/professionals/practice/pdfs/gl0090.pdf* [Accessed August 4, 2009].

80. Hilaire ML, Cross LB, Eichner SF. Treatment of migraine headaches with sumatriptan in pregnancy. Ann Pharmacother 2004;38:1726–30.

81. Ramsay JR, Rostain AL. Adult ADHD research: current status and future directions. J Atten Disord 2008;11(6):624–7.

82. Murphy P. Cognitive functioning in adults with attention-deficit/hyperactivity disorder. J Atten Disord 2002;5(4):203–9.

83. Linnet KM, Dalsgaard S, Obel C, Wisborg K, Henriksen TB, Rodriguez A, et al. Maternal lifestyle factors in pregnancy risk of attention deficit hyperactivity disorder and associated behaviors: review of the current evidence. Am J Psychiatry 2003;160(6):1028–40.

84. Humphreys C, Garcia-Bournissen F, Ito S, Koren G. Exposure to attention deficit hyperactivity disorder medications during pregnancy. Can Fam Physician 2007;53(7):1153–5.

85. Ilett KF, Hackett LP, Kristensen JH, Kohan R. Transfer of dexamphetamine into breast milk during treatment for attention deficit hyperactivity disorder. Br J Clin Pharmacol 2007;63(3):371–5.

86. Morale MC, Serra PA, L'Episcopo F, Tirolo C, Caniglia S, Testa N, et al. Estrogen, neuroinflammation and neuroprotection in Parkinson's disease: glia dictates resistance versus vulnerability to neurodegeneration. Neuroscience 2006;138(3):869–78.

87. Henderson VW. The neurology of menopause. Neurologist 2006;12(3):149–59.

88. Lang AE, Lozano AM. Parkinson's disease. First of two parts. N Engl J Med 1998;339(15):1044–53.

89. Lang AE, Lozano AM. Parkinson's disease. Second of two parts. N Engl J Med 1998;339(16):1130–43.

90. Lees A. Alternatives to levodopa in the initial treatment of early Parkinson's disease. Drugs Aging 2005; 22(9):731–740.

91. Golbe LI. Parkinson's disease and pregnancy. Neurology 1987;37(7):1245–1249.

92. Hagell P, Odin P, Vinge E. Pregnancy in Parkinson's disease: a review of the literature and a case report. Mov Disord 1998;13(1):34–8.

93. Ott BR, Owens NJ. Complementary and alternative medicines for Alzheimer's disease. J Geriatr Psychiatry Neurol 1998;11(4):163–73.

94. Bonner LT, Peskind ER. Pharmacologic treatments of dementia. Med Clin North Am 2002;86(3):657–74.

95. Doggrell SA, Evans S. Treatment of dementia with neurotransmission modulation. Expert Opin Investig Drugs 2003;12(10):1633–54.

25

Mental Health

Tekoa L. King, Ruth Johnson, and Vivian Gamblian

Chapter Glossary

Acute stress disorder The development of acute anxiety, dissociative symptoms, decreased emotional responsiveness within 1 month of a traumatic event that was experienced as a terrifying event. Individuals with acute stress disorder have at least one symptom of PTSD in addition to heightened anxiety and a variety of symptoms.

Anorexia nervosa An eating disorder characterized by low body weight, disturbed body image, and obsessive fear of gaining weight. Anorexia nervosa is a psychiatric disorder.

Anxiolytics Drugs used to treat anxiety. Most are sedative-hypnotic drugs from the barbiturate or benzodiazepine class.

Binge-eating disorder An eating disorder that does not meet the full criteria for anorexia or bulimia.

Bipolar I Also known as manic depression or bipolar affective disorder. Characterized by one or more episodes of abnormally elevated mood. Bipolar I is the classic cyclic expression of manic moods followed by depression. Persons with bipolar I can also experience mixed episodes.

Bipolar II Bipolar disorder with more frequent and intense depressive symptoms when compared to the occurrences of manic episodes. Manic episodes are hypomania rather than actual manic episodes.

Bipolar not otherwise specified A mood disorder with bipolar features that do not fit another bipolar category.

Bulimia nervosa Eating disorder characterized by recurrent binge eating, which is followed by compulsive behaviors. The most common is self-induced vomiting.

Cyclothymia Hypomania with periods of depression that do not meet criteria for major depressive episodes.

Desensitization Resistance of a receptor to agonist neurotransmitters or agonist drugs. Desensitization is the reason initial side effects gradually disappear.

Down regulated The actual disappearance of a receptor on the postsynaptic nerve so that nerve becomes less able to be stimulated by agonist neurotransmitters or agonist drugs.

Dysthymia Mildest form of unipolar depression that is chronic. Characterized by low-level depression and lack of enjoyment in life or pessimism, but ability to function is unimpaired.

Floppy baby syndrome Syndrome noted at birth that has the following characteristics: hypothermia, lethargy, hypotonia, poor respiratory effort, and difficulty feeding. Associated with maternal use of benzodiazepines shortly before birth.

Generalized anxiety disorder (GAD) Excessive anxiety and worry about life circumstances that are difficult to control. The anxiety is unrealistic, generalized, and persistent. It is present on more days than not over a 6-month period.

Hypertensive crisis Rapid rise in blood pressure accompanied by tachycardia. Symptoms include headache, neck pain, chest pain, nausea and vomiting, and sometimes seizures. Although rare, intracranial hemorrhage and cardiac arrest can result.

Kindling A process by which repeated stimuli sensitize the brain to react when the stimulus is reapplied. This concept is used to explain the progression of mental illness that becomes worse over time.

Mania From the Greek *uavia*, which means "to rage or be furious." Mania is a condition of extreme elevated or irritated mood and the behaviors associated with this mood. May be characterized by grandiose thoughts or a flood of good ideas. Most often associated with bipolar disorder. Mania is a continuum of intensity with hypomania (mild mania) at one end and mania with psychotic features at the other end.

Manic episode Period of days to weeks marked by unusually high energy, euphoria, hyperactivity, or impaired judgment.

Mental disorder A behavioral or psychological syndrome that occurs and is associated with distinct disability or significantly increased suffering. There is no single definition for the precise boundaries for the concept of mental disorder.

Monoamine oxidase (MAO) Enzyme that degrades neurotransmitters intracellularly, thereby decreasing the amount of neurotransmitter that can be released into the synapse.

Obsessive-compulsive disorder A form of anxiety disorder characterized by involuntary intrusive thoughts.

Panic disorder A form of anxiety disorder characterized by recurring severe panic attacks.

Phobia A form of anxiety disorder characterized by irrational, persistent fear of specific situations, persons, activities, or items.

Posttraumatic stress disorder (PTSD) A form of anxiety disorder that develops after exposure to a traumatic event or highly unsafe experience. PTSD is characterized by reliving a traumatic event, avoiding it, numbing, and feeling all keyed up.

Psychosis From the Greek *psyche*, which means "mind" or "soul," and *osis*, which means "abnormal condition." Psychosis is a state of delusional thinking that is characterized by hallucinations or delusional beliefs and/or disordered thinking. May be accompanied by unusual behavior and personality changes. Impaired ability to manage activities of daily living is present.

Psychotropics Term for all psychoactive drugs that are used to treat mental illness.

Selective serotonin reuptake inhibitors (SSRIs) Class of antidepressants that inhibit reuptake of serotonin into the presynaptic cell, which increases the amount of serotonin in the synapse. SSRIs have a weak affinity for norepinephrine and dopamine receptors.

Serotonin-norepinephrine reuptake inhibitors (SNRIs) Class of antidepressants that inhibit reuptake of serotonin and of norepinephrine into the presynaptic cell, which increases the amount of serotonin and norepinephrine in the synapse.

Serotonin syndrome A clinical triad of mental status changes, autonomic hyperactivity, and neuromuscular abnormalities caused by excess serotonin in the synapses in the central nervous system. Serotonin syndrome is a predictable adverse drug reaction secondary to excess serotonin in neural synapses within the CNS and periphery. *Serotonin toxicity* is the preferred term, but it is not yet used widely in clinical practice.

Sleepdriving Driving while not fully awake after taking a sedative-hypnotic and having no memory of the event.

Mental Health and Mental Disorders

What is mental health? According to the World Health Organization, "Mental health is a state of well-being in which the individual realizes his or her own abilities, can cope with the normal stresses of life, can work productively and fruitfully, and is able to make a contribution to his or her community."[1] In contrast, the term **mental disorder** refers to all diagnosable conditions characterized by alterations in thinking, mood, and/or behavior. Although the terms *mental illness* and *mental disorder* are synonymous, *mental disorder* is the preferred term. Mental disorders are more common than you might think. An estimated 26.2% of adults in the United States suffer from a diagnosable mental disorder.[2]

The overall rates of mental disorders in men and women are roughly equal; however, there is a striking gender difference in the patterns of illness. Women are twice as likely as men to suffer from depression, anxiety, and **posttraumatic stress disorder** (PTSD).[3] Perinatal depression affects roughly 8–11% of women in the first postpartum year, and women comprise 90% of the population of individuals who have an eating disorder.[4] Women are also more likely than men to have suicide attempts but less likely than men to die by suicide.[5] Additionally, the course of some disorders in women is often different than the course of the same disorder in men. Bipolar disorder is more likely to appear later in life, have a seasonal pattern of mood disturbance, and be associated with comorbid conditions in women compared to men.[6,7] This chapter focuses on psychotropic medications and how they can be used effectively in primary women's healthcare practice. The emphasis is on depression and anxiety, the two most common mood disorders frequently seen in primary care practice.

Treatment of Psychiatric Conditions in Primary Care

Mental disorders are relatively common in the general population, but psychiatric providers who treat these disorders are in short supply, especially those with prescriptive authority. More than half of the persons treated for depression in the United States are treated by a primary care provider.[8] Mental disorders are often episodic in nature and likely to reoccur throughout a woman's lifetime; thus, distorted reasoning or diminished functioning may be first noted by a primary clinician. Prompt intervention can prevent symptoms from worsening and lessen the impact of illness. In addition, women who refuse referral to a specialist may more readily accept treatment from their primary provider. Women who have one of the following disorders may be successfully cared for by a primary care provider who can offer medication and supportive counseling: situational anxiety, mild anxiety disorders, acute stress, unipolar depression without suicidal ideation, and sleep disorders.

Treatment of women's mental disorders in the primary care setting should take place within a practice structure that provides for consultation and collaboration with appropriate psychiatric providers and referral for specialized care when indicated. In some states, only psychiatrists may prescribe medications. In most states, advanced practice psychiatric nurses and psychiatric nurse practitioners (PNPs) may also prescribe. Two states, New Mexico and Louisiana, allow certain psychologists to prescribe psychotropic medications.

Referral to a Psychiatric Specialist

A number of situations require referral to a psychiatric specialist, even if a woman requests that her care be managed in the primary setting. Box 25-1 lists some indications for referral to a mental health specialist. Individual practices should have a list of disorders or symptomatology

---

Box 25-1 Criteria for Referral to a Mental Health Specialist

- The individual is displaying signs of suicidal intent.

- There seems to be a risk of harm to others, or the individual expresses intent to harm another person.

- There are symptoms of psychosis such as self-denigrating auditory hallucinations or somatic delusions.

- There is evidence of severe physical deterioration of the patient: significant weight loss, severe psychomotor retardation or agitation.

- The individual has depression and needs treatment for substance abuse.

- The individual's history suggests bipolar disorder.

- The individual is so disabled by his or her mental disorder that he/she is unable to leave his/her home, look after his/her children or fulfill other activities of daily living.

- Diagnostic uncertainty: The primary care clinician requires the expertise of secondary care to confirm a diagnosis or implement specialist treatment.

- The individual is on multiple medications.

- The primary care clinician feels that the therapeutic relationship with the patient has broken down.

- The primary care interventions and voluntary/nonstatutory options have been exhausted.

- A particular psychotropic medication is required (e.g., clozapine [Clozaril], lithium [Lithobid], or donepezil [Aricept]).

- The individual requests a referral.

Source: World Health Organization 2001.[1]

that require psychiatric consultation and a protocol for managing the transfer of care in that setting.

If a woman is thought to be unable to keep herself or her family safe, the situation becomes a medical emergency. This includes any episode of psychosis or mania wherein the woman's insight is poor and the risk of harm correspondingly high. Particularly during the postpartum period, the risk of successful suicide or infanticide is increased, and hospitalization may be necessary.[9] If a woman appears to pose a danger to herself or others, the clinician becomes responsible for ensuring her safety, which may require committing her for inpatient evaluation and informing authorities if others are in danger. The healthcare professional has a legal duty to inform others and protect them from harm, as specified in each state's statutory code.

Examples of conditions that require psychiatric treatment and/or psychotropic drugs that have significant side effects include severe major depression, especially suicidal thoughts with or without a plan; bipolar disorder, especially **bipolar I** disorder; psychotic disorders, including schizophrenia and postpartum psychosis; **anorexia nervosa**; and **bulimia nervosa**. Psychotropic medication for these disorders should be prescribed by psychiatric clinicians who are experienced in the management of these conditions and the drugs used to treat them. Balancing the complexities of the medications used with the inherent instabilities of these disorders is beyond the purview of primary care practice.

Conversely, the primary care provider can offer valuable assistance in several ways to help women with psychiatric conditions that require care by a psychiatric provider. In contrast to the intensely client-focused process of individual psychotherapy, primary clinicians who are accustomed to family-centered care can bolster a woman's decision making by involving her chosen family members in planning her treatment.

If mental disorders worsen with hormonal shifts, the primary care provider can tailor treatment to regulate or suppress ovulatory cycles, which can optimize the action of psychotropic medications. The primary care provider can also monitor for the drug–drug interactions that can occur when psychotropic drugs and hormonal products are used concomitantly. Some psychotropic drugs have teratogenic potential, and if the prescriber is unaware of a woman's fertility status, the primary clinician can provide effective contraceptive counseling. Finally, primary care providers can offer treatment for comorbid conditions, with special emphasis on monitoring for drug–drug interactions.

The cumulative effects of mental disorders tend to worsen over the course of a lifetime. In the neurologic process known as **kindling**, each episode of illness deepens the damage and leaves the individual increasingly vulnerable to more severe symptoms in response to the next stressor.[10,11] A setback that merely causes a few weeks of insomnia for a 30-year-old may incapacitate the same woman at age 50. Aggressive intervention at the onset of every episode is the best way to prevent future disability, and it is here too that the primary care clinician is uniquely positioned to help women mitigate disease progression.

Psychotropic Medications

Medications used to treat psychiatric disorders are called **psychotropics**, a catch-all term for of a broad array of pharmacologic agents. The psychotropic medications are increasingly prescribed for a variety of conditions that are managed by primary care providers. Whether prescribed alone or in combination with hormonal products, psychotropics are becoming first-line treatment for perimenstrual disorders and midlife symptoms such as vasomotor instability and disordered sleep. Thus clinicians who do not intend to use these medications to treat mental disorders will need to be familiar with their use for other women's healthcare needs.

Differential Diagnosis

The diagnosis of mental disorders relies on clinical information, beginning with a complete history and physical examination that focuses on the emotional and somatic symptoms presented.[12] The history should include a detailed list of medications being taken because some medications have neuropsychiatric side effects. Comorbid conditions can also be the cause of depression. Hypothyroidism, Cushing's disease, and cobalamin deficiency can induce depression, whereas other chronic disorders such as diabetes and cardiovascular disease are associated with depression.

It is important to screen patients for a history of **manic episodes** that might indicate a diagnosis of bipolar disorder. Individuals with bipolar disorder may present with depression, but it is theorized that treatment of persons with bipolar disorder with antidepressants can precipitate a manic episode and exacerbate the bipolar disorder. Therefore use of one of the standardized screening tools is essential when screening for mood disorders in primary care settings.[13]

Several validated screening tools such as the Primary Care Evaluation of Medical Disorders (PRIME-MD) and

754 CHAPTER 25 Mental Health

Edinburgh Postnatal Depression Scale are available to help establish the diagnosis of many mental disorders.[13-16] The PRIME-MD was the first tool developed that actually diagnoses specific disorders using the DSM-IV diagnostic criteria. The PRIME-MD is a 26-item, self-administered questionnaire that screens for depression, eating disorders, anxiety, alcohol abuse, and somatoform disorder. This tool takes about 8 minutes to complete, which makes it too long for most primary care settings. The Patient Health Questionnaire (PHQ) is a shorter version of PRIME-MD that has similar diagnostic validity.[14] Other tools that screen specifically for depression or anxiety are available and the Mood Disorder questionnaire, a 15-item self-report assessment of bipolar symptoms based on the DSM-IV criteria, is also available for use in clinical practice.[13,19]

Diagnostic criteria most often used in practice are delineated in the *Diagnostic and Statistical Manual of Mental Disorders*, 4th edition (DSM-IV).[17] A complete approach to assessment, screening for risk factors, and treatment is outside the scope of this chapter. The interested reader is referred to primary care texts and the DSM-IV manual.[17,18]

Drugs That Have Neuropsychiatric Side Effects

Some medications and medical conditions can cause symptoms of mental disorders (Table 25-1). The medications that are most often associated with depression are glucocorticoids, interferon, propranolol (Inderal), and oral contraceptives.

Treatment Options and Informed Consent

Historically, the only treatment for mental disorders was psychotherapy and/or institutionalization. Interventions such as lobotomy and electroconvulsive therapy had limited success rates. Current evidence regarding the

Table 25-1 Selected List of Medications with Neuropsychiatric Side Effects

Drug Generic (Brand)	Neuropsychiatric Effects	Drug Generic (Brand)	Neuropsychiatric Effects
Acyclovir (Zovirax)	Depression	Dextromethorphan	Psychosis
Adrenocorticoids	Anxiety, panic attack, depression, hallucinations, mania, psychoses	Famotidine (Pepcid)	Depression
		Fluoroquinolone antibiotics	Depression, psychosis
Amphetamines	Psychosis		
Anticholinergic agents	Psychosis	Hormonal preparations	Depression
Anticonvulsants	Depression	Interferon	Depression
Antidepressants such as SSRI, SNRI, TCAs	Suicidal ideation	Isoniazid (INH)	Delirium, psychosis
		L-dopa	Psychosis
Antihistamines*†	Agitation, anxiety, nervousness, confusion, hallucinations	Methyldopa	Depression
		Methylphenidate (Ritalin, Concerta)	Suicidal thoughts, toxic psychosis
Barbiturates	Depression, suicidal ideation, phobias, violent behavior (paradoxical effect of some sedatives)	Metoclopramide (Reglan)	Extrapyramidal effects, dystonic reaction
Benzodiazepines	Depression, psychosis	Nifedipine	Depression
Beta-blockers	Anxiety, agitation, nervousness	Nizatidine (Axid)	Depression
Bromocriptine (Parlodel)	Depression	Oxybutynin (Ditropan)	Drowsiness, hallucinations, cognitive impairment
Calcium channel blockers	Depression		
Carbamazepine (Tegretol)	Depression	Phenytoin (Dilantin)	Depression
Cimetidine (Tagamet)	Confusion, delirium, depression, hallucinations, mania, paranoia	Pramipexole (Mirapex)	Anhedonia, depression
		Propranolol (Inderal)	Depression
Clonazepam (Klonopin)	Depression	Ropinirole (Requip)	Anhedonia, depression
Cold medicines containing phenylpropanolamine	Psychosis	Scopolamine	Psychosis
		Statins	Depression
Corticosteroids	Psychosis, mood disorders, and/or deliriums	Thiazide diuretics	Depression
		Valproic acid	Depression
Dextromethamphetamine (Desoxyn)	Psychomotor agitation, obsessive behaviors, paranoia, psychosis	Verapamil	Depression

SSRI = selective serotonin reuptake inhibitor; SNRI = serotonin-norepinephrine reuptake inhibitor; TCA = tricyclic antidepressant.
* Agents that contain pseudoephedrine can cause anxiety, nervousness, mania, and rarely paranoia.
† Agents that contain phenylpropanolamine can cause confusion, delirium, depression, hallucinations, mania, and rarely paranoia.

effective treatment of psychiatric conditions supports a combination of medication plus psychotherapy, which is more effective than either approach alone.[20] The growth of pharmacologic therapies has exploded in the last 40 years, and today, pharmacologic interventions are credited with improving quality of life for many individuals with mental disorders.

When discussing drug treatment options, risks, and benefits, it is important to remember that mental disorders by definition impair thought processes and can interfere with both memory and reasoning.[21] Secondly, most psychotropic medications have side effects and drug–drug interactions that are clinically significant and should be reviewed as part of the informed consent process. Considerations prior to initiating therapy include review of FDA black box warnings; the effects of drugs during pregnancy, as nearly 50% of all pregnancies in the United States are unintended; and disclosure of off-label use if the drug does not have FDA approval for the disorder being treated[22] (Table 25-2).

Table 25-2 Psychotropic Medications with FDA Black Box Warnings to Be Inserted

Medications Generic (Brand)	FDA Black Box Warnings	Monitoring Recommendations Related to Black Box Warning
Amphetamines	High abuse/diversion potential, drug dependence, sudden death, serious cardiovascular adverse events	Do not administer for long periods of time.
Anticonvulsants	Increased risk of sucidal thoughts	Monitor for notable changes in behavior that could indicate the emergence of worsening suicidal thoughts or depression.
Atypical antipsychotics: All	Increased risk of mortality in elderly patients treated for dementia-related psychosis	Contraindicated for persons with dementia-related psychosis.
Bupropion (Wellbutrin)	Suicidality in children, adolescents, and young adults up to age 25 years	Close observation for suicidal thinking or unusual behavior.
Carbamazepine (Tegretol)*	Aplastic anemia, agranulocytosis	Complete blood count and platelet count should be obtained prior to initiating treatment and yearly afterward.
Conventional antipsychotics: All	Increased mortality in elderly with dementia-related psychosis	Contraindicated for persons with dementia-related psychosis.
Dexmethylphenidate (Focalin)	Chronic abuse can lead to tolerance and dependence, frank psychosis (especially with intravenous use)	Give with caution to persons with a history of drug dependence. Careful supervision required during drug withdrawal.
Droperidol	Increased risk of mortality in elderly patients treated for dementia-related psychosis Unexpected cardiovascular deaths may occur at normal therapeutic doses (QT prolongation and torsades de pointes)	Baseline and periodic ECG and serum potassium during therapy. If baseline QTc is ≥ 450 msec, do not initiate therapy in females. Contraindicated for use with drugs that are CYP2D6 inhibitors and drugs that prolong QT interval. Contraindicated for persons with history of cardiac arrhythmias or congenital long QT syndrome.
Haloperidol (Haldol)	Increased mortality in elderly with dementia-related psychosis, sudden death, QT prolongation, torsades de pointes (especially if given intravenously or in high doses)	Baseline and periodic ECG and serum potassium during therapy. If baseline QTc is ≥ 450 msec, do not initiate therapy in females. Contraindicated for use with drugs that are CYP2D6 inhibitors and drugs that prolong QT interval. Contraindicated for persons with history of cardiac arrhythmias or congenital long QT syndrome.
Lamotrigine (Lamictal)	Serious dermatologic reactions requiring hospitalization including Stevens-Johnson syndrome; incidence 0.8% in persons with bipolar disorder	Discontinue at first sign of a rash. Discontinuation of treatment may not prevent rash from becoming life threatening or permanently disabling.
Methylphenidate (Concerta, Ritalin, Daytrana, Metadate)	Chronic abuse can lead to tolerance and dependence, frank psychosis (especially with intravenous use)	Give with caution to persons with a history of drug dependence. Careful supervision required during drug withdrawal.
Monoamine oxidase inhibitors (MAOIs)	Suicidality in children, adolescents, and young adults up to age 25 years	Close observation for suicidal thinking or unusual behavior.

(continues)

Table 25-2 Psychotropic Medications with FDA Black Box Warnings to Be Inserted (*continued*)

Medications Generic (Brand)	FDA Black Box Warnings	Monitoring Recommendations Related to Black Box Warning
Nefazodone (Serzone)	Suicidality in children, adolescents, and young adults up to age 25 years	Close observation for suicidal thinking or unusual behavior.
Selective serotonin reuptake inhibitors (SSRIs)	Suicidality in children, adolescents, and young adults up to age 25 years	Close observation for suicidal thinking or unusual behavior.
Selegiline (Eldepryl)	Suicidality in children, adolescents, and young adults up to age 25 years	Close observation for suicidal thinking or unusual behavior.
Serotonin-norepinephrine reuptake inhibitors (SNRIs)	Suicidality in children, adolescents, and young adults up to age 25 years	Close observation for suicidal thinking or unusual behavior.
Trazodone (Desyrel)	Suicidality in children, adolescents, and young adults up to age 25 years	Close observation for suicidal thinking or unusual behavior.
Tricyclic Antidepressants	Suicidality in children, adolescents, and young adults up to age 25 years	Close observation for suicidal thinking or unusual behavior.
Thioridazine (Thorazine)	Increased mortality in elderly with dementia-related psychosis, prolonged QT interval, torsades de pointes	Baseline and periodic ECG and serum potassium during therapy. If baseline QTc is $\geq$ 450 msec do not initiate therapy. Contraindicated for use with drugs that are CYP2D6 inhibitors and drugs that prolong QT interval. Contraindicated for persons with history of cardiac arrhythmias or congenital long QT syndrome.
Valproic acid (Depakote, Depakene)	Teratogenicity, hepatotoxicity, pancreatitis	Check baseline liver function tests prior to initiating treatment and yearly afterward. Warn of signs of pancreatitis.

Source: Adapted with permission from Frank B et al. 2008.[21]

Neurobiology of Mental Disorders

While psychotropic medications have been used empirically for many years, it is only recently that research has identified the specific actions of particular medications on human neurochemistry. Since the 1990s, studies have focused on interactions with neurotransmitters. Norepinephrine, dopamine, and serotonin are three neurotransmitters that modulate mood. Table 25-3 summarizes the agonist functions of neurotransmitters involved in mental disorders and how psychotropic drugs stimulate these effects. Norepinephrine, dopamine, and serotonin are monoamines derived from amino acids tryptophan or L-tyrosine. In addition to these three, the two amino acid neurotransmitters, glutamate and gamma aminobutyric acid (GABA), play a role in mental disorders. Figure 25-1 illustrates the actions and relationships among the three primary neurotransmitters.

Neurotransmitters have complex and interrelated effects on many physiologic functions; however, they have a relatively simple life cycle. The life cycle is as follows:

1. All of these neurotransmitters are synthesized in a presynaptic neuron.
2. They are released into the synaptic space where they have an agonist or antagonist action on the postsynaptic neuron.

3. The neurotransmitters are moved from the synaptic space back into the presynaptic neuron. This action is referred to as "reuptake," and it is dependent upon a protein transporter on the presynaptic neuron cell membrane.
4. Once they are back in the presynaptic neuron, the neurotransmitters are either enzymatically degraded or recycled into vesicles for release into the synaptic space again.

The drugs that affect these neurotransmitters alter one of these steps (Figure 25-2).

The Monoamine-Deficiency Hypothesis

The norepinephrine and serotonin nerves originate deep in the brain and spread out over most of the entire brain. One of the earliest theories proposed for why antidepressants work is the monoamine-deficiency hypothesis. According to this theory, persons with depression have a deficiency of the monoamines norepinephrine and serotonin. The theory is overly simple and does not account for the complex interactions between the norepinephrine and serotonin systems or the role of other players such as genetics, stress hormones, and reproductive hormones. This theory, however, has been an important foundation for much of the initial research on mood disorders and

Table 25-3 Biologic Function of Key Neurotransmitters

Neurotransmitter	Function	Adverse Effects
Acetylcholine*	Controls skeletal muscle movement and smooth muscle of parasympathetic system	Dry mouth, blurred vision, constipation, ataxia, increased body temperature, urinary retention
Dopamine	Movement, GI motility, primitive emotions	EPS, increased prolactin levels, psychosis, insomnia, psychomotor agitations
GABA	Presynaptic inhibition slows nerve conduction and transmission, CNS depressant	None known
Histamine	Bronchoconstriction, vasodilation, gastric acid secretion, smooth muscle relaxation	Sedation, hypotension, weight gain, allergic symptoms
Norepinephrine	Memory, information processing, emotions, psychomotor function, blood pressure, heart rate, bladder emptying	Tachycardia, tremors, sexual dysfunction
Serotonin	Appetite and eating behaviors, regulates anxiety, movements, GI motility, sexual function, sleep	Sexual dysfunction, anxiety, obsessions and compulsions, headache, hypotension

* Acetylcholine is antagonized by psychotropic drugs, so in this instance the effects of inhibiting acetylcholine are manifest and are generally referred to as "anticholinergic effects."

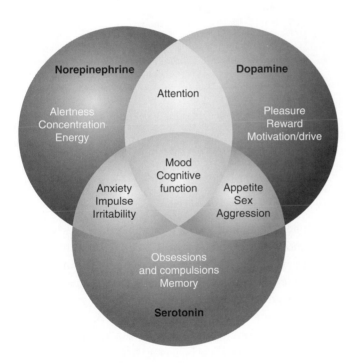

Figure 25-1 Role of dopamine, norepinephrine, and serotonin.

continues to be evaluated as new technologies allow novel methods of assessing brain function.

Role of Gender

The fact that women are twice as likely as men to have major depression suggests there is a biologic difference in the underlying neuropathology of this disorder. However, biologic mechanisms responsible for gender differences in mental disorders are just beginning to be elucidated. The complex interplay between genetic predisposition, psychosocial events such as role stress or victimization, and disadvantaged social status plays a role as well, but the specific influence of each of these various factors has not yet been determined. Women are most susceptible to developing a mental disorder during the childbearing years, and the drugs used to treat these disorders appear to work somewhat differently in women compared to men. Estrogen and progesterone, which control major reproductive transitions such as menstruation, childbirth, and menopause, are associated with an increased occurrence and/or intensity of some mood disorders.[7,23,24]

Role of Genetics

Although there is a clear association between stressful life events and depression, the role of genetic polymorphisms has remained elusive.[25] Noted associations between specific genetic polymorphisms and an increased risk for mental disorders has guided research efforts. Unfortunately, these associations have not been replicated in subsequent studies, and a meta-analysis that compared the effect of stressful life events and the presence of the variation of the serotonin transporter gene confirmed that stressful life events confer a significant risk for developing depression but the incidence of the genetic variation was no different in persons with depression when compared to persons without depression.[25] More work is needed in this area.

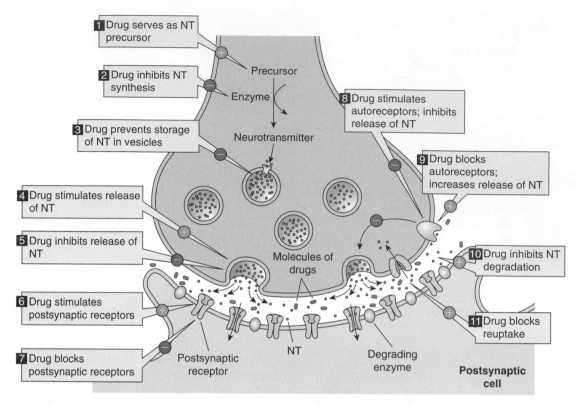

NT = Neurotransmitter; + = Augmentation that stimulates or facilitates transmission;
− = Process that inhibits transmission of the neurotransmitter.

Figure 25-2 The effect of psychotropic drugs on neurotransmitter action. *Source:* Reprinted with permission from Meyer JS 2005.[75]

Overview of Mental Disorders

There are two widely used classification schemes for mental disorders. The International Classification of Diseases (ICD-10) is produced by the World Health Organization, and the DSM-IV is produced by the American Psychiatric Association. The two schemes are largely comparable, and the DSM-IV is the taxonomy preferred by most mental health practitioners in the United States. The DSM categories mood disorders, anxiety disorders, sleep disorders, and eating disorders are addressed in this chapter. Substance abuse disorders are addressed in Chapters 8 and 9. Personality disorders, schizophrenia, psychotic disorders, delirium, and impulse control disorders require psychiatric management and are not addressed. Before describing these mental disorders, a few definitions are in order.

Mania is a state of elevated, expansive, or irritable mood that is characterized by rapid speech, grandiosity, decreased need for sleep, impulsive behavior, and racing thoughts. Mania can appear during an episode of bipolar disorder, and it can be triggered by the use of some medications,

notably the antidepressants if they are inappropriately prescribed for an individual who appears depressed but has an underlying bipolar disorder. Mania can occur simultaneously with depressive thoughts; a woman in such a mixed state is at particularly high risk for suicide.[26] Use of corticosteroids can sometimes induce a manic reaction.

Psychosis is a state of delusional or deeply disorganized thought that is not based in reality, often accompanied by paranoid or hyperreligious beliefs. Extreme states of mania can include psychotic thinking, indicating a dangerous situation that requires immediate intervention. Both manic and psychotic states can be symptoms of a mental disorder, yet psychosis is a rare but potential effect of some psychotropic medications as well. Most importantly, both require prompt intervention and psychiatric management to protect both a woman with psychosis and her family.

Mood Disorders

The mood disorders comprise a set of conditions wherein a disturbance in one's emotional mood is the primary underlying feature. Premenstrual dysphoric disorder is classified as "a depressive disorder not otherwise specified" in the DSM-IV manual and is listed in an appendix as a condition that needs more study. Premenstrual dysphoric disorder is reviewed in Chapter 30 of this book.

The mood disorders that most frequently affect women are depression and the bipolar spectrum disorders. The depressive disorders are further subclassified based on the primary symptomatology. Examples include **dysthymia**, major depressive disorder (MDD), minor depression, atypical depressive disorders, postpartum depression, and seasonal affective disorder. Depression affects women often enough that clinicians should screen for depressive symptoms routinely in the course of regular healthcare visits.[27] For women who are pregnant or postpartum, specialized screening and assessment tools have been developed and translated into several languages.[13,28]

Bipolar Disorders

Bipolar disorder was formerly called "manic depression." Today, bipolar disorders are subclassified as bipolar I, **bipolar II**, **cyclothymia**, and **bipolar disorder not otherwise specified**, which is frequently referred to as "bipolar disorder NOS."

Anxiety Disorders

Anxiety disorders often coexist with depression. The lifetime prevalence of anxiety disorders is 28.8%, which means approximately one in four individuals will have an anxiety disorder at some point.[3] The incidence in women is higher than in men. **Generalized anxiety disorder** (GAD), **panic disorder**, and PTSD are common anxiety disorders that affect women. The term *anxiety* is used to describe pathologic fears and anxieties.

Sleep Disorders

Insomnia is defined as difficulty falling asleep or difficulty staying asleep, or nonrefreshing sleep for a person who has the opportunity to sleep for 7 to 8 hours. Insomnia frequently accompanies other disorders; it is an independent risk factor for mood disorders, and it always compounds or worsens comorbid conditions. Approximately 50% of individuals with chronic insomnia have depression or another mental disorder, and insomnia is more common in women than in men.[29] In addition, sleep deprivation is believed to be the proximal trigger of postpartum mania and psychosis, so preventing sleep loss in the initial postpartum period is a key initial intervention.[30-32] In general, treating insomnia is often the first step in helping an individual with a mental disorder.

Primary sleep disorders include restless legs syndrome, periodic limb movement disorder, and obstructive sleep apnea. Specific treatments for restless legs syndrome are addressed in Chapter 24. Secondary insomnia is the insomnia that occurs as a comorbid condition when a medical or mental disorder is present. Successful treatment of the underlying condition may not treat the insomnia, and therefore insomnia is treated as an independent disorder when it occurs in an individual who has an additional medical condition.

Eating Disorders

The three primary eating disorders are anorexia nervosa, bulimia nervosa, and **binge-eating disorder**. An additional category called "eating disorder not otherwise specified" is used to refer to individuals who have an eating disorder that does not meet the full criteria for anorexia or bulimia. Both anorexia and bulimia are further divided. Anorexia is categorized as binge–purge subtype or restricting subtype. Bulimia includes purging and nonpurging subtypes.[33]

Overview of Psychotropic Drugs

Just like the conditions they treat, psychotropic medications are categorized in several ways. They may be identified according to their original use (e.g., anticonvulsants, antipsychotics), by their chemical structure (e.g., tricyclics, tetracyclics), intended chemical action (e.g., monoamine oxidase inhibitors), or a combination term (e.g., anticonvulsant mood stabilizers). Sometimes the manufacturer invents a category de novo—such as **selective serotonin reuptake inhibitor** (SSRI) or **serotonin-norepinephrine reuptake inhibitor** (SNRI)—and it is incorporated into general usage among the professionals to whom it is marketed. This chapter uses the terminology that is most generally used by mental health professionals, a lexicon that may vary slightly from the terms used by neurologists, internists, or researchers who refer to the same medications.

Mood Disorders

Major depressive disorder (MDD) is a relapsing, remitting disease. Approximately 5–10% of persons seen in a primary care setting meet the DSM-IV criteria for major depression, and 10% meet the criteria for minor depression.[34] The lifetime incidence of depression in the United States is 12% in men and 20% in women.[35] Approximately 50% of the individuals who take an antidepressant will respond partially to the initial medication used. However only 30% of those treated will experience a complete remission with use of one drug alone.[36,37] The criteria for diagnosing depression are listed in Box 25-2. Prescribing antidepressants requires a familiarity with their side effect and adverse effect profiles. Although the medications described in this chapter are generally well tolerated, they can, albeit rarely, trigger a life-threatening illness.

Pharmacologic Treatment of Depression: Antidepressants

Antidepressant medications are one of the most frequently prescribed classes of medications in the United States[38] (Table 25-4). In addition to being used to treat depression, antidepressants are increasingly being used to treat several other disorders including perimenstrual disorders; they are also being used to treat vasomotor symptoms and sleep disturbances, as an aid to smoking cessation, and as an adjunct in the management of chronic pain conditions such as vulvodynia and migraine.

Mechanism of Action

Antidepressants generate a panoply of effects within the body, and they have a complicated mechanism of action that has important clinical implications. These drugs have an immediate effect on inhibiting reuptake of serotonin or norepinephrine (or both) into the presynaptic cell, but clinical remission of depression does not occur for the first 2–3 weeks after treatment is initiated.

Box 25-2 Criteria for Diagnosis of Major Depressive Disorder

In order for one to diagnose major depressive disorder (MDD), five or more of the following symptoms must be present every day during a 2-week period and represent a change from previous functioning. Symptoms must include one of the first two criteria, must cause significant distress or impairment in daily functioning, and cannot be the effect of a medication, drug abuse, medical condition such as thyroid abnormalities, or uncomplicated bereavement.

1. Depressed mood most of the day.

2. Markedly diminished interest or pleasure in all or most activities most of the day.

3. Significant weight loss when not dieting or sudden weight gain (change of > 5% of body weight in 1 month), or large increase or decrease in appetite.

4. Insomnia or excessive sleeping nearly every day.

5. Psychomotor agitation or restlessness or slowness of movement that is observable by others.

6. Fatigue or loss of energy nearly every day.

7. Feelings of worthlessness or excessive or inappropriate guilt (may be delusional).

8. Indecisiveness or diminished ability to think or concentrate.

9. Recurrent thoughts of death or of suicide.

Note: Major depressive disorder cannot be diagnosed if:

A. The person has a history of a manic, hypomanic, or mixed episode that is the direct result of medication or physiologic effects of a medical condition. Manic episodes are symptoms of bipolar disorder.

B. Symptoms are not better accounted for by a schizoaffective disorder, nor are they superimposed on a schizophrenic or psychotic disorder.

Source: American Psychiatric Association 2000.[17]

Table 25-4 Classification of Antidepressant Drugs

Category	Examples Generic (Brand)	FDA-Approved Use	Off-Label Uses
Atypical	Bupropion (Wellbutrin, Wellbutrin SR, Wellbutrin XL, Zyban)	Major depression Smoking cessation	Depression, smoking cessation, ADHD adjunct, mood stabilizer, panic
Monoamine oxidase inhibitors (MAOI)	Phenelzine (Nardil), tranylcypromine (Parnate)	Depression	Dysthymia, panic disorder, bulimia, chronic pain
Serotonin-norepinephrine reuptake inhibitors (SNRIs)	Venlafaxine (Effexor, Effexor XR)	Depression, panic, generalized anxiety, social anxiety disorders	Similar to SSRIs; may be more useful with pain syndromes
	Duloxetine (Cymbalta)	Depression, generalized anxiety disorder, diabetic peripheral neuropathy	Similar to SSRIs; may be more useful with pain syndromes
	Mirtazapine (Remeron)	Depression	Sedative at low doses
	Trazodone (Desyrel)	Depression	Hypnotic
Selective serotonin reuptake inhibitors (SSRIs)	Fluoxetine (Prozac, Sarafem), Sertraline (Zoloft), Paroxetine (Paxil), Fluvoxamine (Luvox), Citalopram (Celexa), Escitalopram (Lexapro)	Individual drugs approved for various types of depressive and anxiety disorders	Depression, anxiety, eating disorders; migraine prophylaxis; smoking cessation; vasomotor symptoms; chronic pain; premature ejaculation
Tricyclics (TCAs)	Imipramine (Tofranil), Nortriptyline (Pamelor), Amitriptyline (Elavil), Doxepin (Sinequan), Clomipramine (Anafranil)	Depression	Depression, anxiety disorders; bulimia; migraine prophylaxis; chronic pain syndromes; insomnia

The physiology that explains this clinical puzzle is not yet proven in humans. However, the theorized mechanism of action underlies current therapeutic recommendations and guidelines for care and is therefore useful to know: When treatment begins, the antidepressant causes an increase in serotonergic or norepinephrine actions throughout the body, and most of the early side effects such as gastrointestinal upset, headache, and jitteriness are attributable to this neurotransmitter rush. After approximately 2 weeks, the postsynaptic neurons that have receptors for these neurotransmitters begin to decrease their receptiveness—called **desensitization**. In addition, some of these receptors are **down regulated**, which is the term that describes the actual disappearance of the receptor protein on the postsynaptic neuron membrane. When desensitization and down-regulation occur, the troublesome side effects recede or disappear. Because desensitization and down-regulation eliminate the negative feedback systems that initiate reuptake of the neurotransmitter into the presynaptic neuron, the concentration of the neurotransmitter within the synaptic space increases, and effectiveness of the medication begins to become apparent.

Animal studies suggest that continued use of antidepressant medication causes changes in gene expression that eventually result in the proliferation of new nerve cells in the hippocampus, an area of the brain that has been identified as a site of atrophy during depressive illness. This phenomenon may also explain why antidepressants take several weeks to become effective, since their therapeutic action may depend on the time required for the regrowth of neurons.

Most antidepressants are equally effective for treating depression. Their differences are primarily in their individual side effect profiles, which are secondary to their effect on different neurotransmitters. Side effects of commonly used antidepressants are summarized in Table 25-5.

Initiation of Therapy

Before a clinician prescribes an antidepressant, one critical clinical assessment must be made. Women whose depression is part of a bipolar mood disorder usually present for treatment while they are depressed and exhibit the same clinical picture as women with unipolar depression.[40] Bipolar disorder requires treatment with mood-stabilizing drugs, not antidepressant medication, even if depression is the presenting problem. Antidepressant drugs can worsen the course of bipolar illness and increase the risk of a manic episode, impulsive behavior or agitation, and rapid-cycling bipolar disorder. These adverse effects are more likely to occur in women.[41] Perhaps more seriously, antidepressants can induce suicidal ideation or psychosis in an individual with bipolar disorder. Some instances of suicidal thinking

Table 25-5 Antidepressant Drugs: Side Effects

Drug Generic (Brand)	Anticholinergic	Sedation	Gastrointestinal Distress	Weight Gain	Orthostatic Hypotension	Cardiac Arrhythmias
Monoamine Oxidase Inhibitors						
Phenelzine (Nardil)	1+	2+	1+	2+	2+	Unknown
Tranylcypromine (Parnate)	1+	1+	1+	2+	2+	1+
Serotonin Norepinephrine Reuptake Inhibitors						
Duloxetine (Cymbalta)	1+	1+	1+	1+	0	1+
Venlafaxine (Effexor)	1+	1+	1+	1+	0	1+
Selective Serotonin Reuptake Inhibitors						
Citalopram (Celexa)	0	1+			0	0
Escitalopram (Lexapro)	0	0			0	0
Fluoxetine (Prozac, Sarafem)	0	0	3+	0	0	0
Fluvoxamine (Luvox)	0	0			0	0
Paroxetine (Paxil)	1+	1+	3+	0	0	0
Sertraline (Zoloft)	0	0	3+	0	0	0
Tricyclic Antidepressants						
Amitriptyline (Elavil)	3+	3+	0	3+	3+	3+
Clomipramine (Anafranil)	3+	3+	0		2+	3+
Despiramine (Norpramin)	1+	3+	0	1+	2+	3+
Doxepin (Sinequan)	3+	3+	0	3+	2+	2+
Imipramine (Tofranil)	3+	2+	1+	3+	3+	3+
Nortriptyline (Pamelor)	1+	3+	0	1+	1+	3+
Second-Generation Tricyclic Antidepressants						
Amoxepine (Asendin)	2+	2+	0	1+	2+	2+
Bupropion (Wellbutrin)	1+	0	1+	0	0	1+
Maprotiline (Ludomil)	2+	3+	0	2+	2+	2+
Mirtazepine (Remeron)	1+	2+			2+	1+
Other						
Nefazodone (Serzone)	0	2+	1+	1+	3+	1+
Trazodone (Desyrel)	0	3+	1+	1+	3+	1+

0 = absent or rare; 1+ = weak activity; 2+ = moderate activity; 3+ = high activity.

and behavior associated with antidepressant medication treatment may actually be secondary to the prescribing clinician's failure to recognize that the individual's depression is part of a bipolar illness.[42] Clues that a woman may have an underlying bipolar illness can appear in a carefully taken history, as shown in Table 25-6.

Once the diagnosis of major depressive disorder is made, there are a few clinically important effects common to different antidepressants. First, all antidepressant medications have a black box warning required by the FDA since 2004 that describes an increased risk of suicidal thinking and behavior in children, adolescents, and young adults up to the age of 25 years who are prescribed these drugs. Counseling prior to initiation of therapy and early monitoring after initiation of therapy is focused on suicidality, safety, and efficacy. Second, antidepressants do not take effect quickly. During the first 2 weeks of

treatment, side effects including gastrointestinal upset, headache, irritability, sleepiness, orthostatic changes, or difficulty sitting still (akathisia) may be prominent. An individual starting an antidepressant may need encouragement to continue taking the medication, and the initial dose may need to be reduced until the side effects begin to dissipate. If a woman reports feeling great and reports a markedly decreased need for sleep within a few days of initiating treatment, emerging hypomania should be suspected, and she should be followed closely or referred for a psychiatric consultation.

Treatment of depression occurs in three phases. The acute phase (first 6–12 weeks) focuses on attaining remission. The maximum effect of an initial dose is usually evident by 8–12 weeks, and if the symptoms are not sufficiently relieved, the dose can be increased at this time. The continuation phase (4–9 months) is directed at

Table 25-6 Signs and Symptoms That Suggest Bipolar Disorder

Personal History*	Family History†
Onset of depressive illness before age 18‡	Relatives diagnosed with manic depression or bipolar disorder‡
History of agitation or irritability while taking antidepressant medication‡	Children diagnosed with attention or impulse-control disorders
History of suicide attempt(s)‡	Relatives who have been hospitalized for psychiatric illness
A previous episode of postpartum psychosis	Relatives who have attempted or completed suicide
History of unsuccessful trials of multiple antidepressant medications	Relatives with substance abuse problems, including alcohol
Episodes of impulsive behavior: excessive spending, unsafe sexual practices or unplanned pregnancies, substance abuse, legal troubles	Family members who have had shifting moods—periods of low mood, low energy, and increased isolation alternating with episodes of great ideas, high energy and drive, or irritability and rage
Diminished insight and poor judgment about the risks of such behavior	
Previous episodes of perceived high achievement, diminished need for sleep and food, or irritability that the woman describes as her normal or good mood	

* Family members may be able to give a more complete history.
† Includes all blood relatives as in any genetic history.
‡ The strongest predictors of bipolar diagnosis.

preventing relapse. It is recommended that the individual continue to take the medication for at least 6 months after complete remission of the illness. Ending treatment sooner increases the likelihood of a relapse within the year.[43] The maintenance phase (6 months to years) is focused on prevention of a reoccurrence or new episode of major depression.

Monoamine Oxidase Inhibitors (MAOIs)

The monoamine oxidase inhibitors (MAOIs) were the first antidepressant drugs to be discovered, and as is typical of medical discoveries, the discovery was an accident. This class of drugs was first used to treat tuberculosis, and as a serendipitous finding, it was found to elevate mood. There was a great deal of initial excitement when the mood-elevating effects were noted, but unfortunately, the MAOIs have some serious adverse effects. They were supplanted first by the tricyclics and later by the SSRIs and SNRIs. The MAOIs appear to be the most efficacious for individuals with atypical or resistant depression and/or anxiety and are prescribed only by mental healthcare specialists. The primary care clinician may occasionally encounter a person with longstanding mental illness who is taking a medication regimen that includes an MAOI.

Mechanism of Action

The MAOI drugs irreversibly inhibit **monoamine oxidase**, which is the enzyme responsible for degrading norepinephrine, dopamine, and serotonin after they are returned into the presynaptic neuron. When monamine oxidase is inhibited, more neurotransmitter becomes available for release by the presynaptic neuron. Because the effect is irreversible, the duration of this action can continue for up to 3 weeks after discontinuation of the drug. For this reason, a washout period of at least 14 days is recommended between discontinuing an MAOI and starting another antidepressant or between discontinuation of the MAOI and resumption of normal diet.

The Story of Cheese and Monoamine Oxidase Inhibitors

Many clinicians know that individuals taking MAOIs cannot eat many foods, but why is this? Monoamine oxidase breaks down tyramine in the liver. Tyramine is a naturally occurring amine found in cheeses, meats, red wine, and pickled foods, and tyramine releases norepinephrine from the presynaptic neuron into the neural synapse.[44,45] When monoamine is inhibited and the individual eats foods that have tyramine, elevated tyramine causes elevated norepinephrine levels in the synaptic spaces of peripheral adrenergic neurons, which results in a **hypertensive crisis**. Individuals who take MAOI drugs should adhere to a low-tyramine diet, as shown in (Table 25-7). There is one exception, which is the new transdermal formulation of selegiline (Emsam). Approved for treatment of MDD by the FDA in 2006, the lowest dose of transdermal selegiline can be used without dietary restrictions.[46]

Side Effects/Adverse Effects

The most common side effects of MAOIs are insomnia and overeating, which causes weight gain. Dizziness, daytime

Table 25-7 Dietary Guidelines for Persons Taking Oral Monoamine Oxidase Inhibitors*†

Foods That Are Allowed	Prohibited Foods	Limited-Intake Foods
All fresh, canned, or frozen vegetables except the few listed in the next column Canned or bottled beers and alcohol	Aged cheeses Alcoholic beverages: beer, red wine, sherry, vermouth Avocado Bananas Broad bean pods Fermented foods (tofu, tempeh) Figs, canned or overripe Licorice Liver Marmite Meats that are canned, aged, smoked, or processed—sausage, bologna, salami, pepperoni, herring, anchovies, sardines Monosodium glutamate Protein extracts—may need to avoid soups made with meat bouillon cubes Raisins Sauerkraut Snails Soy sauce and teriyaki Tap and unpasteurized beer Yeast products—marmite	Alcoholic beverages—some red wines Buttermilk Chocolate Coffee Cottage cheese Cream cheese Milk Peanuts Poultry Ricotta cheese Sour cream Vacuum-packed pickled fish Yogurt

* The list of specific foods that should be avoided and those that can be eaten in small amounts is variable as the amount of tyramine and individual response is not absolutely known. Thus, individuals taking MAO inhibitors should consult with a dietician or clinician who has expertise in this field.
† Transdermal MAOI preparations do not require dietary restrictions, but other precautions apply.

somnolence sedation, headache, movement problems, constipation, anorgasmia, and orthostatic hypotension are also possible.

The MAOI drugs increase the amount of norepinephrine in the presynaptic neurons of the peripheral autonomic nervous system just as they do in the CNS. Thus MAOIs can precipitate a hypertensive crisis if taken in overdose. The hypertensive crisis is most likely to occur, however, as a drug–drug interaction with other drugs that increase the synaptic concentration of norepinephrine or a drug–food interaction with foods that are high in tyramine.

Drug Interactions with MAOIs

MAOIs are associated with multiple drug–drug interactions that fall into one of the following two categories: those that can precipitate a hypertensive crisis and those that cause **serotonin syndrome** (Table 25-8). The clinical picture of serotonin syndrome includes gastrointestinal upset, chills, shakes, increased muscle rigidity or jerking, confusion, restlessness, and delirium, and it may progress to rhabdomyolysis, pulmonary hypertension, and coma (serotonin syndrome is discussed in more detail in Chapter 4).

When given in combination with an MAOI drug, alpha-adrenergic agonists that cause vasoconstriction and sympathomimetic drugs that cause an increase in heart rate can precipitate severe vasoconstriction and hypertension. Decongestants that contain phenylephrine and oxymetazoline and some cold medications should be avoided by persons taking MAOIs. Topically applied nasal sprays usually do not generate sufficient systemic action to be contraindicated in an otherwise healthy individual.

When MAOIs are taken concomitantly with cold medications that contain dextromethorphan or antihistamines, the combination causes high synaptic concentrations of serotonin and the resultant serotonin syndrome.

Table 25-8 Selected Drugs and Herbs That Are Contraindicated for Individuals Taking Monoamine Oxidase Inhibitors*

Increased Risk of Hypertensive Crisis	Increased Risk of Serotonin Syndrome
Antihypertensives	Alcohol
Decongestants and over-the-counter cold remedies	Amphetamines
Ephedrine (ma huang, ephedra)	Antihistamines
Methamphetamine	Bupropion (Wellbutrin)
Pseudoephedrine	Buspirone (BuSpar)
Phenylephrine	Dextromethorphan
Ritodrine (Yutopar)	Guanethidine (Ismelin)
Stimulants, both legal and illegal	Lithium (Lithobid)
Terbutaline (Brethine)	Meperidine (Demerol)
	Monoamine oxidase inhibitors
	SSRIs, especially fluoxetine (Prozac)
	St. John's wort
	Triptans
	Trazodone (Desyrel)
	Tricyclic antidepressants
	Venlafaxine (Effexor)

* This table is not comprehensive as new information is being generated on a regular basis.

Tricyclic Antidepressants

The tricyclic antidepressants (TCAs) are so called because their chemical structure features three rings of atoms. This class of drugs, like the MAOIs, affects several neurotransmitters, which makes them highly effective but also highly likely to generate adverse effects. This class of drugs is subdivided by their chemical makeup into the tertiary amines and secondary amines. The tertiary amines are generally not used as primary antidepressants but can be used at low doses to enhance the efficacy of other antidepressants. Examples of tertiary amines include imipramine (Tofranil) and amitriptyline (Endep). Examples of secondary amines in clinical use include desipramine (Norpramin), which is the active metabolite of imipramine, and nortriptyline (Pamelor). The tetracyclic antidepressants are closely related to the tricyclic antidepressants. Examples include mirtazapine (Remeron), Amoxapine (Asendin), and maprotiline (Deprilept). All the TCAs appear equally effective. Their differences are based on the side effect profile.

Mechanism of Action

The tricyclics bind to presynaptic transport proteins and thereby inhibit reuptake of neurotransmitters that are in the synapse. The TCAs are not discriminating; they bind to the transport proteins for a host of neurotransmitters. TCAs inhibit acetylcholine, histamine, and some alpha-adrenergic receptors. Some TCAs are better at blocking the transport protein for norepinephrine versus the transport protein for other neurotransmitters, and some are more selective for the serotonin transport protein. These differences do not affect their antidepressant efficacy, but they do affect the incidence and pattern of side effects.

TCAs are metabolized in the liver by several CYP450 enzymes. Genetic polymorphisms affect metabolism, which translates clinically into the noted wide variation in blood levels of TCAs. Some have proposed genotyping for CYP2D6 prior to initiating therapy with TCAs to identify poor metabolizers and ultrametabolizers, which could then facilitate individualized dosing. However, this recommendation has not been adopted into clinical practice yet despite the FDA-approved AmpliChip CYP450 test that genotypes for CYP2D6 and CYP2C19.[25,47]

Side Effects/Adverse Effects

The most common side effects of TCAs relate to the anticholinergic effects secondary to increased acetylcholine concentrations in the neural synapse and include dry mouth, urinary retention, constipation, dizziness, impaired memory, and confusion. Sedation and weight gain are related to histamine increase, and orthostatic hypotension is secondary to blockade of the reuptake of alpha-adrenergic neurotransmitters.

The adverse effects of TCAs are the problems that really limit their use. The alpha-adrenergic blockade in combination with blockade of fast sodium channels in myocardial cells increases the risk of cardiac arrhythmias and prolonged QT interval. In addition, the TCAs have a narrow therapeutic window and are reliably lethal if an overdose is taken.

Drug–Drug Interactions

TCAs are involved in many drug–drug interactions (Table 25-9). Desipramine (Norpramin) and nortriptyline (Pamelor) are the least likely drugs in this class to cause drug–drug interactions.[48]

Clinical Considerations

Despite potential serious adverse effects, the TCAs remain useful for some individuals. TCAs are often prescribed for resistant, melancholic depression and can be used to treat chronic pain. Although women of reproductive age tend to respond more readily to the SSRI drugs than to TCAs, postmenopausal women often respond better to TCAs.[49] The tricyclics are not habituating and can be used by persons with a history of substance abuse problems. These drugs should be prescribed by a mental health specialist.

Selective Serotonin Reuptake Inhibitors (SSRIs)

Selective serotonin reuptake inhibitors (SSRIs) are by far the most commonly prescribed antidepressants. Fluoxetine (Prozac) was the first drug designed to act on a single neurotransmitter, serotonin. Since its introduction into clinical practice in 1987, fluoxetine has revolutionized the treatment of depression as a clean drug with a single targeted neurochemical action and therefore limited adverse effects. Today, the SSRIs are all in the top 30 drugs as measured by number of prescriptions dispensed per year in the United States. Over time, additional SSRI drugs have been refined in an attempt to decrease the side effect profile and

Table 25-9 Selected Drug–Drug Interactions of Tricyclic Antidepressants*

Interacting Drug(s) Generic (Brand)	Effect
Amoxapine (Asendin)	Increased risk for extrapyramidal effects
Antiarrhythmic drugs	Increased risk of prolonged QT syndrome
Anticholinergics	Increased anticholinergic response and adverse reactions
Astemizole (Hismanal)	Increased risk of prolonged QT syndrome
Barbiturates	Enhanced barbiturate response
Bupropion (Wellbutrin)	
Calcium channel blockers	Increased TCA levels and increased risk of cardiotoxicity
Cannabis	Increased risk of cardiotoxicity, tachycardia, light-headedness, confusion, mood lability, and delirium
Carbamazepine (Tegretol)	Increased blood levels of carbamazepine
Cimetidine (Tagamet)	Increased TCA levels and increased risk of cardiotoxicity
Clonidine (Catapres)	Decreased antihypertensive effect of clonidine and increased risk of CNS depression
CNS depressants (including alcohol)	Increased CNS depression, increased TCA levels, increased risk of cardiotoxicity
Disulfiram	Increased TCA levels and increased risk of cardiotoxicity
Fluoroquinolones	Risk of arrhythmias
Fluoxetine (Prozac)	Increased TCA levels and increased risk of cardiotoxicity
Haloperidol (Haldol)	Increased risk for extrapyramidal effects
MAOIs	Hyperpyretic crises, severe seizures, convulsions, hypertensive episodes, and death
Methylphenidate (Ritalin)	Increased TCA levels and increased risk of cardiotoxicity
Metoclopramide (Reglan)	Increased risk for extrapyramidal effects
Reserpine (Serpalan)	Increased risk for extrapyramidal effects
St. John's wort	Reduced blood levels of TCAs
Sympathomimetics	Hypertension, risk of arrhythmias
Thyroid medications	Increased antidepressant response and cardiac arrhythmias

TCA = tricyclic antidepressants.
* This table is not comprehensive as new information is being generated on a regular basis.

expand their usefulness. The SSRIs used to treat depression include citalopram (Celexa), escitalopram (Lexapro), fluvoxamine (Luvox), fluoxetine (Prozac), paroxetine (Paxil), and sertraline (Zoloft) (Table 25-10).

All of the SSRI drugs have been approved by the FDA for the treatment of depression. The drug manufacturers have sponsored studies to gain FDA approval of SSRIs for the treatment of other disorders. For example, sertraline (Zoloft) is now approved to treat PTSD, and escitalopram (Lexapro) is approved to treat generalized anxiety disorder. However, the studies usually test the drugs against placebo and not against each other, so all of the SSRIs have proven efficacy in these studies. Therefore, the clinician's first choice of SSRI for a given woman may be based on various other factors besides effectiveness.

Mechanism of Action of SSRIs

As their name implies, SSRI drugs increase the concentration of serotonin in the synapse by inhibiting its reuptake into the presynaptic cell. There are several receptors for serotonin (5-HT_1 through 5-HT_{15}). Each drug in the SSRI family has a slightly different side effect profile based on its action on different serotonin receptors and the elimination half-life of the drug.

Fluoxetine (Prozac) is typically somewhat energizing and is associated with uncomfortable side effects more often than the other SSRIs with the exception of fewer anticholinergic effects.[50] Fluoxetine is typically taken in the morning and can help with focus and attention. Fluoxetine has the longest half-life and may reach a steady state within days of starting the drug; similarly, it tends to wear off gradually and does not appear to have untoward effects when tapering the dose down. Sertraline (Zoloft) is often sedating, especially in the early weeks of treatment, and it is usually taken at night for its hypnotic effect. Paroxetine (Paxil) has a half-life of less than 24 hours and may induce serotonin discontinuation syndrome before the next daily dose is due.

Side Effects/Adverse Effects

While usually well tolerated, SSRIs can cause nausea, headache, jitteriness, dizziness, anhedonia, sweating, photosensitivity, and strange, vivid dreams. These effects generally decrease after a few weeks of treatment, and initial doses can be low until these effects begin to subside. Weight gain or loss, if any, may occur early or late in treatment. Sexual side effects, including decreased libido and delayed orgasm, tend not to decrease over time. Paroxetine is associated with the greatest amount of weight gain and sexual dysfunction, whereas sertraline (Zoloft) is associated with diarrhea more often than are the other SSRIs.

SSRIs may cause suicidal ideation but not completed suicide in children, adolescents, and young adults < age 25.[51] Conversely, they decrease suicide ideation in adults. These drugs have an FDA black box warning that states there is an increased risk of suicidal thoughts in persons

Table 25-10 Selective Serotonin Reuptake Inhibitors, Serotonin Norepinephrine Reuptake Inhibitors, and Atypical Antidepressants Used in Primary Care Settings

Name Generic (Brand)	Dose	Elimination Half-Life	Clinical Considerations
Selective Serotonin Reuptake Inhibitors			
Citalopram (Celexa)	20–60 mg/day	36 h	May help with sleep quality.
Escitalopram (Lexapro)	5–20 mg/day	35 h	Same as citalopram.
Fluoxetine (Prozac, Sarafem)*	20–80 mg/day	3–6 days	Tends to be stimulating; take in AM and consider a sleep aid at night.
Fluvoxamine (Luvox)	50–300 mg/day	15–26 h	
Paroxetine (Paxil, Paxil CR)	20–60 mg qd Give in divided doses	24–31 h	Tends to be sedating; stimulates weight gain; withdrawal syndrome can be severe.
Sertraline (Zoloft)	50–200 mg/day	24–26 h	Tends to be sedating; take at night.
Serotonin Norepinephrine Reuptake Inhibitors			
Duloxetine (Cymbalta)	Cymbalta: 30–60 mg qd Time-release capsule	12 h	May cause nausea, appetite loss, somnolence, insomnia.
Venlafaxine (Effexor)	Effexor: 37.5–150 mg bid Effexor XR: 37.5–300 mg qd	5 h	May cause hypertension, increased intraocular pressure, mydriasis.
Tricyclic Antidepressants			
Amitriptyline (Elavil)	25–100 mg qd, usually hs	10–15 h	The TCAs are considered dirty drugs—i.e., with multiple effects on neurotransmission; used for insomnia, pain syndromes, anxiety, and SSRI-resistant depression. Lethal in overdose.
Other			
Bupropion (Wellbutrin)	225–450 mg/day in divided doses SR 200 mg bid XL 450 mg qd	21 h ± 9 h	Can cause seizures. Contraindicated in those with seizure disorders and those who take meds erratically.
Mirtazapine (Remeron)	15–60 mg qd	37 h	Lower doses can cause somnolence, weight gain.

* Luteal phase dosing may be effective for treating premenstrual syndrome fluoxetine (Prozac) weekly 90 mg taken once per week.

< 25 years of age.[21] If an individual has an underlying bipolar illness, antidepressant therapy can induce mania or suicidality.

SSRI overdose can cause serotonin syndrome, but SSRIs have a wide therapeutic index. Most individuals who overdose will have mild symptoms of generalized toxicity such as nausea and vomiting, dizziness, blurred vision, tachycardia, and rarely CNS toxicity.[52]

Serotonin Discontinuation Syndrome

Serotonin discontinuation syndrome (or serotonin withdrawal syndrome) is not well understood but appears to be related to the adaptation neural cells undergo during therapy with SSRIs. This adaptation leaves the brain unable to quickly adjust to the absence of the drug. Typical symptoms include dizziness, tremor, confusion, vertigo, and an electric shock feeling in the brain. Paroxetine is often given in twice daily doses to prevent this, and discontinuing the drug must be done very gradually to avoid withdrawal effects. Fluoxetine (Prozac) is the least likely SSRI to cause discontinuation syndrome.

Drug–Drug Interactions

The SSRIs are primarily metabolized via the CYP450 enzyme system, and are generally CYP450 enzyme inhibitors that cause increased blood levels of other drugs metabolized by the CYP450 enzyme system. These drugs are associated with a wide variety of drug–drug interactions (Table 25-11). Fluoxetine (Prozac) and paroxetine (Paxil) have the most CYP450 drug–drug interactions, whereas sertraline (Zoloft) and citalopram (Celexa) are the least likely SSRIs to induce drug–drug interactions with coadministered drugs. SSRIs are also highly protein bound and can compete for binding sites. This is the mechanism by which SSRIs increase plasma levels of diazepam (Valium), valproate (Depakote, Depakene), and anticoagulants.

Table 25-11 Selected Drug–Drug Interactions Associated with Selective Serotonin Reuptake Inhibitors*

Drug Generic (Brand)	Effect
Antiarrhythmic medications	Increased risk of cardiac arrhythmias.
Anticoagulants	Increased risk of bleeding with fluoxetine (Prozac), paroxetine (Paxil).
Benzodiazepines	Increased blood levels of benzodiazepines leading to sedation, confusion. Most noted with fluvoxamine (Luvox) and fluoxetine (Prozac).
Beta-blockers	Increased levels of beta-blockers causing bradycardia and ECG abnormalities with fluoxetine (Prozac) and fluvoxamine (Luvox).
Bupropion (Wellbutrin)	Increased risk of seizure.
Buspirone (BuSpar)	Enhanced effect of SSRI with fluoxetine (Prozac).
Calcium channel blockers	Increased blood levels of calcium channel blockers and hypotension.
Carbamazepine (Tegretol)	Increased blood levels of carbamazepine and toxicity with fluoxetine (Prozac), sertraline (Zoloft), and fluvoxamine (Luvox).
Cimetidine (Tagamet)	Increased blood levels of paroxetine (Paxil), citalopram (Celexa), and venlafaxine (Effexor).
Clozapine (Clozaril)	Increased blood levels of clozapine and risk of seizures with fluvoxamine (Luvox).
Cyclosporine (Sandimmune, Neoral)	Increased blood levels of cyclosporine.
Dextromethorphan	Visual hallucinations with fluoxetine (Prozac).
Diazepam (Valium)	Decreased clearance of diazepam with fluvoxamine (Luvox), sertraline (Zoloft).
Digoxin (Lanoxin)	Increased levels of digoxin and digoxin toxicity.
Haloperidol (Haldol)	Increased blood levels of haloperidol and extrapyramidal symptoms with fluoxetine (Prozac) and fluvoxamine (Luvox).
Insulin	Fluvoxamine (Luvox) can decrease blood glucose levels with fluoxetine (Prozac).
Lithium (Lithobid)	Neurotoxicity, confusion, ataxia, seizures with fluoxetine (Prozac) and increased serotoninergic effect with fluvoxamine (Luvox) that causes seizures, nausea, tremor.
MAOIs	Serotonin syndrome, potentially fatal. Hypertensive crisis with all SSRIs.
Methadone (Dolophine)	Fluvoxamine (Luvox) causes increased blood levels of methadone.
Nefazodone (Serzone)	Increased blood level of nefazodone and anxiety.
Phenytoin (Dilantin)	Increased blood levels of phenytoin and toxicity with fluoxetine (Prozac).
Theophylline (Theo-Dur)	Increased blood levels of theophylline and anxiety.
Tolbutamide (Orinase)	Fluvoxamine (Luvox) can decrease blood glucose levels.
Tranquilizers	Increased blood levels of tranquilizer.
Trazodone (Desyrel)	Increased blood level of trazodone and anxiety with fluoxetine (Prozac).
Tricyclic antidepressants	Increased TCA blood levels and cardiac arrhythmias with all SSRIs.
Valproate (Depakote, Depakene)	Increased blood levels of valproate with fluoxetine (Prozac).
Venlafaxine (Effexor)	Increased blood levels of venlafaxine.

* This table is not comprehensive as new information is being generated on a regular basis.

Although still a rare occurrence, the incidence of serotonin syndrome is rising as the use of serotonergic drugs becomes more popular.[53] SSRI use can induce serotonin syndrome when added to other serotonergic drugs and substances. Drugs that can cause serotonin syndrome are listed in Table 25-12.[54-56] An SSRI should not be prescribed until 2 weeks after any MAOI antidepressant has been discontinued.

SSRIs increase the risk of gastrointestinal hemorrhage, and if they are combined with aspirin or nonsteroidal anti-inflammatory drugs, this risk is further increased, although the absolute numbers of individuals affected is low.[57]

Clinical Considerations

In choosing an initial SSRI, a legitimate factor to consider is cost to a woman. Many insurance plans have a first-choice list that requires an individual to try the cheapest drug before the plan will pay for a more expensive one. Unless there is a strong objection to the insurer's preference, it can be a reasonable and cost-effective place to start.

A peculiarity of pharmacologic treatment is that blood relatives often respond similarly to the same medications, even if their diagnoses are different. Conversely, unrelated persons with similar symptoms often need different medications. If members of a woman's family are taking

Table 25-12 Drug Categories Associated with Serotonin Syndrome

Category	Drugs Generic (Brand)
Anticonvulsants	Valproate (Depakene)
Antidepressants	All agents, either singly or in combination
Antiemetics	Ondansetron (Zofran), metoclopramide (Reglan), granisetron (Kytril)
Antiepileptic drugs	Lithium (Lithobid), valproate (Depakene)
Antihistamines	Chlorpheniramine (Chlor-Trimeton)
Antimigraine agents	Triptans such as sumatriptan (Imitrex, Imigran), rizatriptan (Maxalt), naratriptan (Amerge, Naramig), zolmitriptan (Zomig), eletriptan (Relpax), almotriptan (Axert, Almogran in UK), and frovatriptan (Frova, Migard)
Antiparkinson pharmaceuticals (dopaminergic agents)	Amantadine (Symmetrel), levodopa (Sinemet or Kinson)
Atypical antipsychotic drugs	Clozapine (Clozaril), olanzapine (Zyprexa), risperidone (Risperdal), quetiapine (Seroquel), ziprasidone (Geodon), aripiprazole (Abilify), and paliperidone (Invega)
Botanics/herbs	St. John's wort, yohimbine, dietary supplements containing tryptophan, *Panax ginseng*
CNS stimulants	Amphetamines including methylphenidate (Ritalin)
Cough/cold remedies	Oral decongestants, dextromethorphan
Drugs of abuse	Cocaine, ecstasy, LSD
L-tryptophan	Increases serotonin synthesis
Opiates	Opiates such as meperidine (Demerol), tramadol (Ultram), fentanyl (Duragesic), pentazocine, and propoxyphene in any formulation including patches
Triptans	Sumatriptan (Imitrex), naratriptan (Amerge), almotriptan (Axert), eletriptan (Relpax)

psychotropic medication, it is helpful to know what drugs have been helpful and other things being equal, to start with that regimen.

SNRI Drugs: Venlafaxine (Effexor) and Duloxetine (Cymbalta)

Several newer antidepressants are designed to enhance both serotonin and norepinephrine action. Manufacturers claim that these drugs can become effective faster than SSRIs. The two SNRIs in clinical use are venlafaxine (Effexor) and duloxetine (Cymbalta). Depending on a woman's symptoms, history of treatment, cost, or availability, an SNRI may be chosen for first-line treatment. Venlafaxine (Effexor) and duloxetine (Cymbalta) are FDA approved for treating depression. Venlafaxine is more efficacious than other SSRIs and SNRIs, but the effect is modest (remission rates are 5–10% lower than the remission rates associated with other antidepressants), yet this drug is more likely to be discontinued secondary to side effects than are the other SSRIs or SNRIs.[58]

Mechanism of Action

The SNRI drugs inhibit the reuptake of serotonin and norepinephrine in the neuronal synapse. Some also inhibit reuptake of dopamine.

Side Effects/Adverse Effects

Side effects are similar to those of the SSRI drugs, and similarly, they tend to fade with time. SNRI drugs appear to be more toxic in overdose than SSRIs. Adverse effects of SNRIs include excess sweating, asthenia, or syndrome of inappropriate antidiuretic hormone secretion. Venlafaxine (Effexor) and duloxetine (Cymbalta) may cause hypertension, and therefore blood pressure should be monitored during therapy. As with other antidepressants, the SNRI drugs may trigger mania, suicidal thoughts, or seizures, and they carry the same FDA black box warning that is printed on the labels of SSRIs. Withdrawal symptoms can be significant, so doses may need to be tapered down over months.

Drug–Drug Interactions

In general, Venlafaxine (Effexor) can cause serotonin syndrome if combined with lithium (Lithobid), moclobemide (Aurorix, Manerix), fluoxetine (Prozac), and mirtazapine (Remeron). Venlafaxine has also been associated with severe arrhythmias in individuals who are poor metabolizers of CYP2D6. Duloxetine (Cymbalta) is a moderate inhibitor of CYP2D6 and should be used with caution by individuals who take TCAs, antipsychotics, or type 1C antiarrhythmic drugs.[59]

Clinical Considerations

Venlafaxine (Effexor) and duloxetine (Cymbalta) often are helpful for women whose illness includes somatic symptoms or chronic pain. Both drugs are available as time-release pills that can be taken once daily, and unlike mirtazapine (Remeron), they tend to be nonsedating. Like the SSRIs, the SNRIs take time to become effective. The same precautions and course of treatment apply to them as to other antidepressants.

Other Antidepressant Medications

Bupropion (Wellbutrin)

The atypical antidepressant bupropion (Wellbutrin, Zyban) has several characteristics that make it a popular first-line choice for many individuals or for women who have experienced unfavorable side effects with other antidepressants. Bupropion is not sedating and may improve attention and alertness; it does not cause weight gain or loss of sexual desire; and it may take effect more quickly than other antidepressants. It has also been used (under the brand Zyban) to help decrease the craving for nicotine, which is discussed in more detail in Chapter 8.

Although bupropion has been used empirically for years, its exact mechanism of action remains uncertain; its effect is presumed to be related to inhibition of pre-synaptic dopamine and norepinephrine reuptake transporters.[60] Bupropion has no serotonin activity and thus, has none of the side effects associated with serotonin agonists.

Bupropion can cause seizures. It is contraindicated for individuals with known or suspected seizure disorders and is relatively contraindicated for women with paroxysmal conditions such as migraine. A woman who has difficulty remembering her medication or who takes medication on an irregular schedule because of varying work hours may be at increased risk for seizures with bupropion. When restarting the medication, the dose should be tapered up to the prior dose to minimize seizure risk. Bupropion may cause insomnia or other conditions related to excessive neural activation.

Bupropion should be used cautiously with other drugs that lower seizure thresholds, including other antidepressants, antiparkinson drugs, and some antipsychotics.

While bupropion can be useful as an antidepressant, it does not help anxiety. However, bupropion can be helpful in treating a panic disorder.[44] Bupropion is available in a number of brand-name preparations with varying elimination half-lives. Wellbutrin is administered in divided doses three times a day, and Wellbutrin SR and Zyban are given twice a day. Bupropion extended release (Wellbutrin XL) is a product that is effective over a 24-hour period, with no significant peak plasma level and a maximum dose of 450 mg per day. It can be used for individuals who cannot remember to take a second dose of medicine.

Trazodone (Desyrel) and Mirtazapine (Remeron)

Trazodone (Desyrel) and mirtazapine (Remeron) are antagonists for the subtype 5-HT$_2$ serotonin receptor. However, the major metabolite of trazodone is an agonist for several of the serotonin receptor subtypes. Trazodone and mirtazapine are also potent antihistamines, which accounts for the side effects of dry mouth and sedation. Other side effects include orthostatic hypotension and dissociative feelings. There are a few case reports of cardiac arrhythmias developing in individuals taking trazodone, but the mechanism is unclear. Likewise, mirtazapine can increase cholesterol levels in some individuals. Mirtazapine often is taken at bedtime to enhance sleep; it is an unusual medication in that it tends to produce its strongest side effects at low doses. The sleepiness and weight gain that are common when starting mirtazapine usually disappear as the dose is raised. Mirtazapine is available in generic form.

Bipolar Disorder

Bipolar disorder is a chronic and recurrent mental disorder. The lifetime prevalence is approximately 4%.[61] Elevated mood is the cardinal sign that distinguishes bipolar disorder from depression, manic episodes that alternate with depression is the leading cause of impairment and death in individuals with bipolar disorder. The diagnosis of bipolar disorder in primary care settings is difficult. Affected individuals rarely report manic episodes, and a single cross-sectional interview may not elicit the history needed to identify the manic and depressive symptoms. Longitudinal contact with an individual and/or interviews with family members can help identify information that will aid diagnosis. Treatment is the purview of mental health specialists, therefore only a brief introduction to the disorder is included in this chapter. The interested reader is referred to reviews of the topic.[13,42,58,62,63]

Mood-stabilizing drugs are the mainstay of pharmacologic treatment of bipolar I and bipolar II disorders; these drug include lithium (Lithobid) and the antiepileptic drug valproate (Depakote, Depakene). Other antiepileptic drugs and/or antipsychotic medications that reduce the risk of a manic episode can also be used to treat bipolar disorder.

The current controversy is about the addition of antidepressants to help individuals who are not sufficiently treated with a mood-stabilizing drug. The assumption that antidepressants can cause a manic event or more rapid cycling has been an important clinical key point in practice and in this chapter so far. However, the actual induction of mania when an individual with bipolar illness takes an antidepressant is controversial and the subject of current study.[63,64]

There are approximately 10 drugs that are FDA approved for treating bipolar disorder. Monotherapy with a mood stabilizer is usually the initial therapeutic regimen, followed by the addition of an antidepressant or antipsychotic for individuals who have psychotic features.

Lithium

Lithium has been used to treat mania since the Greek physician Galen recommended that patients with mania bathe in alkaline springs and drink the water (which contained lithium). The metal lithium, the lightest metal in the periodic table of the elements, was discovered in 1817 and was noted to have mood stabilizing properties in the late 1800s when it was used to treat gout. In 1949 the Australian psychiatrist John Cade proposed using lithium to treat mania. Its mechanism of action remains unknown. Various preparations of lithium salts are used to treat bipolar disorders, particularly for persons with predominantly manic symptoms. Lithium has a narrow therapeutic window and plasma levels should be monitored approximately monthly once stable.

Side Effects/Adverse Effects

The side effects of lithium are numerous and onerous. Nausea and vomiting, diarrhea, and muscle tremor are common initial problems that are usually treated with dose changes and taking the medication at night. Headache, poor memory, confusion, acne, weight gain, and impaired motor performance are common side effects of lithium (Lithobid).

Lithium can affect the kidney in two ways. Tubular dysfunction reduces the kidney's ability to concentrate urine so polyuria with its companions, polydipsia and nocturia, occur in 15–40% of individuals taking lithium.[65] This is the most common renal complication of lithium therapy. If addressed early, it is reversible once the drug is discontinued, but it can become irreversible once structural damage occurs.[66] Although rare, the glomerular filtration rate will decline if glomerular dysfunction develops.

Lithium also concentrates in the thyroid gland where it induces the formation of thyroid antibodies and subsequent development of hypothyroidism and goiter. Lithium-induced hypothyroidism is much more likely to occur in women compared to men and occurs in approximately 14% of persons who use lithium.[67] Dehydration or heat stress can elevate lithium blood levels and produce toxic effects that include somnolence, cardiac arrhythmias, seizure, and kidney or liver damage. Rarely, lithium can trigger suicidal thoughts.

Drug–Drug Interactions

Lithium is involved in numerous drug–drug interactions. Use of lithium with other drugs that affect kidney function are particularly concerning. All diuretics and NSAIDs should be used with caution while monitoring kidney function to avoid additive effects. Drugs that can elevate serum lithium levels include metronidazole (Flagyl), NSAIDs, ketamine, ACE inhibitors, thiazides, methyldopa (L-dopa), diuretics, and many antibiotics. Agents that speed lithium metabolism and excretion include the bulk-forming laxatives, caffeine, and propranolol (Inderal).

Antiepileptic Drugs

Antiepileptic drugs (AEDs) that may be used as mood stabilizers include phenytoin (Dilantin), carbamazepine (Tegretol), and valproic acid (Depakote, Depakene). Newer agents include gabapentin (Neurontin), pregabalin (Lyrica), lamotrigine (Lamictal), oxcarbazepine (Trileptal), and topiramate (Topamax). While all of the anticonvulsants inhibit seizure activity, not all of them are used as mood stabilizers. Gabapentin (Neurontin) and pregabalin (Lyrica), for example, were developed to treat neuropathic pain, and their role in bipolar disorder is relatively new. Lamotrigine has been associated rarely with Stevens-Johnson syndrome, especially with rapid changes in serum levels or overdose. Each of the antiepileptic drugs has a unique side-effect profile. General pharmacologic management of these drugs is reviewed in Chapter 24.[68,69]

Other Biologic Treatments for Mood Disorders

Electroconvulsive Therapy

Both the old word *electroshock* and the modern term *electroconvulsive therapy* (ECT) can sound ominous to women and their clinicians alike. But as currently practiced—under light general anesthesia and without generalized seizure activity—the brief electrical stimulation of focused areas of the brain can provide relief of severe and otherwise intractable psychiatric illness. In the United States, ECT is most often used when multiple medication trials have failed or when an individual's medical condition precludes risking the interactions of multiple medications. ECT can also produce symptom relief more rapidly than pharmaceuticals, sometimes after a single treatment, in the face of severe symptoms.

Light Therapy

Bright light exposure is most familiar as a treatment for seasonal affective (mood) disorders. However, it is increasingly being used as an adjunct treatment to improve mood and stabilize circadian rhythms in nonseasonal mood disorders and other diagnoses.[70] Bright light exposure has been studied in combination with medication, manipulation of sleep-wake cycles, melatonin, and aerobic exercise and found to be helpful and well tolerated. Bright light therapy has been known to elevate mood to the point of irritability and hypomania, so it should be used with the same precautions as antidepressant medications.

Complementary and Alternative Therapies

Essential Fatty Acids

The essential fatty acids have been studied as a treatment for psychiatric illness, notably in the mood disorders and schizophrenia.[71] In addition, numerous studies have examined the possible effectiveness of omega-3 fatty acid supplementation, given in the form of fish oil, to treat neurodegenerative diseases and impulse-control

disorders including suicidal behavior.[72] While essential fatty acid treatment appears to be helpful as either primary or adjunctive treatment in a variety of disorders, standardized sources and doses for specific situations have yet to be developed.

Herbal Preparations: St. John's Wort

The plant *Hypericum perforatum* (or St. John's wort) produces flavonoids in its buds that may be used to self-treat depressive symptoms, despite controlled trials that do not find such preparations to be more helpful than placebo.[73] Although substances isolated from St. John's wort have been extensively studied to determine potential mechanisms of action, their exact effects on neurotransmission are not clear. An additional concern is that St. John's wort products appear to interact with a variety of commonly prescribed medications including anti-inflammatory agents such as ibuprofen; some antibiotics; cardiovascular drugs including digoxin (Lanoxin), warfarin (Coumadin), and nifedipine (Procardia); CNS agents including antidepressants, benzodiazepines, and opiates; hypoglycemic drugs; oral contraceptives; proton pump inhibitors; allergy medications; and certain statins.[74] Clinicians should regard *Hypericum* preparations with the same cautions accorded to any other drug category and consider risks and potential benefits carefully.

Anxiety Disorders: Acute and Posttraumatic Stress Disorder

Anxiety disorders are at least as common as mood disorders, but anxious women are likely to be overlooked and underdiagnosed by primary care providers. Anxiety disorders include generalized anxiety disorder, panic disorder, **obsessive-compulsive disorder**, **phobias**, **acute stress disorder**, and PTSD. The suffering caused by panic, phobias, and generalized anxiety disorder can be disabling. Obsessive-compulsive illness is one of the very few modern indications for psychosurgery. The anxiety disorders often require specialized multidisciplinary treatment that is beyond the scope of this chapter. However, primary care providers for women can provide crucial treatment—and effective prophylaxis—to women who are exposed to traumatic events.

Drugs used to treat anxiety are called **anxiolytics**. Barbiturates and benzodiazepines are the classic sedative-hypnotics that are also anxiolytics (Table 25-13). These drugs enhance the effects of GABA, the primary

Table 25-13 Anxiolytic Medications

Category Generic (Brand)	Typical Dose	Effects and Use	Clinical Considerations
Antihistamines			
Diphenhydramine (Benadryl)	25–50 mg PO up to tid.	Sedating, calming, antiemetic	Tolerance may develop in 1–2 wks of regular use.
Hydroxyzine (Vistaril, Atarax)	25–100 mg PO or IM.	Sedating, calming, antiemetic	Avoid intravenous use.
Antidepressants			
SSRIs	Usually require higher doses to treat anxiety than depressive disorders. May have slower onset of action.	Long-term treatment or prophylaxis of anxiety disorders, including OCD, PTSD, phobias, panic	The woman may need short-term symptom relief until SSRI begins to be effective.
TCAs	Usually require higher doses to treat anxiety than depressive disorders.	Often helpful for sleep or chronic pain as well as anxiety	Woman may need short-term symptom relief. Postmenopausal women may respond better to TCAs than to SSRIs.
Benzodiazepines			
Midazolam (Versed)	1–2 mg by slow IV push over at least 2 minutes.	Very short acting agent with rapid tolerance and potential rebound symptoms	Used acutely for calming severely agitated individuals.
Lorazepam (Ativan)	0.5–2.0 mg PO up to tid prn acute panic or anxiety.	Short acting, rapid tolerance	Most often used for occasional panic attacks or acute anxiety. Avoid use in those with substance history.
Clonazepam (Klonopin)	0.5–2 mg PO up to tid.	Intermediate-acting anxiolytic, mood stabilizer	May be less habituating than shorter-acting drugs. Avoid use in those with substance history.
Beta-Blockers			
Propranolol (Inderal)	10–40 mg PO up to tid. May be taken prn.	Decreases autonomic arousal; used for stage fright and other phobic situations	Early data suggest use may prevent PTSD in susceptible individuals. See text for regimen.

inhibitory neurotransmitter throughout the CNS. The result is general reduced neuron excitability. The oldest known anxiolytic is alcohol. But as one author states, "It is difficult to administer in accurate doses, and has a very poor therapeutic index. It has no medical use."[75]

Barbiturates

Barbiturates are divided into those that are ultrashort acting, short/intermediate acting, or long acting. Although barbiturates readily induce sleep, this sleep has less rapid eye movement (REM) sleep and is ultimately not restful. The anxiolytic effects are accompanied by adverse cognitive effects such as cloudy mentation, impaired thinking, and loss of judgment.

The story of secobarbital illustrates the fate of this class of drug. For many years barbiturates were used to treat epilepsy, temporary insomnia, and as a preoperative agent prior to use of general anesthesia. The adverse effects include lethal overdoses. In 1963 Marilyn Monroe died from an overdose of chloral hydrate and the barbiturate pentobarbital (Nembutal). In 1969 Judy Garland died from an overdose of secobarbital (Seconal), and in 1970 Jimmy

Hendrix died from an overdose of secobarbital. The publicity from these deaths brought the dangers of these drugs to the public's attention. Over time, the barbiturates have been replaced by benzodiazepines. Today, barbiturates are rarely used for therapeutic purposes, and in 2001, Eli Lilly, the largest manufacturer, discontinued production of secobarbital. Some of these agents are still available and currently used for rare indications such as induced coma following traumatic brain injury, physician-assisted suicide, and death penalty executions.[76,77]

Benzodiazepines

Benzodiazepines are the only class of regularly used prescription drugs that have a popular song dedicated to the drug. "Mother's Little Helper," composed by Keith Richards and Mick Jagger in 1967, referred to a little yellow pill that assisted women of that era, also known as diazepam (Valium). Postmarketing widespread use of diazepam in the early 1960s revealed its addictive properties.

Most anxiety disorders are treated with benzodiazepines for ameliorating acute symptoms while waiting for antidepressants to become effective. The benzodiazepines are used short term only because they can be addicting, and they can cause depression. These drugs are often used as sleep aids and are discussed in more detail in the section on sleep disturbances later in this chapter.

Acute Stress Disorder Versus Posttraumatic Stress Disorder

Women frequently seek help in coping with a traumatic event, whether it is the loss of a loved one, a difficult birth, or a life-threatening illness. Although the residual distress from these events is often referred to as PTSD, disabling symptoms that begin within 1 month after the event are more accurately classified as acute stress disorder.

Hypervigilance, a constant state of autonomic arousal, is the hallmark of anxiety produced by traumatic stress. A woman with stress-related anxiety may feel edgy and irritable or emotionally numb and be unable to focus or concentrate on tasks. In extreme cases, she may dissociate from reality and feel as if she were an observer in her own life, unable to engage with others. Disordered sleep, either insomnia or unrefreshing hypersomnia, is almost universal, and dreams may be especially troubling.

Recommended treatment of acute stress disorder includes benzodiazepines, a combination of antidepressants reviewed earlier in this chapter and short-term psychotherapy. Acute stress symptoms generally begin to resolve, sometimes as soon as a few days after the traumatic experience, but a significant minority of persons will continue to suffer for over a month after the danger has passed. At that time, the illness can be reclassified as PTSD.

It can be difficult to predict who will develop PTSD, even among persons who have been exposed to the same trauma. Risk factors for developing acute or posttraumatic stress include a previous stress response to a traumatic experience, particularly in childhood; a history of anxiety or mood disorder; and a lack of social support and community. Diagnostic criteria for PTSD are listed in Box 25-3.

Box 25-3　Diagnostic Criteria for Posttraumatic Stress Disorder

Diagnostic criteria for posttraumatic stress disorder (PTSD) include a history of exposure to a traumatic event meeting two criteria from (A) and symptoms from each of three symptom clusters: (B) intrusive recollections, (C) avoidant/numbing symptoms, and (D) hyperarousal symptoms. A fifth criterion (E) concerns duration of symptoms, and a sixth (F) assesses functioning.

Criterion A: Stressor

The person has been exposed to a traumatic event in which both of the following have been present:

1. The person has experienced, witnessed, or been confronted with an event or events that involve actual or threatened death or serious injury, or a threat to the physical integrity of oneself or others.

2. The person's response involved intense fear, helplessness, or horror. In children, it may be expressed instead by disorganized or agitated behavior.

Criterion B: Intrusive Recollection

The traumatic event is persistently reexperienced in at least one of the following ways:

1. Recurrent and intrusive distressing recollections of the event, including images, thoughts, or perceptions. In young children, repetitive play in which themes or aspects of the trauma are expressed may occur.

2. Recurrent distressing dreams of the event. In children, there may be frightening dreams without recognizable content.

3. Acting or feeling as if the traumatic event were recurring (includes a sense of reliving the experience, illusions, hallucinations, and dissociative flashback episodes, including those that occur upon awakening or when intoxicated). In children, trauma-specific reenactment may occur.

(continues)

Box 25-3 Diagnostic Criteria for Posttraumatic Stress Disorder *(continued)*

4. Intense psychological distress at exposure to internal or external cues that symbolize or resemble an aspect of the traumatic event.

5. Physiologic reactivity upon exposure to internal or external cues that symbolize or resemble an aspect of the traumatic event.

Criterion C: Avoidant/Numbing

Persistent avoidance of stimuli associated with the trauma and numbing of general responsiveness (not present before the trauma), as indicated by at least three of the following:

1. Efforts to avoid thoughts, feelings, or conversations associated with the trauma.

2. Efforts to avoid activities, places, or people that arouse recollections of the trauma.

3. Inability to recall an important aspect of the trauma.

4. Markedly diminished interest or participation in significant activities.

5. Feeling of detachment or estrangement from others.

6. Restricted range of affect (e.g., unable to have loving feelings).

7. Sense of foreshortened future (e.g., does not expect to have a career, marriage, children, or a normal life span).

Criterion D: Hyperarousal

Persistent symptoms of increasing arousal (not present before the trauma), indicated by at least two of the following:

1. Difficulty falling or staying asleep

2. Irritability or outbursts of anger

3. Difficulty concentrating

4. Hypervigilance

5. Exaggerated startle response

Criterion E: Duration

Duration of the disturbance (symptoms in B, C, and D) is more than 1 month.

Criterion F: Functional Significance

The disturbance causes clinically significant distress or impairment in social, occupational, or other important areas of functioning.

Specify if:

Acute: if duration of symptoms is less than 3 months

Chronic: if duration of symptoms is 3 months or more

Specify if:

With or without delay onset: Onset of symptoms at least 6 months after the stressor

Source: American Psychiatric Association 2000.[17]

Pharmacotherapy for Acute Stress Disorder and Posttraumatic Stress Disorder (PTSD)

Pharmacotherapy can help prevent the emergence of post-traumatic stress disorder (PTSD). Sound, restful sleep is vital to healing the neural damage caused by trauma. Sleep time should be aggressively protected, with medication sufficient to produce at least 5 consecutive hours of sleep each night, plus 3–4 additional hours. The benzodiazepines, especially clonazepam (Klonopin), tend to be helpful because these drugs also combat the anxiety that is prominent after a trauma, but they may cause retrograde amnesia that can interfere with the psychotherapy process. Antidepressants are also used to treat PTSD, but full efficacy may take up to 8 weeks.

Recent studies support the routine use of propranolol (Inderal), an inexpensive beta-blocker, to prevent the development of PTSD.[78] Propranolol blocks beta-adrenergic neurotransmission, the fight or flight response that leads to the neurochemistry of hypervigilance and chronic anxiety. It has also been used to treat the reemergence of PTSD symptoms in persons who have experienced repeated traumas.

This last treatment, in particular, appears to have great potential for preventing the long-term disability connected with exposure to traumatic events. Neither benzodiazepines nor antidepressants have been shown to be helpful in prevention of PTSD; they appear useful only in treating concomitant symptoms. Propranolol is readily available in generic form and is generally very well tolerated and not habit forming. It can be acceptable to women who would not ordinarily like the idea of taking psychiatric medication or sleeping pills.

Sleep Disturbances

Insomnia occurs more frequently in women than in men and is commonly associated with the menstrual cycle, pregnancy, postpartum, and of course, menopause. Approximately 60% of women report having insomnia during the menopausal transition years. In addition, sleep disorders may be related to the development of chronic medical conditions and/or changes in psychosocial factors that occur with aging.

Primary sleep disturbances such as sleep apnea or narcolepsy are possible primary sleep disturbance diagnoses. Sleep disturbance can also be a symptom of another medical condition such as hyperthyroidism, restless leg syndrome, periodic leg movement disorder, depression,

or substance abuse. The relationship between sleep disturbance and depression is a good example of how sleep disturbances affect one's health. This relationship is probably bidirectional in that sleep disturbances make depression worse and the reverse is also true. Therefore, identifying and treating insomnia or sleep disturbances can be an important primary or adjunct therapy for a range of conditions. Because sleep problems often have both a medical and behavioral component, both need to be addressed to ensure a clinical response.

Several medications can cause sleep disturbances. Nicotine and caffeine are well-known stimulants. Bronchodilators, central nervous system stimulants, pseudoephedrine, methyldopa (Aldomet), beta blockers, alpha blockers, and cholinesterase inhibitors are all stimulants that can interfere with sleep. Less well known are the sleep disturbances caused by some medications that are sedating. Opiates, SSRIs, SNRIs, MAO inhibitors, and bupropion (Wellbutrin) alter sleep patterns and can cause sleep that is not restful.

Once a diagnosis has been made and treatment is determined to be necessary, there are is a large number of non-pharmacologic and pharmacologic therapies to treat sleep disturbances. Nonpharmacologic therapies may be preferred, but they are slower to take effect, many clinicians are not aware of how to use them, there are few studies that have documented the efficacy of these interventions, and insurance does not often reimburse for them. Nonetheless, behavioral therapies such as stimulus control and sleep restriction during the day appear to be as efficacious as some of the medications used in the short term, and more efficacious for long-term treatment. Other nonpharmacologic therapies that are often recommended for which there is limited evidence of efficacy are mediation, hypnotherapy, and biofeedback.

Drugs that facilitate sleep can be used to treat sleep disorder and sleep deprivation that is associated with conditions such as acute grief reactions, mid-life sleep disturbances, perimenstrual insomnia, and postpartum. Although there are many medications used to treat sleep disturbances, the FDA has approved only a small number of medications for this indication, and most of them are approved for a duration of less than 35 days (eszopiclone [Lunesta] is the exception). Today, trazodone (Desyrel) is the most commonly prescribed medication for treating insomnia (Table 25-14).

Hormone therapy deserves special mention. Hormone therapy has traditionally been recommended for menopause-related insomnia; however, it has limited efficacy when

Table 25-14 Selected Sleep Aids

Category Generic (Brand)	Typical Dose (mg)	Overdose Risk	FDA Pregnancy Category	FDA Approved for Treating Insomnia	Clinical Considerations
*OTC Antihistamines**			B	N/A	Rapid tolerance to drug.
Diphenhydramine (Benadryl)	25–100	Low	C	N/A	Duration 6–8 h. Sedation, mildly anxiolytic, anticholinergic effects. No evidence of effectiveness for insomnia.
Doxylamine (Unisom)	25–100	Low	C	N/A	Sedation, mildly anxiolytic.
Prescription-Only Antihistamines					
Hydroxyzine (Vistaril, Atarax)	25–100	Low	C	No	Paradoxic CNS stimulation may occur.
Benzodiazepines					
Alprazolam (Xanax)	0.5–1.0	Moderate	D	No	Strongly habituating, short acting with acute withdrawal. Multiple drug–drug interactions.
Clonazepam (Klonopin)	0.5–2.0	Moderate	D	No	Acts as a mood stabilizer. Contraindicated for persons with acute narrow-angle glaucoma or hepatic failure.
Diazepam (Valium)	2–10	Moderate	D	No	Long acting and can cause next-day sedation; has active metabolite. Contraindicated for persons with myasthenia gravis or narrow-angle glaucoma.
Flurazepam (Dalmane)	15–30	Moderate	X	Yes	Long acting and can cause next-day sedation; has active metabolite.
Lorazepam (Ativan)	0.5–2.0	Moderate	D	No	Short to medium acting. Often used for occasional panic attacks. Initial dose should not be > 2 mg; strongly amnesic during initial doses, but tolerance to this develops quickly. Contraindicated for persons with narrow-angle glaucoma, sleep apnea, myasthenia gravis.
Oxazepam (Serax)	15–30	Moderate	D	No	Short-acting metabolite of diazepam. Slow onset of action; used for persons with difficulty maintaining sleep. Moderate amnesic effects. Contraindicated for persons with myasthenia gravis, COPD, hepatic dysfunction.
Quazepam (Doral)	7.5–30	Low	X	Yes	Intermediate acting. Mechanism similar to Z-drugs; fewer side effects than other benzodiazepines. Active metabolites excreted into breast milk; should not be used by lactating women.
Temazepam (Restoril)	7.5–30	Moderate	X	Yes	Intermediate acting. Indicated for severe insomnia. Hypnotic effect decreases number of nightly awakenings. Contraindicated for persons with sleep apnea, narrow-angle glaucoma, myasthenia gravis, hepatic dysfunction.
Triazolam (Halcion)	0.25–0.5	Moderate	X	Yes	Short acting and high potency. Indicated for sleep initiation. High incidence of psychiatric side effects, rebound insomnia, amnesia.
Tricyclic Antidepressants					
Amitriptyline (Elavil)	25–100	High	C	No	Commonly prescribed during pregnancy and lactation.
Doxepin (Sinequan)	25–100	High	D	No	Most often used for sleep initiation. Anticholinergic side effects. Do not mix oral concentrate with carbonated beverages.
Trazodone (Desyrel)	25–200	Low	C	No	Duration typically 8 h, minimal morning drowsiness.

(continues)

Table 25-14 Selected Sleep Aids (*continued*)

Category Generic (Brand)	Typical Dose (mg)	Overdose Risk	FDA Pregnancy Category	FDA Approved for Treating Insomnia	Clinical Considerations
Nonbenzodiazepines					The Z drugs.
Eszopiclone (Lunesta)	5–10	Low	C	Yes	Superior efficacy for treating perimenopause and menopausal insomnia (compared to placebo). No limitation on duration of use. Risk of traveler's amnesia.
Zaleplon (Sonata)	5–10	Low	C	Yes	Ultrashort acting, duration = 4 h. Reports of habituation with long-term use. Multiple drug–drug interactions.
Zolpidem (Ambien)	5–10	Low	B	Yes	Short acting. Indicated for inducing sleep. Risk of traveler's amnesia.[†]
Zolpidem ER (Ambien CR)	12.5	Low	B	Yes	Intermediate acting. Helpful for sleep initiation and maintenance. Risk of traveler's amnesia.[†]
Selective Melatonin Receptor Agonist					
Ramelteon (Rozerem)	8	Low	C	Yes	Short acting. Approved for insomnia characterized by difficulty with sleep onset. No limitation on duration of use. Is not a scheduled drug by DEA.

OTC = over-the-counter; COPD = chronic obstructive pulmonary disease; DEA = Drug Enforcement Administration.

* Effect of antihistamines for sleep may also result in decreased milk production.

[†] Traveler's amnesia is the term that describes memory loss of flight or travel when one of these sleep aids is used during the trip.

objective measures of sleep are studied, and the various estrogen and progesterone components have differential effects on sleep. Hormone therapy is recommended for treatment of menopause-related vasomotor symptoms including night sweats and may have an indirect positive effect on sleep via this mechanism of action, but it is not used to treat primary sleep disorders. Similarly, antidepressants can have an indirect effect on sleep via improvements in menopausal symptoms such as vasomotor symptoms, mood swings, or pain and are considered a possible option for women who do not want to use hormone therapy.

Antihistamines

The antihistamines diphenhydramine (Benadryl) and doxylamine (Unisom) are widely available over the counter (OTC), and many women prefer to try one of them before accepting a prescription sleep aid. As their name implies, antihistamines block the action of the neurotransmitter histamine, and their anticholinergic side effects include sedation and dry mouth. Although antihistamines can be effective for short-term or occasional use, they tend to lose their effectiveness as hypnotics within a week or 2.

For a sleep-threatening situation that continues longer, a woman may need a prescription from another drug category.

Benzodiazepines

The benzodiazepine receptor agonists fall into two categories: (1) those that are prescription hypnotics, which include alprazolam (Xanax), clonazepam (Klonopin), diazepam (Valium), flurazepam (Dalmane), lorazepam (Ativan), temazepam (Restoril), and triazolam (Halcion); and (2) those that act at benzodiazepine receptors but have a nonbenzodiazepine structure, which include eszopiclone (Lunesta), zaleplon (Sonata), and zolpidem (Ambien).

Benzodiazepines often are used for sleep, especially when a woman also has anxiety, because they are anxiolytic agents. All benzodiazepines are schedule IV controlled substances and require a written prescription because of their risk for addiction, as well as their value as street drugs. The risk for addiction appears to be highest for persons with a preexisting substance abuse problem or psychiatric disorder. For most individuals, benzodiazepines can be very helpful in providing restful sleep, calming anxiety, and treating occasional panic attacks.

Benzodiazepines are often categorized by their half-life into short, intermediate, or long acting. The short-acting benzodiazepines such as alprazolam (Xanax) are most associated with dependence because they take effect quickly and wear off suddenly, causing withdrawal symptoms including shakiness, nausea, and rebound anxiety. The longer-acting clonazepam (Klonopin) has some mood-stabilizing effect and tends to be metabolized slowly, without rebound effects. Diazepam (Valium) is another long-acting benzodiazepine whose calming effect can last for several days.

Side effects of benzodiazepines include ataxia, daytime sedation, cognitive impairment, motor incoordination, memory loss, and rebound insomnia. All of these effects are more pronounced in the elderly. Occasional paradoxic effects of benzodiazepines can include increased anxiety, suicidal thoughts, and mania. This group often needs ongoing increases in doses to obtain the desired effect. In 2007, the FDA requested that manufacturers of all benzodiazepines include language on the medication label about risks for allergic reactions and complex sleep behaviors including **sleepdriving**. Benzodiazepines must be tapered slowly after prolonged use to avoid rebound effects. Finally, these drugs are rarely lethal when used alone, but overdoses can be lethal if they are taken concurrent with alcohol or other CNS depressants.

Most benzodiazepines are metabolized in the liver via the CYP450 enzyme system and are subject to high plasma levels if taken concomitantly with CYP450 inhibitors such as azole antibiotics, clarithromycin (Biaxin), and erythromycin (E-mycin). Omeprazole (Prilosec) increases plasma levels of diazepam. Conversely, CYP450 inducers such as rifampin (Rifadin), phenytoin (Dilantin), and carbamazepine (Tegretol) can decrease effectiveness of the benzodiazepine. Of import is the potential combination of antidepressants and alprazolam (Xanax). Depression is often accompanied by insomnia, and if both of these drugs are taken together, the plasma levels of alprazolam can be increased by 100%.

Nonbenzodiazepines: The "Z Drugs"

The search for the perfect sleep medication has led to the development of several new brand-name drugs in recent years. These agents are heavily advertised in the popular media. Zolpidem (Ambien) was the first nonbenzodiazepine introduced, followed by zaleplon (Sonata) and eszopiclone (Lunesta). In 2009, the FDA approved zolpidem tartrate (Ambien CR) for treating insomnia. The nonbenzodiazepines, which are informally referred to as the "Z drugs," are structurally different from the benzodiazepine drugs, and although they are agonists for the same GABAergic receptors in the central nervous system, they are specific for one GABA receptor configuration, which is why they have fewer adverse effects and side effects.

Side effects include somnolence, headache, dizziness, nausea, rebound insomnia, and anterograde amnesia. Tapering the dose may mitigate the rebound insomnia effect. It is believed that the nonbenzodiazepines do not cause dependence or some of the other troubling side effects, but postmarketing research is not yet conclusive and these drugs are popular as illegal recreational drugs secondary to their euphoria effect.

The "Z drugs" are metabolized via CYP450 enzymes in the liver and are therefore subject to several drug–drug interactions. Like benzodiazepines, CYP450 inhibitors can increase plasma levels and therapeutic effects, while CYP450 inducers can interfere with efficacy. Dose reductions many be required if accompanied by erythromycin (E-mycin), ketoconazole (Nizoral), or cimetidine (Tagamet), whereas the dose may need to be increased if rifampin (Rifadin) is being administered.

There has been no research on the safety of the non-benzodiazepines during pregnancy and lactation. Their FDA Pregnancy Category B rating is based on this lack of data, not on their proven safety.

Tricyclic Antidepressants

The tricyclic group of antidepressants contains two drugs that are often used for sleep. Amitriptyline (Endep) may be familiar to women's health clinicians because it has long been used for the treatment of gynecologic pain conditions. At slightly higher doses, it can also be helpful to induce sleep. Doxepin (Sinequan) is another TCA that is used more often for sleep than for depression. Both amitriptyline and doxepin are available as inexpensive generic preparations.

The tetracyclic antidepressant trazodone (Desyrel) is often the first-line hypnotic prescribed by psychiatric clinicians. Trazodone's most notorious side effect is its ability to cause, rarely, priapism among men, and it has been cited as a possible factor in case reports of clitoral pain among women.[79] However, its overall safety and effectiveness make it a useful hypnotic, especially in those with a history of substance abuse.

Complementary and Alternative Therapies for Insomnia

Many women are interested in using natural aids to help restore normal sleep cycles. Recent research on the endocrine hormone melatonin indicates that it may be helpful in regulating circadian rhythms and restoring a normal sleep–wake cycle. Melatonin is produced by the pineal gland, depending on input from the photoreceptor cells of the retinohypothalamic system, and is synthesized from serotonin and its precursor tryptophan. Melatonin is produced exclusively at night and appears to act on wakefulness and arousal in ways that have yet to be fully identified. It is available as an over-the-counter food supplement, and some persons find it effective in inducing sleep or relieving the discomforts of jet lag. Melatonin has not been studied for its safety in pregnancy and lactation.

Eating Disorders

Eating disorders have been long recognized. Bulimia was known among ancient peoples. Anorexia is categorized as binge–purge subtype or restricting subtype. Bulimia includes purging and nonpurging subtypes.[33] It has been estimated that as many as 5% of persons with anorexia nervosa will ultimately develop bulimia nervosa.[80] Thus, unlike some conditions such as hypertension that is based on quantitative laboratory measures, diagnosis of these eating disorders can be challenging.

Even the term *eating disorder* may be misleading. Women who have anorexia nervosa rarely have true anorexia or loss of appetite, but instead perceive themselves as overweight and exercise rigid control to decrease intake. Those individuals with bulimia nervosa or binge-eating disorder also have skewed body perception and tend to eat normally, but have periods of loss of control when they overeat. For most individuals, eating disorders first occur during adolescence.

The etiology is under intense study. One theory suggests that these conditions are similar to substance abuse or addiction.[81] Psychological intervention remains the most common strategy for treatment, although effectiveness is of question. Most pharmacologic agents that are used for women with these conditions are adjunctive to behavior psychology or psychotherapy. The primary use of drugs is for women while they are hospitalized but may be continued after discharge. The most commonly used agents appear to be antidepressants, although some clinicians have prescribed stimulants or drugs such as agents associated with changes in gastric emptying on a case-by-case basis.

Studies of antidepressant treatments for women with anorexia nervosa were reviewed by Claudino et al. in 2006. These researchers conducted a systematic review and found major methodological flaws in the studies published. They were able to include only seven studies for review, acknowledging the lack of rigor. Four placebo-controlled trials failed to find that antidepressants improved weight gain, and although there were some isolated findings suggesting amineptine (Survector) and nortriptyline (Pamelor) have potential use, the research flaws precluded any recommendation of use.[82]

A stronger link has been found between the use of antidepressants and bulimia nervosa. A systematic review of 19 studies comparing antidepressants and placebo included 6 trials with TCAs (imipramine [Tofranil], desipramine [Norpramin], and amitriptyline [Elavil]), 5 with SSRIs (fluoxetine [Prozac]), 5 with MAOIs (phenelzine [Nardil], isocarboxazid [Marplan], moclobemide [Aurorix, Manerix], and brofaromine [Consonar]) and 3 with other classes of drugs (mianserin [Norval], trazodone [Desyrel], and bupropion [Wellbutrin]). There was no single drug of choice and agents in all drug categories demonstrated effectiveness in remission of binge episodes (pooled RR = 0.87; 95% CI, 0.81–0.93; $P < .001$). However, individuals taking the pharmacologic agents were more likely to drop out of the studies because of side effects than those on placebo therapy. Dropouts were more common among those on TCAs when compared to placebo than those on fluoxetine (Prozac); however, no evidence was found that one class of antidepressant should be chosen over others based on efficacy and tolerability overall.[83]

Binge eating has been treated with a wide variety of antidepressants. The basis of the choice of the drug category is the assumption that there is an association between binge eating disorder and depression. A review of publications from 1980–2006 found that 10 out of 14 studies associated the condition with depression, although none were rigorously conducted.[84]

In summary, although eating disorders have been recognized for years, effective treatments remain elusive. The primary care provider may care for women who are using psychotropic agents as long-term therapy for these conditions.

Antipsychotic Drugs

The antipsychotic or neuroleptic drugs were developed to treat psychotic conditions such as schizophrenia. Antipsychotics target dopamine receptors in the brain to varying degrees and are grouped as high potency, intermediate potency, or low potency, depending on their affinity to various neurotransmitter receptors.

The first-generation antipsychotics—including haloperidol (Haldol), chlorpromazine (Thorazine), prochlorperazine (Compazine), promethazine (Phenergan), and perphenazine (Trilafon)—have a high incidence of extrapyramidal side effects (EPS) involving the neurons in the spinal cord that govern reflexes, locomotion, and complex movements. EPS include dystonias, parkinsonism, and tardive dyskinesia, and their severity has led to the development of second- and third-generation agents that are referred to as the novel or atypical antipsychotics. These newer agents, mostly developed within the last 15 years, have more favorable side effect profiles and have been found to be useful beyond the treatment of psychosis.

The novel antipsychotics are often used to stabilize mood and calm the racing thoughts of mania or to boost the action of antidepressants. The drugs are also used for psychotic episodes of PTSD, chronic self-harm, and impulsive or aggressive behavior. In very low doses, several antipsychotics are used as hypnotics. Despite their improved tolerance, novel antipsychotics have a number of significant risks that disproportionately affect women.

Most of the novel antipsychotics—clozapine (Clozaril), olanzapine (Zyprexa), quetiapine (Seroquel), ziprasidone (Geodon), and risperidone (Risperdal)—can be associated with significant weight gain and development of metabolic syndrome. Clozapine and olanzapine are particularly likely to cause an increase in appetite. The newest antipsychotic, aripiprazole (Abilify), is often prescribed for women because it is usually weight neutral, but long-term studies remain to be done. Baseline serum values for glucose tolerance, electrolytes, prolactin levels, thyroid, and liver function should be established and followed along with waist measurements and body mass index. Clozapine also requires frequent monitoring of white blood cell and granulocyte counts so that doses can be titrated to minimize risk of agranulocytosis.

Some drug side effects can be mistaken for symptoms of anxiety; dizziness, fainting, nausea, and palpitations may actually be caused by arrhythmias associated with QT prolongation. Anticholinergic drug effects can reduce peristalsis and cause constipation and dry mouth or blurred vision.

The novel antipsychotics, notably risperidone (Risperdal), can cause hyperprolactinemia, particularly in women who have been pregnant before. Breast engorgement and galactorrhea, amenorrhea, changes in libido, and hirsutism have been reported. If amenorrhea is prolonged, bone density should be monitored. Providers may discuss changing to another agent to prevent osteoporosis the specialist as indicated. Exogenous estrogen therapy may potentiate the hyperprolactinemic effect of antipsychotics.

Hormonal Products and Women with Mental Illness

The gonadal steroids affect neurotransmission. Clinicians who prescribe estrogen or progesterone products must consider that these agents potentially affect the mental status of women who use them, and they can affect the efficacy of psychotropic medications used by women with mental disorders. Primary care providers can work collaboratively with the mental health prescriber to review possible medication interactions when prescribing hormone preparations or contraception for women who take psychotropic drugs. Table 25-15 summarizes some of the clinically relevant interactions.[67]

Table 25-15 Interactions of Psychotropic Medications and Combination Oral Contraceptives

Effects of Psychotropic Drugs on Combination Oral Contraceptives		Effects of Oral Contraceptives on Psychotropic Drugs	
Drugs That *Decrease* COCs Effectiveness	**Drugs That *Increase* COC Effectiveness**	**Drugs with *Increased* Serum Levels in the Presence of COCs**	**Drugs with *Decreased* Serum Levels in the Presence of COCs**
***Antiepileptic Mood Stabilizers**†:**	***Antidepressants:***	Lamotrigine (Lamictal)	***Some Benzodiazepines:***
Carbamazepine (Tegretol)	Fluoxetine (Prozac)	SSRI antidepressants	Lorazepam (Ativan)
Lamotrigine (Lamictal)	Paroxetine (Paxil)	Tricyclic antidepressants	Oxazepam (Serax)
Oxcarbazepine (Trileptal)	Sertraline (Zoloft)		
Phenobarbital (Luminal)	Trazodone (Desyrel)		***Anticonvulsant-Mood Stabilizer:***
Phenytoin (Dilantin)	Venlafaxine (Effexor)	***Some Benzodiazepines:***	Lamotrigine (Lamictal)†
Primidone (Mysoline)		Alprazolam (Xanax)	
Topiramate (Topamax)		Diazepam (Valium)	
Stimulant:			
Modafinil (Provigil)			

* Antiepileptic drugs that do not appear to affect COC effectiveness include valproic acid (Depakote, Depakene) and gabapentin (Neurontin).
† Antiepileptic drugs are known teratogens; neural tube defects are among their effects. Women of childbearing age who take these medications should also take 3–4 milligrams of folic acid daily in case of contraceptive failure.

Drug interactions with combination oral contraceptives (COCs) have been studied more extensively than with other hormone preparations.[85,86] COCs appear to potentiate the effects of SSRI and TCA antidepressants.[87] While the SSRI antidepressants, TCAs, venlafaxine (Effexor), and possibly trazodone (Desyrel) appear to increase the plasma concentrations of COCs.

Oral contraceptives have also been studied as antidepressants themselves and as adjuncts to other medication, with varying outcomes.[88] Perhaps the most encouraging use of oral contraceptives as psychotropics is to stabilize hormone levels to prevent premenstrual worsening of depression.[88]

Psychotropic Drugs During Pregnancy and Postpartum

The reproductive years of a woman's life are the years when she is at highest risk for being diagnosed with a psychiatric disorder. In fact, women are statistically more likely to be hospitalized for mental illness during the year following childbirth than at any other time in life. Depression, anxiety, and bipolar disorder all affect women of childbearing years disproportionately, and many women have a preexisting illness treated with medications when they conceive. Between 10% and 25% of pregnant women meet clinical criteria for major depression.[89]

The Risks of Untreated Mental Illness During Pregnancy

Untreated maternal mental illness poses a number of significant risks to both mother and fetus. Major depression during pregnancy has been associated with pregnancy loss, intrauterine growth restriction, preterm birth, and increased use of cigarettes and alcohol.[90,91] Multiple studies have documented that depressed women are more likely to use substances of abuse to attempt suicide, and they are less likely to take care of themselves or obtain prenatal care.[90,91]

The research on pregnancy outcomes in women with depression is difficult to interpret with surety. It is possible that the physiology of maternal depression can adversely affect fetal growth and development, resulting in poor neonatal outcomes. It seems plausible that the dysregulation of the hypothalamic-adrenal-pituitary axis that has been observed in depressed and anxious women may lead to a disruption in placental blood flow; animal studies suggest that such stress affects fetal brain development and behavioral difficulties after birth.[92,93]

Among women who discontinue pharmacologic treatment of their mental illness during pregnancy, approximately 75% will relapse, usually in the first trimester.[94] Maternal mental illness during pregnancy has also been found to be the strongest predictor of mental illness postpartum. The depression and anxiety that affect 10–15% of women in the early weeks after childbirth can seriously impair a mother's ability to care for her family. Infants of depressed mothers tend to develop impaired cognitive and interpersonal dysfunction that continues into childhood; children of anxious mothers also exhibit behavioral problems.[90]

Risks of Psychotropic Medications During Pregnancy

When compared to the documented risks of untreated mental illness during pregnancy, information on the relative risk of psychotropic medications care is less than robust. Healthcare professionals seeking to advise women must rely largely on case studies, observational studies in which the observers are not blinded to the medication status of the subjects, and retrospective studies that rely on maternal or clinician recall.

All psychotropics need to be evaluated for both for their ability to cause birth defects and for the ability to adversely affect fetal growth and development. The risk of fetal malformations is gestational age specific. For example, exposure between conception and 32 days can affect the neural tube, exposure between 21 and 56 days may affect heart development, and exposure between days 42 and 63 after conception can adversely affect development of the lip and palate. Craniofacial abnormalities can occur during the full first trimester of pregnancy.

Selective Serotonin Reuptake Inhibitors in Pregnancy

Public concerns have been noted regarding possible toxicity or withdrawal syndromes in infants who were exposed to antidepressants late in pregnancy. In 2004, the FDA began requiring warnings to be added to the packaging of antidepressants about the potential for serious adverse neonatal events. It should be kept in mind, however, that the supposed symptoms of newborn exposure to antidepressants are largely the same problems as those noted in the infants of depressed mothers. Studies comparing infants of medicated mothers with infants of unmedicated mothers do not take into account the possible effects of maternal illness.[95]

In 2005, paroxetine (Paxil) was found in two unpublished epidemiological studies to be associated with an increased risk for congenital cardiac malformations.[96] One of these, using Swedish national registry data, found a 2% incidence in cardiac malformations compared to a 1% incidence in the registry as a whole. Another, using a US insurance claims database, found a rate of 1.5% of cardiac malformations in the paroxetine-exposed group compared with 1% in the group exposed to other antidepressants.[97] Using these data, the FDA issued a public health advisory recommending that women and their clinicians consider discontinuation of paroxetine during pregnancy and requested that the drug's manufacturer change the pregnancy category of paroxetine from C to D.[96] Seven months later, the FDA issued another public health advisory regarding SSRI use after 20 weeks' gestation because a retrospective case control study linked use of an SSRI in later gestation with an increased risk of persistent pulmonary hypertension of the newborn, an increase of about six times compared to the unexposed control group (RR 6.1; 95% CI, 2.2–16.8).[97]

Since the studies used by the FDA in their recommendation were published, two large retrospective case control studies found a small, significant association between sertraline (Zoloft) and cardiac septal defects and between paroxetine (Paxil) and right ventricular outflow tract obstruction defects.[98] The other study found no overall association between SSRIs and congenital heart defects but did note that anencephaly, craniosynostosis, and omphalocele appeared more often in infants with an in-utero exposure to SSRIs when compared to infants who were not exposed.[99] These two studies took pains to note that absolute risks of congenital malformations with first trimester SSRI use are very small—for example, even if the association between paroxetine and right ventricular outflow tract obstruction is confirmed in future research, an exposed fetus would have approximately a 1 in 500 chance of developing the disorder (99.8% unaffected).[98,99] One literature review and one meta-analysis of first-trimester SSRI exposure have both found evidence of a small increased risk for cardiac malformations with paroxetine (Paxil).[100,101] However, the authors of the meta-analysis found that infants of women who received any SSRI during pregnancy had a greater than twofold incidence of echocardiograms in the first year of life compared to unexposed infants (OR 2.1; 95% CI, 1.5–2.9) and that the associations seen in the literature may be, in fact, due to detection bias.[101]

Regarding the association between SSRI use later in pregnancy and persistent pulmonary hypertension of the newborn, it is important to recognize that the background rate of persistent pulmonary hypertension is quite low, at 1 to 2 per 1000 live births.[97] Even if the association is confirmed, with a sixfold increase in relative risk for SSRI use after 20 weeks, it would be expected that 98.8% of exposed neonates would not have persistent pulmonary hypertension.[97] However, this condition is very serious, even life threatening (mortality rates of 10–20% despite treatment). Additional risks to the neonate exposed during late pregnancy to SSRIs include self-limiting, usually mild neurobehavioral alterations (RR 3.0; 95% CI, 2.0–4.4),[102] which persist in some babies up to 2 weeks of age. This disorder is characterized by neonatal jitteriness, hypertonia, feeding difficulties, tachypnea, and rarely seizures and respiratory distress (1 in 313 exposed babies developed symptoms requiring interventions other than supportive care, such as intubation).

The clinician is challenged to provide thorough, informed consent and to help women balance the risks associated with untreated depression in the mother (including suicide and neonatal behavioral and developmental alterations) with as-yet-uncertain levels of risk to the fetus from use of antidepressants. Women who choose to continue SSRIs in pregnancy may need dose adjustments as clearance increases in late pregnancy. If a woman and her clinician have decided that the benefits of SSRI use outweigh the risks in her individual case, it is important to ensure that the dose is therapeutic, since otherwise risks are incurred without adequately managing the woman's symptoms.

Serotonin Norepinephrine Reuptake Inhibitors in Pregnancy

Pregnancy safety data on the SNRI venlafaxine (Effexor) are limited, and information on duloxetine (Cymbalta) is even more limited. One study of 150 subjects found no increased risk for major malformations in association with venlafaxine use.[102] However, the manufacturer cites neonatal neurobehavioral alterations like those found with SSRIs as a potential risk with venlafaxine.

Tricyclic Antidepressants in Pregnancy

Pharmacologic treatments for depression other than the SSRIs include tricyclic antidepressants (TCAs). These drugs have not been associated with congenital anomalies. But these drugs are not widely used in pregnancy due to side effect profiles that limit tolerability in many women. When a TCA is desired, desipramine (Norpramin) and nortriptyline (Pamelor) may be preferred in pregnancy due to lessened anticholinergic effects. However, neonatal abstinence effects such as jitteriness, irritability, and rarely seizures have also been reported for tricyclic antidepressants used in pregnancy, and rebound cholinergic hyperactivity in the newborn has occurred resulting urinary retention and functional bowel obstruction.[103]

Bupropion During Pregnancy

Bupropion (Wellbutrin) is chemically unique among antidepressant classes, and although research for human pregnancy is limited, that which is available is reassuring. The pregnancy registry data for bupropion include 909 outcomes over nearly 10 years and do not show an increased risk for major congenital malformations. The registry consensus states that it is not yet possible to detect specific patterns of malformations and that the drug should be used only if benefits outweigh the possible risks. In general, fewer data are available regarding the safety of bupropion compared to the SSRIs.

St. John's Wort in Pregnancy

Almost no data exist regarding use of *Hypericum perforatum* (St. John's wort) in pregnancy. No mutagenic effects have been found in animal studies, and there is very little research of its use in human pregnancy.[104] The mechanism of action includes inhibition of reuptake of serotonin, dopamine, and norepinephrine, which suggests that St. John's wort might share similar effects as those caused by SSRIs.

Anxiety Disorders During Pregnancy

Maternal anxiety disorders may be more prevalent than major depression in pregnancy, and a history of anxiety disorders may be more predictive of postpartum depression than a prior history of depression.[104] SSRIs are also a common treatment for anxiety disorders. Other treatments used in anxiety disorders include benzodiazepines, tricyclic antidepressants, venlafaxine (Effexor), buspirone (BuSpar), hydroxyzine (Vistaril), and certain phenothiazines such as trifluoperazine (Stelazine).

Benzodiazepines During Pregnancy

Older studies of the benzodiazepine drugs—lorazepam (Ativan), alprazolam (Xanax), clonazepam (Klonopin), diazepam (Valium), and oxazepam (Serax)—suggested a risk of oral clefts when taken in the first trimester. More recent studies have conflicting results.[105] Based on the research done to date, benzodiazepines increase the risk for oral clefts, but the absolute increase is very small, from 6 in 10,000 to 7 in 10,000 infants.[106] Benzodiazepine use in pregnancy may be associated with preterm labor and low birth weight, but this finding has not been corroborated.[107,108] It is certain that newborns exposed to benzodiazepines in utero do undergo a withdrawal syndrome. **Floppy baby syndrome** is present in the immediate postpartum period, and subsequent withdrawal symptoms can continue for up to 3 months. The effect of benzodiazepines on long-term neurobehavioral development is not known.

Buspirone (BuSpar) has little data regarding use in pregnancy, and, therefore, it should not be used or it should be used with caution despite its classification of FDA Pregnancy Category B. Although animal data suggest there is little risk, published data regarding human exposure are extremely limited. Hydroxyzine (Vistaril) is an effective agent for short-term relief of anxiety during pregnancy. Women with severe anxiety disorders who are unresponsive to SSRIs and/or hydroxyzine are candidates for benzodiazepine therapy and may be best served by choosing clonazepam (Klonopin). Unlike diazepam (Valium) and lorazepam (Ativan), human data on clonazepam suggest low risk during pregnancy. Case reports of fetal and neonatal toxicity have been reported, but data thus far do not support clonazepam as a major human teratogen.

Bipolar Disorder: Lithium

Pregnancy in the context of bipolar disorder is a particular pharmacologic challenge, as commonly used pharmacotherapeutics (with the exception of first-generation antipsychotics) are either known to be teratogenic or have very little data regarding use in pregnancy (Box 25-4). Lithium is a first-line drug for both acute and maintenance treatment and is associated with a small absolute risk of human cardiovascular malformations. In utero exposure to lithium in the first trimester is associated with ventricular hypoplasia and Ebstein's anomaly, in which the tricuspid valve is downwardly displaced. The increased relative risk is 10 to 20 times that seen in the general population. Although the relative risk is increased substantially, the condition is uncommon, and, therefore, the absolute risk of this event becomes approximately 1 to 2 in 1000 pregnancies.[109,110]

No changes in prenatal growth have been noted in fetuses exposed to lithium, and there is no evidence for developmental delay in children whose mothers took lithium during pregnancy. There have been cases of fetal and neonatal lithium toxicity, however. Lithium levels in the fetus are approximately equivalent to levels found in the mother. Signs of lithium toxicity in the neonate include floppy baby syndrome, thyroid abnormalities, cyanosis, hypotonia, and diabetes insipidus. Incidence rates are not available from prospective studies. Most of these symptoms resolve as the lithium is renally excreted, which may take 1 or 2 weeks in the infant.

Box 25-4 Case Study: Use of Lithium During Pregnancy

GF is a 38-year-old G1P0 with a long history of bipolar disorder who presented for her initial prenatal visit at 7 weeks' gestation. She was stabilized and functioning well for the past 10 years at the same dose of lithium carbonate (Lithobid), 500 mg orally three times a day. This pregnancy was unplanned, but GF and her husband were delighted; the couple had been married for 7 years, and despite inconsistent use of contraception, this was their first pregnancy. GF was concerned because she had heard that lithium can harm her baby. However, in the years before she began lithium treatment, she had several severe manic episodes followed by significant depressive episodes, including at least one suicide attempt. She was essentially asymptomatic after reaching her maintenance dose on lithium and wanted to know if she should stop taking her medication once she became pregnant.

GF was counseled that the primary teratogenic risk associated with lithium is for cardiac abnormalities. At 7 weeks' gestation, cardiac development had already been essentially completed. She was counseled that she had approximately a 998 of 1000 chance of having a baby unaffected by Ebstein's anomaly. She was prescribed a multivitamin containing 400 mcg of folic acid and began regular prenatal care. She was offered a perinatal ultrasound and fetal echocardiogram at 18 weeks, which she accepted. She decided to continue both her lithium and her pregnancy and was able to maintain stable moods throughout the third trimester on her usual dose. Her fetal echocardiogram and ultrasound were found to be normal. At 36 weeks, weekly lithium serum levels were assessed and were found to be in the therapeutic range. When she entered labor at 39 weeks, her lithium was discontinued. Eighteen hours later, she gave birth to a healthy male with Apgar scores of 7 and 9, who was appropriate for gestational age at 7 pounds, 6 ounces. Lithium was restarted the next morning at 500 mg orally twice a day and was then titrated using serum lithium levels for the first 4 days postpartum. GF continued her lithium in the postpartum period and maintained a stable mood other than mild baby blues on day 3. She was discharged with her son on day 4.

Maternal toxicity may also occur, particularly during labor, if maternal dosing requirements have increased over the course of pregnancy to maintain therapeutic levels. A prudent choice is to withhold lithium once labor starts and reduce the dose immediately postpartum to that used preconceptionally, and to monitor lithium levels every few days in the immediate postpartum period.[110]

Bipolar Disorder: Antiepileptic Drugs

Antiepileptic drugs, primarily valproate (Depakote) and carbamazepine (Tegretol), have been used effectively to stabilize mood in bipolar disorder, but both increase the likelihood of neural tube disorders and other congenital malformations among women with epilepsy. It is recommended that women who take these medications during pregnancy supplement folic acid at 4 milligrams a day.[67] However, a retrospective case control study examining the effects of folate supplementation (in a multivitamin formulation) in the first trimester of pregnancy in women who also used carbamazepine (Tegretol), phenytoin (Dilantin), phenobarbital (Luminal), or primidone (Mysoline) found no decrease in the risk for congenital anomalies in the group that supplemented compared to those who did not.[111]

Valproate (Depakote, Depakene) is a known human teratogen and, along with spina bifida occurring in 1 to 2 percent of babies exposed between 17 and 30 days after fertilization, a characteristic pattern of minor facial abnormalities has also been observed; urogenital tract malformations and alterations in the digits are also associated with valproate and valproic acid.[11] Valproate appears also to have neurobehavioral effects in children; those exposed in utero have a higher incidence of lower IQ scores and need for special education. Neonatal abstinence symptoms are also seen in newborns whose mothers take valproate during pregnancy, with higher incidences corresponding to higher doses of valproate in third trimester.[67]

Carbamazepine (Tegretol) exposure in utero is associated with a 1% risk of spina bifida. Carbamazepine is a folic acid antagonist and is associated with an increased risk of minor craniofacial defects, fingernail hypoplasia, and, in some studies but not in others, developmental delay. Carbamazepine (Tegretol) has also been associated with vitamin K deficiency, which potentially increases the risk of neonatal bleeding; women who take carbamazepine are often advised to supplement with an additional 20 mg of vitamin K daily during pregnancy.[67]

Lamotrigine (Lamictal) has recently been approved for mood stabilization, and monotherapy with lamotrigine does not appear to pose a major risk for fetal loss or congenital malformations.[67,103] No data to date suggest neurobehavioral effects of lamotrigine, but human data for pregnancy are limited.

Antipsychotic Drugs During Pregnancy

First-generation antipsychotic agents such as chlorpromazine and prochlorperazine have been used effectively in pregnancy as both acute antimania treatments and monotherapies or adjunctive therapies for bipolar disorder. There is no evidence that these agents have teratogenic effects, though neonates exposed in utero to these agents may have a transient extrapyramidal symptom, which is followed by normal motor development.[67] Atypical antipsychotics such as risperidone (Risperdal), olanzapine (Zyprexa), quetiapine (Seroquel), ziprasidone (Geodon), and aripiprazole (Abilify) have not been studied enough to determine risks for the fetus or neonate with in utero exposure.

Antidepressant Medications During Lactation

Antidepressants have been the subject of more published studies on breastfeeding than any other category of medication. The effects of these drugs on the breastfeeding infant are reviewed in Chapter 38. The majority of studies focus on the SSRIs, and the most extensive studies have been undertaken with sertraline (Zoloft). Neither maternal milk concentration nor infant serum levels appear to consistently correlate with infant difficulties. Anecdotal reports of problems are generally limited to digestive upsets or general fussiness that resolves when the medication or breastfeeding is finished.[112]

Treating the Mature Woman

Although mental illness is most likely to be diagnosed during the childbearing years, two other time periods in a woman's life cycle are associated with vulnerability to psychiatric conditions.

The years just prior to menopause are a time of particular risk for new-onset mental illness.[113] Treatment during these years requires a three-pronged approach that includes ensuring sleep, improving mood, and reducing vasomotor symptoms.[114] Primary care clinicians are ideally positioned to ensure that all three aspects of treatment are addressed to achieve optimal health for their clients.

Treating elderly women presents a number of challenges.[115] Advancing age, comorbid conditions, and use of other medications make medicating psychiatric illness more complex. Drugs are often metabolized more slowly, increasing the risk of toxic reactions, and side effects are often more prominent in older clients. When psychotropic medications are added to a regimen that includes treatment of other conditions common in old age, drug interactions are a serious concern. Geriatric psychopharmacology is still an emerging field, with limited information available on the use and safety of medications that have chiefly been studied in younger populations. Primary care clinicians need to be particularly cautious and work closely with other prescribers when treating older women.

Conclusion

Women's primary healthcare providers are a vital resource in the identification and treatment of mental illness. By integrating the care of women's minds with the care of their bodies, primary clinicians can help women achieve healthy outcomes.

References

1. World Health Organization. World health report 2001—mental health: new understanding, new hope. Geneva, Switzerland: World Health Organization, 2001.

2. Kessler RC, Chiu WT, Demler O, Walters EE. Prevalence, severity, and comorbidity of twelve-month DSM-IV disorders in the National Comorbidity Survey Replication (NCS-R). Archives of General Psychiatry 2005;62(6):617–27.

3. Kessler RC, Berglund PA, Demler O, Jin R, Merikangas KR, Walters EE. Lifetime prevalence and age-of-onset distributions of DSM-IV disorders in the National Comorbidity Survey Replication. Arch Gen Psychiatry 2005;62(6):592–600.

4. Gaynes BN, Gavin N, Meltzer-Brody S, Lohr KN, Swinson T, Gartlehner G, et al. Perinatal depression: prevalence, screening accuracy, and screening outcomes. Evid Rep Technol Assess (Summ) 2005;119:1–8.

5. Weissman MM, Bland RC, Canino GJ, Grenwald S, Hwu HG, Joyce PR, et al. Prevalence of suicide ideation and suicide attempts in nine countries. Psychol Med 1999;29(1):9–17.

6. Arnold LM. Gender differences in bipolar disorder. Psychiatr Clin North Am 2003;26(3):595–620.

7. Cohen LS. Gender-specific considerations in the treatment of mood disorders in women across the life cycle. J Clin Psychiatry 2003;64(suppl 15):18–29.

8. Hing E, Cherry DK, Woodwell DA. National Ambulatory Medical Care Survey: 2004 Adv Data 2006; June 23;374:1–33.

9. Oates M. Perinatal psychiatric disorders: a leading cause of maternal morbidity and mortality. Br Med Bull 2003;67:219–29.

10. Weiss SR, Post RM. Kindling: separate vs shared mechanisms in affective disorders and epilepsy. Neuropsychobiology 1998;38(3):167–80.

11. Manber R, Kraemer HC, Arnow BA, Trivedi MH, Rush AJ, Thase ME, et al. Faster remission of chronic depression with combined psychotherapy and medication than with each therapy alone. J Consult Clin Psychol 2008;76(3):459–67.

12. Johnson R. Mental illness in primary women's health care. In Hackley B, Kriebs JM, Rousseau ME, eds. Primary care of women: a guide for midwives and women's health providers. Sudbury, MA: Jones and Bartlett, 2007:249–312.

13. Das AK, Olfson M, Gameroff MJ, Pilowsky DJ, Blanco C, Feder A, et al. Screening for bipolar disorder in a primary care practice. JAMA 2005;293:956–63.

14. Linzer M, Spitzer R, Kroenke K, Williams JB, Hahn S, Brody D, et al. Gender, quality of life, and mental disorders in primary care: results from the PRIME-MD 1000 study. Am J Med 1996;101(5):526–33. PubMed PMID: 8948277.

15. Spitzer RL, Kroenke K, Linzer M, Hahn SR, Williams JB, deGruy FV 3rd, et al. Health-related quality of life in primary care patients with mental disorders. Results from the PRIME-MD 1000 Study. JAMA 1995;274(19):1511–7.

16. Rickels MR, Khalid-Khan S, Gallop R, Rickels K. Assessment of anxiety and depression in primary care: value of a four-item questionnaire. J Am Osteopath Assoc 2009;109(4):216–9.

17. American Psychiatric Association. Diagnostic and statistical manual of mental disorders, 4th ed., text revision [DSM-IV-TR]. Washington, DC: American Psychiatric Association, 2000.

18. Hackley B, Kriebs JM, Rousseau ME. Primary care of women: a guide for midwives and women's health providers. Sudbury, MA: Jones and Bartlett, 2007.

19. Lang AJ, Norman SB, Means-Christensen A, Stein MB. Abbreviated brief symptom inventory for use as an anxiety and depression screening instrument in primary care. Depress Anxiety 2009;26(6):537–43.

20. Wise DD, Felker A, Stahl SM. Tailoring treatment of depression for women across the reproductive lifecycle: the importance of pregnancy, vasomotor symptoms, and other estrogen-related events in psychopharmacology. CNS Spectr 2008;13(8):647–62.

21. Frank B, Gupta S, McGlynn DJ. Psychotropic medications and informed consent. A review. Ann Clin Psychiatry 2008;20:87–95.

22. Finer LB, Henshaw K. Disparities in rates of unintended pregnancy in the United States, 1884 and 2001. Perspect Sex Reprod Health 2006;38:90–6.

23. Accort E, Freeman MP, Allen JB. Women and major depressive disorder: clinical perspectives on causal pathways. J Womens Health 2008;17:1583–600.

24. Halbriech U, Kahn L. Role of estrogen in the aetiology and treatment of mood disorders. CNS Drugs 2001;15:791–817.

25. Seeringer A, Kirchheiner J. Pharmacogenetics-guided dose modifications of antidepressants. Clin Lab Med 2008;28(4):619–26.

26. Goldberg JF, McElroy SL. Bipolar mixed episode: characteristics and comorbidities. J Clin Psychiatry 2007;68(10):e25.

27. Sanders LB. Assessing and managing women with depression: a midwifery perspective. J Midwifery Womens Health 2006;51(3):185–92.

28. Beck CT, Gable RK. Postpartum depression screening scale: Spanish version. Nurs Res 2003;52(5):296–306.

29. Hamblin JE. Insomnia: an ignored health problem. Prime Care 2007;34:659–74.

30. Sharma V, Mazmanian D. Sleep loss and postpartum psychosis. Bipolar Disord 2003;5(2):98–105.

31. Sharma V, Smith A, Khan M. The relationship between duration of labour, time of delivery, and puerperal psychosis. J Affect Disord 2004;83(2–3):215–20.

32. Ross LE, Murray BJ, Steiner M. Sleep and perinatal mood disorders: a critical review. J Psychiatry Neurosci 2005;30(4):247–56.

33. Wilfley DE, Bishop ME, Wilson GT, Agras WS. Classification of eating disorders: Toward DSM-V. Int J Eat Disord 2007;40:S123–2.

34. Kessler RC, McGonagle KA, Swartz M, Blazer DG, Nelson CB. Sex and depression in the National Comorbidity Survey 1: lifetime prevalence, chronicity and recurrence. J Affect Disord 1993;29:85–96.

35. Kessler RC, Berglund PA, Demler O, Jin R, Koretz D, Merikangas KR, et al. The epidemiology of major depressive disorder. JAMA 2003;289:3095–105.

36. Arroll B, Macgillivray S, Ogston S, Reid I, Sullivan F, Williams B, et al. Efficacy and tolerability of tricyclic antidepressants and SSRIs compared with placebo for treatment of depression in primary care: a meta-analysis. Ann Fam Med 2005;3(5):449–56.

37. Rush AJ, Trivedi MH, Wisniewski SR, Nierenberg AA, Stewart JW, Warden D, et al. Acute and longer-term outcomes in depressed outpatients requiring one or several treatment steps: a STAR*D report. Am J Psychiatry 2006;163(11):1905–17.

38. National Center for Health Statistics. Health, United States, 2008 with chartbook. Hyattsville, MD, 2009. Available from: *http://cdc.gov/nchs/data/hus/hus08 .pdf#097* [Accessed August 17, 2009].

39. Mahew MM. Initial choice of antidepressant. JNP 2009; 7:538–40.

40. McElroy SL. Bipolar disorder: special diagnostic and treatment considerations in women. CNS Spectr 2004; 9(8)(suppl 7):5–18.

41. Yildiz A, Sachs GS. Do antidepressants induce rapid cycling? A gender specific association. J Clin Psychiatry 2003;64:814–8.

42. Muzina DJ, Kemp DE, McIntyre RS. Differentiating bipolar disorders from major depressive disorders: treatment implications. Ann Clin Psychiatry 2007; 19(4):305–12.

43. Trivedi MH, Lin EH, Katon WJ. Consensus recommendations for improving adherence, self-management, and outcomes in patients with depression. CNS Spectr 2007;12(8)(suppl):1–27.

44. Pollack MH. The pharmacotherapy of panic disorder. J Clin Psychiatry 2005;66(suppl 4):23–7.

45. Stahl SM, Felker A. Monoamine oxidase inhibitors: a modern guide to an unrequited class of antidepressants. CNS Spectr 2008;13(10):855–70.

46. Nandagopal JJ, DelBello MP. Selegiline transdermal system: a novel treatment option for major depressive disorder. Expert Opin Pharmacother 2009;10(10): 1665–73.

47. de Leon J, Armstrong SC, Cozza KL. Clinical guidelines for psychiatrists for the use of pharmacogenetic testing for CYP450 2D6 and CYP450 2C19. Psychosomatics 2006;47(1):75–85.

48. Gillman PK. Tricyclic antidepressant pharmacology and therapeutic drug interactions updated. Br J Pharmacol 2007;151(6):737–48.

49. Kornstein SG, Shatzberg AF, Thase ME, Yonkers KA, McCullough JP, Keitner GI, et al. Gender differences in treatment response to sertraline versus imipramine in chronic depression. Am J Psychiatry 2000; 157(9):1445–52.

50. Brambilla P, Cipriani A, Hotopf M, Barbui C. Side-effect profile of fluoxetine in comparison with other SSRIs, tricyclic and newer antidepressants: a meta-analysis of clinical trial data. Pharmacopsychiatry 2005;38(2):69–77.

51. Barbui C, Esposito E, Cipriani A. Selective serotonin reuptake inhibitors and risk of suicide: a systematic review of observational studies. CMAJ 2009; 180(3):291–7.

52. Boyer EW, Shannon M. The serotonin syndrome. N Engl J Med 2005;352(11):1112–20. Review. Erratum: N Engl J Med 2007;356(23):2437.

53. Isbister GK, Bowe SJ, Dawson A, Whyte IM. Relative toxicity of selective serotonin reuptake inhibitors (SSRIs) in overdose. J Toxicol Clin Toxicol 2004; 42:277–85.

54. Rusniak DE, Sprague JE. Toxin-induced hyperthermic syndromes. Med Clin North Am 2005;89(6):1277–96.

55. Gnanadesigan N, Espinoza RT, Smith R, Israel M, Reuben DB. Interactions of serotonergic antidepressants and opioid analgesics: is serotonin syndrome going undetected? J Am Med Dir Assoc 2005; 6(4):265–9.

56. Nelson LS, Erdman AR, Booze LL, Cobaugh DJ, Chyka PA, Woolf Ad, et al. Selective serotonin reuptake inhibitor poisoning: an evidence-based consensus guideline for out-of-hospital management. Clin Toxicol (Phila) 2007;45(4):315–32.

57. Loke YK, Trivedi AN, Singh S. Meta-analysis: gastrointestinal bleeding due to interaction between selective serotonin uptake inhibitors and non-steroidal anti-inflammatory drugs. Aliment Pharmacol Ther 2008;27(1):31–40.

58. Thase ME. Are SNRIs more effective than SSRIs? A review of the current state of the controversy. Psychopharmacol Bull 20081;41(2):58–85.

59. Spina E, Santoro V, D'Arrigo C. Clinically relevant pharmacokinetic drug interactions with second-

generation antidepressants: an update. Clin Ther 2008; 30(7):1206–27.

60. Foley KF, DeSanty KP, Kast RE. Bupropion: pharmacology and therapeutic applications. Expert Reve Neurother 2006;6(9):1249–65.

61. Belmaker RH. Treatment of bipolar depression. N Engl J Med 2007;356:1771–22.

62. Cruellar AK, Johnson SL, Winters R. Distinctions between bipolar and unipolar depression. Clin Psych Rev 2005;25:307–39.

63. Howland RH. Induction of mania with serotonin reuptake inhibitors. J Clin Psychopharmacol 1996;16: 425–7.

64. Grunze HC. Switching, induction of rapid cycling, and increased suicidality with antidepressants in bipolar patients: fact or overinterpretation? CNS Spectr 2008; 13(9):790–5.

65. Movag KLL, Baumgarten HGM, Leufkens JHM, Van Laarhoven JHM, Egberts ACG. Risk factors for the development of lithium-induced polyuria. Br J Psychiatry 2003;182:319–23.

66. Young AH, Hammond JM. Lithium in mood disorders: increasing evidence base, declining use? Br J Psychiatry 2007;191:474–6.

67. Burt VK, Rasgon N. Special considerations in treating bipolar disorder in women. Bipolar Disord 2004; 6:2–13.

68. Andrade C, Thyagagarajan S. The influence of name on the acceptability of ECT: the importance of political correctness. J ECT 2007;23(2):75–7.

69. Pinette MG, Santarpio C, Wax JR, Blackstone J. Electroconvulsive therapy in pregnancy. Obstet Genecol 2007;110(2 pt):465–6.

70. Terman M. Evolving applications of light therapy. Sleep Med Rev 2007;6:497–507.

71. Lin PY, Su KP. A meta-analytic review of double-blind, placebo-controlled trials of antidepressant efficacy of omega-3 fatty acids. J Clin Psychiatry 2007; 68(7):1056–61.

72. Song C, Zhao S. Omega-3 fatty acid eicosapentaenoic acid. A new treatment for psychiatric and neurodegenerative diseases: a review of clinical investigations. Expert Opin Investig Drugs 2001;16(10): 1627–38.

73. Kaper S, Volz HP, Moller HJ, Dienel A, Kiesser M. Continuation and long-term maintenance treatment with *Hypericum* extract WS(R) 5570 after recovery from an acute episode of moderate depression—a double-blind, randomized, placebo-controlled long-term trial. Eur Neuropsychopharmacol 2008;11:803–13.

74. Di YM, Li CG, Xue CC, Zhou SF. Clinical drugs that interact with St. John's wort and implication in drug development. Curr Pharm Des 2008;14(17): 1723–42.

75. Meyer JS, Quenzer LF. Psychopharmacology drugs, the brain, and behavior. Sunderland, MA: Finauer Associates, 2005.

76. Rurup ML, Buiting HM, Pasman HR, van der Maas PJ, van der Heide A, Onwuteaka-Philipsen BD. The reporting rate of euthanasia and physician-assisted suicide: a study of the trends. Med Care 2008;46(12):1198–202.

77. Bassin SL, Bleck TP. Barbiturates for the treatment of intracranial hypertension after traumatic brain injury. Crit Care 2008;12(5):185.

78. Taylor F, Cahill L. Propranolol for reemergent post-traumatic stress disorder following an event of retraumatization: a case study. J Trauma Stress 2002;15(5): 433–7.

79. Medina CA. Clitoral pripism: a rare condition presenting as a cause of vulvar pain. Obstet Gynecol 2002; 100(5 pt 2):1089–91.

80. Kaye WH, Walsh BT. Psychopharmacology of eating disorders. In Davis KL, Charney D, Coyle JT, Nemeroff C, eds. Neuropsychopharmacology: the fifth generation of progress. Philadelphia, PA: Lippincott Williams & Wilkins, 2002,1676–83.

81. Davis C, Carter JC. Compulsive overeating as an addiction disorder. A review of theory and evidence. Appetite 2009, June 11:1–8.

82. Claudino AM, Hay P, Lima MS, Bacaltchuk J, Schmidt U, Treasure J. Antidepressants for anorexia nervosa. Cochrane Database Syst Rev 2006(1):CD004365.

83. Bacaltchuk J, Hay PPJ. Antidepressants versus placebo for people with bulimia nervosa. Cochrane Database Syst Rev 2003(3):CD003391.

84. Araujo DM, Fonseca GD, Nardi AE. Binge eating disorder and depression: a systematic review. World J Biol Psychiatry 2009, June 10:1–9.

85. Westlund TL, Parry BL. Does estrogen enhance the antidepressant effect of fluoxetine? J Affect Disord 2003;77(1):81–92.

86. Cohen LS, Soares CN, Poitras JR, Prouty J, Alexander AB, Shifren JL. Short-term use of estradiol for depression in perimenopausal and postmenopausal women: a preliminary report. Am J Psychiatry 2003; 160(8):1519–22.

87. Gentile S. The role of estrogen therapy in postpartum psychiatric disorders: an update. CNS Spect 2005; 10(12):944–52.

88. Joffe H, Petrillo L, Viguera AC, Gottschall H, Soares CN, Hall JE, Cohen LS. Treatment of premenstrual worsening of depression with adjunctive oral contraceptive pills: a preliminary report. J Clin Psychiatry 2007;68(12):1954–62.

89. American College of Obstetricans and Gynecologists. Use of psychiatric drugs during pregnancy and lactation. Obstet Gynecol 2007;110:1179–98.

90. Wisner KL, Sit DK, Hanusa BH, Moses-Kolko EL, Bogen DL, Hunker DF, et al. Major depression and antidepressant treatment: impact on pregnancy and neonatal outcomes. Am J Psychiatry 2009;166(5):557–66.

91. Marcus SM. Depression during pregnancy: rates, risks and consequences—Motherisk Update 2008. Can J Clin Pharmacol 2009;16(1):e15–22.

92. Weinberg M, Tronick E. The impact of maternal psychiatric illness on infant development. J Clin Psychiatry 1998;59(suppl 2):53–61.

93. Perlstein T, Howard M, Salisbury A, Zlotnick C. Postpartum depression. Am J Obstet Gynecol 2009; 200:357–64.

94. Marcus SM, Heringhuasen JE. Depression in childbearing women complicates pregnancy. Prim Care Clin Office Pract 2009;36:151–65.

95. Cole JA, Ephross SA, Cosmatos IS, Walker AM. Paroxetine in the first trimester and the prevalence of congenital malformations. Pharmacoepidemiol Drug Saf 2007;16(10):1075–85.

96. US Food and Drug Administration. FDA public health advisory: paroxetine. 2005. Available from: *http:// www.fda.gov/Safety/MedWatch/SafetyInformation/ SafetyAlertsforHumanMedicalProducts/ucm151239 .htm* [Accessed August 17, 2009].

97. Chambers CD, Hernandez-Diaz S, Van Marter LJ, Werler MM, Louik C, Jones KL, et al. Selective serotonin reuptake inhibitors and persistent pulmonary hypertension of the newborn. N Engl J Med 2006;354:579–87.

98. Louik C, Lin AE, Werler MW, Hernandez-Diaz S, Mitchell AA. First-trimester use of selective serotonin-reuptake inhibitors and the risk of birth defects. N Engl J Med 2007;356:2675–82.

99. Alwan S, Reefhuis J, Rasmussen SA, Olney RS, Friedman JM. Use of selective serotonin-reuptake inhibitors in pregnancy and the risk of birth defects. N Engl J Med 2007;356:2684–92.

100. Bellantuono C, Migliarese G, Gentile S. Serotonin reuptake inhibitors in pregnancy and the risk of major malformations: a systematic review. Hum Psychopharmacol 2007;22:121–8.

101. Bar-Oz B, Einarson T, Einarson A, Boskovic R, O'Brian L, Malm H, et al. Paroxetine and congenital malformations: meta-analysis and consideration of potential confounding factors. Clin Ther 2007;29:918–26.

102. Einarson A, Fatoye B, Sarkar M, Lavigne SV, Brochu J, Chambers C, et al. Pregnancy outcome following gestational exposure to venlafaxine: a multicenter prospective controlled study. Am J Psychiatry 2001;158:1728–30.

103. Eberhard-Gran M, Eskild A, Opjordsmoen S. Treating mood disorders during pregnancy: safety considerations. Drug Safety 2005;28:695–706.

104. Moretti ME, Maxson A, Hanna F, Koren G. Evaluating the safety of St. John's wort in human pregnancy. Reprod Toxocol 2009;28:96–9.

105. Austin MP, Priest SR. Clinical issues in perinatal mental health: new developments in the detection and treatment of perinatal mood and anxiety disorders. Acta Psychiatrica Scandinavica 2005;112:97–104.

106. Frias GL, Gilbert-Barnes E. Human teratogens: current controversies. Adv Pediatr 2008;55:171–211.

107. Altshuler LL, Cohen L, Szuba MP, Burt VK, Gitlin M, Mintz J. Pharmacologic management of psychiatric illness during pregnancy: dilemmas and guidelines. Am J Psychiatry 1996;153:592–606.

108. Wikner BN, Stiller CO, Bergman U, Asker C, Kalen B. Use of benzodiazepines and benzodiazepine receptor agonists during pregnancy: neonatal outcome and congenital malformations. Pharmaco Epidemiol Drug Safety 2007;16:1203–10.

109. Ward S, Wisner KL. Collaborative management of women with bipolar disorder during pregnancy and postpartum: pharmacologic considerations. J Midwifery Womens Health 2007;52:3–13.

110. Giles JJ, Bannigan JG. Teratogenic and developmental effects of lithium. Curr Pharm Des 2006;12: 1531–41.

111. Hernandez-Diaz S, Werler MM, Walker AM, Mitchell AA. Folic acid antagonists during pregnancy and the risk of birth defects. N Engl J Med 2000;343: 1608–14.

112. Ragan K, Stowe, ZN, Newport DJ. Use of antidepressant and mood stabilizers in breast-feeding women. In Cohen LS, Nonacs RM, eds. Course of psychiatric illness during pregnancy and the postpartum, in

mood and anxiety disorders during pregnancy and postpartum. Washington, DC: American Psychiatric Publishing Inc., 2005:112–34.

113. Cohen LS, Soares CN, Vitonis AF, Otto MW, Harlow BL. Risk for new onset of depression during the menopausal transition: the Harvard study of moods and cycles. Arch Gen Psychiatry 2006;63(4):385–90.

114. Zubenko GS, Sunderlan T. Geriatric psychopharmacology: why does age matter? Harv Res Psychiatry 2000;7(6):311–3.

115. Naranjo CA, Hermann N, Mittmann N, Bremmer KE. Recent advances in geriatric psychopharmacology. Drugs Aging 1995;7(3):184–202.

Skin
You do hold us in
with your blemishes and freckles
and the funny way you
zipper our scrapes and cuts.
Even your method of draping
blue-black curtains over our bruises
catches amazement. Up and down the slopes of our bodies,
under our armpits, between our toes,
we want your rind to surround us
with a suede tough enough to live in.
REPRINTED WITH PERMISSION
FROM CJ STEVENS

Chapter Glossary

Acne A dermatologic condition primarily of the sebaceous skin glands characterized by papules, pustules, or comedones. This condition is more properly termed *acne vulgaris* to differentiate from other, less common types of acne.

Actinic keratosis A premalignant skin condition with multiple crusty patches. Also termed *AK* and *solar keratosis*.

Alopecia A condition in which hair is lost from some or all parts of the body. This primarily affects the scalp.

Alopecia areata Hair loss in a specific area.

Alopecia universalis Hair loss over entire body.

Androgenic alopecia Alopecia that occurs secondary to increased androgen levels. Also called female pattern baldness.

Calcineurin inhibitors Immunosuppressant agents that are theorized to act by selectively inhibiting inflammation through action on T-cell activation.

Carbuncle A skin infection composed of a cluster of boils (furuncles). This infection most frequently is caused by *Staphylococcus aureus*.

Cellulitis An acute spreading dermatologic bacterial infection characterized by significant edema, erythema, and pain.

Cosmeceutical A word coined from the terms *cosmetic* and *pharmaceutical* that is used for agents that have therapeutic effects as well as promote attractiveness.

Dermatophytes A parasitic infection of the skin. An example is athlete's foot.

Eczema Inflammatory dermatologic process that is characterized by pruritus, erythema, and lesions that may be encrusted and scaly.

Furuncle Skin infection commonly involving hair follicle and also called a boil.

Hirsutism From Latin *hirsutus*, which means "shaggy," an excessive hair growth in females in areas where hair is normally minimal or absent. Hirsutism refers to a male pattern of hair distribution in a woman.

Humectant Ingredient that absorbs water and promotes maintenance of moisture on skin.

Intertrigo Rash or inflammation of the body folds or intertriginous areas of the skin.

Keratinocytes Epidermal cells that synthesize keratin.

Langerhans cells Dendritic skin cells that transport antigens to lymph nodes.

Melanin Skin pigment produced by special cells (melanocytes).

Melanocytes Cells located in the bottom layer (the stratum basale) of the skin's epidermis that produce melanin.

Merkel cells Cells found in the middle layers of the skin around hair follicles. Cancer originating among these cells, Merkel cell carcinoma, tends to be highly aggressive.

Onychomycosis Fungal infection of the nails on either fingers or toes.

Psoriasis Skin condition caused by overgrowth of keratinocytes and resulting in patchy, thickened skin.

Pyoderma Skin condition with purulent-filled lesions.

Retinoids Natural or synthetic derivative of vitamin A and widely used in pharmacotherapeutics in dermatology.

Seborrheic keratoses Wartlike, benign skin lesions.

Solar lentigo; *plural*: **lentigines** Flat, pigmented lesions on sun-exposed skin. Also known as senile lentigo.

Sun protection factor (SPF) A measure of how much ultraviolet radiation (sunlight) is required to produce a burn on skin that is protected with sunscreen. A sunscreen with an SPF factor of ≥ 15 is recommended by the American Academy of Dermatology.

Telangiectasia Dark red, elevated skin lesions caused by chronic dilation of capillaries.

Telogen effluvium Acute loss of hair. Follicles are normal but growth is disturbed. Occurs secondary to hormonal stress or exposure to some medications.

Ultraviolet (UV) radiation Rays from the sun that are invisible to the naked eye but capable of skin damage and photoaging.

Xerosis Dry skin.

Introduction

Although the skin is often described as the largest organ of the body, accounting for 15% of an adult's body weight, it is frequently ignored when general health is considered. Equally, when skin problems are identified, many clinicians rapidly refer the person to a dermatologist. Although there are skin conditions that require the evaluation and management skills of a specialist, there are many skin conditions that a primary care clinician can diagnose and treat. This chapter addresses common skin findings that women's health clinicians see in primary care settings.

Anatomy and Physiology of the Skin

The skin is composed of the epidermis, dermis, and hypodermis (also referred to as subcutaneous tissue). Among the functions of the skin are protection, temperature regulation, sensation, and metabolism (especially for vitamin D). In addition to variations of color and texture, skin is subject to normal maturational changes, allergic stimuli, injury, and infection.

The epidermis is formed by stratified layers of squamous epithelial cells and functions primarily as a protective covering (Figure 26-1). As **keratinocytes**, the dominant

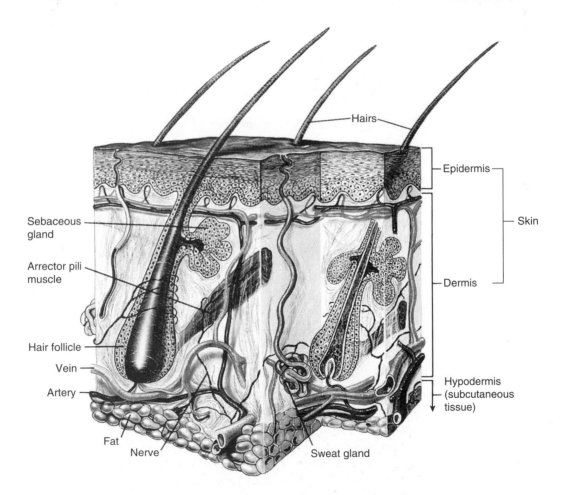

Figure 26-1 The skin and its anatomic components. *Source:* Clark RK 2005.[102]

cell type, move up through the layers of epidermis, they progressively acquire more keratin, harden, and die. The outer layer of dead and dying cells becomes abraded and is shed, a process known as desquamation. Other cells found in the epidermis are **melanocytes**, **Langerhans cells**, and **Merkel cells**. Melanocytes are the source of pigment, **melanin**, which the melanocyte transfers to the keratinocyte via melanosomes that move along the dendrite of the melanocyte to the keratinocyte. The melanin offers protection against ultraviolet radiation. Langerhans cells are macrophages; they respond to antigens on the skin and facilitate recognition by lymphocytes. Merkel cells are sensory receptors.

Divided by a thin basement membrane from the epidermis, the dermis is the source of elasticity in skin and is composed of collagen, elastin, and ground substance, all derived from fibroblasts. Macrophages present in the dermis assist in prevention of infections. The dermis also is the most superficial vascular layer. Thickness varies with location on the body and is the most variable component of the skin. Below the dermis is a layer of subcutaneous fatty tissue.

Various appendages to the skin arise from the subcutaneous and dermal layers. These include sweat glands, sebaceous glands, and hair follicles. Both sweat glands and sebaceous glands are exocrine in nature—discharging their products (sweat and sebum) directly through ducts onto the skin. The sweat glands serve to assist in temperature regulation as well as to discard salts and waste products such as ammonia. Sebaceous glands secrete an oily substance, sebum, which lubricates skin. Table 26-1 lists terms and descriptions for common skin manifestations.

Skin Changes and Women

Skin changes throughout women's lifetimes. Likewise, many skin disorders are age-specific, and the drugs used to treat skin disorders have different clinical effects in persons of different ages.

Dermatology for Pregnant and Lactating Women

Before treating a woman of childbearing age, consideration should always be given to her reproductive status. Questions about last menstrual period, contraceptive methods used, risk of conception, and lactation status are essential parts of the history. The severity of a dermatologic condition, whether treatment is medically necessary or elective, and real or perceived risks to the fetus and newborn all

Table 26-1 Terms and Descriptions for Common Skin Manifestations

Term	Description
Type	
Macule	Flat, well-circumscribed change in skin color
Nodule	Solid lesion that may involve dermis or subcutaneous tissue, larger in size than a papule
Papule	Solid superficial raised lesion, less than 1 cm
Plaque	Solid, superficial raised lesion, ≥ 1 cm in diameter
Vesicle	Fluid-filled lesion at epidermal surface, less than 0.5 cm
Wheal (urticaria)	Raised edematous tissue, involving the epidermis or dermis, irregular in size, shape, and color
Color	
Brown	Hypermelanosis
Red	Erythema, violaceous, purpura (does not blanch)
White	Leukoderma, hypomelanosis
Other colors	Also can be characteristic of various conditions or diseases
Appearance	
Crusting	Dried serum, blood, or pus covering a lesion
Excoriation	Skin torn or irritated by scratching
Fissure	Linear tear in epidermis/dermis
Scaling	Accumulated epidermal tissue
Thickening	In relationship to surrounding tissue
Ulcer	Loss of epidermis and part of dermis, usually round or oval
Shape	
Annular	Central clearing surrounded by a raised lesion
General	Linear, oval, round, clustered
Reticulated	Lacy
Serpentine	Snakelike, curving

affect the decision whether to treat during pregnancy and lactation.

Skin undergoes changes during pregnancy that may affect the course of dermatologic problems. Sebaceous gland secretions increase, with a variable effect on acne and other skin eruptions. Increased sweat gland function can cause skin irritation or rashes. The increased vascular dilation that occurs with pregnancy may facilitate absorption of topical medications so that more is absorbed compared to the amount absorbed during the nonpregnant state. Pregnancy can also result in striae gravidarum, which mark areas of thinned skin.

Throughout this chapter, the effects of drugs administered during pregnancy are referred to by the Food and Drug Administration (FDA) pregnancy categories. As of this writing, the FDA is planning a new system of categorization, although the new categories have not yet been adopted.

Lactation categories are less well defined than the FDA pregnancy categories and include more latitude than many clinicians are truly comfortable with. In general, the

American Academy of Pediatrics (AAP) resources, online sources such as Reprotox, as well as any of several texts focusing on pregnancy and lactation, are useful references. The AAP has published a list of safety ratings of common medications for lactating women.[1] Its most current list was published in 2001, thus, many newer drugs are not addressed. However, the AAP materials include several useful principles regarding prescribing a drug for a breastfeeding mother, including verifying the necessity of treatment, choosing the drug that is safest or least likely to cause harm, and timing the dosing immediately after feedings in order to minimize transfer to the infant.[1] As with pregnancy, the absence of clinical trials means that many drugs have little or no evidence on which to base a recommendation. When possible, discussion of individual agents will include information about known safety during pregnancy and lactation.

Skin Changes in the Elderly

As the population in the United States becomes older, geriatric dermatology is becoming a specialty in health care. Intrinsic aging refers to normal changes associated with maturation, while extrinsic aging is produced by outside factors such as the environment. Photoaging refers to the damage done to skin over a lifetime of exposure to **ultraviolet (UV) radiation** in sunlight. The normal skin aging process for women includes hormonal changes as well as possible skin damage from exposure to weather, sunlight, and smoking.

As skin thins and dries, it becomes less elastic, and wrinkles develop. Receptors for estrogen, progesterone, and androgens all exist in the skin. Following menopause, decreases in estrogen extend to receptors in both fibroblasts and keratinocytes.[2] Skin collagen also decreases with the loss of sex steroid stimulation, causing thinning and weakening of the tissue. Compared with photo-damaged skin, intrinsic skin aging is characterized by thinner, more lax tissue, finer lines, and fewer pigment changes.[3] Topical medications can be less well absorbed by aged skin.

Although the provision of exogenous hormones can reverse hormonally driven changes, it has no effect on extrinsic causes of skin aging such as sun damage, like **solar lentigines** and **telangiectasia**.[4] Smoking also accelerates skin aging and wrinkling. In addition to these problems, xerosis (dry skin) and pruritus are common among older women.[5] The loss of subcutaneous fat coupled with decreased collagen leaves surface blood vessels less protected and increases the risk of bruising. Dilated small blood vessels produce spider veins, particularly on the face and lower extremities.

A variety of additional changes occur with aging skin, regardless of type. Melanocytes tend to decline by up to 15% per decade, while Langerhans cells decrease in both density and responsiveness. Some conditions, such as xerosis, pruritus, and eczema are more common among the elderly. The immune response is decreased, and wound healing is delayed.[6] Some diseases such as diabetes mellitus and HIV have dermatologic expression that confounds diagnosis and treatment.

The skin changes associated with aging affect response to medications. Fewer lipids affect absorption of some topical medications. Decreased vascularity and increased keratin inhibits absorption of topical medications. Kidney and liver function decline with age, which further delays metabolism of medications.

As individuals live longer, chronic diseases become more common. These chronic conditions may include diseases of the skin. In this chapter, when appropriate, drug information specific to caring for the elderly is included.

Sun Damage and Photoaging

Skin color is defined by photo types, a measure of tanning ability. These range from I (pale, white, never tans) to VI (dark brown or black, never burns). Skin color is relevant not only for ease of vitamin D synthesis but for risks of photoaging and other skin damage. In general, more darkly pigmented skin is thicker and more elastic in nature.

Exposure to ultraviolet (UV) radiation, whether from the sun or from artificial light tanning sources, causes long-term damage to the skin. In addition, prolonged exposure to the sun is associated with an increased risk for developing melanoma. UV refers to high-frequency, short wavelength light, not within the visible spectrum of the human eye and is divided into categories UVA, UVB, and UVC; based on the length of the light waves. UVA reaches the earth's surface consistently unaffected by atmospheric condition or location on the planet. Approximately 10% of UVB reaches the earth's surface. The amount of UVB that reaches the earth's surface is affected by latitude and elevation, degree of cloud cover, and proximity to industrial areas. UVC is absorbed by the atmosphere, including ozone, oxygen, carbon dioxide, and water vapor. Both UVA and UVB produce tissue injury. UVA penetrates more deeply into the skin, while UVB primarily affects the upper skin layers and is the cause of sunburns. The mechanisms by which UV affects the skin include breakdown of collagen, promotion of free radicals, interference with intracellular repairs, and suppression of immune responses.

Among the visible effects of skin damage are pigment changes (freckles, liver spots), wrinkling, **actinic keratoses**, and **seborrheic keratoses**. Actinic keratosis, a premalignant lesion, can be found in more than half of light-skinned elderly women living in sunny climates.[7] UV exposure is a major factor in the development of skin cancers—melanoma, basal cell, and squamous cell carcinomas.

Sunscreens and Sunblocks

Sunblocks reflect light and provide a barrier to 99% of the UV light. Common ingredients in sunblocks are titanium dioxide and zinc oxide, which are inert and not absorbed into the skin. A sunscreen is any topical product applied to the skin that blocks ultraviolet (UV) radiation. Sunscreens provide short-term protection against burns, the long-term effects of photoaging, and the development of skin cancers.

Sunscreens block differing amounts of UVA and UVB. The **sun protection factor** (SPF) refers to the length of time sun exposure can be extended without burning (Box 26-1). SPF 15 blocks approximately 93% of radiation; an SPF of 50 blocks more than 98%. Regular reapplication of any sunscreen is necessary. To block UVA, a broad-spectrum sunscreen with multiple components is necessary.

Sunscreens are classified as a drug by the United States FDA. Common ingredients in sunscreens include dibenzoyl methanes, cinnamates, salicylates, benzophenone, and para-aminobenzoic acid (PABA), which has derivatives padimate A and O and glyceryl PABA that can be added as well.[8] Benzophenone and dibenzoyl methanes are effective against UVA.

Contact dermatitis, photoallergic responses, and urticaria may occur following exposure to sunscreen ingredients, although these reactions are less common with newer preparations that do not contain PABA, methyl PABA, or benzophenone-10. There is the possibility of decreased vitamin D absorption with prolonged use of sunscreens; but evidence does not support an increase in osteoporosis or other adverse effects related to potential disturbance of vitamin D synthesis.[9]

Choice of a sunscreen should be based on possible allergic reactions to the screening agent or the vehicle, acceptability of the texture and other characteristics of the product, and degree of sun protection needed. Broad-spectrum agents that protect against both UVA and UBV should be recommended. Topical PABA has minimal absorption and is probably safe for use in pregnancy and lactation, although there is no human research available. There is some suggestion that PABA-free sunscreens may induce fewer allergic reactions, and therefore, are better for the elderly who tend to be at risk for allergies.

Box 26-1 Principles for Using a Sunscreen or Sunblock

The sun protection factor (SPF) is a measure of how long it takes to burn when exposed to UVB radiation when the skin is protected by a sunscreen. Let's assume the average person receives a mild sunburn after 20 minutes without sunscreen. Multiplying the SPF number by the number 20 gives an estimate of how many minutes one can stay in the sun with the sunscreen applied without burning. When 20 minutes is multiplied by SPF 15, this suggests that one application would provide this person with 5 hours of protection.

There are indications for more frequent applications, including fair skin, swimming, and perspiring. When in doubt, reapply.

Application should be on all skin that is exposed, including lips, ears, and neck.

Pay attention to expiration dates that should be printed on products—but if not apparent, the shelf life usually is 3 years.

Look for ingredients that block UVA radiation. The American Academy of Dermatology recommends using a broad-spectrum sunscreen that lists one of these active ingredients: octinoxate, octisalate, oxybenzone, benzophenone, and methyl anthranilate; for sunblock, look for the active ingredients titanium dioxide, iron oxide, or zinc oxide. The American Academy of Dermatology Seal of Recognition is on the labels of sunscreens that have been approved by this organization.

General Considerations

Identifying Skin Changes

Skin changes are described in terms of type, color, shape, distribution, and appearance. The importance of assessing these characteristics in forming a diagnosis and planning treatment cannot be overstressed. Careful consideration is critical. For example, a linear vesicular lesion on a woman's cheek is likely to be caused by an allergic response, such as exposure to poison ivy. Conversely, multiple lesions clustered on the cheek suggest an herpetic etiology.

Dermatologic Reactions to Medications

Many medications produce responses in the skin and/or mucous membranes. Some of these are side effects, while others represent allergic responses or damage to the tissue. These changes are distinguished by type of lesion, location and pattern, timing, and duration. The skin changes may be localized or general, present only on a limited area of the body or broadly, or cause hair loss, itching, or a sunburn rash. In many cases, removal of the allergen and supportive care to ease symptoms is the only intervention; in others, medical treatment, such as the application of a cortisone cream or sunblock may be required. Examples of the types of skin changes and medications associated with each are listed in Table 26-2.

Topical Therapy in Dermatology

Unlike pharmacotherapeutics used to treat conditions in other body systems, many of the treatments recommended for dermatologic conditions are topical. For some women, use of a topical agent may be more acceptable than an oral therapy. When compared to oral therapy, topical agents frequently have much lower levels of systemic absorption, plasma concentration, and bioavailability. Topical administration avoids the first-pass effect of oral therapy, in which passage through the gastrointestinal system into the portal circulation and liver blunts the bioavailability of medications. The choice of a vehicle for topical drugs controls the degree and speed of absorption. In particular, transdermal patches provide a steady dose of medication without peaks and troughs. These pharmacokinetic effects become important in order to limit side effects. During pregnancy and lactation, use of an agent less well absorbed into the bloodstream decreases fetal or infant exposure.

Table 26-2 Examples of Dermatologic Reactions to Medications

Drug or Drug Categories—Generic (Brand)	Dermatologic Reaction	Clinical Picture
Anticoagulants Antimetabolites Norethindrone	Alopecia	Hair loss
Androgenic agents Contraceptive hormones Corticosteroids	Acneform	Cysts, pustules
Bacitracin (Neosporin) Chlorhexidine (Hibiclens)	Contact dermatitis	Papular, localized to area of exposure
Barbiturates Epinephrine Iodine Penicillin Phenytoin (Dilantin) Sulfas Tetracyclines	Fixed eruptions	Nodules in a single location with reexposure to a medication
Quinidine (Quinaglute) Thiazides	Lichenoid	Firm scaling plaques
Anticonvulsants Barbiturates Insulin Salicylates Sulfas Tetracyclines	Morbilliform	Separated, edematous, erythematous papules
Antihistamines Diuretics Fluoroquinolones NSAIDs Sulfas Thiazides Tricyclic antidepressants	Photosensitization	Erythema with papules, edema, blistering in exposed areas
Anticoagulants Corticosteroids Penicillin Sulfas	Purpura	Red or purple discoloration from bleeding under the skin
Vancomycin (Vancocin) Other antibiotics producing powerful antihistamine responses	Red man syndrome	Flushing, pruritus accompanied by hypotension and muscle weakness
NSAIDs Penicillins Phenytoin (Dilantin) Sulfas	Stevens-Johnson syndrome	Papules, bullae, and vesicles, including mucous membrane lesions occurring within weeks of exposure to the allergen
Barbiturates Meperidine (Demerol) Nitrofurantoin (Macrobid) Penicillin Tetracyclines	Urticaria	Raised skin wheals

Delivery of medication topically involves a variety of factors including both active and inactive components of a topical agent, degree of adherence to the skin, level of absorption, and general moisturizing or drying effect

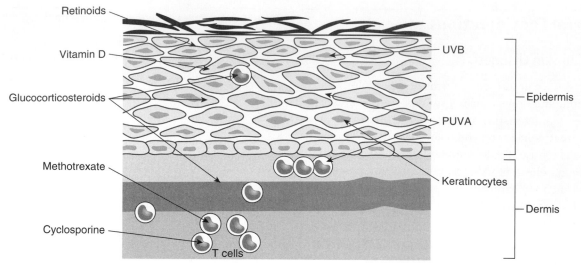

The skin is a multicellular organ containing numerous cells and structures as well as circulating T cells that are targets for dermatologic drugs.

Figure 26-2 Skin as a pharmacologic target.

of the medication on different components of the skin's layers as illustrated in Figure 26-2. Tolerability of topical medications is dependent on skin type, thickness, and sensitivity, and is generally assessed by degree of erythema, dryness, peeling, or other adverse local effects.

Both the active medication and the vehicle in which it is administered can affect the tolerability of a medication. Table 26-3 lists some common inactive components or vehicles associated with topical preparations.

The rule of nines provides a way to characterize the relative surface area to be treated. Originally developed as a method of describing the percentage of body surface injured by burns, it can also be used in describing the distribution of skin lesions or area to be treated (Figure 26-3).

Skin Lesions

Actinic keratosis, a precancerous condition found on exposed skin, is the result of UV damage. The appearance is flat, dry, and variable in color. About 1–5% of all actinic keratoses proceed to squamous cell carcinoma. Actinic keratosis can be removed surgically or treated medically. One of several products, including 5-fluorouracil (5-FU), imiquimod (Aldara), or retinoids can be used to treat actinic keratosis medically.

Imiquimod (Aldara)

Imiquimod (Aldara) is a topical immune modulator that acts by inducing interferons alpha and gamma, tumor necrosis factor, and interleukin. A single packet is applied two to three times a week for up to 16 weeks. During use of imiquimod, sun exposure should be avoided. Adverse effects include erythema, oozing and swelling of tissue, and scaly or crusted skin in the treated area. Two studies have found that three-times weekly application for 4 weeks, with 4-week rest between treatment cycles, cleared all lesions in 50–69% of individuals.[10] In one of these studies, 75% of those in remission continued to be free of lesions at the 12-week period.[11] Animal studies have demonstrated increased pregnancy risks, resulting in an FDA Pregnancy Category C rating. There is no information about the use of imiquimod during lactation. Imiquimod has been suggested as a possible substitute for surgery for melanomas when elderly women are poor surgical candidates. A randomized trial comparing imiquimod to 5-FU and cryosurgery found that sustained remission of lesions over 12 months was present in 73% of individuals receiving imiquimod, versus 33% using 5-FU and 4% who had cryosurgery.[12]

5-Fluorouracil (5-FU)

5-Fluorouracil (5-FU) is available in several formulations—a 5% cream, 2% solution, 1% cream or solution, or

Table 26-3 Vehicles Used for Topical Medications

Cream	An emulsion of oil in water, absorbs well, lubricating.
Emulsion	Stable mixtures of oil, water, and surfactant; often categorized as water in oil or oil in water; microemulsions commonly used with cosmetics.
Foam	Gas bubbles suspended in substance to enhance spread of agent.
Gel	Water or alcohol based with polymer as thickener; less well absorbed than other agents.
Lotion	Suspended powder in water or water and oil, easy to apply, cooling; less potency than creams, gels, or ointments.
Oil	Viscous liquid or liquefiable substance that often is used as a vehicle for botanicals or other agents. Easily spread on skin, may form protective cover, although it is thinner than cream or ointment so it does not remain as stable as those vehicles.
Ointment	Oil-based, thick, adherent to skin, lubricating. Most effective medium for hydration and absorption, so the potency of a drug will be highest when it is formulated in an ointment.
Paste	Semisolid preparations containing a high proportion of finely powdered material.
Powder	A solid that has been pulverized into tiny loose particles to be combined with a pharmacologic agent and spread on skin.
Soaks	Agent dissolved in water; least hydrating of all vehicles.
Solution	Dissolved substance in water, alcohol, or glycol; more drying than other agents, although more hydrating than soaks or lotions.
Spray	Drugs in the form of dispersed droplets contained in water or other liquid and delivered via a dedicated device in a fine mist.
Tape	An occlusive dressing with medication (e.g., steroid) impregnated within the tape.

Note: In general, drying preparations are for use in acute inflammation, and hydrating preparations are for chronic inflammation.

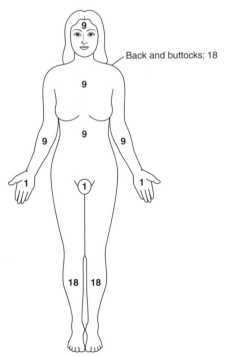

On an adult, the relative proportions are:
Head 9%
Chest front 9%
Abdomen front 9%
Back and buttocks 18%
Each arm 9%
Each leg 18% (9% front, 9% back)
Each palm 1%
Groin 1%

Figure 26-3 The rule of nines.

0.5% micronized cream. This agent blocks DNA synthesis within cells to prevent proliferation. The 5% cream is applied twice daily for up to 6 weeks. The micronized cream is applied once daily. Inflammatory responses may be induced with application of 5-FU. A comparison of daily versus weekly dosing found twice-daily treatment to be significantly more effective ($P = .01$) 24 weeks after treatment.[13] Contraindications include hypersensitivity and pregnancy. 5-FU is teratogenic in humans. It is to be avoided during breastfeeding due to its disruption of genetic and protein synthesis.

Skin Cancers

Nonmelanoma skin cancers, including both basal and squamous cell tumors, are managed by cancer specialists. Surgical treatment is considered standard. For individuals who wish to avoid surgery or who are medically fragile, such as some elderly, the use of topical chemotherapy may be considered as described for actinic keratosis management.

Dermatitis

The term *dermatitis* includes a variety of skin conditions, ranging from allergic responses to infectious processes. This section includes a discussion of xerosis, pruritus, atopic dermatitis (eczema), contact dermatitis, psoriasis, **acne** vulgaris, acne rosacea, and intertrigo. Bacterial skin infections are addressed in a separate section.

Xerosis (Dry Skin)

Xerosis is the condition of extreme skin dryness. The appearance of the skin is dry, flaky, roughened, or cracked. The skin may be irritated and the woman most likely experiences chronic itching. In persons prone to atopic dermatitis, xerosis may precipitate recurrences of the atopic dermatitis. Dehydration, or decreased water storage in the stratum corneum of the skin, also precipitates the symptoms. Aging, excessive washing, and exposure to extreme weather conditions can also further contribute to the problem.

Basic therapy for xerosis is the application of an emollient or moisturizer for xerosis. Creams are the most common formulation. Emollients provide a barrier to protect and sooth the skin, including those that are petroleum based. Moisturizers differ from other emollients in that they may have an added **humectant**–an ingredient that absorbs water thereby moisturizing the area to which the humectant is applied. Products containing urea (e.g., Aqua Care, Carmol) or ammonium lactate (e.g., Lac-Hydrin) are commonly recommended.[14] The most common side effect of the use of emollients and moisturizers is stinging or other skin sensations. True allergies are uncommon.

Aqua Care and Carmol are over-the-counter (OTC) preparations of 10% urea, which acts as a humectant. The lotion is applied twice daily. Carmol-HC, available by prescription, contains hydrocortisone to decrease inflammation and should be used only for inflammatory skin conditions. Preparations that contain hydrocortisone are FDA Pregnancy Category C (animal studies indicate teratogenetic potential of steroids); no information about breast milk transfer is available. Urea/hydrocortisone products are commonly used for elderly women and no special considerations have been noted.

Ammonium lactate (Lac-Hydrin 12%) cream or ointment is available by prescription and over the counter as AmLactin 12%. The two formulations have the same ingredients. It is applied twice daily to affected areas. Improvement should be expected within 1 week. Application to the face or to abraded skin should be avoided due to increased absorption. This agent is FDA Pregnancy Category B. Minimal absorption would be expected and the risk during breastfeeding with topical application is low; however, there is inadequate evidence to ensure safety. No specific recommendations or cautions appear to be associated with use of the drug among older women.

Pruritus

Itching commonly is related to a variety of skin conditions as well as many systemic diseases. There are many etiologies of pruritus including irritation of the skin, neurologic responses to disease, and psychologic responses to a stressful situation. In every case, itching should not be treated without an assessment of possible causes. If there is no apparent dermatologic source of the irritation, laboratory testing should include at least a complete blood count, assessment of thyroid, liver and kidney function, and blood glucose.[15] This general panel will assist in identifying infectious, endocrine, and metabolic causes underlying the symptoms. Other possible screens would include stool samples for ova and parasites indicating a helminthic condition or imaging to identify malignant processes such as lymphoma.[6]

Treatment of pruritus includes topical therapy, with antihistamines (e.g., diphenhydramine [Benadryl gel]), emollients, low-potency steroids, calamine, camphor or menthol, or anesthetics (e.g., pramoxine [PrameGel, ProctoFoam]) recommended for temporary relief. Herbal or botanic remedies (e.g., witch hazel, chamomile, aloe vera) and nutritional supplementation with vitamins D and E and linoleic acid are also used.[16] Further recommendations are discussed in association with specific conditions.

Eczema

Eczema is the product of both genetic influences and inflammatory responses. This condition generally is seen initially in early childhood and often is associated with a personal or family history of childhood asthma. As many as 17% of the American population has symptoms of eczema or atopic dermatitis.[17] Of those, approximately one quarter have chronic symptoms without remission.[5] Criteria for the diagnosis include dry pruritic skin, primarily in flexural areas (e.g., elbow, neck creases), often thickened and with pronounced texture. Vesicles may or may not be present.[18] When signs of infection are present, topical or oral antibiotics usually are prescribed, and the woman to whom it is prescribed is referred for follow-up with a dermatologist.

In addition to medication management, counseling should include information about identifying and avoiding environmental stimuli and allergens that cause symptoms, treatment of secondary infections, and use of antihistamines for symptomatic relief. Table 26-4 lists common antihistamine choices; the newer nonsedating products may be preferred for daytime use. Antihistamine dosing may need to be at the upper end of the range for best effect.

In one study, skin lubrication to reduce dryness reduced the need for corticosteroid treatment up to 50%.[19] A thick cream or ointment should be recommended, rather than a

Table 26-4 Antihistamines for Relief of Pruritus

Name Generic (Brand)	Dose	Side Effects	Selected Drug Interactions		Contraindications	FDA Pregnancy Category
Sedating						
Chlorpheniramine maleate (Chlor-Trimeton)	4 mg orally at bedtime	Drowsiness, decreased mental capacity, dry mouth	Procarbazine (Matulane)	Potentiate CNS depression	Hypersensitivity	C based on animal studies
			Phenytoin (Dilantin) Fosphenytoin	Increased toxicity of phenytoin		
			Belladonna (anticholinergic activity increased)	Potentiate anticholinergic activity		
Diphenhydramine hydrochloride (Benadryl)	25–50 mg PO three times daily to four times daily	Drowsiness, decreased mental capacity, dry mouth	Alcohol and other CNS depressants including opiate	Potentiate CNS depression	Hypersensitivity to antihistamines	B
			MAO inhibitors (increase drying effect)	Potentiate anticholinergic activity		
Hydroxyzine (Vistaril, Atarax)	25 mg orally three times daily to four times daily	Drowsiness, allergic response, tremor, headache, rash	Procarbazine (Matulane) (CNS depression)		Hypersensitivity, early pregnancy	C based on animal studies
Nonsedating						
Cetirizine (Zyrtec)	10 mg orally	Drowsiness, nervousness, dry mouth, dry skin, nausea, allergic reaction, seizure, irregular heartbeat	High-dose theophylline (Theo-Dur)	Decrease cetirizine clearance	Hypersensitivity, use with caution in those with liver or kidney insufficiency	B
Fexofenadine (Allegra)	60 mg twice daily		Ketoconazole (Nizoral)	Potentiate fexofenadine	Hypersensitivity, use with caution in those with liver or kidney insufficiency	C based on animal studies
			Erythromycin (E-mycin)	Potentiate fexofenadine		
			Aluminium magnesium antacids	Decrease fexofenadine		
Loratadine (Claritin)	10 mg orally daily	Drowsiness, nervousness, dry mouth, dry skin, nausea, allergic reaction, seizure, irregular heartbeat	Cimetidine (Tagamet)	Potentiate loratadine	Hypersensitivity, use with caution in those with liver or kidney insufficiency	B
			Amiodarone (Cordarone)	Prolongation of QT interval torsade de pointes		

lotion. Since lotions have more water in their mixture than creams, they are more likely to dehydrate the skin. Common hydrating products that can be recommended include dimethicone, glycerin, colloidal oatmeal, and petrolatum. Generic versions of all these products are available; common brand names include Cetaphil (dimethicone and glycerin); Eucerin (colloidal oatmeal, glycerin, and lanolin among other components); and Aquaphor (petrolatum product).

Atopic Dermatitis

Atopic dermatitis is a chronic relapsing form of eczema. Treatments for atopic dermatitis include topical and oral steroids that reduce the inflammatory process; topical and oral calcineurin inhibitors; and ultraviolet light therapy. A dermatologist or other provider skilled in the management of skin diseases should manage all of these agents with the exception of the topical preparations.

Topical Steroids

Topical glucocorticoids can be prescribed in several levels of potency (class I–VII) with class I being most powerful. Use of topical steroids produces significant relief for up to 80% of those using them.[20] When choosing a prescription, both the strength of the medication and the carrier (e.g., ointment, lotion, solution) should be considered.

In general, the most potent drugs should be prescribed by a dermatologist, although they are included in Table 26-5 for the sake of completeness. The lowest effective potency and dose should be prescribed initially for acute treatment, based on degree of eczematous symptoms. Factors in drug choice include the location of the lesion on the body (thinner areas of skin absorb more of the drug); the presence of skin damage that increases absorption through the exposed dermis; and the amount of tissue to be covered. Thin areas of skin are more susceptible to side effects of the drug. Areas where skin touches skin also absorb more of the drug. In general, larger skin areas and thinner-skinned areas (such as the face and genitals) are treated with milder preparations. All corticosteroids, both oral and topical, are FDA Pregnancy Category C drugs, based on adverse effects in animal studies. Glucocorticoids are considered

Table 26-5 Topical Steroids—Least to Most Potent by Class

Potency (I Is Most Potent)	Generic Name	Brand Names/Percent Active Ingredient/Vehicle
VII	Hydrocortisone widely available as generic	LactiCare/1.0-AC/lotion LactiCare/2.5-AC/lotion
		Hytone/2.5/cream, lotion, ointment
	Hydrocortisone acetate	Epifoam/1.0
VI	Desonide	DesOwen/0.05/cream, lotion
	Flurandrenolide	Cordran SP/0.025/cream
	Fluocinolone acetonide	Capex/0.01/shampoo Derma-Smoothe/0.01
	Prednicarbate	Aclovate/0.05/cream, ointment
	Triamcinolone acetonide	Aristocort A/0.025/cream
V	Betamethasone valerate cream	Betatrex/0.1/cream
	Clocortolone pivalate	Cloderm/0.1/cream
	Desonide	DesOwen/0.05/ointment Tridesilon/0.05/ointment
	Fluocinolone acetonide	Synalar/0.025/cream Synemol/0.025/cream
	Flurandrenolide	Cordran SP/0.05/cream Cordran/0.5/ lotion Cordran/0.025/ointment
	Hydrocortisone butyrate	Locoid/0.1/cream Locoid Lipocream/0.1/ointment, solution
	Hydrocortisone valerate	Westcort/0.2/cream
	Triamcinolone acetamide	Aristocort/0.1/cream Kenalog/0.1/cream, lotion
IV	Amcinonide	Cyclocort/0.1/cream
	Betamethasone valerate	Luxiq/0.12/foam
	Fluocinolone acetonide	Synalar/0.025/ointment
	Flurandrenolide	Cordran/0.05/ointment
	Mometasone furoate	Elocon/0.1/cream, lotion
	Prednicarbate	Dermatop-E/0.1/ointment
	Triamcinolone acetonide	Aristocort A/0.1/ointment Kenalog/0.1/ointment

Potency (I Is Most Potent)	Generic Name	Brand Names/Percent Active Ingredient/Vehicle
III	Amcinonide	Cyclocort/0.1/cream, lotion
	Betamethasone dipropionate	Alphatrex/0.05/cream, ointment Diprosone/0.05/cream, lotion
	Betamethasone valerate	Betatrex/0.1/ointment
	Fluticasone propionate	Cutivate/0.005/ointment
	Mometasone furoate	Elocon/0.1/ointment
	Triamcinolone acetonide	Aristocort A/0.5/cream Kenalog/0.5/cream
II	Amcinonide	Cyclocort/0.1/ointment
	Augmented betamethasone dipropionate	Diprolene AF/0.05/cream
	Betamethasone dipropionate	Diprosone/0.1/aerosol Diprosone/0.05/ointment
	Desoximetasone	Topicort/0.25/cream
	Diflorasone diacetate	Psorcon-E/0.05/cream, ointment
	Fluocinonide	Lidex –E 0.05 Lidex/0.05/cream, gel, ointment, solution
	Halcinonide	Halog/0.1/cream, ointment, solution Halog-E/0.1/cream
	Mometasone furoate	Elocon/0.1/ointment
I	Augmented betamethasone dipropionate	Diprolene/0.05/gel, lotion, ointment
	Clobetasol propionate	Cormax/0.05/cream, ointment, scalp solution Olux/0.05/foam Temovate-E/0.05/cream Temovate/0.05/gel, ointment
	Diflorasone diacetate	Psorcon/0.05/ointment
	Flurandrenolide	Cordran/0.05/tape
	Halobetasol propionate	Ultravate/0.05/cream, ointment

Note: Steroid class varies by preparation (e.g., cream versus lotion) and by percentage of active ingredient, even for products with the same generic or trade name. The prescriber should be attentive to both to avoid error.

compatible with lactation, although some agent is found in breast milk after the drug is consumed orally. Therefore, topical use, with the exclusion of application on the nipples, is preferable.

The evidence from a 2005 systematic review supports the use of once-daily steroid therapy as being similar in effectiveness to more frequent dosing, more cost effective, and less likely to produce adverse effects. However, the authors found that differences in pricing and potency made direct comparisons of products difficult.[21]

Side Effects/Adverse Effects

Over time, use of high-potency topical steroids can cause atrophy of the skin, striae, hypopigmentation, decreased immune function in the skin cells, worsening rosacea and facial telangiectasia, and rare cases of glaucoma following periocular use. Adrenal suppression is an uncommon, albeit serious, effect of topical preparations. Allergic responses to the medication or the vehicle are contraindications to topical use.

In addition to their daily use as first-line management of acute symptoms, topical steroids can be applied once or twice weekly as therapy for maintenance. Berth-Jones et al. evaluated fluticasone (Cutivate) as twice-weekly maintenance dosing and found the cream preparation more effective than ointment; both were more effective than use of an emollient alone in preventing recurrences during a 20-week trial. In that study,[22] persons who used cream were 5.8 times less likely to experience a recurrence than emollient (95% CI, 3.1–10.8; $P <$ .0001) and persons who used ointment were 1.9 times less likely to experience a recurrence than emollient (95% CI, 1.2–3.2; $P =$ .01).

Although oral glucocorticoids can be used for the treatment of particularly severe flares, they are not discussed in depth in this chapter because systemic steroids should not be prescribed in primary care practice, except by those experienced in the management of steroid therapy. Risks of long-term oral steroid use include adrenal insufficiency, decreased bone density, glaucoma, diabetes, and mood changes, among others.

Calcineurin Inhibitors

Calcineurin inhibitors are immune suppressants that inhibit cytokines and reduce inflammation. These drugs bind to intracellular proteins that combine with calcineurin to inhibit cytokine release and thus the activation of T cells. Tacrolimus (Protopic ointment) is similar in

efficacy to high-potency steroids; pimecrolimus (Elidel) is milder in effect.[23] Topical tacrolimus and pimecrolimus usually are prescribed when steroids are not effective in reducing symptoms or when they are not well tolerated. In contrast to the topical steroids, these pharmaceuticals do not increase the risk of skin damage or glaucoma. When using 0.1% tacrolimus for persistent facial or periocular lesions, studies have demonstrated marked reduction of symptoms.[24] Tacrolimus 0.03% has also been shown to be effective, but over time, participants in this study noticed a reduction in improvement with treatment at this lower dose.[25]

Studies also have evaluated the effectiveness of tacrolimus when a steroid, such as betamethasone, is added. Small studies reported by Nakahara et al.[26] and by Furue et al.[27] found relative improvement in symptoms with the steroid-calcineurin inhibitor combination, particularly with regard to skin thickening and lichenification. Furue and colleagues demonstrated effectiveness of tacrolimus plus a glucocorticoid over a 6-month trial of twice weekly maintenance therapy.[27] When combination topical therapies are applied, the steroid is applied first, and the second preparation is applied 15 minutes later so that the vascular dilating effects of the steroid enhances absorption of the second medication.

These agents are not innocuous. In 2006, the FDA issued black box warnings that these drugs are associated with an increased risk of lymphoma and skin cancer with prolonged use. The label includes this information and the FDA has issued a medication guide that should be given to the patient with every prescription. These two drugs should be used as a second-line therapy only if other therapies have failed and should be used for a short time only. Table 26-6 provides prescribing information about these agents.

Both tacrolimus and pimecrolimus are FDA Pregnancy Category C drugs because of inadequate evidence of safety, and similarly safety during breastfeeding is unknown. For the elderly, calcineurin inhibitors generally are effective and have fewer side effects or adverse effects when compared to steroids.

Contact Dermatitis

When dermatitis is caused by direct exposure or contact with a substance, the individual can have an allergic response or an irritant response. The pattern of symptoms of contact dermatitis of either type can be similar, but treatment should be coupled with identification of the trigger substance to avoid recurrences (Box 26-2).

Table 26-6 Topical Calcineurin Inhibitors

Drug Generic (Brand)	Formulation and Dose	Side Effects/Adverse Effects	Contraindications	FDA Pregnancy Category
Pimecrolimus (Elidel)	1% cream twice daily—for eczema, contact dermatitis Apply to affected area in a thin layer	Side effects: Skin irritation, burning, erythema, pharyngitis, flulike symptoms, headache Adverse effect: Increased risk of cancer	Allergy Not approved for long-term use	C
Tacrolimus (Protopic)	0.1% ointment twice daily (0.03% ointment is available for pediatric use and can be used if needed) Apply to affected area in a thin layer	Side effects: Skin irritation, burning, erythema, pharyngitis, flulike symptoms, headache Elevated liver enzymes Adverse effect: Increased risk of cancer	Allergy Not approved for long-term use	C

Box 26-2 A Case of Itchy Palms

An old myth exists that says if the palm of the right hand is itchy, then it foretells that money is coming, but do not scratch it as that stops any payments. If it is the left palm that is itchy, then money will be needed to be paid, so continue to scratch. This case study concerns a woman who had bilateral itchy palms.

KJ is a 30-year-old woman who presented with an irregular, erythematous, highly pruritic rash on the palms of her hands. She currently is taking multivitamins and combination oral contraceptives and finished a course of metronidazole (Flagyl) for treatment of trichomonas vaginalis 3 days ago. She denies any significant health conditions.

One of the major challenges in treatment of persons with dermatologic symptoms is first obtaining the correct diagnosis. Since this woman is being treated with metronidazole, one condition to be included in a differential diagnosis is that of drug side effects. However, in this case, metronidazole is most likely to be associated with fixed drug reactions that most commonly occur up to 8 hours after drug exposure. The site of the hands is a possible site for the reaction to metronidazole, but the timing makes it unlikely.

Palmar rashes also are associated with treponemal infections. This woman is sexually active, has had a sexually transmitted disease (trichomonas vaginalis), and therefore, screening for syphilis is indicated. Rocky Mountain spotted fever also was a possibility, but essentially was ruled out by questioning her.

After taking a careful history and conducting a physical exam, it became apparent that KJ had contact dermatitis.

She currently is working as a produce manager at a supermarket and spends much of her day placing food on displays, including nonorganics that have had pesticides. A common consumer mistake is to use a topical antihistamine in a situation like this. However, irritated skin often does not well absorb the drug and the woman may actually experience more irritation. Alternatively, a systemic antihistamine is a very reasonable option.

KJ responded well to an over-the-counter hydrocortisone cream and nighttime diphenhydramine hydrochloride (Benadryl). Within 24 hours, she noticed an improvement in the rash. Her test for syphillis was found to be negative.

KJ was advised to use protection when touching produce in the future, and it was suggested that she discuss issues of pesticides with her company in order to prevent similar situations with coworkers and potential problems for consumers.

The classic skin allergy is the one occurring after exposure to poison ivy, which, like several other plants, produces urushiol, a powerful allergen. Other common allergies include nickel, chemicals, and preservatives found in clothing and household products as well as antibiotics and topical steroids. The primary symptom of an allergic response is intense itching, accompanied by erythema in the exposed area, papules, and vesicles or oozing with a severe response. Although most allergic dermatitis is caused by an acute exposure, chronic exposure to an irritating substance may lead to the development of similar symptoms.

Treatment for mild allergic responses includes identification and removal of allergen, drying agents, soothing lotions such as calamine (a liquid mixture of zinc oxide and iron) or Aveeno (a combination of colloidal oatmeal, glycerin, and allantoin), and topical steroid creams of moderate potency. Topical antihistamines are frequently offered for relief of the pruritus, although they often are ineffective.

The choice of therapy can be made empirically based on location, the severity of symptoms, and the woman's preference. More severe events may require an oral steroid, either as a dose pack of methylprednisolone (Medrol) or as a tapered prednisone dose (Box 26-3). Oral steroids generally should be taken with food in the morning. Adrenal insufficiency is a significant risk of prolonged steroid therapy; both higher doses and longer regimens may induce the effect. Oral prednisone should not be given for more than 7 days without reducing the dose sequentially (tapering), to avoid triggering adrenal insufficiency. A common dose for a tapered regimen is prednisone 40 mg orally for 5 days, then 20 mg for another 5 days. Hypotension, dehydration, hypoglycemia, and mental confusion are symptoms of acute adrenal insufficiency.

Unlike allergic responses, irritants are more likely to be substances to which there is chronic exposure. As abrasion or chemicals damage skin, the resultant inflammatory response produces the symptoms. While itching may occur, pain, redness, dryness and fissures are the more common symptoms. A systematic review by Saary et al. found some research findings to recommend the use of barrier creams, such as those with the silicon polymer dimethicone (e.g., Cetaphil, Remedy Skin Repair, Johnson's baby cream), lipid rich moisturizers, cotton glove liners, and the use of fabric softeners as strategies to control irritants and prevent skin reactions.[28] However, these authors suggested that larger studies needed to be conducted to determine the efficacy of these products.

Psoriasis

Psoriasis is a chronic skin disorder, affecting both genders and all races. In the United States, the incidence is approximately 2–3%, with onset most common between ages 15 years and 20 years, with a second peak after age 55 years.[29] In psoriasis, overgrowth of keratinocytes and accompanying inflammation occur as a result of a breakdown in the immune system, in which T cells are stimulated and migrate to skin tissue.[21] Normally, it takes approximately a month for skin cells to mature and shed. For women with psoriasis, the cells may mature in a few days, and since the lower layer of skin cells divides more rapidly than normal, dead cells accumulate in thick patches on the epidermis. Several genes that predispose one to develop psoriasis have been identified, as well as environmental triggers that stimulate the onset of symptoms. Among the factors associated with psoriasis are skin infections or injury, medications, stress, and alcohol use. In particular, smoking appears to increase the likelihood of a psoriasis diagnosis.[30]

Plaque psoriasis is the most common type of psoriasis, comprising about 80% of all diagnoses. This condition is characterized by reddened papules and plaques with distinctly outlined silvery, flaking patches of skin, presenting symmetrically. The elbows, knees, and scalp are commonly affected; palms and soles may also be affected. Inverse psoriasis is found in folds of skin, such as the axillae and antecubital and popliteal fossae. Guttate psoriasis generally appears after streptococcal infections and appears as erythematous papules spread across the trunk and extremities.[31] Guttate psoriasis generally has a limited course.

Treatment of psoriasis is determined both by type and severity. Mild psoriasis (< 3% of body surface) can be treated in a stepwise fashion beginning with topical medications. More severe presentations, especially those covering more than 10% of the body surface, should be referred to a dermatologic specialist. The progression of therapy is from topical treatments, light therapy with sunlight or UV radiation, to systemic treatment. Guttate psoriasis is generally treated with UVB light therapy, although long-term antibiotics have been considered, given the relationship of disease onset to skin infections. Either penicillin VK, 1 gram/day or erythromycin 1 gram/day can be given for

---

Box 26-3 Prescribing a Methylprednisolone (Medrol) Dose Pack

Day 1: Six 4-mg tablets

Day 2: Five 4-mg tablets

Day 3: Four 4-mg tablets

Day 4: Three 4-mg tablets

Day 5: Two 4-mg tablets

Day 6: One 4-mg tablet

up to 14 days. There is no evidence that treatment beyond the usual course of antibiotics improves outcomes.[32]

Topical therapy for psoriasis includes many modalities. Topical steroids (Table 26-5), often combined with emollients to soften the skin and create a barrier, are the first line of therapy. The retinoids, agents that are discussed in depth in the section on acne, can be an alternative, as can calcipotriene (Dovonex), salicylic acid creams or ointments, and tar products. The calcineurin inhibitors tacrolimus (Protopic) and pimecrolimus (Elidel) (Table 26-6) are used in more delicate tissue areas such as the face and skin-folds or when steroid-sparing regimens are preferred.

Calcipotriene (Dovonex 0.005%)

Calcipotriene (Dovonex 0.005%) a vitamin D preparation, is available by prescription as an ointment or as a solution. This agent is applied once or twice daily to the affected area for up to 8 weeks. Calcipotriene works by slowing skin cell proliferation; the exact mechanism is unknown. Itching, skin irritation, redness, or peeling may occur with use. Hypercalcemia may occur and use of calcipotriene can cause kidney stones to reoccur in susceptible individuals. This medication will produce sensitivity to sunlight. Pigment changes and skin thinning are rare side effects. There is no evidence about the use of calcipotriene while breastfeeding.

Calcipotriene (Dovonex 0.005%) also is available as a combination preparation with betamethasone under the brand name Taclonex; this preparation may work more rapidly to achieve reduction in psoriasis symptoms than either product alone. Douglas et al. demonstrated a 74.4% reduction in lesion thickness over 4 weeks, compared to 61.3% with betamethasone alone ($P = .0001$) and 55.3% with calcipotriene alone ($P = .0001$).[33] This agent should be applied daily for 4 weeks, after which calcipotriene alone can be continued. The maximum weekly dose should be limited to 100 grams.

Calcipotriene (Dovonex 0.005%) is classified as FDA Pregnancy Category C based on fetal risks in animals treated with the medication in oral formulation. Risk to a fetus is unlikely except among those with a hypersensitivity response to vitamin D.[34] Few of the studies of calcipotriene have included individuals older than the age of 75 years. There are no reports of increased allergic reactions in the elderly but such reactions cannot be ruled out.

Salicylic Acid (SalAc, Dermal Zone)

Salicylic acid (SalAc, Dermal Zone, and multiple other brand names), a nonsteroidal anti-inflammatory agent,

is used as a keratinolytic agent, usually in combination with a steroid. For example, the formulation that is marketed as Diprosalic consists of betamethasone and salicylic acid (Diprosalic). The salicylic acid breaks down keratin, thereby improving absorption of the steroidal component. Concentrations of 2–3% in a variety of formulations are available over the counter; higher concentrations are available by prescription. If a woman has used over-the-counter products without complete resolution, a formulation of not greater than 6% can be prescribed. Higher concentrations are destructive of tissue and should not be used for this purpose. Salicylic acid should not be applied to irritated or inflamed skin, as it may worsen the irritation. Persons with bleeding problems, diabetes, and renal or hepatic disease should use nonsteroidal medications with caution. There is no evidence about the safety of topical salicylates in pregnancy or breastfeeding, although systemic salicylates should be avoided.

Coal Tar

Tar, especially coal tar, is used as an occlusive and emollient and slows the proliferation of skin cells. Over-the-counter products range from 0.5% to 5% active ingredient. Psoriasin ointment (2% coal tar in a petrolatum base with other inactive ingredients) and Psoriasin gel (1.25% coal tar in aloe vera gel with other ingredients) are examples of the many products designed for skin application. Shampoos with tar, such as Tegrin, Neutrogena T/Gel, and Denorex are available for scalp treatment. Coal tar has few side effects, although rash, redness, or irritation may occur. Tar increases sun sensitivity; drug interactions include tetracycline and tretinoin. Women should be cautioned about the risk of staining with the use of tar products. The risk of fetal injury from short-term use during pregnancy is minimal.[22] There is no evidence about the safety of tar products in pregnancy and breastfeeding, nor is there evidence that use of this agent should be modified for elderly individuals.

Other Treatments for Psoriasis: Retinoids, Antimetabolites, and Immune Suppressants

Persons with more severe psoriasis may require ultraviolet light therapy, and/or systemic treatment with retinoids, methotrexate (Rheumatrex, Trexall), cyclosporine, or the immunomodulating biologics. These treatments are managed by a dermatologic specialist.

The **retinoids** are vitamin A analogs. Acitretin (Soriatane) is an oral retinoid approved for use in severe psoriasis at a dose of 25–50 mg once daily. These drugs are believed to work by affecting skin cell proliferation and immune regulation, although the exact mechanism of action is unknown. Common side effects include alopecia, skin dryness, and peeling. Alterations in lipid metabolism, pancreatitis, depression, and pseudotumor cerebri are less common serious adverse effects. Tretinoin (Retin-A, Renova), the topical retinoid preparation, is not FDA approved for treatment of individuals with psoriasis.

Methotrexate (Rheumatrex, Trexall) an antimetabolite and antifolate agent, acts to decrease the production of new skin cells by interfering with cellular metabolism. This agent is an FDA Pregnancy Category X drug since it is a teratogen, and thus, it is contraindicated during pregnancy. Methotrexate is a known abortifacient and is linked to a number of birth defects. This drug is listed as cytotoxic by the AAP, and therefore, it is not to be used during lactation. Elderly with normal renal function appear to be able to take methotrexate without difficulty.

Cyclosporine (Sandimmune), an immune suppressant, has been suggested as another treatment. This agent inhibits lymphocytes and thus decreases T-cell infiltration of the dermis. Both methotrexate and cyclosporine have demonstrated similar effectiveness in treating severe psoriasis.[35]

Most studies of cyclosporine use in pregnancy have been among women who have received an organ transplant. Because these women were taking other medications, the specific contribution of cyclosporine to adverse outcomes is unclear. However, there is little evidence of teratogenicity.[22] Cyclosporine is in FDA Pregnancy Category C secondary to the lack of well-controlled studies. However, both the AAP and the World Health Organization (WHO) advise against breastfeeding if a woman is taking cyclosporine. No evidence has been found to deny the healthy elderly the use of cyclosporine; however, it should be used with caution by a woman of any age who has renal disease.

Biologic Immune Modulators

Biologic immune modulators include alefacept (Amevive), adalimumab (Humira), etanercept (Enbrel), and infliximab (Remicade). Biologics act to stimulate the body's immune system and block the production of T cells or tumor necrosis factor alpha, thus affecting the progression of psoriatic plaques. These products are all administered by injection or infusion (e.g., infliximab). Side effects of this class include a flulike syndrome and injection site inflammation. Because this is a relatively new class of medications, long-term effects are not known. All of the members of this class are FDA Pregnancy Category B drugs. As a class, they cannot be ruled out for breastfeeding risks, due to

lack of information. There are no suggestions to treat older individuals differently based on age.

Acne Vulgaris

Acne vulgaris is the term applied to persistent comedones, nodules, or pustules developing from the pilosebaceous follicles. The pathogenesis of acne vulgaris is based on the following four factors: androgen-mediated hyperstimulation of sebaceus gland activity, which causes increased sebum production; hyperkeratinization, which leads to blockage of the follicular gland, which in turn mixes with the sebum to become impacted within the gland; inflammation that occurs when the follicular epithelium around the mass ruptures; and presence of *Propionibacterium acnes*, which is the dominant bacterium that causes acne vulgaris. The degree of inflammation depends on the individual immune responsiveness. Clinically, acne vulgaris can be noninflammatory, which includes open (blackheads) and closed comedones, or inflammatory, which includes pustules and papules. Acne is also categorized as mild, moderate, or severe, which guides recommended treatment options. The head, neck, and upper trunk are the most common locations for eruptions.

Treatment is divided into preventative/drying and antibacterial categories, and is recommended based on the severity of the outbreak. The use of hormonal contraception offers an additional therapeutic option for managing the symptoms of acne in women of reproductive age.

Several authors describe a stepwise recommendation for choosing the appropriate therapy, recommending topical benzoyl peroxide (Benoxyl, Benzagel, and multiple other brand names) and topical retinoids for mild acne, topical antibiotics with or without retinoids in mild to moderate cases, systemic antibiotics for moderate to severe inflammatory disease, and isotretinoin (Accutane) for the most severe cases of nodular acne. The drugs used are based on both disease severity and the effectiveness of treatment.[36] A secondary goal of this treatment structure is to avoid the prolonged or unnecessary use of antibiotics that may induce resistance in *P acnes*.

Treatment of Mild Acne Vulgaris

Benzoyl peroxide acts to dry and peel away the desquamated epidermis, opening the sebaceous glands, as well as being an antimicrobial agent. It is used in both noninflammatory and inflammatory acne. Benzoyl peroxide is the most cost-effective therapy available for mild acne and is as effective as other regimens, although it may have an unacceptable side effect profile of increased skin irritation.[37]

Azelaic acid (Azelex, Finacea) is a dicarboxylic acid, which occurs naturally in the skin. This agent acts to decrease keratin production and is an antibacterial agent that has been shown to be as effective as tretinoin, benzoyl peroxide, or topical erythromycin (Akne-Mycin) in treating mild to moderate acne.[38] Four to six weeks of treatment with either of these agents is required for an improvement in symptoms to be evident.

For both benzoyl peroxide and azelaic acid, a rash or worsening symptoms of skin irritation require that the clinician be notified, as a contact allergy may be developing. Studies are lacking about benzoyl peroxide in pregnancy, thus it is a Pregnancy Category C drug. Data about use among women who are lactating or who are elderly also are not available, but no case reports of harm have been reported.

Retinoids are vitamin A derivatives that act by normalizing keratinocyte development, reducing inflammation, inhibiting immune factors, and decreasing sebum production, thus preventing comedone formation. Topical preparations, including tretinoin (Retin-A), adapalene (Differin), and tazarotene (Tazorac, Avage), have a 40–70% efficacy in reducing comedones and inflammation. Before beginning any topical retinoid treatment, any woman should discontinue other topical treatments. Adapalene is the best tolerated retinoid. Oral isotretinoin (Accutane, Isotone) is reserved for the treatment of severe acne that does not respond to other therapies. Oral isotretinoin is teratogenic in humans and is therefore prescribed under rigidly controlled conditions discussed later in this chapter. Table 26-7 provides a list of topical retinoid preparations.

Adapalene is an FDA Pregnancy Category C agent because of lack of human data. Tretinoin is teratogenic in humans in systemic form. However, the AAP regards it as usually safe while breastfeeding. As a topical agent, tretinoin may be used with caution during pregnancy. Tazarotene is an FDA Pregnancy Category X drug, on the basis of animal evidence, although there is no good human evidence of malformations, and it appears to have similarly low levels of systemic absorption to the other retinoids when used for acne therapy.[39] There is little information about the use of retinoids during lactation; they should be avoided based on the risks associated with use during pregnancy. Use among elderly does not appear to be different than among any adults, but few studies have explored geriatric prescriptions.

Treatment of Moderate Acne Vulgaris

Topical antibiotics, including clindamycin (Cleocin-T, Clinda-Derm), erythromycin (A/T/S 2%, Erycette, Ben-

zamycin), tetracycline (Actisite, Minocin), and metronidazole (Flagyl) are widely available in generic formulations and are used for the treatment of mild to moderate acne. Benzoyl peroxide and azelaic acid usually are included with the antibiotics since both also demonstrate antimicrobial effects. Table 26-8 lists the doses and adverse effects of these drugs.

Combinations of benzoyl peroxide and clindamycin or erythromycin are more effective than either agent used individually, both in decreasing inflammatory lesions and in overall improvement as assessed by both providers and consumers.[40] Similarly, combination therapy with clindamycin/tretinoin gel (Ziana gel) has superior results than when either component is used individually to treat moderate acne. A report of two randomized trials found improved reduction in both inflammatory ($P = .005$) and noninflammatory ($P = .0004$) lesions.[41] Ozolins et al. compared five topical and oral regimens for management of mild to moderate acne.[42] In this study, benzoyl peroxide/erythromycin combination topical treatment was as effective as either oral oxytetracycline or minocycline and more cost effective.

The use of a combination product for 6–8 weeks is now standard practice. With the exception of benzoyl peroxide and azelaic acid, antimicrobial therapy for acne, whether topical or oral, carries a risk of increasing antibiotic resistance. Individual antibiotic products carry a higher risk of resistance developing when used alone due to selective pressure.

Clindamycin cream (Cleocin-T, Clinda-Derm) is a lincosamide antibiotic. It is bacteriostatic, interfering with bacterial protein synthesis. Used topically for acne, it is directly antibacterial, with small likelihood of side effects other than local irritation. Results can take 12 weeks to be apparent.

Metronidazole gel (Flagyl gel) is a nitroimidazole, approved for use in rosacea, although it can also be prescribed for acne vulgaris. The metabolites of this drug are active and bactericidal. Contraindications to oral metronidazole include anticoagulant therapy, since it potentiates the effect of warfarin (Coumadin) (See Chapter 11 for more information about this drug). The topical gel should be used with caution in women with a history of clotting disorders based on the risks of the oral medication. While complications are less likely with a topical preparation, metronidazole can easily be avoided by using another approved topical treatment. In general, metronidazole gel is used for 3 weeks before improvement typically is seen, and the skin will continue to improve for as much as 6 months after treatment is discontinued.

Table 26-7 Retinoid Therapy

Drug Generic (Brand)	Dose	Formulations	Side Effects/Adverse Effects	Contraindications	FDA Pregnancy Category
Acitretin (Soriatane)	Oral	25–50 mg daily with main meal	Hair loss, skin dryness and peeling, night blindness, alterations in lipid metabolism, pancreatitis, depression, pseudotumor cerebri.	Hypersensitivity. Pregnancy, impaired liver/kidney function, elevated lipid levels, current use of methotrexate or tetracyclines.	X
Adapalene (Differin gl)	Apply 1–2 times daily, thin layer	Gel: 0.3% Cream, solution: 0.1%	Side effects: Photosensitivity, local skin irritation including redness, edema, peeling skin, dryness, itching.	Hypersensitivity. Use with caution with other potentially irritating products or open skin lesions.	C
Micronized isotretinoin	Oral	0.4 mg/kg daily	Dry skin, lips, eyes; itching; photosensitivity; peeling; decreased night vision; vascular fragility (nose bleeds or bleeding gums); nausea; vomiting or diarrhea; stomach pain. Adverse effects: Chest pain, vasculitis, hyperglycemia, thyrotoxicosis, lipid abnormalities, inflammatory bowel disease, pancreatitis, leukocytopenia, anemia, headache, musculoskeletal pain.	Hypersensitivity. Pregnancy.	X
Isotretinoin (Accutane)	Oral	0.5 mg/kg to 1.0 mg/kg daily in divided doses with food Maximum total dose: 120–150 mg/kg	Side effects: Dry skin, lips, eyes; itching; photosensitivity; peeling; decreased night vision; vascular fragility (nose bleeds or bleeding gums). Adverse effects: Elevated triglycerides, hepatotoxicity, hearing loss, pancreatitis, pseudotumor cerebri. Anemia, tachycardia, depression, headaches, jaundice, nausea, vomiting or diarrhea, stomach pain, rectal bleeding, loss of appetite.	Hypersensitivity. Pregnancy. Use with caution by persons with paraben allergy, diabetes, depression, liver disease, cardiac disease, asthma.	X
Tazarotene (Tazorac)	Apply 1–2 times daily	Gel: 0.05%, 0.1% Cream: 0.05%	Side effects: Photosensitivity. Skin irritation including redness, edema, peeling skin, itching. Adverse effects: Hyperlipidemia.	Hypersensitivity. Weak evidence for teratogenicity. Use with caution with irritated or open skin.	X
Tretinoin* (Retin-A, Renova, Avita cream)	Apply daily at bedtime	Cream or gel: 0.01%, 0.025%, 0.05% Solution: 0.05%	Side effects: Photosensitivity, local skin irritation including redness, edema, peeling skin. Adverse effects: Leukocytosis.	Hypersensitivity. Not in pregnancy or with skin lesions or sunburn. Avoid extreme weather.	C
Tretinoin* (Retin-A micro)	Apply daily at bedtime	Gel: 0.04%, 0.1% Active ingredient encapsulated in microspheres	Side effects: Photosensitivity, local skin irritation including redness, edema, peeling skin. Adverse effects: Leukocytosis.	Hypersensitivity. Not in pregnancy or with skin lesions or sunburn. Avoid extreme weather.	D

* Tretinoin is available in an oral format for use *only* to treat acute promyelocytic anemia.

Most topical antibiotics are considered safe during pregnancy. However, because tetracycline taken orally is an FDA Pregnancy Category X drug, topical preparations of tetracycline or oxytetracycline should be avoided in pregnancy. There is little known about breastfeeding considerations with topical antibiotics. Typically, the recommendations follow the recommendations for oral therapy.

Oral Antibiotics

Erythromycin (E-Mycin) and tetracyclines are used to treat moderate to severe acne or when simpler treatments have failed. The tetracyclines cause less antibiotic resistance than erythromycin and are, therefore, favored as first-line therapy.[43] Table 26-9 lists many of the antibiotics used for skin conditions, including those used for

Table 26-8 Topical Antimicrobials

Drug Generic (Brand)	Dose	Formulations	Side Effects/Adverse Effects	Contraindications	FDA Pregnancy Category
Azelaic acid (Azelex, Finacea)	Apply twice daily	Cream: 20% Gel: 15%	Itching, stinging, burning, may cause hypopigmentation Adverse effect: lentigo maligna	Hypersensitivity	B
Bacitracin (Baciguent)	One to three times daily	Ointment	Contact dermatitis	Hypersensitivity; use with caution in myasthenia gravis	C
Benzoyl peroxide	Facial wash one to two times daily Cannot be used simultaneously with retinoids	Gel: 2.5%, 5%, 10% 5% mixed with glycolic acid Solution: 5% mixed with erythromycin	Local irritation, photosensitivity, dryness Bleaching agent; avoid hair and clothing	Hypersensitivity	C
Clindamycin (Cleocin-T)	Apply twice daily	Gel, lotion, solution: 10%	Dry skin, redness, peeling itching, oiliness Rarely with topical application: gastrointestinal upset, diarrhea, colitis, shortness of breath	Hypersensitivity History of ulcerative colitis or antibiotic-associated colitis	B
Erythromycin (Erycette, A/T/S 2%, Benzamycin)	One to two times daily	Gel, ointment: 2% Solution: 1.5%, 2%	Stinging, burning, dryness, peeling, redness	Hypersensitivity	B
Mupirocin (Bactroban)	Ointment: 2% three times daily	MRSA colonization	Burning, itching, headache, nausea, rash	Hypersensitivity	B
Neomycin (Myciguent)	One to three times daily	Ointment	Skin irritation, burning, rash, ototoxicity	Hypersensitivity. Use caution with impaired renal function	C
Polymyxin B/neomycin (Neosporin cream)	10,000 units/gram; 3.5 mg/gram respectively; one to three times daily	Cream	Skin irritation, rash, allergic response	Hypersensitivity Myasthenia gravis	C
Polymyxin B/Bacitracin/ neomycin (Neosporin ointment)	400 units/gram; 3.5 mg/ gram and 5000 units/ gram respectively; one to three times daily	Ointment			
Tetracycline	Twice daily	Ointment: 1%, 3% Solution: 2.2 mg/mL	Dryness, irritation, redness, edema	Hypersensitivity	D

acne. The table includes dose ranges, uses, side effects, and warnings.

Among members of the tetracycline family used for acne are tetracycline, minocycline (Minocin), and doxycycline (Vibramycin). These bacteriostatic antibiotics can be used to treat a broad spectrum of gram-positive and gram-negative bacteria. Anti-infective agents are discussed in more detail in Chapter 11. The tetracycline drugs inhibit the inflammatory properties of normal bacterial flora, an action that contributes to their benefit in treating acne.[44] This drug category is considered bacteriostatic because it interrupts protein synthesis. Subantimicrobial doses of doxycycline have been shown to be effective for treating moderate acne; in one study the reported total decrease in lesions was 52% versus 18% with placebo (P = .01).[45]

The tetracyclines are players in many drug–drug interactions, the most common of which are listed in Table 11-9. When tetracyclines are taken in conjunction with agents that have calcium, magnesium, aluminum, or iron, the absorption of tetracycline is inhibited, and thereby the effectiveness is decreased. Sustained-release forms of doxycycline (Atridox) and minocycline (Solodyn) are now available and may have fewer gastrointestinal effects for some women.

Erythromycin (E-Mycin) is used in the treatment of moderate acne. This macrolide antibiotic has a fairly narrow spectrum and is commonly prescribed in conjunction with benzoyl peroxide. Generally, this agent is prescribed orally in enteric-coated tablets because the base drug is broken down rapidly in the stomach. Erythromycin is an

Table 26-9 Oral Antibacterials Used in Dermatology

Drug Generic (Brand)	Dose Range	Indication	Side Effects/Adverse Effects	Contraindications	FDA Pregnancy Category
Macrolides					
Azithromycin (Zithromax)	500 mg × 1 then 250 mg daily × 5 days	MRSA	Side effects: Diarrhea nausea Adverse effects: Severe allergic response including anaphylaxis or Stevens-Johnson syndrome	Hypersensitivity; use caution with pneumonia, impaired liver or kidney function or prolonged QT interval.	B
Erythromycin	250–750 mg twice daily	Acne	Side effects: Gastrointestinal upset Adverse effects: Decreased liver function, anaphylaxis, cardiac dysrhythmia; diarrhea may indicate _C difficile_	Hypersensitivity, current use.	B-oral
Lincosamide					
Clindamycin hydrochloride (Cleocin)	150–450 mg every 6 hours	MRSA	Side effects: Rash, diarrhea, nausea Adverse effects: Jaundice, pseudomembranous colitis	Hypersensitivity. Simultaneous use of erythromycin. Use with caution with history of colitis, atopy.	B
Cephalosporins					
Cefaclor (Ceclor, Ceclor CD)	250–500 mg every 8 hours ER-375 mg every 12 hours	Skin or subcutaneous infections	Nausea, diarrhea, rash, arthralgia	Hypersensitivity; use caution with penicillin sensitivity, history of colitis.	B
Cefadroxil monohydrate (Duricef)	1 g every day	Skin or subcutaneous infections	Diarrhea, nausea, rash	Hypersensitivity; use caution with penicillin sensitivity, history of colitis.	B
Cephalexin (Keflex)	250 mg every 6 hours or 500 mg every 12 hours	Skin or subcutaneous infections	Nausea, diarrhea, increased liver enzymes	Hypersensitivity; use caution with penicillin sensitivity, history of colitis.	B
Fluoroquinolones					
Ciprofloxacin (Cipro)	400–750 mg orally, every 8–12 hours	Adverse skin infections	Side effects: Rash, diarrhea, nausea, dizziness, headache, tendinitis Adverse effects: Peripheral neuropathy	Hypersensitivity; use caution with alkaline urine, seizure disorder, renal impairment, excessive sunlight.	C
Levofloxacin (Levaquin)	500–750 mg daily	Adverse skin infections	Side effects: Nausea, diarrhea, constipation, headache, hypoglycemia Adverse effects: Prolonged QT interval, liver failure, anemias, tendon rupture, acute renal failure	Hypersensitivity; use caution with CNS disorders, steroid use, diabetes, impaired renal function.	C
Penicillins					
Amoxicillin/ clavulanate (Augmentin)	250 mg every 8 hours or 500 mg q 12 hours	_Staphylococcus aureus, Escherichia coli, Klebsiella_ spp.	Nausea, diarrhea, vaginitis, headache, transient elevation of liver functions, transient anemia	Hypersensitivity; use with caution in liver dysfunction; contraindicated if prior liver symptoms with Augmentin.	B
Dicloxacillin sodium (Dynapen)	250–500 mg every 6 hours	_Staphylococcus_	Nausea, GI upset (take 1 hour before or 2 hours after eating)	Hypersensitivity to drug or to cephalosporins.	C
Sulfonamides					
Trimethoprim-sulfamethoxazole (Bactrim)	1 DS twice daily	MRSA	Side effects: GI distress, urticaria, rash Adverse effects: Aplastic anemia, agranulocytosis, hepatic disease	Hypersensitivity. Pregnancy at term. Folate deficiency. Use with caution in those with G6PD, asthma.	C

(continues)

Table 26-9 Oral Antibacterials Used in Dermatology (*continued*)

Drug Generic (Brand)	Dose Range	Indication	Side Effects/Adverse Effects	Contraindications	FDA Pregnancy Category
Tetracyclines					
Doxycycline (Vibramycin, Atridox)	100 mg twice daily	Acne vulgaris			D
	50–100 mg twice daily	Acne rosacea	Side effects: Photosensitivity Lightheadedness, vertigo, GI upset, diarrhea, vaginitis Adverse effects: pseudotumor cerebri, hepatotoxicity, CNS symptoms	Hypersensitivity. Warnings: In pregnancy, fetal tooth damage and possible bone damage. Use with caution in those with renal or liver impairment or SLE.	
	100 mg twice daily day for 7 days	MRSA			
Minocycline (Minocin, Solodyn)	100 mg twice daily	Acne vulgaris Acne rosacea MRSA			D
Tetracycline	250–500 mg twice daily	Acne vulgaris Acne rosacea			D

MRSA = methicillin-resistant staphylococcus aureus.

FDA Pregnancy Category B drug and is compatible with breastfeeding.

The concern that antibiotics decrease the effectiveness of oral contraceptive interactions appears to be based on conflicting evidence. Overall, although pregnancy rates are higher than perfect use predictions in women who take tetracyclines while using oral contraceptives, the failure rates are well within the values expected in normal use of oral contraceptives.[46] The literature on unintended pregnancies in women taking both antibiotics and oral contraceptives is sparse at best. Archer reports that pharmacokinetic data do not support this association, with the exception of rifampin (Rifadin).[47]

Metabolism of most antibiotics occurs in the liver via the CYP450 enzyme pathway. Erythromycin inhibits CYP3A4 and CYP1A2, which places them in the position of being involved in many drug–drug interactions (Table 11-6). One of the most common drug–drug interactions involves erythromycin (E-Mycin) and carbamazepine (Tegretol). The effect of erythromycin on the enzymes that metabolize carbamazepine is substantial, and carbamazepine toxicity can occur. These two drugs should not be taken concurrently. Drug–herb interactions involving erythromycin also are possible.[48] Providers are advised to both ask women about their use of complementary and alternative medications and to check for possible interactions between those products and prescribed medications.

Treatment of Severe Acne Vulgaris: Isotretinoin (Accutane)

Oral isotretinoin (Accutane) is a naturally occurring vitamin A metabolite that is the only acne vulgaris treatment that acts to correct all four pathologic mechanisms. Persons who need isotretinoin treatment will be cared for by a dermatologist or other provider skilled in the management of severe acne. This pharmaceutical causes major birth defects if taken by pregnant women and has serious adverse reactions that can affect the individual who uses it. Clinicians who prescribe isotretinoin, wholesalers who distribute it, pharmacists who dispense it, and persons who take it are required by the FDA to be part of a risk management program called iPLEDGE[49] (Box 26-4).

Isotretinoin is very lipophilic, and absorption is enhanced if taken with a meal high in fat. Given the high risk of congenital abnormalities when isotretinoin is taken during pregnancy, women of childbearing age who take isotretinoin are counseled to use two methods of birth control simultaneously, and they are advised that they should not donate blood while taking this medication.

Common side effects of isotretinoin (Accutane) include muscle aches, which occur in approximately 16% of persons who take this drug, dryness of the eyes, and dry skin and oral mucosa. Adverse effects include hyperlipidemia, an increased risk of depression, rarely psychosis or suicidal ideation, pseudotumor cerebri (especially if the agent is used in conjunction with tetracyclines), pancreatitis, hepatotoxicity, irritable bowel syndrome, decreased night vision, and hearing loss.

Isotretinoin is metabolized by the CYP450 enzymes. Clinically significant drug–drug interactions occur if it is taken concurrently with carbamazepine (Tegretol), vitamin A, methotrexate (Rheumatrex, Trexall), or a tetracycline. There may be a decreased efficacy of any hormonal contraceptive method, although this effect is individual and variable.[50]

The most important contraindication is pregnancy because the risk of congenital malformations is high and includes craniofacial, cardiac, and central nervous system

Box 26-4 Isotretinoin (Accutane)

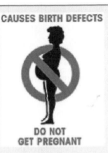

CAUSES BIRTH DEFECTS

DO NOT
GET PREGNANT

Isotretinoin (Accutane) was developed as a chemotherapeutic drug. It is an established cancer treatment even today because isotretinoin kills rapidly dividing cells, a hallmark characteristic of cancer cells.

In the 1930s, high doses of vitamin A were used to treat acne. The pharmaceutical company Hoffman-La Roche conducted multiple studies and eventually created isotretinoin, which is a retinoid or vitamin A derivative. Isotretinoin was approved by the FDA in 1982 for treatment of acne.

Isotretinoin's lethal action on dividing cells became obviously problematic during pregnancy. The first report of an infant born with malformations that appeared to be secondary to maternal use of isotretinoin was published in 1983. In 1984, the FDA issued a black box warning that recommended use of contraception 1 month prior to initiation of therapy and evidence of a negative pregnancy testing prior when the drug was prescribed.

Over time, additional adverse effects were revealed. In 2007, the FDA issued an additional black box warning that recommends users of isotretinoin be monitored for signs of depression or suicide ideation. In addition, pregnancies continued to occur among users of isotretinoin despite use of educational handouts and voluntary participation in voluntary risk management programs.

Today all parties involved in prescribing this drug must register with the iPLEDGE program. The iPLEDGE program is a computer-based risk management program that helps prescribers and individuals who take the drug comply with monthly requirements that are reported to the program. Wholesalers, pharmacists, healthcare providers who prescribe isotretinoin, and the individuals who take this drug participate in the program's reporting requirements. All women who use isotretinoin are required to:

1. Register with the iPLEDGE program and access it monthly to reply to questions about the program's requirements.

2. Obtain baseline liver function values and two negative pregnancy tests before receiving the first prescription.

3. Use two forms of contraception for 1 month prior to starting therapy, during therapy with isotretinoin, and for 2 months after discontinuing the drug. The primary contraceptive agent must be tubal sterilization, partner's vasectomy, hormonal contraception (combined oral contraceptives or patch, vaginal ring, or implantable device). The secondary contraceptive must be a latex condom, diaphragm, cervical cap, or vaginal sponge.

4. Sign a patient information consent form.

5. Review the medication guide and present evidence of a recent pregnancy test with negative results each month when the prescription is renewed. No more than a 30-day supply is prescribed.

6. Fill the prescription within 7 days of a negative pregnancy test and within 30 days of being issued the prescription.

7. Avoid donating blood until 1 month after the drug is discontinued.

8. Agree not to share the drug or obtain it over the Internet.

injuries.[51] Additional contraindications include breastfeeding and not using contraception.

There is no evidence available about the effect of isotretinoin during lactation. Current studies, especially among the elderly, are being conducted to explore if any association exists between isotretinoin and behavioral changes, decrease in folate, and even potential increase in degenerative diseases. However, no strong evidence of such associations is available at this time.

Oral Contraceptives

The use of combination oral contraceptives to treat moderate acne is based on their ability to suppress androgen expression through increased sex hormone binding globulin. Ethinyl estradiol/triphasic norgestimate (Ortho Tri-Cyclen), 20 mcg ethinyl estradiol/levonorgestrel (Alesse), and ethinyl estradiol/drospirenone (Yaz) all have FDA-approved indications for the treatment of acne; but other combined oral contraceptives with similarly low androgen-progesterone ratios have similar overall effects.[52] Triphasic norgestimate/ethynyl estradiol has been shown to reduce both total lesions (mean reduction 46.4% versus 33.9% with placebo; P = .001) and inflammatory lesions (mean reduction 51.4% versus 34.6%; P = .01).[53] Both drospirenone-containing contraceptives and contraceptives containing 20 mcg ethinyl estradiol have been demonstrated to have similar benefits.[54,55] At this time, the effect of other nonoral combined hormonal contraceptive products on acne has not been studied.

Acne Rosacea

In contrast to acne vulgaris, acne rosacea is predominately a problem for middle-aged and older adults. This condition is limited to the central face and occasionally the neck, and can be identified by its limited location. In the initial stages, central facial redness, telangiectasias, and increased flushing are seen. With recurrent exacerbations, the lesions will resemble the papules and pustules of acne vulgaris, but lack comedones. Chronic steroid use can produce a rash identical to that of rosacea.

Unlike the treatment of acne vulgaris, in which combination topical medications are preferred, the use of single-agent topical metronidazole or azelaic acid is the first line of therapy. Topical azelaic acid's mechanism of action is unknown; it is primarily excreted unchanged via the kidneys. Metronidazole 1% gel can be used on a once-daily basis; it is recommended that other formulations be used twice daily, although there is evidence that once-daily 0.75% cream is equally as effective as the 1% gel (P = .76; 95% CI for treatment difference was −15%, 17%).[56] Azelaic acid 15% gel is used twice daily and is equally effective as metronidazole.[57] Benzoyl peroxide can be added to the regimen if necessary, although the drying effect may be unacceptable. As with adolescent acne, 4–6 weeks are required for the benefits to be apparent. When initial therapy is ineffective, or the lesions are severe, tretinoin cream can be added and the dose increased over several weeks from 0.025% cream three times weekly to a maximum of 0.1% cream nightly.

The use of the tetracycline antibiotics in treating rosacea is well established, and any agent within the class can be used. Del Rosso et al.[58] evaluated a low anti-inflammatory-dose regimen of doxycycline (Adoxa) 40 mg day and found it to be as effective as higher doses, with less risk of promoting antibiotic resistance than the higher doses. Similarly, Sanchez et al. compared an antimicrobial dose of tetracycline (20 mg twice daily) plus metronidazole 0.75% lotion twice daily for 12 weeks followed by doxycycline monotherapy, to metronidazole gel/placebo followed by placebo. The use of oral doxycycline in subclinical doses proved effective for treatment without promotion of resistance or altering normal flora elsewhere in the body (P < .01 compared to metronidazole/placebo at 8, 12, and 16 weeks).[59] Use of these drugs during pregnancy and lactation and among the elderly were previously discussed.

Intertrigo

Intertrigo is a term used to describe a rash or inflammation of the body folds or intertriginous areas of the skin. Also commonly called chafing, intertrigo most frequently occurs in areas of warm, moist skin. A diaper rash is an intertrigo, as are rashes experienced by individuals who are overweight, suffer from diabetes, or use prosthetic devices against their skin. The elderly, especially those with incontinence, are at increased risk for intertrigo.[60] This condition may have a bacterial, fungal, or viral infection associated with it, especially if there is broken skin that allows entry of the offending agent. Discussion of secondary infections and their treatments can be found in the sections following.

Treatment of simple intertrigo includes protectants such as petroleum jelly or astringents like zinc oxide cream. If an infection is suspected, therapy should be specific to the agent in question. For example, persistent intertrigo infections tend to be fungal, so antifungal azole creams such as clotrimazole 1% are among the most often employed. Other treatments include palliative use of glucocorticoid over-the-counter cream for symptoms. Protectants and creams used to treat intertrigo tend to be water resistant, so it is suggested to apply them using a vehicle such as tissue or towel to avoid difficulty washing them from hands. Additional advice to a woman with intertrigo should include using antibacterial soap, using washcloths and clothes made of natural fibers, and maintaining a normal body mass index (BMI).

Bacterial Skin Infections

Bacterial skin infections can range from **pyodermas** (surface lesions) to **cellulitis**. These conditions primarily are caused by *Staphylococcus aureus*, less commonly by

Streptococci species. *Pseudomonas aeruginosa* and *Candida* spp. can be the etiologic agents for additional causes. Impetigo is a term commonly applied to describe shallow vesicles and pustules that develop in scattered areas of the face and extremities and that crust before healing. Folliculitis refers to infections at the hair follicle, characterized by redness and pustule development. **Furuncles** are nodules that form following folliculitis. **Carbuncles** (boils) are subcutaneous abscesses; the term carbuncle is used when large lesions or groups of boils appear.

Infections limited to the epidermis and dermis, such as folliculitis, can be treated with topical antibacterials. Over-the-counter products can be used for occasional mild recurrences of bacterial infections. These products include bacitracin, neomycin, or a combination product such as polymyxin B/neomycin sulfate (Neosporin). Mupirocin (Bactroban) is commonly prescribed because it has little cross-resistance, due to a unique mechanism of action in which it binds to RNA during bacterial protein synthesis. Severe or persistent infections can be treated with oral antibiotics. Whenever skin infections do not resolve following use of a first-line treatment, the possibility of methicillin-resistant *Staphylococcus aureus* (MRSA) should be considered.

Furuncles and Carbuncles

Bacterial skin infections can be managed initially with warm soaks to promote drainage; surgical incision and drainage may be needed if the lesions are large or do not improve. When antibiotic therapy is used, dicloxacillin (Dynapen), which is penicillinase resistant, is FDA approved to treat *Staphylococcus* infections and should be the first choice. A 7- to 10-day course usually is an adequate treatment course. Cephalexin (Keflex) and other first-generation cephalosporins can be used to treat most gram-positive organisms and gram-negative aerobes. Persistent infections and women with immune compromise should be treated with a second- or third-generation cephalosporin, and parenteral treatment should be considered. Clindamycin (Cleocin) or erythromycin (E-Mycin) are the drugs of choice for uncomplicated skin and subcutaneous infections for those who are penicillin or cephalosporin allergic.[61] Carbuncles represent a deeper and more extensive infection and require longer courses of therapy at doses in the high end of the dosing range for that drug.

Cellulitis

Deeper infections of the soft tissue, which appear as poorly demarcated, swollen, erythematous, tender areas, are termed cellulitis. Skin disruption coupled with skin colonization or infection predispose to cellulitis. Beta-hemolytic streptococci and *S aureus* microbes are the most common pathogens.[62] Women with significant cellulitis should be evaluated for parenteral therapy in the hospital setting.

Methicillin-Resistant *Staphylococcus Aureus*

Methicillin-resistant *Staphylococcus aureus* (MRSA) can either colonize or infect. Screening for MRSA colonization is not routine but can be done in communities where there is a high incidence of infection. When colonization is identified and treatment is appropriate, pseudomonic acid A, commonly known as mupirocin ointment (Bactroban), can be used. The ointment is applied to the lower nares, the most common carrier location, for a week.

Community acquired MRSA (CA-MRSA), unlike its nosocomial cousin, typically manifests as pustules, boils, and open infectious lesions. An MRSA skin lesion may be erythematous and painful, with or without drainage. When culturing skin lesions, it is essential to specify that sensitivities are desired even if the identified species is MRSA. Many laboratories have not yet recognized that agents other than vancomycin (Vanocin) are available for treatment of skin disease from CA-MRSA.

Empiric therapy for CA-MRSA, whether diagnosed or suspected, can include clindamycin (Cleocin), the long-acting tetracyclines doxycycline (Adoxa) and minocycline (Minocin), and trimethoprim-sulfamethoxazole (Bactrim), among others. None of these treatments are FDA approved specifically for MRSA, but each has been reported to have efficacy against CA-MRSA.[63]

Clindamycin hydrochloride (Cleocin), a bacteriostatic lincosamide, is metabolized via CYP450 enzymes in the liver. This drug is associated with a higher risk of *Clostridium difficile* colitis than other antibiotics, and individuals should be cautioned to report any gastrointestinal disturbance and not to self-medicate to treat diarrhea. The drug interacts with kaolin, a component of some antidiarrheals, which will decrease the effectiveness of clindamycin.[64]

The long-acting tetracyclines, doxycycline (Vibramycin, Atridox), and minocycline (Minocin, Solodyn), should not be used as first-line therapy unless sensitivity is documented because a high rate of antibiotic resistance has developed, particularly among gram-positive aerobes, including *S aureus*. The tetracyclines are poorly metabolized and are excreted unchanged. Drug–drug interactions can be found in Table 11-9. Absorption of tetracyclines is decreased when they are administered simultaneously with antacids and iron-containing compounds.

Trimethoprim-sulfamethoxazole often abbreviated as TMP-SMX or TMP-SMZ (Bactrim, Septra) is a combination of an antibacterial sulfonamide and a folic acid inhibitor. Its use as a treatment for MRSA is based on limited data, although it usually it is employed when other agents are contraindicated. TMP-SFX should not be given to women who have folate deficiency. Multiple drug–drug interactions have been reported. Cyclosporin, methotrexate, warfarin, and thiazide diuretics should not be taken concomitantly with sulfonamides. Use with tricyclic antidepressants and antiseizure medications causes an increased risk of cardiotoxicity and should be avoided. Phenytoin (Dilantin) toxicity can occur when phenytoin is used with TMP-SMX. Oral antidiabetic medications may have greater hypoglycemic effect when administered concurrently with TMP-SMX.

Fungal Skin Infections

Dermatophytes

Tinea corporis, tinea cruris, and tinea pedis are superficial skin infections caused by **dermatophytes** (*Trichophyton* spp., *Microsporum* spp.). They are spread through direct inoculation, including autoinoculation, and through fomites such as bed sheets or towels that carry scales shed from the lesions.

Tinea corporis (ringworm) initially appears as a flat, reddened area. As the infection spreads across the skin, the appearance is annular with a raised, scaly edge and central clearing. Isolated papules may remain in the central area. Tinea cruris is found in the groin area. Initially it may have a moist, reddened appearance. Subsequently, central hyperpigmentation and a raised, papular, flaking edge develop. Occasionally intense pruritus is associated with the infection. Both tinea corporis and tinea cruris are treated with topical antifungals for a period of 2–4 weeks. The use of corticosteroids should be discouraged, as these agents may further irritate the skin, resulting in the development of pustular lesions.[65]

Tinea pedis (athlete's foot) is found in the intertriginous spaces on the feet. This condition is prone to secondary bacterial infections if left untreated. An inflammatory response at the site of infection suggests the need for antibacterial as well as antifungal therapy. Any of the various topical antifungals are efficacious. They can be procured over the counter or by prescription. Most topical antifungals are applied twice daily for 4–6 weeks (Table 26-10).

All the topical antifungals have the same mechanisms of action; they attack the fungal cell wall. Severe or widespread infection can be treated with oral ketoconazole (Nizoral), itraconazole (Sporanox), or fluconazole (Diflucan) weekly for at least 4 weeks. Tinea pedis is likely to recur; women should be cautioned to maintain good hygiene and dry feet carefully after showering.

Tinea Versicolor

Tinea versicolor (also known as pityriasis versicolor) is a chronic infection with lesions primarily found on the trunk, neck, and arms. The causative agent of the fungus is *Malassezia* spp. The lesions are round or oval and slightly raised and may be hypopigmented or hyperpigmented, depending on the skin type. In persistent cases, the lesions may coalesce into large patches. Onset is most common in adolescents and young adults. Following treatment, the skin will remain relatively less able to tan until the skin cells have gone through a complete replacement cycle. Relapses after treatment are common, particularly in summer and in warmer moist climates. Individuals should be reassured that the condition is not related to hygiene and is not communicable to others.

Treatment for tinea versicolor is with a topical antifungal, usually ketoconazole 2% cream by prescription, or miconazole (Monistat) or clotrimazole dermal (Lotrimin). Dermal and vaginal preparations differ in the vehicle used, to reflect differences in absorption from various tissues. The choice of medication can be based on how large an area needs treatment. The prescription-only products come in a larger tube than the OTC products. Ketoconazole is used once daily for 2 weeks, while the OTC products are used twice daily. Selenium sulfide shampoo (Selsun Blue) can be recommended, particularly if the affected area extends above the hair line.

Oral therapy with ketoconazole (Nizoral) as a 400-mg single dose or 200 mg daily for 7–10 days are equally effective,[66] as is itraconazole (Sporanox) 200 mg daily for 5–7 days, which has a clinical cure rate of 94%.[67] The significant adverse effects profile of oral medications limits their advisability except in severe infections. However, some women may prefer oral therapy for ease of treatment. The rate of healing following use of oral preparations is similar to the rate of healing of topical preparations. Intermittent oral dosing with itraconazole 400 mg once a month has been shown to prevent relapses. Mycological cure was 88% versus 57% with placebo ($P < .001$).[68]

Table 26-10 Antifungals

Drug	Route of Administration/Dose	Side Effects	Contraindications	FDA Pregnancy Category
Ciclopirox (Penlac, Loprox)	Topical gel 0.77%, shampoo 1% Gel applied qd for onychomycosis	Irritation, redness at site of application	Hypersensitivity; use caution with diabetes, immune suppression.	B
Clotrimazole (Lotrimin, Gyne-Lotrimin)	Topical-cream, lotion, solution Apply twice daily	Skin irritation, erythema	Hypersensitivity.	B
Clotrimazole/ betamethasone dipropionate (Lotrisone)	Topical cream Apply twice daily	Skin irritation, edema, erythema, secondary infection, paresthesia	Hypersensitivity.	C
Econazole nitrate 1% (Spectazole)	Topical cream: Apply once or twice daily	Itching, erythema	Hypersensitivity.	C
Fluconazole (Diflucan)	Oral 100 mg, 150 mg, 200 mg 150 mg PO once a week for 4 weeks	Rash, nausea, vomiting, elevated liver enzymes	Hypersensitivity.	C
Griseofulvin (Gris PEG, Fulvicin)	Oral: 330 mg daily for onychomycosis	Rash, urticaria, edema, paresthesia, nausea, diarrhea, headache	Hypersensitivity. Development of leukopenia or hepatic toxicity. Interacts with warfarin. Many drug interactions.	Not for use in pregnancy
Itraconazole (Sporanox)	Oral: 200 mg PO qd for one week in divided dose (100 mg PO bid) Increase by 100 mg/day if needed Max dose is 400 mg/day	CHF, photosensitivity, rash including Stevens-Johnson syndrome, lipid abnormalities, GI symptoms, pseudomembranous colitis, hepatotoxicity, anaphylaxis, headache, dizziness, neuropathy	Hypersensitivity, pregnancy, congestive heart failure, renal or liver disease. Many drug interactions.	C
Ketoconazole (Nizoral)	Topical 2% cream or shampoo Oral: 200–400 mg daily	Pruritus, abdominal pain, nausea, vomiting Hepatotoxicity (rare) Anaphylaxis (rare)	Hypersensitivity.	C
Miconazole (Monistat)	Topical 2% cream	Pruritus	Hypersensitivity.	C
Nystatin (Mycostatin)	Topical cream, ointment, powder: Apply twice daily		Hypersensitivity.	B
Selenium sulfide (Selsun Blue)	Topical: Once daily for 7 days	Skin irritation	Hypersensitivity. Inflammation warning: Not for use during pregnancy.	C
Terbinafine hydrochloride (Lamisil)	Topical: 1% gel, cream, solution Oral: 250 mg daily (onychomycosis only)	Headache, GI, itching, taste disturbance Severe skin reactions, including Stevens-Johnson syndrome, hepatotoxicity	Hypersensitivity; use caution with kidney or liver disease, lupus, immunodeficiency.	B

CHF = congestive heart failure; GI = gastrointestinal.

Seborrheic Dermatitis

Seborrheic dermatitis appears as reddened, flaky, occasionally greasy skin on the scalp, face, especially in the naso-labial folds, and chest. Like tinea versicolor, it is associated with *Malassezia* spp. rather than dermatophytes. This condition is chronic and requires persistent treatment to control symptoms. A variety of products are effective, including selenium sulfide shampoo (Selsun Blue) and topical antifungals such as ketoconazole (Nizoral) and terbinafine (Lamisil).[69] These products are applied twice daily to the affected areas, and their use is preferred to topical corticosteroids, since use may be prolonged. Tea tree oil and cinnamic acid have antifungal properties and have potential value, although more research is needed to assess the effectiveness of these complementary therapies.[69]

Pimecrolimus cream (Elidel) and tacrolimus cream (Protopic) are pharmaceuticals that have an immune modulating effect.[70] Pimecrolimus cream has demonstrated effectiveness in the management of severe facial seborrheic dermatitis when applied twice daily for several weeks (*P* = .0156; 95% CI, 0.129–1.197 compared to vehicle alone). A small study of tacrolimus found 61% reported total clearance of symptoms during use.[71] Prophylaxis to prevent recurrences can be provided with ketoconazole shampoo weekly or topical miconazole (Monistat) twice a month.[69]

Oral terbinafine (Lamisil) has been shown to defer recurrences for up to 3 months.[72] Oral itraconazole 200 mg taken on 2 consecutive days monthly has been shown to be an effective maintenance regimen. A small study demonstrated absence of recurrence over a 12-month period using this regimen.[73] Itraconazole persists in tissue due to its lipophilic nature; additionally, it exhibits anti-inflammatory action.

Onychomycosis

Onychomycosis is a fungal infection of the nail and nail bed. Dermatophytes and *Candida* spp. are the most common organisms involved. Onychomycosis is often a secondary infection following tinea pedis.[74] Treatment should be managed by a dermatologist or skin specialist, because severe adverse events can occur when an individual is placed on long-term oral antifungals. Topical preparations are unlikely to be useful in this condition in the form of monotherapy. Ciclopirox (Penlac) has been used for mild to moderate cases and is applied to the affected nail daily; once weekly, the nail is cleaned with alcohol to remove the buildup. Treatment duration can last 6 to 12 months.[75] Ciclopirox inhibits intracellular transport of proteins and disrupts DNA and RNA synthesis. Itraconazole (Sporanox), fluconazole (Diflucan), and terbinafine (Lamisil) all can be prescribed based on efficacy and cost in individual cases. The typical course of treatment is 6 weeks for fingernail infections and up to 12 weeks for toenail infections. Combination therapy using ciclopirox for several months in combination with a standard course of terbinafine, an oral antifungal, has been shown to improve outcomes significantly (mycological cure rate 88.2% combination therapy, 64.7% terbinafine only, *P* = .05).[76]

Topical Antifungal Therapy for Fungal Skin Infections

The imidazole and triazole antifungals act primarily by disrupting the fungal cell membrane with secondary actions including inhibition of lipid synthesis and of exudative/peroxidative enzyme activity. These agents are only minimally absorbed. Whenever treatment with a topical antifungal agent is reasonable, it should be preferred to the oral regimen.

Oral Antifungal Therapy for Fungal Skin Infections

Many individuals prefer the convenience associated with oral therapy. However, the oral antifungals have significant adverse events associated with their use. These medications are metabolized in the liver, with primarily renal excretion. Monitoring liver function tests is a common recommendation, as hepatitis is one of the major risks. The azoles, in particular, have many drug interactions, primarily related to drug metabolism. A selected list of drug–drug interactions can be found in Table 11-18. One author lists them among the red flag drugs responsible for up to 80% of clinically significant drug interactions.[77] Women taking these medications orally need to know to remind all their providers that the drug has been prescribed.

Ectoparasites and Skin Infestations

Scabies (*Sarcoptes Scabiei*)

Scabies (*Sarcoptes scabiei*) is a common skin infestation caused by a microscopic mite that can be found worldwide. Infection is associated with crowding, sharing personal items such as clothing, and close physical contact. Older persons and anyone who has a weakened immune system is at risk of severe infestation. Healthcare workers are often exposed in the work setting. Symptoms include the appearance of burrows, particularly on the webbing between digits and in intertriginous areas or areas where there is constriction from clothing and severe itching. Intense irritation and itching as a result of hypersensitivity to the mites may lead to open sores. Symptoms take 4 or more weeks to develop following first exposure as sensitization occurs. With reinfection, irritation may begin within 24 hours of exposure. Itching tends to be most severe at night and may cause sleep disturbances. Severe infestations in the elderly and immune compromised persons may develop into crusted, or Norwegian, scabies.

Symptoms may persist for several weeks after effective treatment. Following resolution of the hypersensitivity reaction, persistent symptoms are associated with failure to complete treatment, overtreatment, resistance, and reinfection. Overtreatment resulting in an allergic reaction may be treated with an antihistamine, resistance with emollients, and restricted dosing to the recommended amount, and reinfection requires retreatment with improved health counseling and/or a different product.[78]

Treatment for scabies includes cleaning of all personal clothing, household linens, and surfaces (such as furniture) with which the infected person has had contact within the prior 3 days. Items that cannot tolerate hot water washing such as fabric should be sealed in a plastic bag for 2 weeks, dry cleaned, or placed in a hot dryer for > 30 minutes. Furniture and carpets must be vacuumed and the vacuum bag immediately discarded. Unaffected family members need not be treated prophylactically.

Pharmacologic Treatments for Scabies

Permethrin cream 5% (Elimite), Lindane (Kwell), and crotamiton (Eurax) are the three drugs approved by the FDA for treating scabies. Permethrin cream is the recommended first-line topical therapy. It is applied to the entire body below the neck for 8–14 hours before washing thoroughly. A repeat dose may be applied in 14 days if living mites persist. Permethrin kills mites and lice by disrupting nerve cell membranes. Allergy to chrysanthemum plants is a contraindication to the use of permethrin because it is a derivative of the plant. Irritation, itching, or erythema may be exacerbated after treatment. The Cochrane systematic analysis that includes 20 small trials identified permethrin as the most effective topical agent, compared to lindane (Kwell) or Crotamiton (Eurax).[79] Permethrin cream is an FDA Pregnancy Category B drug. Treatment with permethrin is safe during breastfeeding as there is minimal absorption after topical application. There are no reports of special consideration needed for use of permethrin cream among the elderly.

Crotamiton 10% cream or lotion (Eurax) is applied from the neck down; a second application is applied 24 hours later. Washing is delayed for 48 hours after the second dose. It is not as effective as permethrin.

Lindane 1% cream (Kwell) is only recommended today as a second-line therapy because of potential side and adverse effects. Lindane acts as a CNS stimulant and an environmental pollutant. Since it has a long half-life, its use in the environment is of considerable concern, and it has been banned as a pesticide in more than 50 countries and some states such as California. This agent has demonstrated neurotoxicity in humans and is contraindicated for persons with seizure disorders and those with skin lesions that would increase absorption. The FDA has a black box warning notifying consumers of the risk of neurotoxicity.

Lindane is an FDA Pregnancy Category B drug based on animal studies and its risk during lactation is unknown. However, neither lindane (Kwell) nor ivermectin (Stromectol) is recommended for pregnant or lactating women or young children. Compared with other available treatments,

they have an unacceptably high risk of neurologic injury. Moreover, there is an increased risk of neurotoxicity among the elderly where compared to younger cohorts with the use of lindane, so the agent also should be avoided for older women.[80]

Malathion 0.5% lotion (Ovide) is suggested by the CDC but is less effective than permethrin. Like permethrin, malathion acts on the nervous system of lice and mites. A contact hypersensitivity reaction can occur following use of malathion. Use of heat to dry hair or exposure to open flames should be avoided as the lotion is flammable. Malathion is an FDA Pregnancy Category B drug. Minimal absorption with topical use indicates that it is likely to be safe for breastfeeding. This agent has no reported special issues for the elderly.

Oral ivermectin (Stromectol) can be used to treat severe cases and those distinguished by open crusted lesions (Norwegian scabies). As with the other products used for treatment of mites, it is a neurotoxin, although there are indications that it does not cross the blood–brain barrier unless it is used for long periods or at high doses. Risks of neither seizures nor aplastic anemia, albeit possible, are thought to be significant when ivermectin is used as directed for scabies, however, both may be seen with prolonged use. Ivermectin should be avoided during pregnancy and lactation. Use of ivermectin by the elderly is controversial as some studies have suggested increased risk of death with prolonged use for the older individual, but other studies do not have the same findings.[81]

Treatment of crusted scabies requires two to three oral doses of ivermectin (Stromectol), usually in conjunction with topical permethrin or lindane, and it may also require use of a keratolytic agent and vigorous scrubbing prior to topical treatment.[78] All current sexual partners and family members with whom the woman has had close, prolonged, personal contact also should be treated.

Lice (*Pediculus Humanus Capiti, Pediculus Humanus Corporis*, and *Phthirus Pubis*)

Pediculosis humanus capitis (head lice), *Pediculus humanus corporis* (body lice), and *Phthirus pubis* (crab lice or pubic lice) are most commonly transmitted via sexual contact, although sharing linens, clothing, or towels may cause nonsexual transmission. Usually, the afflicted woman will report noticing either nits (white egg cases) or moving lice, or she will experience genital itching. Permethrin 1% lotion (Nix) and pyrethrin with piperonyl butoxide (Rid) are FDA approved for treating head lice, and both are available as OTC preparations

(Table 26-11). Resistance to this class of drugs has been increasing. Accordingly, women should be instructed to observe carefully for incomplete resolution or recurrences. Pyrethrin/piperonyl butoxide is an FDA Pregnancy Category C drug. In 2009, the FDA approved benzyl alcohol lotion for treatment of head lice.

Malathion 0.5% lotion (Ovide) applied for 8–12 hours and ivermectin (Stromectol) 250 mg/kg orally in a single dose can be used as alternatives to permethrin or pyrethrin/piperonyl butoxide if there is hypersensitivity to the first-line therapies, but they are not desirable first-line therapy. Lindane is only used in cases of resistance, when the need outweighs the risks.[69] Repeat treatment in 1 week is advisable to eradicate eggs that may have hatched after treatment, because none of the drugs used is completely ovicidal. Household cleaning and treatment of sexual partners is similar to that for scabies. Whole house fumigation is not required.

Lice found in the hair or eyelashes and body lice are transmitted through close contact, or sharing combs, brushes, or clothing with an infected person. Itching usually is the first symptom. Treatment with permethrin or pyrethrin is the first-line therapy. An Israeli study that compared a natural remedy made up of ylang-ylang, coconut, and anise oils to a control spray that included several pediculicides found them to be equally effective in treating pediatric head lice (92.3% versus 92.2% cure rate).[82]

Table 26-11 Treatments for Scabies and Lice

Drug Generic (Brand)	Dose	Side Effects/Adverse Effects	FDA Pregnancy Category
Benzyl alcohol (Ulesfia)*	Head lice: 5% lotion—apply for 10 minutes then wash off and reapply for 10 minutes, then wash off. May repeat in 1 week if needed.	Side effects: Irritation to skin and numbness at site of application.	B
Crotamiton (Eurax)*	Scabies: 10% cream—apply to whole body from neck down. Leave for 24 hours then wash off before reapplying for a second dose. Wash off the second dose 48 hours after application.	Side effects uncommon. Adverse effects: Severe allergic reactions, rare.	C
Ivermectin (Stromectol)	Scabies or lice: 3-mg tablets. 200 mcg/kg orally repeated in 14 days and second dose 14 days later if needed. Absorption improved if taken with a fatty meal.	Adverse effects: Seizures, muscle spasm, aplastic anemia.	C
Lindane (Kwell)*†	Scabies or lice: 1% lotion or cream—apply in a thin coat to whole body from neck down for 8–12 h and then rinse off. Not recommended for first-line therapy.	Adverse effects: Seizures, muscle spasm, aplastic anemia.	B, but not recommended for pregnant women
Malathion (Ovide)†	Scabies or lice: For treating lice, apply for 8–12 h to hair and scalp, let dry. Lotion is flammable—do not use electrical heat sources like hair dryer or curlers when applying this lotion or apply it near open flames.	Side effects rare, may induce stinging to the skin or scalp. Adverse effects: Severe allergic reactions, rare.	C
Permethrin (Elimite)*	Scabies: 5% cream—apply then rinse off after 8–14 h followed by a second administration 1 week after the first application.	Side effects: Itching and stinging on application.	B
Permethrin lotion (Nix)†	Lice: Apply to the affected area and wash off after 10 minutes. Will continue to kill newly hatched lice for several days. May reapply in 9–10 days. Treatment failure common secondary to increasing resistance.	Side effects uncommon. Adverse effects: Severe allergic reactions, rare.	B
Pyrethrin/butoxide (RID)†	Lice: Apply to affected area and leave on for 5 minutes. Rinse off and reapply in 5–10 days because pyrethrins only kill live lice and do not kill the eggs.		C

* Correct application is critical. The individual should be instructed to take a warm bath or shower, dry off thoroughly, then apply the medication to the whole body excluding face, nose, and mouth. The scalp and groin should be included in the application. Mucosal surfaces should be avoided.
† Prior to treatment, the person should remove clothing that might become wet or stained. Apply medication and leave in place per instructions for that drug. Do not use a crème rinse or combination shampoo/crème rinse prior to applying medication to hair. Do not rewash hair for 1–2 days after applying medication. Comb dead lice and nits out of hair using a fine-tooth comb. Machine wash and dry clothing, bed linens, and other items that have been worn or used during the 2 days prior to treatment. Use a high-heat drying cyle. Soak combs and brushes in hot water (≥ 130°F) for 5 minutes. Vacuum floor and furniture. Do not use fumigant sprays.

Fleas and Ticks

Fleas and ticks are common pests in households where animals live and in outdoor areas across the United States. Most individuals will notice flea bites on the ankles and lower calves; ticks may attach to any part of the body that is exposed. The common flea species are primarily the cause of irritation, although some species can transmit diseases. Bubonic plague is a flea-borne illness, and cases have been reported, albeit rarely, in the United States. Ticks are primarily a source of painful sores at the site of a bite, and can cause a number of illnesses in humans; among the most common are Lyme disease and Rocky Mountain spotted fever.

Lyme disease is the single most common tick-borne disease in the United States. When a tick can be reliably identified as *Ixodes scapularis* and has been attached for more than 36 hours, a single 200-mg dose of doxycycline (Vibramycin) can be given as prophylaxis within 72 hours in areas with high incidence of Lyme disease.[83]

Occasionally, humans, like pets, will develop an allergic dermatitis in response to flea bites. Treatment includes topical lotions such as those discussed earlier for pruritus and topical antibiotics for secondary infection.

Prevention is the best way to deal with possible exposure to fleas and ticks in the outdoors. N, N-diethyl-m-toluamide (DEET) can be found in many bug repellent formulations at 20% or greater concentrations. It can safely be applied to the skin and will last for several hours. Permethrin-containing products can be applied to clothing, but not to skin, to prevent bug bites.

The key to treating both flea and tick infestations is treatment of the house and of pets, which are the common hosts and often the source of human exposure. Veterinary products and household fumigation products for fleas can be easily obtained.

Other Insect and Arachnoid Stings and Bites

Bees, wasps, spiders, bedbugs, and other small animals can produce irritating stings or bites. Unless a person is severely allergic, the management focuses on removing any stinger left behind by a flying insect and treating the symptoms of pain or itching. Ice may relieve the initial painful reaction; antipruritics should then be applied, and a mild painkiller such as acetaminophen or ibuprofen given. Diphenhydramine (Benadryl) or a similar antihistamine may relieve the body's allergic response.

Persons who are aware that they have severe allergies to insect or spider bites should have a prescription for an epinephrine 1:1000 0.3-mg auto-injector (Epi-Pen) and carry it with them at all times.

Minor Burns

Burns are graded by degree of damage to the skin and by the extent of body coverage. First-degree burns are superficial, and the skin remains intact. These burns usually are initially treated with ice or cold water to decrease heat, a mild painkiller, and the use of a topical anesthetic spray such as benzocaine or an herbal product (Box 26-5). Aloe vera gel can be applied for relief of pain and heat three to four times daily, as can tea tree oil, which is applied two to three times daily for pain relief. A meta-analysis of aloe vera studies found a reduction in mean healing time compared to healing time of those in a control group ($P = .006$); however, as the authors noted, the lack of standardization

---

Box 26-5 Gone But Not Forgotten: Butter for Burns

In years past, when a kitchen mishap resulted in a minor burn, the first action was to put some butter on it to soothe and promote healing. Today it is known that there are no research findings that support that action, and, conversely, butter can be harmful. Coating a burn with a greasy layer tends to prolong the heat of the burn, whereas ice or aloe vera bring a cooling effect that stabilizes the burn. Butter also may provide a ready medium for a secondary infection.

It remains unclear why butter was the recommendation of this old wives' tale except that it is readily available in most kitchens, where many burns occur. Other suggested remedies have included milk, toothpaste, and tomatoes, although no evidence exists to their effectiveness either. A few studies have been conducted with honey that appear to be promising, but honey needs more data for recommendation. Until and unless data are reported about alternatives for treatment of minor burns, ice, aloe vera, and topical anesthetics are first-line treatments, and food in the kitchen should be reserved for nutritional consumption.

of products makes evaluation difficult.[84] Propolis, a resinous mixture that honeybees collect from trees, is believed to have effects including immune modulation and antioxidant, anti-inflammatory, and antibacterial properties.[85] There is no evidence to determine the safety of propolis supplements during pregnancy or breastfeeding, and some products may contain high alcohol content.

Second-degree burns include blistering and are partial-thickness burns. In addition to keeping the area clean and dry and leaving the blister intact, topical medication can be used as for first-degree burns. A topical antibiotic can be applied to open areas to prevent secondary bacterial infection. Third-degree, full-thickness burns have damage that extends below the skin and require expert treatment to decrease scarring and risk of infection. The percentage of body surface affected also contributes to burn severity and decision making about office versus hospital treatment.

Silver sulfadiazine cream 1% (Silvadene) is a topical sulfa antimicrobial used to treat both second- and third-degree burns. This cream is applied one to two times a day to the affected area in a thin coat. Side effects include irritation or burning at the site, rash, or skin discoloration. More serious adverse events, such as hypersensitivity, skin damage, urinary problems, leukopenia, and bleeding have been reported. Silver sulfadiazine is an FDA Pregnancy Category B drug; however, the potential for neonatal kernicterus associated with any sulfa drug limits use in late pregnancy. WHO identifies silver sulfadiazine (Silvadene) cream as safe during breastfeeding. No special considerations have been reported for use by the elderly.

▌ Topical Anesthetics

Applications of anesthetic medication to the skin are used for conditions that range from minor burns to cuts and scrapes to surgical procedures. These agents can be considered for use in place of infiltrated anesthetics such as lidocaine 1% (Xylocaine). Topical application may produce an analgesic rather than anesthetic effect, because the absorption is limited in comparison to injection. Topical anesthetics should be applied only to intact skin to prevent excessive absorption. Application of topical anesthetics to the eye or to mucous membranes should be avoided as absorption is increased from these tissues. The minimal amount needed to induce loss of feeling should be applied, and prolonged or frequent use should be discouraged. Mild skin irritation and burning on application are common side effects. Common drug interactions include decreased

antibacterial potency in sulfa drugs and increased cardiovascular risk for persons taking St. John's wort, although it is unclear to what degree these risks are present with correct use of topical treatments.

Eutectic mixture of local anesthetics (EMLA) cream was the first topically applied anesthetic in general use. This drug is available over the counter in some countries. One to two grams per 10 square centimeter area are applied. A drawback to the use of EMLA is the long time period (1 hour) between application and effective anesthesia and the necessity of an occlusive covering during that period. Systematic toxicity is rare, as is hypersensitivity. However, skin diseases that disrupt the epidermis will increase absorption.[86] There are no reports of adverse effects in women who are pregnant, lactating, or elderly. Lidocaine is available as cream, gel, or spray solution in concentrations up to 5%.

A lidocaine patch (Lidoderm) also is available for management of pain from herpes zoster and for chronic pain in various anatomic locations. It is applied for up to 12 hours daily on intact skin followed by 12 hours off before reapplying. Serious allergic responses to the lidocaine patch that may require emergency care include itching, shortness of breath, swelling, dizziness, faintness, tremor, tinnitus, and slowed pulse.

Liposomal carriers are phospholipid-based materials that promote absorption of the anesthetic agent through the skin. A systematic review of 25 randomized, controlled trials found that liposome-encapsulated lidocaine, tetracaine, and liposome-encapsulated tetracaine are at least as effective as EMLA and offer lower-cost alternatives.[87] Liposome-encapsulated lidocaine and EMLA were comparable, using qualitative pain scores. Tetracaine and liposome-encapsulated tetracaine were more effective than EMLA using weighted mean difference in 100-mm visual analogue scale scores. However, other studies have found EMLA is more effective. These differences may be secondary to different research methodologies rather than clinically significant differences.[88]

A gel or solution made of lidocaine, epinephrine, and tetracaine (LET) can also be used for minor laceration repairs. LET should not be applied to any part of the body with end arterial supply, such as the nose or fingers, due to possible damage from vasoconstriction. Application to large areas or to mucous membranes increases the risk of central nervous system or cardiovascular toxicity. Following onset of action, a local injection of anesthetic can be used for longer-acting relief. Both LET and EMLA have been demonstrated to be effective pretreatments for laceration repairs in small studies.[89] Tetracaine HCl cream

(Pontocaine) or gel has PABA as a metabolite. Persons with hypersensitivity reactions to PABA, found in many sunscreens, should not use tetracaine products. Sulfa drugs used at the same time may have decreased antibacterial effect.

Benzocaine 20% spray (Endocaine, Hurricaine) can be recommended for over-the-counter relief of minor cuts, stings, sunburn, and similar pain. This spray can be applied three to four times daily, spraying from a distance of 12 inches. It is intended for short-term use; used externally on intact skin, the risk of hypersensitivity or allergic response is minimal.

The use of topical anesthetics during pregnancy and lactation is considered safe. As a group, they have minimal absorption into the circulation. Similarly, there have been no special considerations recommended for the elderly using topic anesthetics.

▌ Drugs, Cosmetics, and Esthetics

Drugs Versus Cosmetics

Up until this point, this chapter primarily has focused on multiple dermatologic conditions that benefit from a variety of pharmacologic treatments. However, there are a myriad of lotions, creams, and oils used solely for cosmetic reasons. Yet often it is unclear whether or not an individual agent is a drug or a cosmetic. Legally, this question has been answered in the United States by the FDA. In 1938, the United States Congress passed the Federal Food, Drug, and Cosmetic (FDC) Act, which has enabled some degree of regulation of cosmetics.

Drugs and cosmetics are defined according to the intended use. Cosmetics are products used to clean, beautify, and promote appearances without affecting physical structures or functions. Cosmetics include moisturizers, lipsticks, powders, hair dyes, and perfumes, among an expansive list of items. Such agents have a long history of use, back to the most ancient societies. Today there is a finite number of large, multinational companies that dominate the cosmetic marketplace, but an almost infinite number of points of sales including supermarkets, department stores, and sometimes even gas stations.

The modern woman is bombarded with advertisements that carefully suggest therapeutic or positive effects of using a cosmetic without actually stating such. Companies tend to be meticulous about their claims since they are legally restricted regarding what they can print about health benefits of a cosmetic. It is illegal to make drug claims for a cosmetic. However, cosmetics are not held to the same standards as drugs, which are described as agents used to treat disease, prevent disease, or physically affect bodily structures or functions. For example, cosmetics do not require premarketing approval as long as they do not include any ingredients from a short list of prohibited items such as harmful chemicals. These agents do require ingredients to be listed in order of most to least on the label, but proprietary interests allow the list to be general enough that competitors cannot duplicate it; no differentiation between active and inactive ingredients is required, and thus, the label is not always useful to consumers. Cosmetics also frequently use terms that are not standardized, such as *natural* or *hypoallergenic*.

Most importantly, cosmetics are not always innocuous. Among the ancient Egyptians and Romans, cosmetics impregnated with lead and mercury were popular, with resulting long-term untoward effects. Today there are controversies about the safety of several cosmetic additives, especially phthalates and parabens.

Phthalates are chemicals such as dimethyl phthalate (DMP), diethyl phthalate (DEP), and Di-n-butyl phthalate (DBP) that are used to prolong fragrances and keep nail polish from chipping, among other effects. Unfortunately, phthalates may be endocrine disruptors and associated with an increased, albeit low absolute, risk of genital malformations.[90] Controversy exists as to whether these chemicals should be removed from cosmetics, as well as from plastics, where they commonly appear. Parabens are chemicals that act as preservatives with antibacterial and antifungal properties. They often are added to shampoos, moisturizers, personal lubricants, and spray tans. Yet these agents likely are weak xenoestrogens, and there is controversy about whether or not they have a role in increasing the risk of breast cancer.[91] Since federal regulations are limited regarding cosmetics, several consumer groups have been created and disseminate information about increased risks with specific agents.

In addition to the risk of harm, cosmetics pose the risk of being ineffective. As noted, cosmetics often imply but do not state effectiveness. Most individuals are challenged to find data about which skin product is superior to another in terms of decreasing wrinkles, increasing skin firmness, or eradicating blemishes. In large part, the cosmetic marketplace remains a *caveat emptor* (buyer beware) situation.

Cosmeceuticals

A **cosmeceutical** is a cosmetic skin product with pharmaceutical properties. The United States federal government does not recognize the term *cosmeceutical*. Cosmeceutical is a portmanteau first coined in the 1970s and is finding its way into the popular vocabulary. Agents often mentioned as cosmeceuticals include nutritional supplements such as antioxidant vitamins as well as FDA prescription drugs like retinoids. Other frequently named cosmeceuticals include oral ingestion of phytoestrogenic foods and other botanicals.[92] Among the most common botanicals are pomegranates, grape seed, horse chestnut, chamomile, comfrey, allantoin, and aloe. Some research has been conducted, but rigorous clinical trials with use of these agents for specific dermatology reasons have not been reported.

The growth of cosmeceuticals has underscored the evolution of a new field in dermatology itself. A quarter of a century ago, facial rejuvenation was the turf of cosmetic surgeons and plastic surgeons. These professionals were educated in subspecialties within the field of surgery. Today, dermatologists may limit their practices to cosmetics and medical aesthetics (also called esthetics). These clinicians and other providers who care for women are able to employ pharmacologic agents to treat issues such as wrinkles and facial hair.

Wrinkles and Frown Lines

More than 50 years ago, botulinum toxin type A was found to block acetylcholine release at the neuromuscular junction and inhibit a muscle from contracting for a period of several months. Toward the end of the 20th century, reports emerged about using this agent for ophthalmic treatments including strabismus. Side effects were found to include softening of skin and decreasing creases and wrinkles. In 1989, the FDA approved use of botulinum toxin for eradicating frown lines. The initial brand was named Botox, which has become a household name because it is frequently used by popular celebrities. An alternative brand, Dysport, received FDA approval in late 2008. Both agents are composed of *Clostridium botulinum* toxin A, although concentrations are slightly different.

Botulinum toxin is the most lethal poison yet discovered.[93] Although the dose used for cosmetic purposes poses little risk, there have been several cases of botulism, or botulinum poisoning primarily from misuse by untrained individuals. In 2009, the FDA announced the plans for a mandatory boxed warning of potential adverse effects suggestive of botulism. This warning will apply to both Botox and Dysport for all their indications, including cosmetic reasons, cervical dystonia, and hyperhidrosis.

Botox cosmetic is available in a single-use vial to be reconstituted only with 0.9% sterile, nonpreserved saline (100 units in 2.5 mL saline) prior to intramuscular injection. The approved dose is 4 units per 0.1 mL at each of the five injection sites on the forehead for a total dose of 20 units per 0.5 mL. Cosmetic use of botulinum toxin generally is repeated every 3–4 months. Drug interactions are possible with other agents such as curare, but not commonly used drugs. This agent is considered an FDA Pregnancy Category C drug because of lack of studies, and similarly, there are no data about transfer into breast milk. The drug is FDA approved only for individuals younger than 65 years of age, primarily because there were too few older individuals in the preapproval clinical trials.

Other treatments for wrinkles include injectable fillers to soften deep folds in the skin. In 2006, the FDA approved an agent of hyaluronic acid with the brand name of Juvéderm. This drug is used predominantly to fill smile lines and to augment lips, especially as they lose shape during aging. All hyaluronic acid fillers are absorbed within 6–9 months, requiring repeated treatments. An alternative nonanimal hyaluronic acid filler is Restylane, which is used in the same manner. Restylane is a gel created from *Streptococcus* bacteria. Safety in pregnancy and breastfeeding, and among women under the age of 18 remains unknown. There are no documented special considerations for older women.

Hirsutism

Hair growth occurs in three phases: anagen (growth), catagen (involution and transition between growth and resting), and telogen (resting phase).[94] On the scalp, anagen lasts about 3 years and telogen lasts approximately 3 months. The hair follicles are not in the same cycle at the same time so humans continually lose and regrow hair. Most humans have approximately 5–15% of hair in telogen at any one time. **Hirsutism**, or excessive hair growth, occurs when the anagen phase is extended and hair follicles are abnormally enlarged. Hirsutism can be an indication of a pathologic condition such as polycystic ovary syndrome, Cushing's syndrome, and prolactin disorders, or it may be idiopathic and a simple cosmetic concern. Because hirsutism develops secondary to androgen action on hair follicles, disorders characterized by excessive androgen production must be ruled out before making the diagnosis of idiopathic hirsutism. Several medications can cause hirsutism (Table 26-12).[95]

Nonpharmacologic treatments include bleaching, shaving, laser, and electrolysis. OTC chemical depilatories work but often cause skin irritation. Pharmacologic treatments for hirsutism include medications directed at the

Table 26-12 Selected List of Drugs That Cause Hirsutism and Alopecia

Drugs That Cause Hirsutism Generic (Brand)	Drugs That Cause Alopecia Generic (Brand)
Anabolic steroids	Isotretinoin (Accutane)
Danazol (Danocrine)	Amiodarone
Glucocorticoids	Angiotensin-converting enzyme inhibitors
Metoclopramide (Reglan)	Anticoagulants
Methyldopa (Aldomet)	Antifungal drugs
Phenothiazines	Acyclovir (Zovirax)
Phenytoin (Dilantin)	Beta-blockers (propranolol and metoprolol)
Progestins	Carbamazepine (Tegretol)
Reserpine (Serpasil)	Chemotherapeutic agents
Testosterone	Heparin
	Ibuprofen (Advil)
	Isoniazid (INH)
	Lamotrigine
	Levodopa
	Lithium (Lithobid)
	Lopid (Gemfibrozil)
	Naproxen (Aleve)
	Phenytoin (Dilantin)
	Spironolactone (Aldactone)
	Tricyclic antidepressants
	Valproic acid (Depakene)

underlying pathology and medications that are specific for treating excessive hair growth.

Eflornithine (Vaniqa) was initially studied as a chemotherapeutic agent, but found to have greater value in the treatment of African trypanosomiasis and potential use as part of a treatment regimen to reduce the incidence of recurrence of colon polyps. In the area of dermatology, however, eflornithine has been found to inhibit unwanted facial hair growth by irreversibly inhibiting ornithine decarboxylase, an enzyme involved in controlling hair growth and proliferation.[95]

Eflornithine is marketed under the brand name Vaniqa as a cream with a formulation of 13.9%. This cream is used as an adjunct in combination with nonpharmacologic methods of treatment. The cream is applied in a thin layer to the face and under the chin twice daily with 8 hours elapsing between each application. After being rubbed in thoroughly, the medication is to remain for at least 4 hours without washing. Hair growth returns approximately 8 weeks after the drug is discontinued. In clinical trials, older women obtained positive results similar to those obtained by younger women with use of eflornithine (Vaniqa).

Eflornithine (Vaniqa) rarely causes side effects, but those reported include swollen patches of skin, headache, ingrown hairs, and itching, burning, or tingling rash. Contact dermatitis, nausea, and herpes simplex are rare. Eflornithine has no known drug–drug interactions. Eflornithine is an FDA Pregnancy Category C drug because there is a lack of information, and likewise, information is lacking about use during breastfeeding.

Other medications that can slow or stop hair growth include oral contraceptives and the antiandrogens spironolactone (Aldactone) and flutamide (Eulexin). Oral contraceptives are often the first drug of choice for women of reproductive age who do not want to become pregnant.[96] The two antiandrogen drugs are not approved for treatment of hirsutism and are therefore used off-label for this purpose. Treatment with antiandrogens is slow and takes approximately 18 months for full efficacy. Individuals using flutamide need to have liver function monitored. Spironolactone can cause hyperkalemia, but it is a rare side effect. Spironolactone and flutamide are FDA Pregnancy Category D drugs.

Ketoconazole (Nizoral) is also effective for treating hirsutism but has severe side effects including alopecia, abdominal pain, and hepatotoxicity. Ketoconazole is reserved for persons who have not responded to other drugs. Persons taking ketoconazole will need liver function tests on a regular basis while using this medication.

Alopecia

Alopecia, or thin hair, is known to occur in persons who have a genetic predisposition for hair loss; this often occurs during times of significant stress. **Alopecia areata** refers to hair loss in specific areas; **alopecia universalis** is the term used when hair loss occurs over the entire body (e.g., as associated with chemotherapy), and **telogen effluvium** is a sudden loss of hair in which the follicles are normal but growth is disturbed.

The etiology of alopecia often is elusive and may be a function of androgenicity, aging, genetics, metabolic disease, or anxiety, or it may be simply idiopathic. In cases when etiology is known, treatment of the underlying cause, e.g., diabetes, may positively affect the hair loss or thinning. Telogen effluvium occurs when a number of follicles enter telogen prematurely and then shed their follicles. Drugs, fever, parturition, major illness, anorexia, and anemia can cause telogen effluvium. Table 26-12 lists drugs that can cause hair loss.[97] Hair loss typically starts 2–3 months after the inciting event. Regrowth follows and usually takes several months. **Androgenic alopecia**, also called female pattern baldness, is hair loss that occurs in the presence of androgen dihydrotestosterone, which increases as women age. Androgenic alopecia is caused by progressive shortening of the anagen stage and is the most common etiology of alopecia.[98]

The majority of hair regrowth cosmetics are found in the form of shampoos or conditioners and occasionally oral formulations. Among the most popular OTC brands is Nioxin, a line of hair products that propose to act as an antiandrogenic. However, no research supports its use for hair thinning or alopecia. Hair Genesis is a brand containing saw palmetto, a botanical with some preliminary findings that suggest it may be more effective than placebo.[99]

Medications for alopecia affect the hair follicle via non-hormonal mechanisms or they modify the action of androgen on the hair follicle by altering production, transport, or metabolism of androgens. Minoxidil (Rogaine) is an agent that is effective for stopping or slowing hair loss and promoting hair growth in men and women, primarily those with androgenically associated hair loss. Minoxidil (Rogaine) prolongs anagen stage and causes follicles at rest to grow. In a study published in 1994, women who used 2% minoxidil were up to twice as likely to report hair regrowth when compared to a control group of women who used a placebo agent.[100] Minoxidil (Rogaine) is FDA approved for OTC use in a 5% formulation for men and 2% formulation for women and men.[101] It is found in various vehicles such as spray, foam, or liquids, and the recommended dose is 1 mL/spray twice daily. The mechanism of action remains unknown.

The most common side effect of minoxidil (Rogaine) is itching on the scalp and dryness that is probably secondary to the drying effect of the propylene glycol that is in the formulation.[97] Minoxidil is a vasodilator and a powerful antihypertensive agent. If taken orally, it can cause dizziness and cardiac arrhythmias. New hair growth will be lost when minoxidil is discontinued. Minoxidil (Rogaine) is in FDA Pregnancy Category C because animal studies found reduced fertility and increased absorption by the intrauterine conceptus in the case of rabbits. The drug is excreted in breast milk, and safety is unknown.

Finasteride (Propecia) and dutasteride (Avodart) act by inhibiting type II 5-alpha-reductase, the enzyme that converts testosterone to dihydrotestosterone (DHT). These agents are not FDA approved to treat hair loss in women and are more commonly used in Europe compared to frequency of use in the United States.[97] Both these agents are FDA Pregnancy Category X drugs, and both are known to cause birth defects in reproductive organs, especially in male fetuses. Since these agents may be absorbed topically, women are warned not to touch or cut the tablets, even if they do not ingest them. In order to minimize fetal risks, most clinicians do not recommend either of these agents for women. It is unknown whether or not these drugs can be found in breast milk. There is no evidence as to whether or not these drugs are of value for postmenopausal women with thinning hair.

Hair regrowth is not limited to the scalp. In late 2008, the FDA issued approval of bimatoprost ophthalmic solution 0.03% (Allergan) to treat inadequate eye lashes. Bimatoprost first was used for management of borderline glaucoma. However, when this prostaglandin analogue was used, a side effect of increased eyelash length, thickness, and darkness was found. This agent is packaged as a 3-mL bottle with sterile applicators and directions for one application nightly. Side effects and adverse effects include conjunctivitis, reversible darkening of the eyelid skin, and potential irreversible increased brown pigmentation of the iris. Once the agent is discontinued, the eyelashes will return to pretreatment condition within a few weeks or months. Use by a woman who is pregnant or lactating has not been adequately studied.

Solar Lentigines, Freckles, and Other Areas of Hyperpigmentation

Skin whiteners have been popular for centuries. Mercury was once used, to the detriment of many unsuspecting individuals. Today, areas of hyperpigmentation can be treated with other agents. Alpha hydroxy acids (AHAs) are naturally occurring or synthetic acids. In concentrations between 5% and 10%, these agents are found over the counter. Higher concentrations require prescriptions, and concentrations of more than 50% are used for chemical peels by a professional. Although there is some evidence that AHA can decrease hyperpigmentation, there is a risk of side effects that may include increased photosensitivity and even increase the risk of hyperpigmentation. AHAs may be found in creams, lotions, and peels. These agents generally act as exfoliant and have been suggested also to treat mild wrinkles secondary to photoaging.

Hydroquinone (Esoterica, Solaquin) is an agent that is known to inhibit melanin production. Available over the counter in a 2% concentration or by prescription as a 4% concentration, this drug often is inappropriately called a skin bleaching agent. However, it does not bleach but instead disrupts hyperpigmentation due to melanin. Although there are concerns regarding carcinogenicity of the drug, there are few reported side effects with topical use, although it may increase the risk of photosensitivity. The usual dose is to apply cream twice daily to the affected area. No safety data have been reported for use by a woman who is pregnant or breastfeeding.

Today the market for cosmetics and cosmeceuticals is burgeoning. It may seem incongruous to the primary care provider who is accustomed to using drugs for therapeutic agents that women, as well as men (should the provider also care for them), may request prescriptions or recommendations for cosmetic reasons. Individuals may have an increased sense of health when not concerned about appearance. However, even medications for cosmetic reasons have potential risks, and the issue of informed consent for these agents, as well as all others, is paramount.

▌Conclusion

In addition to providing a protective covering for our bodies, the skin serves a number of metabolic and sensory functions. The breadth of conditions that affect the skin, ranging from normal maturation to injury to allergy or infections, presents a challenge for women's healthcare providers. Correct diagnosis begins with an accurate description of the lesion or skin disturbance, whether the onset is acute or chronic, and what predisposing factors may be present. Many of the conditions described in this chapter can be treated in the ambulatory setting if the provider is willing to use assessment skills. Confidence to recognize and manage common skin problems is an essential instrument today in the delivery of primary care to women.

References

1. American Academy of Pediatrics Committee on Drugs. The transfer of drugs and other chemicals into human milk. Pediatrics 2001;108(3):776–89.
2. Raine-Fleming NJ, Brincat MP, Muscat-Baron Y. Skin aging and menopause. Am J Clin Dermatol 2003; (46):371–8.
3. Fisher GJ, Kang S, Varani J, Bata-Czorgo Z, Wan Y, Datta S, et al. Mechanisms of photoaging and chronological skin aging. Arch Dermatol 2002;138:1462–70.
4. Schmidt JB, Binder M, Macheimer W, Kainz C, Gitsch G, Bieglmayer C. Treatment of skin aging symptoms in perimenopausal females with estrogen compounds: a pilot study. Maturitas 1994;20(1):25–30.
5. Roberts W. Dermatologic problems of older women. Dermatol Clinics 2006;24:271–80.
6. Farage MA, Miller KW, Elsner P, Maibach HI. Functional and physiological characteristics of aging skin. Aging Clin Exp Res 2008;20(3):195–200.
7. Salasche S. Epidemiology of actinic keratoses and squamous cell carcinoma. J Am Acad Dermatol 2000; 42:S4–7.
8. Rigel DS. The effect of sunscreen on melanoma risk. Dermatol Clin 2002;20(4):601–6.
9. Lautenschlager S, Wulf HC, Pittelkow MR. Photoprotection. Lancet 2007;370:528–37.
10. Stockfleth E, Sterry W, Carey-Yard M, Bichel J. Multicentre, open-label study using imiquimod 5% cream in one or two 4-week courses of treatment for multiple actinic keratoses on the head. Br J Dermatol 2007;157(suppl 2):41–6.
11. Rivers JK, Rosoph L, Provost N, Bissonette R. Open-label study to assess the safety and efficacy of imiquimod 5% cream applied once daily three times per week in cycles for treatment of actinic keratoses on the head. J Cutan Med Surg 2008;12(3):97–111.
12. Krawtchenko N, Roewert-Huber J, Ulrich M, Mann I, Sterry W, Stockfleth E. A randomized study of topical 5% imiquimod vs. topical 5-fluorouracil vs. cryosurgery in immunocompetent patients with actinic keratoses: a comparison of clinical and histologic outcomes including 1-year follow-up. Br J Dermatol 2007;157(suppl 2):34–40.
13. Jury CS, Ramraka-Jones VS, Gudi V, Herd RM. A randomized trial of topical 5% 5-fluorouracil (Efudix cream) in the treatment of actinic keratoses comparing daily versus weekly treatment. Br J Dermatol 2005;153(4):808–10.
14. Loden M. Role of topical emollients and moisturizers in the treatment of dry skin barrier disorders. Am J Clon Dermatol 2003;4(11):771–88.
15. Heymann WR. Itch. J Am Acad Dermatol 2006; 54(4):705–6.
16. Millikan LE. Alternative therapy in pruritus. Dermatol Ther 2003;16:175–80.
17. Hanefin JM, Reed ML, Eczema Prevalence and Impact Working Group. A population-based survey of eczema prevalence in the United States. Dermatology 2007; 18(2):82–91.
18. Williams, HC. Clinical practice. Atopic dermatitis. N Engl J Med 2005;352:2314–24.
19. Lucky AW, Leach AD, Laskazruski P, Wench H. Use of an emollient as a steroid sparing agent in the treatment of mild to moderate atopic dermatitis in children. Pediatr Dermatol 1997;14:321–4.

20. Hoare C, Li Wan Po A, Williams H. Systematic review of treatments for atopic eczema. Health Technol Assess 2000;4:1–191.

21. Green C, Colquitt JL, Kirby J, Davidson P. Topical corticosteroids for atopic eczema: clinical and cost effectiveness of once-daily vs. more frequent use. Br J Dermatol 2005;152:130.

22. Berth-Jones J, Damstra RJ, Golsch S, Livden JK, Van Hooteghem O, Allegra F, et al. Twice weekly fluticasone propionate added to emollient maintenance treatment to reduce risk of relapse in atopic dermatitis: randomised, double blind, parallel group study. BMJ 2003;326:1367.

23. Ashcroft DM, Dimmock P, Garside R, Stein K, Williams HC. Efficacy and tolerability of topical pimecrolimus and tacrolimus in the treatment of atopic dermatitis: meta-analysis of randomised controlled trials. BMJ 2005;330:516–21.

24. Kawakami T, Soma Y, Morita E, Koro O, Yamamoto S, Nakamura K, et al. Safe and effective treatment of refractory facial lesions in atopic dermatitis using topical tacrolimus following corticosteroid discontinuation. Dermatology 2001;203:32–7.

25. Sugiura H, Uehara M, Hoshino N, Yamaji A. Long-term efficacy of tacrolimus ointment for recalcitrant facial erythema resistant to topical corticosteroids in adult patients with atopic dermatitis. Arch Dermatol 2000;136:1062–3.

26. Nakahara T, Koga T, Fukagawa S, Uchi H, Furue M. Intermittent topical corticosteroid/tacrolimus sequential therapy improves lichenification and chronic papules more efficiently than intermittent topical corticosteroid/emollient sequential therapy in patients with atopic dermatitis. J Dermatol 2004;31:524–8.

27. Furue M, Terao H, Moroi Y, Koga T, Kubota Y, Nakayama J, et al. Dosage and adverse effects of topical tacrolimus and steroids in daily management of atopic dermatitis. J Dermatol 2004;31:277–83.

28. Saary J, Qureshi R, Palda V, DeKoven J, Pratt M, Skotnicki-Grant S, et al. A systematic review of contact dermatitis treatment and prevention. J Am Acad Dermatol 2005;53:845.

29. National Guidelines Clearinghouse, Psoriasis. Available from: *http://guideline.gov/summary/summary.aspx?ss=15&doc_id=8260* [Accessed October 30, 2009].

30. Lebwohl M, Callen JP. Obesity, smoking and psoriasis. JAMA 2006;295(2):208–10.

31. Lebwohl M. Psoriasis. Lancet 2003;361:1197–204.

32. Owen CM, Chalmers RJG, O'Sullivan T, Griffiths CEM. Antistreptococcal interventions for guttate and chronic plaque psoriasis. [Systematic review]. Cochrane Database Syst Rev 2000;(2): CD001976.

33. Douglas WS, Poulin Y, Decroix J, Ortonne JP, Mrowietz U, Gulliver W, et al. A new calcipotriol/betamethasone formulation with rapid onset of action was superior to monotherapy with betamethasone dipropionate or calcipotriol in psoriasis vulgaris. Acta Dermato-Venereologica 2002;82(2):131–5.

34. Lam J, Polifka JE, Dohil MA. Safety of dermatologic drugs used in pregnant patients with psoriasis and other inflammatory skin diseases. J Am Acad Dermatol 2008;59(2):295–315.

35. Heydendael VMR, Spuls PI, Opmeer BC, de Borgie CAJM, Reitsma JB, Goldschmidt WFM, et al. Methotrexate versus cyclosporine in moderate-to-severe chronic plaque psoriasis. N Eng J Med 2003;349: 658–65.

36. Haider A, Shaw JC. Treatment of acne vulgaris. JAMA 2004;292:726–35.

37. Ozolins M, Eady EA, Avery A, Cunliffe WJ, O'Neill C, Simpson NB, et al. Randomised controlled multiple treatment comparison to provide a cost-effectiveness rationale for the selection of antimicrobial therapy in acne. Health Technol Assess 2005;9(1):iii–212.

38. Graupe K, Cunliffe WJ, Gollnick HP, Zaumsell RP. Efficacy and safety of topical azelaic acid (20 percent cream): an overview of results from European clinical trials and experimental reports. Cutis 1996;57 (suppl 1):20–35.

39. Menter A. Pharmacokinetics and safety of tazarotene. J Am Acad Dermatol 2000;43(2 pt 3):S31–5.

40. Leyden JL, Hickman JG, Jarratt MT, Stewart DM, Levy SF. The efficacy and safety of a combination benzoyl peroxide/clindamycin gel compared with benzoyl peroxide alone and a benzoyl peroxide/erythromycin combination product. J Cutan Med Surg 2001;5(1):37–42.

41. Leyden JJ, Krochmal L, Yaroshinsky A. Two randomized, double-blind, controlled trials of 2219 subjects to compare the combination clindamycin/tretinoin hydrogel with each agent alone and vehicle for the treatment of acne vulgaris. J Am Acad Dermatol 2006;54:73–81.

42. Ozolins M, Eady EA, Cunliffe WJ, Li Wan Po A, O'Neill C, Simpson NB, et al. Comparison of five antimicrobial regimens for the treatment of mild to

moderate inflammatory facial acne vulgaris in the community: randomised controlled trial. Lancet 2004;364:2188–95.

43. Cooper AJ. Systematic review of propionibacterium acnes resistance to systemic antibiotics. Med J Aust 1998;169:259–61.

44. Webster G, del Rosso JQ. Anti-inflammatory activity of tetracyclines. Dermatol Clin 2007;25:133–5.

45. Skidmore R, Kovach R, Walker C, Thomas J, Bradshaw M, Leyden J, et al. Effects of subantimicrobial-dose doxycycline in the treatment of moderate acne. Arch Dermatol 2003;139:459–64.

46. Dickinson BD, Altman RD, Nielsen NH, Sterling ML, for the Council on Scientific Affairs, American Medical Association. Drug interactions between oral contraceptives and antibiotics. Obstet Gynecol 2001; 98(5, pt. 1):853–60.

47. Archer JSM, Archer MD. Oral contraceptive efficacy and antibiotic interaction: a myth debunked. J Am Acad Dermatol 2002;46(6):917–23.

48. Pai MP, Momary KM, Rodvold KA. Antibiotic drug interactions. Med Clin North Am 2006;90:1223–55.

49. Food and Drug Administration. Isotretinoin (marketed as Accutane) capsule information. Available from: *http://www.fda.gov/Drugs/DrugSafety/PostmarketDrug SafetyInformationforPatientsandProviders/ucm094305 .htm* [Accessed September 27, 2009] and *https:// ipledgeprogram.com/* [Accessed May 7, 2009].

50. Hendrix CW, Jackson KA, Whitmore E, Guidos A, Kretzer R, Liss CM, et al. The effect of isotretinoin on the pharmacokinetics and pharmacodynamics of ethinyl estradiol and norethindrone. Clin Pharmacol Ther 2004;75(5):464–75.

51. Berard A, Azoulay L, Koren G, Blais L, Perrault S, Oraichi D. Isotretinoin, pregnancies, abortions, and birth defects: a population-based perspective. Br J Clin Pharmacol 2007;63(2):196–205.

52. Huber J, Walch K. Treating acne with oral contraceptives: use of lower doses. Contraception 2006; 73(1):23–9.

53. Redmond GP, Olson WH, Lippman JS, Kafrissen ME, Jones TM, Jorizzo J. L. Norgestimate and ethinyl estradiol in the treatment of acne vulgaris: a randomized, placebo-controlled trial. Obstet Gynecol 1997;89(4):615–22.

54. Thorneycroft IH, Gollnick H, Schellschmidt I. Superiority of a combined contraceptive containing drospirenone to a triphasic preparation containing norgestimate in acne treatment. Cutis 2004;74: 123–30.

55. Winkler UH, Ferguson H, Mulders JAPA. Cycle control, quality of life and acne with two low-dose oral contraceptives containing 20 µg ethinyl estradiol. Contraception 2004;69:469–76.

56. Dahl MV, Jarrat, M, Kapla, D, Tuley MR, Baker MD. Once-daily topical metronidazole cream formulations in the treatment of the papules and pustules of rosacea. J Am Acad Dermatol 2001;45:723–30.

57. Maddin S. A comparison of topical azelaic acid 20% cream and topical metronidazole 0.75% cream in the treatment of patients with papulopustular rosacea. J Am Acad Dermatol 1999;40:961.

58. Del Rosso J, Webster GF, Jackson M, Rendon M, Rish P, Torok H, et al. Two randomized phase III clinical trials evaluating anti-inflammatory dose doxycycline (40 mg doxycycline, USP capsules) administered once daily for treatment of rosacea. J Am Acad Dermatol 2007;56:791–802.

59. Sanchez J, Somolinos AL, Almodovar PI, Webster G, Bradshaw M, Powala C. A randomized, double-blind, placebo-controlled trial of the combined effect of doxycycline hyclate 20 mg tablets and metronidazole 0.75% topical lotion in the treatment of rosacea. J Am Acad Dermatol 2005;53:791–807.

60. Farage MA, Miller KW, Berardesca E, Maibach HI. Incontinence in the aged: contact dermatitis and other cutaneous consequences. Contact Dermatitis 2007;57(4):211–7.

61. Rayner C, Munckhof WJ. Antibiotics currently used in the treatment of infections caused by *Staphylococcus aureus*. Internal Med J 2005;35(suppl 2): S1–16.

62. Roberts S, Chambers S. Diagnosis and management of *Staphylococcus aureus* infections of the skin and soft tissue. Internal Med J 2005;35(suppl 2):s97–105.

63. Gorwitz RJ, Jernigan DB, Powers JH, Jernigan JA, and participants in the CDC-convened experts' meeting on the management of MRSA in the community: summary of an experts' meeting convened by the Centers for Disease Control and Prevention. 2006. Available from: *http://.cdc.gov/ncidod/dhqp/ar_mrsa_ca.html* [Accessed September 27, 2009].

64. Fleisher D, Cheng L, Yuji Z, Pao LH, Karim A. Drug, meal and formulation interactions influencing drug absorption after oral administration: clinical implications. Clin Pharmacokinet 1999;36(3):233–54.

65. Gupta RA. Management of superficial fungal infections. Am J Clin Dermatol 2004;5(4):227–37.

66. Fernandez-Nava HD, Laya-Cuadra B, Tianco EA. Comparison of single dose 400 mg versus 10-day 200 mg daily dose ketoconazole in the treatment of tinea versicolor. Int J Dermatol 1997;36(1):64–6.

67. Del Rosso JQ, Gupta AK. The use of intermittent itraconazole therapy for superficial mycotic infections: a review and update on the 'one week' approach. Int J Dermatol 1999;36(S2):28–39.

68. Faergemann J, Gupta AK, Al Mofadi A, Abanami A, Shareaah AA, Marynissen G. The efficacy of itraconazole in the prophylactic treatment of pityriasis (tinea) versicolor. Arch Dermatol 2002;138:69–73.

69. Gupta AK, Nicol K, Batra R. The role of antifungal agents in the treatment of seborrheic dermatitis. Am J Clin Dermatol 2004;5(6):417–22.

70. Warshaw EM, Wohlhuter RJ, Liu A, Zeller SA, Wenner RA, Bowers S, et al. Results of a randomized, double-blind, vehicle-controlled efficacy trial of pimecrolimus cream 1% for the treatment of moderate to severe facial seborrheic dermatitis. J Am Acad Dermatol 2007;57(2):257–64.

71. Meshkinpour A, Sun J, Weinstein G. An open pilot study using tacrolimus ointment in the treatment of seborrheic dermatitis. J Am Acad Dermatol 2003; 49:145–7.

72. Scapparo E, Quadri G, Virno G, Orific C, Milani M. Evaluation of the efficacy and tolerability of oral terbinafine (Dsakil) in patients with seborrhoeic dermatitis. A multicentre randomized, investigator-blinded, placebo-controlled trial. Br J Dermatol 2001;144:854–7.

73. Baysal V, Yildrim M, Ozcanli C, Ceyhan AM. Itraconazole in the treatment of seborrheic dermatitis: a new treatment modality. Int J Dermatol 2004;43(1):63–6.

74. Haneke E, Roseeuw D. The scope of onychomycosis: epidemiology and clinical features. Int J Dermatol 1999;38(suppl 2):7–12.

75. Baran R, Kaoukhov A. Topical antifungal drugs for the treatment of onychomycosis: an overview of current strategies for monotherapy and combination therapy. J Eur AcacDermatol Venereol 2005;19:25–9.

76. Avner S, Nir N, Henri T. Combination of oral terbinafine and topical ciclopirox compared to oral terbinafine for the treatment of onychomycosis. J Dermatolog Treat 2005;16:327–30.

77. Berranco VP. Update on clinically significant drug interactions in dermatology. J Am Acad Dermatol 2006;54(4):676–84.

78. Chosidow O. Scabies. N Engl J Med 2006;354(16): 1718–27.

79. Strong M, Johnstone PW. Interventions for treating scabies. Cochrane Database Syst Rev 2007(2):000320.

80. Wooltorton E. Concerns over lindane treatment for scabies and lice. CMAJ 2003;168(11):1447.

81. Diazgranados JA, Costa JL. Deaths after ivermectin treatment. Lancet 1997;349:1698.

82. Mumcuoglu KY, Miller J, Zamir C, Zentner G, Helbin V, Ingber A. The in vivo pediculocidal efficacy of a natural remedy. Israel Med Assoc J 2002;4(10):790–3.

83. Wormser GP, Dattwyler RJ, Shapiro ED, Halperin JJ, Steere AC, Klempner MS, et al. The clinical assessment, treatment, and prevention of Lyme disease, human granulocytic anaplasmosis, and babesiosis: clinical practice guidelines by the Infectious Diseases Society of America. Clin Infect Dis 2006;43:1089–134.

84. Maenthaisong R, Chaiyakunapruk N, Niruntraporn S, Kongkaew C. The efficacy of aloe vera used for burn wound healing: a systematic review. Burns 2007;33(6):713–8.

85. Sforcin JM. Propolis and the immune system: a review. J Ethnopharmacol 2007;113(2):1–14.

86. Huang W, Vidimos A. Topical anesthetics in dermatology. J Amer Acad Dermatol 2000;43(2):286–98.

87. Eidelman A, Weiss JM, Lau J, Carr DB. Topical anesthesia for dermal instrumentation: a systematic review of randomized controlled trials. Ann Emerg Med 2005;46:343–51.

88. Friedman PM, Fogelman JP, Nouri K, Levine VJ, Ashinoff R. Comparative study of the efficacy of four topical anesthetics. Dermatologic Surg 1999; 25(12):950–4.

89. Singer AJ, Stark MJ. LET versus EMLA for pretreating lacerations: a randomized trial. Acad Emerg Med 2001;8(3):223–230.

90. Kamrin MA. Phthalate risks, phthalate regulation, and public health: a review. J Toxicol Environ Health B Crit Rev 2009;12(2):157–74.

91. Darbre PD, Harvey PW. Paraben esters: review of recent studies of endocrine toxicity, absorption, esterase and human exposure, and discussion of potential human health risks. J Appl Toxicol 2008;28(5):561–78.

92. Dweck AC. The internal and external use of medicinal plants. Clin Dermatol 2009;27(2):148–58.

93. Barbano R. Risks of erasing wrinkles: buyer beware. Neurology 2006;67:E17–8.

94. Paus R, Costarelis G. Biology of hair follicles. N Engl J Med 1999;341:491–502.

95. Hunter MH, Carek PJ. Evaluation and treatment of women with hirsutism. Am Fam Physician 2003;67:2565–72.

96. Blume-Peytavi U, Hahn S. Medical treatment of hirsutism. Dermatol Thera 2008; 21(5):329–39.

97. Shapiro J. Hair loss in women. N Engl J Med 2007;357:1620–30.

98. Camacho-Martines F. Hair loss in women. Sem Cutan Med Surg 2009;28:19–32.

99. Prager N, Bickett K, French N, Marcovici G. A randomized, double-blind, placebo-controlled trial to determine the effectiveness of botanically derived inhibitors of 5-alpha-reductase in the treatment of androgenetic alopecia. J Altern Complement Med 2002 Apr;8(2):143–52. Erratum in: J Altern Complement Med 2006 Mar;12(2):199.

100. Bandaranayake I, Mirmirani P. Hair loss remedies-separating fact from fiction. Cutis 2004;73:107–14.

101. DeVillez RL, Jacobs JP, Szpunar CA, Warner ML. Androgenetic alopecia in the female: treatment with 2% topical minoxidil solution. Arch Dermatol 1994;130:303–7.

102. Clark RK. Anatomy and physiology: understanding the human body. Sudbury, MA: Jones and Bartlett Publishers, 2005.

27

Otic and Ophthalmic Disorders

Patrick J. M. Murphy and Therese M. Horan

"The best and most beautiful things in the world cannot be seen or even touched. They must be felt with the heart."

HELEN KELLER

Chapter Glossary

Acute otitis media Inflammation of the middle ear. The word *otitis* is Greek for *inflammation of the ear.*

Aqueous humor The watery fluid that circulates in the anterior and posterior chambers of the eye.

Cerumen Earwax.

Choroid Vascular dark brown membrane that lies between the retina and the sclera. Anteriorly, the choroid differentiates into the ciliary body.

Ciliary body A blood-rich ring of tissue that encircles the lens and is composed of the ciliary muscles and ciliary processes. The ciliary processes contain the capillaries that secrete the aqueous humor.

Ciliary muscle Muscle that encircles the lens and controls the shape of the lens.

Closed-angle glaucoma Condition that occurs when the pupil dilates to such an extent that the iris leans against the cornea and blocks outflow of aqueous humor.

Conjunctivitis Commonly called "pink eye," an inflammation of the conjunctiva.

Cornea The transparent anterior part of the eye that allows light to pass through it to the lens.

Cycloplegic drugs Drugs that paralyze the ciliary body and prevent the lens from changing shape. They are used during eye examinations.

Exophthalmos Bulging of the eye anteriorly out of the orbit.

Fixed-dose combination A medication that contains two different drugs, usually a beta-blocker and prostaglandin analog, in one formulation.

Glaucoma A group of disorders characterized by vision loss that is secondary to damage to the optic nerve. This damage occurs when pressure in the aqueous humor increases and interferes with the blood flow to the optic nerve.

Intraocular pressure The pressure created by the aqueous humor.

Iris The colored muscular tissue behind the cornea that contains the opening or pupil in the middle that allows light into the lens.

Lens A transparent crystalline curved structure located directly behind the iris and pupil. The lens is attached to the ciliary body by ligaments.

Miosis Constriction of the pupil.

Miotics Drugs that cause constriction of the pupil.

Mydriasis Excessive dilation of the pupil.

Nystagmus Involuntary eye movement.

Open-angle glaucoma Increased intraocular pressure that results from a blockage in the trabecular meshwork or Schlemm's canal.

Ophthalmia neonatorum Gonorrheal conjunctivitis that occurs when a neonate passes through the birth canal of a mother infected with *N. gonorrhea.*

Otalgia Ear pain or earache.

Otitis externa Inflammation of the external ear canal.

Retina The light-sensitive tissue lining the inner surface of the eye, exposed to the aqueous humor.

Schlemm's canal The canal that delivers aqueous humor from the anterior chamber of the eye into the systemic circulation.

Sclera The fibrous protective outer layer of the eye. Also known as the white of the eye.

Sympathomimetic mydriatic drugs Drugs that cause the iris radial muscle to contract, which results in pupil dilation. Sympathomimetic mydriatics do not paralyze the ciliary muscle and consequently do not prevent lens movement or refocusing during the examination.

Trabecular meshwork Tissue in the eye that is located near the ciliary body and drains the aqueous humor into Schlemm's canal.

Introduction

The use of pharmaceuticals to treat disorders affecting the eye and ear often involves specialized approaches to pharmacotherapy. Although many of the medications discussed in this chapter are presented in detail in other chapters, the route of administration, pharmacokinetics, and pharmacodynamics of a drug may all be modified when used to treat an ophthalmic or otic condition. Ophthalmic medications are frequently used to treat **glaucoma**, **conjunctivitis**, and dry eye. Drugs used for otic disorders include treatments for **acute otitis media** and **otitis externa**.

Structure of the Eye

Medications used to treat ophthalmic disorders primarily act in the anterior chamber of the eye, affecting the **ciliary body**, **trabecular meshwork** and **Schlemm's canal**, **iris**, and **aqueous humor**. First, a brief review of the anatomy of the eye is in order (Figure 27-1).

The eye is an irregular sphere. The wall of the eye has three layers: the **sclera**, **choroid**, and **retina**. The sclera is the outermost layer; it is made of tough, white connective tissue and surrounds the sphere of the eyeball except for where the **cornea** lies. The choroid is a vascular, dark brown membrane that lies between the retina and the sclera. Anteriorly, the choroid differentiates into the ciliary body. The ciliary body surrounds the **lens** and is composed of the **ciliary muscle** that controls the shape of the lens and the ciliary processes that contain the capillaries, which secrete the fluid that makes up the aqueous humor. The lens is a transparent crystalline curved structure located behind the iris and pupil. The lens is attached to the ciliary body by ligaments.

Aqueous humor is the watery fluid that circulates in the anterior and posterior chambers of the eye. The aqueous humor transports oxygen and nutrients to the lens and cornea, facilitates the removal of wastes, and maintains the convex shape of the cornea. It is secreted by the ciliary processes in the posterior chamber, traverses around the iris and through the pupil into the anterior chamber, and is ultimately drained into the venous system primarily through the trabecular meshwork and Schlemm's canal.

Under normal physiologic conditions, an intraocular pressure of 10–20 mm Hg results from the presence of aqueous humor. A constant intraocular pressure is maintained as the rate of aqueous humor production by the ciliary body is equivalent to the rate of drainage through the trabecular meshwork. Antiglaucoma medications are

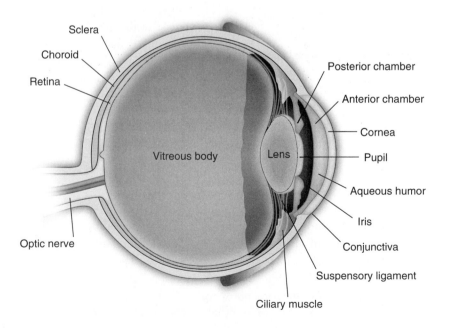

Figure 27-1 Anatomy of the eye.

able to decrease intraocular pressure by either decreasing aqueous humor production or increasing aqueous humor outflow. While the majority of outflow occurs through Schlemm's canal, a fraction (< 20%) of the aqueous humor drains through the iris root (i.e., the uveoscleral pathway), which is subject to pharmacotherapeutic modulation.

Autonomic Nervous System Innervation

Regions of the eye are innervated by both the sympathetic and parasympathetic nervous systems. Activation of muscarinic cholinergic receptors in the ciliary muscle causes contraction, thus focusing the lens for near vision, while activation of muscarinic receptors in the iris sphincter muscle results in pupil constriction, also called **miosis**. Drugs that cause pupil constriction are called **miotics**. Contraction of the ciliary muscle leads to increased opening of pores in the trabecular meshwork that increases aqueous humor outflow and subsequently reduces intraocular pressure. Alpha$_1$ adrenergic receptor activation in the iris radial muscle causes muscle contraction, resulting in **mydriasis** or excessive dilation of the pupil, which facilitates increased outflow of aqueous humor. Aqueous humor outflow may also be increased in the uveoscleral pathway by activation of the sympathetic nervous system. Beta$_1$- and beta$_2$-adrenergic receptors are present on the ciliary epithelium that covers the ciliary processes, and their stimulation facilitates aqueous humor secretion. Inhibition of beta receptors decreases secretion, leading to a lowering of intraocular pressure.

The eye produces a wide range of pharmacokinetically significant enzymes, including acetylcholinesterase, carbonic anhydrase, catechol-O-methyltransferase (COMT), and monoamine oxidase (MAO), all of which affect drug metabolism. Several medications discussed later in this chapter are metabolized by these enzymes, either from an active drug to an inactive metabolite or from an inactive prodrug to an active compound.

Effects of Ocular Physiology on Pharmacokinetic Properties

The pharmacokinetics of topically administered ophthalmic medications deserves special comment. Most are prepared in an aqueous formulation and absorbed into the tear film and epithelium via passive diffusion. Hydrophobic gels and ointments may be used to extend the duration a medication is present on the eye surface. Following topical administration, high concentrations of ophthalmic drugs amass in the aqueous humor and are subsequently distributed through the trabecular meshwork.

Box 27-1 Administration of Topical Ophthalmic Medications

1. Prior to administration, wash hands with soap and water.

2. If the medication is formulated as a suspension, thoroughly shake the bottle.

3. The dropper tip should be treated as a sterile applicator, and it should not touch the eye or come into contact with any surface.

4. With the head tilted back, depress the lower eyelid and gently squeeze the dropper releasing one drop into the eye at a time, then rest with the eyes closed for at least 1–2 minutes before administering the next drop of the same medication.

5. Excess medication can be wiped away from the eye with a clean tissue.

6. In order to allow maximum absorption, 10–15 minutes should transpire between topical administrations of different medications.

They may be absorbed into the bloodstream through the nasal mucosa and systemically distributed throughout the body. Topically administered ophthalmic drugs that are absorbed into the bloodstream through this pathway bypass first-pass metabolism in the liver, which may lead to the accumulation of pharmacologically significant serum drug concentrations. Gentle eyelid closure following drug application increases drug exposure to the eye and decreases systemic absorption. Instructions for administering topical ophthalmic medications are presented in Box 27-1.

Glaucoma

Glaucoma includes a collection of ophthalmic disorders characterized by visual field loss and optic nerve damage. The term glaucoma comes from the Greek word *glaukos*, which means "bluish gray." The term was first used by Hippocrates in referring to the color of the cornea when increased intraocular pressure exists.[1] Glaucoma is often secondary to elevated intraocular pressure caused by impaired outflow of aqueous humor in the anterior chamber. Glaucoma is the leading cause of preventable blindness in the United States and is most common in women and men older than 60 years of age.[2] The initial diagnosis of glaucoma is made by an ophthalmologist.

The two principle forms of glaucoma are **open-angle glaucoma** and **closed-angle glaucoma** (Figure 27-2). Primary open-angle glaucoma accounts for > 90% of glaucoma and is the leading cause of blindness among African Americans. It is estimated that approximately 2.47 million persons in the United States suffer from glaucoma and

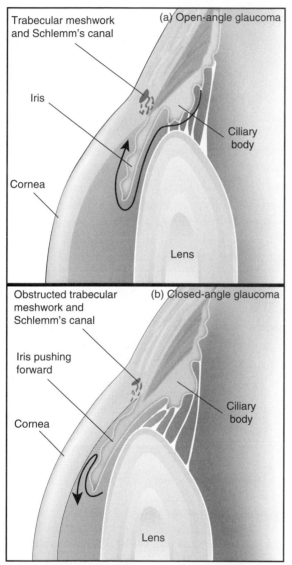

Aqueous humor movement is represented by the arrow. In open-angle glaucoma (a), the trabecular meshwork and Schlemm's canal are accessible. In closed-angle glaucoma (b), the iris occludes the trabecular meshwork and Schlemm's canal, preventing aqueous humor outflow.

Figure 27-2 Illustration of impaired aqueous humor flow in open-angle glaucoma and closed-angle glaucoma.

130,450 of them are legally blind secondary to this disease.[3] Glaucoma is six times more prevalent in African Americans than in Whites, and African Americans are more likely than Whites to develop blindness.[3]

Glaucoma is a chronic and often bilateral disorder that may be painless and progress undiagnosed for years until peripheral vision loss begins to occur. Open-angle glaucoma results from a blockage in either the trabecular meshwork or Schlemm's canal, which prevents aqueous humor outflow and drainage. In contrast to closed-angle glaucoma, the pupil does not dilate or cause a blockage of aqueous humor circulation. Open-angle glaucoma may also develop in persons with disorders such as diabetes mellitus, eye surgery, and hypertension. Closed-angle glaucoma is also referred to as narrow-angle glaucoma. Closed-angle glaucoma develops when the pupil dilates to such an extent that the iris abuts the cornea and blocks outflow of aqueous humor through Schlemm's canal. This disorder is more common in Asians and Asian Americans. Acute closed-angle glaucoma is an emergent condition that develops rapidly, may cause exceptional pain, and can lead to complete and irreversible blindness if untreated within 5 days.

The primary risk factor for both forms of glaucoma is increased **intraocular pressure**.[4] Although it is an important consideration, elevated intraocular pressure measured by tonometry is not in itself definitive for diagnosing chronic glaucoma. A person with primary open-angle glaucoma may be asymptomatic and have an intraocular pressure within normal limits (i.e., 10–20 mm Hg). Individuals may have an extremely elevated intraocular pressure (> 30 mm Hg) but no evidence of optic nerve damage. Genetic testing may assist in screening, and age and family history of glaucoma are additional established risk factors.[5]

Open-Angle Glaucoma Pharmacotherapy

The goal of therapy for open-angle glaucoma is to inhibit disease progression and further optic nerve damage by decreasing intraocular pressure.[6] Open-angle glaucoma is typically managed with topical applications such as eye drops; ointments; and emulsions of beta-adrenergic receptor blockers, which will be referred to as beta-blockers in this chapter; prostaglandin analogs; carbonic anhydrase inhibitors; and alpha$_2$ agonists, all of which decrease intraocular pressure by decreasing aqueous humor volume.[7,8] As discussed later in this chapter, the medications decrease intraocular pressure by either inhibiting aqueous humor production or by increasing outflow. Although not curative, long-term pharmacotherapy for open-angle glaucoma can decrease or prevent further nerve damage.

For an initial course of treatment, it is desirable to have intraocular pressure decreased by approximately 20% from the baseline.[9] In persons exhibiting normotensive glaucoma or advanced optic neuropathy, intraocular pressure should be reduced by ≥ 30% of the baseline intraocular pressure.[8] If single-agent drug therapy is not sufficient to lower intraocular pressure to target levels, switching to an alternate medication or combination drug therapy should be considered. Intraocular pressure should be measured in each eye and managed independently.

The two most commonly identified first-line treatment regimens utilize monotherapy of either a beta-blocker or prostaglandin analog.[6] Beta-blockers are efficacious and have been used as antiglaucoma drugs for more than 20 years, but prostaglandins appear to be equally efficacious and have a better side effect profile.[10] In either case, the lowest efficacious dose of medication should be used after assessing for any individual contraindications for specific agents. If both beta-blockers and prostaglandin analogs are contraindicated, a carbonic anhydrase inhibitor or alpha$_2$ agonist should be considered as a second-line agent.

The evaluation period for an initial treatment is performed over 2–4 months because some medications require 6–8 weeks to produce maximum therapeutic effects. Individuals should be reevaluated for therapeutic response and experienced side effects after 2–4 weeks of treatment, at which time the dose may be adjusted or an alternate first-line medication may be prescribed. If subsequent reevaluation indicates the adjustment in treatment produced unacceptable side effects or an insufficient decrease in intraocular pressure, it is possible to modify the dose, the drug, or consider selecting a second-line medication.

Multidrug pharmacotherapy typically involves 2–4 topically administered medications from different drug classes. In addition to **fixed-dose combinations**, a single-agent beta-blocker is often prescribed with either a prostaglandin or carbonic anhydrase inhibitor.[11] Multidrug treatment regimens, although efficacious, have several potential drawbacks including expense, inconvenience of administration, and additive side effects, all of which should be considered and discussed before being prescribed.

Closed-Angle Glaucoma Pharmacotherapy

Acute closed-angle glaucoma treatment often requires an initial medical and subsequent surgical approach. Initial pharmacotherapy is used to facilitate pupil constriction and mitigate intraocular pressure-associated pain. The goal of subsequent laser or conventional ophthalmic surgery is to increase the flow of fluid and decrease intraocular pressure. Pharmacotherapy includes rapidly acting, systemically administered osmotic diuretics as well as topically administered ocular medications used in treating open-angle glaucoma (e.g., beta-blockers, prostaglandins, and carbonic anhydrase inhibitors). Topical medication should be continued to manage intraocular pressure until surgery can be preformed.

Ocular Hypertension and Normotensive Open-Angle Glaucoma

There is considerable debate as to whether an individual who lacks optic nerve damage should be treated exclusively due to a finding of an abnormally high intraocular pressure. Approximately two thirds of persons with elevated intraocular pressure do not exhibit visual impairment. These individuals are referred to as having ocular hypertension. While some healthcare providers recommend drug therapy for anyone whose intraocular pressure is > 21 mm Hg, others prefer to carefully monitor an asymptomatic person until her intraocular pressure measures > 28–30 mm Hg or signs of visual field change are reported. The Early Manifest Glaucoma Trial demonstrated that early treatment decreases disease progression by half (hazard ratio = 0.50; 95% CI, 0.35, 0.71).[12,13]

In contrast, 10–15% of persons displaying glaucoma-associated optic nerve damage possess an intraocular pressure within normal limits (baseline < 21 mm Hg). Persons displaying this normal-tension glaucoma have nonetheless been shown to benefit from treatments targeting intraocular pressure reduction, showing a decrease in the progression of visual field loss.[9] Therapeutic goals and treatment approaches for managing ocular hypertension and normotensive open-angle glaucoma pharmacotherapy are comparable to primary open-angle glaucoma.

Glaucoma Over the Life Span

Studies investigating glaucoma and lifetime estrogen and progesterone exposure—including pregnancies, deliveries, menstruation years, and the use of oral contraceptives—have not found a significant correlation or increased risk for elevated intraocular pressure.[14] A cross-sectional cohort study evaluating the association between the consumption of fruits and vegetables and the presence of glaucoma in older women found that a higher intake of certain fruits and vegetables showed a decreased glaucoma risk of up to 69% (odds ratio 0.31; 95% CI, 0.11–0.91).[15]

Antiglaucoma Drugs

Pharmacotherapy for both open-angle glaucoma and closed-angle glaucoma is directed at decreasing intraocular pressure by altering aqueous humor production or outflow (Table 27-1). Currently, there are five major classes of drugs used for the treatment of glaucoma, which include (1) beta-adrenoreceptor antagonists, (2) prostaglandin analogues (3) carbonic anhydrase inhibitors (4) cholinergics (acetylcholine receptor agonists), and (5) adrenoceptor agonists.[10] Beta-adrenergic receptor blockers have been the most frequently used topical treatment, but recently, prostaglandin analogs have increasingly replaced beta-blockers.[16]

Prostaglandin analogs are equally efficacious and possess better tolerated side-effect profiles. Carbonic anhydrase inhibitors, alpha$_2$ adrenergic receptor agonists, nonselective sympathomimetics, cholinergic and anticholinesterase miotics, and osmotic diuretics all may be utilized depending on the individual condition. The different mechanisms of actions of these drug classes permit therapeutically advantageous combination drug therapy when monotherapy is insufficient. The profound difference in time frame disease progression—5–15 years for primary open-angle glaucoma versus 1–5 days for acute closed-angle glaucoma—necessitates differences in treatment methodologies and relative urgency.

Table 27-1 Antiglaucoma Medications

Drug Generic (Brand)	Formulation and Dose	Clinical Considerations	FDA Pregnancy Category
Beta$_1$ Receptor Antagonists			
Betaxolol (Betoptic)	0.5% solution or 0.25% suspension 1–2 drops bid	Avoid abrupt withdrawal Ocular irritation, dry eyes, and conjunctivitis; increased risk of bradycardia and hypotension; tolerance may develop.	C*
Levobetaxolol (Betaxon)	0.5% solution 1 drop bid		C*
Mixed Beta$_1$/Beta$_2$ Adrenergic Antagonists			
Timolol (Timoptic)	0.5% solution or 0.25% solution 1 drop qd or bid 0.5% gel or 0.25% gel 1 drop qd	For all beta$_1$/beta$_2$-acting drugs: Contraindicated in persons with bradycardia and atrioventricular heart block; use with caution in persons with asthma or COPD; carteolol produces least ocular burning, metipranolol produces greatest ocular burning.	C*
Carteolol (Ocupress)	1% solution 1 drop bid		C*
Levobunolol (Betagan)	0.5% solution 1 drop qd or bid 0.25% suspension 1 drop bid		C*
Metipranolol (OptiPranolol)	0.3% solution 1 drop bid		C*
Prostaglandin F$_{2\alpha}$ Analogs			
Latanoprost (Xalatan)	0.005% solution 1 drop qd	Localized irritation, redness, and hyperemia; administer in evening to decrease sensation of ocular pain; harmless iris discoloration; lengthening and darkening of eyelashes; latanoprost produces greatest iris discoloration; hyperemia occurs more commonly with bimatoprost and travoprost.	C
Travoprost (Travatan)	0.004% solution 1 drop qd		C
Bimatoprost (Lumigan)	0.03% solution 1 drop qd		C
Unoprostone (Rescula)	0.15% solution 1 drop qd or bid		C
Carbonic Anhydrase Inhibitors: Topical Formulations			
Brinzolamide (Azopt)	1% suspension 1 drop bid or tid	Produce substantially fewer systemic side effects than oral formulations; localized irritation, taste distortion; more ocular stinging with dorzolamide. All carbonic anhydrase inhibitors are sulfonamides and are contraindicated for persons with a sulfa allergy.	C
Dorzolamide (Trusopt)	2% solution 1 drop bid or tid		C
Carbonic Anhydrase Inhibitors: Oral Formulations			
Acetazolamide (Diamox)	Tablets: 125 mg, 250 mg 250 mg q 6–24 h	Fatigue and paresthesias; myopia, appetite loss, GI disturbances, blood dyscrasias, kidney stones; dichlorphenamide less well tolerated than others. All carbonic anhydrase inhibitors are sulfonamides and are contraindicated for persons with a sulfa allergy.	C
Methazolamide (Neptazane)	Tablets: 50 mg 50–100 mg bid or tid initially then 25–50 mg for maintenance bid or tid		C
Dichlorphenamide (Daranide)	Tablet: 50 mg 50–100 mg bid initially then 25–50 mg qd to tid for maintenance dose		C

(continues)

Table 27-1 Antiglaucoma Medications (*continued*)

Drug Generic (Brand)	Formulation and Dose	Clinical Considerations	FDA Pregnancy Category
Combination Medications			
Dorzolamide/timolol (Cosopt)	2%/0.5% solution 1 drop bid	Similar to once-daily administration of latanoprost. Give 10 min apart if given with other eye drops.	C
Alpha₂ Receptor Agonists			
Apraclonidine (Iopidine)	1% solution, 0.5% solution 1 drop bid or tid	Localized irritation, hyperemia, headache; hypotension. Apraclonidine indicated for short-term use only. Respiratory arrest and fatigue (greatest concern in children with brimonidine).	C
Brimonidine (Alphagan)	0.15% solution, 0.1% solution 1 drop bid or qid		B
Nonselective Sympathomimetics			
Dipivefrin (Propine)	0.1% solution 1 drop qd or bid	Contraindicated in closed-angle glaucoma; mydriasis; systemic effects including increased heart rate, blood pressure, and arrhythmias.	B
Epinephryl Borate (Eppy/N)	2% solution, 0.25% solution 1–2 drops qd or bid		C
Direct-Acting Cholinergic Receptor Agonists (Cholinergic Miotics)			
Carbachol (Carboptic)	3% solution 2.25% solution 1.5% solution 0.75% solution 1 drop bid or tid	Myopia, headaches, irritation, and red eye; bradycardia and bronchospasm; should be avoided by persons with iritis or asthma.	C
Pilocarpine (Isopto Carpine)	2% solution 0.5% solution 1 drop q 4–12 h		C
Anticholinesterase Inhibitors (Anticholinesterase Miotics)			
Echothiophate (Phospholine)	0.25% solution 0.03% solution 1–2 drops qd or bid	Myopia, headache; bradycardia, and bronchospasm; has potential to promote cataract formation.	C
Osmotic Diuretics (Only for Acute Closed-Angle Glaucoma)			
Glycerin (Ophthalgan)	50% solution 75% solution	Peripheral edema, electrolyte imbalances, tremors, dizziness, headaches, use with caution if renal impairment or cardiovascular disease.	C
Mannitol (Osmitrol)	20% solution		C

* Contraindicated during second and third trimesters of pregnancy.

Beta-Adrenergic Receptor Antagonists (Beta-Blockers)

Beta-adrenergic receptor antagonists have been the drugs of choice for treating primary open-angle glaucoma.[17] These agents decrease aqueous humor production in the ciliary body, thus lowering intraocular pressure. They may be used as part of the initial management of acute closed-angle glaucoma. The six topically administered medications approved for use in treating glaucoma include the beta₁-selective drugs betaxolol (Betoptic) and levobetaxolol (Betaxon) and the nonselective beta₁/beta₂ antagonists carteolol (Ocupress), levobunolol (Betagan), metipranolol (OptiPranolol), and timolol (Timoptic).

Beta-blockers inhibit the beta-adrenergic receptors of the ciliary epithelium, which results in a decrease in aqueous humor production, which in turn lowers intra-ocular pressure. Although the overwhelming majority of beta receptors in this tissue are of the beta₂ subtype, the beta₁-selective antagonists have been shown to be equally efficacious, and the exact mechanism of action is not well elucidated. Ophthalmic beta-blockers have a long duration of action, which permits them to be administered as single drops either once or twice daily. They have been shown to decrease intraocular pressure by 20–30% from pretreatment levels.[18] Tolerance to ophthalmic beta-blockers may develop with chronic use. As such, periodic monitoring of intraocular pressure is required, and there is the potential need to switch to a medication of a different class or employ combination drug therapy. Differences between members of the drug class include cost, frequency of administration, and the frequency of systemic side effects.

Side Effects/Adverse Effects

Beta-blockers have relatively minor localized side effects including ocular irritation, dry eyes, and conjunctivitis. These effects are generally equivalent among the six drugs. Relative to other members of the class, carteolol (Ocupress) has been reported to produce the least amount of ocular burning and stinging, while metipranolol has been cited as causing the most.[19] Fewer ocular side effects are typically reported with beta-blockers than with second-line treatment modalities, such as epinephrine or pilocarpine.

Disseminated sympatholytic side effects are possible, due in part to the lack of first-pass metabolism following systemic drug absorption. The nonselective $beta_1/beta_2$ antagonists in particular are contraindicated for persons with bradycardia and atrioventricular heart block and should be used with caution by persons with asthma or chronic obstructive pulmonary disease (COPD). Ophthalmic beta-blockers have the potential to inhibit cardiac $beta_1$ and pulmonary $beta_2$ receptors, and thus may cause or exacerbate these conditions. The $beta_1$-selective drugs betaxolol (Betoptic) and levobetaxolol (Betaxon) are less likely to cause bronchospasm and are the preferred beta-blockers for individuals with asthma or COPD; however, they have been reported to cause greater local irritation. Concurrent use of topical ophthalmic beta-blockers and oral cardiac beta-blockers should be avoided as the combination poses an increased risk of bradycardia and hypotension. Systemic side effects decrease in intensity following the first 2 weeks of therapy.

Pregnancy and Lactation

Currently available evidence suggests beta-blockers are generally safe during pregnancy; however, neonatal hypoglycemia, bradycardia, and arrhythmia have all been reported following maternal use of ophthalmic beta-blockers during pregnancy, at parturition, or during breastfeeding. Expert panel recommendations indicate that beta-blockers, including betaxolol (Betoptic) and timolol (Timoptic), be considered an FDA Pregnancy Category D drug during the second and third trimesters.

Prostaglandin Analogs

Prostaglandin $F_{2\alpha}$ analogs represent a newer drug class and have increasingly become the preferred treatment approach for primary open-angle glaucoma.[19] They may be administered once daily as monotherapy and can reduce intraocular pressure by 40–60%. All four prostaglandin analogs have been shown to be equally efficacious as the beta-blockers and display a generally more favorable side effect profile. The drugs increase the outflow of aqueous humor through the uveoscleral pathway and relaxation of the ciliary muscle. Relaxation occurs by several mechanisms, some of which are not fully understood. Prostaglandin analogs may be given in combination with beta-blockers if either drug alone is unable to sufficiently decrease intraocular pressure.

The four ophthalmic prostaglandin analogs are latanoprost (Xalatan), travoprost (Travatan), unoprostone (Rescula), and bimatoprost (Lumigan). These medications are administered topically once daily and are generally well tolerated with minimal systemic side effects. Latanoprost (Xalatan) was the first member of the class and is the most frequently prescribed of all antiglaucoma medications. Bimatoprost (Lumigan) and travoprost (Travatan) have been shown to be efficacious in African Americans with primary open-angle glaucoma.[20]

Side Effects/Adverse Effects

Prostaglandin analogs are well tolerated and systemic reactions are not common. There are a few notable localized adverse effects, including irritation and redness, the physically harmless discoloration (browning) of the iris, and lengthening and darkening of eyelashes. The discomfort typically dissipates during the first month of therapy and may be further decreased by administering the medication before bedtime. Discoloration of the iris occurs most often with latanoprost (Xalatan) and is often permanent.

The most frequently reported adverse effect of prostaglandin analogs is hyperemia, which typically occurs with bimatoprost (Lumigan) and travoprost (Travatan). Some persons who have an insufficient intraocular pressure reduction following latanoprost treatment have been shown to be responsive to bimatoprost.[21]

Pregnancy and Lactation

There are currently no well-controlled antiglaucoma prostaglandin studies in pregnant women, and they are classified as FDA Pregnancy Category C drugs. An observational study of 11 women indicated no systemic or neonatal side effects as a consequence of topically administered latanoprost.[22] However, given adverse fetal effects in animal studies of latanoprost and known uterine actions of orally administered prostaglandins, the question of whether prostaglandin analogs should be contraindicated during pregnancy is currently unresolved.[23]

Carbonic Anhydrase Inhibitors

Carbonic anhydrase inhibitors are second-line antiglaucoma medications available as for both topical and oral administration. In addition to being used for treating individuals who are not responsive to first-line medications for a chronic condition, carbonic anhydrase inhibitors may also be used in the initial management of acute closed-angle glaucoma as part of multidrug therapy. The medications are also used perioperatively for decreasing intraocular pressure prior to eye surgery. Individuals < 40 years of age experience fewer side effects from the medications than older persons do. While the oral drugs were the first to be developed, the topically administered agents have overwhelmingly replaced them due to their improved side effect profiles. The efficacy of topical carbonic anhydrase inhibitors is similar to that observed with timolol (Timoptic). Like beta-blockers, carbonic anhydrase inhibitors reduce intraocular pressure by inhibiting production of aqueous humor. Carbonic anhydrase is an enzyme found in the epithelial cells of the ciliary processes that converts water and carbon dioxide to bicarbonate. Carbonic anhydrase inhibitors prevent the enzymatic production of bicarbonate necessary for fluid transport and aqueous humor production.

The topical formulations include dorzolamide (Trusopt) and brinzolamide (Azopt). Dorzolamide is more often used, both as a single agent and in combination with other antiglaucoma drugs. Topical carbonic anhydrase inhibitors require twice-a-day or three-times-a-day dosing, which is substantially less convenient than the once-daily dosing offered with prostaglandin analogs and some beta-blockers.

Dorzolamide (Trusopt) is available in a fixed dose formulation with the beta-blocker timolol (Cosopt). Twice-a-day dosing of the dorzolamide/timolol (Cosopt) fixed-combination therapy results in safety and efficacy similar to once-daily administration of latanoprost (Xalatan).[24] Both treatments reduce diurnal intraocular pressure from baseline ($P < .0001$), and there is no statistical difference in intraocular pressure between treatments ($P \leq 0.1$) or any individual adverse event. Dorzolamide/timolol is an FDA Pregnancy Category C drug secondary to documented teratogenic effects in animal studies and should be used with caution during pregnancy.

Side Effects/Adverse Effects

Both topical and oral medications are sulfonamides and are therefore contraindicated in persons with known sulfa allergy. The topically administered carbonic anhydrase inhibitors are generally well tolerated and produce substantially fewer systemic effects than orally administered formulations; however, topical formulations are more likely to cause localized reactions, including eye irritation and the sensation of a bitter taste shortly following drug administration. Incidents of ocular stinging and burning occur less frequently with brinzolamide, due to the neutral pH of the medication.

Oral Formulations

The orally administered drugs include acetazolamide (Diamox), methazolamide (Neptazane), and dichlorphenamide (Daranide). The systemic side effects of the orally administered carbonic anhydrase inhibitors have substantially limited their use, and they are no longer recommended for long-term therapy. They are known to cause effects of the nervous system and may result in fatigue and paresthesias. Additional side effects include myopia, loss of appetite, GI disturbances, blood dyscrasias, and kidney stones. Oral carbonic anhydrase inhibitors have diuretic properties, which may result in an electrolyte imbalance and require monitoring. They cross the placenta and are excreted in breast milk.

Alpha$_2$ Adrenergic Receptor Agonists

Brimonidine (Alphagan) and apraclonidine (Iopidine) are alpha$_2$ adrenergic receptor agonists. These drugs inhibit production of aqueous humor and are used as second-line antiglaucoma therapies. Of the two agents, brimonidine is used more often, either as monotherapy if the individual is unresponsive to first-line open-angle glaucoma treatment or as a component in a multidrug regimen. Its efficacy approaches that of timolol and produces a decrease in intraocular pressure of approximately 15–25%. Brimonidine may also produce a beneficial neuroprotective effect via an unidentified mechanism that is independent of intraocular pressure reduction.[25] Apraclonidine is used only short term and perioperatively for eye surgery. Both medications are administered topically three times daily.

The most common side effects include ocular irritation, red eye, hyperemia, and headache. These drugs produce few systemic cardiovascular effects. Brimonidine (Alphagan) is the more lipophilic of the two agents. Brimonidine crosses the blood–brain barrier and elicits alpha$_2$-mediated effects in the brain, including hypotension and fatigue. The CNS effects of brimonidine are of concern and this drug should be used with caution. Nonetheless, brimonidine is classified as an FDA Pregnancy Category B drug while apraclonidine is classified as FDA Pregnancy Category C. Well-controlled studies in pregnant women have not been completed with either medication.

Nonselective Adrenergic Receptor Agonists (Sympathomimetics)

Activators of the sympathetic nervous system in the eye have been shown to be useful as a third-line antiglaucoma treatment approach capable of lowering intraocular pressure.[26] Paradoxically, a nonselective adrenergic receptor agonist may be used in consort with a beta-adrenergic receptor antagonist to lower intraocular pressure. Adrenergic receptor agonists are presumed to decrease intraocular pressure by increasing uveoscleral outflow and also modifying blood flow to the ciliary body. The most commonly used medication in this class is dipivefrin (Propine).

Dipivefrin (Propine) is a highly soluble prodrug that is administered topically twice daily. Once absorbed into the eye, it is rapidly hydrolyzed by enzymes such as acetylcholinesterase and carbonic anhydrase into the active drug epinephrine. Epinephrine stimulates ophthalmic alpha$_1$ adrenergic receptors causing mydriasis, which results in an increase in aqueous humor outflow.

Side Effects/Adverse Effects

Epinephrine is primarily metabolized by ocular enzymes such as COMT and MAO; however, a pharmacologically significant amount of the drug can enter systemic circulation, which causes an increase in blood pressure, arrhythmias, and tachycardia. Because mydriasis exacerbates closed-angle glaucoma, nonselective adrenergic receptor agonists are contraindicated for persons with this condition.

Cholinergic Receptor Agonists (Cholinergic Miotics)

Activation of muscarinic (M$_3$) cholinergic receptors in the eye causes pupil constriction (i.e., miosis) and contraction of the ciliary muscle, thus stretching the trabecular meshwork and permitting greater outflow of aqueous humor. Topically administered direct-acting cholinergic receptor agonists, also referred to as *cholinergic miotics*, include pilocarpine (Isopto Carpine) and carbachol (Carboptic). Cholinergic miotics mimic the effects of acetylcholine in the eye and have been shown to be efficacious in the management of both open- and closed-angle glaucoma. They were among the first classes of medications to be used to lower intraocular pressure and can reduce intraocular pressure by 20–30%. However, their use has substantially declined with the advent of ophthalmic beta-blockers and prostaglandin analogs.[27] Pilocarpine (Isopto Carpine) is the best tolerated cholinergic miotic. These medications have relatively short half-lives and require administration three or four times per day. The combination therapy of a beta-blocker (metipranolol) and cholinergic miotic (pilocarpine) can produce a synergistic effect.

Side Effects/Adverse Effects

Miotics have several common side effects including myopia, ciliary spasm leading to headaches, irritation, and red eye. Although these drugs generally produce fewer systemic effects than the first-line antiglaucoma medications, the frequency with which persons using them experience discomfort from the localized side effects makes them a second- or third-line medication. Cholinergic miotics should be avoided in persons with iritis due to potential worsening of inflammation. Systemic effects, when present, result in generalized parasympathetic activation and include bradycardia and bronchospasm. As such, these drugs are contraindicated in persons with asthma.

Anticholinesterase Inhibitors (Anticholinesterase Miotics)

Ocular acetylcholinesterase regulates the parasympathetic response in the eye by degrading acetylcholine and thus dissipating muscarinic cholinergic receptor activation. Cholinesterase inhibition prevents acetylcholine degradation through this pathway and allows the neurotransmitter to have a prolonged effect via continued interaction with muscarinic receptors. Anticholinesterase inhibitors consequently may be regarded as indirect-acting cholinergic activators. The one drug in this class used for treating glaucoma is echothiophate (Phospholine). Echothiophate irreversibly inhibits cholinesterases, resulting in an extended duration of action of acetylcholine. It is administered topically once every 12–48 hours and is indicated for treating primary open-angle glaucoma in persons who are not responsive to first- or other second-line drug regimens. Anticholinesterase miotics display intraocular pressure reductions equivalent to those achieved using direct-acting cholinergic miotics.[28]

Echothiophate (Phospholine) shares many therapeutic effects and adverse effects with the direct-acting muscarinic agonists. Myopia and headache may develop, as well as increased systemic parasympathetic activity at high doses. Due to the longer half-life of echothiophate, the drug has a greater potential to promote the formation of cataracts. It is more often used by persons who have had lenses removed.

Osmotic Diuretics

The ophthalmic uses of osmotic diuretics are limited to use for acute closed-angle glaucoma emergencies and preoperatively before eye surgery. They are not used for chronic antiglaucoma therapy. Ophthalmic osmotic diuretics include oral formulations of glycerin (Ophthalgan) and isosorbide (Isordil) and an intravenous infusion of mannitol (Osmitrol). These drugs rapidly lower intraocular pressure by creating an osmotic gradient between intraocular fluid (i.e., both aqueous humor and vitreous humor) and the blood, drawing intraocular fluid from the eye and into the vasculature.[29] These medications produce maximum effects within 0.5–1 hour and should be used with caution by individuals with renal or cardiovascular disease. Side effects include peripheral edema, electrolyte imbalances, tremors, dizziness, and headache.

Cycloplegic and Mydriatic Drugs Used During Eye Examinations

Ophthalmic anticholinergic **cycloplegic drugs** (cycloplegics) and **sympathomimetic mydriatic drugs** (mydriatics) are ophthalmic medications used during diagnostic eye exams and ocular surgery. They are administered topically and act on the autonomic nervous system within the eye. Anticholinergic cycloplegics and sympathomimetic mydriatics both facilitate pupil dilatation (mydriasis). Additionally, anticholinergic cycloplegics paralyze the ciliary muscle and thus prevent the lens from adjusting. All these drugs are used clinically for measurement of refraction, intraocular examination, eye surgery, and adjunctive therapy for anterior uveitis. Because of their differing mechanisms of action, anticholinergic and sympathomimetic drugs may be combined to produce greater mydriasis than that observed with a single agent.

Anticholinergic Cycloplegic Drugs

Anticholinergic cycloplegic drugs inhibit muscarinic receptor activation by blocking their interaction with acetylcholine (Table 27-2). Anticholinergic medications cause mydriasis by blocking muscarinic receptors of the iris sphincter muscle, thus inhibiting iris muscle contraction and preventing reflex pupil constriction during the exam. Mydriasis enables the examiner to more fully observe the interior of the eye. The five topically administered anticholinergic cycloplegics—atropine (Atropisol), cyclopentolate (AK-Pentolate), homatropine (Isopto Homatropine), scopolamine (Isopto Hyoscine), and tropicamide

Table 27-2 Mydriatic and Cycloplegic Drugs

Drug Generic (Brand)	Formulation	Dose	Duration of Action	Clinical Considerations	FDA Pregnancy Category
Anticholinergic Cycloplegic Drugs (Cycloplegics)					
Atropine (Atropisol)	2% solution 1% solution 0.5% solution	1 drop before exam	Long (5–12 days)	Photophobia and blurred vision; closed-angle glaucoma secondary to mydriasis. Classic anticholinergic symptoms (dry mouth, blurred vision, constipation, urinary retention, tachycardia, and mental clouding).	C
Cyclopentolate (AK-Pentolate)	2% solution 1% solution 0.5% solution	1 drop before exam	Short (1 day)		C
Homatropine (Isopto Homatropine)	5% solution 2% solution	1–2 drops before exam	Intermediate (1–3 days)		C
Scopolamine (Isopto Hyoscine)	0.25% solution	1–2 drops before exam	Intermediate (1–3 days)		C
Tropicamide (Mydriacyl)	1% solution 0.5% solution	1–2 drops before exam	Very short (< 1 day)		C
Sympathomimetic Mydriatic Drugs (Mydriatics)					
Phenylephrine (Neo-Synephrine)	10% solution for uveitis 2.5% solution	1 drop before exam	Very short (< 1 day)	Photophobia and intense pain in response to bright light; closed-angle glaucoma secondary to mydriasis. Sympathetic nervous system activation (hypertension, dysrhythmias, tremor, and mental clouding).	C

(Mydriacyl)—have similar efficacies and side effect profiles; however, their durations of action vary.[30]

Side Effects/Adverse Effects

The most common side effects include photophobia secondary to pupil dilation and blurred vision secondary to ciliary muscle paralysis and inhibited lens movement. Mydriasis may cause the iris to occlude the trabecular meshwork, which can precipitate a rapid elevation in intraocular pressure and acute closed-angle glaucoma. At therapeutic concentrations, cycloplegics may be absorbed into systemic circulation and produce both peripheral and CNS effects. Systemic effects present as the classic anticholinergic symptoms of dry mouth, blurred vision, constipation, urinary retention, tachycardia, and mental clouding.

Sympathomimetic Mydriatic Drugs

Phenylephrine (Neo-Synephrine) is a potent, direct-acting alpha$_1$ adrenergic receptor agonist with weak beta-adrenergic receptor activity. It stimulates the iris radial muscle to cause contraction, which results in pupil dilation. Sympathomimetic mydriatics do not paralyze the ciliary muscle and consequently do not prevent lens movement or refocusing during the examination.

Side Effects/Adverse Effects

Sympathomimetic mydriatic drugs, like the anticholinergic cycloplegics, can cause acute closed-angle glaucoma secondary to mydriasis. Additional side effects include photophobia and intense pain in response to bright light. Systemic absorption of phenylephrine may result in sympathetic nervous system activation, resulting in hypertension, dysrhythmias, tremor, and mental clouding.

Drugs That Can Cause Ocular Disorders

Some drugs can cause glaucoma or exacerbate preexisting glaucoma. Others can cause **nystagmus**, blurred vision, optic neuritis, **exophthalmos**, or blurred vision. Interestingly, the eyelids are most frequently involved in drug-induced ocular effects and respond with inflammation or dermatitis.[31] A comprehensive review of drug-induced ocular disorders is not possible; therefore the interested reader is referred to published reviews.[1,31-33] Drugs that can cause ocular disorders are listed in Table 27-3.[34,35]

Conjunctivitis

Conjunctivitis is an inflammation of the mucous membrane that lines the inside surface of the eyelid and surrounding tissue. It is the most common diagnosis in individuals who present with unilateral or bilateral red eyes and accompanying discharge. Acute conjunctivitis can be caused by a bacterial infection, viral infection, or allergic reaction. This disorder is typically benign and self-limiting; however, both viral and bacterial diseases are highly contagious, and all three forms can be quite uncomfortable. Pharmacotherapy for conjunctivitis is directed at the underlying etiology.

Etiologies

Bacterial conjunctivitis is most frequently caused by *Staphylococcus aureus, Streptococcus pneumoniae, Haemophilus influenzae,* and *Moraxella catarrhalis*. It is more often observed in children than in adults. The discharge of bacterial conjunctivitis is purulent and typically globular and opaque. Hyperacute bacterial conjunctivitis is a severe, sight-threatening condition caused by *Neisseria* species that warrants immediate treatment by an ophthalmologic specialist.

Viral conjunctivitis is the more common cause of infectious conjunctivitis, both in children and adults. The discharge of viral conjunctivitis is watery and may produce a burning more than itching sensation. Viral conjunctivitis should not be confused with a sight-threatening ocular cytomegalovirus (CMV) infection, which requires antiviral therapy and is discussed briefly later. The clinical course of viral conjunctivitis typically mirrors that of the common cold with symptoms continuing for 2–3 weeks.

Allergic conjunctivitis is caused by direct contact of allergens to the eye, resulting in IgE activation, mast cell degranulation, and histamine release. Both H$_1$ and H$_2$ histamine receptors are activated in response to histamines, and H$_1$ receptors in particular contribute to the observed conjunctivitis symptoms. Although relatively benign and not sight threatening, up to 20% of the population may be affected annually. Many of these individuals seek pharmacotherapy for symptomatic relief. Those afflicted typically have a history of experiencing seasonal or perennial allergies. Watery discharge and itching sensation often develop.

Pharmacotherapy for Bacterial Conjunctivitis

Although bacterial conjunctivitis is generally self-limiting, drug therapy shortens the clinical course of the disease and

Table 27-3 Drugs That Can Cause Ocular Disorders*

Drug Generic (Brand)	Ocular Disorder
Adrenergic agents used to dilate pupils during eye exams	Angle-closure glaucoma
Allopurinol (Zyloprim)	Retinal hemorrhage
Aminoglycosides	Ptosis, extraocular muscle paresis, papilledema
Amiodarone (Cordarone)	Optic neuropathy
Antihistamines	Narrow-angle glaucoma
Barbiturates	Nystagmus
Beta-adrenergic receptor agonists	Dry eye and increased intraocular pressure
Cimetidine (Tagamet)	Narrow-angle glaucoma
Clomiphene citrate	Blurred vision, light flashes
Clonidine (Catapres)	Myosis
Digoxin (Lanoxin)	Scotomas, optic neuritis
Ethambutol (EMB, Myambutol)	Loss of visual acuity or color vision
Glucocorticoids	Angle-closure glaucoma and cataract following long-term use, exophthalmos, cataracts, cranial nerve palsy, papilledema
Hydralazine (Apresoline)	Lacrimation, blurred vision
Hydrochlorothiazide (Maxzide, Dyazide)	Angle-closure glaucoma
Ibuprofen (Advil)	Altered color vision, blurred vision
Ipratropium bromide (Atrovent)	Angle-closure glaucoma
Isoniazid (INH)	Optic neuritis
Linezolid (Zyvox)	Optic neuropathy
Lithium (Lithobid)	Exophthalmos
Metronidazole (Flagyl)	Myopia
Nifedipine (Procardia)	Periorbital edema or eyelid edema
Opiates	Nystagmus
Phenothiazines	Photo toxic retinopathy, nystagmus, and cataracts
Phenytoin (Dilantin)	Nystagmus
Quinolones	Bull's eye maculopathy
Ranitidine (Zantac)	Narrow-angle glaucoma
Salbutamol (Albuterol)	Angle-closure glaucoma
Selective serotonin reuptake inhibitors (SSRIs)	Angle-closure glaucoma
Sulfonamides	Periorbital edema or eyelid edema, Stevens-Johnson syndrome with acute dry-eye syndrome, phototoxic reaction of eyelid skin
Tamoxifen (Nolvadex)	Retinopathy
Tetracyclines	Conjunctival deposits, myopia, papilledema, phototoxic reaction of eyelid skin
Thiazide diuretics	Yellow coloring of vision, myopia
Topiramate (Topamax)	Angle-closure glaucoma
Tricyclic antidepressants	Disturbance of ocular movement, reduced tear formation
Trimethoprim/sulfamethoxazole (TMX/SMX [Bactrim, Septra DS])	Angle-closure glaucoma
Warfarin (Coumadin)	Retinal hemorrhage
Vitamin A overdose	Ptosis, paresis of extraocular muscles
Vitamin D overdose	Calcium deposits in cornea

* This table is not comprehensive as new information is generated on a regular basis.
Source: Adapted from: Li J et al. 2008[31]; Abdollahi M et al. 2004.[34]

decreases communicable transmission (Table 27-4). A meta-analysis of clinical and microbiologic remission found that topical antibiotics significantly improve early (days 2–5) clinical remission rates (RR = 1.24; 95% CI, 1.05–1.45) and microbial remission rates (RR = 1.77; 95% CI, 1.23–2.54); however, this benefit is marginal for later clinical and microbial remission (days 6–10).[36] A decrease in discharge and less redness and irritation should be noted within 2 days of initiating treatment. Obtaining cultures is seldom necessary, and resistance to first-line pharmacotherapy is generally uncommon.

Table 27-4 Drugs for Treating Bacterial Conjunctivitis

Drugs Generic (Brand)	Formulation	Dose	Clinical Considerations	FDA Pregnancy Category
First-Line Medications				
Erythromycin (Ilotycin)	0.5% ointment	Apply thin layer (1.25 cm) q 4–8 h	Commonly administered to newborns after birth for prophylaxis against *Neisseria*, and *Chlamydia* ocular inoculation during birth.	B
Polymyxin B-trimethoprim drops (Polytrim)	Trimethoprim 1 mg/10,000 units polymyxin B per mL	1–2 drops qid	Preferred treatment during pregnancy. Polymyxin B is effective against gram-negative organisms, and trimethoprim is effective against gram-negative organisms. Side effects are rare.	B
Sulfacetamide (Sulf-10, Sulamyd)	10% solution or 10% ointment	1–2 drops qid of solution Small amount qid and once qh	Contraindicated for persons who have sulfa allergy.	C
Second-Line Medications				
Azithromycin drops (Aza Site)	2.5 mL in 5-mL bottle contains 25 mL of azithromycin and 1% sterile ophthalmic solution	Days 1–2: 1 drop bid Days 3–5: 1 drop qd	Requires less frequent dosing than other antibacterials; significantly more expensive.	B
Bacitracin (AK Tracin)	500 units/g	Apply thin layer (1.25 cm) bid or tid	Local irritation possible.	C
Polymyxin B-bacitracin drops (Polysporin)	5000 U per g of bacitracin/1000 U per g of polymyxin B	1–2 drops q 3–4 hrs for 7 days	Efficacious against gram-positive and gram-negative organisms and non-toxic to epithelial tissue.	C
Fluoroquinolones				
Besifloxacin (Besivance)	0.6% ophthalmic suspension	1 drop in both eyes three times per day for 7 days	Newest fluoroquinolone to be approved for treating conjunctivitis. Bottle needs to be inverted and shaken once before applying drops to eye.	C
Ofloxacin (Ocuflox)	0.3% solution	Days 1–2: 1–2 drops q 3 h Days 3–7: 1–2 drops qid	The fluoroquinolones are indicated for moderate to severe conjunctivitis. Highly effective against gram-negative organisms but lack full coverage against *Streptococcus* coverage. Should not be used less than 4 times per day as suboptimum therapeutic levels encourages antibiotic resistance. Treatment for 5–7 days maximum.	C
Ciprofloxacin (Ciloxan)	0.3% solution	Days 1–2: 1–2 drops q 3 h Days 3–7: 1–2 drops qid		C
Levofloxacin (Iquix)	0.5% solution	Days 1–2: 1–2 drops q 3 h Days 3–7: 1–2 drops qid		C
Gatifloxacin (Zymar)	0.3% solution	Days 1–2: 1–2 drops q 3 h Days 3–7: 1–2 drops qid		C

Common side effects of topical antibacterial drugs include localized irritation and inflammation. The pharmacokinetic profiles of ointments tend to make them good vehicles for drug delivery, but adults tend to prefer drops, as ointments blur vision for 15–20 minutes.

First-line treatments include erythromycin ophthalmic ointment (Ilotycin), sulfacetamide ophthalmic drops (Sulf-10, Sulamyd), and polymyxin B-trimethoprim drops (Polytrim).[37] All three are broad-spectrum antimicrobial drugs that have efficacy against the most common bacterial conjunctivitis pathogens.

Erythromycin is a bacteriostatic inhibitor of protein synthesis. It is administered to newborns as prophylactic treatment against sight-threatening infection from **ophthalmia neonatorum** in the first 2 hours following birth. Prophylactic treatment of the newborn eye against chlamydial and gonorrheal infection is legally mandated in most states in the United States. As resistance to erythromycin increases, there is some concern that erythromycin does not universally prevent either chlamydial or gonorrheal infection, and studies evaluating alternative agents are currently being conducted.[38,39]

Polymyxin B (Polytrim) is a bacterial agent that alters the permeability of bacterial cytoplasmic membrane and thereby promotes leakage of intracellular constituents. Both erythromycin (Ilotycin) and polymyxin B-trimethoprim (Polytrim) are FDA Pregnancy Category B drugs and are preferred topical treatments in pregnancy and for nursing mothers.

Other antibacterial drugs frequently employed in the treatment of conjunctivitis include bacitracin ointment (AK Tracin), sulfacetamide ointment (Sulf-10, Sulamyd), azithromycin drops (ASA Site), or fluoroquinolone drops. Aminoglycoside (e.g., gentamicin) drops are not recommended because of their lack of gram-positive antibacterial spectrum coverage and potential toxicity.

Pharmacotherapy for Viral Conjunctivitis

Treatment for viral conjunctivitis is directed at lessening symptoms and not the underlying pathogen (Table 27-5). Viral conjunctivitis does not require systemic therapy and generally is self-limiting. Ocular irritation may worsen for several days and then improve over the course of

2–3 weeks. Nonantibiotic topical lubricants and antihistamine/vasoconstrictor combined medications may provide symptomatic relief. Prescribing either of these medications is rationally preferred over the unwarranted use of topical antibacterials, which will not expedite healing but may hasten antibiotic drug resistance. Topical treatments may themselves produce irritation and increase redness and discharge.

Pharmacotherapy for Allergic Conjunctivitis

Although the principal intervention for allergic conjunctivitis is avoidance of the causal allergen, pharmacotherapy can play an important role in lessening symptoms. Antihistamines, vasoconstrictors, mast cell stabilizers, and

Table 27-5 Drugs for Treating Noninfectious Conjunctivitis

Drug Generic (Brand)	Formulation	Dose	Clinical Considerations	FDA Pregnancy Category
H_1 Receptor Antagonists (Antihistamines): Oral Formulations				
Fexofenadine (Allegra)	30-mg, 60-mg tablets	60 mg bid	May be preferred if averse to ophthalmic application; slower to act. More likely to elicit systemic effects (e.g., headache, somnolence, xerostomia, and nervousness).	C
Loratadine (Claritin)	10-mg tablets	10 mg qd		B
Desloratadine (Clarinex)	5-mg tablets	5 mg qd		C
Cetirizine (Zyrtec)	5-mg, 10-mg tablets	5–10 mg qd		B
H_1 Receptor Antagonists (Antihistamines): Topical Formulations				
Emedastine (Emadine)	0.05% solution	1 drop qid	Ocular stinging.	B
Levocabastine (Livostin)	0.05% suspension	1 drop qid	Ocular stinging.	C
Vasoconstrictors				
Naphazoline (Clear Eyes)	0.012% solution	1–2 drops qid	Ocular stinging; hypertension; palpitations.	C
Oxymetazoline (Visine LR)	0.25% solution	1–2 drops qid	Ocular stinging; hypertension; palpitations.	C
Phenylephrine (Neo-Synephrine)	0.12% solution	1–2 drops qid	Ocular stinging; hypertension; palpitations.	C
Tetrahydrozoline (Visine Moisturizing)	0.05% solution	1–2 drops qid	Ocular stinging; hypertension; palpitations.	C
Mast Cell Stabilizers				
Cromolyn (Opticrom)	4% solution	1–2 drops q 4–6 h	Ocular stinging.	B
Lodoxamide (Alomide)	0.1% solution	1–2 drops qid	Ocular stinging.	B
Nedocromil (Alocril)	2% solution	1–2 drops bid	Ocular stinging.	B
Pemirolast (Alamast)	0.1% solution	1–2 drops qid	Ocular stinging.	C
Dual-Acting Topical Combination H_1 Receptor Antagonists/Vasoconstrictors				
Pheniramine/naphazoline (Visine-A)	0.3% (pheniramine) and 0.025% (naphazoline)	1–2 drops qid	Ocular stinging; limited to qid administration for less than 2 weeks in order to avoid rebound congestion and hyperemia.	C
Dual-Acting H_1 Receptor Antagonists/Mast Cell Stabilizers				
Olopatadine (Patanol)	0.1% solution	1 drop bid	Stinging and headache.	C
Azelastine (Optivar)	0.05% solution	1 drop bid	Stinging and headache.	C
Epinastine (Elestat)	0.05% solution	1 drop bid	Stinging and headache.	C
Ketotifen (Zaditor)	0.025% solution	1 drop bid or tid	Stinging and headache.	C
Pain Relievers: Topical Nonsteroidal Anti-Inflammatory Drugs (NSAIDs)				
Ketorolac (Acular)	0.5% solution	1 drop qid	Headache, GI pain.	C*

* Contraindicated during third trimester.

artificial tears are all used in a stepwise approach to treatment. Artificial tears lubricate the eye to prevent dry eye and irritation. Vasoconstrictors function as ocular decongestants. Antihistamines and mast cell stabilizers inhibit the allergic response. Although glucocorticoids have well-known anti-inflammatory properties, glucocorticoids are associated with major complications and their use is generally limited to prescription by ophthalmologists.

Therapy for Acute Allergic Conjunctivitis

Topical dual-agent formulations of an antihistamine and vasoconstrictor are highly effective short-term treatments for managing acute episodes. They are available as over-the-counter (OTC) medications. One example is the combination of the antihistamine pheniramine (Neo-Synephrine) and the vasoconstrictor naphazoline (Clear Eyes). The antihistamine blocks the effects of histamine on the H_1 histamine receptors and further blocks constitutive histamine receptor activity. Vasoconstrictors act by activating alpha$_1$-adrenergic receptors in the arterioles of the conjunctiva, producing vasoconstriction and decongestion. Use of a combined antihistamine/vasoconstrictor should be limited to administration four times per day for less than 2 weeks in order to avoid rebound congestion and hyperemia. The combination of antihistamine and a vasoconstrictor in a topical formulation produces better effects than either topical medication alone.

Orally administered second-generation antihistamines such as fexofenadine (Allegra), loratadine (Claritin), desloratadine (Clarinex), and cetirizine (Zyrtec) provide an alternative approach to treating allergic conjunctivitis. They selectively inhibit H_1 histamine receptors and are substantially less sedating than nonselective H_1/H_2 antihistamines. They may be preferred by individuals who are averse to ophthalmic application of drops or ointments; however, oral antihistamines are slower to act and more likely to elicit systemic effects (e.g., headache, somnolence, xerostomia, and nervousness). Artificial tears may also be employed as an adjunct to either oral or topical medications.

Extended Therapy for Seasonal or Perennial Allergic Conjunctivitis

When treatment is necessary for more than 2 weeks or if the individual experiences frequent acute attacks of allergic conjunctivitis, a combination of a topical antihistamine and mast cell stabilizer is preferred.[40] Therapeutic effects may take up to 2 weeks to fully develop, and treatment may begin prophylactically in anticipation of an acute attack (e.g., exposure to a known allergen). Oral second-generation

antihistamines and topical mast cell stabilizers alone are also viable treatment approaches, particularly if administered prophylactically.

The combination of a mast cell stabilizer and antihistamine facilitates blockage of both early and late stages of the allergic response. Mast cell stabilizers prevent mast cell degranulation, thus preventing the initial release of histamine. Antihistamines block the activation of H_1 receptors occurring at the end of the atopy, signaling cascade. The dual-acting drugs such as olopatadine (Patanol), azelastine (Optivar), epinastine (Elestat), and ketotifen (Zaditor) produce both selective histamine H_1 antagonism and mast cell stabilization and are widely used. Of these dual-acting agents, olopatadine (Patanol) is generally regarded as the first-line drug of choice. These medications do not affect alpha$_1$ adrenergic receptors, and they do not produce vasoconstriction. Dosing is typically twice daily, and these agents may produce stinging and headache as adverse effects.

Nedocromil (Alocril), pemirolast (Alamast), and cromolyn (Opticrom) act primarily as mast cell stabilizers with minimal antihistaminergic effects. While these medications are safe and efficacious, they typically require more frequent (i.e., four times a day) dosing and have a prolonged onset of action of 1–2 weeks before therapeutic effects are observed.

The efficacy of oral antihistamines in treating allergic conjunctivitis symptoms is generally less than the efficacy of topical antihistamine/mast cell stabilizer medications; however, the oral medications may be preferred if the individual is additionally experiencing nonophthalmic allergic symptoms, such as sneezing and rhinorrhea associated with seasonal allergic rhinitis. Orally administered second-generation antihistamines have an onset of action of 2–5 days, which is longer than the onset of topical antihistamines, but generally shorter than mast cell stabilizer monotherapy. Oral antihistamines more often produce xerostomia and decreased tear production, which may be treated by use of artificial tears.

If other treatment approaches are unsuccessful, topical nonsteroidal anti-inflammatory drugs (NSAIDs) such as ketorolac (Acular) may be an appropriate alternative to lessen ocular itching. Ketorolac does not improve wound healing and has been shown to be less effective than olopatadine (Patanol). Ketorolac may require up to 2 weeks to achieve maximal efficacy.

Pharmacotherapy for Noninfectious-Nonallergic Conjunctivitis, Dry Eye, and Red Eye

Dry eyes resulting from inadequate levels of tear film are particularly common among women. Nonantibiotic topical artificial tear lubricants are available in an array of OTC formulations, including water-soluble polymer drops and lipid-based nonreactive ointments. As with antibacterial ophthalmic preparations, ointments have a more protracted duration of action but may blur vision. Artificial tears may also be used to counter decreased tear production resulting from oral antihistamines. Persons typically respond well to the use of artificial tears, which can be administered as adjuncts to additional ophthalmic drops or ointments. These medications may be used frequently and produce minimal side effects. The preservatives in these topical medications may cause stinging, which can be remedied by switching products. Preservative-free formulations are also available, albeit more expensive.

Sight-Threatening Ophthalmic Viral Infections

Ganciclovir (Cytovene), trifluridine (Viroptic), and vidarabine (Vira-A) are topically administered antivirals used to treat viral ophthalmic infections. Ganciclovir is

indicated for sight-threatening CMV infections such as CMV retinitis, which may occur in immunocompromised patients. Trifluridine (Viroptic) and vidarabine (Vira-A) are indicated for keratoconjunctivitis and recurrent epithelial keratitis caused by herpes simplex virus types I and II. The drugs are nucleoside analogs that act by inhibiting viral DNA synthesis. The most common side effect is localized burning and discomfort at the site of administration. Only trace amounts of the drugs are systemically absorbed.

Otic Drugs

There are three major divisions of the ear—the outer ear, middle ear, and inner ear. The outer and the middle ear are often involved in conditions requiring pharmacotherapeutic intervention (Figure 27-3). The outer ear consists of the auricle and external auditory canal. It is responsible for collecting sound waves and channeling them to the tympanic membrane. The external auditory canal maintains a level of **cerumen** (earwax) that aids in the protection against microbial infection. The middle ear conveys

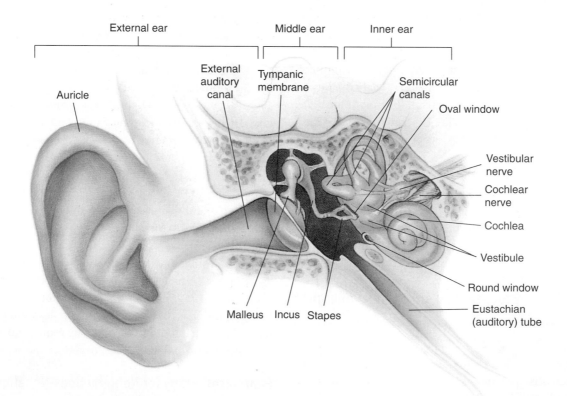

Figure 27-3 Anatomy of the ear. *Source:* Clark RK 2005.[55]

Box 27-2 Application of Otic Drops

The optimal method for applying ear drops is as follows:

1. Treat the dropper tip as a sterile instrument, being cautious not to touch it to the ear or any other surface.

2. Warm the dropper bottle with hands to prevent discomfort and minimize dizziness.

3. Gently clean the external auditory canal as much as possible prior to drop administration.

4. Tilt head to the unaffected side and allow drops to be released. Gently wiggle the ear to allow for improved absorption and distribution within the external auditory canal if desired.

5. Maintain this position for 2–3 minutes following drug administration in order to maximize absorption.

6. If edema in the external auditory canal is inhibiting drop administration, a wick may be used to resolve symptoms more quickly. Discontinue use of the wick once the edema subsides.

7. Visually inspect and clean the canal every 2–5 days.

8. To allow for improved absorption and distribution within the external auditory canal, treat a small plug of cotton with the drops and insert the cotton into the ear.

auditory vibrations from the tympanic membrane to the inner ear. The eustachian tube that connects the middle ear to the nasopharynx is lined with ciliated epithelial cells, which aid in the transit of microbes out of the middle ear. The inner ear includes the semicircular canals and cochlea, which provides balance and the sense organ for hearing.

Otitis media, an infection of the middle ear, is the most common infection of the ear. External otitis, often called swimmer's ear, is seen in persons of all ages. Other conditions that affect the ear and have pharmacotherapeutic treatments include impacted cerumen. Instructions for administering otic drops are presented in Box 27-2.

Acute Otitis Media

The large majority of publications on treatment of otitis media refer to children; thus, the information we have on etiology and treatment is based on data gathered primarily from pediatric populations. Acute otitis media is an infectious disease caused by a bacteria, virus, or mixed combination of pathogens and frequently occurs following an upper respiratory infection. The microbes that are most often implicated in the etiology of acute otitis media are *Streptococcus pneumoniae* (> 40%), *H influenzae* (> 20%), and *M catarrhalis* (> 10%).[41] Acute otitis media is clinically diagnosed by a sudden onset of symptoms that include ear pain (otalgia), fever, irritability, sleeplessness, purulent discharge, middle ear effusion, and signs of middle ear inflammation. Systemic and local symptoms of acute otitis media typically last 1–3 days in individuals receiving antibacterial pharmacotherapy. Symptoms last slightly longer if antibacterial drugs are not used. Middle ear effusion may not subside for several weeks following successful acute otitis media resolution. The increase in antibiotic resistance and question about when it is appropriate to prescribe antibacterial drugs for acute otitis media has been the subject of substantial debate[42] (Table 27-6). Factors to weigh in considering observation in lieu of antibacterial pharmacotherapy include age, diagnostic certainty (i.e., certain versus presumed acute otitis media diagnosis), severity of illness, and assurance of follow-up.

Otalgia is a common symptom of acute otitis media, and management of acute otitis media should include assessment for pain. Regardless of whether antibacterial drugs are used, treatment for pain should commence promptly. Standard analgesics include ibuprofen (Advil), acetaminophen (Tylenol), and codeine. Homeopathic remedies, naturopathic herbal extracts, and external application of heat or cold have all been proposed as alternative approaches to palliative care, but their clinical efficacy is yet to be determined. However, one observational study that compared the outcomes of homeopathic remedies and conventional medications for acute respiratory and ear complaints found that both were equally efficacious at 7 days, the homeopathic group had a quicker response to treatment, and the conventional medication group reported more adverse drug reactions.[43] When antibacterial treatment is determined to be appropriate, administration of high-dose amoxicillin is the first-line treatment. Amoxicillin (Amoxil) is a safe and inexpensive narrow-spectrum antibacterial drug with efficacy against the most common acute otitis media pathogens and intermediate-resistant pneumococci. If amoxicillin is not effective, a course of high-dose amoxicillin/clavulanate (Augmentin) is suggested. Three doses of intramuscular ceftriaxone (Rocephin) is an alternate treatment regimen.

Table 27-6 Commonly Used Ear Medications

Drug Generic (Brand)	Dose	Clinical Considerations
Acute Otitis Media		
Amoxicillin (Amoxil)	875 mg po tid × 5 days	First-line treatment.
Amoxicillin/Clavulanate (Augmentin)	875 mg po bid × 7 days	Second-line treatment.
Ceftriaxone (Rocephin)	1 g IM per day × 1–3 days	Third-line treatment for infections that are resistant to amoxicillin.
Trimethoprim/Sulfamethoxazole (Bactrim, Septra)	1 DS tab po bid for 7–10 days	
Azithromycin (Zithromax)	500 mg × 1 dose, then 250 mg per day × 4 days	For persons with penicillin allergy.
Cefuroxime (Ceftin)	500 mg po bid × 7 days	
Otitis Externa		
Ofloxacin (Floxin Otic)	10 drops qd into affected ear × 7 days	Highly effective and least irritating. If systemic antibiotic is needed, ciprofloxacin (Cipro) 500 mg po bid × 7 days. Avoid benzocaine as a topical anesthetic because it can cause an allergic response. Use acetaminophen (Tylenol) or an NSAID for pain relief.
Ciprofloxacin with hydrocortisone (Cipro HC Otic)	3 drops bid × 7 days	Combination antibiotic and steroid decreases inflammation.
Polymyxin B neomycin, hydrocortisone (Cortisporin)	4–6 drops 3 times per day	Do not use if perforated tympanic membrane. Not effective against *P aeruginosa* or *Staphylococcus* spp.

NSAID = nonsteroidal antiinflammatory drug.
Source: Modified from Bouchard ME 2007.[54]

Acute External Otitis

Acute external otitis (i.e., swimmer's ear) is an inflammation of the outer ear typically caused by *Pseudomonas aeruginosa* and *S aureus*, and is secondary to superficial tissue damage and excessive moisture. The infection may infiltrate into tissue surrounding the external auditory canal, requiring more extensive therapy. Persons with external otitis develop sudden otalgia, otic pruritus, impaired hearing, and purulent discharge. Most report decreased symptoms following 3 days of initiating treatment and resolution within 2 weeks.

Topical medications such as ear drops and gentle cleaning typically provide efficacious antibacterial treatment. Three to four drops are administered four times per day for 3 days beyond the cessation of symptoms. Otalgia may be treated with systemic analgesics such as codeine and NSAIDs. Reevaluation is unnecessary unless the symptoms fail to resolve within 2 weeks of treatment.

Superficial otitis externa infections can be treated with a combination of a 2% acetic acid solution and hydrocortisone.[44] Acetic acid inhibits bacterial growth by acidifying the outer ear, creating an inhospitable environment through direct lowering of the pH. The anti-inflammatory effects of hydrocortisone minimize pain and irritation. Acetic acid is inexpensive, efficacious against almost all bacteria, and does not result in otic sensitization. One potential adverse effect of the medication is irritation to the external auditory canal, which may be lessened by hydrocortisone. The combination therapy of acetic acid and hydrocortisone may also be administered prophylactically with minimal adverse consequences.

When acetic acid is too irritating, a combination antibiotic/steroid cream is equally efficacious. Ciprofloxacin with hydrocortisone (Cipro HC Otic) or polymyxin B neomycin/hydrocortisone (Cortisporin) can be used.[45] All otic pathogens are susceptible to fluoroquinolones whereas polymyxin B may be ineffective against *P aeruginosa*, and is known to be ineffective against *Staphylococcus* spp.[46,47] Aminoglycosides (e.g., gentamicin and tobramycin) produce minimal irritation, yet are potentially ototoxic. Fluoroquinolone otic solutions (e.g., ciprofloxacin [Cipro HC Otic]) and ofloxacin drops (Ocuflox) are highly efficacious and produce the least amount of irritation; however, they are the most expensive treatment option and pose the potential risk of accelerating antibacterial drug resistance.

Oral antibacterial therapy should be used if the infection spreads beyond the external auditory canal.

Fluoroquinolones, including ciprofloxacin (Cipro), are prescribed for adults. Systemic administration of fluoroquinolones is contraindicated in individuals < 18 years of age due to the unusual adverse effect of tendon rupture that is associated with this drug.[48]

Impacted Cerumen

When wax builds up and occludes the ear canal, pain and hearing loss can develop. Wax can be softened to aid removal via installation of a wax emulsifier for a few days. Wax emulsifiers can be found over the counter under the brand names Debrox Drops, Murine Ear Drops, and Auro Ear Drops. Wax emulsifiers are composed of glycerine, propylene glycol, and carbamide peroxide. The glycerin softens the cerumen, and the carbimide peroxide releases hydrogen peroxide and oxygen when exposed to moisture. The oxygen has a weak antibacterial effect and the effervescence that occurs from the production of hydrogen peroxide and oxygen has a mechanical effect of loosening the cerumen from the wall of the ear canal.

Drugs That Cause Otic Disorders

Drugs can cause disorders of the ear and hearing. For example, there is a well-known association between aspirin and tinnitus.[49,50] Many drugs can cause ototoxicity through various mechanisms (Table 27-7). Ototoxicity refers to functional impairment and cellular degeneration of the tissues of the inner ear caused by therapeutic agents. The cochlea, vestibulum, and stria vascularis are the primary sites affected. The drugs most likely to be ototoxic are the aminoglycoside antibiotics, macrolide antibiotics, loop diuretics, antimalarials, and platinum-based chemotherapeutic drugs. Drugs that are not ototoxic when taken as monotherapy can sometimes be ototoxic when taken concomitantly with another drug. Ototoxicity is most likely to affect older persons.

Aminoglycoside-induced ototoxicity results from a unique mechanism of action. The aminoglycoside drug binds with available iron and forms a complex. This complex catalyzes the formation of reactive oxygen species, which in turn promote apoptosis and cell death.[51] Although a detailed description of the mechanisms and treatments of drug-induced ototoxicity are beyond the scope of this chapter, the reader can find detailed information in published reviews on the subject.[51-53]

Conclusion

Ocular and otic conditions are common in primary care. Although glaucoma is usually managed by ophthalmology specialists, primary care providers will want to be aware of drugs that can cause ocular or otic adverse effects to best prevent complications from multidrug use. Most ocular and otic conditions are self-limited and resolve without treatment, but these symptoms can also be the harbinger of a rare, serious condition and therefore always require a thorough evaluation prior to prescribing medications.[54]

Table 27-7 Ototoxic Medications—Generic (Brand)*

Antibiotics	Chemotherapeutic Agents
Amikacin (Amikin)	Carboplatin (Paraplatin)
Azithromycin (Zithromax)	Vincristine (Oncovin)
Capreomycin (Capastat Sulfate)	Loop diuretics
Chloramphenicol (Chloromycetin)	Furosemide (Lasix)
Dihydrostreptomycin	Bumetanide (Bumex)
Gentamicin (Garamycin)	Ethacrynic acid (Edecrin)
Erythromycin (E-Mycin)	**Anti-Malarials**
Metronidazole (Flagyl)	Chloroquine (Aralen)
Neomycin (Neo-Fradin Cortisporin, Neosporin)	Hydro chloroquine (Plaquenil)
Streptomycin	Mefloquine (Lariam)
Tobramycin (Nebcin, TobraDex)	Quinacrine (Atabrine)
Vancomycin (Vanocin)	Quinine Sulfate (Qualaquin)

* This table is not comprehensive as new information is generated on a regular basis.

References

1. Tripathi RC, Tripathi BJ, Haggerty C. Drug-induced glaucomas: mechanism and management. Drug Safety 2003;26:749–67.
2. Friedman DS, Wolfs RC, O'Colmain BJ, Klein BE, Taylor HR, West S, et al. Prevalence of open-angle glaucoma among adults in the United States. Arch Ophthalmol 2004;122:532–8.
3. Racette L, Wilson MR, Zangwill LM, Weinreb RN, Sample PA. Primary open-angle glaucoma in blacks: a review. Surv Ophthalmol 2003;48:295–313.
4. Liesegang TJ. Glaucoma: changing concepts and future directions. Mayo Clin Proc 1996;71:689–94.

5. Mansberger SL, Hughes BA, Gordon MO, Spaner SD, Beiser JA, Cioffi GA, et al. Comparison of initial intraocular pressure response with topical beta-adrenergic antagonists and prostaglandin analogues in African American and White individuals in the Ocular Hypertension Treatment Study. Arch Ophthalmol 2007;125: 454–9.

6. Distelhorst JS, Hughes GM. Open-angle glaucoma. Am Fam Physician 2003;67:1937–44.

7. Vetrugno M, Cantatore F, Ruggeri G, Ferreri P, MOntepara A, Quinto A, et al. Primary open angle glaucoma: an overview on medical therapy. Prog Brain Res 2008;173:181–93.

8. Lee DA, Higginbotham EJ. Glaucoma and its treatment: a review. Am J Health Syst Pharm 2005;62:691–9.

9. Comparison of glaucomatous progression between untreated patients with normal-tension glaucoma and patients with therapeutically reduced intraocular pressures. Collaborative Normal-Tension Glaucoma Study Group. Am J Ophthalmol 1998;126:487–97.

10. Marquis RE, Whitson JT. Management of glaucoma: focus on pharmacological therapy. Drugs Aging 2005; 22:1–21.

11. Khouri AS, Realini T, Fechtner RD. Use of fixed-dose combination drugs for the treatment of glaucoma. Drugs Aging 2007;24:1007–16.

12. Leske MC, Heijl A, Hussein M, Bengtsson B, Dong L, Yang Z, EMGT Group. Factors for glaucoma progression and the effect of treatment: the early manifest glaucoma trial. Arch Ophthalmol 2003;121:48–56.

13. Leskea MC, Heijl A, Hyman L, Bengtsson B, Komaroff E. Factors for progression and glaucoma treatment: the Early Manifest Glaucoma Trial. Curr Opin Ophthalmol 2004;15:102–6.

14. Abramov Y, Borik S, Yahalom C, Fatum M, Avgil G, Brzezinski A, et al. Does postmenopausal hormone replacement therapy affect intraocular pressure? J Glaucoma 2005;14:271–5.

15. Coleman AL, Stone KL, Kodjebacheva G, Yu F, Pedula KL, Ensrud KE, et al. Glaucoma risk and the consumption of fruits and vegetables among older women in the study of osteoporotic fractures. Am J Ophthalmol 2008;145:1081–9.

16. Lee DA, Higginbotham EJ. Glaucoma and its treatment: a review. Am J Health Syst Pharm 2005;62:691–9.

17. Soltau JB, Zimmerman TJ. Changing paradigms in the medical treatment of glaucoma. Surv Ophthalmol 2002;47(suppl 1):S2–S5.

18. Mundorf TK, Ogawa T, Naka H, Novack GD, Crockett RS, US Istalol Study Group. A 12-month, multicenter, randomized, double-masked, parallel-group comparison of timolol-LA once daily and timolol maleate ophthalmic solution twice daily in the treatment of adults with glaucoma or ocular hypertension. Clin Ther 2004;26:541–51.

19. Sorensen SJ, Abel SR. Comparison of the ocular beta-blockers. Ann Pharmacother 1996;30:43–54.

20. Noecker RJ, Earl ML, Mundorf TK, Silverstein SM, Phillips MP. Comparing bimatoprost and travoprost in Black Americans. Curr Med Res Opin 2006;22: 2175–80.

21. Bournias TE, Lee D, Gross R, Mattox C. Ocular hypotensive efficacy of bimatoprost when used as a replacement for latanoprost in the treatment of glaucoma and ocular hypertension. J Ocul Pharmacol Ther 2003;19:193–203.

22. De Santis M, Lucchese A, Carducci B, De Santis L, Merola A, Straface G, et al. Latanoprost exposure in pregnancy. Am J Ophthalmol 2004;138:305–6.

23. Fiscella G, Jensen MK. Precautions in use and handling of travoprost. Am J Health Syst Pharm 2003; 60:484–5; author reply 485.

24. Mulaney J, Sonty S, Ahmad A, Stewart JA, Stewart WC. Comparison of daytime efficacy and safety of dorzolamide/timolol maleate fixed combination versus latanoprost. Eur J Ophthalmol 2008;18:556–62.

25. Evans DW, Hosking SL, Gherghel D, Bartlett JD. Contrast sensitivity improves after brimonidine therapy in primary open angle glaucoma: a case for neuroprotection. Br J Ophthalmol 2003;87:1463–5.

26. Widengard I, Maepea O, Alm A. Effects of latanoprost and dipivefrin, alone or combined, on intraocular pressure and on blood-aqueous barrier permeability. Br J Ophthalmol 1998;82:404–6.

27. Gandolfi SA, Rossetti L, Cimino L, Mora P, Tardini M, Orzalesi N. Replacing maximum-tolerated medications with latanoprost versus adding latanoprost to maximum-tolerated medications: a two-center randomized prospective trial. J Glaucoma 2003;12:347–53.

28. Kaplan-Messas A, Naveh N, Avni I, Marshall J. Ocular hypotensive effects of cholinergic and adrenergic drugs may be influenced by prostaglandins E2 in the human and rabbit eye. Eur J Ophthalmol 2003;13:18–23.

29. Hoh ST, Aung T, Chew PT. Medical management of angle closure glaucoma. Semin Ophthalmol 2002;17: 79–83.

30. Fan DS, Rao SK, Ng JS, Yu CB, Lam DS. Comparative study on the safety and efficacy of different cycloplegic agents in children with darkly pigmented irides. Clin Experiment Ophthalmol 2004;32:462–7.

31. Li J, Tripathi RC, Tripathi BJ. Drug-induced ocular disorders. Drug Safety 2008;31:127–41.

32. Santaella RM, Fraunfelder FW. Ocular adverse effects associated with systemic medications: recognition and management. Drugs 2007;67:75–93.

33. Lachkar Y, Bouassida W. Drug-induced acute angle closure glaucoma. Curr Opin Ophthalmol 2007;18: 129–33.

34. Abdollahi M, Shafiee A, Bathaiee FS, Sharifzadeh M, Nikfar S. Drug-induced toxic reactions in the eye: an overview. J Infus Nurs 2004;27:386–98.

35. Li J, Tripathi RC, Tripathi BJ. Drug-induced ocular disorders. Drug Safety 2008;31:127–41.

36. Sheikh A, Hurwitz B. Topical antibiotics for acute bacterial conjunctivitis: Cochrane systematic review and meta-analysis update. Br J Gen Pract 2005;55: 962–4.

37. Hovding G. Acute bacterial conjunctivitis. Acta Ophthalmol 2008;86:5–17.

38. Zar HJ. Neonatal chlamydial infections: prevention and treatment. Paediatr Drugs 2005;7:103–10.

39. Medves JM. Three infant care interventions: reconsidering the evidence. J Obstet Gynecol Neonatal Nurs 2002;31:563–9.

40. Bielory L, Friedlaender MH. Allergic conjunctivitis. Immunol Allergy Clin North Am 2008;28:43,58, vi.

41. Hendley JO. Clinical practice. Otitis media. N Engl J Med 2002;347:1169–74.

42. American Academy of Pediatrics Subcommittee on Management of Acute Otitis Media. Diagnosis and management of acute otitis media. Pediatrics 2004; 113:1451–65.

43. Haidvogl M, Riley DS, Heger M, Brien S, Jong M, Fischer M, et al. Homeopathic and conventional treatment for acute respiratory and ear complaints: a comparative study on outcome in the primary care setting. BMC Complement Altern Med 2007;7:7.

44. Sander R. Otitis externa: a practical guide to treatment and prevention. Am Fam Physician 2001;63: 927–36, 941–2.

45. van Balen FA, Smit WM, Zuithoff NP, Verheij TJ. Clinical efficacy of three common treatments in acute otitis externa in primary care: randomised controlled trial. BMJ 2003;327:1201–5.

46. Dohar JE, Roland P, Wall GM, McLean C, Stroman DW. Differences in bacteriologic treatment failures in acute otitis externa between ciprofloxacin/dexamethasone and neomycin/polymyxin B/hydrocortisone: results of a combined analysis. Curr Med Res Opin 2009; 25:287–91.

47. Drehobl M, Guerrero JL, Lacarte PR, Goldstein G, Mata FS, Luber S. Comparison of efficacy and safety of ciprofloxacin otic solution 0.2% versus polymyxin B-neomycin-hydrocortisone in the treatment of acute diffuse otitis externa. Curr Med Res Opin 2008;24: 3531–42.

48. Kowatari K, Nakashima K, Ono A, Yoshihara M, Amano M, Toh S. Levofloxacin-induced bilateral Achilles tendon rupture: a case report and review of the literature. J Orthop Sci 2004;9:186–90.

49. Cazals Y. Auditory sensori-neural alterations induced by salicylate. Prog Neurobiol 2000;62:583–631.

50. Seligmann H, Podoshin L, Ben-David J, Fradis M, Goldsher M. Drug-induced tinnitus and other hearing disorders. Drug Safety 1996;14:198–212.

51. Rybak LP, Ramkumar V. Ototoxicity. Kidney Int 2007;72:931–5.

52. Roland PS. New developments in our understanding of ototoxicity. Ear Nose Throat J 2004;83:15–6; discussion 16–7.

53. Yorgason JG, Fayad JN, Kalinec F. Understanding drug ototoxicity: molecular insights for prevention and clinical management. Expert Opin Drug Safety 2006;5:383–99.

54. Bouchard ME. Common conditions of the eye and ear. In Hackley B, Kriebs J, Rousseau ME, eds. Primary care of women: a guide for midwives and women's health providers. Sudbury, MA: Jones and Bartlett Publishers; 2007:339–82.

55. Clark RK. Anatomy and physiology: understanding the human body. Sudbury, MA: Jones and Bartlett Publishers; 2005.

"Having cancer gave me membership in an elite club I'd rather not belong to."

GILDA RADNER (1946–1989), AMERICAN ACTRESS

28
Cancer

Joyce King and Lori Smith

Chapter Glossary

Adjuvant therapy Treatment that is administered after curative surgical intervention or radiation therapy in women who have a high rate of disease recurrence.

Apoptosis Process of programmed cell death.

Brachytherapy Implantation of radiation seeds in close proximity to malignant tumor.

Breast-ovarian cancer syndrome Tumor suppressor genes that encode for proteins that help repair DNA. The BRCA-1 and BCRA-2 proteins bind to DNA to repair double-strand breaks.

Carcinogen Agent that can cause cancer.

Carcinogenesis The process by which normal cells are transformed into cancer cells.

Combination chemotherapy Use of multiple chemotherapeutic agents, often with effects at various points within the cell cycle in an attempt to increase effectiveness.

Control A goal when cure is unable to be attained. The goal is to put a woman's cancer into a remission.

Cure Remission of signs and/or symptoms over a prolonged period of observation. For example, cancer cure rates often are reported in increments such as a 5-year period.

Debulking Surgical removal of as much as possible of a malignant tumor for specific cancers such as brain and ovarian cancer, wherein all of the malignant cells cannot be removed. Debulking often is preceded by pharmacologic treatments to reduce the tumor size or neoadjunctive therapy. Also known as cytoreduction.

Dysplasia Disorganization of tissue architecture and structural variability caused by disordered cellular proliferation. Full thickness epithelial dysplastic involvement is referred to as carcinoma in situ.

Hereditary nonpolyposis colorectal cancer (HNPCC) syndrome Syndrome marked by genetic mutations in the DNA mismatch repair pathway. The DNA mismatch repair genes identify and repair mismatches of DNA bases during DNA replication. They are sometimes referred to as the "spell-checking system" of DNA. Also known as Lynch syndrome.

Hydatidiform mole Condition in which trophoblastic cells that normally would form the placenta proliferate and develop hyperplasia and generalized swelling. No fetus is present. A hydatidiform mole can be complete or partial.

Hyperplasia Tissue with an increase in cellular number.

MicroRNA genes Single-stranded RNA molecules that regulate gene expression. These RNA strands usually down regulate gene expression.

Monoclonal antibodies Monospecific antibodies that are clones of a single parent cell, which are produced using recombinant technologies. When monoclonal antibodies are used as a pharmacologic agent, their names always end in "-mab."

Neoplasia Excessive abnormal growth of tissue. This term is a synonym for the word *tumor*.

Oncogene The mutated form of proto-oncogenes. A gene becomes an oncogene when it becomes capable of turning a normal cell into a cancer cell. For an oncogene to cause cancer, an additional step is usually required, which could be a mutation in another gene or an environmental factor such as a viral infection.

Palliation Relief of disease symptoms and provision of optimum quality of life for the duration of a woman's life. Women with widespread metastatic disease for whom cure or control is not an option qualify for palliative treatment.

Performance status A method used to describe/quantify the general well-being of an individual. Several different instruments are available and are used to address such issues as whether or not chemotherapy should be able to be tolerated and the need for dosing adjustments; such instruments are even used as a measure of quality of life in various randomized, controlled trials.

Progression New lesions or at least 25% increase in measurable disease.

Proto-oncogenes The genes that code for proteins that regulate cell growth or cell differentiation. When a mutation occurs in a proto-oncogene, it can become an oncogene.

Stable disease Less than 50% decrease in a tumor or less than 25% increase in all measurable disease.

Staging The process of determining how much cancer is in the body and where it is located. Staging is associated with prognosis and provides guidance for the development of a treatment plan. Common elements of staging include location of the primary (original) tumor, tumor size and number of tumors, lymph node involvement (whether or not the cancer has spread to the nearby lymph nodes), and presence or absence of metastasis.

Tumor burden Referring to the size of a tumor, amount of cancer in the body, or the number of cancer cells. Also known as tumor load.

Tumor suppressor genes Genes that encode for proteins that promote apoptosis or inhibit progression of the cell cycle. For example, if DNA is damaged, the cell should not divide. Tumor suppressor proteins repair DNA damage. If tumor suppressor genes are inhibited, the repair work does not occur and the damaged cell will continue to replicate.

Women and Cancer

Cancer has no prejudice with regard to age, race, ethnicity, or gender. More than a half million women are diagnosed with cancer annually, and more than one quarter of a million women will die each year as a result of cancer. Although there is an overall improvement in the survival rates of persons diagnosed with cancers during the years 1996–2009 compared to those diagnosed between the years 1975–1979, the improvement is less pronounced among women than men[1] (Figure 28-1).

For women, breast cancer is the most frequently diagnosed cancer, while lung cancer is the most common cancer that causes death. The most common cancer of the female genital tract is endometrial cancer, which accounts for approximately 6% of cancers affecting women. Other gynecologic malignancies include cancers of the cervix, fallopian tube, ovary, peritoneum, vagina, and vulva, as well as gestational trophoblastic disease.[1] Breast cancer, although not restricted to women, is considered a woman's cancer in this context.

Oncology is the quintessential specialty. Primary care clinicians may provide treatment for a woman with an upper respiratory infection without referring her to an infectious disease specialist, prescribe a pharmaceutical agent for an individual with post-Thanksgiving gastritis without sending her to a gastrointestinal center, or even prescribe a mild sedative for a woman's occasional episode of insomnia without the need for a sleep clinic. Primary care providers routinely and appropriately screen for cancer. Yet there is no such entity as a touch of cancer. When cancer is found, specialists in oncology provide the expert care.

Although management of cancer is directed by an oncology team, general health care often remains the purview of the primary provider. For example, a woman with breast cancer certainly should not forgo her routine Pap test. A cancer survivor can have a urinary tract infection as can any other woman. A pregnant woman can develop cancer and still have needs congruent with pregnancy. This chapter provides an overview of chemotherapy and summarizes information about important cancers that affect women with a focus on information important for the primary care provider. Helping to manage side effects of chemotherapy can be an important contribution of the primary care clinician.

Characteristics of Neoplastic Cells

The term **neoplasia** is from the Latin *neo*, for "new," and Greek *plasis*, for "molding" or "growth," to form a term for "new growth," which is used to describe tissues that demonstrate excessive growth that is not consistent with normal growth patterns. The term *neoplasia* is used interchangeably with the term *tumor*, and tumors may be classified as benign, malignant, or borderline malignant. Histologic diagnosis is of utmost importance in determining the presence of malignancy. The primary differentiation between benign tumors, also called solid

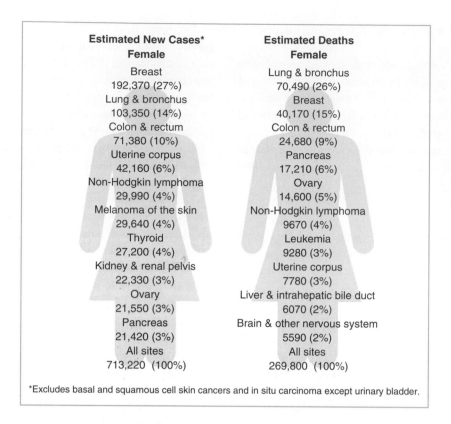

Estimated New Cases* Female	Estimated Deaths Female
Breast 192,370 (27%)	Lung & bronchus 70,490 (26%)
Lung & bronchus 103,350 (14%)	Breast 40,170 (15%)
Colon & rectum 71,380 (10%)	Colon & rectum 24,680 (9%)
Uterine corpus 42,160 (6%)	Pancreas 17,210 (6%)
Non-Hodgkin lymphoma 29,990 (4%)	Ovary 14,600 (5%)
Melanoma of the skin 29,640 (4%)	Non-Hodgkin lymphoma 9670 (4%)
Thyroid 27,200 (4%)	Leukemia 9280 (3%)
Kidney & renal pelvis 22,330 (3%)	Uterine corpus 7780 (3%)
Ovary 21,550 (3%)	Liver & intrahepatic bile duct 6070 (2%)
Pancreas 21,420 (3%)	Brain & other nervous system 5590 (2%)
All sites 713,220 (100%)	All sites 269,800 (100%)

*Excludes basal and squamous cell skin cancers and in situ carcinoma except urinary bladder.

Figure 28-1 Leading sites of new cancer cases and death for women—2009 estimates. *Source:* Modified with permission from the American Cancer Society. Cancer Facts and Figures 2009. Atlanta: American Cancer Society, Inc.

tumors, and the malignant tumors, also termed *cancer*, is that benign tumors do not invade adjacent tissues. Malignant tumors are able to proliferate, invade, and metastasize to distant sites or organs.

Carcinogenesis means "creation of cancer." No single etiology that causes cancer has been identified. Carcinogenesis probably requires both a predisposition to the disease and a specific sequencing of exposures to **carcinogens**.[2] Many substances have carcinogenic effects, and there are several drugs used to treat one disorder that are known to be carcinogenic in either high doses or after prolonged exposure. Examples includealkylating agents (leukemia), anabolic steroids (liver cancer), estrogens (reproductive organ cancers), coal tars (skin cancer), and immunosuppressive drugs (lymphoma and skin cancer).

Normal cell growth is determined by growth-stimulating signals as well as by the space available. These cells undergo a signaling process called **apoptosis**, which initiates the process of cellular death.[3] Malignant cells do not respond to the signals promoting apoptosis, and thus, they achieve a type of immortality that allows them to continue to replicate indefinitely while the host lives.

Normal cells tend to stop growing after approximately 50 generations of cellular division, whereas malignant cells lack this characteristic.[3] Depending on histologic type, malignant cells can spread locally or via the lymphatic and circulatory systems.

The abnormal behavior of malignant cells is most likely associated with alterations in **oncogenes**, **tumor suppressor genes**, or **microRNA genes**.[4] A **proto-oncogene** is a normal gene that codes for proteins involved in cell growth and cell division. A small mutation can alter the proto-oncogene and change it to an oncogene, which then causes malignant cells to grow. Tumor suppressor genes are responsible for retarding cellular division, repairing DNA errors, and triggering apoptosis. Thus, when a mutation of tumor suppressor genes occurs, cells are able to divide rapidly, DNA remains altered, and cellular death is delayed. MicroRNA genes code for a single RNA strand that regulates gene expression.

Sometimes cells develop abnormal characteristics that are not malignant but may develop into malignancies. An example of this type of precursor lesion is high-grade cervical **dysplasia**, which has the propensity to develop into squamous cell carcinoma. Unopposed estrogen exposure can lead to atypical endometrial **hyperplasia**, another precursor lesion associated with endometrial cancer.[3] Regarding epithelial ovarian cancer, there is no single precursor lesion identified to date; however, there has been research that has suggested that ovarian inclusion cysts and atypical endometriosis may play a role in the development of certain ovarian cancer histologies.

Genetics and Cancer

Cancer is a genetic disorder. Although the vast majority of cancers are secondary to a genetic mutation in somatic cells, approximately 5–10% of all cancers are secondary to genetic mutations that are inherited. These disorders are referred to as familial cancer syndrome or hereditary cancer. Genetic predisposition has long been recognized as having a role in the development of cancer. Two cancer susceptibility syndromes account for the majority of inherited gynecologic cancers—the **breast-ovarian cancer syndrome** and the **hereditary nonpolyposis colorectal cancer (HNPCC) syndrome**, which is also called Lynch syndrome.[5] Approximately 10% of ovarian cancer cases and 5–7% of breast cancer cases are due to genetic alterations in the BRCA-1 and BCRA-2 genes.[6,7] Alterations in the MSH2, MLH1,

PMS1, PMS2, and MSH6 genes have been identified in families whose members develop hereditary nonpolyposis colorectal cancer (HNPCC) syndrome.[5] HNPCC syndrome is responsible for 2–7% of colorectal cancers, yet the lifetime risk of colorectal cancer in an individual with HNPCC is approximately 80% and the lifetime risk of developing endometrial cancer is approximately 30–50%.[6] HNPCC syndrome increases the risk that a woman will develop cancer of the endometrium, ovary, colon, or other gastrointestinal organs. Women who have a BRCA-1 or BCRA-2 mutation have a 35–60% lifetime risk of developing ovarian cancer.[5]

Breast-ovarian cancer syndrome and HNPCC syndrome are inherited in an autosomal dominant pattern.[6] If not exposed to a carcinogen, a woman who has the mutation in BRCA-1 or BRCA-2 may never develop an occult cancer, although she retains a 50% chance of passing on the genetic mutation to her children.

The Cell Cycle

All cells, normal and malignant, must undergo a four-step sequential cellular replication to survive[8] (Figure 28-2). During the mitotic (M) phase, cellular division occurs. During the postmitotic, G_1 phase, continued cellular

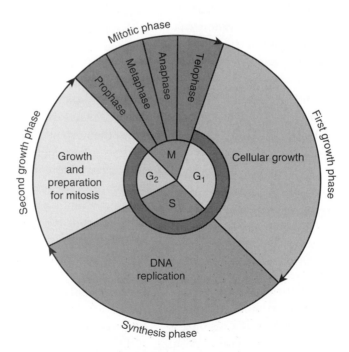

M = Mitotic phase; G_1 = Initial growth phase; G_0 is period of quiescence; S = DNA synthesis; G_2 = Second growth phase.

Figure 28-2 The cell cycle.

activity, RNA synthesis, and DNA repair occur. At this time, the cell can either differentiate and enter the G_0, resting phase, or it can continue the cell cycle. If the cell enters G_0 (period of quiescence), it may reenter the cell cycle at a later time. The S or synthesis phase is the time in which DNA replication takes place. Following the S phase, a cell enters the G_2 phase, a short period in time when a cell has twice the amount of DNA found in a normal cell. From the G_2 phase, a cell reenters the M phase and completes the cell cycle.

Cell Cycle-Specific Drugs

Drugs that are cell cycle specific are frequently used for treating gynecologic malignancies. Cell cycle-specific drugs are chosen because they act on the cell during phases G through M, a time when a cell undergoes proliferation. Examples of cell cycle-specific agents include etoposide (VP-16), which acts during the G_2 phase, methotrexate and 5-fluorouracil (Adrucil) that affect the S phase, and vinca alkaloids that halt mitosis and are active during the M phase.

Cell Cycle-Nonspecific Drugs

Cell cycle-nonspecific agents act on cells during any stage of the cell cycle.[9] Examples of such drugs include cisplatin (Platinol), carboplain (Paraplatin), cyclophosphamide (Cytoxan), doxorubicin (Adriamycin), and mitomycin (Mutamycin).[9] During the treatment of a particular gynecologic malignancy, **combination chemotherapy** may be used, utilizing both cell cycle-specific and nonspecific agents. Combination chemotherapy allows for simultaneous treatment of cells during differing phases of the cell cycle and has been shown to be more efficacious than single-agent therapy alone.[8]

▌General Considerations for Use of Chemotherapeutics

There are three main, albeit different, goals when treating women with gynecologic malignancies—**cure**, **control**, and **palliation**. Treatment goals are dependant on multiple factors including stage at diagnosis, tumor histology, **performance status**, age, comorbidities, overall health status, and the woman's desire for treatment.

Staging of cancer is of particular importance in caring for women with cancer. Staging is a standardized method of evaluating the extent of cancer in the body. Staging also provides information about prognosis, which can guide treatment. Two organizations provide guidance for staging gynecologic cancers. The International Federation of Gynecologists and Obstetricians (FIGO) and the American Joint Committee on Cancer (AJCC) publish staging criteria for gynecologic cancers.[9,10]

Staging usually is categorized by numbers 0-IV and most often is subcategorized by TNM levels to denote such issues as tumor size (T), lymph node involvement (N), and metastasis (M).[11] Staging can also be divided into a clinical stage and a pathologic stage. The clinical stage is based on physical examination, radiologic studies, and endoscopy. In other words, clinical staging is based on all the information available prior to surgery and histologic analysis. Pathologic staging is based on the results of biopsy and results of surgery. Although staging remains important, information such as hormone sensitivity of the tumor, pathology of the sentinel nodes, and risk status also influence the plan of treatment for an individual woman.

Choice of the specific chemotherapeutic agent is increasingly being directed by evidence-based research. The National Comprehensive Cancer Network (NCCN) is an alliance of 21 cancer centers that develops evidence-based guidelines for specific cancers.[12] These guidelines are constantly updated as the results of clinical trials become available. Because of the complexity involved in developing the best plan for an individual, treatment cannot be standardized. This chapter discusses commonly used chemotherapeutic agents without reference to specific regimens.

All the normal routes of administration are used when treating gynecologic malignancies with chemotherapeutic drugs. Side effects experienced are directly related to the route of administration. One unusual route of administration is intraperitoneal, wherein the chemotherapeutic agent is placed directly into the peritoneal cavity, which enables maximal exposure of the tumor to high concentrations of the agent.

Drug resistance can be a major obstacle when using chemotherapeutic agents.[13] Two types of drug resistance exist—acquired resistance and intrinsic resistance. Acquired resistance is secondary to a biochemical change in the cancer cells that occurs subsequent to the specific chemotherapeutic agent.[13] Intrinsic resistance occurs when a tumor fails to respond to initial treatment with the cytotoxic agent. Tumors can display pleiotropic resistance, or multiple drug resistance, to one or more single agents or drug classes, compromising the action of certain chemotherapeutic agents.[13]

Dose intensity refers to the amount of drug delivered over time and is calculated in a standard regimen measurement such as mg/m^2/week.[14] Dose intensity is known to influence successful treatment of gynecologic malignancies, thus maximizing long-term outcomes and overall survival rates of certain malignancies.[14]

The goal of surgical cytoreduction, or **debulking**, is to decrease the amount of **tumor burden** by removing a sizeable portion of cancerous tumors, with the aim of removing it in its entirety or leaving only a small amount of residual disease behind. An increase in overall survival

rates has been directly correlated with the volume of residual disease left after surgery.[3]

Chemotherapeutic Drug Classes

Chemotherapeutic drugs are classified on the basis of their mechanism of action or chemical structure.[15] Sometimes the classification is based on the original plant source from which the drugs are derived. Chemotherapeutic drugs used to treat gynecologic cancers are listed in Table 28-1.

Alkylating Agents

Alkylating agents chemically interact with DNA to cause arrest of mitosis during metaphase by forming single- or

Table 28-1 Selected Cytotoxic Agents, Pharmacologic Class, Indications, and Major Toxicities

Drug Generic (Brand)	Indication	Major Toxicities
Alkylating Agents		
Altretamine (Hexalen)	Recurrent ovarian cancer	All alkylating agents are toxic to tissues that have a high growth fraction; therefore these drugs may have toxic effects on bone marrow, resulting in neutropenia, thrombocytopenia, and anemia. These agents are also toxic to the GI mucosa and to germinal epithelium. Other toxic effects include hair loss and nausea and vomiting.
Carboplatin (Parplatin)	Cervical, endometrial, EOC, GC, GTD, vaginal vulvar	
Cisplatin (Platinol)	Cervical, endometrial, EOC, GC, GTD, vaginal vulvar	
Melphalan (Alkeran)	Cervical, EOC	
Oxaliplatin (Eloxatin)	EOC	
Thiotepa (Thioplex)	Breast, ovarian, or bladder cancer	
Chlorambucil (Leukeran)	EOC, GTD	Mesna is used to decrease hemorrhagic cystitis risk with ifosfamide and cyclophosphamide.
Ifosfamide (Ifex)	Cervical, EOC, sarcoma	
Cyclophosphamide (Cytoxan, Norsar)	Breast cancer, ovarian cancer, and several other malignancies	Cyclophosphamide can also cause acute hemorrhagic cystitis; renal damage can be reduced by adequate hydration.
Plant Alkaloids		
Docetaxel (Taxotere)	Breast, EOC	Significant neutropenia very common. Severe hypersensitivity (hypotension, bronchospasm, generalized rash) can occur. Fluid retention that causes generalized edema, dyspnea at rest, pleural effusion, and/or pronounced abdominal distention can also occur. Other side effects include anemia, nausea, diarrhea, stomatitis, fever, and neurosensory symptoms (paresthesias, pain). Etoposide can cause peripheral neuropathy following repeated infusions (may not be reversible). Etoposide is also associated with hypotension, bradycardia, second- and third-degree heart block, and rarely fatal myocardial infarction. Muscle and joint pain have also occurred. Hair loss, nausea and vomiting, diarrhea, and mucositis are common.
Etoposide (Etopophos, VePesid)	EOC, GTD, GC, sarcoma	
Paclitaxel (Taxol, Onxol)	Ovarian, breast, endometrial	
Vinblastine (Velban)	Breast, GC, GTD	
Vincristine (Oncovin)	Breast, GC, GTD	
Vinorelbine (Navelbine)	EOC, cervical	

(continues)

Table 28-1 Selected Cytotoxic Agents, Pharmacologic Class, Indications, and Major Toxicities (*continued*)

Drug Generic (Brand)	Indication	Major Toxicities
Topoisomerase-1 Inhibitors		
Irinotecan (Camptosar)	EOC	Bone marrow suppression is the dose-limiting side effect (neutropenia occurs in 98% of those treated). Other side effects include hair loss, nausea, vomiting, diarrhea, stomatitis, abdominal pain, and headache.
Topotecan (Hycamtin)	Ovarian cancer	
Hormonal Agents		
Anastrozole (Armidex)	Breast cancer	Aromatase inhibitor. The most common side effects associated with anastrozole are hot flashes, vaginal dryness, musculoskeletal pain, and headache, but they are usually mild.
Exemestane (Aromasin)	Breast cancer	Aromatase inhibitor. Exemestane's most common side effects are fatigue, nausea, hot flushes, depression, and weight gain.
Fluoxymesterone (Halotestin)	Breast cancer	The doses of these drugs, when used for breast cancer, are high; therefore virilization is a common side effect. Adverse effects include severe hypercalcemia.
Testosterone	Breast cancer	
Testolactone (Teslac)	Breast cancer	
Fulvestrant (Faslodex)	Breast cancer	The most common side effects are GI disturbances, hot flushes, headaches, pharyngitis, and bone and back pain.
Letrozole (Fermara)	Breast cancer	Aromatase inhibitor. Letrozole's most common side effects are musculoskeletal pain and nausea.
Megestrol acetate (Magace)	Endometrial, breast, ESS	Thromboembolism is uncommon. There is no increased risk for endometrial cancer.
Raloxifene (Evista)	Breast cancer	Selective estrogen receptor modulator. Side effects are similar to tamoxifen, although raloxifene does not increase the risk for endometrial cancer.
Tamoxifen (Nolvadex)	Breast cancer, EOC	Selective estrogen receptor modulator. The most common side effects are hot flashes, fluid retention, vaginal discharge, nausea, vomiting, and irregular vaginal bleeding. Increased risk of thromboembolic events (e.g., deep vein thrombosis, pulmonary embolism, and stroke). Tamoxifen acts as an estrogen agonist in the uterus, increasing the risk for endometrial cancer.
Toremifene (Fareston)	Metastatic breast cancer	Major toxicities are similar to tamoxifen.
Monoclonal Antibody		
Bevacizumab (Avastin)	EOC	The major adverse effect is cardiac damage that can lead to ventricular dysfunction and congestive heart failure. Many individuals experience flulike symptoms during the first infusion. Infrequently, some persons may have a serious hypersensitivity reaction.
Trastuzumab (Herceptin)	Metastatic breast cancer	Trastuzumab does not cause bone marrow suppression or hair loss.
Antimetabolites		
Capecitabine (Xeloda)	Metastatic colorectal and breast cancer	Severe diarrhea is common and can be dose limiting. Other common side effects include nausea and vomiting, stomatitis, and numbness, tingling, pain, swelling, and erythema of the palms and soles. Can cause leucopenia, but severe bone marrow suppression is uncommon. Hair loss has not been reported.
Fluorouracil (5-FU)	Colon, rectal, breast, stomach, and pancreatic cancer	The most common dose-limiting toxicities are neutropenia and oral and GI ulceration. Other side effects include hair loss, hyperpigmentation, and neurologic deficits.
Gemcitabine (Gemzar)	Recurrent ovarian cancer and uterine sarcomas	Main dose-limiting response if myelosuppression occurs, especially neutropenia. Gastrointestinal effects such as nausea, vomiting, diarrhea, and mucositis. Pulmonary adverse effects are rare but reported. Flu-type syndrome reported in some women.

(*continues*)

Table 28-1 Selected Cytotoxic Agents, Pharmacologic Class, Indications, and Major Toxicities (*continued*)

Drug Generic (Brand)	Indication	Major Toxicities
Hydroxyurea (Hydrea)		This drug inhibits the production of DNA. Side effects include nausea and vomiting, diarrhea, constipation, mucositis, and myelosuppression. Concern that hydroxyurea can increase the risk of leukemia limits use, although studies that corroborate this association are lacking.
Methotrexate (Rheumatex, Trexall)	Gestational trophoblastic disease and noncancers such as ectopic pregnancy and rheumatoid arthritis.	Minimal side effects at therapeutic doses. At high doses, may have fatal bone marrow toxicity, renal toxicity, and cerebral dysfunction. Should be avoided with women with renal insufficiency because it is excreted through the kidneys.
Antitumor Antibiotics		
Actinomycin D (Dactinomycin)	Gestational trophoblastic disease	May be used in combination therapy. Myelosuppression is main effect that causes changes in dosing. GI toxicity, alopecia, and skin ulceration secondary to action as vesicant have been reported.
Bleomycin (Mithracin)	Ovarian cancer	Main toxic effects are pulmonary adverse effects including pneumonitis, especially among the elderly. Rashes also are common, but neutropenia is not a common effect.
Doxorubicin (Adriamycin)	Endometrial cancer	Cardiotoxicity is most pronounced among women over the age of 70 and with cumulative dosing. GI side effects tend to be mild, but alopecia is to be expected.
Liposomal doxorubicin (Doxil)	Recurrent epithelial ovarian carcinoma	Minimal GI, alopecia, and cardiotoxicity effects. Increased risk of stomatitis and PPE for women using this drug compared to others in same drug category.
Mitomycin-C (Mutamycin)		Myelosuppression is main effect that causes changes in dosing. GI toxicity, alopecia, and skin ulceration secondary to action as vesicant have been reported.

EOC = epithelial ovarian carcinoma; EES = endometrial stromal sarcoma; GC = germ cell tumor; GTD = gestational trophoblastic disease.

double-strand breaks of DNA.[8] These drugs are cell cycle nonspecific.[8] Cross resistance to other drugs within this class is common because the alkylating agents have similar mechanisms of action.[8]

Antitumor Antibiotics

Antitumor antibiotics are a class of chemotherapeutic drugs that are isolated during the fermentation process of naturally occurring fungi such as the *Streptomyces* species.[8] This class of drug, which is cell cycle nonspecific, causes free radical formation that damages DNA, RNA, and proteins. They also cause metal ion chelation and tumor cell membrane alteration.

Antimetabolites

Antimetabolites are a cell cycle-specific class of drug that acts on proliferating cells, primarily during the S phase.[3] These agents are useful when treating tumors that exh-

ibit a pattern of accelerated growth, characteristically with short doubling times and large growth fractions. A longer duration of exposure to the drug is generally more effective when treating tumors with antimetabolites because of their cell cycle-specific mechanism of action. This class of chemotherapeutic agents is further subclassified into purine analogs, fluorinated pyrimidines, ribonucleotide reductase inhibitors, and folic acid antagonists.[8]

Although methotrexate is a chemotherapeutic drug, it is not exclusively used to treat cancers. This agent is used to treat a woman with rheumatoid arthritis or a woman with an ectopic pregnancy. This agent has a predilection for the rapidly dividing cells of early pregnancy and is a known antifolate drug. Because it is an antifolate, some clinicians suggest that women supplement their diets with folate. However, folate might decrease the efficacy of the drug, and because the effect of folate is unclear, supplementation is controversial.

Plant Alkaloids

There are several alkaloid drugs derived from different plants that have different mechanisms of action and are sometimes classified on the basis of their mechanisms of action versus their plant origin. The Madagascar periwinkle *Catharanthus roseus* is used to derive vinca alkaloids such as vinblastine (Velban).[16] These agents cause mitotic arrest at metaphase. Extracts of the roots and rhizomes of the *Podophyllum peltatum*, alternately known as the mandrake plant, compose the cytotoxic agent epipodophyllotoxin (Etoposide, VP-16). These drugs block the cell cycle in the late S phase by causing damage to the DNA. Taxanes, such as paclitaxel (Taxol) and docetaxel (Taxotere), are derived from the bark of the *Taxus brevifolia* and *Taxus baccata*, respectively.[17] These drugs are mitotic spindle inhibitors that interfere with mitosis.

Topoisomerase-1 Inhibitors

Topoisomerase-1 is an enzyme that is necessary for DNA replication, repair, and transcription. When this enzyme activity is blocked by topoisomerase-1 inhibitors, DNA strands break and cell death occurs.[15] Topoisomerase-1 inhibitors are cell cycle specific. Examples of this class of drug used in the treatment of gynecologic malignancies are topotecan (Hycamptin) and irinotecan (Camptosar), both of which are derived from the wood stem of the *Camptotheca acuminate* tree.[15]

Hormonal Agents

Hormonal agents are used in the treatment of certain gynecologic malignancies, such as ovarian and endometrial carcinomas, as well as cancer of the breast. Hormones have multiple mechanisms of action. Some are used to cease production of a specific hormone naturally produced by the human body, while others block hormone receptors on the surface of the tumor cell. Other hormonal agents are used to substitute inactive chemically similar agents in place of the active hormone. Hormonal agents used to treat cancer include progestins, antiestrogens, aromatase inhibitors, and selective estrogen receptor modulators (SERMs).

Monoclonal Antibodies

In 1893, W. B. Coley published an article advocating the treatment of cancer with injections of killed bacteria.[18] Coley noticed that individuals with solid tumors who subsequently developed a high fever and bacterial infe-ction caused by *Streptococcus pyrogenes* often had a regression of the cancerous tumor. He postulated that induction of the immune system by the bacterial infection facilitated or caused an immune response against the tumor. Coley invented an infusion of killed bacteria called Coley's toxins that successfully induced remissions in several patients with severe tumors. The advent of radiotherapy eclipsed this initial foray into immunotherapy, and it was not again pursued until late in the 20th century.

Today, cancer immunotherapy is the subject of a large number of research investigations. In 1997, the Food and Drug Administration (FDA) approved the first **monoclonal antibody** for use in cancer and brought immunotherapy back into play in the war against cancer. Monoclonal antibodies are a form of passive immunization.[19] They are tumor-specific antibodies that can be effective for a short duration of time, and they must be provided in large amounts. There are two types of monoclonal antibodies used—naked and conjugated. Naked monoclonal antibodies lack drug or radioactive substance attachment, whereas conjugated monocolonal antibodies are attached to a chemotherapeutic agent, radioactive substances, or toxins.[19] The standard chemotherapeutic drugs interfere with mitosis, DNA synthesis, and DNA repair systems. The immunotherapeutic agents use immune response processes to retard tumor growth and/or induce apoptosis. The different mechanisms of action have correspondingly different side effects and adverse effects.[20]

Examples of monoclonal antibodies used in the treatment of gynecologic malignancies include trastuzumab (Herceptin) and bevacizumab (Avastin), which are used to treat breast cancer. Trastuzumab is used in the treatment of breast cancer characterized by an overexpression of the human epidermal growth factor receptors (HER1 through HER4). These transmembrane receptors normally regulate cell growth and survival when they are activated.[21] Trastuzumab binds to the HER2 receptor and prevents activation of its agonist effect.[21] Bevacizumab (Avastin), a monoclonal antibody, binds to VEGF, a substance necessary for the production of new blood vessels, in an attempt to halt angiogenesis.[22]

Breast Cancer

According to the American Cancer Society, the 5-year survival rate in women diagnosed with localized breast cancer has increased from 80% in the 1950s to 98%

today, with some variation based upon staging of the cancer[10,24] (Table 28-2). This improvement in survival time has been attributed to earlier detection through screening as well as to improved treatments. Prognosis is improved if tumors are ≤ 2.0 cm in size, the lymph node biopsies are negative, the tumor cells are well differentiated, and the tumors are estrogen receptor positive and HER2 negative.

Surgery and radiotherapy are used to treat tumors in the breast, chest wall, and regional lymph nodes while chemotherapy drugs and hormonal agents are used as **adjuvant therapy** to reduce metastasis and recurrences.[24] Trastuzumab (Herceptin) is recommended as adjuvant therapy for women with HER2-positive invasive breast cancer.[21] The National Comprehensive Cancer Network publishes clinical practice guidelines that list current recommended regimens for treating breast cancer.[25]

The majority of breast cancers express estrogen receptors that facilitate cell growth when estrogen binds to the receptor. For women whose tumors are estrogen receptor positive, agents that inhibit the growth of breast tumors by competitive antagonism of estrogen at its receptor site generally are recommended to reduce the likelihood

of recurrence and to prolong disease-free survival. The standard hormonal treatment is the estrogen antagonist, tamoxifen (Nolvadex).

The mechanism of action of tamoxifen is complex since SERMs have partial estrogen-agonist effects as well act as estrogen-antagonist effects. The agonist effects can have additional benefits such as prevention of bone loss in postmenopausal women, but they can also be detrimental given the effects that increase the risk of estrogen-related uterine cancer and thromboembolism.[26,27] Aromatase inhibitors can be an alternative to tamoxifen (Nolvadex). These drugs suppress estrogen levels in postmenopausal women by inhibiting aromatase, the enzyme responsible for the synthesis of estrogen from androgenic substrates in peripheral tissues. Unlike tamoxifen, aromatase inhibitors have no agonist activity.[28] Therefore, aromatase inhibitors are not associated with adverse estrogenic effects, but they also lack the agonist effect on bone.

Chemoprevention

There is no question that prevention of a disease is far better than treatment. Due to the incidence of breast cancer and its response to chemotherapy, research has been conducted in the area of chemoprevention of breast cancer. Although this method seems promising, some major clinical questions continue to exist about use of chemotherapeutics to decrease the risk of the disease as described in Box 28-1.[29,30]

Table 28-2 Breast Cancer Staging

Stage	Description	5-Year Survival
0	Carcinoma in situ. No tumor is regional lymph nodes. No distant metastases.	99%
I	Tumor is less than or equal to 2 centimeters. No tumor is regional lymph nodes. No distant metastases.	92%
IIA	No evidence of primary tumor or tumor less than 5 centimeters. No tumor in regional lymph nodes. No distant metastases.	82%
IIB	Tumor is more than 2 cm and/ or more than 5 cm without tumor in regional lymph nodes and no distant metastases.	65%
IIIA	Invasive cancer but no evidence of primary to movable or fixed ipsilateral nodes. No distant metastases.	47%
IIIB	Tumor extends to chest wall, may include primary tumor. No distant metastases.	44%
IV	Any primary tumor involvement. Any nodal involvement. Distant metastases.	14%

Sources: Greene FL et al. 2002[10]; Singletary SE et al. 2006.[11]

▌Cervical Cancer

Human papilloma virus (HPV) infection is the most important risk factor for the development of both preinvasive and/or invasive cervical cancer. In 2006, the FDA approved the use of human papilloma quadrivalent (types 6, 11, 16, and 18) recombinant vaccine (Gardasil) for the use in girls and women aged 9–26. Detailed information about HPV is available in Chapter 23. The clinical practice guidelines and staging criteria published by FIGO are the criteria most frequently used to stage cervical cancers.[9] Table 28-3 describes the FIGO staging system.

Chemotherapy is used for the treatment of cervical cancer in two scenarios. It is used as primary treatment for women who present with stage IVB or recurrent disease, as well as in women with stage IIB, III, or IVA

Box 28-1 To Treat or Not to Treat: The Role of Chemoprevention

Treatment of cancer, albeit important, is of less value than primary prevention of the disease. After more than 20 years of use as chemotherapy, tamoxifen was approved by the FDA for use as a chemopreventive agent in 1998 for breast cancer. In 2007, raloxifene (Evista) joined as the second selective estrogen receptor modulator with that indication. For both drugs, studies found that the risk of breast cancer was reduced by more than 40% among postmenopausal women at high risk. Unfortunately, neither drug is without side and adverse effects.

Some authorities suggest choosing raloxifene because thromboembolic events and endometrial hyperplasia occur less often than with tamoxifen. In either case, major questions remain unanswered regarding how to characterize high risk; which women benefit the most from chemoprevention; how long these agents should be used; and how long protection lasts. Assuming these questions are answered and the side/adverse effect profiles of these agents are improved, chemoprevention may join other prophylactic regimens such as folic acid to prevent neural tube defects.

Table 28-3 Cervical Carcinoma Staging

Stage	Description	5-Year Survival Rate
Stage I	The carcinoma is strictly confined to the cervix.	> 95%
IA	Diagnosed only by microscopy, no visible lesions.	
IB	Visible lesion or a microscopic lesion with > 5 mm of depth or horizontal spread of > 7 mm.	Approximately 90%
Stage II	Invasion beyond the cervix but not to the pelvic wall or to lower third of vagina.	Approximately 75–78%
IIA	Involves upper two thirds of vagina but no parametrial invasion.	
IIB	Parametrial invasion.	
Stage III	Tumor extends to pelvic wall and/or invades the lower third of vagina and/or causes hydronephrosis or nonfunctioning bladder.	Approximately 50%
IIIA	Extension to the lower one third of vagina but no extension to pelvic wall.	
IIIB	Extension to pelvic sidewall or hydronephrosis.	
Stage IV	Mucosal involvement of bladder or rectum, or distant disease.	Approximately 20–30%
IVA	Tumor invades mucosa of bladder or rectum and/or extends beyond the true pelvis.	
IVB	Distant metastasis.	

Sources: Benedet JL et al. 2000[9]; Greene FL et al. 2002.[10]

in conjunction with radiation therapy.[30] With the exclusion of the 5–10% of women who experience complete response to single-agent therapy, response rates are generally short lived.

Endometrial Cancer

The most common gynecologic malignancy in the United States is endometrial carcinoma, which accounts for 6% of all cancers affecting women.[1] Ninety percent of women with endometrial cancer initially present with vaginal bleeding, most commonly in the postmenopausal period.[31] In the United States, uterine sarcomas represent less than 5% of uterine cancers and include malignant mixed mullerian tumors, leiomyosarcomas, and other classifications such as endometrial stromal sarcomas. FIGO staging of endometrial cancers is presented in Table 28-4.

Most women with endometrial cancer present with early endometrial cancer (stage I), which is treated surgically with a hysterectomy; however, for women who present with advanced or metastatic disease, radiation, **brachytherapy**, or radiation seed implantation with or without surgery or chemotherapy may be recommended.

Gestational Trophoblastic Disease

Gestational trophoblastic disease (GTD) is a spectrum of diseases that include benign **hydatidiform moles**, malignant moles, and gestational trophoblastic neoplasia. The different GTD disorders are classified on the basis of histology and malignant or nonmalignant characteristics (Table 28-5). Although the etiology remains uncertain, at some early point in the pregnancy, trophoblastic cells that normally would form the placenta proliferate and villous stroma becomes edematous. The latter changes

Table 28-4 Endometrial Carcinoma and Ovarian Carcinoma Staging

Stage	Endometrial Cancer Description	Ovarian Cancer Description
Stage I	*Endometrial Involvement*	*Growth Limited to the Ovaries*
IA	Tumor limited to the endometrium	One ovary; no ascites; capsule intact; no tumor on external surface
IB	Invasion to less than 50% of the myometrium	Two ovaries; no ascites; capsule intact; no tumor on external surface
IC	Invasion to more than 50% of the myometrium	One or both ovaries with surface tumor, ruptured capsule, or ascites or peritoneal washings with malignant cells
Stage II	*Endocervical/Stromal Involvement*	*Pelvic Extension*
IIA	Endocervical glandular involvement	Involvement of the uterus and/or tubes
IIB	Cervical stromal invasion	Involvement of other pelvic tissues
IIC		IIA or IIB with factors as in IC
Stage III	*Metastasis*	*Peritoneal Implants Outside Pelvis and/or Positive Retroperitoneal or Inguinal Nodes*
IIIA	Tumor invades serosa or adnexa or positive peritoneal cytology	Grossly limited to true pelvis; negative nodes; microscopic seeding of abdominal peritoneum
IIIB	Vaginal metastasis	Implants of abdominal peritoneum ≤ 2 cm; nodes negative
IIIC	Metastasis to the pelvic or para-aortic lymph nodes	Abdominal implants > 2 cm and/or positive retroperitoneal or inguinal nodes
Stage IV	*Metastasis Outside Pelvis*	*Distant Metastasis*
IVA	Tumor invasion of bladder and/or bowel mucosa	
IVB	Distant metastasis including intra-abdominal and/or inguinal lymph nodes	

Sources: Benedet JL et al. 2000[9]; Greene FL et al. 2002.[10]

become the grapelike clusters that characterize a hydatidiform mole. Hydatidiform moles are categorized as either complete hydatidiform mole or incomplete hydatidiform mole based on the degree and extent of the changes. Complete and partial hydatidiform moles can develop into nonmetastatic or metastatic gestational trophoblastic neoplasia.[32]

Gestational Trophoblastic Neoplasia

Complete hydatidiform moles are the types most likely to develop gestational trophoblastic neoplasia (GTN).

The most common GTN tumors are invasive moles and gestational choriocarcinoma, based on characteristics of the disease. Invasive moles involve penetration of the myometrium but tend not to metastasize to distant organs. Chemotherapy is highly effective, and cure rates range between 80% and 100% depending on the extent of the disease.[33] Choriocarcinoma, however, usually develops systemic metastases if not aggressively treated early.

Once GTN is diagnosed, surgical treatment in the form of a hysterectomy is a common first-line treatment. Chemotherapy is recommended with or without surgery. For women with low-risk disease, the most common chemotherapeutic agent is methotrexate (Trexall), although some oncologists will use pulsed actinomycin D (Dactinomycin). Women who have high-risk GTN (e.g., older than 40 years, $\geq$ hCG 10^5, diagnosed with multiple metastases) are treated with combination chemotherapy.

A woman who has one molar pregnancy has a 1–2% risk of another. Pregnancy after chemotherapy has not been found to have an increased risk of adverse outcomes.[34]

Ovarian Cancer

In the United States, epithelial ovarian cancer (EOS) is the fifth leading cause of cancer death and the leading cause of death from a gynecologic malignancy.[1] Symptoms of the disease are vague, which makes diagnosis challenging. The most common symptoms include bloating, pelvic/abdominal pain, urinary changes (frequency/urgency), early satiety, and difficulty eating. Most women (75%) have stage III or IV disease at initial diagnosis (Table 28-4), and overall, approximately 40% of women diagnosed with the disease will be cured.[35] Ovarian cancer is initially treated surgically with a total hysterectomy and bilateral oophorectomy. Ovarian malignancies are comprised of multiple histopathologic subtypes. Upon final histopathologic diagnosis, an appropriate treatment plan is individualized for each woman who has been diagnosed.

A number of cytotoxic agents can be used for treating epithelial ovarian cancer. The most active agents are platinum compounds, such as cisplatin and carboplatin. Women are considered platinum sensitive if they experience disease **progression** more than 6 months after initial treatment with a platinum agent. Women who are considered platinum resistant have (1) disease

Table 28-5 Gestational Trophoblastic Tumors

Tumor Type	Description	Benign Versus Malignant
Hydatidiform mole	Placental villi swollen in fluid filled clusters. Hydatidiform moles are not cancerous, but they can develop into gestational trophoblastic neoplasia (GTN). Hydatidiform moles are subdivided into two categories—partial and complete.	A hydatidiform mole is considered malignant when serum beta hCG levels continue to rise after surgical removal (assuming a normal pregnancy is not present). This occurs in approximately 15% of hydatidiform moles.
Partial hydatidiform mole	Partial hydatidiform moles occur when two sperm fertilize an egg. The tumor contains some fetal tissue but no fetus. Partial moles are completely removed via surgery.	Incidence of GTN is 2–3%.
Complete hydatidiform mole	A complete hydatidiform mole develops when 1 or 2 sperm fertilize an egg that does not have maternal DNA. This hydatidiform mole is completely paternal genetic material, and there is no fetal tissue. Approximately 20% of complete moles will have persistent tissue remaining following surgery that develops into an invasive mole if not treated.	The incidence of GTN is 18–30%.
Gestational Trophoblastic Neoplasia (GTN)		
Invasive mole	Hydatidiform mole that grows into the uterine myometrium. Invasive moles occur in approximately 20% of women who have a hydatidiform mole.	Invasive moles are malignant. Approximately 15% metastasize to distant organs, usually the lungs.
Choriocarcinoma	Choriocarcinoma can develop de novo in other organs such as ovaries or chest. Most often associated with a complete hydatidiform mole.	Highly metastatic if untreated.
Placental-site trophoblastic tumor and epithelioid trophoblastic tumor	Rare gestational trophoblastic neoplasms. Unlike choriocarcinoma, these trophoblastic tumors can develop long after a gestational event.	Approximately 15–25% become malignant with distant metastases.

hCG = human chorionic gonadotropin.
Source: Berkowitz RS, Goldstein DT 2009.[33]

progression while on an initial platinum-based chemotherapy regimen, (2) continued **stable disease** while on initial treatment, or (3) relapse within 6 months of a combination regimen.

Vulvar and Vaginal Cancer

Vaginal and vulvar cancers are the least common gynecologic malignancies. Squamous cell carcinomas comprise 85% of vaginal cancers and are known to commonly metastasize to the lungs and liver. Conversely, adenocarcinoma represents 15% of vaginal cancers and is most often seen in women ages 17–21 years, with common sites of metastasis being the lungs and supraclavicular and pelvic lymph nodes.[36] Less commonly occurring vaginal cancers include melanoma, sarcoma, and adenosquamous types. Women with a history of in utero diethylstilbestrol (DES) exposure commonly present with vaginal adenosis, which rarely progresses into a vaginal adenocarcinoma.[37] Although rare, the clear cell type of vaginal cancer occurs in women with a history of in utero DES exposure and

generally in those who are under the age of 30 years[35] (Box 28-2).

Vulvar cancer can occur at any age but is most often seen in women who are postmenopausal.[3] Many vulvar cancers are preceded by condylomas or dysplasias, and HPV is the causative factor in the development of many genital tract malignanies.[38] Cellular types include basal cell, verrucous carcinoma, sarcoma, histocytosis X, and malignant melanoma. Treatment options for both vulvar and vaginal cancers are dependant on the cellular classification and stage of the disease and include surgery, radiation, and/or chemotherapy.

Major Chemotherapeutic Side Effects and Adverse Effects

Chemotherapeutic agents have an array of toxic side effects and adverse effects that are collectively referred to as chemotherapy toxicities. In general, highly proliferative cells, such as those in the gastrointestinal tract and bone marrow, are the cells that in addition to tumor cells are most affected.[39]

Box 28-2 Gone But Not Forgotten: Diethylstilbestrol (DES)

Diethylstilbestrol (DES) is a nonsteroidal estrogen that was discovered more than 7 decades ago in England. In the early 1940s, this drug received FDA approval as a treatment for gonorrhea, atrophic vaginitis, and menopause, as well as a lactation suppression agent. Gradually the drug gained popularity for off-label use to treat threatened abortion and as a prophylactic intervention for women with a history of previous spontaneous abortion. In 1947, this indication was added to the list by the FDA. By the mid 1950s, research found that DES was not effective to prevent pregnancy loss, yet the drug continued to be used, although the number of prescriptions decreased. The peak years of use were between 1941 and 1971.

Many agents have been discovered to be ineffective and disappeared from the market. Although use of DES in early pregnancy disappeared, lifetime effects of the drug have been discovered. Not only do women who took the pharmaceutical have an increased risk of breast cancer, but the agent was discovered to have teratogenic effects. Offspring now are commonly called DES daughters and DES sons or those with second-generation exposure. Perhaps most significantly, DES daughters have an increased risk of vaginal adenocarcinoma, a relatively rare cancer. DES daughters not only have increased risk of vaginal carcinoma, but have an increased risk of breast cancer, clear cell cancers of the cervix and vagina, infertility, and pregnancy complications such as preterm birth. Long-term effects for DES sons suggest increased risks of epididymal cysts, hypospadias, and perhaps autoimmune disorders. Research continues to be ongoing regarding the second generation as these individuals age. Research today on the third generation suggests that it is possible DES will continue to plague families as the children of DES daughters and DES sons may have untoward perinatal outcomes. However, longitudinal studies are needed to determine if there are third generation effects and establish how much longer this drug that is gone will remain unforgotten.

Myelosuppression results in varying degrees of cytopenia including anemia, neutropenia, and thrombocytopenia. Bone marrow suppression becomes evident after mature blood components are normally removed from the system. White blood cells, especially neutrophils, have the shortest life span (6–12 hours), which is why neutropenia is the most common form of myelosuppression. Platelets normally live 5–10 days, and when they are used up, thrombocytopenia can become evident. Red blood cells normally live about 120 days, but there are many ways an individual with cancer can become anemic in addition to bone marrow suppression, and anemia is therefore a common problem. All of the epithelial cells that line the gastrointestinal tract have a rapid turnover time.

Mucositis and diarrhea are both manifestations of chemotherapy-associated gastrointestinal toxicities. These side effects and adverse effects are most likely to be the symptoms a primary care clinician can help treat. The Multinational Association of Supportive Care in Cancer, an international coalition of professional associations in oncology, regularly meets and updates clinical practice guidelines for care of chemotherapy side effects and adverse effects.[40]

All of the symptoms reviewed here can be secondary to any number of disorders. Therefore, the first step in evaluating an individual on chemotherapy who presents with one of the following symptoms is to identify and treat other causes before using agents specifically recommended for chemotherapy toxicities.

Fatigue

One of the most common and distressing side effects of cancer and cancer treatment is fatigue, which can be secondary to anemia, depression, pain, or the cancer itself. There have been multiple randomized trials of various drug therapies for fatigue.[41] A Cochrane meta-analysis of 27 randomized trials found that methylphenidate (Ritalin) and erythropoietin have a modest positive effect on cancer-related fatigue, but paroxetine (Prozac) and progestational steroids are no better than placebo.[41]

Anemia

Despite the fact that red blood cells have a longer life span than other blood components, anemia is the most common hematologic abnormality in persons receiving chemotherapy.[42] Chemotherapeutic drugs cause anemia by reducing the number of circulating erythrocytes, but additional etiologies include malnutrition secondary to mucositis, hemolysis, renal dysfunction, and bone marrow metastases. Many women are already anemic when chemotherapy is first initiated. If anemia does develop, the first step is to determine the etiology and correct it if possible. If the cause is determined to be myelosuppression, anemia can be treated with iron supplementation, a blood transfusion, or an erythropoiesis-stimulating drug.[43]

Erythropoietin, which is produced in the kidney, regulates red blood cell production. In 1993, the FDA approved the use of human recombinant erythropoietin-stimulating agents such as epoetin alfa (Procrit, Eprex, and Epogen) for the treatment of chemotherapy-induced anemia.[43] Initial studies and a meta-analysis found that erythropoietin-stimulating agents increase hemoglobin levels, decrease the need for blood transfusion, and reduce fatigue.[44] Unfortunately, many recent studies have found that epoetin alfa (Procrit, Eprex, and Epogen) increases the risk of thromboembolic disease, promotes tumor growth, and may be associated with decreased survival.[44]

In 2007, the FDA issued a black box warning for erythropoietin that cautions about the potential for tumor promotion and thromboembolic events. An FDA advisory panel in 2008 recommended that this drug be used at the lowest dose feasible and only for individuals with a hemoglobin level < 11 g per deciliter.[45]

Neutropenia

Neutrophils are phagocytes that are highly important in immune function and infection prevention. Depending on the chemotherapeutic agent used, neutropenia generally occurs 6–12 days after drug administration and in most cases the person with neutropenia recovers within 21–24 days.[3] In persons receiving chemotherapy, neutropenia and the more serious febrile neutropenia occur in 24% and 14%, respectively.[46] Neutropenia is the most common dose-limiting factor in adjusting chemotherapy dose schedules. Agents such as carboplatin (Paraplatin) and paclitaxel (Taxol) have higher incidences of neutropenia due to their myelosuppressive characteristics.

The development of neutropenia increases the risk of developing certain bacteria and fungal infections that can potentially be life threatening. If a woman receiving chemotherapy has a one-time oral temperature of 101.0°F (38.3°C) or a fever of 100.4°F (38°C) for more than 2 hours, she should be evaluated for possible infection. The treatment of neutropenia is largely empirical. Common bacterial infections are those that affect the skin, such as *Staphylococcus aureus* and infections involving the gastrointestinal tract, such as *Escherichia coli* or *Klebsiella pneumoniae*. Fungal infections such as *Candida* and *Aspergillus* are common among women with neutropenia who have been treated with antibiotics, and these infections require prompt treatment with the usual antifungal drugs.

Granulocyte colony-stimulating factor (G-CSF) and granulocyte-macrophage colony-stimulating factor (GM-CSF) are naturally occurring growth hormones involved in the maturation of blood cell components, available as filgrastim (Neupogen) or pegfilgrastim (Neulasta); these agents stimulate the production of neutrophils. GM-CSF, which is available as sargramostim (Leukine), stimulates production of neutrophils, eosinophils, monocytes, and macrophages.[47] Both agents reduce the duration and severity of neutropenia, and current national guidelines from the National Comprehensive Cancer Network recommend that they be used prophylactically for persons whose risk of developing neutropenia is > 20%.[44] Side effects and adverse effects of pegfilgrastim are bone pain, urticaria, angioedema, anaphylaxis, sickle cell crisis, acute respiratory distress syndrome (ARDS), splenomegaly, and rare splenic rupture that may be fatal. Pegfilgrastim is considered to be an FDA Pregnancy Category C drug because evidence of teratology exists in animals, although no teratogenic effects have been reported among humans. Caution should be used in women who are breastfeeding while receiving pegfilgrastim, because it is unknown if the medication is excreted in breast milk. Pegfilgrastim is contraindicated for persons who are hypersensitive to *E coli*-derived proteins, pegfilgrastim, or filgrastim.

Thrombocytopenia

Individuals with platelet counts < 20,000/mm³ have a significantly increased risk of spontaneous hemorrhage.[3] Common hemorrhagic sites are the skull and the gastrointestinal tract.[3] Women with thrombocytopenia may experience abdominal or extremity petechiae, epistaxis, oral bleeding (gingival), hematuria, rectal bleeding, or bloody stools. Women with excessive bruising or vaginal bleeding should also be evaluated for thrombocytopenia. Oprelvekin (Neumega), which is synthetically derived interleukin-11, is administered prophylactically to prevent thrombocytopenia. Oprelvekin stimulates bone marrow production of megakaryocytes, the precursor of platelets.

The most commonly occurring adverse events associated with oprelvekin (Neumega) include neutropenic fever, syncope, atrial fibrillation, fever and pneumonia, edema, dyspnea, tachycardia, conjunctival infection, palpitations, atrial arrhythmias, and pleural effusions.[47,48] Postmarketing reports of allergic reactions include anaphylaxis, optic disc edema, ventricular arrhythmia, capillary leak syndrome, renal failure, and injection site reactions.[48]

Alopecia

Contrary to popular belief, some chemotherapeutic drugs do not cause hair loss. Alopecia is generally experienced when using chemotherapeutic agents such as cisplatin (Platinol), cyclophosphamide (Cytoxan), doxorubicin (Adriamycin), and paclitaxel (Taxol). There are no interventions identified to prevent alopecia. Hair loss often is patchy, and upon regrowth, hair may be different in character or color. Even when alopecia is expected, it can happen quickly over a few days but does not happen immediately after the first dose of chemotherapy. This gives women time to plan ahead and be fitted for wigs if desired.

Nausea and Vomiting

Approximately 70–80% of all persons who are undergoing chemotherapeutic treatment will experience nausea and/or vomiting, with nausea more frequent than emesis. Women are more likely than men to experience chemotherapy-induced nausea and vomiting, a side effect associated with significant deterioration in quality of life for affected individuals.[49] The five classifications of chemotherapy-induced nausea and vomiting are (1) acute, (2) delayed, (3) anticipatory, (4) breakthrough, and (5) refractory. Emesis occurring within 24 hours of chemotherapy is referred to as acute and generally occurs within the first 7 hours after chemotherapy.[50] Delayed emesis occurs 24 hours after the administration of a chemotherapeutic agent and can persist for 72 to 96 hours after treatment. If a woman has previously experienced emesis during or after the administration of chemotherapy, she might experience anticipatory emesis, which can occur at any time before, during, or after an antineoplastic agent is administered.[8] When nausea and/or vomiting occur despite administration of antiemetics, it is termed *breakthrough nausea and vomiting*. Refractory nausea and vomiting occur during subsequent chemotherapy cycles when antiemetic therapy has failed in earlier cycles.

Chemotherapeutic drugs have an inherent emetogenicity that varies among agents. This emetogenicity is the primary consideration in forming treatment plans to eradicate or mitigate nausea and vomiting. The drugs are assigned to one of four classifications, which were updated in 2004 by the Multinational Association of Supportive Care in Cancer[49,51] (Table 28-6). There has been significant progress in finding the pharmacologic agents that best mitigate these symptoms. Vomiting can be prevented in 70–80% of individuals who receive a chemotherapy drug with high emetic potential via the use of a serotonin antagonist, neurokinin-1 receptor antagonist, and steroid in combination.[52]

Table 28-6 Emetogenicity of Chemotherapeutic Drugs

High (> 90%)*	Moderate (30–90%)*	Low (10–30%)*	Minimal (< 10%)*
Intravenous			
Carmustine	Carboplatin	5-Fluorouracil	2-Chlorodeoxyadenosine
Cisplatin	Cyclophosphamide < 1500 mg/m²	Bortezomib	Bevacizumab
Cyclophosphamide 1500 mg/m²	Cytarabine > 1 g/m²	Cetuximab	Bleomycin
Dacarbazine	Daunorubicin	Cytarabine 100 mg/m²	Busulfan
Mechlorethamine	Doxorubicin	Docetaxel	Fludarabine
Streptozotocin	Epirubicin	Etoposide	Vinblastine
	Idarubicin	Gemcitabine	Vincristine
	Ifosfamide	Methotrexate	Vinorelbine
	Irinotecan	Mitomycin	
	Oxaliplatin	Mitoxantrone	
		Paclitaxel	
		Pemetrexed	
		Topotecan	
		Trastuzumab	
Orally Administered			
Hexamethylmelamine	Cyclophosphamide	Capecitabine	6-Thioguanine
Procarbazine	Etoposide	Fludarabine	Chlorambucil
	Imatinib		Erlotinib
	Temozolomide		Gefitinib
	Vinorelbine		Hydroxyurea
			L-phenylalanine mustard
			Methotrexate

* Percentage = The risk of vomiting if no antiemetic drug is administered.
Source: Adapted from Antiemetic Subcommittee of the Multinational Association of Supportive Care in Cancer 2006.[51]

The mechanism of action underlying chemotherapy-induced nausea and vomiting is fairly straightforward. Chemotherapeutic drugs stimulate the enterochromaffin cells in the gastrointestinal tract to release serotonin. Once serotonin binds to serotonin receptors, the vagal afferent pathway is stimulated, which activates the vomiting center in the central nervous system. The areas of the brain where the vagal pathway terminates have receptors for several neurotransmitters that have roles in the emetic response. These neurotransmitters include neurokinin-1, serotonin, histamine, and dopamine.[49] There are several pharmacologic options for treating each type of chemotherapy-induced nausea and vomiting. Commonly used drugs and doses are listed in Table 28-7.

The antiemetic that has most recently been approved by the FDA for treating chemotherapy-induced nausea and vomiting is aprepitant (Emend), which is a neurokinin-1 receptor antagonist. Aprepitant inhibits both acute and delayed emesis when given in combination with ondansetron (Zofran) and dexamethasone (Decadron).[53,54]

Aprepitant has the potential to alter circulating plasma concentrations of multiple drugs due to its actions as a substrate, moderate inducer of CYP2C9, and moderate inhibitor of CYP3A4.[55] Drug–drug interactions are possible, and therefore this drug should be administered by a clinician who is knowledgeable about the properties of aprepitant. Care should also be taken when administering aprepitant with warfarin. Supplemental contraception has been advocated for women using hormonal contraceptive methods while taking aprepitant because of potential increased metabolism of the oral contraceptive hormones.

Table 28-7 Antiemetic Drugs for Treating Nausea and Vomiting Associated with Chemotherapy Treatment

Drug Generic (Brand)	Dose*
Serotonin Antagonists	
Dolasetron (Anzemet)[†]	100 mg IV (infused over 30 seconds) 1 hour prior to chemotherapy.
Granisetron (Kytril)[†]	10 mcg/kg IV (infused over 30 seconds) 30 minutes prior to chemotherapy; only on the day that chemotherapy is given. Transdermal patch available.
Ondansetron (Zofran)[†]	24 mg IV 30 minutes prior to chemotherapy. 8 mg PO q 8 hours × 1–3 days after chemotherapy for delayed emesis.
Palonosetron (Aloxi)[†]	0.25 mg IV (infused over 30 seconds) 30 minutes prior to chemotherapy.
Tropisetron (Navoban)[†]	5 mg IV or PO.
Dopamine Antagonists	
Droperidol (Inapsine)	
Metoclopramide (Reglan)[†]	1–2 mg/kg IV (infuse over 1–2 minutes) 30 minutes prior to chemotherapy.
Prochlorperazine (Compazine)[†]	5–10 mg (PO, IM, IV) 3–4 times a day PRN.
Promethazine (Phenergan)	12.4–25 mg (PO, IM, IV) q 4–6 hours.
Glucocorticoids	
Dexamethasone (Decadron)*	The most efficacious dose of steroid use with serotonin antagonists has not been standardized; however, researchers have suggested that a single dose of 8 mg is adequate when used with the serotonin antagonist.
Cannabinoids	
Dronabinol (Marinol)[†]	5–7.5 mg/m² PO q 24 hours PRN.
Nabilone (Cesamet)[†]	1–2 mg PO 3–4 times a day PRN.
Neurokinin-1 Inhibitors	
Aprepitant (Emend)[† §]	Aprepitant and fosaprepitant are used in combination with other antiemetics. 125 mg PO 1 hour prior to chemotherapy followed by 80 mg PO on the second and third days following chemotherapy.
Fosaprepitant (Emend)[§]	Fosaprepitant is the prodrug of aprepitant. 115-mg dose given IV.
Benzodiazepines	
Lorazepam (Ativan)	Used as adjunct rather than primary drug for anticipatory or delayed nausea and vomiting.
Midazolam	Rapid onset of action.

* May vary depending on whether chemotherapeutic agent is considered highly or moderately emetogenic.
[†] Moderate to high therapeutic index.
[‡] Low therapeutic index.
[§] Aprepitant/fosaprepitant is a substrate, inducer, and inhibitor of several CYP450 enzymes. Drug–drug interactions can occur with a number of drugs that might be used concurrently. More information is available from Hesklith PJ 2008.[49]
Sources: Adapted from Hesketh PJ 2008[49] and Dando TM et al. 2004.[53]

Mucositis or Stomatitis

Approximately 40% of women undergoing primary chemotherapeutic management of cancer will experience such oral side effects with each cycle due to slowed basal epithelium regeneration. The buccal and labial mucosa, oral soft palate and floor, and the ventral surface of the tongue are the most commonly observed areas affected, and symptoms occur approximately 5–7 days after chemotherapy administration (Box 28-3).

Due to its desiccant effects, milk of magnesia (MOM) should be avoided. Cold liquids and ice chips may be implemented for comfort. Pharmacologic management may include the use of 2% viscous lidocaine or a 50/50 mixture of attapulgite/diphenhydramine (Kaopectate/Benadryl) to be used as needed.[56] Systemic analgesics can be used to minimize pain.[57] The Multinational Association of Supportive Care in Cancer guidelines for treating oral mucositis were updated in 2004 and revised in 2007.[58,59]

Diarrhea

Diarrhea can be a consequence of disorders such as malnutrition, irritable/inflammatory bowel syndrome, malabsorption, medications, or infection, and it can also be experienced by persons undergoing chemotherapy. There are several different etiologies of diarrhea, which are linked to specific chemotherapy drugs.[60] For example, some drugs decrease intestinal enzyme production, which results in osmotic diarrhea. When a woman presents with diarrhea, an evaluation for an underlying cause other than chemotherapy and evaluation for dehydration or electrolyte imbalance is the first step in diagnosing and treating her condition.[61] If hospitalization is not indicated, loperamide (Imodium) is usually the first pharmacologic agent recommended, followed by octreotide (Sandostatin).[61] Octreotide is associated with significant side effects and is only used when loperamide is not effective. Medications such as diphenoxylate-atropine sulfate (Lomotil) and tincture of opium (Paregoric) can also be used, although the latter is increasingly difficult to find through local pharmacies.

Constipation

Constipation, like all other chemotherapy side effects, can be a result of underlying medical conditions, medications, or the chemotherapy drugs. The most serious complication associated with constipation is bowel obstruction. Additional symptoms of bowel obstruction include nausea, vomiting, abdominal distention, decreased/no flatus, decreased/no bowel movements, and crampy abdominal pain. Unless contraindicated, medications such as psyllium (Metamucil), senna (Senokot), bisacodyl (Dulcolax), docusate sodium (Colace), glycerine suppository, magnesium hydroxide (milk of magnesia), lactulose (Chronulac), or sorbitol and sodium phosphate (Fleet's enema) are reasonable treatments for constipation.

Palmar-Plantar Erythrodysesthesia

Palmar-plantar erythrodysesthesia (PPE), also known as hand-foot syndrome, is a cutaneous skin reaction characterized by painful erythematous plaques on the hands or feet. Initial symptoms are usually tingling in the hands or feet followed by swelling, tenderness, pain, intense erythema with blanching between joints, and perhaps

---

Box 28-3 A Case of Stomatitis

CC is a 61-year-old woman who is receiving chemotherapy for the treatment of breast cancer. After her third treatment, she presented to her primary care provider reporting difficulty eating due to painful sores in her mouth and throat. The diagnosis of oral mucositis (i.e., stomatitis) was made.

Stomatitis is a common complication of chemotherapy because many of the chemotherapeutic agents alter the integrity of the mucosa, the normal microbial flora of the oral cavity, salivary quantity, and epithelial maturation. This can result in not only pain and dysphagia, but can alter the nutritional status of the woman and increase her risk for infection. CC was assessed for local infections such as esophageal candidiasis, and no infections were discovered.

Oral hygiene and dietary modification such as eating foods that require little or no chewing and avoiding acidic, spicy, salty, coarse, or dry food items were recommended. Over-the-counter mucosal coating agents such as Pepto Bismol were suggested to her. CC reported that the palliative agents were helpful. Had they not relieved the discomfort, topical agents such as anesthetics, analgesics, or topical opioids could have been the next treatments of choice.

desquamation. Pain relief and superinfection prevention are the main goals when treating women with PPE.[3]

Hypersensitivity Reactions

Approximately 5% of women treated for a gynecologic malignancy will have some form of hypersensitivity reaction to the agent used during treatment. Allergic reactions are most notably experienced during the first or second cycle and generally occur within the first few minutes of beginning the infusion. Hypersensitivity reactions to platinum occurs in approximately 5–20% of persons treated, and it has been reported that 12% of individuals exposed to carboplatin (Paraplatin) may experience an allergic reaction. Hypersensitivity reactions to other chemotherapy agents are rare.

Nephrotoxicity and Neurotoxicity

Many chemotherapeutic agents and their metabolites are excreted renally, and therefore the renal system and urinary tract are at risk of injury. The two most common chemotherapeutic agents associated with neurotoxicity are cisplatin and paclitaxel. Manifestations of neurotoxicity include peripheral neuropathy, autonomic dysfunction, ototoxicity, retinal toxicity, and seizures. Peripheral neuropathy is the most common neurotoxicity. Symptoms are generally described as stocking-glove distribution parasthesias of the feet, legs, arms, and hands, which can ultimately result in loss of deep tendon reflexes (DTR) and vibratory sensation.

Antiseizure medications such as gabapentin (Neurontin), topiramate (Topamax), pregabalin (Lyrica), carbamazepine (Tegretol), and phenytoin (Dilantin) are effective for the treatment of nerve pain with medication-related side effects being drowsiness and dizziness. Topical lidocaine patches may also be used, in which a woman places the patch over the area of most severe pain. Tricyclic antidepressants, such as amitriptyline (Elavil) and nortriptyline (Pamelor), have also been used to treat peripheral neuropathy.

Chemo Brain

It has estimated that after chemotherapy, more than 30% of women experience a noticeable decrease in cognition.[62] This frustrating and often anxiety-providing condition has several different names, including postchemotherapy cognitive impairment, chemo brain, and chemo fog. Breast cancer survivors were the first to report chemo brain symptoms such as decreased concentration and memory after chemotherapy.

Risk factors to assist in identifying which women are most likely to develop the condition are not well established. The etiology for chemo brain is elusive, particularly since cognitive changes also may be confounded by other factors such as anesthesia, age, menopause, and other medications. Potential causes have been suggested to include vascular injury, autoimmune responses, and even shrinkage of certain sections of the brain.[63,64] Treatments have been suggested to include psychotherapy, nutritional supplements, and various pharmaceuticals. However, effectiveness has not been reliably demonstrated for any specific intervention. Fortunately, chemo brain is a time-limited event, although full resolution may not occur for several years.

Drug–Drug Interactions

Combination chemotherapy is chosen carefully because of the potential of adverse drug to drug interactions. For example, use of cisplatin (Platinol) and methotrexate (Trexall) can result in renal damage as both these agents are excreted by the kidney. Sequencing of cisplatin and paclitaxel can be synergistic or antagonistic, depending upon which drug is administered first.[65] These factors are well considered by the oncology team determining the best chemotherapy treatments for a woman.

In the primary care arena, selected drug interactions are more common among chemotherapeutic agents and nutritional supplements or medications used for comorbid conditions.[66] Some of the potentially adverse reactions may be secondary to good intentions. Although use of antioxidants may be an attempt to advance healthy habits, chemotherapeutics that act by destruction of DNA theoretically may have decreased effectiveness when taken with antioxidants such as vitamin A, C, or E. Sometimes drugs needed for one condition, such as depression, may potentially interfere with chemotherapeutics. For example, controversy exists about selective serotonin reuptake inhibitors (SSRIs) potentially reducing the effectiveness of concomitant administration of tamoxifen. Not all SSRIs are problematic, and more research is necessary in this area.[67] Table 28-8 lists selected drug interactions with chemotherapeutic agents.

Table 28-8 Selected Drug–Drug Interactions Between Chemotherapeutic Agents and Other Drugs*

Chemotherapeutic Agent Generic (Brand)	Other Drug Generic (Brand)	Potential Risk
Cisplatin (Platinol)	Ondansetron (Zofran)	Reduced plasma concentration of cisplatin
Cisplatin (Platinol)	Phenytoin (Dilantin)	Reduced plasma concentration of phenytoin
Cyclophosphamide (Cytoxan, Nosar)	Quinolones	Mucositis may alter absorption of quinolones
Cyclophosphamide (Cytoxan, Nosar) Fluorouracil (5-FU)	Hydrochlorothiazide (Dyazide)	Increased risk of chemotherapy-induced neutropenia
Fluorouracil (5-FU)	Phenytoin (Dilantin)	Increased plasma concentration of phenytoin
Fluorouracil (5-FU)	Cimetidine (Tagamet)	Increased plasma concentration of fluorouracil
Fluorouracil (5-FU)/ capecitabine (Xeloda)/ etoposide (Etophos, VePesid)/carboplatin (Paraplatin)/paclitaxel (Taxol, Onxol)/ gemcitabine (Gemzar)	Warfarin (Coumadin)	Increased bleeding
Tamoxifen (Nolvadex)	Warfarin (Coumadin)	Increased bleeding
Tamoxifen (Nolvadex)	SSRIs	Decreased efficacy of tamoxifen

*This table is not comprehensive as new information is being generated on a regular basis.
Source: Riechelmann RP et al. 2007.[66]

Reproductive Considerations

Chemotherapy-Induced Ovarian Failure

Chemotherapy-induced ovarian failure may be caused by the administration of certain chemotherapeutic agents. Factors related to the development of this toxicity include age, agent used total cumulative dose, and length of time since treatment. Sterility may be temporary or permanent and should be discussed in great detail with a woman and her partner. Alkylating agents have been found to be fertility damaging, and chemotherapeutic agents such as busulfan (Busulfex), melphalan (Alkeran), cyclophosphamide (Cytoxan), nitroureas, cisplatin (Platinol), chlorambucil (Leukeran), mechlorethamine (Mustargen), carmustine (BiCNU), lomustine (CeeNu), cytarabine (Cytosar-U), ifosfamide (Ifex),

vinblastine (Velban), and procarbazine (Matulane) are known to be gonadotoxic.[68,69]

An evolving approach to fertility conversation involves several techniques such as cryopreservation of ovarian tissue, oocytes, and embryos. A successful autotransplantation of cryopreserved ovarian cortical tissues has been reported. However, at this time, such interventions are considered experimental, and more research is needed before it becomes common practice.[70]

Chemotherapy During Pregnancy

A concern unique to women is a cancer diagnosis during pregnancy. Chemotherapy may be recommended if delay in treatment until after birth is not prudent and pregnancy termination is not desired. When caring for a pregnant woman with cancer, a multidisciplinary team that includes an oncologist, perinatologist, and neonatologist is needed to coordinate care and to improve the outcome for both the mother and the fetus/neonate. The decision to use chemotherapy during pregnancy must always be balanced against the effect of treatment delay on maternal survival.

If possible, chemotherapy should be avoided during the first trimester since most chemotherapy agents administered during this time increase the incidence of spontaneous miscarriages, fetal death, and major malformations. Use of chemotherapy in the second and third trimesters appears to be relatively safe, although there is an increase in the risk of fetal growth restriction.[3] It is recommended that low-molecular-weight and highly diffusible drugs (e.g., antimetabolites) be avoided as these drugs have properties that favor transfer across the placenta from mother to fetus. Chemotherapy should not be given near term because spontaneous delivery may occur before the bone marrow has recovered, increasing the risk for hemorrhage and infection due to the potential of maternal neutropenia and thrombocytopenia.[3] Chemotherapy administered shortly before delivery results in the presence of the drugs in the newborn, who may have limited ability to metabolize and excrete drugs due to immaturity of the liver and kidneys; this is especially true for premature infants.[3]

Breastfeeding is contraindicated while undergoing chemotherapy. Neonatal neutropenia has been reported in an infant whose mother was being treated with cyclophosphamide (Cytoxan). The amount of drug that passes into breast milk is variable and related to the dose and timing of chemotherapy. For most chemotherapy agents, no specific breastfeeding information is available, although concerns exist, and, therefore, it is recommended that they are avoided.

Care of the Cancer Survivor

Once a woman has cancer, she is forever changed. Some may be reminded of the disease every day because of scars on their bodies secondary to surgery or radiation. Others are reminded of the disease because they become economically disadvantaged because of the cost of treating the disease out of pocket, potential loss of income, and potential loss of future insurance secondary to pre-existing disease. All women who have experienced cancer have faced an issue of their vulnerability to a potentially fatal disease, even those who had one of the more easily cured cancers.

In 2009, the National Cancer Institute published estimates that there are more than 11 million cancer survivors in the United States, three times the number in 1970.[1] Cancer survivors will seek care from primary care providers. Women who have had cancer are as likely as any others to have various health needs. In the vast majority of cases, treatments will be the same for women who have had cancer as well as those who have not. However, for those women whose cancers have a hormonal component, pregnancy and use of perimenopausal hormones present special challenges.

Pregnancy After Cancer

Much has been accomplished in the treatment of childhood cancers. Most cancers for a young child or adolescent consist of radiation, chemotherapy, and sometimes surgery. The Childhood Cancer Survivor Study reported that there was an increased risk of premature ovarian failure for those who had cancer when compared to their siblings (8% versus 0.8%; RR = 13.21; 95% CI, 3.26–53.51; $P < .001$). Among the more than 1900 women in the study who had more than 4000 births, the only adverse pregnancy outcome reported was small for gestational age. There was no increased risk in congenital anomalies among childhood cancer survivors.[71]

Women who have had gynecologic malignancies have developed cancer at a later age and more often develop ovarian failure than those who had childhood cancers. However, there are some women who retain fertility in this subgroup, especially women with premenopausal breast cancer, which often has a hormonal component. Some women may opt not to pursue conception, but for those who do, the data are limited. Among the considerations is whether or not pregnancy itself will increase risk of recurrence, although anecdotal reports appear reassuring.[72] Pregnancy concerns that have been suggested include potential increase in risk of preterm birth or intrauterine growth restriction, although congenital anomalies secondary to previous treatments appear to be remote, and there are not enough data to estimate the risks of these events. Guidelines from Canada recommend that women who become pregnant after breast cancer can breastfeed successfully.[73] Although it is impossible to conduct large RCTs for cancer survivors who become pregnant, this area needs much more study in order to provide reasonable information for those women who are considering pregnancy.

Use of Perimenopausal Hormones

Menopause and the controversies about use of hormones are discussed in detail in Chapter 34. However, for cancer survivors for whom such pharmacologic intervention is recommended, hormone therapy is even more controversial. In general, women who have receptor-positive estrogen or progesterone cancers often have been counseled against using hormones. However, rigorous studies have been few.

Since breast cancer is the most frequently diagnosed gynecologic malignancy, it is logical that the best studies have been conducted among women posttreatment of breast cancer. A randomized clinical trial called HABITs was conducted to explore whether women of any type receptor status, who had been treated for breast cancer were more likely to have recurrences when treated with perimenopausal hormones. Of the 221 women in the hormone therapy arm, 39 developed a new breast cancer, whereas 17 of the 221 in the control group experienced such an event (HR = 2.4; 95% CI, 1.3–4.2). Cumulative incidences were 22.2% in the hormone therapy arm and 8.0% in the control arm at the 5-year point. The study was halted early because of these findings, which indicate hormone therapy is not to be recommended for women who are breast cancer survivors.[74] Although this study was limited to survivors of breast cancer, limited data exist regarding women with other types of cancers and hormone therapy.

Complementary and Alternative Therapy

Complementary and alternative medicine (CAM) often is used to treat cancer- and chemotherapy-related symptoms. Studies have shown that acupuncture may be a helpful adjunct for pain management ($P < .0001$),[75] for decreasing nausea and vomiting ($P < .001$),[76] and for reducing fatigue associated with cancer treatment.[77]

A review of 11 randomized clinical trials support the use of therapeutic touch, a form of energy healing, for the treatment of pain and anxiety.[78] Meditation practices such as transcendental meditation, mindfulness meditation, and yoga may reduce anxiety, stress, and depression, although studies with cancer symptom management are lacking.[79]

Alternative treatments for nausea and vomiting are perhaps the best studied. Ginger root preparations may reduce nausea and vomiting, although the ideal dose has not been determined.[80] A review of four randomized clinical trials suggests that Huangqi compounds (*Astragalus membranaceus* root) can reduce the proportion of persons who experience chemotherapy-induced nausea and vomiting. In addition, these compounds were associated with a decrease in the incidence of leukopenia and an increase in the number of T-lymphocytes.[81]

Although the researchers found no evidence of harm arising from the use of these compounds, individuals should be cautioned about the use of botanicals because of mounting evidence of botanical–drug interactions.[79] There are reports of drug–herb interactions with *Hypericum perforatum* (St. John's wort) and *Allium sativum* where the herb behaves as a CYP450 inhibitor or inducer, which potentiates toxicity or decreases chemotherapy effectiveness.[82] The use of antioxidants is controversial. There is limited human research but many preclinical studies that indicate vitamins E, C, and coenzyme Q10 are beneficial for reducing tumor size and chemotherapy-related toxicities.[82]

Conclusion

Gynecologic malignancies alter one's life path irrevocably. All healthcare providers involved in the care of woman with a gynecologic malignancy can be knowledgeable about evaluation and management of some of the side effects experienced during treatments. Working collaboratively to care for women may not only assist individuals during the treatment process, but it can also add to the support a woman with one of these disorders so clearly needs.

References

1. American Cancer Society. Cancer facts and figures, 2009. Atlanta GA:ACS, 2009.

2. Sherman ME. Theories of endometrial carcinogenesis: a multidisciplinary approach. Mod Pathol 2000; 13:295–308.

3. Berek JS, Hacker NF. Practical gynecologic oncology. Philadelphia: Lippincott Williams & Wilkins, 2009.

4. Croce CM. Oncogenes and cancer. N Eng J Med 2008; 358:502–11.

5. Kehoe SM, Kauff ND. Screening and prevention of hereditary gynecologic cancers. Semin Oncol 2007; 34(5):406–10.

6. Frank TS, Critchfield GC. Hereditary risk of women's cancers. Best Pract Res Clin Obstet Gynaecol 2002; 16(5):703–13.

7. Lu KH. Hereditary gynecologic cancers: differential diagnosis, surveillance, management and surgical prophylaxis. Fam Cancer 2008;7(1):53–8.

8. Rubin SC. Chemotherapy of gynecologic oncology, 2nd ed. Philadelphia, PA: Lippincott Williams & Wilkins, 2004.

9. Benedet JL, Bender H, Jones H 3rd, Ngan HY, Pecorelli S. FIGO staging classifications and clinical practice guidelines in the management of gynecologic cancers. FIGO Committee on Gynecologic Oncology. Int J Gynaecol Obstet 2000;70(2):209–62.

10. Greene FL, Page DL, Fleming ID, Fritz A, Balch CM, Haller DG, et al. AJCC cancer staging manual, 6th ed. Verlag, NY: Springer, 2002.

11. Singletary SE, Connolly JL. Breast cancer staging: working with the sixth edition of the AJCC cancer staging manual. Ca Cancer J Clin 2006;56:37–47.

12. National Comprehensive Cancer Network. Clinical practice guidelines in oncology Available from: *http://nccn.org/professionals/physician_gls/f_guidelines.asp* [Accessed September 30, 2009].

13. Wilson TR, Johnston PG, Longley DB. Anti-apoptotic mechanisms of drug resistance in cancer. Curr Cancer Drug Targets 2009;9(3):307–19.

14. Lyman GH. Impact of chemotherapy dose intensity on cancer patient outcomes. J Natl Compr Canc Netw 2009;7(1):99–108.

15. Espinosa E, Zamora P, Feliu F, Baron MG. Classification of anticancer drugs: a new system based on therapeutic targets. Can Treat Rev 2003;29:515–23.

16. Noble RL. The discovery of the vinca alkaloids—chemotherapeutic agents against cancer. Biochem Cell Biol 1990;68(12):1344–51.

17. Efferth T, Li PC, Konkimalla VS, Kanina B. From traditional Chinese medicine to rational cancer therapy. Trends Mol Med 2007;8:353–61.

18. Coley WB. The treatment of malignant tumors by repeated inoculations of erysipelas: with a report of ten original cases. Am J Med Sci 1893;10:487–511.

19. Schuster M, Nechansky A, Kircheis R. Cancer immunotherapy. Biotechnol J 2006;1(2):138–47.

20. Ma WW, Adjei AA. Novel agents on the horizon for cancer therapy. CA Cancer J Clin 2009;59(2):111–37.

21. Hudis CA. Trastuzumab—mechanism of action and use in clinical practice. N Engl J Med 2007;357(1):39–51.

22. Weiner LM, Dhodapkar MV, Ferrone S. Monoclonal antibodies for cancer immunotherapy. Lancet 2009; 373:1033–40.

23. American Cancer Society. Cancer facts & figures 2007–2008. 2007. Available from: *http://cancer.org/downloads/STT/BCFF-Final.pdf* [Accessed September 30, 2009].

24. Zeigler J, Citron M. Dose-dense adjuvant chemotherapy for breast cancer. Cancer Nurs 2006;29:266–72.

25. Hind D, Ward S, De Nigris E, Simpson E, Carroll C, Wyld L. Hormonal therapies for early breast cancer: systematic review and economic evaluation. Health Technol Assess 2007 Jul;11(26):iii–iv, ix–xi, 1–134.

26. McArthur HL, Hudis CA. Adjuvant chemotherapy for early-stage breast cancer. Hematol Oncol Clin N Am 2007;21:207–22.

27. Fisher B, Jeong JH, Bryant J, Anderson S, Dignam J, Fisher ER, et al. Treatment of lymph-node-negative, oestrogen-receptor-positive breast cancer: long-term findings from National Surgical Adjuvant Breast and Bowel Project randomized clinical trials. Lancet 2004;364:858–68.

28. Smith IA, Dowsett M. Aromatase inhibitors in breast cancer. NEJM 2003;348:2431–42.

29. Cummings SR, Tice JA, Bauer S, Browner WS, Cuzick J, Ziv E, et al. Prevention of breast cancer in postmenopausal women: approaches to estimating and reducing risk. J Natl Cancer Inst 2009;101(6):384–98.

30. Thomsen A, Kolesar JM. Chemoprevention of breast cancer. Am J Health Syst Pharm 2008;65(23):2221–8.

31. Moore DH. Neoadjuvant chemotherapy for cervical cancer. Exprt Opin Pharmacother 2003;4(6):859–67.

32. Espindola D, Kennedy KA, Fischer EG. Management of abnormal uterine bleeding and the pathology of endometrial hyperplasia. Obstet Gyn Clin 2007;34(4): 717–37.

33. Berkowitz RS, Goldstein DP. Molar pregnancy. N Engl J Med 2009;360:1639–45.

34. Lok CA, van der Houwen C, ten Kate-Booij MJ, van Eijkeren MA, Ansink AC. Pregnancy after EMA/CO for gestational trophoblastic disease: a report from The Netherlands. BJOG 2003;110(6):560–6.

35. Jemal A, Siegel R, Ward E, Hao Y, Xu J, Thun MJ. Cancer statistics, 2008. CA Cancer J Clin 2008;58: 71–96.

36. Herbst AL, Robboy SJ, Scully RE, Poskanzer DC. Clear cell adenocarcinoma of the vagina and cervix in girls: analysis of 170 registry cases. Am J Obst Gynecol 1974;119(5):713–24.

37. Hammes B, Laitman CJ. Diethylstilbestrol (DES) update: recommendations for the identification and management of DES-exposed individuals. J Midwifery Womens Health 2003;48(1):19–29.

38. zur Hausen H. Papillomaviruses causing cancer: evasion from host-cell control in early events in carcinogenesis. J Natl Cancer Inst 2000;92(9):690–8.

39. Worthington HV, Clarkson JE, Eden OB. Interventions for preventing oral mucositis for patients with cancer receiving treatment. Cochrane Database Syst Rev 2006(2):CD000978.

40. Multinational Association of Supportive Care in Cancer. *http://www.mascc.org/mc/page.do?sitePageId=86969&orgId=mascc* [Accessed September 30, 2009].

41. Minton O, Stone P, Richardson A, Sharpe M, Hotopf M. Drug therapy for the management of cancer related fatigue. Cochrane Database Syst Rev 2008(1): CD006704.

42. Aapro MS, Link H. September 2007 update on EORTC guidelines and anemia management with erythropoiesis-stimulating agents. Oncologist 2008; 13(suppl 3):33–6.

43. Blau CA. Erythropoietin in cancer: presumption of innocence? Stem Cells 2007;25:2094–7.

44. Bohlius J, Wilson J, Seidenfeld J, Piper M, Schwarzer G, Sandercock J, et al. Erythropoietin or darbepoetin for patients with cancer. Cochrane Database Syst Rev 2006(3):CD003407.

45. Khuri FR. Weighing the hazards of erythropoiesis stimulation in patients with cancer. N Eng J Med 2007; 356:2445–348.

46. Crawford J, Dale DC, Lyman GH. Chemotherapy-induced neutropenia. Cancer 2004;100:228–37.

47. Lyman GH, Shayne M. Granulocyte colony-stimulating factors: finding the right indication. Curr Opin Onc 2007;19:299–307.

48. Smith JW 2nd. Tolerability and side-effect profile of rhIL-11. Oncology (Williston Park) 2000;14(9) (suppl 8):41–7.

49. Hesketh PJ. Chemotherapy-induced nausea and vomiting. N Engl J Med 2008;358(23):2482–94.

50. Navari RM. Pathogenesis-based treatment of chemotherapy-induced nausea and vomiting—two new agents. J Support Oncol 2003;1(2):89–103.

51. Antiemetic subcommittee of the Multinational Association of Supportive Care in Cancer (MASCC). Prevention of chemotherapy- and radiotherapy-induced emesis: results of the 2004 Perugia International Antiemetic Consensus Conference. Ann Oncol 2006;17:20–8.

52. Jordan K, Schmoll HJ, Aapro MS. Comparative activity of antiemetic drugs. Crit Rev Oncol Hematol 2007; 61(2):162–75.

53. Dando TM, Perry CM. Aprepitant: a review of its use in the prevention of chemotherapy-induced nausea and vomiting. Drugs 2004;64(7):777–94.

54. Chawla SP, Grunberg SM, Gralla RJ, Watt DG, Roila F, de Wit R, et al. Establishing the dose of the oral NK 1 antagonist aprepitant for the prevention of chemotherapy induced nausea and vomiting. Cancer 2003; 97(9):2290–300.

55. Shadle CR, Lee Y, Majumdar AK, Petty KJ, Gargano C, Bradstreet TE, et al. Evaluation of potential inductive effects of aprepitant on cytochrome P4503A4 and 2C9 activity. J Clin Pharmacol 2004;44(3): 215–23.

56. Harris DJ, Eilers J, Harriman A, Cashavelly BJ, Maxwell C. Putting evidence into practice: evidence-based interventions for the management of oral mucositis. Clin J Oncol Nurs 2008;12(1):141–52.

57. Lalla RV, Sonis ST, Peterson DE. Management of oral mucositis in patients who have cancer. Dent Clin North Am 2008;52(1):61–77.

58. Keefe DM, Schubert MM, Elting LS, Sonis ST, Epstein JB, Raber-Durlacher JE, et al. Mucositis Study Section of the Multinational Association of Supportive Care in Cancer and the International Society for Oral Oncology. Updated clinical practice guidelines for the prevention and treatment of mucositis. Cancer 2007;109(5):820–31.

59. Rubenstein EB, Peterson DE, Schubert M, Keefe D, McGuire D, Epstein J et al. Clinical practice guidelines for the prevention and treatment of cancer therapy-induced oral and gastrointestinal mucositis. Cancer 2004;100(9)(suppl):2026–46.

60. Gibson RJ, Keefe DM. Cancer chemotherapy-induced diarrhoea and constipation: mechanisms of damage and prevention strategies. Support Care Cancer 2006; 14(9):890–900.

61. Richardson G, Dobish R. Chemotherapy induced diarrhea. J Oncol Pharm Pract 2007;13(4):181–98.

62. Reid-Arndt SA. Breast cancer and "chemobrain:" the consequences of cognitive difficulties following chemotherapy and the potential for recovery. Mo Med 2009;106(2):127–31.

63. Nelson CJ, Nandy N, Roth AJ. Chemotherapy and cognitive deficits: mechanisms, findings, and potential interventions. Palliat Support Care 2007;5(3): 273–80.

64. Inagaki M, Yoshikawa E, Matsuoka Y, Sugawara Y, Nakano T, Akechi T, et al. Smaller regional volumes of brain gray and white matter demonstrated in breast cancer survivors exposed to adjuvant chemotherapy. Cancer 2007;109(1):146–56.

65. Chabner B, Longo DL. Cancer chemotherapy and biotherapy: principles and practice, 4th ed. Philadelphia, PA: Lippincott Williams & Wilkins, 2005.

66. Riechelmann RP, Tannock IF, Wang L, Saad ED, Taback NA, Krzyzanowska MK. Potential drug interactions and duplicate prescriptions among cancer patients. J Natl Cancer Inst 2007;99(8):592–600.

67. Lash TL, Pedersen L, Cronin-Fenton D, Ahern TP, Rosenberg CL, Lunetta KL, et al. Tamoxifen's protection against breast cancer recurrence is not reduced by concurrent use of the SSRI citalopram. Br J Cancer 2008;99(4):616–21.

68. Howell S, Shalet S. Gonadal damage from chemotherapy and radiotherapy. Endocrinol Metab Clin North Am 1998;27(4):927–43.

69. Goodwin PJ, Ennis M, Pritchard KI, Trudeau M, Hood N. Risk of menopause during the first year after breast cancer diagnosis. J Clin Oncol 1999;17(8): 2365–70.

70. Chang HJ, Suh CS. Fertility preservation for women with malignancies: current developments of cryopreservation. J Gynecol Oncol 2008;19(2):99–107.

71. Green DM, Sklar CA, Boice JD Jr, Mulvihill JJ, Whitton JA, Stovall M, et al. Ovarian failure and reproductive outcomes after childhood cancer treatment: results from the Childhood Cancer Survivor Study. J Clin Oncol 2009;27(14):2374–81.

72. Chabbert-Buffet N, Uzan C, Gligorov J, Delaloge S, Rouzier R, Uzan S. Pregnancy after breast cancer: a need for global patient care, starting before adjuvant therapy. Surg Oncol 2009;E1–9.

73. Helewa M, Lévesque P, Provencher D, Lea RH, Rosolowich V, Shapiro HM. Breast Disease Committee and Executive Committee and Council, Society of Obstetricians and Gynaecologists of Canada. Breast cancer, pregnancy and breastfeeding. J Obstet Gynaecol Can 2002;24(2):164–80.

74. Holmberg L, Iversen OE, Rudenstam CM, Hammar M, Kumpulainen E, Jaskiewicz J, et al., HABITS study group. Increased risk of recurrence after hormone replacement therapy in breast cancer survivors. J Natl Cancer Inst 2008;100(7):475–82.

75. Alimi D, Rubino C, Pichard-Learndri E, Dubreuil-Lemaire ML, Hill C. Analgesic effect of auricular acupuncture for cancer pain: a randomized, blinded, controlled trial. J Clin Oncol 2003;21:4120–6.

76. Shen J, Wenger N, Glaspy J, Hays RD, Albert PS, Choi C, et al. Electroacupuncture for control of myeloablative chemotherapy-induced emesis: a randomized controlled trial. JAMA 2000;284:2755–61.

77. Vickers AJ, Straus DJ, Fearon B, Cassileth BR. Acupuncture for postchemotherapy fatigue: a phase II study. J Clin Oncol 2004;22:1731–35.

78. Spence JE, Olson MA. Quantitative research on therapeutic touch: an integrative review of the literature 1985–1995. Scand J Caring Sci 1997;11:183–90.

79. Mansky PJ, Wallerstedt DB. Complementary medicine in palliative care and cancer symptom management. Cancer J 2006;12:425–31.

80. Boon H, Wong J. Botanical medicine and cancer: a review of the safety and efficacy. Expert Opin Pharmacother 2004;5:2485–501.

81. Taixiang W, Munro AJ, Guanjian L. Chinese medical herbs for chemotherapy side effects in colorectal cancer patients. Cochrane Database Syst Rev 2005(1): CD004540.

82. Hardy ML. Dietary supplement use in cancer care: help or harm. Hematol Oncol Clin North Am 2008;22 (4):581–617.

V
Gynecology

Most discussions of the etymology of the term *gynecology* note that the word indicates the study of women, or the study of diseases of women. However, current connotation is the branch of health care involving women and conditions associated with reproductive organs. These conditions are not always pathologic. For example, "Contraception and Reproductive Health" not only addresses potential side and adverse effects associated with hormonal contraceptives but also the growing list of noncontraceptive benefits of such drugs.

Of course, some gynecologic conditions are abnormal. "Pelvic and Menstrual Disorders" reviews infections and menstrual irregularities, among others. Many disparate conditions presented in this chapter use the same drugs as remedies. "Vaginal Conditions" addresses the management of vaginal infections as well as changes due to hormonal milieus that benefit from targeted treatments. "Vulvar Disorders" includes changes in pigmentation as well as symptoms such as pruritus that can cause major concerns to women. Another issue for women involves sexual dysfunction, which may be treated by pharmacologic agents and is perhaps caused by other medications; these agents are discussed in "Sexual Dysfunction." The last chapter in this section, "The Mature Woman," discusses a normal condition in which women will find themselves spending a third of their lives, namely postmenopause, and drugs used by those women.

29
Contraception and Reproductive Health

Patricia Aikins Murphy

◈ Chapter Glossary

Barrier contraceptive methods Physical devices such as condoms, sponges, and diaphragms that generally are used with spermicides for increased effectiveness.

Biphasic formulations Combined oral contraceptives in which two separate doses of the ethinyl estradiol or the progestin component are delivered during the 21 days of active pills.

Combined hormonal contraceptives Contraceptive methods (e.g., pills, patches) that contain both an estrogen and a progestin.

Combined oral contraceptives (COCs) Contraceptive pills that have a combination of estrogen and progestin as the primary components.

Effectiveness How well a method works under real-life conditions. Synonym for *typical use*.

Efficacy How well a method works when used consistently as prescribed. Synonym for *perfect use*.

Emergency contraception The use of oral hormonal contraceptives (in various formulations) that are taken within 5 days of having unprotected intercourse to prevent pregnancy. Also called postcoital contraception or the morning-after pill.

Ethinyl estradiol (EE) The estrogen used in the majority of oral contraceptive formulations.

Extended cycling Use of combined oral contraceptives for longer than 21 days to prevent menses.

Fecundity The ability to reproduce or state of fertility.

Implantable contraceptives Long-term hormonal contraceptives that are placed, or implanted, into a woman for continuous release over a period of years.

Injectable contraceptives Long-term progestins that are administered by injection and provide contraceptive protection for several weeks.

Intrauterine contraceptive Products (also called devices or systems) that reside *in situ* intrauterinely and provide contraceptive methods for several years. These products may be inert or impregnated with a progestin.

Kaplan Meier A statistical method that calculates a separate rate for each month of use as opposed to an entire study period. This calculation is preferred over the Pearl Index by scientific journals.

Medical Eligibility Criteria for Contraceptive Use Publication from the World Health Organization that is based on evidence-based research regarding initiation and/or continuation of various contraceptives for women with conditions (e.g., postpartum conditions) or diseases (e.g., thromboembolic disease).

Method failure A pregnancy that occurs despite perfect use of a method.

Mini pill A term originally designating progestin-only pills. Now falling into disuse because of common misconception that it may apply to any low-dose contraceptive pill. Current preferred term is *progestin-only pill* or *POP*.

Monophasic formulations Combined oral contraceptives in which there is a single dose of the ethinyl estradiol and the progestin component delivered during the 21 days of active pills.

Pearl Index A calculation in which the number of pregnancies is divided by total woman-years of exposure to pregnancy risk. Although it is used by the FDA, the Pearl Index is based on assumptions that call its use into question.

Perfect use How well a method works when used consistently as prescribed. Synonym for *efficacy*.

Plan B A form of emergency contraception that contains levonorgestrel only. Plan B is packaged as two tablets each containing 0.75 mg of levonorgestrel. The two tablets are taken within 72 hours of unprotected intercourse. They can be taken together at one time or as a divided dose 12 hours apart.

Progestin-only pills (POPs) Hormonal contraceptives that do not have an estrogen component. Of value for women who experience significant estrogen-related side effects.

Spermicide Chemical agent that kills sperm as its contraceptive mechanism of action. In the United States, the only spermicide marketed is nonoxynol-9 (N-9).

Transdermal contraceptive patch A contraceptive method that provides delivery of hormones through a transdermal product. Currently each contraceptive patch is to be used for 1 week; after 3 weeks there is a patch-free week.

Triphasic formulations Combined oral contraceptives in which there are three separate dosing levels of either the ethinyl estradiol and/or the progestin component during the 21 days of active pills.

Typical use How well a method works under real-life conditions. Synonym for effectiveness.

User failure A pregnancy that results from an error by the individual using a contraceptive method. Methods that are coital dependent (e.g., condoms) or require frequent interventions (e.g., daily administration) tend to have more user failures than long-term methods that require little attention by a woman such as intrauterine devices.

Vaginal contraceptive ring A hormonally impregnated ring that provides contraceptive protection when placed intravaginally. A single ring is used for 3 weeks, followed by a ring-free week.

Yuzpe regimen A form of emergency contraception that uses brand name COCs and taking a specified number of pills (Table 29-5).

Introduction

An interest in controlling fertility is as old as history, and women have practiced contraception since ancient times. Observations that animals grazing on certain plants did not reproduce likely led to use of the same herbs and plants used to prevent conception among women.[1] The Kahun and Ebers papyrus writings from ancient Egypt, centuries before the Christian era, discuss the contraceptive use of vaginal suppositories made of wool and soaked in acacia, dates, or honey, or suppositories made of crocodile dung, gum, or honey.[2] Hippocrates wrote that the seeds of the plant Queen Anne's lace (wild carrot) prevented pregnancy when eaten.[3] In other eras and regions of the world, women used sea sponges moistened with lemon juice or vinegar, or half of a lime or lemon used in a similar manner to a cervical cap or diaphragm. Penile sheaths made of linen or animal intestines were used in ancient Egypt, Greece, and Rome, although perhaps more for decoration, but writings from at least the 16th century describe the protective function of condoms.[4] Tampons or pessaries of crushed roots, seaweed or beeswax, and the application of oils to the vagina and cervix have also been used.[2]

As society moved into the more industrial ages, contraceptive devices began to be manufactured from rubber, and with the development of technology for the vulcanization of rubber in the mid-1800s, manufacture of condoms and womb veils (earlier versions of today's diaphragms and cervical caps) increased dramatically until the 1873 Comstock Act outlawed their dissemination in the United States.[2]

The roots of modern hormonal contraception began in the early 20th century. Estrogens were administered to animals in order to prevent pregnancy after mating in the 1920s.[5] By the 1930s, synthetic estrogens were developed and used to treat various gynecological disorders, and the ovulation-disrupting properties of the drugs were noted.[6] In the early 1940s, Russell Marker synthesized progesterone from a Mexican plant that was allegedly used by indigenous people as a contraceptive, and shortly after, in the 1950s, Carl Djerassi developed orally active progestins. With financial support from the wealthy widow Katherine McCormick, a group of scientists that included Gregory Pincus and John Rock began the work that led to development of the modern oral contraceptive pill. This chapter reviews the various methods of contraception, the mechanism(s) of action, pharmacology, evidence for safety and effectiveness, and clinical issues such as side effects and availability.

Prevention of Pregnancy

Definition of Pregnancy

Since 1978, the US Department of Health and Human Services (DHHS) has defined pregnancy as "the period of time from confirmation of implantation through any of the presumptive signs of pregnancy, such as missed menses, or via a medically acceptable pregnancy test, until the expulsion or extraction of the fetus."[7] The American College of Obstetricians and Gynecologists similarly defines pregnancy as "The state of a female after conception and until termination of the gestation," noting that "conception is the implantation of the blastocyst. It is not synonymous with fertilization."[8] Some states have defined pregnancy differently, generally as part of legislation to control abortion,[9] and some women personally define pregnancy as starting at conception, but the accepted medical definition remains as defined by DHHS and the American College of Obstetricians and Gynecologists.

Efficacy and Effectiveness of Contraceptive Methods

Not every act of intercourse results in a pregnancy. Becoming pregnant depends on many factors, and contraceptive agents act on many of these factors. The establishment of a pregnancy is a process that takes several days. First ovulation must occur. Fertilization is the process by which a single sperm penetrates the layers of an egg or oocyte to form a new cell. This can take up to 24 hours and usually occurs in the fallopian tubes. There is only a narrow window (12–24 hours) within which the egg can be fertilized after ovulation; otherwise the egg dissolves. Implantation of the fertilized egg in the uterine lining begins around day 5 after fertilization, and implantation is usually complete by day 14. As noted previously, pregnancy is considered to have begun when the fertilized ovum is completely implanted in the uterine lining. Studies estimate that between one third and one half of all fertilized eggs are never fully implanted, and after implantation, approximately 15% of pregnancies end in spontaneous abortion (miscarriage).[9]

The risk of pregnancy from a single act of intercourse is low. Researchers estimate that if 100 women have unprotected intercourse during week 2 or 3 of their menstrual cycle, only approximately 8 will become pregnant that month. A number of other factors also affect **fecundity** (the physiologic ability to reproduce). For example, older women are less fecund than younger women; this decline in fecundity begins in the late 20s for women and a similar decline begins in the late 30s for men.[10] Thus, all methods of contraception will appear to reduce the risk of pregnancy better among older (less fecund) couples. In addition, studies have reported differences in the risk of pregnancy according to a woman's motivation to avoid pregnancy in contrast to simply spacing pregnancies. Relationship status, sexual activity, adherence to the method, and accuracy of pregnancy reporting all affect the reported risk of pregnancy.

The term **efficacy** refers to how well a method works when used consistently as prescribed. Failure rates related to a method's efficacy occur even when the method is used perfectly and are termed **method failures**. The term **effectiveness** refers to how well a method works in conditions of typical use. Failure rates related to effectiveness include all pregnancies that occur whether the method is or is not used properly. All methods have inherent method failure rates; thus, not all failures are **user failures**.

Contraceptive Failure Rates

Pregnancy (failure) rates for all contraceptive methods decrease over time; most failures are concentrated in early usage of the method, in part because the more fertile women will have earlier failures, and women who do not use a contraceptive method consistently will also get pregnant sooner. Failure rates for contraceptive methods are calculated in two ways.

The **Pearl Index**, named after biologist Richard Pearl, has remained popular for decades in part because of its simplicity in calculations. This index reflects the number of pregnancies divided by total woman-years of exposure to pregnancy risk. A lower Pearl Index reflects a lower chance of getting pregnant unintentionally. The Pearl Index is based on an assumption that the risk of pregnancy is constant, an assumption in contrast to the aforementioned information. Essentially, the longer a woman is involved in a study that evaluates a particular method of contraception, the lower the Pearl Index rating will be. Comparing studies of different lengths is inappropriate statistically. For example, a Pearl Index of 1200 woman-years of exposure to pregnancy risk can indicate 1200 women followed for 1 year or 120 women followed for 10 years each. Moreover, the index only addresses accidental pregnancy, not the number of women lost to follow-up, experiencing adverse reactions, or dissatisfied with the method. Many clinicians assume that the highest possible Pearl Index is 100 and that would indicate 100% of women in the study conceived in the first year. However, if all the women in the study conceived in the first month, the Pearl Index would be 1200 or above. Thus, the Pearl Index is not considered the best measure of contraceptive efficacy, but it has long been the FDA standard for new drug applications.

The **Kaplan Meier** rate calculates a separate rate for each month of use as opposed to the entire study period. With this method, it is possible to derive 6- or 12-month cumulative failure rates that include discontinuation for all reasons including pregnancy. This calculation is preferred by scientific journals.

Much of the data from which these failure rates are derived come from clinical trials. Clinical trials attempt to enroll typical or average women. It is important to remember that such trials often exclude women under the age of 18 (due to informed consent restrictions), and may also exclude older women, women with health problems, and women who are overweight or obese. Such women all need contraception, but unless they are included in the clinical trials, data addressing effectiveness in these groups are lacking. Due to ethical concerns, contraceptive trials are done without a placebo group; if comparisons are included, they are generally comparisons to known contraceptives and may be retrospective, based on previously published data.

WHO Medical Eligibility Criteria for Contraceptive Use

In 2000, the World Health Organization published a series of evidence-based family planning guidelines, *Medical Eligibility Criteria for Contraceptive Use*. The document, now in its third edition,[11] provides guidance for the safe use of contraceptive methods by providing a summary of the main recommendations of an expert working group, representing 36 participants from 18 countries, agencies, and organizations. The recommendations are based on current research, clinical, and epidemiological data.

The WHO Medical Eligibility Criteria classify health conditions into one of four categories that inform either the initiation or continued use of the particular contraceptive.[11] These guidelines generally are accepted by experts in the field of family planning as standards for the management of contraception. The categories are:

1. A condition for which there is no restriction for the use of the contraceptive method, and the method can be used in any circumstances.
2. A condition where the advantages of using the method generally outweigh the theoretical or proven risks. The method can generally be used, but careful follow-up is indicated.
3. A condition where the theoretical or proven risks usually outweigh the advantages of using the method. Use of the method is not usually recommended unless other more appropriate methods are not available or not acceptable. If there are no resources for the close follow-up, the method should probably not be used.
4. A condition that represents an unacceptable health risk if the contraceptive method is used. The contraceptive method should not be used.

Clinical Management of Contraceptive Methods: WHO Practice Recommendations

Despite widespread use of contraceptive methods, contemporary clinical management of common side effects and adverse events generally is not evidence based. Strategies for managing problems are often extrapolated from older studies of methods no longer in use (such as hormonal contraceptives with higher doses of contraceptive steroids), theoretical concerns that have not been confirmed in clinical practice, or on empirical management strategies that reflect the opinions of individual providers but have not been scientifically evaluated. In addition, practice is also based on medical-legal concerns as evidenced in manufacturers' package inserts, and on evidence from clinical trials that, as noted previously, may not include women who are representative of all users of hormonal contraception.

The World Health Organization convened a second working group to provide guidance on the use of contraceptive methods once they are determined to be medically appropriate. This group addressed the evidence for specific management questions,[12] which are summarized in the text that follows.

Hormonal Contraception

Hormonal contraceptives interfere with the cascade of events that result in ovulation and fertilization. Therefore, a brief review of those events is in order. At the beginning of each menstrual cycle counting day 1 as the first day of menstrual flow, low levels of estrogen and progesterone permit secretion of gonadotropin releasing hormone (GnRH) from the hypothalamus, which, in turn, stimulates release of follicle stimulating hormone (FSH) from the pituitary. A cohort of follicles in the ovary will respond to FSH with accelerated growth and secretion of estrogen. Estrogen levels rise, and when the level exceeds a threshold, it triggers release of luteinizing hormone (LH) by the pituitary. Ovulation occurs within 36 hours after the onset of the LH surge, and then follicle walls collapse. Most of the progesterone produced during the cycle is secreted over the next several days, with progesterone levels peaking about 8 days after ovulation. Rising estrogen levels stimulate proliferation of the uterine endometrium, and progesterone produces a secretory endometrium—changes that are important for implantation of a fertilized egg. When conception does not occur, the thickened endometrium loses its hormonal support, becomes ischemic, and is shed during menstruation.

In addition to the events of ovulation, the capacity for conception is also affected by changes in cervical mucus. The rapidly increasing estrogen production by the dominant follicle causes an increase in thin, watery cervical mucus secretion that facilitates sperm transport, whereas rising progesterone after ovulation changes cervical mucus to a thick and sticky consistency that inhibits sperm.

Hormonal contraception includes combination hormonal contraceptives that are formulated as pills, a transdermal patch, and an intravaginal ring. Progestin-only hormonal contraceptives are formulated as pills, injectable agents, and a unique agent that is implanted subcutaneously.

Combination Hormonal Contraceptives

Combined hormonal contraceptive pills are the most commonly used method of reversible contraception in the United States[13]; they are used by 11.6 million women. Most users are younger than 30 years of age.[13] More recently, alternative delivery systems (transdermal and intravaginal) have expanded options for women choosing combination hormonal methods. It should be noted that there are no evidence-based recommendations for starting a particular pill or method other than WHO medical eligibility.

Mechanism of Action

A review of the mechanism of action of estrogens and progestin can be found in Chapter 14. The main mechanism of action of the combination hormonal contraceptive methods is prevention of ovulation. This phenomenon occurs via inhibition of gonadotropin release from the pituitary that interferes with the normal cascade of events that leads to ovulation. The estrogen component of the pill primarily inhibits release of FSH, and the progestin component inhibits release of LH. Low levels of estrogen and progestin also inhibit proliferation of the endometrium, and progestins contribute to the formation of inhospitable cervical mucus. The hormones are theorized also to inhibit the ability of the sperm to fertilize an egg and to delay sperm transport through the reproductive tract.

Most of the contraceptive effect comes from the progestin component of hormonal contraceptives due to the blocking of the LH surge. The estrogen component offers additional contraceptive efficacy by inhibiting the development of a dominant follicle. Estrogen also stabilizes the endometrium to provide better cycle control (less unscheduled bleeding) and potentiates the action of progestins. Thus, the addition of estrogen allows reductions in progestin dose.

Oral Products

Combined oral contraceptives (COCs) available in the United States are packaged in blister pack containers that have 21 or 28 pills. One pill is taken every day, and because the doses range throughout the 28-day cycle, each package is designed to dispense one dose every day. The majority of COCs available in the United States have **ethinyl estradiol** (EE) as the estrogen component. Mestranol, which is metabolized to ethinyl estradiol, continues to be found in a few formulations, but most formulations in the United States contain 20–35 mcg EE. A few formulations contain 50 mcg EE, but these are no longer commonly prescribed (Table 29-1). Metabolism of ethinyl estradiol varies significantly from woman to woman; thus some women will experience side effects from the same dose that does not produce side effects in another person (Box 29-1).

Oral contraceptive progestins available in the United States include the estranes (norethindrone, norethindrone acetate, ethynodiol diacetate), the gonanes (norgestrel, levonorgestrel, desogestrel, norgestimate), and a 17 α-spironolactone derivative, drospirenone (Figure 29-1). Most authorities assert that the clinical effects of the various progestins in contemporary hormonal contraceptives are essentially the same; doses of the different progestins have been adjusted to account for their differing biologic effects, and for most women, clinical differences are minimal.[14] However, individual differences in progestin metabolism may lead to differences in side effects and preferences for certain progestins, although the differences cannot be predicted in advance. A Cochrane meta-analysis suggested that the use of gonanes may be associated with a better bleeding profile and less self-discontinuation (RR = 0.71; 95% CI, 0.55–0.91).[15]

Early formulations of the pill contained higher doses of both hormones; estrogen doses were 3–4 times higher and progestins 10 times higher than currently used formulations. High rates of undesirable side effects and cardiovascular complications led to attempts to drive the doses lower. With today's lower doses, there is evidence that suppression of ovarian activity is less complete than with higher dose formulations, and it is likely that

Table 29-1 Oral Contraceptive Formulations Available in the United States

Product	Estrogen Dose per Tablet	Progestin Dose per Tablet	Active/Hormone-Free Intervals*	Other
Progestin-Only Pills				
Camilla, Errin, Jolivette, Micronor, Nora-BE, Nor-QD	n/a	0.35 mg norethindrone	None (continuous)	
Ovrette	n/a	0.075 mg norgestrel	None (continuous)	
20-mcg Pills				
Alesse, Aviane, Lessina, Levlite, Lutera	20 mcg ethinyl estradiol	0.1 mg levonorgestrel	21/7 days	
Lybrel	20 mcg ethinyl estradiol	0.09 mg levonorgestrel	365/0 days	
Loestrin-24 Fe	20 mcg ethinyl estradiol	1 mg norethindrone acetate	24/4 days	75 mg ferrous fumarate × 7 days
Junel 1/20, Loestrin-FE 1/20, Microgestin 1/20	20 mcg ethinyl estradiol	1 mg norethindrone acetate	21/7 days	
Junel 1/20 Fe, Loestrin-FE 1/20, Microgestin 1/20 Fe	20 mcg ethinyl estradiol	1 mg norethindrone acetate	21/7 days	75 mg ferrous fumarate × 7 days
Yaz	20 mcg ethinyl estradiol	3 mg drospirenone	24/4 days	
30-mcg Pills				
Cryselle, Lo-Ogestrel, Lo-Ovral	30 mcg ethinyl estradiol	0.3 mg norgestrel	21/7 days	
Levlen, Levora, Nordette, Portia	30 mcg ethinyl estradiol	0.15 mg levonorgestrel	21/7 days	
Jolessa, Quasense, Seasonale	30 mcg ethinyl estradiol	0.15 mg levonorgestrel	84/7 days	
Junel 1.5/30, Loestrin 1.5/30, Microgestin 1.5/30	30 mcg ethinyl estradiol	1.5 mg norethindrone acetate	21/7 days	
Junel 1.5/30 Fe, Loestrin 1.5/30 FE, Microgestin 1.5/30 Fe	30 mcg ethinyl estradiol	1.5 mg norethindrone acetate	21/7 days	75 mg ferrous fumarate × 7 days
Apri, Desogen, Ortho-Cept, Reclipsen	30 mcg ethinyl estradiol	0.15 mg desogestrel	21/7 days	
Yasmin	30 mcg ethinyl estradiol	3 mg drospirenone	21/7 days	
35-mcg Pills				
Necon 1/35, Norethin 1/35, Norinyl 1 + 35, Nortrel 1/35, Ortho-Novum 1/35	35 mcg ethinyl estradiol	1 mg norethindrone	21/7 days	
Brevicon, Modicon, Necon 0.5/35, Nortrel 0.5/35	35 mcg ethinyl estradiol	0.5 mg norethindrone	21/7 days	
Balziva, Ovcon 35	35 mcg ethinyl estradiol	0.4 mg norethindrone	21/7 days	Also available as a chewable tablet.
MonoNessa, Ortho-Cyclen, Previfem, Sprintec	35 mcg ethinyl estradiol	0.25 mg norgestimate	21/7 days	
Demulen 1/35, Kelnor, Zovia 1/35	35 mcg ethinyl estradiol	1 mg ethynodiol diacetate	21/7 days	
Phased Formulations				
Kariva, Mircette	20 mcg ethinyl estradiol × 21 days; 10 mcg ethinyl estradiol × 5 days	0.15 mg desogestrel × 21 days	21/2/5 days	
Seasonale	0.03 mg ethinyl estradiol	0.15 mg levonorgestrel		
Seasonique	30 mcg ethinyl estradiol × 84 days; 10 mcg ethinyl estradiol × 7 days	0.15 mg levonorgestrel	84/7 days	

(continues)

Table 29-1 Oral Contraceptive Formulations Available in the United States (*continued*)

Product	Estrogen Dose per Tablet	Progestin Dose per Tablet	Active/Hormone-Free Intervals*	Other
Estrostep-FE	20 mcg ethinyl estradiol × 5 days 30 mcg ethinyl estradiol × 7 days 35 mcg ethinyl estradiol × 9 days	1 mg norethindrone acetate × 21 days	7/7/7/7 days	75 mg ferrous fumarate × 7 days
Ortho Tri-Cyclen Lo	25 mcg ethinyl estradiol × 21 days	0.18 mg norgestimate × 7 days 0.215 mg norgestimate × 7 days 0.25 mg norgestimate × 7 days	7/7/7/7 days	
Cesia, Cyclessa, Velivet	25 mcg ethinyl estradiol × 21 days	0.1 mg desogestrel × 7 days 0.125 mg desogestrel × 7 days 0.150 mg desogestrel × 7 days	7/7/7/7 days	
Enpresse, Tri-Levlen, Triphasil-28, Trivora	30 mcg ethinyl estradiol × 6 days 40 mcg ethinyl estradiol × 5 days 20 mcg ethinyl estradiol × 10 days	0.05 mg levonorgestrel × 6 days 0.075 mg levonorgestrel × 6 days 0.125 mg levonorgestrel × 10 days	6/5/10/7 days	
Ortho Tri-Cyclen, Trinessa, Tri-Previfem, Tri-Sprintec	35 mcg ethinyl estradiol × 21 days	0.18 mg norgestimate × 7 days 0.215 mg norgestimate × 7 days 0.25 mg norgestimate × 7 days	7/7/7/7 days	
Ortho-Novum 7/7/7, Necon 7/7/7, Nortrel 7/7/7	35 mcg ethinyl estradiol × 21 days	0.5 mg norethindrone × 7 days 0.75 mg norethindrone × 7 days 1 mg norethindrone × 7 days	7/7/7/7 days	
Aranelle, Leena, Tri-Norinyl	35 mcg ethinyl estradiol × 21 days	0.5 mg norethindrone × 7 days 1 mg norethindrone × 7 days 0.5 mg norethindrone × 7 days	7/7/7/7 days	
Ortho-Novum 10/11, Necon 10/11	35 mcg ethinyl estradiol × 21 days	0.5 mg norethindrone × 10 days 1 mg norethindrone × 11 days	10/11/7 days	
Jenest	35 mcg ethinyl estradiol × 21 days	0.5 mg norethindrone × 7 days 1 mg norethindrone × 14 days	7/14/7 days	
50-mcg Pills				
Ortho-Novum 1/50, Necon 1/50, Norinyl 1/50	50 mcg mestranol[†]	1 mg norethindrone		
Ogestrel, Ovral	50 mcg ethinyl estradiol	0.5 mg norgestrel		
Demulen 1/50, Zovia 1/50	50 mcg ethinyl estradiol	1 mg ethynodiol diacetate		
Ovcon 50	50 mcg ethinyl estradiol	1 mg norethindrone		

* Can eliminate hormone-free interval by starting a new pack right away.

[†] Mestranol must be converted to ethinyl estradiol in the body. Animal studies have suggested that mestranol is weaker, but this is not confirmed in human studies.

Source: Speroff L & Darney PD 2005.[54]

contemporary dosing cannot be lowered further without engendering an unacceptable reduction in efficacy. Variations in the formulations introduced in recent years are intended to minimize the total hormonal load while maximizing ovarian suppression and effective management of common side effects. **Monophasic formulations** maintain the same dose of EE (20, 30, or 35 mcg) and progestin for 21 days, followed by 7 days of a hormone-free interval. Many brands provide inert or placebo pills for this interval. Some formulations add iron to the pills taken during the placebo week. Newer monophasic formulations extend the time active pills are taken or reduce the hormone-free interval. **Biphasic formulations** provide two separate doses of the EE or the progestin component over 21 days, followed by a hormone-free interval. These regimens were developed to reduce the total steroid dose over the 21 days of active pills while maintaining adequate cycle control and reducing breakthrough bleeding. Biphasic formulations begin with a lower progestin dose for the first 1–10 days of the active pill cycle, followed by a

Box 29-1 The Troublesome Side Effects

JN is a 26-year-old woman who initiated combined oral contraceptive pills 2 months ago. She calls her provider to report that she is taking the pills without missing any, but she has frequent nausea and is experiencing intermenstrual bleeding/spotting. She is requesting to switch to another pill with fewer problems.

JN clearly is seeking relief from troublesome symptoms she attributes to the oral contraceptives. Unless they are addressed, it is possible that JN may discontinue the method entirely, and even potentially risk pregnancy. In the past, women often have been told that unpredictable bleeding may occur for up to 3 months after initiation; yet with the lower-dose agents commonly used today, some irregular bleeding may occur for up to 6 months, and thus JN needs this information. Empirically based advice such as taking pills at bedtime to decrease nausea have little evidence to support them, but they can be mentioned as there is little risk involved. However, there is no clinical evidence that another combined oral contraceptive brand will be a remedy for irregular bleeding and/or nausea. Although there are many brand names, there are relatively few formulations to which she could be switched. Counseling JN about the normalcy of these early side effects may help her continue the method, especially since it is a highly effective one. However, after counseling, JN may consider another contraceptive method entirely. In that case she should be informed that all hormonal contraceptives, which are the most effective contraceptive methods, involve irregular bleeding at some point.

higher progestin dose for the remainder of the 21 days. **Triphasic formulations** also modulate the hormone dosing over the 21-day interval by providing three different doses. Some formulations change only the EE dose, some change just the progestin dose, and some alter both over the course of 21 days (Table 29-1).

Studies have shown that with a 7-day hormone-free interval, FSH begins to increase on cycle day 3 to 4, permitting follicular growth. The reinitiation of pharmacologically active pills causes the follicles to degenerate.[15] Newer formulations are designed to shorten the hormone-free interval with the aim of increasing suppression of ovarian activity. There is one 21/2/5-day regimen (Kariva, Mircette) that has 2 hormone-free days followed by 5 days of a very low dose of EE (10 mcg). Two brands (Yaz and Loestrin-24 Fe) have a 24-4 cycle (4 hormone-free days).

Some of the newest formulations eliminate the monthly 7-day hormone-free interval, offering a withdrawal bleeding episode once every 3 months (Seasonale and Seasonique). When the hormone-free interval exceeds 7 days, the chance of follicle growth and possible breakthrough ovulation appear to be higher,[16] and there is some evidence that continuous hormone use will more effectively prevent ovarian follicle development and ovulation.[17] However, there are no large-scale studies that report improvement in efficacy based on variations of combined oral contraceptive regimens.

Note that specially formulated products are not necessary to eliminate or shorten the hormone-free interval; women can be instructed to start a new package of pills immediately after finishing the active pills in one pack to achieve the same effect. The only disadvantage to this method is that over each 12-week period, instead of three packages of oral contraceptive, a woman will need to purchase four packages, an action that may cause problems with insurance reimbursement. Similarly, shortening the hormone-free interval to 2–4 days does not require dedicated products. A monthly bleeding episode is not physiologically necessary in women using hormonal contraception, and many women appreciate the convenience, although some others may prefer a monthly bleeding even when they understand that it is not a natural menstrual cycle.[18,19]

Transdermal Products

Only one **transdermal contraceptive patch** product (Ortho Evra) is available in the United States. Transdermal delivery of contraceptive hormones avoids hepatic first-pass metabolism, allowing for lower total hormone doses than oral formulations that are metabolized in the liver before reaching the systemic circulation. Transdermal delivery also avoids gastrointestinal symptoms related to pill ingestion and provides a more steady-state release of hormones than the typical peaks and troughs that occur with daily ingestion of a pill. However, transdermal delivery does not counteract the estrogen-induced increase in sex hormone-binding globulin, which results in lower levels of free testosterone; thus the patch is expected to be similar to oral contraceptives with respect to beneficial effects on acne.

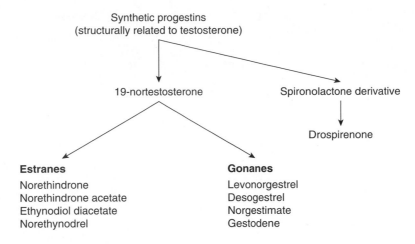

Figure 29-1 Progestins used for contraception.

Dosing Considerations

The transdermal product is a thin, beige patch approximately 4.5 cm square. The patch has an outer protective layer of polyester, an adhesive layer that contains the medication, and a protective liner that is removed prior to application. This product is placed on clean, dry skin of the buttock, abdomen, upper outer arm, or upper torso; it should not be placed over irritated or infected skin. The patch should not be placed on the breasts, not because of known risks, but to avoid any risks, real or imagined, of an association with breast cancer. The user should be certain not to apply the patch over lotion, cream, oil, or other substances that could interfere with adherence. Each patch is designed to be worn for 7 days; a month's supply contains three patches (21 days of hormone dosing). Each patch delivers 20 mcg of EE and 150 mcg of norelgestromin (the primary active metabolite of norgestimate) daily into the systemic circulation. After 3 weeks of use, or three patches, a 7-day hormone-free week is advised according to package labeling, although eliminating or shortening the hormone-free interval can be considered as off-label use. Pharmacokinetic parameters are similar at the various recommended placement sites, and serum levels remain stable under varied conditions of heat, humidity, and exercise.

Hormone levels for contraceptive efficacy are reached after 48 hours[20]; forgetting to restart the patch after a hormone-free interval of several days raises the risk of unintended pregnancy, as is true with oral contraceptives. Should intercourse occur more than 7 days after the end of the hormone-free period, it should be considered unprotected intercourse and emergency contraception is recommended. Once the patch is reapplied, typical clinical recommendations are to use a backup contraceptive method for 7 days, although the exact length of time this is needed is not clear. During the second and third weeks of patch use, being 1-2 days late in placing a new patch does not substantially increase the risk of unintended pregnancy. If a patch is partially or completely detached, adequate contraceptive hormone levels cannot be assured (Figure 29-2). If the patch adheres well after reapplication, it can be used; otherwise it should be replaced. Use of a backup contraceptive method or emergency contraception may be indicated if the period of detachment is unknown or exceeds 1–2 days (Figure 29-3).

Pharmacokinetics

The pharmacokinetics of transdermal delivery systems that have 20 mcg of EE in each patch are different than the pharmacokinetics of the 20-mcg EE pill, and therefore, they cannot be compared despite having the same dose of EE. In fact, pharmacokinetic studies have shown that the area under the curve and average concentration at steady state for EE are approximately 60% higher in women using the patch than in women using an oral contraceptive containing 35 mcg EE. On the other hand, the peak concentrations of EE are approximately 25% lower in women using the patch.[21,22] Whether these pharmacokinetic differences affect the risk of serious adverse events is not known. Increased estrogen exposure may increase the risk of adverse events, including venous thromboembolism,

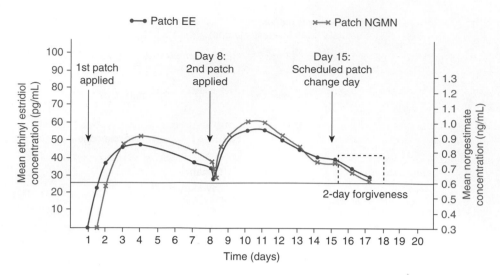

Figure 29-2 Transdermal contraceptive patch and dosing reserve beyond 7 days for Norgestimate and Ethinyl Estradiol. *Source:* Reprinted with permission from Abrams LS, Skee D, Natarajan J, Wong F. An overview of the pharmacokinetics of a contraceptive patch. Int J Gyn Obstet 2000;70 (suppl 2) B78–B82.

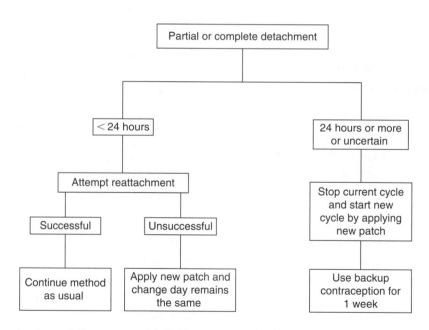

Figure 29-3 Algorithm for management of partial or completely detached transdermal contraceptive patch.

but existing studies have not consistently demonstrated an association.[23,24] Some clinicians are hesitant to recommend extended or continuous use of the patch due to these higher levels of hormones, but there are no evidence-based data available about this practice.

Intravaginal Rings

One **vaginal contraceptive ring** product (NuvaRing) is available in the United States. The flexible ring is made of ethylene vinyl acetate (a plastic used in many medical products) and has an outer diameter of 54 mm and is approximately 4 mm thick. The ring is inserted in the vagina and left there for 3 weeks. Maximum serum concentrations of hormones are reached approximately 1 week after insertion of the ring, and then concentrations decrease over time. After a 7-day hormone-free interval (or sooner if a shorter hormone-free interval is desired), the ring is removed and a new one is inserted. Contraceptive hormones are embedded in the ring and deliver 15 mcg EE and 120 mcg etonogestrel (which is derived from desogestrel) daily across the vaginal mucosa and into the systemic circulation. The ring releases the hormones in steady concentrations throughout the day, avoiding hepatic first-pass metabolism and gastrointestinal interference with absorption, and thus allows lower doses to be used. Note that contraceptive pills can occasionally be administered vaginally as well, for example in women with significant nausea and vomiting. Similar efficacy results if the pill is inserted vaginally and absorbed via the vaginal mucosa as if the pill is taken orally, and the woman will have a reduction in side effects.[25,26]

Some women remove the ring during intercourse or for other reasons during the 21-day hormonal period; if it is removed for more than 3 hours, it should be replaced and backup contraception used for the next 7 days.[27] Studies of ovarian function during NuvaRing use indicate that it takes several days after removing the ring for a dominant follicle to develop[28]; thus, the longer the hormone-free interval, the higher the risk of ovulation. The vaginal ring has been studied in the context of **extended cycling** or continuous use.[29] When the ring is used in extended cycles of 49 days, 91 days or year-round patterns, many women will have an increase in unscheduled spotting days as compared to the standard 28-day cycle (3 weeks of use followed by 7 hormone-free days). However, the amount of bleeding is small and may be tolerable for women who wish to avoid menstrual periods.

Initiation of Combined Hormonal Contraceptives

Traditionally, hormonal contraceptives have been initiated with a menstrual period, either on the first day, the fifth day, or the Sunday following the onset of bleeding. The rationale for this approach was to rule out pregnancy, to initiate hormones before follicle development, and to reduce unscheduled bleeding. In addition, the risk of ovulation within the first 5 days of the menstrual period is low; after 5 days, ovulation may not be effectively suppressed, and 7 days of continuous contraceptive hormone use may be needed to prevent ovulation.[12]

An alternative, Quick Start, allows for beginning the hormonal contraceptive at any point in the cycle as long as the woman is not pregnant. This approach takes advantage of the woman's motivation to begin contraception and eliminates the need for complicated instructions about when to start the method. Quick starting a hormonal contraceptive method does not increase unscheduled bleeding or spotting in the initial cycle.[30] A woman interested in Quick Start should be assessed for possible pregnancy and/or the need for emergency contraception and advised to use backup contraception for the first week. She should be advised to have a pregnancy test if she does not have a withdrawal bleeding episode during the first hormone-free interval or within 3 weeks after she starts extended cycling. There is no evidence that taking contemporary hormonal contraceptives in very early pregnancy is associated with adverse effects.

Missing Doses

Inconsistent use of combination hormonal contraceptives is a major cause of unintended pregnancy. If a woman misses an active pill, she should take a hormonal pill as soon as possible. Missing three or more active 30- to 35-mcg EE pills or two or more 20-mcg or less EE pills requires additional protection until she has 7 continuous days of pill use to prevent ovulation.[12] Frequently, pill packs are marked with days of the week; in this case the woman may choose to discard missed pills. It is not necessary to double up. Vomiting and diarrhea are presumed to have similar effects on contraceptive efficacy as missing pills, and similar precautions should be advised for women who have a gastrointestinal illness.[12]

Efficacy of Combination Hormonal Contraceptives

For women using combination hormonal contraceptives, **perfect use** (following instructions perfectly) will result in an estimated three pregnancies in 1000 women (0.3% pregnancy rate). More **typical use** results in a pregnancy rate of approximately 8%[31,32] or about 1 in 12 women. These estimates are drawn primarily from experience with oral contraceptives. Long-term experience with transdermal and vaginal delivery systems is scanty, but early trials suggest that effectiveness is at least as good as with oral formulations, and theoretically, reducing opportunities to forget pills should improve effectiveness. However, if transdermal patches are detached (completely or partially) or the ring is removed and not replaced within 3 hours, the effective hormone dose can be reduced, possibly compromising effectiveness.

Drug/Herb–Drug Interactions

The cytochrome P450 enzymes (CYP450) represent a large family of enzymes involved in the metabolism of drugs. The cytochrome P450 3A4 (CYP3A4) subfamily is one of the most important enzymes in this group and has been documented as responsible for approximately 60% of P450-mediated metabolism of therapeutic drugs,[33] including contraceptive steroid hormones. Enhanced CYP activity (induction) results in a more rapid metabolic rate and may decrease plasma concentrations and diminish therapeutic effect of medications. Because low-dose and very-low-dose contraceptive steroids are the most commonly prescribed hormonal contraceptives, any agent that could induce, even slightly, more rapid metabolism of these steroids raises the theoretical risk of contraceptive failure and unintended pregnancy (Box 29-2). Transdermal and transvaginal delivery does not avoid the drug–drug or drug–herb interactions that arise from alterations in hepatic metabolism of contraceptive steroids.

Antiseizure medications such as phenobarbital (Luminal), phenytoin (Dilantin), and carbamazepine (Tegretol) induce the CYP450 system. Pharmacokinetic data link use of these drugs to decreased contraceptive steroid levels,[34] and case reports have implicated these drugs in contraceptive failures,[35] although more reliable data are lacking. The antibiotic rifampin (Rifadin) is a potent inducer of CYP3A4, and its effect on reducing levels of contraceptive steroids has been well characterized.[36] Many herbs and natural compounds isolated from herbs have also been identified as substrates, inhibitors, and/or inducers of various CYP enzymes,[37] and St. John's wort in particular has been shown to induce metabolism of contraceptive hormones.[38] See Chapter 4 for more details about drug–drug interactions.

The Effect of Obesity on Effectiveness of Hormonal Contraceptives

There has been growing concern that obesity may affect the efficacy of hormonal contraceptives. More than 25 years ago, Boden reported a cluster of low-dose oral contraceptive failures among relatively heavy women.[39] More recently, Holt[40] found that women in the highest weight quartiles (> 70.5 kg/> 155 pounds) had an increased risk of oral contraceptive failure. This ranged as high as a relative risk of failure of 4.5 for users of very-low-dose pills. Brunner[41] used data from the National Survey of Family Growth to correlate self-reported body

---

Box 29-2 A Challenge in Primary Care

NB, a 17-year-old nulligravida, is being seen for a regular visit, and she requests pills for contraception. Her past history includes a diagnosed seizure disorder that is controlled with phenytoin (Dilantin). Her last seizure was 6 months ago, and she is under the continuing care of a neurologist. Her physical examination is unremarkable, including normal vital signs including BMI.

Prescribing combination oral contraceptives is challenging in this situation. Combination oral contraceptives (COCs) will not cause a physiological change in her seizure disorder. The issue is one of drug–drug interactions. Contraceptive efficacy of oral contraceptives can be decreased if taken concurrently with phenytoin; therefore, contraceptive failure is more likely than if she did not take the agent. In addition, phenytoin is not metabolized as rapidly and serum levels increase when these two drugs are taken concomitantly; therefore, serum levels of phenytoin can become excessive. The same issues theoretically apply to the use of the transdermal patch (Ortho Evra) and ring (NuvaRing).

However, NB is at risk for an unwanted pregnancy as well as possible teratogenic effects from the antiepileptic medication. Depot medroxyprogesterone acetate (Depo-Provera) may be a reasonable option for JN, especially since it can also decrease seizure activity. If prescribed, as for all adolescents, she should receive counseling about dietary and exercise options to increase bone density. Although JN is nulliparous, that alone is not a contraindication to an intrauterine contraceptive agent. Therefore JN can also be offered the choice of one of the intrauterine devices.

Consultation with this woman's neurologist may be of great value. Nonenzyme-inducing antiepileptic agents (e.g., gabapentin [Neurontin] and pregabalin [Lyrica]) do not appear to have the same drug–drug interactions associated with phenytoin. Should the seizure activity be controlled with the use of these drugs, she may be able to use her first choice, combination oral contraceptives.

weight with conception occurring during oral contraceptive use and found that women with a body mass index of ≥ 30 had a nearly twofold increased risk of contraceptive failure compared to the risk of contraceptive failure in women who have a normal BMI. Other studies found overweight and obese women had nearly twice the odds of having an unintended pregnancy than women with normal BMIs[41,42] and two national surveillance systems showed a twofold to threefold increase in apparent contraceptive failure based on increasing BMI.[43] However, the most recent population-based study[44] found no effect of obesity on hormone contraceptive effectiveness. It is important to note that these assessments depend on self-reported weight and recall of contraceptive use at the time of conception months after the event in order to judge the presence or absence of an association, and large prospective studies directly addressing this hypothesis need to be conducted in order to answer the question.

In one prospective clinical trial of the transdermal patch, 5 of the 15 pregnancies reported occurred in the 3% of users who weighed over 198 pounds.[45] This trial included women who weighed approximately 35% more than ideal body weight (not typical for clinical trials, where women outside the range of normal body weight are often excluded). Note that weighing 130% or more of ideal body weight is considered overweight but not obese for women. FDA-approved product labeling for the patch now warns that "contraceptive effectiveness may be decreased in women weighing over 198 pounds."

In summary, there are no directed prospective studies on the association between weight or body mass index and contraceptive failure, nor are there evidence-based guidelines for management. Some authorities have suggested prescribing pills with 35 mcg of estrogen as the failure rate appears to be less than those with lower estrogen levels, but this has not been evaluated in clinical studies.[46] Without good data on the relationship between BMI and contraceptive failure, the clinician can be perplexed when confronted with a woman desiring the transdermal patch and weighing less than 198 pounds, but with a BMI of 30. However, even if there is some decrease in efficacy, the absolute failure (pregnancy) rates are very low when compared to other methods.

WHO Medical Eligibility

Combination hormonal contraceptives are in WHO category 1 or 2 for most conditions, except for the conditions listed in Table 29-2. Women with conditions that affect the skin beneath the patch (such as psoriasis or eczema) should not use it due to uncertainty about absorption of the medication.

Adverse Effects of Hormonal Contraceptives

Many adverse effects attributed to hormonal contraceptives over the decades, such as altered glucose tolerance, cholecystitis, and liver tumors, were associated with higher hormone levels and occur rarely with contemporary low-dose formulations. The most concerning adverse effects associated with combined hormonal contraceptives used today are related to thrombotic events such as myocardial infarction and stroke. Contemporary low-dose hormonal contraceptives do not appreciably increase these risks in healthy women who do not smoke and who do not have underlying endothelial damage from hypertension or who do not have other cardiovascular risk factors.[47,48] Migraineurs with aura have a higher risk of ischemic stroke that is compounded by use of estrogen-containing contraceptives.[49] Thus, appropriate selection using the WHO eligibility criteria of women for whom it is safe to use hormonal contraceptives is important to reduce the incidence of these adverse effects.

When compared to women who do not use hormonal contraceptive methods, the risk of thromboembolism is higher among combined hormonal contraceptive users. An event usually occurs within the first 2 years of use and is often associated with an underlying inherited coagulation disorder. This elevation in risk is generally thought to be due to the estrogen component, with the higher doses (80 and 100 mcg EE) in early birth control pill formulations associated with a sixfold increase in the risk of venous thrombosis.[50] As the doses of estrogen have dropped, so has the incidence of thromboembolism, although it is important to note that simultaneously with the advent of lower dose formulations, practice guidelines called for better screening and not prescribing hormonal contraceptives for women with cardiovascular risk.[14] Nonetheless, the use of hormonal contraceptives containing estrogen produces at least a threefold increase in the risk of thromboembolism.[14] Some studies implicated the newer progestins desogestrel, norgestimate, gestodene (not available in the United States), and drospirenone in the development of venous thromboembolism.[51,52] These findings were subsequently reevaluated in a number of reports, and any observed increase in risk due to newer

Table 29-2 WHO Medical Eligibility* Categories 3 and 4 Cautions for Combined Oral Contraceptives

Condition	Eligibility Category Warning	Clinical Considerations
Postpartum	Category 3 for the first 21 days after delivery	
Breastfeeding	Category 4 from birth to 6 weeks postpartum Category 3 from 6 weeks to 6 months postpartum	
Smoking	If age 35 or older: category 3 for less than 15 cigarettes a day; category 4 if 15 cigarettes or more daily	
Cardiovascular risk factors	Current (or a history of) ischemic heart disease or stroke: category 4 Complicated valvular heart disease (for example, with pulmonary hypertension or a history of bacterial endocarditis): category 4 Hypertension or multiple risk factors that raise a risk of cardiovascular events (older age, diabetes, hypertension): category 3 or 4, depending on history Known hyperlipidemias should be assessed for their severity and the presence of other cardiovascular risk factors.	
Coagulopathies	A history of (or current) deep vein thrombosis, pulmonary embolism, or a known thrombogenic mutation such as factor V Leiden or protein C or S deficiencies: category 4 Any prolonged immobilization (such as after major surgery): category 4	A family history of DVT or PE in a first-degree relative is listed as category 2. Varicose veins and superficial thrombophlebitis are not contraindications to use.
Migraine headaches	< age 35, if migraines without aura may initiate combined hormonal contraceptives (category 2), but continuation warrants careful assessment of risk and benefit (category 3). Age 35 or older: category 3 or 4	The risk of stroke is higher in women with migraines if they use hormonal contraceptives.
Breast cancer	Current breast cancer: category 4 Past history of cancer but no evidence of disease for 5 years: category 3	
Diabetes	Diabetes with evidence of nephropathy, retinopathy, neuropathy, or other vascular disease, or diabetes of more than 20 years' duration: category 3 or 4	
Cholecystitis	Current gallbladder disease (even if it is controlled on medical treatment) or a history of cholestasis on hormonal contraceptives: category 3	Asymptomatic gallbladder disease or that treated by cholecystectomy is category 2. A history of pregnancy-related cholestasis is also listed as category 2.
Liver disease	Active hepatitis, benign or malignant liver tumors, and cirrhosis of the liver: category 4	

* Eligibility categories are as follows:
  1. No restriction for the use of the contraceptive method.
  2. Advantages of using the method generally outweigh the theoretical or proven risks.
  3. Theoretical or proven risks usually outweigh the advantages of using the method.
  4. The method should not be used.

Note: Combination hormonal contraceptives are in WHO category 1 or 2 for most conditions.
Source: World Health Organization 2004.[11]

progestins was determined to be either so small as to be not meaningful or the result of bias and confounding in the original studies.[14]

Women with a known risk for developing thromboembolism should not take COCs. Certain conditions, such as factor V Leiden mutation, may account for many cases of venous thromboembolism in COC users. Because the incidence of these events is very small, approximately 4–5 cases per 100,000 women per year,[53] screening for such disorders would require testing large numbers of healthy women to detect an uncommon condition to prevent a

very small number of events. Most experts do not recommend screening for these inherited disorders unless the woman or a close family member has had a history of unexplained thromboembolism.[54]

In 2005, the FDA updated its approved labeling for the Ortho Evra contraceptive patch to warn healthcare providers and women that this product exposes those using it to higher levels of estrogen than most birth control pills. While higher estrogen doses are associated in general with an increased risk of thrombotic events, the actual clinical implications of these pharmacokinetic findings for the patch are unclear. As a result, investigations of the frequency of venous thromboembolism (VTE) among patch users were initiated. In 2006, the FDA added information to the Ortho Evra labeling indicating that two studies examining the risk of VTE in users of the contraceptive patch yielded conflicting results.

Increases in angiotensin II and aldosterone activity associated with estrogens and progestins may increase blood pressure in susceptible individuals. If due solely to the estrogen component, the effect is reversible on discontinuing the contraceptives.

Drospirenone has antimineralocorticoid activity, and contraceptives containing this progestin should not be prescribed to women taking other potassium-sparing drugs such as ACE inhibitors, certain diuretics, or chronic use of nonsteroidal anti-inflammatory drugs (NSAIDs), without assessing potassium levels.

Common Side Effects

Side effects occur frequently in combination hormonal contraceptive users, but not always because of the product. A double-blind, placebo-controlled trial showed that many side effects traditionally thought to be due to the hormone content of the birth control pill occurred with the same frequency in pill and placebo users.[55] Side effects listed in pill packaging (and read by consumers) list those side effects experienced by pill users during clinical trials; these may or may not have been related to the pill use during that time period. Thus complaints of side effects should not be automatically attributed to contraceptive hormones, but should be evaluated and managed appropriately. There are few evidence-based data on management of side effects determined to be related to the contraceptive product. In general, most of the side effects will disappear within the first months of use as the woman adjusts to the different hormone levels. Changing to another product to alter the hormone dosing is an option if expectant management fails; individual patterns in drug metabolism may make certain formulations more tolerable for individual women even if larger studies do not show an overall benefit.

Altered bleeding patterns, such as spotting and breakthrough bleeding, are common in the first few months of use as the endometrium adjusts to hormone dose. From 10% to 30% of users will have unscheduled bleeding in the first month of use; 10% or fewer will experience this by the third month. Smokers will have even higher rates of unscheduled bleeding, especially if they use pills with 20 mcg of EE.[54] Forgetting to take pills is also associated

with spotting and bleeding. Withdrawal bleeding during the hormone-free interval may be less or absent with contemporary low-dose hormonal contraceptives.

Breast tenderness is another common complaint in the first few months of hormonal contraceptive use and is likely related to both estrogen and progestin components. Lower doses of EE produced fewer symptoms in one study.[56] Users of the transdermal patch are more likely to experience breast tenderness than women using oral formulations.[57] Increased vaginal discharge in some women is likely due to the estrogen component, but there is no evidence that combination hormonal contraceptives increase risk of vaginal infections. Use of the contraceptive ring is not associated with cervical or cytological abnormalities or bacteriological changes in vaginal flora, even though women may report increased discharge.

Some women will experience a worsening of acne or hirsutism, but in general hormonal contraceptives decrease androgen production and increase sex-hormone binding globulins, which bind testosterone and androgen, thus reducing free testosterone that influences acne and hirsutism. Some oral contraceptive formulations have FDA indications for treatment of acne (Ortho Tri-Cyclen, Estrostep, Yaz) but all combined hormonal contraceptives act in a similar fashion and should be effective in treating acne.[58] Occasional headaches are common complaints in women who use hormonal contraceptives. New onset, severe, or worsening headaches need to be evaluated promptly. Nausea is often related to the estrogen component of the hormonal contraceptive. Many clinicians advise women who experience nausea to take their pills at bedtime, yet there is no evidence that this is of value, although it also does no harm. The nausea may be a local gastric effect or operate at the level of the central nervous system. Progestins may contribute to decreased peristalsis, constipation, or bloating.[59] In most cases, the symptoms resolve after a few months of use.

Vomiting and diarrhea (for example, with gastroenteritis) may interfere with absorption of contraceptive steroids, and such illness has been associated with contraceptive failures.[60] Women should be advised to use backup contraception during and for a week after such an illness or consider emergency contraception, if appropriate.

Depression, mood alterations, and changes in libido are occasionally reported by women. There is no evidence of an overall increased risk of clinical depression in hormone users; however, it is important to remember that depression is common in reproductive-aged women in general. Some women may experience a decrease in libido due to lower levels of free testosterone.[61,62] Two studies have suggested a small beneficial effect of drospirenone-containing hormonal contraceptives on symptoms of premenstrual syndrome and premenstrual dysphoric disorder,[63,64] and in 2006, Yaz (a combined oral contraception with drospirenone and 24-day dosing) received the first FDA approval given to a COC for treatment of premenstrual dysphoric disorder.

Skin changes such as darkened patches on the face called chloasma may result due to estrogen stimulation of melanocytes; this coloration may fade when estrogen is discontinued, but may not fade completely. These changes may develop in users of the transdermal patch under the patch site as well.

Weight change (especially weight gain) often is attributed to combined hormonal contraceptive use. A number of different studies have shown that oral contraceptive use is not associated with any more weight change than that typically seen in women in the United States who do not use hormonal contraceptives. Nonetheless, individual women may have a particular response to the hormone component of contraceptives, and reducing the hormone dose or progestin may help. Weight gain due to fluid retention may be minimized by the use of preparations containing drospirenone.

Cost and Availability

All combined hormonal contraceptives are prescription products. There can be a wide range in the pricing, but, in general, a 1-month supply often costs over $40. Generic alternatives are available for most oral formulations, but not for the patch or the ring. Insurance coverage for contraceptive products is not universal.

Progestin-Only Hormonal Contraceptives

As noted, many of the serious and concerning adverse events associated with hormonal contraceptives are related to the estrogen component. Breastfeeding women are advised to avoid estrogen-containing contraceptives for several months after childbirth. Thus progestin-only contraceptives may be an important option for many women. Progestin-only pills are sometimes referred to as **mini pills**, but this term risks being confused with very-low-dose pills and should be avoided. The preferred term is **progestin-only pills** (POPs).

Mechanism of Action

Most of the contraceptive effect of all hormonal contraceptives comes from the progestin component. Progestins have a negative feedback effect on the hypothalamic-pituitary axis and suppress the LH surge necessary for ovulation.[14] Ovulation is not uniformly prevented in users of POPs, however, and many women will have regular cycles while taking the medication (regular menses being a sign of ovulatory activity). Other contraceptive effects of the progestin-only agents may be more important than suppression of the LH surge.[14] Progestins thicken cervical mucus to inhibit sperm migration. In order to maintain this mechanism of action, it is important that the pill be taken at the same time every day, as the cervical mucus effect wanes within 24 hours. Progestins also produce a thinly developed endometrium, which may inhibit implantation, and they are associated with irregular and unpredictable bleeding and amenorrhea.

Initiation

Women can begin progestin-only pills at any time they are reasonably certain they are not pregnant. The women should be assessed for the need for emergency contraception, and if there are any doubts about a possible early pregnancy, a pregnancy test can be done 2–3 weeks after beginning the contraceptive. Forty-eight hours of POP use will produce contraceptive effects on cervical mucus.[12]

Efficacy

In the first year of use, the probability of pregnancy is estimated to be similar between users of POPs and users of COCs (0.3% for perfect use and 8% for typical).[31,32] One older study indicated slightly higher pregnancy rates for POP users[65] than COC users. Women who are fully breastfeeding enjoy the highest efficacy (nearly 100%) due to the hormonal effects of lactation that also provide some contraceptive benefit. Missing POPs is a prime reason for unintended pregnancy. Expert opinion is that missing a pill by 3 hours or more creates a risk of unintended pregnancy due to diminishing of the cervical mucus effect; a woman who misses a pill should take it as soon as possible and abstain from sex or use additional protection for 48 hours to permit resumption of the cervical mucus effect.[12] Vomiting and diarrhea are presumed to have the same effect as missing pills.[12]

WHO Medical Eligibility

Use of progestin-only oral contraceptives falls into WHO medical eligibility category 1 or 2 for most conditions. The exceptions are listed in Table 29-3. Concomitant use of drugs or herbs that induce liver enzymes (thus increasing metabolism and clearance of the hormone) may reduce efficacy of POPs. When a woman is concomitantly taking rifampin and anticonvulsants that induce the P450 liver enzyme system, the WHO medical eligibility category is 3 for progestin-only pills and progestin-containing implants. Because the dose of progestin is much higher in progestin-only injectables, these agents remain WHO medical eligibility category 2 contraceptives when concomitant use of medications that induce CYP3A4 are used.

Adverse Effects

Serious adverse effects are unlikely in women who take progestin-only hormonal contraceptive pills, and those that occur are generally secondary to allergic reactions to progestins. However, progestin-only methods in general raise concerns about an increased likelihood of ectopic pregnancy should a contraceptive failure occur. This is due to thickening of mucus and slowing of tubal motility, which could theoretically contribute to a tubal pregnancy. Because the use of POPs is effective in preventing pregnancy, the *overall* rate of ectopic pregnancy in POP users is not increased above what is expected (approximately 2%), but if a woman taking POPs becomes pregnant, the likelihood that the pregnancy is ectopic is approximately 10%.[59] One study reported a threefold increased risk of developing diabetes among Latina women diagnosed with gestational diabetes who were breastfeeding and using POPs after delivery. The mechanism of this association is unclear.[66]

Common Side Effects

Breast tenderness, headaches, changes in vaginal discharge, and other minor side effects may be experienced by any hormonal contraceptive user. A variety of treatments such as dietary restrictions and botanical treatments have been suggested to treat the side effects, but data on efficacy are lacking.

Approximately 40% of women taking POPs will have normal ovulatory cycles; most will have irregular periods of bleeding or spotting, or amenorrhea.[67] The addition of estrogen in combined hormonal contraceptives reduces

Table 29-3 WHO Medical Eligibility* Categories 3 and 4 Cautions for Progestin-Only Contraceptives

Condition	Eligibility Category Warning	Clinical Considerations
Breast cancer	Current breast cancer: category 4 History of breast cancer: category 3	
Postpartum	Less than 6 weeks postpartum: category 3	This is due to concerns about ingestion of hormones by the neonate. There are few effects on lactation or infant health and growth. There are no data on progestogen effects on brain and liver development.
Coagulopathies	Current deep vein thrombosis: category 3	
Cardiovascular disease	Current ischemic heart disease or stroke: category 3	
Migraines	Migraine with aura: category 3	
Liver disease	Active hepatitis, severe cirrhosis, or liver tumors (benign or malignant): category 3	
Additional Criteria of Progestin-Only Injectables		
Diabetes	Diabetes with nephropathy, retinopathy, neuropathy, other vascular disease or diabetes of > 20 years' duration: category 3	
Hypertension	Multiple risk factors for arterial cardiovascular disease, or HTN ≥ 160 or diastolic ≥ 100, or in hypertensive women with vascular disease: category 3	This is because their effects may persist for some time after discontinuation.
Unexplained vaginal bleeding	Until the cause has been evaluated: category 3	This applies to the use of injectables and implants, which may aggravate the bleeding.

* Eligibility categories are as follows:
  1. No restriction for the use of the contraceptive method.
  2. Advantages of using the method generally outweigh the theoretical or proven risks.
  3. Theoretical or proven risks usually outweigh the advantages of using the method.
  4. The method should not be used.

Note: Progestin-only contraceptives are in WHO category 1 or 2 for other conditions.

Source: World Health Organization 2004.[11]

irregular bleeding. Irregular bleeding does not cause any harm nor signal any pathology, but if it is bothersome, the woman can be switched to a COC, providing COCs are not contraindicated for her.

Cost and Availability

Progestin-only pills are less commonly prescribed and less likely to be stocked by pharmacies. They are more expensive than COCs.

Progestin-Only Injectables

There are two **injectable contraceptives** available in the United States; both are progestin-only methods. Depot medroxyprogesterone acetate (DMPA) is marketed as Depo-Provera, which contains 150 mg DMPA and is given as a deep intramuscular injection every 12 (range of 11–13) weeks. In 2005, a new formulation (the so-called *mini depo*) began to be marketed as Depo-SubQ Provera.[68] This agent is a medroxyprogesterone acetate injectable suspension that is given as a subcutaneous injection. Aside from the lower dose, the subcutaneous delivery system allows for the potential for self-injection, rather than needing to visit a provider's office for injections. There is no evidence that the incidence of common side effects is reduced, and the newer formulation may not be covered by all insurance plans.

Mechanism of Action

As noted previously, the contraceptive effect of progestins is a negative feedback effect on the hypothalamic-pituitary axis and promotes suppression of the LH and FSH peaks necessary for ovulation. They also thicken cervical mucus to inhibit sperm migration and produce endometrial changes, which may inhibit implantation, but are associated with irregular and unpredictable bleeding and amenorrhea.

Initiation

Injectable contraception is labeled for initiation with a menstrual period. The injection can be given up to day 7 of the menstrual cycle[12] due to the low risk of ovulation in the first week after a menses has occurred.[12] The Quick Start method can be used, but because amenorrhea is an expected side effect of the method, women should be carefully assessed for pregnancy and advised to have a pregnancy test 2–3 weeks after initiation if there is any concern about the possibility of unintended pregnancy.

Injectables cannot be discontinued as oral contraceptives can, in the event that pregnancy is diagnosed.

Efficacy

DMPA is extremely effective; the probability of pregnancy is approximately 0.3% in perfect users and 3% in typical users.[31,32] In three clinical studies, no pregnancies were detected among 2,042 women using DMPA subcutaneously (Depo-SubQ Provera 104) for up to 1 year; thus it is likely that the efficacy will be similar to DMPA when the subcutaneous formulation achieves wider use.

Product labeling recommends reinjection every 11 to 13 weeks. If more than 13 weeks has elapsed, another method of contraception should be used until reinjection, and emergency contraception should be considered if unprotected intercourse occurs. Some studies of the 150-mg intramuscular formulation have suggested that contraceptive efficacy is maintained for at least 14 weeks, and the WHO Expert Working Group considers the risk of ovulation to be minimal within 2 weeks of the scheduled repeat injection (at 12 weeks)[12]; in fact, some women will not resume ovulation for several months after discontinuing injectable contraceptives. However, these events cannot be predicted and standard clinical recommendations are that efficacy wanes if reinjection is delayed.

WHO Medical Eligibility

The WHO medical eligibility for use of progestin-only injectables is the same as the eligibility for progestin-only contraceptive pills with three additional restrictions that are listed in Table 29-3.

Adverse Effects

As noted previously, progestin-only methods raise concerns about an increased likelihood of ectopic pregnancy should a contraceptive failure occur. Injectables are extremely effective at preventing pregnancy, which makes the likelihood of ectopic pregnancy very low.

In 2004, the FDA announced the addition of a black box warning to the labeling of Depo-Provera contraceptive injection, noting that prolonged use of injectables may result in the loss of bone density. The warning states that prolonged use of the drug may result in significant loss of bone density and that the loss is greater the longer the drug is administered. It further states that this bone density loss may not be completely reversible after discontinuation of the drug. The warning states that a woman should only use Depo-Provera contraceptive injection as a long-term birth control method (for example, longer than 2 years) if other birth control methods are inadequate for her.

Recent reevaluations of data about bone density suggest that the black box warning may be too strict or at least overinterpreted. Bone loss does not appear to be permanent. Findings of lower bone density have *not* been linked to osteoporosis or fractures. Bone mineral density in former adult DMPA users is similar to that of those women who have never used DMPA.[69,70] Bone mineral density is also similar in postmenopausal women regardless of whether they are former users of DMPA or never used DMPA. In adolescents, recovery of bone mineral density is substantial within 12 months of stopping DMPA.[71] This pattern resembles that of the relationship between bone mineral density and lactation. Spinal bone mineral density declines by 4% during 6 months of breastfeeding but recovers after lactation. There is no evidence that women who have breastfed have more osteoporosis or fractures.

A Cochrane review[72] also found that DMPA (Depo-Provera) was related to lower bone mineral density, but there are no data to assess whether this loss is related to fractures. Since bone density is a surrogate marker for fracture (it addresses bone quantity, not bone quality), its validity in the setting of contraceptive use risk is unknown.[73] In 2006, WHO issued a statement[74] on hormonal contraception and bone health. Its experts said there should be no restriction on the use of DMPA in women ages 18–45 who are otherwise eligible to use the method. For women younger than 18 years and women older than 45 years, the advantages generally outweigh the theoretical safety concerns about fracture risk. Some authorities suggest prescribing menopausal hormone replacement doses of estrogen for perimenopausal women using DMPA to control hot flashes, maintain bone, and reduce the increased bleeding associated with endometrial atrophy.[59]

Common Side Effects

Unscheduled bleeding is common in the first cycle or two of use of progestin-only injectables; heavy and/or prolonged bleeding are common. Heavy bleeding can be treated with oral estrogen (2 mg estradiol or 1.25 mg conjugated estrogens) or a nonsteroidal anti-inflammatory agent daily for 7 days,[54] although the WHO Expert Working Group determined that these interventions were likely to be of only short-term or limited benefit.[12]

Some women note marked weight gain when using DMPA. As noted, progestins may contribute to decreased peristalsis, constipation, or bloating. However, women using DMPA appear to gain on average 5–6 pounds in the first year, and up to 14 pounds over 4 years of use.[75] This gain is more than is found among users of progestin implants or COCs. The weight is likely related to an effect in increasing appetite (rather than fluid retention), and seems to be more common in overweight adolescents and certain ethnic groups.[76-78] There is no evidence that increased body weight adversely affects the efficacy of DMPA.[46]

Cost and Availability

A single dose of DMPA costs an estimated $75 for up to 13 weeks of contraception. A single dose of the subcutaneous formulation costs approximately $20 more. There may also be a fee associated with providing the injection.

Progestin-Only Implants

Implantable contraceptives are small rods or capsules containing a progestin. They are inserted under the skin of the upper arm and continuously release the hormone into the circulation. They have the advantage of not being coitus dependent, not requiring daily or periodic action on the part of the user, and they are highly effective. The first implantable contraceptive that was developed was Norplant, which contained six small, flexible capsules, each of which had 36 mg levonorgestrel. This implant was approved for 5 years of continuous use. Jadelle, or Norplant II, has two capsules each containing 150 mg of levonorgestrel. Neither of these currently is marketed in the United States. Other implants are in development or available in other countries.

Implanon is the only implant currently available in the United States. Implanon consists of one capsule containing 68 mg etonogestrel and provides contraceptive protection for 3 years. The capsules are not radio opaque but can be localized with ultrasound.

Mechanism of Action

Implanon effectively inhibits ovulation. In clinical trials, the earliest evidence of ovulation after appropriate insertion of Implanon occurred in the third year of use. Etonogestrel levels in the serum reach a level compatible with ovulation inhibition within 8 hours.[79] Increased viscosity of cervical mucus likely is the reason that even with evidence of returned ovulation, pregnancy is still prevented. As is true of all progestin-only contraceptives, the endometrial effect is associated with irregular bleeding or amenorrhea. Once removed, serum levels of etonogestrel fall rapidly and are undetectable within a week.[80]

Initiation

Implants are intended to be placed during a menstrual period in order to rule out pregnancy. Although some clinicians might consider the Quick Start method, implants cannot be discontinued as quickly as other hormonal contraceptives should an unintended pregnancy be diagnosed after initiation. Thus, it is imperative to place the implant when there is little probability of pregnancy.

Efficacy

Clinical trials that preceded FDA approval reported no pregnancies in women who used Implanon. Since approval and more widespread use, there have been a number of unintended pregnancies reported. Some are likely method failures, including those related to interactions with other medications, and some are related to failure to properly insert the device according to recommendations. The estimated method failure rate is approximately 1 per 1000 insertions. There is no evidence for decreased efficacy in overweight women, but women who weighed over 130% of ideal body weight were not included in the pre-approval clinical trials. However, serum concentrations of etonogestrel are inversely related to body weight[81]; thus the possibility of a modest decrease in efficacy exists.

WHO Medical Eligibility

Eligibility considerations are the same for users of implants as for those using POPs (Table 29-3). The additional restrictions are that use before evaluation of unexplained vaginal bleeding is a category 3 situation. Insertion of an implant will likely aggravate the bleeding.

Adverse Effects

As previously noted, progestin-only methods raise concerns about an increased likelihood of ectopic pregnancy should a contraceptive failure occur. Implanon has very high contraceptive efficacy, which makes the likelihood of ectopic pregnancy very low overall.

Common Side Effects

Ovarian follicular activity is not inhibited as well as ovulation is, and benign follicular cysts of the ovary can occur with any progestin-only method. Hormonal side effects such as breast pain, headaches, dizziness, acne, and mood swings have been reported for less than 12% of users in clinical trials. Conversely, acne improved in 61% of users in one study,[82] and dysmenorrhea improved in 91% of users.

With the absence of ovulation, irregular bleeding activity is common. Amenorrhea is the most common pattern, but any pattern of frequent, irregular, prolonged bleeding or spotting is possible, and the patterns are unpredictable over time. Nonsteroidal anti-inflammatory drugs and oral estrogen have been recommended to treat heavy bleeding, but there are limited data about effectiveness of these interventions.[12]

Cost and Availability

Implants require a substantial initial financial outlay for the device (~ $500) and clinician visits for insertion and removal. Averaged over 3 years of potential use, the cost is less than that of 3 years of other hormonal contraceptive methods.

Postpartum Contraception—Using Hormonal Methods

Initiation of a hormonal contraceptive method postpartum is another area of some controversy, often involving off-label use. The WHO medical eligibility tables do not consider estrogen-containing methods for a breastfeeding woman category 2 contraceptives until after 6 months because estrogen is thought to decrease milk supply in lactating women. However, many clinicians will prescribe such with admonishments to increase maternal fluids and infant feedings, although data on this practice with regard to maintaining milk supply are lacking. The WHO medical eligibility tables also note that COCs, injectables, patches, and rings should not be prescribed prior to 21 days postpartum for nonbreastfeeding women because of hypercoagulability seen during pregnancy, but package inserts for such agents generally specify 4 weeks (28 days).

POPs are considered category 3 contraceptives for breastfeeding women less than 6 weeks postpartum and are in category 1 for breastfeeding women who are 6 weeks or more postpartum or nonbreastfeeding women of any status. More details about postpartum contraception can be found in Chapter 37.

Intrauterine Contraception

Intrauterine contraceptive devices are among the most effective contraceptive methods in use today. These small devices are inserted into the uterus by a trained clinician. Once inserted, the devices are not coitus dependent, nor do they require daily action on the part of the user for contraceptive effect. They provide 5–10 years of effective contraception, depending on the device. They are the most popular method of contraception worldwide, after sterilization.

The Gräfenberg ring was first developed in Germany in 1909, and the Ota device in Japan in the 1930s. Lippes designed a loop with an attached string to allow checking to ensure the device was in place and to enable easy removal. The Lippes Loop became one of the most widely used intrauterine devices (IUDs). Another device, the Dalkon Shield, was associated with increased risk of pelvic infection and septic abortion in women who became pregnant. The Dalkon Shield IUD was withdrawn from the US market in 1974. Although the Dalkon Shield IUD had a unique design flaw that led to the increased risk of pregnancy and infection, use of IUDs in general declined after the device was removed from the market most likely due to the public erroneously extrapolating bad press about the Dalkon Shield IUD to all IUDs.

Recent years have seen renewed interest in intrauterine contraception. Early IUDs were made primarily of inert materials, but contemporary intrauterine contraceptives include additional active materials that are intended to improve efficacy. Two devices currently are available in the United States. The copper IUD (ParaGard T380A) is a T-shaped polyethylene device. The body is wound with 176 mg of copper wire, and each of the arms has a copper collar with approximately 68-mg copper. The levonorgestrel intrauterine contraceptive/system (Mirena), also a T-shaped polyethylene frame, has a reservoir around the stem that contains 52 mg of the progestin levonorgestrel. The reservoir is covered by a silicone membrane. Levonorgestrel is released into the uterine cavity at a rate of 20 mcg/day.

Mechanism of Action

Multiple mechanisms of action are likely to operate with intrauterine contraception. The primary action is prefertilization—inhibition of sperm, changes in tubal transport, or destruction of the ovum. Essentially, IUDs work primarily to prevent sperm and ovum from meeting. There may be some postfertilization effects, although all contraceptive action is thought to occur before implantation.[83] The copper-containing IUDs inhibit sperm function via the release of copper ions in the uterine and tubal fluids and also alter cervical mucus.[14] Changes in the endometrium may also inhibit sperm migration; copper IUDs increase the number of leukocytes in the endometrium, producing a chronic inflammatory response in the endometrium.

The levonorgestrel-releasing systems (initially termed a *system* rather than a *device* due to the release of the hormone levonorgestrel, although more recently the manufacturer is using the term *intrauterine contraceptive*, abbreviated as IUC) produce atrophy of the endometrial glands, which may inhibit sperm survival. The progestin effect decreases endometrial thickness and secretions while thickening cervical mucus, which may alter sperm penetration. Some studies have suggested that the use of intrauterine contractive devices can lower the risk of endometrial cancer (most likely due to endometrial changes)[84,85] and possibly cervical cancer,[86] but definitive studies are lacking. The progestin-releasing system also has several medical uses; for example, treating heavy uterine bleeding from fibroids or heavy menses, as well as protection of the endometrium as part of hormone therapy in menopause.

Initiation

Intrauterine contraception is an option for most reproductive-aged women. Many clinicians are familiar with it as an option only for parous women, but in 2005 the FDA approved the copper IUD for use in nulligravid and nulliparous women aged 16 and older. Nulligravid women may have a higher risk of expulsion (Box 29-3). Women with allergy to any of the constituents of the device (copper, progestin) should not use that IUD. Intrauterine contraception is not contraindicated for women who have a history of sexually transmitted infection (STI), but women at continued high risk for acquiring STIs may not be the best candidates.[11] Devices may be inserted up to day 7 of the cycle.[12] Prophylactic antibiotics are not needed for insertion of intrauterine contraceptive devices in healthy women.[87]

Efficacy

The ParaGard device is FDA approved for 10 years of continuous use. In the first year of use, the pregnancy rates are less than 1% (0.7 per 100 women), and pregnancy rates fall even lower in years 2 through 10. The levonorgestrel intrauterine contraceptive (Mirena) device currently is approved for 5 years of use. Typical use pregnancy rates in the first year are also less than 1%, and the cumulative 5-year pregnancy rates are 0.7 per 100 women. These rates rival those of tubal sterilization.[31,32] Should a woman become

Box 29-3 A Case of the Missing Strings

MB is a 38-year-old G 3 P2103 who comes into your office for a visit reporting she can't find the strings of her ParaGard since just before her last menses. Her last menstrual period started 5 days ago and was normal in character and amount. Her history reveals that she has hypertension treated with medications. She expelled a previous intrauterine contraceptive device several years ago and then used combination oral contraceptives (COCs) until she became hypertensive. Two months ago she had a ParaGard inserted. Her physical examination is normal except for a body mass index (BMI) of 36 and a blood pressure of 138/80. Upon pelvic examination, the IUD strings are not visible, nor is the device felt during the bimanual examination.

Although pregnancy is unlikely, most clinicians would perform a test to provide reassurance to the clinician and woman alike. Regarding possible expulsion, the provider should not attempt to blindly explore the uterine cavity in a quest to find the intrauterine device. However, gentle rotation of a cotton tipped applicator in the cervical os may locate the strings if they have simply curled within the cervical os. If the strings cannot be located, a sonogram should be obtained. If the ParaGard is visualized *in situ* on sonogram with a fundal position, there should be a discussion with MB about her desires. Fundal placement provides contraceptive protection, but she will be unable to verify appropriate placement, which may be concerning, especially since she already has expelled one IUD. If she chooses to have the IUD removed, it should be done under ultrasound visualization.

Alternative contraceptive options for MB are limited if she does not want to choose condoms or one of the barrier methods. Hypertension and obesity incur an increased risk for cardiovascular disease, yet those conditions also can negatively influence a pregnancy, which is a possible consequence of using some of the less effective methods. MB might consider a progestin-only method such as a POP or implant. Depot medroxyprogesterone acetate (Depo-Provera) should be avoided because of the side effect of weight gain. MB might also opt for permanent sterilization for herself or her partner.

pregnant when using an intrauterine contraceptive device, the risks of miscarriage, preterm birth, and infection are substantial, and if the device can be easily removed, it should be.[12]

WHO Medical Eligibility

Intrauterine contraceptive options are in WHO category 1 or 2 except for the conditions listed in Table 29-4. There is a small increase in the incidence of pelvic infection in IUD users that is limited to the first 20 days after insertion, and is likely related to preexisting infection or contamination during the insertion process.

The relationship between IUDs and ectopic pregnancy is often misconstrued. The high contraceptive efficacy of IUDs makes the likelihood of ectopic pregnancy very low, and IUD usage decreases the risk of ectopic pregnancy overall by 90%.[88] However, should a pregnancy occur while a woman has an IUD *in situ*, she should be evaluated for an ectopic pregnancy as the risk in an individual pregnancy is higher for her than for a woman not using an IUD who gets pregnant. That being said, the cumulative rate of ectopic pregnancy over 12 years in a large multicenter international investigation was only 0.4 per 100 woman-years.[89] Should a woman become pregnant with the IUD in place, the IUD should be removed to reduce the risk of miscarriage, septic abortion, and preterm labor.[11]

Concerns that IUD use could lead to tubal infertility were evaluated in a study[90] that demonstrated that tubal infertility is strongly associated with previous chlamydia infection; IUDs in isolation are not associated with infertility. Whether the IUD string can contribute to ascending pelvic infection in women who acquire a sexually transmitted infection is unknown, but current WHO guidelines do not mandate IUD removal in women diagnosed with an STI.[11]

Common Side Effects

Copper-containing IUDs are associated with increased menstrual blood flow and cramping. Blood loss increases by approximately 55% in copper IUD users.[91] Over several years of use, serum ferritin levels may drop; in women at high risk of iron deficiency anemia, assessment and possible supplementation may be warranted.[12,92] Use of nonsteroidal anti-inflammatory drugs or prostaglandin synthesis inhibitors effectively treats the cramping and can also treat heavy menses.[12] Treatment should begin at the onset of menses and continue for 3 days.

Tabe 29-4 WHO Medical Eligibility* Categories 3 and 4 Cautions for Intrauterine Contraception

Condition	Eligibility Category Warning	Comment
Postpartum	48 h to 4 wk postpartum: category 3 Recent puerperal or pelvic infection: category 4	
Pelvic disease	Any anatomical distortion of the uterine cavity: category 4 Unexplained uterine bleeding: category 4 until a diagnosis is established Malignant disease that might require frequent cervical or uterine procedures: category 4	Proper placement may not occur in cases of anatomical distortion.
Sexually transmitted infection	Current or recent STD: delay IUD insertion	Women at increased risk for acquiring STIs are not the best candidates for the method.
Liver disease	Progestin-releasing system not advised in women with active liver disease, liver tumors, current or history of breast cancer, current DVT, or current ischemic heart disease or stroke, or migraine with aura.	Concerns related to the possibility of systemic progestin effects and hypoestrogenic effects that may result in decreased HDL levels.

* Eligibility categories are as follows:
1. No restriction for the use of the contraceptive method.
2. Advantages of using the method generally outweigh the theoretical or proven risks.
3. Theoretical or proven risks usually outweigh the advantages of using the method.
4. The method should not be used.

Note: Intrauterine contraceptive devices and systems are within WHO category 1 or 2 for other conditions.
Source: World Health Organization 2004.[11]

The progestin-releasing systems are associated with frequent spotting for the first several months of use, followed by very light menses or amenorrhea. There are no data on effective treatment options; the administration of estrogen may interfere with the desired atrophic effect on the endometrium and is therefore not recommended as a treatment for irregular bleeding in this situation. Benign follicular cysts of the ovary can occur with any progestin-only method and have been observed among levonorgestrel intrauterine contraceptive/system (Mirena) users. Hormonal side effects such as breast pain, headaches, dizziness, acne, and mood swings also have been reported.

Cost and Availability

Intrauterine contraception costs include the device (approximately $350–$400), as well as the clinician visit for insertion. Removal requires a clinician visit as well. Although the initial outlay may seem sizable, when averaged over 5–10 years of potential use, intrauterine devices are among the most cost effective of contraceptive methods.

Spermicides

Spermicides are chemical substances used as contraceptives; they are intended to inactivate or kill sperm in the woman's reproductive tract, thus preventing fertilization. According to the 2002 National Survey of Family Growth, approximately 26% of women of reproductive age report ever using a spermicidal product as a sole method of birth control, but reported usage is concentrated in older age groups. Current use of spermicide as a sole contraceptive method is so low that it is not reported separately.[93] In Title X family planning clinics, an estimated 1–5% of women reported using nonoxynol-9 (N-9) formulations as their sole method of contraception.[94]

All spermicides currently marketed in the United States contain N-9. There are other products and spermicides available in other countries (menfegol, benzalkonium chloride, octoxynol), and some can be obtained via the Internet. Because spermicides share many characteristics with vaginal microbicides, and a woman-controlled contraceptive method also could reduce risk of sexually transmitted infections, a great deal of research and development is currently under way in regard to microbicides-spermicides. Dozens of potential spermicide-microbicides are in development and several are being studied in clinical trials. These include surfactants that disrupt the cell membranes of sperm and some pathogens, like N-9 (discussed later), octoxynol-9, menfegol, and benzalkonium chloride, and a compound known as C31G (Savvy). Buffering agents maintain acidity in the vagina in the presence of alkaline seminal fluid (a compound called BufferGel is in clinical trials). New products are likely to become available in the United States shortly.

Mechanism of Action

N-9 and similar spermicides are surfactants, designed to dissolve lipids in the sperm cell membrane, thus inactivating or killing the sperm. Because they are toxic to cell membranes, they also have the potential to disrupt cervical and vaginal epithelium. They may also alter vaginal flora, predisposing users to urinary tract infections.[95] There are various formulations for delivering the spermicide, including jellies, foams, creams, or soluble films. Vaginal suppositories and tablets that are designed to melt or foam after insertion are also available. These contain carbon dioxide, which forms bubbles to help disperse the product.

Spermicides can be used alone or with other barrier devices such as condoms, diaphragms, or cervical caps. Different formulations may need different amounts of time for dispersion of the N-9 product. For example, film or suppositories need time (approximately 10–15 minutes) to melt. Duration of activity once the agent is inserted in the vagina also is unclear. Some product instructions state that protection will last for 6–8 hours, although Speroff[54] warns that tablets and suppositories may have only 1 hour of effectiveness.

Doses of N-9 are generally 50–150 milligrams per dose. The contraceptive sponge contains approximately 1000 mg of N-9, but after being moistened, the sponge gradually releases 125–150 mg of spermicide over 24 hours of use. General instructions for use are the same for all N-9 products, although all of the products were on the market before FDA oversight was instituted and the package instructions are not necessarily evidence based.

A spermicide that acts as a buffering agent (Buffer-Gel) has recently been studied in clinical trials. In the natural acidity of the vagina, acid-sensitive sperm are immobilized and the alkalinity of semen acts to counter this effect. Buffering compounds maintain the acidic environment in the vagina and provide a contraceptive effect. Such products, however, are not yet available in the United States.

Efficacy

There are few well-done studies of the contraceptive effectiveness of spermicides alone. Typical-use 6-month pregnancy rates in well-designed studies ranged from 10% up to 28%,[96,97] which would extrapolate to 12-month failure rates of 18–39%. These studies compared N-9 in various formulations (film, tablets, suppositories, and gels), without other physical barriers. Formulations containing at least 100 mg of N-9 had lower pregnancy rates. Spermicides used alone are less effective in preventing pregnancy than other contraceptive methods, but use of spermicide continues to remain superior to using no method.

WHO Medical Eligibility

Spermicides are listed as WHO category 1 contraceptives for nearly all circumstances with the following exceptions. Spermicides are listed as category 2 contraceptives for women with cervical cancer awaiting treatment because frequent or high doses of N-9 can cause cervical irritation or abrasions. In addition, spermicides are listed as category 4 contraceptives for women at high risk of acquiring HIV or who have HIV infection or AIDS. This is because repeated and high-dose use of N-9 has been associated with genital lesions that may facilitate acquisition of HIV.

Adverse Effects

N-9 is an irritant in human tissue, and frequent use is associated with increased reports of vaginal irritation. The risk of damage to epithelial tissue in the vagina increases with frequency of use and dose. Despite assumptions that the surfactant activity might also disrupt other organisms and possibly prevent sexually transmitted infection, N-9 does not reduce this incidence of STIs among sex workers or women attending STI clinics,[98] and in fact may even increase the risk of HIV acquisition in high-risk women, although the etiology of this association remains unclear.[99]

The FDA recently required package labeling to state that N-9 does not provide protection against infection from HIV or other sexually transmitted diseases.[100] Contraindications for the use of N-9–based spermicides are: (1) N-9 should not be used for purpose of STI protection; (2) N-9 should not be used by women with multiple daily acts of intercourse; (3) N-9 should not be used by women at high risk for HIV acquisition; (4) N-9 should not be used rectally. However, for women at low risk of HIV acquisition, N-9 is an appropriate contraceptive option and is in fact intended to be used with other female barriers such as diaphragms and condoms.

Common Side Effects

Data from clinical trials describe the likelihood of developing certain genital infections over a period of 6–7 months of use. There is a 13–17% risk of developing a yeast infection, 8–12% probability of developing bacterial vaginosis, and a 19–27% chance of having general vulvovaginal irritation. Urinary tract symptoms have been reported among 11–15% of women using N-9 spermicides (although less than 6% are urinary tract infection by culture). Because these studies had no comparison groups, it is not clear if the rates are different from the general population of sexually active, contracepting women.[96]

Cost and Availability

Spermicides containing N-9 are widely available over the counter. These agents do not require a prescription or provider visit. Advantages for women include accessibility, personal control, and low cost. They are coitus-dependent in that they must be applied immediately prior to each act of intercourse.

Physical Barriers

Spermicides are often used in conjunction with **barrier contraceptive methods**, intended to prevent sperm from entering the upper reproductive tract where fertilization occurs. Barriers include male and female condoms and vaginal and cervical barriers. Some barriers are both physical and chemical barriers (such as the vaginal sponge) in that they also deliver a spermicide. Physical barriers are made of substances that may have some adverse effects in some users.

Mechanism of Action

Many condoms and other barriers are made of latex, an agent manufactured from a milky fluid obtained from the rubber tree (*Hevea brasiliensis*). The natural rubber proteins may induce latex allergy. Alternatives are natural skin condoms (made from lamb intestines) and synthetics (such as polyurethane). Lea's shield and FemCap, which are vaginal and cervical barrier devices, are latex free and composed of medical-grade silicone. The sponge that is available in the United States is made of polyurethane foam; the sponge also functions as a reservoir for 1000 mg of N-9, which is gradually released over 24 hours; it is somewhat less effective for multiparous women. Effective use assumes that the individual has both knowledge and dexterity required to properly use/insert and remove the devices.

WHO Medical Eligibility

Latex and polyurethane condoms are WHO category 1 contraceptives in all instances except the case of latex allergy. Nonlatex physical barrier devices have not been associated with allergic reactions.

Adverse Effects

Symptoms of latex allergy include irritant contact dermatitis, allergic dermatitis, and generalized hypersensitivity including anaphylaxis.

Common Side Effects

Spermicide-related side effects may occur with any of these devices if they are used in conjunction with the chemical agents. Diaphragms have been associated with an increased risk of urinary tract infection.

Cost and Availability

Condoms can be purchased over the counter; the latex condoms are cheaper than synthetic and natural skin condoms. Diaphragms must be fit by a clinician and thus the cost includes the fitting visit as well as the device. Lea's shield and FemCap are available through Planned Parenthood clinics and certain providers.

Emergency Contraception

Emergency contraception (EC) is a woman's only reliable option for preventing pregnancy after unprotected intercourse. There are two methods, which include insertion of a copper-containing IUD or a short course of oral contraceptive steroid hormones taken within 72 hours of unprotected intercourse. The latter is the much more commonly used method and is available over the counter for women age 18 and over.

Oral Emergency Contraception

Possibly the first documented case of oral **emergency contraception** was in the mid-1960s when physicians in the Netherlands gave estrogens to a 13-year-old girl who had been raped.[101] Initially, high-dose estrogens, either ethinyl estradiol (5 mg per day for 5 days) or diethyl stilbestrol (DES), became the standard for postcoital contraception (generally offered in cases of rape).[101]

In the 1970s, Yuzpe and colleagues published results of their studies on a combination of estrogen and progestin (levonorgestrel) as postcoital contraception; this regimen replaced the high-dose estrogen and DES formulations that were used originally. At approximately the same time, research began on progestin-only postcoital contraceptives. Kesseru[102] investigated using various doses of levonorgestrel as an ongoing postcoital method, instructing participants to take a tablet within 3 hours after intercourse. Women could use the method as often as necessary (up to 2 years for some).[5]

Oral EC may be one of two different types. The first, also known as the **Yuzpe regimen**, contains EE and levonorgestrel; the second contains levonorgestrel only. The Yuzpe method has been prescribed for decades and can be followed by taking a specified number of pills from specific brands of oral contraceptives (Table 29-5).

Table 29-5 Oral Contraceptives That Can Be Used for Emergency Contraception in the United States*

Brand	Company	Pills per Dose[†]	Ethinyl Estradiol per Dose (mcg)	Levonorgestrel per Dose (mg)[‡]
Progestin-only pills: take one dose[†]				
Plan-B	Barr/Duramed	2 white pills	0	1.5
Combined progestin and estrogen pills: take two doses 12 hours apart				
Alesse	Wyeth-Ayerst	5 pink pills	100	0.50
Aviane	Barr/Duramed	5 orange pills	100	0.50
Cryselle	Barr/Duramed	4 white pills	120	0.60
Enpresse	Barr/Duramed	4 orange pills	120	0.50
Jolessa	Barr/Duramed	4 pink pills	120	0.60
Lessina	Barr/Duramed	5 pink pills	100	0.50
Levlen	Berlex	4 light-orange pills	120	0.60
Levlite	Berlex	5 pink pills	100	0.50
Levora	Watson	4 white pills	120	0.60
Lo/Ovral	Wyeth-Ayerst	4 white pills	120	0.60
Low-Ogestrel	Watson	4 white pills	120	0.60
Lutera	Watson	5 white pills	100	0.50
Lybrel	Wyeth-Ayerst	6 yellow pills	120	0.54
Nordette	Wyeth-Ayerst	4 light-orange pills	120	0.60
Ogestrel	Watson	2 white pills	100	0.50
Ovral	Wyeth-Ayerst	2 white pills	100	0.50
Portia	Barr/Duramed	4 pink pills	120	0.60
Quasense	Watson	4 white pills	120	0.60
Seasonale	Barr/Duramed	4 pink pills	120	0.60
Seasonique	Barr/Duramed	4 light-blue-green pills	120	0.60
Tri-Levlen	Berlex	4 yellow pills	120	0.50
Triphasil	Wyeth-Ayerst	4 yellow pills	120	0.50
Trivora	Watson	4 pink pills	120	0.50

Notes: * Plan-B is the only dedicated product specifically marketed for emergency contraception. Alesse, Aviane, Cryselle, Enpresse, Jolessa, Lessina, Levlen, Levlite, Levora, Lo/Ovral, Low-Ogestrel, Lutera, Lybrel, Nordette, Ogestrel, Ovral, Portia, Quasense, Seasonale, Seasonique, Tri-Levlen, Triphasil, and Trivora have been declared safe and effective for use as ECPs by the US Food and Drug Administration. Worldwide, about 50 emergency contraceptive products are specifically packaged, labeled, and marketed. Levonorgestrel-only ECPs are available either over the counter or from a pharmacist without having to see a clinician in 50 countries.
[†]The label for Plan B says to take one pill within 72 hours after unprotected intercourse, and another pill 12 hours later. However, recent research has found that both Plan B pills can be taken at the same time. Research has also shown that all of the brands listed here are effective when used within 120 hours after unprotected sex.
[‡] The progestin in Cryselle, Lo/Ovral, Low-Ogestrel, Ogestrel, and Ovral is norgestrel, which contains two isomers, only one of which (levonorgestrel) is bioactive; the amount of norgestrel in each tablet is twice the amount of levonorgestrel.
Source: Reprinted with permission from The Emergency Contraception Web site (not-2-late.com).

In 1998, a dedicated product for emergency contraception (Preven), containing EE and levonorgestrel, was approved by the US FDA. Preven is no longer marketed because it was found to be less effective and has more side effects than levonorgestrel alone.

Plan B, a levonorgestrel-only emergency contraceptive, was approved in 1999, and approximately 3 million packages of levonorgestrel (Plan B) were sold in the United States and Canada by prescription after it was approved and marketed. Levonorgestrel (Plan B) was approved in the United States as an over-the-counter medication in 2006; however,

a prescription is still required for women under the age of 18. These age limits mandate its availability to be behind-the-counter in order for dispensing pharmacies to ensure the woman is over the age of 18. Levonorgestrel (Plan B) is the only EC that is available over the counter in the United States and other countries. It is labeled to be taken as two doses of 0.75 mg each, 12 hours apart, within 72 hours of unprotected intercourse. Both consumers and providers occasionally still call emergency contraception "the morning after pill"; however, this is a misnomer because these agents can be taken up to 72 hours after unprotected intercourse.

Mifepristone (Mifeprex), an antiprogesterone used for medication abortion and originally known as RU 486, also has been evaluated as a postcoital contraceptive. This agent is not approved for use as a postcoital contraceptive in the United States and is only available through clinicians or facilities providing medication abortion.

Mechanism of Action

How oral EC works is not entirely clear, and the mechanism of action may depend on when in the menstrual cycle it is taken. It is hypothesized that the high levels of hormones from the EC regimen, when taken around the time of ovulation, blunt the luteinizing hormone (LH) surge required for ovulation; thus an egg will not be released. However, it is statistically unlikely that the method could be as effective as it appears to be if interference with ovulation were the only mechanism of action. Other effects are hypothesized if ovulation has already occurred, including thickening of cervical mucus, slowing of tubal motility, interference with sperm transport, deficient luteal function, and changes in endometrium making it inhospitable to implantation.[103,104] Observations that a dose of estrogen and levonorgestrel caused changes in the endometrium that interfered with implantation led to the Yuzpe regimen, but recent studies have not supported an effect of altered endometrial receptivity that interferes with implantation.[5,68,105]

Dosing Considerations

EE and levonorgestrel are components of approved combination oral contraceptives. The current maximum dose of EE in the most commonly used products is 35 mcg. The current maximum dose of levonorgestrel in the commonly prescribed products is 0.15 mg per day (although hormonal contraceptives with higher doses may be available, they are not typically prescribed). For emergency contraception using the Yuzpe regimen, the dose is typically 200 mcg EE and 1 mg levonorgestrel divided into two doses taken 12 hours apart.[5] There are currently no dedicated EC products of this type available in the United States, but the regimen can be given using typical combination OCs (Table 29-5). While this regimen can be used if levonorgestrel-only methods are not available, the latter method is preferable because it is more effective and has fewer side effects. For levonorgestrel-only EC (Plan B), the dose recommended is 1.5 mg/day, taken either in a single dose or divided in two doses taken 12 hours apart. It is recommended that levonorgestrel (Plan B) be taken within 72 hours of having unprotected intercourse, although some

experts suggest it will continue to be effective up to 5 days after unprotected intercourse.

Efficacy

Postcoital hormonal contraception reduces the risk of pregnancy from approximately 8% to 1–2%, depending on the regimen used. This represents a 75% to 89% reduction in the risk of pregnancy following a single act of unprotected sex.[106,107] Oral EC prevents pregnancy during the days between intercourse and implantation; it is ineffective after implantation has occurred. Efficacy is best if EC is taken as directed as soon as possible after unprotected intercourse. In one study with the Yuzpe regimen, there were no significant differences in pregnancy rates (which ranged from approximately 1.5% to 2.25%) whether the regimen was begun on day 1, 2, or 3 after unprotected intercourse.[108] However, in the large World Health Organization trials,[109] efficacy was significantly and inversely related to time since unprotected coitus for both the Yuzpe regimen and levonorgestrel-only pills. Pregnancy rates were 0.5% and 1.5% if the pills were taken at 12 or 24 hours, respectively, and were 3–4% if the pills were taken on day 3.

Studies done by the World Health Organization have shown that levonorgestrel (Plan B) is an effective and well-tolerated regimen for postcoital contraception.[110] However, these current labeling recommendations (two doses taken 12 hours apart) create opportunity for missed second doses and possible decreased efficacy. A study found that a single dose of 1.5 mg (two 0.75-mg tablets taken together) is of equal efficacy with no increase in side effects.[111] Thus a single levonorgestrel dose of 1.5 mg can substitute for two 0.75-mg doses 12 hours apart; if using the United States-marketed levonorgestrel (Plan B) product, both doses can be taken at once.

Studies have examined whether other progestins (such as norethindrone) can be used as emergency contraception and suggest that such products are also somewhat effective.[112] However, there are no dedicated EC products using progestins other than levonorgestrel.

WHO Medical Eligibility

Table 29-6 describes the WHO eligibility criteria for emergency contraceptive use.[11] Note that the guidelines do not distinguish between levonorgestrel-only and combined oral contraception. Since the duration of use for EC purposes is so much less than for continued use of oral contraceptives, any potential for adverse effects is likely to have little clinical impact.[11]

Adverse Effects

Serious adverse effects following use of EC are unlikely given the short duration of use. Clinically significant reduction in bioavailability with CYP450 enzyme inducers is unreported, but given case reports of women using levonorgestrel-containing hormonal contraceptive implants who have experienced breakthrough pregnancies while concomitantly treated with CYP450 enzyme-inducing antiseizure medications, the possibility may exist.[113] Thus the possibility of drug–herb interactions with emergency contraception should be considered. Some authorities recommend increasing the dose, although studies are lacking to identify the appropriate dose change.[114]

The toxicologic profile of levonorgestrel is similar to other progestins. These steroids are generally nontoxic, even in high doses, when administered over a short period of time.[115] A number of studies of the risk of teratogenesis when COCs are inadvertently taken in early pregnancy have shown no increase in risk to the fetus. Concerns have been voiced that an EC failure may raise the risk of ectopic pregnancy due to effects on thickening reproductive tract mucus and slowing tubal motility, but there are no data to date that support this concern.[116] Given the vast number of women who have used EC, an increased risk of ectopic pregnancy is unlikely; in fact, use of EC may be protective against ectopic pregnancy because it prevents pregnancy effectively.

Common Side Effects

A study of over 2000 administrations demonstrated that levonorgestrel-only regimens used in emergency contraceptive doses are very well tolerated.[115] The Yuzpe regimen is associated with nausea (50% of women) and vomiting (nearly 19% of women). In comparison, the levonorgestrel-only formulation is associated with nausea in 23.1% of women taking it, and vomiting occurs in 5.6% of women taking levonorgestrel (Plan B).[110] Standard antiemetics can be used by women who experience nausea and vomiting with emergency contraceptive pills. Due to side effects associated with antiemetics, routine antiemetic prophylaxis is not recommended but should be offered if appropriate. Two hours is probably sufficient for absorption of the hormone dose, and no repeat dosing is needed if vomiting occurs after this time.[12]

Cost and Availability

Pharmacy availability of levonorgestrel (Plan B) is not universal, and there are documented instances of pharmacists refusing to provide the product.[117]

Table 29-6 WHO Medical Eligibility* Criteria for Oral Hormonal Emergency Contraception

EC Regimen	Recommended Dosage	Instructions for Use	WHO Eligibility[†]
Levonorgestrel only (Plan B)	1.5 mg levonorgestrel	Take in two doses of 0.75 mg each, 12 hours apart, or take 1.5 mg (both tablets) at once.	1[‡]
Yuzpe regimen[§]	200 mcg ethinyl estradiol plus 1 mg levonorgestrel	Take in two doses 12 hours apart, beginning as soon as possible after unprotected intercourse.	1[‡]

* Eligibility categories are as follows:
1. No restriction for the use of the contraceptive method.
2. Advantages of using the method generally outweigh the theoretical or proven risks.
3. Theoretical or proven risks usually outweigh the advantages of using the method.
4. The method should not be used.

[†] WHO criteria do not distinguish between levonorgestrel only and combined oral contraceptives used as emergency contraception.

[‡] Exceptions are women with a history of severe cardiovascular complications or angina, those with migraine, and those with severe liver disease. For these women, the regimen is a category 2 contraceptive.

[§] No dedicated product currently available in the United States. Dosages are approximate, depending on which oral contraceptives are used.

Source: World Health Organization 2004.[11]

Intrauterine Device for Emergency Contraception

Intrauterine contraceptive devices are discussed in more detail elsewhere in this chapter, but it is important to include the copper-bearing devices in this section as they can be used for postcoital contraception by being inserted up to 5 days after an episode of unprotected intercourse. This use was first reported by Lippes and Tatum in 1976.[118]

Mechanism of Action

The copper in the intrauterine device has toxic effects on ovum and sperm; thus its effectiveness in inhibiting fertilization is immediate following insertion. The copper IUD, as a secondary mode of action, may prevent implantation if fertilization has already occurred.

Efficacy

In a review of 20 studies and over 8000 insertions, the failure rate for copper IUD insertion as a postcoital contraceptive was estimated at 0.1%.[119] This is far lower than the failure rate for the Yuzpe and progestin-only regimens.

WHO Medical Eligibility

The WHO criteria for the use of the copper IUD as a postcoital contraceptive are the same as the recommendations for its use as a contraceptive in general. It is listed as a WHO medical eligibility category 3 contraceptive for women at high risk of acquiring an STI (this would apply to women who have been raped), and a category 1 contraceptive for women at low risk for STIs.

Side Effects/Adverse Effects

Adverse effects and side effects are the same as the effects listed in the section on intrauterine contraception.

Cost and Availability

Copper-bearing intrauterine contraceptive devices are more expensive than oral emergency contraception. Some clinicians or programs also require testing for STIs prior to insertion of the IUD. The advantage, however, is that the device provides excellent continuing long-term contraception for 10 years, and thus, it may be the best form of EC for some individuals.

Medication Abortion

For women with unintended pregnancy, termination of the pregnancy is an option. Surgical abortion may not be available for many women, or medication options may be preferred. There are three drugs currently used in the United States for medical termination of a pregnancy.

Mechanism of Action

Mifepristone (Mifeprex) is an antiprogestin and blocks the action of progesterone, which is necessary for the maintenance of pregnancy. Thus, mifepristone will cause the uterine lining to shed. Methotrexate (Trexall) is an antimetabolite that interferes with the growth of rapidly dividing cells and is used to treat certain conditions such as neoplastic disease, psoriasis, and rheumatoid arthritis. It is sometimes used to terminate a pregnancy. Methotrexate (Trexall) acts on the cytotrophoblast rather than the embryo and is effective in treating extrauterine pregnancies. Misoprostol (Cytotec) is a prostaglandin analog that produces a softening of the cervix and uterine contractions, which result in the expulsion of uterine contents. Misoprostol is approved for the prevention and treatment of stomach ulcers.

Dosing and Efficacy

In 2000, the US FDA approved the use of mifepristone in conjunction with misoprostol for the termination of early pregnancy. The FDA-approved regimen (based on older research) calls for oral dosing with 600 mg of mifepristone, followed 2 days later by 400 mcg of misoprostol taken orally to terminate a pregnancy of no more than 49 days' gestation. A number of alternate, evidence-based regimens are also used in the United States. In most, the dose of mifepristone is 200 mg orally. Misoprostol is then administered orally (400 mcg) or vaginally (800 mcg) 1, 2, or 3 days later (depending on institutional protocols). Following this regimen, 95% of women will abort completely but success is somewhat less in women who have a more advanced gestation. Effective termination of pregnancies up to 63 days' gestation has been demonstrated.[120]

Methotrexate (Trexall) is generally given by injection (50 mg/m²), followed by administration of vaginal misoprostol (Cytotec) 3–7 days later. If the pregnancy is less than 49 days' gestational age, 95% of women using this method will abort completely, but in 20–30%, it may take longer than the mifepristone regimen (as long as 1–5 weeks).[120]

There is no standard protocol for use of misoprostol (Cytotec) alone for termination of early pregnancy, and it is not approved for this use. Studies have evaluated several dosing regimens, most providing 600–800 mcg vaginally at periodic intervals, with efficacy ranging from 65% to 90%.[120]

Contraindications

Use of mifepristone (Mifeprex) is contraindicated in the following situations: the woman has a confirmed or suspected ectopic pregnancy, history of allergy to mifepristone; chronic use of corticosteroids; chronic adrenal failure; coagulopathy or current therapy with anticoagulants; and inherited porphyria. Methotrexate (Trexall) is contraindicated in women with a history of allergy or intolerance to methotrexate, coagulopathy or current severe anemia, acute or chronic renal or hepatic disease, acute inflammatory bowel disease, or uncontrolled seizure disorders. Misoprostol is contraindicated in women with a history of allergy. Intrauterine devices should be removed before medication abortion regimens are begun.

Side Effects/Adverse Effects

Reported side effects of medication abortion regimens are sometimes difficult to distinguish from the abortion itself, but include nausea, vomiting, diarrhea, dizziness, headache, fever, chills, and cramping. In some cases, the abortion may be incomplete, or the uterine bleeding following abortion may be prolonged; approximately 2–10% of women will require intervention for these events.[121] Additional side effects of methotrexate (Trexall) include oral ulcers. Uterine and abdominal pain are managed with analgesics and opiates.

There is no evidence that mifepristone (Mifeprex) is associated with birth defects in the case of failed abortion, but methotrexate (Trexall) has been associated with birth defects when given in high doses, and misoprostol (Cytotec) is associated with a birth defect known as Mobius syndrome, although the causal relationship is unclear and the actual risk is low.

From 2003 to 2006, there were reports of five deaths associated with medication abortion. These were attributed to infection with *Clostridium sordelli*, a gram-positive, toxin-producing anaerobe. Clostridial toxic shock syndrome has been known to occur in women with genital tract infections; the actual risk is unknown but presumed to be rare.[122] Some providers eliminated vaginal dosing of misoprostol in response to these deaths, although it is not clear that contamination from the gastrointestinal tract was responsible for the infection; others maintain vaginal dosing due to evidence of improved efficacy at certain gestational ages. Another death in a woman undergoing medication abortion occurred from an undiagnosed ectopic pregnancy; the actual risk of such a complication is low, estimated at approximately 0.02%.[123]

Hormonal Contraception for Men

There are no hormonal contraceptive methods currently available for men in the United States. In part, this is because development of hormonal contraceptives for men must target the continuous production of sperm over a period of several weeks, as opposed to targeting ovulation and a defined fertile period in women. Research on hormonal control of male fertility has evaluated the contraceptive efficacy of interfering with hormonal support necessary for the development, maturation, function, and transport of sperm. Suppression of LH and FSH in men via administration of a progestin inhibits the production of sperm in the testes. However, testosterone production is also inhibited, and most regimens being studied require adding additional synthetic testosterone to reverse adverse effects on libido and ejaculatory function.[124] A nonhormonal derivative of cottonseed oil (gossypol) has been studied in China, and it appears to effectively suppress sperm production without effects on testosterone; however, it is associated with a number of side effects.[125]

Conclusion

There are a number of pharmacologic options for contraception available for women in the United States. Nonetheless, of the 6 million pregnancies that occur each year, approximately half (48%) are unintended. Half of those unintended pregnancies occur among couples who were actively practicing contraception; the remainder occurs among couples who were not using a birth control method at the time of conception.[126,127] Couples who stop a contraceptive method often increase their risk of unintended pregnancy by substituting a less effective method or no method at all; approximately 80% either fail to use a substitute contraceptive or adopt one that is less effective.[128,129]

Given that approximately 1 million pregnancies a year result from contraceptive misuse and discontinuation, identification of women in need of contraceptive options is a critically important responsibility of clinicians. Counseling on contraceptive options, assisting women with selection of appropriate methods, and follow-up to ensure persistence with a method or a method change if indicated should improve the efficient and continued use of contraception. The best contraceptive method is one that the woman wants and the one that she will be able to use successfully.

References

1. Riddle JM. Contraception and abortion from the ancient world to the Renaissance. Cambridge, MA: Harvard University Press, 1992.
2. Tone A. Devices and desires: a history of contraceptives in America. New York: Hill & Wong, 2001.

3. Skuy P. Tales of contraception. Toronto, Ontario, Canada: Janssen-Ortho, Inc., 1995.

4. Parisot J. Johnny come lately: a short history of the condom. London: Journeyman Press, 1987.

5. Ellertson C. History and efficacy of emergency contraception: beyond Coca-Cola. Fam Plann Perspect 1996;28(2):44–8.

6. Wallach M, Grimes DA. Modern oral contraception. Totowa, NJ: Emron, 2000.

7. DHHS Code of Federal Regulations 45CFR46.203. In Services DoHaH, ed.; 1978.

8. Hughes EC. Gametogenesis and fertilization. In ACOG, ed. Obstetric-gynecologic terminology. Philadelphia, PA: Davis, 1972.

9. Benson Gold, R. The implications of defining when a woman is pregnant. 2005. Available from: *www.guttmacher.org/pubs/tgr/08/2/gr080207.html* [Accessed February 2, 2008].

10. Dunson DB, Colombo B, Baird DD. Changes with age in the level and duration of fertility in the menstrual cycle. Hum Reprod 2002;17(5):1399–403.

11. WHO. Medical eligibility criteria for contraceptive use, 3rd ed. Geneva, Switzerland: World Health Organization, 2004.

12. WHO. Selected practice recommendations for contraceptive use, 2nd ed. Geneva, Switzerland: World Health Organization, 2005.

13. Mosher WD, Martinez GM, Chandra A, Abma JC, Willson SJ. Use of contraception and use of family planning services in the United States: 1982–2002. Adv Data 2004;(350):1–36.

14. Speroff L, Fritz MA. Clinical gynecologic endocrinology and infertility, 7th ed. Philadelphia, PA: Lippincott Willams & Wilkins, 2005.

15. Sulak PJ, Scow RD, Preece C, Riggs MW, Kuehl TJ. Hormone withdrawal symptoms in oral contraceptive users. Obstet Gynecol 2000;95(2):261–6.

16. Elomaa K, Rolland R, Brosens I, Moorrees M, Deprest J, Tuominen J, et al. Omitting the first oral contraceptive pills of the cycle does not automatically lead to ovulation. Am J Obstet Gynecol 1998;179(1):41–6.

17. Birtch RL, Olatunbosun OA, Pierson RA. Ovarian follicular dynamics during conventional vs. continuous oral contraceptive use. Contraception 2006;73(3):235–43.

18. Miller L, Notter KM. Menstrual reduction with extended use of combination oral contraceptive pills: randomized controlled trial. Obstet Gynecol 2001;98 (5, pt 1):771–8.

19. Sulak PJ, Kuehl TJ, Ortiz M, Shull BL. Acceptance of altering the standard 21-day/7-day oral contraceptive regimen to delay menses and reduce hormone withdrawal symptoms. Am J Obstet Gynecol 2002; 186(6):71142–9.

20. Burkman RT. The transdermal contraceptive system. Am J Obstet Gynecol 2004;190(suppl 4):S49–S53.

21. van den Heuvel MW, van Bragt AJ, Alnabawy AK, Kaptein MC. Comparison of ethinylestradiol pharmacokinetics in three hormonal contraceptive formulations: the vaginal ring, the transdermal patch and an oral contraceptive. Contraception 2005;72(3):168–74.

22. US Food and Drug Administration. Ortho Evra (norelgestromin/ethinyl estradiol) information. 2008. Available from: *www.fda.gov/cder/drug/infopage/orthoevra/default.htm* [Accessed February 2, 2008].

23. Jick SS, Kaye JA, Russmann S, Jick H. Risk of nonfatal venous thromboembolism in women using a contraceptive transdermal patch and oral contraceptives containing norgestimate and 35 microg of ethinyl estradiol. Contraception 2006;73(3):223–8.

24. Cole JA, Norman H, Doherty M, Walker AM. Venous thromboembolism, myocardial infarction, and stroke among transdermal contraceptive system users. Obstet Gynecol 2007;109(2, pt 1):339–46.

25. Coutinho EM, Mascarenhas I, de Acosta OM, Flores JG, Gu ZP, Ladipo OA, et al. Comparative study on the efficacy, acceptability, and side effects of a contraceptive pill administered by the oral and the vaginal route: an international multicenter clinical trial. Clin Pharmacol Ther 1993;54(5):540–5.

26. Ziaei S, Rajaei L, Faghihzadeh S, Lamyian M. Comparative study and evaluation of side effects of low-dose contraceptive pills administered by the oral and vaginal route. Contraception 2002;65(5):329–31.

27. Organon. [Nuvaring package insert]. Available from: *http://www.nuvaring.com/Authfiles/Images/309_76063.pdf* [Accessed June 29, 2009].

28. Mulders TM, Dieben TO, Bennink HJ. Ovarian function with a novel combined contraceptive vaginal ring. Hum Reprod 2002;17(10):2594–9.

29. Miller L, Verhoeven CH, Hout J. Extended regimens of the contraceptive vaginal ring: a randomized trial. Obstet Gynecol 2005;106(3):473–82.

30. Westhoff C, Morroni C, Kerns J, Murphy PA. Bleeding patterns after immediate vs. conventional oral contraceptive initiation: a randomized, controlled trial. Fertil Steril 2003;79(2):322–9.

31. Trussell J. Choosing a contraceptive: efficacy, safety and personal considerations. In Hatcher RA, Trussell J, Nelson AL, Cates W Jr, Stewart F, Kowal D, eds. Contraceptive technology, 19th ed. New York: Ardent Media, 2008:19–41.

32. Summary table of contraceptive efficacy. 2007. Available from: *www.contraceptivetechnology.org/table.html* [Accessed February 2, 2008].

33. Raucy JL. Regulation of CYP3A4 expression in human hepatocytes by pharmaceuticals and natural products. Drug Metab Dispos 2003;31(5):533–9.

34. Back DJ, Orme ML. Pharmacokinetic drug interactions with oral contraceptives. Clin Pharmacokinet 1990;18(6):472–84.

35. Li AP, Jurima-Romet M. Overview: pharmacokinetic drug–drug interactions. Adv Pharmacol 1997;43:1–6.

36. Back DJ, Breckenridge AM, Crawford FE, Hall JM, MacIver M, Orme ML, et al. The effect of rifampicin on the pharmacokinetics of ethynyl estradiol in women. Contraception 1980;21(2):135–43.

37. Ioannides C. Pharmacokinetic interactions between herbal remedies and medicinal drugs. Xenobiotica 2002;32(6):451–78.

38. Murphy PA, Kern SE, Stanczyk FZ, Westhoff CL. Interaction of St. John's wort with oral contraceptives: effects on the pharmacokinetics of norethindrone and ethinyl estradiol, ovarian activity and breakthrough bleeding. Contraception 2005;71(6):402–8.

39. Boden DC. Unplanned pregnancies and the pill. Med J Aust 1980;1(8):391.

40. Holt VL, Cushing-Haugen KL, Daling JR. Body weight and risk of oral contraceptive failure. Obstet Gynecol 2002;99(5, pt 1):820–7.

41. Brunner Huber LR, Hogue CJ. The association between body weight, unintended pregnancy resulting in a live birth, and contraception at the time of conception. Matern Child Health J 2005:9(4):1–8.

42. Brunner LR, Hogue CJ. The role of body weight in oral contraceptive failure: results from the 1995 national survey of family growth. Ann Epidemiol 2005;15(7):492–9.

43. Brunner Huber LR, Hogue CJ, Stein AD, Drews C, Zieman M. Body mass index and risk for oral contraceptive failure: a case-cohort study in South Carolina. Ann Epidemiol 2006;16(8):637–43.

44. Brunner Huber LR, Toth JL. Obesity and oral contraceptive failure: findings from the 2002 National Survey of Family Growth. Am J Epidemiol 2007;166 (11):1306–11.

45. Zieman M, Guillebaud J, Weisberg E, Shangold GA, Fisher AC, Creasy GW. Contraceptive efficacy and cycle control with the Ortho Evra/Evra transdermal system: the analysis of pooled data. Fertil Steril 2002; 77(2, suppl 2):S13–S18.

46. Speroff L, Andolsek KM. Hormonal contraception and obesity. Dialogues Contraception 2003;8(2):1–4.

47. Tanis BC, van den Bosch MA, Kemmeren JM, Cats VM, Helmerhorst FM, Algra A, et al. Oral contraceptives and the risk of myocardial infarction. N Engl J Med 2001;345(25):1787–93.

48. Rosenberg L, Palmer JR, Rao RS, Shapiro S. Low-dose oral contraceptive use and the risk of myocardial infarction. Arch Intern Med 2001;161(8):1065–70.

49. Chang CL, Donaghy M, Poulter N. Migraine and stroke in young women: case-control study. The World Health Organisation Collaborative Study of Cardiovascular Disease and Steroid Hormone Contraception. BMJ 1999;318(7175):13–8.

50. RCGP. Oral contraceptives, venous thrombosis, and varicose veins. Royal College of General Practitioners' Oral Contraception Study. J R Coll Gen Pract 1978; 28(192):393–9.

51. Spitzer WO, Lewis MA, Heinemann LA, Thorogood M, MacRae KD. Third generation oral contraceptives and risk of venous thromboembolic disorders: an international case-control study. Transnational Research Group on Oral Contraceptives and the Health of Young Women. BMJ 1996;312(7023):83–8.

52. Lewis MA, Heinemann LA, MacRae KD, Bruppacher R, Spitzer WO. The increased risk of venous thromboembolism and the use of third generation progestagens: role of bias in observational research. The Transnational Research Group on Oral Contraceptives and the Health of Young Women. Contraception 1996;54(1):5–13.

53. Vandenbroucke JP, Van der Meer FJ, Helmerhorst FM, Rosendaal FR. Factor V Leiden: should we screen oral contraceptive users and pregnant women? BMJ 1996;313(7065):1127–30.

54. Speroff L, Darney PD. A clinical guide to contraception, 4th ed. Philadelphia, PA: Lippincott Williams & Wilkins, 2005.

55. Redmond G, Godwin AJ, Olson W, Lippman JS. Use of placebo controls in an oral contraceptive trial: methodological issues and adverse event incidence. Contraception 1999;60(2):81–5.

56. Rosenberg MJ, Meyers A, Roy V. Efficacy, cycle control, and side effects of low- and lower-dose oral contraceptives: a randomized trial of 20 micrograms and 35 micrograms estrogen preparations. Contraception 1999;60(6):321–9.

57. Audet MC, Moreau M, Koltun WD, Waldbaum AS, Shangold G, Fisher AC, et al. Evaluation of contra-

ceptive efficacy and cycle control of a transdermal contraceptive patch vs an oral contraceptive: a randomized controlled trial. JAMA 2001;285(18):2347–54.

58. Huber J, Walch K. Treating acne with oral contraceptives: use of lower doses. Contraception 2006;73(1):23–9.

59. Hatcher R, Trussel J, Nelson AL, Cates Jr W, Stewart F, Kowal D, eds. Contraceptive technology, 19th ed. New York: Ardent Media, Inc., 2008.

60. Hansen TH, Lundvall F. Factors influencing the reliability of oral contraceptives. Acta Obstet Gynecol Scand 1997;76(1):61–4.

61. Graham CA, Bancroft J, Doll HA, Greco T, Tanner A. Does oral contraceptive-induced reduction in free testosterone adversely affect the sexuality or mood of women? Psychoneuroendocrinology 2007;32(3):246–55.

62. Graham CA, Ramos R, Bancroft J, Maglaya C, Farley TM. The effects of steroidal contraceptives on the well-being and sexuality of women: a double-blind, placebo-controlled, two-centre study of combined and progestogen-only methods. Contraception 1995;52(6):363–9.

63. Brown C, Ling F, Wan J. A new monophasic oral contraceptive containing drospirenone. Effect on premenstrual symptoms. J Reprod Med 2002;47(1):14–22.

64. Freeman EW, Kroll R, Rapkin A, Pearlstein T, Brown C, Parsey K, et al. Evaluation of a unique oral contraceptive in the treatment of premenstrual dysphoric disorder. J Womens Health Gend Based Med 2001;10(6):561–9.

65. Sheth A, Jain U, Sharma S, Adatia A, Patankar S, Andolsek L, et al. A randomized, double-blind study of two combined and two progestogen-only oral contraceptives. Contraception 1982;25(3):243–52.

66. Kjos SL, Peters RK, Xiang A, Thomas D, Schaefer U, Buchanan TA. Contraception and the risk of type 2 diabetes mellitus in Latina women with prior gestational diabetes mellitus. JAMA 1998;280(6):533–8.

67. Broome M, Fotherby K. Clinical experience with the progestogen-only pill. Contraception 1990;42(5):489–95.

68. ACOG. Emergency contraception. ACOG Pract Bull 2005;69:1–10.

69. Scholes D, La Croix AZ, Ichikawa LE, Barlow WE, Ott SM. Injectable hormone contraception and bone density: results from a prospective study. Epidemiology 2002;13(5):581–7.

70. Petitti DB, Piaggio G, Mehta S, Cravioto MC, Meirik O. Steroid hormone contraception and bone mineral density: a cross-sectional study in an international population. The WHO Study of Hormonal Contraception and Bone Health. Obstet Gynecol 2000;95(5):736–44.

71. Scholes D, LaCroix AZ, Ichikawa LE, Barlow WE, Ott SM. Change in bone mineral density among adolescent women using and discontinuing depot medroxyprogesterone acetate contraception. Arch Pediatr Adolesc Med 2005;159(2):139–44.

72. Lopez LM, Grimes DA, Schulz KF, Curtis KM. Steroidal contraceptives: effect on bone fractures in women. Cochrane Database Syst Rev 2006(4):CD006033.

73. Grimes DA, Schulz KF. Surrogate end points in clinical research: hazardous to your health. Obstet Gynecol 2005;105(5, pt 1):1114–8.

74. d'Arcangues C. WHO statement on hormonal contraception and bone health. Contraception 2006;73(5):443–4.

75. Depo-Provera contraceptive injection patient labeling. 2006. Available from: *www.pfizer.com/files/products/ppi_depo_provera_contraceptive.pdf* [Accessed June 29, 2009].

76. Bonny AE, Britto MT, Huang B, Succop P, Slap GB. Weight gain, adiposity, and eating behaviors among adolescent females on depot medroxyprogesterone acetate (DMPA). J Pediatr Adolesc Gynecol 2004;17(2):109–15.

77. Mangan SA, Larsen PG, Hudson S. Overweight teens at increased risk for weight gain while using depot medroxyprogesterone acetate. J Pediatr Adolesc Gynecol 2002;15(2):79–82.

78. Espey E, Steinhart J, Ogburn T, Qualls C. Depo-provera associated with weight gain in Navajo women. Contraception 2000;62(2):55–8.

79. Croxatto HB, Makarainen L. The pharmacodynamics and efficacy of Implanon. An overview of the data. Contraception 1998;58(6 suppl):91S–7S.

80. Makarainen L, van Beek A, Tuomivaara L, Asplund B, Coelingh Bennink H. Ovarian function during the use of a single contraceptive implant: Implanon compared with Norplant. Fertil Steril 1998;69(4):714–21.

81. Organon. [Implanon (etonogestrel implant) physician's insert]. 2006. Available from: *www.implanon-usa.com/authfiles/images/543_174733.pdf* [Accessed June 29, 2009].

82. Funk S, Miller MM, Mishell DR Jr, Archer DF, Poindexter A, Schmidt J, et al. Safety and efficacy of

Implanon, a single-rod implantable contraceptive containing etonogestrel. Contraception 2005;71(5):319–26.

83. ACOG. Intrauterine device. ACOG Pract Bull 2005;59:1–9.

84. Rosenblatt KA, Thomas DB. Intrauterine devices and endometrial cancer. The WHO Collaborative Study of Neoplasia and Steroid Contraceptives. Contraception 1996;54(6):329–32.

85. Sturgeon SR, Brinton LA, Berman ML, Mortel R, Twiggs LB, Barrett RJ, et al. Intrauterine device use and endometrial cancer risk. Int J Epidemiol 1997; 26(3):496–500.

86. Lassise DL, Savitz DA, Hamman RF, Baron AE, Brinton LA, Levines RS. Invasive cervical cancer and intrauterine device use. Int J Epidemiol 1991;20(4): 865–70.

87. Grimes DA, Schulz KF. Prophylactic antibiotics for intrauterine device insertion: a meta-analysis of the randomized controlled trials. Contraception 1999; 60(2):57–63.

88. Nelson AL. The intrauterine contraceptive device. Obstet Gynecol Clin North Am 2000;27(4):723–40.

89. WHO. Long-term reversible contraception. Twelve years of experience with the TCu380A and TCu220C. Contraception 1997;56(6):341–52.

90. Hubacher D, Lara-Ricalde R, Taylor DJ, Guerra-Infante F, Guzman-Rodriguez R. Use of copper intrauterine devices and the risk of tubal infertility among nulligravid women. N Engl J Med 2001;345(8):561–7.

91. Milsom I, Andersson K, Jonasson K, Lindstedt G, Rybo G. The influence of the Gyne-T 380S IUD on menstrual blood loss and iron status. Contraception 1995;52(3):175–9.

92. Hassan EO, el-Husseini M, el-Nahal N. The effect of 1-year use of the CuT 380A and oral contraceptive pills on hemoglobin and ferritin levels. Contraception 1999;60(2):101–5.

93. Chandra A, Martinez GM, Mosher WD, Abma JC, Jones J. Fertility, family planning, and reproductive health of US women: data from the 2002 National Survey of Family Growth. Vital Health Stat 2005;23(25):1–160.

94. CDC. From the Centers for Disease Control and Prevention. Nonoxynol-9 spermicide contraception use—United States, 1999. JAMA 2002;287(22):2938–9.

95. Scholes D, Hooton TM, Roberts PL, Stapleton AE, Gupta K, Stamm WE. Risk factors for recurrent urinary tract infection in young women. J Infect Dis 2000;182(4):1177–82.

96. Raymond EG, Chen PL, Luoto J, Group ST. Contraceptive effectiveness and safety of five nonoxynol-9 spermicides: a randomized trial. Obstet Gynecol 2004;103(3):430–9.

97. Raymond E, Dominik R. Contraceptive effectiveness of two spermicides: a randomized trial. Obstet Gynecol 1999;93(6):896–903.

98. Wilkinson D, Tholandi M, Ramjee G, Rutherford GW. Nonoxynol-9 spermicide for prevention of vaginally acquired HIV and other sexually transmitted infections: systematic review and meta-analysis of randomised controlled trials including more than 5000 women. Lancet Infect Dis 2002;2(10):613–7.

99. Van Damme L, Ramjee G, Alary M, et al. Effectiveness of COL-1492, a nonoxynol-9 vaginal gel, on HIV-1 transmission in female sex workers: a randomised controlled trial. Lancet 2002;360(9338):971–7.

100. US Food and Drug Administration. FDA mandates new warning for nonoxynol 9 OTC Contraceptive products. 2007. Available from: *www.fda.gov/ bbs/topics/NEWS/2007/NEW01758.html* [Accessed February 2, 2008].

101. Haspels AA. Emergency contraception: a review. Contraception 1994;50(2):101–8.

102. Kesseru E, Larranga A, Parada J. Post-coital contraception with D-norgestrel. Contraception 1973;7: 367–79.

103. Croxatto HB, Devoto L, Durand M, Ezcurra E, Larrea F, Nagle C, et al. Mechanism of action of hormonal preparations used for emergency contraception: a review of the literature. Contraception 2001;63(3):111–21.

104. Ugocsai G, Rozsa M, Ugocsai P. Scanning electron microscopic (SEM) changes of the endometrium in women taking high doses of levonorgestrel as emergency postcoital contraception. Contraception 2002;66(6):433–7.

105. Yuzpe AA. Postcoital contraception. Int J Gynaecol Obstet 1978;16(6):497–501.

106. Trussell J, Rodriguez G, Ellertson C. Updated estimates of the effectiveness of the Yuzpe regimen of emergency contraception. Contraception 1999;59(3): 147–51.

107. Trussell J, Rodriguez G, Ellertson C. New estimates of the effectiveness of the Yuzpe regimen of emergency contraception. Contraception 1998;57(6):363–9.

108. Trussell J, Ellertson C, Rodriguez G. The Yuzpe regimen of emergency contraception: how long after the morning after? Obstet Gynecol 1996;88(1):150–4.

109. Piaggio G, von Hertzen H, Grimes DA, Van Look PF. Timing of emergency contraception with levonorgestrel or the Yuzpe regimen. Task Force on Postovulatory Methods of Fertility Regulation. Lancet 1999;353(9154):721.

110. WHO. Randomised controlled trial of levonorgestrel versus the Yuzpe regimen of combined oral contraceptives for emergency contraception. Task Force on Postovulatory Methods of Fertility Regulation. Lancet 1998;352(9126):428–33.

111. von Hertzen H, Piaggio G, Ding J, et al. Low dose mifepristone and two regimens of levonorgestrel for emergency contraception: a WHO multicentre randomised trial. Lancet 2002;360(9348):1803–10.

112. Ellertson C, Evans M, Ferden S, Leadbetter C, Spears A, Johnstone K, et al. Extending the time limit for starting the Yuzpe regimen of emergency contraception to 120 hours. Obstet Gynecol 2003; 101(6):1168–71.

113. Odlind V, Olsson SE. Enhanced metabolism of levonorgestrel during phenytoin treatment in a woman with Norplant implants. Contraception 1986;33(3):257–61.

114. The Emergency Contraception Web site. 2007. Available from: *http://ec.princeton.edu/questions/ecdilantin.html* [Accessed June 29, 2009].

115. Gainer E, Mery C, Ulmann A. Levonorgestrel-only emergency contraception: real-world tolerance and efficacy. Contraception 2001;64(1):17–21.

116. Trussell J, Hedley A, Raymond E. Ectopic pregnancy following use of progestin-only ECPs. J Fam Plann Reprod Health Care 2003;29(4):249.

117. Cantor J, Baum K. The limits of conscientious objection—may pharmacists refuse to fill prescriptions for emergency contraception? N Engl J Med 2004;351(19):2008–12.

118. Lippes J, Malik T, Tatum HJ. The postcoital copper-T. Adv Plan Parent 1976;11(1):24–9.

119. Trussell J, Ellertson C. Efficacy of emergency contraception. Fertil Control Rev 1995;4(2):8–11.

120. Pymar HC, Creinin MD. Alternatives to mifepristone regimens for medical abortion. Am J Obstet Gynecol 2000;183(suppl 2):S54–S64.

121. Kruse B, Poppema S, Creinin MD, Paul M. Management of side effects and complications in medical abortion. Am J Obstet Gynecol 2000;183 (2 suppl):S65–S75.

122. Beal MW. Update on medication abortion. J Midwifery Womens Health 2007;52(1):23–30.

123. Shannon C, Brothers LP, Philip NM, Winikoff B. Ectopic pregnancy and medical abortion. Obstet Gynecol 2004;104(1):161–7.

124. Brady BM, Anderson RA. Advances in male contraception. Expert Opin Investig Drugs 2002;11(3): 333–44.

125. Coutinho EM. Gossypol: a contraceptive for men. Contraception 2002;65(4):259–63.

126. Finer LB, Henshaw SK. Abortion incidence and services in the United States in 2000. Perspect Sex Reprod Health 2003;35(1):6–15.

127. Martin JA, Hamilton BE, Sutton PD, Ventura SJ, Menacker F, Munson ML. Births: final data for 2002. Natl Vital Stat Rep 2003;52(10):1–113.

128. Rosenberg MJ, Waugh MS. Oral contraceptive discontinuation: a prospective evaluation of frequency and reasons. Am J Obstet Gynecol 1998;179 (3, pt 1):577–82.

129. Trussell J. The cost of unintended pregnancy in the United States. Contraception 2007;75(3):168.

30

Pelvic and Menstrual Disorders

Kerri Durnell Schuiling and Mary C. Brucker

Chapter Glossary

Abnormal uterine bleeding (AUB) Excessive bleeding during menses or bleeding that occurs outside of the normal menstrual cycle bleeding.

Coxibs (COX-2 inhibitors) Drugs that selectively inhibit the COX-2 isoform of cyclooxygenase, thereby inhibiting the production of proinflammatory prostaglandins without inhibiting the COX-1 isoform. The COX-1 isoform is involved in the production of prostaglandins that have a protective function in maintaining gastrointestinal mucosa and other homeostatic functions.

Cyclooxygenase (COX) The enzyme that converts arachidonic acid to prostaglandin.

Down-regulation The process by which a cell decreases the number of cell membrane receptors.

Dysfunctional uterine bleeding (DUB) Abnormal uterine bleeding for which no etiology can be detected.

Dysmenorrhea Painful menstruation wherein the uterine pain interferes with daily activities and/or requires medication.

Flare Exacerbation of symptoms of dysfunctional uterine bleeding that occurs initially when gonadotropin-releasing hormone (GnRH) therapy is started.

Menometrorrhagia Excessive bleeding during both normal cycle menses and menses that result from irregular cycle intervals.

Menorrhagia Heavy bleeding during normal menses.

Metrorrhagia Uterine bleeding during menses that are irregular in cycle interval.

Premenstrual dysphoric disorder (PMDD) Symptoms of premenstrual syndrome that are severe and include a significant emotional component.

Premenstrual syndrome* (PMS) The cyclic appearance of one or more of a large constellation of symptoms just prior to the menses, occurring to such a degree that lifestyle or work is affected, followed by a period of time entirely free of symptoms.

Primary amenorrhea An absence of menses by the age of 14 with accompanying delayed maturation of secondary sex characteristics or absence of menses by age 16 with evidence of secondary sex characteristics.

Primary dysmenorrhea Painful menstruation for which there is no identifiable etiology.

Secondary amenorrhea A cessation of menses in one who previously menstruated regularly and who is not pregnant.

Secondary dysmenorrhea Painful menstruation that is associated with a specific pathologic condition such as endometriosis.

Selective estrogen receptor modulators (SERMs) A class of drugs that act on the estrogen receptor. SERMs act as agonists in a specific tissue and as estrogen antagonists in other tissues. For example, tamoxifen is an estrogen antagonist in breast tissue but an estrogen agonist in uterine tissue.

* Definition from Speroff et al. 2005.[58]

Introduction

If only the Lydia Pinkham remedy were as effective as claimed in the opening quote, this chapter would be the shortest one in the book. Her treatment encompassed a wide variety of ills, including kidney disease, depression, insomnia, gastrointestinal conditions, and others.

However, the majority of individuals who used Lydia Pinkham's tonic were women seeking relief from menstrual disorders, pelvic disease, and/or infertility. Today's healthcare provider is challenged by the number of pharmaceuticals available to treat a woman with any of these conditions.

Menstrual and pelvic disorders are quintessentially women-specific conditions. Unfortunately, they are common conditions, either independently or together. For example, the menstrual disorder of anovulation is intimately associated with female infertility; dysmenorrhea often is part of the constellation of symptoms that occur with chronic pelvic pain. For women with menstrual variations or pelvic disease, therapy may be directed at a single symptom, such as dysmenorrhea. Other times, treatment is needed for a diagnosed condition, such as endometriosis. Often, treatments for different conditions share the same drugs such as analgesics, hormones, and hormone modulators. This chapter focuses on both symptoms and disease conditions involving menstruation, pelvic pain, and infertility. Since infertility is a condition shared by a dyad, male infertility is briefly discussed.

Unlike the other chapters that separately discuss pharmacologic management of women who are pregnant, lactating, or of advanced age in separate sections, the conditions in this chapter generally are exclusive to reproductive-aged women who are neither pregnant nor breastfeeding. However, the clinician should always consider pregnancy, especially if the woman has any menstrual disorders.

Menstrual Disorders

A fallacy exists that all healthy, reproductive-aged women have a 3- to 5-day menses every 28 days. It is well established that cycle frequency and duration of menses varies among women, and it varies over time in an individual woman. Despite variation in frequency and timing, there are menstrual abnormalities that may benefit from pharmacologic intervention. Among these are episodes of dysmenorrhea, abnormal uterine bleeding, amenorrhea, and mood disorders related to the menstrual cycles.

Dysmenorrhea

Simply defined, **dysmenorrhea** means painful menstruation. Most women experience dysmenorrhea at some point during their lives. Dysmenorrhea is categorized as either primary or secondary. **Primary dysmenorrhea** is painful menstruation for which there is no identifiable pathology and usually occurs with the onset of normal ovulatory cycles.[1,2] Generally, the initial onset of primary dysmenorrhea occurs shortly after menarche, and frequently backache, nausea and vomiting, and diarrhea are accompanying symptoms.[3] Primary dysmenorrhea occurs most often among adolescents and young adults.[2-4]

Secondary dysmenorrhea is menstrual pain associated with identifiable pathology. This entity is more likely to present after years of relatively painless menses and often has an acyclic or chronic component.[5,6] Common causes of secondary dysmenorrhea include uterine leiomyomata (also known as fibroid), adenomyosis, endometriosis, and pelvic inflammatory disease.[5] Pharmacologic treatment for dysmenorrhea depends on the etiology, although nonsteroidal anti-inflammatory drugs frequently are used to treat the pain associated with either category.

The painful abnormal uterine cramping that occurs during primary dysmenorrhea is secondary to overproduction of prostaglandins (PG) within the endometrium, with elevated levels of vasopressin potentially also involved.[1,3,4] PGs are paracrine hormones that function as inflammatory modulators. Prostaglandins in the uterine muscle stimulate myometrial contractions and ischemia, thereby producing the classic, cramping pain of dysmenorrhea.[1] Elevated levels of vasopressin can produce dysrhythmic uterine contractions that reduce uterine blood flow causing myometrial hypoxia (Figure 30-1).[3]

Pharmacologic Treatments for Dysmenorrhea

Most conditions are best treated by removing the etiologic stimuli. In the case of dysmenorrhea, antispasmodics have been proposed as potential pharmacologic agents. However, few studies have been conducted with these agents. One clinical trial investigating hyoscine N-butylbromide (Buscopan), an agent used to treat bladder or intestinal spasms, investigated the use of hyoscine N-butylbromide for the treatment of women with dysmenorrhea, but results have not been promising.[7] Therefore, the agents used in the management of primary dysmenorrhea directly address pain relief. Prominent among them are nonsteroidal anti-inflammatory drugs (NSAIDs). Other treatments include combined oral contraceptives, selective estrogen receptor modulators (SERMs), as well as various complementary and alternative therapies.

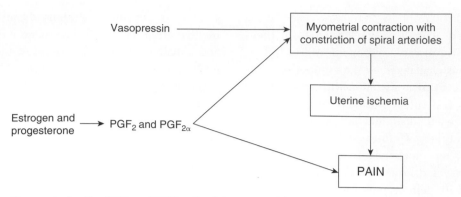

The prostaglandins PGF$_2$ and PGF$_{2\alpha}$ stimulate myometrial contraction and sensitize the afferent nerves to pain, thereby contributing to dysmenorrhea in two ways.

Figure 30-1 Pathophysiology of primary dysmenorrhea.

Nonsteroidal Anti-Inflammatory Drugs

Nonsteroidal anti-inflammatory drugs (NSAIDs) are the most common pharmacologic treatment for dysmenorrhea. Strictly speaking, aspirin (ASA) is a type of NSAID, although it has some unusual properties and will be addressed separately at the end of this section. The NSAIDs are significantly more effective than placebo for treating of dysmenorrhea (OR = 7.91; 95% CI, 5.65–11.09); however, adverse side effects are also common (OR = 1.52; 95% CI, 1.09–2.12).[8] Currently there is insufficient evidence to determine which NSAID is the most effective and safest for treating dysmenorrhea, although ibuprofen (Advil, Motrin, Midol IB) often is considered the gold standard because of its proven effectiveness in providing pain relief, low risk of side effects during short-term use, and wide availability in many inexpensive generic formulations (Box 30-1).[2,8]

In addition to ibuprofen, other NSAIDs commonly used to treat dysmenorrhea include diclofenac potassium (Cataflam), ketoprofen (Orudis, Orudis KT), naproxen (Naprosyn), and naproxen sodium (Aleve). All of the aforementioned agents are available over the counter (Table 30-1).

Although a full description of the mechanism of action of NSAIDs can be found in Chapter 12, there are some functions specific to the reproductive tract. The primary mechanism of action of NSAIDs is inhibition of **cyclooxygenase** (COX), the enzyme that converts arachidonic acid to prostaglandin. When COX is removed from the physiologic pathway, inhibition of PG synthesis occurs, which, in turn, results in decreased hypercontractility of the uterus or decreased dysmenorrhea.[2,4] Several small studies

suggest NSAIDs decrease the volume of the menstrual flow, although reports of this occurrence are subjective and, therefore, not amenable to quantification.[9] NSAIDs also have direct analgesic properties in the central nervous system.[2]

Of the two main isoforms of the COX enzyme, COX-1 and COX-2, COX-1 is synthesized constitutively and, therefore, is present in all tissues at all times. COX-1 generates prostaglandins that are involved in homeostatic maintenance including gastrointestinal mucosal protection, platelet function, regulation of blood flow to the kidney and stomach, and regulation of gastric acid secretion (Figure 12-3).[10,11] COX-2 is inducible. This form of COX mediates pain and inflammation at the site of tissue damage.[10,11]

The therapeutic effects of NSAIDs are due primarily to their ability to inhibit production of COX-2. Since inhibition of COX-1 and COX-2 also can suppress ovulation, NSAIDs are not recommended for use by women who are trying to achieve a pregnancy.[12] NSAIDs are metabolized primarily in the liver, and NSAID metabolites are excreted mainly by the kidneys.

Side Effects/Adverse Effects

The most common side effect of NSAIDs is gastric irritation, which can be somewhat alleviated by taking the medication with food. Serious side effects are gastrointestinal related and include ulceration, gastrointestinal bleeding, and potential perforation. The risks for adverse reactions appear to increase with age and in individuals who have a history of gastrointestinal ulcers, smoking, or alcoholism. Women with the aforementioned history should use

▌Box 30-1 Care for an Adolescent with Dysmenorrhea

A 15-year-old high school student who is healthy and not sexually active comes in to an ambulatory unit. She reports "horrible cramps with my periods" for the last 3 months, requiring that she stay home from school for 1–2 days every month. She does not understand why "this is happening now" and questions what she can do. She experienced menarche 18 months prior to this visit and her menses occur every 28–31 days, lasting 4–5 days. Her best friend had dysmenorrhea, but has noticed that it has lessened since she started taking combined oral contraceptives.

Many adolescents and their parents are perplexed that dysmenorrhea occurs not with menarche, but several months thereafter. Physiologically, this is a normal response since the first year or so after menarche, bleeding is unpredictable and anovulatory. When dysmenorrhea occurs, it generally indicates the presence of ovulation. Therefore, one of the first actions is to provide health counseling and reassurance of normalcy for this young woman. Good health habits such as exercise may be of general benefit for her, although evidence is unclear of its effectiveness for the treatment of dysmenorrhea.

Nonsteroidal anti-inflammatory drugs (NSAIDs) would be the most logical first-line treatment, with ibuprofen (Advil) the agent commonly used. This drug may be initiated shortly before expected menses or with the first sign of pain or bleeding, usually in a dose of 400–800 mg every 6–8 hours. There is lack of evidence that one regimen is superior to the other.

Appropriate to her developmental age, this young woman has a best friend. Therefore, she is asking about combined oral contraceptives (COCs) since her friend is using them. COCs are another reasonable method and may offer noncontraceptive benefits such as decreased dysmenorrhea, improved acne, and potential long-term benefits of protection from endometrial and ovarian cancers. This 15-year-old also may be considering sexual activity and the contraceptive protection with COCs can be of value to her. There is no indication that one brand or type (e.g., monophasic, continuous) is better than another. However, it is of note that most jurisdictions allow adolescents to give personal consent for care only in cases of sexually transmitted diseases, pregnancy, or contraception. Therefore, if this woman is not sexually active or does not desire to be sexually active, parental consent for COCs may be required.

Regardless of which treatment method is chosen, this woman should be told that the menstrual flow may decrease due to the treatment, and that if she does not experience relief within the next 2–3 menses she should return for follow-up.

Table 30-1 Nonsteroidal Anti-Inflammatory Drugs (NSAIDs) Used to Treat Primary Dysmenorrhea

Drug Name Generic (Brand)	Dose/Route	Frequency	Onset/Peak	Duration
Diclofenac potassium (Cataflam)	50 mg PO.	Tid	30 minutes/2–3 hours	8 hours
Ibuprofen (Advil, Motrin, Midol IB)	400 mg PO; 600–800 mg.	q 4–6 hours q 6–8 hours	Varies/1–2 hours	4–6 hours
Ketoprofen (Orudis, Orudis KT)	25–50 mg PO.	q 6–8 hours Maximum dose 300 mg/daily	2–3 hours/6–7 hours	Unknown
Naproxen (Naprosyn)	500 mg PO, then 250 mg PO.	250 mg PO q 6–8 hours up to 1.25 g/daily	1 hour/2–4 hours	6–8 hours
Naproxen sodium (Aleve)	550 mg PO, then 275 mg.	275 mg PO q 6–8 hours up to 1375 mg/daily	1 hour/2–4 hours	7 hours
Naproxen sodium (Naprelan)	Sustained-release formulation 375-mg or 500-mg tablets. Dose is 1000 mg PO.	Once daily	Unknown	Unknown
Acetylsalicylic acid (aspirin)	325–650 mg PO. 500 mg PO. Do not exceed 4 g/day.	q 4 hours; q 3 hours	15–20 min/1–3 hours	3–6 hours

NSAIDs with caution and should avoid them entirely if they have ongoing health problems that increase the risk of gastrointestinal irritation. Women who are using selective serotonin reuptake inhibitors (SSRIs) may be at a moderately increased risk of serious upper gastrointestinal events with concurrent NSAID use and also should use NSAIDs with caution.[13] General contraindications to the use of NSAIDs include kidney impairment, liver disease, and active or chronic inflammation or ulceration of the gastrointestinal tract.

The majority of NSAIDs are nonselective since they inhibit both COX-1 and COX-2. However, the **coxibs**, a newer generation of NSAIDs, are selective COX-2 inhibitors. Because the selective COX-2 inhibitors do not affect COX-1 function, their side effect profile is quite different than the side effects associated with nonselective NSAIDs.

Although initially some COX-2 selective drugs (e.g., celecoxib [Celebrex]) seemed promising for the treatment of dysmenorrhea, their associated cardiovascular risks appear to outweigh the benefits for most women.[14] Rofecoxib (Vioxx) and valdecoxib (Bextra) were withdrawn from the marketplace in 2004 and 2005, respectively, because of their adverse cardiovascular effects. Generally, coxibs are not recommended for the treatment of dysmenorrhea. In addition, little information is available about use of coxibs for lactating women, so alternative NSAID agents should be chosen for the breastfeeding woman experiencing dysmenorrhea.[15]

NSAIDs interact with many drugs as illustrated in Table 12-7, and, therefore, it is critical to know the full details of a woman's pharmacologic history and current use, including prescription medications, over-the-counter products, complementary and herbal preparations, and any illicit drugs. NSAIDs decrease the effectiveness of ACE antihypertensives and may prolong prothrombin time if taken with anticoagulants.[16] Women taking NSAIDs should avoid alcohol use because of an increased risk of gastric irritation when NSAIDs and alcohol are used concomitantly.

Acetylsalicylic Acid (Aspirin)

Acetylsalicylic acid (aspirin) is an NSAID that has properties that are different from other NSAIDs and requires separate discussion. The commonalities shared by aspirin and NSAIDs include analgesic, anti-inflammatory, and antipyretic properties. One major difference is that aspirin inhibits platelet aggregation for the life of the platelet, which accounts for some of the adverse side effects observed. However, this effect is also the reason aspirin is used for other purposes such as cardiovascular protection.[16]

Aspirin is indicated for treatment of mild to moderate pain and may be used to treat dysmenorrhea. If heavy bleeding accompanies the cramping, then aspirin should be avoided because of its antiplatelet effects. Aspirin is contraindicated for anyone with allergies to the agent and should not be used by individuals with bleeding disorders, gastric irritation, or ulcers, or by those who have vitamin K deficiencies.[16] This agent should be used with caution by anyone with asthma, NSAID-induced bronchospasm, or impaired renal function and should never be prescribed if there is suspicion that the individual (especially those ≤ 19 years) has influenza or varicella due to its association with the development of Reye's syndrome. Therefore, adolescents with dysmenorrhea should avoid ASA. Aspirin also should be avoided by persons anticipating surgery within 1 week of taking the medication.

Adverse effects of aspirin include aspirin toxicity, gastric irritation, occult bleeding, and salicylism. A number of drug–drug interactions associated with aspirin exist, such as increased bleeding with oral anticoagulants and increased risk of gastrointestinal ulcers if taken concomitantly with steroids. Salicylates are ototoxic at high blood levels and, therefore, should be discontinued if the individual develops dizziness, tinnitus, or difficulty hearing. Most of the adverse effects of aspirin are associated with long-term use, and the risk for women using aspirin for treatment of dysmenorrhea is low. Information regarding doses can be found in Table 30-1.

Combination Oral Contraceptives

Combination oral contraceptives (COCs) often are used to treat dysmenorrhea because they decrease PG synthesis by the endometrial tissues during menstruation.[2-5,17] More recently marketed continuous COCs also result in fewer days of bleeding and, thus, less opportunity for dysmenorrhea. The off-label use of COCs for dysmenorrhea provides relief for approximately 90% of the women who use them. In a small study of 35 women, when compared with placebo, the women using COCs reported greater pain relief and lost less time from school and work than the women taking placebos.[18] However, despite the results from this small study, data are lacking about the effectiveness of this common treatment. The Cochrane meta-analysis conducted by Proctor et al. was unable to establish whether or not COCs were successful treatment for primary dysmenorrhea.[19] When an NSAID or aspirin is ineffective, COCs may be used as second-line treatment.[17] Further discussion about the mechanisms of action, effects, and contraindications of COCs can be found in Chapter 29.

Selective Estrogen Receptor Modulators

Selective estrogen receptor mediators (SERMs) such as raloxifene hydrochloride (Evista) and tamoxifen citrate (Nolvadex) have been suggested for treatment of dysmenorrhea.[20] Tamoxifen inhibited uterine contractions and ameliorated pain from menstrual cramps in one study.[20] More studies are necessary to determine the safety of prescribing SERMs for dysmenorrhea in the select populations of women for whom NSAIDs or COCs provide no relief. The expense of these agents, as well as the adverse effects of SERMs such as hot flashes, nausea and vomiting, and venous thromboembolism make them an uncommon treatment for dysmenorrhea at this time.

Complementary Therapies in the Treatment of Dysmenorrhea

Women with dysmenorrhea frequently use botanicals to treat the condition, and there are a variety of herbal preparations and formulations marketed for this use. However, there are few well-controlled studies in humans that demonstrate the effectiveness of herbal preparations. Providers unfamiliar with the use of herbs should consult with skilled clinicians such as naturopathic doctors who are nationally certified and licensed to prescribe herbal therapy. Chapter 10 addresses complementary and alternative medicine (CAM) in more detail. A few examples are provided here; however, more research is needed to validate effectiveness, doses, side effects, and contraindications.

A Cochrane meta-analysis of randomized, controlled trials (RCTs) that evaluated the effectiveness of dietary and herbal therapies for the treatment of dysmenorrhea found that the majority of randomized trials assessing the use of CAM for dysmenorrhea evaluated thiamine (vitamin B_1), vitamin B_6 (pyridoxine), vitamin E, magnesium, omega-3 fatty acids (fish oil), and guaifenesin, which is available over the counter in multiple formulations and in many brand names.[21] A list of doses and additional information about use of these therapies is presented in Table 30-2.

Thiamine (Vitamin B₁)

One randomized trial has assessed magnesium versus placebo for treating dysmenorrhea; this trial found that magnesium is more effective than placebo for pain relief and it decreased the need for other medications.[21,22]

There is some suggestion that vitamin B_1 is most useful for women who have a vitamin B_1 deficiency.

Table 30-2 Dietary Supplements and Vitamins Used to Treat Dysmenorrhea

Name Generic (Brand)	Dose	Available Forms
Guaifenesin	2400 mg per day for 2 days*	Tablets
Magnesium (MagMin, Maginex, Magnesiocard)	Unclear	Tablets
Omega-3 fatty acids	2 g/daily	Liquid
Thiamine hydrochloride—vitamin B₁	100 mg/daily	Elixir Injections Tablets
Tocopherol—vitamin E	200 IU bid or 2500 IU daily × 5 days	Capsules Drops Liquid Tablets

* Guaifenesin comes in many formulations including long-acting preparations and combination preparations. Generic tablets that contain guaifenesin only are available in 100-mg, 200-mg, and 400-mg tablets and caplets; extended-release tablets contain 600 mg and 1200 mg; liquid preparations have 100 mg/5mL.

Symptoms of a vitamin B_1 deficiency include muscle cramps, fatigue, and reduced pain tolerance.[1] An open trial conducted more than 50 years ago found that 90% of women given 100 mg of niacin every 2–3 hours twice daily when they were actively cramping reduced symptoms; however, more rigorous study has not been conducted.[23]

Vitamin E (Tocopherols)

Vitamin E relieves dysmenorrhea by inhibiting PG synthesis and promoting vasodilator and uterine muscle relaxation.[3] Ziaei et al. conducted a randomized, placebo-controlled trial in 100 women suffering from dysmenorrhea comparing treatment with 500 IU of vitamin E daily versus placebo for 5 days beginning 2 days before menstruation. Vitamin E was more effective in ameliorating symptoms than the placebo.[24] The same researchers confirmed these findings in another study of a group of 278 adolescents with dysmenorrhea. In this latter randomized controlled trial, the group receiving 200 IU of vitamin E twice daily had a significant reduction in severity and duration of pain from primary dysmenorrhea (0.5 versus 6 on scale; $P > .001$; and 1.6 hours versus 17 hours; $P > .0001$ respectively) and reduced amount of menstrual blood loss (46 mL versus 70 mL; $P > .0001$).[25] A precautionary note about vitamin E supplementation is that it may increase the risk of bleeding especially in women who are taking other medications such as warfarin (Coumadin) or NSAIDs.

Magnesium

Magnesium is theorized to reduce PGs and decrease muscle contractility.[1] In a 6-month double-blind study, 50 patients suffering from dysmenorrhea received a magnesium supplement (Mg 5-longeral).[26] Twenty-one of the 25 women in the magnesium-supplemented group reported a decline in symptoms. In addition, the investigators found a 45% decrease in PGF2 alpha in menstrual blood. The clinical benefits were believed to be due to both the direct muscle relaxant effects of magnesium and inhibition of the biosynthesis of PGF2 alpha.[27] Benassi et al. investigated the therapeutic effect of magnesium among 32 women with primary dysmenorrhea (ages 16–42 years) and found that magnesium (Magnesiocard) in a dose of 5 mmol taken orally three times on the day preceding menstruation and on the first and second day of menstruation had a beneficial therapeutic effect on both back pain and lower abdominal pain in the second and third day of menstruation. Another clinical trial tested the effectiveness of oral magnesium among 30 women with primary dysmenorrhea (average age of 22.6 years).[28] Half the women were given 4.5 mg magnesium pidolate three times daily from the seventh day preceding menstruation until the third day of menstruation. The women assessed pain for six consecutive cycles using a visual analogue scale. There was a significant reduction in visual analogue scores from the first to the sixth cycle on the first day of menstruation. Less pain was shown on days 2 and 3, but results were not statistically significant. The true mechanism of action of magnesium is not known; thus the dose, preparation, and regimen to use in the treatment of dysmenorrhea are unclear, and further studies are needed.[1]

Omega-3 Fatty Acids (Fish Oil)

Diets of women residing in North America include fewer omega-3 fatty acid sources (e.g., oily fish) compared to omega-6 fatty acids (e.g., arachidonic acid).[29] The theoretic mechanism related to the development of dysmenorrhea is an imbalance between omega-3 fatty acids from which anti-inflammatory vasodilator eicosanoids are derived and omega-6 fatty acids that increase inflammatory, vasoconstrictor eicosanoids.[30]

Some studies suggest that fish oil relieves dysmenorrhea better than placebo, and women whose diets are higher in fish n-3 fatty acid have significantly less pain during their menses than those with diets low in the fatty acids.[31,32] A small clinical trial in 42 adolescent women suffering from painful menstruation found that the daily consumption of fish oil (1.8 g of eicosapentaenoic acid [EPA] and 0.72 g of docosahexaenoic acid [DHA]) for 2 months significantly reduced symptoms and the need for ibuprofen.[32] Newer studies suggest that diets higher in omega-3 fatty acids may be protective against dysmenorrhea.[29] As with vitamin E, omega-3 fatty acids may reduce platelet aggregation and thus should be used cautiously in patients taking drugs that have anticoagulant properties.

Omega-3 polyunsaturated fatty acids are potentially potent anti-inflammatory agents, and therefore they may be effective in combating dysmenorrhea. Evidence of their effectiveness against some inflammatory diseases (e.g., rheumatoid arthritis) is strong, but evidence is weak for treatment of others (e.g., inflammatory bowel disease). In summary, omega-3 fatty acids have potential for effectively treating dysmenorrhea because they are effective anti-inflammatory agents and they decrease the production of PGs.[33] More studies are warranted for clarification of effectiveness, as well as for dose and route.[21]

Guaifenesin

Guaifenesin is a common expectorant found in many over-the-counter preparations marketed for treating cough. Guaifenesin is an old drug. It was originally derived from the resin of guaiacum trees and used in the 16th century as an analgesic.[34] Over time, this agent has been used as an analgesic treatment, for improving fertility by way of improving spinnbarkeit of cervical mucus and cervical cellularity, and it has also been used to speed labor by way of its effects on cervical effacement.[34] A small RCT with 25 participants assessed the effects of guaifenesin on dysmenorrhea and suggested that it may be useful. Although the findings were not statistically significant, trending demonstrated that the women in the study preferred using guaifenesin over placebo.[34] The theoretical mechanism of action is that guaifenesin thins secretions, which includes vaginal secretions, perhaps decreasing accompanying dysmenorrhea. However, there are no studies published to date that clearly support its use.

Nonpharmacologic Treatments for Dysmenorrhea

There is a growing body of information about nonpharmacologic treatments for dysmenorrhea such as transcutaneous electrical nerve stimulation (TENS), spinal manipulation, acupuncture, and exercise. These interventions are briefly discussed because they may be used in clinical practice to augment drugs.

TENS is a therapy in which electrodes are placed on the skin, and electrical current that stimulates nerves is passed into the body. Presumably, it is designed to reduce a person's ability to perceive pain signals at the spinal level and not directly from the uterine tissue. According to a Cochrane meta-analysis published in 2002, high-frequency TENS was shown to be more effective than placebo in reducing pain from primary dysmenorrhea.[35] A number of clinical studies published between 1985 and 2007 used TENS for the treatment of dysmenorrhea, with generally positive results.[28,36-40] However, larger, better controlled studies with more objective outcome measures are needed to extend and confirm the results of these studies. Advocates of the chiropractic technique of spinal manipulation (high velocity, low amplitude) feel that dysmenorrhea can result from a mechanical dysfunction in certain vertebrae, which affects the sympathetic nerve supply to the blood vessels to the uterus causing vasoconstriction. This causes a disruption of blood flow to the uterine muscle, resulting in the pain of dysmenorrhea. This technique attempts to increase spinal mobility and improve uterine blood supply. Several clinical trials have been conducted since 1992 with conflicting results.[41] Only a few studies have been conducted evaluating the benefits of acupuncture for the treatment of dysmenorrhea.[42] In 2008, a large, multicenter, randomized, controlled trial was published wherein 179 women were randomized and completed the study.[43] Pain decreased from a score of 6 to 3 based on a numeric rating scale in the acupuncture group after 3 months. This score was maintained for 3–6 months. Pain scores decreased from 6.5 to 5.5 after 3 months in the control group. Few studies have investigated exercise and relaxation training as methods to improve menstrual symptoms in young women with dysmenorrhea, and results have been promising.[44-46] One study showed that topically applied heat at 38.9°C for 12 hours was as effective as ibuprofen in reducing pain in dysmenorrhea.[47]

Menstrual Disorders: Abnormal Uterine Bleeding

Dysmenorrhea is only one of several menstrual disorders. **Abnormal uterine bleeding** (AUB) is a term to denote excessive bleeding during the menses or bleeding that occurs outside the parameters of a normal menstrual cycle.[48] Other terms further define the specific conditions, such as **menorrhagia**, which designates heavy bleeding during the expected time of menses; **metrorrhagia**, which refers to uterine bleeding at irregular periods; and **menometrorrhagia**, which is excessive bleeding both during an expected menses and intermenstrually. A variety of conditions can cause abnormal uterine bleeding including anovulation, systemic disease, reproductive tract pathology (e.g., sexually transmitted infections such as *Chlamydia trachomatis* or gonorrhea), iatrogenic causes (e.g., trauma), and a woman's lifestyle (e.g., illicit drug use, poor nutrition). Some pharmaceuticals have among their side effects a negative influence on normal menses (Table 30-3). Management is directed toward treating the underlying cause of the AUB. If no pathology is identified, the AUB usually is renamed **dysfunctional uterine bleeding** (DUB).

Acute hemorrhage necessitates in-hospital treatment and should be individualized based on etiology and a woman's status. Pharmaceuticals may include some of the agents discussed in treatment of AUB, but customized management options are beyond the scope of this chapter.

Table 30-3 Selected Drugs That Can Cause Abnormal Vaginal Bleeding

Drug Category	Common Drugs Generic (Brand)
Agents commonly abused	Alcohol
	Amphetamines*
	Cannabis
	Heroin
Alkylating agents	Procarbazine
Anticoagulants	Coumadin (Heparin)
Antidepressants	Tricyclics—e.g., amitriptyline (Elavil)*
	MAOI—e.g., phenelzine (Nardil)
Antidopaminergic	Droperidol (Inapsine)
Antihistamines	Cimetidine (Tagamet)*
Antihypertensives	Methyldopa (Aldomet)
	Reserpine (Serpasil)*
Antitubercular agents	Isoniazid (INH)*
Benzodiazepines	Diazepam (Valium)*
Butyrophenone antipsychotics	Haloperidol (Haldol)*
Diuretics	Spironolactone (Aldactone)*
Hormones	Thyroid, estrogens,* progesterones,* testosterones*
Opiates	Morphine*
	Methadone
Phenothiazines	Prochlorperazine (Compazine)
	Chlorpromazine (Thorazine)
	Promethazine (Phenergan)
Sedative/hypnotics	Chlordiazepoxide (Librium)

* Also associated with galactorrhea.

Menstrual Disorders: Dysfunctional Uterine Bleeding

DUB commonly is defined as abnormal bleeding occurring in the absence of uterine pathology. Some experts believe DUB can be one of two types: ovulatory and anovulatory.[49] Pregnancy must first be ruled out in all women of childbearing age who present with uterine bleeding. The goal of treating abnormal bleeding is to normalize the bleeding, correct anemia, prevent/or diagnose early cancer, and restore quality of life.[50] Treatment is either emergent, requiring hospitalization, or it is nonemergent and can be effectively treated in the office setting. This chapter will focus on the latter.

The approach to accurate assessment and treatment of AUB varies according to a woman's reproductive status. A brief description of abnormal bleeding patterns and related etiologies in the context of reproductive status provides a framework for differential diagnosis and the appropriate pharmacologic treatment. For an in-depth discussion, the reader is referred to any of several major texts about women's gynecologic health.

Adolescents

Anovulation is frequently the cause of DUB in adolescent girls aged 13 to 17, particularly in the first year or 2 after menarche. The second most common cause of abnormal bleeding in adolescents is undiagnosed coagulopathies including von Willebrand's disease leukemia, or aplastic anemia.[49] Congenital malformations of the uterus and/or outflow tract may also be the cause of abnormal vaginal bleeding. These conditions become more apparent around the usual time of menarche because menses is early, delayed, or abnormal in character.

Childbearing Age

Complications of pregnancy are commonly the cause of abnormal bleeding in women of childbearing age, which is why it is essential to rule out pregnancy whenever a woman with reproductive potential has AUB.[49] Other causes of AUB during these years include uterine fibroids, endometrial hyperplasia, and anovulation associated with polycystic ovary syndrome as discussed later in the chapter.

Perimenopause

During their 40s and early 50s, many women will experience changes in their menstrual pattern. As the reproductive system begins its normal transition toward menopause anovulation, which can be accompanied by abnormal bleeding patterns, occurs with increasing frequency. Menses that are light (oligomenorrhea) or absent (amenorrhea) are not uncommon. However, menorrhagia, metrorrhagia, and menometrorrhagia are not normal, and further evaluation is warranted. Since ovulation is unpredictable during the perimenopausal period, pregnancy should always be ruled out prior to treatment.

Postmenopause

Postmenopausal bleeding never is considered normal, and cancer must always be considered as a diagnosis. Bleeding may be due to the endometrium becoming atrophic; however, this diagnosis can only be made after verifying that endometrial cancer or other pathologies are not present.

Treatment of Dysfunctional Uterine Bleeding

Overall, anovulatory bleeding is the most common reason for DUB in all age groups. Anovulation is associated with a level of progesterone that is insufficient to offset estrogen stimulation of the endometrium. The result may be uterine hyperplasia, which causes bleeding that is initially shorter than normal and eventually becomes prolonged and heavy as hyperplasia of the endometrium becomes more pronounced. The most common etiological condition for chronic anovulation is polycystic ovary syndrome (PCOS).[48] DUB also may occur with ovulatory cycles, especially in the presence of leiomyomata.

In clinical practice, a progesterone challenge is a commonly used test to determine whether there is appropriate endogenous estrogen production. If a woman has an intact hypothalamus/pituitary/ovarian axis and is not pregnant, vaginal bleeding should result within a few days after cessation of the progesterone. This progesterone withdrawal usually is used to induce bleeding in women who are amenorrheic or to regulate menses when a woman is experiencing abnormal uterine bleeding. If withdrawal bleeding occurs following the administration of a progestogen and the possibility of a pituitary tumor is ruled out, the diagnosis is anovulation, and treatment is as outlined in this section. To administer a progesterone challenge, the clinician can prescribe a variety of agents. Options can be found listed in Box 30-2. If micronized progesterone is used, it should be taken in the evening because it is known

Box 30-2 Progesterone Challenge Test

Indication

In the case of secondary amenorrhea with a negative pregnancy test, a progesterone challenge should result in vaginal bleeding if adequate estrogen is present.

Progesterone Options

1. Medroxyprogesterone (Provera), 10 mg PO qd for 7–10 days

2. Norethindrone (Aygestin), 5 mg PO qd for 7–10 days

3. Progesterone, 5 mg PO qd for 7–10 days

4. Micronized progesterone gel 4% or 8% intravaginal application qod for 6 doses

Interpretation

Withdrawal bleeding that occurs within 2–7 days after last dose validates adequate endogenous estrogen production and signifies the patency of the outflow tract.

to cause drowsiness, and clinicians should remember that this agent is contraindicated for individuals with peanut allergies.

Combined Oral Contraceptives

When a woman is experiencing mild DUB regardless if she is anovulatory or ovulatory, initial treatment typically is a prescription for combination oral contraceptives (COCs). If the bleeding is not acute, the COCs are taken in the same manner as prescribed for contraception as discussed in Chapter 29. Usually after 3 months of treatment with COCs, the endometrium will be of normal thickness and subsequent withdrawal of the progesterone will stimulate a normal bleeding episode.[50] If the flow remains abnormal, further investigation and consultation is necessary.

Women whose bleeding is acute but whose condition overall does not require hospitalization may respond well to relatively high doses of hormones. The usual treatment is a monophasic COC taken every 4–6 hours over a period of 4–7 days, after which the dose is tapered or stopped, and normal withdrawal bleeding usually ensues.[51] Following

this regimen, standard doses are used. All known side effects and contraindications to use of COCs apply when they are used for this purpose.

Cyclic Progestins

Cyclic progestin therapy instead of COCs also may be used to treat menorrhagia associated with chronic anovulation (Table 30-4). If withdrawal bleeding does not occur within 7 days of stopping the progestogen, further evaluation is merited. Women need to be informed that cyclic progestins prescribed as therapy for anovulation do not provide contraception. Contraindications to progestins are discussed in Chapter 14.

Side Effects/Adverse Effects

Common adverse effects associated with use of progestins include headache, breakthrough bleeding, spotting, amenorrhea, bloating, and weight changes. Some women report moodiness. More serious side effects include changes in or loss of vision, cerebrovascular disorders, and increases in blood pressure. If any of the latter signs or symptoms occur, the progestogen should be discontinued immediately. Progestins should not be prescribed if pregnancy is suspected, although there is no documented teratogenic effect.

Table 30-4 Progestin Therapy for Menorrhagia

Drug Generic (Brand)	Dose	Schedule
Aqueous progesterone—progesterone in oil	5–10 mg/day IM × 6–8 days.	Must take on consecutive days.
Depot medroxyprogesterone acetate (Depo-Provera)	150 mg IM.	Administered every 12 weeks.
Levonorgestrel intrauterine contraceptive system (LNG IUS, Mirena)	The LNG-IUS contains 52 mg levonorgestrel at time of insertion.	Effective for contraception for up to 5 years.
Medroxyprogesterone acetate (Provera)	5–10 mg PO/day × 5–10 days.	Start on day 16 or 21 of the menstrual cycle.
Norethindrone acetate (Aygestin)	2.5–10 mg PO.	Start day 5 of cycle and end on day 25.
Oral micronized progesterone (Prometrium Crinone)*	400 mg PO × 10 days.	Take in the evening—may cause drowsiness.

* Contraindicated for persons who are allergic to peanuts.

High-Dose Estrogen

High-dose estrogen usually will abort an acute bleeding episode that is most likely due to anovulation. This agent allows time for evaluation of underlying causes and is not considered a long-term treatment. Nausea is a common side effect of high-dose estrogen; therefore, prescribing an antiemetic may be necessary. Frequently, conjugated equine estrogen (Premarin) is prescribed after the bleeding stops and is followed by the addition of medroxyprogesterone acetate (Provera) for the last 10 days of therapy to initiate withdrawal bleeding. The usual length of treatment is 3 months, after which, if there is no improvement, reevaluation is necessary.[50] Information about doses can be found in Table 30-5.

Studies comparing the efficacy of various doses of estrogens or how best to taper the doses are lacking.[49] High-dose estrogen can precipitate a thromboembolic event and, therefore, is contraindicated in women with a history of thrombosis or family history of idiopathic thromboembolism.

Nonsteroidal Anti-Inflammatory Drugs (NSAIDs)

NSAIDs are effective for treating ovulatory menorrhagia. Menorrhagia may be of sudden onset or a result of several months with heavier bleeding each cycle. First-line pharmacologic therapies for acute bleeding (menorrhagia) usually are NSAIDs. It is theorized that NSAIDs may decrease the amount of bleeding because they inhibit production of specific vasodilator prostaglandins.[51] Controversy exists over when to initiate NSAID therapy in order to decrease bleeding, with some clinicians suggesting women start the agent up to 3 days prior to the onset of the menses and others with the onset of bleeding, while others advocate starting the drugs when menses begins. Evidence is lacking as to which method should be used. Doses are listed in Table 30-6.

Progestins

Systemic progestins, in addition to being useful for the treatment of anovulatory DUB, are also useful for treating ovulatory DUB, although studies suggest their use offers no advantages over other pharmacologic therapies, including NSAIDs, progesterone-releasing intrauterine systems, or danocrine.[52] It generally is conceded that progestogen therapy during days 5–26 of the cycle results in markedly less bleeding.[49] However, women usually find systemic treatment with the accompanying side effects of bloating and moodiness less preferable than nonsystemic systems such as the progesterone-releasing intrauterine system wherein these symptoms are markedly less common. Amenorrhea due to endometrial atrophy almost always occurs with long-term use of continuous progestin therapy.

Progestins are not as effective as estrogen in treating acute bleeding episodes but are effective for long-term treatment for chronic anovulation. Progestins should not be prescribed if the woman believes she may be pregnant.

Progesterone-Releasing Intrauterine Systems

The levonorgestrel-releasing intrauterine system (LNG-IUS) releases levonorgestrel, a potent progestin, in low daily doses into the uterine cavity, thus, directly targeting the endometrium (Table 30-5). As a result, endometrial proliferation is suppressed, which, in turn, significantly decreases menstrual

Table 30-5 Selected Medical Therapies for Menorrhagia

Acute Bleeding	Long-Term/Chronic Management
1. Replete intravascular volume	1. Cyclic MPA 10 mg/day for 10–14 days every 30–40 days
2. *CEE 25 mg IV q 4–6 h as needed followed by CEE 2.5–5 mg PO qid for 2–3 days, then add MPA 10 mg for 10–14 days (continue CEE)	2. Combined contraceptives (oral, patch, ring)
3. COCs bid/tid, then taper	3. Oral micronized progesterone† 300 mg for 10–14 days, every 30–40 days
	4. Depot medroxyprogesterone (Depo-Provera) 150 mg IM every 3 months
	5. Levonorgestrel intrauterine contraceptive system (LNG-IUS)
	6. NSAIDs as needed for pain

CEE = conjugated equine estrogen; MPA = medroxyprogesterone acetate; COC = combined oral contraceptives; NSAIDs = nonsteroidal anti-inflammatory drugs.
* High doses of estrogen can precipitate a thrombotic event and are contraindicated in women with a history of thrombosis or family history of idiopathic venous thromboembolism.
† Contraindicated for persons with an allergy to peanuts.
Source: Reprinted with permission from Faucher M 2006.[50]

Table 30-6 Nonsteroidal Anti-Inflammatory Drugs (NSAIDs) Used to Treat Menorrhagia

Drug Generic (Brand)	Dose
Ibuprofen (Advil)	600–800 mg tid × 3–5 days
Mefenamic acid (Ponstel)	500 mg tid × 3–5 days
Naproxen sodium (Aleve)	550 mg loading dose then 275 mg q 6 hours × 3–5 days

flow. Several studies have found that the levonorgestrel-releasing intrauterine system (LNG-IUS [Mirena]) is an effective treatment for menorrhagia related to anovulation or leiomyomas.[53-56] Studies demonstrate that women using LNG-IUS experienced a marked reduction in bleeding and at 3 months indicated their menstrual flow had become very light. Overall, studies indicate that women were satisfied with the IUS[57] and the method can be cost effective.

Continuous use of the LNG-IUS can effectively suppress endometrial proliferation for up to 5 years.[55] The most common side effects of progesterone-releasing intrauterine systems are related to the levonorgestrel and include mood changes, acne, breast tenderness, hirsutism, and weight change, although these side effects occur to a lesser degree compared to systemic delivery of levonorgestrel.[55] Some intermenstrual spotting, which is a normal side effect frequently experienced with any IUS or IUD, may occur. See Chapter 29 for an in-depth discussion about the indications and contraindications to using an intrauterine agent.

Androgens

Danocrine (Danazol) is a weak androgen that has been found in some studies to be more effective than NSAIDs, progestogens, and COCs for the treatment of women with menorrhagia.[58] A 2007 Cochrane meta-analysis of danocrine for treatment of menorrhagia supports earlier positive findings, but the authors noted that the confidence intervals of the studies reviewed were wide and results imprecise.[59] Women on danocrine also reported more adverse effects compared to NSAIDs or progestogens (OR = 7.0; 95% CI, 1.7–28.2 and OR = 4.05; 95% CI, 1.6–10.2, respectively), including androgenic side effects such as such as hot flashes, hirsutism, and acne, which are not acceptable to most women.[58,59] It appears from current studies that danocrine may be effective to treat dysmenorrhea, but its use is limited because of the side effects.

Gonadotropin-Releasing Hormone Agonists

Gonadotropin-releasing hormone (GnRH) agonists attach to the gonadotropin-releasing hormone receptor in the pituitary, which stimulates the synthesis and release of follicle-stimulating hormone (FSH) and leuteinizing hormone (LH), which then facilitates regulation of the menstrual cycle via their natural biologic function. GnRH agonists are a synthetic form of GnRH. Native GnRH is released in a pulsatile fashion, causing stimulation of the release of gonadotropins. When these agents are administered constantly, first an exacerbation of symptoms, also

called a **flare** effect tends to occur. Within a few weeks, the GnRH receptors retract into the pituitary cell—a process called **down-regulation**. At that point, these drugs effectively suppress pituitary production of FSH and LH, which results in hypoestrogenemia amenorrhea and decreases in uterine and leiomyoma volume.[49,60]

Typically, the GnRH agonists have been used to treat prostatic and breast cancer. They are also useful for the treatment of endometriosis and leiomyomata. The doses used to treat leiomyomata effectively decrease heavy bleeding. Often the formulation is depot, indicating that the drug should be injected or implanted so it is slowly absorbed into the circulation. For example, a depot injection is the intramuscular injection of a drug in an oil suspension that results in the gradual release of the medication over several days. GnRH agonists that effectively treat menorrhagia are leuprolide acetate (Lupron Depot), nafarelin acetate (Synarel), and goserelin acetate (Zoladex).

Leuprolide Acetate

Leuprolide acetate is a luteinizing hormone agonist that occupies pituitary GnRH receptors and desensitizes them.[61] Leuprolide acetate (Lupron Depot) is available in either 3- or 4-month doses. This agent is contraindicated in pregnancy and in women who have undiagnosed vaginal bleeding. It should be used cautiously by women who are lactating. Adverse effects include dizziness, headache, blurred vision, lethargy, peripheral edema, thrombophlebitis, and myocardial infarction. Women on leuprolide may experience urinary frequency and hematuria that may indicate urinary obstruction or other abnormality, and if this occurs, they should be referred to a specialist. Hot flashes, sweats, and bone pain may also accompany use of leuprolide.[61]

Nafarelin Acetate (Synarel)

Nafarelin acetate (Synarel) is a potent GnRH analogue that initially stimulates LH and FSH release from the pituitaryl, whereas prolonged use causes desensitization of the GnRH receptor and then decreased LH and FSH secretion.[61] The desired therapeutic effect is diminished bleeding from endometrial tissue that is no longer stimulated by LH and FSH.

Women who have undiagnosed vaginal bleeding, women who are pregnant, or women who are lactating should not take nafarelin (Synarel). Adverse effects include headaches, sleep disorders, and some dizziness. The androgenic side effects of nafarelin can cause acne, hirsutism, and weight gain. Hypoestrogenic side effects include vasomotor reactions such as hot flashes, sweating, and emotional lability. A significant adverse effect in women who use the drug long term is decreased bone density; therefore, any woman who has osteoporosis or osteopenia should not take nafarelin. Treatment is generally limited to 6 months because of the risk of osteoporosis. If treatment is longer than 6 months, concomitant therapy with low doses of estrogen and progesterone are recommended to prevent bone loss.[49]

Goserelin Acetate (Zoladex)

Goserelin acetate is a potent inhibitor of pituitary gonadotropin secretion. Initial administration produces a rise in FSH and LH that causes an increase in testosterone, which causes a flare reaction. After 2–4 weeks of therapy, women taking goserelin (Zoladex) have lowered serum estradiol levels that effectively reduce the size and function of the ovaries.[62] The uterus and mammary glands also decrease in size.

Goserelin (Zoladex) is contraindicated for women who have undiagnosed vaginal bleeding, are sensitive to any GnRH drugs, or are pregnant or lactating. Adverse effects include insomnia, lethargy, emotional lability, cardiac arrhythmia, nausea, and anorexia. Hot flashes, dysmenorrhea, and urinary tract and vaginal infections have also been reported.

GnRH agonist therapy generally is reserved for episodes of acute menorrhagia caused by leiomyomas. The treatment enables the woman's hemoglobin to return to normal prior to surgery or other types of intervention. Information about doses for GnRH agonist therapy is listed in Table 30-7.

Premenstrual Syndrome and Premenstrual Dysphoric Disorder

Premenstrual syndrome (PMS) is common among women, from adolescence to middle age. The distinct pattern of emotional, cognitive, behavioral, and physical symptoms affiliated with PMS occur during the luteal phase of the menstrual cycle and spontaneously subside within a few days of the onset of menses. A concise definition of premenstrual syndrome (PMS) is offered by Speroff and Fritz "... the cyclic appearance of one or more of a large constellation of symptoms just prior to the menses, occurring to such a degree that lifestyle or work is affected, followed by a period of time entirely free of symptoms."[58]

Table 30-7 Gonadotropin-Releasing Hormone Agonists Used to Treat Menorrhagia*

Drug Generic (Brand)	Dose/Route and Course of Treatment
Goserelin (Zoladex)	The drug is given via implant. To thin the endometrium the following schedule is suggested: One to two 3.6-mg SQ depots 4 weeks apart; surgery is done week 4 after the first dose and within 2–4 weeks after the second dose if two are used.
Leuprolide acetate (Lupron Depot—3 month or 4 month)	Use depot formulation. 3.75 mg IM as a single monthly injection for 3 months or 11.25 mg IM once.
Nafarelin acetate (Synarel)	Primarily used to treat endometriosis; however, its mechanism of action decreases heavy bleeding. 400 mcg/day: one spray (200 mcg) into one nostril in the morning and one spray into the other nostril in the evening. Start treatment between days 2 and 4 of the menstrual cycle. Treatment is recommended for 6 months.

* If anemia is present due to the menorrhagia, iron supplements also are recommended.

Premenstrual dysphoric disorder (PMDD) is a diagnostic label from the American Psychological Association, which describes PMDD as symptoms that are much more severe than those experienced with PMS and includes predominant severity of emotional symptoms.[63] Symptoms experienced by women who have either PMS or PMDD include abdominal bloating and pain, irritability, moodiness, depression, decrease in ability to concentrate, fatigue, headache, and breast tenderness and pain.[63-65] It is estimated that approximately 85% of menstruating women report having one or more of these symptoms, and up to 10% report symptoms so severe they are disabling.[66] Additionally approximately 8% of women who are ovulating experience PMDD.[67]

The etiology of PMS/PMDD remains unclear, but most authorities suspect gonadal hormones are involved because ovulation suppression frequently results in improvement. Initial treatment is often nonpharmacologic; however, if symptoms remain unrelieved, then symptom-specific drugs are prescribed. Treatment is by necessity individualized and symptom specific. Selective serotonin reuptake inhibitors are considered the first-line treatment for PMS/PMDD while drugs such as anxiolytics, ovulation suppressants, and diuretics are recommended for specific symptoms.[68] Additional information about psychotropic drugs can be found in Chapter 25.

Selective Serotonin Reuptake Inhibitors (SSRIs)

Selective serotonin reuptake inhibitors (SSRIs) (fluoxetine [Prozac], paroxetine [Paxil], sertraline [Zoloft], and citalopram [Celexa]) are considered first-line drugs for severe PMS and for PMDD.[68] Fluoxetine can be found in two popular forms: a green and white pill under the brand name Prozac, or a pink and purple tablet directly advertised to consumers under the woman-friendly name of Sarafem. Other than coloring and outside packaging, the agents are the same. It has been suggested that rebranding the drug enables women to avoid any perceived stigma associated with use of antidepressants.[69]

The SSRIs inhibit the serotonin transporter thereby preventing reuptake of serotonin into the presynaptic neuron, which increases the synaptic concentration. Since the symptoms of PMS/PMDD occur during the luteal phase with remittance at the onset of menses, many authorities suggest that treatment can be limited to the luteal phase.[70]

There does appear to be a difference in the involvement of the serotonergic system in PMDD from that of other depressive orders. The response to SSRIs is much more rapid in women with PMDD than in women who have other depressive disorders.[70] The fact that SSRIs are effective for PMDD even when administered only during the luteal phase is yet another distinctive difference. These differences suggest that the underlying cause of PMDD is different than that of other depressive disorders.[70] There is a wide variety of SSRIs that are effective in treating severe PMS and PMDD. Some of the more common SSRIs used to treat PMS/PMDD are discussed here, and information about doses and the extensive drug–drug interactions associated with these drugs are provided in Table 30-8.

Fluoxetine Hydrochloride (Prozac, Sarafem)

Fluoxetine (Prozac, Sarafem) is indicated for the treatment of symptoms such as anger/irritability, depression, and affect lability related to PMDD. When taken during the luteal phase, fluoxetine significantly ameliorates mood-related symptoms associated with PMDD; however, it has little effect on associated physical symptoms such as leg and

Table 30-8 Drugs Used for Treatment of Severe Premenstrual Syndrome (PMS) and Premenstrual Dysphoric Disorder (PMDD)

Drug Generic (Brand)	Category	Indication	Dose	Onset/Peak of Action
Alprazolam (Xanax XR)*	Benzodiazepine	Anxiety and other affective symptoms	PMS dosage: 0.25 mg PO tid. PMDD dosage: 0.375–1.5 mg PO/daily.	30 min/1–2 h.
Bromocriptine mesylate (Parlodel)	Dopamine receptor agonist	Mastalgia	Up to 2.5 mg PO tid.	Varies/1–3 h.
Citalopram hydrobromide (Celexa)	SSRI	Premenstrual dysphoric disorder	20 mg/day PO as a single dose. Increase to 40 mg/day only if clearly needed and patient is not responding. Use just during luteal phase.	Onset is 4 h.
Clomipramine hydrochloride (Anafranil)	Tricyclic antidepressant	All symptoms, anticholinergic effects	25–75 mg/day.	Slow onset.
Fluoxetine hydrochloride (Sarafem)	SSRI	Premenstrual dysphoric disorder	20 mg/day PO starting 14 days prior to menses and continue until first full day of menses. Do not exceed 80 mg/day.	Onset is 6–8 h.
Ibuprofen (Advil)	NSAID	Pain/mastalgia	500–1000 mg/day.	Onset 0.5 to 1 hr, duration 4–6 h.
Paroxetine hydrochloride (Paxil)	SSRI	Premenstrual dysphoric disorder	12.5 mg/day PO as a single dose in the AM. Range 12.5–25 mg/day. May be given daily or just during luteal phase of cycle.	Onset is 5 h.
Sertraline hydrochloride (Zoloft)	SSRI	Premenstrual dysphoric disorder	50 mg/day PO or just during luteal phase of menstrual cycle.	Onset is 4.5–8 h.
Spironolactone (Aldactone)	Diuretic	Water retention	100 mg PO daily.	24–48 h/48–72 h.

* Alprazolam is a controlled schedule C-IV substance.

joint pain.[63] Fluoxetine is contraindicated for individuals with hypersensitivity to the medication. This agent should be used cautiously by women who have impaired liver or renal function, diabetes mellitus, or a history of seizures or suicide attempts. There appears to be a paucity of information about its use during lactation, and fluoxetine is listed by the American Academy of Pediatrics as a drug that may be of concern for use during lactation.[17]

Adverse effects include headache, nervousness, drowsiness, seizures, and dizziness. Hot flashes may occur with use. Dermatologic adverse effects include sweating, rash, pruritus, and contact dermatitis. Gastrointestinal adverse effects include nausea, vomiting, diarrhea, anorexia, dry mouth, and constipation, and some women will notice taste changes. Some women using fluoxetine note an increase in dysmenorrhea, sexual dysfunction in the form of loss of libido, and urinary frequency. Weight changes are not uncommon. Fluoxetine (Prozac, Sarafem) should never be taken with monoamine oxidase inhibitors (MAOIs) or within 14 days of the administration of an MAOI because the this drug–drug reaction can be fatal.[71] Increased serum concentrations of tricyclic antidepressants (TCAs) occur if taken concomitantly with fluoxetine. Smoking decreases the effectiveness of fluoxetine, and this agent should never be combined with alcohol. Avoidance of administering other serotonergic drugs to someone on fluoxetine is critical because of the risk of serotonin syndrome (hypertension, hyperthermia, and mental status changes).

Paroxetine (Paxil)

Paroxetine provides an antidepressant effect and is FDA approved to treat depressive symptoms associated with PMDD.[72] It is contraindicated for anyone who is also using MAOIs or thioridazine (Mellaril). Adverse effects include somnolence, dizziness, insomnia, headache, and sometimes anxiety. Sweating and rash may occur. Nausea, dry mouth, constipation, and diarrhea are notable gastrointestinal side effects.[71]

Paroxetine interacts with digoxin (Lanoxin) and phenytoin (Dilantin) by decreasing the therapeutic effects of these drugs. If paroxetine is used with procyclidine (Kemadrin), tryptophan, or warfarin (Coumadin), it can increase the serum concentrations of these drugs with toxicity as a potential outcome.[71]

Sertraline Hydrochloride (Zoloft)

The therapeutic actions of sertraline (Zoloft) are the same as the effects of all other SSRIs. Sertraline is indicated for treatment of mood-related symptoms of PMDD. It is contraindicated for anyone who has hypersensitivity to SSRIs or specifically to sertraline. The drug should be used with caution by individuals with impaired liver or renal function, during lactation, or by women who are pregnant. Side effects include general CNS effects such as headache, nervousness, drowsiness, insomnia, and fatigue. This drug may cause nausea and vomiting, diarrhea, and dry mouth. Sertraline also may increase the risk of dysmenorrhea.

Sertraline (Zoloft) should never be used with other MAOIs, and at least 14 days should elapse between MAOI and sertraline use. There is a possible risk of abnormal heart rhythms if used with the antipsychotic pimozide (Orap), and these two drugs should not be used concurrently. Food increases the absorption rate of sertraline. If sertraline is taken with St. John's wort, there is risk of a serotonin syndrome.[71]

Citalopram Hydrobromide (Celexa)

Citalopram (Celexa), an SSRI, is used off label to treat PMDD.[58,62] It is contraindicated for anyone who is using MAOIs or other SSRIs and should not be used with pimozide (Orap). It should be used with caution by individuals with hepatic or renal impairment, and side effects are the same as those with other SSRIs.

If citalopram (Celexa) is taken with MAOIs, the serum concentrations of citalopram can increase, which, in turn, increases a risk of toxicity. There should be a 14-day window following cessation of MAOIs prior to administering citalopram. There is a potential for increased citalopram serum concentrations in persons who also are taking azole antifungals or macrolides.[71] There is a possibility of severe adverse effects if used with TCAs, erythromycin (E-Mycin), or beta-blockers. Citalopram may increase the bleeding time of persons on warfarin (Coumadin). Citalopram should never be taken with pimozide (Orap), as this combination can cause fatal heart arrhythmias.

Clomipramine Hydrochloride

Clomipramine (Anafranil) is a TCA. TCAs affect neurotransmitters serotonin and norepinephrine by inhibiting their reuptake into the presynaptic neuron.[71] They are also antagonists of histamine receptors, which contributes to the side effects of weight gain and drowsiness. The TCAs are absorbed in the gastrointestinal tract following oral administration. They are highly lipophilic and protein bound.[71]

These agents are used to treat depression and are less costly than newer drugs such as some of the selective serotonin reuptake inhibitors (SSRIs). However, the side effects of TCAs are more serious than those associated with SSRIs, thus the TCAs are not prescribed as often for PMS/PMDD.

TCAs are contraindicated for anyone with a cardiac disorder because of their direct alpha adrenergic blocking effect.[71] They should be used with caution by women who have glaucoma or urinary incontinence. TCAs should not be prescribed to anyone who is also taking monoamine oxidase inhibitors (MAOIs).[71] These drugs are excreted in small amounts in breast milk, and caution should be used in prescribing a TCA to a breastfeeding mother.

Side effects include sedation and anticholinergic effects such as dry mouth, constipation, urinary hesitancy, and urinary retention. Other side effects include weight gain, drowsiness, and loss of libido. As with all drugs affecting the central nervous system, the dose should be titrated slowly (in either direction). The therapeutic window is very narrow, and, therefore, great caution should be taken in using TCAs for PMDD if depression with suicidal ideology is apparent.

The most significant drug interactions are those that increase the blood levels of the TCA, increasing the risk of toxicity and cardiac arrhythmias. Chapter 25 includes discussion of a number of drug–drug interactions that can occur with TCAs.

Bromocriptine Mesylate (Parlodel) to Treat PMS-Associated Mastalgia

Bromocriptine (Parlodel) is an antiparkinson drug and dopamine receptor agonist. This drug is a semisynthetic ergot derivative that is effective for treating mastalgia.[73] Bromocriptine acts directly on postsynaptic dopamine receptors of the prolactin-secreting cells of the anterior pituitary to inhibit the release of prolactin.[61] Bromocriptine is contraindicated for anyone with hypersensitivity to any ergot alkaloid, severe ischemic heart disease, or peripheral vascular disease and should not be used by lactating women because it decreases production of breast milk. In years past, this agent was used as a lactation suppressant for women in the immediate postpartum period who chose to bottle-feed their infants until the side effects were determined to be too significant when compared to the potential benefits.

Adverse effects of bromocriptine include dizziness, fatigue, hypotension, constipation, diarrhea, vomiting, and abdominal cramping. Bromocriptine may exacerbate symptoms of Raynaud's syndrome. Bromocriptine increases

the blood levels of erythromycin (E-Mycin), which can cause toxic effects of erythromycin. When used concomitantly with phenothiazines, bromocriptine decreases the effectiveness of phenothiazines. An increase in bromocriptine side effects can occur if it is taken concomitantly with sympathomimetics.

Spironolactone (Aldactone) to Treat PMS-Associated Water Retention

Spironolactone (Aldactone) is a potassium-sparing diuretic and aldosterone antagonist that can be used to provide relief from water retention.[74] The use of this agent for the treatment of women with PMS is off label. Spironolactone is contraindicated for anyone with allergies to the drug and for individuals who have hyperkalemia, renal disease, anuria, and by persons who use amiloride (Midamor) or triamterene (Dyrenium).[74] This diuretic should be used with caution during lactation. Spironolactone blocks the effects of aldosterone in the renal tubule, which results in loss of sodium and water while potassium is retained.

Adverse effects include dizziness, headache, drowsiness, cramping, diarrhea, irregular menses or amenorrhea, and sometimes postmenopausal bleeding.[74] Gynecomastia and deepening of the voice have also been reported.[74] The diuretic effect of spironolactone may be decreased when taken with salicylates. Additional drug–drug interactions include increased hyperkalemia if taken with potassium supplements, ACE inhibitors, or in persons who have diets rich in potassium. Increased hypotensive effects may occur if taken with other diuretics.

Alprazolam (Xanax) to Treat PMS-Associated Anxiety

Alprazolam (Xanax) is benzodiazepine and anxiolytic; its mechanism of action is not well understood. New studies suggest an involvement with the GABAergic system.[75] Although its use in treating a woman with PMS/PMDD is off label, alprazolam has been used to treat symptoms of profound anxiety in women suffering from a severe form of either condition.[62] The dose for treating anxiety associated with PMS is less than that for treating the anxiety of PMDD. This drug is potentially addictive and the most commonly abused benzodiazepine; therefore, it is considered a second-line treatment for PMS/PMDD.[68]

Alprazolam is contraindicated for individuals with hypersensitivity to benzodiazepines or those who have acute narrow-angle glaucoma, and it should not be used during lactation since breastfeeding infants whose mothers were using the drug may become lethargic and suffer weight loss. Adverse effects include mild drowsiness, particularly when the drug is initiated; lightheadedness; headache; and restlessness.[62]

Historic but Ineffective Methods of Treatment

Progesterone acetate has been widely prescribed for the treatment of PMS. Unfortunately, few studies demonstrate its effectiveness, and some experts suggest that progesterone actually worsens some of the physical and emotional symptoms associated with PMS.[64] A systematic review of 36 RCTs[76] found no improvement in overall symptoms in women taking progesterone for their PMS, and, therefore, progesterone is not recommended in the treatment of PMS.

COCs are not consistent in their effectiveness for treating PMS or PMD. It is believed that the benefit, if any, is probably due to the estrogen component, and therefore, monophasic pills may be the best choice of treatment if COCs are used to treat PMS.[64] Progesterone-only methods may actually worsen the symptoms associated with PMS in some women, while ameliorating the physical symptoms for others.[64] Overall, their use, particularly for women with severe PMS and those with PMDD, is very limited.

Complementary and Alternative Treatments for PMS and PMDD

Several lifestyle modifications can be suggested to ease many of the problem symptoms of PMS and PMDD, yet data on efficacy are generally lacking, although many have biologic plausibility. Routine exercise improves many symptoms of PMS, possibly by releasing endorphins, which may help to elevate mood. Dietary modifications also have great potential in improving many of the symptoms. Diets high in complex carbohydrates could reduce food cravings, and foods high in tryptophan could elevate brain levels of serotonin and help to improve mood. Reducing sodium consumption could reduce water retention and weight gain. Lowering caffeine in the diet could aid in improving sleep and reduce irritability.

Vitamins and Dietary Supplements

Vitamin supplements including calcium and magnesium have been well studied and reduce many physical symptoms of PMS. Serum levels of calcium are said to fluctuate during the menstrual cycle.[77] Some symptoms of hypocalcemia (depression, muscle cramps, and personality disturbances) mimic those of PMS. Several clinical trials have found calcium supplementation to be effective at reducing PMS symptoms such as anxiety, depression, irritability, mood swings, headache, fluid retention, and menstrual cramps.[77-79] A dose of 1200 mg of calcium carbonate (TUMS) daily in divided doses taken two to four times per day is the typical dose used in most of these trials.

Magnesium levels also fluctuate with the menstrual cycle. Magnesium is involved in many cellular pathways that directly influence PMS. Magnesium deficiency has been linked to PMS.[80] A dose of 200 to 360 mg per day in divided doses during the luteal phase is the typical dose used for treating PMS.[81] A Cochrane meta-analysis that included three small trials comparing magnesium to placebo found magnesium was effective for relieving pain and decreased the need for additional medication.[21] More study is needed to determine an appropriate dose.

A systematic review of the efficacy of pyridoxine (vitamin B$_6$) for treatment of PMS included nine clinical trials (n = 940 women) but found that most of the trials were of low quality. Larger and better designed studies are needed.[82] However, the overall conclusion of this systematic review was that vitamin B$_6$ supplementation improves several PMS symptoms when compared to placebo. The mechanism of pyridoxine's possible benefit is unclear but could relate to its mechanism of action as a necessary cofactor for dopamine production in the brain.

Supplementation with other vitamins such as vitamins E and D have also been investigated for their possible benefits in treating PMS. Two double-blind, randomized studies were carried out in the 1980s and reported that 400 IU vitamin E resulted in significant improvements in several PMS symptoms (compared to a control group that took a placebo).[83,84] Also, women who supplemented their diets with 700 IU of vitamin D daily were shown in one study to have a 40% lower risk of developing PMS.[85] Table 30-9 provides doses and other information about CAM treatments purported to be effective in the treatment of women with PMS or PMDD.

Pelvic Disorders: Pelvic Pain

Dysmenorrhea is pain that accompanies menses, yet some women have pain independent of their menstrual cycles. The diagnosis of pelvic pain is challenging because the nature of the pain can be diffuse and difficult to localize.

Table 30-9 Complementary and Alternative Treatments for Premenstrual Syndrome and Premenstrual Dysphoric Disorder

Agent	Dose	Symptoms Relieved
Nutritional Supplements		
Calcium carbonate	1200–1600 mg/day	Negative mood, water retention, and food cravings
Magnesium	200–500 mg/day taken either cyclically or only during luteal phase	Bloating
Vitamin B$_6$	25–100 mg/day	Mastalgia, swollen breasts, pain, bloating, and depression
Herbal		
Chasteberry (*Vitex agnus castus*)	20–40 mg/day	Breast engorgement and core symptoms
Evening primrose oil	500 mg/day to 1000 mg tid	Breast tenderness
St. John's wort (*Hypericum perforatum*)*	300 mg/day	Mood disturbances

* Rare but severe phototoxicity reported with use. Significant drug reactions can also occur, including reduced levels of birth control pills, theophylline, cyclosporine, antiretroviral drugs, digoxin, buspirone, and carbamazepine.

At some time or another during life, both men and women are likely to experience pelvic pain. Pelvic pain is a symptom, not a disease, and it may be due to a variety of causes such as gastrointestinal conditions or, for men, chronic prostatitis. However, in women, pelvic pain also may be a symptom of disorders within the reproductive tract.

Pelvic pain is subdivided into two types: acute and chronic. Regardless of type of pelvic pain or underlying pathology, the first consideration always should be adequate pain relief for the woman. In many situations, nonpharmacologic pain relief strategies and analgesics as described in detail in Chapter 12 can be employed, especially for relief if the woman is undergoing necessary examinations to identify the exact causative factor.

Acute Pelvic Pain

The common diagnoses associated with acute pelvic pain are listed in Table 30-10. Because pelvic pain may be caused by infections (e.g., urinary tract), muscle strain, or other factors, most pharmacotherapeutic interventions for conditions related to acute pelvic pain are discussed in specific chapters elsewhere in the text. For example, obstetrical/gynecologic causes of acute pelvic pain include ectopic

pregnancy (Chapter 35) or salpingitis associated with pelvic infections (Chapter 23). Some etiologies, such as ovarian torsion, require surgical intervention.

Chronic Pelvic Pain

Chronic pelvic pain is an enigmatic symptom that may signal one of several pathologies, or, perhaps, no discernible entity at all. Yet it is listed as the main indication for 12% of hysterectomies performed in the United States.[86] There are suggestions that chronic pelvic pain often may be misdiagnosed. In one study, more than one third of women presenting with a diagnosis of chronic pelvic pain had irritable bowel syndrome.[87] Some women with painful bladder syndrome or interstitial cystitis are first evaluated for chronic pelvic pain. These urinary tract disorders are discussed in more depth in Chapter 22.

The generally accepted definition of chronic pelvic pain relates to duration as opposed to intensity. Three months of pain is usually the time required for persistent pain to be termed chronic, although some sources mandate a 6-month period, and the pain may be of constant low-level intensity or of varying degrees of discomfort.[88,89] The woman may describe pain as originating in a variety of areas, including the vagina, uterus, bladder, gastrointestinal tract, or spine.

Pharmacologic Therapy for Pelvic Pain: Goserelin (Zoladex)

Currently the most common interventions for pelvic pain include laparoscopy, which is performed to assess and exclude serious pathology, as well as analgesics, hormonal therapy, and surgery to interrupt nerve pathways as methods

Table 30-10 Differential Diagnoses for Acute Pelvic Pain

Category	Differential Diagnosis
Complication of pregnancy	Ectopic pregnancy
	Abortion
Infections	Pelvic inflammatory disease, including tubo-ovarian abscess
Ovarian disorders	Ovarian cysts (hemorrhagic, functional, neoplastic)
	Ovarian torsion
Referred pain from other conditions	Gastrointestinal conditions, including appendicitis, bowel obstruction, diverticulitis, irritable bowel syndrome, urinary tract conditions (e.g., cystitis, pyelonephritis, ureteral lithiasis)
Musculoskeletal conditions	Hematoma
	Hernia

for treatment of pain. A review by Stones et al.[90] included 14 randomized, controlled trials that focused on pain relief and increase in quality of life. The participants included women with chronic pelvic pain but without primary dysmenorrhea, endometriosis, chronic pelvic inflammatory disease, or irritable bowel syndrome. Although counseling and a multidisciplinary approach demonstrated value, among the pharmaceuticals used, only medroxyprogesterone acetate (MPA) and goserelin (Zoladex) appeared to be of value. MPA reduced pain (OR = 2.64; 95% CI, 1.33–5.25; n = 146), but the benefit no longer was apparent when reevaluated following 9 months of therapy. Additional information about MPA and other progestins can be found in Chapters 14 and 29.

Goserelin (Zoladex) is a GnRH analogue that is chemically similar to native GnRH but possesses an extended half-life. The usual dose is 3.6 mg administered subcutaneously as an implant every 28 days. Goserelin rapidly binds to the GnRH receptor cells in the pituitary gland, leading to an initial increase in production of luteinizing hormone and thus an initial increase in the production of corresponding sex hormones and a flare effect that can be worse than the original symptoms. However, after 2–3 weeks, production of LH is reduced due to receptor down-regulation. In the trial conducted by Soysal et al., goserelin provided a longer duration of pelvic pain relief than did MPA (*P* = .0001; n = 47).[91]

Goserelin is not widely used for several reasons: the flare effect, overall expense, and the fact that this drug can be used for 6 months only. Thus, there is no clear and effective single pharmaceutical known to date that a clinician can prescribe for chronic pelvic pain. Most women suffering from chronic pelvic pain are treated for specific symptoms, such as dysmenorrhea or infertility or subfertility, which may respond to pharmacologic treatments.

Infertility

Women with pelvic pain and/or abnormal menstrual conditions also commonly experience infertility. Infertility is defined as failure to achieve a pregnancy after 12 months of frequent unprotected intercourse. Infertility has many causes, of which the majority (55%) are attributed to female factors, 35% attributed to male factors, and 10% for which the cause is unexplained.[58] Ovulatory disorders are an identified cause of female infertility, and PCOS is the most common cause of oligo-ovulation and anovulation.[92]

The successful treatment of infertility is continuously improving with new methods and new drugs being discovered annually. Many of the drugs are extremely potent and have serious side effects necessitating specific guidelines to assure the woman's safety and to avoid superfecundity. It is recommended that clinicians who are not specialists in infertility collaborate and consult with specialists in the field of infertility before prescribing any fertility regimen.

Infertility and Thyroid Disorders

A causal relationship exists between hypothyroidism in women and resulting infertility because thyroid deficiency can cause ovulatory dysfunction.[93,94] Controversy exists over whether women considering conception should be screened for thyroid insufficiency.[95] The American Association of Clinical Endocrinologists (AACE) recommends that all women considering conception be screened for thyroid dysfunction; whereas the American College of Obstetricians and Gynecologists (ACOG) and the United States Preventive Services Task Force (USPSTF) recommend that only women who are symptomatic for thyroid dysfunction should be screened for thyroid disorders.[96-98] Signs of hypothyroidism include menstrual irregularities both in cycle regularity and bleeding patterns. For women with hypothyroidism, a euthyroid status usually is achieved with thyroxine supplementation, and generally, spontaneous ovulatory cycles will resume.[93]

Synthetic thyroid replacement compounds are used instead of natural hormones because the bioavailability of the natural compounds varies.[99] Thyroid hormone is contraindicated for women with acute myocardial infarct (MI). These drugs decrease the effectiveness of digitalis. Thyroid levels need to be monitored when thyroid replacement drugs are prescribed. Additional information about thyroid and pharmacologic treatments can be found in Chapter 19.

Infertility and Amenorrhea

Amenorrhea is categorized as either primary or secondary. **Primary amenorrhea** is defined as an absence of menses by the age of 14 with accompanying delayed maturation of secondary sex characteristics, or absence of menses by age 16 with evidence of secondary sex characteristics. **Secondary amenorrhea** is the term used for women who have a cessation of menses, previously menstruated regularly, and are not pregnant. Once pregnancy is ruled out in a woman with amenorrhea, then a prolactin level, a thyroid-stimulating hormone level, and a progesterone challenge are the usual diagnostic steps in determining the cause of the amenorrhea.

Pharmacologic Treatments for Infertility

Ovulatory disorders account for 30–40% of all cases of female infertility.[93] However, ovulatory induction and superovulation are the most widely used treatments for infertility, especially since well-established agents have existed for the last several decades.[92,100] Ovarian stimulation is accomplished by either the administration of exogenous gonadotropins or augmenting endogenous FSH with clomiphene citrate (Clomid).[100] Table 30-11 contains common doses and other information about fertility drugs. The World Health Organization (WHO) and the European Society for Human Reproduction and Embryology developed a classification system of ovulatory disorders that assists in the identification of associated health risks and defining options for treatment (Box 30-3).

Clomiphene Citrate

Clomiphene citrate (Clomid, Milophene, Serophene) is an estrogen agonist/antagonist and has been the first line of treatment for ovulatory disorders for more than 40 years, resulting in a fecundity rate of 15%.[100] Clomiphene citrate is indicated for treatment of ovulatory failure in women with normal liver function and normal endogenous estrogen levels. Clomiphene citrate (Clomid) decreases the number of available estrogen receptors, which falsely signals the hypothalamus and pituitary to increase FSH and LH secretion. This action, in turn, stimulates the ovary.[62 (p. 450)]

Table 30-11 Fertility Drugs

Drug Generic (Brand)	Dose/Route and Course of Treatment
Clomiphene citrate (Clomid, Milophene, Serophene)	Treatment of ovulatory failure: Initial treatment: 50 mg PO × 5 days started anytime if no recent bleeding or on fifth day of cycle if uterine bleeding occurs. Second course: If ovulation does not occur after first course, administer 100 mg/day PO for 5 days; start this course as early as 30 days after previous one. Third course: Repeat second course regimen, and if no response, further treatment with clomiphene is not recommended. Treatment of male sterility: 50–400 mg/day PO for 2–12 months (controversial).
Letrozole (Femara)	2.5–5 mg/daily for 5 days.
Human menopausal gonadotropin (hMG)	Ovulation induction: 75 IU/day SQ, increase by 37.5 IU/day after 14 days; may increase again after 7 days. Do not exceed 35 days of treatment.
Follitropin alpha (Gonal-F)	Follicle development: 150 IU/day on days 2 or 3 and continue for 10 days. In women whose endogenous gonadotropin levels are suppressed, initiate at 225 IU/day SQ. Adjust dose after 5 days based on patient response. Dose should be adjusted no more than every 3–5 days and by no more than 75–150 IU at each adjustment. Maximum dose 450 IU/day. Given in conjunction with hCG. Spermatogenesis: 150 IU SQ 3 ×/week in conjunction with hCG. May increase to 300 IU prn 3 ×/week prn. May administer up to 18 months for adequate effect.
Follitropin beta (Follistatin)	Ovulation induction: Same as for follitropin alpha. Follicle development: 150–225 IU/day SQ or IM for at least 4 days of treatment. Adjust dose based on ovarian response. Given in conjunction with hCG.
Menotropins* (Pergonal, Humegon, Menopur, Repronex)	225 units IM; then 150 units/day × 10 days up to maximum of 450 units IM/day for no longer than 12 days.
Human chorionic gonadotropin (hCG) (Chorex-5, Chorex-10, Choron 10, Pregnyl, Profasi)	5000–10,000 units IM, 1 day following the last dose of menotropins.

hCG = human chorionic gonadotropin.
* To achieve ovulation, menotropins must be followed with administration of hCG.

Box 30-3 World Health Organization Classification of Anovulation

WHO class 1: Hypogonadotropic hypogonadal anovulation (hypothalamic amenorrhea)

Women in this category have low or low-normal serum follicle-stimulating hormone (FSH) concentrations and low serum estradiol concentrations due to decreased hypothalamic secretion of gonadotropin-releasing hormone (GnRH) or pituitary unresponsiveness to GnRH.

WHO class 2: Normogonadotropic normoestrogenic anovulation

Women in this category may secrete normal amounts of gonadotropins and estrogens. However, FSH secretion during the follicular phase of the cycle is subnormal. This group includes women with polycystic ovary syndrome (PCOS). Some ovulate occasionally, especially those with oligomenorrhea.

WHO class 3: Hypergonadotropic hypoestrogenic anovulation

The primary causes of hypergonadotropic hypoestrogenic anovulation are premature ovarian failure (absence of ovarian follicles due to early menopause) and ovarian resistance (follicular form).

Hyperprolactinemic anovulation

The women in the hyperprolactinemic anovulation category are anovulatory because hyperprolactinemia inhibits gonadotropin and therefore estrogen secretion; they may have regular anovulatory cycles, but most have oligomenorrhea or amenorrhea. Their serum gonadotropin concentrations are usually normal.

Source: World Health Organization 1973.[136]

Clomiphene citrate is contraindicated for any woman who suspects she is pregnant, has AUB of undetermined etiology, an ovarian cyst, uncontrolled renal or thyroid dysfunction, or organic intracranial lesions. It should be used with caution during lactation. Women taking clomiphene citrate should be informed it can cause abdominal bloating, nausea, visual disturbances, insomnia, and ovarian hyperstimulation.

Clomiphene Citrate Challenge Test

Because a number of women today are delaying childbearing, an increasing number are presenting with infertility due to advancing age and diminished ovarian reserve. There are a number of tests used to determine ovarian reserve; however, currently the best documented test of ovarian reserve is the clomiphene citrate challenge test.[101] A daily dose of 100 mg of clomiphene citrate is administered from day 5 to day 9 of the menstrual cycle. An abnormal test is indicated by the absence of FSH suppression.[101,102] Tests of ovarian reserve are often used to predict failure of in vitro fertilization because an abnormal clomiphene citrate challenge test is associated with a significant reduction in pregnancy rates in women who have an infertility diagnosis.[103]

Aromatase Inhibitors

Aromatase inhibitors have become an increasingly popular first step for ovarian stimulation and may replace clomiphene citrate in the future.[92] Inhibition of aromatase leads to a decrease in estrogen production, which increases the secretion of FSH; this stimulates the ovaries, which results in follicular development.[100] Letrozole (Femara) is the most widely used aromatase inhibitor.[100] Letrozole produces a thicker endometrium, has better pregnancy rates, and costs less than clomiphene citrate.[100] Side effects include hot flashes, headache, depression, and sometimes vaginal bleeding. Women should not use this drug if there is any suspicion of pregnancy or impaired liver function. Myocardial infarct and thromboembolism are the major adverse reactions to aromatase inhibitors.

Gonadotropin-Releasing Hormone (Leuprode)

Synthetically produced gonadotropin-releasing hormone (Leuprolide) may be used to stimulate ovulation. If the woman has functional pituitary activity and an ovary to produce a luteinizing hormone (LH) surge, GnRH can be used in pulsatile doses to stimulate ovulation.

Menotropins

Menotropins (Pergonal, Humegon, Repronex) are a combination of FSH and LH that is derived from urine of menopausal women. Menotropins are also referred to as human menopausal gonadotropin (hMG) because these products are extracted from the urine of menopausal women then standardized for LH and FSH content. Menotropins (Pergonal, Humegon, Repronex) are used to produce ovarian follicle development and to stimulate ovulation when followed by administration of hCG.[62 (p. 452)] These agents are useful for treating male infertility, and when used in conjunction with hCG for at least 3 months, they can induce spermatogenesis.

The greatest risks associated with FSH analogs are multiple births and arterial thromboembolism. Adverse effects include dizziness, nausea, vomiting, and abdominal bloating. Ovarian enlargement may be a sign of ovarian hyperstimulation syndrome. The drug should be discontinued if there are any signs or symptoms of ovarian hyperstimulation. Severe symptoms may require hospitalization and removal of excess fluid in the abdominal cavity. If a woman taking any of the FSH analogues experiences abdominal bloating and pain she should seek care immediately.

Menotropins are ineffective if the woman has primary ovarian failure; thus, if she has a high gonadotropin level (which is indicative of primary ovarian failure), these agents are contraindicated. Menotropins also are contraindicated for women who have overt thyroid or adrenal dysfunction, AUB of unknown etiology, or polycystic ovary syndrome, or if pregnancy is suspected. Adverse effects include dizziness, arterial thromboembolism, nausea, vomiting, abdominal bloating, and ovarian hyperstimulation syndrome. Table 30-11 provides information about doses.

Follitropins

Follitropin alpha (Gonal-F) and follitropin beta (Follistim) are recombinant DNA synthetically manufactured FSH. Follitropins do not have LH or contaminant urinary proteins and there is more batch-to-batch consistency in these products. Follitropins have a greater stimulatory effect on ovarian follicles and slightly higher pregnancy rate compared to menotropins. These drugs are also cheaper and more available than menotropins.

Human Chorionic Gonadotropins (hCG)

Human chorionic gonadotropin (hCG) (Chorex-5, Profasi) is used to stimulate ovarian function and to stimulate the corpus luteum to produce progesterone and androgens.[62 (pp. 451-452)] To induce ovulation, hCG is administered the day following the last dose of menotropins. This drug should be used with caution by women who have epilepsy, migraines, asthma, cardiac disease, renal disease, or by those who are breastfeeding. Human chorionic gonadotropin is contraindicated in women with known sensitivity to chorionic gonadotropins, precocious puberty, or any androgen-dependent carcinoma. If there is any suspicion the woman is pregnant, hCG should not be used.

Complementary and Alternative Therapies for Infertility

Glyceryl Guaiacolate

Guaiacol glyceryl ether (Guaifenesin, Robitussin) is an expectorant used to treat upper respiratory infections and pulmonary disease. Some experts suggested it might be useful in the treatment of infertility because of its ability to thin secretions.[104,105] A few small studies that evaluated the use of guaiacol glycerol ether treating infertility have been performed.[105] All of the 40 participants in the seminal study done in 1982 had cervical mucous abnormalities and were trying to achieve a pregnancy. Each woman was treated with 200 mg guaifenesin orally three times daily beginning at day 5 until her temperature rise indicated ovulation occurred. No other treatment was provided. After 6 months, 23 of the women showed marked improvement in their cervical mucous penetrability. Of these 23 women, 15 achieved a pregnancy. Some clinicians suggest that women use guaifenesin concurrently with clomiphene citrate.[105] The recommended dose is guaifenesin 600 mg orally twice a day begun 5 days prior to ovulation and stopping once ovulation occurs. If a woman is taking clomiphene, it is suggested she begin guaifenesin the day after her last dose of clomiphene. It is possible that guaifenesin will have the same thinning effect on men with thick semen; however, studies to confirm this are lacking.

Vitamin C

Vitamin C is involved in recycling vitamin E and glutathione. Glutathione plays a role in the development of the zygote. Glutathione is present in the oocyte and in the tubal fluid. In one randomized, control trial, vitamin C supplementation at a dose of 750 mg per day was given to women with luteal phase defects and this treatment resulted in improved pregnancy rates.[106] In another randomized, controlled trial enrolling 620 women, high doses of vitamin C supplementation (1, 5, or 10 grams per day) were given during the luteal phase to women undergoing in vitro fertilization preembryo transfer.[107] No differences in pregnancy rate or implantation rates were observed.

Multivitamins

Multivitamin supplementation was associated with less infertility due to anovulation in an observational study of healthy women (n =18,555) who were followed for 8 years.[108] The women who took multivitamins had approximately a one third lower risk of developing ovulatory infertility compared to nonmultivitamin users. Women taking B vitamins (B_1, B_2, B_6, B_{12}, folic acid, and niacin) at least three times a week had a decrease in ovulatory infertility. It is thought that folic acid may be the most influential vitamin influencing infertility.

One small study provides evidence that dehydroepiandrosterone (DHEA) may be useful for women with infertility.[109] Five women with unexplained infertility and lack of response to gonadotropin stimulation received DHEA (80 mg/day) for 2 months. All five women showed enhanced responsiveness to gonadotropin and had increased plasma estradiol levels.

Male Infertility

Although this text is focused on care of women, infertility relates to both male and female partners. Male factor is the sole cause of infertility in 35% of infertile couples, and it may be a contributing factor in many more cases. Infertility in men is caused by many factors including anatomic or structural problems, abnormal sperm production or function, or sexual, hormonal, and genetic conditions. Other causes of male infertility include erectile dysfunction and decreased testosterone production. Treatment depends on the cause of the infertility, and unfortunately, with few exceptions, male infertility is not amenable to medical treatment. Studies suggest that genetics are more frequently the cause of infertility in men. This section focuses on medications that are occasionally used to treat male infertility.

Clomiphene Citrate (Clomid)

Clomiphene acts on the hypothalamic-pituitary axis to increase serum levels of LH, FSH, and testosterone, and it is commonly used by some clinicians to treat idiopathic oligospermia, asthenospermia, and teratospermia. However, most studies show that the use of clomiphene to treat male infertility leads to little if any improvement in sperm parameters and shows no improvement in pregnancy rates.[110] Many experts question its use.

Testosterone

Androgens such as testosterone sometimes are advocated in the treatment of male infertility due to idiopathic oligospermia, asthenospermia, and teratospermia. The theory is that testosterone stimulates spermatogenesis directly by increasing intratesticular androgen concentrations and indirectly by causing a rebound increase in pituitary gonadotropin secretions. However, studies on the use of testosterone to improve male fertility have had conflicting results. Interestingly, many men with fertility problems indicate they have used testosterone supplements to improve their fertility.

Gonadotropins

Hypogonadotropic hypogonadism can be effectively treated with GnRH. First, hyperprolactinemia or a hypothalamic or pituitary lesion must be ruled out prior to beginning GnRH therapy. GnRH treatment has to be titrated to the individual to be successful. Exogenous GnRH therapy is costly and cumbersome, and spermatogenesis may take up to 2 years.

An alternative treatment for hypogonadotropic hypogonadism is to use hCG 1000–2500 IU twice a week with the dose titrated to maintain serum testosterone and estradiol levels within normal range.[93] Treatment with hCG is then combined with hMG at a dose of 150 IU three times weekly.[93]

Polycystic Ovary Syndrome: Menstrual Disorders and Infertility

Polycystic ovary syndrome (PCOS) is the most common known cause of anovulation, with its accompanying menstrual irregularities affecting between 5% and 8% of all women.[92,111] PCOS is a multifaceted disorder, and central to its pathogenesis are hyperandrogenemia and hyperinsulinemia, which are targets for treatment.[111] Hyperandrogenemia causes hirsutism, alopecia, acne, virilization, and menstrual irregularity and infertility. Women with PCOS are frequently overweight, which is believed to be due to insulin resistance that accompanies the syndrome. If an obese woman desires a pregnancy and is diagnosed with PCOS, she is first encouraged to lose weight. Weight loss has been shown to reverse the deleterious effects of obesity, and often ovarian function improves.[112]

PCOS is associated with a classic ovarian morphology.[113] The polycystic ovary has 12 or more follicles measuring 2–9 mm in diameter and/or increased ovarian volume to more than 10 cm³. The diagnosis of PCOS may be made on the basis of only one ovary having the aforementioned appearance.[114] The focus of this section is on pharmacologic treatment to restore ovulation and fertility in women with PCOS.

Clomiphene Citrate

Clomiphene citrate (Clomid) remains the first line of intervention for medically induced ovulation in women with PCOS. A functional hypothalamus-pituitary-ovarian axis is required for clomiphene citrate to be effective. It is believed clomiphene citrate binds and inhibits stimulation of estrogen receptors in the hypothalamus, which decreases the normal hypothalamus-estrogen feedback loop.[93] This increases the GnRH levels, which in turn increases pituitary secretion of gonadotropins and promotes ovarian follicle development. Unfortunately among obese women with PCOS and insulin resistance, the success rate of clomiphene citrate alone is relatively low.[93]

Metformin Hydrochloride

Metformin hydrochloride (Fortamet, Glucophage, Riomet) is a member of a group of hypoglycemia-inducing drugs used for treating diabetes mellitus. Metformin acts primarily by decreasing hepatic glucose production and increasing glucose utilization in peripheral tissues.[92,111] More details on these agents are found in Chapter 18. Insulin-sensitizing agents such as metformin may be used prior to administration of clomiphene citrate, administered at the same time as clomiphene citrate, or prescribed as monotherapy for women with PCOS who are resistant to clomiphene citrate.[93] Ovulation rates increase in women with PCOS who use metformin (Glucophage).[111] Metformin is available in short- and long-acting formulations.

Metformin is contraindicated for women who have heart problems, type 1 diabetes, renal disease, or conditions predisposing to renal dysfunction, liver disease, and serious hepatic impairment. The safety of this agent is not established in lactation. Adverse effects of metformin include diarrhea, abdominal bloating, nausea, and a metallic taste. Anorexia can occur. The most serious adverse effect is lactic acidosis.

Studies comparing the use of clomiphene citrate alone, metformin alone, and clomiphene citrate with metformin found that the combined regimen of clomiphene citrate and metformin significantly increase the success of ovulation induction when compared to clomiphene citrate or metformin alone.[115-117] Information about doses is provided in Table 30-12.

Thiazolidinediones

Thiazolidinediones (TZDs) are insulin sensitizers that act by improving insulin sensitivity and affecting adipocyte gene expression[111] (Table 30-13). Initially, these drugs were used to treat type 2 diabetes, then it became apparent they could be effective in inducing ovulation in women with PCOS. The first TZD introduced was troglitazone (Rezulin), which was eventually removed from the market secondary to a risk of fatal liver failure (1/50,000).[93,111] Two newer TZDs, rosiglitazone (Avandia) and pioglitazone (Actos) show promise, although there is a question of possible adverse cardiovascular events associated with use of these agents. The FDA released a black box warning in 2007 mandating that the labels of these drugs state that they are associated with an increased risk of heart attack and/or angina.

Rosiglitazone Maleate (Avandia)

Rosiglitazone (Avandia) resensitizes peripheral tissues to insulin, decreases hepatic glucogenesis, and increases glucose transport to muscle. Rosiglitazone is used off-label to increase ovulatory frequency in women with PCOS. Rosiglitazone is contraindicated for women who have allergies to TZDs, type 1 diabetes, ketoacidosis, or who are lactating. Adverse effects include headache, hypoglycemia, hyperglycemia, diarrhea, and liver injury. Some individuals have reported sinusitis and rhinitis with its use. Rosiglitazone interacts with gemfibrozil (Lopid) and will increase serum concentrations of rosiglitazone if they are taken together. Serum glucose levels of women taking this drug need consistent monitoring.

Pioglitazone (Actos)

Pioglitazone (Actos) is an antidiabetic pharmaceutical that acts by binding to insulin receptors and making them more responsive to insulin, thus lowering blood glucose and improving the action of glucose.[62 (p. 396)] It is used off label as an ovulatory induction agent in women with PCOS. Pioglitazone (Actos) is contraindicated for anyone with allergies to TZDs, who has type 1 diabetes or ketoacidosis, or who is lactating. Adverse effects include headache, aggravated diabetes, diarrhea, and liver injury. There exists a theoretical risk of decreased effectiveness of hormonal contraceptives with the use of pioglitazone.

Aromatase Inhibitors

Aromatase inhibitors such as letrozole (Femara) are being used with increasing frequency and increasing success as a first-line treatment for anovulation. Although there are studies confirming that the use of clomiphene citrate with metformin is superior to clomiphene citrate alone and that letrozole is superior to clomiphene citrate alone,

Table 30-12 Metformin Therapy With and Without Clomiphene Citrate for Ovulation Induction in Women with Polycystic Ovary Syndrome (PCOS)

Drug Generic (Brand)	Treatment Regimen	Monitoring
Metformin (Glucophage)	Confirm normal liver and renal function. Do pregnancy test when indicated. Initiate therapy as follows: 500 mg once/day with breakfast for 4 days 500 mg twice/day with breakfast and dinner for 4 days 500 mg with breakfast and 1000 mg with dinner for 4 days and thereafter—1000 mg twice a day at breakfast and dinner	If using metformin alone, evaluate serum progesterone levels weekly to detect occurrence of ovulation. Ovulation may take up to 2 months.
Metformin (Glucophage) with clomiphene citrate (Clomid)	Add clomiphene at the usual starting dosage of 50 to 100 mg once/day from days 5–9 when the full dose of metformin has been reached if spontaneous ovulation has not occurred. If ovulation does not occur, clomiphene citrate can be increased incrementally by 50 mg once/day in subsequent cycles.	Home LH detection kits can be used to detect ovulation and time intercourse. If the combination of metformin and clomiphene does not induce ovulation, the diagnosis should be reviewed again by an infertility expert.

Source: Burney R et al. 2007.[93]

Table 30-13 Thiazolidinediones (TZD) Regimen for Ovulation Induction in Women with Polycystic Ovary Syndrome

Drug Generic (Brand)	Dose/Route	Onset	Peak
Rosiglitazone maleate (Avandia)	4 mg/daily PO or divide into two doses. If adequate response is not observed in 8–12 weeks, increase to 8 mg/daily PO. Combination therapy with metformin (Glucophage): 4 mg/daily PO added to the established dose of metformin; may be increased after 12 weeks to 8 mg/daily PO.	Rapid	1.3–3.5 h
Pioglitazone (Actos)	15–30 mg/day PO as a single dose. If adequate response is not seen, may increase dose to maximum of 45 mg/day. Combination therapy with metformin (Glucophage): 15–30 mg/daily PO added to established dose of metformin. If hypoglycemia occurs, reduce the dose of metformin.	Rapid	2–4 h

there are no studies that have evaluated the combination of metformin with letrozole.[118] The potential benefit of the latter combination is that it would provide insulin control along with an increase in FSH secretion and regular ovulation and menstruation.

Endometriosis: Pelvic Pain and Infertility

Endometriosis is a condition that is associated with chronic pelvic pain and dysmenorrhea as well as infertility. The classic definition of endometriosis, also termed *adenomyosis externa*, is the presence of endometrial tissue outside of the endometrial cavity (Figure 30-2). Adenomyosis is a separate condition that is characterized by the presence of endometrial glands and stroma within the myometrium, although symptoms and pharmacologic treatments are similar for both conditions. Endometriosis often is associated with primary or secondary infertility, although the most common initial symptom is pelvic pain. The pelvic pain may be specific to dyspareunia, or include severe dysmenorrhea. Most women with severe endometriosis are cared for by gynecologists who have expertise in this area.

Endometriosis has been a known gynecologic entity since the 1920s, and it is estimated that 10% of adult women suffer from the condition. Yet much about endometriosis remains unknown. For example, the etiology of the condition is subject to a variety of hypotheses including retrograde menstruation, polygenic causes, or autoimmune influences, among others. A physical examination is often nonspecific, although a tender nodule at the uterosacral

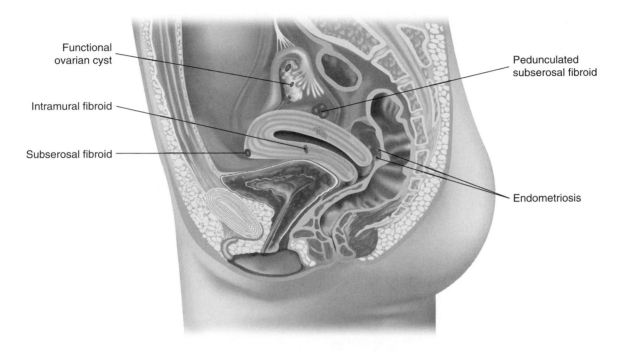

Figure 30-2 Pelvic sites associated with pelvic pain. *Source:* Adapted from Schuiling KD et al. 2006.[137]

---

ligament may be pathognomonic. The only definitive diagnosis is one made during surgery.

Even surgical diagnosis of endometriosis and visual determination of degree of endometriosis does not always correlate to the degree of pain a woman experiences or the risk of infertility. The American Society for Reproductive Medicine has a classification system based on size, location of endometriomas, depth, extent of adhesions, and ovarian/tubal enclosure or obliteration to allow better documentation of the degree of the disease.[62 (p. 228)] However, some women with minimal disease still may have significant problems of infertility, pain, or recurrence.

Although the degree of disease may or may not be clinically relevant, some researchers have evaluated interventions that cause disease regression. Others have concentrated on the two most common symptoms associated with endometriosis, namely pelvic pain and subfertility/ infertility. Ironically, one of the most basic interventions to promote regression of the disease process treatment of pain is to attain pregnancy. Pregnancy, with its accompanying endometrial quiescence, will delay progression of the disease and may retard pain, although recurrence is common. Yet subfertility/infertility precludes this treatment for many if not most women. However pregnancy is not always desirable, which makes this particular intervention available to a limited number of women with endometriosis.

The pharmacologic agents most frequently used to promote endometrial quiescence include hormonal contraception such as combined oral contraceptives and medroxyprogesterone acetate (MPA, Depo Provera). If a woman desires treatment of endometriosis-associated infertility, MPA usually is avoided because of length of amenorrhea after discontinuation. These two drug categories specifically are used to treat endometriosis: a synthetic testosterone and various GnRH agonists.

Danocrine (Danazol)

Danocrine (Danazol) is a derivative of 17 alpha ethinyl testosterone, which has multiple antigonadotropin properties that create a high androgen/low estrogen environment hostile to endometrial growth. Danocrine was the first drug to be FDA approved for use in treatment of endometriosis. Danocrine is a fat-soluble drug that increases androgens and decreases secretion of endogenous estradiol. Gonadotropin levels are usually not changed, although LH may be slightly elevated. Because danocrine changes the hormonal milieu, pregnancy is prevented, but the drug is not intended to be a contraceptive. Danocrine has been primarily used to treat fibrocystic breast disease or menorrhagia although this is off-label use. Danocrine is metabolized in the liver and should be used with caution by women with liver compromise. The usual treatment regimen for danocrine is to initiate therapy with a dose of 800 mg daily in four divided doses and, if used for pain relief and satisfactory response is attained, to continue at 200–800 mg daily in two to four divided doses.

Although danocrine (Danazol) has been available for more than 3 decades, its use appears to be diminishing because of side effects that make it relatively unattractive to women. The androgenic adverse effects include amenorrhea, acne, weight gain, hirsutism, and for a few women, a masculine-sounding voice. Most treatment regimens are limited to 6 months in an attempt to minimize the side effects. More clinicians prescribe GnRH analogues for endometriosis instead of danocrine.

GnRH Analogues

GnRH analogues such as leuprolide acetate (Lupron), buserelin (Suprefact), and nafarelin (Synarel) are nonsteroidal agents that suppress ovarian estrogen production. Although these agents tend to initially cause a flare effect or an increase in untoward symptoms, down-regulation occurs because of the continuous administration, and, ultimately, a reversible state of hypogonadism results.

Table 30-14 summarizes some of the most recent reviews of randomized clinical trials for treatment of endometriosis and its symptoms.[119-124] Pharmacologic treatment for endometriosis is often combined with surgical intervention. The most common surgery is ablation of endometrial implants (so-called powder burns) and lysis of adhesions, although the long-term effectiveness of pharmacologic and surgical treatments is not well established. Recurrence rates are estimated to be as high as 40% over a 5-year period. Many women with severe disease ultimately have a hysterectomy and bilateral salpingo-oophorectomy for definitive treatment.

Leiomyomata (Uterine Fibroids): Menstrual Disorders, Pelvic Pain, and Infertility

Leiomyomata is the most common benign tumor found in women. The incidence of uterine fibroids is estimated to be as high as 35% among normal, healthy women, with 50% of them asymptomatic.[125]

As women age, the uterus and ovaries naturally decrease in size, as do uterine leiomyomata. Therefore, many fibroids are never problematic to a woman unless they are incidental findings during a physical exam, imaging studies, or surgery.

However, for the 50% of women who do experience symptoms associated with fibroids, the condition can range from being a minor problem to a major, life-altering condition. The most common symptoms include dysmenorrhea, DUB, and pelvic pain. Fibroids also are associated with subfertility/infertility.[126]

Table 30-14 Summary of Cochrane Systematic Reviews of Pharmacologic Treatments for Women with Endometriosis

Pharmacologic Treatment	Focus	Number of Trials	Findings
Presurgical/postsurgical hormonal suppression[119]	To determine if hormonal treatments benefit surgical outcome	11 with 3397 women	Insufficient evidence to support presuppression/postsuppression.
Combined oral contraceptives (COCs) versus GnRH analogue[120]	To determine if COCs decrease pain associated with endometriosis	1 with 57 women	Limited data; both relieved pain equally well. Goserelin only studied for 6 months. GnRH useful for dysmenorrhea by inducing amenorrhea; COCs successful.
Nonsteroidal anti-inflammatory drugs (NSAIDs) versus placebo[121]	To investigate effectiveness of NSAIDs with pain associated with endometriosis	1 with 24 women	Inconclusive evidence.
Ovulation suppression and later pregnancy[122]	To evaluate if ovulation suppression benefits subfertile/infertile women	23 with 3043 women	No evidence of benefit in the use of ovulation suppression in subfertile women with endometriosis who wish to conceive, and since ovulation is stopped for the time or treatment, fertility may be further reduced.
Danazol for subfertility[124]	To determine if danazol is effective in treating infertility	2 with 71 women	Most commonly prescribed drug for endometriosis but no evidence that it increases rate of pregnancy or live births.

Black women of any age are more likely than women of other races and ethnicities to have multiple and larger fibroids that are symptomatic. The incidence of fibroids peaks during the perimenopausal years and, thus, women tend to seek care for the condition more often during this period.[127]

Treatment of Leiomyomata

Initial treatment of a woman with fibroids is a symptom-targeted approach. Women with dysmenorrhea usually are treated with analgesics. In addition to dysmenorrhea, fibroids can cause DUB. Previously, there were concerns that fibroids were estrogen-dependent and use of combined oral contraceptives would cause growth of the uterine tumor. However, today's COCs actually have been linked to a reduction in the development of symptomatic fibroids,[128] and there is no indication that use of COCs for treatment of women with menorrhagia results in an increase in fibroid size. The LNG intrauterine system has been found to be effective to decrease bleeding for women with fibroids as well as those without, but not to decrease the size of the fibroid and other associated symptoms such as pelvic pressure and pain.[129-131]

Both current COCs and the LNG-IUS use low-dose amounts of hormones. Inhibition of hormonal production, either with estrogen or progesterone or both, has been theorized as effective treatments for fibroids. GnRH agonists were first suggested as a method to decrease the size of fibroids and, therefore, the symptoms associated with them. However, GnRH agonists have potent side effects, and women often were faced with a Hobson's choice between the effects of the fibroids and the side effects of the treatment. Today, GnRH is more commonly used to decrease the size of the fibroid in anticipation of an easier operative intervention. A course of therapy for 3–4 months prior to either a myomectomy or a hysterectomy is associated with shorter operative time, smaller incisions,

increased operative options (e.g., vaginal hysterectomy versus abdominal), and less blood loss.[125]

Selective estrogen receptor modulators (SERMs) have been used by some researchers for treatment of fibroids. Tamoxifen (Nolvadex) and raloxifene (Evista) have been suggested due to their antiestrogen properties, but more research is needed to assess the efficacy of these agents.[132]

Mifepristone (Mifeprex, formerly RU486) is an antiprogestin that is a progesterone receptor modulator. This agent, combined with misoprostol, is used as a medical abortifacient and is discussed in more depth in Chapter 29. However, as a progesterone receptor modulator, mifepristone can decrease the size of fibroids. In 2004, a systematic review was published that evaluated the use of mifepristone for treatment of symptoms associated with uterine fibroids. Six trials were identified (n = 66 women). Mifepristone did reduce the volume of the leiomyomas. It also decreases the incidence of dysmenorrhea, menorrhagia, and pelvic pressure. Unfortunately, 28% of the 36 women screened by endometrial biopsy demonstrated the presence of endometrial hyperplasia, causing routine use of the drug to be called into question.[133] A more recent randomized trial published in 2008 found similar positive results for use of mifepristone and symptoms of fibroids with use of either 5 or 10 mg per day, with only a 2% risk of endometrial hyperplasia. This study suggests that the risk of endometrial hyperplasia, although still present, is dose dependent.[134] Several other novel progesterone receptor modulators, including asoprisnil, onapristone, and ulipristal, are being investigated as possible therapies for future treatment of fibroids.[135]

A hysterectomy is the definitive treatment for leiomyomata, yet a woman may choose a myomectomy in order to maintain possible fertility. Uterine artery embolization is less invasive than abdominal myomectomy, although no type of surgery for fibroids has been found to be a clear cure for fibroid-related subfertility. Table 30-15 summarizes systematic reviews regarding treatments for fibroids.

Table 30-15 Summary of Cochrane Systematic Reviews of Interventions for Women with Fibroids

Intervention	Focus	Number of Trials	Findings
Preoperative GnRH analogue therapy for fibroids before surgery[125]	To determine if GnRH analogues shrink leiomyomata in order to have less invasive surgeries	26 trials; some subgroups of trials analyzed separately	Significant reduction of size when GnRH is administered 3–4 months before surgery. In treatment group, women more likely to have less risk of anemia, reduced operating time, increased number of vaginal versus abdominal hysterectomies. Limited data on myomectomy and postoperative fertility. Financial implications of treatments were not included.
SERMs for treatment of leiomyomata[132]	To determine whether or not SERMs are useful for treatment of fibroids	3 trials of small size	Because trials are small, and some are of poor quality, no conclusions were reached and more studies are recommended.

Additional reviews of the use of acupuncture, herbal preparations, and other pharmaceuticals like danocrine currently are under way.

Conclusion

Women can have a variety of gynecologic conditions and symptoms. Prominent among them are menstrual disorders, pelvic disease, and infertility. Several conditions such as endometriosis, polycystic ovarian syndrome, and fibroids are distinct entities with shared gynecologic symptoms. In most cases, pharmacologic treatments are targeted to the symptoms, and many of the pharmacologic treatments overlap. Often definitive studies are lacking regarding efficacy of treatments. However, the advent of designer drugs that mimic normal endogenous agents and development of new delivery systems such as intrauterine systems may herald research opportunities from which future treatments will emerge. Until the unlikely day that a Lydia Pinkham–type all-encompassing treatment is found, modern healthcare providers need to be aware of multiple pharmaceuticals for the multiple gynecologic symptoms that women may experience.

Ballad of Lydia Pinkham

Let us sing (let us sing) of Lydia Pinkham
The benefactress of the human race.
She invented a vegetable compound,
And now all papers print her face,

O, Mrs. Brown could do no housework,
O, Mrs. Brown could do no housework,
She took three bottles of Lydia's compound,
And now there's nothing she will shirk,

Mrs. Jones she had no children,
And she loved them very dear.
So she took three bottles of Pinkham's
Now she has twins every year.

References

1. Doty E, Attaran M. Managing primary dysmenorrhea. J Pediatr Adolesc Gynecol 2006;19:341–4.
2. Harel Z. Dysmenorrhea in adolescents and young adults: etiology and management. J Pediatr Adolesc Gynecol 2006;19:363–71.
3. Dawood MY. Primary dysmenorrhea: advances in pathogenesis and management. Obstet Gynecol 2006; 108:428–41.
4. French L. Dysmenorrhea. Am Fam Physician 2005; 71:285–91.
5. Proctor M, Farquhar C. Diagnosis and management of dysmenorrhoea. BMJ 2006;332:1134–8.
6. Ryan GL, Stolpen A, Van Voorhis BJ. An unusual cause of adolescent dysmenorrhea. Obstet Gynecol 2006;108:1017–22.
7. de los Santos AR, Zmijanovich R, Perez Macri S, Marti ML, Di Girolamo G. Antispasmodic/analgesic associations in primary dysmenorrhea double-blind crossover placebo-controlled clinical trial. Int J Clin Pharmacol Res 2001;21:21–9.
8. Marjoribanks J, Proctor ML, Farquhar C. Nonsteroidal anti-inflammatory drugs for primary dysmenorrhoea. Cochrane Database Syst Rev 2003;(4): CD001751.
9. Lethaby A, Augood C, Duckitt K, Farquhar C. Nonsteroidal anti-inflammatory drugs for heavy menstrual bleeding. Cochrane Database Syst Rev 2007; (4):CD000400.
10. Lema MJ. Introduction: The role of coxibs in pain management. J Pain Symptom Manage 2003;25:3–5.
11. Weberschock TB, Muller SM, Boehncke S, Boehncke WH. Tolerance to coxibs in patients with intolerance to non-steroidal anti-inflammatory drugs (NSAIDs): a systematic structured review of the literature. Arch Dermatol Res 2007;299:169–75.
12. Gaytan M, Morales C, Bellido C, Sanchez-Criado JE, Gaytan F. Non-steroidal anti-inflammatory drugs (NSAIDs) and ovulation: lessons from morphology. Histol Histopathol 2006;21:541–56.
13. Helin-Salmivaara A, Huttunen T, Gronroos JM, Klaukka T, Huupponen R. Risk of serious upper gastrointestinal events with concurrent use of NSAIDs and SSRIs: a case-control study in the general population. Eur J Clin Pharmacol 2007;63:403–8.
14. DeMaria AN, Weir MR. Coxibs—beyond the GI tract: renal and cardiovascular issues. J Pain Symptom Manage 2003;25:S41–9.
15. American Academy of Pediatrics Committee on Drugs. Transfer of drugs and other chemicals into human milk. Pediatrics 2001;108:776–89.
16. Burke A, Smyth E, FitzGerald G. Analgesic-antipyretic and antiinflammatory agents: pharmacotherapy of gout. In Brunton L, Lazo J, Parker K, eds. Goodman & Gilman's the pharmacological basis of therapeutics, 11th ed. New York: McGraw Hill, 2006:653–70.

17. Harel Z. Dysmenorrhea in adolescents and young adults: from pathophysiology to pharmacological treatments and management strategies. Expert Opin Pharmacother 2008;9:2661–72.

18. Hendrix SL, Alexander NJ. Primary dysmenorrhea treatment with a desogestrel-containing low-dose oral contraceptive. Contraception 2002;66:393–9.

19. Proctor ML, Roberts H, Farquhar CM. Combined oral contraceptive pill OCP as treatment for primary dysmenorrhoea. Cochrane Database Syst Rev. 2001;(2):CD002120. DOI: 10.1002/14651858. CD002120.

20. Pierzynski P, Swiatecka J, Oczeretko E, Laudanski P, Batra S, Laudanski T. Effect of short-term, low dose treatment with tamoxifen in patients with primary dysmenorrhea. Gynecol Endocrinol 2006; 22(12):698–703.

21. Proctor ML, Murphy PA. Herbal and dietary therapies for primary and secondary dysmenorrhoea. Cochrane Database Syst Rev. 2001;(2):CD002124. DOI: 10.1002/ 14651858.CD002124.

22. Gokhale LB. Curative treatment of primary (spasmodic) dysmenorrhoea. Indian J Med Res 1996;103: 227–31.

23. Hudgins AP. Vitamin C and niacin for dysmenorrhea therapy. West J Surg Obstet Gynecol 1954; 12:610–1.

24. Ziaei S, Fughihzadeh S, Sohrabuand F, Lamyian M, Emamgholy T. A randomized placebo-controlled trial to determine the effect of vitamin E in the treatment of primary dysmenorrhea. BJOG 2001; 108:1181–3.

25. Ziaei S, Zakeri M, Kazemnejad A. A randomized controlled trial of vitamin E in the treatment of primary dysmenorrhea. BJOG 2005;112:466–9.

26. Seifert B, Wagler P, Dartsch S, Schmidt U, Nieder J. Magnesium—a new therapeutic alternative in primary dysmenorrheal. Zentraldl Gynakol 1989; 111(11): 755–60.

27. Fontana-Klaiber H, Hogg B. Therapeutic effects of magnesium in dysmenorrhea. Schweiz Rundsch Med Prax 1990;79(16):491–4.

28. Benassi L, Barletta FP, Baroncini L, Bertani D, Filippini F, Beski L, et al. Effectiveness of magnesium pidolate in the prophylactic treatment of primary dysmenorrhea. Clin Exp Obstet Gynecol 1992;19(3):175–9.

29. Sampalis F, Bunea R, Pelland M, Kowalski O, Duguet N, Dupuis S. Evaluation of the effects of Neptune Krill Oil on the management of premenstrual syndrome and dysmenorrhea. Alternative Med Rev 2003;8:171–9.

30. Saldeen P, Saldeen T. Women and omega-3 fatty acids. Obstet Gynecol Surv 2004;59:722–30.

31. Deutch B. Menstrual pain in Danish women correlated with low n-3 polyunsaturated fatty acid intake. Eur J Clin Nutr 1995;49:508–16.

32. Harel Z, Biro FM, Kottenhahn RK, Rosenthal SL. Supplementation with omega-3 polyunsaturated fatty acids in the management of dysmenorrhea in adolescents. Am J Obstet Gynecol 1996;174:1335–8.

33. Calder PC. N-3 polyunsaturated fatty acids, inflammation, and inflammatory diseases. Am J Clin Nutr 2006;83:1505S–19S.

34. Marsden JS, Strickland CD, Clements TL. Guaifenesin as a treatment for primary dysmenorrhea. J Am Board Fam Pract 2004;17:240–6.

35. Proctor ML, Smith CA, Farquhar CM, Stones RW. Transcutaneous electrical nerve stimulation and acupuncture for primary dysmenorrhoea. Cochrane Database Syst Rev 2002;(1):CD002123.

36. Tugay N, Akbayrak T, Demirturk F, Karakaya II, Citak K, Ozge T, et al. Effectiveness of transcutaneous electrical nerve stimulation and interferential current in primary dysmenorrhea. Pain Med 2007;8:295–300.

37. Lewers D, Clelland JA, Jackson JR, Varner RE, Bergman J. Transcutaneous electrical nerve stimulation in the relief of primary dysmenorrhea. Phys Ther 1989;69:3–9.

38. Dawood MY, Ramos J. Transcutaneous electrical nerve stimulation (TENS) for the treatment of primary dysmenorrhea: a randomized crossover comparison with placebo TENS and ibuprofen. Obstet Gynecol 1990;75:656–60.

39. Milson I, Hedner N, Mannheimer C. A comparative study of the effect of high intensity transcutaneous nerve stimulation and oral naproxen on intrauterine pressure and menstrual pain in patients with primary dysmenorrhea. Am J Obstet Gynecol 1994;170(1):123–9.

40. Kaplan B, Rabinerson D, Lurie S, Peled Y, Royburt U, Neri A. Clinical evaluation of a new model of transcutaneous electrical nerve stimulation device for management of primary dysmenorrhea. Gynecol Obstet Invest 1997;44(4):255–9.

41. Kokjohn K, Schmid DM, Triano JJ, Brennan PC. The effect of spinal manipulation on pain and prostaglandin levels in women with primary dysmenorrhea. J Manipulative Physiol Ther 1992;15:279–85.

42. White AR. A review of controlled trials of acupuncture for women's reproductive health care. J Fam Plan Reprod Health Care 2003;29(4):233–6.

43. Witt CM, Reinhold T, Brinkhaus B, Roll S, Jena S, Willich SN. Acupuncture in patients with dysmenorrhea: a randomized study on clinical effectiveness and cost-effectiveness in usual care. Am J Obstet Gynecol 2008;198:166.e1, 166.e8.

44. Israel RG, Sutton M, O'Brien KF. Effects of aerobic training on primary dysmenorrhea symptomatology in college females. J Am College Health 1985;33:241–4.

45. Golub LJ, Menduke H, Lang WR. Exercise and dysmenorrhea in young teenagers: a 3-year study. Obstet Gynecol 1968;32:508–11.

46. Ben-Menachem M. Treatment of dysmenorrhea: a relaxation therapy program. Int J Gynaecol Obstet 1980;17:340–2.

47. Akin MD, Weingund KW, Hengehold DA, Goodale MB, Hinkle RT, Smith RP. Continuous low-heat topical heat in the treatment of dysmenorrhea. Obstet Gynecol 2001;97:343–9.

48. Fazio SB, Ship AN. Abnormal uterine bleeding. South Med J 2007;100:376, 382; quiz 383, 402.

49. Meniru G, Hopkins M. Abnormal uterine bleeding. In Curtis M, Overhold S, Hopkins M, eds. Glass' office gynecology, 6th ed. rev. Philadelphia, PA: Lippincott Williams & Wilkins, 2006:176–201.

50. Faucher M, Schuiling K. Normal and abnormal uterine bleeding. In Schuiling K, Likis F, eds. Women's gynecologic health. Sudbury, MA: Jones and Bartlett, 2006:507–32.

51. Grimes DA, Hubacher D, Lopez LM, Schulz KF. Nonsteroidal anti-inflammatory drugs for heavy bleeding or pain associated with intrauterine-device use. Cochrane Database Syst Rev 2006;(4):CD006034.

52. Lethaby A, Irvine G, Cameron I. Cyclical progestogens for heavy menstrual bleeding. Cochrane Database Syst Rev 2008;(1):CD001016.

53. Kriplani A, Singh BM, Lal S, Agarwal N. Efficacy, acceptability and side effects of the levonorgestrel intrauterine system for menorrhagia. Int J Gynaecol Obstet 2007;97:190–4.

54. Lethaby AE, Cooke I, Rees M. Progesterone or progestogen-releasing intrauterine systems for heavy menstrual bleeding. Cochrane Database Syst Rev 2005;(4):CD002126.

55. Sitruk-Ware R. The levonorgestrel intrauterine system for use in peri- and postmenopausal women. Contraception 2007;75(6 suppl):S155–60.

56. Varma R, Sinha D, Gupta JK. Non-contraceptive uses of levonorgestrel-releasing hormone system (LNG-IUS)—a systematic enquiry and overview. Eur J Obstet Gynecol Reprod Biol 2006;125:9–28.

57. Lethaby AE, Cooke I, Rees M. Progesterone or progestogen-releasing intrauterine systems for heavy menstrual bleeding. Cochrane Database Syst Rev 2005;(4):CD002126. DOI: 10.1002/14651858.CD002126. pub2 Cyclic progestins vs IUS—finding IUD better accepted by women. Cochrane 2008; (January 23): CD001016.

58. Speroff L, Fritz M. Clinical gynecologic endocrinology and infertility, 7th ed. Baltimore: Lippincott Williams & Wilkins, 2005.

59. Beaumont H, Augood C, Duckitt K, Lethaby A. Danazol for heavy menstrual bleeding. Cochrane Database Syst Rev 2007;(3):CD001017.

60. Bradley LD. Abnormal uterine bleeding. Nurse Pract 2005;30:38,42, 45–49; quiz 50–51.

61. Parker KL, Schimmer BP. Pituitary hormones and their releasing factors. In Brunton L, Lazo J, Parker K, eds. Goodman & Gilman's the pharmacological basis of therapeutics, 11th ed. New York: McGraw Hill, 2006:1489–510.

62. Schorge JO, Schaffer JI, Halvorson LM, Bradshaw KD, Cunningham FG. Williams Gynecology. New York: McGraw Hill, 2008.

63. Halbreich U, O'Brien PM, Eriksson E, Backstrom T, Yonkers KA, Freeman EW. Are there differential symptom profiles that improve in response to different pharmacological treatments of premenstrual syndrome/premenstrual dysphoric disorder? CNS Drugs 2006;20:523–47.

64. Dickerson LM, Mazyck PJ, Hunter MH. Premenstrual syndrome. Am Fam Physician 2003;67:1743–52.

65. Johnson SR. Premenstrual syndrome, premenstrual dysphoric disorder, and beyond: a clinical primer for practitioners. Obstet Gynecol 2004;104:845–59.

66. American College of Obstetricians & Gynecologists. Premenstrual syndrome (ACOG Practice Bulletin No. 15). Washington, DC: ACOG, 2000(April).

67. Wittchen HU, Becker E, Lieb R, Krause P. Prevalence, incidence and stability of premenstrual dysphoric disorder in the community. Psychol Med 2002; 32:119–32.

68. Kaur G, Gonsalves L, Thacker HL. Premenstrual dysphoric disorder: a review for the treating practitioner. Cleve Clin J Med 2004;71:303,5, 312–3, 317–8, passim.

69. Greenslit N. Pharmaceutical branding: identity, individuality, and illness. Mol Interv 2002;2:342–5.

70. Freeman EW. Luteal phase administration of agents for the treatment of premenstrual dysphoric disorder. CNS Drugs 2004;18:453–68.

71. Baldessarini RJ. Pharmacotherapy of psychosis and mania. In Brunton L, Lazo J, Parker K, eds. Goodman & Gilman's the pharmacological basis of therapeutics, 11th ed. New York: McGraw Hill, 2006:461–500.

72. Jarvis CI, Lynch AM, Morin AK. Management strategies for premenstrual syndrome/premenstrual dysphoric disorder. Ann Pharmacother 2008; 42:967–78.

73. Sanders-Bush E, Mayer SE. 5-Hydroxytryptamine (Serotonin): receptor agonists and antagonists. In Brunton L, Lazo J, Parker K, eds. Goodman & Gilman's the pharmacological basis of therapeutics, 11th ed. New York: McGraw Hill, 2006:297–316.

74. Jackson EK. Diuretics. In Brunton L, Lazo J, Parker K, eds. Goodman & Gilman's the pharmacological basis of therapeutics, 11th ed. New York: McGraw Hill, 2006:737–69.

75. Singh A. Kumar A. Protective effect of alprazolam against sleep deprivation-induced behavior alternations and oxidative damage in mice. Neurosci Res 2008;60(4):372–9.

76. Wyatt K, Dimmock P, Jones P, Obhrai M, O'Brien S. Efficacy of progesterone and progestogens in management of premenstrual syndrome: systematic review. BMJ 2001;323:776–80.

77. Thys-Jacobs S, Ceccarelli S, Bierman A, Weisman H, Cohen MA, Alvir J. Calcium supplementation in premenstrual syndrome. J Gen Intern Med 1989; 4:183–9.

78. Thys-Jacobs S, Starkey P, Bernstein D, Tian J. Calcium carbonate and the premenstrual syndrome: effects on premenstrual and menstrual symptoms. Am J Obstet Gynecol 1998;179:444–52.

79. Penland JG, Johnson PE. Dietary calcium and magnesium effects on menstrual cycle symptoms. Am J Obstet Gynecol 1993;168:1417–23.

80. Quaranta S, Buscaglia MA, Meroni MG. Pilot study of the efficacy and safety of a modified release magnesium 250 mg tablet (Sincromag) for the treatment of premenstrual syndrome. Clin Drug Investig 2007;27:51–8.

81. Umland EM, Weinstein LC, Buchanan EM. Menstruation-related disorders. In Dipiro JT, Talbert RL, Yee GC, Matzke GR, Wells BG, Posey LM, eds. Pharmacotherapy: a pathophysiologic approach. McGraw-Hill Publishing Company, 2008:1465–84.

82. Wyatt KM, Dimmock PW, Jones PW, O'Brien PM. Efficacy of vitamin B6 in the treatment of premenstrual syndrome: systematic review. BMJ 1999; 318:1375–81.

83. London RS, Murphy L, Kitlowski KE, Reynold MA. Efficacy of alpha-tocopherol in the treatment of the premenstrual syndrome. J Reprod Med 1987;32(6):400–4.

84. London RS, Sundaram GS, Murphy L, Goldstein PJ. The effect of alpha-tocopherol on premenstrual symptomatology: a double-blind study. J Am Coll Nutr 1983;2(2):115–22.

85. Bertone-Johnson ER, Hankinson SE, Bendih A, Johnson SR, Willett WC, Manson JE. Calcium and vitamin D intake and risks of incident premenstrual syndrome. Arch Intern Med 2005;165:1246–52.

86. Song A, Advincula A. Adolescent chronic pelvic pain. J Pediatr Adolesc Gynecol 2005;18:371–7.

87. Williams RE, Hartmann KE, Sandler RS, Miller WC, Savitz LA, Steege JF. Recognition and treatment of irritable bowel syndrome among women with chronic pelvic pain. Am J Obstet Gynecol 2005;192(3):761–7.

88. Howard FM. Chronic pelvic pain. Obstet Gynecol 2003;101:594–611.

89. Haugstad GK, Haugstad TS, Kirste UM, Leganger S, Klemmetsen I, Malt UF. Mensendieck somatocognitive therapy as treatment approach to chronic pelvic pain: results of a randomized controlled intervention study. Am J Obstetrics Gynecol 2006; 194:1303–10.

90. Stones W, Cheong YC, Howard FM. Interventions for treating chronic pelvic pain in women. Cochrane Database Syst Rev 2000;(4):CD000387.

91. Soysal ME, Soysal S, Vicdan K, Ozer S. A randomized controlled trial of goserelin and medroxyprogesterone acetate in the treatment of pelvic congestion. Hum Reprod 2001;16(5):931–9.

92. Urman B, Yakin K. Ovulatory disorders and infertility. J Reprod Med 2006;51:267–82.

93. Burney R, Schust D, Yao M. Infertility. In Berek J, ed. Berek & Novak's gynecology, 14th ed. Philadelphia, PA: Lippincott Williams & Wilkins, 2007:1185–275.

94. Trokoudes KM, Skordis N, Picolos MK. Infertility and thyroid disorders. Curr Opin Obstet Gynecol 2006;18:446–51.

95. Wier FA, Farley CL. Clinical controversies in screening women for thyroid disorders during pregnancy. J Midwifery Womens Health 2006;51:152–8.

96. Baskin HJ, Cobin RH, Duick DS, Gharib H, Guttler RB, Kaplan MM, et al. American Association of Clinical Endocrinologists medical guidelines for

clinical practice for the evaluation and treatment of hyperthyroidism and hypothyroidism. Endocr Pract 2002;8:457–69.

97. American College of Obstetricians & Gynecologists. Thyroid disease in pregnancy (Technical Bulletin No. 37). Washington, DC: ACOG, 2002.

98. *Screening for Thyroid Disease*, Topic Page. January 2004. U.S. Preventive Services Task Force. Agency for Healthcare Research and Quality, Rockville, MD. http://www.ahrq.gov/clinic/uspstf/uspsthyr.htm [Accessed July 10, 2009].

99. Farwell AP, Braverman LE. Thyroid and antithyroid drugs. In Brunton L, Lazo J, Parker K, eds. Goodman & Gilman's the pharmacological basis of therapeutics, 11th ed. New York: McGraw Hill, 2006:1524.

100. Kafy S, Tulandi T. New advances in ovulation induction. Curr Opin Obstet Gynecol 2007;19:248–52.

101. Hendriks DJ, Mol BW, Bancsi LF, te Velde ER, Broekmans FJ. The clomiphene citrate challenge test for the prediction of poor ovarian response and non-pregnancy in patients undergoing in vitro fertilization: a systematic review. Fertil Steril 2006;86:807–18.

102. Bukulmez O, Arici A. Assessment of ovarian reserve. Curr Opin Obstet Gynecol 2004;16:231–7.

103. Tobar Hicks AB, Fox MD, Sanchez-Ramos L, Kaunitz AM, Freeman MF. Clinical characteristics of patients with an abnormal clomiphene citrate challenge test. Am J Obstet Gynecol 2003;189:348, 352; discussion 352–3.

104. Check JH. Diagnosis and treatment of cervical mucus abnormalities. Clin Exp Obstet Gynecol 2006; 33:140–2.

105. Check JH, Adelson HG, Wu CH. Improvement of cervical factor with guaifenesin. Fertil Steril 1982; 37:707–8.

106. Henmi H, Endo T, Kitajima Y, Kitjima Y, Manase K, Hata H, et al. Effects of ascorbic acid supplementation on serum progesterone levels in patients with a luteal phase defect. Fertil Steril 2003;80:459–61.

107. Griesinger G, Franke K, Kinast C, Kutzelnigg A, Riedinger S, Kulin S, et al. Ascorbic acid supplementation during luteal phase in IVF. J Assist Reprod Genetics 2002;4:164–8.

108. Chavarro JE, Rich-Edwards JW, Rosner BA, Willett WC. Use of multivitamins, intake of B vitamins, and risk of ovulatory infertility. Fertil Steril 2008; 89:668–76.

109. Casson PR, Lindsay MS, Pisarska MD, Carson SA, Buster JE. Dehydroepiandrosterone supplementation augments ovarian stimulation in poor responders: a case series. Hum Reprod 2000;15(10):2129–32.

110. Bhasin S. Approach to the infertile man. J Clin Endocrinol Metab 2007;92:1995–2004.

111. Dronavalli S, Ehrmann DA. Pharmacologic therapy of polycystic ovary syndrome. Clin Obstet Gynecol 2007;50:244–54.

112. Bhathena RK. Therapeutic options in the polycystic ovary syndrome. J Obstet Gynaecol 2007;27:123–9.

113. Anderson, C. Hyperandrogenic disorders. In Schuiling K, Likis F, eds. Women's gynecologic health. Sudbury, MA: Jones and Bartlett, 2006:533–60.

114. Balen AH, Laven JS, Tan SL, Dewailly D. Ultrasound assessment of the polycystic ovary: international consensus definitions. Hum Reprod Update 2003;9:505–14.

115. Khorram O, Helliwell JP, Katz S, Bonpane CM, Jaramillo L. Two weeks of metformin improves clomiphene citrate–induced ovulation and metabolic profiles in women with polycystic ovary syndrome. Fertil Steril 2006;85:1448–51.

116. Neveu N, Granger L, St-Michel P, Lavoie HB. Comparison of clomiphene citrate, metformin, or the combination of both for first-line ovulation induction and achievement of pregnancy in 154 women with polycystic ovary syndrome. Fertil Steril 2007;87:113–20.

117. Palomba S, Pasquali R, Orio F Jr, Nestler JE. Clomiphene citrate, metformin or both as first-step approach in treating anovulatory infertility in patients with polycystic ovary syndrome (PCOS): a systematic review of head-to-head randomized controlled studies and meta-analysis. Clin Endocrinol (Oxf) 2009;70:311–21.

118. Lanham MS, Lebovic DI, Domino SE. Contemporary medical therapy for polycystic ovary syndrome. Int J Gynaecol Obstet 2006;95:236–41.

119. Yap C, Furness S, Farquhar C. Pre and post operative medical therapy for endometriosis surgery. Cochrane Database Syst Rev 2004;(3):CD003678.

120. Davis L, Kennedy SS, Moore J, Prentice A. Modern combined oral contraceptives for pain associated with endometriosis. Cochrane Database Syst Rev 2007 Jul 18;(3):CD001019.

121. Allen C, Hopewell S, Prentice A. Non-steroidal anti-inflammatory drugs for pain in women with endometriosis. Cochrane Database Syst Rev 2005 Oct 19;(4):CD004753.

122. Hughes E, Brown J, Collins JJ, Farquhar C, Fedorkow DM, Vanderkerckhove P. Ovulation suppression for

endometriosis. Cochrane Database Syst Rev 2007 Jul 18;(3):CD000155.

123. Jacobson TZ, Barlow DH, Koninckx PR, Olive D, Farquhar C. Laparoscopic surgery for subfertility associated with endometriosis. Cochrane Database Syst Rev 2002;(4):CD001398.

124. Hughes E, Brown J, Tiffin G, Vandekerckhove P. Danazol for unexplained subfertility. Cochrane Database Syst Rev 2007 Jan 24;(1):CD000069.

125. Lethaby A, Vollenhoven B, Sowter M. Pre-operative GnRH analogue therapy before hysterectomy or myomectomy for uterine fibroids. Cochrane Database Syst Rev 2001;(2):CD000547.

126. Divakar H. Asymptomatic uterine fibroids. Best Pract Res Clin Obstet Gynaecol 2008 August;22(4): 643–54.

127. Gupta S, Jose J, Manyonda I. Clinical presentation of fibroids. Best Pract Res Clin Obstet Gynaecol 2008 August;22(4):615–26.

128. Huber JC, Bentz EK, Ott J, Tempfer CB Non-contraceptive benefits of oral contraceptives. Expert Opin Pharmacother 2008 September;9(13):2317–25.

129. Gunes M, Ozdegirmenci O, Kayikcioglu F, Haberal A, Kaplan M. The effect of levonorgestrel intrauterine system on uterine myomas: a 1 year followup study. J Minim Invasive Gynecol 2008 November-December;15(6):735–8.

130. Bahamondes L, Bahamondes MV, Monteiro I. Levonorgestrel-releasing intrauterine system: uses and controversies. Expert Rev Med Devices 2008 July;5(4):437–45.

131. Kaunitz AM. Progestin-releasing intrauterine systems and leiomyoma. Contraception 2007 June;756(suppl): S130–3.

132. Wu T, Chen X, Xie L. Selective estrogen receptor modulators SERMs for uterine leiomyomas. Cochrane Database Syst Rev 2007 Oct 17;(4):CD005287.

133. Steinauer J, Pritts EA, Jackson R, Jacoby AF. Systematic review of mifepristone for the treatment of uterine leiomyomata. Obstet Gynecol 2004 June;103(6): 1331–6.

134. Carbonell Esteve JL, Acosta R, Heredia B, Pérez Y, Castañeda MC, Hernández AV. Mifepristone for the treatment of uterine leiomyomas: a randomized controlled trial. Obstet Gynecol 2008;1125:1029–36.

135. Chwalisz K, DeManno D, Garg R, Larsen L, Mattia-Goldberg C, Stickler T. Therapeutic potential for the selective progesterone receptor modulator asoprisnil in the treatment of leiomyomata. Semin Reprod Med 2004 May;22(2):113–9.

136. World Health Organization. Advances in fertility regulation. World Health Organ Tech Rep Ser 1973;1–42.

137. Schuiling KD, Likis FE. Women's gynecologic health. Sudbury, MA: Jones and Bartlett Publishers, 2006.

"We were worried about what we think about vaginas, and even more worried that we don't think about them. There's so much darkness and secrecy surrounding them—like the Bermuda triangle. Nobody ever reports back from there."

EVE ENSLER, *THE VAGINA MONOLOGUES*

Chapter Glossary

Atrophic vaginitis A condition that often accompanies a low estrogen milieu and is characterized by pale, smooth vaginal walls. Women with atrophic vaginitis may report vaginal burning and dyspareunia.

Bacterial vaginosis A disruption in the normal vaginal flora so that there is a decrease in the usual number of hydrogen peroxide-producing lactobacilli. Often abbreviated as BV, this is the most common of the vaginal conditions.

Candidiasis A fungal overgrowth. The *Candida* species are the most common etiological agents for vaginal candidiasis.

Desquamative inflammatory vaginitis A vaginal condition most often experienced by perimenopausal women and characterized by burning and dyspareunia. Frequently abbreviated as DIV, this condition is diagnosed by exclusion and treated empirically.

Lactic acid A byproduct of metabolism of glycogen and a common inhabitant of a healthy vagina that assists in maintaining the acidic environment.

Leukorrhea Thin or thick white vaginal discharge that results from congestion of the vaginal mucosa.

Trichomonas vaginalis The etiologic organism for trichomoniasis. Often used as a synonym for trichomoniasis.

Trichomoniasis (*Trichomonas* vaginitis) A vaginal condition caused by *Trichomonas vaginalis* that is sexually transmitted. Of questionable clinical significance, there exists controversy about treatment for women who are asymptomatic. Can be abbreviated as TV.

Vulvovaginal candidiasis A common type of fungal infection, located in the vulva and/or vagina and usually abbreviated as VVC.

Vaginal Conditions

Uncomfortable vaginal discharge is a common reason for primary healthcare visits. This symptom usually is related to one of three conditions, including **bacterial vaginosis** (BV), ***Trichomonas* vaginitis**, or **vulvovaginal candidiasis** (VVC). It is important that a correct diagnosis be made so the individual receives the most appropriate treatment.[1] This chapter reviews treatment of these conditions, in addition to two other conditions that women may experience: atrophic vaginitis and desquamative vaginitis. Vaginal discharges that are symptoms of sexually transmitted infections are addressed in Chapter 23. Table 31-1 reviews the differential diagnosis of common vaginal disorders.

The Vaginal Ecosystem

Vaginal secretions are composed of a mixture of shed vaginal epithelium, cervical mucus, vaginal transudate, and scant material from the Skene's and Bartholin's glands. This combination provides physiologic lubrication for a woman. Normal vaginal secretions usually are clear or cloudy and nonirritating in nature, although they may leave a yellow cast on clothing after drying. These secretions occur in response to the hormonal milieu of the woman and increase in amount around ovulation, during the premenstrual period, during pregnancy, and when sexual arousal occurs. The increased amount often is termed **leukorrhea** and classically is described as a thin or thick white vaginal discharge that results from congestion of the

Table 31-1 Differential Diagnosis of Common Vaginal Disorders

	Normal	Bacterial Vaginosis	Trichomonas Vaginitis	*Candida* Monilia	Chemical Allergic	Atrophic Vaginitis
Etiology	Occasional vaginal secretions	Disproportionate overgrowth of bacteria	Protozoa	*Candida* species	Allergens/ chemical irritants, but may be unknown	Low estrogenic milieu (e.g., perimenopause, breastfeeding)
Color of vaginal secretions	Clear or cloudy	Gray/white	Yellow/green	White/yellow	Clear or cloudy	Gray/yellow
Odor	None	Fishy	Malodorous	Sometimes yeasty	None	None
Consistency of vaginal secretions	Usually thin	Thin, homogenous	Frothy	Thick plaques	Usually thin	Watery, sticky
Complaint(s)	Variable amount	Malodorous discharge, pruritus	Pruritus, burning dyspareunia	Pruritus, burning dyspareunia	Burning, tenderness, dyspareunia	Dyspareunia, burning
Physical	No abnormalities	Pooling of discharge at introitus	Erythema, edema	Erythema, vaginal plaques, excoriation	Erythema, edema	Pale, pink vagina, little rugation
pH	3.8–4.5	> 4.5	5.2–7.0	3.8–4.5	3.8–4.5	5.5–7.0
Microscopic findings	No pathology	Clue cells	Trichomonads	Pseudohyphae, few lactobacilli	No pathological organism	No clear pathogen
Clinical considerations	Education, reassurance		Remember to treat partner.	Look to ameliorate predisposing conditions.	Treat palliatively; remove allergen.	Consider strategies to increase endogenous lubrication.

vaginal mucosa. Leukorrhea is typically a sign of health of the vaginal ecosystem and does not require treatment.

The epithelial cells of the vagina contain glycogen. When glycogen is metabolized, lactic acid is produced as one of the byproducts. **Lactic acid** maintains the normal acidity within the vagina. Usually there are multiple asymptomatic microbes in the vagina, including *Lactobacilli acidophilus, Staphylococcus epidermidis,* and *Corynebacteria,* as well as anaerobic microorganisms, like *Peptostreptococcus, Bacteroides,* and anaerobic lactobacilli. There often are 5–15 different species of bacteria and normal inhabitants of a vagina may include a few microorganisms that can be pathologic in larger amounts. These microbes include, for example, *Escherichia coli,* various *Candida* species, and *Mobiluncus.*

Any ecosystem may become out of balance, and the vagina is no exception. Thus, an overgrowth of some normal inhabitants or transmission of a sexually transmitted infection (STI) can result in discomfort to a woman. Vaginal infection is a common self-diagnosis and a frequent reason for women to seek healthcare services.

Bacterial Vaginosis

Bacterial vaginosis (BV) is the most common cause of vaginal discharge[2] and one of the most frequent causes of infection in women of reproductive age.[3] Normally, the vagina

of a reproductive-aged woman is colonized with lactobacilli that produce substances such as hydrogen peroxide, lactic acid, and bacteriocins that maintain the pH of the vagina in an acidic range, usually between 3.8 and 4.5. A lower pH is a hostile environment for bacteria other than the lactobacilli. If the pH of the vagina rises to a more alkaline environment, an overgrowth of anaerobic and facultative bacteria may occur. This overgrowth can predispose a woman to the development of BV.[1,4] Therefore, women should avoid practices such as douching that may alter the normal acidic pH of the vagina.[5] There may or may not be symptoms associated with the presence of BV.[2] If symptoms are present, the two most common are foul odor (often described as fishy) and vaginal irritation.[6]

BV is more common in women who smoke and in African Americans compared to women who are Asian or Caucasian. BV has been associated with postoperative infection after gynecologic procedures.[3] In a study conducted by Blackwell et al., 28% of asymptomatic women screened for BV prior to pregnancy termination were found to have BV.[7] This alteration in vaginal flora is also more common in lesbian and bisexual women than in heterosexual women, and if present, is usually found in both partners.

Treatment of Symptomatic Bacterial Vaginosis

Treatment of BV should be offered to ameliorate symptoms, prevent infectious complications after genito-urinary procedures, and to reduce the risk of acquiring other genital infections. There is some evidence that women with BV have a higher risk of acquiring chlamydia and/or HIV infection.

The Centers for Disease Control and Prevention (CDC) recommends that all symptomatic women be tested for BV and, if this test is positive, that they either take metronidazole (Flagyl) or clindamycin (Cleocin, Clindesse)[8] (Table 31-2).

The overall cure rate for BV using the medications recommended by the CDC is 70%.[8] The most common medication used is metronidazole (Flagyl).

Metronidazole (Flagyl) is a synthetic antimicrobial agent in the nitroimidazole class. It is effective against protozoa such as **Trichomonas vaginalis**, as well as the bacteria that cause bacterial vaginosis. Metronidazole is selective for anaerobic bacteria that contain an agent that reduces metronidazole to its active metabolite within the organism. The mechanism of action is DNA breakage and cell death, which is initiated when the active metabolite of metronidazole binds to the bacterial DNA (Figure 31-1).

Metronidazole has a low molecular weight and limited binding to serum proteins. Resistance is almost nonexistent. This drug can be administered orally or intravaginally

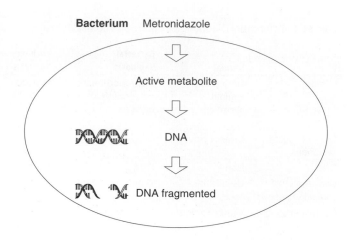

Figure 31-1 Mechanism of action of metronidazole (Flagyl).

in a topical formulation. The bioavailability is approximately 90% following oral absorption. When administered intravaginally, low serum levels (approximately 2% of the serum level found with a 500-mg oral dose) are obtained. Metronidazole is metabolized in the liver via hydroxylation and eliminated via the kidney. The half-life is approximately 8 hours.

Dosing Considerations

Other doses of metronidazole (Flagyl), such as a one-time dose of 2 grams given orally, or other medications such as ofloxacin (Floxin) 200 mg administered orally twice daily have been shown to have "similar cure rates at 2 weeks after treatment, but have higher relapse rates after that 2-week timeframe."[1] Women who are HIV positive should be treated with the same regimen as those who are HIV negative.[8]

Since the CDC guidelines were published in 2006, oral tinidazole (Tindamax) has been approved by the FDA for treatment of BV.[9] A double-blinded, placebo-controlled trial of 235 women reported by Livengood et al. found no statistically significant different outcomes for women treated with tinidazole 1 gram daily for 5 days versus women treated with tinidazole 2 grams daily for 2 days (cure rate of 36.8% versus 27.4%, respectively), although both were superior to the 5.1% cure found among women using the placebo.[10]

Treatment of Asymptomatic Bacterial Vaginosis

Treatment of women who are asymptomatic is more controversial as the incidence of adverse outcomes in women with BV is not readily apparent. Women with asymptomatic BV

Table 31-2 Recommended Treatment of Bacterial Vaginosis

Drug—Generic (Brand)	Dose	Duration
Treatment for Uncomplicated BV		
Metronidazole (Flagyl)	500 mg PO bid	7 days
Metronidazole gel 0.75% (Flagyl)	One applicator daily intravaginally	5 days
Clindamycin cream 2% (Cleocin)	One applicator daily intravaginally	7 days
Alternate Regimens for Uncomplicated BV		
Metronidazole (Flagyl)	2 g PO as one-time dose	Single dose
Clindamycin (Cleocin)	300 mg PO bid	7 days
Clindamycin ovules (Cleocin)	100 g PO qd	3 days
Treatment During Pregnancy		
Metronidazole (Flagyl)	500 mg PO bid	7 days
Metronidazole (Flagyl)	300 mg PO tid	7 days
Clindamycin (Cleocin)	300 mg PO bid	7 days
Treatment for Recurrent BV		
Metronidazole (Flagyl)	500 mg PO	10–14 days
Metronidazole gel 0.75% (Flagyl)	One applicator daily intravaginally	10 days*
Tinidazole (Tindamax)	500 mg PO bid	14 days†

BV = Bacterial vaginosis.
* Followed by twice-weekly applications for 4–6 months.
† Off-label use.
Sources: From Alfonsi GA et al. 2004[17]; Baylson FA et al. 2004[18]; CDC 2006[8]; Soper DE 2005.[16]

who are undergoing surgical abortion or hysterectomy may be treated prior to the procedure to decrease the incidence of postoperative infection.[8] Treatment is not recommended for male partners of women who receive treatment for BV because there is no indication that treatment of a male partner influences successful treatment of the woman. Treatment of asymptomatic women with BV undergoing in vitro fertilization remains controversial. In general, it is not recommended that treatment be given to women who are asymptomatic, unless as prophylactic treatment prior to gynecologic procedures as aforementioned; however, this recommendation may change.[1,8] Research on the relationship between treating asymptomatic BV and reducing the incidence of infection with chlamydia is ongoing.[11]

Bacterial Vaginosis in Pregnancy

The CDC recommends that all symptomatic pregnant women receive treatment for BV; however, treatment of asymptomatic women is not recommended.[12] Recent recommendations from the US Preventive Services Task Force also support treating symptomatic women but not asymptomatic women.[13] Historically, it was assumed that BV might be a risk factor for preterm delivery based on the concept of infection as an etiology for many preterm births. However, when Nygren et al. reviewed the literature on treatment of asymptomatic and symptomatic pregnant women with BV, there was no evidence to support treatment of asymptomatic pregnant women with BV whether or not they were at high risk for preterm birth.[14] Alternatively, there were conflicting data about the efficacy of treating pregnant women at high risk for preterm birth who had symptomatic BV. Contrary to the expected outcome, two of the clinical trials reviewed found that women with symptomatic BV who were treated for the condition actually had an increased incidence of preterm birth.[14]

When a clinician chooses to not follow the current CDC recommendations and treats asymptomatic women who are pregnant, a follow-up examination for cure should occur at 1 month following treatment.[8] The recommended pharmacologic treatment is provided in Table 31-2. In the past, it was recommended that treatment with metronidazole (Flagyl) be withheld during the first trimester of pregnancy. However, studies have failed to find teratogenic effects of metronidazole when used during the first trimester, and the agent is an FDA Pregnancy Category B medication.[8,12]

Most drugs consumed by a breastfeeding mother are excreted into the breast milk in small amounts, usually less than 5% of the maternal dose. However, metronidazole is concentrated in breast milk, and approximately 20% of the ingested dose is excreted into breast milk.[15] Although there have not been any reports of adverse outcomes in breastfeeding infants of mothers who received metronidazole, because of the limited studies and the probability of neonatal gastric distress, the CDC recommends that women who are lactating withhold breastfeeding during treatment and for 12–24 hours after consuming the last dose of metronidazole.[8,15] During this time frame, the breastfeeding mother should express breast milk and discard it.

Recurrent Bacterial Vaginosis

As many as 70% of women who have experienced an episode of BV report a recurrence of the condition.[16] By using the most effective treatment during the initial episode of BV, the rate of recurrence should be decreased.[10] The regimen of metronidazole (Flagyl) 500 mg orally twice daily for 7 days has been associated with the lowest rate of recurrence.[12] Although the CDC guidelines discuss the problem of recurrent BV, no long-term therapies are recommended and it is suggested that women with recurrent BV be followed by specialists in the area.[8] Others have recommended a variety of treatment plans to address the issue of recurrent BV. See Table 31-2.[1,16-18] No studies have found a regimen that is effective enough to be recommended for treatment of recurrent BV.

▌ Trichomoniasis

Trichomoniasis or *trichomonas* vaginitis is one of the most common nonviral sexually transmitted infections (STIs). Additional information about STIs can be found in Chapter 23. *Trichomonas* vaginitis is caused by the protozoan, *T vaginalis*. As many as 50% or more cases are theorized to be asymptomatic.[19] When symptoms are present, they most often consist of vulvar itching and a malodorous vaginal discharge.[7]

Treatment of Trichomoniasis

Trichomoniasis is almost exclusively transmitted sexually and may increase the risk of acquiring other STIs such as HIV. In observational studies, the presence of trichomoniasis increased the risk for acquiring HIV by approximately twofold.[19] Recommended treatment options are listed in Table 31-3. Treatment regimens are for both men and women. Women infected with HIV should be treated

Table 31-3 Treatment of Trichomoniasis

Drug—Generic (Brand)	Dose	Duration
Treatment for Uncomplicated Trichomoniasis		
Metronidazole (Flagyl)	2 g PO	Single dose
Metronidazole (Flagyl)	500 mg PO bid	7 days
Tinidazole (Tindamax)	2 g PO	Single dose
Treatment During Pregnancy*		
Metronidazole (Flagyl)	2 g PO	Single dose
Treatment for Recurrent Trichomoniasis		
Metronidazole (Flagyl)	500 mg PO bid	7 days
Tinidazole (Tindamax)	2 g PO	Single dose
Treatment for Treatment Failures		
Metronidazole (Flagyl)	2 g PO daily	5 days
Tinidazole (Tindamax)	2 g PO daily	5 days

* Recommended only for women who are symptomatic.
Source: From CDC 2006.[8]

according to the same regimen as those women who are HIV negative[8] (Box 31-1).

The most common pharmacotherapeutic agent used to treat trichomoniasis is metronidazole (Flagyl). The mechanism of action of this agent against protozoa remains unclear. It has been proposed that the drug facilitates the development of extensive vacuoles in the parasite and, depending on the drug concentration, is highly lethal. Treatment with topical formulations, such as metronidazole gel, has been shown to be less efficacious than oral therapy. This may be due to the fact that trichomonads can reside in the urinary tract as well as the crypts of the vagina.[1,8] The single 2-gram oral dose of metronidazole is the CDC recommended first-line therapy. Cure rates are more than 90% after this single-dose treatment.[19]

Although there is the possibility of metronidazole resistance, it is rare. Resistance to metronidazole is reported to occur in 1–3% of *T vaginalis* isolates.[19] If the infection is resistant to the standard recommended dose of metronidazole, the CDC recommends metronidazole 500 mg orally for 7 days or tinidazole (Tindamax) 2 grams as a one-time oral dose. If these fail, consider the treatment of either metronidazole or tinidazole 2 grams daily for 5 days or directly consult with the CDC.[8]

Treating Asymptomatic Trichomoniasis

There is no debate regarding treatment of women who are symptomatic with trichomonas vaginitis. The disease can negatively affect quality of life. However, treatment of asymptomatic women with trichomonas is controversial.[19]

Trichomoniasis is a sexually transmitted infection, and as such, for years there has been an aggressive approach to treating all women with the condition, regardless of symptoms, as well as their partners. Although clinical significance of an asymptomatic infection was elusive, some authorities felt that at least pregnant women should be treated in an attempt to decrease prematurity and low-birth-weight infants.[19] Even though observational studies suggested that trichomoniasis was associated with these neonatal outcomes, no randomized, controlled studies have demonstrated that treatment during pregnancy changed the perinatal outcome.[7] Moreover, one large study identified an increased likelihood of preterm birth among women who were treated for trichomoniasis, creating the question of whether or not treatment actually may induce harm.[19]

Since treatment of the asymptomatic pregnant women has been called into question, the concept of treating all women with trichomoniasis has been challenged. Unlike other sexually transmitted infections, trichomoniasis has not been linked to infertility or long-term sequela for men or women. In an era of evidence-based care, the question "what harm does the presence of trichomoniasis do?" has been asked. Certainly all women who are symptomatic should receive treatment to relieve discomforts and their partners treated to minimize reinfection. Although some studies have suggested that trichomoniasis may increase the risk for acquiring HIV for women exposed to the virus, all women should be counseled to engage in safe sex practices. Therefore, many healthcare providers no longer screen all women routinely for vaginitis and avoid facing the controversy of deciding to treat or not to treat the asymptomatic woman.

Trichomoniasis and Pregnancy

There is no evidence that treating women who are pregnant with asymptomatic *T vaginalis* will decrease the incidence of preterm birth. One large, randomized, controlled trial found increased rates of preterm births among asymptomatic women with trichomoniasis who were treated with metronidazole (19% versus 10.7%; RR = 1.8; 95% CI, 1.2–2.7; *P* = .004) compared to asymptomatic women with BV who were not treated.[20] Therefore, the CDC recommends that only pregnant women who are symptomatic be treated for trichomoniasis.[8] Table 31-3 lists the CDC recommended treatment. As previously stated, the CDC guidelines recommend that women should withhold breastfeeding during treatment and for 12–24 hours after consuming the last dose of metronidazole.[8]

Box 31-1 Treatment of Trichomonas

WF is a 25-year-old woman who reports burning and vaginal pruritus. Her last normal menstrual period was 3 weeks ago, and she says she usually uses condoms for birth control. A vaginal examination revealed a yellow-green discharge that was positive for flagellated protozoa upon microscopic visualization. The diagnosis is trichomoniasis. There is no question that WF should be treated since she is symptomatic.

The most common treatment is 2 grams of oral metronidazole (Flagyl). However, there are issues other than a simple prescription to consider. With rare exception, trichomoniasis is a sexually transmitted infection. When one sexually transmitted infection is diagnosed, the clinician should screen for others. Moreover, trichomoniasis often obscures other vaginal discharges and conditions. Gonorrhea and chlamydia cultures are indicated.

In years past, metronidazole (Flagyl) would have been avoided until the woman's next menses in an attempt to avoid exposing a fetus to this agent in the first trimester of pregnancy. Today, recognizing that no teratogenicity has been linked with this drug and it is an FDA Pregnancy Category B drug, there is no reason to ask WF to uncomfortably wait for her next menses.

Metronidazole is associated with a disulfiram effect, although the frequency is likely to be uncommon. However, since it can be avoided entirely by not ingesting alcohol with the drug, WF should be advised not to drink alcoholic beverages for several days after use of metronidazole. The most common side effects of metronidazole (Flagyl) are gastrointestinal, such as nausea, vomiting, and unpleasant taste. In an attempt to minimize these effects, some clinicians prescribe the drug as 1 gram followed by 1 gram 12 hours later. Reports suggest that this may be associated with similar cure rates as the single 2-gram dose, but it should be recognized that the use of 2 grams administered in a divided dose is not formally recommended by the Centers for Disease Control and Prevention.

Note that because trichomonas may be found in the urinary tract of the woman, metronidazole gels are not indicated for treatment even though the organism was noted in a vaginal smear. Such gels are reserved for treatment of bacterial vaginosis, a condition localized to the vagina where the topical agent can be of value.

WF's partner(s) should be treated with the same dose of metronidazole that is prescribed for WF. Treatment of partners may be outside the scope of practice of some providers of women's care and may necessitate a referral. The woman should be counseled to avoid unprotected intercourse until both WF and her partner have completed the treatment; otherwise the treated partner may be reinfected.

Finally, no follow-up is needed unless WF's symptoms do not resolve within the next 1–2 weeks. At that time, a subsequent examination is likely to find another condition previously obscured. Resistance to metronidazole is rare.

Recurrent Trichomoniasis

Treatment recommendations for recurrent infection can be found in Table 31-3. If these treatments fail, it is recommended that clinicians consult a specialist and that susceptibility testing be done. Both consultation and susceptibility testing are available from the CDC.[8]

Vulvovaginal Candidiasis

Vulvovaginal candidiasis (VVC) is a common cause of vaginitis, and up to 75% of women of reproductive age will have at least one episode.[1] VVC is also known as candida vaginitis or yeast vaginitis. More than 90% of all cases are caused by the organism *Candida albicans*, but other species of *Candida*, such as *glabrata*, *tropicalis*, and *krusei* have also been implicated as the cause of VVC. These latter species may be more resistant to common treatments.[8] *Glabrata* is known to have decreased susceptibility to the azole-containing drugs, and both *C glabrata* and *C krusei* have strains that are resistant to fluconazole (Diflucan).[21,22]

VVC is classified as uncomplicated or complicated depending on symptoms, frequency of occurrence, implicated organism, response to treatment, and general health of the host (e.g., immunocompromised)[3] (Table 31-4). Symptoms, if present, usually include vulvar itching and irritation, painful urination, and vaginal discharge.[1,8]

The majority of vaginal infections are treated with topical preparations of antifungal medications or antibiotics that are inserted into the vagina, although there are a few indications for orally administered antifungal drugs or antibiotics. The most commonly used antifungal drugs are either imidazoles (e.g., miconazole [Monistat], clotrimazole [Gyne-Lotrimin]), or triazoles (fluconazole [Diflucan]).

Treatment of Uncomplicated Vulvovaginal Candidiasis

Most cases of uncomplicated VVC are caused by *C albicans* and can be adequately treated with a short course of one of the topical azole drugs, such as butoconazole (Mycelex), clotrimazole (Gyne-Lotrimin), miconazole (Monistat), tioconazole (Monistat 1-Day), and terconazole (Terazol-3) (Table 31-5).

Table 31-4 Classification of Vulvovaginal Candidiasis

Uncomplicated Vulvovaginal Candidiasis	Complicated Vulvovaginal Candidiasis
Sporadic or infrequent vulvovaginal candidiasis or	Recurrent vulvovaginal candidiasis or
Mild to moderate vulvovaginal candidiasis or	Severe vulvovaginal candidiasis or
Etiology likely to be *C albicans* or	Nonalbicans candidiasis or
Nonimmunocompromised women	Women with uncontrolled diabetes, debilitation, or immunosuppression or those who are pregnant

Sources: Reprinted with permission from Mashburn J 2006[1]; information from CDC 2006.[8]

All the topical drugs work by interfering with the normal action of ergosterol, a critical component of fungal cell membranes. Polyene antifungals (e.g., nystatin [Mycostatin] or itraconazole [Sporanox]) are less frequently used today, but can be employed to treat vaginitis. These drugs bind with sterols (especially ergosterol) in the fungal cell membrane to facilitate leakage and ultimate breakdown of the cell wall. The antifungals imidazole and triazole inhibit the CYP450 enzyme 14 alpha-demethylase, inhibiting the conversion of lanosterol to ergosterol, which is necessary for fungal cell membrane synthesis (Figure 31-2).

There is no evidence that any specific azole offers better cure rates than the others when treating *C albicans*.[23] Cost and availability of the drug should be considered when recommending one drug over the other. Treatment of partners is not warranted in women with uncomplicated VVC.

Boric acid has been shown to be an effective treatment for nonalbicans species, in the form of a 600-mg suppository or capsules administered per vagina once daily for 14 days.[24] When boric acid is used, women should be counseled to keep it away from children and pets since oral ingestion can be fatal.

Many of the topical azole drugs are available over the counter without prescription. Women should be cautioned about using over-the-counter treatments without confirmation of the diagnosis of VVC.[1] At least one study using culture-proven diagnoses found that only 33% of women

Table 31-5 Recommended Treatment for Vulvovaginal Candidiasis

Intravaginal Agents	Brand Name	Dose	Duration
Butoconazole 2% cream	Mycelex 3	5 g intravaginally qhs	3 days*
Butoconazole 2% sustained release	Gynazole-1	5 g intravaginally qhs	Single dose
Clotrimazole 1% cream	Gyne-Lotrimin-7 Mycelex-7	5 g intravaginally qhs	7–14 days*†
Clotrimazole 100-mg vaginal tablet	Gyne-Lotrimin-7	1 tablet intravaginally qhs	7 days
Clotrimazole 100-mg vaginal tablet	Gyne-Lotrimin-7	Place 2 suppositories tablet qhs	3 days
Clotrimazole 500-mg vaginal tablet	Gyne-Lotrimin	1 tablet intravaginally qhs	Single dose
Miconazole 2% cream	Monistat-7	5 g intravaginally qhs	7 days*†
Miconazole 100-mg suppository	Monistat-7	1 suppository intravaginally qhs	7 days*
Miconazole 200-mg suppository	Monistat-3	1 suppository intravaginally qhs	3 days*
Nystatin 100,000-unit vaginal tablet	Mycostatin	1 tablet intravaginally qhs	14 days
Tioconazole 6.5% ointment	Monistat 1-Day Vagistat 1	5 g intravaginally qhs	Single dose*
Terconazole 0.4% cream (45 g)	Terazol-7	5 g intravaginally qhs	7 days†
Terconazole 0.8% cream (30 g)	Terazol-3	5 g intravaginally qhs	3 days
Terconazole 80-mg suppository	Terazol-3	1 suppository intravaginally qhs	3 days
Oral Agents			
Fluconazole	Diflucan	150-mg oral tablet qhs	Single dose

* Over the counter.
† Recommended during pregnancy.
Sources: Reprinted with permission from Mashburn J 2006[1]; information from CDC 2006.[8]

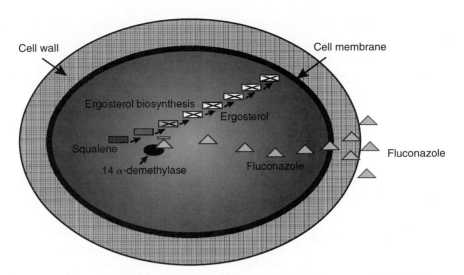

Fluconazole (Diflucan) inhibits 14 α-demethylase, which is one of the fungal CYP450 enzymes that facilitates an essential step in converting squalene to ergosterol (a component of the fungal cell membrane). The result is accumulation of 14 α-methyl sterols within the fungus and a weakened cell membrane.

Figure 31-2 Mechanism of action of fluconazole (Diflucan).

Box 31-2 Technique for Administering Vaginal Cream or Tablet

1. Load the applicator to the fill line with cream.

   Or

   Unwrap the tablet, wet it with warm water, and place it in the applicator.

2. Lie down with knees drawn up.

3. Gently insert the applicator high into the vagina.

4. Withdraw the applicator and discard if it is disposable, or wash it with soap and rinse well with water.

5. To keep the medication from getting on your clothing, wear a mini-pad or panty liner.

6. Wear underwear with cotton crotches.

7. Do not use tampons or douche.

8. Avoid intercourse until course of therapy is completed.

Box 31-3 Vulvovaginal Candidiasis: Indications and Contraindications for Self-Treatment

Self-treatment of *Candida* infections are best reserved for women who:

- Are at least 12 years of age.

- Have previously had a professionally diagnosed episode of vulvovaginal candidiasis.

Women should seek professional care for the vaginal infection if they:

- Have a foul-smelling vaginal discharge.

- Experience pain in lower abdomen, back, or shoulder.

- Are diabetic, pregnant, or have/suspect having HIV.

- Are febrile.

- Do not experience relief or improvement within 3 days or have reoccurrence of symptoms within 2 months.

who self-diagnose VVC actually had VVC.[25] Overusage of the antifungal drugs could lead to drug resistance in the future. Guidelines for use of vaginal medications are found in Box 31-2, and guidelines for self-treatment are found in Box 31-3.

Another treatment option is oral fluconazole (Diflucan) 150 mg as a single dose. Fluconazole is available by prescription only and has cure rates comparable to azole treatments.[8] The fluconazole option is more expensive, and because this drug has significant drug–drug interactions, it is not usually recommended for first-line treatment. However there is no significant difference in efficacy when topical agents are compared to treatment with fluconazole.

Fluconazole is an FDA Pregnancy Category C drug due to teratogenicity found in rats and rabbits when high doses were used. These congenital anomalies were theorized to be due to inhibition of estrogen synthesis. No controlled studies of the effects of fluconazole during pregnancy have been conducted with women, nor has any clear association been found between use of the drug by pregnant women and teratogenic effects in the fetus or newborn.

Treatment of Complicated Vulvovaginal Candidiasis

Complicated VVC cases are most often caused by *C albicans*. These cases will respond favorably to the azole medications as well but require a longer period of therapy than the 1- to 3-day therapy recommended for uncomplicated VVC.

The optimal treatment of nonalbicans VVC is unknown. Ray et al. reported that women who have diabetes and develop VVC present more often with *C glabrata* than *C albicans*.[21] Their study found that infections in the participants with the *glabrata* strain responded more favorably to treatment with boric acid 600 mg suppositories administered once daily for 14 days when compared to treatment with a single oral dose of fluconazole (Diflucan) 150 mg (63.6% versus 28.6%, respectively; *P* = .01). The CDC recommendations for treatment are listed in Table 31-6.

VVC frequently occurs during pregnancy. When VVC is diagnosed in a pregnant woman, it automatically should be considered complicated VVC. The treatment for VVC during pregnancy is a topical azole for 7 days.[8]

Recurrent Vulvovaginal Candidiasis

Recurrent VVC affects fewer than 5% of women each year, and VVC is termed recurrent if the woman experiences four or more symptomatic episodes per year.[7] The recommended treatment options are found in Table 31-6. The CDC 2006 Sexually Transmitted Diseases Treatment Guidelines state that in the case of a woman who has recurrent VVC, treatment of male partners "... may be considered in women who have recurrent infection."[8] In addition, male partners with balanitis often benefit from topical antifungal treatment.[8] Fluconazole (Diflucan) is the most common drug used and is administered orally. Fluconazole is safe to use by breastfeeding women but has many drug–drug interactions and is contraindicated if the woman must take some medications that interact with fluconazole.

Table 31-6 Treatment of Recurrent VVC, Severe VVC, and Nonalbicans VVC

Drug	Brand Name	Dose	Length of Therapy
Treatment for Recurrent VVC			
Topical azole	(Mycelex, Gyne-Lotrimin, Monistat	Daily	7–14 days
Fluconazole	Diflucan	100, 150, or 200 mg q 3 days	3 doses
Maintenance Therapy			
Fluconazole	Diflucan	100, 150, or 200 mg PO	Weekly for 6 months
Clotrimazole	Gyne-Lotrimin	200 mg intravaginally	Weekly for 6 months
Clotrimazole	Gyne-Lotrimin	500 mg intravaginally	Weekly for 6 months
Severe VVC			
Topical azole	Mycelex, Gyne-Lotrimin, Monistat	Daily	7–14 days
Fluconazole	Diflucan	150 mg PO	2 doses 72 hours apart
Nonalbicans VVC			
Nonfluconazole drug	Amphotericin B	Oral or topical	7–14 days
Boric acid gelatin capsule		600 mg intravaginally	14 days*

VVC = vulvovaginal candidiasis.
* May be found in health-food stores.
Source: CDC 2006.[8]

Adverse Effects of Azole Drugs

Topical azoles may cause mild and self-limiting local skin reactions such as burning or irritation. Women who use condoms or diaphragms for contraception and are prescribed topical azoles need to be educated that many of these products are oil based and may weaken latex. Therefore, they should refrain from intercourse during therapy or use another method of contraception.[3]

Oral azoles have been known to cause elevated liver enzymes, so it is recommended that appropriate baseline laboratory values be obtained when the drug is to be used for long-term therapy. These agents may also cause nausea, headache, and abdominal pain.[8]

Drug–Drug Interactions

Oral azoles are known to be inhibitors of some of the important CYP450 enzymes and substrates for others.[26] Azoles can, therefore, precipitate dangerous drug interactions,

Table 31-7 Selected Azole Drug–Drug Interactions*

Antifungal—Generic (Brand)	In Combination with—Generic (Brand)	Clinical Effect and Mechanism	Suggested Clinical Management
Itraconazole (Sporanox) Ketoconazole (Nizoral)	Antacids H$_2$-receptor antagonism (e.g., cimetidine [Tagamet]) Didanosine (oral) (Videx) Proton pump inhibitors (e.g., omeprazole [Prilosec]) Sucralfate (Carafate)	Decreased serum concentration of azole by decreased dissolution/absorption of solid dosage form.	Avoid combination of these agents in general. Take antacids within 2 hours of oral azole therapy.
Fluconazole (Diflucan) Itraconazole (Sporanox) Ketoconazole (Nizoral)	Carbamazepine (Tegretol) Isoniazid (INH) Phenobarbital (Luminal) Phenytoin (Dilantin) Rifampin (Rifadin)	Decreased serum concentration of azole by induction of cytochrome-P450 mediated metabolism of azole.	Use alternative agents and avoid concomitant use of these drugs.
All antifungals	Cisapride (Propulsid) Disopyramide (Norpace)	Prolonged QT interval.	Contraindicated combination.
Fluconazole (Diflucan) Itraconazole (Sporanox) Ketoconazole (Nizoral)	Cyclosporin (Neoral)† Digoxin (Lanoxin)† Dofetilide (Tikosyn)† Ergotamine (Cafergot)† Lovastatin (Mevacor)† Pimozide (Orap)† Quinidine (Cardioquin)†	Increased serum concentration of coadministered drug or metabolite of that drug via CYP450 inhibition with potential toxic effects.	Contraindicated combinations.
Fluconazole (Diflucan) Itraconazole (Sporanox) Ketoconazole (Nizoral)	Alprazolam (Xanax) Busulfan (Myleran) Carbamazepine (Tegretol)‡ Cyclophosphamide (Endoxana) Diltiazem (Cardizem) Isoniazid (INH) Loratadine (Claritin) Methylprednisolone (Medrol)‡ Midazolam (Versed)‡ Oral hypoglycemic agents (e.g., metformin [Glucophage]) Phenytoin (Dilantin)‡ Protease inhibitors (e.g., saquinavir [Invirase], ritonavir) Rifabutin (Mycobutin)‡ Rifampin (Rifadin)‡ Sulfonylureas† Tacrolimus (Protopic)‡ Theophylline (Theo-Dur)‡ Triazolam (Halcion)‡ Vincristine (Oncovin) Warfarin (Coumadin)	Increased serum concentration of coadministered drug or metabolite of that drug via CYP450 inhibition.	Avoid concomitant use if possible. Severity of possible interaction is drug dependent. Consult prescribing information of each drug to address interaction severity.

* This table is not comprehensive. New information is being identified on a regular basis.
† Contraindicated if taking itraconazole or ketoconazole secondary to toxic levels of coadministered drug.
‡ Can cause moderately severe adverse reactions secondary to high plasma levels of coadministered drug.

and it is essential to know which medications (prescription and nonprescription) a woman is taking prior to prescribing an azole medication so that a drug interaction is avoided. There are some drug–azole combinations that are contraindicated, and a list of these combinations can be found in Table 11-18. In addition, Table 31-7 provides a partial list of clinically significant azole drug–drug interactions.

Alternative Therapies for Vaginitis

Alternative Therapies for Bacterial Vaginosis

Bacterial vaginosis has been recognized to self-cure in some women. Carey and the NIH Maternal Fetal Network researchers found that 77.8% were cured in a large, randomized, clinical trial of women with asymptomatic BV during pregnancy. However, of the 966 who were treated with a placebo, 37.4% were cured, illustrating the phenomenon of natural resolution of the condition.[27] This natural cure of BV makes it difficult to assess the effectiveness of various remedies without a randomized, controlled trial. For example, capsules of goldenseal, tracheal, and garlic have been suggested as treatments, but there is no evidence to support their use.

Alternative Therapies for Trichomoniasis

Peeled garlic wrapped in gauze and placed intravaginally every 12 hours has been suggested as a way of relieving vaginitis symptoms associated with trichomoniasis. Douching with a boric acid vinegar solution has also been suggested, as well as douching twice daily with a solution containing calendula, goldenseal, and echinacea.[28] No studies have been found that assess the efficacy of these treatments.

Alternative Therapies for Vulvovaginal Candidiasis

The use of yogurt administered either orally or intravaginally has been anecdotally reported to decrease yeast colonization. The active ingredient in yogurt is lactobacillus, and the theory is that adding or increasing the number of lactobacillus in the vagina will cause a competitive inhibition of candida species. Several studies have evaluated the use of lactobacillus capsules and/or yogurt with mixed findings regarding the efficacy in curing infection.[29-33] To date, some strains of lactobacillus have demonstrated ability to colonize in the vagina and prevent growth of *Candida* in the in vitro studies and some human studies; however, clinical trials have had mixed results.[32] A study performed by Pirotta and colleagues failed to demonstrate an improvement in the incidence of postantibiotic vulvovaginitis among 235 women who were given either oral or vaginal forms of lactobacillus. When compared with placebo, the odds ratio for having a positive vaginal swab after oral or vaginal lactobacillus treatment was not statistically significant (OR for oral treatment 1.06; 95% CI, 0.58–1.94; OR for vaginal treatment 1.38; 95% CI, 0.75–2.54).[31] The minimum amount of yogurt containing active cultures that one needs to consume in order to decrease vulvovaginitis symptoms is not known. Not all yogurt contains active cultures.[31]

Peeled, crushed garlic wrapped in gauze and placed intravaginally has been recommended as a treatment for *Candida*. Garlic is known to have antifungal properties as well as antiviral properties. There have been in vitro studies that show promising results for treating *Candida* vaginitis with garlic, but no in vivo trials have been conducted.[34]

Gentian violet is a purple dye that has antifungal properties and has been used to treat vaginal yeast infections as well as thrush in the neonates and is perhaps the oldest known treatment for yeast infections, although studies on efficacy are lacking. It is no longer available over the counter without a prescription. A 0.05% or 1% solution of gentian violet is "painted" on the walls of the vagina using a large cotton swab and can stain clothing, so use of cotton pads or throwaway panties is recommended during treatment. No studies that compare the effectiveness of gentian violet to the effectiveness of other drug treatments have been conducted. Gentian violet can also be painted on the nipples of breastfeeding women to treat candidal infections of the breasts; it is safe for the infant but will cause the infant's lips to turn purple.[35]

Other nonpharmacologic treatments include behaviors or activities to decrease moisture in the vaginal area and thus help to prevent recurrences of vulvovaginitis. For example, women often are counseled to wear loose-fitting pants and underwear/pantyhose with cotton crotches.[28] However, no randomized, controlled trials have been published that have evaluated these common interventions, although they do no harm.

In summary, there is some evidence from in vitro studies and observational studies that lactobacillus and garlic are effective treatments for VVC, but no clinical trials that have proven effectiveness have been conducted. Gentian violet has been recommended for many decades and is assumed to be both safe and effective, but again, no clinical trials have been performed.

Atrophic Vaginitis

Atrophic vaginitis is seen most frequently among women experiencing decreased estrogen production, a condition that most commonly occurs in women who are perimenopausal, postmenopausal, or lactating.[36] Atrophic vaginitis is characterized by decreased vaginal lubrication and elevated vaginal pH. Other symptoms include genital itching and burning as well as urinary frequency and pain. It is estimated that 10–40% of women will have symptoms of atrophic vaginitis after menopause. Only 20–30% of women who are symptomatic will seek therapy for their symptoms. Over time this condition may lead to sexual dysfunction.[37]

Treatment of Atrophic Vaginitis

Lubrication with moisturizing agents helps to decrease symptoms and discomfort, especially in those women who do not desire to, or are unable to, use estrogen therapy.[37] These lubricants include Astroglide, K-Y, Replens, and Zestra. Aci-Jel is a water-dispersible acid jelly that contains acetic acid with a formulated pH of 3.9–4.1 and may be used to help restore the normal pH of the vagina.[31] In theory, restoring the normal acidic pH of the vagina should relieve symptoms of atrophic vaginitis.

Estrogen therapy can be used to replace the loss of estrogen in women with atrophic vaginitis and is administered either locally (vaginal) or orally. Estrogen therapy promotes revascularization of the vaginal epithelium and restores the normal pH of the vagina that decreases symptoms of atrophy.[37] Vaginal estrogen therapy should be used for women whose only symptom of decreased estrogen is atrophic vaginitis. The oral medication increases the blood level of estrogen and, therefore, provides relief from vasomotor symptoms. Oral estrogen therapy is warranted if vasomotor symptoms are present.

Desquamative Inflammatory Vaginitis

Desquamative inflammatory vaginitis is an uncommon syndrome that is characterized by a profuse vaginal discharge accompanied by vaginal irritation, burning, and dyspareunia, especially among perimenopausal women. The predominant lactobacilli flora of the vagina is replaced with gram-positive coccobacilli, usually group B *Streptococcus*.[13] Often the diagnosis of desquamative inflammatory vaginitis occurs only after the more common conditions have been ruled out. Sobel reported the results of empirically treating 51 women who had desquamative inflammatory vaginitis with 2% clindamycin suppositories every night for 14 nights, and improvement was reported in more than 95% of those treated in a retrospective review of charts. If women are perimenopausal, additional treatment with estrogen therapy may aid in maintaining remission.[38] The noticeable difference between desquamative inflammatory vaginitis and atrophic vaginitis is that desquamative inflammatory vaginitis does not respond to estrogen therapy alone.[13]

Allergic Reactions

In 30% of cases of genital tract symptoms, no infectious agents are identified. Irritants such as spermicides (nonoxynol-9), latex, sanitary pads, douches, soaps, perfumes, antifungal drugs, female barrier contraceptives, and condoms may cause an allergic reaction with vaginitis symptoms.[13] The causative agent should be identified so its use can be stopped and the woman can be treated with antihistamines and/or steroids as appropriate.

Conclusion

Approximately 10 million visits to healthcare providers per year are made by women seeking treatment of a vaginal issue. Usually the symptoms are related to one of the three main causes of vaginal discharge, bacterial vaginosis, **candidiasis**, or trichomoniasis. Most of the cases of these infections will respond to appropriate therapy. It is important for healthcare providers to correctly identify the cause of the symptoms and prescribe the diagnosis-specific recommended therapy.[1]

References

1. Mashburn J. Etiology, diagnosis, and management of vaginitis. J Midwifery Womens Health 2006;51: 423–30.
2. Klebanoff MA, Schwebke JR, Zhang J, Nansel TR, Yu KF, Andrews WW. Vulvovaginal symptoms in women with bacterial vaginosis. Obstet Gynecol 2004;104:267–72.
3. Beigi RH, Austin MN, Meyn LA, Krohn MA, Hillier SL. Antimicrobial resistance associated with the treatment of bacterial vaginosis. Am J Obstet Gynecol 2004;91:1124–9.
4. Ness RB, Hillier SL, Kip KE, Soper DE, Stamm CA, McGregor JA, et al. Bacterial vaginosis and risk of pelvic inflammatory disease. Obstet Gynecol 2004;104:761–9.
5. Zhang J, Hatch M, Zhang D, Shulman J, Harville E, Thomas AG. Frequency of douching and risk of bacterial vaginosis in African American women. Obstet Gynecol 2004;104:756–60.
6. Weir E. Bacterial vaginosis; more questions than answers. Can Med Assoc J 2004;171:448–501.
7. Blackwell AL, Thomas PD, Wareham K, Emery SJ. Health gains from screening for infection of the lower genital tract in women attending for termination of pregnancy. Lancet 1993;342(8865):206–10.
8. Centers for Disease Control and Prevention. Sexually transmitted diseases treatment guidelines 2006. Centers for Disease Control and Prevention. MMWR Recomm Rep 2006;55(RR-11):1–95.

9. Nailer MD, Sobel JD. Tinidazole for bacterial vaginosis. Exp Rev Antiinfec Ther 2007;5:343–8.

10. Livengood CH III, Ferris DG, Wiesenfield HC, Hillier S, Soper D. Effectiveness of two tinidazole regimens in treatment of bacterial vaginosis. Obstet Gynecol 2007;110(2):302–9.

11. Schwebke JR, Desmond R. A randomized trial of metronidazole in asymptomatic bacterial vaginosis to prevent the acquisition of sexually transmitted diseases. Am J Obstet Gynecol 2007;196:517.e1–517.e6.

12. Burtin P, Taddio A, Einarson TR, Koren G. Safety of metronidazole in pregnancy: a meta analysis. Am J Obstet Gynecol 1995;172(2, pt 1):530–9.

13. US Preventive Services Task Force. Screening for bacterial vaginosis in pregnancy to prevent preterm delivery: US Preventive Services Task Force recommendation statement. Ann of Intern Med 2008;148:214–9.

14. Nygren P, Rongwei F, Freeman M, Klebanoff M, Guise, JM. Evidence of the benefits and harms of screening and treating pregnant women who are asymptomatic for bacterial vaginosis: an update review for the US preventive Services Task Force. Ann Intern Med 2008;148:220–33.

15. Einarson A, Koren G. Can we use metronidazole during pregnancy and breastfeeding? Can Fam Phys 2000;46:1053–4.

16. Soper DE. Taking the guesswork out of diagnosing and managing vaginitis. Contemporary OB/GYN 2005; 50:32–9.

17. Alfonsi GA, Shlay JC, Parker S. What is the best approach for managing recurrent bacterial vaginosis? J Fam Prac 2004;53:650–2.

18. Baylson FA, Nyirjesy P, Weitz MV. Treatment of recurrent bacterial vaginosis with tinidazole. Obstet Gynecol 2004;104:931–2.

19. Sobel JD. What's new in bacterial vaginosis and trichomonas? Infect Dis Clin N Am 2005;19:387–406.

20. Klebanoff MA, Carey JC, Hauth JC, Hillier SL, Nugent RP, Thom EA, et al. National Institute of Child Health and Human Development Network of Maternal-Fetal Medicine Units. Failure of metronidazole to prevent preterm delivery among pregnant women with asymptomatic *Trichomonas vaginalis* infection. N Engl J Med 2001;345:487–93.

21. Ray D, Goswami R, Banerjee U, Dadwal V, Goswami D, Mandal P, et al. Prevalence of *Candida glabrata* and its response to boric acid vaginal suppositories in comparison with oral fluconazole in patients with diabetes and vulvovaginal candidiasis. Diabetes Care 2007;30:312–17.

22. Shorr AF, Lazarus R, Sherner JH, Jackson WL, Morrel M, Fraser VJ, et al. Do clinical features allow for accurate prediction of fungal pathogenesis in bloodstream infections? Potential implications of the increasing prevalence of non-albicans candidemia. Crit Care Med 2007; 35:1077–83.

23. Sobel JD. Vulvovaginal candidiasis. Lancet 2007;369: 1961–71.

24. Sobel JD, Chaim W, Nagappan V, Leaman D. Treatment of vaginitis caused by *Candida glabrata*: use of topical boric acid and flucytosine. Am J Ob Gyn 2003;189:1297–1300.

25. Ferris DG, Nyirjesy P, Sobel JD, Soper D, Paveletic A, Litaker MS. Over-the-counter antifungal drug misuse associated with patient-diagnosed vulvovaginal candidiasis. Obstet Gynecol 2002;99:419–25.

26. Yu DT, Peterson JF, Seger DL, Gerth WC, Bates DW. Frequency of potential azole drug-drug interactions and consequences of potential fluconazole drug interactions. Pharmacoepidemiol Drug Safety 2005;14: 755–67.

27. Carey JC, Klebanoff MA, Hauth JC, Hillier SL, Thom EA, Ernest JM, et al. Metronidazole to prevent preterm delivery in pregnant women with asymptomatic bacterial vaginosis. National Institute of Child Health and Human Development Network of Maternal-Fetal Medicine Units. N Engl J Med 2000;342:534–40.

28. Fogel CI. Gynecologic infections. In Schuiling KD, Likis FE, eds. Women's gynecologic health. Sudbury, MA: Jones and Bartlett, 2006:403–19.

29. Watson C, Calabretto H. Comprehensive review of conventional and non-conventional methods of management of recurrent vulvovaginal candidiasis. Aust NZ J Obstet Gynecol 2007;47:262–72.

30. Neafsey PJ, Donat D. Bugs, drugs, and yogurt. Home Health Nurse 2005;23:13–5.

31. Pirotta M, Gunn J, Chondros P, Grover S, O'Malley P, Hurley S, et al. Effect of lactobacillus in preventing post-antibiotic vulvovaginal candidiasis: a randomized controlled trial. BMJ 2004;329(7465):548.

32. Falagas ME, Betsi GI, Athanasiou S. Probiotics for prevention of recurrent vulvovaginal candidiasis: a review. J Antimicrob Chemother 2006;58(2):266–72. [Epub 2006 Jun 21].

33. Jeavons HS. Prevention and treatment of vulvovaginal candidiasis using exogenous *Lactobacillus*. J Obstet Gynecol Neonatal Nurs 2003;32:287–96.

34. Van Kessel K, Assefi N, Marrazzo J, Eckert L. Common complementary and alternative therapies for yeast

vaginitis and bacterial vaginosis: a systemic review. Obstet Gynecol Surv 2003;58:351–58.

35. Mayo Clinic Drugs and Supplements. Gentian violet (vaginal route). Available from: *http://www.mayoclinic .com/health/drug-information/DR600725* [Accessed January 27, 2009].

36. Palmer AR, Likis FE. Lactational atrophic vaginitis. J Midwifery Womens Health. 2003;48(4):282–4.

37. Bachman GA, Nevadunsky NS. Diagnosis and treatment of atrophic vaginitis. Am Fam Physician 2000; 61:3090–6.

38. Sobel JD. Desquamative inflammatory vaginitis: a new subgroup of purulent vaginitis responsive to topical 2% clindamycin therapy. Am J Obstet Gynecol. 1994; 171:1215–20.

32
Vulvar Disorders

Teri Stone-Godena

"The widespread practice of mislabeling female genitalia is almost as astounding in its implications as is the silence that surrounds this fact. . . . What new meaning might Freud's concept of "penis envy" take on, if we consider the fact that in his lifetime the words "clitoris," "vulva" and "labia" were not included in the dictionary and, in this country the only word in Webster's dictionary for female genitalia was "vagina"? Who decides what words are in the dictionary and what is real?"

HARRIET GOLDHOR LERNER, *THE DANCE OF DECEPTION*, 1994

 Chapter Glossary

Acanthotic Thickening of the epidermis.

Acne inversa Another term for hidradenitis suppurativa.

Allodynia Light touch.

Behçet's syndrome A syndrome of unknown etiology characterized by recurrent genital ulcerations that are painful and lead to scarring.

Desiccant A drying agent.

Extramammary Paget's disease Cutaneous adenocarcinoma that is classified based on source of the primary lesion.

Folliculitis Inflammation of hair follicles that occurs primarily where hairs are subjected to trauma such as buttocks, perineal area, thighs, and inguinal area.

Furuncle Commonly called a boil, this is an accumulation of purulent and dead material usually around a hair follicle. A cluster of furuncles can form interconnections and are then termed *carbuncles*. Severe cases of furuncles may result in abscesses.

Guttate A term used particularly with psoriasis to describe lesions that are droplike in appearance.

Hidradenitis suppurativa Also known as Verneuil's disease or acne inverse, this condition is characterized by chronic, painful, inflamed, suppurative lesions of the apocrine glands. This orphan disease may be found on the vulva as manifested by furuncles.

Inflammatory dermatosis Contact dermatitis of the genital skin that exhibits lesions that may include simple erythema, edema, vesicles, or scaling.

Lichen planus An inflammatory condition that includes lesions and papules on mucous membranes such as the vulva. Although etiology is unknown, there is a strong suggestion that the condition is autoimmune.

Lichen sclerosus A relatively rare condition whose etiology remains unknown, but which is manifested by dermatological lesions that often result in scarring on and around the vulva.

Lichen simplex chronicus Another term for squamous cell hyperplasia.

Molluscum contagiosum A benign poxvirus that causes lesions, including genital lesions.

Pediculosis Small insects that can cause genital infestation, often called pubic lice or crabs.

Psoriasis A skin condition characterized by inflamed skin patches and excessive skin production. This condition can occur over various areas of the body, including the vulva.

Seborrheic dermatitis A papulosquamous condition associated with flaking of the skin that often is found on the adult scalp in the form of dandruff, but also can be a vulvar condition.

Squamous cell hyperplasia Also known as lichen simplex chronicus, this skin condition can occur on the vulva and is characterized by thickened skin secondary to an itch-scratch-itch cycle experienced by a person. Squamous cell hyperplasia generally is benign, although when atypia is found, it is classified as vulvar intraepithelial neoplasia.

Verneuil's disease Another term for hidradenitis suppurativa.

Vulvar intraepithelial neoplasia (VIN) An intraepithelial lesion of the vulva that has various degrees of atypia. The basement membrane is normal, therefore the lesion is not invasive.

Vulvodynia A condition characterized by pain or burning in the vulva.

Vulvar Conditions

Some conditions affecting the vulva have a readily identifiable etiology and well known evidence-based treatments whereas others are not easily categorized or treated. When pathophysiology is not well understood, it is difficult to develop treatment strategies. Although the majority of the conditions discussed in this chapter are a manifestation of a disease affecting other parts of the body, such as psoriasis, lichen planus, and Behçet's syndrome, other diseases are specific to the vulva, such as vulvodynia. Where diseases affecting multiple organs are concerned, only treatments for the vulvar conditions will be discussed in this chapter. Genital herpes and warts caused by human papillomavirus are reviewed in Chapter 23.

Folliculitis

Folliculitis is inflammation of hair follicles occurring primarily on portions of the body where hairs are subjected to trauma. Lesions can be found on the scalp, neck, and face as well as buttocks, perineal area, and the thighs and groin. The most common cause of folliculitis is the bacteria *Staphylococcus aureus*, although persons who have been on suppressive antibiotics for other conditions are susceptible to fungal folliculitis. In addition, hot tub folliculitis, a less common form of the disorder caused by *Pseudomonas aeruginosa*, thrives in inadequately chlorinated warm water. Rarely, folliculitis can occur following occlusion of the area. When this situation occurs, it is common to find that no organisms are found in the fluid found around the hair follicle, resulting in a sterile culture.[1-3]

Folliculitis affects all age groups and ethnicities. Certain practices encourage the process. Folliculitis begins with damage to hair follicles. Shaving, waxing, plucking, electrolysis, and wearing tight clothes abrade hair follicles and cause microscopic breaks in integrity of the skin at the base of the hair. Hair follicles can be irritated or blocked by common substances like sweat, cocoa butter, or makeup; or more uncommon agents like machine oils, tar, and creosote, which are components of some medications used to treat psoriasis. Additional information on dermatology can be found in Chapter 26. Long-term use of antibiotics or steroid creams may eliminate healthy flora and encourage more virulent bacteria or fungi to grow. Having an infected cut, scrape, or surgical incision in a vulnerable area can enable the spread of the bacteria or fungi to nearby hair follicles. Individuals who are immunocompromised secondary to conditions such as diabetes or AIDS can have less ability to fight infection in general. Use of a hot tub, whirlpool, or swimming pool that is not properly treated with chlorine allows bacteria to have close approximation to vulnerable hair follicles.[3] Once injured, follicles are more likely to become infected by bacteria entering the break in the skin as the hair regrows. These lesions usually are similar to red papules or pimples with a hair in the center of each one. However, some lesions may be pustular, and these commonly cause itching or burning. If the infection involves the deep part of the follicle, it results in a painful **furuncle**. Recurrent folliculitis in the same follicle can result in scarring or hair loss.

Differential diagnosis should include consideration of impetigo, heat rash, scabies, insect bites, herpesvirus, and keratosis pilaris. Definitive diagnosis is usually by history and physical examination. When laboratory analysis is necessary to exclude other possible etiologies, the most common lab tests include Gram staining and culture of a fluid sample, a herpesvirus culture, and, rarely, a punch biopsy of the lesion. Often individuals are treated empirically.

Treatment of Folliculitis

Treatment of mild folliculitis includes keeping the area clean and dry since the lesions generally heal spontaneously within approximately 2 weeks. Warm compresses made with 1 tablespoon of white vinegar to 1.3 cups of warm water or Burow's solution (5% aluminum subacetate) applied for 5–10 minutes, three to six times per day may help relieve itching. No studies support the efficacy of vinegar, but it has been used as an antipruritic since Roman times.

If the infection is more severe or recurrent, antibiotic or antifungal cream or systemic antibiotics may be used. Mupirocin 2% (Bactroban) is applied topically (Table 32-1). As a general rule, it is advisable to verify that topical treatments do not contain alcohol. Ointments rarely have alcohol, but some creams may contain the irritant. Since the nares are a known source of *S aureus*, some authorities recommend applying mupirocin to the nares during treatment of the perineum to eliminate the carrier state. Mupirocin as a sole treatment for perineal carriage of *S aureus* has not been demonstrated to be efficacious, but one study recommended concurrent treatment as an option.[4]

Table 32-1 Treatments for Folliculitis

Drug Generic (Brand)	Adult Dosage	Contraindications	Clinical Considerations and Selected Drug–Drug Interactions	FDA Pregnancy Category
Mupirocin (Bactroban)	2% applied topically three or four times daily for 14 days.	Hypersensitivity.	None	B
Dicloxacillin	250–500 mg PO four times daily for 14–21 days.*	Hypersensitivity, penicillin allergy.	Decreases effectiveness of oral contraceptives anticoagulants. Probenecid and disulfiram may increase penicillin levels.	B
Cephalexin (Keflex)	250–500 mg PO four times daily for 10–14 days.*	Hypersensitivity, penicillin allergy.	Increases nephrotoxicity of aminoglycosides.	B
Clindamycin (Cleocin)†	150–300 mg/dose PO every 6–8 hours for 10–14 days.* Topical: apply 2% lotion sparingly over affected area.	Documented hypersensitivity, regional enteritis, ulcerative colitis, hepatic impairment, antibiotic-associated colitis.	Adjust dose in severe hepatic dysfunction; associated with possibly fatal colitis from overgrowth of *Clostridium difficile*. Topical agent can cause dryness and burning. Antidiarrheals may delay absorption. Erythromycin may antagonize. May prolong neuromuscular blockade from tubocurarine.	B
Trimethoprim-sulfamethoxazole (Bactrim, Septra)	160 mg TMP/800 mg SMZ PO every 12 hours for 10–14 days.	Hypersensitivity, megaloblastic anemia. Third trimester pregnancy. G-6-PD deficiency.	Discontinue if rash or sign of adverse reaction. Obtain CBC frequently; discontinue if hematologic changes occur. Caution in folate deficiency renal or hepatic impairment. Warfarin may increase PT. Dapsone and phenytoin may increase blood levels of both. Methotrexate may cause bone marrow suppression.	B
Erythromycin (E-Mycin, EES, Ery-Tab) (Emgel, Erycette topically)	250 mg erythromycin stearate/base (or 400 mg ethylsuccinate) every 6 hours PO, or 500 mg every 12 hours. Alternatively, 333 mg PO every 8 hours; increase to 4 grams per day for 10–14 days.* Topical: apply at bedtime or twice daily until clear.	Hypersensitivity, megaloblastic anemia.	Caution in liver disease; estolate formulation may cause cholestatic jaundice; GI side effects are common. Discontinue if nausea, vomiting, malaise, abdominal colic, or fever occur. May increase toxicity of theophylline, digoxin, carbamazepine, and cyclosporine; may potentiate warfarin. Increased risk of rhabdomyolysis with lovastatin and simvastatin; decreases metabolism of repaglinide.	B
Ciprofloxacin (Cipro)	250–750 mg PO every 12 hours for 10–14 days.*	Hypersensitivity.	Need increased water consumption. Antacids reduce serum level. Caffeine, cyclosporin, theophylline, digoxin increase toxicity. Warfarin may increase PT.	C

CBC = complete blood count; PT = prothrombin time.
* Duration of therapy dependent on severity of infection.
† Effective against *Staphylococcus* and *Streptococcus*.

The systemic drug of choice for treatment of *S aureus* is dicloxacillin (Dynapen), which is prescribed for 14–21 days depending on the severity of the infection. For a woman who has a penicillin allergy without cross-sensitivity to cephalosporins, a first-generation cephalosporin may be employed. When a true penicillin allergy is known, clindamycin (Cleocin) or two double-strength trimethoprim-sulfamethoxazole (Bactrim, Septra) may be taken twice a day for 7–14 days if the individual has a body weight of < 80 kg; for those with body weights ≥ 80 kg, the double-strength trimethoprim-sulfamethoxazole may be taken three times a day.[2] Only one randomized, controlled trial has demonstrated effectiveness of trimethoprim-sulfamethoxazole (Bactrim or Septra). However, a large body of anecdotal evidence, case studies, or small, open label studies support the use.[5,6] When treating folliculitis among pregnant women, caution should be exercised in prescribing sulfa-based drugs (i.e., trimethoprim-sulfamethoxazole [Bactrim or Septra]) during the third trimester because sulfonamides ingested close to the time of birth can be associated with newborn jaundice and hemolytic anemia. No reports of adverse effects have been noted in infants whose lactating mothers take sulfonamides for a short time, generally 2 weeks or less.

Although homeopathic treatments are not FDA approved, many individuals use them based on the principle that like cures like or the law of similars. Highly diluted substances are administered, and one example is Folistitin, a treatment that is purported to relieve symptoms of folliculitis. Folistitin is taken as 15 drops in a glass of water, twice daily for 40 days and has no known contraindications. However, there are no data regarding its effectiveness.

Prevention consists of using antibacterial soap, good hand washing technique, wearing loose clothing, avoiding oils on the skin, and avoiding public hot tubs and other risky behaviors. Since folliculitis is increased among obese individuals, weight loss may be associated with a decrease in incidence.

Lichen Sclerosus

Lichen sclerosus of the vulva is the most common of the vulvar dermatoses, accounting for 40% of vulvar lesions. Lichen sclerosus is a chronic, progressive disease of unknown etiology. Since it has been noted in greater incidence among Whites and found in clusters in families, there exists a supposition of a genetic predisposition. The overall prevalence of lichen sclerosus in the general gynecology population is 2%, and the distribution is bimodal, with 15% of cases among prepubescent children, and the remainder is found among postmenopausal women. This bimodal distribution leads some to theorize that the disorder is due to hypoestrogenic states.[7] Lichen sclerosus is found more often among females, with a female to male ratio of 6:1. Penile lichen sclerosus, although very rare, is found almost exclusively in uncircumcised males. Extracellular matrix glycoprotein antibodies (ECM-1) have been noted in 75–80% of lichen sclerosus lesions, and up to 20% of persons with lichen sclerosus have a concomitant thyroid dysfunction, so current research is focused on an autoimmune etiology.[8]

Lesions of lichen sclerosus are found anywhere on the vulva, but not in the vagina. Lichen sclerosus lesions are usually symmetrical and white, with rough, thin, parchment paper-like crinkled patches usually termed *plaques*. Inflammation and altered fibroblast function in the papillary dermis lead to fibrosis of the upper dermis and cause epidermal atrophy. Changes in appearance of labial, perineal, and perianal areas along with introital narrowing may be termed *keyhole*, *hourglass*, or *figure of 8*. The atrophy leads to fissures, ulcers, submucosal hemorrhages, and pigmentation changes. Areas may be depigmented or hyperpigmented. These patches may be confused with squamous cell carcinoma, extramammary Paget's disease (rare), vitiligo, chronic inflammatory dermatoses, psoriasis, or squamous cell hyperplasia, and, since 5% of women who have had lichen sclerosus are at risk for developing squamous cell carcinoma, the diagnosis of lichen sclerosus requires a biopsy[9] (Table 32-2).

Lichen sclerosus does not cause cancer, but the scarred, damaged tissue from long-term lichen sclerosus is more vulnerable to dysplastic changes. External tissue shrinkage and destruction can lead to the assumption of the labia minora into the labia majora, introital stenosis, chronic pain, and sexual dysfunction. Despite extensive damage, only approximately 50% of women with lichen sclerosus report symptoms of pruritus vulvae, dyspareunia, vulvodynia, and sometimes dysuria or genital bleeding. Tissue damage cannot be reversed, but to prevent further damage, the disease should be treated regardless of symptomatology.[10]

Treatment of Lichen Sclerosus

Treatment of lichen sclerosus usually includes use of topical ultrapotent topical steroids. A leading vulvovaginal disorders clinic at the University of Michigan uses clobetasol propionate 0.05% (Temovate) topically, twice daily for a

Table 32-2 Treatments for Lichen Sclerosus

Drug Generic (Brand)	Adult Dosage	Contraindications	Clinical Considerations and Selected Drug–Drug Interactions	FDA Pregnancy Category
Clobetasol propionate (Temovate)	0.05% cream or lotion: apply thin layer once daily for 1 month then pulse dose for 1 month, 2 consecutive days of the week, off 5 days.	Hypersensitivity, paronychia, cellulitis, impetigo, angular cheilitis, erythrasma, erysipelas, rosacea, perioral dermatitis, acne.	Systemic absorption may occur and produce reversible HPA-axis suppression with potential for glucocorticoid insufficiency after withdrawal of treatment; do not use in skin with decreased circulation; can cause atrophy of groin, face, and axillae; if infection develops and is not responsive to antibiotic treatment, discontinue until infection is under control.	C
Triamcinolone (Kenalog, Aristocort)	0.1% ointment: apply thin film twice or three times daily until favorable response, or 1 cc injected intralesionally with bupivacaine once every 3–6 months.	Hypersensitivity or concomitant fungal infection.	Cushing syndrome from systemic absorption if used over prolonged period, over large area, or with occlusive dressings. Avoid more than 40-mg injection weekly.	C
Isotretinoin (Accutane)	40–50 mg PO every day for 4 months.	Hypersensitivity, pregnancy.	May decrease night vision; associated with irritable bowel syndrome, hepatitis; diabetics have difficulty with glycemic control. Avoid exposure to ultraviolet light; mood swings. Can be very irritating to vulvar tissues. Toxicity with vitamin A administration; pseudotumor cerebri or papilledema with tetracyclines. May reduce levels of carbamazepine.	X
Tacrolimus (Protopic)	0.1% ointment: apply to affected areas twice daily for 2–6 wk.	Hypersensitivity; ointments can lead to maceration in skin folds; not recommended in immunocompromised persons.	No interactions reported.	C

month and then daily for 2 months[11] (Box 32-1). Regarding treatment after the initial 3 months of therapy, there is debate among experts whether long-term steroids are indicated. Some researchers recommend using clobetasol on an as-needed basis, or for mild cases, a medium potency steroid such as triamcinolone (Kenalog, Aristocort). Chapter 26 provides more details on use of steroids in dermatology.

Hormones have been used for lichen sclerosus treatment in the past, but both testosterone and progesterone have not been found to be superior to placebos in clinical trials.[12] Retinoids may provide relief for some women who cannot tolerate steroids.[13] Vitamin A is necessary for epithelial cell differentiation. Retinoids, which are vitamin A derivatives, increase epidermal proliferation and regulate growth and differentiation of keratinocytes.[14] Retinoids are most appropriately used by providers familiar with their

use, and if they are used for reproductive-aged women, they should be limited to women using highly effective forms of contraception since they are contraindicated during pregnancy. While no studies exist on the effect of systemic retinoids in lactation, vitamin A is excreted in breast milk, and the presence of isotretinoin would be expected, so the same caution would apply as during pregnancy. During pregnancy and lactation, steroids may be substituted for retinoids if needed. Periodic pregnancy tests should be performed during retinoid use.

On the assumption lichen sclerosus is immune moderated, some researchers have found success with the use of topical immunomodulators, especially tacrolimus (Protopic), a macrolactam that inhibits the action of interleukin (IL2) by stimulating helper T cells.[15] The FDA issued a public health advisory in 2005 regarding a potential cancer risk from use of tacrolimus ointment (Protopic), advising it

Box 32-1 Case Study: Lichen Sclerosus

A 58-year-old woman reports that approximately 3 months ago she acquired a new sexual partner. Over the next several weeks she noted that intercourse was increasingly uncomfortable. She attributed the dyspareunia to vaginal dryness secondary to her postmenopausal state and began using lubricants. However, the topical agents were not of value and the dyspareunia continued. Within the last few weeks she began experiencing mild burning and increasing itching of the vulva.

Her past history includes two healthy, full-term pregnancies and births. She currently routinely takes a multiple vitamin, low-dose aspirin because of a family history of cardiovascular disease, and levothyroxine for mild hypothyroidism diagnosed last year. She has never used estrogen therapy. She and her partner are using condoms for sexually transmitted infection (STI) protection.

Upon physical examination, this woman's vulva is marked by a pale, almost white, patch of skin around the introitus. Some areas of redness on the edges are apparent with irritation suggestive of scratching dry skin. This woman has lichen sclerosus. She has a thyroid dysfunction, which is relatively common among women with lichen sclerosus. Not only does she have symptoms suggestive of the condition, but her physical examination provides a clinical picture of lichen sclerosus. A biopsy could be performed for confirmation although she may be treated empirically. This woman should be reassured that lichen sclerosus is not cancerous.

Several different options exist for treatment. Since her condition is mild, one potential option is prescription of clobetasol propionate 0.05% to be used as needed once or twice a day on her vulva. A 15- or 30-gram tube of medication should be sufficient as it should be applied sparingly. Oral diphenhydramine hydrochloride (Benadryl) can be recommended at bedtime for its antihistamine and sedative effects. Relief is likely to be gradual. A follow-up visit in 2–3 months should enable the provider to assess whether or not the therapy has been successful. This woman also should be counseled that the condition, even if resolved, may reoccur.

be used only when other treatments fail or cannot be tolerated. Some clinicians combine tracrolimus and clobetasol propionate in a pulsatile fashion, such as 2 weeks of using one followed by 2 weeks of using the other.

Based on the hypothesis that cyclosporine (Sandimmune), an immunomodulator, might be as effective in the treatment of lichen sclerosus as it has been in the treatment of psoriasis, two small, open-label trials investigated the use of oral cyclosporine for treatment of severe lichen sclerosus.[16] The seven participants all experienced improvement of their lesions within 4 weeks and all had clearance by 12 weeks. Three individuals experienced minor side effects, which did not lead to discontinuation of the drug. Larger studies need to establish if these findings continue. However, when compared to standard steroid treatments, none of the alternatives have been reported to work as quickly or as effectively and all are significantly more expensive.

When lichen sclerosus causes significant vulvar discomfort, a sedative may be used for the first 2 weeks of treatment until the effect of the steroids is noted. Oral antihistamines, doxepin topical cream 5% (Zonalon), doxepin 25–75 mg nightly and tricyclic antidepressants

(e.g., amitriptyline 10–25 mg nightly with increases up to, but not exceeding 150 mg) may be prescribed when pruritus is severe.[8] Tricyclics are contraindicated with pregnancy and lactation, and the use of doxepin should be limited to the topical form. When pharmacologic treatments fail or when a stenotic introitus or deep fissuring is present, a perineoplasty may offer relief.[17] Emollients such as Aquaphor (active ingredient petroleum) or Cetaphil (active ingredient antifungal/antibacterial triclosan) may be useful in keeping tissue soft. Counseling should include discussions of the chronic nature of the disease and the potential for malignancy in the target area. All topical steroids, emollients, and immunomodulators are safe for use in pregnancy and with lactation.

Squamous Cell Hyperplasia

Squamous cell hyperplasia is sometimes known as **lichen simplex chronicus**, although it is not a distinct entity but is a skin change resulting from an itch-scratch-itch cycle. By the time squamous cell hyperplasia develops, the original trigger, whether it was lichen sclerosus, eczema, candida, psoriasis, chemical irritants, or allergens may no longer be discernible. Lesions appear similar to lichen sclerosus in the early stages but without the loss of skin folds or shrinkage. Histologically, the lesions are distinct from those of lichen sclerosus.[18] With lichen sclerosus, the epidermis thins. Squamous cell hyperplasia causes thickening of the epidermis. The thickening may be a response to chronic pruritus. When infection is suspected, aerobic bacterial and fungal or viral cultures can be helpful in identifying a causative organism. Because of the similarity between squamous cell hyperplasia lesions and invasive squamous cancer, lesions should be biopsied. Squamous cell cancer has been noted adjacent to areas of squamous cell hyperplasia. However, for a woman who does not have squamous atypia on a biopsy nor a history of lichen sclerosus, squamous cell hyperplasia is associated with minimal malignant potential. When atypia is found, it usually is the result of a human papillomavirus (HPV) infection and is classified as **vulvar intraepithelial neoplasia** (VIN).[19]

Burning, extreme itching, pain, and tenderness are hallmarks of squamous cell hyperplasia. Classically, the lesions are red or pink, raised, **acanthotic**, and leathery; and they may be asymmetrical. An overlying gray-white keratin layer covers the lesions. While an infectious agent or irritant may be the source of the skin changes, it is unclear whether there is an autoimmune or hormonal component. The peak incidence is among women in their sexual maturity. VIN is rarely found among pubertal or young women, and is found twice as often among premenopausal women as it is in those who are postmenopausal.[20]

Treatment of Squamous Cell Hyperplasia

Treatment of squamous cell hyperplasia begins with removing the source of the itching and breaking the itch-scratch-itch cycle. Infection, if present, needs to be treated with appropriate antibiotics. The oral route is more efficacious than topical antibiotics but can result in worsening of symptoms if fungal overgrowth results. Therefore, when using antibiotics to treat a woman with an infection, periodically the provider should add an antifungal agent for prophylactic use. No single antifungal treatment has shown to be superior compared to another. Suggestions include using a 100-mg dose of oral fluconazole (Diflucan), a single dose vaginal preparation every 3 days, a 3-day vaginal preparation, or a 150-mg dose of oral fluconazole every 7 days. Irritants such as laundry detergents, soap with additives, and perfumes should be identified and removed. Mild to moderate disease can be treated with short-term medium potency steroids such as triamcinolone used as an ointment or intralesional injection used for 2–4 weeks.[21] Some authors recommend steroids with concomitant use of crotamiton as an antipruritic.[18] For severe disease, an ultrapotent steroid (clobetasol propionate [Temovate, Dermovate] 0.05%) can be applied topically for 2–4 weeks then replaced with triamcinolone (Kenalog, Aristocort).[21]

Systemic sedating antihistamines like diphenhydramine (Benadryl) or hydroxyzine (Atarax) or amitriptyline (Elavil) 10–40 mg taken orally at bedtime have met with success in the treatment of several disorders in which pruritus is a presenting issue[11] (Table 32-3). Amitriptyline use should be limited to nonpregnant/nonlactating women as there has been reported animal teratogenicity and use in lactation is considered to be of potential concern, although no studies provide strong evidence to confirm or refute human risks during pregnancy and lactation.

Lichen Planus

Lichen planus, an acute or chronic inflammatory lesion of the skin and mucous membrane, is of unknown etiology but is likely to be an autoimmune disease. Rarely found in children or the elderly, the peak incidence for lichen planus is among women aged 30–60, suggesting a role for hormones in the disease.[21]

The lesions of lichen planus are erosive and can resemble lichen sclerosus, HPV, syphilis, chancroid, Behçet's syndrome, or pemphigus. These lesions may range from white papules or plaques to homogenously white epithelium or erosions surrounded by white epithelium (lacy pattern) and are found on the genitals, in the mouth, and on the scalp. While lichen sclerosus is not found in the vagina, lichen planus lesions begin in the vestibule and can obliterate the vagina.[20] Both lichen sclerosus and lichen planus can cause scarring, leading to obliteration of the vagina, labia minora, and the clitoral hood. Hair loss and pruritus may be present and contact bleeding and dyspareunia are common. Diagnosis is by biopsy.[18]

Treatment of Lichen Planus

No treatments for lichen planus have been evaluated by randomized clinical trials and many drugs are used off label. As underlying infection is common, antibiotics are a first-line treatment. Antibiotic treatment is most effective by mouth and initiated in the early, erosive stages of lichen planus. Antibiotics with anti-inflammatory properties can be used long term and include doxycycline (Vibramycin)

Table 32-3 Antihistamines Used to Treat Pruritus of Squamous Cell Hyperplasia

Drug Generic (Brand)	Adult Dosage	Contraindications	Clinical Considerations and Selected Drug–Drug Interactions	FDA Pregnancy Category
Antiinflammatory Agents				
Triamcinolone (Kenalog, Aristocort)	0.1% ointment: apply thin film bid/tid until favorable response or injected intralesionally with bupivacaine every 3–6 months.	Hypersensitivity or concomitant fungal infection.	Cushing syndrome from systemic absorption if used over prolonged period, over large area, or with occlusive dressings. Avoid more than 40 mg injection weekly.	C
Clobetasol propionate (Temovate, Dermovate)	0.05%: apply thin layer once daily for 1 month then pulse dose for 1 month, 2 consecutive days of the week, off 5 days.	Hypersensitivity, paronychia, cellulitis, impetigo, angular cheilitis, erythrasma, erysipelas, rosacea, perioral dermatitis, acne.	Systemic absorption may occur and produce reversible HPA-axis suppression with potential for glucocorticoid insufficiency after withdrawal of treatment; do not use in skin with decreased circulation; can cause atrophy of groin, face, and axillae; if infection develops and is not responsive to antibiotic treatment, discontinue until infection is under control. No reported interactions.	C
For Pruritus				
Diphenhydramine (Benadryl)	25–50 mg PO at bedtime.	Hypersensitivity.	Do not operate machinery or drive. May cause constipation, dry mouth. Increases anticholinergic effects of MAO inhibitors.	B
Amitriptyline (Elavil)	10–40 mg at bedtime, increase weekly to maximum 150 mg.	Pregnancy; recent myocardial infarction.	Potentiates effects of alcohol and MAO inhibitors.	C
Doxepin (Zonalon)	25–75 mg po at bedtime or 5% cream topically at bedtime or up to three times daily.	Hypersensitivity; narrow angle glaucoma.	Do not operate machinery or drive. Do not use longer than 8 days. Potentiates MAO inhibitors.	C

MAO = monoamine oxidase.

and clindamycin (Cleocin) (Table 32-4). When antibiotics are used, it is helpful also to treat lichen planus with an antifungal agent every 3–7 days (see the section on treatment of squamous cell hyperplasia). For extensive disease, oral steroids such as prednisone (Deltasone, Sterapred) may be necessary until skin healing begins, at which time topical steroids should be used.[18]

Emollients (e.g., petroleum jelly, mineral oil, olive oil) may have some therapeutic value in keeping the tissue soft. If topical steroids are desired, the initial one should be an ultrapotent one such as clobetasol (Temovate, Dermovate) 0.05%, and it may be used for 2 weeks then tapered to a medium-potency steroid like topical or intralesional triamcinolone acetonide.[19] In observational studies, hydrocortisone suppositories in the form of Anusol HC 25 mg have been shown to be effective in the treatment of vaginal lichen planus. One half of a suppository is inserted in the vagina twice a day for 2 months, then daily for two months.[20,21] Some authorities recommend continuing the treatment indefinitely using 1–3 suppositories per week

while others have noted no further improvement after the first 4 months.[21,22] For recalcitrant lichen planus, tacrolimus 0.1% (Protopic) can be applied externally as an ointment twice a day, and tacrolimus 0.1% vaginal suppositories can be made by a compounding pharmacist by mixing 2 mg of tacrolimus with 2 grams of an inert base.[23] This suppository can be used nightly for 2 months.

Some authors recommend using vaginal dilators during treatment to decrease the risk of scarring.[17] A dilator can be lubricated with a mild to medium potency steroid such as hydrocortisone. As the upper third of the vault is most prone to scarring, the dilator must be inserted fully into the vagina. Dilators may come in the form of instruments specifically designed for the purpose, although a plastic speculum or even nonmedical items can be covered with condoms and used.

Alternative treatments include dapsone, an antibacterial used in the treatment of Hansen's disease; as well as antimetabolites such as methotrexate (Rheumatrex), cyclosporine (Neoral, Sandimmune), cyclophosphamide

Table 32-4 Treatments for Lichen Planus

Drug Generic (Brand)	Adult Dosage	Contraindications	Clinical Considerations and Selected Drug–Drug Interactions	FDA Pregnancy Category
Doxycycline (Vibramycin)	100 mg twice daily for 7–10 days.	Hypersensitivity, hepatic dysfunction.	Photosensitivity with exposure to ultraviolet light. Fanconi-like syndrome with outdated drugs. Permanent discoloration of teeth if intrauterine exposure or exposure during childhood to age 8; contraindicated for pregnant women and young children. Bioavailability decreases with use of antacids. Decreases effectiveness of oral contraceptives. Increases antithrombogenic effects of anticoagulants.	D
Clindamycin (Cleocin)	150–300 mg/dose PO every 6–8 hours. Topical: apply 2% lotion sparingly over affected area.	Documented hypersensitivity, regional enteritis, ulcerative colitis, hepatic impairment, antibiotic-associated colitis.	Adjust dose in severe hepatic dysfunction; associated with possibly fatal colitis from overgrowth of *Clostridium difficile*. Topical can cause dryness and burning. Antidiarrheals may delay absorption. Erythromycin (E-mycin) may antagonize. May prolong neuromuscular blockade from tubocurarine (Jexin, Tubarine).	B
Prednisone (Deltasone)	30–60 mg/day PO for 4–6 wk followed by gradual taper.	Hypersensitivity.	Adrenal crisis with abrupt discontinuation; hyperglycemia, edema, osteonecrosis, myopathy, peptic ulcer disease, hypokalemia, osteoporosis, psychosis, myasthenia gravis, growth suppression, infections may occur. Acetaminophen, alcohol, NSAIDs, amphotericin B, carbonic anhydrase inhibitors, and antacids decrease absorption. Anticoagulants, tricyclic agents, antidiabetic agents, antithyroid hormones, estrogens, digitalis (Lanoxin), diuretics, ephedrine, folic acid, immunosuppressants, potassium supplements, and ritodrine (Yutopar) cause pulmonary edema.	B
Clobetasol (Temovate, Dermovate)	Apply thin layer once daily for 1 month then pulse dose for 1 month, 2 consecutive days of the week, off 5 days.	Hypersensitivity, paronychia, cellulitis, impetigo, angular cheilitis, erythrasma, erysipelas, rosacea, perioral dermatitis, acne.	Systemic absorption may occur with reversible hypothalamus–pituitary–ovarian axis suppression and potential for glucocorticoid insufficiency after withdrawal of treatment; do not use in skin with decreased circulation; can cause atrophy of groin, face, and axillae; if infection develops and is not responsive to antibiotic treatment, discontinue until infection is under control. No interactions reported.	C
Hydrocortisone (Anusol HC)	1/2 of a 25-mg (2.5%) suppository vaginally twice daily for 2 months then daily for 1 month.	Hypersensitivity, serious infections, fungal infections, varicella.	Administration of live virus vaccines. Do not use with occlusive dressings. No interactions reported.	C
Tacrolimus (Protopic)	0.1% ointment: apply to affected areas twice daily for 2–6 wk.	Hypersensitivity; ointments can lead to maceration in skin folds; not recommended in immunocompromised persons.	No interactions reported.	C
Dapsone (Avlosulfon)	50–100 mg daily PO.	Hypersensitivity, G6PD disease.	Screen for G6PD disease. Blood dyscrasia with folic acid antagonists. Decreased effectiveness with rifampin (Rifadin).	C
Methotrexate (Rheumatrex)	7.5–25 mg/week PO/SC.	Hypersensitivity, alcoholism, hepatic insufficiency, immunodeficiency syndromes, blood dyscrasias, leukopenia, thrombocytopenia, significant anemia, renal insufficiency.	Photosensitivity reaction, hepatotoxicity, fibrosis, cirrhosis, bone marrow suppression. Monitor CBC monthly and liver and renal function q 1–3 months during therapy. Discontinue if significant drop in CBC. Aminoglycosides, charcoal decrease absorption. Folic acid decreases response. Probenecid, salicylates, procarbazine (Matulane), and sulfonamides, including TMP-SMZ (Bactrim, Septra), increase effects. Etretinate (Tegison) may increase hepatotoxicity.	X

CBC = complete blood count; TMP-SMZ = trimethoprim/sulfamethoxazole.

(Neosar, Cytoxan), and azathioprine (Imuran), which are used in the treatment of psoriasis and Behçet's syndrome.[18] These drugs are more expensive and entail greater risks; therefore, they generally are reserved for use by a specialist in vulvar diseases. Retinoids have been reported to be effective in the treatment of oral lesions but have not been associated with improvement of vulvovaginal disease. Retinoids, such as antimetabolites, are known teratogens, or FDA Pregnancy Category X drugs. Therefore, since there is a lack of associated improvement and an increased risk, these agents have no place in the treatment of vulvar lichen planus.[18,20]

Psoriasis

Psoriasis is a chronic disorder affecting 2% of the population. The precise pathophysiology is not known, but a genetic predilection is suspected, since 30% of the population with psoriasis report a family member with the disease. This condition can affect persons of all ages but causative stimulus may be different by age. In young persons, infections with streptococci often precipitate an outbreak. In older patients the more common stimulants are drugs (e.g., NSAIDs, beta-blockers, and lithium), stress, and exposure to cold.[24]

Symptoms include pruritus and soreness. Genital and nongenital sites such as flexor surfaces, scalp, and crural folds can be affected. The appearance of the lesions may vary widely, but usually are bilateral and symmetric. These lesions may be red or pink, sharply demarcated plaques or **guttate** (droplike) lesions with elevated silver scales, or they may be scabbed over or moist and oozing. When found in the vulvar region, the lesions usually begin on the thigh and spread upwards, most commonly affecting the outer labia to the groin folds and up to the mons pubis. Individuals with psoriasis often have pitting of the nail beds. Since the lesions may assume different forms and may be confused with other disorders, definitive diagnosis must be by biopsy.[24]

Treatment of Psoriasis

Similar to lichen sclerosus, no cure exists for psoriasis. However, there are a variety of treatment regimens, many with years of varying degrees of success, but many are not appropriate to vulvar tissue. Topical agents include tar emulsion and topical calcipotriene (vitamin D_3). These agents may be used on the thighs and mons but are not recommended for tender vulvar tissue. Ultrapotent steroids

often are used to decrease the inflammation. Steroids work rapidly but become less effective over time and can cause tissue atrophy. Tazarotene (Tazorac), a retinoid gel, is FDA approved for psoriasis (Table 32-5). A pea-sized amount is applied to a lesion (an area the size of an open hand) nightly. Care should be taken to keep the medication limited to the plaques. Retinoids are absorbed through the skin and are teratogenic, so women using them must use an effective form of birth control such as hormonal contraceptives or intrauterine systems. Tacrolimus, an immune modulator, has been used on the inguinal area, but with the recent FDA warning discussed previously, it should be used by a specialist familiar with its use. Severe psoriasis may be treated with systemic therapies including methotrexate, cyclosporine, and oral retinoids. These treatments are best prescribed by a specialist in vulvar diseases and are contraindicated during pregnancy or lactation. For women with vulvar psoriasis who have lesions over 20% or more of their bodies, systemic therapy is indicated and should be managed by an expert in dermatology. Emulsions for comfort may accompany any of the other therapies.

Hidradenitis Suppurativa

Hidradenitis suppurativa, also known as **Verneuil's disease** or **acne inversa**, is one of the orphan diseases. In other words, there is no consensus about its name, pathogenesis, prevalence, or treatment. The condition is characterized by chronic, painful, inflamed, suppurative lesions of the apocrine glands. Lesions arise when a defect in the follicular epithelium of a hair follicle is aggravated by friction, from sweat, heat, stress, tight clothing, or hormonal changes. Boillike, often malodorous, nodular lesions form with sinus tracts between them and the surface. Inflammation, infection, and extension to the subcutaneous tissue follow. Healing is associated with scarring.

Hidradenitis suppurativa is reported among 1–4% of the population. Perhaps because it resembles other lesions, the average time from onset to diagnosis is 8 years.[25,26] Obesity is not an etiologic agent, but has been found to be an aggravating factor.[25] Thirty-eight percent of those with the disorder report a family history, suggesting genetics may be involved.[27] The disease more often affects women than men with a ratio of 4:1 and occurs almost exclusively between puberty and age 40, lending support to a hormonally mediated etiology, although the link is unclear. Flares are associated with women with shorter menstrual cycles and longer menstrual flow, but also have been noted to begin with the

Table 32-5 Treatments for Psoriasis

Drug Generic (Brand)	Adult Dosage	Contraindications	Clinical Considerations and Selected Drug–Drug Interactions	FDA Pregnancy Category
Calcipotriene (Dovonex)	Apply thin film to area bid until lesions respond.	Hypersensitivity, hypercalcemia.	May irritate skin. No interactions reported.	C
Clobetasol (Temovate, Dermovate)	Apply thin layer once daily for 1 month then pulse dose for 1 month, 2 consecutive days of the week, off 5 days.	Hypersensitivity, paronychia, cellulitis, impetigo, angular cheilitis, erythrasma, erysipelas, rosacea, perioral dermatitis, acne.	Systemic absorption may occur with reversible hypothalamus–pituitary–ovarian-axis suppression, potential glucocorticoid insufficiency after withdrawal of treatment; do not use in skin with decreased circulation; can cause atrophy of groin, face, and axillae; if infection develops and is not responsive to antibiotic treatment, discontinue until infection is under control. No interactions reported.	C
Tazarotene (Tazorac)	0.05%–0.1% cream or gel: apply to the area once daily at bedtime.	Hypersensitivity, pregnancy.	May irritate skin. Thiazides, tetracyclines, fluoroquinolones, sulfonamides, phenothiazines.	X
Tacrolimus (Protopic)	0.1% ointment: apply to affected areas twice daily for 2–6 weeks.	Hypersensitivity; ointments can lead to maceration in skin folds; not recommended in immunocompromised persons.	No interactions reported.	C

onset of combined oral contraceptive use.[28] There are two reports associating smoking with increased incidence of the disease.[26] Complications of hidradenitis suppurativa include local or systemic infection, anemia from chronic infection, arthritis, lymphedema, fistulae, and frustration and depression.[29]

Diagnosis of hidradenitis suppurativa is based on clinical presentation. The disease is present in discrete portions of the anatomy—the axillae, inframammary, and the genito-anal area, which includes genitofemoral creases, gluteal folds, perianal area, and mons pubis. The disease is chronic and recurring and progresses through three stages (Table 32-6).

Laboratory testing generally is not needed for diagnosis. If a woman is febrile, a complete blood count or chemistry panel may produce supportive evidence, and a culture of the drainage may direct antibiotic choice, particularly since a common bacterial infection is *Pseudomonas* from the bowel. In perianal disease, biopsy may be indicated to differentiate among hidradenitis suppurativa, Crohn's disease, and cancer.[30]

No single treatment has been supported by any randomized, controlled trial. Antibiotics are used routinely, though many lesions are bacteria free and tend to heal in the same amount of time whether treated with antibiotics or left untreated.[28] Wide local excision to remove damaged tissue with healing by secondary intention has been

shown to be the treatment associated with the longest term improvement. One study reported findings of 106 participants who had suffered from hidradenitis suppurativa. In this research, the disease was present for a mean of 7 years, and 90% of the subjects had multiple lesions and underwent wide excision of the lesions. Ultimately the participants were followed for 36 months postoperatively. The complication rate was 17.8% with the majority of complications minor, such as suture disruption, postoperative bleeding, and hematoma. Wound infection occurred in only 3.7% of participants. The rate of recurrence of lesions in the operated areas was 2.5%.[31]

In general, treatment is tailored to the severity of the lesions. Stage 1 lesions often are managed with nonpharmacologic measures. In one study, 45% of those with the condition reported heat, exercise, and sweat aggravated their symptoms. However, hydrotherapy in the forms of warm, moist compresses and/or swimming relieved the symptoms for approximately one third of those afflicted.[32] Stage 2 lesions require medical or surgical treatment. Stage 3 lesions are most appropriately managed with an invasive intervention. Radiotherapy is being investigated as a treatment option. In Frolich's study of 231 patients, 38% reported complete relief from their symptoms after radiotherapy, and another 40% reported improvement. The long-term side effects of radiotherapy are not yet known. Cryotherapy has resulted in relief in a small series of

Table 32-6 Staging of Hidradenitis Suppurativa and Usual Treatments

Stage	Description	Nonpharmacologic Treatment	Pharmacologic Treatment
1	Single or multiple nodular lesions form without sinus tracts or scars.	Hydrotherapy. Warm compresses. Stress management. Weight loss.	Antibacterial soap.
2	Recurrent single or multiple lesions in widely spread areas form with tracts, and fibrosis.	Hydrotherapy. Warm compresses. Stress management. Weight loss.	Antibiotics for infections (culture directed): Dicloxacillin 250–500 mg four times daily for 10–14 days based on severity. Doxycycline (Dynapen) 100 mg PO twice daily for 7–10 days based on severity. Clindamycin (Cleocin) topical apply sparingly to area twice daily for 7–10 days. Zinc gluconate 90 mg daily. Clobetasol (Clobex, Temovate) apply sparingly to area daily for 14 days. NSAIDs as needed for discomfort. Antitissue necrosing factor-α as infliximab (Remicade) two infusions at 5 mg/kg. Antiandrogens in the form of drospirenone (Yasmin) one tablet daily.
3	Lesions form in multiple, scattered, broad areas with multiple tracts and scars.	Warm compresses. Exposure to light and air.	Antibiotics for infections (culture directed) as listed for stage 2.

patients, but significant pain and prolonged healing were major drawbacks to the method.[33]

Some association appears to exist between acne and hidradenitis suppurativa, so the antibiotics used in the treatment of acne are often used in the treatment of hidradenitis suppurativa.[34] While systemic antibiotics are commonly used, the only randomized, controlled trial of such agents revealed topical clindamycin (Cleocin) was not statistically different from systemic tetracycline (Sumycin) for the treatment of axillary hidradenitis suppurativa.[35] Various organisms have been isolated from hidradenitis suppurativa lesions including *Staphylococcus*, *Escherichia coli*, and beta-hemolytic *Streptococcus*. Axillary hidradenitis suppurativa is more commonly infected with *Staphylococcus* and is better treated with antistaphylococcals such as dicloxacillin (Dynapen) and clindamycin (Cleocin). For perineal hidradenitis suppurativa, broad-spectrum coverage is needed, and doxycycline (Vibramycin, Adoxa) and minocycline (Minocin) are commonly used antibiotics.[32] Minocycline, a tetracycline derivative, has been associated in staining of teeth and should be avoided during pregnancy and lactation.

Zinc salts have been used in the treatment of dermatoses. The salts activate natural killer cells and stimulate phagocytosis by granulocytes. In France, a small pilot study was conducted for 22 individuals who were primarily in stage 2 hidradenitis suppurativa. The participants were treated initially with 90 mg of zinc gluconate orally per day for 4 months. As symptoms abated, the dosage was reduced by 15 mg every 2 months. Success was defined as 6 months of no new or recurrent lesions with total follow-up for 2 years. Eight of the 22 participants experienced complete remission, and 14 experienced partial remission. One person discontinued treatment due to nausea and vomiting, while three others had gastrointestinal side effects but continued the program. The dosage of zinc was higher than routinely used in the treatment of dermatoses.[36] Although the size of the study precludes wide generalizability, zinc supplements might be an attractive, inexpensive option and require further exploration.

Because of the association between hidradenitis suppurativa and hormonal changes, antiandrogens have been suggested as potential treatments. In case reports, two individuals were reported to improve with the use of finasteride (Proscar), but another, larger series demonstrated no improvement.[34,37] In 1986, cyproterone (Cyprostat, Cyproterone, Procure), a synthetic derivative of 17-hydroxyperogesterone and an androgen receptor antagonist with weak progestational and glucocorticoid activity, was combined with ethinyl estradiol and used successfully in a controlled trial. However, later studies have not shown the cyproterone to be consistently useful, and this agent is not approved for use in the United States.[34] In the 1980s, hidradenitis suppurativa was thought to be a disease of abnormal keratinization, and retinoids were trialed as treatment. Most studies demonstrated isotretinoin (Accutane) works well on acne but not on hidradenitis suppurativa.[38] There also are significant fertility risks of prescribing a teratogenic agent during the peak of a woman's reproductive life; therefore, it should not be used in the treatment of hidradenitis suppurativa. Current research is being conducted on corticosteroids and immunomodulators. Topical and injectable triamcinolone is being investigated, although there are no large clinical trials to date precluding this drug from consideration as first-line treatment. ACTH, azathioprine, and cyclosporin have all been used experimentally with some preliminary favorable results.[34,39]

Hidradenitis suppurativa often accompanies Crohn's disease, an autoimmune disease. Thus, there is growing evidence that hidradenitis suppurativa may be an autoimmune disease itself. Drugs used for other autoimmune disorders are being investigated for use with hidradenitis suppurativa. The most promising research is in the area of antitumor necrosis factor (TNFα) drugs. Etanercept (Enbrel) and infliximab (Remicade) are FDA-approved drugs for rheumatoid arthritis and Crohn's disease and are currently being studied in the United States and Europe for hidradenitis suppurativa. The numbers of participants in these studies have been small and not randomized, but among a select group (24 participants in total) there was reported dramatic relief.[40] A nonrandomized, open-label, uncontrolled study has been completed in Greece and is awaiting publication, and 40 individuals have enrolled in an ongoing clinical trial in the United States.[41]

Even with the variety of drugs available for treatment, 24% of participants in one study reported that nothing helped.[28] For many, even with successful treatment of lesions, new lesions often develop, resulting in a cycle of exacerbation-remission-exacerbation. Counseling is a critical adjunct to providing medical or surgical treatment.[42] Women need to understand the condition is a chronic condition unassociated with poor hygiene.

Inflammatory Dermatosis

Inflammatory dermatosis or contact dermatitis of the genital skin can be initiated by friction from tight clothes, physical activities like bicycle riding, chemical irritation from urine or stool, perfumed personal hygiene products, and excessive washing, especially with harsh soaps.[43] Any age group can experience inflammatory dermatosis, but the elderly are particularly vulnerable. After menopause, mucosa is thinned and tissue is less elastic and easily traumatized. Those who may have difficulty with removing waste products from the skin when toileting, such as persons who are obese or those with limited mobility, are particularly prone to inflammatory dermatosis. Diagnosis is usually by history and physical examination. Lesions may vary from simple erythema and edema to the presence

of vesicles or bullae, or if severe, lichenification (scale formation) or erosion with exudates and crusting.[44]

Evaluation should include cultures to rule out a yeast or staphylococcal infection. Treatment begins with removing the source of irritation. Incontinence should be managed with treatment based on severity and type of incontinence as discussed in detail in Chapter 22. The vulva and anus should be rinsed with plain water after each episode of toileting and the area given an opportunity to dry out. If adult diapers or other occlusive clothing are used, they should be changed frequently. Zinc oxide ointment, ointment with vitamins A and D, or petroleum jelly will help provide a protective barrier to the inflammatory agent.[43] Burow's solution, containing aluminum acetate dissolved in water, may provide symptomatic relief.[44] A mild steroid such as triamcinolone acetonide (Kenalog cream 0.1%) will decrease inflammation. Common sense advice tends to prevail even though randomized, controlled trials are not available. For example, if the inflammation is from prolonged contact with friction-producing garments or activities, the contact should be avoided. Soaps coming in contact with the genital area should be free of perfumes and additives. Underwear should be loose, all cotton, and washed in hot water and dried using high heat. After prolonged exercise, the genital area should be thoroughly cleansed and rinsed.

Behçet's Syndrome

Behçet's syndrome is a disease named after a Turkish dermatologist, Hulusi Behçet, who, in 1937, described a syndrome of recurrent oral aphthous ulcers, genital ulcerations, and uveitis leading to blindness. Although the cause of the disease is unknown, it has become recognized as a multisystemic inflammatory disease with painful ulcerations with erythematous borders and yellow bases, beginning first in the oral cavity but affecting many parts of the body, especially the uvea of the eye and the genital area. Rarely found among individuals of western European or African descent, this syndrome most commonly affects those of eastern Mediterranean or Asian origin.[41] The mouth and genital ulcers are generally painful and recur in crops (many shallow ulcers at the same time). They range in size from a few millimeters to 20 millimeters in diameter. The mouth ulcers occur on the gums, tongue, and inner lining of the mouth. The genital ulcers occur on the scrotum and penis of males and vulva of women and can leave scars. Diagnosis is determined by the international criteria or the Duffy criteria, both of which are

Table 32-7 Criteria for Diagnosis of Behçet's Syndrome

International Criteria	Duffy Criteria

Recurrent oral ulcerations (≥ 3 episodes in a 12-month period) plus two of any of the following:
Recurrent genital ulcerations
Eye lesions:
    Anterior uveitis
    Posterior uveitis
Cells in the vitreous
Retinal vasculitis
Skin lesions:
    Erythema nodosum
    Pseudo folliculitis
    Papulopustular lesions
Acneiform nodules (in a postadolescent not taking corticosteroids)
Positive pathergy test. The pathergy test includes piercing the skin of the forearm with a blunt, sterile needle. The test is positive if after 24–48 hours, a small pustule develops.[51]
	Presence of recurrent aphthous ulcerations plus any two of the following:
	Genital ulcers
	Uveitis
	Cutaneous pustular vasculitis
	Synovitis
	Meningoencephalitis
	Exclusion of inflammatory bowel disease, systemic lupus erythematosus (SLE), Reiter syndrome, and herpetic infections.[52]

Source: Adapted from O'Duffy JD 1990.[46]

summarized in Table 32-7.[45,46] The differential diagnosis includes herpesvirus and Crohn's disease.

Although C-reactive protein and erythrocyte sedimentation rates may be elevated, and 30% of women with Behçet's syndrome will have antiphospholipid antibodies, there are no specific laboratory tests diagnostic for Behçet's syndrome. Viral cultures can rule out hidradenitis suppurativa.

Treatment of Behçet's Syndrome

Colchicine is effective for genital lesions among individuals with Behçet's syndrome. A double-blind trial of colchicine administered to 116 persons with Behçet's syndrome confirmed colchicine may be useful in the treatment of women with genital lesions. Kaplan-Meier analysis showed the treated group had statistically significant improvement at $P = 0.004$ compared to the untreated group.[47] Topical anesthetics are generally ineffective.[48] Mild to moderate strength topical steroid gels and creams and intralesional triamcinolone often are prescribed for small lesions. For larger lesions, systemic steroids (e.g., prednisone) are more effective[45,49] (Table 32-8). Recent studies suggest that thalidomide (Thalomid) may be of benefit for certain individuals with Behçet's syndrome in treating and preventing ulcerations of the mouth and genitals. Side effects of thalidomide include promoting abnormal development of fetal growth, nerve injury (neuropathy), and hypersedation. Thalidomide should only be prescribed by a specialist familiar with the use of the drug and clearly

avoided for women of reproductive age because of known teratogenic effects.[50]

Antimetabolites and interferon should be reserved for persons whose condition does not respond following a course of prednisone. The treatment program should be managed by a dermatologist or gynecologist with extensive experience with the drugs. In Japan, pentoxifylline (Trental), a drug used in the treatment of peripheral artery disease, has been suggested to heal lesions. Pentoxifylline is an FDA Pregnancy Category C drug due to some animal problems at extremely high doses, although no teratogenicity has been suggested for humans. The agent decreases viscosity of blood, increasing circulation to the area, and healed ulcers remained healed for up to 29 months.[51]

Some persons with mild lesions have noted improvement with the use of an herbal remedy called Canker Rid, which is a byproduct of honey bee products. There have been no randomized trials of this product, and caution should be used by diabetics and those with bee allergies.

■ Molluscum Contagiosum

Molluscum contagiosum is caused by a benign poxvirus. Found more commonly among children, a person in any age group can acquire the disorder. Since the late 1980s there has been an increase in the incidence of this disorder, primarily in the sexually active population and in HIV immunocompromised individuals.[52,23] The virus is communicable through direct contact with someone who has the lesion or contact with a surface that has been in contact with mature lesions, such as a towel, exercise mats, or equipment.[53] The lesions have a predilection for skin already inflamed by psoriasis or eczema. The lesions proceed through three stages of development and are often found on flexor surfaces. Among adult women, the genital area is most commonly affected. Initially lesions are often described as tiny goose bumps (cutis anserina), often 20 or more concentrated in a 3-cm diameter. However, within a few days to weeks, the lesions evolve into molelike lesions, which are usually pale, 2–6 mm in diameter, and umbilicated. The final stage occurs after about several weeks when the lesions appear similar to pimples about to erupt.[53]

The core of the lesion contains a white, waxy substance. Diagnosis is usually by examination of the characteristic lesions, but DNA analysis can be performed if diagnosis is unclear. Within each cluster of molluscum there are usually 1–2 dominant lesions that appear to control the growth of

Table 32-8 Treatments for Behçet's Syndrome

Drug Generic (Brand)	Adult Dosage	Contraindications	Clinical Considerations and Selected Drug–Drug Interactions	FDA Pregnancy Category
Colchicine	1–2 mg per day in 3–4 divided doses	Hypersensitivity. Renal, hepatic disease.	Gastrointestinal discomfort at higher doses. Alopecia at higher doses.	X
Prednisone (Deltasone, Sterapred, Orasone)	15 mg/day, with tapering to 10 mg/day after 1 week and discontinuation over a 2- to 3-week period.	Hypersensitivity.	Adrenal crisis with abrupt discontinuation. Hyperglycemia, edema, osteonecrosis, myopathy, peptic ulcer disease, hypokalemia, osteoporosis, psychosis, myasthenia gravis, growth suppression; infections may occur. Acetaminophen (Tylenol), alcohol, NSAIDs, amphotericin B (Fungizone), carbonic anhydrase inhibitors, and antacids decrease absorption. Anticoagulants, tricyclics, antidiabetic agents, antithyroid hormones, estrogens, digitalis (Lanoxin), diuretics, ephedrine, folic acid, immunosuppressants, potassium supplements, and ritodrine (Yutopar) cause pulmonary edema.	B
Cyclosporine (Sandimmune, Neoral)	5 mg/kg/day PO based on ideal body weight.	Hypersensitivity. Uncontrolled hypertension. Malignancies.	Carbamazepine (Tegretol), phenytoin (Dilantin), isoniazid (INH), rifampin (Rifadin), and phenobarbital (Luminal) decrease drug concentrations. Azithromycin (Zithromax), azoles, nicardipine (Cardene), erythromycin (E-mycin), verapamil (Calan), grapefruit juice, diltiazem (Cardizem), aminoglycosides, acyclovir (Zovirax), amphotericin B (Fungizone), and clarithromycin (Biaxin) increase toxicity. With lovastatin (Mevacor), causes acute renal failure, rhabdomyolysis, myositis, and myalgias.	C
Azathioprine (Imuran)	100–150 mg/day PO	Hypersensitivity. Pregnancy; lactation. Low levels of serum thiopurine methyl transferase (TPMT).	Caution with liver and renal impairment; check TPMT level prior to therapy. Monitor liver, renal, and hematologic function. Toxicity with allopurinol. Leucopenia with ACE inhibitors. Increases methotrexate (Rheumatrex, Trexall) metabolites. Decreases effects of anticoagulants, neuromuscular blockers, and cyclosporine (Neoral).	D

other lesions. Eliminating the dominant lesion seems to be the key to curing the disorder. Molluscum is self-limiting and not associated with cancer or long-term morbidity; but resolution may take up to 2 years and autoinoculation can occur, so treatment is recommended.

Treatment of Molluscum Contagiosum

No FDA-approved medications exist for treatment of molluscum contagiosum, but several drugs have been used for years. Some of these treatments emerged from treatment of condylomata acuminata. Commonly used treatments include these chemicals: podophyllin derivatives, trichloroacetic acid 85%, cantharidin solution, or the antiviral topical cream imiquimod (Aldara) 5% (Table 32-9). Destructive procedures such as curettage, evisceration, cryosurgery, and tape stripping are also performed to eradicate this disorder.

Imiquimod 5% cream (Aldara) is a potent topical immunomodulatory agent that is FDA approved for the treatment of condylomata acuminatum. Imiquimod works by inducing high levels of IFN-α and other cytokines locally. It has been used for more than a decade to treat molluscum contagiosum. Well tolerated, imiquimod has had no known systemic or toxic effects, although application site irritation is common. No one treatment regimen has been supported by a randomized, controlled trial, but in one small, open-label clinical trial, imiquimod cream was applied to the affected area nightly 5 nights a week, left on the lesions 8–10 hours, then rinsed or washed off. More than 80% of the subjects experienced either complete clearance or a greater than 50% reduction in lesions in 9 weeks, although cure can take up to 4 months.[54]

Podophyllin (Pododerm) is a caustic **desiccant**. A 25% suspension of podophyllin in a tincture of benzoin or alcohol may be applied to molluscum once a week. Podophyllotoxin is derived from the roots and rhizomes of *podophyllum* (Mandrake), a member of the juniper family found throughout North America. The precise mechanism of action of the drug is unknown, but the alcoholate drug is cytotoxic, causing tissue necrosis by arresting cellular

Table 32-9 Treatments for Molluscum Contagiosum

Drug Generic (Brand)	Adult Dosage	Contraindications	Clinical Considerations and Selected Drug–Drug Interactions	FDA Pregnancy Category
Podophyllotoxin (Podofilox, Condylox)	0.5% topical gel apply bid for 3 days, discontinue for 4 days then repeat for a maximum 4 cycles.	Hypersensitivity.	Local skin reaction. Headache.	C
Trichloroacetic acid	Apply to lesions sparingly, repeat in 1–2 weeks.	Hypersensitivity.	Use sparingly. Avoid sun. No interactions reported.	C
Cantharidin solution (Cantharone)	Single application once per month.	Hypersensitivity.	Use sparingly.	C
Imiquimod (Aldara)	Apply to lesions 3 times per week.	Hypersensitivity.	No interactions reported.	C
Tretinoin (Retin-A)	Apply nightly.	Hypersensitivity.	Use sparingly. Toxicity with benzoyl peroxide, salicylic acid, spices, and lime.	X

division in metaphase and antiproliferative by preventing DNA synthesis; these processes lead to cell failure and erosion of tissue. Some of the listed side effects include severe erosive damage in adjacent normal skin that may cause scarring and systemic effects such as peripheral neuropathy, renal damage, adynamic ileus, leucopenia, and thrombocytopenia. This treatment should only be applied by a health professional. Podophyllotoxin (Podofilox, Condylox) is a more stable form of podophyllin. This self-applied agent is composed of only the biologically active portion of the compound. The treatment is application of 0.05 mL of 5% cream or gel in lactate-buffered ethanol twice a day for 3 days.

Podophyllin contains two mutagens, quercetin and kaempherol, and many clinicians avoid the use of the drug during pregnancy. Podophyllin and a similar agent, podophyllotoxin, have been reported as teratogens, although the evidence is controversial. Therefore, the manufacturers have stated that these agents are contraindicated during pregnancy and lactation.[55] Cantharidin (Cantharone, Cantharone Plus), a 0.9% solution of collodion and acetone, is a blister-inducing agent used with some success in the treatment of molluscum contagiosum. A synthetic version of a substance produced by several insect species to protect their eggs, cantharidin has a long history of use in Eastern and folk medicine. The precise mechanism of action is unclear, but it involves intraepithelial blistering and lysis of the skin.[56] Applied in the same fashion as podophyllin (carefully and sparingly) to the dome of the lesion, the solution is left in place for at least 6 hours before washing and applying a bandage. The bandage should be removed after 24 hours. Cantharidin should be tested on a single lesion before treating large numbers of lesions. This

treatment is repeated every week until the lesions clear, usually 1–3 treatments.[57]

Trichloroacetic acid, or less commonly, bichloracetic acid, eliminates molluscum by destroying proteins in the cells. It is provider applied in the same fashion as podophyllin, weekly for three applications; tricholoroacetic acid is most commonly used prior to prescribing home treatment with imiquimod.

All of the burning or blistering agents work best on moist tissue but still can burn healthy surrounding tissue, so application should be preceded by protecting the adjacent tissue with a waterproof barrier such as petroleum jelly. If burning is intolerable after application, sodium bicarbonate can be applied immediately to the tissue to inactivate the burning.

Cimetidine (Tagamet) is a histamine 2 receptor antagonist used in the treatment of ulcers and heartburn. Cimetidine is known to stimulate T lymphocyte production important in controlling viral infections. One uncontrolled study showed resolution in 9 of 13 participants. In this study, the dosage was 40 mg/kg/day orally in two divided doses for 2 months.[58] The authors recommended further placebo-controlled, double-blind studies be completed to determine the efficacy of cimetidine in treating molluscum contagiosum. Because cimetidine interacts with many systemic medications, anyone who uses the agent should have all other medications routinely reviewed.

Tretinoin (Retin-A) 0.05–0.1% cream has been used off label in the treatment of molluscum contagiosum. It is applied twice daily to the lesions for 10–14 days. Erythema at the site of removed lesions is a common side effect. As an FDA Pregnancy Category X drug, this treatment should be reserved for those women who are not at risk for pregnancy, such as women who are postmenopausal or using a highly effective form of birth control.[59]

Pediculosis

Pediculosis is sometimes called pubic lice or crabs, which are small jumping insects that live in pubic hair and feed on the blood of the host. Spread through intimate contact or through bedding and clothing infested with lice, approximately 6 million cases are diagnosed each year in the United States.[60,61] Itching is intense and scratching can result in spreading the lice to other parts of the body. Black specks may be noted on the bed linens, and hives or reddened areas may be noted on the area infested with lice. Diagnosis of lice is by history and/or physical examination. The lice are visible to the naked eye; adults are the size of a pinhead, oval in shape, and grayish, but appearing reddish-brown when full of blood from their host. Nits, or the eggs, also are visible, usually observed clinging to the base of the hair.[1]

Treatment of Pediculosis

Treatment of lice is with lotions or shampoos containing one of several ingredients. Permethrin 1% (Nix, Elimite) and pyrethrins with piperonyl butoxide (RID) are available over the counter and are preferred drugs for treatment of pubic lice.[59] Details of how to use these medications can be found in Chapter 26.

The most potent pediculicide is lindane, a neurotoxic agent that is available by prescription only and contraindicated during pregnancy and while nursing and for children under age 2 years (Table 32-10). Lindane causes liver, kidney, and brain damage in laboratory animals. One dose of lindane pollutes 6 million gallons of water. Because of the human and environmental risks, products containing lindane cannot be purchased in California since 2002, and it is no longer a first-line treatment in many areas of the United States. In 2003, the US FDA issued a public health advisory, also known as a black box warning, to appear on lindane products, which explains the proper use and potential adverse effects of the drug, and it developed a medication guide that pharmacists are required to distribute when filling a prescription for lindane.[62] The content of the FDA black box warning and description of how to use lindane are described in more detail in Chapter 26.

Less commonly used for treatment of pubic lice is a scabicide, crotamiton. Crotamiton, marketed as Eurax in the United States, is available by prescription only, and the mechanism of action is unknown. The drug is applied nightly for 2 consecutive nights and washed off 24 hours after the second application. Crotamiton is an FDA Pregnancy Category C drug because of lack of studies. Since more specific, safer drugs currently exist, crotamiton has little role in the treatment of pubic lice. Crotamiton also is used as an antipruritic, but diphenhydramine (Benadryl) or calamine lotion are safer choices for itching until the lice are eliminated.[60]

Regardless of which treatment is used, manufacturers recommend washing the infested area and toweling dry

Table 32-10 Treatments for Pediculosis

Drug Generic (Brand)	Adult Dosage	Contraindications	Clinical Considerations and Selected Drug–Drug Interactions	FDA Pregnancy Category
Lindane*	Shampoo: apply to dry pubic hair and surrounding areas; allow to set for 4 min, lather for 4 min, then rinse; repeat in 7 days prn.	Hypersensitivity. Neonates.	Caution with seizures. Do not apply to eyes, face, or mucous membranes. Penetrates human skin and may cause CNS toxicity. See black box warning. Oil-based hairdressings may increase toxicity.	C
Permethrin (Elimite, Nix)	Apply topically to affected area; leave 5–10 min, then rinse.	Hypersensitivity.	May exacerbate redness, swelling, and itching, at least temporarily. No interactions reported.	B
Crotamiton (Eurax)	Apply thin layer to affected area.	Hypersensitivity.	Avoid urethral meatus. No interactions reported.	C

* Lindane has a black box warning that details contraindications and proper use. In addition, a medication guide for users must be dispensed with any prescription for this medication.

before applying and thoroughly saturating the hair with lindane 1% shampoo, permethrin 1% cream, or pyrethrin shampoo. Lindane is left on for 4 minutes and permethrin or pyrethrins with piperonyl butoxide are left on for 10 minutes, after which time it should be thoroughly rinsed off with water and the area dried with a clean towel. Even after treatment, dead nits will still be attached to hair shafts. Nits may be removed with fingernails or a fine-toothed comb. Clean underwear, clothing and bed clothing should be used, and retreatment in 7–10 days is recommended to ensure all nits have been killed.[59] Because the eggs may live up to 6 days, it is important to apply the treatment for the time recommended on the package for all of these agents.[61]

To prevent self-reinfection and transmission to others, anyone with whom an infested individual has come into close contact, including family and close friends as well as sex partners, needs to be treated. All clothing and bedding used within 3 days of first finding the lice should be dry cleaned or washed in very hot water (125–130°F). If washing clothing and bedding, the laundered items then need to be dried at a high setting for at least 20 minutes and ironed to rid them of any lice. Pubic lice die within 24 hours of being separated from the host.

Seborrheic Dermatitis

Seborrheic dermatitis is a papulosquamous condition associated with flaking of the skin.[1] Most commonly found in sebum-rich areas such as the scalp, the disorder is termed cradle cap among infants and dandruff among adults. In its form as dandruff, it is estimated that approximately 15–20% of the population has seborrhea.[63] Seborrhea can be found elsewhere on the body such as the face or areas with creases, such as the groin, although the incidence is much lower (2–3%). Seborrhea on parts of the body other than the scalp is not found in the prepubescent population.[64] Usually seen in adults ages 30–60, the peak incidence for seborrhea is around age 40. As with many of the dermatologic disorders, the etiology is unknown. Hormones are thought to play a role as seborrhea is rarely seen outside infancy until well into adulthood. Another etiology that has been suggested is that a normal inhabitant of the skin, a lipophilic fungus of the *Malassezia* genus, *Pityrosporum ovale* is a catalyst.[53] The theory for this etiology is supported by the fact that seborrhea frequently responds to antifungal therapy. Seborrheic dermatitis is associated with normal levels of *Malassezia* but an abnormal immune response. Helper T cells, phytohemagglutinin and concanavalin stimulation, and antibody titers are depressed compared with those of control subjects.[63]

Seborrhea increases with changes in temperature and humidity (peaking in winter and early spring) and is made worse by scratching. Persons with neurologic diseases such as epilepsy or Parkinson's disease are noted to have seborrhea at a higher rate than persons who do not have these disorders. Persons who have HIV/AIDS have an increased incidence of seborrheic dermatitis, approaching 85%.[65] This distribution has raised speculation about multiple origins of the disorder. Various medications may cause flares or induce seborrheic dermatitis. Some of these medications include organic gold compounds, buspirone (Buspar), cimetidine (Tagamet), ethionamide (Trecator SC), griseofulvin (Grisovin), haloperidol (Haldol), interferon alfa (Intron A, Roferon-A), lithium (Eskalith), methyldopa (Aldomet), and various phenothiazines.

Diagnosis usually is made by history and finding the lesions in areas of high sebum on physical examination. With exfoliative erythroderma, a skin biopsy may be necessary, and a fungal culture can be used to rule out tinea capitis.[1]

Skin lesions appear as greasy scaling over red, inflamed skin. Hypopigmentation is seen in persons of darker color. Infectious eczematoid dermatitis, with oozing and crusting, suggests secondary infection.[1]

Treatment of Seborrheic Dermatitis

Treatment of seborrheic dermatitis varies with the age group and the location of the lesions and is focused on symptomatic relief versus cure. The only treatment with FDA approval is ketoconazole (Nizoral) 2%, which is applied to the area twice daily for 4 weeks.[66] Ketoconazole is an FDA Pregnancy Category C drug due to lack of studies. Treatment for adults with seborrhea in folds and creases consists of comfort measures such as Burow's solution for topical relief from itching. Low to moderate potency steroid lotions may be used 1–2 times per day to decrease inflammation during an acute flare but are felt to exacerbate flares if used chronically. Alternatives include immunomodulatory calcineurin inhibitors such as pimecrolimus or tacrolimus, sulfur or sulfonamide combinations, or propylene glycol.[67] Systemic ketoconazole or fluconazole (Diflucan) may be valuable if seborrheic dermatitis is severe or unresponsive or if there is evidence of a fungal overgrowth. Treatment with ultraviolet light improves seborrheic lesions, which is the likely explanation for improvement of the condition during the summer.[68] Tea tree oil has been proposed as a natural treatment for seborrheic dermatitis and is the active ingredient in many dandruff shampoos.[69] However, since it is an essential oil, there is the risk of contact dermatitis, especially if a strong solution is applied to the area.[70] One report noted an increase in gynecomastia in prepubertal boys who used tea tree oil, although underlying etiology is unclear.[71]

Prevention consists of frequent removal of sebum with soap and water. Zinc- or coal tar-containing shampoos, zinc soap, or benzoyl peroxide washes are also helpful in controlling seborrhea.[1] Education includes cautioning the person to rinse thoroughly after application of these agents and to apply moisturizer to the area. Individuals should be warned that these agents may bleach clothing and bed linens.

Extramammary Paget's Disease

Extramammary Paget's disease is cutaneous adenocarcinoma that may be classified based on source of the primary lesion. Approximately 75–90% of cases are histologically diagnosed as adenocarcinoma in situ. A rare form of cancer, Paget's disease accounts for only 1–2% of vulvar cancers.[53] The pathogenesis remains controversial. Histologically, the lesions from mammary and extramammary Paget's disease are identical, and the physical examination should include an evaluation of the breasts and other areas rich in apocrine glands. Although the disease can involve areas other than the vulva, this chapter focuses on extramammary Paget's disease of the vulva. A disease of senescence, the peak incidence occurs among Caucasian females in their 60s.[72] Symptoms include intense pruritus, irritation, a weeping or bleeding lesion, and rarely pain. Lesions can appear well defined, moist, and white (macerated) or reddish tan and scaling.[73] These manifestations can appear infiltrated, eroded, or similar to an ulcerated plaque. The differential diagnosis for extramammary Paget's disease includes psoriasis, contact dermatitis, fungal infections, lichen sclerosus, intraepithelial neoplasia, and melanoma.[1] Any vulvar lesion in a postmenopausal woman is suspicious and should be diagnosed by biopsy. There is no pharmacologic treatment for Paget's disease. Treatment is surgical, with wide excision recommended.[53] The recurrence rate is about 30% with the average time for recurrence being 2–3 years, so after surgery women should be followed carefully.[74]

Vulvodynia

Vulvodynia is the diagnosis when a woman has pain or burning in the vulva (Figure 32-1) of more than 3 months' duration, which cannot be explained by any specific, clinically identifiable disorder.[75] Vulvodynia may be generalized or focal, unilateral or bilateral, constant or sporadic, provoked or nonprovoked. Dyspareunia may or may not be a feature, but intercourse can trigger pain. **Allodynia** (light touch) is a hallmark of this disorder. Women may report tight pants, sitting for prolonged periods, or even the movement of pubic hair provoking pain. Some women have symptoms of a urinary tract infection with a sterile urine culture. Others report hyperalgesia, an increased response to a stimulus that is normally painful. This disorder (or multiple disorders) is thought to occur in up to 16% of women at some time during their lives.[76]

Vulvodynia is a diagnosis of exclusion and is usually established through history, although laboratory testing including biopsy may be performed to exclude other causes. One theory of vulvar pain is that an abnormal pain arc develops between the spinal cord and the brain. Trauma (chemicals, injury, or disease) initiates a pain response, and after the trauma is removed, the pain receptors continue to respond as if the trauma is ongoing.[62] The trauma may not have been noted consciously by the woman. Another theory is that the pain is nociceptive from repeated, long-term trauma.[77] The cells themselves develop an abnormal pain response. Estrogen is thought to affect sensory perception, and alteration in estrogen may be associated with vulvodynia.[78] This etiology might explain why dysesthetic or essential vulvodynia begins about the time of menopause.

Provoked vestibulodynia, a subset of vulvodynia limited to the vulvar vestibule, found during reproductive years, may have a different pathophysiology. Primary vestibulodynia occurs with first intercourse, first tampon insertion, or other initial contact of pressure or friction against the vestibule. Secondary vestibulodynia occurs after a pain-free interval.[69] Secondary vestibulodynia has a peak incidence in women in their mid-30s.[76] Triggers may include a prolonged bout with a vaginal infection or childbirth, even if the birth is a cesarean delivery. Some women spontaneously develop pain without a readily observable trigger. Because the etiology is unknown, diagnosis can take up to 5 years and treatments are largely based on anecdote, small series of cases, or expert opinion.[76]

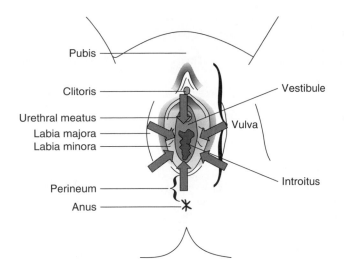

• Apply gentle pressure with cotton swab to sites surrounding the introitus (1 o'clock thru 12 o'clock positions). Ask woman to rate the severity of pain she experiences at each site.

• Pain is typically most severe in posterior vestibule between 5 and 7 o'clock positions.

Figure 32-1 Cotton-tipped application to elicit allodynia.
Source: Slide courtesy of NVA presentation: Vulvodynia: Integrating current knowledge into practice. © 2005.

Treatment of Vulvodynia

As with squamous cell hyperplasia, breaking the cycle is the first step in treatment. Lidocaine (Xylocaine) application has been theorized to be therapeutic by desensitizing the nerve fibers. Topical anesthetics prior to intercourse and vaginal examinations allow penetration without pain. When applied only to the vestibule, anesthetics do not alter vaginal or clitoral sensation. Used nightly, a 4–5% lidocaine ointment (Topicaine) has been associated with gradually diminishing pain in some women.[79] EMLA, which is the generic and brand name for a eutectic mixture of local anesthetic, contains lidocaine and prilocaine. While EMLA has been demonstrated to be as effective as lidocaine in dermatologic surgery, the disadvantage of the drug is that it is available by prescription only and costs more than twice as much as an equivalent amount of lidocaine alone. Lidocaine provides relief within 15 minutes and requires no occlusive dressing. EMLA takes from 45 to 90 minutes for peak effect and requires an occlusive dressing. The prilocaine in EMLA has been associated rarely with methemoglobinemia.

A newer drug, LMX 4, is a 4% lidocaine solution reported to have a similar pain relief profile to EMLA and a cost equivalent to EMLA but requiring less time to act and no occlusive dressing. LMX 4 is limited in that its half-life is only 50% that of EMLA.[80] The muscles enervating the vulva in women with vulvodynia have been shown to be hypertonic. Botulinum toxin (Botox) has been used successfully to paralyze the muscles, breaking the pain response.[81]

Tricyclic antidepressants are among the best researched treatments for neurogenic pain (Table 32-11). The precise mechanism of action is unknown. The amount of medication needed for pain relief is less than the amount used for the treatment of depression, and the side effects are fewer. Amitriptyline (Elavil) begins with a dosage of 25 mg at bedtime for 1 week, then gradual increase until symptoms improve.[82] Nortriptyline (Aventyl) is usually prescribed as 10 mg at bedtime for 3–4 days with gradual increase every 3–4 days until symptoms improve. Most researchers recommend maintaining the therapeutic dosage for 6 months before considering tapering.[82] When discontinuing, decrease the dosage by half every 3–4 days. There is poor evidence regarding use of tricyclic antidepressants during pregnancy and lactation. In general, most authorities suggest avoiding their use. Women using tricyclics should be using a reliable method of birth control. Tricyclics should be prescribed by a provider skilled in their use.

In 2008, Boardman and colleagues published the results of a study of 51 women with vulvodynia who were treated for a minimum of 8 weeks with topical gabapentin. The pain score was significantly decreased from 7.26 to 2.49 (Mean change = −4.77; 95% CI, −5.47 to −4.07). They reported that 80% of women reported at least a 50% improvement in pain scores and an increase in sexual function. Fourteen percent of the subjects discontinued the treatment regimen. These researchers found that topical gabapentin was well tolerated and associated with significant pain relief for these women with vulvodynia.[83]

Table 32-11 Medication Options for Vestibulodynia*

Drug— Generic (Brand)	Initial Dosage	Continuing Dosage	Side Effects	Clinical Considerations
Oral Agents				
Amitriptyline (Elavil)	25 mg at bedtime for 7 nights then increase every 3–4 nights until symptoms improve.	50–150 mg at bedtime. Average needed is 60 mg at bedtime. When discontinuing drug, decrease by half every 3 to 4 days.	Dry mouth Constipation Weight gain Sedation	Tricyclic antidepressants are contraindicated in pregnancy and lactation. Alcohol consumption should not exceed 1 drink per day.
Nortriptyline (Aventyl)	10 mg at bedtime for 3–4 nights then increase every 3–4 nights until symptoms improve.	50–150 mg at bedtime. Average needed is 60 mg at bedtime.	Dry mouth Constipation Weight gain Sedation	See amitriptyline.
Gabapentin (Neurontin)	300 mg at night for 3 nights, then 300 mg twice daily for 3 days; increase by 300 mg every 3 days until symptoms improve.	Maximum of 1200 mg 3 times daily. Average needed is 1500 mg daily in divided doses.	Nausea Drowsiness Dizziness Anorgasmia[43]	Off-label use. Safety in pregnancy and lactation has not been established. Antacids may reduce absorption.
Topical Agents				
Lidocaine 5%	Pea-sized amount to painful area.	Increase to amount needed for comfort.	Prolonged use may cause drying of tissue	Store away from light and moisture.
EMLA	Pea-sized amount to painful area.	Increase to amount needed for comfort.	Redness, burning	Requires 30 minutes to work.
Injectable Agents				
Triamcinolone in bupivacaine	2 mL of a 3 mg/mL solution with 1 mL bupivacaine 0.25–0.5%.	May increase to 3 mL of triamcinolone.	Mild burning with injection	

EMLA = eutectic mixture of lidocaine and prilocaine.
* Currently no medications are FDA approved for the treatment of vestibulodynia. Medications commonly used in treatment were developed for other purposes and represent an off-label use.
Source: Reprinted with permission from Stone-Godena M 2006.[75] Sources include Dworkin RH et al. 2003[77]; McKay M 1993[82]; and Zolnoun DA et al. 2003.[79]

Other treatments reviewed in the literature without consensus or strong evidence include use of antiseizure medications, yoga, hypnotherapy, pelvic muscle physical therapy, and psychotherapy.[75]

As with any vulvar disorder, hygiene measures provide comfort and imbue a woman with some control over her condition. A healthy diet provides support to the immune system, and emotional support encourages the woman to continue to explore treatment options until she finds one that works for her.

Conclusion

Millions of women suffer with vulvar pain or lesions. It is a private and public health issue. While some lesions are easily identified, many lack clear etiology or definitive treatment. Frustration with finding answers has caused many women to either abandon hope for relief or to lose productive hours of their lives seeking relief. Access to

qualified providers and well-documented methods of relief are critical to health. It is incumbent on women's health providers to foster optimism in women in their care and to continue to lobby for research dollars toward finding causes and cures of the various pain syndromes.

References

1. Kelly P. Folliculitis and the follicular occlusion tetrad. In Bolognia JL, Jorizzo JL, Rapini RP, eds. Dermatology, St. Louis, MO: Mosby, 2003:553–66.

2. Hammock LA, Barrett TL. Inflammatory dermatoses of the vulva. J Cutan Path 2005;32:604–11.

3. Yo Y, Cheng AS, Wang L, Dunne WM. Hot tub folliculitis or hot hand foot syndrome caused by *Pseudomonas aeruginosa*. J Am Acad Derm 2007;57:596–600.

4. Wertheim HFL, Verveer J, Boelens HA, van Belkum A, Verbrugh HA, Vos MC. Effect of mupirocin treatment

on nasal, pharyngeal and perineal carriage of *Staphylococcus aureus* in healthy adults. Antimicrob Agents Chemother 2005;49:1465–7.

5. Stevens D, Bison A, Chambers H, Everett ED, Dellinger P, Goldstein EJC, et al. IDSA practice guidelines for the diagnosis and management of skin and soft tissue infections. Clin Infect Dis 2005;41:1373–80.

6. Markowitz N, Quinn EL, Saravoltz LD. Trimethoprim-sulfamethiazole compared with vancomycin for the treatment of *Staphylococcus aureus* infections. Ann Intern Med 1992;117:390–2.

7. Goldstein AT, Marinoff SC, Christopher K, Srodon M. Prevalence of vulvar lichen sclerosus in a general gynecology practice. J Reprod Med 2005;50:477–80.

8. Chan I, Oyama N, Neill SM, Wojnarowska F, Black MM. Characterization of IgG autoantibodies to extracellular matrix protein 1 in lichen sclerosus. Clin Exp Dermatol 2004;29:499–505.

9. Smith YR, Haefner HK. Vulvar lichen sclerosus: pathophysiology and treatment. Am J Clin Dermatol 2004;5:105–25.

10. Cooper SM, Gao XC, Powell JJ, Wojnarowska F. Does treatment of vulvar lichen sclerosus influence its prognosis? Arch Dermatol. 2004;140:709–12.

11. Haefner HK, Colins ME, Davis GD, Edwards L, Foster DC, Hartmann ED, et al. The vulvodynia guideline. J Low Gen Tract Dis, 2005;9:40–51.

12. Bornstein J, Heifetz S, Kellner Y, Stolar Z, Abramovici H. Clobetasol dipropionate 0.05% versus testosterone propionate 2% topical application for severe vulvar lichen sclerosus. Am J Ob Gyn 1998;178(80):790–4.

13. Bousema MT, Romppanen U, Geiger M, Baudin M, Vaha-Eskeli K, Vartiainen J, et al. Acitretin in the treatment of severe lichen sclerosus et atrophicus of the vulva: a double blind, placebo controlled study. J Am Acad Dermatol 1994;30:225.

14. Marill J, Idres N, Capron C, Nguyen E, Chabot G. Retinoic acid metabolism and mechanism of action: a review. Curr Drug Metab 2003;4:1–10.

15. Assman T, Becker-Wegerich P, Grewe M, Megahed M, Ruzicka T. Tacrolimus ointment for the treatment of vulvar lichen sclerosus. J Am Acad Dermatol 2003;48:935–7.

16. Bulbul Baskan E, Turan H, Tunali S, Toker SC, Sarcaoglu H. Open label trial of cyclosporine for vulvar lichen sclerosus. J Am Acad Dermatol 2007; 57:276–8.

17. Rouzier R, Haddad B, Deyrolle C, Pelisse M. Perineoplasty for the treatment of introital stenosis related to vulvar lichen sclerosus. Am J Ob Gyn 2002;186:49–52.

18. Larrabee R, Kylander D. Benign vulvar disorders: identifying features, practical management of non-neoplastic conditions and tumors. Postgrad Med 2001;201:151–64.

19. Jimenez-Ayala M, Jimenez-Ayala B. Terminology for vulvar cytology based on the Bethesda system. Acta Cyto 2002;26:505–15.

20. Ball SB, Wojnarowska F. Vulvar dermatoses: lichen sclerosus, lichen planus and vulval dermatitis/ lichen simplex chronicus. Semin Cutan Med Surg 1998;17:182–8.

21. Clark TJ, Etherington IJ, Luesley DM. Response of vulvar lichen sclerosus and squamous cell hyperplasia to graduated topical steroids. J Reprod Med 1999;44:958–62.

22. Byrd JA, Davis M, Rogers R. Recalcitrant symptomatic vulvar lichen planus response to tacrolimus. Acta Derm 2004;140:715–20.

23. Lewis F. Patient education for vulval lichen planus. International Society for the Study of Vulvovaginal Diseases. 2006. Available from: *http://www.issvd.org/ document_library/VULVAR%20LICHEN%20PLANUS .doc* [Accessed June 26, 2009].

24. MacDonald A, Burden AD. Psoriasis: advances in pathophysiology and management. Postgrad Med J 2007;83:690–7.

25. Revuz J. Medical treatments of hidradenitis suppurativa: a new paradigm. Dermatology 2007;215:95–6.

26. Jemec GBE. Hidradenitis suppurativa. J Cutaneous Med Surg 2003;7:47–56.

27. Von der Werth JM, Williams HC, Raeburn JA. The clinical genetics of hidradenitis suppurativa revisited. Br J Dermatol 2000;142:947–53.

28. Von der Werth JM, Williams HC. The natural history of hidradenitis suppurativa. J Eur Acad Dermatol Venereol 2000;14:389–92.

29. Jansen I, Altmeyer P, Piewig G. Acne inversa (alias hidradenitis suppurativa). J Eur Acad Dermatol Venereol 2001;15:532–40.

30. Krbec, A. Current understanding and management of hidradenitis suppurativa. J Am Acad Nurse Pract 2007;19:228–34.

31. Rompel R, Petres J. Long-term results of wide surgical excision in 106 patients with hidradenitis suppurativa. Dermatol Surg 2000;26:638–43.

32. Shah N. Hidradenitis suppurativa: a treatment challenge. Am Fam Physician 2005;72:1547–52.

33. Bong JL, Shalders K, Saihan E. Treatment of persistent painful nodules of hidradenitis suppurativa with cryotherapy. Clin Exp Dermatol 2003;28:241–4.

34. Plewig G, Steger M. Acne inversa alias acne triad, acne tetrad or hidradenitis suppurativa. In Mars S, Plewig G, eds. Acne and related disorders. London, England: Martin Dunitz, 1991:345–57.

35. Jemec GBE, Wendelboe P. Topical clindamycin versus systemic tetracycline in the treatment of hidradenitis suppurativa. J Am Acad Dermatol 1998;39:971.

36. Brocard A, Knol A, Khammari A, Dréno B. Verneuil's disease and zinc: a new therapeutic approach—a pilot study. Dermatology 2007;214:325–7.

37. Farrell AM, Randall VA, Vafaee T, Dawber RP. Finasteride as a therapy for hidradenitis suppurativa. Br J Dermatol 2007;215:41–4.

38. Boer J, VanGemert MJ. Long term results of isotretinoin in the treatment of 68 patients with hidradenitis suppurativa. J Am Acad Dermatol 1999;40:73–6.

39. Rose RF, Goodfield MJD, Clark SM. Treatment of recalcitrant hidradenitis suppurativa with oral cyclosporin. Clin Exp Dermatol 2006;31:154–5.

40. Fernandez-Vozmediano JM, Armario-Hita JC. Infliximab for the treatment of hidradenitis suppurativa. Dermatology 1999;141:1138–9.

41. Howes RJ, Barlow M. The evidence base and rationale for the use of anti TNFα biologic drugs for the treatment of hidradenitis suppurativa: an advocacy report from the Hidradenitis Suppurativa Foundation Inc. Available from: *www.hs-foundation.org/pdf/HSF_Biologics_Research.pdf* [Accessed January 26, 2009].

42. Wolkenstein P, Loundou A, Barrau K, Auquier P, Revuz J. Quality of life impairment in hidradenitis suppurativa: a study of 61 cases. J Am Acad Dermatol 2007;56:621–3.

43. Margesson LJ. Contact dermatitis of the vulva. Dermatol Ther 2004;17:20–7.

44. Bauer A. Vulvar dermatoses-irritant and allergic contact dermatitis of the vulva. Dermatology 2005; 210:143–9.

45. The International Study Group for Behçet's Disease, Evaluation of diagnostic ('classification') criteria in Behçet's disease—towards internationally agreed criteria. Rheumatology 1992;31:299–308.

46. O'Duffy JD. Behçet's syndrome. N Engl J Med 1990;322:326–8.

47. Yurdakul S, Mat C, Tuzun Y, Ozyazgan Y, Hamuryudan V. A double-blind trial of colchicine in Behçet's syndrome. Arthritis Rheum 2001;44:2686.

48. Alpsoy E. Behçet's disease: treatment of mucocutaneous lesions. Clin Exp Rheumatol 2005;23:532–9.

49. Mat C, Yurdakul S, Uysal S, Gogus F, Ozyazgan Y, Uysal O, et al. A double-blind trial of depot corticoster-

oids in Behçet's syndrome. Rheumatology (Oxford) 2006;45:348.

50. Hamuryudan V, Mat C, Saip S, Yilmaz O, Siva A, Yurdakaul S, et al. Thalidomide in the treatment of the mucocutaneous lesions of the Behçet syndrome. A randomized, double-blind, placebo-controlled trial. Ann Intern Med 1998;128:443.

51. Anandarajah A. American College of Rheumatology, annual scientific meeting: advances in the treatment of connective tissue diseases. Future Rheumatology 2007;2:379–84.

52. Billstein SA, Mattaliano VJ Jr. The "nuisance" sexually transmitted diseases: Molluscum contagiosum, scabies, and crab lice. Med Clin North Am 1990;74: 1487–1505.

53. Habif TP. Clinical dermatology, 4th ed. St. Louis, MO: Mosby, 2004:242–5.

54. Hengge UR, Esser S, Schultewolter T, Behrendt C, Meyer T, Stockfleth E, et al. Self-administered topical 5% imiquimod for the treatment of common warts and molluscum contagiosum. Br J Dermatology 2000;143:1026–31.

55. Weiner CP, Buhimschi C. Drugs for pregnant and lactating women. Philadelphia, PA: Churchill Livingstone, 2004:801–2.

56. Moed L, Shwayder T, Chang MW. Cantharid revisited. Arch Dermatol 2001;137:1357–60.

57. Silverburg NB, Sidbury R, Mancini AJ. Childhood molluscum contagiosum: experience with cantharidin therapy in 300 patients. J Am Acad Dermatol 2000; 43:503–7.

58. Dohil M, Prendiville JS. Treatment of molluscum contagiosum with oral cimetidine: clinical experience on 13 patients. Pediatric Dermatol 1996;13:310–2.

59. Centers for Disease Control. Sexually transmitted diseases treatment guidelines. 2006 MMWR Morb Mortal Wkly Rpt 51;RR:61–9.

60. Wendel K, Rompalo A. Scabies and pediculosis pubis: an update of treatment regimens and general review. Clin Infect Dis 2002;35(suppl 2):146–51.

61. Chosidow O. Scabies and pediculosis. Lancet 2000; 355:819–26.

62. Oaklander AL. The pathology of pain. Neuroscientist 1999;5:302–15.

63. Schwartz RA, Janusz CA, Janniger CK. Seborrheic dermatitis: an overview. Am Fam Physician 2006;74:125–30.

64. Gupta AK, Bluhm R. Seborrheic dermatitis. J Eur Acad Dermatol Venereol 2004;18:13.

65. Cowley NC, Farr PM, Shuster S. The permissive effect of sebum in seborrheic dermatitis: an explanation

of the rash in neurological disorders. Br J Dermatol 1990;122:71–6.

66. Pierard GE, Pierard-Franchimont C, Van Cutsem J, Rurangirwa A, Hoppenbrouwers ML, Schrooten P, et al. Ketoconazole 2% emulsion in the treatment of seborrheic dermatitis. Int J Dermatol 1991;30:806.

67. Cunha PR. Pimecrolimus cream 1% is effective in seborrheic dermatitis refractory to treatment with topical corticosteroids. Acta Derm Venereol 2006;86:69–70.

68. Wikler JR, Janssen N, Bruynzeel DP, Nieboer C. The effect of UV-light on *Pityrosporum* yeasts: ultrastructural changes and inhibition of growth. Acta Derm Venereol 1990;70:69–71.

69. Satchell AC, Sauraje, A, Bel C, Barnetso RS. Treatment of dandruff with 5% tea tree oil shampoo. J Am Acad Dermatol 2002;47:852.

70. Knight TE, Hausen BM. Melaleuca oil (tea tree oil) dermatitis. J Am Acad Dermatol 1994;30:423.

71. Henley DV, Lipson N, Korach KS, Bloch CA. Prepubertal gynecomastia linked to lavender and tea tree oils. N Engl J Med 2007;356:479.

72. Parker LP, Parker JR, Bodurka-Bevers D, Deavers M, Bevers MW, Shen-Gunther J, et al. Paget's disease of the vulva: pathology, pattern of involvement, and prognosis. Gynecol Oncol 2000;77:183–9.

73. Piura B, Rabinovich A, Dgani R. Extramammary Paget's disease of the vulva: report of five cases and review of the literature. Eur J Gynaecol Oncol 1999;20:98–101.

74. Mehta NJ, Torno R, Sorra T. Extramammary Paget's disease. South Med J 2000;93:713–5.

75. Stone-Godena M. Vulvar pain syndromes: vestibulodynia. J Midwifery Womens Health 2006;51:502–9.

76. Harlow BL, Stewart BG. A population based assessment of chronic unexplained vulvar pain: have we underestimated the prevalence of vulvodynia? J Am Med Women's Assoc 2003;58:82–8.

77. Dworkin RH, Backonja M, Rowbotham MC, Allen RR, Argoff CR, Bennett GJ, et al. Advances in neuropathic pain: diagnosis, mechanisms and treatment recommendations. Arch Neurol 2003;60:1524–30.

78. Smith PG. Effects of estrogen on peripheral pain pathways. In Vulvodynia-Toward understanding a pain syndrome. Bethesda, MD: National Institute of Child Health and Human Development, April 14–15, 2003:27–8.

79. Zolnoun DA, Hartmann KE, Steege JF. Overnight 5% lidocaine ointment for treatment of vulvar vestibulitis. Obstet Gynecol 2003;102:84–7.

80. Friedman P, Mafong E, Friedman E, Geronemus R. Topical anesthetics update: EMLA and beyond. Amer Soc Dermatol Surg 2001;27:1019–26.

81. Gunter J, Brewer A, Tawfik O. Botulinum toxin A for vulvodynia: a case report. J Pain 2004;5:238–40.

82. McKay M. Dysesthetic ("essential") vulvodynia: treatment with amitriptyline. J Repro Med 1993;38:9–13.

83. Boardman LA, Cooper AS, Blais LR, Raker CA. Topical gabapentin in the treatment of localized and generalized vulvodynia. Obstet Gynecol 2008; 112(3):579–85.

"Sex is something you do, sexuality is something you are."

ANNA FREUD

33
Sexual Dysfunction

Jennifer G. Hensley and Mary C. Brucker

Chapter Glossary

Arousal disorder The persistent or recurring inability to attain or maintain adequate sexual excitement, causing personal distress. It may be experienced as lack of subjective excitement or lack of genital (lubrication/swelling) or other somatic responses. Also known as female sexual arousal disorder (FSAD).

Desire disorder Disorder that is subcategorized as either a hypoactive sexual desire disorder (HSDD) or sexual aversion disorder.

Dyspareunia Recurrent or persistent genital pain associated with sexual intercourse. A pain disorder.

Female sexual dysfunction (FSD) A sexual dysfunction that meets DSM-IV-TR criteria for a sexual disorder that includes both dysfunction and marked distress. There are four subclassifications: desire, arousal, orgasm, and pain. Also called female sexual disorder.

Hypoactive sexual desire disorder The persistent or recurring deficiency (or absence) of sexual fantasies/thoughts and/or receptivity to sexual activity that causes personal distress.

Libido The primary sexual appetite; feelings that motivate a person to obtain sex and focus his or her attention on that goal.

Noncoital genital pain Recurrent or persistent genital pain induced by noncoital sexual stimulation. A pain disorder.

Orgasmic disorder The persistent or recurrent difficulty, delay in, or absence of attaining orgasm following sufficient sexual stimulation and arousal that causes personal distress. May be a primary or secondary condition.

Pain disorder A female sexual pain disorder that includes one of the following: dyspareunia, vaginismus, or noncoital pain.

Sexology The study of sexuality.

Sexual aversion disorder The persistent or recurrent phobic aversion to and avoidance of sexual contact with a sexual partner which causes personal distress.

Sexual dysfunction Disturbance in sexual functioning involving one or multiple phases of the sexual response cycle or pain associated with sexual activity.

Sexual health State of physical, emotional, mental, and social well-being related to sexuality. Integration of somatic, emotional, intellectual, and social aspects in ways that are positively enriching and that will enhance personality, communication, and love.

Vaginismus Recurrent or persistent involuntary spasms of the musculature of the outer third of the vagina that interfere with vaginal penetration and which cause personal distress. A pain disorder.

Sources: American Psychiatric Association 2000[7]; Clayton AH 2007[20]; World Health Organization 2008.[56]

Introduction

All humans are sexual beings. Not only is sex necessary for continuation of the species, but sexual health is an integral component of a person's general health. Yet sexuality often is shrouded in taboos. The United States has deep

Puritan roots, and many women may be reticent to express sexual concerns. However, as the baby boomers of the sexual revolution age, they are likely to be healthier than their parents were at a similar age and have high expectations of continued sexual activity. Moreover, some pharmaceuticals have been developed that treat erectile dysfunction for men of all ages and potentially cause both positive and negative reactions for female partners, while other medications have adverse sexual effects that can cause women to seek care. Therefore, an increasing number of women are sharing sexual concerns with their primary care providers.

The conditions most frequently reported by women include decreased sexual desire, difficulty with orgasm, and dyspareunia. In order to address these issues, the provider first should be aware of what is known and unknown about normal sexuality.

History of Sexology in the United States

Sexology, or the scientific study of sexuality, came of age in the United States in the 20th century with the work of Alfred Kinsey, who is commonly called the father of sexology. In 1938, Kinsey, a zoologist at Indiana University, was asked to conduct a class on sex for women who were married or considering marriage. Realizing there was a paucity of scientifically based information, Kinsey and his

team conducted 18,000 face-to-face, in-depth interviews with women and men on sex. Results were published in *Sexual Behavior in the Human Male* and *Sexual Behavior in the Human Female* in 1948 and 1953, respectively. These reports allowed public review of sex in the United States, once a taboo subject. The Kinsey Institute for Research in Sex, Gender, and Reproduction, which was founded in 1947, continues the study of human sexuality today.[1]

While the average person might have initially considered Kinsey's work simply titillating, Masters and Johnson's work was biologically directed and well integrated within the scientific community. In 1966, Masters and Johnson published *Human Sexual Response*, which detailed the physiology of the normal sexual response.[2] In this book, the scientists described the following four phases of sexual response: excitement, plateau, orgasm, and resolution. These phases were assumed to occur in a linear progression. Although their work was covered extensively by the public press, perhaps most importantly, their findings were incorporated in all forms of formal healthcare education. Forty years later, this remains the predominant model used to explain normal sexual response. Table 33-1 summarizes changes associated with the phases of sexual response according to the model of Masters and Johnson.

Although the Masters and Johnson model remains the one most commonly used, other sexual response models have emerged from other experts in sexology such as

Table 33-1 Masters and Johnson Model for Female Sexual Response

Excitement	Plateau	Orgasm	Resolution
Initial arousal	Full arousal, preorgasm		Postorgasm
Vaginal lubrication	The outer 1/3 of the vagina swells and the opening narrows by 1/3; referred to as the orgasmic platform	Serotonin, oxytocin, and other smooth-muscle contracting agents resulting in discharge of accumulated sexual intensity as rhythmic muscular contractions of the uterus, outer 1/3 of the vagina, anal sphincter, and clitoris occur	If continued sexual stimulation and interest, multiorgasmic response
Inner 2/3 of vagina expands			Or return to unaroused state
Cervix and uterus pulled forward			Muscles relax and vasocongestion dissipates with loss of orgasmic platform; uterus returns to resting state; vagina shortens in width and length; clitoris returns to normal size and position
Labia majora become flatter and move outwards in nulliparas. Labia majora increases in size in parous women	Inner 2/3 of vagina expands as uterus is elevated; called tenting		
Labia minora of vagina enlarge	Clitoris withdraws into the clitoral hood		
Clitoral gland, clitoral glans becomes swollen	Labia minora engorge and enlarge and can triple in size	Probable release of female ejaculate from Bartholin's glands remains unclear	Breasts decrease in size and areola and nipples flatten
Nipples become erect and breasts slightly increase in size	Labia minora change color due to vasocongestion and precede orgasm	Heart rate, respiratory rate, and blood pressure at highest values	Breathing, heart rate, and blood pressure return to normal
Increased sexual tension above unaroused state	Areola and breasts enlarge		
Some increase in heart rate, respiratory rate, blood pressure and muscle tension	Blotchy skin pattern may be seen as sex flush	Other muscles such as buttocks or feet may involuntarily contract	
Blood flow to genitals increases	Increased muscle tension		
Vasocongestion of the skin, called "sex flush," occurs in 50–75% of women	Further increase in heart rate, respiratory rate, and blood pressure		

Source: Masters WH et al. 1966.[2]

Kaplan; Reed; Whipple and Brash-McGreer; and Basson and are summarized in Table 33-2.[3-6] Kaplan's linear model has been used with Masters and Johnson's model as the basis for categorization of female sexual dysfunction in the *Diagnostic and Statistical Manual*, 4th edition (Text Revision) (DSM-IV-TR).[7] The DSM-IV-TR, extensively used for both clinical categorization and reimbursement, has been criticized because it exclusively focuses on psychiatric issues related to female sexual dysfunction without regard to organic causes.[7,8]

Another researcher, Basson, diverged from the linear model of Masters and Johnson by proposing a circular model. Basson's model, as illustrated in Figure 33-1, often is preferred in clinical practice because it includes the effect of intimacy on sexual response, both positively and negatively.[8] Sexual response in women is far more complex than can be described in a linear or circular model because physiologic, psychologic, social, and cultural factors play interrelated roles as well. However, these models provide

some understanding of the female sexual response, which the clinician can use as a basis for diagnosing and treating female sexual dysfunction.

Open discussion of sex was taboo a century ago. Kinsey's publications as well as Masters and Johnson's provided a venue for individuals to speak and think more freely about sex. The sexual revolution in the United States, which began in the mid-1960s, coincided with political activism, feminism, and marketing of combined oral contraceptives. The latter was a watershed event as women became free to explore their sexuality, unfettered by fear of pregnancy.

The year 1998 ushered in its own sexual revolution when sildenafil (Viagra) was approved as a treatment for male erectile dysfunction. More midlife couples became capable of intercourse. Unwittingly, this created sexual problems for some women who previously had ceased sexual relations.[9] Some women found they had vaginal atrophy and coitus was difficult, thus they requested assistance

Table 33-2 Comparison of Models of Female Sexual Response

Researchers	Year(s)	Type	Summary
Masters and Johnson[2]	1966	Linear	Excitement—plateau—orgasm—resolution
Kaplan[3]	1976	Linear-triphasic	Desire—excitement—orgasm Condensed the model of Masters and Johnson and added desire
Reed[4]	Unknown	Nonlinear	Seduction—sensations—surrender—reflection Reflection allows the participant to decide if the experience was positive or negative, which adds to or detracts from future sexual experiences
Whipple and Brash-McGreer[5]	1997	Nonlinear	Seduction—sensations—surrender—reflection—seduction Expands on Reed's unpublished model
Basson[6]	2001	Circular	Emotional intimacy—sexual stimuli—sexual arousal—arousal and sexual desire—emotional and physical satisfaction—back to emotional intimacy

Sources: Masters WH, Johnson VE 1966[2]; Kaplan HS 1976[3]; Kammerer-Doak D, Rogers RG[4]; Sugrue DP et al. 2001[5]; Basson R 2000.[6]

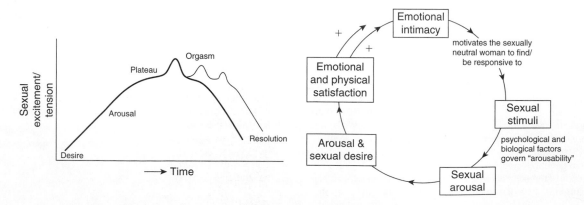

Figure 33-1 Traditional sex response cycle of Masters and Johnson alongside intimacy-based female sex response cycle. *Source:* Reprinted with permission from Basson R 2001.[6]

in restoring vaginal integrity for intercourse. The American Association of Retired Persons reported that their organization experienced a substantial increase in adults seeking information about sex from 1999 to 2004.[10]

Normal Reproductive and Sexual Physiology

Puberty is the process of physical maturation that makes reproduction possible. The neurohormonal trigger that heralds the onset of puberty and development of secondary sexual characteristics is unknown. The hypothalamic-pituitary-ovarian axis becomes functional at puberty.[11,12] In girls, the onset of puberty is typically between 8–13 years. At this time, an increased production of gonadotropin-releasing hormone from the hypothalamus causes gonadotropins from the pituitary to stimulate the ovaries. The ovaries respond with production of estrogen, which initiates dramatic changes in the female body.

Estrogen causes cellular proliferation of all female sexual organs. Over time, this twentyfold increase in estrogen production will lead to development of stroma tissue, the ductal system and adipose deposition in the breast; differentiation of cuboidal to squamous cells capable of mucous production in the vagina; and cellular proliferation and enlargement of the vagina, cervix, uterus, fallopian tubes, and ovaries. The vaginal epithelium becomes mature and thick, and rugation can be seen.

The mean age of menarche is 13 years.[12] Prior to puberty and menarche, it is normal for female infants to touch and stimulate their genitals and toddlers to exhibit curiosity toward differences between sexes.[13-16] Sexual arousal is believed to occur secondary to classical conditioning, i.e., stimulus/response.[16] Positive experiences reinforce the value of the arousal, whereas negative responses do not. Masturbatory activities in childhood, alone or with peers, is not uncommon.[15] Adolescents may actively engage in sexual experimentation, which can lead to untoward consequences such as sexually transmitted infections or unwanted pregnancies.[14,16] Many factors, including biology, family, culture, and society play into adolescents' determinations of their sexual identities.[16] Adult women actively engage in sexual activities for procreation, intimacy, and physiologic release. Women past menopause are no less interested in their sexuality and sexual expression than are younger women.[17]

Two basic physiologic reactions occur during female sexual response, vasocongestion as blood engorges the genitals and breasts, and neuromuscular tension as energy is built up in the nerves and muscles.[2] The total response, however, is multifactorial, responding to neurotransmitters and hormones at both the central and peripheral levels. Estrogen, testosterone, progesterone, and oxytocin act centrally to excite sexual desire and arousal while prolactin acts as an inhibitor. Neurotransmitters and other cellular messengers such as dopamine, norepinephrine, melanocortins, nitric oxide, vasoactive intestinal peptide, and cyclic guanosine monophosphate act peripherally to enhance sexual desire and sexual excitement via vasocongestion and neuromuscular tension. Serotonin appears to have an inhibitory effect peripherally.[18] Figures 33-2 and 33-3 illustrate the excitatory and inhibitory effects of these neurotransmitters.

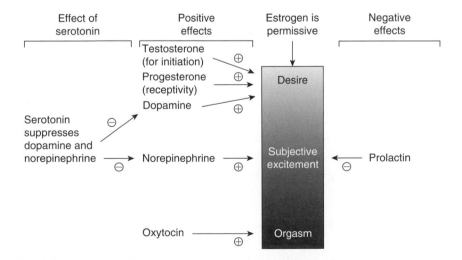

Figure 33-2 Central effect of sex hormone on female sexual response.

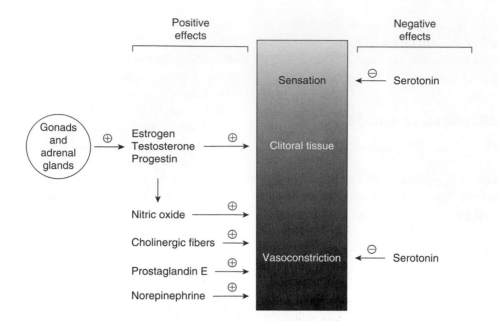

Figure 33-3 Peripheral effects on sexual function. *Source:* Adapted with permission from Clayton AH 2003.[20]

As with the hormonal trigger that initiates puberty, the exact mechanism for menopause is not completely understood. As normal aging occurs, the body responds more slowly to hormones, neurotransmitters, and chemical messengers that affect vasocongestion and neuromuscular tension. This can lead to a disruption in the sexual response during perimenopause and postmenopause. The mean age of menopause is 51 years, although perimenopause usually begins up to 7 years prior.[11]

Female Sexual Dysfunction

Even with knowledge about sexual behaviors and physiology of sexual response, providers continue to be challenged in caring for women with sexual dysfunction. Each woman is unique, and there is little consensus on what defines normal for an individual woman's sexual response.[19] Multiple factors such as age, physical health, emotional status, relationships (past and present), sexual expectations religious/cultural background, and a woman's individual beliefs are some of the factors that affect sexual health as illustrated in Figure 33-4. For example, some women tolerate occasional anorgasmia without concern, whereas for others it is cause for an emergent visit to a healthcare professional. If the sexual condition

is not distressing to the woman, there is no problem or dysfunction.[20]

Unlike hypertension or hypercholesterolemia wherein exact laboratory tests confirm a diagnosis, **female sexual dysfunction** essentially is self-described or self-diagnosed. A woman seeking care already has recognized that she has a **sexual dysfunction**. The ability to self-diagnose may be empowering to women, but it also may have other implications. For example, women may believe the popular press suggests that women should always be sexually responsive and even sexy. Such a concept implies that any variation requires treatment.

Some authorities have suggested that female sexual dysfunction does not exist as a distinct condition, but is instead the direct result of the medicalization of sex.[21] It has been suggested that the term *female sexual problem* may be preferred to the more medical term *dysfunction* or *disorder*.[22]

Although it has limitations, the DSM-IV-TR criteria provide the most commonly used criteria for female sexual dysfunction and a lexicon for use in diagnosis, treatment, and research. In this system, a female sexual dysfunction is a sexual condition including both dysfunction and marked distress to the individual. Four classifications exist—**desire disorders**, **arousal disorders**, **orgasmic disorders**, and **pain disorders**, all requiring personal distress before the diagnosis is made. Desire disorders are

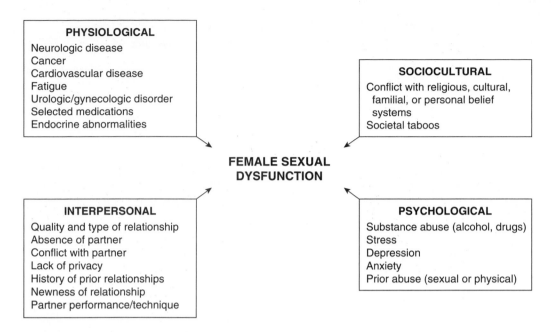

PHYSIOLOGICAL
Neurologic disease
Cancer
Cardiovascular disease
Fatigue
Urologic/gynecologic disorder
Selected medications
Endocrine abnormalities

SOCIOCULTURAL
Conflict with religious, cultural,
    familial, or personal belief
    systems
Societal taboos

**FEMALE SEXUAL
DYSFUNCTION**

INTERPERSONAL
Quality and type of relationship
Absence of partner
Conflict with partner
Lack of privacy
History of prior relationships
Newness of relationship
Partner performance/technique

PSYCHOLOGICAL
Substance abuse (alcohol, drugs)
Stress
Depression
Anxiety
Prior abuse (sexual or physical)

Figure 33-4 Factors affecting female sexual disorder.

subclassified as **hypoactive sexual desire disorder** or **sexual aversion disorders**, and in both conditions, women lack normal sexual fantasies/thoughts/receptivity. Desire disorders are often termed low libido. **Libido** is a term that is difficult to define since sexual desire is personal, and a normal level is not only elusive but likely impossible to codify. Arousal disorders or female sexual arousal disorders include the inability to attain or maintain sexual excitement. Orgasm disorder includes difficulty, delay, or absence of attaining orgasm. The last category, pain disorder, is subcategorized into **dyspareunia**, **vaginismus,** and **noncoital genital pain**. These categories also are used in the reports of most studies on sexuality, including evaluation of treatments. Other descriptors of note, in addition to the DSM-IV-TR criteria, include the use of terms for length of time of condition (primary [lifelong] or secondary [acquired]); for when it occurs (situational or generalized); and for the degree of distress (mild, moderate, or marked).[23]

Prevalence of Female Sexual Dysfunction

Even with the use of the DSM-IV-TR, the diagnosis of female sexual dysfunction is difficult at best. Therefore, determination of prevalence of these conditions is equally challenging. An *overall* rate of sexual dysfunction in women of up to 43% is reported in the following three large studies: (1) a US national probability sample of women aged 18–59 years (N = 1749) from 1992, reanalyzed in 1999 using latent class analysis[24]; (2) an international survey of women aged 40–80 years in 29 countries (N = 13,882)[25]; and (3) a national probability sample of women aged 57–85 years (N = 1550).[26] A cross-sectional, population-based survey of adult women over 18 years in the United States (N = 31,581) revealed a lower rate of sexual dysfunction in women (12–22%) when they were asked if the dysfunction was *accompanied by personal distress.*[27]

In all, the most frequently reported symptoms include low libido/lack of interest in sex, inability to orgasm, and problems with vaginal lubrication. The prevalence of each condition increased with age, poor health, and depression. Prevalence of specific categories of female sexual dysfunction is found in Table 33-3, based on a review of the literature over a 10-year period. The authors note that many studies lacked methodological rigor and consistent use of DSM-IV-TR criteria, which accounts for large differences in reported percentages.[28] Thus, concerns related to female sexual dysfunction could be underreported.

Diagnosis of Female Sexual Dysfunction

Women may suffer from hypoactive sexual desire disorder, female sexual arousal disorder, female orgasmic disorder, sexual pain from dyspareunia, or a combination of all (Figure 33-5). Acquired hypoactive sexual desire disorder can develop as a result of surgical menopause, which can be diagnosed with the use of a simple survey.

Table 33-3 Prevalence of Female Sexual Disorders

Condition	Prevalence
Sexual Desire Disorders	
Hypoactive sexual desire disorder (HSDD)	5–46%
Sexual aversion disorder	Rare
Arousal Disorder	
Female sexual arousal disorder	6–21%
Orgasmic Disorder	
Female orgasmic disorder	5–42%
Pain Disorders	
Dyspareunia among premenopausal women	3–46%
Dyspareunia among peri/postmenopausal women	9–21%
Vaginismus	0.5–30%

Source: Simons JS and Carey MP 2001.[28]

Table 33-4 Selected Medical Conditions That Affect Female Sexual Dysfunction

Condition	Sexual Function Affected
Depression	Desire
Diabetes	Arousal and orgasm
Thyroid disease	Desire
Cardiovascular conditions	Arousal
Neurologic disorders	Arousal and orgasm
Androgen insufficiency	Desire
Estrogen deficiency	Arousal

Sources: Basson R and Schultz WW 2007[29]; Kingsberg SA and Janata JW 2007.[56]

Etiologies of Female Sexual Dysfunction

Menopause, natural or surgical, and antidepressants are the major contributors to sexual concerns. Other medical conditions, including those listed in Table 33-4, also may have a negative association with sexual functioning.[28,29]

In addition, the pharmaceuticals used to treat some medical conditions can negatively affect sexual function. Pharmaceutical agents associated with sexual dysfunction are listed in Table 33-5.

Natural or Surgical Menopause

Life expectancy for women has increased to approximately 80 years of age, and it is estimated that women will live one third of their lives after natural menopause. As women age, sexual concerns can be attributed to declining ovarian hormones, poor health, and/or the side effects of

medications.[11] The most commonly performed gynecologic surgery in the United States, a hysterectomy with bilateral salpingo-oophorectomy, confers immediate surgical menopause. For younger women, this may signal a dramatic decrease in estrogen levels and cause a clinical presentation of vasomotor symptoms and sexual dysfunction.[30]

Estradiol (E_2), the major estrogen produced by the ovary during reproductive years, is responsible for vaginal lubrication and maintenance of vaginal epithelium. As ovarian function declines, estradiol production decreases, and the woman may experience vaginal dryness with resultant itching and burning that can lead to dyspareunia. The vaginal epithelium atrophies; the walls become pale and dry. Vaginal blood flow diminishes, lubrication decreases and the pH rises as lactobacilli that are fed by estrogen-rich epithelium disappear. The vagina shortens in width

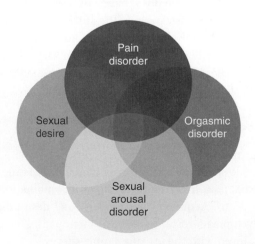

Figure 33-5 Overlap of female sexual dysfunctions.

Table 33-5 Selected Medications That Can Cause Female Sexual Dysfunction

Drug Class	Medication	Area of Sexual Dysfunction
Antidepressants and mood stabilizers	SNRIs and SSRIs	Desire, arousal, and orgasm
	Tricyclic antidepressants	Desire and arousal
	MAOIs	Arousal
	Antipsychotics	Desire and orgasm
	Benzodiazepines	Desire, arousal, and orgasm
Antiepileptics	Carbamazepine (Tegretol)	Desire
	Phenytoin (Dilantin)	Desire
Antihypertensives	Beta-blockers	Desire and arousal
	Alpha-blockers	Desire versus arousal
	Diuretics	Desire
Cardiovascular agents	Lipid-lowering agents	Desire
	Digoxin	Desire

SNRI = serotonin/norepinephrine reuptake inhibitor; SSRI = selective serotonin reuptake inhibitor
Sources: Basson R and Schultz WW 2007[29]; Kingsberg SA and Janata JW 2007.[55]

and length.[31] Eventually, pain and bleeding can occur with insertion of a speculum or penis into the vagina. Exogenous estrogen, systemically or locally, may be required to treat symptomatic women.

Testosterone is necessary for normal ovarian function during the reproductive years. Testosterone is produced by the adrenal glands and ovaries and from peripheral conversion of pro-androgens; 98–99% is bound to sex hormone-binding globulin (SHBG) or albumin. Pro-androgens include dehydroepiandrosterone sulfate (DHEA-S), androstenedione, dehydroepiandrosterone (DHEA), and dihydrotestosterone, which are produced in the adrenal glands and/or ovaries and are peripherally converted to testosterone. Although necessary for sexual desire in men, the role of testosterone in female **sexual health** is less clear.[32] Testosterone levels in postmenopausal women, natural or surgical, appear to decline as a result of the normal aging process, not because of the decline in ovarian function.[32]

Administration of exogenous estrogen for contraception or menopausal symptoms increases sex-hormone binding globulin. As sex-hormone binding globulin increases, it binds more testosterone, which results in less circulating testosterone available to receptors located throughout the body, in particular the brain and genitalia. Use of exogenous hormones during the reproductive years for contraception, such as combined oral contraceptives (COCs), can increase sex-hormone binding globulin, bind testosterone, and potentially lower libido. Despite the lack of evidence regarding its role in sexual health, menopausal women who take exogenous testosterone have reported a positive effect on sexual desire, arousal, and orgasm.[32]

Antidepressants and Sexual Depression

Antidepressants are among the most commonly prescribed pharmaceuticals in the United States. Reports of sexual dysfunction while taking selective serotonin reuptake inhibitors (SSRIs) have been reported in up to 80% of those surveyed.[33,34] Hypoactivity of monoamine neurotransmitters in the brain, particularly serotonin and norepinephrine, have been postulated as part of the complex pathophysiology of depression. Medications that inhibit reuptake of these neurotransmitters, such as SSRIs and serotonin norepinephrine reuptake inhibitors (SNRIs), are used for treatment of depression. Women successfully treated with antidepressants who are in remission may begin to feel better only to then experience sexual problems.

When SSRIs were initially marketed in the early 1990s, the decrease in overall side effects compared to the tricyclic and monoamine oxidase inhibitor antidepressants led to a belief that these agents also had few sexual side effects.[34]

However, the true incidence of sexual dysfunction in women who take SSRIs varies from a small percentage up to 80%; sexual dysfunction is dose dependent and includes decreased desire, arousal, and orgasm.[31,32] Conversely, SNRIs, such as bupropion (Wellbutrin), or tetracyclic antidepressants, such as mianserin (Bolvidon), do not appear to have as many sexual side effects.[35,36]

SSRIs are theorized to interfere with normal sexual response via serotoninergic, dopaminergic, and anticholinergic pathways, as well as mechanisms that utilize nitric oxide and prolactin as shown in Figures 33-2 and 33-3. The SSRIs inhibit uptake of serotonin and dopamine.[36] Serotonin is known to have an inhibitory effect on sexual arousal while dopamine has an excitatory effect. More available serotonin in the neural synapse and less available dopamine leads to decreased desire, decreased arousal, and difficulty achieving orgasm. Elevated levels of serotonin and decreased dopamine also trigger increased levels of prolactin, which further inhibits dopamine. Serotonin may impede the vasocongestive phase of sexual response with anticholinergic effects by blocking acetylcholine necessary for local vasodilation of the clitoral veins as well as being a potent inhibitor of the vasodilator nitric oxide.[34] These factors contribute to sexual problems, dysfunction, and the possibility of a sexual function disorder.

Treatment for Sexual Dysfunction

Treatment for female sexual dysfunction will depend upon the disorder, whether it is hypoactive sexual desire disorder, female sexual arousal disorder, female orgasm disorder, or a pain disorder due to dyspareunia. In an era of evidence-based care, the first line of treatment should be based upon randomized, controlled trials that have established safety and efficacy. However, for female sexual dysfunction, female sexual arousal disorder, and female orgasmic disorder, the final determination of success remains with the woman. To date, few of the published studies account for powerful confounding variables such as the impact of the relationship with the partner(s) on female sexual dysfunction (e.g., male sexual dysfunction; length of relationship; multiple partners; female partners), environment (e.g., new environment), or others. Therefore, the following data on testosterone and sildenafil (Viagra) should be considered within the context of these limitations.

Estrogen for Vaginal Conditions

Estrogen therapy administered via one of several routes may be offered to women who experience troublesome vasomotor symptoms around the time of natural or surgical menopause for the shortest amount of time necessary.[37] Women who have an intact uterus and who take estrogen will need additional progestin to prevent endometrial hyperplasia. Hormone therapy is addressed in detail in Chapter 34.

The vaginal epithelium responds to both systemic and local preparations of estrogen. In severe cases of vaginal atrophy, use of both topical and systemic estrogen preparations may be necessary for a time to restore vaginal epithelium. Vaginal atrophy is associated with aging but also can occur in lactating women whose hormonal milieu is changed while breastfeeding. Although systemic estrogen is effective, topical estrogens are more commonly used.

A Cochrane systematic review examined 19 trials with 4162 women and found that vaginal preparations of estrogen (ring, cream, tablet) all were effective in treating vaginal atrophy.[38] The ring appeared to offer women the greatest satisfaction, especially since it was inserted and remained in situ for several weeks compared to daily use of a vaginal pill or cream preparation. The large majority of women treated with local vaginal estrogen reported improvement in symptoms related to vaginal atrophy. Studies that have evaluated the estrogen patch suggest it has a similar effect on vaginal atrophy as do other topical formulations. Currently, additional progestin is not necessary for the woman who has an intact uterus and who uses topical estrogen, unless she begins to bleed. However, there are no safety data on the use of local estrogen for longer than 12 consecutive months.[31,38]

Contraindications

As with any estrogen, there are contraindications, which are listed in Table 34-4. Contraindications include a history of current or previous estrogen-dependent cancer, pregnancy, or undiagnosed vaginal bleeding. Table 33-6 provides a list of commonly used pharmaceuticals containing estrogen.

Testosterone for Sexual Dysfunction

A Cochrane systematic review examined 23 trials with 1957 women in which various formulations of testosterone were used. In general, it was found that the addition of testosterone improved sexual function in postmenopausal women, although there were limitations that confounded some of the trials.[39] All of the studies included testosterone as an adjunct to estrogen that was administered with or without progesterone. Testosterone was used for no more than 26 weeks.

Exogenous testosterone appears to improve sexual functioning for women experiencing hypoactive sexual desire

Table 33-6 Estrogen Preparations for Treatment of Vaginal Atrophy

Drug Generic (Brand)	Vaginal Formulation	Dose	Regimen
Conjugated equine estrogens (Premarin)	Cream*	0.625 mg per 2 grams of cream	2 grams daily for 2 wks, then 1–2 grams 1–3 ×/wk
Estradiol 0.1% (Estrace)	Cream*	0.1 mg per 2 grams of cream	2 grams daily for 2 wks, then 1–2 g/day × 1–2 wk, then 1–2 grams 1–3 ×/wk
Estradiol (Estring)	Ring	2 mg	Will provide 0.75 mg/d over 90 days
Estradiol acetate (Femring)	Ring	12.4 or 24.8 mg	Will provide 0.5–1.0 mg/d over 90 days
Estradiol hemihydrate (Vagifem)	Tablet	25 mcg	1 tablet daily for 2 wks, then 1 tablet 2 ×/wk

* Creams may be applied vaginally and/or to vulva.

disorder after surgical menopause[32] as well as women who have experienced natural menopause.[39] Several studies reported use of testosterone replacement via a transdermal patch for menopausal women experiencing low sexual desire. All studies were limited in length to 6 months. Overall, it appears a minimum of 300 mcg/day of testosterone administered via a transdermal patch is necessary for improvement of sexual well-being. Long-term use of testosterone replacement has not been studied.

In 2005, three studies revealed that testosterone replacement in the form of a transdermal patch that administered 300 mcg per day, in addition to estrogen replacement, offered a statistically significant increase in sexual well-being. Braunstein et al. studied 447 women, divided into four groups of approximately the same number; all women were taking estrogen therapy. Over the 24-week period, the various groups added a testosterone transdermal patch that delivered 150 mcg, 300 mcg, or 400 mcg per day. No significant differences were reported comparing the estrogen-only group to the women using the 150 mcg/day testosterone patch. However, the women in both the 300-mcg/day and 450-mcg/day testosterone patch had significant improvement.[40]

Similarly, Simon et al. conducted a study of 562 women, divided into two groups. Their study was also conducted over a 24-week period. One group received estrogen alone while the other received estrogen replacement plus 300 mcg/day of testosterone in the form of a transdermal patch. Women using the patch experienced a statistically significant increase in sexual activity ($P = .0003$).[41]

Buster et al. used a 300-mcg/day testosterone transdermal patch and subdivided 533 women into two groups of approximate equal size; one group was on estrogen only and the other was on estrogen plus the testosterone patch. They found sexual activity was increased among women in the testosterone patch group from a mean 0.73 episodes per 4 weeks to 1.56 episodes per week (*P* = .001).[42]

In 2008, Davis et al. conducted a randomized, placebo-controlled, multicenter trial that included 841 women who had experienced natural or surgical menopause and who reported low sexual desire. None of the participants were receiving hormone replacement. They were divided into these three groups: placebo, 150 mcg, or 300 mcg/day of testosterone delivered via transdermal patch. The groups were followed for treatment efficacy for 24 weeks with a follow-up for safety at 52 weeks. Use of the 300 mcg/day testosterone patch resulted in statistically significant improvements from baseline in several domains of sexual functioning (desire, arousal, orgasm, and pleasure), among other areas (including decreased distress and concerns), in women with natural or surgically induced menopause; use of the 150 mcg/day testosterone patch resulted only in significant positive changes in desire and decreased distress.[43] Significant results also included an increase in the number of sexual episodes per month for women receiving 300 mcg/day of testosterone (2.1) versus placebo (0.7); whereas the difference in number of sexual episodes per month in the 150 mcg/day of testosterone group versus the placebo group was not significant. Although the number of sexual episodes in the 300 mcg/day testosterone patch was 1.4 times more per month compared to the placebo group, like other studies in this area, this one failed to report women's opinions of the meaningfulness of these sexual changes.[44]

The studies on transdermal testosterone used a patch that Proctor and Gamble anticipated marketing in the United States as Intrinsa. The Food and Drug Administration has not yet approved the agent, most recently requesting more information, especially about adverse effects. Now there are indications Proctor and Gamble may divest itself of its pharmaceutical branch, and future studies and marketing plans for Intrinsa are unclear.

Side Effects, Adverse Effects, and Contraindications

For any woman considering testosterone, side effects such as acne, hirsutism, unfavorable changes in HDL levels, clitoromegaly, and deepening of the voice need be addressed. Topical testosterone is preferred over oral testosterone to avoid a first bypass through the liver; this results in fewer untoward androgenic side effects. Women with liver disease should not use testosterone. Table 33-7 lists testosterone

preparations for HSDD. Box 33-1 lists the guidelines established by North American Menopause Society for the use of testosterone.

Sildenafil Citrate (Viagra) for Female Sexual Dysfunction

Although not FDA approved for women with sexual dysfunction, the phosphodiesterase type 5 inhibitor (PDE5I) sildenafil citrate (Viagra) has shown promising results, especially for women with hypoactive sexual arousal disorder and female orgasmic disorder secondary to antidepressant use.[45,46] Sildenafil is approved for use for male erectile dysfunction and acts by allowing smooth muscle relaxation and vasocongestion of the genitalia, improving genital blood flow and the sexual-response cycle.[46] At the cellular level, the nitric oxide-cyclic guanosine monophosphatase pathway (cGMP) is necessary for a woman to experience smooth muscle relaxation, vasodilation, and engorgement of the clitoris. Nitric oxide activates guanylate cyclase, which increases levels of cGMP. Phosphodiesterase type 5 breaks down cGMP, decreasing the effect of nitric oxide on vasodilation. Sildenafil, a PDE5I, increases cGMP, allowing nitric oxide to vasodilate smooth muscle, leading to clitoral engorgement. Sildenafil was first proposed as a treatment for angina pectoralis, and the vasodilating effect on genitalia was an incidental finding.[47]

Table 33-7 Testosterone Preparations for Hypoactive Sexual Desire Disorder

Drug Generic (Brand)	Formulation	Formulation	Dosing
Esterified estrogens and methyltestosterone (Estratest)	Tablet	1.25 mg and 2.5 mg	Daily or cyclically, 3 wks on and 1 wk off; reassess q 6 months; women with a uterus must also take a progestin.
Esterified estrogens and methyltestosterone (Estratest HS)	Tablet	0.625 mg and 1.25 mg	Daily or cyclically, 3 wks on and 1 wk off; reassess every 6 months; women with a uterus must also take a progestin.
Testosterone (Androderm)	Transdermal patch	2.5 mg and 5 mg	1.5–4 mg twice a week.
Testosterone 1% (AndroGel)	Gel	5 grams (5 mg)	3 mg/day.
Testosterone enanthate	Injectable	75 mg and 150 mg	IM monthly.

Box 33-1 Clinical Guidelines from North American Menopause Society 2005 Major Recommendations on Use of Testosterone by Postmenopausal Women

Postmenopausal women may be candidates for testosterone therapy if they present with symptoms of decreased sexual desire associated with personal distress and have no other identifiable cause for their sexual concerns.

Testosterone therapy without concomitant estrogen therapy cannot be recommended, because there are no data on the safety and efficacy of testosterone therapy in women not using concomitant estrogen.

Laboratory testing of testosterone levels should be used only to monitor for supraphysiologic testosterone levels before and during therapy, not to diagnose testosterone insufficiency. Laboratory assays are not accurate for detecting testosterone concentrations at the low values typically found in postmenopausal women, and no testosterone level has been clearly linked to a clinical syndrome of hypoandrogenism or testosterone insufficiency. Oral methyltestosterone cannot be measured by standard assays.

Testosterone values vary from laboratory to laboratory. In assessing results of testosterone testing, clinicians should use the reference ranges provided by the testing laboratory.

The simplest and most readily available clinical estimate of free testosterone is the free testosterone index, calculated from total testosterone and sex hormone-binding globulin (SHBG).

The Sodergard equation for free testosterone uses total testosterone, SHBG, and albumin. Although it is a more complex formula, it provides a more accurate calculation than the free testosterone index. It is an option to consider if the testing laboratory can provide the calculation.

Salivary testing is not considered to be a reliable measure of testosterone levels.

Before initiating testosterone treatment, baseline profiles for serum lipids and liver function tests should be established and retesting at 3 months considered. If levels are stable, annual testing is advised.

Testosterone therapy should be administered at the lowest dose for the shortest time that meets treatment goals.

Testosterone transdermal patches and topical gels or creams may be preferred over oral products based on their avoidance of first-pass hepatic effects documented with oral formulations. However, only oral and intramuscular testosterone products for women are currently government approved.

Pellet and intramuscular testosterone formulations have a risk of excessive dosing. Also, administration may be uncomfortable.

Testosterone products formulated specifically for men provide excessive doses for women and should not be used unless doses are reduced considerably and blood testosterone levels are monitored closely for supraphysiologic levels.

Custom-compounded testosterone products should be used with caution because the dosing may be more inconsistent than it is with government-approved products.

There are insufficient data for any conclusions to be made regarding the efficacy and safety of testosterone therapy exceeding 6 months.

Therapeutic monitoring of testosterone therapy should include subjective assessments of sexual response, desire, and satisfaction as well as evaluation for potential adverse effects.

If adverse events are observed with testosterone therapy, dose reductions are advised. If the adverse events do not diminish with lower doses, therapy should be discontinued.

(continues)

> **Box 33-1** Clinical Guidelines from North American Menopause Society 2005 Major Recommendations on Use of Testosterone by Postmenopausal Women (*continued*)
>
> Contraindications of testosterone therapy are focused primarily on those associated with estrogen therapy. However, testosterone therapy should not be initiated in postmenopausal women with breast or uterine cancer or with cardiovascular or liver disease.
>
> Counseling regarding the potential risks and benefits of testosterone use and the limitations of formulations not government approved should be provided before initiating therapy.
>
> *Source:* Reprinted with permission from North American Menopause Society 2005.[34]

There is biologic plausibility for the use of sildenafil (Viagra) for women because of its effect on vasocongestion. However, most of the studies on the agent either are case reports, small studies, or animal research.[48-50] Off-label use of sildenafil for women with hypoactive sexual arousal disorder, female sexual arousal disorder, and female orgasmic disorder has had favorable anecdotal results.

In 2003, Berman et al. reported on the use of sildenafil (Viagra) for treatment of female sexual dysfunction in a 12-week, double-blind, placebo-controlled, multicenter study.[51] An adjustable oral dose of 25 mg to 100 mg of sildenafil versus placebo 1 hour before anticipated sexual activity was used to treat 202 postmenopausal women (whose menopause was either natural or surgically induced) with female sexual arousal disorder. All women were taking hormone therapy, either estrogen alone or estrogen and a progestin. Women with sexual arousal disorder who received sildenafil (Viagra) had significant improvement compared to women who were taking placebo on the two primary efficacy end points, increased sensation/feeling in the genital area during intercourse or stimulation (OR = 2.14; 95% CI, 1.14–4.03; *P* = .017), and increased satisfaction with intercourse and/or foreplay (OR = 2.24; 95% CI, 1.16–4.32; *P* = .015). Women with female sexual arousal disorder and without concomitant hypoactive sexual arousal disorder had results that were statistically more significant; women with hypoactive sexual arousal disorder alone did not appear to benefit from sildenafil.[45]

In 2008, Nurnberg et al. investigated the use of sildenafil (Viagra) for women with antidepressant use–associated female sexual dysfunction. This randomized, controlled trial was relatively small (N = 49) and relatively short (8 weeks), with a 22% attrition rate in each group. Sildenafil was dosed at 25–50 or 100 mg by mouth 1 hour prior to attempting sexual arousal. The group taking sildenafil reported a greater overall sexual response and less sexual dysfunction (RR = 0.8; 95% CI, 0.6–1.0; *P* = .001).[46-50] The most common side effects included flushing, nasal congestion, dyspepsia, and transient visual disturbances.[46]

Contraindications

Contraindications to the use of sildenafil (Viagra) include heart disease, use of nitrates, liver or kidney disease, and peptic ulcer disease. Interactions with the following agents need to be considered, and doses may need to be adjusted: alpha-blockers, antifungals, bosentan (for pulmonary hypertension), CYP3A4 inhibitors (e.g., grapefruit, fluoxetine [Prozac]), etravirine (antiretroviral), HMG-CoA reductase inhibitors (statins), macrolide antibiotics, protease inhibitors, sapropterin (for phenylketonuria), organic nitrates, high-fat meals, alcohol, and St. John's wort. FDA warnings for all PDE5Is on the market include the possibility of a sudden decrease or loss of hearing or eyesight that may be permanent.

There is no evidence that use of dopamine agonists (buspirone or amantadine) or adjunctive bupropion (Wellbutrin) therapy help with SSRI-induced hypoactive sexual arousal disorder, female sexual arousal disorder, or female orgasmic disorder.[52-54] Switching classes of antidepressants, however, may be beneficial.

Herbal Aphrodisiacs

For centuries, potent sexual effects have been attributed to various botanical and herbal combinations. In fiction, be it books, television, or film, women surreptitiously receive these agents in a drink or food and become overwhelmed with sexual desire. Actually, aphrodisiacs are more myth than reality.

The word *aphrodisiac* is derived from Aphrodite, the Greek goddess of love. However, there is no standard definition of an aphrodisiac. Most so-called aphrodisiacs are targeted at men, particularly those with erectile dysfunction. Tiger penis and rhinoceros horns are two commonly mentioned, albeit ineffective, treatments. Oysters, rich in zinc, have been suggested aphrodisiacs perhaps because zinc deficiency is related to male impotency. Prior to the advent of sildenafil (Viagra), yohimbine hydrochloride and melanocortin receptor agonists were available for prescription for erectile dysfunction, but these agents have been replaced largely by sildenafil and tadalafil (Cialis).

The internet contains advertisements for a large number of aphrodisiacs specifically for women. Most of these agents are focused on increasing desire. Scents with pheromones, lubricants with warming sensations, chocolate food items, and a large variety of supplements are sold to women. However, no large, randomized, controlled trials support their use. Box 33-2 describes the classic aphrodisiac, Spanish fly.

Conclusion

Basson wrote, "Augmenting the biologic basis for a woman's sexual responsivity will require concurrent attention to its psychologic basis."[6] The female sexual response is complex and not defined by physiology alone. An increasing number of women are seeking care for sexual concerns. Women will appreciate the clinician who considers their sexual health during routine health visits.

Box 33-2 Gone but Not Forgotten—Spanish Fly

The powder of the Spanish fly has been suggested to be a powerful aphrodisiac, able to drive men and women wild with sexual desire. In reality, the fly is a beetle in the genus *Cantharis*, sometimes called a *cantharide*. Cantharides irritate a male's urethra, with subsequent inflammation causing an erection of the penis. There is no indication that it affects sexual desire for either gender, and it can have major toxic effects, especially on the kidneys. Spanish fly is illegal in the United States, although some herbal agents using a similar name may contain pepper, ginseng, or other ingredients.

References

1. The Kinsey Institute. Mission statement. Available from: *www.indiana.edu/~kinsey/resources/sexology.html* [Accessed December 6, 2008].
2. Masters WH, Johnson VE. Human sexual response. New York: Bantam, 1966.
3. Kaplan HS. The new sex therapy. New York: Brunner-Routledge, 1976.
4. Kammerer-Doak D, Rogers RG. Female sexual function and dysfunction. Obstet Gynecol Clin North Am 2008;35(2):169–83, vii.
5. Sugrue DP, Whipple B. The consensus-based classification of female sexual dysfunction: barriers to universal acceptance. J Sex Marit Therapy 2001;(27):221–6.
6. Basson R. Female sexual response. The role of drugs in the management of sexual dysfunction. Obstet Gynecol 2001; 98:350–3.
7. American Psychiatric Association. Diagnostic and statistical manual for mental disorders. 4th ed., text rev: DSM-IV-TR. Washington, DC: American Psychiatric Press, 2000.
8. Basson R, Berman J, Burnett A, Derogatis L, Ferguson D, Fourcroy J, et al. Report on the international consensus development conference on female sexual dysfunction: definitions and classifications. J Urol 2000; 163:888–93.
9. Association of Reproductive Health Professionals. ARHP clinical proceedings: women's sexual health in midlife and beyond. Washington, DC: Association of Reproductive Health Professionals, May 2005:1–25.
10. AARP. The magazine, TNS NFO Atlanta. Sexuality at midlife and beyond: 2004 update of attitudes and beliefs. Washington, DC: AARP, 2005.
11. Katz VL, Lentz GM, Lobo RA, Gershenson DM. Comprehensive gynecology, 5th ed. Philadelphia, PA: Mosby-Elsevier, 2007:75.
12. Gajdos ZK, Hirschhorn JN, Palmert MR. What controls the timing of puberty? An update on progress from genetic investigation. Curr Opin Endocrinol Diabetes Obes 2009;16(1):16–24.
13. Fonseca H, Greydanus DE. Sexuality in the child, teen and young adult: concepts for the clinician. Prim Care Clin Off Prac 2007;34:275–92.
14. Erickson EH. Identity: Youth and crisis. New York: Norton, 1968:30.
15. Brown RG, Brown JD. Adolescent sexuality. Prim Care Clin Office Pract 2006;33:373–90.

16. Abel GG, Coffey L, Osborn CA. Sexual arousal patterns: normal and deviant. Psychiatr Clin North Am 2008;31:643–55.

17. Ginsberg TB. Aging and sexuality. Med Clin N Am 2000;90:1025–36.

18. Clayton A. Sexual function and dysfunction in women. Psych Clinics of North Am 2003;26:673–82.

19. Rosen RC, Barsky JL. Normal sexual response in women. Obstet Gynecol Clin North Am 2006;33:515–26.

20. Clayton AH. Epidemiology and neurobiology of female sexual dysfunction. J Sex Med 2007; 4(suppl 4): 260–68.

21. Graham CA. Medicalization of women's sexual problems: a different story? J Sex Marital Ther 2007; 33(5): 443–7.

22. Wood JM, Koch PB, Mansfield PK. Women's sexual desire: a feminist critique. J Sex Res 2006;43(3):236–44.

23. Basson R, Leiblum S, Brotto L, Derogates L, Fourcroy J, Fugl-Meyer K, et al. Revised definitions of women's sexual dysfunction. J Sex Med 2004;1(1):40–8.

24. Laumann EO, Paik A, Rosen RC. Sexual dysfunction in the United States: prevalence and predictors. JAMA 1999;281(6):537–44.

25. Laumann EO, Nicolosi A, Glasser DB, Paik A, Gingell C, Moreira E, et al. Sexual problems among women and men aged 40–80 y: prevalence and correlates identified in the global study of sexual attitudes and behaviors. Intern J Impotence Res 2005;17:39–57.

26. Lindau ST, Schumm LP, Laumann EO, Levinson W, O'Muirheartaigh C, Waite LJ. A study of sexuality and health among older adults in the United States. NEJM 2007;357(8):762–74.

27. Shifren JL, Monz BU, Russo PA, Segret A, Johannes CB. Sexual problems and distress in United States women. Obstet Gynecol 2008;112(5):970–7.

28. Simons JS, Carey MP. Prevalence of sexual dysfunctions: results from a decade of research. Arch Sex Behav 2001;30(2):177–219.

29. Basson R, Schultz WW. Sexual sequelae of general medical disorders. Lancet 2007;369:409–24.

30. Wu JM, Wechter ME, Geller EJ, Nguyen TV, Visco AG. Hysterectomy rates in the US, 2003. Obstet Gynecol 2007;110:1091–5.

31. The North American Menopause Society. Position statement: the role of local vaginal estrogen for treatment of vaginal atrophy in postmenopausal women: 2007 position statement of the North American Menopause Society. J North Am Menopause Soc 2007;14(3):357–69.

32. The North American Menopause Society. Position statement: the role of testosterone therapy in postmenopausal women: position statement of the North American Menopause Society. J Menopause: North Am Menopause Soc 2005;12(5):497–511.

33. Montejo-Gonzalez AL, Liorca G, Izquierdo JA, Ledesma A, Bousono M, Calcedo A, Carrasco JL, et al. SSRI-induced sexual dysfunction: fluoxetine, paroxetine, sertraline, and fluvoxamine in a prospective, multicenter and descriptive clinical study of 344 patients. J Sex Marital Ther 1997;23(3):176–94.

34. Rosen RC, Lane RM, Menz M. Effects of SSRIs on sexual function: a critical review. J Clin Psychopharm 1999;19(1):67–85.

35. Dolberg OT, Klag E, Gorss Y, Schreiber S. Relief of serotonin selective reuptake inhibitor induced sexual dysfunction with low-dose mianserin in patients with traumatic brain injury. Psychopharmacology 2002;161: 404–7.

36. Baldessarini RJ. Pharmacotherapy of psychosis and mania. Goodman & Gilman's the pharmacological basis of therapeutics, 11th ed. New York: McGraw Hill, 2006:441–500.

37. The North American Menopause Society. Position statement: estrogen and progesterone in postmenopausal women: July 2008 position statement of the North American Menopause Society. Menopause: J North Am Menopause Soc 2008;15(4):584–603.

38. Suckling J, Lethaby A, Kennedy R. Local oestrogen for vagina atrophy in postmenopausal women. Cochrane Database Syst Rev 2006 Oct 18;(4):CD001500.

39. Somboonporn W, Davis S, Seif MW, Bell R. Testosterone for peri- and menopausal women. Cochrane Database Syst Rev 2005 Oct 19;(4):CD004509.

40. Braunstein GD, Sundwall DA, Katz M, Shifren JL, Buster JE, Simon JA, et al. Safety and efficacy of a testosterone patch for the treatment of hypoactive sexual desire disorder in surgically menopausal women: a randomized, placebo-controlled trial. Arch Intern Med 2005;165:1582–9.

41. Simon J, Braunstein G, Nachtigall L, Utian W, Katz M, Miller S, et al. Testosterone patch increases sexual activity and desire in surgically menopausal women with hypoactive sexual desire disorder. J Clin Endocrinol Metab 2005;90:5226–33.

42. Buster JE, Kingsberg SA, Aguirre O, Brown C, Breaux JG, Buch A, et al. Testosterone patch for low sexual desire in surgically menopausal women: a randomized trial. Obstet Gynecol 2005;105:944–52.

43. Davis SR, Moreau M, Kroll R, Bouchard C, Panay N, Gass M, et al. Testosterone for low libido in postmenopausal women not taking estrogen. N Engl J Med 2008;359:2005–17.

44. Heiman JR. Treating low sexual desire—new findings for testosterone in women. N Engl J Med 2008; 359:2047–9.

45. Berman JR, Berman LA, Toler SM, Gill J, Haughie S for the Sildenafil Study Group. Safety and efficacy of sildenafil citrate for the treatment of female sexual arousal disorder: a double-blind, placebo controlled study. J Urol 2003;170:2333–38.

46. Nurnberg HG, Hensley PL, Heiman JR, Croft HA, Debattista C, Paine S. Sildenafil treatment of women with antidepressant-associated sexual dysfunction. JAMA 2008;300(4):395–404.

47. Cavalcanti Al, Bagnoli VR, Fonseca AM, Pastore RA, Carsoso EB, Paixao JS, et al. Effect of sildenafil on clitoral blood flow and sexual response in postmenopausal women with orgasmic dysfunction. Int J Gynecol Obstet 2008;102:115–9.

48. Carson CC, Lure TF. Great drug classes: phosphodiesterase type 5 inhibitors for erectile dysfunction. BJU Int 2005;96:257–80.

49. Riley A, Scott E, Boolell M. The enhancement of vaginal vasocongestion by sildenafil in healthy premenopausal women. J Womens Health Gend Based Med 2002;11(4):357–65.

50. Angulo J, Cuevas P, Cuevas B, Bischoff E, Sáenz de Tejada I. Vardenafil enhances clitoral and vaginal blood flow responses to pelvic nerve stimulation in female dogs. Int J Impot Res 2003;15(2):137–41.

51. Berman JR, Berman LA, Toler SM, Gill J, Haughie S, for the Sildenafil Study Group. Safety and efficacy of sildenafil citrate for the treatment of female sexual arousal disorder: a double-blind, placebo controlled study. J Urol 2003;170(6 pt 1):2333–8.

52. Michelson D, Bancroft J, Targum S, Kim Y, Tepner R. Female sexual dysfunction associated with antidepressant administration: a randomized, placebo-controlled study of pharmacologic intervention. Am J Psychiatry 2000;157:239–43.

53. Masand PS, Ashton AK, Gupta S, Frank B. Sustained-release bupropion for selective serotonin reuptake inhibitor-induced sexual dysfunction: a randomized, double-blind, placebo-controlled, parallel-group study. Am J Psychiatry 2001;158:805–7.

54. DeBattista C, Solvason B, Poirier J, Kendrick E, Loraas E. A placebo-controlled, randomized, double-blind study of adjunctive bupropion sustained release in the treatment of SSRI-induced sexual dysfunction. J Clin Psychiatry 2005;66:844–8.

55. Kingsberg SA, Janata JW. Female sexual disorders: assessment, diagnosis and treatment. Urol Clin North Am 2007;34(4):497–506.

34
The Mature Woman

Nancy A. Carroll, Susan E. Davis Doughty, Mary Ellen Rousseau, and Mary C. Brucker

✛ Chapter Glossary

17 β-estradiol See *estradiol*.

Abnormal uterine bleeding (AUB) Excessive and or erratic bleeding; a condition that often occurs among perimenopausal women.

Androgens Hormones that are produced in the ovary, adrenal glands, and in fat and muscle tissue where it is converted to estrone. Androgens affect female libido, body habitus, muscle development, energy, and sense of well-being. The adrenal androgens dehydroepiandrosterone (DHEA) and androstenedione decline with age regardless of menopausal status. Testosterone levels do not change during the menopausal transition, but later decline slowly.

Bioidentical hormone therapy Hormone products that are molecularly the same as the hormones naturally present in the body.

Bisphosphonates Drugs that reduce bone resorption by decreasing osteoclast activity.

BMD T-score A measure of bone density. Comparison of the participant's results to the mean peak bone mineral density of a normal, young, same-gender population. A T-score under −2.5 constitutes osteoporosis.

BMD Z-score A measure of bone density. Comparison to a reference population of the same age, gender, and ethnicity. A Z-score of −2 indicates something other than age is causing the low bone mass.

Bone mineral density (BMD) A surrogate marker for bone strength. It is measured by dual-energy X-ray absorptiometry (DEXA) and expressed as grams of mineral per volume. BMD evaluations are made at the hip, femoral neck, and spine. Results are reported as standard deviations from the mean of a reference population.

Dehydroepiandrosterone (DHEA) Androgen produced by the adrenal gland.

Endometrial hyperplasia Condition that occurs when endometrial tissue proliferates excessively. It is most likely to occur in settings where estrogen stimulates the endometrial glands and there is a deficiency of progesterone, which inhibits estrogen's effect on this tissue. Endometrial hyperplasia is a risk factor for the development of endometrial cancer.

Estradiol (E2, 17 β-estradiol) The most biologically active human estrogen of the reproductive age; ovarian in origin.

Estrogen therapy (ET) The use of estrogen alone, without a progestogen, for treatment of postmenopausal symptoms.

Estrone (E1) The dominant circulating estrogen in postmenopause. It is derived primarily from aromatization of androstenedione.

Final menstrual period (FMP) The date of menopause identified after 12 months of no menses.

Hormone therapy (HT) Estrogen with progestogen therapy. It replaces the older term, *hormone replacement therapy (HRT),* which implied *replacement,* whereas HT in much lower doses than produced by the reproductive ovary HT may also represent estrogen with testosterone, but usually is reserved for estrogen plus progesterone.

Osteoblasts Bone building cells located on the surface of the bone; they are immature bone cells in their inactive form.

Osteoclasts Cells that are necessary for reduction of bone volume. They migrate to bone surfaces and promote bone breakdown that later is filled by osteoblast activity.

Osteocytes Mature bone cells that regulate response to stress and mechanical load in part by communication with other osteocytes and osteoblasts. They arise from osteoblasts trapped in bone matrix.

Osteopenia Low bone mass, diagnosed when the T-score falls between −1.0 and −2.5. A T-score under −2.5 constitutes osteoporosis.

Osteoporosis From the Greek word for "porous bone," a condition characterized by low bone mass and microarchitectural deterioration of bone tissue, leading to enhanced bone fragility and consequent increase in fracture risk.

Perimenopause Period of time around menopause that begins with elevated levels of FSH and changes in the length of the cycle. It ends with the FMP, determined retrospectively after 12 months of amenorrhea. Also known as stage −2 into stage +1 using the STRAW continuum.

Phytoestrogens Botanicals including isoflavones and lignins that are often used for management of menopausal symptoms with or without hormones.

Polypharmacy Concomitant use of several drugs. This term is used when more drugs are prescribed than are clinically warranted.

Progestin Hormones with the properties of progesterone, including both synthetic progestational agents (progestogens) and progesterone.

Selective estrogen receptor modulators (SERMs) Estrogen agonists and antagonists, acting like a weak estrogen in some tissues and as an estrogen blocker in others. SERMs are bone preserving.

Sex hormone binding globulin (SHBG) A serum protein produced in the liver that binds both estrogens and androgens, making them unavailable. Oral estrogens have been shown to increase SHBG, causing a decline in bioavailable testosterone.

Stages of reproductive aging workshop (STRAW) A structure of seven stages to describe the menopausal transition.

Thermo-neutral zone A neutral temperature threshold above which sweating occurs, and below which, shivering occurs. The thermo-neutral zone narrows during perimenopause.

Vasomotor symptoms Also referred to as hot flashes, the second most frequently reported symptom after AUB. They increase during perimenopause and are most frequent and intense in the first 2 years after the FMP.

Vulvodynia Chronic vulvar pain (especially on penetration) experienced by up to 15% of the female population.

▌ Introduction

Until the 20th century, many women did not live long enough to reach menopause or suffer the chronic diseases that often accompany aging. For millennia, women died long before menopause, from communicable diseases and complications from reproduction, a situation that unfortunately continues today in some developing nations. A baby girl born in the United States in 1900 had an average life expectancy of 48.3 years,[1] whereas her counterpart born in 2005 has a life expectancy of 80.4 years and should not only reach menopause, but spend the last third of her life in the postmenopausal period. This increase in life expectancy is secondary to a number of factors, including improved nutrition and sanitation and increased knowledge about both healthy habits and risky behaviors. Individuals older than 65 years of age comprise the fastest growing segment of population today in the United States. By the year 2040, senior citizens will account for almost one fourth of the residents in the United States.[2]

The use of medications also has positive influences on life expectancy. Compared to men, women are more likely to live longer, and it is a rare senior citizen of either gender who does not take regular medication for prophylactic reasons (e.g., aspirin to prevent a second cardiac event) or to treat chronic diseases (e.g., an antihypertensive for chronic hypertension). Frequently, individuals use drugs for both reasons, and occasionally add agents to treat acute conditions such as coughs and infections. In general, prescribing for older women requires balancing evidence of effectiveness and safety derived from clinical trials that were conducted with younger subjects, extrapolation of information based on the physiology of the elderly, practical considerations, and the desire of the individual.[3]

Many mature women simultaneously use multiple agents, including prescription and over-the-counter pharmaceuticals. In a study of community-based individuals, women who were ≥ 65 years of age had the highest overall prevalence of drug use, with 12% taking at least 10 medications and 23% reporting taking at least five prescription drugs.[4] Women in nursing homes are estimated to use even more drugs because their medical conditions require such care.

Polypharmacy, or use of multiple drugs concomitantly, is an issue of special concern for the elderly. Some individuals have several chronic conditions, and multiple drugs may work synergistically for therapeutic benefits. However, especially when multiple prescribers are involved, a woman may have drugs from providers who are unaware that she is taking different agents, with a resulting increased risk of adverse effects and drug–drug interactions. Conversely, some drugs may be underused among the elderly, and associated factors have not been well studied.[5] Vaccines for influenza and pneumococcal infections are recommended, but often not received. Antidepressants can be either overused or underused among older women, even though depression is often reported.

Pharmacology and Aging

The physiology of aging presents special considerations for prescribing drugs. Pharmacokinetics and pharmacodynamics can be profoundly influenced by the physiologic changes that occur as a woman ages.[5]

Absorption

Drugs that depend upon an acidic environment for absorption, such as ketoconazole (Nizoral), cefuroxime (Ceftin), and various antivirals, have decreased effectiveness in the age-related higher pH of the stomach, which is due to atrophy of the parietal cells. Older individuals also tend to have a reduced rate of gastric emptying, less blood flow to the small intestine, and decreased surface area of the intestine. All of these factors may further decrease absorption of drugs. Fortunately, factors involved in drug absorption rarely are clinically important, especially since most modern drugs have wide therapeutic indices.

Distribution

The volume of distribution of drugs is also affected over time. As persons age, muscle often is replaced with fat. This increase in fat increases allows for a larger volume of distribution of lipophilic agents and may extend the half-life for elimination. Extracellular and intracellular spaces have less body water, which results in a concentration of some water-soluble drugs in both blood and tissues. The decrease in serum albumin levels is documented, but the clinical significance of lower serum concentrations of albumin is unclear.

Metabolism

Changes in the liver are of major significance. Hepatic mass and blood flow decrease with age, and some agents have reduction of hepatic metabolism and clearance. Due to the marked variability in metabolic changes, individual titration may be required, even for some pharmaceuticals used as maintenance doses. Among agents with reported reduced hepatic metabolism are anti-inflammatory drugs like naproxen (Aleve); cardiovascular drugs such as nifedipine (Procardia), propranolol (Inderal), and verapamil (Calan); estrogen; and psychoactive drugs such as diazepam (Valium).

Excretion

Similar to hepatic changes, renal mass, tubular function, and renal blood flow also decrease as a woman ages. As early as the age of 30, some women experience a drop in creatinine clearance, even though creatinine levels may remain in the normal range. Various agents have been found to have reduced renal elimination because of these factors. These drugs include antibiotics such as ciprofloxacin (Cipro), gentamicin (Garamycin), and nitrofurantoin (Macrobid); cardiovascular agents such as captopril (Capoten), digoxin (Lanoxin), and lisinopril (Zestril, Prinivil); diuretics such as furosemide (Lasix) and hydrochlorothiazide (Maxzide, Dyazide); as well as other agents including cimetidine (Tagamet), lithium (Eskalith, Lithobid), and methotrexate (Trexall, Rheumatrex). Therefore, it is suggested that elderly individuals have regular assessment of renal function and drug use be reviewed at every point of contact with a provider.

Pharmacodynamics

When compared to younger women, mature women may experience unpredictable larger or smaller drug concentrations at the site of action. The changes in effects on cellular and organ function may be due to a variety of factors, most prominently pathophysiology of organ systems. Some individuals become more sensitive to certain agents as they age, including morphine, warfarin (Coumadin), and angiotensin-converting enzyme (ACE) inhibitors. Production of active metabolites (e.g., benzodiazepines) among the elderly may be an additional factor in causing increased sedation.

Drug–Drug Interactions

Polypharmacy presents an important risk for adverse drug–drug interactions in this population. Alternatively, women should not be denied appropriate therapy simply because of age. A good rule of thumb is that mature women should be treated when needed, with the lowest effective doses and monitored regularly for therapeutic and adverse effects, although it may be argued that this approach is warranted for all women regardless of age.[6]

Most of the chapters in this book focus on drugs for specific conditions and address use of the agents among the elderly. The reader is directed to the chapter of interest for specific drugs. Age-specific conditions such as menopause and osteoporosis are discussed in this chapter.

Transition to Menopause

Meno is derived from the Greek word for month, and *pause* is derived from the Greek word for pauses, or halt. *Menopause* is the technical term for a point at which menses and fertility cease. All healthy women make the transition to menopause, but each will experience this physiologic passage in a unique way. The shift from the reproductive phase of life begins in a woman's mid- to late forties and continues for several years. The average age of natural menopause, approximately 51.4 years, has remained constant for the last several hundred years despite improvements in nutrition and health care.[6]

Most women experience the transition to and through menopause as a normal part of life. An individual woman's experience will be influenced by her beliefs about aging, her lifestyle, culture, and menopause-related symptoms.

For some women, menopause occurs when there is finally time to focus on relationships and personal interests and presents few problems. In 1996, a study in the United Kingdom of more than 8000 women aged 45–54 years of age reported that the majority of women surveyed had a symptom of menopause (e.g., vasomotor and atrophic symptoms). However, only 22% perceived them as problematic to any degree.[7] Other women undergo this transition at a time when they are still parenting teenagers, caring for their own parents, working outside of the home, and feeling stressed by multiple responsibilities. Similar menopausal symptoms can be perceived as one more part of a chaotic life. In addition, a few women may experience severe symptoms that negatively influence their quality of life.

Stages in the Reproductive Cycle

In 2001, a multidisciplinary conference focused on menopause and research derived from the TREMIN Research Program, previously known as the TREMIN Trust, the world's largest repository of data on menstruation.[8] Named the **Stages of reproductive aging workshop** (STRAW), this conference offered a framework that is useful for describing the menopausal transition.[9] The STRAW continuum includes seven stages—five occurring before menopause and two after (Figure 34-1). All women do not progress linearly. Some women may skip a stage entirely, while others slip in and out of adjacent categories.

Stages:	−5	−4	−3	−2	−1	0	+1	+2
Terminology:	Reproductive			Menopausal transition			Postmenopause	
	Early	Peak	Late	Early	Late*		Early*	Late
				Perimenopause				
Duration of stage:	Variable			Variable		(a) 1 yr	(b) 4 yrs	Until demise
Menstrual cycles:	Variable to regular	Regular		Variable cycle length (> 7 days different from normal)	≥ 2 skipped cycles and an interval of amenorrhea (≥ 60 days)	Amen × 12 months	None	
Endocrine:	Normal FSH	↑ FSH		↑ FSH			↑ FSH	

Final menstrual period (FMP) — 0

Recommended staging system.
* Stages most likely to be characterized by vasomotor symptoms, follicle-stimulating hormone (FSH) increase, and amenorrhea. Stage +1 is subdivided into segment "a" for first 12 months after FMP and "b" for next 4 years.

Figure 34-1 Stages of reproductive aging workshop (STRAW). *Source:* Reprinted with permission from Soules MR et al. 2001.[9]

The first three stages of STRAW occur during the reproductive years. These stages are divided into *early reproductive*, or –5 (when cycles may be either variable or regular, and follicle-stimulating hormone [FSH] levels indicate ovarian responsiveness), *peak reproductive*, or –4 (regular cycles and FSH indicative of responsive ovaries), and *late reproductive*, or –3 (when cycles remain regular but FSH levels rise).

The next two stages encompass the time of *menopausal transition*, or **perimenopause**, and lead to the **final menstrual period** (FMP). The FMP is the date of menopause, but cannot be noted as such until 12 months afterward, making menopause a retrospective diagnosis. During both of these stages, there are elevated levels of FSH and an increased number of irregular cycles. In stage –2, the *early transition*, cycle interval shortens by 7 days or more. At least two skipped cycles define stage –1, the *late transition*. The FMP occurs at stage 0. The *early postmenopause*, stage +1, encompasses the first 4 years after the FMP. Late postmenopause, stage +2, continues from that time until the woman's death.[9] This section focuses on both early and late menopausal transition, stages –2 and –1, leading up to the FMP. Pharmacologic management of menopausal symptoms most commonly involves the use of hormones. Therefore, a brief review of the reproductive hormones and hormone receptors is in order. Additional information can be found in Chapter 14.

Hormones in Flux: An Overview of Estrogen and Progesterone for the Mature Woman

Changes in the central nervous system's control of the ovaries and accelerated ovarian follicular atresia or cell death precede menopause. The follicles that are left this late in the reproductive years are likely to be resistant to follicle-stimulating hormone (FSH). As their numbers decline in the presence of FSH resistance, the pituitary increases secretion of FSH in an attempt to promote ovulation. An FSH level of ≥ 40 mIU marks the end of the menopausal transition when a woman can expect no more menses. Changes in endogenous hormones as well as hormonal therapy can interfere with the clinical usefulness of FSH testing, so the best marker for menopause simply is 12 months after the FMP.[10]

Initially, ovarian follicular development may be sustained. On occasion, more than one follicle can be recruited per cycle, which stimulates ovarian production of estrogen and causes elevated levels of **17 β-estradiol**, which is also called **estradiol** or **E2**.[10] Besides thickening the endometrium, increased E2 secretion may lead to the growth of uterine fibroids and menorrhagia, as well as symptoms of breast tenderness, bloating, and irritability.

Later in the transition, the remaining ovarian follicles become more resistant to FSH and luteinizing hormone (LH). Ovulation usually is erratic, and the levels of E2 can fluctuate widely. When estrogen levels are low because of the failure of follicular development, ovulation may not occur, resulting in lack of a corpus luteum. Without a corpus luteum, there is inadequate progesterone to allow the endometrial lining to be converted to secretory tissue. Although irregular or unpredictable bleeding usually is a normal part of the perimenopause transition, when it occurs it should be evaluated to rule out endometrial polyps and development of **endometrial hyperplasia**, which is associated with an increased risk for uterine cancer. Irregular bleeding is the most frequently reported sign of the transition to menopause.[11]

As follicles become increasingly unresponsive to FSH, E2 levels decline, and women continue to experience irregular bleeding, ultimately culminating in permanent amenorrhea. Vasomotor symptoms and vaginal dryness may precede or coincide with the last menstrual period.[8] **Estrone** (E1), by default, becomes the dominant circulating estrogen derived primarily from aromatization of androstenedione. Obese women have higher levels of estrone, with adipose tissue as a primary source.[12]

Women in the perimenopausal and postmenopausal stages continue to produce ovarian **androgens**, but not in the same amount as in earlier years. Although androgens often are thought of as male hormones, they have been shown to affect female libido, body habitus, muscle development, energy, and sense of well-being. Since androgens are precursors of estrogen, androgens have an important role for postmenopausal women. Androgens are produced in the ovary, adrenal glands, and peripherally by substrate conversion to become the weakest estrogen, estrone (E1).

The adrenal androgens, **dehydroepiandrosterone** (DHEA) and androstenedione, decline with age regardless of menopausal status, or even gender.[10] Testosterone levels of ovarian origin do not change appreciably during the menopausal transition, but later decline slowly over time. This demonstrates the appreciable role postmenopausal ovaries continue to play in women past their menopause. At any given point, only 1–2% of testosterone is unbound and, therefore, metabolically active. The remainder is tightly attached to **sex hormone binding globulin** (SHBG). Oral estrogens have been shown to increase SHBG, causing a decline in bioavailable testosterone.[11]

Hormone Receptors

Proteins found in the fluid within the cell or the cytosol bind to sex hormones and transfer the hormone into the cell nucleus. Two distinct hormone receptors, ER-α and ER-β, have been identified for estrogen. Concentrations of the receptors vary in different tissues, with more ER-α receptors in the reproductive tissue and liver, and more ER-β receptors in bone, blood vessels, and lungs.[13] Both types of receptors are found in the ovary and central nervous system and are discussed in more detail in Chapter 14. Estrogen receptors bind to a variety of substances, or ligands, which vary in their affinity for ER-α and ER-β. Both estrogen receptors bind to 17 β-estradiol, but the weaker phytoestrogens found in some plants and foods seem to have a higher affinity for ER-β.[14]

The response to ligand binding to an estrogen receptor is complex and initiates a series of steps that involve coactivators or corepressors. This phenomenon is the origin of the term **selective estrogen receptor modulators** (SERMs). These agents can cause an antagonist effect in one tissue but stimulate an agonist effect in different tissue when bound to the estrogen receptor (Chapter 14). For example, the drug tamoxifen (Nolvadex) is an antagonist in breast tissue, associated with decreased risk of breast cancer but a partial agonist in uterine tissue, associated with an increased risk of endometrial cancer.

Progesterone receptors (PRs) also are subtyped in a similar fashion. PR-α and PR-β are found in most tissues, with PR-α dominant in the ovary and uterus and PR-β in the breast. Progesterone agonists and antagonists are currently being evaluated in many drug trials. Mifepristone (RU 486, Mifeprex) is the only progesterone product available and is used primarily for labor induction, missed abortion, and pregnancy termination.

Recently, a new class of drugs called selective progesterone receptor modulators (SPRMs) have been identified. These agents are progesterone receptor ligands with mixed agonist/antagonist properties has been described. In the future, progesterone antagonists with mixed properties may be helpful in treating menopausal uterine fibroids as well as endometriosis and cancer.[15]

Hormone Therapy for Primary Prevention of Chronic Conditions: Panacea or Poison?

Symptoms of potential concern to mature women during perimenopause include a decline in fertility and irregular uterine bleeding. As the transition evolves (from stage −2 to stage −1), more women note vasomotor symptoms (hot flashes), vaginal dryness, genitourinary symptoms such as

dyspareunia or pruritus, and sleep disturbances, although the relationship between these symptoms and menopause is not always clear.[6] Each of these conditions will be addressed later in the chapter. However, it is difficult to discuss care of the perimenopausal or menopausal woman without first discussing use of hormones, especially because these drugs often have been prescribed for multiple reasons, including as a general panacea.

Estrogen therapy was first advocated in the 1960s (Box 34-1).[16-19] Later, the finding that unopposed estrogen could be carcinogenic caused a rapid decrease in use of the agent. However, when progesterone was added to the regimen to counteract estrogen's effect on uterine endometrium, the formulations prescribed were renamed hormone replacement therapy (HRT) and slowly began to regain popularity. More than 68 million prescriptions for conjugated estrogens Premarin or Prempro, the two most commonly used formulations, were written in the year 2000.[20]

Today the word *replacement* is falling into disuse because hormone formulations of estrogen and progesterone do not replace hormones to the premenopausal levels. The term **hormone therapy** (HT) currently is preferred to designate estrogen and progestin therapy, although a few authorities use the notation E + P. The abbreviation ET is

---

Box 34-1   Estrogen-Deficient State: Gone But Not Forgotten

Estrogen products for the treatment of menopausal symptoms were first approved by the FDA in 1941 and became popular by the 1960s following the publication of Robert Wilson's book, *Feminine Forever*.[16,17] Wilson, a gynecologist, described menopause as an estrogen-deficient state and promoted the use of estrogen for treatment of multiple symptoms, some of which were likely to be secondary to aging and not specific to menopause. Wilson's work was widely disseminated and pharmaceutical companies marketed the products before the 1962 amendments to the Food Drug and Cosmetics Act required demonstrable safety. By 1975, it was clear that unopposed estrogen therapy was associated with a significantly increased risk for endometrial hyperplasia and endometrial cancer (fivefold increased risk after 3 years of therapy).[18,19] Until it was discovered that the addition of a progestin could decrease the endometrial risk, hormonal use fell into disfavor.

used for **estrogen therapy** alone. In this chapter, HT and ET will be used throughout. Although the term *hormone* may refer to a wide variety of agents including thyroid and growth hormones, for the sake of simplicity in this chapter, it is used to refer to estrogen and progesterone.

Over the last several decades, questions have emerged about the indications, effectiveness, and safety of the use of hormones. Many of the early studies such as the Nurses' Health Study, were exclusively observational. However, large, randomized trials now have been conducted, some with unexpected findings.[21-26] Table 34-1 offers a brief review of major studies on postmenopausal hormones published in various journals. Prominent among them is the Women's Health Initiative.

A Watershed Study: The Women's Health Initiative

Observational data, especially from the large Nurses' Health Study, suggested that women using hormones not only had a decrease in menopausal symptomatology, but perhaps more importantly, a decrease in cardiovascular events. By the mid-1990s, many clinicians were prescribing hormones prophylactically for mature women, in a similar way aspirin is recommended for cardiac protection. This widespread use, combined with other assumed advantages and risks of estrogen, was the impetus for a large, randomized clinical trial (RCT) in the United States called the Women's Health Initiative (WHI). The WHI was composed of several smaller studies, including a primary prevention study to evaluate the role of hormones in cardiac disease prevention.[27]

Participants who had undergone a hysterectomy were given 0.625 mg conjugated equine estrogen (CEE, Premarin) or a placebo daily. These women comprised the ET arm of this randomized, controlled placebo trial.[28] Women with a uterus received 0.625 mg CEE plus 2.5 mg medroxyprogesterone acetate (MPA; Prempro) or placebo daily and were part of the HT arm of the WHI trial.[27]

Table 34-1 Hormone Trials with Postmenopausal Women

Trial Name	Year	Type of Study	Number and Type of Subjects	Study Intention	Major Findings, Journal Reporting
PEPI[21]	1991	RCT	875 postmenopausal; 32% previous hysterectomy	Effects of HT on CHD risk factors	Three groups: CEE alone, CEE plus 2.5, 10 MPA, CEE plus 200 mg micronized progesterone. Found increased HDL, decreased LDL and fibrinogen. Micronized progesterone had less blunting of estrogen lipid benefit than MPA. No effect on BP.
WHI HT[22]	1993	RCT	16,608 postmenopausal age 50–79, majority 10 years after FMP	Primary cardiac protection	Studied women on CEE plus MPA versus placebo and women on CEE only. Found increased risk of MI, DVT, CVA, and breast cancer. Decreased risk of colon cancer and hip fracture. No evidence of cardiac protection.
WHI ET[23]	1993	RCT	10,739 all without uterus	Primary cardiac protection	Studied CEE only versus placebo or CEE plus MPA. Found small increased risk of CVA. Placebo group had nonsignificant higher risk of breast cancer than CEE group. No evidence of cardiac protection.
Million Woman Study (UK)[41]	1996	Observational	1,084,110 aged 50–64	HT, ET influence on risk of various conditions	Studied ET and HT according to report by more than 1 million women over the age of 50 (approximately 25% of the age population). Found HT current users increased risk of breast cancer by 100%; ET current users increased risk 30%. Risk increased with duration of treatment. Study ongoing with additional research being published on various conditions such as HT and gallbladder risk.
HERS[25]	1998	RCT	2763 postmenopausal and post-MI	Secondary cardiac protection	Studied CEE/MPA group versus placebo among women who had experienced a cardiac event. Found increased risk of second MI, 2–3 × risk DVT, increased gallbladder disease.
HOPE[26]	2001	RCT	2805 postmenopausal; mean age 53	Risk involved with lower dose HT	Studied CEE 0.625; MPA 0.5–2.5 or placebo. Found HT, even lower dose, had decreased hyperplasia, more amenorrhea. Typical dose had improved bone density. No difference: hot flashes, atrophic vagina, lipid effect among groups.

CHD = coronary heart disease; MI = myocardial infarction; HDL = high-density lipoprotein; LDL = low-density lipoprotein; BP = blood pressure; DVT = deep vein thrombosis; CVA = cerebrovascular accident.
Sources: The Writing Group for the PEPI 2001[21]; Manson JE et al. 2003[22]; Anderson G et al. 2004[23]; Beral V et al. 2004[24]; Hulley S et al. 1998[25]; Pickar JH 2003[26]; Beral V et al. 1996.[41]

The WHI HT study had an early termination after 5.2 of the planned 8 years, when it became apparent that HT failed to provide primary prevention of coronary heart disease (CHD) and the increase in invasive breast cancer exceeded the preset stopping point (breast cancer hazard ratio [HR] = 1.26; 95% CI, 1.00–1.59).[27] The breast cancer finding became media news around the world with little discussion of what was the more surprising finding, namely the failure of HT to provide cardiac protection. HT also was associated with some risks, including an increased incidence of thrombotic/ischemic stroke after 2 years of therapy. Although studies prior to the WHI found a higher risk of ovarian cancer mortality among women who used postmenopausal estrogen therapy for more than 10 years,[29] in the WHI no such finding was found among women who used HT. The latter may be explained by the small number of ovarian cancer cases.[30]

Beneficial effects of HT also were found, including a decrease of 37% in the incidence of colon cancer (HR = 0.63; 95% CI, 0.43–0.92) and a 24% decrease in hip fractures (HR = 0.66; 95% CI, 0.45–0.98).[27] However, the overall global index of risk versus benefit showed no statistical significance.[30] Because of the publicity in the popular press about the cancer risks involved with the use of hormones, it is helpful for prescribers to appreciate the absolute numbers (Table 34-2) of adverse effects instead of the relative risks that are most often quoted in media reports about the WHI.[17,27]

It is notable that the WHI exclusively studied women taking either placebo alone, CEE alone, or CEE and MPA. Experts are undecided if the results can be extrapolated to other hormone formulations, although the North American Menopause Society (NAMS) suggests that in the absence of data, the results of one estrogen or progesterone should be generalized to other estrogens and/or progesterones.[29]

Differences also were found between those women treated with HT and those on ET. Similar to the HT trial, the ET trial also was ended early after 6.8 years, when an increased risk of stroke was found in the absence of apparent benefit for the risk of CHD.[23] A trend was found toward a slightly lower, albeit not statistically significant, rate of breast cancer risk in the ET treatment arm of the study.[30]

At this time, there continues to be ongoing adjudication of the WHI data. A subgroup analysis of the WHI trials of women aged 50–59 indicated there was a reduced risk of CHD among women who took ET alone or who were themselves less than 10 years from the FMP, although no statistically significant findings have been reported.[30] The issues needing further study include differentiating between oral and nonoral HT, the effects of nonoral HT, the effects of androgens, as well as the effects on trust of women in the healthcare system.[11,31]

Cancer and Hormones: Reality or Public Scare?

Estrogen is said to be a known carcinogen because of the relationship between the agent and endometrial cancer. However, the exact relationships with other cancers remain more elusive. A review of 51 population observational studies from the 1980s and 1990s noted an increase in breast cancer risk among current and recent users of HT when compared to nonusers. This risk essentially decreased 5 years after discontinuation of HT.[32] The HT arm of the WHI study also found an increase in the risk of invasive breast cancer, and the breast cancers diagnosed were more advanced than the breast cancers diagnosed in women taking the placebo.[33] However, women in the ET arm did not have an increased risk of breast cancer during the first 7 years of follow-up.[34] Six types of breast cancer were evaluated among users and nonusers of HT and ET as part of the Million Women Study, and the global

Table 34-2 Summary of Women's Health Initiative Estrogen Plus Progestin (HT) Study

Outcome Measure	Hazard Ratio and 95% Confidence Interval for HT vs No HT	Women Using HT (CEE + MPA) Events per 10,000 Person-Years	Women on Placebo Events per 10,000 Person-Years	Absolute Risk (HT vs No HT in 10,000 Women over 1 Year)
Invasive breast cancer	1.26 (1.00–1.59)	38	30	8 more women affected
Coronary heart disease	1.29 (1.02–1.63)	37	30	7 more women affected
Cerebrovascular accident/stroke	1.41 (1.07–1.85)	28	21	8 more women affected
Venous thromboembolism*	2.11 (1.58–2.52)	34	16	8 more women affected
Hip fractures	0.66 (0.45–0.98)	10	15	5 fewer women affected
Colorectal cancer	0.63 (0.43–0.92)	10	16	6 fewer women affected

* Includes deep vein thrombosis and pulmonary embolism.
Sources: Adapted from Rousseau ME 2002[17]; Rossouw JE et al. 2002.[27]

risk was significantly increased among all current users, although the risk was lower among women with higher body mass index.[35] Interestingly, none of these studies found an increase in cancer mortality among the women who developed breast cancer.

Another area of controversy is whether women who are breast cancer survivors should take ET or HT. Several short-term studies conducted for less than 5 years found no increase in recurrence of breast cancer.[36,37] A review of 15 studies with more than 1400 breast cancer survivors and almost 2000 women without such a history failed to find any increase in cancer recurrence with HT. Research today is finding that breast cancer is not a single disease, but rather a group of molecularly distinct neoplastic disorders.[38] It is likely that as research develops, so will a greater understanding of hormonal influences on breast cancer.

Ovarian cancer is another major cancer that affects women. Several observational studies had suggested that use of estrogen is associated with an increased risk of ovarian cancer for women who used this agent for 10 or more years.[39,40] The results from the Million Women Study reported that women currently using ET or HT had an increased risk of developing ovarian cancer and dying from the disease compared with nonusers, although the increased risk disappeared after hormone use stopped.[41] The WHI failed to find a statistical association between use of hormones and ovarian cancer, although there may not have been adequate time because the duration of the study was less than 10 years.[30]

▌ Pharmacologic Management of Hormones

Initiating Hormones: Indications

Hormone therapy, whether it is ET or HT, offers documented relief for hot flashes, night sweats, sleep problems related to hot flashes, and vaginal discomforts. Women who suffer with these symptoms usually seek advice. Once starting HT, relief often is afforded within days for hot flashes. Vaginal conditions may be associated with sexual problems, both of which are likely to be relieved with hormonal use, although improvement for vaginal problems may take as long as 2 months. Pharmaceuticals should be offered to women who have distressing symptoms to improve quality of life. Some women need professional support to allay fears and risks about using hormones.

Known Risks and Benefits

The case for and against use of hormones has become increasingly controversial as more data have emerged. After the WHI trial was published, it was recommended that use of hormones should be restricted for relief of the known symptoms, which only included hot flashes and vaginal symptoms. Currently the FDA approves use of hormones for severe vasomotor symptoms, treatment of moderate to severe vulvar/vaginal symptoms, and prevention of postmenopausal osteoporosis.[42] However, before using hormones for prevention of osteoporosis, other options should be considered because of the risk profile associated with these agents. Table 34-3 summarizes benefits and risks to the use of hormones.

Contraindications

Significant contraindications exist to the use of hormones and are listed in Table 34-4. Contraindications usually can be evaluated through a thorough health history, a complete physical exam, and a screening mammography. Even though there is some controversy about the association between hormone use and cancer, many breast cancers are hormone dependent, so it is generally agreed that women with known or suspected cancer of the breast should not take hormones. Ovarian and endometrial cancers also may be hormonally dependent, thus precluding the use of steroidal hormones. Known heart disease including coronary heart disease, stroke, and history of thromboembolic disease are contraindications. Hormones are contraindicated for women with a history of biliary tract disease as well as liver disease. Estrogen is metabolized through the liver, and if there is compromised liver function, serum estrogen levels can become dangerously high.

Table 34-3 Risks and Benefits of the Use of Hormones

Potential Risks	Potential Benefits
Breast cancer	Relief of vasomotor symptoms
Endometrial cancer*	Reduced risk of colorectal cancer
Stroke	Reduced risk of coronary heart disease potentially among healthy women in early STRAW stages†
Venous thromboembolism	Reduced risk of dementia
	Reduced risk of diabetes mellitus
	Reduced risk of osteoporosis and osteoporosis-related fractures

*In women with an intact uterus treated with estrogen alone.
† Controversial.

Use of a Risk Profile

Creation of an individualized risk profile is advisable before using hormones for treatment for menopausal symptoms to evaluate a woman's cardiovascular and breast cancer risks as illustrated in Table 34-5. The woman and her healthcare provider should discuss whether the woman might be willing to assume specific risks, especially given the impact of menopausal symptoms on her specific quality of life. Women may differ in their choices after discussing the risks and benefits in light of a personal health history and the seriousness of symptoms. Because many of the risks of ET and HT are well documented, a fully informed consent for their use must be obtained and included in the health record prior to initiating therapy.

Table 34-4 Contraindications to Use of Hormones

Absolute Contraindications to Estrogen Use	Absolute Contraindications to Progestogen Use
Known or suspected cancer of the breast	Active thrombophlebitis or thromboembolic disease
Known or suspected estrogen-dependent neoplasia	Liver dysfunction or disease
History of uterine or ovarian cancer	Known or suspected cancer of the breast
History of coronary heart disease or stroke	Undiagnosed abnormal genital bleeding
History of biliary tract disorder	Pregnancy
Undiagnosed abnormal genital bleeding	
History of active thrombophlebitis or thromboembolic disease	

Formulations and Route

A number of hormone therapy options exist for postmenopausal women. Table 34-6 provides the doses, various potencies, and routes of different formulations of hormones used for HT and ET. All formulations are equally effective in treating menopausal symptoms and preserving bone density. Some women prefer synthetic hormones or hormones from plant products to CEE, as the latter is derived from pregnant mare urine, hence the brand name Premarin.

Table 34-5 Risk Profile to Consider Prior to Initiating Hormones

Cardiovascular Risk	Breast Cancer Risks
Age: over 50/postmenopausal	Increases with aging
CRP elevated	Nulliparous
HDL/C:LDL/C ratio greater than 2.1	First pregnancy after 30
Sedentary lifestyle	First-degree relative with diagnosis
Elevated waist:hip ratio	Breast density increased
HDL below 50	Atypia diagnosed by breast biopsy
LDL over 130	Alcohol use in excess of 2 drinks per day
Triglycerides over 150	Low vegetable and fruit diet
First-degree relative with MI before age 50	Lack of exercise/obesity
Hypertension	Radiation exposure
Diabetes	Menarche before 12
Active smoking	Menopause after 53
	Active smoking
	Female gender

MI = myocardial infarction.

Table 34-6 FDA-Approved Hormones

Product Generic (Brand)	Formulations	Indications
Estrogen (oral)		
Synthetic conjugated estrogens (Cenestin)	0.3 mg, 0.45 mg, 0.625 mg, 0.9 mg, 1.25 mg	Vasomotor/vaginal symptoms
Synthetic conjugated estrogens (Enjuvia)	0.3 mg, 0.45 mg, 0.625 mg, 0.9 mg, 1.25 mg	Vasomotor/vaginal symptoms
Estradiol—micronized (Estrace)	0.5 mg, 1 mg, 2 mg	Vasomotor/vaginal symptoms
Estradiol acetate (Femtrace)	0.45 mg, 0.9 mg, 1.8 mg	Vasomotor/vaginal symptoms
Esterified estrogens (Menest)	0.3 mg, 0.625 mg, 1.25 mg, 2.5 mg	Vasomotor/vaginal symptoms
Estropipate (Ogen)	0.625 mg, 1.25 mg, 2.5 mg	Vasomotor/vaginal symptoms
Estropipate (Ortho-Est)	0.625 mg, 1.25 mg	Vasomotor/vaginal symptoms
Conjugated equine estrogens (Premarin)	0.3 mg, 0.45 mg, 0.625 mg, 0.9 mg, 1.25 mg, 2.5 mg	Vasomotor/vaginal symptoms
Estrogen (transdermal)		
Estradiol (Alora)	0.025, 0.05, 0.075, 0.1 mg per day	Vasomotor/vaginal symptoms
Estradiol (Climara)	0.025, 0.0375, 0.05, 0.06, 0.075, 0.1 mg per day	Vasomotor/vaginal symptoms
Estradiol (Divigel)	0.25, 0.5, 1 mg/packet	Vasomotor/vaginal symptoms
Estradiol (Elestrin)	0.87g/pump	Vasomotor/vaginal symptoms

(continues)

Table 34-6 FDA-Approved Hormones (*continued*)

Product Generic (Brand)	Formulations	Indications
Estradiol (Esclim)	0.025, 0.0375, 0.05, 0.075, 0.1 mg per day	Vasomotor/vaginal symptoms
Estradiol (Estraderm)	0.05, 0.1 mg per day	Vasomotor/vaginal symptoms
Estradiol (Estrasorb)	1.74 g/pouch	Vasomotor/vaginal symptoms
Estradiol (EstroGel)	1.25 g/pump	Vasomotor/vaginal symptoms
Estradiol (Menostar)	0.014 mg per day	Vasomotor/vaginal symptoms
Estradiol (Vivelle)	0.05, 0.1 mg per day	Vasomotor/vaginal symptoms
Estradiol (Vivelle-DOT)	0.025, 0.0375, 0.05, 0.075, 0.1 mg per day	Vasomotor/vaginal symptoms
Estrogen (vaginal)		
Estradiol (Estrace)	0.01% (0.1 mg/g)	Vaginal symptoms
Estradiol (Estring)	7.5 mcg/24 hours	Vaginal symptoms
Estradiol (Femring)	0.05 mg per day, 0.1 mg per day	Vaginal symptoms Vasomotor symptoms
Conjugated equine estrogens (Premarin)	0.625 mg/g	Vaginal symptoms
Estradiol (Vagifem)	25 mcg	Vaginal symptoms
Progestogen (oral)		
Norethindrone acetate (Aygestin)	5 mg	Prevent endometrial hyperplasia
Progesterone—micronized (Prometrium)	100 mg, 200 mg twice daily	Prevent endometrial hyperplasia
MPA (Provera)	2.5 mg, 5 mg, 10 mg	Prevent endometrial hyperplasia
Combined estrogen and progestogen (oral)		
Estradiol/norethindrone acetate (Activella)	1 mg/0.5 mg	Vasomotor/vaginal symptoms
Estradiol/drospirenone (Angeliq)	1 mg/0.5 mg	Vasomotor/vaginal symptoms
Norethindrone acetate + ethanol estradiol (Femhrt)	0.5 mg/2.5 mcg, or 1 mg/5 mcg	Vasomotor/vaginal symptoms
Estradiol 3 tablets, then estradiol/norgestimate 3 tablets, repeat (Prefest)	1 mg; then 1 mg/0.09 mg, repeat	Vasomotor/vaginal symptoms
Conjugated equine estrogens 14 tablets; then conjugated estrogens/MPA 14 tablets (Premphase)	0.625 mg; then 0.625 mg/5 mg	Vasomotor/vaginal symptoms
Conjugated equine estrogens/MPA 28 tablets (Prempro)	0.3 mg/1.5 mg; 0.45 mg/1.5 mg; 0.625 mg/2.5 mg; 0.625 mg/5 mg	Vasomotor symptoms
Combined estrogen and progestogen (transdermal)		
Estradiol/levonorgestrel (Climara Pro)	Delivers 0.045 mg/0.015 mg per day	Vasomotor/vaginal symptoms
Estradiol/norethindrone acetate (CombiPatch)	Delivers 0.05 mg/0.14 mg per day, or 0.05 mg/0.25 mg per day	Vasomotor/vaginal symptoms
Estrogen + androgen (oral)		
Esterified estrogens/methyl testosterone (Estratest H.S.)	0.625 mg/1.25 mg	Vasomotor/vaginal symptoms
Esterified estrogens/methyl testosterone (Estratest)	1.25 mg/2.5 mg	Vasomotor/vaginal symptoms

MPA = medroxyprogesterone acetate.

Few clinically significant differences exist between estrogens. Although there is no method to identify which specific agent or formulation is best suited for individual women, the different pharmacokinetics involved in the routes are worth consideration.

The oral route often is preferred because women are comfortable taking pills. Estrogen delivered orally has a greater effect on the liver secondary to the first-pass effect, which delivers high concentrations via the portal circulation. Estrogen stimulates hepatic production of sex hormone-binding globulin, triglycerides, high-density lipoprotein (HDL), and clotting factors, which are, therefore, increased in women who take oral formulations. Nonoral hormones offer the advantage of elimination of the first-pass hepatic effect thus diminishing peaks and nadirs of the drug, maintenance of more stable serum hormone levels, and prevention of the gastrointestinal-tract conversion of more potent estradiol to the weaker estrone as well as other gastrointestinal side effects.[43] Transdermal and vaginal preparations are preferred in certain clinical situations such as for women with hypertension, hypertriglyceridemia, and the individual who is at risk for cholelithiasis, as listed in Box 34-2.[44]

Box 34-2   Potential Indications for Nonoral Routes for Hormone Therapy

Therapy

Decreased libido

Depression

Gallbladder disease

GI dysfunction

Hypertension also contraindicated in nonoral products

Increased triglycerides

Migraines sensitive to hormones

Nicotine addiction

Symptoms do not respond to oral therapy

Type 2 diabetes

Woman's preference for nondaily regimen such as a transdermal patch

Note: Skin redness or itch at site of transdermal patches is an indication to switch to a transdermal gel.

Source: John SC et al. 2007.[44]

Box 34-3   To Treat or Not to Treat: Are Progestins Needed with Topical Estrogens

For women posthysterectomy who use estrogen therapy or hormone therapy, a progestin is unnecessary because there is no risk of endometrial hyperplasia or cancer. When a woman with an intact uterus takes estrogen orally or transdermally, a progestin is added to counter abnormal endometrial growth.[47] However, there exists a controversy about the need for a progestin when a woman uses a topical estrogen such as creams and rings for vaginal atrophy. The North American Menopause Society has stated that when low-dose estrogen is used vaginally at doses approved for the indication of vaginal atrophy, a progestin is not needed as serum estrogen levels are not high enough to adversely affect the endometrium.[48-50] However, some authorities disagree and note that topical estrogens are readily absorbed through the vaginal mucosa and for some women can result in appreciable blood levels, especially when the estrogen is used for periods longer than a year.[42] Until clear evidence is published, professionals are left to use their own clinical acumen in regard to this controversy.

Dosing Considerations

NAMS recommends using the lowest dose of hormones necessary to relieve symptoms.[29] Estrogen doses are based on self-reported symptom relief, but occasions for serum evaluation do exist, including early onset of menopause symptoms younger than age 40 and vasomotor symptoms refractory to hormones.[45,46] The following are approximate equivalent daily doses: conjugated equine estrogen (0.3–0.625 mg) = micronized 17 β-estradiol (0.5–1 mg) = transdermal estradiol (14–100 mcg).[42]

When a woman takes exogenous estrogen, serum estradiol levels of 60–120 pg/mL are considered to be in a therapeutic range and reflect adequate dosing. However, symptom report tends to be as accurate as serum estradiol levels. This is particularly true since CEE is the most frequently used estrogen. CEE is primarily converted to estrone in the liver, and serum estradiol is therefore an inadequate marker of CEE levels. In general, if sleeping and hot flashes are improved, the medication appears effective and the dose adequate.

Serum progestin levels have not been studied. However, in practice, progesterone formulations are used to counteract possible endometrial hyperplasia in women who have an intact uterus. In this setting, unexplained uterine bleeding or withdrawal bleeding prior to day 7 after onset of progestin therapy use may be considered a suggestion of inadequate progestin therapy, and further evaluation is suggested to rule out endometrial hyperplasia. Comparable progestin choices to offset the estrogen effect on the endometrium include MPA at 2.5 mg daily or 5 mg for 10–12 days per month, micronized progesterone at 100 mg daily or 200 mg for 10–12 days per month, norethindrone at 0.35 mg daily or 5 mg for 10–12 days per month, or levonorgestrel at 0.075 mg daily. Use of a progestin to counteract endometrial hyperplasia in women who use topical estrogen agents varies in clinical practice[42,47-50] (Box 34-3).

Topical progestins have not been found to adequately oppose estrogen simulation of the endometrium.[48] Because the lowest therapeutic doses of progestins have not been determined in long-term trials, it is essential to monitor unexplained vaginal bleeding in women who are taking hormone formulation.[51]

Prescription Regimens

Many different regimens can be used when prescribing ET or HT. These patterns include varying doses, modes of administration, and various kinds of estrogens or progesterone. The use of lower hormonal doses is associated with a reduced risk of irregular bleeding and breast tenderness, adverse effects that have been cited as obstacles to the use of hormones. Women using lower ET or HT doses experience 50% lower rates of irregular bleeding and breast tenderness compared with women using standard doses.

Often a woman will have a preference for one type of hormone therapy. After an initial trial, if problems occur, a change may be indicated. Clinical outcomes of symptom management, endometrial protection from hyperplasia as evidenced by no unscheduled bleeding, and side effects are the keys to making the best choice.

The initial hormone regimens used CEE alone for the first 25 days of the calendar month. In 1975, two studies found that women using estrogen alone were found to have a ninefold increased incidence of endometrial cancer.[52,53] Thereafter, progestins were added to protect the endometrium from overstimulation by estrogen. Medroxyprogesterone acetate (MPA, Provera), the first progestin available, was taken on days 15–25 of the month. This was to emulate the menstrual cycle with 3 weeks on and 1 week off. Some women had vasomotor symptoms and heavy bleeding on the hormone-free days. Today it is common to prescribe the estrogen product without stopping, then adding a progestin the first 12–10 days of the calendar month. When prescribed in this manner, women usually bleed after the last progestin tablet. If bleeding begins before the 7th day of the progestin, there is concern that the amount of progestin is not adequate. In this situation an ultrasound of the uterine lining or an endometrial biopsy is indicated.

Vaginal bleeding is a major reason why women discontinue hormones. Unscheduled bleeding is problematic for some women, although others do not like even scheduled bleeding. Prescribing a low daily dose of HT may achieve amenorrhea following a few months of breakthrough bleeding. Adequate teaching about what to expect depending on how the hormones are taken is essential. Abnormal bleeding whether between periods or simply unpredicted bleeding necessitates careful monitoring of the endometrium with ultrasound or endometrial biopsy.

Some women have a difficult time with medroxyprogesterone acetate, the most commonly prescribed progestin. This agent can cause cyclic weight gain, decreased libido, headache, bloating, and feelings of depression. Other options include micronized progesterone (Prometrium) and norethindrone acetate (Aygestin), which often are better tolerated. Some women choose not to take any progestin because of side effects. Annual endometrial biopsies for women who cannot tolerate the use of progesterone are recommended, but studies are lacking on the efficacy, safety, and cost of this approach.

If a woman is in early STRAW stage +1a, within only 6 months after her last menstrual period, she is likely to have erratic spotting for up to 6 months if placed on a continuous-combined regimen, followed by amenorrhea (Table 34-7). Many women do well on a cyclic regimen of daily estrogen, adding progestin for the first 12 days of the month.[53] With this method, most women will usually have a withdrawal bleed after the combined estrogen/progesterone dose days (after calendar day 12), which becomes shorter and lighter with time.

Pulsed progestin therapy uses estrogen daily, with progestin dosed intermittently in cycles of 3 days on and 3 days off without interruption. This pulsed dosing may decrease the incidence of erratic spotting that can accompany continuous progestin exposure. The brand Prefest was designed with this sequence, but studies were only conducted for 1 year. Thus, more data have yet to be reported with this regimen.[54]

Continuous-cyclic (sequential), long-cycle HT (e.g., CEE 0.625 mg daily with MPA 10 mg or 5 mg for 14 days every 3 months) lessens exposure to progestin, which may promote protection against the risk of breast cancer.[27] Studies addressing this intermittent progestin use added to standard doses of daily estrogen (0.625 mg CEE per day) have found no evidence of endometrial hyperplasia after 1 year of therapy.[30]

Table 34-7 Hormone Regimens

Regimen	Estrogen	Progestin
Cyclic	Days 1–25	Last 10–14 days of ET cycle*
Cyclic-combined	Days 1–25	Days 1–25*
Continuous-cyclic (sequential)	Daily	10–14 days every month
Continuous-cyclic (sequential) long-cycle	Daily	14 days every 2–6 months
Continuous-combined	Daily	Daily
Intermittent-combined (pulsed-progestogen; continuous-pulsed)	Daily	Repeated cycles of 3 days on, 3 days off

* Most prescriptions include a daily estrogen to avoid the symptoms that arise the week off the hormone. Continuous combined or continuous cyclic are most frequently prescribed.

Side Effects/Adverse Effects

Use of estrogen products has both nuisance and serious side effects. The side effects include vaginal bleeding or spotting, nausea, headache/migraine, mood changes, glucose intolerance, and libido changes. Serious symptoms include breast, ovarian, and endometrial cancers, cholestatic jaundice, gallbladder disease, pancreatitis, hypertension, and depression.

Progestins are associated with menstrual irregularities, amenorrhea, breast tenderness, weight changes, headache, fluid retention, and abdominal distention. Because of these side effects, some women self-discontinue the agent while maintaining use of estrogen. When women do this, they put themselves at risk of endometrial hyperplasia and endometrial cancer. Progestin products also are associated with adverse effects that include thromboembolism, hypertension, breast cancer, depression, and cholestatic jaundice.

Micronized progesterone has a lower side effect profile than medroxyprogesterone acetate and acts as a somnolent, so it should be taken at bedtime. The third progesterone product is norethindrone acetate found as an individual drug in Aygestin, in an oral combination product like Activella and Femhrt or the transdermal CombiPatch.

Hormonal Influences on Laboratory Testing

Hormones also can confound diagnosis or monitoring of other conditions because of effects on common laboratory tests. Some of these changes are associated with the hepatic changes associated with estrogen, whereas others occur for unknown reasons. Table 34-8 lists changes that may be found among frequently used laboratory tests.[55]

Drug–Drug Interactions

Estrogen can interfere with liver metabolism of many drugs. Estrogen increases metabolism of many drugs, thereby decreasing blood levels. These include lamotrigine (Lamictal), carbamazepine (Tegretol), nevirapine (Viramune), phenytoin (Dilantin), phenobarbital (Luminal), primidone (Mysoline), rifampin (Rifadin), aromatase inhibitors, and ursodiol (Actigall). Estrogens also decrease blood levels of omega 3 acids, thereby minimizing their antihyperlipidemia effect.

In contrast, hepatic metabolism of aripiprazole (Abilify), dasatinib (Sprycel), and lapatinib (Tykerb) is inhibited, which can increase the risk of toxicity.

Estrogen increases the incidence of hyperglycemia when taken with diazoxide (Proglycem), thiazolidinediones

Table 34-8 Changes in Laboratory Values Associated with Hormone Therapy (ET and HT)

Increased Levels	Decreased Levels
Carotene/vitamin A	Alkaline phosphatase, serum
Copper, serum	Folic acid/folate
Cortisol	Follicle-stimulating hormone (FSH)
FTI/free thyroxin index	Luteinizing hormone (LH)
Glucose, blood	Niacin/nicotinic acid
Growth hormone	Phosphorus, inorganic, serum
Hepatic function tests	Partial thromboplastin time/activated PTT
High-density lipoprotein (HDL)	Testosterone
Insulin level	Tri-iodothyronine/T$_3$ resin uptake
Insulin-like growth factor	Vitamin B$_{12}$, serum
Mean corpuscular hemoglobin (MHC)	Zinc, serum
Mean corpuscular hemoglobin concentration (MCHC)	
Mean corpuscular volume (MCV)	
Platelet count	
Prolactin	
Sodium, serum	
Thyroid-binding globulin	
Thyroxin (T$_4$)	
Total iron-binding capacity (TIBC)	
Triglycerides	

(e.g., exenatide or Byetta), and other hypoglycemic agents including metformin (Glucophage).

Erythromycin, fluvoxamine (Luvox), and telithromycin (Ketek) can increase estrogen blood levels. Griseofulvin (Fulvicin), oxcarbazepine (Trileptal), rifampin (Rifadin), and rifapentine (Priftin) may decrease estrogen levels when taken concurrently.

Some drugs interfere with the action of progestins. Agents such as aprepitant (Emend), bexarotene (Targretin), bosentan (Tracleer), carbamazepine (Tegretol), griseofulvin (Grifulvin V), oxcarbazepine (Trileptal), phenytoin (Dilantin), rifabutin (Mycobutin), and rifampin (Rifadin) may result in decreased progestin levels and thus decreased efficacy.

Duration and Discontinuation

Because the risk of breast cancer has been found to increase after 5 years of ET or HT, there is a general consensus to restrict use to less than 5 years, although data are lacking for an exact recommendation.[27] It is rare that women continue to have hot flashes for long after menopause. Despite the risks, women who do continue to have distressing symptoms might wish to continue use for years. The decision to continue therapy should be individualized based on the risk/benefit ratio discussed between the woman and her provider and the belief that continuation is necessary to contribute to quality of life.[48,56,57]

Adherence to taking hormones is not high. Many women stop using it for personal reasons such as not liking to take medicine, feeling hormones are not natural, fear of weight gain, and unacceptable expense. According to a report published in 1999 by Ettinger, it was estimated that 50% of women use hormones for less than a year, 10% only use hormones sporadically, and only 20% continue use for several years.[58] Others never get their initial hormone prescription filled.[58]

When a woman stops ET or HT, symptoms have a 50% chance of recurring, but depending on her age, the vasomotor symptoms may not last long.[19] No specific weaning regimens have proven most effective to avoid rebound symptoms, but many providers typically recommend either lengthening the time between doses or reducing the dose over time. If return of symptoms has compromised quality of life, many women choose to resume hormones at the lowest indicated dose.[29]

Bioidentical Hormone Therapy

The term **bioidentical hormone therapy** refers to products that are molecularly the same as the hormones naturally present in the body. These agents are further divided into two kinds. First are the bioidentical products that are in common use and approved by the FDA. Examples include estradiol (Estrace) and micronized progesterone. The appeal of bioidentical hormones is that they are molecularly the same as those made in the body, produced in the laboratory, and purported to cause fewer side effects than nonbioidentical products.

The second type of bioidentical hormones are obtained by women at selected pharmacies that offer hormones made by compounding various preparations. These agents usually are composed of various amounts of estradiol, estrone, estriol, and natural progesterone. It should be noted that in 2008, the Food and Drug Administration notified compounding pharmacies that estriol is not FDA approved, causing a major controversy as well as accusations that the FDA was subject to undue influence from pharmaceutical companies who manufacture commercial hormone formulations.[59]

Compounded hormones are individualized in amount or route of delivery, such as a sublingual troche or transdermal cream, oral capsules, sublingual tablets, topical gels, creams, and patches. Commonly a product combines all three estrogens (i.e., estradiol, estrone, and estriol). The pharmacists at the select pharmacies compound hormones in smaller doses or different doses than usually are prescribed by providers and dispensed by regular pharmacies. Other products regularly compounded include DHEA and testosterone. Many of these pharmacies offer hormone saliva testing to quantify the amount of hormones in the body that is actually usable by cells. This test is not approved by the FDA.

Topical progesterone in nonprescription form is synthesized by a chemical process using plants such as soybeans and wild yams. The end product is nearly identical to endogenous progesterone, but diosgenin, the precursor of progesterone found in these plants, cannot be converted to progesterone by simple ingestion of the products. Therefore, these products do not afford any protection for the endometrial lining.

One example of a distinct advantage of compounding is a custom compound of oral progesterone for a woman with a peanut allergy who cannot take micronized progesterone in peanut oil. In such cases, it is essential to work with an accredited compounding pharmacy and provide full disclosure to the woman regarding known and unknown risks, benefits, and implications of non-FDA approval.

Most of the products on the market are synthetic hormones including CEE and others as listed on Table 34-7. Frequently used products consist of molecules that are not identical to human estrogen yet offer relief of symptoms and are well tolerated by most women. That said, women may report fewer side effects if they use the bioidentical micronized progesterone instead of medroxyprogesterone acetate. Some formulations such as 17 β-estradiol, with the same molecular structure as ovarian estradiol, usually are well tolerated.

Complementary and Alternative Therapies

It is estimated that as many as 34% of the US population takes herbal remedies or botanicals on a regular basis.[60] Herbs, both singly and in combination, have been used to treat menopausal symptoms. Few randomized, controlled trials have been conducted, and other studies lack from small treatment groups, lack of a control group, and short duration. This leaves the clinician with a less than appropriate knowledge base for caring for women who take herbal preparations as well as the inability to confidently include herbal preparations in their therapeutic formulary. Chapter 10 addresses the subject of complementary and alternative care for various menopausal symptomatology in more detail. The more common treatments briefly are addressed in the following section.

Black Cohosh

Cimicifuga racemosa, or black cohosh, has a long history of use as a remedy for women's health ailments. Black cohosh was used extensively by Native Americans and early American settlers for female complaints and was the main component and active ingredient in Lydia Pinkham's Vegetable Compound, a turn-of-the-century remedy for a host of female complaints ranging from premenstrual syndrome to menopausal discomforts, as mentioned in Chapter 30. This plant was considered to be active because of phytoestrogen like properties; however, it is not clear what the mechanism of action is in relieving menopausal symptoms. Black cohosh is considered nonestrogenic.[61] Herbs are usually taken in small doses, so it can take longer to see a change in symptoms or other side effects.

Black cohosh can be taken as drops; however, the most commonly used preparation is Remifemin, in tablet form. This over-the-counter product is widely used in Germany and has been available for a number of years in the United States through a standardized extract. Appropriate dose for the treatment of menopausal symptoms is Remifemin 40 mg in the form of one tablet twice daily. Some studies report therapeutic effects of black cohosh on hot flashes in 2 weeks, whereas others not for months. Due to lack of information, it is suggested that black cohosh not be used for more than 6 months.[62]

In a recent double-blind, placebo-controlled randomized trial, the Herbal Alternatives for Menopause (HALT) Study, a multiarmed trial of 351 women investigated black cohosh by comparing five distinct groups of women—those using black cohosh, other herbal blends, CEE with or without MPA, or placebo. Black cohosh demonstrated little potential as therapy for relief of vasomotor symptoms.[63] This study, albeit the best publicized, is not the only randomized, controlled trial, and results have been contradictory overall. Thus, controversy remains regarding the effectiveness of black cohosh.

Phytoestrogens

Women are often hesitant to take hormones and feel that the natural sources are a better choice. **Phytoestrogens** are plant-derived compounds and include isoflavones and lignans. Functionally, they can exert both estrogenic and antiestrogenic properties depending on their concentration and the concentration of endogenous sex hormones. Isoflavones include genistein, daidzein, and others. Genistein and daidzein are found in soybeans, soy products, and red clover. Soy products vary in composition and concentration. To promote taste and obtain color-free protein preparations, some processors in the United States essentially remove all of the phytochemicals in the food. Soy products appear to be of potential value for treating mild vasomotor symptoms with short-time use and most likely in food form. More details are found in Chapter 10.

Red clover is a source of isoflavones, and the flower of the plant contains the isoflavones genistein and daidzein. Red clover is marketed as Promensil. Three randomized trials report equivocal results for the treatment of hot flashes.[56,64,65] These agents generally are considered safe if consumed in whole-food products such as soy foods. Isoflavone supplements negate the beneficial effect of aromatase inhibitors for women with breast cancer and should not be used.[18,56]

Other herbal products (Table 34-9) have been proposed as remedies for menopausal conditions. However, evening primrose oil, vitamin E, and ginseng have not been shown to have any positive effect on decreasing hot flashes.[66]

Table 34-9 Herbals Commonly Used for Menopausal Symptom Relief

Product	Usual Dose*	Purpose in Menopause	Clinical Considerations
Black cohosh (*Cimicifuga racemosa*)	20 mg bid (proprietary standardized extract)	Vasomotor symptoms	Multiple products and formulations available Research evidence suggests beneficial effect on menopausal symptoms, benefit similar to estrogen for hot flash relief Safety for use > 6 months not established Product labels frequently recommend much higher does Can potentiate antihypertensives Wide variations in product ingredients, extraction processes, and purity Side effects rare; usually intestinal upset, headache, dizziness, hypotension, or painful extremities; more common with higher doses

(continues)

Table 34-9 Herbals Commonly Used for Menopausal Symptom Relief (*continued*)

Product	Usual Dose*	Purpose in Menopause	Clinical Considerations
Chastetree berry (*Vitex agnus castus*)	Effective dose unknown; hard to find standardized extract	Menstrual irregularity	More popular in Europe than the US; approved in Germany for PMs, mastalgia, and menopause symptoms Often found in combination products Research focuses on PMS symptoms; no data on relief of menopause symptoms Side effects rare; usually headache, intestinal upset
Dong quai (*Angelica sinensis*)	2 capsules bid to tid; usually in combination products	Gynecologic conditions	Widely used in Asia Research found no benefit for menopause symptoms Often in Chinese herb combination products (*Chinese Materia Medica* advises against giving it alone) A "heating" herb, can cause a red face, hot flashes, sweating, irritability, or insomnia Contains coumarin derivatives; contraindicated in those taking warfarin Can cause photosensitivity, hypotension
Evening primrose oil (*Oenothera biennis*)	3–4 g daily in divided doses	Hot flashes Mastalgia	Data show no benefit in treatment versus controls Potentiates risk for seizure if taken with seizure disorder, phenothiazines, and other medications that lower the seizure threshold Side effects include diarrhea and nausea
Ginkgo (*Ginkgo biloba*)	40–80 mg of standardized extract tid	Memory changes	Insufficient research on safety and efficacy Memory changes often related to sleep disturbances, menopausal sleep disturbances frequently related to vasomotor symptoms or other life stressors Side effects include gastrointestinal distress, hypotension; chronic use had been linked with subarachnoid hemorrhage, subdural hematoma, and increased bleeding times
Ginseng (*Panax ginseng*)	1–2 g root daily in divided doses	General "tonic" Improved mood, fatigue	Heavily adulterated Research showed no benefit on menopausal symptoms; showed benefits on well-being, general health, and depression Can cause uterine bleeding, mastalgia Contraindicated with breast cancer, and with monoamine oxidase inhibitors, stimulants, or anticoagulants; may potentiate digoxin and others (multiple drug interactions) Side effects include rash, nervousness, insomnia, hypertension
Kava (*Piper methysticum*)	150–300 mg of root extract daily in divided doses	Irritability Insomnia	Banned in several countries due to hepatotoxicity; thus, not recommended Contraindicated with depression Side effects include gastrointestinal discomfort, impaired reflexes and motor function, weight loss, hepatotoxicity, rash
Licorice root (*Glycyrrhiza glabra*)	5–15 mg of root equivalent daily in divided doses	Menopause-related symptoms	Found in many Chinese herb mixtures No data supporting relief of hot flashes High doses can lead to primary aldosteronism, cardiac arrhythmias, cardiac arrest Contraindicated if hepatic or renal disease, diabetes, hypertension, arrhythmias, hypokalemia, hypertonia, pregnancy, or on diuretics
Passion flower (*Passiflora incarnata*)	3–10 grains daily in divided doses	Sedative	Research shows mixed results in sleep improvement Menopausal sleep disturbances frequently related to vasomotor symptoms or other life stressors
St. John's wort (*Hypericum perforatum*)	300 mg tid (standardized extract)	Vasomotor symptoms Irritability Depression	No data supporting vasomotor relief Research findings support use for depression; there are no clinical trials for menopause Often combined with black cohosh for menopause symptom treatment Interferes with metabolism of many medications that are metabolized in the liver (C450) (e.g., estrogen, digoxin, theophylline); reduces international normalized ratio (INR) levels; not to be used concomitantly with antidepressants, monoamine oxidase inhibitors, or immunosuppressants

(continues)

Table 34-9 Herbals Commonly Used for Menopausal Symptom Relief (continued)

Product	Usual Dose*	Purpose in Menopause	Clinical Considerations
St. John's wort (*Hypericum perforatum*) (continued)			Side effects include photosensitivity, rash, constipation, cramping, dry mouth, fatigue, dizziness, restlessness, insomnia
Valerian root (*Valeriana officinalis*)	300–600 mg aqueous extract 0.5–1 hour before bed (insomnia); 150–300 mg aqueous extract each morning and 300–400 mg each evening (anxiety)	Sedative Antianxiety	Used for insomnia in intermittent dosing; for anxiety with chronic dosing Research showed improvement in sleep and depression/mood scales Side effects include headache, uneasiness, excitability, arrhythmias, morning sedation, gastrointestinal upset, cardiac function disorders (with long-term use)
Wild yam (*Dioscorea villosa*)	Unknown	Menopausal symptoms	Products claim that creams are converted to progesterone; however, the human body cannot concert topical or ingested wild yam into progesterone Research showed no benefit on menopausal symptoms

* Doses vary and differ according to formulation (e.g., tincture, liquid extract, drops, essential oil, etc.).
Sources: Modified from Alexander IM et al. 2006[125]; Data from Decker GM et al. 2001[126]; Gaudet TW 2004[127]; Low Dog T 2004[128]; North American Menopause Society 2004.[129]

Perimenopause and Fertility

The ability to conceive declines 10 or 15 years before the FMP. By the age of 45 years, there is a 50% increase in spontaneous abortions, chromosomal abnormalities, and pregnancy complications such as premature labor in the women who do conceive. If a mature woman desires to become pregnant, and a cycle-day 3 FSH level is elevated, (stage −3, late reproductive on the STRAW scale), she should consider seeking early assistance to enhance fertility. Additional information about infertility treatments can be found in Chapter 30.

The woman who does not desire pregnancy should know that unplanned pregnancy is still possible until after the FMP. Most healthy, perimenopausal woman can use any of the contraceptive methods. In well-screened women, these options include traditional or extended regimens of hormonal methods such as low-dose combination estrogen–**progestin** oral contraceptives, progesterone only oral contraceptives (POPs), injectables, implants, or similar transdermal or ring-delivery products. However, products containing estrogen are not advised for women who smoke or those who have a history of deep vein thrombosis or other major cardiovascular risk factors.[11] In general, a perimenopausal woman should have all options explained, and the best contraceptive method for a healthy perimenopausal woman is the one she chooses and is able to use successfully.

Abnormal Uterine Bleeding (AUB)

The most frequently reported symptom during perimenopause is irregular uterine bleeding. The flow may be heavier or prolonged, there may be spotting between menses, and the interval between cycles may shorten. The term used by NAMS for irregular bleeding during perimenopause is **abnormal uterine bleeding** (AUB) and is defined as bleeding that is abnormal in frequency, severity, or duration and is not the same as the normal irregular menses that occur during perimenopause nor is it bleeding secondary to menopausal hormone therapy. AUB may be treated with a variety of pharmacologic agents that may or may not offer contraceptive effects. Abnormal uterine bleeding is reviewed in detail in Chapter 30 and will be briefly reviewed here.

When evaluating a woman with AUB, it is first important to determine if she is premenopausal, perimenopausal, or postmenopausal. Additional etiologies to explain the irregular bleeding will depend on this initial stratification. A serum FSH may be obtained in women in < 45 years who have irregular menses and/or vasomotor symptoms. However, an FSH between 25 and 40 mIU has little predictive value other than to have an association with irregular menses, which can be elicited in taking the woman's menstrual history. If a woman has an elevated FSH > 25 mIU, the indication is that she has low estradiol levels and is in perimenopause, while an FSH in the normal reproductive range or < 12 mIU suggests additional investigation is needed to rule out thyroid or pituitary conditions as a cause of the irregular menses. Salivary testing has not been proven reliable.

During perimenopause and menopause, the most common etiologies of abnormal uterine bleeding include endometrial polyps, endometrial hyperplasia, leiomyomas, and rarely coagulopathies or carcinoma. Other factors to consider in a differential diagnosis include thyroid disease and liver dysfunction. Any bleeding that occurs at or after 1 year following the final menstrual period requires evaluation, including a pelvic examination, uterine/endometrial assessment, including a possible biopsy, pelvic ultrasound or hysteroscopy, and hormonal testing including thyroid, pituitary, and adrenal evaluation. Although irregular bleeding usually results from anovulation, pregnancy always should be ruled out prior to instituting any other treatments.

The major differential diagnosis is endometrial hyperplasia, which is associated with an increased risk for endometrial cancer. The risk for uterine cancer is based on the histological classification of the hyperplasia: simple (1% risk), complex (5% risk), simple with atypia (10% risk), and complex with atypia (25% risk).[67]

High doses of estrogen can be administered parenterally when a woman is hemorrhaging and in need of hospitalization or specialist care. Although high-dose estrogen can cause thrombosis, it is unlikely because the estrogen is administered only over a few hours to days. Surgical interventions for AUB include endometrial ablation and hysterectomy. These options are second line and generally employed only after pharmaceutical attempts have failed.

Contraceptive Products for Abnormal Uterine Bleeding

All estrogen–progestin contraceptives, including the extended regimen, may be helpful because the progestin therein controls bleeding by leading to an atrophic endometrium. Continuous progestin-only contraceptives, including depot medroxyprogesterone acetate (Depo-Provera, DMPA) or the levonorgestrel-releasing intrauterine system (Mirena IUS),[68] may be good choices, especially for women who are smokers, over the age of 35, have hypertension, or have a history of venous thromboembolism (VTE) when estrogen is contraindicated. DPMA is associated with bone loss among susceptible individuals. If a woman has additional risks for osteopenia and osteoporosis, add-back low-dose estrogen may promote bone protection.[11]

Noncontraceptive Progestin Products for AUB

Table 30-4 provides a summary of noncontraceptive progestin agents that can be used to manage AUB. On these dose schedules, pregnancy protection is not provided, and women should be aware that although subfertility may exist, they still have a risk of pregnancy until the FMP is confirmed. Cyclic oral progestin therapy does not provide contraception but may be valuable for treatment of AUB. Predictable progesterone withdrawal bleeding usually begins within 3–5 days after completion of the progestin. This cycling of progestin is similar to a progesterone challenge as discussed in Chapter 30 and may be continued until no withdrawal bleeding occurs postprogestin.[11]

Nonsteroidal Anti-Inflammatory Drugs

Nonsteroidal anti-inflammatory drugs (NSAIDs) decrease endometrial prostaglandin levels. For some women, NSAIDs have dual advantages of improving dysmenorrhea and decreasing blood loss. Table 30-1 lists doses and prescribing information for use of these agents.

Vasomotor Symptoms

During the perimenopausal period, **vasomotor symptoms**, also called hot flashes or hot flushes, are the second most frequently reported symptom after AUB. Vasomotor symptoms increase during perimenopause and are most frequent and intense in the first 2 years after the FMP. These symptoms usually decline over time, typically lasting 6 months to 5 years after peaking, but rarely persisting for 15 years or longer.[69] Hot flash prevalence rates vary, but are estimated to be experienced by 75% of women during the menopause transition. Climate, diet, lifestyle, and race may play a role. Cigarette smoking increases the likelihood of hot flashes. Most hot flashes are reported to be mild to moderate, although 10–15% of women report severe or very frequent hot flashes. Ninety percent or more of women have hot flashes after bilateral oophorectomy or surgical induction of menopause.[11]

Perimenopausal women may first experience hot flashes in the days immediately before their menses. Many women report that premenstrual hot flashes have a significant impact on quality of life, including sleep disturbances, mood swings, and difficulty concentrating.[70] Approximately 25% of naturally menopausal women in the United States ask their medical care provider for help in dealing with hot flashes.[71,72] Although obese women may have higher levels of circulating estrogen due to peripheral conversion in the adipose tissue, they also may report increased hot flashes related to the insulation related to obesity for reasons unclear at this time.[73,74]

Pathophysiology of Vasomotor Symptoms

Hot flashes occur when estrogen is reduced, but the pathophysiology of this association is not clear. In spite of exhaustive research over years, the cause of vasomotor symptoms is still open to speculation. Since vasomotor symptoms are alleviated by estrogen supplementation, the etiology was once assumed to be estrogen deficiency. Current belief is that hot flashes result when lowered estrogen levels disrupt the hypothalamic thermoregulatory process. Decreased concentrations of circulating serotonin, increased concentrations of circulating norepinephrine, and decreased concentrations of estrogen cause a narrowing of the **thermo-neutral zone**. Temperatures above this neutral threshold cause sweating, and those below cause shivering.[75]

Throughout the reproductive years, estrogen metabolites in the hypothalamus stimulate the production of beta-endorphins. Both estrogen and endorphins act to suppress norepinephrine secretion. But with estrogen in decline, norepinephrine levels climb, which in turn up-regulate serotonin receptors and resets the thermostat. Since a hot flash (sweating, vasodilatation) is a heat-dissipation response, once the thermostat is reset and the thermo-neutral neutral zone shrinks, the flash can be triggered by a very slight increase in core body temperature resulting from subtle changes in the environment.[76] Obese women, especially those with increased abdominal adiposity, are more likely to experience vasomotor symptoms, although the mechanism is not well understood.[12]

Another hormone that may contribute to vasomotor symptoms is cortisol, an adrenal glucocorticoid.[73] Glucocorticoid secretion follows a circadian rhythm, with peak values in the early morning. Serum concentrations at all ages are higher in women than men. Women with severe vasomotor symptoms have higher cortisol levels when compared to women without severe hot flashes. This higher cortisol is attributed to the link between the hypothalamic-pituitary-adrenal (HPA) axis, the hypothalamic-pituitary-ovarian (HPO) axis, and the stress response associated with the menopause transition.

Reproductive hormone influence on cortisol levels diminishes during the later postmenopausal phases.

Nonpharmacologic Treatments for Vasomotor Symptoms

Some women are able to manage vasomotor symptoms in perimenopause with environmental and lifestyle changes, although data about the effectiveness of these modalities tend to be anecdotal. See Box 34-4 for suggested strategies.[11,70]

Pharmacologic Treatments for Vasomotor Symptoms

When hot flashes are problematic enough to require treatment, estrogen-containing pharmaceuticals are the most commonly prescribed agents. First-line therapy usually consists of estrogen-based contraception products for ET or HT.

If hormones are contraindicated, off-label use of some drugs may be considered (Table 34-10), although none have been shown to be as effective as hormones for treatment of vasomotor symptoms.[11] As of this writing, no comparative trials for efficacy have been completed, and there is no safety evidence for long-term use.

Antidepressants

Antidepressants have been shown to decrease hot flashes in women, especially in women who have a history of breast cancer. This is likely the result of alterations of

---

Box 34-4 Strategies for Managing Hot Flashes

Avoid personally perceived hot flash triggers such as hot drinks and alcohol.

Maintain a cool ambient room temperature, especially in the bedroom.

Dress in layers.

Pace respiration during a hot flash (slow, deep, abdominal breathing).

Engage in regular exercise to help maintain a healthy weight and promote better sleep.

Practice regular relaxation supported by music, massage, meditation, or yoga to help deal with anxiety, which is positively associated with hot flashes.

Source: North American Menopause Society 2007.[11]

Table 34-10 Pharmacologic Treatments for Vasomotor Symptoms

Drug Generic (Brand)	Drug Category	Dose	Clinical Considerations
Clonidine (Catapres)	Oral antihypertensive	0.05 mg PO bid to 0.1 mg PO bid	Side effects include hypotension, bradycardia, arrhythmias at high doses, dry mouth, dizziness, constipation, sedation.
Clonidine (Catapres)	Transdermal antihypertensive	0.1 mg PO bid	Gradual taper off necessary to avoid nervousness, headache, agitation, confusion, abrupt hypertension.
Depot medroxyprogesterone acetate (MPA)	Progestogen	150-mg monthly injection or 400- to 500-mg injection every 3 months	Avoid if at risk for osteoporosis. Long half-life problematic if side effects occur. Only FDA approved for contraception.
Fluoxetine (Prozac)	SSRI	20 mg PO qd	May decrease orgasm and/or libido.
Gabapentin (Neurontin)	Anticonvulsant	300–900 mg PO qd to start (100 mg per day if > 65 y)	Bedtime administration to minimize drowsiness during waking hours. Side effects include dizziness, weight gain. Antacids reduce bioavailability.
Medroxyprogesterone acetate (MPA)	Progestogen	20 mg PO qd	Side effects include menstrual irregularities, amenorrhea, depression, fluid retention. Potential association with increased risk of breast and ovarian cancer when used with estrogen.
Megestrol acetate (Megace)	Progestogen	20 mg PO bid	Not recommended for persons with diabetes, thromboembolic disease. Side effects include hypertension, insomnia, anemia, headaches reported.
Methyldopa (Aldomet)	Cardiovascular agents/ antiadrenergic agents, centrally acting	250–500 mg up to bid	Not recommended for persons with hepatitis, cirrhosis, impaired liver function, or those taking MAO inhibitors. Rare association with hemolytic anemia, leucopenia, thrombocytopenia, sedation, headache, hyperprolactinemia.
Paroxetine (Paxil)	SSRI	12.5–25 mg PO qd	Potential drug–drug interaction with tamoxifen (Nolvadex). Paroxetine inhibits CYP2D6, which converts tamoxifen to its active metabolite.
Sertraline (Zoloft)	SSRI	50 mg PO qd	Weight gain, blurred vision.
Venlafaxine (Effexor)	SSRI	37.5–75 mg PO qd	Hypertension, anorexia.

central serotonin or norepinephrine concentrations. Venlafaxine (Effexor) administered 75 mg per day can provide a quick and significant response, but may also cause nausea and vomiting.[77] Paroxetine (Paxil), administered at 10–20 mg per day also have been associated with decreased hot flashes. Desvenlafaxine succinate (Pristiq), a novel serotonin and norepinephrine update inhibitor, also has demonstrated some success.[78] Fluoxetine (Prozac), another SSRI, approved for treatment of depression and premenstrual dysphoric disorder, has also been studied for relief of hot flashes with some modest success.[56,79] Sertraline (Zoloft) does not appear to be effective.

Vasomotor relief usually is accomplished within the first week with SSRIs and serotonin norepinephrine reuptake inhibitors (SNRIs), but any mood benefit may not be observed for 6–8 weeks.[11] Side effects of nausea or sexual dysfunction may become a deterrent to use, although nausea will subside within 2 weeks if medication is taken with food. If drowsiness occurs, bedtime dosing is encouraged.

In all cases, SSRIs and SNRIs may be related to low bone density and fracture, a risk often found among mature women.[11] To minimize side effects, the lowest applicable dose is suggested for 1 week and then raised if necessary. Abrupt cessation of SSRIs and SNRIs may cause anxiety and headache, so women should taper off their dose for a period of at least 2 weeks.

Gabapentin (Neurontin)

Gabapentin (Neurontin) is an anticonvulsant drug that has been studied for relief from hot flashes and that has been used for hot flash relief. Its mechanism is unknown but may be related to modulation of intracellular calcium currents. RCTs, single-arm studies, and one open case series support a significant decrease in hot flashes. For control of seizures or neuropathies, 3000 to 3600 mg per day may be used. For vasomotor symptoms, the dose may be started as low as 100 mg and increased to as much as 900 mg at bedtime.[56]

Clonidine (Catapres)

Clonidine (Catapres) is an antihypertensive drug that has been used for a long time to offer hot flash relief to women who are unable to take hormones or who desire not to. During the 1980s, it was studied in two RCTs, both small, with no more than 29 participants. It was found that given either orally or transdermally, hot flashes were reduced by 47%; however, four women in the clonidine group withdrew because of drug related side effects including nausea, fatigue, headaches, dizziness, and dry mouth. Clonidine (Catapres) lowers blood pressure and heart rate, and pulse rate and arrhythmias have been reported at high doses. Adverse reactions include drowsiness, dizziness, dry mouth, and sedation.[66]

Progestins

Progestins have been used to reduce the incidence of vasomotor symptoms (Box 34-5).[51] Progesterone may be considered if the risk/benefit ratio supports use. In women with a history of breast cancer or endometrial cancer there are no data demonstrating safety. Progestins may contribute substantially to increased cancer risk.[66] Mammographic density is increased with progestin use, which has been linked with a higher breast cancer risk.[79] Medroxyprogester-

one acetate (MPA, Provera), at the dose of 400–500 mg per injection, has been shown to be efficacious when looking for relief from hot flashes in clinical trials.[80] Uterine bleeding can be a common side effect.

Megestrol acetate (Megace) is another oral progestin that has been studied for vasomotor symptom relief and it has been found efficacious. The primary use of megestrol acetate (Megace) is the treatment of metastatic breast cancer. When taking megestrol acetate (Megace) for relief of vasomotor symptoms, it is common that symptoms will not be relieved for up to 4 weeks. Women may use megestrol acetate (Megace) for up to 3 years with few adverse effects, although long-term data are lacking. The primary adverse reaction was bleeding, which occurred upon discontinuation of the therapy.

▍ Sleep Disturbances

Wakefulness, which may begin in perimenopause, is a common postmenopausal symptom. In a national survey in 2007, 46% of US women between the ages of 40 and 54 years and 48% between the ages of 55 and 64 years reported sleep problems, including difficulty falling asleep

---

▍ Box 34-5 Every Woman Has a Story

MM is a 51-year-old woman whose last normal menses was 9 months ago, but she reports irregular menses most of her life. She presents for help coping with hot flashes. They occur both day and night, and she finds they interfere with work and her relationships. She has a ParaGard IUD in situ, a birth control method she has used regularly since the birth of her child many years ago. Her vital signs and basic laboratory findings (including blood glucose value and thyroid stimulating hormone [TSH]) are normal, and her BMI is 34. MM has been a lacto-ovarian vegetarian for the last 4 years.

MM is a perimenopausal woman with significant symptoms that are interfering with activities of daily living. Her history of irregular menses, one pregnancy, and high BMI places her at risk for long periods of unopposed estrogen. By receiving HT that includes a progestin, she will get relief from the vasomotor symptomatology as well as protection from endometrial hyperplasia.

After a discussion of her risks and benefits with HT, MM considered CEE but was concerned about its equine origin. Instead, she chose to take Femhrt, a synthetic product that is a continuous regimen and combines estrogen and progestin with the intention of using the pharmaceuticals for the shortest period possible. General health education for MM included suggestions of nonpharmacologic interventions such as natural fibers for clothing, discussion of achieving and maintaining a healthy weight, and encouraging regular exercise and screening tests including mammograms and colonoscopy. She should be encouraged to continue having the ParaGard in place until she reaches menopause.

or staying asleep, or early waking.[81] These women are more than twice as likely to use prescription sleep aids as younger women.[76,77,81] Sleep problems should be assessed and addressed, especially in view of the new data demonstrating the significant morbidity and mortality that can result from chronic insomnia.[77]

Sleep disturbances often are attributed to vasomotor symptoms, especially if they occur during the first half of the night; sleep apnea, often associated with obesity; restless leg syndrome; and various life stressors including psychiatric conditions. Chronic illnesses such as arthritis, fibromyalgia, respiratory illnesses, allergies, and GI disturbances can also contribute to sleep problems.

Physiology of Sleep Disturbances

The etiology of midlife sleep changes may be related to aging and include nocturnal urination, obesity-related sleep apnea, and chronic pain from arthritis or fibromyalgia. Stress, alcohol abuse, and negative mood likely contribute as well. Hot flashes can trigger wakefulness and are associated with diminished libido and depression.[78]

Lifestyle changes usually are the first-line therapy. Behavioral therapies include the four Rs: **R**egularize bedtime, **R**itualize preparation for sleep, use **R**elaxation techniques, and **R**esist caffeine, alcohol, stimulation, and stress close to bedtime.[11]

Pharmacologic Management of Sleep Disturbances

Medication therapy to help with difficulty falling asleep may be successful with a short-acting nonbenzodiazepine such as zolpidem (Ambien), zaleplon (Sonata), or eszopiclone (Lunesta) (Table 34-11). Another option is ramelteon (Rozerem), a drug that increases melatonin, causes fewer side effects, and is associated with less tolerance than benzodiazepines.[11] NAMS recommends that the use of any of these agents be limited to no more than 3 nights a week to reduce tolerance and dependence.[11]

Although not approved to treat insomnia, estrogen has been shown to improve sleep by decreasing restlessness, awakening, and hot flashes.[78] If not contraindicated, estrogen-containing products that provide contraception or a low-dose estrogen patch may be helpful for sleep disruptions during perimenopause. Women using micronized progesterone, an agent with soporific effects, as part of treatment for AUB, may find that nighttime dosing helps with sleep.

Table 34-11 Medications Used to Treat Sleep Disturbances

Prescription	
Sedatives and hypnotics *(may break a cycle of insomnia, use as a last resort)*	
Short-acting nonbenzodiazepine	
Fewer withdrawal effects, lower addictive tendency, and less decrease in efficacy with time than benzodiazepines. May cause memory loss if awakened or inadequate time in bed for sleep.	
Name	**Duration**
Zolpidem (Ambien) 5 mg, 10 mg	4–5 hours
Ambien CR 6.25 mg 12.5 mg	6–8 hours
Zaleplon (Sonata) 5 mg, 10 mg	1–3 hours
Eszopiclone (Lunesta) 1 mg, 2 mg, 3 mg	6 hours
Benzodiazepines	
To be used no more than three times per week to minimize tolerance and dependence. Next-day sedation and rebound insomnia with discontinuation may occur. High-fat meals delay effect.	
Diazepam (Valium) 2 mg, 5 mg, 10 mg. Avoid with glaucoma.	
Alprazolam (Xanax) 0.25 mg, 0.5 mg, 1 mg, 2 mg. Xanax XR 0.5 mg, 1 mg, 2 mg, 3 mg. Avoid with glaucoma.	
Lorazepam (Ativan) 0.5 mg, 1 mg, 2 mg	
Flurazepam (Dalmane) 15 mg, 30 mg	
Temazepam (Restoril) 7.5 mg, 15 mg, 22.5 mg, 30 mg	
Other drugs	
Ramelteon (Rozerem) 8 mg: a melatonin receptor agonist.	
Indiplon: a hypnotic that promotes morning sleep (in development).	
Trazodone (Desyrel) 50 mg, 100 mg, 150 mg, 300 mg: antidepressant used off-label at sleep aid at doses 25–50 mg.	
Nonprescription	
Tylenol PM, Advil PM	
Contain diphenhydramine HCl as a sleep aid along with the analgesic acetaminophen (in Tylenol only).	
Combined with three or more alcoholic drinks daily may cause liver damage. Daily use may cause rebound wakefulness.	
Herbs *(lacking scientific data to support efficacy)*	
Valerian	Chamomile
Lavender	Hops
Lemon balm	Passion flower
Melatonin, serotonin *(lacking scientific data to support efficacy)*	

Headaches

During perimenopause, headaches can increase in frequency and intensity, especially in women who have suffered previous menstrual headaches. Although there is not a clear association between headaches and menopause, some data suggest progestins, especially medroxyprogesterone acetate (MPA), may precipitate or aggravate a headache. For a woman who needs a progestin but finds headaches increase with the use of a progestin, micronized progesterone may be a better choice since it is bioidentical to the progesterone made by the ovary.

Headaches should be treated during an acute incident and include prevention therapy when they are a chronic problem. Behavioral changes and medications for headaches are discussed in Chapter 24. An extended-regimen estrogen/progestin (monophasic pills) contraceptive that eliminates hormonal fluctuations may be useful for perimenopausal women with histories of headaches related to the menstrual cycle.

Vaginal and Vulvar Symptoms

Changes in the vagina, including dyspareunia, postcoital spotting, and dryness are reported by approximately one third of women in the early postmenopausal period, and up to one half in the later postmenopausal years.[6] As estrogen levels diminish postmenopause, the lining of the vagina becomes thinner and vaginal fluid becomes scant and yellow. Sexual activity may be painful and cause vaginal spotting from microabrasions, which, in turn, also increase the likelihood of acquiring a sexually transmitted infection. Lubricants can help diminish this symptom, but local estrogen may be necessary.

Symptomatic vaginitis may present in both sexually active and inactive women. Not all postmenopausal women experience vulvovaginal symptoms, but for those who do, the vaginal mucosa usually appears pale with decreased elasticity and flattened rugae. For sexually inactive women, the vagina may shorten and narrow. Microscopic evaluation of the vaginal lining reveals an absence of lactobacilli and superficial mucosal cells. Vaginal pH rises toward alkaline, which also increases vulnerability to vaginitis. Additional discussion regarding atrophic vaginitis is found in Chapter 31.

Another common cause of postmenopausal dyspareunia is **vulvodynia**. This chronic vulvar pain, especially on penetration, may linger for days after a sexual encounter. As many as 15% of the female population may experience vulvodynia, but often women with symptoms attribute it to aging and do not report the condition. The etiology of vulvodynia is unknown. Pain often is localized to the vulvar vestibule and can be reproduced with a cotton swab test as an assessment test that should be included in the physical evaluation for dyspareunia. Additional information about vulvodynia is found in Chapter 32.

Nonprescription water-based lubricant (e.g., Astroglide, K-Y Jelly, Gyne-Moistrin, Dura gel, Norform) vaginal sup-

positories may be helpful if dryness is noted during sex in perimenopause. Women should be counseled to avoid non-water-based products (e.g., Vaseline, baby oil, butter, coconut butter, fish oils) because they can irritate the sensitive mucous membrane around and inside the vagina and also may damage condoms if used. Some women find vaginal moisturizers very helpful for reducing vaginal irritation not related to intercourse. Some products include Liquibeads, Replens, and Silken Secret.

Treatment of Vulvovaginal Symptoms

Vaginal symptoms may be corrected with systemic hormones or vaginal estrogen products. A progestin generally is not indicated with local vaginal estrogen therapy although some controversy exists as previously discussed. Regular stimulation from sexual activity promotes blood flow to the vagina, protects the vagina to some degree from atrophy, and supports improved sexual response. Although estrogen receptors are found in the vulva, data have yet to confirm the role of estrogen in vulvar disorders other than a decrease in the overall size of the vulva.[11] For treatment of vulvodynia, more information may be found in Chapter 32.

Sexual Desire and Functioning

Decreased sexual desire has been theorized to affect nearly one half of US women including those at midlife.[45] Despite the large number of women who report these changes, the association between menopausal status and sexual functioning is quite complex and poorly understood.[80] Normal sexual desire remains to be defined, and, thus, any increases or decreases also are subject to discussion. Health, partner's health, sociodemographic factors, psychological variables, lifestyle, and history of sexual dysfunction are likely to be more important than menopausal status itself in desire and arousal.[82]

However, lowered reproductive hormone levels may play a role in midlife libido changes. Declining estrogen levels leading to dyspareunia and sleep disturbance have been found to affect sexual functioning.[83] Decreased arterial blood flow to the labia and clitoris and decreased estrogen effects on the central and peripheral nervous systems (impairing touch and vibration perception) may also be related to sexual functioning.[72] Lowered progesterone does not seem to affect sexual function.

Experts agree that androgens (androstenedione, DHEA, and testosterone) can strongly affect libido. While both estrogens and androgens decrease with age, unlike estradiol there is no abrupt decline in androgens with menopause and the level of estrone remains quite stable. Most testosterone is made by peripheral conversion of DHEA from the adrenal cortex and from androstenedione (not estradiol) produced in the ovaries and adrenal cortex.[84] Hence the ovaries do continue to be a source of testosterone. Alternatively, studies have shown that surgical menopause decreases testosterone by 50%. A negative correlation between the estradiol:testosterone ratio and a positive correlation between midcycle peak testosterone levels and the frequency of sexual activity has been reported in the literature.[82,85] By the time most women reach their 60s, their testosterone levels are one half of what they were before age 40 and strongly bound to SHBG, limiting biologic activity. Additional studies are needed to explore normal sexuality, and then, changes with age and hormonal status should be studied as well.

Treatment of Sexual Dysfunction

Oral estrogen therapy has the effect of reducing bioavailable androgen by increasing SHBG, which binds free testosterone. Thus libido may be negatively impacted. Caution must be exercised because exogenous androgens can increase a woman's risk for cardiac disease, hypertension, and virilization such as hirsutism and changes in voice pitch. A comprehensive sexual history is essential to determine if androgen therapy is indicated.[86] Potential physical, psychological, and social factors amenable to intervention need to be addressed, including depression, anxiety, and fatigue, response to stress, relationship issues, and sexual dysfunction in the partner. Other medications that might affect sexual function must also be taken into consideration.

A large, randomized, double-blind, placebo-controlled clinical trial in which testosterone was administered by transdermal patch found frequency of satisfying sexual activity and desire was significantly increased both in women who were surgically induced postmenopausal and in women who were naturally postmenopausal.[87] The testosterone patch, 300 mcg applied to the abdomen twice weekly, was studied in clinical trials in 2004 by Proctor and Gamble and Watson Pharmaceuticals for women who were surgically postmenopausal. More than 1000 participants reported increased frequency of satisfying sexual intercourse and improved sexual desire over placebo, but the data were inadequate according to the FDA hearing committee that reviewed it. This group expressed concern about adverse effects and requested longer term safety data regarding the risks of heart disease and breast

cancer. Today, the patch, under the brand name Intrinsa, is available by prescription in both Canada and Great Britain.[88] Additional information about testosterone for sexual dysfunction and recommendations from NAMS can be found in Chapter 33.

Currently there are no FDA-approved products for treating sexual dysfunction in postmenopausal women. The only androgen-containing product available in the United States is a combination of esterified estrogens (EE) and methyl testosterone (MT) marketed as Estratest (1.25 mg EE with 2.5 mg MT), and Estratest HS (half strength) (0.625 mg EE with 1.25 mg MT) indicated for vasomotor symptom management unresponsive to estrogen alone. The FDA has indicated it could continue on the market (where it has been for 40 years) while additional FDA-approved studies of testosterone remedies are conducted.[89]

Non-FDA-approved custom compounded preparations of micronized testosterone in oral, transdermal, or intramuscular pellet forms are available by prescription, but no definitive studies have determined absorption and utilization rates. Supraphysiologic levels may be a concern. Topical testosterone USP cream (2%) or ointment applied directly to the vaginal or clitoral area or any skin surface improves libido by anecdotal evidence; however, safety and efficacy remain unclear because of lack of controlled trial data. Topical preparations may stimulate dark hair growth on any skin surface, so the mons pubis is an optional site for application. Clitoral enlargement may occur with topical application. Monitoring for hirsutism and acne is important while evaluating subjective sexual response, and it is estimated that typically a 3-month trial is necessary for receptors to respond.

Cognitive Function and Depression

Labile moods are frequently a symptom of the menopausal transition. Depression may reoccur in up to 10% of women with a history of postpartum depression or previous depressive disorder.[82] However, women without a history of depression are no more or less likely to experience the condition during the menopause than in any other time in the life cycle. Many women present to primary care providers with symptoms before consulting a psychiatrist and deserve an initial assessment for clinical depression in the gynecology setting.

Oftentimes postmenopausal women bemoan losing words in their quick-recall memory bank, only to have these memories magically reappear when they stop chasing them. Study results are equivocal regarding the association between vasomotor symptoms and difficulty with concentration and memory.[28] The abrupt decline in estrogen production that occurs with surgically induced menopause has been suggested to exert an effect on cognition.[90] Reproductive hormones and cortisol all influence brain function; however, the effect of the hormones on concentration, memory, and other cognitive functions is not yet clearly outlined. Memory and cognitive abilities decline with advancing age in both genders and may be independent of hormonal changes.

Treatment of Psychological Symptoms

Physical exams and laboratory tests assist in ruling out medical comorbidity. Side effects of medications must be considered. If depressed mood stems from sleep interruption related to vasomotor symptoms, treating the vasomotor symptoms may constitute adequate treatment for mood as well. Instead of oral formulations, switching to transdermal hormones may minimize peaks and nadirs in levels, thereby stabilizing mood. Progestins may worsen mood, although choosing low-dose continuous oral micronized progesterone may be of benefit in some cases.[91] Antidepressants used to minimize vasomotor symptoms will have the added benefit of help for mood disorders.

Treatment of Cognition Deficits

Observational data suggest that physical and mental activity may benefit memory and help protect against dementia. Study outcomes are inconsistent regarding whether supplements such as the B vitamins, omega-3 fatty acids, gingko biloba, and soy protein are helpful.[11] The effect of hormones on cognitive function is still not clear. Some observational data indicate those taking ET or HT have higher scores on cognitive tests than those women who do not use hormone therapy, but other studies have found the opposite to be true.[92] The WHI Memory Study (WHIMS) investigated cognitive function in women between the ages of 65 and 79 years and found the risk of dementia to be doubled in women using CEE and MPA and increased by one half in women using CEE alone.[93] It is important to note that the women in the WHIMS study population were older than those most likely to use hormones to manage perimenopausal symptoms. For younger women, there is a suggestion that hormone treatments begun early may benefit cognitive skills,[94] although hormones are not FDA approved for this indication.

Bone Health and Aging

Osteoporosis is often thought of as a disease of late menopause. But the seeds of osteoporosis begin when a woman has achieved her greatest bone mass at approximately age 30. Diets high in calcium should be encouraged especially as children, adolescents, and young adults build bone. This is not easy to do when canned soft drinks and coffee are easy options. Milk serves up calcium, along with various nutrients that enhance its nutritional power punch. Young women between ages 20 and 30 years still have an opportunity to increase bone mass, which is of great value as they approach menopause. Unfortunately youth do not often think about their later years.

From age 30 to menopause, women slowly lose bone mass. Interventions to minimize this loss include continuing a high-calcium diet, ingestion of calcium tablets along with vitamin D, and exercise five times a week. With menopause, the slope of the loss of bone mineral density decreases rapidly for about 7 years[95] (Figure 34-2). Diets that are high in calcium and vitamin D should be started or continued, and supplements should be added as needed. Exercise is even more important, and decisions need to be made regarding evaluation and treatment of the individual's bone mass. The use of drugs and an evaluation of the skeleton by dual-energy X-ray absorptiometry (DEXA) scan needs to be determined for individual women.

Osteoporosis is defined as "a disease characterized by low bone mass and micro-architectural deterioration of bone tissue, leading to enhanced bone fragility and consequent increase in fracture risk."[96] Osteoporosis increases among both genders with age, but it is a particular health issue for postmenopausal women, resulting not only in fractures of the hip and spine, but limbs, pelvis, and ribs. Although frequently thought of as a sequela of menopause, osteoporosis also can result from secondary causes, including the use of glucocorticoids for more than 3 months.[11]

Bone is a metabolically active tissue that rebuilds itself. Formation and resorption of bone are in balance during normal bone remodeling. Women build bone into their 20s or early 30s, at which time peak bone mass is reached. Several types of cells compose the healthy bone. **Osteoblasts**, bone-building cells located on the surface of the bone, form osteoid, a protein that ultimately mineralizes to become bone. Osteoblasts also produce prostaglandins that act on the bone. In physiologic terms, osteoblasts are the immature bone cells in their inactive form, and they essentially cover all bone surfaces. **Osteocytes** are derived

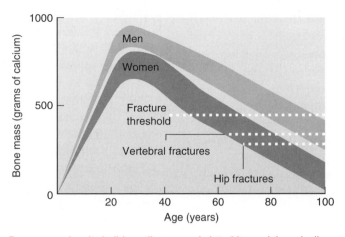

Bone mass density builds until a woman's late 20s, and then declines at a slow rate until menopause. These are times to prepare for menopause by having the highest possible bone mass density by ensuring adequate calcium and vitamin D intake and participating in weight-bearing exercise. For the 6 or 7 years following menopause, bone loss declines most rapidly, as seen above. Women then continue to lose bone mass for the rest of their lives at a slower rate.

Figure 34-2 Changes in bone mass density (BMD) over time. *Source:* Modified from Edlin G et al. 2007.[94]

from osteoblasts that are trapped in bone matrix. Osteocytes are mature bone cells that regulate response to stress and mechanical load in part by communication with other osteocytes and osteoblasts. **Osteoclasts** are necessary for reduction of bone volume. These cells migrate to bone surfaces and promote bone breakdown, which is later filled by osteoblast activity. Bone remolding occurs at different sites in the body and at different points in the bone resorption cycle.

During the postmenopause period, the loss of ovarian estradiol (E2) increases production of cytokines, which in turn promote osteoclast activity. The resultant bone resorption has been blamed for both the rapid bone loss seen in the early postmenopausal years and the slower loss that continues with aging. However, recent studies have found increased bone turnover in women when E2 levels are still in the premenopausal range. During this phase, ovarian inhibins are decreased, and as a consequence FSH is elevated. It is believed that inhibins block the development of osteoblasts. An elevated serum FSH may be a clinical marker that correlates with the initiation of bone loss.[97,98]

Many studies indicate that steady vertebral bone loss begins early, approximately 18 months before the last menstrual period, and continues at a rate of about 3% per

year for approximately 5 years. Bone loss at the hip starts out more slowly, at only about 0.5% per year leading into menopause, but in the years immediately following menopause the loss accelerates to 5–7% per year. This phase of acute bone loss slows after 4–5 years.[99]

It is logical to assume that the longer a woman is exposed to estrogen, the lower her risk of osteoporosis would be. Age at menarche and age at menopause have been shown to influence bone density, but only during the early postmenopausal period. By the time women reach the age of 75, the number of years between the first and last period makes no difference in bone density.[100]

Genetics is credited with up to 80% of the variability in peak bone mass. Fracture rates are greater among Whites than Blacks, with those of Asian and other races in between.[11] Ignoring bone fragility is easy because it is a silent condition until a fracture occurs. However, osteoporosis is pervasive and costly, and therefore, attention to the risk of bone loss is imperative. It is estimated that half of all women over age 50 will have at least one osteoporotic fracture during their life. After age 50, the risk of a fracture doubles every 7 or 8 years. By age 80, most women have lost 30% of their peak bone mass, and during that 9th decade, one out of every three women will have a hip fracture, with a 25% increased risk of mortality within the year following the fracture, and the same percentage will be forced to enter long-term care. Fifty percent will experience significant loss of mobility.[100] Therefore, it is important that osteoporosis be addressed long before it is a clinical issue. Adolescents and young women need information and encouragement to make good choices for bone health later in life, especially since these groups often avoid dairy foods rich in calcium and at the same time are increasingly sedentary. Osteoporosis cannot be corrected with a magic bullet after menopause, so providers need to encourage individuals to make healthy choices for their bones in their diet and exercise.

Bone Mineral Density

Bone mineral density (BMD) is a surrogate for bone strength. It is measured by DEXA, and expressed as grams of mineral per volume. BMD evaluations are made at the hip, femoral neck, and spine. Results are reported as standard deviations from the mean of a reference population.

A **BMD T-score** compares the participant's results to the mean peak BMD of a normal, young, same-gender population. For women, this reference population is White females age 20–29. A normal T-score is above –1.0. **Osteopenia** (low bone mass) is diagnosed when the T-score falls between –1.0 and –2.5. A T-score under –2.5 constitutes osteoporosis.[95] A **BMD Z-score** uses a reference population of the same age, gender, and ethnicity. A Z-score of –2 indicates factors other than age are causing the low BMD.[95]

Fractures

Many risk factors for fracture are not related entirely to BMD. Age and fracture history are examples (Box 34-6). A 75-year-old woman with a T-score of –2.5 has a 10-year fracture risk that is 8–10 times higher than that of a 45-year-old woman with the same T-score. A history of one fracture doubles the risk for another; adjustment for BMD does not significantly affect the prediction.[95]

Unfortunately, a reliable marker to evaluate fracture risk or risk reduction from therapy does not yet exist.[101] It may take 2 years of treatment for the BMD to significantly increase, and some variability may occur because of the relative imprecision of DEXA testing. It is not advised that clinicians use biochemical markers of bone turnover in routine practice because the results vary by food intake, time of day, and lack of assay standardization.[96] It should be noted that the type of fracture is of paramount importance; a fractured wrist is problematic, but a fractured hip or spine directly influences quality of life and potentially even life expectancy.

According to NAMS, there are three parts to fracture prevention, which include (1) slowing or preventing bone loss, (2) reducing nonstructural remodeling, and (3) controlling factors that may lead to falling.[11] Box 34-7 lists fracture risk factors.[102,103]

Nonpharmacologic Treatments

Nonmodifiable risk factors for osteoporosis include age and menopausal status. Although no specific data on risk

---

> ## Box 34-6   Fact or Fiction? A Woman Can Never Be Too Rich nor Too Thin
>
> AM is a 59-year-old woman who experienced menopause at age 53. She has three children ranging in age from 17 to 35. AM reports normal menses during her reproductive years. Her current BMI is 21 and she engages in regular exercise three times a week. Her mother had a hip fracture at age 67 subsequent to a fall and never regained full mobility.
>
> AM has not used any hormone therapy because of concern about side effects and complications. She takes no regular medications, reports drinking two glasses of nonfat milk daily and states she eats a good diet.
>
> AM is at risk for osteoporosis as suggested by her age, low BMI, and mother's hip fracture. She had not had a DEXA scan, and, therefore, one was ordered. Subsequently it was revealed that her T-score was –1.4. In order to treat the osteopenia, she should be encouraged to seek 5–15 minutes of sunlight without sunblock daily, augment her diet with calcium 1500 mg, and vitamin D 1200 mg. An increased weight to normal level and weight-bearing exercise are other positive interventions. AM should return in 6 months to 1 year. If she does not stabilize her BMD, bisphosphonates are likely to be the next recommended therapy.

> ### Box 34-7 Fracture Risk Factors
>
> Advanced age
>
> Alcohol intake > 2 drinks per day
>
> Current smoking any amount
>
> Diet deficient in calcium or vitamin D
>
> Glucocorticoid use for > 3 months
>
> Hip fracture in a parent
>
> Increased risk of falling secondary to impaired vision, dementia, poor health, low physical activity, history of recent falls
>
> Low BMD
>
> Previous fracture as an adult (excluding toe, ankle, finger, face, skull)
>
> Small frame: BMI < 21 or weight < 127 lbs.
>
> *Source:* North American Menopause Society 2007.[103]

reduction are available, changes in lifestyle including exercise, fall prevention, moderation of alcohol intake, discontinuation of smoking, and certain nutritional interventions may reduce fracture risk for many. These interventions are suggested for all women.[11]

Exercise

Weight-bearing exercise is theorized to increase osteoblast activity. Adolescents and young adults who exercise reach a higher peak bone mass. Postmenopausal women who perform strength training usually gain at least moderate amounts of bone mass, whether or not they use ET or HT.[101] Women over the age of 75 years who exercise have been found to build muscle and strength and improve balance. These women have a reduction in the risk of falls compared to those of the same age who do not exercise.[11] Exercise contributes to improved proprioception.

Manipulation of Alcohol Intake

The relationship between alcohol and fractures appears somewhat complex. Compared to individuals who do not imbibe alcohol, persons drinking half to one drink per day have lower hip fracture risk (RR = 0.80; 95% CI, 0.71–0.91). Conversely, persons who drink more than two drinks daily have a higher risk of hip fracture (RR = 1.39; 95%, CI, 1.08–1.79).[104] A similar relationship exists with BMD and femur fractures. This relationship between high levels of alcohol and untoward findings may exist because of increased risk of falls secondary to overuse of alcohol and subsequent impaired balance or potentially because of newer studies suggesting molecular targets within the bone that respond to alcohol at certain doses.[104] NAMS recommends that postmenopausal women not exceed seven drinks per week.[103]

Cessation of Smoking

Numerous studies have shown that compared to nonsmokers, smokers reach menopause an average of 2 years earlier, achieve lower peak bone mass, and lose bone faster.[2] Although the pathophysiology of this relationship is not clear, there is some evidence that smoking is associated with decreased calcium absorption.[105]

Fall Prevention

Nearly 90% of all fractures are the result of a fall, and one third of women over 60 years of age fall at least once a year.[11] Prevention of falls should be paramount for all postmenopausal women.

Nutritional Supplements

Adequate calcium and vitamin D throughout life are critical for reaching and maintaining peak BMD. Evidence is limited about optimal dosing as well as specific effects on fracture.[106] Calcium requirements increase at the time of menopause because absorption and renal conservation, enhanced by estrogen, decline when E2 levels are low. Yet American women obtain less than half the calcium required from their diet. Guidelines for calcium intake suggest 1500 mg daily, including diet, which should be the primary source. To reach that target, women with the average American diet will need 600 mg to 900 mg daily in the form of supplements. Calcium carbonate absorption is enhanced when taken with food, can be found in inexpensive forms, but also has been associated with rare, but severe, cases of hypercalcemia over time. Calcium citrate supplements are well absorbed, even on an empty stomach, and are associated with minimal constipation and gaseousness but tend to be more expensive. Both are better absorbed in divided doses of 500 mg or less at a time with a bedtime dose optimal to cover the time from 3 AM to 6 AM when most of the bone resorption takes place. It has been shown to be safe, but not recommended, for healthy adults to consume up to 2500 mg per day.[103]

Although vitamin D is needed for calcium absorption, vitamin D supplementation alone has failed to demonstrate a reduction in fractures. Sources of vitamin D include sunlight, fortified dairy products, fatty fish, and supplements. Vitamin D has a long half-life, so it is not necessary to take it at the same time as calcium. The National Osteoporosis Foundation recommends 800–1000 IU per day of vitamin D₃ for adults age 50 and older. This amount usually can be reached with a daily vitamin (most contain 400 IU), milk or breakfast cereal fortified with 100 IU, and a calcium supplement that also contains 400 IU.[103]

No clinical trial data have been found to support the use of isoflavones in diet or as supplements for prevention or treatment of osteoporosis.[103] Additional information about vitamins as pharmaceuticals can be found in Chapter 5. Complementary alternative therapies such as isoflavones are discussed in more detail in Chapter 10.

Pharmacologic Management for Osteoporosis

The guidelines from the NAMS recommend adding drug therapy to lifestyle modifications for all postmenopausal women who have any one of the following: (1) history of an osteoporotic vertebral fracture; (2) BMD values diagnostic for osteoporosis (T-scores ≤ −2.5); or (3) BMD values in the range of −2.0 to −2.5 with low weight (either less than

127 pounds or a BMI less than 21), history of postmenopausal fragility fracture, and/or history of a hip fracture in a parent.[103] Many primary care clinicians prefer to refer women to an expert to assist in exploring options for treating osteopenia and osteoporosis. Pharmacologic therapies include hormones, **bisphosphonates**, the SERM raloxifene (used for prevention of breast cancer reoccurrence and contraindicated in women with a history of thromboembolic disease), parathyroid hormone, and calcitonin. With the exception of parathyroid hormone, all are antiresorptive agents that act by decreasing osteoclast activity. In contrast, parathyroid hormone is anabolic and stimulates new bone formation by activating osteoblasts.[103]

No studies have been conducted comparing these options directly against each other in a head-to-head study in regard to fracture reduction. To complicate comparisons further, most studies include varying doses of calcium and vitamin D supplementation in addition to the agents themselves, and the changes in BMD that result do not always correlate with fracture reduction.[11] All these drugs have been found to reduce vertebral fracture. Only three bisphosphonates (alendronate [Fosamax], risedronate [Actonel], and zoledronic acid [Reclast, Zometa]) and estrogen therapy have been found to reduce hip and other nonvertebral fractures in placebo-controlled trials. Table 34-12 provides a list of the larger trials of some of these agents.[107-112]

Drug treatment for fracture prevention is usually long term, and adherence has been shown to be poor.[103] Less frequent dosing regimens (once weekly, monthly or even yearly instead of daily) increase a woman's ability to take the agents therapeutically. For example, a single intravenous infusion of zoledronic acid (Zometa) given at baseline, 12 months, and 24 months has been shown to reduce vertebral fracture by 70% over placebo during a 3-year

Table 34-12 Clinical Trials: Osteoporosis

Trial and Drug Evaluated	N	Dose	Decrease in Vertebral Fracture Risk	Decrease in Nonvertebral Fracture Risk
VERT-1[107] risedronate	2458	5 mg qd	65% after 1 y ($P < .001$) 41% after 3 y ($P = .003$)	39% after 3 y ($P = .02$)
VERT-2[108] risedronate	1226	5 mg qd	61% after 1 y ($P = .06$) 49% after 3 y ($P < .001$)	33% after 3 y ($P = .06$)
HIP[109] risedronate	9331	2.5 and 5 mg qd	Not reported	20% after 3 y ($P = .03$)
FIT-1[110] (1) alendronate	4432	5 mg qd × 2 y then 10 mg qd × 2 y	44% after 4 y ($P = .001$)	12% after 4 y ($P = .13$)
FIT-2[111] alendronate	2027	5 mg qd × 2 y then 10 mg qd × 1 y	47% after 3 y ($P < .001$)	20% after 3 y ($P = .063$)
Alendronate Phase III Osteoporosis Treatment Study[112]	994	5 or 10 mg qd for 3 y 20 mg qd for 2 y, then 5 mg qd for 1 y	Pooled data from all: 48% reduction after 3 y ($P = .03$)	21% after 3 y (P values not significant, not reported)

Sources: Harris ST 1990[107]; Reginster JM et al. 2000[108]; McClung MR et al. 2001[109]; Black DM et al. 1996[110]; Ensrud KB-C et al. 2004[111]; Tonino RM et al. 2000.[112]

period (3.3% versus 10.9%; RR = 0.30; 95% CI, 0.24–0.38). In addition, hip fracture is reduced by 41% over placebo during the 3 years of treatment (1.4% versus 2.5%; RR = 0.59; 95% CI, 0.42–0.83).[96] Cost may be another barrier to adherence, as generics are not widely available.[113]

Estrogen

There is consistent evidence that ET and HT reduce the risk of postmenopausal osteoporotic fracture of both the spine and hip. For example, in the WHI, after 5.2 years, those treated with estrogen plus progestin were found to have reduction in hip fracture (RR = 0.66; 95% CI, 0.45–0.98) and in combined fractures (RR = 0.76; 95% CI, 0.69–0.85).[27] Estrogen prescription drugs may be FDA approved for prevention but are not approved for treatment of osteoporosis. After a careful risk/benefit analysis including consideration of alternatives, ET and HT can be an option for newly menopausal women at high risk of fracture within the upcoming 5–10 years.[11] However, such women must be aware of the risks of ET or HT, including an increase in breast cancer with 5 years of use.[27]

Another study that supported the use of hormones for bone prevention is a large study in which women who had discontinued HT within the previous 5 years demonstrated an increase in hip fractures compared to women who continued to use HT (OR = 1.65; 95% CI, 1.05–2.59). As could be expected, after more than 5 years post-HT

discontinuation, fracture risk equaled never users.[114] Other studies indicate that when ET or HT is used in the early postmenopause (+1 STRAW stage), BMD is maintained and there are fewer fractures than with placebo, even several years after discontinuation.[11]

Bisphosphonates

Bisphosphonates reduce bone resorption by dampening osteoclast activity. Many clinical trials involving both young and old postmenopausal women show a dose-dependent significant increase in BMD at both the spine and hip. Generally, for women with osteoporosis, a 40–50% reduction in vertebral fracture and a 20–25% decrease in fractures at other sites (including hip) can be expected[11] (Figure 34-3).

The 2006 NAMS position statement on osteoporosis management identifies bisphosphonates as the first-line treatment for osteoporosis.[103] The following four bisphosphonates have been approved for treatment of postmenopausal osteoporosis in the United States: alendronate (Fosamax), risedronate (Actonel), ibandronate (Boniva), and zoledronic acid (Reclast, Zometa)[2] (Table 34-13).

Optimal duration of bisphosphonate therapy is not clear. According to NAMS, current evidence is not sufficient to recommend the duration of bisphosphonate use. Protection against fracture was proven during 4 years of alendronate (Fosamax) therapy and 5 years of risedronate,

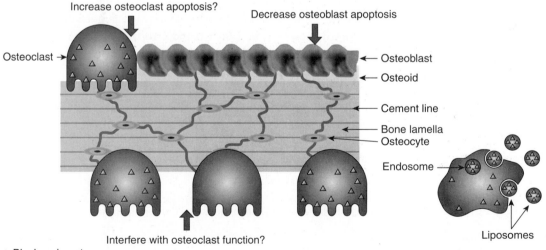

Bisphosphonates (triangles) bind to bone mineral. Osteoclasts release the bound bisphosphonates via acidification and absorb them into the osteoclast. In the osteoclast, the bisphosphonate inhibits farnesyl pyrophosphate synthase, which causes osteoclast apoptosis.

Figure 34-3 Proposed mechanism of action for bisphosphonates.

Table 34-13 Bisphosphonates

Drug Generic (Brand)	Formulation	Dose for Prevention	Dose for Treatment
Alendronate (Fosamax)	Tablet, solution.	5 mg per day or 35 mg/wk	10 mg qd or 70 mg/wk
Alendronate + cholecalciferol (vitamin D$_3$) (Fosamax Plus D)	Combined in single tablet.	NA	70 mg alendronate + 2800 IU vitamin D 3 times weekly
Risedronate (Actonel)	Tablet.	5 mg per day or 35 mg/wk or 75 mg on 2 consecutive days per month or 150 mg/month	
Risedronate plus calcium carbonate (Actonel with Calcium)	Risendronate and calcium packaged together in 28-day supply tablets.	35 mg/wk risedronate taken once weekly day 1, 1250 mg Ca days 2–7 per wk (equivalent to 500 mg elemental Ca)	
Ibandronate (Boniva)	Tablet or intravenous injection (IV).	2.5 mg/day or 150 mg/month	150 mg/month or if given IV, 3 mg every 3 months
Zoledronic acid (Reclast)	Intravenous infusion.	NA	IV 5 mg/year

but this was to be expected because bisphosphonates have long half-lives,[115] and gains in BMD may continue through 7–10 years of treatment.[11,110] Once the bisphosphonate is stopped, continuation of protection varies across the medications. For example, after 4–5 years of alendronate treatment, BMD remains stable or decreases slowly. One year after discontinuing ibandronate, bone loss was the same as seen in nontreated postmenopausal women.[111,112]

Oral bisphosphonates are poorly absorbed and should be taken on an empty stomach before breakfast. Only approximately 0.5% of an oral dose is absorbed. Any food, drink, or medication should be avoided for a minimum of 30 to 60 minutes after taking ibandronate (Boniva).

Side Effects/Adverse Effects

Side effects of oral bisphosphonates center on esophageal and gastric irritation and are worse when dosing guidelines are not followed. Women should be counseled to take each dose with a full glass of water and remain upright for half an hour to promote absorption and decrease gastric adverse effects. The intravenous forms of ibandronate and zoledronic acid (Reclast) do not carry warnings about gastric distress. These parenteral agents are preferable for women with gastritis, reflux, and hiatal hernia. In one study, serious atrial fibrillation was found in 50 of the

3889 participants in the zoledronic acid-treated group versus 20 of the 3876 participants in the control group ($P < .001$).[115]

Flulike symptoms may occur when large doses of either oral or intravenous bisphosphonates are given. Discomfort is usually mild and transient and is most likely with the first dose. Before starting a bisphosphonate, a serum creatinine should be obtained to evaluate glomerular filtration. Therapy should be restricted to women with a level ≥ 30 mL/min. In 2008 the FDA issued an alert noting that bisphosphonates can cause severe muscle, joint, or bone pain that resolves when the drug is discontinued.

Osteonecrosis of the jaw (ONJ) has been reported among individuals using large intravenous doses of bisphosphonates to treat cancer-related bone disease. The incidence of ONJ in people using the lower doses prescribed for osteoporosis is not known but is estimated to be 1:60,000 and 1:100,000. Because the disease often presents as a nonhealing lesion observed after invasive dental work, NAMS recommends an oral exam by the prescriber before starting a bisphosphonate.[11]

There are a number of other pharmacologic options for treatment of osteoporosis that are neither estrogens nor bisphosphonates (Table 34-14). Some of these agents, like SERMS, are first-line therapy.

Table 34-14 Nonestrogens/Nonbisphosphonates for Management of Postmenopausal Osteoporosis

Drug Category	Drug Generic (Brand)	Indication	Formulation	Dose
SERM	Raloxifene (Evista)	Prevention and treatment	Tablet	60 mg qd
Calcitonin	Calcitonin, salmon (Fortical, Miacalcin)	Treatment > 5 years postmenopause	Nasal spray, subcutaneous injection	200 IU qd, 100 IU every other day
Parathyroid hormone	Teriparatide (recombinant human PTH 1–34) (Forteo)	Treatment for those at high fracture risk	Subcutaneous injection	20 mcg qd

Selective Estrogen Receptor Modulators

SERMS are estrogen agonists and antagonists, acting like a weak estrogen in some tissues and as an estrogen blocker in others. The optimal SERM to manage osteoporosis would provide the bone benefits of estrogen without the risks to the endometrium or breast.[11]

Raloxifene (Evista) is the only SERM approved for prevention and treatment of osteoporosis. Raloxifene antagonizes the effects of estrogen on endometrial and breast tissue, but like estrogen, it dampens osteoclastic activity in bone (Table 34-14). Increases in BMD range from 1% to 3%. Results from the Multiple Outcomes of Raloxifene Evaluation (MORE) trial showed that after 36 months of treatment, compared to control subjects, the risk of clinical vertebral fracture in women with low BMD (mean age 67 years) receiving raloxifene 60 mg daily was decreased 30% (RR = 0.7; 95% CI, 0.5–0.8) and for those taking 120 mg daily the benefit was a 50% reduction (RR = 0.5; 95% CI, 0.4–0.7).[116] Side effects include development and/or worsening of vasomotor symptoms, which can be severe, and leg cramps. There was a null effect on cardiovascular disease, although it did have the same risk of venous thromboembolic event as estrogen. In two large trials, raloxifene significantly reduced the incidence of estrogen receptor-positive breast cancer without causing endometrium proliferation[116-120] (Table 34-15).

The optimal length of treatment with SERMS remains unknown, although the BMD increase and breast cancer protection has been shown to continue when women take the drug for as long as 8 years. A decline of 2.4% in BMD was noted within the first year after therapy ended.[116] From another perspective, Mosca et al. studied the effect of raloxifene on the incidence of all strokes, stroke deaths, and venous thromboembolic events. 10,101 women who had or were at risk for coronary heart disease were followed for 5.6 years. While the differences for all strokes did not differ between groups, the women in the raloxifene group versus placebo group had a higher incidence of fatal strokes and venous thromboembolic events.[120] Treatment options for raloxifene should be based on a balance of the potential risks and the possible benefits.

NAMS guidelines suggest raloxifene be considered for young postmenopausal women with osteoporosis whose risk for spine fracture is greater than hip, and for older women with low bone mass.[103] The extraskeletal risks and benefits associated with raloxifene should be factors in the decision.

Calcitonin

Parafollicular cells that surround the thyroid secrete the hormone calcitonin (CT). An increase in serum calcium stimulates the secretion of CT, as does estrogen. Its importance

---

Table 34-15 Randomized Clinical Trials of Raloxifene (Evista)

Study	Year	Study Intention	Major Findings
MORE[116]	1994 4 years N = 7705	Endpoint: (1) determination of the effect of raloxifene on risk of vertebral and nonvertebral fractures in women with osteoporosis; (2) breast cancer incidence.	Data resulted in the approval of raloxifene 60 mg per day for treatment and prevention of osteoporosis; reduced risk of invasive breast cancer by 76% in estrogen + receptor disease.
RUTH[118] trial	1988–2000 N = 10,101 Median 5.6 years	To evaluate the risks and benefits of raloxifene in women with or at risk for CHD. First endpoint is incidence of coronary disease; second is breast cancer.	No difference in incidence of death from coronary causes. The results were also not different in women with established coronary disease; second 44% reduced incidence of estrogen receptor + invasive breast cancer.
CORE[119]	1999, follow-up at years 4 and 8 N = 4011	(1) Determine incidence of invasive breast cancer in response to raloxifene; (2) toxicities associated with raloxifene after 8 years (same women as in the MORE trial).	Raloxifene group had reduced incidence of estrogen receptor + disease invasive breast disease. Data from MORE and CORE showed a reduction of estrogen receptor + breast cancer with raloxifene compared to placebo.
STAR[117]	1999–2004 N = 19,747 Median age 58.5	To compare tamoxifen to raloxifene in postmenopausal women at increased risk of breast cancer. Endpoints: invasive breast cancer, endometrial cancer, CVD, osteoporotic fracture.	No difference for invasive breast cancer; fewer noninvasive cancers (both lobular in situ and ductal carcinoma in situ) in tamoxifen group but did not reach significance; tamoxifen increased endometrial cancer while no such increase with raloxifene.
Mosca[120]	2002–2008 N = 10,101	Evaluate effect of raloxifene on all strokes.	For incidence of *all* strokes, there was no difference between raloxifene and placebo; higher incidence of fatal stroke with raloxifene but no other strokes. Smoking proved to result in greater incidence of stroke.

Sources: Ettinger B et al. 1999[116]; Vogel VG et al. 2006[117]; Mosca L et al. 2001[118]; Siris ES et al. 2005[119]; Mosca L et al. 2009.[120]

in regulating calcium has not been clearly established, and, unlike parathyroid hormone (PTH), an excess or shortage has little effect on calcium homeostasis. The pharmaceutical calcitonin, another osteoclast inhibitor, is not as efficacious as the other options for management of osteoporosis and should be reserved for those women who cannot tolerate a more potent treatment. This agent increases BMD in the 3–5% range and decreases vertebral fracture by 36% after 5 years of use.[11] Calcitonin is approved for treatment, but not prevention of osteoporosis in women at least 5 years postmenopause. This drug also has been found to help decrease bone pain immediately after fracture and may be helpful in treating osteoarthritis. A side effect of the nasal spray is local irritation.

Anabolic Agent: Parathyroid Hormone

The hormone PTH is the major agent in bone remodeling involved in both formation and resorption of bone. This agent also regulates serum calcium through action on the kidneys, bone, and intestine. When used for osteoporosis management, parathyroid hormone (teriparatide [recombinant human PTH 1–34]) is an agent in a class by itself. It stimulates osteoblasts, resulting in substantial increases in bone density. This drug, administered by subcutaneous injection, is approved for up to 2 years of use for adults with high fracture risk.[121] Vertebral fracture risk has been shown to decrease by 65% (RR = 0.35; 95% CI, 0.25–0.88), and BMD of the spine improves with treatment.[107] When treatment ends, there is rapid bone loss.[116] Treatment with alendronate following teriparatide has been found to maintain or improve BMD.[103] The safety of a second course of teriparatide is unknown. NAMS recommends reserving this drug for women with very high risk of fracture and very low BMD (< −3.0 T-score).[103]

The most common side effect of this pharmaceutical is muscle cramps. Hypercalcemia, nausea, and vertigo are experienced infrequently. Contraindications include hypercalcemia, bone metastases, Paget's disease, and prior skeletal radiation (including radiation for breast cancer).[121]

Tibolone (Livial)

Tibolone (Livial) is a synthetic selective tissue estrogenic regulator that affects different tissues in different ways. Tibolone has weak estrogenic, androgenic, and progestational properties. This agent has been available for the last 2 decades in many countries, although not in the United States. Concerns have been expressed about an increased incidence of stroke and abnormal bleeding associated with this drug. In addition, the effects of this agent on actual fractures, breast cancer, and cardiovascular disease remain uncertain.[122]

The Tibolone Histology of the Endometrium and Breast Endpoints Study (THEBES) was conducted among 3240 women receiving either CEE and MPA or tibolone over a period of 2 years. In the CEE/MPA group, there were two cases of endometrial hyperplasia and none in the tibolone group. The incidence of atrophic/inactive endometrium was higher in the tibolone group, giving credence to the safety of tibolone use with regard to the endometrium.[122,123]

However, other studies continue to suggest that there may be an association between tibolone and endometrial activity, as well as other issues. In 2008, results from the LIFT (Long Term Intervention on Fractures with Tibolone) trial were published. This 3-year, randomized, controlled trial with a 2-year extension included 4538 postmenopausal women. Multiple benefits were found, including a decreased risk of vertebral fracture (relative hazard [RH] = 0.55; 95% CI, 0.41–0.74; $P < .001$), decreased risk of nonvertebral fracture, (RH = 0.74; 95% CI, 0.58–0.93; $P = .01$), decreased risk of invasive breast cancer (RH = 0.32; 95% CI, 0.13–0.80; $P = .02$), and a decreased risk of colon cancer (RH = 0.31; 95% CI, 0.10–0.96; $P = .04$). However, women in the tibolone group were twice as likely to experience a stroke than cohorts not using tibolone (RH = 2.19; 95% CI, 1.14–4.23; $P = .02$).[124] Vaginal bleeding was found among 9.5% of the women on tibolone versus 2.5% among women on placebo ($P = .001$) and in contrast to the THEBES trial, endometrial cancer was diagnosed for four of the women on tibolone, but none on placebo. However it was the doubling of the risk of stroke that ultimately caused the trial to be halted prematurely.

Pharmaceuticals for Osteoporosis

Postmenopausal osteoporosis often is an underestimated health concern, especially in slender, White women. As the population ages, osteoporosis will have an enormous impact on public health. Prevention trumps treatment, and should be lifelong, beginning during childhood when adequate calcium, vitamin D, and exercise can help women achieve peak bone mass. Fracture prevention for all women can be nonpharmacologic, focusing on fall prevention, decreasing alcohol and cigarette consumption, and improving diet. Medications for management of osteopenia and osteoporosis have varying effects and side-effect profiles, and specialists are best suited to help women choose a regimen. Optimal duration of therapy has not been clearly determined.

Conclusion

Menopause is a time of mystery, a rite of passage, and a new direction. The woman who is menopausal has the opportunity to find her strong voice and become her true self. Some women dread the onset of menopausal changes, but most travel the road without distress or problems. Often the decade before the menopause is when women experience the most anxiety. This apprehension is lessened for many because menopause is a slow transition; changes happen slowly and sometimes imperceptibly, which relieves women of anticipated stress.

Some of the changes women experience at midlife have more to do with aging, such as decreased skin resilience and turgor, or weight gain than with menopause per se. Other significant changes include relationships—children are leaving home or returning—some of whom are doing well and others who are not. Relationships with spouses must be renegotiated whether or not children are involved. Women find it is a time for reinvestment in themselves as individual women.

Most women experience changes associated with menopause such as vasomotor symptoms and vaginal symptoms. For some women, these symptoms cause great distress, while other women adjust to these symptoms because they are not severe or because the symptoms are accepted as part of the change. For many women, menopausal symptoms cause them to seek health care. In addition to the two symptoms directly related to hormone shifts, women can experience sleep disruption, sexual changes, pain, decreased libido, memory changes, bone loss, and depression during this period of life. Fortunately, pharmacotherapies can offer help for most of these difficulties.

Women have many choices for therapy to treat menopausal or aging symptoms.[129] First and probably the most important is to address lifestyle changes. Second, there are a great many options of drugs. The professional community has a much better understanding about which drug or class of drugs is appropriate for each woman. Women also know much more than they did in past decades. Some women need estrogen alone while others need an estrogen plus progestin product. In some situations, a woman is given a progestin alone. SERMs are used to treat vasomotor symptoms as well as depression. Women may choose to avoid conventional medicines and use bioidentical drugs from a compounding pharmacy or purchase herbs at a health food store. For most women, the symptoms will last 1–3 years. By that time, most women will have stopped treatment. Finally, osteoporosis is a silent but deadly disease that must not be ignored. Women need surveillance, prevention, and sometimes treatment for which there are many options. It is the provider's responsibility to make certain that when conditions occur, the mature woman is diagnosed correctly, on the right drug appropriate for the condition, age-appropriate screening is performed, and health education shared with the woman.

References

1. Centers for Disease Control and Prevention. US Health, 2008. Bethesda, MD: Government Publishing Company, 2009.

2. Hayes BD, Klein-Schwartz W, Barrueto F Jr. Polypharmacy and the geriatric patient. Clin Geriatr Med 2007;23(2):371–90.

3. Jackson SHD, Mangoni AA, Batty GM. Optimization of drug prescribing. Brit J Clin Pharm 2004;57 (3):231–36.

4. Kaufman DW, Kelly JP, Rosenberg L, Anderson TE, Mitchell AA. Recent patterns of medication use in the ambulatory adult population of the United States: the Slone survey. JAMA 2002;287:337–44.

5. Oats JA. The science of drug therapy. In Brunton LL, Lazo JJ, Parker KL, eds. Goodman & Gilman's the pharmacological basis of therapeutics, 11th ed. New York: McGraw-Hill, 2006:117–36.

6. Grady D. Management of menopausal symptoms. N Engl J Med 2006;355:2338–47.

7. Porter M, Penney GC, Russell D, Russell E, Templeton A. A population based survey of women's experience of the menopause. BJOG 1996;103(10):1025–28.

8. Mansfield PK, Carey M, Anderson A, Barsom SH, Koch PB. Staging the menopausal transition: data from the TREMIN research program on women's health. Womens Health Issues 2004;14(6):220–26.

9. Soules MS, Parrott S, Rebar E, Santoro R, Utian N, Woods W, et al. Executive summary: stages of reproductive aging workshop (STRAW). Climacteric 2001; 4(4):267–72.

10. Speroff L, Fritz MA. Clinical gynecologic and endocrinology and infertility, 7th ed. Philadelphia, PA: Lippincott Williams and Wilkins, 2005:639.

11. Menopause practice: a clinician's guide, 3rd ed. Cleveland, OH: North American Menopause Society, 2007.

12. Thurston RS, Sowers MR, Sutton-Tyrrell K, Everson-Rose SA, Lewis TT, Edmundowicz D, et al. Abdominal

adiposity and hot flashes among midlife women. Menopause 2008;15(3):429–34.

13. Moriarty K, Kim KH, Bender JR. Mini review: estrogen receptor-mediated rapid signaling. Endocrinology 2006;147:5557–63.

14. Deroo BJ, Kodrach KS. Estrogen receptors and human disease. J Clin Invest 2006;116:561–70.

15. Chabbert-Buffet N, Meduri G, Bouchard P, Spitz IM. Selective progesterone receptor modulators and progesterone antagonists: mechanisms of action and clinical applications. Hum Reprod Update 2005 May–Jun;11(3):293–307

16. Wilson, R. Feminine forever. New York: Evans, 1996.

17. Rousseau M. Hormone replacement therapy: short-term versus long-term use. J Midwifery Womens Health 2002;47(6):461–70.

18. The North American Menopause Society. Role of pro-gestogens in hormone replacement therapy for post-menopausal women: position statement of the North American Menopause Society. Menopause 2003;10: 113–32.

19. Corson SL, Richart RM, Caubel P, Lim P. Effect of a unique constant-estrogen, pulsed-progestin hormone replacement therapy containing 17B-estradiol and norgestimate on endometrial histology. Int J Fertil 1999;44:279–85.

20. Hackley B, Rousseau, ME. Managing menopausal symptoms after the Women's Health Initiative. J Midwifery Womens Health 2004;49(2):87–95.

21. The Writing Group for the PEPI. Effects of estrogen or estrogen/progestin regimens on heart disease risk factors in postmenopausal women. The Postmeno-pausal Estrogen/Progestin Interventions (PEPI) Trial. JAMA 1995;273(3):199–208.

22. Manson JE, Hsia J, Johnson KC, Rossouw JE, Assaf AR, Lasser NL, et al. Women's Health Initiative Investiga-tors. Estrogen plus progestin and the risk of coronary heart disease. N Engl J Med 2003;349(6):523–34.

23. Anderson G, Limacher M, Assaf AR, Anderson GL, Limacher M, Assaf AR, et al. Effects of conjugated equine estrogen in postmenopausal women with hys-terectomy: the Women's Health Initiative randomized controlled trial. JAMA 2004;291(14):1701–12.

24. Beral V, Bull D, Doll R, Peto R, Reeves G. Collaborative Group on Hormonal Factors in Breast Cancer. Breast cancer and abortion: collaborative reanalysis of data from 53 epidemiological studies, including 83,000 women with breast cancer from 16 countries. Lancet 2004;363(9414):1007–16.

25. Hulley S, Grady D, Bush T, Furberg C, Herrington D, Riggs B, et al. Randomized trial of estrogen plus pro-gestin for secondary prevention of coronary heart dis-ease in postmenopausal women. Heart and Estrogen/ progestin Replacement Study (HERS) Research Group. JAMA 1998;280(7):605–13.

26. Pickar JH, Yeh IT, Wheeler JE, Cunnane MF, Speroff L. Endometrial effects of lower doses of conjugated equine estrogens and medroxyprogester-one acetate: two-year substudy results. Fertil Steril 2003;80(5):1234–40.

27. Rossouw JE, Anderson GL, Prentice RL, LaCroix AZ, Kooperberg C, Stefanick ML, et al. Risks and benefits of estrogen plus progestin in healthy postmenopausal women: principal results from the Women's Health Initiative randomized controlled trial. JAMA 2002; 288:321–33.

28. Sherwin BB. Estrogen and cognitive function in women. Endocr Rev 2003;24:133–51.

29. North American Menopause Society Position State-ment: estrogen and progestogen in peri and post menopausal women: position statement of the North American Menopause Society. Menopause 2007; 14(2):168–82.

30. Hulley S, Grady D. The WHI estrogen alone trial—do things look any better? JAMA 2004;291(14):1771.

31. Huston SA, Jackowski RM, Kirking DM. Women's trust in and use of information sources in the treat-ment of menopausal symptoms. Womens Health Issues 2009;19(2):144–53.

32. Collaborative Group on Hormonal Factors in Breast Cancer. Breast cancer and hormone replacement ther-apy: collaborative reanalysis of data from 51 epidem-iological studies of 52,705 women with breast cancer and 108,411 women without breast cancer. Lancet 1997;350(9084):1047–59.

33. Chlebowski RT, Hendrix SL, Langer RD, Stefanick ML, Gass M, Lane D. Influence of estrogen plus pro-gestin on breast cancer and mammography in heal-thy postmenopausal women: the Women's Health Initiative randomized trial. JAMA 2003;289(24): 3243–53.

34. Stefanick ML, Anderson GL, Margolis KL, Hendrix SL, Rodabough RJ, Paskett ED, et al. Effects of con-jugated equine estrogens on breast cancer and mam-mography screening in postmenopausal women with hysterectomy. JAMA 2006;295(14):1647–57.

35. Reeves GK, Beral V, Green J, Gathani T, Bull D. Hor-monal therapy for menopause and breast cancer risk

by histological type: a cohort study and meta-analysis. Lancet Oncol 2006;7:910–8.

36. Holmberg L, Anderson H. HABITS (hormonal replacement therapy after breast cancer)—is it safe? A randomised comparison: trial stopped. Lancet 2004;363 (9407):453–5.

37. von Schoultz E, Rutqvist LE. Menopausal hormone therapy after breast cancer: the Stockholm randomized trial. J Natl Cancer Inst 2005;97(7):533–5.

38. Sotiriou C, Pusztai L. Gene expression signatures in breast cancer. N Engl J Med 2009;360(8):790–800.

39. Lacey JV Jr, Mink PJ, Lubin JH, Sherman ME, Troisi R, Hartge P, et al. Menopausal hormone replacement therapy and risk of ovarian cancer. JAMA 2002;288 (3):334–41.

40. Rodriguez C, Patel AV, Calle EE, Jacob EJ, Thun MJ. Estrogen replacement therapy and ovarian cancer mortality in a large prospective study of US women. JAMA 2001;285(11):1460–5.

41. Beral V, Million Women Study Collaborators. Ovarian cancer and hormone replacement therapy in the Million Women Study. Lancet 2007;369:1703–10.

42. AACE Menopause Guidelines Revision Task Force. American Association of Clinical Endocrinologists medical guidelines for clinical practice for the diagnosis and treatment of menopause. Endocr Pract 2006;12:315–337.

43. Nachtigall LE. Emerging delivery systems for estrogen replacement: aspects of transdermal and oral delivery. Am J Obstet Gynecol 1995;173:993–7.

44. John SC, Malcolm W. Oral versus non-oral hormone replacement therapy: how important is the route of administration? Ginekol Pol 2007;78(7):514–20.

45. McCoy N, Davidson J. A longitudinal study of the effect of menopause on sexuality. Maturitas 1985;7: 203–10.

46. van der Stege JG, Groen H, van Zadelhoff SJ, Lambalk CB, Braat DD, van Kasteren YM, et al. Decreased androgen concentrations and diminished general and sexual well-being in women with premature ovarian failure. Menopause 2008 Jan-Feb;15(1):23–31.

47. Furness S, Roberts H, Marjoribanks J, Lethaby A, Hickey M, Farquhar C. Hormone therapy in postmenopausal women and risk of endometrial hyperplasia. Cochrane Database Syst Rev 2004;(3):CD000402.

48. Utian WH, Archer DF, Bachmann GA, Gallagher C, Grodstein F, Heiman JR, North American Menopause Society. Estrogen and progestogen use in postmenopausal women: July 2008 position statement of the North American Menopause Society. Menopause 2008;15(4, pt 1):584–602.

49. Hsia J, Langer R, Manson J, Kuller L, Johnson K, Hendrix S, et al. Conjugated equine estrogens and coronary artery disease. Arch Intern Med 2006;166: 357–65.

50. Holzer G, Riegler E, Honigsman H, Farokhnia S, Schmidt JB. Effects and side effects of 2% progesterone cream on the skin of perimenopausal and postmenopausal women: results from a double-blind, vehicle-controlled, randomized study. Br J Dermatol 2005;153:626–34.

51. Lethaby A, Suckling J, Barlow D, Farquhar CM, Jepson RG, Roberts H. Hormone replacement therapy in postmenopausal women: endometrial hyperplasia and irregular bleeding. Cochrane Database Syst Rev 2004;(3):CD000402.

52. Smith DC, Prentice R. Thompson DJ, Herrmann WL. Association of exogenous estrogen and endometrial carcinoma. N Engl J Med 1975;293(23):1164–7.

53. Ziel HF, Finkle WD. Increased risk of endometrial carcinoma among users of conjugated estrogens. N Engl J Med 1975;293(23):1167–70.

54. Bjarnason K, Cerin A, Lindgren R, Weber T. Adverse endometrial effects during long cycle hormone replacement therapy. Scandinavian Long Cycle Study Group. Maturitas 1999;32:161–70.

55. Ettinger B, Selby J, Citron JT, Vangessel A, Ettinger VM, Hendrickson MR. Cyclic hormone replacement therapy using quarterly progestin. Obstet Gynecol 1994;83:693–700.

56. Loose DS, Stancel GM. Estrogens and progesterones. In Brunton LL, Lazo JJ, Parker KL, eds. Goodman & Gilman's the pharmacological basis of therapeutics, 11th ed. New York: McGraw-Hill, 2006:1541–72.

57. Martin KM, Manson JE. Approach to the patient with menopausal symptoms. Endocr Metab 2008;93(12): 4567–75.

58. Ettinger B. Personal perspective of low-dose estrogen therapy for postmenopausal women. Menopause 1999;6:273–76.

59. US Food and Drug Administration. FDA takes action against compounded menopause hormone therapy drugs. 2008. Available from: *http://orwh.od.nih.gov/FDA_ActionHormoneTherapyDrugs.html* [June 23, 2009].

60. Eisenberg DM, Kessler RC, Foster C, Norlock FE, Calkins DR, Delbanco T. Unconventional medicine in the United States: prevalence, costs, and patterns of use. N Engl J Med 1993;328(4):246–52.

61. Albertazzi P. Non-estrogenic approaches for the treatment of climacteric symptoms. Climacteric 2007;2: 115–20.

62. Uebelhack RB, Blohmer JU, Graubaum HJ, Busch R, Gruenwald J, Wernecke KD. Black cohosh and St. John's wort for climacteric complaints: a randomized trial. Obstet Gynecol 2006;107(2, pt 1):247–55.

63. Newton KR, Reed SD, LaCroix AZ, Grothaus LC, Ehrlich K, Guiltinan J. Treatment of vasomotor symptoms of menopause with black cohosh, multi botanicals, soy, hormone therapy, or placebo: a randomized trial. Ann Intern Med 2006;145(12):869–79.

64. Knight DH, Howes JB, Eden JA. The effect of Promensil, an isoflavone extract, on menopausal symptoms. Climacteric 1999;2(2):79–84.

65. Tice JE, Ettinger B, Ensrud K, Wallace R, Blackwell T, Cummings SR. Phytoestrogen supplements for the treatment of hot flashes: the Isoflavone Clover Extract (ICE) Study: a randomized controlled trial. JAMA 2003;290(2):207–14.

66. Society NAM. Treatment of menopause-associated vasomotor symptoms: position statement of the North American Menopause Society. Menopause 2004;11 (1):11–33.

67. Lurain JR. Uterine cancer. In Berek JS, ed. Berek & Novak's gynecology, 14th ed. Philadelphia, PA: Lippincott Williams and Wilkins, 2007:1343–401.

68. Peled Y, Perri T, Pardo Y, Kaplan B. Levonorgestrel-releasing intrauterine system as an adjunct to estrogen for the treatment of menopausal symptoms—a review. Menopause 2007;14(3):550–4.

69. Secor RM, Simon JA. New options for treating the symptoms of menopause. Womens Health Ob-Gyn Ed. 2006(July–August):44–52.

70. Berecki-Gisolf J, Begum N, Dobson AJ. Symptoms reported by women in midlife: menopausal transition or aging? Menopause 2009 Jun 10;[in press].

71. Freeman EW, Sammel MD, Grisso JA, Berlin JA, Grisso JA, Battistini M. Hot flashes in the late reproductive years: risk factors for African American and Caucasian women. J Women Health Gend Based Med 2001;10:67–76.

72. Bachman GA. Vasomotor symptoms in postmenopausal women. Am J Obstet Gynecol 1999;180(3, pt 2): S312–S16.

73. Woods NC, Carr MC, Tao EY, Taylor HJ, Mitchell ES. Increased urinary cortisol levels during the menopausal transition. Menopause 2006;13(2):212–21.

74. Reame NK. Adiposity and hot flashes: one more tree in the forest. Menopause 2008;15(3):408–9.

75. Dalal S, Zhukovsky D. Pathophysiology and management of hot flashes. J Support Oncol 2006;4(7):315–20.

76. Freedman RR, Roehrs TA. Sleep disturbance in menopause. Menopause 2007;14:826–9.

77. Loprinzi CK, Kugler JW, Sloan JA, Mailliard JA, LaVasseur BI, Barton PJ, et al. Venlafaxine in management of hot flashes in survivors of breast cancer: a randomised controlled trial. Lancet 2000;356(9247): 2059–63.

78. Archer DF, Dupont CM, Constantine GD, Pickar JH, Olivier S, Study 319 Investigators. Desvenlafaxine for the treatment of vasomotor symptoms associated with menopause: a double-blind, randomized, placebo-controlled trial of efficacy and safety. Am J Obstet Gynecol 2009;200(3):238.

79. Loprinzi CS, Sloan JA. Perez EA, Quella SK, Stella PJ, Mailliard JA, et al. Phase III evaluation of fluoxetine for treatment of hot flashes. J Clin Oncol 2002;20(6): 1578–83.

80. Loprinzi CL, Levitt R, Barton D, Sloan JA, Dakhil SR, Nikcevich DA, et al. Phase III comparison of depomedroxyprogesterone acetate to venlafaxine for managing hot flashes: North Central Cancer Treatment Group Trial N99C7. J Clin Oncol 2006;24(9):1409–14.

81. National Sleep Foundation. Sleep in America poll. Washington, DC, 2007. Available from: *http://www .sleepfoundation.org/sites/default/files/Summary_Of _Findings%20-%20FINAL.pdf* [Accessed June 26, 2009].

82. Reed SD, Newton KM, LaCroix AZ, Grothaus LC, Ehrlich K. Night sweats, sleep disturbance, and depression associated with diminished libido in late menopausal transition and early postmenopause baseline data from the Herbal Alternatives for Menopause Trial (HALT). Am J Obstet Gynecol 2007;196(6): 593.e1–593.e7.

83. Hachul H, Bittencourt LR, Anderson ML, Haidar MA, Baracat EC, Tufik S. Effects of hormone therapy with estrogen and/or progesterone on sleep pattern in postmenopausal women. Int J Gynaecol Obstet 2008 Dec;103(3):207–12.

84. Gracia CR, Sammel MD, Freeman EW, Liu L, Hollander L, Nelson DB. Predictors of decreased libido in women during the late reproductive years. Menopause 2004;11:144–55.

85. Hallward A, Ellison JM. Antidepressants and sexual function. London: Mosby, 2001:8–9.

86. Meston CM, Derogatis LR. Validated instruments for assessing female sexual function. J Sex Marit Ther 2002;28(suppl):155–64.

87. Basaria S, Dobs AS. Clinical review: controversies regarding transdermal androgen therapy in postmenopausal women. J Clin Endocrinol Metab 2006;91(12): 4743–52.

88. Simon J, Braunstein G, Nachtigall L. Testosterone patch increases sexual activity and desire in surgically menopausal women with hypoactive sexual desire disorder. J Clin Endocrinol Metab 2005;90:5226–33.

89. Sarrel P, Dobay B, Wiita B. Estrogen and estrogen-androgen replacement in postmenopausal women dissatisfied with estrogen-only therapy. J Reprod Med 1998;43:847–56.

90. Phillips SM, Sherwin BB. Effects of estrogen on memory function in surgically menopausal women. Psychoneuroendocrinol 1992;17:485–95.

91. Bjorn I, Bixol M, Strandberg N, Nyberg S, Backstrom T. Negative mood changes during hormone replacement therapy: a comparison between two progestogens. Am J Obstet Gynecol 2000;183:1419–26.

92. Colcombe S, Kramer AF. Fitness effects on the cognitive function of older adults: a meta-analytic study. Psychol Sci 2003;14:125–30.

93. Espeland MA, Rapp SR, Schumaker SA, Brunner R, Manson JR, Sherwin B, et al. For the Women's Health Initiative Memory Study Investigators. Conjugated equine estrogens and global cognitive function in postmenopausal women: Women's Health Initiative Memory study. JAMA 2004;291:2959–68.

94. Bagger YZ, Tanko LB, Alexandersen P, Qin G, Christiansen C. Early postmenopause hormone replacement therapy may prevent cognitive impairment later in life. Menopause 2005;12:12–7.

95. Edlin G, Golanty E. Health and wellness, 9th ed. Sudbury, MA: Jones and Bartlett, 2007:48.

96. Kanis JA and the WHO Study Group. Assessment of fracture risk and its application to screening for postmenopausal osteoporosis. Report of a WHO study group. Osteoporosis Int 1994;4:368–81.

97. Bonjour JP, Theintz G, Law F, Slosman D, Rizzoli R. Peak bone mass. Osteoporosis Int 1994;4(suppl 1):S7–S13.

98. Perrien DS, Achenbach SJ, Bledsoe SE, Wasler B, Suva LJ, Khosla S, et al. Bone turnover across the menopause transition: correlations with inhibins and follicle stimulating hormone. J Clin Endocrinol Metab 2006;9:1848–54.

99. Gallagher JC. Effect of early menopause on bone mineral density and fractures. Menopause 2007;14(3): 567–71.

100. Gerdhem P, Obrant KJ. Bone mineral density in the old age: the influence of age at menarche and menopause. J Bone Miner Metab LJ I 2004;22:372–5.

101. Borer KT. Physical activity in the prevention and amelioration of osteoporosis in women: interaction of mechanical, hormonal and dietary factors. Sports Med 2005;35(9):779–830.

102. Berg KM, Kunins HV, Jackson JL, Nahvi S, Caudhry A, Harris KA Jr, et al. Association between alcohol consumption and both osteoporotic fracture and bone density. Am J Med 2008;121(5):406–18.

103. North American Menopause Society. Position statement. Management of osteoporosis in postmenopausal women: 2006. Menopause 2006;13:340–67.

104. Himes R, Wezeman FH, Callaci JJ. Identification of novo bone-specific molecular targets of binge alcohol and ibandronate by transcriptome analysis. Alcohol Clin Exp Res 1008;32(7):1167–80.

105. Krall E, Dawson-Hughes B. Smoking and bone loss among postmenopausal women. J Bone Miner Res 1991;6(4):331–8.

106. Bischoff-Ferrari HA, Willett WC, Wong JB, Giovannucci E, Dietrich T, Dawson-Hughes B. Fracture prevention with vitamin D supplementation: a meta-analysis of randomized controlled trials. JAMA 2005;293(18): 2257–64.

107. Harris ST. A randomized controlled trial. Vertebral Efficacy with Risedronate Therapy (VERT) Study Group. JAMA 1999;282(14):1344–52.

108. Reginster JM, Minne HW, Sorensen OH, Hooper M, Roux C, Brandi ML, et al. Randomized trial of the effects of risedronate on vertebral fractures in women with established postmenopausal osteoporosis. Vertebral Efficacy with Risedronate Therapy (VERT) Study Group. Osteoporosis Int 2000;11(1):83–91.

109. McClung MR, Geusens P, Miller PD, Zippel H, Bensen WG, Roux C, et al. Hip Intervention Program Study Group. Effect of risedronate on the risk of hip fracture in elderly women: Hip Intervention Program Study Group. N Engl J Med 2001;334(5):333–40.

110. Black DM, Cummings SR, Karpf DB, Cauley J, Thompson D, Nevitt D, et al. Randomised trial of effect of alendronate on risk of fracture in women with existing vertebral fractures. Lancet 1996;348(9050): 1535–42.

111. Ensrud KB-C, Barrett-Connor EL, Schwartz A, Santora AC, Bauer DC, Suryawanshi S, et al. Fracture Intervention Trial Long-Term Extension Research Group. Randomized trial of effect of alendronate continuation versus discontinuation in women with low BMD: results from the Fracture Intervention Trial long-term extension. J Bone Mineral Res 2004 Aug;19(8):1259–69.

112. Tonino RM, Meunier PJ, Emkey R, Rodriguez-Portales JA, Menkes CJ, Wasnich RD. Skeletal benefits of alendronate: 7-year treatment of postmenopausal osteoporotic women. Phase III Osteoporosis Treatment Study Group. J Clin Endocrinol Metab 2000;85(9): 3109–15.

113. Yates J, Barrett-Connor E, Barlas S, Chen Ya-Ting, Miller P, Siris E. Rapid loss of hip fracture protection after estrogen cessation: evidence from national osteoporosis risk assessment. Obstet Gynecol 2004;103(3): 440–6.

114. Zizic T. Pharmacologic prevention of osteoporotic fractures. Am Fam Physician 2004;70(7):1293–300.

115. Black DM, Pierre DD, Eastell R, Reid IR, Boonen S, Cauley JA, et al. Once-yearly zoledronic acid for treatment of postmenopausal osteoporosis. N Engl J Med 2007;356(18):1809–22.

116. Ettinger B, Black DM, Mitland BH, Knickerbocker RK, Nickelsen T, Genant HK, et al. Reduction of vertebral fracture risk in postmenopausal women with osteoporosis treated with raloxifene. JAMA 1999;282: 637–45.

117. Vogel VG, Costantino JP, Wickerham DL, Cronin WM, Cecchini RS, Atkins JN, et al. National Surgical Adjuvant Breast and Bowel Project (NSABP). Effects of tamoxifen vs raloxifene on the risk of developing invasive breast cancer and other disease outcomes: the NSABP Study of Tamoxifen and Raloxifene (STAR) P-2 trial. JAMA 2006;295(23):2727–41.

118. Mosca L, Barrett-Connor E, Wenger NK, Collins P, Grady D, Kornitzer M, et al. Design and methods of the Raloxifene Use for the Heart (RUTH) study. Am J Cardiol 2001;88(4):392–5.

119. Siris ES, Harris ST, Eastell R, Zanchetta JR, Goemaere S, Diez-Perez A, et al. Continuing Outcomes Relevant to Evista (CORE) Investigators. Skeletal effects of raloxifene after 8 years: results from the Continuing Outcomes Relevant to Evista (CORE) study. J Bone Miner Res 2005;20(9):1514–24.

120. Mosca L, Grady D, Barrett-Connor E, Collins P, Wenger N, Abramson BL, et al. Effect of raloxifene on stroke and venous thromboembolism according to subgroups in postmenopausal women at increased risk of coronary heart disease. Stroke 2009;40(1): 147–55.

121. Neer RM, Arnaud CD, Zanchetta JR, et al. Effect of parathyroid hormone on fractures and bone mineral density in postmenopausal women with osteoporosis. N Engl J Med 2001;344:1434–41.

122. Archer DF, Dorin M, Lewis V, Schneider DL, Pickar JH. Effects of lower doses of conjugated equine estrogens and medroxyprogesterone acetate on endometrial bleeding. Fertil Steril 2001;75(6):1080–7.

123. Fuleihan G el-H. Tibolone and the promise of ideal hormone-replacement therapy. N Engl J Med 2008;359:753–75.

124. Cummings SR, Ettinger B, Delmas PD, Kenemans P, Stathopoulos V, Verweij P, et al. LIFT Trial Investigators. The effects of tibolone in older postmenopausal women. N Engl J Med 2008;359(7):697–708.

125. Alexander IM, Andrist LC. Menopause. In Schuiling K, Likis F, eds. Women's gynecologic health. Sudbury, MA: Jones and Bartlett, 2006:249–89.

126. Decker GM, Meyers J. Commonly used herbs: implications for clinical practice. Clin J Onco Nurs 2001 Mar–Apr;5(2):13p.

127. Gaudet TW. CAM approaches to menopause management: overview of the options. Menopause Manage Womens Health Through Midlife Beyond 2004; 13(1):48–50.

128. Low Dog T. CAM approaches to menopause management: the role for botanicals in menopause. Menopause Manage Womens Health Through Midlife Beyond 2004;13(1):51–3.

129. North American Menopause Society. Treatment of menopause-associated vasomotor symptoms: position statement of the North American Menopause Society. Menopause 2004;11(1):11–33.

VI

Pregnancy and Lactation

The last section of this book discusses pharmacology and areas of quintessential women's health. Pregnancy and lactation are specific to women. It would be ideal if all women were so healthy during pregnancy, during childbirth, and while breastfeeding that no drugs were recommended. However, some drugs, such as folic acid, are suggested to promote health. Other agents are used for common conditions such as anemia and various infections. Others are used to stop a medical emergency such as postpartum hemorrhage.

The chapter titled "Pregnancy" discusses the pharmacologic management of a wide variety of conditions that can occur during pregnancy. The pharmacotherapeutic challenge of considering two individuals simultaneously is addressed at length. "Labor" includes discussion of various conditions that may occur during the intrapartum period as well as pain management for women in labor. The following chapter, "Postpartum," acknowledges that healthy women rarely need drugs during this period of time. However, those conditions that are best treated pharmacologically are presented.

There is no controversy that breast is best, but some breastfeeding women have conditions that also are best treated with drugs. "Breastfeeding Mothers" provides a discussion of the challenge involved in choosing the best treatments for the maternal/newborn dyad while promoting the continuation of breastfeeding. The last chapter, "The Newborn," provides a review of pharmacology of the fetus/neonate and a discussion of common therapies for these young individuals.

35
Pregnancy

Laura Manns-James

Chapter Glossary

Embryogenesis The process by which an embryo is formed and develops.

Erythroblastosis fetalis An alloimmune condition that develops in the fetus when maternal IgG antibodies cross the placenta and attack fetal red blood cells. Fetal anemia and fetal hydrops develop as the disease progresses. Erythroblasts are a form of reticulocyte or immature red blood cell that still has a nucleus. The presence of a large number of erythroblasts in the fetal circulation is the basis of the name *erythroblastosis fetalis*.

Fetotoxic Agent that produces toxic effects in a fetus.

Food and Drug Administration (FDA) pregnancy category An assessment of a pharmaceutical's risk of fetal injury based on animal studies, human studies, or both. The FDA mandates that pregnancy categories be assigned, but the decision about which category a drug should be assigned to is made by the drug manufacturer.

Ion trapping A higher concentration of a chemical on one side of a cell membrane against a concentration gradient that would normally equalize. Ion trapping occurs when the ion is altered on one side of the membrane in a way that prevents transport across the membrane.

Placental barrier The layer of placental tissue that separates maternal and fetal circulations. It is not really a barrier, and thus the term is somewhat misleading.

Teratogen Any agent that irreversibly alters growth, structure, or function of a developing embryo or fetus.

Thyrotoxicosis Hypermetabolic clinical syndrome that is the result of serum elevations in thyroid hormones.

Introduction

Pregnant women and their providers are always concerned about the effect of drugs on the developing fetus. Despite this worry, most women use both over-the-counter or prescription drugs during pregnancy.[1] The most common medications used are vitamins, calcium, iron, and analgesics.[2,3] The most common prescription medications used are antidepressants, anxiolytics, antiasthmatics, antibiotics, nonsteroidal anti-inflammatory drugs (NSAIDs), and oral contraceptives and Rho(D) immunoglobulin.[4] Approximately one in every five pregnant women in the United States uses a medication that is classified as **Food and Drug Administration Pregnancy Category** D or X at least once.[5,6]

Medication use during pregnancy has changed a great deal since the thalidomide disaster was made public in 1963.[7] Today women and their care providers are very concerned about drugs that cause birth defects. However, 50% of pregnancies are unintended, and awareness of pregnancy usually occurs after **embryogenesis** has started. In addition, there has been an explosion of new drugs available for treating common conditions, and knowledge of the effect of these drugs in pregnant women is sparse.

The public often assumes that studies done prior to FDA approval identify all possible adverse effects of a drug, including possible birth defects. Unfortunately, the opposite is true. Most rare adverse effects and teratogenic effects are only discovered after the drug is on the market and used by large numbers of individuals, including pregnant women. Several types of studies are required prior to FDA approval. The teratogenic effects or lack of teratogenic effects found in required animal studies cannot be translated to human effects reliably, and the human clinical trials that evaluate efficacy and safety do not include pregnant women.[8,9] Postmarketing reporting of teratogenic effects is not required. Thus clinicians who must balance drug efficacy with drug safety, often do not have enough information to inform their decisions. This chapter summarizes the pharmacokinetic changes of pregnancy and reviews the efficacy and safety of drugs commonly used by pregnant women.

Teratology and Fetotoxic Drugs

Prior to the recognition in 1941 that rubella was a teratogen, the placenta was viewed as a protective barrier that kept the fetus from being exposed to harmful agents.[7] In 1963 it became clear that thalidomide, which was administered to treat nausea, is a potent **teratogen**.[7] It is now known that the placenta is not an impermeable barrier and drugs can be teratogenic.

After the recognition that thalidomide causes limb deformities, concerns about the teratogenesis of drugs increased. In some cases, these fears resulted in drugs being removed from the market that did not have real evidence of fetal harm. In at least one case, a drug that is safe and effective for use during pregnancy is no longer available to women in the United States (Box 35-1).

Teratogens (from the Greek word *teratos*, which means "monster") are agents that irreversibly alter growth, structure, or function of the developing embryo or fetus. Fears about teratogens are common, yet both women and clinicians tend to overestimate teratogenic risk.[10] The background risk for all congenital malformations is approximately 3–4%.[4] Yet ≤ 3% are attributable to drug exposures. There are relatively few drugs that are categorically teratogenic, and this list has remained remarkably consistent and short for several decades, despite the recent explosion of new drugs used in practice. The criteria used to determine that a drug is a teratogen is listed in Box 35-2.[11]

The drugs that can cause fetal harm are categorized as either teratogenic or **fetotoxic** based on the gestational age that exposure occurs. Nicotine is fetotoxic because it does not cause malformations but can cause fetal growth restriction. Ethanol is both a teratogen and a fetotoxic agent because it can cause major malformations (e.g., fetal alcohol syndrome [FAS]) and developmental alterations (e.g., alcohol-related neurodevelopmental disorder [ARND]).[12] Drug effects can be evident at birth, as was the case with the limb abnormalities caused by thalidomide, or appear after a long latency period, which is the story of diethylstilbestrol (DES). Finally, many drugs have a threshold below which no fetal harm occurs. Table 35-1 lists selected known teratogenic and fetotoxic drugs.

Box 35-1 Gone But Not Forgotten: The Bendectin Story

Bendectin, a combination of doxylamine and pyridoxine (vitamin B_6), was approved by the FDA in the 1950s to treat nausea and vomiting of early pregnancy. In the 1970s, lawsuits arose, erroneously claiming that Bendectin caused birth defects. The drug was withdrawn from the US market in 1982 despite evidence that it was a safe and effective medication used by 40% of pregnant women. The manufacturer chose to withdraw Bendectin due to fear of litigation; Bendectin thus became the first "litogen." After Bendectin was withdrawn from the market, hospitalizations of pregnant women for nausea and vomiting doubled in the United States and Canada. To date, no other medication has been approved by the US FDA for the indication of nausea and vomiting of early pregnancy (the drug continues to be available in Canada under the name Diclectin).[19] The Bendectin story illustrates the impact that fear of teratogenic risk, in the absence of evidence, can have on the entire childbearing population of a country.

The formula for Bendectin can be duplicated using doxylamine, marketed over the counter as Unisom, and pyridoxine (vitamin B_6). The original formula included 10 mg each of doxylamine and pyridoxine. An alternative is to take 10 mg pyridoxine and 10 mg doxylamine (Unisom) two to three times per day. 10 mg of doxylamine is roughly 1/2 of a tablet, so many prescribers recommend that women take 10 mg of pyridoxine three times per day and 1/2 tablet of doxylamine (Unisom) in the morning and again at night. It can be difficult to find 10 mg tablets of pyridoxine (Vitamin B_6) and some studies have shown that larger doses improve the efficacy. Therefore, a half of a 25 mg or 50 mg tablet taken twice daily can be substituted for the 10 mg tablet if needed. Doxylamine may cause drowsiness (Unisom is marketed as a sleep aid), and women should be cautioned to avoid driving until they are familiar with how the medication affects their level of alertness. There are two drugs marketed as Unisom. Women who are going to use this over-the-counter formula need to be cautioned to get the Unisom that is doxylamine, which is formed into a tablet, and avoid the Unisom that is phenylhydrine, which is formed as a capsule.

Box 35-2 Criteria for Proof of Human Teratogenicity*

1. Proven exposure to agent at critical time(s) in prenatal development (prescriptions, physicians' records, dates).

2. Consistent findings by two or more epidemiologic studies of high quality

   a. control of confounding factors

   b. sufficient numbers

   c. exclusion of positive and negative bias factors

   d. prospective studies, if possible

   e. relative risk of six or more

3. Careful delineation of the clinical cases. A specific defect or syndrome, if present, is very helpful.

4. Rare environmental exposure associated with rare defect. Probably three or more cases (e.g., oral anticoagulants and nasal hypoplasia, methimazole (Tapazole) and scalp defects).

5. Teratogenicity in experimental animals important but not essential.

6. The association should make biologic sense.

7. Proof in an experimental system that the agent acts in an unaltered state. This is important information for prevention.

* Items 1–3 or 1, 3, and 4 are essential criteria.

Source: Shephard TH 1994.[11]

Table 35-1 Drugs Associated with Birth Defects

Drug Generic (Brand)	Teratogenic or Fetotoxic Effect	Critical Period
Aminoglycosides; e.g., streptomycin, kanamycin	Congenital deafness (eighth cranial nerve damage).	All trimesters
Amiodarone (Cordarone)	Contains iodine and can cause transient fetal hypothyroidism if given in the second or third trimester.	Second and third trimesters
Androgenic steroids; e.g., danazol	Virilization of the female fetus; clitoromegaly and labial fusion.	All trimesters
Angiotensin-converting-enzyme inhibitors	Prolonged renal failure and hypotension in the newborn, decreased skull ossification, renal tubule dysgenesis. First-trimester exposure: increased risk of cardiovascular and nervous system abnormalities.	Second and third trimesters
Angiotensin II receptor blockers	Prolonged renal failure and hypotension in the newborn, decreased skull ossification, renal tubule dysgenesis.	All trimesters
Anticonvulsants; e.g., carbamazepine	Neural tube defects, higher than background risk for several congenital malformations.	First trimester
Antithyroid drugs; e.g., propylthiouracil and methimazole	Fetal and neonatal goiter, fetal hypothyroidism, aplasia cutis with methimazole.	All trimesters
Aspirin	Low dose (80 mg/d): low evidence of harm and some benefit in pregnancies complicated by antiphospholipid antibody syndrome or lupus. High dose (> 150 mg/d): evidence for prolonged gestation, prolonged labor, bleeding complications in the neonate, premature closure of ductus arteriosus, intrauterine growth restriction, increased perinatal mortality.	All trimesters
Benzodiazepines	Early data on oral cleft association is controversial, but because of lipophilic nature, increased risk of neonatal withdrawal.	All trimesters

(continues)

Table 35-1 Drugs Associated with Birth Defects (continued)

Drug Generic (Brand)	Teratogenic or Fetotoxic Effect	Critical Period
Cocaine	Vascular disruption increases likelihood of malformations, placental abruption.	All trimesters
Cyclophosphamide (Cytoxan)	CNS and skeletal defects, fetal growth restriction, cleft palate.	First trimester
Diethylstilbestrol (DES)	Clear cell adenocarcinoma, vaginal adenosis, cervical and uterine abnormalities.	First trimester
Ergot alkaloids	Spontaneous abortion and stillbirth, Möebius syndrome, intestinal atresia, cerebral development abnormalities.	All trimesters
Ethanol	Fetal alcohol syndrome or effects, physical and neurologic/behavioral abnormalities.	All trimesters
Iodine/iodides	Significant absorption following maternal topical, vaginal, or perineal use. Transient hypothyroidism in some newborns. Development of fetal goiter.	All trimesters
Isotretinoin (Accutane)	CNS abnormalities, craniofacial anomalies, conotruncal cardiovascular malformations, thymic defects, branchial-arch mesenchymal-tissue defects, miscellaneous anomalies.	All trimesters
Lindane (Kwell)	Potential for neurotoxicity, convulsions, and aplastic anemia.	All trimesters
Lithium (Lithobid)	Small risk of Ebstein's anomaly (1 to 2 in 1000). Risk for maternal and fetal/neonatal toxicity.	First trimester
Methotrexate (Trexall)	Folic acid antagonist. Used to induce abortion and terminate ectopic pregnancies. Teratogenic and fetotoxic.	First trimester
Mifepristone (Mifeprex)	Antiprogestogen. Used as abortifacient. Not a teratogen in one primate species; human data limited.	All trimesters
Misoprostol (Cytotec)	Prostaglandin E1 analog; Möebius syndrome; potent uterine stimulant that induces abortion in early pregnancy. Used as an illegal abortifacient. Potential teratogen due to vascular disruption and hemorrhage.	All trimesters
Nicotine, carbon monoxide and trace chemicals; cigarettes	Low birth weight, increased risk of sudden infant death syndrome, association with prematurity, increased respiratory illness in the neonate.	All trimesters
Nonsteroidal anti-inflammatory drugs	Postdatism; premature closure of the ductus arteriosus; necrotizing enterocolitis.	Second and third trimesters
Phenytoin (Dilantin)	Fetal hydantoin syndrome: distinct facial abnormalities, anomalies of the digits, hypoplasia and ossification of the distal phalanges. Orofacial clefts; impaired development (physical and mental) and congenital heart defects. Data suggesting transplacental carcinogenicity.	First trimester
Selective serotonin reuptake inhibitors	Controversial: Some data suggest paroxetine (Paxil) is associated with an increased risk for cardiovascular defects, but this finding has not been confirmed. Some question of neonatal withdrawal syndrome.	First and third trimesters
Statins	Data are limited, but suggest intrauterine growth restriction, structural anomalies, and potential increased risk for VACTERL association (a nonrandom association of different birth defects).	All trimesters
Sulfonamides	Increased likelihood hyperbilirubinemia in the neonate.	Second and third trimesters
Tetracycline and doxycycline	Tooth staining, incorporation into bone and tooth matrix. Maternal liver disease. Some evidence of increased risk of other minor malformations.	Second and third trimesters
Thalidomide	Bilateral limb reduction defects; vertebral defects; neural tube defects; facial asymmetry, ocular defects and ear defects, cardiac defects, GI atresia and stenosis; absence of gallbladder and appendix; kidney anomalies, cryptorchidism, double vagina.	First trimester
Trimethoprim	Theoretic risk of neural tube defects, oral clefts, cardiovascular defects and hypospadias. Trimethoprim is a folate antagonist.	First trimester
Valproic acid	Spina bifida 1–2% incidence. Three times the risk of other congenital malformations. Evidence of developmental delay.	First trimester
Vitamin A	Avoid doses greater than 8000 IU/day. Doses greater than 25,000 mg/d are teratogenic and may be lower threshold. Marked deficiency may also cause malformations.	All trimesters
Warfarin (Coumadin)	Embryopathy, spontaneous abortion, stillbirth, prematurity, hemorrhage, central nervous system defects, neonatal death, fetal warfarin syndrome (nasal hypoplasia with depressed nasal bridge; may also have low birth weight, eye defects, hypoplasia of extremities, developmental delays, seizures, scoliosis, deafness, congenital heart disease).	All trimesters

CNS = central nervous system.

Teratogens cause specific birth defects via their effect during a critical period of embryogenesis. Gestation is divided into three distinct critical periods with regard to teratogenesis. In the preimplantation period, which is the time between fertilization and implantation, exposure to a teratogen usually has an all-or-nothing effect on the developing embryo; if the embryo survives the exposure, repair or replacement of affected cells will occur, allowing normal development. The most critical period for teratogenic effects to occur is during the embryonic period (2–9 weeks postfertilization). In the fetal period (the 9th week after fertilization to term), untoward effects of drug exposure can cause fetotoxic effects such as growth restriction, change in size or functioning of certain organs, or developmental and behavioral abnormalities (Figure 35-1).

Studies on Birth Defects

Lack of teratogenicity does not ensure that a drug is safe. There is very little new information about the safety of drugs that are used by pregnant women. Must current knowledge is from pregnancy databases that were compiled more than 40 years ago. The most famous database is probably the Collaborative Perinatal Project. This United States-based prospective study of pregnancy and childhood began in 1959 and continued gathering data until 1974. This project accrued a great deal of information about pregnancy, birth, and childhood; some of this information on use of drugs during pregnancy provided the evidence relied upon today for safety of specific drugs.[13]

The National Birth Defects Prevention Study is the largest ongoing case-control study looking at risk factors

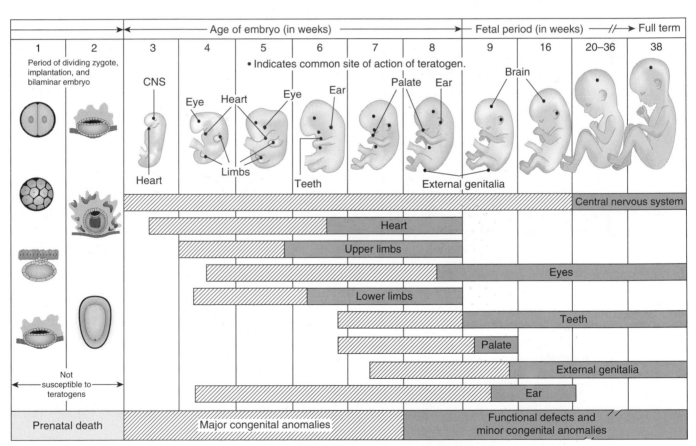

* Patterned area indicates highly sensitive periods when teratogens may induce major anomalies.

Figure 35-1 Critical periods in human development.* *Source:* Adapted with permission from Moore et al. 2007.[127]

and causes of birth defects. Families are identified from registries in eight states. Participants are interviewed, and DNA samples are collected to study the effect of genetics, environment, and their interactions to explore the etiologies of a broad range of birth defects. This study also collects data about drug use in pregnancy that is used to determine drug safety.[14,15]

The other sources of information about the effects of drugs on pregnancy are pregnancy registries that are maintained by drug manufacturers. Because pregnant women are not included in premarketing clinical trials, teratogenic effects do not become evident until a large population is exposed. In other words, teratogenic effects are an ex post facto phenomenon.

Drug Labeling: FDA Pregnancy Categories

In 1979, the US Food and Drug Administration (FDA) developed pregnancy labeling categories that classify drugs by safety categories.[16,17] It is generally assumed that these risk categories (A–X) progressively rank the teratogenic potential of drugs, but this is not true. First, the FDA does not assign a pregnancy category to a pharmacologic agent; rather the categories are assigned by the manufacturer without reference to standard criteria for making the assignations. Secondly, the categories do not address information on severity, dose, or timing of the adverse effect. Additional ambiguities inherent in the FDA pregnancy categories are summarized in Chapter 1. Given these problems, many well-known experts in this field use the FDA categories and then independently rank drugs based on their interpretation of safety in pregnancy.[18] Clinicians can therefore occasionally be presented with two differing

pregnancy categories. The FDA is currently considering significant changes in this system because there are some limitations to the current labeling.

Until new labeling with descriptive narrative regarding risks is available from the FDA, clinicians are advised to consult other sources for meaningful data when making choices regarding prescribing drugs or advising women regarding inadvertent exposures. Two excellent resources, both available on the World Wide Web, include the Motherisk Program based in Toronto, Canada,[19] and the Organization of Teratology Information Services (OTIS), whose Web site includes fact sheets on specific drugs in English, Spanish, and French.[20] Both of these services are available without registration or subscription and are free to users. Motherisk offers a free telephone help line to both clinicians and women.

Pharmacokinetic Changes During Pregnancy

The physiologic changes that occur during pregnancy alter the pharmacokinetics of drugs taken in this period. Changes in absorption, distribution, metabolism, and excretion are summarized in Table 35-2. Absorption of most orally administered drugs is not significantly affected even though intestinal transport time is slowed and gastric pH rises in midgestation. There are some changes with regard to metabolism and clearance that are clinically important. Distribution is the pharmacokinetic process most affected by the pregnant state.

Table 35-2 Pharmacokinetic Changes in Pregnancy

Pharmacokinetic Process	First Trimester	Second Trimester	Third Trimester
Absorption	Decreased with nausea and vomiting.	Longer intestinal transport time may facilitate absorption of hydrophilic drugs. No change in absorption of lipophilic drugs.	
Distribution	No significant changes.	Increased volume of distribution as fetal compartment develops; this may result in lower serum levels and requirements for larger loading doses. Reduction in plasma proteins (especially albumin) plasma expansion begins; may result in higher levels of free drug not bound to albumin.	Further increase in volume of distribution. Plasma expansion peaks at 38 weeks, albumin levels lowest in third trimester; sex steroid hormones compete for albumin binding sites.
Metabolism	No significant changes.	Hepatic enzyme systems affected by rising levels of estrogen and progesterone leading to slower metabolism of some drugs (e.g., caffeine) and faster metabolism of others.	Lower albumin levels mean more unbound drug with potential for periods of more rapid clearance.
Excretion/ clearance	Since glomerular filtration rate increases until peak at 34 gestational weeks, drugs excreted by the kidneys clear more rapidly. Excretion via the lungs is more rapid secondary to increased respiratory rate.		

Metabolism

CYP3A4 and CYP2D6 activity is increased during pregnancy, whereas CYP1A2 is down regulated. Caffeine has a longer half-life during pregnancy because CYP1A2 is less active.[21] Blood flow through the liver during pregnancy is not changed to a large degree, so first-pass effects are not significantly different.[22]

Excretion

The glomerular filtration rate (GFR) increases beginning soon after conception, reaching a peak at 9 to 16 weeks' gestation, then plateaus at a rate approximately 50% higher than prepregnancy at approximately 34 to 36 weeks of gestation. Increased GFR favors faster elimination of drugs that do not require hepatic metabolism, resulting in lower serum concentrations during pregnancy.[23] Drugs such as nicotine, fluoxetine (Prozac), and citalopram (Celexa) may be excreted so easily that decreased therapeutic efficacy can ensue. Reduction in nicotine blood levels may lead to increased maternal smoking or cigarette craving in late pregnancy, whereas lower levels of selective serotonin reuptake inhibitors may require higher or more frequent doses to achieve therapeutic benefits in the third trimester.[24]

Distribution

Drug distribution is dependent on the lipid solubility, tissue affinity, and plasma protein binding characteristics of the drug. During pregnancy, the plasma volume increases by approximately 50%, which lowers serum concentrations of drugs (particularly ionized, unbound drugs). The concentration of albumin in plasma decreases in pregnancy. In addition, plasma levels of steroid hormones such as estradiol and progesterone increase in the later half of pregnancy and these steroids compete for protein-binding sites on albumin and other plasma proteins. Steroid hormones may also displace drugs already bound to plasma proteins. The overall effect is more free drug fraction, which is unbound and metabolically active. Anticonvulsants and serotonin reuptake inhibitors are subject to this phenomenon.

As pregnancy continues, maternal albumin levels decrease while the fetus produces endogenous plasma proteins. This can lead to a concentration gradient favoring increased transport of free drug from mother to fetus. This is the purported mechanism that explains why diazepam (Valium) can be found in higher concentrations in the fetus than in the mother.[8]

The most significant alteration in drug distribution in pregnancy is the development of a new compartment, the fetal-placental-amniotic compartment, into which almost all drugs eventually are distributed to varying degrees. The chance that a drug will cause a fetal malformation is highest in the first trimester during critical periods of embryogenesis; yet drugs are most easily transported across the placenta in the third trimester. Decreased space between maternal and fetal blood and increased maternal and fetal blood that flows through the placenta allows easier transport of most agents as pregnancy progresses.

The Placenta

The fetal circulation is separated from the maternal circulation by the syncytiotrophoblast. Altogether, there are five layers of tissue that make up the **placental barrier** that nutrients must traverse once they are in the maternal blood-filled space of the placenta and in contact with the fetal placental villi. These include (1) the syncytiotrophoblast membrane, (2) the syncytiotrophoblast cell, (3) the syncytiotrophoblast basal membrane, (4) connective tissue of the cytotrophoblast villus, and (5) endothelial cells that line the fetal vessels. This barrier thins as the pregnancy progresses, and in the third trimester, the cytotrophoblast villus tissue becomes discontinuous so the two separate circulations are closer to each other.

The placenta also has several enzyme systems that metabolize some drugs, and the placental cells do express P-glycoprotein, which actively pumps some substrates away from the fetus. Drugs known to be substrates for P-glycoprotein have lower concentrations in the fetal than the maternal circulation.

Overall, the structure and function of the placenta minimizes fetal drug exposure. Most nutrients and wastes move into the fetal compartment via diffusion across the cell membranes that separate the maternal and fetal circulations. Molecules can also be transported via facilitated diffusion, active transport, or pinocytosis (Figure 35-2). Drugs usually have a mass between 250 and 400 daltons, and many diffuse slowly. Drugs that have a molecular weight of < 500 daltons, those that are lipophilic (e.g., antibiotics and anesthetics), and those that are unionized readily diffuse across the placental cell membrane barriers.[4] Larger drugs gain access to the fetal compartment via pinocytosis, and a few drugs with molecular weights > 1000 daltons such as heparin, insulin, oxytocin, thyroid supplements, glyburide, and interferon do not cross into the fetal compartment in any appreciable amount.

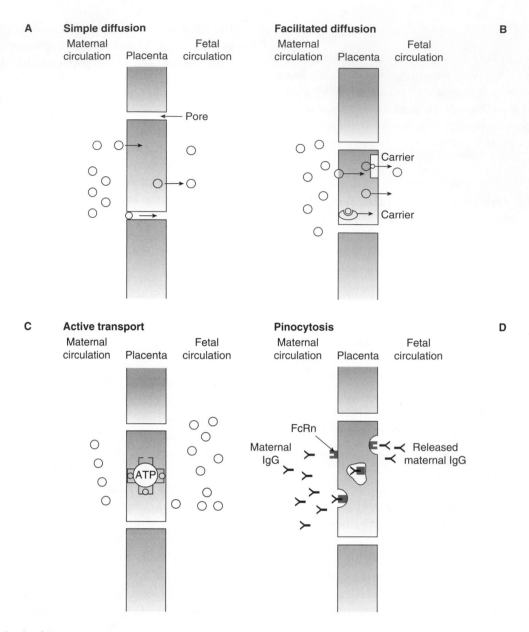

A   Simple diffusion

Maternal circulation   Placenta   Fetal circulation

Pore

Facilitated diffusion   B

Maternal circulation   Placenta   Fetal circulation

Carrier

Carrier

C   Active transport

Maternal circulation   Placenta   Fetal circulation

ATP

Pinocytosis   D

Maternal circulation   Placenta   Fetal circulation

FcRn

Maternal IgG

Released maternal IgG

Figure 35-2 Methods of transporting molecules across the placenta.

The Fetal Compartment

The fetal liver has some capacity to metabolize drugs by about 8–10 weeks postconception. At term, the fetal liver has approximately 30–60% of the CYP450 activity of an adult.

Concentration gradients between maternal and fetal blood affect rates of diffusion, as does a slight difference in maternal and fetal pH. As a result of this pH gradient, weak basic drugs such as opiates can concentrate in the fetal compartment. The slightly acidic environment in

the fetal circulation encourages their ionization, which changes their shape and makes return to the more basic maternal blood more difficult, a phenomenon known as **ion trapping**.

Once a drug is in the fetal compartment, distribution is influenced by the stage of gestation. Prior to skin keratinization at 20 weeks of gestation, amniotic fluid acts as extracellular fluid with drugs diffusing readily across the fetal skin. As development continues, skin permeability decreases significantly, and drugs that enter the fetus must be excreted rather than simply diffused into the amniotic fluid. Drugs that enter the fetal circulation in the umbilical vein can either be metabolized in the liver via the first-pass effect or shunted across the ductus venosus directly to the heart and general circulation. Both the placenta and the fetal liver are capable of some drug metabolism. Ultimately, fetal concentration of most drugs achieve steady state levels is between 50% and 100% of maternal concentration.[22]

Drug Safety for Pregnant Women

Safe prescribing for a pregnant woman begins with an accurate diagnosis of the condition that requires pharmacologic intervention. The goal is to use the lowest effective dose of the drug known to be the safest for the shortest period of time. If several different drugs are equally effective, the one that has been used for the longest and has the most data indicating safety should be chosen.[1] Additional principles for prescribing in pregnancy include avoiding drugs during the first trimester if possible, choosing topical instead of oral formulations if equally effective, and using medications only if the benefit outweighs the risk of the disorder.

Women may start pregnancy already taking a medication for a preexisting condition. These drugs should not be discontinued unless there is a high suspicion or known risk of maternal or fetal harm.[23] Some drugs, such as the antiepileptic agents, have a risk of harming the fetus but may need to be continued during pregnancy for the woman's health. Women who become pregnant while taking one of these agents should be referred to an obstetric specialist for in-depth counseling.

Vitamin and Mineral Supplementation During Pregnancy

Folic Acid

Supplemental folic acid significantly reduces neural tube defects by approximately 50% when taken within 3 months of conception and during the first trimester (RR 0.28; 95% CI, 0.13 to 0.58).[25] The background risk for neural tube defects is 1:1000 in the United States.[26] Women absorb folic acid from supplements (100%) and folic-acid enriched foods (85%) more readily than dietary folate sources (50%).[27] Because closure of the neural tube is normally complete by 28 days after conception, a time many women are not yet aware they have conceived, routine folic

acid supplementation is recommended for all women of childbearing age.[28] The recommended daily dose of supplemental folic acid is 400 micrograms (0.4 mg).[29]

There is a theoretical concern that folic acid supplementation could mask vitamin B_{12} deficiency anemia and allow the neurologic abnormalities associated with vitamin B_{12} deficiency to become permanent. Although there is no evidence that the incidence of vitamin B_{12} deficiency increases in women who take folic acid, doses of ≥ 1 mg/day are not encouraged for routine supplementation.

Women who had a prior pregnancy affected by a neural tube defect are advised take 4 mg of folic acid per day for 1 month prior to conception and through the first 3 months of pregnancy. This recommendation, from the Centers for Disease Control and Prevention (CDC), was based on findings from the Medical Research Council Vitamin Study Research Group that found women with a previous pregnancy affected by a neural tube defect who took 4 mg folic acid daily had a 72% reduction in risk of having a fetus with a neural tube defect in the subsequent pregnancy (RR 0.28; 95% CI, 0.12–0.71).[30] Additional risk factors for a neural tube defect include previous child with an orofacial cleft, family history of neural tube defects, antiepileptic drug use, epilepsy, insulin-dependent diabetes, medically diagnosed obesity, and use of antifolate drugs. However, there is no evidence that high-dose folic acid supplementation will reduce the incidence of neural tube defects in women with these risk factors, and therefore they are advised to take the standard 400 mcg/day dose routinely during the childbearing years and during pregnancy.

Iron

Iron deficiency anemia is the most common micronutrient deficiency in women worldwide. During pregnancy, the maternal need for iron increases from 0.8 mg/day to 6–7 mg/day in the last half of gestation. This extra demand can exhaust iron stores in women who have normal stores prior to becoming pregnant. Because it is difficult to get enough iron from dietary sources, iron supplementation is sometimes recommended. However, routine iron supplementation during pregnancy is controversial. The CDC recommends that all women receive, as primary prevention, 30 mg a day of oral iron supplements starting at the first prenatal visit.[31] The US Preventive Services Task Force, by contrast, recommends screening pregnant women for anemia, but states the evidence is insufficient to recommend routine iron supplementation for women with normal hemoglobin levels.[32] There is consensus that routine iron supplementation is associated with higher hemoglobin and hematocrit values at term and postpartum.[33] However, there is insufficient evidence that iron supplementation in the absence of anemia improves maternal or newborn outcomes.[33,34]

Women who have hemoglobin values < 9.5 g/dL before or during the second trimester have an increased incidence of poor outcomes, and infant iron stores are adversely affected.[33] Iron deficiency in the neonate and young child has negative cognitive and developmental consequences, including decreased motor activity, social interaction, and attention to tasks.[31] Delayed cord clamping has been shown to increase iron stores in the neonate.[33]

Iron supplementation is generally recommended when the hemoglobin and hematocrit are 11 g/dL and 33% in the first and third trimester and 10.5 g/dL and 32% in the second trimester. The CDC recommends that pregnant women who are anemic take 60–120 mg/d of elemental iron orally, and if the anemia does not respond after 4 weeks of treatment, further evaluation is advised to assess iron stores and look for causes of anemia other than iron deficiency. Individuals who smoke and those who live at high altitudes have higher hemoglobin and hematocrit values. Therefore the laboratory value used to define anemia in these populations is 0.3 g/dL higher for hemoglobin and 1% for hematocrit.[33]

Iron-deficient individuals can convert between 50 and 100 mg of ferrous salts daily into hemoglobin, and approximately 25% of oral ferrous salts are absorbed. Absorption of iron in late pregnancy is significantly higher than in the nonpregnant state, reaching potentially 5 mg a day in the third trimester with a diet high in bioavailable iron.[34] When iron supplementation recommended, the various iron preparations of ferrous or ferric salts contain different amounts of elemental iron (Table 5-9). The ferrous salts are more bioavailable than the ferric salts. Additional information about iron supplements can be found in Chapter 5.

Side effects of oral iron supplementation are primarily gastrointestinal and dose related. Constipation, abdominal pain, nausea, and vomiting are the most frequent side effects reported.[35] Women taking ferrous fumarate and intermediate-release ferrous sulfate report uncomfortable side effects most often (56.3% and 53.7%, respectively) followed by slow-release ferrous sulfate (43.3%). Slow-release ferrous sulfate is not recommended because iron is absorbed in the proximal portion of the small intestine of the stomach and the slow-release formulations do not dissolve quickly enough to become bioavailable. Iron administered as ferrous fumarate within a multivitamin preparation and ferric bisglycinate has the fewest side effects (23.7% and 21.2%, $P < .01$) and lower rates of

discontinuation (0.0% and 6.1% due to side effects alone, $P < .05$).[35] Iron is a leading cause of poisoning in young children; as few as 10 iron tablets may be fatal, so keeping iron out of reach of children is extremely important.

Parenteral iron therapy should be reserved only for those persons with documented severe iron-deficiency anemia in pregnancy who cannot tolerate any form of oral iron. Although parenteral iron improves hemoglobin levels more quickly than oral supplements, potential harms include anaphylaxis, thrombosis, tissue staining, and significant pain. More information on parenteral forms of iron can be found in Chapter 16.

Multivitamins

Folic acid and iron are often routinely supplemented in pregnancy in a prenatal multivitamin formulation. The Institute of Medicine's Dietary Reference Intake for pregnancy has a list of Recommended Daily Allowances and Adequate Intakes for multiple micronutrients[36] (Table 35-3). Because large doses of some nutrients in multivitamins can be harmful, women should not take more than the recommended number of pills or capsules per day in an effort to increase their intake of a single micronutrient. Excess vitamin A is teratogenic, but there are no human studies that have determined what level is required for teratogenesis to occur. Conversely, doses < 10,000 mg a day are known to be safe. Excessive vitamin E can theoretically interfere with platelet aggregation and leukocyte function.

Deficiencies in vitamins and elements, particularly zinc, selenium, calcium, vitamin A, folic acid, iodine, iron, magnesium, selenium, and copper have been linked with various pregnancy and neonatal complications, especially in developing countries where nutritional deficiencies are more prevalent and can be severe. There is some evidence that supplementation with multiple micronutrients decreases the number of low-birth-weight infants and small-for-gestational-age infants when compared to placebo. However, this effect is no longer statistically significant when micronutrient supplementation is compared to supplementation with iron and folate.[25]

Calcium

The recommended daily allowance of calcium for nonpregnant and pregnant women is 1000 mg/day and 1300 mg/day for pregnant women younger than age 18. Next to iron, calcium is the nutrient most difficult to obtain in sufficient amounts in a typical US diet. An inverse relationship between dietary intake of calcium and the incidence of hypertensive disorders was first

Table 35-3 Recommended Daily Allowance and Adequate Intakes of Vitamins and Minerals for Pregnant Women, by Age Group

Micronutrient Goals for Pregnancy	Age 14–18	Age 19–30	Age 31–50
Vitamin A mcg/d	750	770	770
Vitamin B$_6$ mg/d	1.9	1.9	1.9
Vitamin B$_{12}$ mcg/d	2.6	2.6	2.6
Vitamin C mg/d	80	85	85
Vitamin D mcg/d	5*	5*	5*
Vitamin E mg/d	15	15	15
Vitamin K mcg/d	75*	90*	90*
Biotin mcg/d	30*	30*	30*
Calcium mg/d	1300*	1000*	1000*
Chloride g/d	2.3*	2.3*	2.3*
Choline mg/d	450*	450*	450*
Chromium mcg/d	29*	30*	30*
Copper mcg/d	1000	1000	1000
Fluoride mg/d	3*	3*	3*
Folate mcg/d	600†	600†	600†
Iodine mcg/d	220	220	220
Iron mg/d	27	27	27
Magnesium mg/d	400	350	360
Manganese mg/d	2.0*	2.0*	2.0*
Molybdenum mcg/d	50	50	50
Niacin mg/d	18	18	18
Pantothenic mg/d	6*	6*	6*
Phosphorus mg/d	1250	700	700
Potassium g/d	4.7*	4.7*	4.7*
Riboflavin mg/d	1.4	1.4	1.4
Selenium mcg/d	60	60	60
Sodium g/d	1.5*	1.5*	1.5*
Thiamin mg/d	1.4	1.4	1.4
Zinc mg/d	12	11	11

Bold = recommended daily allowances (covers nutritional needs of 97% of individuals in this group).
* Adequate intake (believed to cover the needs of those in these groups, but lack of data makes percentage covered uncertain).
† Includes 400 mcg of supplemental folic acid or folic acid from fortified foods.
Source: Adapted from Institute of Medicine 1998.[27]

noted in 1980 in epidemiologic studies. It is theorized that low calcium intake either stimulates the parathyroid gland or renin secretion, thereby causing high blood pressure. Several observational and randomized trials were conducted based on these observations. The effect of calcium supplementation on the incidence of preeclampsia and preterm birth has been evaluated in several randomized trials. In the most recent meta-analysis of randomized controlled trials, calcium supplementation with at least 1 g/day lowered the risk of preeclampsia by half (RR = 0.48; 95% CI, 0.33–0.69; 12 studies, n = 15,206), particularly in women at high risk for

this condition (RR = 0.22; 95% CI, 0.12–0.42; 5 trials, n = 587) and in women with low baseline calcium intake (RR = 0.36; 95% CI, 0.18–0.70; 7 trials, n = 10,154).[37] Women with an adequate dietary intake of calcium had a reduction in the risk of preeclampsia, but the reduction was not statistically significant.[37] The theoretic risk of increased renal stone formation in women who take calcium supplements was not substantiated in these studies.[37]

Calcium may be formulated in several ways with varying amounts of elemental calcium[38] (Table 5-5). Calcium carbonate may be either produced in a laboratory (refined) or mined from limestone derived from fossilized oyster shell (natural source). Dolomite is calcium magnesium carbonate in mineral form. Calcium phosphate or hydroxyapatite is produced from powdered bone (bone meal). Calcium is also bound to organic chelates to produce calcium gluconate, calcium lactate, and amino acid calcium products.

Calcium supplements are dietary supplements and therefore not subject to FDA regulation. A study comparing lead levels[38] in these various preparations found that calcium chelates and refined calcium carbonate had the lowest lead content, followed by dolomite, then calcium carbonate derived from oyster shells (natural source), with bone meal having the highest lead levels. More than half of the natural-source calcium carbonate supplements were shown to have lead levels over the provisional total tolerable daily lead intake of 6 mcg.

The most common adverse effects of calcium supplements are bloating, excess gas, and constipation, and these occur most often with calcium carbonate preparations. Changing to a different calcium preparation such as calcium gluconate and increasing fluid intake usually relieve these symptoms. Calcium citrate may be better absorbed and cause fewer gastrointestinal side effects than other calcium preparations. Taking calcium supplements with a meal increases absorption. Some foods (wheat bran, spinach, and rhubarb) may decrease absorption. Calcium can interfere with absorption of iron and zinc so should be taken separately from other multiple micronutrient or iron supplements in pregnancy.

Therapies Used to Treat Common Gestational Discomforts

Pregnancy, for most women, involves many uncomfortable physiologic changes. The need for relief when these conditions interfere with the ability to maintain normal daily activities is balanced against the risks involved in medical therapy for these conditions. Many of the common discomforts of pregnancy are not managed with pharmacologic agents. For those that are amenable to pharmacologic treatment, choosing the lowest effective dose of the safest medical therapy for the shortest duration is a useful approach, and whenever appropriate, promoting nonpharmacologic comfort measures prior to prescribing a pharmacologic agent is preferred.

Nausea, Vomiting, and Hyperemesis

Approximately 70–85% of women experience nausea in early pregnancy, and 50% vomit.[39] Although this is a well-known and generally benign aspect of pregnancy, at least one famous woman, Charlotte Brontë, is purported to have died from hyperemesis gravidarum. Brontë, the author of *Jane Eyre*, married at age 38 and had a happy but short marriage before she died after several weeks of intractable nausea and vomiting in 1855.[40] Medical historians have long thought that Brontë was in the early part of her first pregnancy and have attributed her symptoms to hyperemesis, although the cause of her death is not known for certain.

Pregnancy-related nausea and vomiting commonly begins at approximately 6–8 weeks' gestation and persists, in the majority of women, until 10–12 weeks.[41] A few women experience pregnancy-related nausea and vomiting until 16 weeks or later. The etiology of nausea and vomiting in pregnancy remains unknown, although there is a positive relationship between high levels of human chorionic gonadotropin (hCG) and increasing severity of nausea and vomiting.

Several different neurotransmitters can stimulate the chemoreceptor trigger zone (CTZ) within the brain that initiates vomiting. The CTZ has receptors for histamine, dopamine, serotonin, opioids, and benzodiazepines. This variety in types of neurotransmitters is fortunate because drugs in several different classes can be used as antiemetics.

Pharmacologic Therapies for Nausea and Vomiting in Pregnancy

Medications proven useful for treating nausea and vomiting of early pregnancy include (1) first-generation, sedating antihistamine-anticholinergics such as doxylamine (Unisom), diphenhydramine (Benadryl), and meclizine (e.g., Antivert, Bonine); (2) dopamine antagonists, metoclopramide (Reglan), and phenothiazines such as promethazine

(Phenergan) and prochlorperazine (Compazine); and (3) serotonin antagonists such as ondansetron (Zofran).[41] A protocol for managing nausea and vomiting that is presented in Table 35-4, and doses of the antiemetic drugs used are listed in Table 35-5.

The first step is to ascertain the severity of nausea and vomiting. The Pregnancy-Unique Quantification of Emesis/Nausea (PUQE) Index is based on only three questions and is a reliable, validated tool for assessing severity of nausea and vomiting of pregnancy.[42]

Women with mild nausea may find sufficient relief from nonpharmacologic interventions such as small, frequent meals, avoiding triggers, and discontinuing prenatal vitamins. Sea-Bands, ginger capsules, and vitamin B_6 all have some effectiveness for minimizing nausea.

Table 35-4 Treatment Options for Nausea and Vomiting During Pregnancy

1. **Mild nausea without vomiting or with occasional vomiting:**
   a. Stop prenatal vitamins with iron; replace with folic acid supplement
   b. Pyridoxine (vitamin B_6) 25 mg PO tid
   c. Ginger 250 mg PO qid
   d. P6 acupressure (Sea-Bands)
   e. Lifestyle counseling

2. **Moderate nausea with mild vomiting ≤ 2 times per day, no dehydration:**
   Pyridoxine 25 mg PO bid–tid and doxylamine (Unisom) 12.5 mg PO qid or at hs only (1/2 tablet)
   If ineffective add one of the following:
   Chlorpromazine (Thorazine) 10–25 mg PO q 4–6 h
   Prochlorperazine (Compazine) 5–10 mg PO q 6–8 h
   Promethazine (Phenergan) 25 mg PO q 4–6 h
   Metoclopramide (Reglan) 5–10 mg PO q 8 h
   Ondansetron (Zofran) 8 mg PO q 12 h
   Use one of the following for breakthrough vomiting as needed:
   Promethazine (Phenergan) 25 mg PR q 4–6 h
   Prochlorperazine (Compazine) 5–10 mg PR q 6–8 h

3. **Nausea and vomiting with dehydration, ketonuria, unable to orally rehydrate:**
   a. Start IV for rehydration
   b. 1 amp multivitamin supplement in first liter and daily thereafter (until able to tolerate oral medications) or 100 mg thiamine IV qd
   c. Dimenhydrinate (Benadryl) 50 mg IV (in 50 mL saline over 20 min) q 4–6 h
   d. ADD one of the following to initial intravenous solution:
      Promethazine 12.5–25 mg IV PB q 4–6 h OR
      Chlorpromazine 25–50 mg IV q 4–6 h OR
      Prochlorperazine 5–10 mg IV q 6–8 h OR
      Metoclopramide 5–10 mg IV q 8 h
      Ondansetron 8 mg IV over 15 min q 12 h
      Droperidol (Inapsine) 0.625 mg IV given slowly

4. **If vomiting is intractable, refer for medical management:**
   Consider methylprednisolone (Solu-Medrol) 15 to 20 mg IV q 8 hr and/or total parenteral nutrition

Source: Adapted from Levichek et al. 2002.[41]

Table 35-5 Doses of Antiemetics Used to Treat Nausea and Vomiting in Pregnancy

Drug Generic (Brand)	Dose	Clinical Considerations	FDA Pregnancy Category
Antihistamines (H₁ Antagonists)			
Diphenhydramine (Benadryl)	50–100 mg q 4–6 h PO/IM/IV	May cause drowsiness. Can be used to offset anxiety caused by metoclopramide or phenothiazines.	B
Dimenhydrinate (Dramamine)	50–100 mg q 4–6 h PO/PR* 50 mg (in 50 mL of saline over 20 min) q 4–6 h IV	May cause drowsiness. Can be used to offset anxiety caused by metoclopramide or phenothiazines.	B
Doxylamine (Unisom)	12.5 mg bid PO or 12.5 mg in AM and 25 mg in PM PO		A
Phenothiazines (Central D₂ Antagonists)			
Prochlorperazine (Compazine)	5–10 mg q 4–6 h PO/IM/IV 25-mg rectal suppository bid	Sedation, anticholinergic effects, dry mouth, dystonic reaction. Maximum dose is 40 mg/day. Hypotension if given IV too quickly.	C
Promethazine (Phenergan)	12.5–25 mg q 4–6 h PO/IM/IV/PR	Sedation, anticholinergic effects, dry mouth, EPS. Hypotension if given IV too quickly.	C
Benzamides (Central and Peripheral D₂ Antagonists)			
Metoclopramide (Reglan)	5–10 mg PO q 8 h PO/IM 1–2 mg/kg IV	EPS, agitation, anxiety, acute dystonic reactions. Give 50 mg diphenhydramine before dose to prevent EPS.	B
Serotonin Antagonists			
Ondansetron (Zofran)	4–8 mg PO tid to qid 4–8 mg over 15 min IV q 12 h May be given 1 mg/h continuously for 24 h	Headache.	B
Butyrophenones			
Droperidol† (Inapsine)	0.625–2.5 mg IV over 15 min then 1.25 mg prn, or 2.5 mg IM Can be given IV continuously at 1–1.25 mg/h	EPS, prolonged QT syndrome. Give 50 mg diphenhydramine before dose to prevent EPS. Reserve for persons who have failed other regimens.	C

* Maximum dose is 200 mg/day if taken concomitantly with doxylamine, 400 mg/day if taken as a single agent.
† To be used only following medical consultation and if other medications have failed to resolve symptoms, secondary to risk for prolonged QT syndrome.

For women with moderate nausea, no vomiting and no evidence of dehydration, pyridoxine (vitamin B₆) at doses of 10–25 mg by mouth taken three times per day significantly improves nausea.[39] There are no adverse effects associated with these doses of pyridoxine, and it is usually the first-line pharmacologic agent recommended.

An over-the-counter formulation of doxylamine (Unisom tablets) can be added to pyridoxine to create the same formulation that constituted Bendectin, which is no longer available in the United States (Box 35-1). Several well-designed studies and meta-analyses have shown that this combination of doxylamine and pyridoxine is both effective and safe.[43-45] There are no reported adverse effects associated with the use of doxylamine/pyridoxine, but it is not very effective as an antiemetic.

Finding the right combination of medication for a woman with moderate to severe nausea and vomiting is often a matter of trial and error (Box 35-3). The first-generation antihistamines are antiemetics, but they can cause drowsiness and more rarely, confusion, blurred vision, dry mouth, or urinary retention. High doses can induce complications of asthma or narrow-angle glaucoma due to their anticholinergic properties. The phenothiazines are particularly effective antiemetics, but they are also dopamine antagonists and may induce extrapyramidal symptoms, excessive sedation, and rarely bone marrow aplasia.[46]

Metoclopramide (Reglan) has both a central and peripheral mechanism of action. This drug is a dopamine antagonist and a serotonin antagonist in the chemoreceptor vomiting center in the central nervous system, and it is also a promotility agent in the gastrointestinal tract. Metoclopramide is usually well tolerated but does cross the blood–brain barrier and can induce extrapyramidal effects. Metoclopramide does not cause sedation, however, and is being used more in the outpatient setting because it is better tolerated than the antihistamines and phenothiazines.

Box 35-3 Normal Nausea or Hyperemesis?

NR, a 26-year-old woman experiencing her second pregnancy, was being seen for an initial visit. Her primary complaint was all-day nausea. She was 8 weeks from her last menstrual period, and had been increasingly nauseated for 2 weeks. She was wearing the Sea-Bands her sister gave her, but they were not helping.

NR does not have a history of a gastrointestinal disorder, eating disorder, or other condition that is associated with nausea and vomiting. She is taking a prenatal vitamin once a day. On exam, NR weighed 122 pounds, which is 4 pounds less than her prepregnancy weight; her urine specific gravity was 1020. The rest of her physical exam was normal, and an office ultrasound revealed a single viable fetus with a crown-rump length consistent with 8 weeks of gestation. Although NR felt very ill, she did not have signs of depression.

NR was not vomiting, and at first glance it may have appeared that she had mild nausea. However, her PUQE index score was 8 because of the number of hours she was nauseated and the number of times she had dry retching. When queried about how she was coping with the nausea, she said she was avoiding eating and drinking so she wouldn't vomit.

The clinician made an initial assessment of moderate nausea with dehydration. She counseled NR about the need for hydration, reviewed the nonpharmacologic interventions, and recommended an IV for hydration and initiation of an antiemetic.

After NR was hydrated and feeling better, she and her clinician discussed antiemetics. A week later, NR was the same weight. She reported the nausea was slightly better and she was able to eat and drink more often. Her urine specific gravity was 1015. NR was comfortable with her progress and did not feel she needed medication. She was seen weekly for another 2 weeks until her symptoms began to subside.

The most expensive yet anecdotally most effective drug is the serotonin antagonist ondansetron (Zofran). Ondansetron is used off label for nausea and vomiting in pregnancy, and there is a paucity of evidence that substantiates efficacy and safety of this drug.[47]

Hyperemesis

Severe nausea and vomiting of pregnancy that begins in the first trimester and causes dehydration, ketosis, and weight loss of ≥ 5% is termed hyperemesis gravidarum. A diagnosis of exclusion, hyperemesis can involve electrolyte disturbance, biochemical (though not clinical) hyperthyroidism, and elevated liver enzymes.

The cornerstones of hyperemesis management are fluid, electrolyte, vitamin replacement, and antiemetic therapy that is usually initiated intravenously. When any of the dopamine antagonists are given intravenously, the risk of inducing extrapyramidal effects is significant, and therefore when these agents are used, 50 mg of diphenhydramine (Benadryl) is administered intravenously concomitantly with the dopamine antagonist.[48]

Rarely, severe thiamine deficiency due to prolonged periods of vomiting will cause Wernicke's encephalopathy, which is manifested by changes in level of consciousness, confusion, ataxia, diplopia, and/or abnormal ocular movements and permanent neurologic sequelae. Wernicke's encephalopathy may be triggered by rapid initiation of intravenous glucose or dextrose, which increases thiamine requirements, so it is essential to replace thiamine prior to initiating intravenous solutions containing glucose in women with severe nausea and vomiting or hyperemesis.[46] Thiamine at 100 mg daily intravenously is recommended.

Benzodiazepines such as lorazepam (Ativan) and diazepam (Valium) have also been used in the treatment of hyperemesis, but there have been few studies and there is no evidence that indicates that these agents are more efficacious than drugs that are known to be safe. There is some evidence that exposure to benzodiazepines in the first trimester can cause oral cleft defects in the fetus, but controversy exists over the validity of these findings.[49] These drugs are heterogenic with regard to their pharmacokinetics, but most are lipophilic and known to enter the fetal compartment fairly easily.

Systemic steroid therapy has been used with some success to treat women with hyperemesis that is unresponsive to other antiemetic therapy.[50] Prednisone or prednisolone are used because these steroids are metabolized quickly by the placenta, whereas dexamethasone readily crosses the placenta and can suppress fetal adrenal function.[50] However, systemic corticosteroids have been shown in four large epidemiologic studies to be associated with a small increased risk for orofacial clefting, and pregnant women should be informed of this risk prior to initiating corticosteroid therapy for hyperemesis or asthma.

Ptyalism

Ptyalism, defined as excessive salivation, can accompany severe nausea and vomiting in pregnancy.[51] The etiology remains unknown, and there has been no real success in developing drugs for symptom relief. The watery, copious saliva begins to flow with the onset of nausea and produces a bad taste in the mouth. It is possible that this excessive salivation may in fact be inability to swallow normal amounts of saliva due to nausea. In the 1940s, belladonna, atropine, and hexamethonium were used to treat the condition. Currently, glucose solutions (e.g., Emetrol), lozenges, candies, fluids, chewing gum, and lifestyle changes such as eating smaller meals more frequently have all been tried but with little evidence of benefit. The condition frequently manifests as early as 2–3 weeks postconception and ceases after delivery, but it may actually increase in intensity after the first trimester.[51] Effective treatment of nausea and vomiting may help. More research is indicated to address this frustrating condition.

Complementary Therapies

Herbal remedies used by pregnant women to alleviate nausea and vomiting include ginger, peppermint, chamomile, and in one report, cannabis.[52] Ginger has been shown in randomized, controlled studies to be more effective than placebo[53] in reducing both nausea and vomiting and equivalent in efficacy to pyridoxine (vitamin B_6). The effective dose of ginger has been shown to be approximately 1 gram per day in 3 or 4 divided doses of dried, powdered rhizome or ginger syrup containing 250 mg ginger administered orally. At this dose, no adverse effects have been observed.[53,54] Peppermint tea may be effective and is probably reasonable but no data on human efficacy or safety are available.

Heartburn

An estimated 30–50% of pregnant women experience heartburn, which is due to an increase in pressure in the abdomen combined with decreased lower esophageal sphincter tone.[55] Symptoms are usually worse after meals and at bedtime. Initially, lifestyle changes such as elevating the bed, eating smaller, more frequent meals, and avoiding food for at least 2 hours before sleep may be useful.

Both tablet and liquid antacids containing magnesium, calcium, or aluminum salts may be used to neutralize stomach acids but should be taken separately from vitamin or iron supplements due to interference with absorption of the latter.[55] Antacids alone relieve heartburn symptoms in 30–50% of pregnant women.[55] Overuse of antacids containing sodium bicarbonate can cause maternal or fetal metabolic alkalosis and fluid overload, and thus should be avoided in pregnancy. More information on antacids can be found in Chapter 21.

Histamine$_2$-receptor antagonists cimetidine (Tagamet), famotidine (Pepcid), nizatidine (Axid), and ranitidine (Zantac) may be prescribed if antacids and lifestyle changes are not sufficient. All of these drugs are in FDA Pregnancy Category B. Cimetidine is known to have potential for multiple drug interactions and thus is not a preferred agent. Ranitidine (Zantac) is usually recommended first because unlike the other drugs in this class, it does not have anti-androgenic activity in animals. Metoclopramide (Reglan), another FDA Pregnancy Category B drug, can also be used to help relieve the symptoms of heartburn. Metoclopramide increases lower esophageal sphincter tone and promotes gastric emptying.

The proton pump inhibitors (PPI) all are FDA Pregnancy Category B drugs, except omeprazole (Prilosec), which is an FDA Pregnancy Category C drug, because of animal studies showing embryonic and fetal mortality. These medications are reserved for severe cases of gastroesophageal reflux disease (GERD), and many clinicians prefer to use them only after the first trimester. Lansoprazole (Prevacid) is the preferred PPI because of its safety profile.

Constipation and Hemorrhoids

Constipation is common during pregnancy, especially in the first trimester as progesterone levels rise and intestinal motility slows. Daily fiber supplements of wheat or bran have been found to increase frequency of defecation (OR 0.19; 95% CI, 0.05–0.67) and soften stools.[56] Stool softeners such as docusate sodium (Colace) are recommended if fiber supplementation is not sufficient.

Hemorrhoids are also common in pregnancy and are managed best with fiber supplementation, increased liquid intake, stool softeners, and topical preparations including anesthetics, glucocorticoids, and phlebotonics. Information on prescribing many of these agents can be found in Chapter 21. Information regarding use of these therapies in pregnancy is extrapolated from the general population, so effectiveness has not been specifically addressed for pregnancy in the majority of cases.[57]

Leg Cramps, Varicose Veins, and Back and Pelvic Pain

Leg pain in pregnancy may be due to muscle cramps or to varicose veins and rarely deep vein thrombosis. Muscle cramps in the legs are poorly understood but occur in approximately half of pregnant women, primarily at night.[58] Leg cramps result from a buildup of lactic and pyruvic acid in the muscles of the leg, perhaps as a result of two potential causes: decreased venous return in later pregnancy, and/or transient nutritional deficiencies related to the changing needs of the developing fetus.

Several remedies have been suggested over time, most commonly calcium supplementation. However, in the one randomized trial conducted to date, calcium has been shown to be similar to placebo in effectiveness for leg cramps.[58] Magnesium supplementation, with 5 mmol in the morning and 10 mmol in the evening may be effective in relieving or reducing the frequency of cramps.[58] Both calcium and magnesium supplementation may be beneficial in pregnancy for other indications, as noted above.

Back Pain and Sciatica

Lower back pain and round ligament pain are the most common musculoskeletal discomforts during the second half of pregnancy. Muscle relaxants are not used in pregnancy, and therefore, there is no easy pharmacologic treatment. The tincture of time and rest with positional support are the best remedies. Pelvic pain and sciatica may occur and tend to worsen as the pregnancy advances. Lower back pain is more common than pelvic pain, affecting up to two thirds of pregnant women, whereas pelvic pain occurs in approximately one in five.[59] Many therapies have been utilized to attempt to ameliorate back pain, including analgesics, hot and cold compresses, rest, physiotherapy, special exercises such as the pelvic tilt, acupuncture, transcutaneous electric nerve stimulation (TENS) units, and specially designed support pillows. Exercise programs (including pelvic tilt), physiotherapy, and acupuncture all are effective in relieving discomfort.[59] Analgesics often used for back pain include topical mentholated or capsicin rubs (over the counter) and acetaminophen (Tylenol). Severe back pain may require opiate analgesia if a woman is unresponsive to the therapies outlined above. There is limited information about human use of cyclobenzaprine (Flexeril), but animal studies and one human surveillance study failed to find evidence of teratogenicity or embryotoxicity in newborns exposed to cyclobenzaprine in the first trimester.

Insomnia

Most women experience changes in sleep patterns during pregnancy secondary to multiple factors including the need to void frequently, the discomfort of advanced pregnancy, and hip or back pain that may require frequent changes of position. Coping with these sleep alterations can be a challenge for pregnant women, particularly those who are balancing responsibilities that make daytime naps impractical. Sleep hygiene education, fluid restriction prior to bedtime, pillows, air mattresses or other supports, and warm packs may help along with traditional remedies such as warm milk and chamomile tea.

Sleep disturbances that do not respond to these measures and interfere with functioning may be managed with short-term pharmacologic agents.[60] Prior to initiation of such agents, it is important to rule out anxiety, depression, mania, or other mental health issues because these disorders can cause insomnia and they are best treated with different pharmacologic agents. Diphenhydramine (Benadryl), hydroxyzine (Vistaril), and doxylamine (Unisom SleepTabs) may be used short term to improve rest in women with insomnia during pregnancy. Zolpidem (Ambien), although an FDA Pregnancy Category B drug, has limited data for use in pregnancy, and if used at all, should be considered second-line therapy.

Pharmacotherapeutics in Pregnancy

Pregnant women are slightly more susceptible to viral illnesses, monilial vaginitis, and urinary tract infection, but just as vulnerable as everyone else to the everyday colds, allergies, and insect bites. Some conditions require alterations of standard treatments that take the unique pharmacokinetics and possible adverse effects on the fetus into account. When a pregnant woman presents with any disorder that is usually treated pharmacologically, the effect of the drug on the fetus is an initial consideration; after that, the effect of the condition on the pregnancy and the effect of pregnancy on the condition are both important considerations.

Allergies and the Common Cold

The common cold is well named because it affects humans more often than any other acute illness and pregnant women are not immune. Caused by a variety of viruses, manifestations include rhinorrhea, fatigue, cough, congestion in the ears and/or nose, sore throat, and a general feeling of illness, along with a possible low-grade fever. A good practice for treating colds during pregnancy is to treat the most bothersome symptom specifically and avoid polypharmacy. Although there are a plethora of cold formulations, most include one of a few ingredients—an antihistamine, decongestant, cough suppressant, expectorant, nasal corticosteroids, and/or an analgesic.

Older, sedating, first-generation antihistamines such as chlorpheniramine (Chlor-Trimeton), diphenhydramine (Benadryl), triprolidine (in Actifed, in combination with pseudoephedrine), and doxylamine (Unisom SleepTabs) can improve symptoms of rhinorrhea and watery eyes and have been studied fairly extensively in pregnancy; no evidence of increased teratogenic risk has been identified.[61] Newer nonsedating, second-generation antihistamines have been studied less extensively in humans. Cetirizine (Zyrtec) is an active metabolite of hydroxyzine (Vistaril) that has been used for many years and is not associated with teratogenicity.[61] Loratadine (Claritin) had been linked with hypospadias; however, the CDC examined data from the Birth Defects Prevention Study and determined that no link could be found between loratadine and second- and third-degree hypospadias.[62] Fexofenadine (Allegra) has shown no evidence of teratogenicity in animals at 47 times the therapeutic level; however human studies are lacking and rats given three times the therapeutic level achieved fewer implantations for pregnancy, and showed increased postimplantation abortions.[61] Decongestants are formulated for both oral and nasal use and may be used during an acute congestive episode. The most common decongestants are phenylephrine (e.g., Neo-Synephrine, AH-CHEW D) and

pseudoephedrine (e.g., Sudafed, Chlor-Trimeton nasal decongestant). Phenylephrine appears safe but some authors suggest it is ineffective for treating nasal congestion. Pseudoephedrine has been associated with a small increased risk of anomalies, particularly gastroschisis. This association has not been confirmed in cohort or large case control studies, and it is possible that the viral illness that caused the upper respiratory infections for which the oral decongestants were used may be responsible for the abdominal wall defects.[61,63] Pseudoephedrine is effective and safe for the fetus after the first trimester.

Nasal decongestants may be safely used during the first trimester if indicated. Nasal decongestants include short-acting phenylephrine (Neo-Synephrine 4-hour, Rhinall), and long-acting (up to 12 hours) oxymetazoline (Afrin spray) and xylometazoline (Otrivin). Both phenylephrine and oxymetazoline have been evaluated for use in pregnancy. One study suggests that higher-than-recommended dosing of oxymetazoline may be of concern and should be used cautiously in women whose placental reserve is potentially compromised (e.g., preeclampsia, chronic hypertension diabetes). Oxymetazoline can cause vasoconstriction via the alpha-adrenergic receptors of the uterine vessels. In women with healthy pregnancies, use as directed should not pose a significant risk.[61]

Another common cold symptom is cough, and although cough medications containing alcohol should be avoided, those containing the cough suppressant dextromethorphan (e.g., Delsym, Robitussin Maximum Strength, Vicks 44 Cough Relief), the expectorant guaifenesin (e.g., Guaifenex LA, Robitussin), and codeine are not associated with untoward fetal effects. Codeine preparations may be indicated for mothers whose sleep is adversely affected.

Nasal corticosteroids have been shown to be the most efficacious agent for allergic rhinitis in the nonpregnant population,[61] and fortunately, human pregnancy data about the inhaled corticosteroids budesonide (Rhinocort AQ) and beclomethasone (Beconase AQ) is reassuring.[61] These agents have little systemic absorption and they may be considered first-line therapy for allergic rhinitis treatment. Intranasal cromolyn sodium (NasalCrom), a mast-cell stabilizer, also has good evidence for use in pregnancy and may be considered as first-line therapy.[61]

Fever and sore throat pain may be treated with acetaminophen (Tylenol), which has a long record of both safety and effectiveness. Nonsteroidal anti-inflammatory drugs (NSAIDs) such as indomethacin (Indocin, Indocin CR), ibuprofen (e.g., Advil, Motrin), and naproxen (e.g., Aleve, Naprosyn) are not associated with teratogenic effects, but NSAIDs can cause premature closure of the fetal ductus arteriosus and should therefore be avoided especially in the third trimester. NSAIDs are currently not recommended for use in pregnancy. Acetylsalicylic acid (aspirin) is also an NSAID, which is contraindicated throughout pregnancy. When acetylsalicylic acid is taken at subtherapeutic doses (< 100 mg/day) no untoward effects will occur. Conversely, when used in therapeutic doses, an increased risk for placental abruption and other bleeding problems becomes evident. Opioid analgesia is not linked with congenital malformations or fetotoxicity.[5]

Bacterial and Viral Respiratory Infections

If clinical judgment suggests antibiotic treatment is required for a woman with acute sinusitis, appropriate choices include amoxicillin-clavulanate (Augmentin), cefprozil (Cefzil), and cefuroxime axetil (Ceftin). Streptococcal pharyngitis requires antibiotic treatment, and penicillin has excellent data for use in pregnancy; although increased clearance of penicillin may require higher or more frequent dosing to achieve similar therapeutic levels as those found among the nonpregnant population. Erythromycin (e.g., E.E.S, Ery-Tab) or azithromycin may also be used; erythromycin estolate (Ilosone) should be avoided due to a 10% incidence of reversible hepatotoxicity in pregnancy, and clarithromycin (Biaxin) has little data regarding use in human pregnancy and would thus not be a first choice, particularly in the first trimester. Limited specific safety data exist for the use of azithromycin (Zithromax, Zmax), but macrolide antibiotics are not known to be human teratogens.

Prior to the availability of antibiotics, pneumonia in pregnancy resulted in mortality rates up to 24%. Pneumonia is a serious illness in pregnancy and usually requires hospitalization and intravenous antibiotics. Current estimates suggest that 0–3% of women who contract pneumonia in pregnancy die from it.[64] Pregnancy does not seem to influence incidence rates. *Streptococcus pneumoniae* and *Haemophilus influenzae* are the most common bacteriologic pathogens that cause pneumonia during pregnancy. Third-generation cephalosporins are effective, and the addition of a macrolide antibiotic such as azithromycin or clarithromycin is recommended for coverage against *Legionella* pneumonia. *Legionella* pneumonia may present similarly to pneumococcal pneumonia but has a higher mortality risk. *Legionella* pneumonia kills up to 6%

of previously healthy persons who receive correct treatment and up to 80% of immunocompromised individuals or ill persons who experience excessive delay in receiving the proper treatment.[64] It has been uncommonly reported in pregnancy. Doxycycline, while a drug of choice in the nonpregnant population, is a tetracycline, and like any tetracycline drug, should be avoided during pregnancy.[64]

Influenza

Prevention remains the most beneficial approach to influenza in pregnancy. Women who develop influenza while pregnant are at increased risk for pneumonia.[65] Pregnant women with influenza A-related pneumonia have a higher mortality rate than nonpregnant women with pneumonia.

Inactivated vaccine is recommended for all women who will be pregnant during influenza season, regardless of trimester. Live, attenuated influenza vaccine (nasal spray vaccine, FluMist) is contraindicated secondary to theoretic concerns regarding fetal risk.[66] Limited data suggest that the immune response to influenza vaccine is similar in pregnant and nonpregnant individuals, and vaccination of pregnant women can provide passive immunity to the infant, which may last through the first 6 months of life.[66]

Antiviral medications used after exposure to influenza, such as amantadine (Symmetrel), rimantadine (Flumadine), oseltamivir (Tamiflu), and zanamivir (Relenza) have limited data for use in pregnancy and are therefore recommended for use only when the potential benefits outweigh the potential risks.[65]

Dental Treatment and Infections

A clinician may be consulted by women and dental care providers regarding various treatments and medications during pregnancy. Local anesthetics such as lidocaine have not been associated with major congenital anomalies. Likewise, dental X-rays during pregnancy have not been found to be associated with any fetal abnormalities.[67] Maternal lead shielding of the abdomen, use of high-speed film, and limiting dental X-rays to bitewing rather than full-mouth series can reduce risk to the fetus while allowing the dental practitioner sufficient information to address acute and chronic problems.[68]

The human mouth may harbor up to 500 species of bacteria, most of which reside transiently and without harming the host. A few types of bacteria cause most acute odontogenic infections, and the drug of choice for the majority is either penicillin, amoxicillin (Amoxil), or amoxicillin-clavulanate (Augmentin). Amoxicillin used to treat a dental infection may be dosed at 500–875 mg every 8–12 hours orally, and the recommended dose of amoxicillin-clavulanate acid at 500–875/125 mg per 8 hours or 500–875/125 mg per 12 hours. Both have good efficacy data for use in pregnancy. Clindamycin (Cleocin) has also been used in dental infections with bone involvement due to better coverage of bone and requires no dosing changes in pregnancy. Treatment length for acute dental infections is typically 7–10 days.[68]

Gastrointestinal Disorders

Gastroesophageal Reflux Disease (GERD)

Women may begin pregnancy with preexisting GERD. For these women, lifestyle changes plus antacids and histamine$_2$-receptor antagonists may not be sufficient to relieve symptoms. The proton pump inhibitors are indicated for GERD symptom control and healing of esophagitis. Their efficacy in pregnancy has not been proven.[55] Omeprazole (Prilosec), lansoprazole (Prevacid), and pantoprazole (Protonix) have been studied prospectively in pregnancy and have not been associated with any increased risk for congenital malformations, with omeprazole having the most exposed subjects.[69] Because of less experience in human pregnancy and less evidence for efficacy, the proton pump inhibitors should be reserved for women whose GERD symptoms do not resolve with lifestyle changes plus antacids and histamine$_2$-receptor antagonists. Women already taking a proton pump inhibitor prior to pregnancy may be continued on their current therapy.

Peptic Ulcers

Peptic ulcer disease and severe GERD symptomatology may be related to infection with the spiral bacterium *Helicobacter pylori*. It is possible that *H pylori* infection may have a role in hyperemesis gravidarum.[70] *H pylori* infections identified in pregnancy can be treated with the triple therapy regimen commonly used in nonpregnant persons, consisting of two antibiotics and a proton pump inhibitor; however, clarithromycin (used as a part of triple therapy) has limited data pertaining to humans and is not a preferred antibiotic agent during pregnancy.

Sucralfate (Carafate) inhibits pepsin activity and is used to treat peptic ulcers. It acts locally at the ulcer site with minimal systemic effects and is poorly absorbed systemically. There is limited information regarding potential teratogenic risk with sucralfate, but preliminary data are reassuring, and fetal toxicity in humans has not been reported. It is an FDA Pregnancy Category B drug.[55]

Misoprostol (Cytotec), a synthetic prostaglandin E1 analog used to protect the gastric lining from NSAID-induced ulcers, is a potent uterine stimulant that acts directly on the myometrium to induce labor; thus it is contraindicated during pregnancy.[71] Using misoprostol in the first trimester has been found to be rarely associated with Moebius sequence malformations (equinovarus with cranial nerve defects), presumably due to vascular disruption due to uterine contractions.[72]

Headache

Migraine

Migraine frequency and severity is influenced by hormonal changes such as pregnancy. Approximately one in five women experience migraine with aura, defined as focal neurologic symptoms that accompany or precede the headache pain. Women with the latter type of headache are less likely to experience decreases in headache episodes during pregnancy than women who experience migraines without aura, a substantial percentage of whom improve markedly during the later part of pregnancy.[73] Migraines may initially worsen in the first trimester, then decrease or even cease in the later part of pregnancy. It is relatively rare for a first migraine to occur during pregnancy, and new onset of headache symptoms should prompt a thorough diagnostic workup to rule out secondary causes.[73]

Therapy for migraine headaches during pregnancy can be prophylactic or abortive agents used to relieve acute symptoms. Many women are able to cope with and reduce migraine symptoms using nonpharmacologic interventions such as rest and ice packs. When these are ineffective and pharmacotherapy is indicated, nonspecific agents with evidence for use in pregnancy include acetaminophen (Tylenol), opiates such as codeine, and caffeine (in limited amounts). Caffeine can cause rebound migraine headaches in some women. A reasonable acute treatment plan includes 1 gram of oral acetaminophen at the first sign of a migraine. Suppositories or injectable opiates may be necessary to abort a severe migraine if the woman is vomiting. Oral opiates may be used if no vomiting is present. Nausea and vomiting that accompany migraine may be treated by the agents recommended for use in nausea and vomiting of early pregnancy.

Triptans or selective serotonin receptor agonists are the standard treatment for nonpregnant individuals. Traditionally, the triptans have been considered contraindicated in pregnancy. The manufacturers maintain three pregnancy registries and there are no reports of teratogenic effects, but because data on safety has been limited, they have not been used in clinical practice. More recently, studies evaluating the effect of triptans in pregnancy have been published, and triptans do not appear to be associated with adverse outcomes with the possible exception of a questionable increase in preterm labor.[74,75] Sumatriptan (Imitrex), the best studied of the selective serotonin receptor agonists, is becoming more frequently used in pregnancy for severe, frequent migraine headaches.

Ergot alkaloids such as caffeine-ergotamine (Cafergot, Wigraine), dihydroergotamine (DHE, Migranal), ergotamine (Ergomar), and methysergide (Sansert) are contraindicated due to abortifacient and teratogenic effects.[73]

Preventive agents that may be considered in pregnancy include propranolol (Inderal) and amitriptyline (Elavil); however, since spontaneous regression in migraine occurs in 80% of women with migraines, and since this improvement is greater than that which can be expected with preventive medication regimens, few women should require preventive therapy during pregnancy, and their use can be reserved for the second and third trimester if required. If propranolol (Inderal) is used daily, it may inhibit conversion of T3 to T4, so monitoring of thyroid status should be initiated.[73]

Sexually Transmitted Diseases

Genital Herpes

Herpes simplex virus infections of the genital area can be caused by either herpes simplex virus type 1 (HSV-1) or type 2 (HSV-2). HSV-2 almost always occurs as a genital pathogen, but HSV-1 can manifest in either the genital area or the circumoral region and also may cause keratoconjuctivitis.[76] Less than 20% of pregnant women who test positive serologically for HSV-2 report a history of having herpes.[77] HSV-1 is becoming a more common genital pathogen and one third to one half of neonatal herpes infections are now caused by HSV-1.[76] Neonatal herpes is usually acquired via vertical transmission during labor and birth. Eighty percent of neonatal HSV infections occur in

newborns of mothers with no reported history of HSV infection. No evidence suggests a time frame after rupture of membranes when cesarean is no longer effective in reduction of transmission.

Treatment of genital herpes in pregnancy is accomplished by use of oral acyclovir (Zovirax) or valacyclovir (Valtrex). Women with a history of genital herpes should be assessed for lesions and prodromal symptoms of herpes outbreak at the onset of labor, and, if present, cesarean birth is recommended.[77] There is some controversy about this recommendation as newborns of mothers who have recurrent herpes usually have some passively acquired immunity and are less likely to become ill.

Suppressive therapy should be offered for these women beginning at 36 weeks of gestation to help reduce the risk of recurrent outbreak at delivery and the need for cesarean birth. Acyclovir has the most data for use in pregnancy, though no adverse effects have been reported with the use of valacyclovir, a prodrug of acyclovir. Valacyclovir gives consistent higher serum concentrations and is dosed only twice a day. Both drugs are in FDA Pregnancy Category B. There are no published data as yet for the use of famciclovir in pregnancy[76] (Table 35-6).

Chlamydia and Gonorrhea

After vaginal infections with *Chlamydia trachomatis* are treated in pregnancy, the CDC recommends that a test of cure be performed 3–4 weeks following treatment with either ampicillin (Principen) (500 mg orally three times a day for 7 days) or a single dose of azithromycin (1 gram by mouth). Women who are allergic to these two medications may alternatively be prescribed erythromycin base (Erythrocin) (500 mg by mouth four times a day for 7 days or 250 mg by mouth four times a day for 14 days)

Table 35-6 Antiviral Therapy for Genital Herpes

Clinical Condition	Acyclovir (Zovirax)	Valacyclovir (Valtrex)
Suppression (starting at 36 weeks gestation)	400 mg PO tid until birth	500 mg PO bid until birth
Recurrent episodes	400 mg PO tid or 800 mg PO bid × 5 d	500 mg PO bid × 3 d or 1 g PO qd × 5 d
Primary episode	400 mg PO tid × 7–10 d (or longer if healing incomplete at 10 days)	1 g PO bid × 7–10 d (or longer if healing incomplete at 10 days)
Disseminated disease	5–10 mg/kg IV q 8 h × 2–7 d, then oral therapy for primary infection to complete 10 days of therapy in total	N/A

or erythromycin ethylsuccinate (EES) (800 mg by mouth four times a day for 7 days or 400 mg by mouth four times a day for 14 days). Erythromycin estolate (Ilosone) is contraindicated due to increased risk for hepatotoxicity in pregnant women.

Gonorrhea during pregnancy should be treated with a single-dose regimen of ceftriaxone (Rocephin) 125 mg intramuscularly or cefixime (Suprax) 400 mg by mouth. If a woman is allergic to cephalosporins, a single intramuscular dose (2 g) of spectinomycin is recommended. If no nucleic acid amplification test results for chlamydia are available to prove negative status, the woman should also be treated with one of the recommended chlamydia treatments in the previous paragraph.

When treating a woman with an infection caused by gonorrhea, chlamydia, or trichomonas, the sexually transmitted nature of the conditions must be acknowledged. Thus, partners also should be referred for testing and treatment, and intercourse avoided for 7 days after single-dose regimens and until treatment is completed in both partners for 7- or 14-day regimens.[78] The clinician should consider testing for syphilis and HIV. State reporting should be performed as appropriate for the condition.

Vaginal Conditions

Candidal Vaginitis

Candidal vaginitis is a common diagnosis in pregnancy, and topical azole antifungals such as butoconazole (Gynazole, Femstat 3), clotrimazole (Gyne-Lotrimin, Mycelex), miconazole (e.g., Monistat, Vagistat), terconazole (Terazol), and nystatin (Mycostatin) are effective treatments for symptomatic yeast infections. The azole antifungals, used topically, are absorbed systemically from the vaginal tract, but data do not support an association with congenital anomalies. Nystatin is poorly absorbed from the vaginal tract and also has no evidence of teratogenicity.

Oral fluconazole (Diflucan) has, despite its FDA Pregnancy Category C classification, been found to be a probable teratogen if used in the first trimester for prolonged periods at high doses (400 mg per day or more). Congenital anomalies found in offspring of women exposed to oral fluconazole for prolonged periods in the first trimester (weeks to months) at doses at or over 400 mg a day included craniofacial abnormalities, skeletal abnormalities, and cardiac malformations.[79] For pregnancies exposed to lower doses of fluconazole, like the single 150 mg oral dose commonly prescribed for vaginal candida, no data suggesting increased levels of congenital anomalies have been identified.[11]

Bacterial Vaginosis and Trichomoniasis

Bacterial vaginosis (BV) is present in up to 20% of pregnant women, and more than half of these women have no symptoms.[78] Bacterial vaginosis is characterized by a shift in normal vaginal flora to a condition in which lactic acid-secreting lactobacilli are decreased or absent, and potentially pathogenic bacteria flourish. In the clinic setting, it is often identified when women report increased vaginal discharge that is malodorous. Microscopy of vaginal secretions reveals clue cells and the relative absence of lactobacilli; the vaginal pH shows an increase in vaginal alkalinity (at or above 4.7), and addition of potassium chloride solution to the vaginal secretions results in a characteristic amine odor (positive whiff test). Current recommendations for the treatment of bacterial vaginosis in pregnancy include 7-day oral regimens of either metronidazole (Flagyl) or clindamycin (Cleocin).

Controversy exists regarding the relationship between bacterial vaginosis and preterm labor. There is considerable evidence that infection and more specifically vaginal microbes play a key role in causing preterm labor. Although women with bacterial vaginosis do have an increased risk of preterm labor, and treatment of the condition does decrease the preterm labor incidence, screening and treatment of women who have bacterial vaginosis but who are asymptomatic does not yield lower rates of preterm birth[80,81] (Box 35-4).

The CDC recommends that women who are at high risk for preterm labor be screened and treated with metronidazole (Flagyl) at the usual nonpregnant dose schedule if bacterial vaginosis or trichomoniasis is diagnosed. In addition, women who are symptomatic should be treated. Oral metronidazole has been evaluated thoroughly and not found to increase likelihood for teratogenesis or fetal toxicity in any trimester.[78] Metronidazole was the cause of some concern in the past for both women and clinicians due to reports of mutagenicity in bacteria and carcinogenicity in rodents and may have been avoided by prescribers due to fear that it was a litogen, but extensive study over 30 years has failed to find evidence of human teratogenicity.[82] Metronidazole is classified as an FDA Pregnancy Category B drug and may be safely used in the first trimester.

Metronidazole (Flagyl) has a bad reputation for another reason. This drug has traditionally been the first-line

Box 35-4   To Treat or Not to Treat: Bacterial Vaginosis

Research interest in bacterial vaginosis (BV) has grown since an association between the condition and preterm birth was identified in the 1990s. Bacterial vaginosis has also been linked with preterm premature rupture of membranes, chorioamnionitis, and postpartum endometritis.

Many studies have been undertaken to ascertain whether treatment of BV in pregnancy is useful in preventing adverse perinatal outcomes. Contradictory findings have led researchers to try to better identify the relationships between BV and these pregnancy complications.

The current debate revolves around several issues, including the value of screening and treatment for asymptomatic BV or the more amorphous intermediate flora, in which some features of BV are present on gram stain but do not meet BV diagnostic criteria; which pregnant women are most likely to benefit from screening and/or treatment; optimal timing for screening and treatment; and what is the best regimen to use. A Cochrane meta-analysis[80] confirmed that antibiotic treatment with clindamycin (Cleocin) or metronidazole (Flagyl) does eradicate BV during pregnancy but antibiotic treatment does not decrease in the risk of preterm birth or preterm prelabor rupture of membranes. However, in women with a prior preterm birth, antibiotic use was not associated with reduction in births < 37 weeks but was associated with a statistically significant reduction in preterm prelabor rupture of membranes (PPROM). The reviewers note that studies were quite heterogenous in design, including timing of treatment, and it is possible that treatment early in pregnancy may yet prove beneficial. At this time, however, there is little evidence supporting routine screening or routine antibiotic treatment for women with asymptomatic bacterial vaginosis.

treatment for trichomoniasis. A meta-analysis[83] of second-trimester antibiotic use found more preterm births in women who used metronidazole as the sole antibiotic (OR 1.31; 95% CI, 1.08–1.58), which raised the concern that perhaps the drug itself has adverse effects. Subsequent studies have had conflicting results. Symptomatic *Trichomonas* infections may be treated with a single oral dose (2 g) of metronidazole, which is as effective as a 7-day course of metronidazole and, in light of the current controversies regarding metronidazole use and preterm birth, may be preferable until further data become available. Metronidazole gel (MetroGel) is not recommended for *Trichomonas* due to inactivity in the bladder and vestibular glands, which may be reservoirs for the trichomonad organism.[78] Tinidazole (Tindamax) has no safety data yet available for use in pregnancy and is thus not recommended.[78]

Intravaginal clindamycin (Cleocin T, Cleocin Vaginal), though effective in women who are not pregnant and possibly effective in improving perinatal outcomes if used early in pregnancy,[84] is not recommended by the CDC due to evidence of increased risk for preterm birth associated with use during the second and third trimesters of pregnancy.[78] Antibiotic treatment should probably be limited to symptomatic women, for the express purpose of symptom relief. The clinician may consider using oral clindamycin to treat bacterial vaginosis in the second and third trimesters until more is known about how metronidazole affects preterm birth risk.

Urinary Tract Infection

Urinary tract infections (UTIs) are the most common bacterial infections in pregnancy. UTIs occur more frequently in pregnancy secondary to ureteral dilatation and increased urinary stasis. Approximately 2–10% of pregnant women have asymptomatic bacteriuria (ASB), 1–4% develop acute cystitis (also referred to as lower urinary tract infection), and 1–2% develop pyelonephritis.[85] ASB predisposes women to pyelonephritis, and if left untreated, 20–40% of women with ASB will develop pyelonephritis.[85] Interestingly, cystitis is not associated with an increased risk for pyelonephritis. All urinary tract infections increase the risk for preterm labor.

Bacterial Organisms

Bacteria that cause UTIs commonly include *Enterobacteriaceae, Escherichia coli, Proteus, Klebsiella, Enterobacter,*

Pseudomonas, Citrobacter, group B *Streptococcus,* and *Staphylococcus saprophyticus.*[85] *E coli* is responsible for 95% of pyelonephritis, yet surveillance data from 2000 found 40% of *E coli* resistant to ampicillin, 20% resistant to trimethoprim/sulfamethoxazole (Bactrim, Septra, TMP/SMX), 4% resistance to ciprofloxacin (Cipro), and only 1% resistant to nitrofurantoin (Macrobid). There is significant geographic variation in the resistance to all the antibiotics in the United States with the pattern of resistance increasing as one travels east to west. The highest prevalence of multidrug resistant phenotypes is on the Pacific Coast. Thus a urine culture with antibiotic sensitivities is especially helpful when choosing an antibiotic for women with a urinary tract infection. Table 35-7 summarizes the antibiotics commonly used to treat urinary tract infections during pregnancy. All antibiotics that the offending organism is not resistant to are effective. A Cochrane review[86] found insufficient evidence for recommending any particular antimicrobial agent or regimen for treatment of uncomplicated symptomatic UTI in pregnancy.

Table 35-7 Antibiotics Used to Treat Urinary Tract Infections During Pregnancy

Antibiotic Generic (Brand)	Dose	Clinical Considerations	Contraindications	FDA Pregnancy Category
Asymptomatic Bacteruria				
Amoxicillin (Amoxil)	500 mg three times/day for 3–7 days	20% resistance overall, but wide geographic variation. Must have susceptibilities before prescribing a beta-lactam. Used to treat GBS without urine culture sensitivities.	Allergy to penicillin.	B
Amoxicillin-clavulanic acid (Augmentin)	250/125 mg four times/day for 3–7 days	20% resistance overall, but wide geographic variation. Must have susceptibilities before prescribing a beta-lactam. Used to treat GBS without urine culture sensitivities.	Allergy to penicillin.	B
Ampicillin (Principen)	500 mg four times/day for 3–7 days	20% resistance overall, but wide geographic variation. Must have susceptibilities before prescribing a beta-lactam. Used to treat GBS without urine culture sensitivities.	Allergy to penicillin.	B
Cephalexin (Keflex)	500 mg four times/day for 3–7 days	Widely used in many regions.	Cross-sensitivity if significant allergy to penicillin exists.	B
Clindamycin (Cleocin)	300 mg twice daily for 3–7 days	Used for treatment of GBS bacteruria in women who are allergic to penicillin.		B
Trimethoprim/sulfamethoxazole DS (Bactrim DS, Septra DS)	160/800 mg twice daily for 3–7 days	Folate antagonist. Adverse effects include fever, rash, photosensitivity, nausea and vomiting, neutropenia, and Stevens-Johnson syndrome.	Contraindicated in first trimester and third trimester for persons with G6PD deficiency and allergy to sulfa.	C
Uncomplicated Urinary Tract Infection (Cystitis)				
Amoxicillin (Amoxil)	500 mg three times/day for 7–10 days	20% resistance overall, but wide geographic variation. Must have susceptibilities before prescribing a beta-lactam. Used to treat GBS without urine culture sensitivities.	Allergy to penicillin.	B
Amoxicillin-clavulanic acid (Augmentin)	250/125 mg four times/day for 7–10 days	20% resistance overall, but wide geographic variation. Must have susceptibilities before prescribing a beta-lactam. Used to treat GBS without urine culture sensitivities.	Allergy to penicillin	B

(continues)

Table 35-7 Antibiotics Used to Treat Urinary Tract Infections During Pregnancy (*continued*)

Antibiotic Generic (Brand)	Dose	Clinical Considerations	Contraindications	FDA Pregnancy Category
Ampicillin (Principen)	500 mg three times/ day for 7–10 days	20% resistance overall, but wide geographic variation. Must have susceptibilities before prescribing a beta-lactam. Used to treat GBS without urine culture sensitivities.	Allergy to penicillin.	B
Cephalexin (Keflex)	500 mg four times/ day for 7–10 days		Cross-sensitivity if significant allergy to penicillin exists.	B
Ciprofloxacin (Cipro)	250 mg twice daily for 3 days			C
Nitrofurantoin (Macrodantin)	100 mg four times/ day for 7–10 days	Urinary antiseptic, concentrates in urine.	Contraindicated for persons with G6PD deficiency. Controversy regarding use near term to avoid hemolytic anemia in an infant with G6PD deficiency.	B
Nitrofurantoin (Macrobid) sustained release	100 mg twice/daily for 7–10 days	Urinary antiseptic, concentrates in urine.	Contraindicated for persons with G6PD deficiency. Controversy regarding use near term to avoid hemolytic anemia in an infant with G6PD deficiency.	B
Trimethoprim/ sulfamethoxazole (Bactrim DS, Septra DS)	160/800 mg twice daily for 7–10 days	Folate antagonist with theoretic increased risk of neural tube defect.	Contraindicated in first trimester and third trimester for persons with G6PD deficiency and allergy to sulfa.	C
Pyelonephritis				
Cefazolin (Ancef)*†	1 to 2 g IV q 6–8 h until afebrile	Hospitalization until afebrile then conversion to oral antibiotics followed by discharge if she remains afebrile.	Cross-sensitivity if significant allergy to penicillin exists.	B
Ceftriaxone (Rocephin)‡	1 to 2 g IV or IM q 24 h until afebrile		Cross-sensitivity if significant allergy to penicillin exists.	B
Cefuroxime (Ceftin)†	0.75 to 1.5 g IV q 8 h until afebrile		Cross-sensitivity if significant allergy to penicillin exists.	B
Gentamicin†	2 mg/kg loading dose, followed by 1.7 mg/kg IV q 8 h until afebrile		Potential ototoxicity.	D
Suppression Therapy				
Nitrofurantoin (Macrodantin)	100 mg at hs	To be used for remainder of pregnancy with monthly cultures.	Contraindicated for persons with G6PD deficiency. Controversy regarding use near term.	B
Postcoital Prophylaxis				
Nitrofurantoin (Macrodantin)	50 mg hs	To be used for remainder of pregnancy.	Contraindicated for persons with G6PD deficiency. Controversy regarding use near term.	B
Other				
Phenazopyridine (Pyridium)	200 mg three times/day as needed for dysuria	May turn urine and contact lenses orange.		B

PCN = penicillin; GBS = group B streptococcus; N&V = nausea and vomiting; NTD = neural tube defect.

* May use with or without gentamicin 2 mg/kg intravenous loading dose then 1.7 mg/kg q 8 h for duration of therapy.

† Conversion to oral agents once afebrile: cephalexin (e.g., Keflex, Keftab) 500 mg PO three or four times/day for total therapy of 14 d or cefuroxime 250 mg twice daily for total therapy of 14 d.

‡ If the woman is ≤ 24 weeks pregnant, healthy, and able to comply with therapy, outpatient therapy can be instituted following hydration, antipyretics, the first intramuscular or intravenous dose of ceftriaxone followed by a second injection 24 hours later, then conversion to oral agents if she is afebrile.

Length of Treatment

There is significant geographic variation in the agent most often used, the length of therapy, and the use of a culture after treatment to establish cure. A 3-day course of antibiotic has demonstrated effectiveness in a nonpregnant population, and there are several studies that have documented this duration is effective for pregnant women with ASB or acute cystitis, but the short course will not usually be recommended until more studies are available.

Follow-Up Culture

A posttreatment culture and monthly cultures thereafter are recommended for women treated for ASB. A single posttreatment of cure is always recommended for women with acute cystitis or pyelonephritis.

Suppressive Therapy

Suppressive therapy is indicated after either pyelonephritis or recurrent cystitis and can be prescribed either as a single postcoital dose or daily therapy regimen. If suppressive therapy is instituted, monthly cultures are recommended.

Medications for UTIs

Trimethoprim/sulfamethoxazole (TMP/SMX) is a sulfonamide that inhibits folate metabolism. Although controversial, at least one controlled, retrospective study found trimethoprim/sulfamethoxazole exposure in the first trimester associated with an increased risk of cardiovascular defects (RR 3.4; 95% CI, 1.8–6.4) and oral clefting (RR 2.6; 95% CI, 1.1–6.1).[87] Women in this study who supplemented with the folic acid were less likely to have an affected infant; cardiovascular defect relative risk was 1.5 (95% CI, 0.6–3.8) compared with 7.7 (95% CI, 2.8–21.7) in women who did not supplement, but the recommendation that TMX/SMX be used with folic acid supplementation has not been adopted in clinical practice. TMP/SMX should be avoided in the first trimester and again in the third trimester as it may increase risk of hyperbilirubinemia in the neonate.[85]

Nitrofurantoin has maintained good activity against *E coli* though it is limited in effectiveness against other gram-negative uropathogens. Nitrofurantoin concentrates solely in urine and is effective for uncomplicated cystitis. Some authors recommend avoiding nitrofurantoin near the end of pregnancy due to an increased risk for hemolytic anemia in individuals who have G6PD deficiency.

The urinary pain reliever phenazopyridine (Uristat, Azo-Stat), which is available over the counter, has not been associated with congenital anomalies. Another OTC product, sodium salicylate and methenamine (Cystex), contains an aspirin derivative and is not recommended for use in pregnancy, although methenamine has not been shown to be associated with birth defects. Conversely, the urinary anesthetic phenazopyridine (Pyridium) is safe for use in pregnancy.

Asymptomatic Bacteriuria

Antibiotic choices for asymptomatic bacteriuria are guided by safety of the agent in pregnancy and the sensitivity of the culture; optimal length of treatment has yet to be determined (Box 35-5). There is evidence to support treatment lengths as short as 1 day or 3 days for initial infections followed by tests of cure 10 days after completion of therapy.[85] Asymptomatic bacteriuria caused by group B *Streptococcus* should be treated with an antibiotic to which the organism is sensitive, and the pregnant woman should receive intrapartum prophylaxis if group B *Streptococcus* is present in any amount on the urine culture.[85]

Cystitis or Lower Urinary Tract Infection

All of the antibiotics used to treat ASB can be used to treat acute cystitis. The only change is the length of therapy. Some authors suggest a 3-day course is sufficient, but this is not universally adopted in practice yet, and the standard 7- to 10-day course is generally recommended.

Pyelonephritis

Pyelonephritis has traditionally been treated with an initial hospitalization for hydration, monitoring for preterm labor, and initiation of intravenous antibiotic therapy. Parenteral cephalosporin agents such as cefazolin (Ancef), with or without gentamicin, cefuroxime (Ceftin), and ceftriaxone (Rocephin), are appropriate first-line agents, and cephalexin (Keflex) may be used as oral continuation therapy for susceptible organisms, with a 10- to 14-day total course recommended.[85]

Outpatient therapy is beginning to replace hospitalization in selected women who are in the first or second trimester of pregnancy, generally healthy, and able to comply with therapy. If this regimen is chosen, ceftriaxone (Rocephin) is administered intravenously or intramuscularly once every 24 hours until the women are afebrile and then followed with an oral agent for 10–12 days.

Box 35-5 Asymptomatic Bacteriuria in Pregnancy

MR is a 22-year-old African American primigravida who presented for her first prenatal visit at 10 weeks' gestation. She denied any problems and was excited about the event. Regular prenatal laboratory testing was performed and all results were normal with the exception of establishing that MR has sickle cell trait and a urine culture that revealed a single gram-negative organism with a colony count of 10^5. MR was called, and it was verified that she had no symptoms of a urinary tract infection.

MR has asymptomatic bacteriuria (ASB), a common condition during pregnancy, particularly among women who have sickle cell trait. ASB may occur at other times in a woman's life, but it is rarely screened for outside of pregnancy. During pregnancy, dilated ureters and increased bladder capacity contribute to a higher risk of ascending infection. ASB usually is treated empirically based on the assumption that the offending organism is *Escherichia coli*. A sensitivity is often not performed for the initial testing. Several drugs may be used, although all have major drug resistance and require monitoring to ascertain therapeutic response. MR received a prescription for nitrofurantoin (Macrodantin) 100 mg nightly for 10 days.

Follow-Up

Two weeks later, MR returned for a repeat culture after completing the medication as prescribed. At that time, her culture was still positive for the single gram-negative organism. She then received a prescription for cephalexin (Keflex) 500 mg four times daily for 10 days. Two weeks after completing the cephalexin regimen, her culture remained positive. She was then placed on suppressive therapy of nitrofurantoin 100 mg nightly for the remainder of the pregnancy, with monthly cultures to verify therapeutic success. MR had a normal vaginal birth of a healthy infant at 41 gestational weeks. Her postpartum urine culture was negative. During the pregnancy, she never developed cystitis or pyelonephritis.

Chronic Medical Conditions

Some chronic medical conditions such as diabetes and hypertension can be exacerbated during pregnancy, whereas others, such as migraines or asthma, may actually improve during pregnancy. In general, women with chronic medical conditions who require ongoing pharmacotherapeutic agents will be managed in pregnancy by an obstetric specialist. However, many of these women will initially present to their primary care provider for care. Initiating therapy and identifying specific concerns can improve the overall care these women receive and facilitate seamless transitions between providers as needed.

Asthma

Asthma affects approximately 4–8% of pregnant women.[88] Women with asthma have higher rates of preeclampsia, preterm birth, intrauterine growth restriction, and perinatal mortality.[88] The strongest associations are between poor asthma control and these adverse outcomes. Interestingly, asthma may improve, remain unchanged, or worsen in pregnancy, and the mechanism that underlies this variability is unknown.

Medications are classified as long-term control medications (e.g., inhaled corticosteroids, long-acting beta agonists, leukotriene modifiers, cromolyn, and theophylline) or rescue therapy that provides immediate relief (e.g., albuterol [Proventil, Ventolin]) (Tables 20-10 through 20-14). A stepwise guide to asthma management in pregnancy is available from the National Institutes of Health[89] (Figure 20-4).

Pregnant women with well-controlled asthma should continue the medications taken prior to pregnancy. The National Asthma Education and Prevention Guidelines recommend stepping down one step when asthma has been well controlled for 3 months, but this is generally not recommended during pregnancy given the adverse outcomes associated with uncontrolled asthma.[88] Short-acting beta agonists such as albuterol (Proventil, Ventolin) have the most data for safety in pregnancy and can be used as needed for quick relief. For mild, persistent asthma, addition of an inhaled corticosteroid at the normal adult dose is recommended. Budesonide (Pulmicort) has been shown to be safe for use in pregnancy. Alternatively, cromolyn sodium (Intal) may be used; cromolyn is not associated with increased congenital anomalies.[11] Other alternatives include leukotriene receptor antagonists such as montelukast (Singulair) or zafirlukast (Accolate) or sustained-release theophylline (Theo-24, Uniphyl). The leukotriene receptor antagonists have very limited data in human pregnancy, yet animal studies have been reassuring. However, long-acting beta agonists are more effective than leukotriene receptor antagonists. Theophylline has been used for many years in pregnancy, but it has a narrow therapeutic index and is associated with many drug–drug interactions.

Moderate persistent asthma may be treated with a low-dose inhaled corticosteroid combined with a longer-acting beta$_2$ agonist such as salmeterol (Advair, Serevent) or formoterol (Foradil). There are limited safety data available for use of the long-acting beta$_2$ agonists in pregnancy, but they are expected to have properties similar to albuterol; salmeterol has been available longer in the United States.

Severe persistent asthma may require oral corticosteroid therapy. Oral corticosteroids are associated with an increased risk of premature birth and preeclampsia.[88] Collaboration with the physician is warranted in moderate or severe asthma, when significant exacerbations of mild asthma occur, and at any time when respiratory distress is present.

Cardiovascular Conditions

Chronic Hypertension

Chronic hypertension increases pregnancy risks for both the mother and the fetus. Chronic hypertension is defined as hypertension that predates pregnancy or by a blood pressure measurement of ≥ 140/90 on two separate occasions at least 6 hours apart presenting prior to the 20th week of pregnancy.[90] In the first half of pregnancy, the normal course of blood pressure is that it usually falls due to normal physiologic changes. Blood pressure may be easier to control without medications or with reduced doses. Decreased peripheral vascular resistance in response to prostacyclin and relaxin and the vasodilatory effects of nitric oxide cause a reduction in diastolic blood pressure to a nadir of 10–15 mm Hg below prepregnant levels at 24–32 weeks. The diastolic pressure then gradually returns to prepregnant levels by term. The systolic

blood pressure remains either stable or decreases slightly as the diastolic decreases occur.

Evidence suggests that women with blood pressures that meet the Seventh Report of the Joint National Committee on Detection, Prevention, Evaluation and Treatment of High Blood Pressure (JNC 7) criteria for stage 1 hypertension (≥ 140/90 but < 160/100) during pregnancy do not benefit from pharmacologic treatment.[90] Conversely, women with blood pressures that meet stage 2 criteria (≥ 160/100) should be treated during pregnancy. Women with proteinuria and/or with serum creatinine levels above 1.4 mg/dL in early pregnancy are at higher risk for neonatal adverse outcomes, particularly if superimposed preeclampsia occurs.[90]

Certain classes of medications used to treat hypertension are known to be fetotoxic, others have never been found to affect the embryo or fetus, and others are equivocal in terms of safety data for pregnancy. Methyldopa (Aldomet), a central α_2-agonist, has been extensively studied in pregnancy and is the most commonly used antihypertensive medication in pregnant women.[91] If used for mild hypertension, the usual dose is 250 mg orally three times a day. For severe hypertension, daily doses are usually 1 to 2 grams a day in four divided doses, which can be increased up to 4 grams a day (1000 mg every 6 hours). If adequate blood pressure control is not achieved with maximal dosing, other medications such as beta-blockers, hydralazine (Apresoline), or nifedipine (Procardia) may be added. Labetalol (Trandate), a combination alpha$_1$-blocker and beta-blocker, is currently utilized more in pregnancy as a first-line therapy for chronic hypertension. Labetalol (Trandate) is better tolerated than methyldopa (Aldomet), which may cause drowsiness, dry mouth, lethargy, liver dysfunction, hemolytic anemia, and postural hypotension.[92] Other beta-blockers have been used during pregnancy but have fewer well-controlled studies compared with labetalol (Trandate). Atenolol (Tenormin) in particular has been associated with fetal growth restriction, lower birth weights, and reduced placental function, so it should be avoided during pregnancy.[93]

Thiazide diuretics are considered first-line therapy in nonpregnant women with hypertension, and as a result, many women who have hypertension become pregnant while taking these agents. Since these agents cause a decrease in plasma volume (the opposite of the normal physiologic plasma expansion, which occurs in pregnancy) and may result in adverse effects such as electrolyte imbalances, hyperglycemia, hyperlipidemia, and neonatal electrolyte imbalance, thrombocytopenia, and small size for gestational age, it is prudent to discontinue thiazide diuretics at the first prenatal visit or preconceptionally. If this is a woman's only antihypertensive medication, she may not need antihypertensive medications for the remainder of her pregnancy due to both physiologic reductions in blood pressure and the recommendation to avoid medicating stage 1 hypertension during pregnancy. Diuretics may be added in late pregnancy if needed to control pulmonary edema, but are otherwise contraindicated later in pregnancy.[94]

Some data regarding clonidine (Catapres), a central alpha$_2$-agonist similar to methyldopa, exist for use in pregnancy. Oral administration in pregnancy is divided into two daily doses of 0.05 mg to 0.15 mg each. Total dose may be increased up to 1.2 mg per day. Abrupt discontinuation can cause significant rebound hypertension and should be avoided. Experience with first-trimester use of clonidine is limited, and its safety during early pregnancy has not yet been confirmed. For this reason, it should not be a first-line agent.

Calcium channel blockers such as nifedipine (Procardia) are used in pregnancy to relax the smooth muscles of the uterus in preterm labor and may also be used to reduce acute severe hypertension. Very limited data related to use of nifedipine in chronic hypertension during pregnancy exist.

Angiotensin-converting enzyme inhibitors (ACEIs) and angiotensin II receptor antagonists (ARBs) are contraindicated in pregnancy due to documented fetotoxic effects in the case of ACEI drugs and similar mechanism of action in the ARBs.[95] Aliskiren (Tekturna), the first in the new drug class of renin inhibitors, would be expected to produce similar fetotoxic effects due to its similar mechanism of action (blockage of angiotensin, thus reducing placental perfusion), and thus should be avoided in pregnancy.[96] ACEIs reduce placental perfusion, resulting in oligohydramnios, fetal and neonatal renal failure, intrauterine growth restriction, and fetal and neonatal death. The oligohydramnios produced by fetal renal compromise may itself lead to limb contractures, pulmonary hypoplasia, persistent patent ductus arteriosus, craniofacial malformations, and death. These effects occur in the second trimester rather than the first trimester, so risks of exposure prior to 12 weeks may be less catastrophic.[90]

▌ Diabetes

Diabetes and impaired glucose tolerance affect 3–6% of pregnancies.[97] Type 1 diabetes, in which the body fails to produce sufficient insulin, most often predates pregnancy, and insulin therapy is required throughout gestation. Type 2 diabetes, in which the body develops resistance to endogenous insulin and relative insulin deficiency, is becoming more common in women of childbearing age.[98] Gestational diabetes is the most common diabetic condition in pregnancy, and it involves both insulin resistance and relative insulin deficiency. Gestational diabetes refers to diabetes diagnosed for the first time during pregnancy. Diabetes that predates pregnancy has been associated with increased risks for congenital anomalies, spontaneous abortion, prenatal morbidity and mortality, and neonatal morbidity. Risks for these complications increase concomitly with maternal glucose levels.[98]

For many years, pharmacologic treatment for type 1 diabetes, both prior to and during pregnancy, has involved the exclusive use of exogenous human insulin (Humulin, Novolin), which remains the treatment of choice for this condition. Recent developments in synthetic insulin analogues have been promising, and these agents are being used more frequently. The best studied insulin analogue for use during pregnancy is insulin lispro (Humalog), a synthetic molecule very similar to human insulin with the exception of the amino acids proline and lysine, which are substituted for one another in adjacent positions on the beta chain of the molecule. It appears (via cord blood studies) that, like human exogenous insulin, insulin lispro crosses the placenta only minimally and may in fact be less transferred than human insulin.[98] The advantages of this agent include increased absorption after subcutaneous injection, which leads to a faster onset of action resulting in better postprandial blood glucose control and less late hypoglycemia.

Insulin lispro has been shown to result in lower hemoglobin A1C levels, lower rates of pregnancy loss, and higher satisfaction from women using it compared with human insulin.[99] There is no evidence to date that insulin lispro results in any increase in the rates of congenital malformations beyond that usually seen in the context of diabetes. A newer insulin analog, insulin aspart (NovoLog), has been studied very minimally during pregnancy and cannot yet be recommended for use. Insulin glargine (Lantus), a long-acting insulin analog, has also not been studied for use in pregnancy, and further studies are needed to determine safety and efficacy.[98] Inhaled human insulin (Exubera) has not been studied for use in pregnancy and is off the market. It is theorized that respiratory changes during pregnancy may lead to altered absorption and duration of action of inhaled human insulin, but this has yet to be determined. Diabetes in pregnancy that requires medication for control is an indication for physician consultation.

Type 2 Diabetes

Women with type 2 diabetes are usually placed on an oral antidiabetic agent that they may be taking when they become pregnant. Hyperglycemia is the primary teratogen in women with diabetes. Oral hyperglycemic agents have not been traditionally used in the United States secondary to the concern that these drugs cross the placenta and could cause fetal hypoglycemia. Conversely, oral hyperglycemic agents are often used in other countries where the incidence of type 2 diabetes is high. The first-generation sulfonylureas, biguanides (e.g., metformin [Glucophage]) and thiazolidinediones cross the placenta readily, but the second-generation sulfonylureas (e.g., glyburide [Micronase]) do not transfer to the fetal compartment in any appreciable amount.

The data linking sulfonylureas and teratogenic effects are contradictory and largely confounded by lack of glycemic control, which exerts an independent teratogenic effect.[100] Metformin (Glucophage) is not associated with teratogenic effects in women with polycystic ovary syndrome, a finding that is reassuring because these women were euglycemic.[101] There are not enough data on possible teratogenic effects of thiazolidinediones to draw conclusions about this class of antihyperglycemic drug.

Both metformin (Glucophage) and glyburide (Micronase) have been evaluated for effectiveness in treating diabetes during pregnancy. Glyburide has been extensively evaluated for treatment of gestational diabetes, which is discussed later in this chapter. The studies on metformin have been problematic. The studies done to date have found an increased risk of preeclampsia and perinatal mortality in women on metformin when compared to women on insulin, but the women on metformin had independent risk factors for these outcomes.[101] Conversely, women with polycystic ovary syndrome who take metformin throughout pregnancy have lower rates of the same adverse outcomes.

Pregnancy itself is a state of insulin resistance that increases as the pregnancy progresses, and most women with type 2 diabetes ultimately need insulin therapy to maintain a euglycemic state. Theoretically, metformin would enhance insulin sensitivity and allow for lower doses of insulin, but studies evaluating metformin for this purpose have not yet been completed.

Thyroid Disorders

Hypothyroidism

Maternal overt clinical hypothyroidism is associated with spontaneous abortion, stillbirth, preeclampsia, placental abruption, and low birth weight, and there is some association between hypothyroidism during pregnancy and subsequent cognitive impairment in the child.[102,103] Treatment of overt hypothyroidism may prevent these problems.

Subclinical hypothyroidism, however, defined as elevated thyroid-stimulating hormone (TSH) in the presence of normal levels of triiodothyronine (T3) and thyroxine (T4), with or without thyroid antibodies,[103] is the subject of current controversy. Some evidence exists that placental abruption and preterm birth, neonatal intensive care admission, and respiratory distress are more common in women with subclinical hypothyroidism compared with euthyroid women.[103] The American Association of Clinical Endocrinologists recommends screening all women who are considering pregnancy and who are pregnant, during the first trimester, for thyroid dysfunction, and it recommends treatment with levothyroxine for women who have subclinical hypothyroidism, overt hypothyroidism, and positive thyroperoxidase antibodies.

The American College of Obstetricians and Gynecologists[104] and the US Preventive Services Task Force[105] do not recommend screening women routinely for thyroid dysfunction during or prior to pregnancy. A recent American College of Obstetricians and Gynecologists publication specifically addresses subclinical hypothyroidism[104] and recommends neither screening nor treatment for subclinical hypothyroidism, since neither has been proven beneficial.

Levothyroxine sodium (Synthroid, Levothroid), a synthetic thyroxine, is the drug of choice in clinical hypothyroidism in pregnancy. When hypothyroidism is identified for the first time in pregnancy, initial doses of levothyroxine should be 1.0 to 2.0 micrograms/kilogram/day, or approximately 100 micrograms a day.[102] TSH is then measured every 6–8 weeks (since pituitary adaptation to new hormone levels takes at least 6 weeks) and levothyroxine is titrated to maintain a TSH between 0.5 and 2.5 milliunits/L. Women with known preexisting hypothyroidism should have a TSH measurement during their first visit since needs for exogenous thyroid hormone typically rise during pregnancy and nearly half of women will need an increase in their daily dose. Several drugs may interfere with levothyroxine absorption and should not be taken at the same time, including drugs commonly used by pregnant women such as ferrous sulfate and aluminum hydroxide antacids.

Hyperthyroidism

Overt hyperthyroidism, most commonly caused by Graves' disease, occurs in approximately 2 in 1000 pregnancies and is associated with pregnancy loss, thyroid storm, preterm birth, preeclampsia, intrauterine growth restriction, and maternal congestive heart failure. The fetus can develop **thyrotoxicosis**, which may be secondary to the disease or to the medications used to treat it. Thioamide drugs, including methimazole (Tapazole) and propylthiouracil (PTU), are available to treat hyperthyroidism in pregnancy; radioablative techniques are contraindicated, and surgery is reserved for failure of medical management.

The agent of choice in pregnancy has traditionally been propylthiouracil based on a belief that, due to increased protein binding of PTU, less placental transfer occurred than with methimazole. Both agents can cause fetal hypothyroidism.[106] In addition, there is an association between methimazole and certain congenital anomalies such as aplasia cutis and esophageal atresia. However both agents cross the placenta equally effectively and it is possible that the malformations noted in newborns exposed to methimazole are related to hyperthyroidism itself rather than the drug, as several studies have found no increased incidence of these or other malformations with use of methimazole.

During pregnancy, new onset of overt hyperthyroidism may require higher dosing than is used for nonpregnant women, and one option is to start propylthiouracil at 300 mg a day or higher. The goal of therapy is to maintain free thyroxine in the upper range of normal, using the lowest effective dose of a thioamide drug. It usually takes 6–8 weeks of therapy to reach the free thyroxine goal, though improvement may be seen as early as 4 weeks.[105] Until further evidence is available, it may be prudent to reserve methimazole for therapy in women who are intolerant of PTU or for whom PTU does not have a therapeutic effect.[106] Initiation of pharmacologic therapies for hypothyroidism or hyperthyroidism in pregnancy should involve physician care.

Therapies for Pregnancy-Specific Conditions

There are a few conditions that require pharmacologic treatment, which only appear during pregnancy. Rh isoim-

munization; gestational hypertension; gestational diabetes; pruritic urticarial papules and plaques of pregnancy (PUPPP); and intrahepatic cholestasis are reviewed in the following sections. With the exception of Rh isoimmunization, these disorders resolve spontaneously after delivery.

Prevention of Rh Isoimmunization

Karl Landsteiner, an Austrian physician, discovered the blood group antigens present on the surface of red blood cells in 1901 and named them A, B, and O.[107] He discovered the rhesus factor antigen in 1937 during experiments using the blood of rhesus monkeys. This discovery won Dr. Landsteiner the Nobel Prize in Medicine, and it set the stage for understanding hemolytic disease of the newborn. The development of an agent that would prevent Rh immunization took another 28 years. The first participants in the clinical trials that assessed the efficacy of Rho(D) immune globulin were Rh-negative male inmates at Sing Sing Prison in Ossining, New York. The trials were successful and Rho(D) immune globulin was first introduced for prevention of Rh isoimmunization in 1968. Today Rho(D) immune globulin (RhoGAM) is obtained from human plasma that is subsequently filtered and screened for infectious diseases, then made in a thimerosal-free formulation available for intramuscular administration.

There are five main rhesus antigens—D, C/c, and E/e, and two genes that encode for these antigens, although the term *rhesus factor* or *Rh factor* usually refers only to the D antigen. An individual can be heterozygous or homozygous for each of the five antigens, but it is the D antigen that triggers an immune response when an individual who does not have the Rh(D) antigen is exposed to blood from an individual who has the Rh-D antigen. The anti-D antibodies are small IgG antibodies that can cross the placenta and lyse fetal red blood cells causing **erythroblastosis fetalis**. The first exposure to significant quantities of fetal blood usually occurs with placental separation at delivery of the first child who is Rh positive. That child will not be adversely affected in utero or develop hemolytic disease of the newborn. Following birth and mixture of maternal and fetal blood, the antibodies develop and remain present in maternal sera. These anti-D antibodies can cause erythroblastosis fetalis in a subsequent pregnancy with an Rh-positive fetus.

Synthetic Rho(D) immune globulin (RhoGAM) is a human γ-globulin concentrate of anti-D antibody that prevents initial isoimmunization in Rh(D)-negative mothers by destroying fetal erythrocytes in the maternal system before maternal antibodies can develop and maternal memory cells become sensitized. This is a classic passive immunization technique. Rho(D) immune globulin (RhoGAM) is administered in the first few days following birth and after any potentially immunizing events such as amniocentesis, or antepartum bleeding episodes.

The standard dose of Rho(D) immune globulin (RhoGAM) is 300 mcg given intramuscularly, which prevents the development of antibodies for an exposure of up to 15 mL of fetal red blood cells. It must be given intramuscularly because trace amounts of other plasma proteins present in the liquid could cause anaphylaxis if administered intravenously.

More than one standard dose of Rho(D)-immune globulin may be required if more than 15 mL of fetal cells entered the maternal circulation—a condition usually seen only following placental trauma such as abruption. A smaller dose of 50 mcg (MICRhoGAM, BayRho-D Mini-Dose) is available for use prior to 12 weeks of gestation and covers exposure of up to 2.5 mL of fetal cells; however, controversy exists regarding the necessity of Rho(D) immune globulin administration in the context of first-trimester nontraumatic spontaneous bleeding.[108]

Rh isoimmunization has been almost completely eradicated following routine use of Rho(D) immune globulin postpartum; however, because a small number of women can become isoimmunized during pregnancy secondary to an occult fetal-maternal bleed in the third trimester, a one-time administration of Rho(D) immune globulin (RhoGAM) during the third trimester was instituted in the late 1970s. After antepartum administration of Rho(D) immune globulin, a low serum anti-D antibody titer (1:4 or less) normally develops, which reflects the presence of the anti-D antibodies injected. Thus the woman will have a weakly positive indirect Coombs test for approximately 12 weeks after Rho(D) immune globulin is given.

Rho(D) immune globulin does cross the placenta and can cause lysis of a few fetal Rh-positive cells, but there is no evidence of harm to the fetus, and although the newborn can have a weakly positive Coombs (direct antibody test), there is no increase in the incidence of anemia, jaundice, hemolytic disease of the newborn, or need for phototherapy.[109]

The primary problem today is limited supply of human donors for the plasma pool that is used to manufacture Rho(D) immune globulin (RhoGAM). Two products that use monoclonal antibody techniques and recombinant human anti-D (MonoRho, ZlB Bioplasma AG) have been developed and appear promising. Both are currently being evaluated for efficacy and safety in premarketing clinical trials.[110] Historically, erythroblastosis fetalis and hemolytic disease of the newborn were common and often fatal. Prior to the development of Rho(D) immune globulin, 16% of Rh(D)-negative women became isoimmunized. Today with the use of antenatal and postpartum prophylaxis, only 1–2% of Rh(D)-negative women become isoimmunized, and these cases are largely due to failure to administer Rho(D) immune globulin (RhoGAM) and the small percentage of women who become sensitized early in pregnancy.

Gestational Hypertension, Preeclampsia, and Eclampsia

The medical management of gestational hypertension, preeclampsia, and eclampsia varies according to the gestational age when detected, the severity of the disease, and the progression thereof. Gestational hypertension is defined as systolic blood pressure ≥ 140 mm Hg and/or diastolic ≥ 90 mm Hg on at least two occasions at least 6 hours apart after the 20th week of gestation, in women known to be normotensive prior to this time and prior to pregnancy.[90] Severe gestational hypertension is defined by blood pressures ≥ a systolic of 160 mm Hg and/or a diastolic ≥ 110 mm Hg.[90] Preeclampsia is defined as gestational hypertension plus proteinuria (300 mg or more in 24 hours).[91] In the absence of proteinuria, preeclampsia should be considered if symptoms such as persistent cerebral disturbances, epigastric or right upper quadrant pain with nausea or vomiting, or thrombocytopenia and abnormal liver enzymes coexist with hypertension.[90,111] Severe preeclampsia is diagnosed if there is severe gestational hypertension with proteinuria, hypertension with severe proteinuria (at least 5000 mg in 24 hours), or if multiorgan involvement is evident (pulmonary edema, oliguria, seizures, thrombocytopenia, abnormal liver enzymes accompanying persistent epigastric or right upper quadrant pain, and/or persistent severe central nervous system symptoms such as headaches, blurred vision, blindness, and altered mental status). Eclampsia is defined as convulsions in a woman who has gestational hypertension or preeclampsia.[90,111] Medications used to treat preeclampsia and eclampsia include magnesium sulfate for seizure prophylaxis and antihypertensives to reduce blood pressure.

To date, there is no clear benefit in treating mild preeclampsia or mild gestational hypertension with antihypertensives, and doing so may mask progression of the disease to severe gestational hypertension or severe preeclampsia.[90,111] Severe hypertension (either a systolic of ≥ 160 mm Hg or a diastolic of ≥ 110 mm Hg) does increase the risk for cerebrovascular complications, and women with severe hypertension should receive antihypertensive medications in the hospital setting. It is not clear which antihypertensive medication provides the most benefit with the fewest adverse effects, and several antihypertensives are available for use.[112]

Prevention of Preeclampsia

Multiple preventive therapies for preeclampsia have been evaluated, and few have shown clear benefit. Calcium, as noted previously, has had some success particularly in women with high risk of preeclampsia and for women with low baseline intake of calcium. Aspirin has also been evaluated for prevention of preeclampsia in one meta-analysis and found to be beneficial in low doses (75 mg/day) for women at risk for preeclampsia. The authors note that higher doses of aspirin may be more effective in preventing preeclampsia, but bleeding risks may rise concurrently.[113] It is not yet clear who will benefit most from aspirin prophylaxis or when prophylaxis should begin, and there are no guidelines recommending use of aspirin or other antiplatelet drugs for prevention of preeclampsia at this time.

Gestational Diabetes

Gestational diabetes is defined as hyperglycemia first diagnosed during pregnancy. Gestational diabetes affects approximately 7% of all pregnant women and is associated with an increased risk for macrosomia, neonatal hypoglycemia, and birth trauma.[114] This disorder is usually managed initially with diet and exercise. If these lifestyle changes are insufficient to maintain adequate glucose control, pharmacotherapy is initiated. Traditionally, insulin has been the drug of choice for treating gestational diabetes. The insulin molecule does not cross the placenta, and therefore, does not cause adverse fetal effects. Two oral antidiabetic agents, sulfonylurea glyburide (DiaBeta, Micronase) and metformin (Fortamet, Glucophage), are increasingly being used—albeit off label—as neither is FDA approved for this indication.

Similarities exist in the pathophysiology of gestational diabetes and type 2 diabetes, which leads one to hope oral agents would be effective. The second-generation sulfonylurea glyburide (DiaBeta, Micronase) has been as extensively studied for use in pregnancy and although it is effective, it is less effective than inuslin.[98,100] Langer et al.[115] randomized 404 pregnant women with gestational diabetes to treatment with glyburide or insulin and found no differences in macrosomia, hypoglycemia, admission to neonatal intensive care units, lung complications, or congenital anomalies between the groups. Of the glyburide group, 4% of women had to be switched to insulin to achieve glucose control goals.

Pruritic, Urticaric Papules and Plaques of Pregnancy (PUPPP)

Primigravidas account for 80% of the women who develop pruritic, urticarial papules and plaques of pregnancy (PUPPP). More than three fourths of the cases become manifest during the third trimester.[116] PUPPP is characterized by itchy papules, which typically begin in the striae of the pregnant abdomen, and these become confluent into plaques with an erythematous base. Lesions may then spread to the buttocks and thighs, and in most women, this is the extent of skin involvement. Healing is spontaneous and complete with no residual scarring after delivery. This condition does not tend to recur. PUPPP occurs exclusively in pregnancy, and etiology is still undetermined.[116]

The mainstay of treatment for PUPPP is topical corticosteroids and antihistamines to relieve symptoms, since the condition poses no known risk to mother or baby. Low-, medium-, and high-potency topical corticosteroids may be used, although caution should be used when using high-potency steroids to avoid nonintact skin and/or durations of treatment beyond 2 weeks, since considerable systemic absorption may occur. This risk is higher with ointments than with creams or lotions. Other topical treatments include calamine, oatmeal (Aveeno), and a lotion made of a mixture of camphor, menthol, and phenol that cools irritated skin (Sarna). Hydroxyzine (Vistaril) may be used in doses of 25 to 100 mg orally every 6 hours, and diphenhydramine (Benadryl) used in doses of 25 to 50 mg may be administered with the same dosing frequency.[117] In refractory cases, oral prednisolone may be needed for a short duration (starting dose of 40 to 60 mg daily and tapered over several days) and is usually effective in resolving PUPPP within days.[116]

Intrahepatic Cholestasis of Pregnancy (ICP)

Intrahepatic cholestasis of pregnancy (ICP) is a pregnancy-specific liver disorder that occurs with varying frequency in different regions and appears to be genetically influenced. In many areas, the incidence is less than 1 in 1000, but the condition may occur in up to 2% of pregnancies in Scandinavia and 6% or higher in Chile. ICP is characterized by pruritus without visible rash (though excoriations may occur) that develops in the last half of pregnancy. Itching is often noted in the palms of the hands and soles of the feet. Elevations in serum aminotransferases (ALT and AST) and bile acids (fasting levels > 10 mmol/L) may be present. Occasionally, jaundice, steatorrhea, and fat malabsorption causing vitamin K deficiency occurs.[118]

The pathophysiology of ICP is complex but essentially involves cholestasis and deposition of bile salts in skin. Elevated estrogen levels in susceptible women alter the balance between sulfation of bile salts, which makes them more water soluble, and glucuronidation. This imbalance adversely affects the metabolism and transport of bile acids, causing accumulation and damage. The condition resolves spontaneously after birth.[119,120]

Although severe sequelae for the mother do not accompany this disease, the elevation in serum bile acids can have profound effects on the fetus. Bile salt values of ≥ 40 mmol/L are associated with term intrauterine fetal demise and stillbirth (1 to 2%), preterm birth (19–60%), and nonreassuring fetal heart rates in labor (22–33%).[120]

Various pharmacotherapies have been tried to reduce symptoms and improve perinatal outcomes. In the past, cholestyramine (Questran, Prevalite), a bile acid sequestrant, has been used to reduce pruritus. While cholestyramine binds bile acids, it also binds fat-soluble vitamins and anionic drugs and can result in low levels of vitamin K, which may increase risks for fetal or maternal hemorrhage.[121]

Ursodeoxycholic acid (Urso, Actigall) is a bile acid found in a traditional Chinese medicine, dried powdered black bear's bile. The latter has been used since approximately 618 AD to treat liver diseases and other disorders. Ursodeoxycholic acid acts by stimulating secretion in impaired hepatocytes, a process that may help eliminate toxic compounds from the diseased liver cells. The agent has a protective effect against apoptosis of liver cells and stimulates drug and steroid metabolism. This drug may protect cholangiocytes from pathologic effects of endogenous bile acids by making bile less toxic.[119] Ursodeoxycholic acid (Urso, Actigall) is superior to both cholestyramine and dexamethasone,[120] though as yet it is not clear that any treatment improves perinatal outcomes from ICP.[120,122] Medications and doses used to treat ICP are listed in Table 35-8.[118]

More recently, dexamethasone (Decadron) has been proposed as a treatment strategy for ICP. Dexamethasone reduces estrogen levels by inhibiting the substrates used for estrogen synthesis by the placenta, which include dehydroepiandrosterone (DHEA) and DHEA sulfate. Dexamethasone may reduce pruritus in some women who do not have a therapeutic response to ursodeoxycholic acid. However, some concerns regarding a possible association between repeated steroid courses and low birth weight, adverse effects on fetal organ growth, and potential abnormal neuronal development make dexamethasone an investigational, second-line treatment at this time.[120,122]

Table 35-8 Pharmacologic Treatments for Intrahepatic Cholestasis of Pregnancy (ICP)

Medication	Dose	Formulation	Mechanism of Action
Chlorpheniramine (Chlor-Trimeton)	4 mg tid	4-mg tablets or 8-mg time-released tablets	Antihistamine
Hydroxyzine (Vistaril)	25–50 mg/day	25- or 50-mg tablets	Antihistamine
Cholestyramine (Questran)*	4 g bid	4 g cholestyramine contained in 9-g powder packet	Bile acid sequestrant that binds bile acids in the gut to facilitate excretion
Ursodeoxycholic acid (Actigall)	900 mg–2 g/day	300-mg tablets	Natural water-soluble bile acid interferes with the nonsoluble bile acids that injure cell membranes, thereby decreasing release of pruritic agents
Dexamethasone (Decadron)	12 mg/day	2-mg, 4-mg, or 6-mg tablets	Glucocorticoid anti-inflammatory effect

* Cholestyramine is not as effective as ursodeoxycholic acid in reducing pruritus. Women treated with cholestyramine should be given supplemental fat-soluble vitamins and vitamin K 10 mg/day.
Source: Adapted with permission from Bruce K et al. 2007.[118]

Venous Thromboembolism

A pregnant woman has a risk for developing a deep vein thrombosis (DVT) that is 2–4 times higher than that of a nonpregnant woman.[123] The incidence of venous thromboembolic disease in pregnancy is estimated to be fairly low, with a combined antenatal and postpartum rate of approximately 1 in 1000 for women under 35, and 2 in 1000 for women over 35. Approximately half of pregnancy-associated DVTs occur in women with thrombophilia, either inherited or acquired. The majority of DVTs in pregnancy (80–90%) occur in the left leg, believed to be due to the crossing of the left iliac vein by the right iliac artery. Most DVTs in pregnant women occur in the iliofemoral vein (70%) rather than the popliteal or other distal locations. Iliofemoral DVTs are more likely to embolize than DVTs in distal sites.[123] DVT is associated with a 15–25% risk for pulmonary embolism, which is the leading cause of pregnancy-related maternal mortality in the USA.[123] DVT is followed by venous insufficiency in approximately 60% of cases. Venous thromboembolism and/or anticoagulant therapy in pregnancy requires physician involvement in this aspect of the woman's care.

Warfarin (Coumadin) is a known human teratogen and, as such, is contraindicated for use during pregnancy. Heparin has a high molecular weight (up to 20,000 daltons) and does not cross the human placenta easily, and for years was the sole drug of choice for venous thromboembolism during pregnancy.[124] Low-molecular-weight heparins (LMWHs) have better absorption, longer half-lives than unfractionated heparin, lower incidences of osteoporosis, and lower incidences of heparin-induced thrombocytopenia. LMWH formulations are now widely used in pregnancy. Of the many LMWHs and heparinoid drugs now available, the following three have been studied the most during pregnancy: dalteparin (Fragmin), enoxaparin (Lovenox), and nadroparin (Fraxiparine, available in Canada but not in the United States).

Low-molecular-weight heparins and unfractionated heparin inhibit different aspects of the clotting cascade. Because LMWHs do not inhibit factor IIa, no change in the partial thromboplastin time (PTT) occurs with these agents, and the PTT is not used to monitor treatment effectiveness.[124] PTT levels may be used to monitor unfractionated heparin (UH), and therapeutic target levels for unfractionated heparin are 1.5 to 2.5 times the average laboratory control value.

Dosing of LMWH depends upon whether the goals of therapy are treatment of an acute DVT (therapeutic dosing) or prevention of a first or recurrent DVT (prophylactic dosing). Because of the longer half-life of LMWH, fewer injections per day are required compared to heparin. Both unfractionated heparin and LMWH heparins are administered parenterally; LMWH for treatment may be initiated either intravenously or subcutaneously. Monitoring of therapeutic levels is not necessary when an LMWH is used prophylactically as long as renal failure and/or increased risk factors for bleeding are not present, and provided that the woman's body weight is between 50 and 90 kg.[124]

LMWH dosing requires twice-daily administration to achieve full anticoagulation, while once-daily dosing is used for prophylaxis. Typical therapeutic and prophylactic doses for unfractionated heparin and LMWH are shown in Table 35-9.[124]

Clinicians sometimes change anticoagulation therapy to a regimen of unfractionated heparin as term approaches, since LMWH's longer half-life (an advantage prior to term) can result in higher risks for bleeding if birth occurs sooner than anticipated, and regional anesthesia may be used sooner after discontinuation of unfractionated heparin compared with LMWH.[125]

Heparin-induced thrombocytopenia is an immunoglobulin-G mediated phenomenon that usually develops 5 to 15 days after beginning heparin therapy; it occurs in 1–3% of anticoagulated individuals. The risk of heparin-induced thrombocytopenia is rare when LMWHs are used. However, if heparin-induced thrombocytopenia occurs during pregnancy when the woman is using unfractionated heparin, a possibility exists for recurrence with LMWH. Therefore, fondaparinux, a pentasaccharide and selective factor Xa inhibitor, is recommended.[126]

Table 35-9 Therapeutic and Prophylactic Doses of Unfractionated Heparin and Low-Molecular-Weight-Heparins

Drug Generic (Brand)	Therapeutic (Initial) Dose for VTE	Prophylactic Dose for VTE
Unfractionated heparin	30,000–35,000 U per 24 h, continuous IV or SQ	Unfractionated heparin SQ bid adjusted to target a midinterval partial thromboplastin test in the therapeutic range
Enoxaparin sodium (Lovenox)	1 mg/kg/day bid SQ or 1.5 mg/kg daily	40 mg daily SQ or 30 mg bid SQ
Dalteparin sodium (Fragmin)	100 IU/kg/day bid SQ	2500 to 5000 IU daily or 2500 IU bid SQ

VTE = venous thromboembolism.
Source: Adapted from Laurent et al. 2002.[124]

Complementary and Alternative Medicine in Pregnancy

Several of the most effective, least hazardous treatments for common conditions and diseases encountered during pregnancy are complementary, rather than allopathic. Effective, safe treatments for nausea and vomiting have been reviewed previously in this chapter. Clinicians and women seek effective, safe remedies for physiologic discomforts in pregnancy, and many are turning to complementary and alternative medicine (CAM) therapies. Although herbal remedies are frequently used by pregnant women, data remain for the most part experiential. Table 35-10 includes a list of herbs commonly recommended for use in pregnancy and a summary of safety information that is available.

Conclusion

Pregnancy, a unique state in the human life span due to the coexistence of two individuals in one physiologic system, continues to be a challenge for the prescribing clinician. Pregnancy is predominantly a normal, healthy stage of the female life span and no pharmacologic treatment

Table 35-10 Herbal Medicines Used in Pregnancy

Name	Also Known As . . .	Indication	Preparation/Dose	Safety Data for Pregnancy
Alfalfa	*Medicago sativa*, lucerne, *Medicago*, phytoestrogen, purple medick	Source of vitamins K, A, C, and E and minerals calcium, potassium, phosphorus, and iron.	Leaves used orally; tablets of 5 to 10 g PO tid.	Contains isoflavonoids with estrogenic effects. Large amounts vitamin K. Possibly unsafe.
Arnica	*Arnica Montana*, arnica flos, arnica flower, leopard's bane, mountain tobacco, wolf's bane	Topical use for inflammation associated with bruises, sprains, aches. Orally, used as an abortifacient.	Flower head: 2 g in 100 mL of water, ointments contain 20–25%.	May inhibit human platelet function. Can cause contact dermatitis and mucous membrane irritation. Likely unsafe (oral or topical).
Basil	*Ocimum basilicum*, common basil, garden basil, sweet basil, St. Joseph's wort	Promotion of circulation before and after childbirth, morning sickness.	Tea: 2–4 g in 150 cc boiling water for 10–15 min; strain. 1 c fresh brewed tea PO bid–tid between meals.	Likely safe when leaves, stems, and flowers used as a spice. Possibly unsafe when used in larger amounts due to estragole in essential oil, which may have mutagenic effects. May cause hypoglycemia.
Black cohosh	*Actaea racemosa*, *Cimicifuga racemosa*, baneberry, black snakeroot, bugbane, bugwort, cimicifuga, rattlesnake root, squaw root	Labor induction.	Rhizome and root tincture. Some use 1 dropperful in 1 oz H$_2$O.	Estrogen-like effects. May cause liver disease. May inhibit cytochrome P450 (CYP2D6), causing drug interactions. No clinical evidence of efficacy for labor induction. Possibly unsafe when used prior to term; may increase miscarriage risk. Observational evidence of safety for mother or fetus.
Blue cohosh	*Caulophyllum thalictroides*, blue ginseng, caulophyllum, papoose root, squaw root, yellow ginseng	Induction of labor.	Rhizome and root.	Likely unsafe. Uterine stimulant. Can induce labor. Constituents may be teratogenic. When used near term, may cause life-threatening neonatal toxicity. Constricts coronary arteries and may decrease oxygenation to the heart.
Catnip	*Nepeta cataria*, catmint, catswort, field balm	Insomnia, GI upset, migraines. Topical: for hemorrhoids to relieve swelling.	Flowering tops. 1–2 tsp in 6 oz boiling water (tea).	May have uterine stimulant properties; avoid using. Likely unsafe.

(continues)

Table 35-10 Herbal Medicines Used in Pregnancy (*continued*)

Name	Also Known As . . .	Indication	Preparation/Dose	Safety Data for Pregnancy
Chamomile	*Matricaria recutita*, blue chamomile, German chamomile, Hungarian chamomile, true chamomile, wild chamomile, sweet false chamomile	Morning sickness, insomnia, restlessness, afterpains postpartum.	1 mL PO tid.	Insufficient reliable information available. May compete with estrogen receptors. Avoid use.
Dandelion	*Taraxacum officinale*, blowball, common dandelion, cankerwort, lion's tooth, swine snout, wild endive	Reduction of anemia, swelling, and as a nutritional supplement.	Tincture of leaves/ root or eat tender leaves in spring. No typical dosage.	Insufficient information available; avoid using in amounts greater than in food. May lower fluoroquinolone levels.
Echinacea	*Echinacea angustifolia*, coneflower, black sampson, comb flower, red sunflower, scurvy root, snakeroot, Indian head	Immunostimulant, treatment for the common cold, treating genital HSV and vaginal candida.	Multiple preparations and dosages.	Possibly safe when used orally, short term. Possibly effective to prevent recurrent vaginal yeast and for the common cold. Increases caffeine concentrations by 30% in nonpregnant population. Inhibits CYPA12 enzymes.
Evening primrose oil	*Oenothera biennis*, EPO, cis-linoleic acid, fever plant, gamma linolenic acid (GLA), linoleic acid	Cervical ripening, prevention of preeclampsia, prevention of postdate pregnancy.	500 mg PO tid × 7 d then PO qd. Others have used capsules intravaginally.	Possibly unsafe when used orally. May increase risk for prolonged rupture of membranes, increased use of oxytocin, arrest of descent, associated with increased rates of vacuum extraction.
Ginger	*Zingiber officinale*, African ginger, black ginger, Indian ginger, Jamaican ginger, race ginger, ardraka	Morning sickness.	250 mg PO qid.	Possibly safe when used orally. More effective than placebo.
Lavender	*Lavandula angustifolia*, common lavender, English lavender, garden lavender, spike lavender, true lavender, French lavender, Spanish lavender	Insomnia, nervousness, aromatherapy for pain and agitation. Soothing facial cloths for labor.	3 drops essential oil in water for topical use.	Insufficient reliable information available.
Nettle	*Urtica dioica*, bichu, common nettle, stinging nettle, small nettle, great stinging nettle	Anemia, poor circulation. Leaves, above-ground parts eaten as cooked vegetable. Leaves contain vitamin C and vitamin K.	Leaf, stem, and root used. Allergic rhinitis dose: 300 mg of leaf extract PO tid.	Likely unsafe due to possible uterine stimulant and abortifacient effects.
Oat straw	*Avena sativa*, cereal fiber, dietary fiber, green oat grass, groats, oat, oat bran, oat fiber, rolled oats	Anxiety, GI upset, skin irritation.	No typical dosing.	Likely safe when used orally.
Pycnogenol	*Pinus pinaster*, French marine/ maritime pine bark extract, condensed tannins	Back, pelvic pain of late pregnancy, hip pain, leg cramps.	30 mg/daily.	Some preliminary clinical research of safety in third trimester, but evidence insufficient.
Red raspberry	*Rubus idaeus*, raspberry, raspberry ketone, *Rubus*	Morning sickness, prevention of miscarriage, facilitating labor and birth, uterine tonic.	Labor facilitation: 2 g dried leaf in 240 mL boiling water × 5 min and straining. Tablets containing 2.4 g daily starting at 32 weeks.	Likely safe when used orally in amounts common in foods. Possibly safe when used orally in medicinal doses in late pregnancy. Likely unsafe when used orally in medicinal doses throughout pregnancy or for self-treatment. Does not seem to reduce the length of labor or decrease need for analgesia.
Valerian	*Valeriana officinalis*, all-heal, Belgium valerian, common valerian, garden heliotrope, tagar	Insomnia, anxiety-associated sleeping disorder.	Root and rhizome. 400–900 mg valerian extract PO up to 2 h before bedtime.	Insufficient reliable information available; avoid using. Potential for interaction with CNS depressants.

may be needed, particularly in a well-nourished woman. When drugs are prescribed, the imperative to avoid unnecessary medications must be balanced against the need to treat conditions that impair the health or well-being of the mother and/or the fetus. The key is to provide individualized pharmacologic care that considers the preexisting health needs of each mother, the evolving development of the fetus, and the challenges that pregnancy itself may pose in the form of preeclampsia and other pregnancy-related conditions and diseases. In a few situations, several pharmacologic agents may be necessary, requiring close consultation between the primary provider and other specialists. The rewards of these ongoing, careful calculations are simple, yet profound—working with women to achieve the best possible outcomes for them and their babies.

References

1. Hansen WF, Peacock AE, Yankowitz J. Safe prescribing practices in pregnancy and lactation. J Midwifery Womens Health 2002;47(6):409–21. Review. PubMed PMID: 12484662.

2. Lee E, Maneno MK, Smith L, Weiss SR, Zuckerman IH, Wutoh AK, et al. National patterns of medication use during pregnancy. Pharmacoepidemiol Drug Saf 2006;15:537–45.

3. Rayburn WF, Amazne A. Prescribing medications safely during pregnancy. Med Clin North Am 2000; 92:1227–37.

4. Buhimschi C, Weiner CP. Medications in pregnancy and lactation. Obstet Gynecol 2009;113:166–88.

5. Andrade SE, Gurwitz JH, Davis RL, Chan KA, Finkelstein JA, Fortman K, et al. Prescription drug use in pregnancy. Am J Obstet Gynecol 2004;191: 398–407.

6. Wen SW, Yang T, Krewski D, Yang Q, Nimrod C, Garner P, et al. Patterns of pregnancy exposure to prescription FDA C, D and X drugs in a Canadian population. J Perinatol 2008;28:324–9.

7. Larimore WL, Petrie KA. Drug use in pregnancy and lactation. Prim Care 2000;27:35–42.

8. Lo WY, Friedman JM. Teratogenicity of recently introduced medications in human pregnancy. Obstet Gynecol 2002;100:465–73.

9. Frederiksen MC. The drug development process and the pregnant woman. J Midwifery Womens Health 2002;47(6):422–5. PubMed PMID: 12484663.

10. Ratnapalan S, Bona N, Chandra K, Koren G. Physicians' perceptions of teratogenic risk associated with radiography and CT in early pregnancy. Am J Roentgenol 2004;182:1107–9.

11. Shephard TH. "Proof" of human teratogenicity [letter]. Teratology 1994;50:97–8.

12. Centers for Disease Control and Prevention. Fetal alcohol spectrum disorders. Available from: *www.cdc.gov/ncbddd/fas/fasask.htm* [Accessed July 8, 2007].

13. Klebanoff MA. The Collaborative Perinatal Project: a 50-year retrospective. Paediatr Perinat Epidemiol 2009;23(1):2–8.

14. Yoon PW, Rasmussen SA, Lynberg MC, Moore CA, Anderka M, Carmichael SL, et al. The National Birth Defects Prevention Study. Public Health Rep 2001; 116(suppl 1):32–40.

15. US Department of Health Education and Welfare, Public Health Service, National Institutes of Health. The Collaborative Perinatal Study of the National Institute of Neurological Diseases and Stroke: the women and their pregnancies. 1972: DHEW Publication No. (NIH) 73-379.

16. Addis A, Sharabi S, Bonati M. Risk classification systems for drug use during pregnancy: are they a reliable source of information? Drug Saf 2000;23:245–53.

17. Food and Drug Administration. Pregnancy labeling. Fed Regist 1979;44:124, 37464–5.

18. Briggs GG, Freeman RK, Yaffe SJ, eds. Drugs in pregnancy and lactation, 8th ed. Philadelphia, PA: Wolters Kluwer/Lippincott Williams & Wilkins, 2008.

19. Motherisk: Treating the mother—protecting the unborn. The Hospital for Sick Children, Toronto, Canada. Available from: *www.motherisk.org/prof/index.jsp* [Accessed November 4, 2007].

20. Organization of Teratology Information Specialists. Available from: *www.motherisk.org/prof/index.jsp* [Accessed November 4, 2007].

21. Tracy TS, Venkataramanan R, Glover DD, Caritis SN. National Institute for Child Health and Human Development Network of Maternal-Fetal-Medicine Units. Temporal changes in drug metabolism (CYP1A2, CYP2D6 and CYP3A activity) during pregnancy. Am J Obstet Gynecol 2005;192(2):633–9.

22. Schoonover LL, Littell CE. Pharmacokinetics of drugs during pregnancy and lactation. In Yankowitz J, Niebyl JR, eds. Drug therapy in pregnancy, 3rd ed. Philadelphia, PA: Lippincott Williams & Wilkins, 2001:5–19.

23. Blackburn ST. Pharmacology and pharmacokinetics during the perinatal period. In Blackburn ST, ed. Maternal, fetal & neonatal physiology: a clinical perspective, 3rd ed. St. Louis, MO: Saunders, 2007: 193–226.

24. Baldessarini RJ, Tarazi FI. Drugs and the treatment of psychiatric disorders: psychosis and mania. In Hardman JG, Limbird LL, eds. Goodman & Gillman's the pharmacological basis of therapeutics, 10th ed. New York: McGraw-Hill, 2001:485–520.

25. Haider BA, Bhutta ZA. Multiple-micronutrient supplementation for women during pregnancy. Cochrane Database Syst Rev 2006(4):CD004905.

26. Mathews TJ. Trends in spina bifida and anencephalus in the United States 1991–2005. Hyattsville, MD: US Department of Health and Human Services, Centers for Disease Control and Prevention, National Center for Health Statistics; 2007.

27. Standing Committee on the Scientific Evaluation of Dietary Reference Intakes, Food and Nutrition Board, Institute of Medicine. Dietary reference intakes: folate, other B vitamins, and choline. Washington, DC: National Academy Press, April 17, 1998. Available at: *www.nap.edu/openbook.php?record_id=6015& page=196* [Accessed November 5, 2007].

28. United States Preventive Services Task Force. Folic acid to prevent neural tube defects, topic page. Rockville, MD: US Preventive Services Task Force, Agency for Healthcare Research and Quality. Available from: *www.ahrq.gov/clinic/uspstf/uspsnrfol.htm* [Accessed September 20, 2009].

29. The Centers for Disease Control and Prevention. Folic acid: Public Health Service recommendations. Available from: *www.cdc.gov/ncbddd/folicacid/recommendations .html* [Acessed September 20, 2009].

30. Medical Research Council Vitamin Study Research Group. Prevention of neural tube defects: results of the Medical Research Council Vitamin Study. Lancet 1991;338:131–7.

31. Centers for Disease Control and Prevention. Recommendations to prevent and control iron deficiency in the United States. MMWR 1998;47:1–29.

32. United States Preventive Services Task Force. Screening for iron deficiency anemia: including iron supplementation for children and pregnant women. 2006. Available from: *www.ahrq.gov/clinic/uspstf/uspsiron .htm* [Accessed November 12, 2007].

33. Pena-Rosas JP, Viteri FE. Effects of routine oral iron supplementation with or without folic acid for women during pregnancy. Cochrane Database Syst Rev 2006 (3):CD004736.

34. Graves BW, Barger MK. A "conservative" approach to iron supplementation during pregnancy. J Midwifery Womens Health 2001;46:159–66.

35. Melamed N, Ben-Haroush A, Kaplan B, Yogev Y. Iron supplementation in pregnancy: does the preparation matter? Arch Gynecol Obstet 2007;276:601–4.

36. Food and Nutrition Board, Institute of Medicine, National Academies. Dietary Reference Intakes (DRIs): recommended intakes for individuals, vitamins and elements. Available from: *www.iom.edu/?id=21381* [Accessed July 21, 2007].

37. Hofmeyr GJ, Atallah AN, Duley L. Calcium supplementation during pregnancy for preventing hypertensive disorders and related problems. Cochrane Database Syst Rev 2006(3):CD001059.

38. Bourgoin BP, Evans DR, Cornett JR, Lingard SM, Quattrone AJ. Lead content in 70 brands of dietary calcium supplements. Am J Public Health 1993;83: 1155–60.

39. Jewell D, Young G. Interventions for nausea and vomiting in early pregnancy. Cochrane Database Syst Rev 2003(4):CD000145.

40. Weiss G. The death of Charlotte Brontë. Obstet Gynecol 1991;78(4):705–8.

41. Levichek Z, Atanackovic G, Oepkes D, Maltepe C, Einarson A, Magee L, et al. Nausea and vomiting of pregnancy: evidence-based treatment algorithm. Motherisk program, The Hospital for Sick Children, 2002. Available from: *http://motherisk.org/prof/updates Detail.jsp?content_id=348#fig1* [Accessed July 22, 2007].

42. Koren G, Boskovic R, Hard M, Maltepe C, Navioz Y, Einarson A. Motherisk-PUQE (pregnancy-unique quantification of emesis and nausea) scoring system for nausea and vomiting of pregnancy. Am J Obstet Gynecol 2002;186(5)(suppl understanding):S228–31.

43. Food and Drug Administration. Determination that Bendectin was not withdrawn for sale for reasons of safety or effectiveness. Fed Regist 1999;64:43190–1.

44. Kutcher JS, Engle A, Firth J, Lamm SH. Bendectin and birth defects. II: ecological analyses. Birth Defects Res A Clin Mol Teratol 2003;67(2):88–97.

45. Magee LA, Mazzotta P, Koren G. Evidence-based view of safety and effectiveness of pharmacologic therapy for nausea and vomiting of pregnancy (NVP). Am J Obstet Gynecol 2002;186(5)(suppl understanding): S256–61.

46. Olsen JC, Keng JA, Clark JA. Frequency of adverse reactions to prochlorperazine in the ED. Am J Emerg Med 2000;18(5):609–11.

47. Einarson A, Maltepe C, Navioz Y, Kennedy D, Tan MP, Koren G. The safety of ondansetron for nausea and vomiting of pregnancy: a prospective comparative study. BJOG. 2004;111(9):940–3. PubMed PMID: 15327608.

48. Vinson DR, Drotts DL. Diphenhydramine for the prevention of akathisia induced by prochlorperazine: a randomized, controlled trial. Ann Emerg Med 2001; 37(2):125–31.

49. Iqbal MM, Sobhan T, Ryals T. Effects of commonly used benzodiazepines on the fetus, the neonate and the nursing infant. Psychiatr Serv 2002;53:39–49.

50. Bondok RS, El Sharnouby NM, Eid HE, Abd Elmaksoud AM. Pulsed steroid therapy is an effective treatment for intractable hyperemesis gravidarum. Crit Care Med 2006;34:2781–3.

51. VanDinter MC. Ptyalism in pregnant women. J Obstet Gynecol Neonatal Nurs 1990;20:206–9.

52. Westfall RA. Uses of anti-emetic herbs in pregnancy: women's choices, and the question of safety and efficacy. Complement Ther Nurs Midwifery 2004; 10:30–6.

53. Borrelli F, Capasso R, Aviello G, Pittler MH, Izzo AA. Effectiveness and safety of ginger in the treatment of pregnancy-induced nausea and vomiting. Obstet Gynecol 2005;105:849–56.

54. Vutyavanich T, Kraisarin T, Ruangsri R. Ginger for nausea and vomiting in pregnancy: a randomized, double-masked, placebo-controlled trial. Obstet Gynecol 2001;97:577–82.

55. Richter JE. Review article: the management of heartburn in pregnancy. Aliment Pharmacol Ther 2005;22:749–57.

56. Jewell DJ, Young G. Interventions for treating constipation in pregnancy. Cochrane Database Syst Rev 2001(2):CD001142.

57. Quijano CE, Abalos E. Conservative management of symptomatic and/or complicated hemorrhoids in pregnancy and the puerperium. Cochrane Database Syst Rev 2005(3):CD004077.

58. Young GL, Jewell D. Interventions for leg cramps in pregnancy. Cochrane Database Syst Rev 2002(1): CD000121.

59. Pennick VE, Young G. Interventions for preventing and treating pelvic and back pain in pregnancy. Cochrane Database Syst Rev 2007(2):CD001139.

60. Pien GW, Schwab RJ. Sleep disorders during pregnancy. Sleep 2004;27:1405–17.

61. Gilbert C, Mazzotta P, Loebstein R, Koren G. Fetal safety of drugs used in the treatment of allergic rhinitis: a critical review. Drug Saf 2005;28:707–19.

62. Moretti ME, Caprara D, Coutinho CJ, Bar-Oz B, Berkovitch M, Addis A, et al. Fetal safety of loratadine use in the first trimester of pregnancy: a multicenter-study. J Allergy Clin Immunol 2003;111:479–83.

63. Källen BA, Olausson PO. Use of oral decongestants during pregnancy and delivery outcome. Am J Obstet Gynecol 2006;194:480–5.

64. Shariatzedeh MR, Marrie TJ. Pneumonia during pregnancy. Am J Med 2006;119:872–6.

65. Beigi R. Pandemic influenza and pregnancy: a call for preparedness planning. Obstet Gynecol 2007;109: 1193–6.

66. The Centers for Disease Control and Prevention. Influenza vaccination in pregnancy: practices among obstetrician-gynecologists—United States, 2003–04 influenza season. MMWR 2005;54:1050–2.

67. Pascal Demoly JD. Comment: managing asthma in pregnancy. Lancet 2005;365:1212–3.

68. Giglio JA, Lanni SM, Laskin DM, Giglio NW. Oral health care for the pregnant patient. J Can Dent Assoc 2009;75(1):43–8.

69. Diav-Citrin O, Arnon J, Shechtman S, Schaefer C, VanTonningen MR, Clementi M, et al. The safety of proton pump inhibitors in pregnancy: a multicentre prospective controlled study. Aliment Pharmacol Ther 2005;21:269–75.

70. Penney DS. *Helicobacter pylori* and severe nausea and vomiting during pregnancy. J Midwif Womens Health 2005;50:418–22.

71. McMahon MJ. Drug therapy for the treatment of gastrointestinal disorders in pregnancy and lactation. In Yankowitz J, Niebyl JR, eds. Drug therapy in pregnancy, 3rd ed. Philadelphia, PA: Lippincott, Williams & Wilkins, 2001:77–99.

72. Gonzalez CH, Marques-Dias MJ, Kim CA, Sugayama SM, Da Paz JA, Huson SM, et al. Congenital abnormalities in Brazilian children associated with misoprostol misuse in first trimester of pregnancy. Lancet 1998;351:1624–7.

73. Fox AW, Diamond ML, Spierings EL. Migraine during pregnancy: options for therapy. CNS Drugs 2005; 19:465–81.

74. Evans EW, Lorber KC. Use of 5-HT1 agonists in pregnancy. Ann Pharmacother 2008;42(4):543–9.

75. Soldin OP, Dahlin J, O'Mara DM. Triptans in pregnancy. Ther Drug Monit 2008;30(1):5–9.

76. American College of Obstetricians & Gynecologists. ACOG Practice Bulletin No. 82. Management of herpes in pregnancy. June, 2007. Obstet Gynecol 2007; 109:1489–98.

77. Baker DA. Consequences of herpes simplex virus in pregnancy and their prevention. Curr Opin Infect Dis 2007;20:73–6.

78. The Centers for Disease Control and Prevention. Sexually transmitted diseases treatment guidelines 2006. Available from: *www.cdc.gov/std/treatment/2006/toc .htm* [Accessed August 2, 2007].

79. King CT, Rogers PD, Cleary JD, Chapman SW. Antifungal therapy during pregnancy. [Review]. Clin Infect Dis 1998;27(5):1151–60. PubMed PMID: 9827262

80. McDonald HM, Brocklehurst P, Gordon A. Antibiotics for treating bacterial vaginosis in pregnancy. Cochrane Database Syst Rev 2007(1):CD000262.

81. Carey JC, Klebanoff MA, Hauth JC, Hillier SL, Thom EA, Ernest JM, et al. Metronidazole to prevent preterm delivery in pregnant women with asymptomatic bacterial vaginosis. National Institute of Child Health and Human Development Network of Maternal-Fetal Medicine Units. N Engl J Med 2000;342(8):534–40.

82. Burtin P, Taddio A, Ariburnu O, Einarson TR, Koren G. Safety of metronidazole in pregnancy: a meta-analysis. Am J Obstet Gynecol 1995;172:525–9.

83. Morency A, Bujold E. The effect of second-trimester antibiotic therapy on the rate of preterm birth. J Obstet Gynaecol Can 2007;29:35–44.

84. Ugwumadu A. Role of antibiotic therapy for bacterial vaginosis and intermediate flora in pregnancy. Best Pract Res Clin Obstet Gynaecol 2007;21:391–402.

85. Le J, Briggs GG, McKeown A, Bustillo G. Urinary tract infections during pregnancy. Ann Pharmacother 2004;38:1692–701.

86. Vazquez JC, Villar J. Treatments for symptomatic urinary tract infections during pregnancy. Cochrane Database Syst Rev 2003(4):CD002256.

87. Hernandez-Diaz S, Werler MM, Walker AM, Mitchell AA. Folic acid antagonists during pregnancy and the risk of birth defects. N Engl J Med 2000;343: 1608–14.

88. Schatz M, Dombrowski M. Asthma in pregnancy. N Engl J Med 2009;360:1862–9.

89. US Department of Health and Human Services, National Institutes of Health. Quick reference from the working group report on managing asthma during pregnancy: recommendations for pharmacologic treatment, update 2004. Available from: *www.nhlbi .nih.gov/health/prof/lung/asthma/astpreg/astpreg_qr .pdf* [Accessed July 28, 2007].

90. US Department of Health and Human Services, National Institutes of Health. The seventh report of the Joint National Committee on the Detection, Prevention, Evaluation, and Treatment of High Blood Pressure, 2003. Available from: *www.nhlbi.nih.gov/guidelines/ hypertension/jnc7full.pdf* [Accessed July 28, 2007].

91. Ghanem FA, Movhed A. Use of antihypertensive drugs during pregnancy and lactation. Cardiovasc Ther 2008;26:38–49.

92. Report of the National High Blood Pressure Education Program Working Group on High Blood Pressure in Pregnancy. Am J Obstet Gynecol 2000;183(1):S1–22.

93. Podymow T, August P. Hypertension in pregnancy. Adv Chronic Kidney Dis 2007;14(2):178–90.

94. Al-Balas M, Bozzo P, Einarson A. Use of diuretics during pregnancy. Can Fam Physician 2009;55(1):44–5.

95. Cooper WO, Hernandez-Diaz S, Arbogast PG, Dudley JA, Dyer S, Gideon PS, et al. Major congenital malformations after first-trimester exposure to ACE inhibitors. N Engl J Med 2006;354:2443–51.

96. Alwan S, Reefhuis J, Rasmussen SA, Olney RS, Friedman JM. Use of selective serotonin-reuptake inhibitors in pregnancy and the risk of birth defects. N Engl J Med 2007;356:2684–92.

97. Tuffnell DJ, West J, Walkinshaw SA. Treatments for gestational diabetes and impaired glucose tolerance in pregnancy. Cochrane Database Syst Rev 2003(3): CD003395.

98. Homko CJ, Reece EA. Insulins and oral hypoglycemic agents in pregnancy. J Matern Fetal Neonatal Med 2006;19:679–86.

99. Bhattacharyya A, Brown S, Hughes S, Vice PA. Insulin lispro and regular insulin in pregnancy. QJM 2001;94:255–60.

100. Merlob P, Levitt O, Stahl B. Oral antihypoglycemic agents during pregnancy and lactation. Pediatr Drugs 2002;4:755–60.

101. Feig DS, Briggs GG, Koren G. Oral antidiabetic agents in pregnancy and lactation: a paradigm shift? Ann Pharmacother 2007;41:1174–80.

102. Casey BM, Leveno KJ. Thyroid disease in pregnancy. Obstet Gynecol 2006;108:1283–92.

103. Weir FA, Farley CL. Clinical controversies in screening women for thyroid disorders during pregnancy. J Midwifery Womens Health 2006;51:152–8.

104. ACOG Committee Opinion No. 381. Subclinical hypothyroidism in pregnancy. Obstet Gynecol 2007; 110:959–60.

105. US Preventive Services Task Force. The guide to clinical preventive services 2007: recommendations from the US Preventive Services Task Force. Available from: *www.ahrq.gov/Clinic/pocketgd07/pocketgd07.pdf* [Accessed November 25, 2008].

106. Chattaway JM, Klepser TB. Propylthiouracil versus methimazole in treatment of Graves' disease during pregnancy. Ann Pharmacother 2007;41:1018–22.

107. Wegmann A, Glück R. The history of rhesus prophylaxis with anti-D. Eur J Pediatr 1996;155(10):835–8.

108. Hannafin B, Lovecchio F, Blackburn P. Do Rh-negative women with first-trimester spontaneous abortions need Rh immune globulin? Am J Emerg Med 2006; 24:487–9.

109. Jones ML, Wray J, Wight J, Chilcott J, Forman K, Tappenden P, et al. A review of the clinical effectiveness of routine antenatal anti-D prophylaxis for rhesus-negative women who are pregnant. BJOG 2004; 111(9):892–902.

110. Kumpel BM. Lessons learnt from many years of experience using anti-D in humans for prevention of RhD immunization and haemolytic disease of the fetus and newborn. Clin Exp Immunol 2008;154(1):1–5.

111. Sibai B, Dekker G, Kupferminc M. Pre-eclampsia. Lancet 2005;365:785–99.

112. Magee LA, Cham C, Waterman EJ, Ohlsson A, Von Dadelszen P. Hydralazine for treatment of severe hypertension in pregnancy: meta-analysis. BMJ 2003; 327:1–10.

113. Duley L, Henderson-Smart DJ, Meher S, King JF. Antiplatelet agents for preventing pre-eclampsia and its complications. Cochrane Database Syst Rev 2007 (2):CD004659.

114. Nicholson W, Bolen S, Whitkob CT, Neale D, Wilson L, Bass E. Benefits and risks of oral diabetes agents compared with insulin in women with gestational diabetes. Obstet Gynecol 2009;113:193–205.

115. Langer O, Conway DL, Berkus MD. A comparison of glyburide and insulin in women with gestational diabetes mellitus. N Engl J Med 2000;343:1134–8.

116. Ahmadi S, Powell FC. Pruritic urticarial papules and plaques of pregnancy: current status. Australas J Dermatol 2005;46:53–60.

117. Brzoza Z, Kasperska-Zajac A, Oles E, Rogala B. Pruritic urticarial papules and plaques of pregnancy. J Midwifery Womens Health 2007;52:44–8.

118. Bruce K, Watson S. Management of intrahepatic cholestasis of pregnancy: a case report. J Midwifery Womens Health 2007;52:67–72.

119. Beuers U. Drug insight: mechanisms and sites of action in ursodeoxycholic acid in cholestasis. Nat Clin Pract Gastroenterol Hepatol 2006;3:318–28.

120. Glantz A, Marschall H-U, Lammert F, Mattsson L-A. Intrahepatic cholestasis of pregnancy: a randomized controlled trial comparing dexamethasone and ursodeoxycholic acid. Hepatology 2005;42: 1399–405.

121. Kondrackiene J, Beuers U, Kupcinskas L. Efficacy and safety of ursodeoxycholic acid versus cholestyramine in intrahepatic cholestasis of pregnancy. Gastroenterology 2005;129:894–901.

122. Diac M, Kenyon A, Nelson-Piercy C, Girling J, Cheng F, Tribe RM, et al. Dexamethasone in the treatment of obstetric cholestasis: a case series. J Obstet Gynecol 2006;26:110–4.

123. Ginsburg JS, Bates SM. Management of venous thromboembolism during pregnancy. J Thromb Haemost 2003;1:1435–42.

124. Laurent P, Dussarat G, Bonal J, Jego C, Talard P, Bouchiat C, et al. Low molecular weight heparins: a guide to their optimal use in pregnancy. Drugs 2002; 62:463–77.

125. Harnett MJ, Walsh ME, McElrath TF, Tsen LC. The use of central neuraxial techniques in parturients with Factor V Leiden mutation. Anesth Analg 2005; 101:1821–3.

126. Greer IA. Anticoagulants in pregnancy. J Thromb Thrombolysis 2006;21:57–65.

127. Moore KL, Persaud TVN. The developing human: clinically oriented embryology, 8th ed. Philadelphia, PA: Elsevier, 2007.

> *"I understood once I held a baby in my arms, why some people have the need to keep having them."*
>
> SPAULDING GRAY

> *"Anyone who thinks women are the weaker sex never witnessed childbirth."*
>
> ANONYMOUS

36
Labor

Nancy K. Lowe and Tekoa L. King

✦ Chapter Glossary

Actin Double helix protein strand that provides the scaffold to which myosin binds to create muscle contraction.

Active phase of labor The period of the first stage of labor of maximal rate of cervical dilatation. Usually between 3–5 cm and approximately 8–9 cm.

Beta-sympathomimetics Drugs that mimic the effects of catecholamines such as epinephrine or norepinephrine. Also called beta agonists. The drug in this class used to treat preterm labor is terbutaline.

Cervical ripening Process by which the cervix softens via the breakdown of collagen fibrils. Ripening is the first step in the process of cervical effacement and dilatation.

Corticotrophin-releasing hormone (CRH) Hormone synthesized by the placenta, decidua, amnion, and myometrium. CRH plays a role in both maintaining uterine quiescence during pregnancy and in determining the time of onset of labor.

First stage of labor The period of labor between the onset of regular painful contractions and when the cervix is fully dilated or 10 cm.

Intrathecal A synonym for intraspinal. The intrathecal space is the space in the spinal cord where the spinal fluid resides.

Latent phase of labor The period of time between the initial onset of painful uterine contractions and the phase of rapid cervical dilatation. The latent phase of labor is usually over when the cervix is between 3 and 5 cm, but the precise cervical dilatation is variable. The length of the latent phase of labor is also more variable in timing in that it can last a few hours or several hours.

Myosin The primary contractile protein in muscle. Made of two heavy chains, two light chains, and a globular head that protrudes from the filament. The myosin head binds to actin, which forms a cross-bridge and structural change that results in shortening or muscle contraction.

Myosin light-chain kinase (MLCK) A kinase is an enzyme that modifies a protein by adding a phosphate group to the protein. Myosin light-chain kinase (MLCK) phosphorylates the myosin light chain, which converts myosin from an active to an inactive state. MLCK is able to make this structural change to myosin only after forming a bond with calmodulin. In turn, the MLCK-calmodulin complex occurs when intracellular calcium is present.

Oxytocin Peptide hormone that is made in the hypothalamus and released by the pituitary. Oxytocin has many functions, one of which is to produce an increase in intracellular calcium in myometrial cells, which initiates muscle contraction during labor.

Parturition The process of expelling a newborn and placenta from the uterus into the vagina and out of the body. Commonly referred to as labor and delivery or childbirth.

Prodromal labor A prolonged latent phase of labor wherein contractions are regular and painful but not associated with cervical dilatation. A latent phase of labor that is > 20 hours in a primigravida is considered prolonged, and one that is > 14 hours is considered prolonged in a multigravida.

Second stage of labor Interval between complete dilatation of the cervix and birth of the infant. Characterized by maternal pushing efforts and descent of the fetus in the birth canal.

Third stage of labor Period of time from delivery of infant to delivery of placenta.

Tocolytics Drugs used to suppress or inhibit premature labor. From Greek word *tocos*, which means "for childbirth," and *lytic*, which means "capable of dissolving."

Transition phase of labor A period during labor wherein the cervix does not dilate as quickly as it does earlier in the active phase. Usually occurring when the cervix is dilated between 8 and 10 cm, this is the time when the fetus internally rotates and begins to descend. Although the term is often used and is also called a deceleration phase, there is controversy about whether a deceleration phase actually exists and further controversy about what cervical dilatation is present when it occurs, if it does exist.

Introduction

The focus of this chapter is on drugs that may be indicated for use during labor, with the exception of those used to treat anxiety or nausea. The majority of the drugs discussed are those used to induce and/or stimulate labor and others required for the prevention or treatment of common complications of childbirth. Therefore, an understanding of the physiology of uterine function during labor and birth is required for safe prescribing of these medications.

Parturition Physiology Overview

Biologically, **parturition** is the process of producing offspring and includes all of its attendant physiologic mechanisms, particularly those that lead to the eventual expulsion of the fetus from the mother. Although virtually all maternal organ systems are involved in the physiology of reproduction, the primary focus of parturition physiology is the uterus as the environment that supports fetal development and sustenance, and the organ responsible for fetal expulsion. The uterus is a remarkable organ that has the ability to accommodate itself to the presence of the growing fetus through growth and myometrial quiescence and to expel the fetus on cue through the processes of labor and birth.

The uterine phases of parturition are designated as Phase 0 through Phase 3 and conceptually illustrated in Figure 36-1.[1] The majority of pregnancy, designated as parturition Phase 0, is characterized by extensive uterine growth and inhibition of myometrial activity through the actions of a host of endogenous substances including progesterone, prostacyclin (PGI$_2$), relaxin, parathyroid hormone-related peptide (PTHrP), and nitric oxide. Generally, these substances inhibit myometrial contraction by inhibiting calcium (Ca^{2+}) release from intracellular stores or reducing **myosin light-chain kinase** (MLCK) activity. During Phase 0, the cervix normally remains rigid and unyielding.[2]

During Phase 1 of parturition, the myometrium is activated in preparation for labor and birth, and the uterine cervix softens to allow eventual dilatation and fetal passage. Myometrial activation occurs through the synthesis of a group of contraction-associated proteins (CAPs) that act within the uterus to enable the myometrium to exert strong, synchronous contractions.[3] CAPs are one of three types: (1) those that facilitate the interaction between **actin** and **myosin** molecules in the myocyte to cause myometrial contraction, (2) those that lower the depolarization threshold of myocytes to increase the excitability of the myometrium (e.g., oxytocin and prostaglandin-F receptors), and (3) those that provide the intercellular

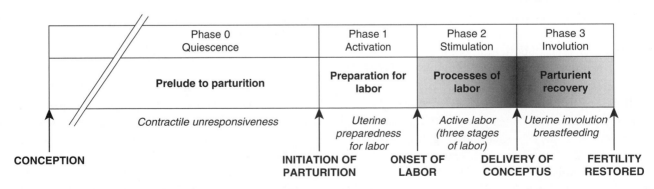

		Phase 0 Quiescence	Phase 1 Activation	Phase 2 Stimulation	Phase 3 Involution
		Prelude to parturition	**Preparation for labor**	**Processes of labor**	**Parturient recovery**
		Contractile unresponsiveness	*Uterine preparedness for labor*	*Active labor (three stages of labor)*	*Uterine involution breastfeeding*
CONCEPTION			**INITIATION OF PARTURITION**	**ONSET OF LABOR**	**DELIVERY OF CONCEPTUS**	**FERTILITY RESTORED**

Figure 36-1 Uterine phases of parturition. *Source:* Reprinted with permission from Cunningham FG et al. 2007.[41]

connectivity of myocytes necessary for synchronous uterine contractions (e.g., gap junctions created by multimers of connexin-43).[3,4]

Phase 2 of parturition (corresponding to the clinical stages of labor) is the stimulation phase characterized by synchronous and progressively more intense uterine contractions that effect cervical effacement and dilatation, fetal descent, and, in concert with the active bearing down efforts of the mother, eventual birth of the fetus and placenta.[2] These strong, myometrial contractions are stimulated by endogenous uterotonins such as prostaglandins and oxytocin.

Finally, parturition Phase 3 is the period of postpartum uterine involution characterized by tonic uterine contractions influenced by neuroendocrine-released **oxytocin** in response to suckling of the infant at the mother's breast. As described by Young,[5] these uterine phases occur over months (Phase 0), to days (Phase 1 involving up-regulation of the contractile proteins), to hours (Phase 2, the process of labor and birth), to minutes (Phase 3 with the transition from phasic to tonic contraction).

Mechanisms of Initiation and Progression of Labor

The precise trigger that causes the onset of progressive labor remains elusive. Although many maternal and fetal mechanisms have been identified in various animal models and are believed to have some relevance to the events of human parturition, considerable research is needed to integrate the rapidly expanding knowledge into a complete picture of the fetal and maternal roles in the initiation of human labor.[6] As expressed by Smith, investigations into the mechanisms of human parturition have led to the realization that "human parturition is a distinctly human event."[3, p. 271] In humans, the timing of birth is most closely associated with placental expression of the gene for **corticotrophin-releasing hormone** (CRH) production, suggesting a placental clock as the determining factor. Current understanding suggests that powerful positive feed-forward systems in both mother and fetus stimulate a progressively and rapidly increasing rate of placenta CRH production in late gestation.[3]

In their review of fetal signals and the mechanisms of parturition, Challis and colleagues conclude that human birth "involves a series of amplifying, positive feed-forward cascades involving cytokines, prostaglandins and steroid modulator hormones."[4, p. 492] The key feature of the progression from Phase 0 to Phase 1 of parturition is myometrial activation. This activation process is most likely precipitated by interactions of the fetal genome with maternal tissue, including increased CRH production through (1) a growth pathway stimulating activation through uterine stretch, and (2) an endocrine/paracrine pathway characterized by increasing fetal-hypothalamic-pituitary-adrenal (HPA) axis activity and production of fetal cortisol.[2] Increased placental production of CRH drives increased fetal cortisol production, fetal pulmonary maturation, proinflammatory amniotic fluid proteins and phospholipids, and myometrial receptor expression. Placental CRH also drives progressive increases in maternal cortisol production and estrogen synthesis via corticotrophin stimulation of the maternal adrenals. Both fetal and maternal cortisol stimulate continued increase in placental CRH production. As labor nears, local myometrial CRH receptors change from a form favoring relaxation to a form favoring a contractile pathway. These factors combine through a number of independent activating pathways to precipitate labor and birth in a robust fashion.[3]

Physiology of Cervical Ripening and Dilatation

Fibrous connective tissue dominates in the cervix and is composed of an extracellular matrix (collagen, elastin, and proteoglycans) and a cellular portion (smooth muscle and fibroblasts, epithelium, and blood vessels).[7] **Cervical ripening** or softening occurs during the final 3–4 weeks of pregnancy in response to local and hormonal agents that create a bioactive catabolic environment causing extensive remodeling of the extracellular matrix.[2,8]

Although the precise biochemical mechanisms are not completely understood, cervical ripening is characterized by the breakdown of collagen fibrils, an increase in collagen solubility, and increased quantities of glycosaminoglycans binding large amounts of water. Ripening begins the process of cervical effacement and dilatation so that, on average, the cervix is approximately 50% effaced and 2 centimeters dilated at the onset of labor, although wide individual differences are observed clinically. When labor commences, a sharp rise in cervical concentration of hyaluronic acid causes the tissue to swell and the cervix to become more distensible. The cervical collagen framework weakens further, allowing the progressive passive dilatation of the cervix.[8] Dilatation primarily occurs in response to pressure exerted by the fetal presenting part during uterine contractions. As the cervix continues to efface during labor, the internal os is taken up laterally, becoming indistinguishable from the lower uterine segment, a phenomenon that suggests the internal os may be the location of maximal cervical softening.

Physiology of Uterine Activity

The uterus is truly a remarkable visceral smooth muscle organ, since it exhibits tone and phasic contractions, both without significant nerve control. Similar to other smooth muscle, the myometrium can exert substantial force with relatively little energy expenditure, generate force in any direction within the cell, and exhibit significantly greater shortening than striated skeletal muscle. Uterine growth, initially due to myometrial hyperplasia, primarily results from extensive and remarkable myometrial hypertrophy in response to hormonal (progesterone and estrogen) and mechanical influences. This hypertrophy is associated with increases in oxytocin receptor proteins and the number of myocytes expressing oxytocin receptors as gestation advances toward term.[5,9]

Control of Myometrial Activity

Although uterine muscle agonists such as oxytocin and prostaglandins are powerful modulators of uterine contraction, uterine smooth muscle is myogenic and able to contract without nervous or hormonal input.[10] The uterine source of the phasic contractions characteristic of labor remains unidentified. Potential mechanisms that initiate and propagate uterine contractions include (1) specialized myometrial cells within a heterogeneous population of smooth muscle cells acting as pacemakers, (2) specialized interstitial cells acting as electrical pacemakers similar to Cajal cells in the gastrointestinal tract, (3) an electrical syncytium created by gap junctions that link myocyte to myocyte, (4) a metabolic syncytium allowing a group of cells to act as a local pacemaker, and (5) a hydrodynamic stretch activation mechanism that facilitates organ-level communication and myocyte recruitment to create a coordinated uterine contraction.[5]

Mechanisms of Myometrial Contraction

Uterine contraction is structurally dependent upon the interaction between actin and myosin that is regulated by the calcium-sensitive enzyme MLCK.[11] Actin is a polymerized double-helical strand comprising the thin filaments. Myosin comprises the thick filaments of smooth muscle and is a hexamer of two heavy chain subunits ($\sim$ 200 kDa) and two pairs each of 20- and 17-kDa light chains molecularly arranged as a double helix tail (two spirally wrapped heavy chains) with a double head at one end (two light chains to each free head). Depolarization of the myometrial cell membrane opens the voltage-sensitive calcium channels allowing calcium ion influx and the release of calcium ions from sarcoplasmic reticulum stores within the cell.[10] The binding of intracellular calcium to calmodulin forms a calcium-calmodulin complex that activates the essential enzyme MLCK, which in turn phosphorylates the regulatory myosin light chains to initiate binding with actin. The functional structural complex actinomycin converts the chemical energy of adenosine triphosphate (ATP) into the mechanical energy of contraction[11] (Figure 36-2). From an organ-level perspective, uterine contractions of labor are characterized by a descending propagation of the contractile wave from the uterine fundus toward the lower uterine segment, and a longer duration and greater strength of contraction in the fundus. These characteristics serve to push the fetus toward the cervix creating the mechanical force of cervical effacement and dilatation, and, in combination with maternal efforts, eventual birth.

Clinically, labor is divided into three stages. The **first stage of labor** is the time from the onset of regular, painful contractions to complete cervical dilatation. This stage is often subdivided into the **latent phase of labor**, **active phase of labor**, and deceleration or **transition phase of labor**. The **second stage of labor** commences when the cervix is fully dilated and ends with the birth of the infant. The **third stage of labor** starts at birth and ends when the placenta is delivered.

The remainder of this chapter reviews drugs used to treat common complications of parturition and those used for prophylactic purposes. These include drugs used to inhibit uterine contractions; facilitate cervical ripening and simulate uterine contractions for induction and augmentation of labor; and treat intrapartum infection, preeclampsia, eclampsia, and acute postpartum hemorrhage. In addition, prophylactic management of group B *Streptococcus* (GBS), infective endocarditis, human immunodeficiency virus, and threatened preterm birth are reviewed.

Preterm Labor Tocolytics

The diagnosis of preterm labor is one of the most challenging clinical problems in the care of pregnant women, although its potential endpoint, preterm birth (any birth before 37 completed weeks from the first day of the last menstrual period), is more precisely defined.[12,13] Preterm birth is the single most important contributor to infant morbidity and mortality.[14,15] In 2004, 36.5% of all infant deaths were due to preterm-related causes,[15] and in 2006, 12.8% of all live-born infants in the United States were

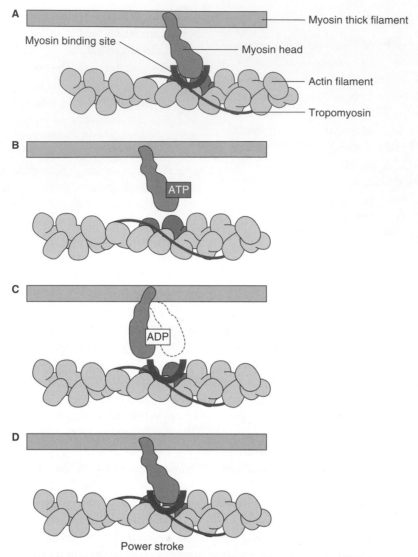

(A) Attached: At the start of the cycle, the myosin head is attached to the myosin binding site on the actin filament. **(B) Recharging:** A molecule of ATP binds to a large cleft at the back of the myosin head which causes a slight change in the conformation of the myosin binding site which reduces the affinity the myosin head has for the myosin binding site. **(C) Cocked:** The cleft on the myosin head closes around the ATP, which causes a large shape change so that the head is displaced along the actin filament by a distance of approximately 5 nm. **(D) Force-generating:** As ATP is hydrolyzed to ADP, the myosin head once again binds tightly to the next myosin binding site on the actin filament and in this process the myosin head essentially ratchets along the actin filament, creating the muscle contraction.

Figure 36-2 Uterine muscle contraction.

preterm with the highest rates seen in non-Hispanic Black infants (18.4%).[16] Although multiple gestations are associated with a significantly higher risk of preterm birth, 10.8% of all live-born singleton infants were preterm in 2004.[17] The American College of Obstetricians and Gynecologists (ACOG) estimates that preterm labor precedes 40–50% of preterm births and that preterm labor is the most common cause of hospitalization during pregnancy.[18]

Unfortunately, other than historic risk factors such as previous preterm birth, there are no methods of effectively screening the general obstetric population for risk of preterm birth. In those women at historic high risk, ultrasonographic assessment of cervical length, fetal fibronectin (fFN) testing, or a combination of these may help to determine those women at high risk for preterm labor.[19,20] In both high-risk women and women experiencing symptoms of preterm labor, the clinical usefulness of data obtained from these assessments is primarily in terms of their negative predictive value.

The complex etiology of preterm labor and birth is reflected in its epidemiologic risk factors, which include multiple gestation, history of preterm birth, bleeding in the second trimester of pregnancy, genitourinary tract infection, African American race, young maternal age (< 18 years), low maternal body mass index, cigarette smoking, and frequent contractions during the current pregnancy.[12] The pathogenic pathways have been summarized as activation of the maternal/fetal hypothalamus-pituitary axis (HPA), inflammation, decidual hemorrhage, and pathologic uterine distention resulting in preterm rupture of the membranes, preterm labor, or both. ACOG defines preterm labor as "regular contractions that occur before 37 weeks of gestation and are associated with changes in the cervix."[18] More precisely and as traditionally defined, preterm births are those that occur between 20 weeks and 36⁶/₇ weeks' gestation.[12] Common maternal signs and symptoms include pelvic pressure, increased vaginal discharge, backache, menstrual-like cramps, and painful or painless contractions that are persistent.[12]

Prevention of preterm labor has been an elusive goal. At this time it is recommended that women with a singleton pregnancy who have a history of preterm birth or preterm premature rupture of membranes in a prior pregnancy be offered progesterone therapy at the beginning of the second trimester. Progesterone is available as a 100-mg vaginal suppository or a 200-mg micronized progesterone vaginal gel. Randomized trials using 250 mg of 17α-hydroxy-progesterone caproate administered intramuscularly once a week found a decrease in the preterm delivery in this population of women who have a high risk of recurrent preterm birth. This formulation is not available commercially but can be made by a compounding pharmacy. Although progesterone therapy is recommended by ACOG, none of these formulations has been FDA approved for this indication.

Tocolysis is the use of drugs to inhibit myometrial contractions[21] (Box 36-1). Once the diagnosis of preterm labor has been made, the advisability of prolonging the pregnancy has been evaluated, and the decision to attempt to stop preterm labor contractions by drug therapy has been made, the provider can choose one of several **tocolytics**. Tocolytics include beta-sympathomimetic drugs, calcium channel blockers, prostaglandin or cyclooxygenase inhibitors, and magnesium sulfate. Specific therapeutic regimens are described in Table 36-1 and illustrated in Figure 36-3. Contraindications to tocolysis are listed in Table 36-2. The reader is referred to the excellent discussion by Iams and Romero of full clinical protocols for the various tocolytic options.[13]

Box 36-1   Gone But Not Forgotten: Pharmacologic Use of Alcohol as a Tocolytic

In the 1970s, alcohol was a commonly accepted treatment to inhibit labor. Women at term who were having prodromal labor or simply frequent Braxton-Hicks contractions often were referred to a bar close to the hospital for a therapeutic drink in order to relax. The assumption was that, like morphine, alcohol would either cause uterine quiescence or labor would continue in a more effective pattern.

For women with symptoms of preterm labor that included early or advanced cervical dilatation, alcohol was as a tocolytic of note. It was stated that alcohol inhibited release of endogenous oxytocin and also promoted myometrium relaxation. In addition, it was reported that alcohol use was as effective as beta-adrenergic drugs and/or NSAIDs.[99] When used as a tocolytic for preterm labor, alcohol was administered intravenously. Women experienced similar effects to oral ingestion including intoxication and potential alcohol poisoning followed by hangovers when it was discontinued. Managing the care of an inebriated pregnant woman presented major challenges to hospital units, sometimes requiring the woman to be restrained in bed even while she experienced alcohol-induced hallucinations and projectile vomiting. Overall, the use of alcohol as a tocolytic was a less-than-satisfying method for women and providers alike. Alcohol also was found to be associated with aspiration pneumonia because of effects of alcohol on the gastric mucosa.[100] However, there were no reported cases of fetal alcohol syndrome (FAS) associated with use of the agent for inhibition of term or preterm labor.

With the growing public health campaign about alcohol abstinence to avoid FAS, it became confusing and difficult to advocate for the use of an agent with known intrapartum complications and for which other options existed. Alcohol as a tocolytic fell into disuse, and today most women would be astounded if their providers even suggested a glass of wine as treatment of prodromal labor.

Table 36-1 Tocolytic Treatment of Preterm Labor

Drug Generic (Brand)	Dose	Maternal Side Effects	Fetal Side Effects	Contraindications
Beta-Sympathomimetics				
Terbutaline* (Brethine)	Single subcutaneous injection of 0.25 mg (May consider repeating every 1 to 6 hours if maternal heart rate < 130 beats per minute)	Cardiovascular: flushing, tachycardia, palpitations, hypotension, arrhythmia, chest pain, myocardial ischemia, shortness of breath, pulmonary edema, adult respiratory distress syndrome Metabolic: hyperglycemia, hypokalemia Nervousness, nausea, or vomiting	Tachycardia, hyperinsulinemia Fetal hyperglycemia, neonatal hypoglycemia, hypocalcemia, hypotension Ileus	Known or suspected cardiac disease, hyperthyroidism, diabetes mellitus, or convulsive disorders.
Calcium Channel Blockers				
Nifedipine (Procardia)	Loading dose: 30 mg orally; or 10 mg orally, repeated every 20 minutes if contractions persist up to 3 doses (30 mg) Then 10–20 mg orally every 4–6 hours	Transient hypotension, tachycardia, headache, flushing, dizziness, nausea, palpitations, edema	None known	Cardiovascular disease or hemodynamic instability. Do not combine with beta-sympathomimetic drugs.
Prostaglandin or Cyclooxygenase (COX) Inhibitors				
Indomethacin	Loading dose: 50 mg orally or 50–100 mg by rectal suppository Then 25–50 mg orally every 6 hours, for 48–72 hours	Gastritis, nausea, proctitis with hematochezia, impairment of renal function, increased postpartum hemorrhage, hypertension	Oligohydramnios, premature constriction of ductus arteriosus, necrotizing enterocolitis, intraventricular hemorrhage	Gestation ≥ 32 weeks. Presence of fetal growth restriction or oligohydramnios. History of asthma, urticaria, or allergic-type reactions to aspirin or other nonsteroidal anti-inflammatory drugs.
Magnesium Sulfate				
Magnesium sulfate	Loading dose: 4–6 g intravenously over 30 minutes Then 1–4 g per hour by continuous intravenous infusion titrated beginning at 2 g per hour and increasing by 1 g per hour up to 4 g until tocolysis achieved	Flushing, nausea and vomiting, diplopia, blurred vision, headache, lethargy, ileus, hypocalcemia, muscle weakness, pulmonary edema, cardiac arrest	Hypotonia, lethargy, bone demineralization	Poor renal function.

* Terbutaline is the only tocolytic that can be administered subcutaneously.
Sources: Adapted from Iams JD et al. 2004[12]; Iams JD et al. 2007[13]; ACOG 2003[18]; Ables AZ et al. 2005.[26]

The primary goals of tocolytic therapy are to arrest labor and delay birth long enough to initiate prophylactic corticosteroid therapy when indicated for stimulation of fetal lung maturity (discussed later in this chapter) and arrange for maternal/fetal transport to a perinatal tertiary care hospital if indicated. Admittedly, the use of currently available tocolytics remains controversial because, overall, these drugs have not been successful in improving perinatal outcomes.[22] The primary problem may be that tocolytics only attempt to stop the uterus from contracting rather than treating the specific cause of the preterm labor.[21]

Beta-Sympathomimetics

Beta-sympathomimetics have been prescribed widely for the treatment of preterm labor for more than 30 years and were once the most frequently used tocolytic agents.[12] Beta$_2$-adrenoreceptor agonist tocolytics, commonly called beta agonists, such as ritodrine (Yutopar) and terbutaline (Brethine), produce smooth muscle relaxation by increasing intracellular production of cyclic adenosine monophosphate (cAMP) resulting in inactivation of MLCK, thereby inhibiting the interaction of actin and myosin.[11,21,23] The first and only drug approved by the US Food and Drug

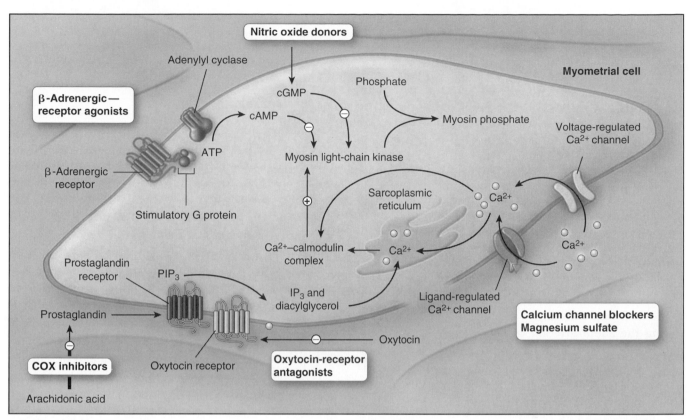

COX = cyclooxygenase; PIP$_3$ = phosphatidylinositol triphosphate; IP$_3$ = inositol triphosphate; cAMP = cyclic AMP; gAMP = cyclic guanosine monophosphate.

Figure 36-3 Sites of action of commonly used tocolytic drugs. *Source:* Reprinted with permission from Simhan HN et al. 2007.[21]

Table 36-2 Contraindications to Tocolysis

Maternal	Fetal
Abruption	Chorioamnionitis
Cardiac disease	Gestational age > 36 6/7 weeks
Chorioamnionitis	Intrauterine fetal demise
Hemorrhage	Intrauterine fetal growth restriction
Intolerant to tocolytics	Lethal anomaly
Pulmonary hypertension	
Severe preeclampsia	

Administration (FDA) for tocolysis was ritodrine in 1980.[21] Ritodrine was withdrawn from the market in 1998 and is not available in the United States today.

In 1998, the FDA issued an advisory regarding the subcutaneous infusion of terbutaline, warning that its effectiveness and safety had not been established and alerting practitioners that "the continuous administration of subcutaneous terbutaline sulfate has not been demonstrated to be effective and is potentially dangerous."[24] Since this advisory was issued, the use of terbutaline as a tocolytic has waned in the United States and often is limited to single-dose therapy for the initiation of acute tocolysis. However, others support the usefulness of terbutaline as both an acute and maintenance tocolytic.[23] It also is commonly used as part of intrauterine fetal rescue and resuscitation in the event of uterine tetany during labor and to promote uterine quiescence during external fetal version procedures.

As described in Table 36-1, maternal and fetal cardiovascular and metabolic physiology can be dramatically affected by terbutaline due to the ubiquitous nature of the beta-adrenergic receptor, cross-reactivity of β_1 and β_2 receptors, and the free passage of the drug across the placenta resulting in fetal serum concentrations equivalent to maternal concentrations.[23,25] Peak serum concentration is reached in 20–30 minutes after subcutaneous injection, and the serum half-life is estimated at 3 hours. These estimates have not been evaluated in pregnant women.

Calcium Channel Blockers

Calcium channel blockers promote uterine relaxation by decreasing the influx of calcium ions into myometrial cells through the voltage-dependent calcium channels and the release of intracellular calcium to inhibit MLCK activity and hence myometrial contraction.[12,21] Because these drugs are nonspecific, the same effect is seen in cardiac, vascular, and nonvascular smooth muscle. Nifedipine (Procardia) has been most widely studied as a tocolytic agent and has less effect on the cardiac conduction apparatus than older drugs such as verapamil (Isoptin, Covera-HS).[26] Nifedipine has an onset of action of less than 20 minutes administered orally and 1–5 minutes administered sublingually with a half-life of approximately 1.3 hours.[27] A review of the safety of these drugs as tocolytics concluded that they should not be combined with intravenously administered beta agonists due to an increased risk of pulmonary edema, and should not be used in the presence of maternal cardiovascular compromise or multiple gestations. Blood pressure should be monitored frequently for the development of hypotension during the administration of immediate-release tablets, and women should be cautioned not to chew these tablets.[28] Lyell et al. have suggested that intravenously hydrating women with 500 mL of lactated Ringer's solution prior to nifedipine administration may ameliorate the risk of significant hypotension.[29]

Prostaglandin or Cyclooxygenase (COX) inhibitors

Cyclooxygenase (COX) is an enzyme responsible for the formation of specific prostaglandins. There are several isoforms of cyclooxygenase. COX-1 and COX-2 are enzymes necessary for the biosynthesis of prostaglandins critical in parturition. The nonspecific COX inhibitor indomethacin (Indocin), a nonsteroidal anti-inflammatory drug (NSAID), is the most commonly used tocolytic in this drug class and has been the subject of a number of small clinical trials. Indomethacin inhibits uterine contractions by reducing the synthesis of prostaglandins.[12] As noted by Iams and Romero, a Cochrane review found that compared to placebo, indomethacin (Indocin) produced a reduction in birth at < 37 weeks' gestation, increased birth weight, and increased gestational age.[13] However, authors of another review found insufficient evidence to support the safety of indomethacin tocolysis in relation to neonatal outcomes.[29] The potential for serious adverse fetal effects such as constriction of the ductus arteriosus, neonatal pulmonary hypertension, intraventricular hemorrhage, and oligohydramnios have led to recommendations that indomethacin tocolysis be limited after 32 weeks' gestation and be avoided in growth-restricted fetuses or in the presence of oligohydramnios.[30] It does not appear that the use of indomethacin tocolysis at less than 34 weeks' gestation

increases the risk of adverse neonatal outcomes.[29] Peak serum levels of indomethacin are reached within 2 hours of administration with a mean half-life of approximately 4.5 hours.[31]

Magnesium Sulfate

Magnesium sulfate is currently the most popular tocolytic in the United States. It is theorized to inhibit myometrial contractility by hyperpolarizing the plasma membrane and competing with intracellular calcium to inhibit MLCK activity,[21] although its precise mechanism of action as a tocolytic is unknown.[12] Despite the popularity of magnesium sulfate as a tocolytic in the United States, authors of a Cochrane systematic review concluded that the agent is ineffective in either delaying or preventing preterm birth, provides no benefit to the fetus or neonate, and is associated with more pediatric mortality.[32] In addition, magnesium sulfate is associated with a significantly increased profile of maternal morbidity due to physiologically distressing and potentially serious side effects as presented in Table 36-1.[29] There is increasing support for discontinuing the use of magnesium sulfate as a tocolytic agent.[21,32]

The role for antenatal magnesium sulfate therapy as a neuroprotective agent that works to prevent cerebral palsy in the preterm fetus also has been explored.[33] Animal studies have suggested that magnesium reduces ischemia-induced cellular injury in the fetal brain and also reduces neurologic morbidities. Several randomized clinical trials that were specifically designed to assess the neuroprotective effects of magnesium sulfate have been conducted to date, and the Cochrane collaboration has published a meta-analysis.[34] This body of research has found that magnesium sulfate does reduce the incidence of cerebral palsy and does not increase the risk of death in preterm infants less than 32 weeks who survive.[34] However, the clinical significance of these findings, which were statistically significant, is controversial. Magnesium sulfate is also associated with an increased risk of death in preterm infants. Thus, it is unclear if the neuroprotective effect for surviving infants is well balanced against the increased risk of death in other preterm infants. At the time of this writing, use of magnesium sulfate for neuroprotection is not universally recommended.

Because magnesium is exclusively excreted by the kidneys, adequate renal function (urine output ≥ 100 mL per hour) is essential for safe administration. Acute magnesium toxicity is evidenced by a sudden decline in blood pressure and respiratory paralysis. Frequent monitoring of maternal respiratory effort and patellar deep tendon reflexes is essential for the early recognition of overdose. In the event of respiratory arrest, 10–20 mL of a 5% solution of calcium gluconate is an effective antidote.

Efficacy of Tocolytics

As summarized by Iams and Romero,[13] meta-analyses of the effects of tocolytic agents indicate that delivery can be delayed by an average of 2–7 days with use of calcium channel blockers and for up to 48 hours with beta-sympathomimetics. Calcium channel blockers have the most favorable risk-to-benefit ratio. Further, there is insufficient evidence that the effectiveness of COX inhibitors and magnesium sulfate is ineffective in delaying delivery.

Although the oxytocin antagonist atosiban has a similar effectiveness profile as calcium channel blockers, the FDA has not approved the drug for use in the United States. The goals of tocolytic therapy are to provide time for maternal transport if needed, and for GBS and steroid prophylaxis. Tocolytic therapy is discontinued when contractions have ceased or occur less frequently than four per hour without cervical change. There is no evidence that continued tocolysis after acute management prolongs pregnancy or reduces the rate of preterm birth.[13]

Table 36-3 Indications, Contraindications, and Special Considerations* to Induction of Labor

Indications	Contraindications	Clinical Considerations*
Abruptio placentae	Vasa previa or complete placenta previa	One or more previous low-transverse cesarean deliveries
Chorioamnionitis	Transverse fetal lie	Breech presentation
Fetal demise	Umbilical cord prolapse	Maternal heart disease
Pregnancy-induced hypertension	Previous transfundal uterine surgery (classical uterine incision)	Multifetal pregnancy
Premature rupture of membranes	Active genital herpes infection	Polyhydramnios
Postterm pregnancy		Presenting part above the pelvic inlet
Maternal medical conditions		Severe hypertension
Fetal compromise (e.g., severe fetal growth restriction, isoimmunization)		Abnormal fetal heart rate patterns not necessitating emergent delivery
Preeclampsia, eclampsia		

* These situations are not absolute contraindications to induction but are clinical situations requiring special attention and vigilance.
Sources: Adapted from ACOG 1999[38]; Battista LR et al. 2007.[36]

Induction and Augmentation of Labor

Induction of labor is the medical procedure of artificially stimulating the uterus to contract in a rhythmic manner prior to the onset of spontaneous labor with the goal of a vaginal birth.[34] Induction of labor is one of the fastest growing medical procedures in the United States, having more than doubled in frequency over the past 2 decades, with increasing evidence that its growth is due to non-medical indications.[35] Particularly, increases in induction for postdate pregnancies (more than 40 completed weeks) in contrast to postterm pregnancies (more than 42 completed weeks) and elective reasons seem to be primary contemporary influences.[35,36] Despite these trends, induction of labor should be considered a therapeutic option only when the benefits of birth outweigh the risks of continuing the pregnancy to mother or fetus and there is no contraindication to vaginal birth.[35,37] Identified medical indications for induction of labor and contraindications to the procedure as identified by ACOG and others are listed in Table 36-3.[35,37,38]

Induction of labor is most problematic for nulliparous women since it is associated with an approximately twofold increased risk of operative birth via cesarean section.[35,39] The risk of iatrogenic prematurity with subsequent significant neonatal complications such as respiratory distress syndrome mandate that the gestational age is rigorously evaluated and documented prior to the decision to attempt labor induction.[35] Further, Wahl[40] has hypothesized that exogenous oxytocin administered during labor induction may be linked to the later development of autism in children. Although this hypothesis requires rigorous research evaluation, it has support from coincident and molecular perspectives.

Medical induction of labor has two components: (1) cervical ripening and (2) induction of contractions. When induction of labor is indicated, cervical readiness for labor is evaluated by pelvic examination and determination of a Bishop score (Table 36-4).

Prostaglandins for Cervical Ripening

In 1930, two American gynecologists, Kurzok and Lieb, discovered that strips of human uterine muscle would relax when exposed to semen. A few years later, Von Euler identified the active material and named it *prostaglandin*.

Table 36-4 Bishop Score to Determine Cervical Readiness for Labor

Pelvic Evaluation Component	Score*			
	0	1	2	3
Dilatation of cervix (cm)	Closed	1–2	3–4	≥ 5
Effacement of cervix (%)	0–30	40–50	60–70	≥ 80
Station of presenting part†	–3	–2	–1, 0	+1, +2
Cervical consistency	Firm	Medium	Soft	
Position of cervix	Posterior	Midposition	Anterior	

* Score for each of the five components of the cervix are added to obtain the total score.
† Station determined on a –3 to +3 scale.

Prostaglandins are local or paracrine endocrine agents that exert their effect locally and are then metabolized locally. This is an issue pharmacologically because it is hard to make a prostaglandin formulation that works when given orally or systemically. Prostaglandin receptors are always present in myometrial tissue, which is why prostaglandins can be used to induce labor throughout pregnancy, whereas oxytocin is dependent upon the up-regulation of receptors in myometrial tissue just before and during labor in order to exert its uterotonic effects.

For women with an unfavorable cervix (total Bishop score < 6) for whom induction of labor is medically indicated, pharmacologic methods of cervical ripening include administration of synthetic prostaglandin E_1 (misoprostol) or prostaglandin E_2 (dinoprostone) (Table 36-5). These

Table 36-5 Drugs for Induction and/or Augmentation of Labor

Drug Generic (Brand)	Dose and Route	Contraindications and Clinical Considerations
*Cervical Ripening Prostaglandin Agents**		
Dinoprostone; prostaglandin E_2† (Prepidil and Cervidil)	Cervical gel (Prepidil): 0.5 mg (in 2.5 mL syringe) inserted into the endocervix May repeat in 6–12 hours Maximum of three doses (1.5 mg) in 24 hours	Contraindicated if abnormal fetal heart rate pattern. Woman should remain recumbent for 30 minutes to prevent leakage; oxytocin may be initiated ≥ 6 hours after insertion; electronically monitor uterine activity and fetal heart rate prior to and for 2 hours after insertion. Disadvantage is that it cannot be easily removed in the event of uterine hyperstimulation or abnormal fetal heart rate pattern.
	Vaginal insert (Cervidil): 10-mg slow release at 0.3 mg/hour Remains in place until active labor begins or for 12 hours	Oxytocin may be initiated ≥ 30 minutes after insert removal; electronically monitor uterine activity and fetal heart rate prior to and after placement until ≥ 15 minutes after insert removal.
Misoprostol; prostaglandin E_1 (Cytotec)	25–50 mcg intravaginally 100-mcg oral tablet is broken into four 25-mcg pieces or two 50-mcg pieces (alternately a 200-mcg oral tablet is broken into four 50-mcg pieces)	Contraindicated in women with a scarred uterus due to prior cesarean delivery. Oxytocin may be initiated ≥ 4 hours after last dose of misoprostol; electronically monitor uterine activity and fetal heart rate prior to and after placement for 2–4 hours. Disadvantage is that it cannot be easily removed in the event of uterine hyperstimulation or abnormal fetal heart rate pattern.
Induction or Augmentation Agent		
Oxytocin (Pitocin)	10 units in 500–1000 mL of normal saline or lactated Ringer's solution (some use 60 units in 1000 mL or 30 units in 500 mL to simplify arithmetic calculation of dose) *Low-dose regimen:* 0.5–1.0 mU per minute, increased by 1–2 mU per minute at 30- to 60-minute intervals or 1.0–2.0 mU per minute, increased by 1–2 mU per minute at 15- to 30-minute intervals *High-dose regimen:* 6 mU/minute, increased by 6 mU/minute at 15-minute intervals (maximum dose 40 mU per minute)	Administer via infusion pump to provide continuous, precise dose control via piggyback to nonmedicated intravenous infusion line; continuous electronic monitoring of uterine activity and fetal heart rate required; never administer in an electrolyte-free solution. Risk of water intoxication (hyponatremia) due to the antidiuretic effect of oxytocin. Symptoms do not usually appear until the plasma sodium level is < 125 mEq/L. High-dose regimen is a labor augmentation protocol for nulliparous women in spontaneous active labor in the context of 1-to-1 nursing care.

* May also lead to uterine contractions and the induction of labor.
† Dinoprostone preparations are considerably more costly than misoprostol ($75–$150 per dose compared to < $1).

drugs are not contraindicated in the presence of maternal asthma as is prostaglandin $F_{2\alpha}$, which can produce significant bronchospasm.[41] These agents may be used following or in combination with a number of nonpharmacologic mechanical cervical ripening methods such as stripping the fetal membranes during a vaginal examination, hygroscopic endocervical dilators, or placement of a balloon catheter above the internal cervical os.

The most frequent complication of prostaglandin administration is uterine hyperstimulation; hence attentive monitoring of uterine activity and fetal status during administration is essential. It is important to note that only dinoprostone is approved by the FDA for use as a cervical ripening agent, although ACOG acknowledges the apparent safety and effectiveness of misoprostol for this purpose.[37] Since the use of cervical ripening agents is frequently associated with the onset of labor, the distinction between cervical ripening and induction may become blurred and indistinguishable.[36] In women with a favorable Bishop score > 6, most induction methods will stimulate the onset of uterine contractions. Due to the significantly increased risk of uterine rupture in women with a prior cesarean birth, the use of prostaglandins is contraindicated for women planning vaginal birth after cesarean (VBAC).[42]

Oxytocin for Induction of Labor

In 1909, Sir Henry Dale discovered oxytocin as a substance from the posterior pituitary. He named oxytocin using the Greek words *tokos* (to give birth) and *oxus* (which means quick). Fifty years later, the biochemist Vincent du Vigneaud succeeded in synthesizing oxytocin and won the Nobel Prize in Chemistry for the discovery. Today, medical induction of uterine contractions is accomplished via intravenous administration of synthetic oxytocin. Oxytocin causes uterine contractions sufficient for delivery, but it is a poor cervical ripener and therefore best used for induction when the cervix is favorable.

Although there are considerable variations in reports of the biologic half-life of oxytocin, it is now generally agreed that the half-life is between 10 and 12 minutes and that continuous intravenous oxytocin infusion is associated with a linear increase in plasma oxytocin concentration reaching a steady state in about 40 minutes.[43,44]

Oxytocin is a powerful drug that may quickly hyperstimulate the uterus. The most frequent adverse effect of oxytocin, hyperstimulation, or tachysystole, is defined as > 5 uterine contractions in 10 minutes, averaged over a 30-minute period.[45] Uteroplacental perfusion may be compromised in these situations, leading to fetal heart rate decelerations or bradycardia and neonatal acidemia

at birth.[46] Frequent assessment of uterine activity and fetal well-being is required during the administration of oxytocin. Although institutional policies often dictate continuous electronic fetal monitoring (EFM) during oxytocin administration, there are no data to indicate that EFM is essential to adequate ongoing fetal assessment or the monitoring of uterine response.

Oxytocin is administered via an electronic infusion pump to carefully control the titration of oxytocin dose. This intravenous infusion should be connected via a secondary intravenous line that is piggybacked into the primary intravenous line in close proximity to the catheter's entrance into the woman's skin. These measures improve safety by decreasing the amount of oxytocin that will be administered if the infusion must be suddenly discontinued due to hyperstimulation or fetal compromise and protecting the integrity of the primary intravenous line.

Unfortunately, neither the optimal oxytocin administration regimen nor the maximum oxytocin dose has been established through research or agreed-upon expert opinion, although the two most common approaches are a low-dose or a high-dose regimen as presented in Table 36-5 and Table 36-6.[35] Advocates of high-dose oxytocin note that labors tend to be more rapid, and failure of induction less common than with low doses, whereas advocates of low-dose oxytocin regimens point out that hyperstimulation rates and abnormal fetal heart rate patterns are less common, while the progress of labor is similar. In addition to the low-dose versus high-dose oxytocin controversy, other unresolved safety concerns are if the length of time of infusion is related to outcomes, if there is a maximum dose of oxytocin that should not be exceeded, if oxytocin should be administered in a pulsatile rather than continuous infusion to more closely mimic a physiologic pattern, and what the relationship is of epidural anesthesia to the dosing of oxytocin.[47] Despite these questions, institutional standardization of the dilution and

Table 36-6 Oxytocin Protocol—Four Steps to Improving Patient Safety

Step 1—Dilution	10 units of oxytocin in 1000 mL of normal saline (2.5 units of oxytocin in 250 mL of normal saline) Resultant concentration is 10 mU per mL
Step 2—Initial dose	2 mU per minute Infusion 12 mL per hour
Step 3—Incremental increase	Increase by 2 mU per minute (12 mL per hour) every 45 minutes until adequate labor
Step 4—Maximum dose	16 mU per minute (96 mL per hour)

Source: Adapted with permission from Hayes EJ et al. 2008.[44]

dosing regimen for intravenous oxytocin is one important strategy to improve patient safety. Hayes and Weinstein[44] have proposed a four-step approach of dilution, initial dose, incremental increase, and maximum dose for the safe administration of oxytocin presented in Table 36-6.

Because of the antidiuretic properties of oxytocin and the physiologic maternal adaptations to pregnancy and labor, water intoxication, a form of hyponatremia, is one of the most severe adverse effects of oxytocin administration, albeit relatively rare.[48] The risk of this complication can be reduced by administering oxytocin only in isotonic intravenous solutions such as lactated Ringer's solution, avoiding high doses of oxytocin for prolonged periods of time, and limiting large volume boluses of intravenous fluids.[47] In addition, maternal intake and output should be closely monitored.

Central nervous system, gastrointestinal, and musculoskeletal system symptoms of water intoxication usually do not appear until the serum sodium levels fall below 125 mEq/L. Mild symptoms may include apathy, lethargy, headache, nausea and vomiting, muscle cramps, and diminished deep tendon reflexes. More severe symptoms are confusion and disorientation to seizures, coma, tentorial herniation, and death.[48] The clinician must remember that the fetus and/or newborn infant of a woman with hyponatremia also is at significant risk of water intoxication.

Augmentation of Labor with Oxytocin

Pharmacologic augmentation of labor also is accomplished with intravenous synthetic oxytocin administration. Its use has also increased dramatically over the past 20 years with the concomitant increase in the use of epidural analgesia during labor.[49] The most common non-pharmacologic methods of augmentation are amniotomy (surgical rupture of the fetal membranes) and manual or breast-pump–induced nipple stimulation to induce the endogenous release of oxytocin.

Medical augmentation of labor is a decision based on the clinical evaluation of the adequacy of uterine activity to promote cervical dilatation and the pace of cervical dilatation. Dystocia or abnormal labor is commonly categorized as protraction (slower-than-normal progress) or arrest disorders.[50] While the *diagnosis* of dystocia may be iatrogenic in origin, the etiology of true dystocia may be the result of one or more abnormalities of the cervix, uterus, maternal pelvis, or fetus. Although it is beyond the scope of this chapter to review the critical aspects of this important clinical evaluation, the clinician must be cognizant of this fundamental responsibility in the diagnosis and management of dystocia.

Complementary and Alternative Methods Used for Cervical Ripening and Labor Induction

There are several herbs that have putative uterotonic effects, which are used to induce labor. Black cohosh and blue cohosh are reviewed in Chapter 10. Neither blue nor black cohosh has proven benefit. There are case reports of perinatal stroke and myocardial infarction associated with ingestion of black and blue cohosh, and they should be avoided. Black cohosh has not been evaluated scientifically, and therefore, no recommendations about efficacy or safety are available. Homeopathic doses of these agents appear to be safe, but again, there is no proven benefit to date. Red raspberry leaves have been recommended for general uterine tone during labor. Red raspberry leaves have no effect on initiating or augmenting labor but appear to be safe. Evening primrose is the other herb that may be used to induce labor. It has been evaluated in one small retrospective study and does not appear to shorten gestation.

Castor oil is a stimulant laxative that is an FDA Pregnancy Category X drug because it can cause uterine contractions. The purported mechanism of action is irritation of the gastrointestinal tract that subsequently stimulates the uterus to contract; however, there is some evidence that ricinoleic acid, the active component of castor oil, actually enters the systemic circulation and has a direct effect on the uterus, causing coliclike, uncoordinated contractions. Ricinoleic acid can transfer to the fetus and it is theorized to cause meconium passage. In addition, castor oil consistently causes nausea and diarrhea. Thus the lack of proven efficacy in combination with unpleasant side effects and theoretic adverse effects suggest castor oil should not be used.

Chorioamnionitis

Chorioamnionitis (i.e., intra-amniotic infection [IAI], amnionitis, intrapartum infection, amniotic fluid infection) is inflammation or infection of the placenta and of the fetal membranes.[51,52] Chorioamnionitis may be a clinical, histologic, or subclinical diagnosis. Risk factors for clinical IAI are low parity and maternal bacterial vaginosis, and the intrapartum factors of long labor, prolonged rupture of membranes, multiple vaginal examinations during labor, internal fetal monitoring, and long duration of monitoring.[51,53] Clinical IAI occurs in 1–2% and up to 15% of term and preterm births, respectively.[52] Generally an ascending polymicrobial infection, clinical IAI is manifested by maternal fever, maternal or fetal

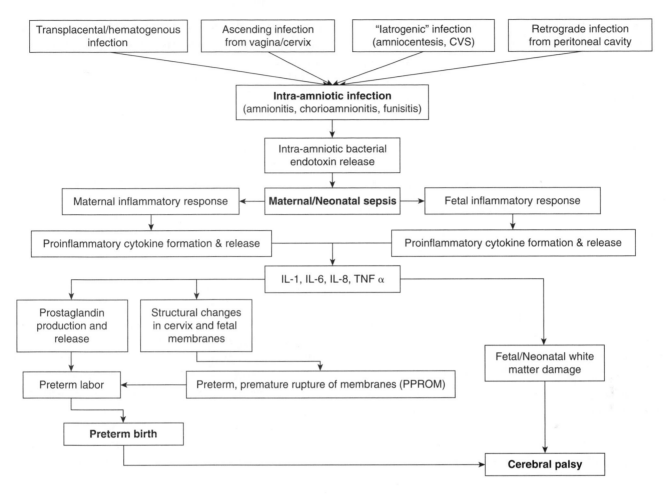

Figure 36-4 Pathogenesis and consequences of intra-amniotic infection. *Source:* Adapted with permission from Fahey JO 2008.[53]

tachycardia, foul smelling amniotic fluid, uterine tenderness, and leukocytosis (> 15,000 with a left shift). Clinical IAI is highly associated with preterm birth before 30 weeks' gestation and preterm premature rupture of the membranes[54] (Figure 36-4). At term, dysfunctional labor, particularly decreased uterine contractility that may be unresponsive to oxytocin augmentation, and an increased incidence of cesarean section are common occurrences following the development of chorioamnionitis. Neonatal risks include a higher incidence of respiratory distress syndrome, intraventricular hemorrhage, and periventricular leukomalacia in preterm infants, and of neonatal sepsis, hypoxic-ischemic encephalopathy, and cerebral palsy in both preterm and term infants.[54]

Clinical IAI is treated with broad-spectrum intravenous antibiotics and efforts to stimulate the progression of labor and eventual birth, although arbitrary time limits are not associated with improved maternal or neonatal outcomes.[51] Antibiotic therapy is designed to cover a wide range of gram-positive and gram-negative organisms that also covers anaerobic and aerobic organisms. Table 36-7 lists common antibiotic regimens that combine a beta-lactam and aminoglycoside for the treatment of clinical IAI. If a cesarean section birth occurs, coverage for anaerobic bacteria such as clindamycin (900 mg intravenously) or metronidazole (15 mg/kg intravenously over 30 to 60 min) should be administered at the time of cord clamping. Although antibiotics may be continued postpartum until the woman is afebrile and asymptomatic for 24 hours, a single postpartum intravenous administration of each drug at its next scheduled dose is equally effective.[55]

Preeclampsia/Eclampsia

Preeclampsia/eclampsia remains a significant concern for maternal morbidity and mortality. Criteria for the diagnosis of preeclampsia include hypertension (blood pressure

Table 36-7 Antibiotic Regimens for the Intrapartum Treatment of Intra-amniotic Infection

Antibiotic	Dose
Combination Therapies:	
Ampicillin (Principin) and gentamicin (Garamycin)	2 g ampicillin every 6 hours and 2 mg/kg loading dose then 1.5 mg/kg every 8 hours gentamicin or single dose of 5.1 g/kg gentamicin once daily
Piperacillin/tazobactam (Zosyn)	3.375 g of piperacillin every 6 hours and 1.5 g of tazobactam every 6 hours
Cefazolin (Ancef) and gentamicin (Garamycin)	1 g cefazolin every 8 hours and 2 mg/kg loading dose then 1.5 mg/kg gentamicin every 8 hours or single dose of 5.1 g/kg gentamicin once daily
Single-Agent Therapies:	
Ampicillin-sulbactam (Unasyn)	3 g every 6 hours
Ticarcillin-clavulanic acid (Timentin)	3.1 g every 6 hours
Cefoxitin (Mefoxitin)	2 g every 8–12 hours
Cefuroxime (Ceftin)	1.5 g every 8 hours
If Penicillin Allergic:	
Vancomycin (Vanocin)	500 mg every 6 hours
Erythromycin (E-mycin)	1 g every 6 hours
Clindamycin (Cleocin)	900 mg every 8 hours
Add One of These Agents if Cesarean Section Performed:	
Clindamycin (Cleocin)	900 mg every 8 hours or single dose 900 mg at cord clamping
Metronidazole (Flagyl)	500 mg every 6 hours

Source: Reprinted with permission from Fahey JO 2008.[53]

Table 36-8 Diagnostic Criteria for Severe Preeclampsia

Once Preeclampsia Is Diagnosed, It Is Considered Severe Preeclampsia if One or More of the Following Criteria Also Is Present:

1. Blood pressure of ≥ 160 mm Hg systolic or ≥ 110 mm Hg diastolic on two occasions at least 6 hours apart while the woman is on bed rest
2. Proteinuria of ≥ 5 g in a 24-hour urine specimen, or ≥ 3+ on two random urine samples collected at least 4 hours apart
3. Oliguria of < 500 mL in 24 hours
4. Cerebral or visual disturbances
5. Pulmonary edema or cyanosis
6. Epigastric or right upper-quadrant pain
7. Impaired liver function
8. Thrombocytopenia
9. Fetal growth restriction

Source: Adapted from ACOG 2006.[56]

≥ 140/90 after 20 weeks of gestation in a woman with no history of hypertension) and proteinuria (≥ 0.3 g protein in a 24-hour urine specimen). Primarily a syndrome of first pregnancy, the incidence of preeclampsia is estimated at 5–8%.[56] Severe preeclampsia is currently diagnosed according to criteria presented in Table 36-8 and defined by ACOG in 2002.[56] Medical treatment of severe preeclampsia during the intrapartum period is aimed at preventing convulsions, reducing blood pressure, and maintaining renal and uterine perfusion.

Eclampsia is diagnosed with new onset grand mal seizures and/or unexplained coma among women with signs and symptoms of preeclampsia that occur antepartum, intrapartum, or postpartum.[56] Most cases of postpartum eclampsia occur within 48 hours of birth, although isolated cases have been reported as long as 23 days postpartum. The estimated incidence of eclampsia in western countries ranges from 1 in 2000 to 1 in 3500 pregnancies.[57] The hallmark for the diagnosis of pregnancy-related convulsions as eclampsia is hypertension, although its pathogenesis is unknown.

Unfortunately, the spectrum of signs prior to the onset of eclamptic convulsions may range from severe hypertension, severe proteinuria, and generalized edema to absent or minimal hypertension, no proteinuria, and no edema. Approximately 20% of women with eclampsia have no premonitory signs or symptoms prior to the onset of convulsions.[57] More than 90% of cases occur after 28 weeks' gestation, with molar degeneration of the placenta the most common etiology of those cases that occur before this time. Management of eclampsia includes measures to prevent maternal injury and support respiratory and cardiovascular functions followed by medical therapy to prevent recurrent convulsions and reduce blood pressure to a safe range without inducing hypotension.

Figure 36-5 presents a treatment flow diagram for the two primary goals of drug therapy for severe preeclampsia and/or eclampsia. Intravenous magnesium sulfate is administered to prevent initial or recurrent seizures, while antihypertensives (hydralazine, labetalol, or nifedipine) are used to reduce the maternal blood pressure to a safe range. In his 2005 review,[57] Sibai recommends a hypertension treatment goal to maintain blood pressure between 140 and 160 mm Hg systolic and between 90 and 110 mm Hg diastolic.

Magnesium sulfate has a narrow therapeutic window. The therapeutic range for magnesium sulfate seizure prophylaxis is between 4.8 and 9.6 mg/dL. Magnesium is excreted renally, and unless the woman has renal compromise, serum magnesium levels do not need to be obtained. Symptoms of magnesium toxicity include absence of deep tendon reflexes (although this sign is unreliable in women with epidural analgesia/anesthesia), somnolence, respiratory depression, and cardiac arrest. If respiratory depression occurs, calcium gluconate 1 g (10 mL of a 10% solution) should be given intravenously over 3 minutes. Calcium gluconate should be readily available, labeled,

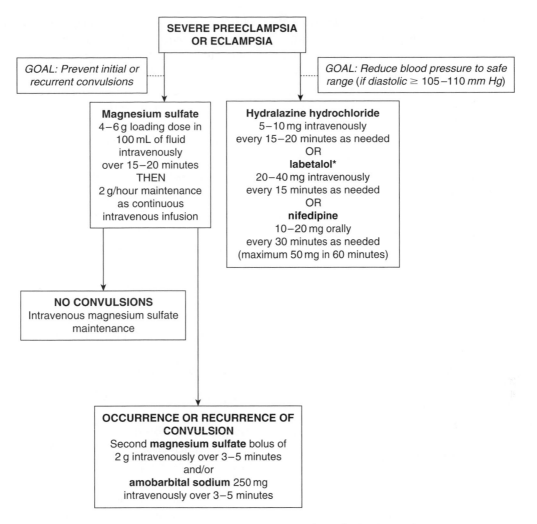

Figure 36-5 Drug therapy by treatment goals for severe preeclampsia and/or eclampsia.

and kept at the bedside ready for use during magnesium sulfate administration.

Immediate Postpartum Hemorrhage

Postpartum hemorrhage (PPH) most commonly occurs immediately after birth and is most frequently due to uterine atony. Other etiologies include retained placental fragments, trauma (laceration or uterine rupture), or bleeding disorders. Postpartum hemorrhage is defined as > 500 cc blood loss during a vaginal birth or > 1000 cc during a cesarean birth. Despite these definitions, nearly half of all women are thought to shed more than 500 cc during a normal vaginal birth.[58]

PPH is more common in women with a hyperdistended uterus (macrosomia, multiple gestation, or hydramnios), a prolonged or very rapid labor, chorioamnionitis, or a history of uterine atony and PPH. Women also are more prone to PPH if they have received oxytocin for the induction or augmentation of labor, magnesium sulfate during labor, or general anesthesia for birth.

Authors of a Cochrane review concluded that active management of the third stage of labor is associated with reduced blood loss, PPH, and prolonged third stage of labor.[59] Active third-stage management (defined as a package of interventions including administration of a prophylactic oxytocic with or immediately after the infant's birth, early clamping and cutting of the umbilical cord, and controlled cord traction to facilitate placental delivery) is, however, associated with increased maternal nausea and vomiting, and, if ergometrine is the oxytocic used, maternal hypertension. The effect of this active management package, particularly early cord clamping, on the newborn has not been sufficiently studied. Since many women in the United States have intravenous fluids infusing at the time of birth, a common practice is the addition of 10–20 units of oxytocin to the hanging fluid bag run at a brisk infusion rate after the birth. If either of these approaches is taken, the clinician must be absolutely certain that there is not an undiagnosed multiple pregnancy.

Management of PPH due to uterine atony includes intravenous fluids, drug therapy, emptying the bladder, and preparation for possible blood transfusion, uterine tamponade procedures, or surgical intervention. Table 36-9 presents first- and second-line drug therapy for the treatment of PPH.[60] Pitocin administered intravenously in solution (never to be administered undiluted as an intravenous bolus) or intramuscularly is widely accepted as the first-line therapy for immediate PPH. However, clinicians must be aware that women who have received oxytocin prior to delivery for induction or augmentation of labor may be less responsive to postpartum oxytocin due to saturation of myometrial oxytocin receptors.

Methylergonovine Maleate (Methergine)

Methylergonovine maleate (Methergine) is often the second drug choice if oxytocin (Pitocin) fails to stop a postpartum hemorrhage that is secondary to uterine atony. The adverse effects (ergotism) have been known since at least 600 BC. Ergotism or St. Anthony's fire is a syndrome of burning and gangrene in limbs or extremities, central nervous system disturbances, abortion, and, ultimately, death. It is caused by a fungus, *Claviceps purpura*, that grows on rye. Epidemics of ergotism were frequent in the Middle Ages. In 1582, ergot was used to speed labor, but this practice was stopped in the early 1800s because ergot too often causes uterine rupture, stillbirth, and maternal death.

Today, the ergot alkaloids methylergonovine maleate (Methergine, which is a semisynthetic version) and ergonovine maleate (Ergotrate, which is a naturally derived byproduct of the rye fungus) are used to prevent or stop postpartum hemorrhage. Ergot alkaloids are alpha-adrenergic agonists, and therefore they initiate contraction of vascular smooth muscle in both arteries and veins. Contraction of uterine muscle exhibits as an increase in force and frequency such that the contraction becomes tetanic. Methylergonovine maleate (Methergine) is contraindicated in the presence of maternal hypertension since its vasoconstrictive action may cause sudden severe hypertension.

Misoprostol (Cytotec)

Two prostaglandins are used when oxytocin and/or methylergonovine maleate are not effective. Prostaglandin $F_{2\alpha}$ (Hemabate) is contraindicated with asthma due to the risk of bronchial spasm. Misoprostol (Cytotec), a PGE_1 analogue, is currently the most effective drug therapy for acute postpartum hemorrhage. This drug is used off label because it is not FDA approved for this indication. Contraindications include allergy, active cardia, and pulmonary or hepatic disease, and it should be used with caution in women with asthma.

Table 36-9 Uterotonics for Immediate Postpartum Hemorrhage Due to Uterine Atony

Drug Generic (Brand)	Dose and Route	Contraindications	Side Effects
First-Line Therapy			
Oxytocin (Pitocin)	20–40 U in 1000 mL of normal saline or lactated Ringer's solution run continuously or 10 U intramuscular injection	Never give undiluted as a bolus injection	Cramping Water intoxication (hyponatremia)
Second-Line Therapy			
Misoprostol (Cytotec)	800 mcg per rectum, one dose (range 400–1000 mcg)		Diarrhea and abdominal pain
Methylergonovine maleate (Methergine)	0.2 mg intramuscular injection May repeat in 5 minutes Thereafter every 2–4 hours	Hypertension	Cramping Nausea and vomiting Hypertension, seizure, and/or headache
15-methyl-$F_{2\alpha}$-prostaglandin (Hemabate)	0.25 mg intramuscular injection May repeat every 15–90 minutes up to eight doses	Asthma or active cardiac, pulmonary, renal, or hepatic disease	Vomiting and diarrhea, nausea, temperature elevation
Dinoprostone (Prostin E_2)	20 mg vaginal or rectal suppository May repeat every 2 hours	Hypotension	Vomiting and diarrhea, nausea, temperature elevation

Nitroglycerine for Retained Placenta

An emerging therapy for the treatment of retained placenta when it is the etiology of PPH is 1 mg sublingual[61] or ≤ 200 mcg intravenous[62] nitroglycerine. Due to the hemodynamic vasodilating effects of nitroglycerine that may significantly decrease maternal blood pressure, precautions include the presence of a large bore intravenous line, hemodynamic monitoring, and sufficient skilled staffing to manage hypotension.

Chemoprophylaxis During Parturition

There are several disorders that women in labor have an increased risk for, or that are more likely to infect the fetus during the labor and birth process. Consequently, there are several antibiotics used for prophylaxis in labor.

Antibiotic Prophylaxis in Labor: Group B *Streptococcus*

Systematic efforts to prevent perinatal GBS disease through intrapartum antibiotic prophylaxis began in the 1990s as the condition emerged as the leading infectious cause of neonatal morbidity and mortality.[63] Although the majority of women with genital tract GBS colonization are asymptomatic, the organism is responsible for both early newborn onset (first week of life) and late-onset (> 1 week to about 3 months of age) infant infections. GBS infection in infants appears most commonly as septicemia or pneumonia and less commonly as meningitis, osteomyelitis, or septic arthritis.[63] The *CDC Guidelines for the Prevention of Perinatal Group B Streptococcal Disease* were last revised in 2002, and it is expected that a revised edition that has small changes in the doses of antibiotics used will be available in 2010. As outlined in Figure 36-6, these

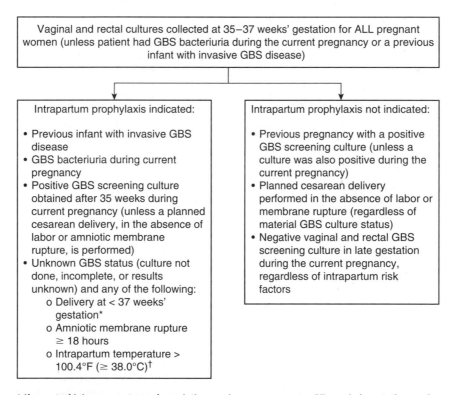

* If onset of labor or rupture of amniotic membrane occurs at < 37 weeks' gestation and there is a significant risk for preterm delivery (as assessed by the clinician), a suggested algorithm for GBS prophylaxis management is provided in Schrag SR et al. 2002.[63]

† If amnionitis is suspected, broad-spectrum antibiotic therapy that includes an agent known to be active against GBS should replace GBS prophylaxis.

Figure 36-6 Centers for disease control and prevention GBS universal screening algorithm. *Source:* Schrag SR et al. 2002.[63]

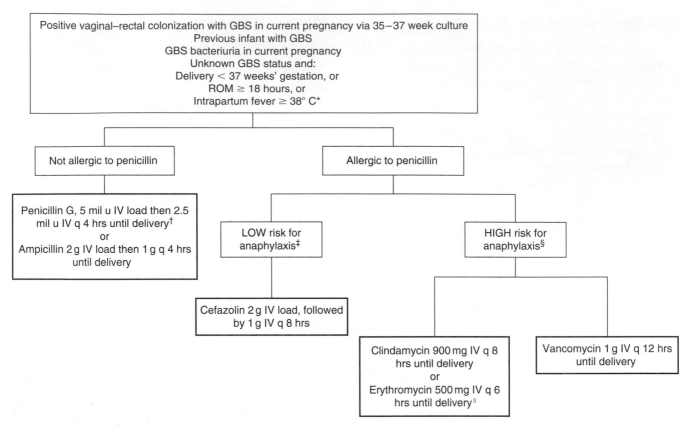

GBS = group B streptococcus; ROM = rupture of membranes.

* Broad-spectrum agents that include an agent effective against GBS should be used for treatment of chorioamnionitis.

† It is anticipated that the recommended dose of penicillin will change to 6 million units loading dose and 3 million units for ongoing doses until delivery in 2010. Readers should check the Centers for Disease Control and Prevention Web site for the most recent recommendations for the dose of penicillin.

‡ Persons with a history of rash only.

§ Persons who have experienced an immediate hypersensitivity reaction.

‖ Resistance to erythromycin is often associated with resistance to clindamycin. If a strain is resistant to either antibiotic, it may have inducible resistance to the other.

Figure 36-7 Antibiotic regimen for group B streptococcus prophylaxis in labor. *Sources:* Adapted with permission from Jolivet R 2002[64]; Schrag S et al. 2002.[63]

guidelines are based on the central principle of universal screening of all pregnant women for vaginal and rectal GBS colonization at 35 to 37 weeks' gestation, unless a woman has had GBS isolated from her urine in any concentration at any point during the current pregnancy. Figure 36-7 presents the CDC recommendations for intrapartum antibiotic prophylaxis regimens to prevent perinatal GBS disease.[64] When the serum penicillin levels of fetuses exposed to fewer than 4 hours of intrapartum prophylaxis were compared to those who were exposed for longer duration, higher levels were found in those

exposed for fewer than 4 hours[65] (Box 36-2). Fetal concentration of penicillin increased linearly after the loading dose, reaching peak levels at approximately 1 hour. Finally, the clinician must remember that the antibiotics recommended for GBS prophylaxis are not the recommended treatment for chorioamnionitis that were previously discussed. Anecdotal reports suggest that some providers who attend out-of-hospital births use oral penicillin formulations or other treatments for GBS-positive women, although data are lacking on the effectiveness of such regimens.

> ### Box 36-2 Intrapartum Antibiotic Prophylaxis for GBS
>
> LN is a 22-year old primigravida at 37 weeks and 2 days' gestation with a negative past health history and a healthy pregnancy. LN is allergic to penicillin. When queried about her allergy during a prenatal visit, she stated that she got a rash after taking Ampicillin (Principen) as a child and has not had any subsequent exposures to penicillin.
>
> LN's allergy is most likely the classic "Ampicillin rash," which is actually an allergic reaction to impurities in the drug. This is not a Type 1 hypersensitivity reaction that puts her at risk for anaphylaxis or angioedema. Because the incidence of cross-reactivity between penicillin and cephalosporins is low and she does not have a history of a true penicillin allergy, a cephalosporin is the best choice for GBS prophylaxis when she is in labor if her vaginal–rectal culture is positive for GBS.
>
> The culture is obtained at this visit. LN's practitioner does not request sensitivities or note that she is allergic to penicillin. She could order sensitivities to determine of this particular GBS isolate is sensitive to erythromycin (E-mycin) or clindamycin (Cleocin), but obtaining sensitivities in this situation would be an unnecessary cost.
>
> LNs culture was positive for GBS. She came to the in-hospital birth center in active labor at 40 weeks and 4 days. An intravenous (IV) catheter was placed in LN's left forearm, 1000 mL lactated Ringer's (LR) solution hung, and 2 g of cefazolin (Ancef) as a loading dose followed by 1 g 6 hours later for asymptomatic GBS prophylaxis was administered. LN's labor progressed normally and she gave birth to a 3650 g (8 pounds, 1 ounce) male infant with Apgar scores of 7 and 9 under pudendal anesthesia. The postpartum and neonatal courses of mother and son were uneventful and they were discharged at 23 hours. The infant did well.

Infective Endocarditis

In 2007, the American Heart Association released a new clinical guideline, *Prevention of Infective Endocarditis*.[66] Although infective endocarditis is a life-threatening condition, the American Heart Association expert panel reinforced the assertion of the 1997 guidelines that most cases of infective endocarditis are the result of randomly occurring bacteremias acquired from routine daily activities rather than attributable to invasive procedures. The most important aspect of these new guidelines for obstetrical care is that vaginal and cesarean births are conditions for which antibiotic prophylaxis is *not* recommended *regardless of predisposing risk factors* for infective endocarditis. The central principle is that "antibiotic prophylaxis solely to prevent infective endocarditis is not recommended for GU or GI tract procedures."[66, p. 13] Therefore, childbearing women, regardless of cardiac risk, should not receive intrapartum antibiotics as infective endocarditis prophylaxis.

Antiretroviral Prophylaxis in Human Immunodeficiency Virus-Infected Women

The transmission of human immunodeficiency virus type 1 (HIV-1) from mother to fetus/infant is substantially reduced through a multifaceted approach recommended by the US Public Health Service that includes:

1. Universal prenatal screening
2. Antenatal combined antiretroviral prophylaxis beginning at ≤ 28 weeks' gestation for women who are HIV infected and do not require immediate antiretroviral therapy for their own health
3. Scheduled cesarean section birth for women who have HIV RNA levels > 1000 copies/mL at term following 3 hours of preoperative intravenous zidovudine (AVT, ZDV, Retrovir) prophylaxis
4. Intrapartum intravenous zidovudine prophylaxis for all HIV-infected women regardless of their antepartum regimen with a loading dose of intravenous zidovudine (AVT, ZDV, Retrovir) of 2 mg/kg administered intravenously over 1 hour, followed by a maintenance dose of 1 mg/kg/hr as a continuous infusion until delivery
5. Discontinuation of antepartum stavudine administration during labor
6. Continuation of oral antiretroviral regimen components other than stavudine and zidovudine during labor
7. Rapid HIV antibody testing in labor on admission for women of unknown HIV status followed by intravenous zidovudine administration if the initial test is positive

8. The avoidance of breastfeeding

9. Risk-determined neonatal antiretroviral prophylaxis and follow-up[67]

Because of the rapid evolution of HIV management recommendations, practitioners should consult the AIDS information Web site of the National Institutes of Health on a regular basis for the most current information.

Corticosteroid Prophylaxis for Women in Preterm Labor

There is widespread agreement that the most beneficial medical treatment for women in preterm labor is the administration of corticosteroids to accelerate fetal pulmonary maturation. A single course of antenatal steroids for all women at risk of giving birth before 34 weeks' gestation has been the standard of care since the 1994 National Institutes of Health Consensus Conference.[68] Antenatal corticosteroids are associated with significant reductions in neonatal death, respiratory distress syndrome, intraventricular hemorrhage, necrotizing enterocolitis, and early systemic infections in the neonate without increasing maternal risk of death, chorioamnionitis, or puerperal sepsis.[69] Further, antenatal corticosteroids are effective in reducing neonatal morbidity and mortality for women with premature rupture of membranes and pregnancy-related hypertension syndromes.

Women at risk of preterm birth between 23 and 34 weeks' gestation are candidates for corticosteroid treatment.[70] The two commonly used regimens are detailed in Table 36-10. Current evidence suggests the benefits of antenatal corticosteroids are optimal if 48 hours or more has elapsed between the initial dose and birth. Further, the benefits appear to decline after 7 days, and repeat dosing may be considered *if a significant risk of preterm birth remains*. Although repeat dose(s) of corticosteroids are believed to reduce the occurrence and severity of neonatal lung disease and the risk of serious health problems in the first few weeks of life, critics have questioned the data analyses on which these recommendations have been made,[71] and repeat doses are associated with reduced birth weight and head circumference at birth.[72] Although betamethasone (Celestone) has gained popularity as the drug of choice due to beliefs that it has a higher gain and lower risk profile,[73,74] a recent double-blinded trial showed that the two drugs, betamethasone (Celestone) and dexamethasone (Decadron), were equivalent in reducing the rates of most major neonatal morbidities and mortality. Dexamethasone was superior in reducing the rate of intraventricular hemorrhage with a reported absolute risk reduction by 11.3% (95% CI, 2.7–11.9%).[75] It should be noted that dexamethasone is more widely available globally and has lower cost. Corticosteroids may cause maternal glucose intolerance with transient hyperglycemia in nondiabetic and increased insulin requirements in diabetic women and also may predispose pregnant women to pulmonary edema.[76]

Drug therapy during parturition and its various complications whether for therapeutics or prophylaxis should be approached cautiously. All pharmacologic agents carry significant risks of both maternal and fetal adverse effects despite their potential to treat, ameliorate, or prevent some adverse processes or outcomes that may be associated with the normal physiologic process of labor and birth. Appropriate clinical judgment requires a healthy respect for the integrity of the maternal–fetal unit and the physiology of parturition, and a healthy skepticism of the potential for drugs to provide benefit that exceeds their attendant risks.

Analgesia and Anesthesia During Labor

Relief for the pain of labor has been desired since antiquity. Prior to the 1700s, pain and suffering were seen as signs of sin, and therefore, endurance was the only recourse women had. During the Enlightenment, pain became viewed as natural phenomena that could potentially be controlled. Since then, methods of abrogating the pain in labor have been the continued preoccupation of childbearing women, anesthesia providers, and clinicians who care for women in labor.

When drugs are used to treat labor pain, they are evaluated for several effects, which include (1) the efficacy of pain relief, (2) side effects or adverse effects for the woman, (3) side effects or adverse effects for the fetus, and (4) side effects or adverse effects on the progress of labor.

Table 36-10 Corticosteroid Prophylaxis to Promote Fetal Maturation in Preterm Labor

Drug Generic (Brand)	Dose
Betamethasone (Celestone)	12 mg intramuscular (6 mg each of betamethasone acetate and betamethasone sodium phosphate) Two doses 24 hours apart
Dexamethasone (Decadron)	6 mg intramuscular Every 12 hours for four doses

Strategies for ameliorating labor pain can be divided into the following three general categories: (1) those that attempt to remove or diminish the painful stimuli such as regional anesthesia; (2) those that provide sensory stimulation that competes with and inhibits painful awareness such as transcutaneous electric nerve stimulation (TENS), intradermal water injections, and acupressure; and (3) techniques that modify the individual's reaction and perception of pain such as hypnosis, prepared childbirth, and the use of doulas. Opioids have two of these effects in that they both diminish painful stimuli and modify the perception of pain.[77,78]

The nonpharmacologic methods have varied evidence for safety and efficacy. This topic has been extensively reviewed and will not be discussed in this chapter. The interested reader is referred to the published systematic reviews.[77-80]

Physiology of Labor Pain

Pain during the first stage of labor is secondary to cervical dilatation and progressive ischemia within the uterine muscle. These pain signals are transferred to the spinal cord via C and A-delta afferent nerve fibers that enter the spinal cord between L1 and T10. The pain is usually a dull, cramping, visceral pain that may radiate to the lower back or legs. Pain during the second stage of labor is additionally from pelvic floor distention, transmitted to the spinal cord via the pudendal nerve, and entering the spinal cord at the level of S4 through S2. This pain is usually sharp and somatic. The fibers enter the spinal cord through the dorsal horn, and then they cross the spinal cord to enter the ascending nerve bundles in the spinothalamic tract. These nerves terminate in the cortex of the brain.[81] There are three general types of pain that women experience in labor—abdominal pain, contraction-related back pain, and continuous low back pain. All women experience abdominal pain. A seminal survey of a small group of multipara and primipara women conducted by Melzak et al. in the 1980s found that 74% experience contraction-related back pain, and 33% have continuous low back pain.[82]

Role of Stress Response

The classic fight or flight response is a physiologic response to stress that enables the body to cope by increasing the heart rate, the blood pressure, and shunting blood away from the nonvital organs to the brain, lungs, and skeletal muscles. The one aspect of this response that may be particularly problematic for the laboring woman is that the release of catecholamines that orchestrates the stress response also causes blood to be shunted from the uterus. So the question for laboring women is how much stress is too much stress? Although there are no clinical studies that have addressed this question adequately, the theory is that women who are excessively anxious or afraid will release higher levels of catecholamines, which then slows their labors.[83-86]

Sedatives and Hypnotics

Barbiturates, phenothiazines, and benzodiazepines all have sedative/hypnotic effects. The ones used to treat women in labor are barbiturates and phenothiazines. Benzodiazepines are contraindicated because they have some amnesic effects in the pregnant woman and they are associated with neonatal depression (Table 36-11).

Historically, a barbiturate such as secobarbital (Seconal) was given to control anxiety and promote sleep for women experiencing long **prodromal labor**. These drugs do not have any analgesic effect. Barbiturates are highly lipophilic, so they cross the placental barrier easily and quickly. The half-life of barbiturates is quite long, so a single dose given in early labor can cause decreased motor tone and difficulty breastfeeding in the neonate for up to 48–72 hours after birth. Today, barbiturates are contraindicated for laboring women.

Phenothiazines continue to be used to treat prolonged latent phase of labor in combination with an opioid. The opioid inhibits uterine contractions and the phenothiazine counteracts the nausea that opioids can produce. A combination of promethazine (Phenergan) and morphine given either intramuscularly or intravenously is one standard

Table 36-11 Sedative/Hypnotics for Prolonged Latent Phase of Labor

Drug Generic (Brand)	Dose	Clinical Considerations
Promethazine (Phenergan)	50 mg IV or IM	Associated with a reduction in FHR variability but no effect on labor progress and association
Hydroxyzine hydrochloride (Vistaril)	50–100 mg IM	Painful IM injection; cannot be given IV No effect on labor progress Associated with neonatal depression
Prochlorperazine (Compazine)	25 mg PR or 5–10 mg IV or IM or 5–10 mg PO	Given with morphine sulfate for sleep during prolonged latent phase

FHR = fetal heart rate.

regimen. Hydroxyzine (Vistaril), which is actually an antihistamine, can also be used, but unlike promethazine, hydroxyzine cannot be given intravenously and must be administered orally or intramuscularly. Neither promethazine nor hydroxyzine has known adverse effects on the fetus/newborn or the progress of labor.

The actual effect of phenothiazines on pain is controversial. In the two randomized trials that have been published, pain was not significantly reduced in women who were administered meperidine (Demerol) and promethazine (Phenergan) when compared to women who were given meperidine (Demerol) and placebo.[86,87] This is a subtle but important point because when one administers a drug that decreases anxiety and one that inhibits pain, the woman will exhibit less pain behavior and may be tranquil, which leads one to conclude that the sedative potentiates the pain relief of the opioid. However, sedation can prevent the woman from communicating her actual level of pain. Although anecdotally the pain relief potentiation theory appears sound, it has not been evaluated scientifically. The use of this combination may be useful in certain situations such as latent labor or the administration of preoperative medications. Sedative/ hypnotics in combination with opioids should not be used to treat moderate or severe pain.

Opioids

The severe pain associated with active labor requires stronger analgesics (Table 36-12). Opioids are the only agents used systemically to mitigate the pain of active labor and they have been used for centuries. Opioids produce incomplete analgesia and have significant side effects of clinical import.[87]

The opioids are categorized by their effect on the various opioid receptors (Chapter 12). Meperidine (Demerol), fentanyl (Sublimaze), and morphine are pure mu agonists, whereas butorphanol (Stadol) and nalbuphine (Nubain) are mixed agonist/antagonists. The effect of these drugs on the respective opioid receptors accounts for the clinical effect. For example, when an agonist binds to the mu opioid receptor, the result is slowed gastrointestinal motility, nausea and vomiting, respiratory depression,

Table 36-12 Opioid Doses for Management of Pain During Active Labor

Opioid Generic (Brand)	IM Dose (Dose/Peak/Duration)	IV Dose (Dose/Peak/Duration)	Agonist Effect	Maternal Side Effects	Fetal/Neonatal Effects
Fentanyl (Sublimaze)	50–100 mcg/ 1–2 h/1–2 h Maximum dose usually 500–600 mcg	50–100 mcg/ 3–5 min/1–2 h Maximum dose usually 500–600 mcg	Pure agonist at mu receptor,* kappa receptor,[†] sigma receptor,[‡] and delta receptor[§]	Short acting less effective than morphine or meperidine (Demerol) but very few side effects noted	None reported
Meperidine[‖] (Demerol)	75 mg/40–50 min/2–4 h	75–80 mg/5 min/2–4 h	Pure agonist at mu and kappa receptors	N and V, urinary retention Respiratory depression, sedation	Respiratory depression 1–4 hours after dose; effect is independent of dose Neonatal developmental depression 20–60 hours after last dose
Morphine[‖]	10 mg/1–2 h/2–4 h	2.5–5 mg/20 min/2–4 h	Pure agonist at mu and kappa receptors	Pruritus, N and V, urinary retention, respiratory depression	↓ FHR variability Cumulative effect respiratory depression
Butorphanol (Stadol)	2 mg/30–60 min/3–4 h	1–2 mg/30 min/2–4 h	Kappa agonist and sigma agonist	Ceiling effect	Transient pseudo-sinusoidal FHR pattern
Nalbuphine (Nubain)	10–20 mg/30–60 min/2–4 h	10–20 mg/30 min/2–4 h	Mu antagonist and kappa partial agonist	Ceiling effect	Transient pseudo-sinusoidal FHR pattern

FHR = fetal heart rate.
* Mu-receptor stimulation causes slowed gastrointestinal motility, nausea and vomiting, respiratory depression, spinal and supraspinal analgesia, sedation, urinary retention, pruritus, and euphoria.
[†] Kappa-receptor stimulation causes sedation, spinal analgesia, and miosis.
[‡] Sigma-receptor stimulation causes dysphoria, hallucination, and mydriasis.
[§] Delta-receptor stimulation causes spinal and supraspinal analgesia.
[‖] Morphine causes more pruritus and urinary retention when administered epidurally or intrathecally. Maternal respiratory depression can be a late effect in epidurally administered morphine sulfate secondary to slow uptake into CNS.

analgesia, sedation, and euphoria. Agonists that bind to the kappa receptor elicit sedation and analgesia but no nausea or vomiting. The agonists/antagonists are chosen because they cause less nausea and vomiting and less sedation secondary to mu receptor antagonism but continue to cause analgesia secondary to the kappa agonist effect.

All opioids are lipophilic and cross the placental barrier easily. These drugs all reach equilibrium between maternal and fetal circulations. Opioids are weak bases and subject to ion trapping in a fetus with acidemia, an effect that is important to remember if newborn resuscitation is needed.

In general the opioids do not affect labor progress in the active phase.[87] Morphine is used to abolish contractions in women who are experiencing a prolonged latent phase, and the putative mechanism is that morphine stops uncoordinated contraction activity. If the woman is actually in the active phase of labor when morphine is given, labor will progress unimpeded.

Meperidine (Demerol)

Meperidine (Demerol) has been the most frequently used opioid for treating labor pain worldwide. Meperidine has been studied extensively and has recently fallen out of favor, for good reason. Today, it can be stated definitively that meperidine should not be used to treat women in the active phase of labor. First, this drug does not appear to provide effective pain relief. When women are queried about their satisfaction with meperidine, over half report that it did not mitigate labor pain effectively.[87]

The half-life of meperidine (Demerol) in the fetus is between 13 and 26 hours, and thus, neonatal depression can occur several hours after birth. In addition, meperidine has active metabolites that are the presumed etiology of altered neurobehavioral tests in the newborn up to 3 days after birth. Thus the acute newborn effects appear related to the dose of meperidine given in labor and the delayed newborn affects are probably secondary to the active metabolite normeperidine. The host of clinical implications includes lower Apgar scores, difficulty establishing breastfeeding, and decreased neonatal alertness.[87]

Fentanyl (Sublimaze) and Morphine

The two mu-opioid receptor antagonists increasingly used for laboring women in the United States today are fentanyl (Sublimaze) and morphine. Fentanyl is given intravenously or subcutaneously several times as

needed. There are anecdotal reports of using fentanyl as a continuous intravenous drip in a patient-controlled intravenous setup, and there is one randomized controlled trial of this method of administration.[87] Patient-controlled analgesia (PCA) appears to increase patient satisfaction in general, but the one study that evaluated fentanyl for treating labor pain did not find any difference between PCA and intermittent bolusing.[87] Fentanyl is often placed in the epidural space along with local anesthetics to augment the effects of regional analgesia. Morphine administered intramuscularly or intravenously is used to treat the prolonged latent phase of labor. Morphine is also often placed in the epidural catheter as an adjunct for pain relief following a cesarean birth or extensive perineal laceration.

Butorphanol (Stadol) and Nalbuphine (Nubain)

Butorphanol and nalbuphine exhibit antagonism to the mu receptor and kappa agonists. They are often used in settings where epidural analgesia is not available or desired. The primary clinical consideration to remember when using these agents is that they are contraindicated for persons who have a history of drug abuse/addiction. This is because the mu antagonism can elicit withdrawal symptoms in this situation.

Naloxone (Narcan)

Naloxone (Narcan) is the opioid antagonist used to reverse the respiratory depression effect of opioids in the newborn. Naloxone is an antagonist to all the opioid receptors. Naloxone can be given intravenously or intramuscularly and comes in the following three formulations: 0.02 mg/mL, 0.4 mg/mL, and 1 mg/mL. The dose is 0.01 mg/kg of body weight. The effect following an intravenous dose should be evident in 1–2 minutes, and the peak effect will occur in 5–15 minutes. The onset of action following an intramuscular dose is 2–5 minutes, and the peak effect is in 5–15 minutes.[88]

Naloxone (Narcan) should be administered within the confines of a clinical protocol that dictates the required supervision and assessment of vital signs and should not be used routinely.[88] If the dose is insufficient, respiratory depression can reoccur when the naloxone wears off. If more than one dose is needed, the infant should be closely monitored.

Naloxone is also used to counter the intense pruritus associated with intrathecal morphine. When this is required, the analgesic effect is also blocked and the woman will need additional systemic analgesia. Naloxone will induce withdrawal effects in a person who is opioid dependent and is therefore contraindicated for individuals with a history of opioid abuse.

Regional Analgesia

In 1957, Virginia Apgar published an article comparing regional anesthesia to general anesthesia and found that babies born to mothers who had regional anesthesia were more vigorous than those who were born to mothers given general anesthesia for delivery. This finding generated a powerful incentive to refine the regional anesthetic procedure and in essence brought us to where we are today.

Epidural analgesia is the most popular form of regional analgesia for labor pain in the United States today. Other regional techniques include spinal anesthesia for cesarean section, pudendal block for perineal laceration repair, and rarely paracervical block to relieve the pain of the late first stage or second stage of labor. Epidurals and spinals are initiated and managed by anesthesia personnel; however, a general understanding of the technique and thorough understanding of the effects are important for all clinicians who care for women in labor. Pudendal blocks are less complicated and are used by obstetric providers. Paracervical blocks are infrequently used secondary to their association with fetal bradycardia and are not reviewed here.

Various local anesthetics are used in regional blocks, and all have the same basic mechanism of action that is reviewed in detail in Chapter 12. The important consideration for laboring women when a regional block is initiated with a local anesthetic is the accidental injection into the bloodstream, which results in a rapid systemic toxicity reaction or the inadvertent intrathecal injection, which results in a very rapid initiation of the regional block, hypotension, respiratory depression, and loss of consciousness. Signs and symptoms of both intervascular and intrathecal injections are reviewed in Chapter 12.

Anatomy of the Epidural Space

The epidural space surrounds the meninges; i.e., the dural and subarachnoid membranes that in turn surround the spinal cord. It is bounded posteriorly (toward the back) by the ligamentum flavum and is commonly defined as divided into an anterior space in the front and dorso-lateral spaces on the sides of the spinal cord. The anterior epidural space is very narrow because of the proximity of the dura. This space is widest posteriorly, and the width varies with the vertebral level ranging from 1–1.5 mm at C5 to 5–6 mm at L2. The anterior space or portion is

frequently divided by membranes or connective tissue[89] (Figure 36-8).

There are several anatomic structures within the epidural space including nerve root ganglia that traverse the epidural space, which is why local anesthetics work when placed there. Fat extends throughout the epidural space. Fat itself has great affinity for drugs with high lipid solubility (such as bupivacaine). Uptake of drug into fat competes with vascular and neural uptake. Large, valveless veins that communicate with the occipital venous systems within the cranium superiorly and the uterine and iliac veins inferiorly are also present in the epidural space. Drugs placed in the epidural space will diffuse into the maternal circulation via the epidural vessels in a quantity that is dependent upon the lipid solubility and concentration.

Epidurals

Epidurals are categorized by the technique of drug administration and the type of medication used. The technique can be an intermittent bolus, continuous infusion, or patient-controlled epidural anesthesia (PCEA). Additionally, a newer technique that combines an initial **intrathecal** injection of fentanyl (Sublimaze) to provide a walking epidural followed by a regular epidural placement later, called combined spinal-epidural (CSE), is increasingly popular.

Local anesthetic placed in the epidural space is the most common application of epidural analgesia. These agents inhibit infusion of sodium ions into the neural cell, which effectively blocks nerve transmission. This block affects all nerves that the local anesthetic reaches, thus both a sensory and motor block is the result. Both sensory and motor blocks can vary from minimal to complete (which is used for cesarean section) depending on the dose and concentration of anesthetic that is injected.

Epidural analgesia is associated with many side effects and a few rare adverse effects. These effects can be subdivided into (1) those that are secondary to the technique of anesthetic placement, (2) maternal and fetal effects, and (3) effects on labor progress. The technique is generally quite safe, and adverse effects that are caused by epidural catheter placement are exceedingly rare. Inadvertent dural puncture can cause a spinal headache that appears in the first 24 hours after birth. Misplacement and injection of epidural doses into the intrathecal space can cause a high spinal and maternal respiratory depression. Systemic toxicity reactions can occur if the anesthetic is inadvertently injected into the circulation instead of the epidural space. Epidural abscess or hematoma are also possible adverse outcomes of catheter placement.

A Epidural analgesia

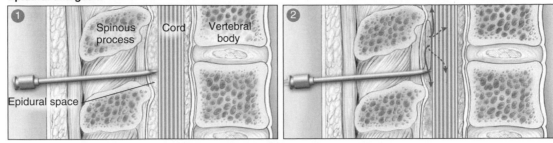

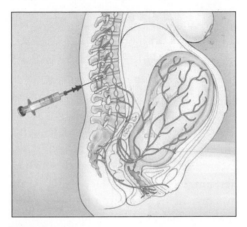

B Combined spinal–epidural analgesia

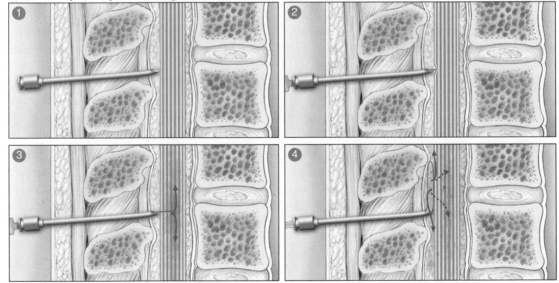

(A1) Epidural analgesia: A catheter is placed into the lumbar epidural space. After the desired intervertebral space (e.g., between L3 and L4) has been identified and infiltrated with local anesthetic, a hollow epidural needle is placed in the intervertebral ligaments. These ligaments are characterized by a high degree of resistance to penetration. In contrast, the epidural space has a low degree of resistance. **(A2)** When the anesthesiologist slowly advances the needle while feeling for resistance, he or she recognizes the epidural space by a sudden loss of resistance as the epidural needle enters the epidural space. An epidural catheter is advanced into the space to administer solutions of a local anesthetic, opioids, or a combination. **(B1) Combined spinal–epidural analgesia:** The lumbar epidural space is identified with an epidural needle. **(B2)** A very thin spinal needle is introduced through the epidural needle into the subarachnoid space. Correct placement can be confirmed by free flow of cerebrospinal fluid. **(B3)** A single bolus of local anesthetic, opioid, or a combination of the two is injected through this needle into the subarachnoid space. **(B4)** The needle is removed and a catheter is advanced into the epidural space through the epidural needle. When the single-shot spinal analgesic wears off, the epidural catheter can be used for the continuation of pain relief.

Figure 36-8 Epidural and combined spinal–epidural analgesia technique. *Source:* Reprinted with permission from Eltzschig HK et al. 2003.[89]

The effect of regional analgesia on the mother and her fetus as well as the effect on the progress of labor has been the subject of both controversy and extensive review. Readers who care for women in labor are referred to several summary analyses that address these controversies.[89-95] The systematic review by Mayberry et al. summarizes the evidence for managing common side effects of regional analgesia.[95]

Intrathecal or Walking Epidural

The walking epidural is not really an epidural as the drug (Fentanyl) is administered intrathecally where it directly affects the opioid receptors on the spinal cord and creates an analgesic effect without interfering with motor function. Drugs injected into the intrathecal space do not diffuse into the maternal bloodstream as there are no blood vessels within the spinal canal, so this technique does prevent the opioid from crossing the placenta. The duration of analgesia from one intrathecal injection is approximately 3–5 hours. This is administered as a one-time dose only because puncture to the dura can cause spinal fluid to leak, which results in a spinal headache. Although an intrathecal dose of fentanyl does not alleviate the pain of very active labor as well as local anesthetics in the epidural space, it does work better than intravenous opioids, and unlike the use of local anesthetics in the epidural space, there is no motor block so women can walk or move about unimpeded.

Pudendal Block

A pudendal block involves placement of 10–15 mL of 1% lidocaine (Xylocaine) transvaginally just behind the ischial spines bilaterally. This placement effectively blocks transmission of the afferent fibers in the pudendal nerve, which initiates anesthesia of the perineum. Pudendal blocks are most often used for repair of perineal lacerations. The primary adverse effects are inadvertent intravascular injection. Proper technique to ensure the needle is not placed in a blood vessel is used to prevent this complication.

Paracervical Block

A paracervical block can be obtained by injecting local anesthetic into the submucosal area just underneath the vaginal mucosa in both fornices beside the cervix. This placement instills anesthetic around Frankenhäuser's ganglion, which contains visceral sensory nerves from the uterus, cervix and upper vagina. The technique can be effective in mitigating pain of the first stage of labor for approximately 40–90 minutes. Paracervical blocks are associated with a relatively high incidence of fetal bradycardia that occurs in approximately 15% of parturients following placement of the anesthetic into the paracervical space.[96] The bradycardia occurs within 2–10 minutes and can last for 10–30 minutes and is the primary reason paracervical block is rarely used in obstetrics today.

Inhaled Anesthetics

Inhaled anesthetics were the first anesthetics used by women in labor. In 1853, Queen Victoria used chloroform to ease the pain of her eighth birth (Prince Leopold), and this act effectively started obstetric anesthesia and analgesia. Once the public became aware of her choice, the social elite demanded the same, and widespread use of chloroform and ether for managing labor pain was the result.[95]

As is true today with postmarketing research, once these agents were used in a large general population, the adverse effects quickly became apparent. Postpartum hemorrhage, prolonged labor, and neonatal asphyxia limited continued use of these agents, and by the early 1900s, they were replaced with systemic agents.

Today the one inhaled anesthetic used by laboring women in nitrous oxide.[97] Although only a few hospitals have nitrous oxide available, use is increasing because it is safe and effective and has minimal side effects or adverse effects.[98] The nitrous oxide is mixed in a 50/50 mixture with oxygen. The woman holds the mask over her face and breathes the gas mixture intermittently. She will obtain best results if she takes a few deep inhalations just before the contraction starts so that the nitrous oxide effect coincides with the peak of the contraction. The onset of action occurs in approximately 50 seconds. Nitrous oxide can cause dysphoria and sedation that is more pronounced if the gas effect occurs when there is no contraction pain.[98]

In summary, the drugs chosen to abrogate the pain of labor are institution and provider specific. There is wide variability in what analgesic agents are available in different birth settings, some of which is based on the availability of nurse-anesthetists and anesthesiologists. Individual practitioners tend to be most comfortable with one drug or technique and predominately rely on that drug. There are no national guidelines that address labor analgesia.

However, each woman is unique, each labor is unique, and there is no single pharmacologic agent that is useful for everyone. Therefore it is important that clinicians be knowledgeable about a variety of nonpharmacologic and pharmacologic methods available to help women through labor and birth.

Conclusion

Very few drugs are used for women during parturition. Pregnant women in developed nations are generally healthy, and obstetric providers are cautious about exposing a pregnant woman and her fetus to adverse drug effects. However, the drugs that are used for this population can be lifesaving, and clinicians caring for women during labor and birth often need to make complicated judgments quickly; thus, a thorough knowledge of the drugs discussed in this chapter is an important component of clinical acumen and clinical practice.

References

1. Challis JRG. Mechanism of parturition and preterm labor. Obstet Gynecol Survey 2000;55:650–60.
2. Gibb W, Lye SJ, Challis JRG. Parturition. In Neill J, Wassarman P, eds. Knobil and Neill's physiology of reproduction. Vol 2. Amsterdam, Netherlands: Elsevier, 2006:2925–74.
3. Smith R. Parturition. N Eng J Med 2007;356:271–83.
4. Challis JRG, Bloomfield FH, Bocking AD, Casciani V, Chisada H, Connor K, et al. Fetal signals and parturition. J Obstet Gynaecol Res 2005;31:492–9.
5. Young RC. Myocytes, myometrium and uterine contractions. Ann N Y Acad Sci 2007;1101:72–84.
6. Bernal AL. Overview of current research in parturition. Exp Physiol 2001;86:213–22.
7. Ludmir J, Sehdev HM. Anatomy and physiology of the uterine cervix. Clin Obstet Gynecol 2000;43:433–9.
8. Bauer M, Mazza E, Nava A, Zeck W, Eder M, Bajka M, et al. In vivo characterization of the mechanics of human uterine cervices. Ann N Y Acad Sci 2007;1101: 186–202.
9. Monga M, Sanborn BM. Biology and physiology of the reproductive tract and control of myometrial contraction. In Creasy RK, Resnik R, Iams JD, eds. Maternal-fetal medicine: principles and practice, 5th ed. Philadelphia, PA: Saunders, 2004:69–78.
10. Wray S, Kupittayanant S, Shmygol A, Smith RD, Burdyga T. The physiological basis of uterine contractility: a short review. Exper Physiol 2001;86:239–46.
11. Bernal AL. Mechanisms of labour—biochemical aspects. BJOG 2003;110(suppl 20):39–45.
12. Iams JD, Creasy RK. Preterm labor and delivery. In Creasy RK, Resnik R, Iams JD. Maternal-fetal medicine: principles and practice, 5th ed. Philadelphia, PA: Saunders, 2004:623–62.
13. Iams JD, Romero R. Preterm birth. In Gabbe SG, Niebyl RJ, Simpson JL, eds. Obstetrics: normal and problem pregnancies, 5th ed. Philadelphia, PA: Churchill Livingstone Elsevier, 2007:668–712.
14. Lumley J. Defining the problem: the epidemiology of preterm birth. BJOG 2003;110(suppl 20):3–7.
15. Mathews TJ, MacDorman MF. Infant mortality statistics from the 2004 period linked birth/infant death data set. Natl Vital Stat Rep 2007;55(14):1–32.
16. Hamilton BE, Martin JA, Ventura SJ. Births: preliminary data for 2006. Natl Vital Stat Rep 2007;56(7):1–18.
17. Martin J, Hamilton BE, Sutton PE, Ventura SJ, Menacker F, Kirmeyer S. Births: final data for 2004. Natl Vital Stat Rep 2006;55(1):1–34.
18. ACOG Practice bulletin number 43: management of preterm labor. 2006 compendium of selected publications. Washington, DC: American College of Obstetricians and Gynecologists, 2003:673–81.
19. ACOG Practice bulletin number 31: assessment of risk factors for preterm birth. 2006 compendium of selected publications. Washington, DC: American College of Obstetricians and Gynecologists, 2001:366–73.
20. Chandiramani J, Shennan A. Preterm labour: update on prediction and prevention strategies. Curr Opin Obstet Gynecol 2006;18:618–24.
21. Simhan HN, Caritis SN. Prevention of preterm delivery. N Eng J Med 2007;357:477–87.
22. Terrien J, Marque C, Germain G. What is the future of tocolysis? Eur J Obset Gynecol 2004;117S:S10–4.
23. Lam F, Gill P. Beta-Agonist tocolytic therapy. Obstet Gynecol Clin North Am 2005;32:457–84.
24. United States Food and Drug Administration. Warning on use of terbutaline sulfate for preterm labor. JAMA 1998;279:9.
25. Caritis S. Adverse effects of tocolytic therapy. BJOG 2005;112(suppl 1):74–8.
26. Ables AZ, Romero AM, Chauhan SP. Use of calcium channel antagonists for preterm labor. Obstet Gynecol Clin North Am 2005;32:519–25.
27. Oei SG. Calcium channel blockers for tocolysis: a review of their role and safety following reports of

serious adverse events. Eur J Obset Gynecol 2006;126: 137–45.

28. Papatsonis DNM, Lok CAR, Bos JM, van Geijn HP, Dekker GA. Calcium channel blockers in the management of preterm labor and hypertension in pregnancy. Eur J Obset Gynecol Reprod Biol 2001;97:122–40.

29. Lyell DJ, Pullen K, Campbell L, Ching S, Druzin ML, Chitkara U, et al. Magnesium sulfate compared with nifedipine for acute tocolysis of preterm labor: a randomized controlled trial. Obstet Gynecol 2007; 110:61–7.

30. Loe SM, Sanchez-Ramos L, Kaunitz AM. Assessing the neonatal safety of indomethacin tocoloysis: a systematic review with meta-analysis. Obset Gynecol 2005;106:173–9.

31. Vermillion ST, Robinson CJ. Antiprostaglandin drugs. Obstet Gynecol Clin North Am 2005;32:501–17.

32. Crowther CA, Hiller JE, Doyle LW. Magnesium sulphate for preventing preterm birth in threatened preterm labour. Cochrane Database Syst Rev 2002;(4): CD001060.

33. Grimes DA, Nanda K. Magnesium sulfate tocolysis: time to quit. Obstet Gynecol 2006;108:986–9.

34. Doyle LW, Crowther CA, Middleton P, Marret S, Rouse D. Magnesium sulphate for women at risk of preterm birth for neuroprotection of the fetus. Cochrane Database Syst Rev 2009;(1):CD004661.

35. Briggs GG, Wan SR. Drug therapy during labor and delivery, part 2. Am J Health-Syst Pharm 2006;63: 1131–9.

36. Battista LR, Wing DA. Abnormal labor and induction of labor. In Gabbe SG, Niebyl RJ, Simpson JL, eds. Obstetrics: normal and problem pregnancies, 5th ed. Philadelphia, PA: Churchill Livingstone Elsevier, 2007: 322–43.

37. Sanchez-Ramos L. Induction of labor. Obstet Gynecol Clin North Am 2005;32:181–200.

38. ACOG committee opinion number 228: induction of labor with misoprostol. 2006 compendium of selected publications. Washington, DC, American College of Obstetricians and Gynecologists, 1999:101–2.

39. Lowe NK. A review of factors associated with dystocia and cesarean section in nulliparous women. J Midwifery Womens Health 2006;52:216–28.

40. Wahl RUR. Could oxytocin administration during labor contribute to autism and related behavioral disorder? A look at the literature. Med Hypoth 2004;63:456–60.

41. Cunningham FG, Leveno KJ, Bloom SL, Hauth JC, Gilstrap III LC, Wenstrom KD. Williams obstetrics, 22nd ed. New York: McGraw-Hill, 2007.

42. Lyndon-Rochelle M, Holt VL, Easterling TR, Martin DP. Risk of uterine rupture during labor among women with a prior cesarean delivery. N Eng J Med 2001;345:3–8.

43. Arias F. Pharmacology of oxytocin and prostaglandins. Clin Obstet Gynecol 2000;43:455–68.

44. Hayes EJ, Weinstein L. Improving patient safety and uniformity of care by a standardized regimen for the use of oxytocin by a standardized regimen for the use of oxytocin. Am J Obstet Gynecol 2008;198:622.e1–7.

45. Macones GA, Hankins GDV, Spong CY, Hauth J, Moore T. The 2008 National Institute of Child Health and Human Development workshop report on electronic fetal monitoring. Obstet Gynecol 2008;112: 661–6.

46. Bakker PCAM, Durver PHJ, Kuik DJ, van Geijn HP. Excessive uterine activity over the course of labor is associated with neonatal academia at birth. Am J Obstet Gynecol 2007;196:313.e1–6.

47. Smith JG, Merrill DC. Oxytocin for induction of labor. Clin Obstet Gynecol 2006;49:594–608.

48. Ophir E, Solt I, Odeh M, Bornstein J. Water intoxication—a dangerous condition in labor and delivery rooms. Obstet Gynecol Surv 2007;62:731–8.

49. Mayberry LJ, Clemmens D, De A. Epidural analgesia side effects, co-interventions, and care of women during childbirth: a systematic review. Am J Obstet Gynecol 2002;186:S81–93.

50. ACOG practice bulletin number 49: dystocia and augmentation of labor. Obstet Gynecol 2003;102:1445–54.

51. Gibbs RS, Sweet RL, Duff WP. Maternal and fetal infectious disorders. In Creasy RK, Resnik R, Iams JD. Maternal-fetal medicine: principles and practice, 5th ed. Philadelphia, PA: Saunders, 2004:741–801.

52. Edwards RK. Chorioamnionitis and labor. Obstet Gynecol Clin North Am 2005;32:287–96.

53. Fahey JO. Clinical management of intraamniotic infection and chorioamnionitis: a review of the literature. J Midwif Womens Health 2008;53:227–35.

54. Hermansen MC, Hermansen MG. Perinatal infections and cerebral palsy. Clin Perinatol 2006;33:315–33.

55. Edwards RK, Duff P. Single additional dose postpartum therapy for women with chorioamnionitis. Obstet Gynecol 2003;102:957–61.

56. ACOG practice bulletin number 33. Diagnosis and management of preeclampsia and eclampsia. 2006 compendium of selected publications. Washington, DC: American College of Obstetricians and Gynecologists, 2006:444–52.

57. Sibai BM. Diagnosis, prevention, and management of eclampsia. Obstet Gynecol 2005;105:402–10.

58. Francois KE, Foley MR. Antepartum and postpartum hemorrhage. In Gabbe SG, Niebyl RJ, Simpson JL, eds. Obstetrics: normal and problem pregnancies, 5th ed. Philadelphia, PA: Churchill Livingstone Elsevier, 2007:456–85.

59. Prendiville WJP, Elbourne D, McDonald SJ. Active versus expectant management in the third stage of labour. Cochrane Database Syst Rev 2000(3):CD000007.

60. ACOG Practice Bulletin Number 76: postpartum hemorrhage. Obstet Gynecol 2006;108:1039–47.

61. Bullarbo M, Tjugum J, Ekerhovd E. Sublingual nitroglycerin for management of retained placenta. Internat J Gynecol Obstet 2005;91:223–32.

62. Chedraui PA, Insuasti DF. Intravenous nitroglycerin in the management of retained placenta. Gynecol Obstet Invest 2003;56:61–4.

63. Schrag S, Gorwitz R, Fultz-Butts K, Schuchar A. Prevention of perinatal group B streptococcal disease: revised guidelines from CDC. MMWR 2002;51 (RR-11):1–22.

64. Jolivet RR. Early-onset neonatal group B streptococcal infection: 2002 guidelines for prevention. J Midwif Womens Health 2002;47:435–66.

65. Barber EL, Zhao G, Buhimschi IA, Illuzzi JL. Duration of intrapartum prophylaxis and concentration of penicillin G in fetal serum at delivery. Obstet Gynecol 2008;112:265–70.

66. Wilson W, Taubert KA, Gewitz M, Lockhart PB, Baddour LM, Levinson M, et al. Prevention of infective endocarditis: guidelines from the American Heart Association. Circulation 2007;116(15):1736–54.

67. Mofenson LM. U.S. Public Health Service Task Force Perinatal HIV Guidelines Working Group. Recommendations for use of antiretroviral drugs in pregnant HIV-1-infected women for maternal health and interventions to reduce perinatal HIV-1 transmission in the United States. MMWR 2002;51(RR18):1–38. Available from: *http://www.cdc.gov/mmwr/preview/mmwrhtml/rr5118a1.htm* [Accessed September 30, 2009].

68. National Institutes of Health Consensus Development Statement. Effect of corticosteroids for fetal maturation on perinatal outcomes. Am J Obstet Gynecol 1995; 183:246–52.

69. Roberts D, Dalziel SR. Antenatal corticosteroids for accelerating fetal lung maturation for women at risk of preterm birth. Cochrane Database Syst Rev 2006; (3):CD004454.

70. ACOG committee opinion number 273. Antenatal corticosteroid therapy for fetal maturation. 2006 compendium of selected publications. Washington, DC: American College of Obstetricians and Gynecologists, 2002:11–22.

71. Gates S, Brocklehurst P. Decline in effectiveness of antenatal corticosteroids with time to birth: real or artifact? BMJ 2007;335:77–9.

72. Crowther CA, Harding JE. Repeat doses of prenatal corticosteroids for women at risk of preterm birth for preventing neonatal respiratory disease. Cochrane Database Syst Rev 2007;(2):CD003935.

73. Jobe AH, Soll RF. Choice and dose of corticosteroid for antenatal treatments. Am J Obstet Gynecol 2004;190:878–81.

74. Murphy KE. Betamethasone compared with dexamethasone for preterm birth: a call for trials. Obstet Gynecol 2007;110:7–8.

75. Elimian A, Garry D, Figueroa R, Spitzer A, Wiencek V, Quirk JG. Antenatal betamethasone compared with dexamethasone (Betacode trial): a randomized controlled trial. Obstet Gynecol 2007;110:26–30.

76. Mercer BM. Assessment and induction of fetal pulmonary maturity. In Creasy RK, Resnik R, Iams JD. Maternal-fetal medicine: principles and practice, 5th ed. Philadelphia, PA: Saunders, 2004:451–63.

77. Simkin P, O'Hara M. Non-pharmacologic relief of pain during labor: systematic reviews of five methods. Am J Obstet Gynecol 2002;186:S131–59.

78. Simkin P, Bolding A. Update on Nonpharmacologic approaches to relieve labor pain and prevent suffering. J Midwifery Womens Health 2004;489–505.

79. Abboud TK. Management of pain in parturition: the opoids. Female Patient 1994;19:29–36.

80. Smith CA, Collins CT, Cyna AM, Crowther CA. Complementary and alternative therapies for pain management in labour. Cochrane Database Syst Rev 2006; 18(4):CD003521.

81. Lowe NK. The pain and discomfort of labor and birth. JOGNN 1996;25(1):82–92.

82. Melzack R, Schaffelberg D. Low-back pain during labor. Am J Obstet Gynecol 1987;156(4):901–5.

83. Lederman RP, Lederman E, Work B Jr, McCann DS. Anxiety and epinephrine in multiparous women in labor: relationship to duration of labor and fetal heart rate pattern. Am J Obstet Gynecol 1985 Dec 15; 153(8):870–7.

84. Lagercrantz H, Slotkin TA. The "stress" of being born. Sci Am 1986;254(4):100–7.

85. Lederman RP, Lederman E, Work BA Jr, McCann DS. The relationship of maternal anxiety, plasma catecholamines, and plasma cortisol to progress in labor. Am J Obstet Gynecol 1978 Nov 1;132(5):495–500.

86. Zsigmond EK, Patterson RI. Double-blind evaluation of hydroxyzine hydrochloride in obstetric analgesia. Anesth Analg 1967;46:275–80.

87. Bricker L, Lavender T. Parenteral opioids for labor pain: a systematic review. Am J Obstet Gynecol 2002; 186:S94–109.

88. Guinsburg R, Wyckoff MH. Naloxone during neonatal resuscitation: acknowledging the unknown. Clin Perinatol 2006;22:121–32.

89. Eltzschig HK, Lieberman ES, Camann WR. Regional anesthesia and analgesia for labor and delivery. N Engl J Med 2003;348(4):319–32.

90. Lieberman E, O'Donoghue C. Unintended effects of epidural analgesia during labor: a systematic review. Am J Obstet Gynecol 2002;186(5)(suppl nature): S31–68.

91. Leighton BL, Halpern SH. The effects of epidural analgesia on labor, maternal, and neonatal outcomes: a systematic review. Am J Obstet Gynecol 2002;186(5) (suppl nature):S69–77.

92. Torvaldsen S, Roberts CL, Bell JC, Raynes-Greenow CH. Discontinuation of epidural analgesia late in labour for reducing the adverse delivery outcomes associated with epidural analgesia. Cochrane Database Syst Rev 2004(4):CD004457.

93. Anim-Somuah M, Smyth R, Howell C. Epidural versus non-epidural or no analgesia in labour. Cochrane Database Syst Rev 2005(4):CD000331.

94. Brancato RM, Church S, Stone PW. A meta-analysis of passive descent versus immediate pushing in nulliparous women with epidural analgesia in the second stage of labor. J Obstet Gynecol Neonatal Nurs 2008;37(1):4–12.

95. Mayberry LJ, Clemmens D, De A. Epidural analgesia side effects, co-interventions, and care of women during labor: a systematic review. Am J Obstet Gynecol 2002;186:S81–94.

96. Rosen M. Paracervical block for labor analgesia. A brief historic review. Am J Obstet Gynecol 2002; 186:S127–30.

97. Bishop J. Administration of nitrous oxide in labor: expanding options for women. J Midwifery Womens Health 2007;52:308–9.

98. Rosen M. Nitrous oxide for relief of labor pain: a systematic review. Am J Obstet Gynecol 2002;186: S110–27.

99. Niebyl JR, Blake DA, Johnson JW, King TM. The pharmacologic inhibition of premature labor. Obstet Gynecol Surv 1978;33(8):507–15.

100. Greenhouse BS, Hood R, Hehre FW. Aspiration pneumonia following intravenous administration of alcohol during labor. JAMA 1969;210(13):2393–5.

37
Postpartum

Mary Ann Rhode

Chapter Glossary

Baby blues Also called maternity or puerperal blues, this designates a transitory period of sadness that usually resolves spontaneously.

Hunting reaction The body's automatic, protective periodic vasodilation alternating with vasoconstriction by the autonomic nervous system as it hunts for equilibrium while attempting to prevent tissue damage.

Kleihauer-Betke Laboratory test used to ascertain how much fetal hemoglobin is in the maternal circulation. Usually performed after birth on women who are Rh(D)-negative to determine the required dose of Rho(D) immune globulin (RhoGAM).

Lactogenesis A series of cellular changes whereby mammary cells change from nonsecretory to secretory. There are two stages of lactogenesis. During the first stage, colostrum is produced and secreted. During the second stage, lactose is generated and copious amounts of breast milk are made.

Multimodal analgesia Also known as balanced analgesia, an approach to analgesia that uses concurrent administration of different classes of analgesics, each of which relieves pain by a different mechanism.

Postpartum depression (PPD) A puerperal mood disorder characterized by multiple depressive symptoms, anxiety, insomnia, and anhedonia.

Postpartum psychosis Major psychiatric condition that occurs during the postpartum period and usually includes a disassociation from reality as characterized by hallucinations. Infanticide and/or suicide are potential events that are linked with this disorder.

Preemptive analgesia Analgesia administered prior to surgery and as a means to reduce postoperative pain and postoperative analgesic, especially opiate, use.

Puerperium A synonym for postpartum.

Rosette test Qualitative laboratory test that detects D-antigen-positive RBCs in the maternal circulation. If the rosette test is positive, a Kleihauer-Betke test can be performed to determine the amount of fetal hemoglobin present in the maternal circulation. If negative, one ampule or 300 mcg Rho(D) immune globulin should be adequate.

Sitz baths From the German for *sit*, hydrotherapy of the body between the waist and the thighs. Also called hip baths. May be warm or ice cold.

Introduction

The postpartum period is a unique part of a woman's life, during which the most commonly occurring situations rarely require pharmacologic intervention. Although this chapter addresses the **puerperium**, some caveats must be noted. Many of the research studies that today's interventions are based upon were conducted decades ago. Postpartum is an area that aches for more rigorous, modern evidence, especially evidence that supports or refutes routine interventions. Also, this chapter discusses management of the postpartum woman who has given birth within 2–3 days and is generally still in a hospital. This approach was chosen since more than 90% of women in the United States give birth in hospitals. However, it should be noted that the principles of postpartum care and pharmacology remain regardless of whether or not the woman is in an in-hospital or out-of-hospital birth setting.

In the postpartum period, comfort measures often work well and minimize or eliminate the need for pharmacologic agents. Women who are not heavily medicated have more opportunities to accomplish essential tasks of the postpartum. Conversely, women who are appropriately medicated for discomforts that are not relieved by comfort measures have more energy to care for their infants when pain is reduced. Negotiating the fine line between overreliance on drugs and undermedication requires careful assessment and appropriate management by care providers. Yet there are few research studies regarding the effectiveness of comfort measures or pharmacologic agents, even though the latter are routinely ordered. A closer look at medications commonly used in the postpartum period, many of them over-the-counter agents, may facilitate the delivery of individualized care.

Physiologic Changes During the Postpartum Period

The puerperium, or postpartum period, is a time of rapid change physiologically. During this 6- to 8-week period women experience an involution of the uterus, **lactogenesis**, or initiation of lactation, and multiple endocrine changes as the body returns to a nonpregnant state.[1-4]

Motility in the gastrointestinal system is slowed in the immediate postpartum period. By the 10th postpartum day, the circulating blood volume has diminished secondary to urinary diuresis and returns to the normal prepregnant volume. Cardiac output increases in the immediate postpartum period, but then slowly declines until it reaches a nonpregnant state around 2 weeks postpartum. Bladder capacity has increased volume and occasionally decreased sensitivity that can result in urinary retention. Anatomic changes of pregnancy such as dilatation of ureters may take several months to resolve. Other changes that take several months include the resolution of the pregnancy-enlarged thyroid and the predisposition to higher postprandial glucose levels. These metabolic functions become normal by 8–12 weeks postpartum.

Considerations Prior to Prescribing Drugs in the Postpartum Period

Fortunately most pharmacologic agents have wide therapeutic ranges, and puerperal changes, although dramatic, rarely require modifications in dosing or choice of drugs. Drugs used to treat pathologic conditions such as diabetes and hypothyroidism may require some changes. In addition, prescribing drugs to lactating women requires careful assessment of the transfer of drugs to the newborn via breast milk.

Other factors need to be considered when ordering or administering medications to women during the postpartum period. Parity is important. First-time mothers may have minimal experience with discomforts that might require the use of medication. Second-time mothers are frequently surprised they are experiencing afterpains, since they did not have them after the first baby and often worry that these pains indicate something is wrong. In addition, the postpartum woman differs significantly from the nonpregnant or even pregnant woman physiologically and psychologically. She has a newborn for whom she must assume care. Treatment of her symptoms should be designed to minimize side effects that can limit a woman's ability to care for a newborn. All of these variables beg for true individualization of care in a medical environment that, for the most part, views this part of a woman's life as routine.

Pain

Postpartum women can experience pain from several different anatomic sites. Nipple pain, perineal pain due to trauma and/or edema, uterine pain, backache, painful hemorrhoids, and pain from a full bladder all require different interventions. Relieving the underlying problem is the first step in pain management. For those for whom pain medication becomes necessary, the analgesics listed in Table 37-1 are appropriate for various types of postpartum pain and may be used selectively in conjunction with available complementary alternative therapies.[5-12] It is important to remember that some women do not know ibuprofen is the generic name for Motrin or Advil, or that Tylenol and acetaminophen are the same medication. Thus it is important to educate women about these analgesics prior to sending them home with a prescription for one of them. Lack of knowledge can lead to inadvertent overdosing or unnecessary costs for a family who fills a recommended prescription for ibuprofen, not realizing they already have it at home under another name.

Postpartum Perineal Pain

A study published in 2004 reported perineal pain among postpartum women in one of three groups: (1) women who

Table 37-1 Analgesics Commonly Used in the Postpartum Period

Drug Generic (Brands)	Formulations	Indication and Dose	Recommendations for Lactation	Clinical Considerations
NSAIDs				
Acetaminophen (Tylenol)	325 mg, 500 mg	Mild to moderate pain 500 mg q 4–6 h with max 4 g/day	Compatible with breastfeeding.	Total acetaminophen daily dose should not exceed 3250 mg/day. Toxic metabolite, N-acetyl-p-benzoquinone-imine, present only in acute overdose or when maximum dose is exceeded over a prolonged period of time. Assist users to identify presence of acetaminophen in OTC combination medications to avoid exceeding maximum dose.
Ibuprofen (Motrin, Advil)	200, 400, 600 mg	Mild to moderate pain 600 mg q 6 h	Compatible with breastfeeding.	
Ketorolac tromethamine (Toradol)	15, 30, 60 mg for IM dose 10 mg for PO dose	Short-term treatment for postoperative pain 60 mg IM × 1 dose	Compatible with breastfeeding.	Can reduce opiate use by 25–45% and lower side effects attributable to opiate medications. One study of 10 mothers found that between 0.16% and 0.40% of the total daily maternal dose was excreted in breast milk. Switch to alternative analgesics as soon as possible. Side effects include GI ulcerations, bleeding, perforation, and postoperative bleeding. Use with caution if impaired maternal renal function or hypertension.
Codeine Combination Products				
Acetaminophen (Tylenol)/codeine	Tylenol with codeine No. 2: 300 mg acetaminophen/ 15 mg codeine Tylenol with codeine No. 3: 300 mg acetaminophen/ 30 mg codeine Tylenol No. 4: 300 mg acetaminophen/60 mg codeine	Moderate pain relief Tylenol No. 3 q 4–6 h	Compatible with breastfeeding.	Codeine is metabolized to morphine. Potential for abnormally high levels in breast milk of ultrarapid metabolizers of codeine. Choose lowest effective dose for shortest period of time. Mother to watch for increased sleepiness (more than usual), difficulty breastfeeding or breathing, or decreased tone in newborn.
Oxycodone/ acetaminophen (Percocet, Magnacet)	Percocet: 2.5/325 mg, 5/325 mg, 7.5/325 mg Magnacet: 5/400, 5/400; 7.5/400 mg	Moderate pain 1–2 tablets q 4–6 h Max dose of acetaminophen is 3250 mg/day	Limited human data.	Anecdotal information suggests probable compatibility with breastfeeding, although monitoring for neonatal sedation suggested. Percodan is oxycodone with aspirin and should be prescribed with caution in lactating women due to a theoretic risk of Reye syndrome and metabolic acidosis in the nursing infant.
Hydrocodone bitartrate and acetaminophen (Vicodin, Lortab, Lorcet)	Vicodin 5 mg/500 mg Lortab 2.5/500, 5/500, 7.5/500 Lorcet Plus 7.5 mg/650 mg Lorcet 10/650	Moderate pain 1–2 tablets q 4–6 h	No human data.	Anecdotal information suggests probable compatibility with breastfeeding. Report of hydrocodone excretion in breast milk in two cases. Infants received an estimated 3.1% and 3.7% of the maternal weight-adjusted dosage. Concluded moderate dosages of hydrocodone appear acceptable during breastfeeding, but more data are needed to determine the maximum safe dosage.
Morphine				
Morphine sulfate, opiate agonist analgesic	Several formulations for intravenous administration	Severe pain 5–10 mg IM or IV	Compatible with breastfeeding.	Additional opioids or sedatives should not be used. When placed in PCA or PCEA, patient-controlled dosing is continued until the woman is tolerating oral medications. All administration routes have the potential for clinically significant amounts of opiate in breast milk.
Meperidine (Demerol)	50, 100 mg/mL	Severe pain 50–100 mg IM q 1–3 h	Compatible with breastfeeding.	Use in breastfeeding mothers not recommended because of reports of neonatal sedation. Meperidine has active metabolites.

PCA = patient-controlled analgesia; PCEA = patient-controlled epidural analgesia; OTC = over the counter.
Sources: Koren G et al. 2006[5]; Windle ML et al. 1989[7]; Clark JH et al. 1981[8]; Anderson PO et al. 2007[9]; Pavy TJG et al. 2001[10]; Montgomery A et al. 2006.[11]

had an intact perineum; (2) those with a first- or second-degree laceration; and (3) those with an episiotomy. At day 1, the pain was 75%, 95%, and 97%, respectively, and by day 7, pain was still present with reported percentages of 38%, 60%, and 71%, respectively.[13]

When perineal pain is present, the goal is to increase maternal comfort and decrease edema. No optimal method for episiotomy or laceration repair has yet been identified.[14,15] Most practices traditionally employed for postpartum perineal care are not evidence based, and both non-pharmacologic and pharmacologic methods are often used in tandem.[16]

Perineal Splinting and Perineal Floor Exercises

Perineal splinting, or supporting the perineum with the fingers while having a bowel movement, can be suggested for women with a very edematous perineum. Although somewhat awkward to perform, case reports suggest this maneuver decreases pain that is secondary to Valsalva pushing efforts. Perineal floor exercises or Kegel's exercises may be useful in mobilizing edema and reducing pain. A prospective study of 198 women that evaluated the effects of intensive versus routine pelvic floor exercises found significantly fewer women in the intensive exercise group reporting perineal pain at 3 months ($P < .01$). No differences in stress incontinence, dyspareunia, or timing of resumption of intercourse were noted when the outcomes of women in the intensive group were compared to the outcomes of women who did not perform these measures.[17]

Application of Cold and Heat

Ice applied to the perineum immediately postpartum appears to minimize edema and increase comfort by reducing inflammation, decreasing capillary permeability, and reducing nerve conduction velocity. Ice should be applied intermittently; e.g., left in place for 20 to 30 minutes, and then removed for 30 to 60 minutes. Prolonged contact renders the therapy ineffective due to the **hunting reaction**, an automatic, protective periodic vasodilation alternating with vasoconstriction wherein the autonomic nervous system hunts for equilibrium while attempting to prevent tissue damage. Fortunately, most types of ice packs used in the postpartum period will melt or reach room temperature in approximately 30 minutes. Unless ice packs are immediately replaced when warm, the time interval of treatment probably avoids the hunting reaction in most cases. Ice therapy is useful for the first 24–48 hours, after which warm, moist heat, to draw blood flow to the area and mobilize edema, is more helpful.

Severe perineal pain and painful hemorrhoids may be treated with ice **sitz baths**. The idea of sitting down in a basin of ice water is unappealing and some women automatically reject the idea. The proper technique is to start with lukewarm water and gradually add crushed ice to the water. Analgesia from ice sitz baths can last for several hours.[18] A Cochrane review of the use of postpartum local cooling treatments found limited evidence supporting the effectiveness of cold sitz baths on the basis trials that had small sample sizes.[19]

The use of heat immediately after trauma or injury is inadvisable.[20,21] Moreover, many women voice an increase in discomfort from edema and throbbing pain. Appropriately, the use of warm sitz baths has declined. Postpartum women report comfort from warm baths or whirlpool baths, possibly because such immersion affects the whole body rather than just the perineum, or because relief of other sore muscles from second stage pushing is enough to distract women experiencing mild perineal discomfort. Additional studies are needed in the area of perineal pain and healing in order to develop evidence-based interventions in the future.

Herbal Sitz Bath Additives

Many over-the-counter herbal preparations are advertised for use either in sitz baths, for irrigation while urinating, or for perineal compresses. Botanicals such as calendula, comfrey, yarrow, rosemary, lavender, sage, uva ursi, garlic, myrrh, and shepherd's purse all have been proposed for use either individually or in combination with other herbs. These herbs are said to have either an astringent, antiseptic, or anti-inflammatory effect or a combination of the three. Randomized, controlled studies of lavender oil, salt, and a chlorhexidine gluconate/cetrimide (Savlon) concentrate found no statistically significant difference in pain relief associated with the use of these additives.[22] It is possible that sitz bath additives are effective, but they have not been adequately studied. These additives may simply provide a more pleasant experience during the postpartum recovery process.

Ointments, Compresses, Anesthetic Sprays, and Suppositories

Ointments, compresses using various solutions, and anesthetic sprays are often used for relief from perineal discomfort or pain. Most of these preparations have either not been studied or the only research is older and less rigorous in design.[23-27]

A randomized, controlled comparison of witch hazel compresses, ice, and pramoxine/hydrocortisone foam

(Epifoam) found no difference in pain relief among the three analgesics and no difference in timing of resumption of intercourse, wound healing, or resolution of perineal pain.[28] Similarly, a randomized, double-blind, placebo-controlled trial that compared 5% lidocaine ointment with a placebo found no significant reduction in pain using the lidocaine ointment.[29]

In summary, a Cochrane review of eight randomized clinical trials concluded that evidence for effectiveness of topically applied local anesthetics used to treat perineal pain is not compelling.[30] Another Cochrane review of the use of nonsteroidal anti-inflammatory (NSAID) rectal suppositories found two randomized, controlled trials that compared analgesic rectal suppositories with placebo. The women who received NSAID suppositories were less like to experience pain in the first 24 hours after birth (RR = 0.37; 95% CI, 0.10–1.38; 2 trials, 150 women) and requested less supplemental analgesia (RR = 0.31; 95% CI, 0.17–0.54; 1 trial, 89 women) than those in the placebo group.[31] However, suppositories have not been adopted much in the United States.

Use of topical steroids has decreased due to the concern that topical steroid use can impair wound healing. The use of sulfonamide vaginal creams, dimethyl sulfoxide (DMSO), and proteolytic enzymes from the papaya plant, which are consumed orally, have also been proposed, but evidence is lacking about the value of these agents in reducing postpartum perineal pain.

Compresses may be made from solutions such as magnesium sulfate solution (Epsom salts) by soaking sterile gauze pads in the chosen solution. Witch hazel (*Hamamelis virginiana*) compresses (Tucks) are the most commonly used, commercially available compresses. Witch hazel is an astringent and an anti-inflammatory agent in which the main active ingredient is tannin. The currently used distillation process removes the tannin, so today's commercially prepared witch hazel relies on the 14% alcohol content for the astringent action. Infusions (made from leaves and stems by pouring boiling water over the firm plant material such as bark, root, or nuts simmered in water for 20 minutes) of witch hazel do contain tannin. Although anecdotal reports advocate the use of witch hazel, there is little or no research on its effectiveness.

Arnica (*Arnica montana*) has been suggested for use in reducing postoperative pain, muscle aches, bruising, hemorrhoids, and edema. This agent is available as a homeopathic preparation and as an herbal product. The homeopathic preparation, taken orally, contains a minute amount of natural product in concert with the homeopathic principles of exposure to small amounts of agents. Research demonstrating the effectiveness of homeopathic arnica is inconclusive.[32] Herbal arnica, available commercially as a cream or ointment, is more potent and has been proposed for postpartum use on sore perineal or leg muscles.[33] There is little evidence about the effectiveness of topical arnica, and little information is available about the amounts of arnica absorbed when used topically, so use by women who are breastfeeding is discouraged. Topical use in high concentrations or for prolonged periods of time may cause blistering or scarring; therefore, use on broken skin or mucous membranes is not recommended.

Hemorrhoidal Pain

Postpartum women are predisposed to hemorrhoid development due to pressure during vaginal delivery, constipation, relaxation of the smooth muscles in vein walls, and impaired with blood return, which is secondary to increased pressure from the pregnant uterus, and finally, trauma sustained during birth adds additional risk factors.

Nonpharmacologic methods to control hemorrhoidal pain include ice packs, ice sitz baths, and digitally reinserting hemorrhoids into the rectum. Prevention or correction of constipation, advocating the use of side-lying position, and proper toileting habits and positions that minimize pushing pressure on the hemorrhoids during defecation are useful. Warm water sitz baths help relieve irritation and pruritus, possibly by relaxation of the internal anal sphincter.[34] A meta-analysis of seven controlled trials found that increasing dietary fiber significantly reduces episodes of bleeding from hemorrhoids (RR = 0.50; 95% CI, 0.28–0.68).[35]

Severe hemorrhoidal pain may require oral pain medication and topical analgesics with added corticosteroids to reduce pain, inflammation, and itching. Topical corticosteroids decrease inflammation by suppression of the migration of polymorphonuclear leukocytes and reversal of increased capillary permeability. Other over-the-counter preparations have not been shown to be efficacious, but are reported as useful by many women. Typically, these topical medications contain substances that have a vasoconstrictive and/or protective effect. These agents are not designed for long-term use, and little scientific evidence as to their benefits exists. Agents available for use in treatment of hemorrhoid symptoms are listed in Table 37-2.[35,36] In the absence of thrombosed hemorrhoids or rectal fissures, hemorrhoid pain will decrease over time, even without treatment. Additional information regarding treatment of hemorrhoids can be found in Chapter 21.

Nipple and Breast Pain

Nipple pain is difficult to treat with pain medication alone as it is often due to incorrect latch-on and/or removal of the nursing infant.[37] Early assistance with breastfeeding to ensure correct positioning can help prevent nipple trauma. Some nipple tenderness is to be expected. Research has shown that nipple tenderness should peak at approximately the third postpartum day and then begin to subside by the fifth postpartum day.[38] Even though multiple treatments, both nonpharmacologic and pharmacologic, have existed for millennia for nipple and breast pain, evidence is still scant and studies are ongoing. Intolerable nipple pain is never normal and requires careful evaluation.

A wide variety of topical creams, ointments, and gels are available without prescription and are commonly used for sore nipples. This group includes petrolatum, lanolin, beeswax, and glycerin-based products, hydrogel products, and antiseptic products. Many women find the use of these products comforting. Nipple care products are considered harmless but can be costly, and their use

Table 37-2 Pharmacologic Agents Used for Relief of Hemorrhoidal Pain

Drug Category Generic (Brand)	Mechanism of Action	Preparations Available	Clinical Considerations
Local anesthetics: benzocaine, benzyl alcohol, dibucaine, dyclonine, lidocaine, pramoxine, tetracaine (Nupercainal, Tronolane)	Block nerve conduction. For relief of pain, irritation, pruritus.	Spray, ointment, cream forms available OTC in concentrations of 0.5%, 1%, and 2.5%. Use of 1% preparation recommended.	Use longer than 1 week may result in contact dermatitis. Considered compatible with breastfeeding. Systemic effects are unlikely when used according to directions.
Steroids: hydrocortisone (Anucort-HC, Anusol-HC, Anusol HC-1, Cortaid intensive therapy, Cortizone-10 maximum strength, Dermtex HC, Nupercainal hydrocortisone cream, Preparation H hydrocortisone, Tucks anti-itch, Westcort)	Anti-inflammatory, lysosomal membrane stabilization, antimitotic and vasoconstrictive properties.	Aerosol, cream, ointment, gel, rectal suppository forms available over the counter in 0.2–2.5% concentrations.	Use longer than 1 week may result in mucosal atrophy. Compatible with breastfeeding. OTC products with hydrocortisone are not recommended by the FDA for anorectal use.
Fiber supplement laxatives	Promote easy passage of stool and decrease straining.	See Table 37-5.	Fiber supplementation reduces incidence of bleeding episodes. Aim for dose of 20–30 g/day.
Astringent/protectant/ vasoconstriction products: (Preparation H ointment, Tucks medicated wipes) contain astringents, protectants, or vasoconstrictors	Reduce trauma to tissues, promote hygiene.	Cream, ointment, gel, suppositories, medicated wipes.	Avoid excessive or aggressive wiping with harsh toilet tissue or use of astringent cleaners. Products listed as extra strength or maximum strength usually include a local anesthetic such as pramoxine 1%.
Astringents: calamine, hamamelis water—also known as witch hazel— zinc oxide	Coagulate proteins in surface skin cells, resulting in decreased cellular volume. Leaves a thin layer protecting underlying tissue. Decrease inflammation and irritation by decreasing mucus and secretions.	Cream, ointment.	Witch hazel for external use only.
Protectants: aluminum hydroxide gel, calamine, coco butter, cod liver oil, glycerin (external use only), shark liver oil, white petrolatum, hard fat, mineral oil, petrolatum, topical starch	Prevent water loss from the stratum corneum and decrease inflammation by forming a physical barrier.	Cream, ointment.	External use only.
Vasoconstrictors: ephedrine sulfate, epinephrine, phenylephrine HCl	Stimulate alpha-adrenergic receptors in vasculature and promote constriction of blood vessels to reduce swelling.	Creams, ointment.	External use only.

Sources: Alonso-Coello P et al. 2005[35]; Barnes CL et al. 2002.[36]

does not prevent cracks from developing. Only warm water, hydrogel products (for use on damaged, noninfected skin only), and purified lanolin have been shown to actually reduce soreness, with some suggestion that the hydrogel products may be the most effective of the three.[39] Applying expressed breast milk to nipples and allowing it to dry has been suggested to result in less nipple pain than wet compresses or air drying alone.[40]

Products that need to be removed from the nipple in order to limit infant exposure should be avoided because the process of removal may increase irritation and skin damage as opposed to treating the nipple. One of the most commonly used ointments, A and D ointment, does not need to be removed prior to nursing because it contains limited amounts of vitamins A and D. Cracked nipples may be treated with a compounded medication composed of betamethasone and mupirocin (Bactroban); however, RCTs that have evaluated their effectiveness are lacking at this time.

Breast Engorgement

Breast engorgement usually peaks in 3 to 5 days postpartum and usually subsides within the next 24 to 36 hours.[41] Years ago a variety of drugs were used to suppress lactation in women who did not want to breastfeed, but these agents had limited effectiveness and adverse side effects[42] (Box 37-1).

Treatments to mitigate the pain of breast engorgement include heat application, cold application, cabbage leaf compresses or cabbage leaf extract cream, breast massage and milk expression, ultrasound, breast pumping, and anti-inflammatory medications.[42] A meta-analysis of studies on postpartum breast engorgement found no difference in outcomes between treatment and control groups for cabbage leaves, cold packs, gel packs, oxytocin, or ultrasound treatments.[42] However, when compared to placebo, both serrapeptase (Danzen), an anti-inflammatory agent derived from silkworms, and a bromelain/trypsin complex significantly improved the total symptoms of engorgement (OR = 3.6; 95% CI, 1.3–10.3 and OR = 8.02; 95% CI, 2.8–23.3 respectively).[42] Serrapeptase has been used for more than 30 years in Europe and Japan, but is not FDA approved in the United States, and bromelain/trypsin can be obtained as a nutritional supplement.

Postoperative Cesarean Section Incision Pain

There is wide variation in the intensity of postoperative incision pain experienced by women who have had a cesarean section birth. Several studies have found an

---

Box 37-1 Gone But Not Forgotten: Lactation Suppressants

Bottle-feeding mothers often ask about the use of lactation suppressants, usually prompted by an older family member who remembers the use of such agents in the past. Lactation suppressants were frequently ineffective, caused rebound engorgement after a course of therapy was completed, and increased the risk for thromboembolic vents, convulsions, cerebral edema, and myocardial infarctions. In 1978, the FDA Advisory Committee for Reproductive Health Drugs recommended that approval be withdrawn for the use of estrogen-containing drug products for suppression of postpartum breast engorgement. The medications in question were diethylstilbestrol (Stilbestrol), chlorotrianisene (Tace), testosterone enanthate (Delatestryl), and estradiol valerate (Deladumone). The latter was the only injectable preparation.

Bromocriptine mesylate (Parlodel), an ergot derivative, was also used for lactation suppression. However, between June of 1993 and November of 1998, approval was gradually discontinued for use of all the lactation suppressant medications, including bromocriptine. As of this writing, no drugs have FDA approval as a lactation suppressant.

Source: Oladapo OT, Fawole B 2009.[115]

---

association between postoperative cesarean section pain and chronic pelvic pain.[43]

Postoperative cesarean section incision pain traditionally has required use of the opiate pain medications listed in Table 37-1. Routes for opiate medication administration include oral, intramuscular, intravenous, intrathecal, and epidural. The intravenous route has largely replaced intramuscular analgesia. Both intravenous patient-controlled analgesia (PCA) and patient-controlled epidural analgesia (PCEA) may be used and appear more efficacious than when the drugs are requested by the woman and then administered by a provider.[44]

Changes in obstetric practice such as allowing early intake of oral fluids and solids after cesarean section has also led some to question a primary reliance on traditional postcesarean pain management strategies that limit a woman's movement which can result in higher rates of nausea, vomiting, pruritus, urinary retention, constipation, and respiratory depression.[45]

Preemptive Analgesia

Preemptive analgesia refers to analgesia administered prior to surgery. This technique is being investigated as a means to reduce postoperative pain and postoperative opiate use via inhibition of central sensitization and the pain processing system.[46,47] Local anesthetics, opioids, and NSAIDs all can be used for preemptive analgesia. Studies on placement of local anesthetics preincision before cesarean section have been conflicting, so use of this technique is not widespread. However one randomized, controlled study that combined preincisional bupivacaine, intrathecal morphine, and oral ibuprofen plus acetaminophen reported significantly reduced postoperative pain ($P < .0001$) when compared with PCA morphine followed by oral acetaminophen plus codeine.[48] A meta-analysis of postoperative epidural analgesia studies including but not limited to cesarean section concluded that epidural analgesia, regardless of analgesic agent, provides better postoperative analgesia ($P < .01$) when compared to parenteral opiates, including PCA-controlled analgesia.[49]

Multimodal Analgesia

Multimodal analgesia, or balanced analgesic regimens, i.e., the concurrent administration of different classes of analgesics, has been found to be more effective than single agents.[48,50] Because each class of analgesics relieves pain via a different mechanism, they potentiate each other when administered together. NSAID use is associated with a 30–50% opiate-sparing effect for either systemic- or neuraxial-administered opiates.[51]

Ketorolac (Toradol) is an NSAID that is used intravenously either prior to surgery or for 24 hours after cesarean section.[10,52] Intramuscular ketorolac has been found to be as effective as intramuscular meperidine ($P < .05$) although less effective than epidural morphine.[10]

Scheduled Dosing

Scheduled dosing rather than as-needed dosing may also be more effective, especially for individuals who have severe pain. Administration of medications at fixed intervals to postoperative patients is mentioned by several authors as a strategy that increases a woman's satisfaction.[44] Relatively new devices that continuously infuse local anesthetic (bupivacaine or ropivacaine) directly into the incision site (e.g., On Q Pain Buster Post-op Relief System) can take advantage of both scheduled dosing and a multimodal analgesic regimen. Although no significant difference in pain scores between groups using a continuous local anesthetic infusion system infusing either bupivacaine or normal saline was noted in a randomized trial, women in the bupivacaine group used less postoperative morphine.[52] A small, randomized trial of women postcesarean section compared routine care with a group that was given a continuous infusion of ropivacaine (Naropin) into the incision. These investigators found that the women in the ropivacaine group had significantly reduced pain due to movement and reduced need for additional analgesics ($P < .01$) as well.[53]

Neuraxial Morphine Installation

Single-dose preservative-free morphine sulfate (Duramorph PF) placed into the neuraxial space is used widely by anesthesia providers immediately after cesarean section, as part of a multimodal approach to pain relief. Neuraxial morphine provides pain relief for long periods without loss of motor, sensory, or sympathetic function.

Generalized pruritus and urinary retention are common side effects. Women who receive neuraxial morphine need a Foley catheter to effectively drain the bladder for the first 24 hours after birth. Side effects, in general, respond to naloxone administration, which should be readily available whenever this technique is used. However, naloxone will inhibit the pain-relieving effect in addition to resolving side effects, so it is used as a last resort when pruritus is markedly uncomfortable. The neuraxial route produces negligible maternal plasma levels of morphine and is compatible with breastfeeding.

Neuraxial administration can cause acute respiratory depression and/or respiratory arrest or delayed respiratory depression for up to 24 hours, so the use of neuraxial morphine requires observation in an environment with personnel skilled in resuscitation. Most institutions require that all pain medication be ordered by the anesthesia staff overseeing the patient during the first 24 postoperative hours.[54] Women who have a depleted blood volume or who are administered other drugs such as phenothiazines or general anesthetics have an increased risk of significant hypotension. Dysphoric reactions and toxic psychoses are possible.

Management of Postoperative Pain for Women on Methadone

Women who are on methadone maintenance are a unique subset of individuals who require extra help in controlling postcesarean section pain. These women can require up to 70% more opiate medication following cesarean section when compared to the medication requirements of women who are not on methadone. Unfortunately, these women may be the least likely to receive adequate pain relief based on misconceptions of care providers regarding their pain relief needs.[55] The usual daily oral methadone dose should be resumed as soon as possible after delivery. Opioid antagonists or mixed antagonist/agonists should not be administered to women who are on methadone maintenance because these agents can trigger withdrawal symptoms.

Treatments for Gas Pains

Thomas et al., in an era in which early ambulation was not common, studied the effects of several regimens, including various combinations of low gas-producing foods, simethicone, rocking, and bisacodyl suppositories for relief of gas pains.[56] Rocking for 60 minutes or more a day (possibly the equivalent of contemporary early ambulation) reduced gas pains. Simethicone use combined with rocking was no more effective than simethicone alone. Bisacodyl suppositories used independently were even less effective.[56]

Afterpains

Approximately 50% of primiparas and 86% of multiparas experience uterine cramping or afterpains, with multiparas describing afterpains as more severe.[57] Cramping during breastfeeding also increases as parity increases.[58] Therefore, an analgesic prior to nursing can be useful and is perhaps and interesting example of preemptive analgesia (Box 37-2). Uterine cramping is theorized to be due to prostaglandin release, a myometrial stimulant. Discomfort rarely lasts more than 2 or 3 days. Afterpains are often subjectively felt as back pain, a fact that can be confusing to new mothers. Common alternative methods for relief of afterpains can provide relief in up to 40% of women.[57] Nonsteroidal anti-inflammatory drugs are particularly effective in reducing afterpains due to their antiprostaglandin properties.[59,60]

Effect of Methylergonovine on Afterpains

In the past, 0.2 mg of methylergonovine (Methergine) was administered routinely every 4 hours for six doses to minimize bleeding. It was not uncommon for women to refuse to take the methylergonovine or to surreptitiously discard it because of the increased pain they experienced. This

---

Box 37-2 Caution with Codeine

MR is a 20-year-old primigravida who had a prolonged labor, and a forceps delivery was performed. She had a midline episiotomy with a fourth-degree extension.

At 20 hours postpartum, she had significant perineal edema and requested pain medication. Acetaminophen 325 g/codeine 30 mg (Tylenol No. 3) was ordered to be administered orally every 4 hours, but MR's pain was not well controlled on this regimen. The dose was changed to acetaminophen 325 mg/codeine 60 mg (Tylenol No. 4) to be given orally every 4 hours, and that dose improved pain control but she was not pain-free. MR planned to breastfeed but her nurse stated MR was having difficulty initiating breastfeeding because both she and her infant were very drowsy much of the time. The infant appeared to have poor tone.

This woman is a member of an ethnic group that has a 16–28% incidence of a specific CYP2D6 genotype that metabolizes codeine very rapidly to its active metabolite, morphine. Her drowsiness may be due to a lengthy and difficult labor or it may be a sign that she is an ultrarapid metabolizer of codeine, which leads to higher than expected maternal serum and breast milk morphine levels. It was important that all available alternative comfort measures be utilized to minimize her need for opiate medication.

Because the sedation effect of codeine was inhibiting MR's ability to care for herself and her infant, there were several choices that could be made. Her medication order could be changed to a non–codeine-containing medication such as propoxyphene/acetaminophen (Darvon) or hydrocodone (Dilaudid), which is not metabolized via the CYP enzyme system and does not have an active metabolite. An NSAID could also be added to the regimen so she could have the benefit of multimodal analgesia.

practice was discontinued when research demonstrated that blood loss with the methylergonovine regimen was not statistically different from blood loss in untreated women. Subsequently, anecdotal reports were made of the need for decreased analgesia since cramping produced by methylergonovine could be severe. Intramuscular methylergonovine can be used as an adjunct to oxytocin to reduce excessive bleeding due to atony immediately postpartum. Women will appreciate providers who anticipate the impending need for pain medication when administering methylergonovine.

Postpartum Infections

Fever in the postpartum period can be secondary to urinary tract infection, endomyometritis, mastitis, surgical site infection (cesarean delivery incision, episiotomy, or perineal lacerations), and more rarely pelvic abscess, anesthesia complications, or deep vein thrombosis. Causes unrelated to pregnancy such as appendicitis or viral syndrome are also possible.

Since 1935, postpartum febrile morbidity has been defined by the United States Joint Commission on Maternal Welfare as an oral temperature of ≥ 38.0°C (100.4°F) on any 2 of the first 10 days postpartum or 38.7°C (101.6°F) or higher during the first 24 hours. Isolated, single fever spikes < 38.7°C that occur during the first 24 hours are common and do not require treatment.[61,62]

Urinary Tract Infection

Asymptomatic bacteriuria is present in as many as 17% of women on the first postpartum day, with spontaneous resolution in approximately 75% by the third postpartum day.[63,64] Symptomatic urinary tract infections are the most common cause of postpartum febrile illness in the postpartum period. Risks include previous urinary tract infection, catheterization, sterile vaginal exams during labor, and trauma to the bladder and/or urethra during labor and birth.[65]

Choice of therapeutic agent is based on the specific organism involved, but because women have an increased risk for developing pyelonephritis during this time, treatment is started empirically before urine culture results are available. The pathogens found in postpartum women are the same pathogens that cause urinary tract infections in pregnancy and in nonpregnant women; therefore, a 3-day course of trimethoprim/sulfamethoxazole (Bactrim,

Septra) is the antibiotic regimen of choice unless the woman has an allergy to sulfa or resides in an area that has significant resistance to trimethoprim/sulfamethoxazole. This agent causes eradication of pathogens and cure in approximately 94% of cases.[63] If trimethoprim/sulfamethoxazole is contraindicated, a 3-day course of ciprofloxacin (Cipro) or a 7-day course of nitrofurantoin (Macrodantin, Macrobid) can be substituted.

Trimethoprim/sulfamethoxazole (Bactrim, Septra) should not be given to breastfeeding mothers whose infants have hyperbilirubinemia or who have known G6PD deficiency. Because even a small amount of nitrofurantoin (Macrodantin, Macrobid) can cause a hemolytic reaction, it should not be prescribed to individuals who have a risk for G6PD deficiency. Trimethoprim/sulfamethoxazole and nitrofurantoin are considered compatible with breastfeeding by the American Academy of Pediatrics.[64] Ciprofloxacin (Cipro) is also considered compatible with breastfeeding by the American Academy of Pediatrics but is not the first choice. Fluoroquinolone use during lactation has been controversial because juvenile animal studies found an association between fluoroquinolones and cartilage damage.

Pyelonephritis is usually treated with hospitalization and ciprofloxacin (Cipro) or a combination of ampicillin (Principen) and gentamicin (Garamycin) administered intravenously until the fever and acute symptoms have subsided.

Endometritis

Postpartum endometritis, also called endomyometritis, is a polymicrobial infection of several gram-positive or gram-negative aerobes and anaerobes. Many risk factors for endometritis exist, with cesarean delivery, especially nonelective cesarean delivery, being the most prominent. Endometritis onset can occur early (within 48 hours) or late (up to 6 weeks) in the postpartum period. Antibiotic treatment is initiated on the basis of fever and clinical symptoms such as uterine tenderness, foul-smelling lochia, chills, and lower abdominal pain. At present, a treatment regimen of clindamycin (Cleocin) (900 mg every 8 hours) and gentamicin (Garamycin) (1.5 mg/kg every 8 hours for women with normal renal function) administered intravenously is considered the gold standard and is often the control regimen for clinical trials of other treatment regimens.[66] Fever should resolve within 48 to 72 hours of treatment, and the antibiotics should be discontinued once the woman has been afebrile for 24 hours if she had a vaginal birth and after 48 hours if she had a cesarean section. Oral antibiotic therapy after intravenous therapy is not indicated.[67]

Episiotomy Dehiscence

The incidence of episiotomy dehiscence is approximately 0.1–2.1%.[68] Predisposing factors include infection, human papillomavirus, cigarette smoking, morbid obesity, and coagulation disorders. Superficial breakdown and localized redness is treated with expectant management and perineal care. If purulent drainage and/or systemic symptoms are present, antibiotic treatment, debridement, and rerepair will be performed. Formerly, repair was delayed for several months to allow the wound to granulate and heal, which posed a significant hardship for the woman without clear benefits. However, early repair is safe and effective.[68] The preoperative protocol includes intravenous antibiotics, removal of all sutures, debridement of necrotic tissue, sitz baths several times daily, and scrubbing of the wound twice daily with a povidone iodine- (Betadine-) impregnated scrub brush.

Mastitis

Mastitis, or inflammation of the breast(s), refers to a spectrum of conditions that develop most commonly between 2 and 3 weeks postpartum. However, mastitis can occur anytime from 5 days to 1 year postpartum. The most common etiologic organism is *Staphylococcus aureus*, although other organisms include group A and B streptococci, *Haemophilus influenzae*, and *Haemophilus parainfluenzae*. Breast abscess formation is associated with delay of antibiotic treatment and abrupt weaning during an episode of mastitis. Risk factors for mastitis include fatigue, cracked nipples, plugged/blocked ducts, ample milk supply, engorgement, and milk stasis.

Increased fluids, bed rest, frequent breastfeeding, moist heat applications, and nonopioid analgesics usually are instituted at the first signs of mastitis. Antibiotics are indicated if fever is present or if no improvement is seen in afebrile women after 12–24 hours.

Treatment options for the various stages and types of mastitis are listed in Table 37-3.[69,70] Antibiotic treatment for less than 10 to 14 days is associated with recurrent mastitis. Vitamin E-rich sunflower,[71] echinacea,[72] and vitamin C[73] have also been mentioned as being helpful in prevention or treatment of mastitis, although scientific evidence is lacking.

Postpartum Depression

Puerperal changes often are discussed solely from a physiologic point of view. However, it is increasingly apparent that the psychologic health of a woman can be at risk during this period of time. The vast majority of new mothers experience some degree of sadness and moodiness in the first 10 days after giving birth, with the peak incidence at 5 days postpartum and usual resolution within 48 to 72 hours.[74] For years this has been called the **baby blues**, postpartum blues, and maternity blues. Regardless of semantics, the blues are recognized as a condition that generally resolves with restorative sleep. The etiology of this transitory depression is unknown, but it may be related to the changing hormonal milieu. However, sleep deprivation is an obvious putative etiology.

Postpartum Depression

Postpartum depression (PPD) can occur any time within the first year postpartum and affects approximately 13% of all new mothers. This condition has been recognized for centuries. The gynecologist Tortula from the medical school at Salerno wrote the following in the 11th century: "If the womb is too moist, the brain is filled with water and the moisture running over to the eyes, compels them to involuntarily shed tears." PPD is a condition that shares some of the same symptoms as the blues but has more severe forms.

PPD is defined as a major depressive disorder that occurs within 1 month of childbirth. PPD is not recognized by the Diagnostic and Statistical Manual of Mental Disorders (DSM-IV) as distinct from major depressive illness; thus, the criteria for diagnosing PPD are the same criteria used to diagnose depression in nonpregnant individuals. However, many of these symptoms are common normal sequela of childbirth and therefore, in clinical practice, the diagnosis of PPD can be challenging. Symptoms of depression include depressed mood, lack of pleasure or interest, insomnia, excessive sleeping, diminished concentration, weight loss, agitation, feelings of worthlessness or inappropriate guilt, anxiety, changes in libido, eating disturbances, difficulty in performing activities of daily living, and thoughts of death or suicide.[75]

Although there is no simple, single diagnostic instrument for PPD, the Edinburgh Postnatal Depression Scale often is used both in research and clinical sites. A score of more than 12 on this scale is used as indication

Table 37-3 Pharmacologic Treatments for Mastitis

Disorder	Antibiotics	Antifungal*	Other Therapy
Blocked duct/nipple blebs	Mupirocin 2% ointment (not cream) if blocked pore (bleb) opened.	Only if recurrent or persistent then culture nipple/areola, bleb if present and milk. Fluconazole: (Diflucan) 200–400 mg daily for 2–3 weeks or until blocked duct has resolved for 1 week. Consider undiagnosed maternal IgA deficiency.	If no improvement within 24–48 hours, then order therapeutic ultrasound 2 watts/cm², continuous, for 5 minutes once a day to the affected region. It may be repeated once the next day. Lecithin one tablespoon per day or 1200 mg 3–4 times per day can be used to prevent or treat recurrences. If recurrent, have mother limit saturated fats and increase rest. Lecithin can also be rubbed into a bleb to soften it.
Noninfectious mastitis	If symptoms do not resolve within 12–24 hours, then treat for infectious mastitis as below.	None.	Hot compresses, massage of affected area, frequent milk removal on affected side.
Infectious mastitis	Dicloxacillin (Dynapen) 500 mg qid for 10–14 days or cephalexin (Keflex) 500 mg qid for 10–14 days. If penicillin allergic, use clindamycin 300 mg qid or erythromycin 250 mg or 500 mg qid for 10–14 days.	If indicated based on cultures or the development of burning breast pain.	As noted for noninfectious mastitis above. Cultures of milk and nipple indicated for maternal acute illness, failure to respond to treatment, high suspicion of MRSA, bilateral mastitis. Infant may need to be treated concurrently particularly if group A or B Streptococcus suspected.
Recurrent mastitis	Culture and treat as appropriate for 14–30 days.	Culture and treat as appropriate for 14–30 days.	Low dose erythromycin or clindamycin may be given on a daily or weekly basis. Consider cultures and treatment with nasal mupirocin (Bactroban) if S aureus carrier state suspected.
Ductal infections	Culture and treat for at least 14 days. Can empirically start treatment with clindamycin 300 mg qid or sulfamethoxazole-trimethoprim (Bactrim) double strength bid.	Treat with antifungals if any signs of yeast on infant. First line. Fluconazole: fluconazole (Diflucan) 200–400 mg as one dose followed by 100–200 mg daily for 2–3 weeks or until symptoms have resolved for 1 week. Ketoconazole (Nizoral) may also be used.	Sterilize any object that comes in contact with maternal breast, breast milk, or infant mouth; e.g., pumping parts, bottles, pacifiers, toys. Consider other family members as carriers if yeast is recurrent.
Nipple infections	Mupirocin 2% ointment (not cream): 15 grams or polymyxin B sulfate (Bacitracin) If no improvement, culture and treat based on sensitivity results or treat empirically for yeast. Apply mupirocin or polymyxin after each nursing or pumping.	Nystatin (Nilstat) Neonate: 100,000 units/mL. Place 1 mL in cup, then swab inside of infant's mouth qid. Use 2 mL qid for older infants. Have infant drink what is left. Maternal: May treat topically with nystatin (Nilstat) suspension or with cream. Apply cream or suspension after each nursing. Allow suspension to air dry or if using cream, rub in small amount. Gentian violet 1% in 10% alcohol can be applied to the infant's mouth with a cotton swab before feeding so the nipple will be coated during the feeding. Use daily for 4–7 days. Apply clotrimazole cream (Gyne-Lotrimin) after each feeding/pumping and rub in well.	The following topical treatment, Dr. Newman's "All purpose nipple ointment" (APNO) will treat bacterial and yeast infections. APNO is compounded and contains mupirocin 2% ointment (not cream) 15 grams. Betamethasone 0.1% ointment (not cream): 15 grams Add miconazole powder to formulate a final concentration of 2% miconazole. If miconazole is unavailable, substitute clotrimazole powder added so the final concentration is 2% clotrimazole. Sparingly apply APNO after each feeding and use until nipple soreness has dissipated.
Abscess (puerperal)	Outpatient: Dicloxacillin (Dynapen) 500 mg PO qid for 10–14 days or clindamycin (Cleocin) 300 mg PO qid. Inpatient: Nafcillin or oxacillin 2.0 g every 4 hours IV or cefazolin 1.0 g every 6 hours IV or vancomycin 1.0 g every 12 hours IV.	If indicated based on cultures or the development of burning breast pain.	I and D (incision and drainage) or use ultrasound-guided needle for aspiration. Send aspirate or discharge for culture. Infants may continue nursing on affected side unless the area of incision involves the areola. May want to treat infant concurrently if S aureus or streptococcal disease is present.

MRSA = methicillin-resistant staphylococcus aureus. * If Candida is suspected or diagnosed, mother and infant must be treated concurrently even if one is asymptomatic.
Source: Reprinted with permission from Betzhold CM 2007.[70]

that the woman probably has PPD.[76] The *Postpartum Depression Predictors Inventory Revised* also is being proposed as a useful screen.[76] Several risk factors are associated with PPD. Prominent among them is a previous history of depression, including previous postpartum mood disorder. Other risk factors include high anxiety during pregnancy, stressful life events, previous premenstrual dysphoria, poor social support, marital conflict, and young maternal age.[77,78]

Untreated depression is associated with multiple adverse infant outcomes including heightened arousal and poor self-regulation in infancy, negative maternal-infant interactions, impaired child development, and poor cognitive function. It is not clear if treatment of PPD improves infant development, but given the serious effects of untreated disease, most research in this area has focused on identification of effective therapies.

Studies have been conducted in which women at risk for postpartum depression were treated prophylactically with antidepressants during pregnancy. However, these studies were small and not of rigorous design, so prophylaxis with antidepressants was not proven effective nor determined to be ineffective.[77]

Psychotherapeutic treatments have a decisive but modest effect in improving symptoms of postpartum depression yet long-term evaluation of therapy is lacking.[78] Interpersonal psychotherapy, cognitive-behavioral therapy, psychodynamic therapy, supportive counseling, and psychoeducation have been evaluated and found to be effective. Although therapy in conjunction with antidepressants has proven efficacy, it is unclear exactly which combination of interventions is best for a particular individual.[79]

Prior to initiating treatment with an antidepressant, it is critical that postpartum depression be diagnosed accurately and other disorders ruled out. Symptoms of depression are also symptoms of bipolar disorder, and antidepressants can trigger a manic episode if the problem is bipolar disorder rather than depression. Assessment for suicidality or thoughts of harming the infant are indications of possible postpartum psychosis and require immediate psychiatric evaluation and probable hospitalization for inpatient care.

Multiple antidepressants can be used for women with PPD (Table 37-4). If the individual has successfully used an antidepressant prior to pregnancy, that agent should be restarted.[80] For women who are naïve to antidepressant therapy, selective serotonin reuptake inhibitors are generally the first choice as they have low toxicity and are easy to administer. Fluoxetine (Prozac) was one of the first used and remains a mainstay. Tricyclic antidepressants are also effective but have more undesirable side effects. Although head-to-head drug studies to determine a single first-line agent that is most effective are lacking, sertraline (Zoloft) is often recommended for initial therapy if the woman has no prior history of antidepressant use because it has negligible effects on the newborn. Chapter 25 provides additional details about the pharmacologic effects of antidepressants and suggested patient education when initiating antidepressant therapy.

The drug regimen for treating postpartum depression occurs in three phases: acute initial dosing, continuation dosing, and maintenance dosing. Because women during the postpartum period are especially sensitive to the side effects of these drugs, they are usually started at half the recommended starting dose for the first 4 days then increased weekly until full remission is evident. It is generally recommended that drug therapy continue for 9–12 months, at which time the drug is gradually titrated down and discontinued. Maintenance treatment is recommended for persons who have had more than three episodes of major depression within three years.

Use of antidepressants during lactation is an important issue. No data suggest that any of the aforementioned agents are contraindicated for the breastfeeding dyad. Table 37-4 summarizes the effects of commonly used antidepressants on a breastfeeding infant. More information can be found in Chapter 38.

Nonpharmacologic treatments that have been proposed include dietary manipulation, such as increased omega 3 acids, protein, B vitamins, St. John's wort, kava, traditional Chinese medicine, massage, and acupuncture.[78] Although there have been small studies evaluating these techniques, overall, evidence of effectiveness remains lacking. The interested reader is referred to reviews of the topic.

Postpartum Psychosis

Postpartum psychosis is an entity distinct from the blues or postpartum depression. Postpartum psychosis occurs in 1 in 500 mothers. This disorder has a rapid onset and usually appears in the first 2 weeks after giving birth. A woman with this condition experiences hallucinations and delusions and may report hearing voices. Any woman who has serious compulsions to harm herself or her child/ children should immediately receive expert psychiatric

Table 37-4 Pharmacologic Treatment for Postpartum Depression

Drug Generic (Brand)	Starting Dose	Maintenance Dose and Maximum Dose	Clinical Considerations	Implications for Breastfeeding
Serotonin Selective Reuptake Inhibitors (SSRIs)				
Citalopram (Celexa)	10–20 mg/day	20–40 mg/day Max dose is 60 mg/day	SE: nausea, vomiting, dizziness Few drug–drug interactions	May produce detectable serum levels in some infants Case reports of newborn somnolence reported
Escitalopram (Lexapro)*	10 mg/day	5–20 mg/day	Active metabolite of citalopram and has the same SE, however escitalopram is more potent and generally better tolerated	Case reports of newborn somnolence reported
Fluoxetine (Prozac)*	10–20 mg/day	20 mg/day Max dose is 80 mg/day	Long half-life of both drug and active metabolite SE: dizziness, nausea, anorexia, anxiety, sexual dysfunction	Serum level in infant similar to equivalent serum level in adult in infants who are symptomatic Case reports of colic, irritability, poor feeding, and drowsiness
Fluvoxamine (Luvox)*	50 mg/day	50–100 mg bid Max dose is 300 mg/day	No active metabolites SE: Can be sedating, nausea common, sexual dysfunction Drug–drug interactions with Coumadin (warfarin)	Levels not detected in infant. No adverse effects have been reported
Paroxetine (Paxil)*	10–20 mg	20 mg/day in divided doses Max dose is 60 mg/day	No active metabolites SE: more anticholinergic effects than other SSRIs, sedating, sexual dysfunction Avoid use in adolescents Serum levels increased by cimetidine (Tagamet)	Low or undetectable levels in infant serum No adverse effects reported
Sertraline (Zoloft)*	25–50 mg/day	50–100 mg/day Max dose is 200 mg/day	Weakly active metabolite SE: not sedating, diarrhea Bioavailability increased with food	Low or undetectable levels in infant serum No adverse effects reported
Tricyclic Antidepressants				
Amitriptyline (Elavil)	25–50 mg/day	25–100 mg/day Max dose is 300 mg/day	SE: Highly sedating, and anticholinergic effects	Low or undetectable levels in infant serum No adverse effects reported
Desipramine (Norpramin)	25–50 mg/day	50–200 mg/day Max dose is 300 mg/day	SE: Sedation, weight gain, anticholinergic effects, orthostatic hypotension May be activating and therefore usually given at night Baseline ECG recommended[†]	Low or undetectable levels in infant serum No adverse effects reported
Nortriptyline (Aventyl, Pamelor)*	10–25 mg/day	75–100 mg/day Max dose is 150 mg/day	Twice as potent as other TCAs SE: Sedation, weight gain, anticholinergic effects, orthostatic hypotension Baseline ECG recommended[†]	Low or undetectable levels in infant serum No adverse effects reported
Other				
Bupropion (Wellbutrin SR, Zyban)*	100 mg bid	150 mg bid Max dose is 400 mg in divided doses	Active metabolite SE: agitation, dry mouth, headache dizziness, nausea, No sexual side effects Increased risk of seizure for persons with bulimia. Dosing must titrate up.	Low or undetectable levels in infant serum No adverse effects reported

(continues)

Table 37-4 Pharmacologic Treatment for Postpartum Depression (*continued*)

Drug Generic (Brand)	Starting Dose	Maintenance Dose and Maximum Dose	Clinical Considerations	Implications for Breastfeeding
Mirtazapine (Remeron)	15 mg/day	15–45 mg/day Max dose is 45 mg/day	SE: dry mouth, somnolence, nausea, dizziness Low incidence of sexual dysfunction Administer at night	Unknown
Nefazodone (Serzone)*	50–100 mg/day	200 mg bid Max dose is 600 mg/day	SE: dry mouth, somnolence, nausea, dizziness	Few case reports of adverse effects in newborn (premature infant)
Selective norepinephrine reuptake inhibitors				
Venlafaxine (Effexor)	37 mg bid	75 mg bid Max dose is 375 mg/day in divided doses	SE: hypertension, diaphoresis, anxiety, headache, jitteriness, nausea, insomnia, sexual dysfunction Particularly helpful for refractory depression	Undetectable or low serum levels of drug Metabolite is measurable at levels similar to those in adults. Drug level may be higher in breast milk than in maternal serum
Venlafaxine (Effexor, Effexor SR)	37.5–75 mg qid	150 mg/day Max dose is 225 mg/day	SE: hypertension, diaphoresis, anxiety, headache, jitteriness, nausea, insomnia, sexual dysfunction Particularly helpful for refractory depression	Undetectable or low serum levels of drug Metabolite is measurable at levels similar to those in adults. Drug level may be higher in breast milk than in maternal serum

SE = side effects; SSRI = selective serotonin reuptake inhibitor.
* Multiple drug–drug interactions because it is an inhibitor of CYP450 enzymes.
† If the ECG shows conduction defects, consider a nontricyclic antidepressant.

intervention, including admission for inpatient care and the use of antipsychotic pharmacologic agents.[81,82]

Anemia

The two most common reasons for anemia in the postpartum period are preexisting iron deficiency anemia and acute blood loss at the time of delivery.[83] It is important to distinguish between the two. Women with chronic iron deficiency anemia may be in any of three stages of iron deficiency: iron depletion (iron stores are low but hemoglobin levels are adequate), iron deficiency without anemia (low serum iron and transferrin saturation), or iron deficiency anemia with low hemoglobin levels. Examination of the initial prenatal hemoglobin/hematocrit values, the values obtained during late second trimester, and the values obtained on admission in labor can provide a picture of the severity and duration of anemia. The need for postpartum iron supplementation can be identified based on these values, even before knowing the amount of blood loss after delivery (Table 37-5).

A woman with high prenatal hemoglobin/hematocrit values, presumably adequate iron stores, and a large blood loss may recover well without additional iron supplementation or with a shorter course of supplementation than a woman who had iron deficiency anemia prior to birth. Multiparous women, particularly those with short intervals between pregnancies, are more likely to have depleted iron stores, as are women with multiple fetuses, wherein the demand for iron during pregnancy is higher than normal. Women who have declined to take iron preparations during pregnancy due to gastrointestinal side effects should be reminded that both vitamins and iron are often better tolerated in the nonpregnant state.

Postpartum blood tests for anemia can be misleading. Absolute levels are variable due to level of hydration, the amount of blood loss, preexisting hemoglobin levels, altitude (higher normal values at higher altitudes), and timing of the blood draw after birth. Nelson found that no single timed hematocrit determination in the first 24 hours after delivery detected the maximum drop in hemoglobin or hematocrit in most women. He recommended that postpartum hematocrits be obtained no sooner than 16 hours after birth unless clinically necessary.[84] Several authors have argued that a routine postpartum hematocrit is unnecessary for a clinically stable woman assuming she had an estimated blood loss of less than 500 mL after a vaginal birth.[85] In addition,

Table 37-5 Examples of Varying Needs for Postpartum Iron Supplementation After Vaginal Birth

Woman's Gravidity/Parity	G2 P1001 Hgb/Hct	G5 P4004 Hgb/Hct	G1 P0000 Hgb/Hct	G1 P0000 Hgb/Hct	G3 P1011 Hgb/Hct	G3 P2002 Hgb/Hct
Initial prenatal hematocrit/hemoglobin	40.4/13.9	32.4/10.9	41.4/14.4	39.5/13.0	32.3/10.2	26.7 /8.9
Antepartum ferritin/transferrin saturation values	Not indicated	Not indicated	Not indicated	Not indicated	Not indicated	Decreased ferritin, increased transferrin
Prenatal hematocrit/ hemoglobin at 26–28 weeks	38.8/13.0	30.8/10	39.1/14.3	38.1/13.2	30.8/10	27.8/9
Admission hematocrit/ hemoglobin	41.6/14.0	32.1/10.9	41.0/14.0	39.0/13.4	29.3/9.7	29.1/9.7
Estimated blood loss greater than 500 mL?	No	No	Yes	Yes	Yes	No
Postpartum orthostatic symptoms present?	No	No	No	Yes	Yes	No
Postpartum hematocrit/ hemoglobin	Not indicated, unlikely to change management plan	Not indicated, unlikely to change management plan	34.3/10.8	27.9/9.3	20.3/6.9	Not indicated, unlikely to change management plan
Postpartum iron supplementation?	Not needed.	Yes, correct preexisting chronic anemia.	Acute anemia without evidence of preexisting iron deficiency. Iron in prenatal vitamins and diet may be sufficient to correct anemia.	Yes, correct significant acute anemia.	Yes, correct both chronic and acute anemia. Blood transfusion may be considered if severe orthostatic symptoms persist.	Yes, continue iron supplementation started antepartum to correct chronic but improving iron deficiency anemia. Monitor for improvement.

postpartum hematocrit levels are not reliable markers for the need for postpartum iron supplements and correlate poorly with postpartum serum ferritin levels. When necessary, differential diagnosis of anemia should wait until blood parameters return to normal nonpregnant values 1–3 weeks after the birth.

The usual recommended dose for maximal rate of hemoglobin regeneration is 150–200 mg of elemental iron daily, taken in divided doses to minimize side effects. Iron absorption can vary greatly between individuals. As a woman recovers from anemia, the rate of change in hemoglobin levels slows. Rebuilding iron stores is a slow process that may take up to a year, with various sources recommending from 3 to 12 months of therapy after hematocrit/hemoglobin levels return to normal. It is clear that further research to determine reliable indicators for postpartum iron supplementation and best dose schedules to enhance compliance would be beneficial.

Orange juice, meat, poultry, and fish enhance dietary iron absorption while cereals, tea, red wine, and milk inhibit it.[86] Iron is best absorbed between meals, but ferrous

supplements may need to be taken with food to minimize gastric upset.

There are many different formulations of iron available. Iron can cause bothersome gastrointestinal side effects such as heartburn, nausea, abdominal cramps, constipation, and diarrhea. The most common side effect is constipation. In one double-blind study, in which ferrous sulfate, ferrous gluconate, ferrous fumarate, and placebo were given in identically appearing tablets, there were no significant differences in gastrointestinal symptoms between the different iron salts.[86]

Several strategies to improve a woman's ingestion of ferrous supplements are available.[87,88] Generally, ferrous sulfate (325-mg tablets with 65 mg of elemental iron) is the lowest cost, but it often is the least tolerated. However, side effects may be diminished by encouraging women to start the medication incrementally; e.g., one tablet every 3 days for a week, increasing to one tablet every 2 days for a week, and then finally, one tablet or more daily. Different types of iron preparation may be tried if one type is not tolerated. Lowering the dose may also decrease side effects. Enteric-coated or prolonged-release preparations are not recommended because the reduction in side effects is accompanied by less absorption. Combination products increase costs, side effects, or both. Since iron preparations are primarily over-the-counter medications, it is important to know the woman's funding source. Writing a prescription for an over-the-counter medication can incur a charge for filling the prescription and cost of a copayment that may exceed the actual over-the-counter cost.

Common Discomforts in the Postpartum Period

Backache

Approximately 25% of women have persistent pregnancy-related lumbopelvic pain after giving birth, and 5% of women have lumbopelvic pain that is serious enough to require medical attention.[60] There are two types of back pain that must be differentiated. Pelvic girdle pain is pain between the posterior iliac crest and gluteal fold near the sacroiliac crests and/or pain over the symphysis. Pelvic girdle pain is associated with pregnancy. It is generally more severe during pregnancy and regresses postpartum. The putative etiology is excessive mobility of the pelvic joints. Lumbar or low back pain may be exacerbated during pregnancy but tends to become worse postpartum if it persists.

Factors associated with persistent lumbopelvic pain are presence of back pain before pregnancy, presence of back pain during pregnancy, physically heavy work, and multiple pregnancies.[60] Treatment of women with lumbopelvic pain is an area in which both alternative methods and short-term use of medications can be helpful. Physical therapy and acupuncture have documented effectiveness. Pelvic stabilizing exercises and pelvic belts are frequently recommended.

NSAIDs are efficacious for relieving discomfort from low back pain. Muscle relaxants are not commonly used because there are limited human data about use of muscle relaxants by lactating women. In addition, spasmolytics such as diazepam (Valium) can cause sedation, which may be dangerous for a woman who is caring for a newborn.

Local discomfort at the site of placement of continuous lumbar epidural anesthesia is also common, simply due to the local anesthetic injection and pressure on tissues when palpating for correct placement. A brief explanation of the cause for this discomfort and duration of this local tenderness usually is sufficient to reassure new mothers. As with any injury, heat may be applied after 24–48 hours to promote healing.

Constipation

Constipation is a common postpartum condition and occurs secondary to lax abdominal muscles, hormonal effects on the intestine during pregnancy, inadequate fluid and fiber intake, decreased physical activity, decreased anal sensitivity, use of perinatal opiate analgesia, and avoidance of bowel movements due to real or anticipated perineal pain. Gastroenterologists recommend first asking a woman to self-define the term constipation. It may be useful to help distinguish between decreased frequency of bowel movements or hardened stools for a day or two that is a common consequence of minimal solid food intake during labor. Reassurance that sutures, if present, are sturdy and reviewing comfort measures can be helpful. Women should be encouraged to increase fluids and choose high fiber foods the first few days after birth. After the initial postpartum recovery period, regular exercise should also be encouraged to correct or prevent constipation. These measures are preferable to laxative use and provide information to women to promote healthy lifestyle decisions for themselves and their families.

Of special note during the puerperium is the use of emollients or stool softeners (Table 37-6). Docusate sodium (Col-ace) is an over-the-counter medication. Docusate sodium capsules are administered orally and dissolve in the stomach. Rectal administration is also possible, in conjunction with a saline or oil retention enema. Docusate sodium, a relatively large, water-soluble, anionic molecule, passes unaltered through the gastrointestinal tract and is absorbed in small amounts from the duodenum and jejunum and is then excreted in bile. The various docusate salts are indicated for women in whom straining is contraindicated rather than for their laxative effect. They also are commonly ordered for women who have sustained third- or fourth-degree lacerations so the woman can avoid putting pressure on the sutures, although there is no clear evidence for this intervention.

Pharmacokinetic parameters of docusate sodium have not been determined and the exact mechanism of docusate is unknown, but research indicates two possible mechanisms. Docusate decreases surface tension, allowing water and lipids to penetrate and soften feces. Second, water and electrolyte secretion is stimulated in the colon, which may account for most of the laxative effect noted.

Table 37-6 Treatments for Constipation Used During the Postpartum Period

Name Generic (Sample Brands)	Mechanism of Action/Indication	Clinical Considerations
Emollients/Lubricants (Stool Softeners)		
Docusate sodium (Colace, Surfak)	Unknown mechanism; probably reduces surface tension, allowing fluids to penetrate fecal mass.	Effects noted in 1–3 days. Softens stools without increasing frequency.
Mineral oil	Coats the bowel and stool mass with waterproof film to keep moisture in the stool. Used when straining is contraindicated.	May interfere with absorption of nutrients, vitamins, and oral contraceptives. Prolonged use in pregnancy may cause severe bleeding in the newborn. Do not take concurrently with docusate sodium (Colace).
Bulk Producing		
Psyllium seed (Fiberall, Fibro-Lax, Fibro-XL, Genfiber, Hydrocil instant; Konsyl-D; Konsyl easy mix; Konsyl orange; Konsyl; Metamucil plus calcium; Metamucil smooth texture; Metamucil; Modane bulk; Reguloid; Serutan), natural fiber therapy	Absorb water, increase stool bulk.	May cause gas or bloating when first started. Must be taken with at least 250 cc of fluid to rinse any remaining particles from the throat and esophagus to avoid choking or difficulty breathing as the product swells. Some products contain aspartame, dextrose, or sucrose. Sugar-free preparations contain phenylalanine.
Methylcellulose (Citrucel, Fiber ease)	Absorb water, increase stool bulk.	Must be taken with at least 250 cc of fluid to rinse any remaining particles from the throat and esophagus to avoid choking or difficulty breathing as the product swells. Effects noticed in 12–72 hours. Theoretically may bind with nitrofurantoin (Macrodantin) and interfere with absorption.
Calcium polycarbophil (Fiberall tablets, FiberCon)	Absorb water, increase stool bulk.	Calcium polycarbophil may cause less gas and bloating due to less bacterial degradation
Stimulants		
Anthraquinones Cascara sagrada Senna (ExLax) Senna and docusate (Senokot) Aloe (casanthranol)	GI stimulant, purgative.	Likely to cause gastrointestinal cramping. Effects in newborns are unknown because there are few reports available in the literature. Increased incidence of diarrhea in the newborn has been suggested. Considered compatible with breastfeeding per the American Academy of Pediatrics.
Castor oil Bisacodyl (Dulcolax, Doxidan)	Stimulates enteric nerves to cause colonic contractions.	Onset of action is 6–10 hrs when taken orally and 15–60 minutes when administered rectally as a suppository.

* Laxative use for longer than 7 days is not recommended without professional assessment.

Increased concentrations of cyclic adenosine monophosphate (cAMP) are found in mucosal cells of the colon after administration of docusate. This finding suggests involvement of G protein-based second messenger receptors. Via a second messenger system, the permeability of mucosal cells is altered and active ion secretion is stimulated, which produces increased fluid within the colon. The usual dose of docusate is 50–360 mg each day, with wide variation in dose that can be tailored to the severity of the condition and therapeutic response. If stool softeners are indicated, higher doses may be needed at first. Response can be expected in 1–3 days.

Theoretically, stool softeners may improve absorption of many oral medications. Therefore, some clinicians avoid concurrent administration with oral drugs with narrow therapeutic indices such as theophylline (Theo-Dur) and

lithium (Lithobid). Additional discussion of this topic may be found in Chapter 21.

The few doses of docusate routinely given to women who do not have extensive lacerations may be of no use, unnecessarily contributing to hospital costs, and giving the false impression that laxative use is always necessary after having a baby.[89] Nonpharmacologic measures to avoid constipation such as ambulation, high fiber diet, and adequate fluid intake in these women are probably more efficacious.

Urinary Retention

Postpartum urinary retention is a possible complication of the puerperium. The incidence of this condition is difficult to ascertain as there is no standardized definition, but it has been estimated to be between 0.5% and 14%. The most commonly agreed upon diagnosis is inability to spontaneously urinate within the first 6 hours postpartum. Most urologists agree that residual bladder volumes of less than 50 mL are normal; however, volumes of more than 200 mL are abnormally high. Amounts in between are subject to debate.[64] Risk factors for postpartum urinary retention include cesarean birth, instrumental delivery, and prolonged labor (Box 37-3).

Treatment of postpartum urinary retention generally is nonpharmacologic. A woman is catheterized, often intermittently, and usually recovery is spontaneous within 24 hours.[65] Occasionally urinary retention may persist for several days, and in this situation the primary treatment is either self-catheterization or placement of an indwelling Foley catheter that is removed after several days. Because frequent or indwelling catheters increase the risk for urinary tract infection, some clinicians add prophylactic anti-infectives such as nitrofurantoin (Macrodantin), but this recommendation is not universal.

Vaginal Dryness

Due to the altered hormonal status during breastfeeding, many women experience some vaginal dryness with intercourse, similar to the atrophic vaginitis experienced by postmenopausal women. For the majority of women, use of a water-based lubricant will alleviate this discomfort. Over-the-counter treatments include water-based lubricants such as Astroglide, K-Y Jelly, Gyne-Moistrin, and Duragel. Vaginal suppositories also may be used. Conversely, women should avoid non–water-based products such as petroleum jelly (Vaseline) or A&D ointment because they can be irritating to vaginal mucosa and also weaken the integrity of condoms. Vaginal moisturizers such as Liquibeads, Replens, and Silken Secret may decrease vaginal dryness. In severe cases, a short-term, 1- to 3-week course of an estrogen vaginal cream (e.g., Premarin or Estrace) may be needed to control symptoms, although a more rapid return of ovulation and decreased milk production are possible with estrogen use.[90]

Medications Used During the Postpartum Period

Although the majority of postpartum women are healthy, breastfeeding women are as prone to minor health problems as the rest of the population. One of the most common questions from breastfeeding mothers is what to take for cold or allergy symptoms. Use of a normal saline nasal spray and humidifier in addition to sufficient fluid intake will usually be enough to ensure adequate relief from congestion symptoms. Women should be counseled to use single-entity medications instead of combination products whenever possible.

Common Cold

It is important to remember that breast milk is a secretion. If a woman is in need of an antihistamine for allergy symptoms or respiratory infections, the antihistamine also may diminish her milk supply by decreasing prolactin levels. If an antihistamine is required, the lowest effective dose should be used for the shortest period of time, and additional actions such as drinking more fluids and feeding the baby often can minimize the medication effect on milk supply. It has been suggested that pseudoephedrine is a lactation suppressant. Use of topical decongestant sprays, when necessary, may be a better choice than oral preparations. Additional information about drugs and lactation can be found in Chapter 38.

Vitamin Supplementation

Women who have been taking prenatal vitamins during pregnancy often will ask how long they should continue the vitamins postpartum.

Although it is uncommon in developed countries for a woman's diet to be deficient enough to lower vitamin levels in her milk, breastfeeding women generally are encouraged to continue prenatal vitamins as long as they are breastfeeding even though evidence that this improves outcomes in developed countries is limited. Research has focused primarily on individual nutrients such as iron, vitamin A, vitamin D, and vitamin B[12].

Research shows that one third of lactating women do not meet their folate requirements from diet alone, based on mandated levels of folic acid fortification.[88] In general, vitamin supplementation during the postpartum period is recommended only for women who have restricted diets or medical conditions wherein vitamins are part of the therapeutic regimen.[91]

Immunobiologics

Vaccines and immune globulins are two types of immunobiologics that may be prescribed for women in the immediate postpartum period (Table 37-7)[92-95] unless there is a specific indication based on personal exposure, potential for occupational exposure, or imminent international travel.

Killed or attenuated vaccines are compatible with breastfeeding. Live vaccines such as smallpox vaccine and nasal influenza vaccine should not be given to breastfeeding women or to household contacts of breastfeeding women. Specific data regarding the use of most vaccines in breastfeeding women are generally unavailable. In some regions and institutions, postpartum women are identified vehicles for advancing local public health recommendations for specific immunizations. Some examples include facilities that provide routine pneumococcal vaccines. However, the most common immunologics are rubella vaccine for women who are rubella nonimmune, Rho(D) immune globulin (RhoGAM) and the tetanus, diphtheria, and pertussis (Tdap) vaccine, which is now recommended for all postpartum women who were not previously vaccinated.

Table 37-7 Immunobiologics Most Commonly Administered in the Postpartum Period

Immunobiologic	Indication	Type	Route/Dose	Clinical Considerations
Hepatitis B vaccine (Energix-B, Recombivax HB)	Preexposure or postexposure for those at risk or if required for school or work	Noninfectious, purified surface antigen vaccine	> 19 y: 20 mcg/ 1.0 mL IM given as a three-dose series at 0, 1, and 6 months	If a series has been started, it is not necessary to start the series over if all doses are not administered on schedule. Just resume the series. First dose of series is recommended for newborns prior to hospital discharge.
Trivalent inactivated influenza vaccine	Influenza season, nonvaccinated mother	Inactivated virus vaccine	Single IM dose	Vaccination recommended prior to hospital discharge in unvaccinated mothers during influenza season (October to March).
Rubella vaccine	Nonimmune or equivocal rubella status	Live, attenuated virus vaccine	Single SQ dose	Virus or virus antigen may be found in breast milk, but no reported adverse effects or symptoms of clinical disease in infants have been found. Side effects include mild fever, transient lymphadenopathy, transient rash (lasting 7–10 days), arthralgias, or transient arthritis (commencing 1–3 weeks after vaccination and lasting 1–3 weeks).
Rho(D) immune globulin (human) (RhoGAM)	Nonsensitized Rh-negative mother with Rh-positive newborn or a newborn who tests weakly D positive	Immune globulin	Intramuscular Usual dose is 300 mcg that will suppress an immune response to 15 mL or less of Rh(D)-positive red blood cells	Given within 72 hours postpartum. Available in prefilled, single-dose syringes. Contraindicated if Rho(D)-positive or Du-positive, or previously sensitized to Rho(D) or Du antigens.
Tdap: Tetanus toxoid Diphtheria toxoid Acellular pertussis vaccine booster (Adacel)	Postpartum women who have not previously received Tdap	Combination toxoid and vaccine	Single IM dose 0.5 mL	May be given concurrently with hepatitis B and trivalent inactivated influenza vaccine. 2-year interval between last tetanus vaccination and Tdap is recommended.

Since administration of all immunobiologics may cause hypersensitivity in some individuals, 20 minutes of observation after administration is advised.
Sources: Tingle AJ et al. 1985[92]; CDC 2006[93]; CDC 2006[94]; CDC 2007.[95]

Rho(D) Immune Globulin (Human) (RhoGAM)

Rho(D) immune globulin (RhoGAM) given within 72 hours after delivery reduces the incidence of Rh sensitization from 12–13% to 1–2%[96] (Figure 37-1). If Rho(D) immune globulin also is administered at 28 weeks' gestation, the incidence is reduced even further to 0.1–0.2%.[97] Information regarding the effectiveness of Rho(D) immune globulin administered after 72 hours is limited, but the vaccine should be administered beyond the 72-hour window if necessary because the 72-hour time frame was initially based on the basic clinical trial, and few studies have evaluated delayed administration. An exception was one study that reported isoimmunization in approximately 50% of subjects when given Rho(D) immune globulin was given 13 days after exposure.[98]

Prior to postpartum administration, testing to detect fetal-maternal hemorrhage greater than that covered by a single dose of the globulin is required by the American Association of Blood Banks. Several tests may accomplish this. The **rosette test** is a qualitative test that can detect a fetal-maternal hemorrhage of about 10 mL. The rosette test may not be reliable if the newborn is weak D-positive. If the rosette test is positive or if the newborn is weak D-positive, quantitative tests must be done to determine the correct dose. These tests include the enzyme-linked antiglobulin test (ELAT) and flow cytometry HbF assay; although both of these tests are also not appropriate for detecting weak D fetal-maternal hemorrhage.

The **Kleihauer-Betke** acid-elution test may be used in all instances.[99] The Kleihauer-Betke test is considered less accurate and less reproducible than flow cytometry, but flow cytometry is a more expensive test. Women who have received an antepartum dose of Rho(D) immune globulin within 3 weeks of delivery do not need a postpartum dose. Testing for fetal-maternal hemorrhage is recommended in those women. It is possible for a large enough number of Rh-positive fetal red blood cells to cross the placenta into the maternal circulation late in pregnancy to cause a positive antiglobulin test for weak D (Du). Rho(D) immune globulin should be administered in the absence of documented maternal Rh status.

Since Rho(D) immune globulin (RhoGAM) is derived from human blood, this agent may pose a problem for subsets of the population, e.g., Jehovah's Witnesses, who refuse to receive blood because of religious convictions. However, not all women ascribing to the religion actually will refuse blood products. A study of 61 women who stated that they were Jehovah's Witnesses revealed that 50.1% would not accept any type of blood, but the rest would.[100] Therefore, each woman, regardless of stated religion, should be approached individually and provided with full information. In cases where women will refuse anti-D serum on the basis of religious beliefs, those traditions should be upheld.

Rubella Vaccine

A theoretic possibility exists that Rho(D) immune globulin (RhoGAM) will interfere with the development of antibodies to live vaccines, such as rubella vaccine, when given concurrently. However, if indicated, rubella vaccination should be administered to women receiving Rho(D) immuneglobulin. Whenever two vaccinations are given at the same time, it is recommended that the two vaccinations be given in separate anatomic sites and if possible, rubella titers should be tested 3 months postpartum to verify immunization. Measles vaccine is associated with febrile episodes. Traditional postpartum practice requires administration of rubella vaccine just prior to discharge to

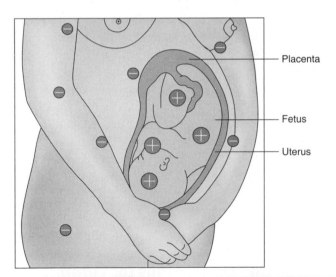

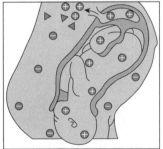 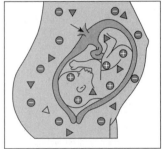

⊕ = RH + RBCs
⊖ = RH(D)-negative RBCs
△ = anti-D antibodies

Figure 37-1 Process of Rh isoimmunization.

avoid a febrile response that could be confused with puerperal morbidity. Evidence-based support for this practice is lacking. In 2001, the CDC revised its recommendations to state that women who receive a rubella vaccine should be counseled to avoid pregnancy for 28 days, not 3 months.[101]

Tdap Vaccine (Adacel)

Tdap (Adacel) administration in the postpartum period has been receiving increased attention due to the rising incidence of adult pertussis. Research has identified the mother as the source in 32% of infant pertussis infection cases, and cases of adult pertussis are increasing.[102,103] Administration prior to pregnancy is preferred, and today postpartum administration for women who have not received this vaccine is recommended.[92]

Contraception

Ideally, desired methods of contraception, if any, should have been discussed prior to delivery. However, it is common to meet postpartum women who are unclear about what contraceptives are available or undecided on their choice. Those women will need a review of available methods, including the risks and benefits of each relative to their needs and lifestyle.

Resumption of sexual intercourse, and thus, risk of pregnancy is subject to personal desires of the woman and her partner, as well as cultural mores. There is no evidence-based recommendation. Ovulation occurs around 10 weeks postpartum in bottle-feeding women. Although the first menses tends to be anovulatory, a woman cannot depend upon that as a contraceptive alert. Therefore, for women desiring a method of postpartum contraception, it is recommended that a method be started during the third week postpartum for partially breastfeeding and bottle-feeding women. Women who are breastfeeding exclusively and who are amenorrheic are eligible to use the Lactational Amenorrheic Method (LAM). LAM is highly effective for these women for up to 6 months.

All postpartum women desiring contraception should have a clear, preferably written, plan for when to start the method they have chosen, where to obtain their chosen method, and where to obtain follow-up care. This information is particularly important for women without insurance or whose insurance may expire in the near future. They are often the least likely to know what

low-cost resources are available for annual well-woman exams and family planning. Women who would like to use any of the natural family planning methods should be referred for classes to maximize the effectiveness of their chosen method. Lack of knowledge plays a role in diminished effectiveness of all contraceptive methods. Chapter 29 provides additional information about contraception.

Combined Oral Contraceptives

Hematologic changes responsible for the hypercoagulable state of pregnancy return to normal by 3 weeks after delivery, although the manufacturer's package inserts included with oral contraceptives usually recommend waiting for 28 days postpartum before taking the first pill. After this time, estrogen-containing contraceptive methods are considered safe for women who do not have any other contraindications for their use. Specifics concerning each method of contraception are found in Table 37-8.[104,105]

Breastfeeding women using combined oral contraceptives breastfeed for a mean of 3.7 months versus 4.6 months by control subjects.[105] Breastfeeding women desiring an estrogen-containing contraceptive should be made aware that use of any estrogen-containing contraceptive will decrease milk quantity. An interim method that will not interfere with milk production, such as the progestin-only pill, depot-medroxyprogesterone acetate (Depo-Provera), single-rod contraceptive implant (Implanon), or a barrier method should be encouraged. Women also can be educated regarding the lactational amenorrhea method and how to maximize its effectiveness.

Restarting Medications for Chronic Medical Conditions

Women with chronic conditions such as epilepsy, thyroid disease, hypertension, depression, thromboembolic disease, and diabetes will usually be counseled during pregnancy about appropriate use of usual medications during labor and after birth. In the postpartum period, it is rare that a previously used medication is contraindicated. However, several studies have shown significantly lower breastfeeding rates in women with medical conditions, presumably because their care providers were not aware of recommendations for medication use during lactation.[107,108] An overview of information concerning

Table 37-8 Use of Reversible Contraceptive Methods in the Postpartum Period

Contraceptive Method	Postpartum Timing of Initiation and Precautions	
	Breastfeeding Mother	**Nonbreastfeeding Woman**
Lactational amenorrhea	Requirements for maximum effectiveness are: amenorrhea, exclusive or near exclusive breastfeeding at regular intervals, < 6 months after birth, no substitute pacifiers or bottles.	Not applicable.
Fertility awareness or natural family planning methods Detectable fertility signs or hormonal changes are unlikely < 4 weeks after birth	Cervical mucus changes indicating fertility are considered reliable during lactation but methods may be less effective than when not breastfeeding. Detectable fertility signs or hormonal changes are unlikely less than 6 weeks after delivery. Can be used after three regular menses.	Considered more reliable than calendar-based methods. Can be used after fertility signs are noted. Can be used after three regular menses.
Condoms	Use of a lubricant compatible with condoms may be necessary in some breastfeeding women.	May be used safely.
Diaphragm/cervical cap	Unsuitable for use until uterine involution is complete, about 6 weeks after birth.	Unsuitable for use until uterine involution is complete, about 6 weeks after birth.
Spermicides (nonoxynol 9)	Contraindicated if previous allergy to nonoxynol 9.	Contraindicated if previous allergy to nonoxynol 9.
Combination oral contraceptives, patch (Evra), ring (NuvaRing)	Not recommended for women < 6 weeks postpartum. 6 weeks to 6 months postpartum risks usually outweigh advantages since use may diminish quantity of breast milk. > 6 months after birth, advantages usually outweigh risks.	May be used < 21 days after birth if advantages outweigh risks. No restrictions on use > 21 days postpartum.
Progestin-only oral contraceptives	< 6 weeks after birth, risks usually outweigh advantages due to lack of data on effects of progestin exposure via breast milk on neonatal brain and liver development. > 6 weeks postpartum, no restrictions on use.	May be safely used immediately after delivery.
Etonogestrel-releasing contraceptive implant (Implanon)	May insert 4 weeks after delivery. No data are available for use < 4 weeks.	May insert at 21–28 days after delivery. If > 4 weeks after birth, exclude pregnancy and recommend use of a nonhormonal method for 7 days after insertion.
Depot-medroxyprogesterone acetate DMPA (Depo-Provera)	4–6 weeks after birth recommended by manufacturer. May enhance milk production.	4–6 weeks after birth recommended by manufacturer.
Copper intrauterine device	< 48 hours after birth, advantages may outweigh risks. 48 hours to 4 weeks, risks usually outweigh advantages. No restriction after 4 weeks postpartum.	Same as for breastfeeding women. Lowest expulsion rates after 4 weeks in both breastfeeding and bottle-feeding women.
Levonorgestrel intrauterine device	< 4 weeks after birth, advantages may outweigh risks. No restriction after 4 weeks.	Same as for breastfeeding women. Lowest expulsion rates after 4 weeks in both breastfeeding and bottle-feeding women.

continued use of selected medications in postpartum women with coincidental medical conditions is provided in Table 37-9.[109-114]

Conclusion

While most providers are sympathetic to the needs of new mothers and want to keep them safe and make them comfortable, this relatively brief period in a woman's life cycle has not attracted the same interest and scientific inquiry as other life phases. Disease states, pregnancy, and labor have been more pressing or perhaps more interesting subjects for research. Far too many postpartum practices are in place simply because that's the way it has always been done. While more research is now being conducted, there is still room for improvement.[18] For the most part, women have done well, perhaps because the postpartum period is a normal event, designed to be uncomplicated. Women may do even better when evidence-based practice guides more of the care they receive after having a baby and leaves them free to be mothers.

Table 37-9 Postpartum Considerations for Medications to Treat Women with Selected Medical Conditions

Commonly Used Medications (Brand)	Clinical Considerations Regarding Transition to Postpartum Use/Precautions/Use in Breastfeeding
Diabetes	
Insulin	Insulin requirements are significantly lower in the first postpartum week compared with preconception requirements and remain significantly lower over the first 2 postpartum months. Not secreted in breast milk. Safe for breastfeeding.
Sulfonylureas: Tolbutamide (Orinase) Glyburide (Micronase) Glipizide (Glucotrol)	Tolbutamide compatible with breastfeeding. Other sulfonylureas are less well studied. Glyburide and glipizide are highly protein-bound and unlikely to pass into breast milk.[110]
Alpha-glucosidase inhibitors: Acarbose (Precose)	Low bioavailability, large molecular size and water soluble. Unlikely to be excreted into breast milk in clinically significant amounts.[110]
Biguanides: Metformin (Glucophage)	Nonsignificant amounts in breast milk. Compatible with breastfeeding.
Thiazolidinediones: Rosiglitazone (Avandia) Pioglitazone (Actos)	No studies done to date that have evaluated the passage of thiazolidinediones into breast milk. Thiazolidinedones associated with risk for lactic acidosis and hepatotoxicity.
Epilepsy	
Sedative drugs: Phenobarbitol (Luminal) Mysoline (Primidone) Benzodiazepines, such as: Carbamazepine (Tegretol) Diazepam (Valium) Lorazepam (Ativan) Alprazolam (Zanax) Oxcarbazepine (Trileptal) Phenytoin (Dilantin) Lamotrigine (Lamictal) Valproate (Depakote) Topiramate (Topamax) Gabapentin (Neurontin)	The best AED is the one that effectively controls seizures prior to pregnancy, using monotherapy and lowest possible drug dose. However, higher teratogenicity associated with valproate makes it less desirable for use. Changing drugs at any time, antepartum or postpartum, exposes the fetus or newborn to an additional drug and should be avoided when possible. Hormonal contraceptive failure may occur with AEDs that are inducers of the hepatic cytochrome P450 system, such as carbamazepine, phenytoin, phenobarbital, primidone, topiramate, and oxcarbazepine. If AED dose has been changed during pregnancy, consider a return to prepregnancy dose during the first few weeks postpartum. AEDs are not contraindicated during breastfeeding. Carbamazepine and phenytoin are preferred choices for women who are breastfeeding. The sedative AEDs may cause infant irritability, sleepiness, and failure to thrive, so the infant needs to be monitored closely if sedative AEDs are prescribed. Phenobarbital, primidone, and benzodiazepines are found in neonatal plasma for several days; infants of mothers receiving these medications prior to birth should be monitored for sedation and possibly neonatal withdrawal syndrome. Although valproate is considered compatible with breastfeeding, there is a potential for fatal hepatotoxicity in breastfed children younger than 2 years. Primidone should be avoided with breastfeeding.
Hypertension	
Beta-blockers: Propranolol (Inderal) Metoprolol (Lopressor) Labetalol (Normodyne)	Listed medications have lowest transfer into breast milk. Atenolol (Tenormin), nadolol (Corgard), and sotalol (Betapace) are excreted in higher amounts that can lead to hypotension, bradycardia, and tachypnea in infants.
Thiazide diuretics	Excreted in small amounts into breast milk. Do not suppress lactation.
ACE inhibitors	Use with caution in first few weeks postpartum in breastfeeding women due to possible effects on neonate's kidneys.
Hyperthyroidism	
Beta-blockers: Propranolol (Inderal)	Beta-blockers are used to mitigate moderate to severe acute symptoms, and then use is decreased as symptoms resolve due to reports of occasional cases of neonatal growth restriction when prescribed for breastfeeding women. Thyroid storm precipitated by labor, infection, preeclampsia, or cesarean section is rare.
Thionamides: Propylthiouracil (PTU) (preferred) Methimazole (Tapazole)	Compatible with breastfeeding. Despite being compatible, in a prospective, observational cohort study, only 44.4% of women receiving propylthiouracil (PTU) breastfed versus 83.3% women no longer requiring propylthiouracil (PTU) and control subjects ($P < .1$). Advice and attitude of physicians toward breastfeeding during propylthiouracil (PTU) therapy was the only significant predictor ($P = .017$) of the decision to breastfeed.[95] Probable association of methimazole with fetal developmental abnormalities such as choanal or esophageal atresia.
Radioactive iodine	Radioactive iodine is contraindicated in pregnancy and breastfeeding.

(continues)

Table 37-9 Postpartum Considerations for Medications to Treat Women with Selected Medical Conditions (*continued*)

Commonly Used Medications (Brand)	Clinical Considerations Regarding Transition to Postpartum Use/Precautions/Use in Breastfeeding
Hypothyroidism	
Levothyroxine	Most women will need dose reduced to prepregnancy levels after delivery; measure serum TSH 4–6 weeks later.
Thromboembolic Disease	
Unfractionated heparin	Safe for use in lactation due to high molecular weight that does not transfer into milk easily. Any heparin transferred into breast milk would be destroyed in intestines of the baby.
Warfarin (Coumadin)	Considered safe in pregnancy. Possibly associated with prolonged prothrombin time in some infants. Infants should be monitored for signs and symptoms of bleeding.

Sources: Spencer JP et al. 2001[110]; Saez-de-Ibarra L et al. 2003[109]; Tran TA et al. 2002[111]; Kuhnz W et al. 1988[112]; Kaplan MM 1996[113]; Abalovich M et al. 2007.[114]

References

1. Blackburn S. Maternal, fetal and neonatal physiology, 3rd ed. New York: Elsevier, 2007:153.

2. Gibbs RS, Karlan BY, Haney AF, Nygaard IE. Danforth's obstetrics and gynecology. 10th ed. Philadelphia, PA: Lippincott Williams & Wilkins, 2008.

3. Briggs GG, Freeman RF, Yaffee SF. Drugs in pregnancy and lactation: a reference guide to fetal and neonatal risk, 7th ed. Philadelphia, PA: Lippincott Williams & Wilkins, 2005.

4. American Academy of Pediatrics. The transfer of drugs and other chemicals into human milk. Pediatrics 2001; 108(3):776–89.

5. Koren G, Cairns J, Chitayat D, Gaedigk A, Leeder SJ. Pharmacogenetics of morphine poisoning in a breast-fed neonate of a codeine-prescribed mother. Lancet 2006;368(9536):704.

6. USFDA Alert. Information for healthcare professionals: use of codeine products in nursing mothers. MedWatch, August 17, 2007. Available from: *http://www.fda.gov/Drugs/DrugSafety/PostmarketDrugSafetyInformationforPatientsandProviders/DrugSafetyInformationforHeathcareProfessionals/ucm084282.htm* [Retrieved September 13, 2009].

7. Windle ML, Booker LA, Rayburn WF. Postpartum pain after vaginal delivery: a review of comparative analgesic trials. J Repro Med 1989;34(11):891–5.

8. Clark JH, Wilson WG. A 16-day-old breast-fed infant with metabolic acidosis caused by salicylate. Clin Pediatr (Phila) 1981;20:53.

9. Anderson PO, Sauberan JB, Lane JR, Rossi SS. Hydrocodone excretion into breast milk: the first 2 reported cases. Breastfeed Med 2007;2(1):10–4.

10. Pavy TJG, Paech MJ, Evans SF. The effect of intravenous ketorolac on opioid requirement and pain after cesarean delivery. Anesth Analg 2001;92:1010–4.

11. Montgomery A, Hale T. Academy of Breastfeeding Medicine Clinical Protocol No. 15: Analgesia and anesthesia for the breastfeeding mother. Breastfeed Med 2006;1(4):271–7.

12. Miller E. The World Health Organization analgesic ladder. J Midwifery Womens Health 2004;49(6):542–5.

13. Macarthur AJ, Macarthur C. Incidence, severity, and determinants of perineal pain after vaginal delivery: a prospective cohort study. Amer J Obstet Gynecol 2004;191(4):1199–204.

14. Leeman LM, Rogers RG, Greulich B, Albers LL. Do unsutured second-degree perineal lacerations affect postpartum functional outcomes? J Am Board Family Med 2007;20(5):451–7.

15. Kettle C, Hills RK, Ismail KMK. Continuous versus interrupted sutures for repair of tears. Cochrane Database Syst Rev 2007(4):CD000947.

16. Calvert S, Fleming V. Minimizing postpartum pain: a review of research pertaining to perineal care in childbearing women. J Adv Nurs 2000;32(2):407–15.

17. Sleep J, Grant A. Pelvic floor exercises in postnatal care—the report of a randomized controlled trial to compare an intensive exercise regimen with the programme in current use. Midwifery 1987;3(4):158–64.

18. Rhode MA, Barger M. Perineal care: then and now. J Nurse-Midwifery 1990;35(4):220–30.

19. East CE, Begg L, Henshall NE, Marchant P, Wallace K. Local cooling for relieving pain from perineal trauma sustained during childbirth. Cochrane Database Syst Rev 2007(4):CD006304.

20. Tejirian T, Abbas MA. Sitz bath: where is the evidence? Scientific basis of a common practice. Dis Colon Rectum 2005;48(12):2336–40.

21. Barclay L, Martin N. A sensitive area (care of the episiotomy in the post-partum period). Aust J Adv Nurs 1983;1(1):12–9.

22. Dale A, Cornwell S. The role of lavender oil in relieving perineal discomfort following childbirth: a

blind randomized clinical trial. J Adv Nurs 1994;19 (1):89–96.

23. Meyer H. Postpartum care of the perineum: the use of a topical anesthetic spray. J La State Med Soc 1964;116(6):221–2.

24. Harrison RF, Brennan M. Evaluation of two local anaesthetic sprays for the relief of post-episiotomy pain. Curr Med Res Opin 1987;10:364–9.

25. Goldstein PJ, Lipman M, Luebehusen J. A controlled clinical trial of two local agents in postepisiotomy pain and discomfort. Southern Med J 1977;70(7):806–8.

26. Bouis PJ, Martinez LA, Hambrick TL. Epifoam (hydrocortisone acetate) in the treatment of postepisiotomy patients. Curr Ther Res 1981;30(6):912–6.

27. Greer IA, Cameron AD. Topical pramoxine and hydrocortisone foam versus placebo in relief of post partum episiotomy symptoms and wound healing. Scott Med J 1984;29:104–6.

28. Moore W, James DK. A random trial of three topical analgesic agents in the treatment of episiotomy pain following instrumental vaginal delivery. J Obstet Gynaecol 1989;10:35–9.

29. Minassian VA, Jazayeri A, Prien SD, Timmons RL, Stumbo K. Randomized trial of lidocaine ointment versus placebo for the treatment of postpartum perineal pain. Obstet Gynecol 2002;100(6):1239–43.

30. Hedayati H, Parsons J, Crowther CA. Topically applied anaesthetics for treating perineal pain after childbirth. Cochrane Database Syst Rev 2007(4):CD 00075320-100000000-03233.

31. Hedayati H, Parsons J, Crowther CA. Rectal analgesia for pain from perineal trauma following childbirth. Cochrane Database of Syst Rev 2005(2):CD004223.

32. Mathie RT. Homeopathy for trauma. 2007. Available from: *http://www.library.nhs.uk/cam/viewResource .aspx?resID=261605&code=3d539eb1889f3a1444786 1323a0ddd96* [Accessed October 22, 2009].

33. Clark D. Herbs for postpartum perineum care: part one. Midwifery Today.com. 2005. Available from: www .midwiferytoday.com/articles/herbspostperineum1 .asp [Accessed September 13, 2009].

34. Shafik A. Role of warm-water bath in the anorectal conditions. The "thermosphincteric reflex." J Clin Gastroenterol 1993;16:304.

35. Alonso-Coello P, Guyatt G, Heels-Ansdell D, Johanson JF, Lopez-Yarto M, Mills E, et al. Laxatives for the treatment of hemorrhoids. Cochrane Database Syst Rev 2005(4):CD004649.

36. Barnes CL, Scates AC, Fine JS. Treatment of hemorrhoids. US Pharm 2002;22(8):1–9.

37. Shultz KM, Hill PD. Prevention of and therapies for nipple pain: a systematic review. JOGNN 2006;34(4):428–37.

38. Ziemer MM, Pigeon JG. Skin changes and pain in the nipple during the first week of lactation. JOGNN 1993;22(3):247–56.

39. Dodd V, Chalmers C. Comparing the use of hydrogel dressings to lanolin ointment with lactating mothers. JOGNN 2003;32:486–94.

40. Akkuzu G, Taskin L. Impacts of breast-care techniques on prevention of possible postpartum nipple problems. Prof Care Mother Child 2000;10(2):38–41.

41. Lauwers J, Swisher A. Counseling the nursing mother, 4th ed. Sudbury, MA: Jones and Bartlett, 2005.

42. Snowden HM, Renfrew MJ, Woolridge MW. Treatments for breast engorgement during lactation (Cochrane Review). In The Cochrane Library. Oxford: Update Software 2002(3).

43. Lavand'homme P. Postcesarean analgesia: effective strategies and association with chronic pain. Curr Opin Anaesthesiol 2006;19:244–8.

44. World Health Organization. Cancer pain relief. Geneva, Switzerland: WHO, 1986:51.

45. Davis KM, Esposito MA, Meyer BA. Oral analgesia compared with intravenous patient-controlled analgesia for pain after cesarean delivery: a randomized controlled trial. Am J Obstet Gynecol 2006;194(4):967–71.

46. Ke RW. A preemptive strike against surgical pain. Contem Ob Gyn 2001;46(1):65–70.

47. Ke RW, Portera SG, Bagous W, Lincoln SR. A randomized, double-blinded trial of preemptive analgesia in laparoscopy. Obstet Gynecol 1998;92(6):972–5.

48. Rosaeg OP, Lui ACP, Cicutti NJ, Bragg PR, Crossan ML, Krepski B. Peri-operative multi-modal pain therapy for caesarean section: analgesia and fitness for discharge. Can J Anaesth 1997;44(8):803–9.

49. Block BM, Liu SS, Rowlingson AJ, Cowan AR, Cowan JA, Wu CL. Efficacy of postoperative epidural analgesia: a meta-analysis. JAMA 2003;290(18):2455–64.

50. Pasero C. Multimodal balanced analgesia in the PACU. J Perinaesthesia Nsg 2003;18(4):265–8.

51. Lowder JL, Shackelford DP, Holbert D, Beste TM. A randomized, controlled trial to compare ketorolac tromethamine versus placebo after cesarean section to reduce pain and narcotic usage. Am J Obstet Gynecol 2003;189(6):1559–62.

52. Givens VA, Lipscomb GH, Meyer NL. A randomized trial of postoperative wound irrigation with local anesthetic for pain after cesarean delivery. Am J Obstet Gynecol 2002;186(6):1188–91.

53. Fredman B, Shapiro A, Zohar E, Feldman E, Shorer S, Rawal N, Jedeikin R. The analgesic efficacy of patient-controlled ropivacaine instillation after cesarean delivery. Anesth Analg 2000;91:1436–40.

54. Meyer M, Wagner K, Benvenuto A, Plante D, Howard D. Intrapartum and postpartum analgesia for women maintained on methadone during pregnancy. Obstet Gynecol 2007;110:261–6.

55. Thomas L, Ptak H, Giddings LS, Moore L, Oppermann C. The effects of rocking, diet modifications, and anti-flatulent medication on postcesarean section gas pain. J Perinatal Neonatal Nurs 1990;4(3):12–24.

56. Horlocker TT, Burton AW, Connis RT, Hughes SC, Nickinovich DG, Palmer CM, et al. Practice guidelines for the prevention, detection, and management of respiratory depression associated with neuraxial opioid administration. American Society of Anesthesiologists Task Force on Neuraxial Opioids. Anesthesiology 2009;110(2):218–30.

57. Murray A, Holdcroft A. Incidence and intensity of postpartum lower abdominal pain. Br Med J 1989; 298:1619.

58. Holdcroft A, Snidvongs S, Cason A, Dore CJ, Berkley KJ. Pain and uterine contractions during breast feeding in the immediate post-partum period increase with parity. Pain 2003;104:580–96.

59. Windle ML, Booker LA, Rayburn WF. Postpartum pain after vaginal delivery: a review of comparative analgesic trials. J Repro Med 1989;34(11):891–5.

60. Gutke A, Ostgaard HC, Oberg B. Predicting persistent pregnancy-related low back pain. Spine 2008; 33(12):E386–93.

61. Filker R, Monif G. The significance of temperature during the first 24 hours postpartum. Obstet Gynecol 1979;53(3):358–61.

62. Mantha VR, Vallejo MC, Ramesh V, Phelps AL, Ramanathan S. The incidence of maternal fever during labor with intermittent than with continuous epidural analgesia: a randomized controlled trial. Int J Obstet Anesth 2008;17(2):123–9.

63. Marraro RV, Harris RE. Incidence and spontaneous resolution of postpartum bacteriuria. Am J Obstet Gynecol 1977;128(7):722–3.

64. Yip SK, Sahota D, Pang MW, Day L. Postpartum urinary retention. Obstet Gynecol 2005;106(3):602–6.

65. Evron S, Dimitrochenko V, Khazin V, Sherman A, Sadan O, Boaz M, et al. The effect of intermittent versus continuous bladder catheterization on labor duration and postpartum urinary retention and infection: a randomized trial. J Clin Anesth 2008;20(8): 567–72.

66. French LM, Smaill FM. Antibiotic regimens for endometritis after delivery. Cochrane Database Syst Rev 2004(4):CD001067.

67. Livingston JC, Llata E, Rinehart E, Leidwanger C, Mabie B, Haddad B, et al. Gentamicin and clindamycin therapy in postpartum endometritis: the efficacy of daily dosing versus dosing every 8 hours. Am J Obstet Gynecol 2003;188(1):149–52.

68. Ramin SM, Gilstrap LC. Episiotomy and early repair of dehiscence. Clin Obstet Gynecol 1994;37(4):816–23.

69. Almeida OD, Kitay DZ. Lactation suppression and puerperal fever. Am J Obstet Gynecol 1986;154(4): 940–1.

70. Betzhold CM. An update on the recognition and management of lactational breast inflammation. J Midwifery Womens Health 2007;52:595–605.

71. Filteau SM, Lietz G, Mulokozi G, Bilotta S, Henry CJ, Tomkins AM. Milk cytokines and subclinical breast inflammation in Tanzanian women: effect of dietary red palm oil or sunflower oil supplementation. Immunology 1999;97:595–600.

72. Binns SE. Light-mediated antifungal activity of Echinacea extracts. Plant Med 2000;66(3):241–4.

73. Wambach KA. Lactation mastitis: a descriptive study. J Hum Lact 2003;19(1):24–34.

74. Dennis CL, Ross LE, Herxheimer A. Oestrogens and progestins for preventing and treating postpartum depression. Cochrane Database Syst Rev 2004(4): CD001690.

75. Wisner KL, Parry BL, Piontek CM. Postpartum depression. N Engl J Med 2002;347(3):194–9.

76. Oppo A, Mauri M, Ramacciotti D, Camilleri V, Banti S, Borri C, et al. Risk factors for postpartum depression: the role of the Postpartum Depression Predictors Inventory-Revised (PDPI-R): Results from the Perinatal Depression-Research & Screening Unit (PNDReScU) Study. Arch Womens Ment Health 2009;12(4):239–49.

77. Howard LM, Hoffbrand S, Henshaw C, Boath L, Bradley E. Antidepressant prevention of postnatal depression. Cochrane Database Syst Rev 2005(2): CD004363.

78. Dennis C-L, Hodnett E. Psychosocial and psychological interventions for treating postpartum depression. Cochrane Database Syst Rev 2007(4):CD006116.

79. Affonso DD, Domino G. Postpartum depression: a review. Birth 2007;11(4):231–5.

80. Hoffbrand SE, Howard L, Crawley H. Antidepressant treatment for post-natal depression. Cochrane Database Syst Rev 2001(2):CD002018.

81. Sharma V. Treatment of postpartum psychosis: challenges and opportunities. Curr Drug Saf 2008;3(1): 76–81.

82. Spinelli MG. Postpartum psychosis: detection of risk and management. Am J Psychiatry. 2009;166(4): 405–8.

83. Schindler AM. Isolated neonatal hypomagnesaemia associated with maternal overuse of stool softener. Lancet 1984;2(8406):822.

84. Wisniewski PM, Wilkinson EG. Postpartum vaginal atrophy. Am J Obstet Gynecol 1991;165(4, pt 2): 1249–54.

85. Buetler E. Disorders of iron metabolism. In Lichtman MA, Kipps TJ, Kaushanshky K, eds. Williams Hematology, 7th ed. New York: McGraw-Hill Medical, 2006.

86. Nelson GH, Donnell S, Griffin G, Nelson RM. Timing of postpartum hematocrit determinations. Southern Med J 1980;73(9):1202–4.

87. Petersen LA, Lindner DS, Kleiber CM, Zimmerman MB, Hinton AT, Yankowitz J. Factors that predict low hematocrit levels in the postpartum patient after vaginal delivery. Am J Obstet Gynecol 2002;186(4): 737–44.

88. Andrews NC. Iron deficiency and related disorders. In Greer JP et al., eds. Wintrobe's clinical hematology, 11th ed. vol 1. Philadelphia, PA: Lippincott Williams & Wilkins, 2004.

89. Bonnar J, Goldberg A, Smith JA. Do pregnant women take their iron? Lancet 1969;1:457.

90. Sherwood KL, Houghton LA, Tarasuk V, O'Connor DL. One-third of pregnant and lactating women may not be meeting their folate requirements from diet alone based on mandated levels of folic acid fortification. J Nutr 2006;136(11):2820–6.

91. Weiss R, Fogelman Y, Bennett M. Severe vitamin B_{12} deficiency in an infant associated with a maternal deficiency and a strict vegetarian diet. J Pediatr Hematol/Oncol 2004;26(4):270–1.

92. Tingle AJ, Chantler JK, Kees HP, Paty DW, Ford DK. Postpartum rubella immunization: association with development of prolonged arthritis, neurological sequelae, and chronic rubella viremia. J Infect Dis 1985;152(3):606–12.

93. Centers for Disease Control and Prevention. Preventing tetanus, diphtheria, and pertussis among adults: use of tetanus toxoid, reduced diphtheria toxoid and acellular pertussis vaccine recommendations of the Advisory Committee on Immunization Practices (ACIP) United States. MMWR Recomm Rep 2006; 55(RR-17):1–37.

94. Centers for Disease Control and Prevention. General recommendations on immunization: recommendations of the Advisory Committee on Immunization Practices (ACIP). United States, December 1, 2006. MMWR 2006;51(RR-2):1–48.

95. Centers for Disease Control and Prevention. Recommended adult immunization schedule. United States, October 2007-September 2008. MMWR 2007; 56(41):Q1–4.

96. Freda VJ, Gorman JG, Pollack W, Bowe E. Prevention of Rh hemolytic disease-ten years' clinical experience with Rh immune globulin. New Engl J Med 1975;292:1014–6.

97. Bowman JM, Chown B, Lewis M, Pollock JM. Rh isoimmunization during pregnancy: antenatal prophylaxis. Can Med Assoc J 1978;118:623–7.

98. Samson D, Mollison PL. Effect on primary Rh immunization of delayed administration of anti-Rh. Immunol 1975;28:349–57.

99. Hogan LS. Weak D effect on estimating fetal-maternal hemorrhage: a case study. Clin Lab Sci 1998;11(4):204.

100. Gyamfi C, Berkowitz RL Responses by pregnant Jehovah's Witnesses on health care proxies. Obstet Gynecol 2004;104:541–4.

101. Centers for Disease Control and Prevention. Revised ACIP recommendation for avoiding pregnancy after receiving a rubella-containing vaccine. MMWR 2001; 50(49):1117.

102. Bisgard KM, Pascual FB, Ehresmann KR, Miller CA, Cianfrini C, Jennings CE, et al. Infant pertussis: who was the source? Pediatr Infect Dis J 2004;23: 985–9.

103. McIntyre P, Wood N. Pertussis in early infancy: disease burden and preventive strategies. Curr Opin Infect Dis 2009;22(3):215–23.

104. Medical eligibility criteria for contraceptive use. Reproductive health and research, 3rd ed. Geneva, Switzerland: World Health Organization, 2004.

105. King J. Contraception and lactation. J Midwifery Womens Health 2007;52:614–20.

106. Aljazaf K, Hale TW, Ilett KF, Hartmann PE, Mitoulas LR, Kristensen JH, et al. Pseudoephedrine: effects on milk production in women and estimation of infant exposure via breast-milk. Br J Clin Pharmacol 2003; 56:18–24.

107. Lee A, Moretti ME, Collantes A, Chong D, Mazzotta P, Koren G, et al. Choice of breastfeeding and physicians' advice: a cohort study of women receiving propylthiouracil. Pediatrics 2000;106(1, pt 1):27–30.

108. Ito S, Moretti M, Liau M, Koren G. Initiation and duration of breast-feeding in women receiving antiepileptics. Am J Obstet Gynecol 1995;172(5):881–6.

109. Saez-de-Ibarra L, Gaspar R, Obesso A, Herranz L. Glycaemic behaviour during lactation: postpartum practical guidelines for women with type 1 diabetes. Practical Diabetes Int 2003;20(3):271–5.

110. Spencer JP, Gonzalez LS, Barnhart DJ. Medications in the breast-feeding mother. Am Fam Physician 2001;64(1):119–26.

111. Tran TA, Leppik IE, Blesi K, Sathanandan ST, Remmel R. Lamotrigine clearance during pregnancy. Neurology 2002;59:251.

112. Kuhnz W, Koch S, Helge H, Nau H. Primidone and phenobarbital during lactation period in epileptic women: total and free drug serum levels in the nursed infants and their effects on neonatal behavior. Dev Pharmacol Ther 1988;11:147.

113. Kaplan MM. Management of thyroxine therapy during pregnancy. Endocr Pract 1996;2:281.

114. Abalovich M, Amino N, Barbour LA, Cobin RH, De Groot LJ, Glinoer D, et al. Management of thyroid dysfunction during pregnancy and postpartum: an endocrine society clinical practice guideline. J Clin Endocrinol Metab 2007;92(8)(suppl):S1–47.

115. Oladapo OT, Fawole B. Treatments for suppression of lactation. Cochrane Database Syst Rev 2009(1): CD005937.

116. Dodds P, Hans AL. Distended urinary bladder drainage practices among hospital nurses. Appl Nurs Res 1990;3(2):68–9.

38
Breastfeeding Mothers

Thomas W. Hale

⊹ Chapter Glossary

Absolute infant dose (AID) An estimate of the drug concentration in milk (per mL), which is calculated by multiplying the volume of breast milk ingested per day by either the maximum or average concentration of drug in breast milk per day.

Colostrum The liquid produced and secreted by lactocytes prior to lactogenesis. Colostrum has limited fat but has high amounts of maternal immunoglobulins necessary for initiation of the infant's immune system.

Dopamine agonists Drugs whose actions mimic dopamine. Dopamine agonists are prolactin antagonists and inhibit milk production.

Dopamine antagonists Drugs that inhibit dopamine by preventing the usual effect it has in maintaining prolactin storage within the lactotrophs in the pituitary gland. When dopamine is inhibited, prolactin is released from the pituitary.

Galactogogue Drug that induces milk production.

Human *ether-a-go-go*-Related gene (HERG) A gene that encodes for the potassium ion channel that repolarizes the current in the cardiac action potential. Many drugs can bind to this channel and alter its function, which results in a prolonged QT interval.

Lactocytes Epithelial cells within the alveoli of the breast. The lactocytes produce and secrete human milk.

Lactogenesis I Stage of mammary gland development when the lactocytes have the ability to produce and secrete colostrum. This stage ends when lactogenesis II starts.

Lactogenesis II Onset of breast milk secretion, which occurs about 40 hours after birth.

Milk/plasma (M/P) The ratio of the concentration of drug in breast milk to the concentration in maternal plasma. This ratio is a quantification of the amount of drug that is transferred into the breast milk based on the amount that is bioavailable in the maternal plasma.

OCT1 and OCT2 organic cation transporters Organic efflux transporters that are responsible for the hepatic and renal transport of metformin (Glucophage). They have been found in alveolar tissue, which is why metformin does not remain in breast milk even if it diffuses into this compartment initially.

Plasma glycoprotein A gene that encodes for a protein that extends across the cell plasma membrane and functions as an efflux pump. The presence of plasma glycoprotein explains why some drugs are present in breast milk in lower-than-expected concentrations.

Relative infant dose (RID) An estimate of the weight-normalized infant dose of drug relative to the mother's dose of the drug.

Introduction

Human milk is the infant's first and perfect choice for protection against infectious disease during the first year of life except for a few very rare situations. Not only is it perfectly suited for the infant's gastrointestinal tract, but its numerous growth factors in breast milk enhance growth and maturation of the infant's relatively permeable gastrointestinal tract. Breast milk components also modify the bacterial environment that is best suited for the gastrointestinal (GI) tract of the infant, enhancing the growth of bifidus bacterium and reducing the growth of hazardous bacteria.

The mother benefits from breastfeeding as well. Women who breastfeed have enhanced weight loss and a major reduction in breast cancer risk compared to women who do not breastfeed. Numerous studies now suggest that the longer a mother breastfeeds, the greater the reduction in risk of breast cancer.[1,2] While recent studies have clearly suggested that the number of women who choose to breastfeed is rising (approximately 72% currently initiate breastfeeding in the United States), the number of women who discontinue breastfeeding to take a medication because of advice from their healthcare professional is simply too high. Surveys in other countries indicate that 90–99% of women will receive some medication during the first week postpartum, and virtually all will consume medications throughout the breastfeeding period.[3,4] In Scandinavia, the use of medications is a major reason why women discontinue breastfeeding prematurely, and 17–25% of breastfeeding women report having taken a medication during the 2 weeks prior to discontinuing breastfeeding.

While the drugs used early postnatally primarily include analgesics, methylergonovine (Methergine), antihypertensives, and sedatives, many other new mothers are now taking antidepressants, antipsychotics, antiepileptics, antibiotics, steroids, and medications from many other drug categories. Hence, the number of medications that an infant is exposed to appears to be rising. Because so many women ingest medications during the early neonatal period, one of the most common questions encountered in pediatrics and obstetrics concerns the effects of various drugs in breastfeeding mothers.

Almost invariably, professionals simply review the package insert and often advise the mother to not breastfeed without having done a thorough study of the literature to find the true answer. More often than not, advice to discontinue breastfeeding is inaccurate. Most mothers could easily continue to breastfeed their infants and take the medication without risk to the infant.

In the past 20 years, a proficient understanding of the kinetics of drug entry into human milk has emerged. Most of the physiochemical properties that facilitate transfer into milk (e.g., molecular weight, pKa, lipophilicity) are known today and well understood. This chapter describes the physiology and anatomy of the breast, reviews the biochemistry of milk production, details the transfer of medications into human milk, and discusses the implications of

this transfer for the infant. The objective of this chapter is to provide the busy clinician with data showing that, on average, most medications are quite safe to use in breastfeeding mothers. Indeed, the Academy of Pediatrics[5] and others[6] have published compendiums that provide data on the relative safety of many medications. But many newer medications have not yet been studied, and some background on the pharmacokinetics of drug entry into human milk is in order. Therefore, this chapter will also provide the clinician with methods one can use to properly evaluate the safety of using medications in breastfeeding mothers, and even to evaluate medications for which data are lacking. It is always important to remember that breastfeeding is incredibly important to the health and well-being of young infants. Recommending that a mother discontinue breastfeeding to take a medication is almost never required and should only be done as a last resort.

The Alveolar Subunit and Breast Milk Production

Whereas the anatomy of the human breast is to some degree well understood, there are still many biologic principles of human milk synthesis that are poorly understood. Figure 38-1 provides an illustration of the anatomy of the breast including the ductal system. Milk ducts start in the nipple and then migrate backward into the breast fat pads, terminating into extensive lobular-alveolar clusters (grapelike), as illustrated in Figure 38-2. Each alveolus is lined with a single layer of polarized secretory epithelial cells called **lactocytes** that are uniquely capable of synthesizing human milk. The alveoli are then surrounded by a basketlike network of specialized smooth muscle cells called the *myoepithelial cells*. These specialized smooth muscle cells have receptors of oxytocin, and when alveoli are stimulated by the release of oxytocin from the pituitary, milk is forced out of the alveoli into the terminal ductal system near the nipple.

During pregnancy, lactocytes are small in size and poorly functional, largely due to high circulating levels of progesterone. The initial fluid secreted by the lactocytes is called **colostrum**, and production of colostrum is referred to as **lactogenesis I**. Colostrum has limited fat and volume, but during this stage of development, large intercellular gaps exist, and numerous components from the maternal plasma compartment are able to leak into colostrum. These components include immunoglobulins (IgG, IgA, IgM, and IgE),

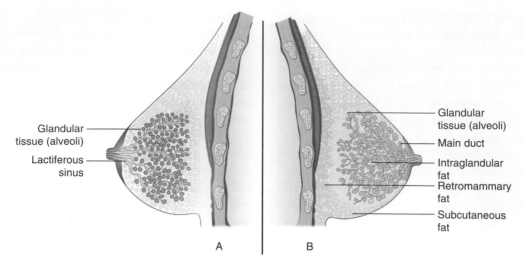

A. Traditional schematic diagram of the anatomy of the breast. The main milk ducts below the nipple are depicted as dilated portions or lactiferous sinuses, and the glandular tissue is deeper within the breast.
B. Schematic diagram of the ductal anatomy of the breast based on recent finding. Milk ducts are small and branch a short distance from the base of the nipple. The ductal system is erratic, and glandular tissue is situated directly beneath the nipple.

Figure 38-1 A schematic drawing of the anatomy of the human breast.
Source: Reproduced with permission. Copyright Medela. Inc.

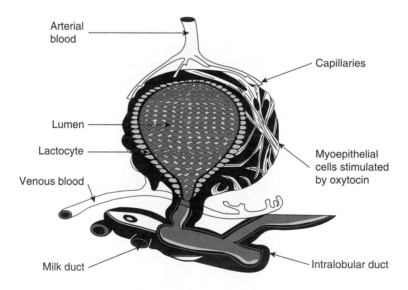

Figure 38-2 Structure of the alveolar subunit with blood supply and milk-creating lactocytes.
Source: Modified from Vorherr H. The breast: morphology, physiology and lactation. New York, 1974, Academic Press.

macrophages, leukocytes, and numerous other cellular components from the maternal circulation. Colostrum is incredibly important to the infant's new GI tract because it provides numerous growth factors, such as IGF-1 and maternal antibodies that suppress hazardous bacterial growth and promote beneficial bacterial colonization.

After delivery of the placenta, maternal estrogen and progesterone levels drop to baseline prepregnancy levels. This generally occurs by approximately 40 hours postpartum. When the plasma levels of these two hormones fall, their inhibitory effect on prolactin ceases and **lactogenesis II** occurs. Prolactin dramatically stimulates the lactocytes to produce milk. During this terminal growth phase, lactocytes connect to one another via an apical junctional complex that functions to inhibit direct paracellular exchange of substances from the maternal compartment into the breast milk compartment.

Prolactin is the driving force behind milk synthesis, along with other hormones, such as estrogen, thyroid hormones, and perhaps many others. Much of the physiology and release of prolactin production by the pituitary is to some degree understood. Less well known is how prolactin actually stimulates or supports milk synthesis by the lactocyte in the breast. Thus, when evaluating drug use in breastfeeding mothers, one must always first evaluate the effect the drug may have on milk production.

Drugs That Inhibit Milk Production

Because infant weight gain and development are directly linked to milk production and milk volume, even modest changes in milk supply can have profound effects on the breastfeeding infant. Thus, the use of various medications that affect prolactin levels will have profound effects on milk synthesis and infant development.

Estrogen and Progesterone

Drugs that may suppress prolactin release include the estrogens and potentially the progestins. Estrogens have been found clinically to profoundly reduce milk synthesis,[7] and these agents have been used to reduce severe postpartum engorgement for some mothers.[8] Unfortunately, although commonly accepted, the scientific support for this clinical result is difficult to find. Nevertheless, even the World Health Organization strongly warns against the use of oral contraceptives by breastfeeding mothers.[9] Breastfeeding mothers should be strongly advised to avoid estrogen-containing birth control products. In addition, progestins used early postnatally (first 48 hours) could theoretically impede the activation of the lactocytes by prolactin. Although strong evidence for this effect is missing in research done to date, it is grounded on good theory and knowledge of the biology. Mothers should be advised to avoid progestin-only products for the first 4–6 weeks postpartum. Even when initiated after 6 weeks postpartum, some mothers report a reduction in milk synthesis when using progestin-only contraceptives. Therefore, virtually any hormonal product, estrogen, progestin, or testosterone may suppress lactation, and women should be told that this is the case during prenatal and/or postpartum contraception counseling.

Bromocriptine (Parlodel)

Bromocriptine (Parlodel) is a **dopamine agonist** and a prolactin antagonist. This agent has been used in the past to reduce engorgement and inhibit milk production, although it was associated with numerous cases of cardiac dysrhythmias, stroke, intracranial bleeding, cerebral edema, convulsions, and myocardial infarction.[10-13] A newer analog, cabergoline (Dostinex), has fewer side effects and is considered safer for impeding milk synthesis.[14,15] Doses of 1 mg administered orally early postpartum will completely inhibit lactation. For established lactation, 0.25 mg given orally twice daily for 2 days has been found to completely inhibit lactation.[16,17]

Pseudoephedrine (Sudafed)

In one study published in 2003, the nasal decongestant pseudoephedrine (Sudafed) was shown to suppress milk production.[18] Studies are still preliminary, but mothers should be cautious using pseudoephedrine, particularly if they are at late-stage lactation (> 8 months) or have a poor milk supply. Box 38-1 provides a list of common medications that may inhibit milk production.

Box 38-1 Drugs That May Inhibit Breast Milk Production

Generic (Brand)

Bromocriptine (Parlodel)

Cabergoline (Dostinex)

Estrogen

Ergotamine (Cafergot)

Progestins

Pseudoephedrine (Sudafed)

Testosterone

Bupropion (Wellbutrin)*

* The risk to a newborn from exposure to bupropion via breast milk is theoretical.

Drugs That Stimulate Milk Production

The majority of mothers who produce insufficient milk do so as a result of poor management, including infrequent emptying of the breasts, major engorgement, poor latch, or other factors that can be avoided early postpartum. In many of these mothers, milk production may be recovered by proper management, including in some instances the use of various galactagogues including some dopamine antagonists.

However, milk production is a complex process, much of which is poorly understood. During pregnancy, breast tissue should enlarge significantly under the influence of progesterone and estrogen. These hormones stimulate growth and development of the ductal and alveolar system in the breast. Lack of breast tissue growth is foreboding for full development of lactogenesis II. Although assessment of breast growth should be part of the routine physical evaluation of mothers wishing to breastfeed, there are other etiologies of failed lactogenesis II that include thyroid dysfunction, pituitary disorders, retained placental tissue, and gestational ovarian theca lutein cysts.

Among those women who do not experience breast enlargement during pregnancy, milk production may be poor and is probably nonrecoverable, even with high levels of prolactin and frequent emptying of the breasts. Other women who have undergone lactogenesis II, even with significant development of breast tissue and higher levels of prolactin, still cannot produce sufficient quantities of milk for reasons that are less well understood. In addition, while it is true that elevated levels of prolactin are required for adequate production of milk, higher levels of prolactin do not necessarily increase production.[19] Prolactin is considered permissive of lactation and only slightly elevated levels will permit milk production to continue unabated.

Prenatal prolactin levels initially are quite high, and over the next 6 months after birth, these levels drop significantly almost to normal ranges, even though milk production levels are virtually unchanged.[20] Thus, as long as the levels of prolactin are slightly higher than baseline (at least 50–70 ng/mL), most mothers can continue to produce large quantities of milk. However, as prolactin levels drop too low or are near prepregnancy (20–30 ng/mL) levels, the production of milk suffers.

In women who have low prolactin levels, dopamine antagonist medications that inhibit dopamine receptors in the hypothalamus such as metoclopramide (Reglan) or domperidone (Motilium) can be used as galactagogues. Prolactin is stored in the lactotrophs of the pituitary under the powerful influence of dopamine. If dopamine is blocked, then prolactin is released from the lactotrophs and enters the plasma compartment. Dopamine antagonists dramatically stimulate maternal prolactin levels and, therefore, milk production. Other dopamine antagonists, such as risperidone (Risperdal), chlorpromazine (Thorazine), and other phenothiazine neuroleptics, are all well known to stimulate milk production, even in males, resulting in clinical gynecomastia. The two drugs most commonly used to stimulate milk production are the dopamine antagonists metoclopramide (Reglan)[21-23] and domperidone (Motilium),[24,25] which is not available in the United States.

Metoclopramide (Reglan)

Metoclopramide (Reglan) can in some cases profoundly stimulate milk production as much as 100%. Metoclopramide stimulates release of prolactin.[26] However, it is difficult, if not impossible, to predict which women will respond with elevated milk synthesis. Theory would suggest this agent is most useful for mothers whose prolactin levels were originally high but have dropped.

The prolactin-stimulating effect of metoclopramide is dose related. The standard dose required for efficacy is 10–15 mg given orally three times per day for a maximum of 30–45 mg/day.[26] Milk production normally responds quickly with the mother noticing significant increases of milk volume within 24–48 hours. The dose of metoclopramide present in milk is small, ranging from 28 to 157 mcg/L in the early puerperium.[23] This dose is far less than the clinical dose administered directly to infants (800 mcg/kg/d) for other conditions.

Side Effects/Adverse Effects

While milk synthesis may rebound efficiently, metoclopramide does cross the blood–brain barrier, and a drug-induced depression is common in mothers who consume this drug for more than 3 weeks. Other side effects of metoclopramide include extrapyramidal symptoms and gastric cramping. Aside from these side effects, millions of mothers have used this product to stimulate milk synthesis.

Domperidone (Motilium)

Domperidone (Motilium) is another dopamine antagonist used outside the United States that stimulates prolactin levels. It is apparently safer since it does not penetrate the blood–brain barrier. However, domperidone is not available in the United States other than via compounding pharmacies. Numerous studies show that domperidone stimulates milk production very well.[24,27,28] Milk levels of domperidone are extraordinarily low, only 1.2 ng/mL.[27] Even this amount of the drug in milk is not well absorbed, as the oral bioavailability of domperidone is less than 17%.

Side Effects/Adverse Effects

Unfortunately, domperidone is an antagonist to the **Human ether-a-go-go-Related gene** (HERG) potassium channel receptor. Because the HERG potassium channel repolarizes the cardiac action potential, use of domperidone may, under extraordinary conditions, cause minor arrhythmias. While the FDA has issued a black box warning that recommends domperidone not be used to stimulate milk production, the world community has largely ignored its warning. Domperidone still remains the preferred galactagogue used internationally.

Because the milk supply is dependent on an elevated prolactin level, the precipitous withdrawal of these galactagogues may result in a significant loss of milk supply. A slow taper of the drug is generally recommended over several weeks to a month to prevent loss of milk supply. Unfortunately, some mothers may require these drugs for long periods of time to maintain milk synthesis.

Passage of Drugs Across the Alveolar Epithelium

The passage of drugs, protein, and lipids across the apical membrane of the alveolar cell and into breast milk is not well understood. It is clear, however, that the transport of these agents is tightly controlled by the alveolar cell and the physiochemistry of the medications involved. The pathways for drug entry into milk are illustrated in Figure 38-3. Drug transfer into human milk is largely a result of equilibrium forces between the maternal plasma and the milk compartment. As maternal plasma levels rise, the medication is subsequently forced over into the milk compartment. While there are a few transport processes (influx transporters) for a few drugs (e.g., ranitidine [Zantac], nitrofurantoin [Macrobid], acyclovir [Zovirax], and iodine), few drugs enter milk by active transport, but instead simply diffuse across the alveolar bilayer membranes from an area of higher concentration (maternal plasma) to an area of lower concentration (milk). Thus, drugs maintain a close equilibrium with the plasma com-

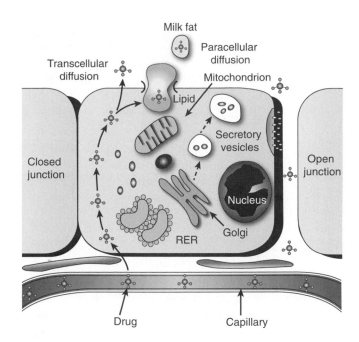

Figure 38-3 Diagrammatic representation of the various pathways for drug transfer into the human milk compartment.
Source: Reprinted with permission from Hale TW & Hartmann PE 2007.[123]

partment diffusing into and out of milk as a function largely of the maternal plasma level.

Molecular Weight of the Drug

The passive diffusion of medication across a lipid bilayer is largely determined by the molecular weight of the compound. The lower the molecular weight (< 500 daltons), the more likely the drug is to transfer into human milk. Drugs larger than 800 daltons seldom attain clinically relevant amounts in milk. Any drug much larger than 1000 daltons is unlikely to enter milk in clinically relevant levels. Alternatively, a medication such as lithium (Lithobid), with no protein binding and a low molecular weight of 6.94 daltons, readily enters the milk compartment and can achieve high levels in milk. Very large molecules, such as heparin (12,000–15,000 daltons), are largely excluded from breast milk. It is now apparent that many of the IgG preparations such as infliximab (Remicade) and etanercept (Enbrel) are virtually excluded from the milk compartment as well.

Lipid Solubility of the Drug

The lipid content of milk is high, ranging from 2.3% in foremilk to as high as 8% in hindmilk. The lipophilicity of the drug is measured by its octanol:water partition coefficient ($log_{10}P$). The more lipid soluble a drug, the better able it is to penetrate through the lipid bilayer of the cell membrane of the lactocytes and become concentrated in the milk compartment. Such drugs are often those that penetrate the blood–brain barrier and produce high levels in the central nervous system (CNS); the antidepressant mirtazapine (Remeron) is a classic example. The concentration of mirtazapine in hindmilk (high lipid content) is 2.3 times higher than in foremilk (low lipid content). Thus, if a drug is active in the CNS, it may produce higher levels in breast milk as well.

Milk pH and Drug pKa

The pKa of a drug is a unique physicochemical property that controls its ionization state when in solution. If the pH of the solution in which the drug exists is the same as its pKa, then 50% of the drug exists ionized and 50% exists nonionized. As the pH of the solution is changed, the state of ionization changes as well. If the drug is relatively unionized at a pH of 7.4 in the plasma, once it enters the milk (pH = 7.2), it may become more ionized and, thus, trapped in the milk compartment. In general, drugs with a pKa higher than 7.4 may become significantly trapped in the milk compartment.[29]

Protein Binding

It is well known that most drugs travel in plasma bound to albumin or other plasma proteins. Those with high binding affinity have difficulty diffusing out of the plasma compartment. Thus, only the free drug is available to transfer into peripheral compartments. This is especially true with respect to milk. Drugs with high maternal protein binding almost invariably produce lower levels in breast milk. Warfarin sodium (Coumadin), which is 99% bound, is virtually excluded from milk. Other highly protein-bound drugs, such as celecoxib (Celebrex), an NSAID, are found in low levels in milk.[30] Conversely, drugs with no protein binding, such as lithium (Lithobid), are found in higher levels in milk.

Bioavailability of Drugs in Mother and Infant

The absorption of medications by the infant is a function of the dose administered to the mother, the bioavailability of the drug in the mother, and the amount transferred into human milk. The bioavailability of a medication refers to the proportion of a dose that reaches the systemic circulation after its administration. Classically, this term is used when referring to drugs administered by all routes except intravenous because bioavailability is 100% when administered intravenously. Drugs administered orally are absorbed into the portal circulation of the gut and then pass through the liver prior to their delivery to the general circulation. Often the liver sequesters and metabolizes many drugs, thus eliminating their systemic effect. This is particularly true of opiates (e.g., morphine), which are largely eliminated from the circulation during their first pass through the liver.

While little is known about the oral absorption or bioavailability of medications in infants, there are apparently many similarities, particularly after the first month of life.[31] In neonates, gastric emptying time is delayed and intestinal absorption irregular and even limited in some cases. Slower intestinal absorption tends to be advantageous, as this would tend to keep drug plasma concentrations lower in the infant.[32] Medications presented to the infant in breast milk can, in rare instances, produce gastrointestinal symptoms of diarrhea or constipation. Diarrhea has been reported in some infants exposed to antibiotics or 5-aminosalicylic acid products. But most medications must be systemically absorbed into the infant's plasma compartment to produce untoward effects. Usually, those medications with poor oral bioavailability in adults are also poorly absorbed in infants.

Thus, for breastfeeding mothers, using medications that have poor oral bioavailability is recommended as it ultimately reduces the infant's exposure to untoward effects. Table 38-1 lists a number of medications that are poorly bioavailable and are ideal for breastfeeding mothers simply because they are poorly absorbed even in infants.

Milk/Plasma Ratio

The ratio of the concentration of drugs in breast milk to that in maternal plasma is known as the **milk/plasma** (M/P) ratio (Figure 38-4). The primary use of M/P is in quantifying the extent of drug transfer into milk and giving some indication of the underlying mechanisms. Clinically, it has no or little role unless one knows the absolute level of drug in the maternal plasma compartment at the time of measuring the M/P ratio. Ultimately, it is the concentration of a drug in milk (C_{milk}) that is the determinant of infant exposure, which in turn can be used to assess safety. Thus, one should avoid the use of M/P ratios unless they are exceedingly low. With the exception of iodine, most other drugs with high M/P ratios often fail to attain clinically relevant doses via breast milk.

Table 38-1 Maternal Medications That Are Safe for the Breastfed Infant Secondary to Decreased Bioavailability

Drug Generic (Brand)	Molecular Weight (Daltons)	Oral Bioavailability in Adults	Clinical Considerations
Albuterol and related inhaled beta adrenergic agonists	239	Insignificant	Systemic absorption minimal; inactivated by first-pass uptake in liver. Administered via inhalation.
Budesonide (Rhinocort)	430	10.7% orally	Poor oral absorption. High first-pass uptake in liver.
Ceftriaxone (Rocephin)	555	Not absorbed orally	Administered IV.
Etanercept (Enbrel)	51,235	Not absorbed	Decomposed in gut by proteases. Administered SC.
Fluticasone (Flonase)	500	< 0.5%	Administered via inhalation; systemic absorption minimal.
Gentamicin (Garamycin) and related aminoglycosides	478	Insignificant	First-pass hepatic inactivation. Intravenous only.
Heparin	12,000–15,000	Not absorbed	Unabsorbed; decomposed in GI tract.
Infliximab (Remicade)	144,190	Not absorbed	Decomposed by gut proteases. Only available IV.
Interferon-α and interferon-β	22,500–28,000	Not present in milk or absorbed	Decomposed by gut pH and protease enzymes. Administered SC.
Lansoprazole (Prevacid)	369	80% (enteric coated)	Unstable at low pH. Extensive metabolism by hepatic enzymes.
Omeprazole (Prilosec)	345	30–40% (enteric coated)	Unstable at low pH. Half-life is about 1–1.2 hours.
Pantoprazole (Protonix)	405	77% (enteric coated)	Unstable at low pH. Rapidly metabolized by hepatic enzymes.

$$\text{Milk/Plasma Ratio} = \frac{C_{Milk}}{C_{Plasma}}$$

Figure 38-4 Milk/plasma ratio formula.

Active Transport of Medications Into and Out of Breast Milk

While most drugs transfer into milk largely as a function of equilibrium forces between the maternal plasma and milk compartment, there are a few drugs where the milk/plasma ratio is significantly elevated to a degree that is far more than would be expected by passive diffusion. These drugs are being transported by various transporters. Such drugs include nitrofurantoin (Macrodantin, Macrobid) (M/P = 6),[33] acyclovir (Zovirax) (M/P = 4.1),[34] ranitidine (Zantac) (M/P = 6.7–23.77),[35] and iodine (M/P = 23).[36,37] While these drugs may be concentrated in milk, with the exception of iodine, they normally do not attain ranges that have clinical effect. Iodine, on the other hand, is transported so extensively that clinically hazardous ranges have been noted.[36] Therefore, with the exception of iodides, most of the aforementioned drugs that are actively

transported into human milk are actually quite safe for use by breastfeeding mothers.

It is also possible that active transport out of the breast milk compartment could exist. For example, **plasma glycoprotein** is a gene extensively expressed in intestinal epithelium, the blood–brain barrier, hepatocytes, and renal tubules. The plasma membrane that this gene codes for is an efflux transporter that actively transports drugs out of cells. This plasma membrane has been located in either apical or basolateral epithelial membranes as well.[38] Metformin (Glucophage) provides an example. Assuming a passive diffusion model, theoretic calculations of the transfer of metformin into human milk would suggest an M/P ratio of 2.93.[39] However, the clinically observed M/P ratio in three studies have reported much lower M/P values (0.63, 0.35, and 0.46, respectively) and a flat milk concentration-time profile.[39-41] The lower observed M/P ratios may indicate an active efflux transporter, pumping metformin out of milk and back into the plasma compartment.[41] Apparently, metformin is a substrate for the **OCT1 and OCT2 organic cation transporters**. The OCT1 efflux transporter is also expressed in human mammary gland epithelium.[42]

Calculation of Infant Dose

Ultimately, the evaluation of risk to the infant depends on the dose of medication the infant receives during the period of exposure to the medication.[43] There are two ways of calculating this dose, one is the **absolute infant dose** (AID), and the other is the **relative infant dose** (RID).[44]

Absolute Infant Dose

The AID (Figure 38-5) is an estimate of the drug concentration in milk (per mL) multiplied by the volume of milk received each day, where C_{max} is equal to the maximum concentration of drug in milk or where $C_{average}$ is the average concentration of drug in milk throughout the dosing period.

This method assumes that the volume of milk received each day is known, and this is its weakest point. Many sources now use a value of 150 cc/kg/day as an estimate of milk delivery to infant per day as many mothers do not actually know the volume of milk they feed to the infant each day. The use of C_{max} almost always leads to an overestimate of the actual infant dose. When $C_{average}$ is available, it is significantly more accurate clinically.

Relative Infant Dose

The RID (Figure 38-6) provides an estimate of the weight-normalized dose relative to the mother's dose. The measurement is the most useful method for assessing drug safety in breastfeeding mothers and their infants, and it is commonly used in many reviews and textbooks in this field.

This method provides the clinician with a good estimate of how much of the mother's dose of the drug is actually transferred to the infant daily on a dose-per-weight basis. The RID tells the clinician what percent of the mother's dose is transferred to the infant during a particular dosing interval. Interpretation of the relative risk in this method is dependent on a notional safe level of concern. This level of concern was suggested by Bennett in 1966 to be a cutoff value of 10% of the mother's dose.[45] Doses higher than this were considered more risky, and thus, doses less than 10% are considered relatively safe. This level has been widely accepted in the literature. But in reality, this level of concern still depends on the relative toxicity of the drug. Medications that are extremely hazardous would require much lower values than the 10% level (e.g., methotrexate, other anticancer agents).

Risk–Benefit Analysis

Unfortunately, infants have little to gain from exposure to medication via milk, but they do have much to gain from continued breastfeeding. If a technique to reduce exposure, particularly to hazardous drugs, is required, a mother may briefly interrupt breastfeeding, use alternative and safer drugs, postpone treatment until the infant is less sensitive, or in rare cases, use formulas while pumping and discarding her milk. Each case must be individually assessed, taking into account the importance of therapy, the timing of

$$AID = \text{Drug concentration in milk } (C_{max} \text{ or } C_{average}) \times \text{Volume of milk received/day}$$

Figure 38-5 Absolute infant dose.

$$RID = \frac{\text{Dose infant} \left(\frac{mg/kg}{day} \right)}{\text{Dose mother} \left(\frac{mg/kg}{day} \right)}$$

Dose infant = dose in infant/day

Dose mother = dose in mother/day

Figure 38-6 Relative infant dose.

therapy, the choice of medications, the ability of the infant to tolerate the medication, and the overall toxicity of the drug itself.

Predisposing Infant Factors

Virtually all medications taken by breastfeeding mothers will attain at least a minimum level in their breast milk; however, most often this is a subclinical level. The ability of the infant to adjust and maintain homeostasis while exposed to varying quantities of drug is largely a function of the infant's metabolic status. All infants should be categorized as low, moderate, or potentially at risk for the medication of interest. Infants at low risk are generally older infants (6–18 months) who can metabolize and handle drugs efficiently. Moderate-risk infants are those less than 4 months who suffer from various metabolic problems, such as complications from the delivery, apnea, GI anomalies, hepatitis, or other metabolic problems. Infants at higher risk are newborn or premature infants, infants who are unstable, or infants with poor renal output.

In summary, the ultimate evaluation of the safety of drugs in breast milk depends on three major factors, including (1) the amount of medication present in the breast milk, (2) the oral bioavailability of the medication in the infant, and (3) the ability of the infant to clear the medication if absorbed. Even though there are numerous studies reviewing the levels of drugs in breast milk and their bioavailability, the ability of the infant to clear most medications is still highly variable and requires close evaluation by the attending clinician.

The following sections describe the transfer of many drugs and drug classes into human milk. While sometimes the actual levels in milk can be predicted using kinetics, nothing is superior to actual studies in breastfeeding mothers. Many drugs have been studied in the last 30 years, and these data are in part listed below by drug category.

Analgesics

Analgesics compose the most commonly used agents by breastfeeding mothers and are used most commonly early postpartum. Table 38-2 provides the relative infant dose and compatibility of most analgesics and anti-inflammatory drugs.

Aspirin

Aspirin levels in milk are generally quite low, approximately 0.1–0.4% of the maternal dose. Used briefly and in low doses, aspirin probably poses little risk to a breast-fed infant. Unfortunately, the relative risk of Reye syndrome remains unknown as a function of the dose of aspirin or even the age of infant. Most cases of Reye syndrome occur among adolescents, using therapeutic doses of aspirin (650 mg or more). Current practice suggests low-dose (81 mg) aspirin is likely to be compatible with breastfeeding.

Acetaminophen (Tylenol)

Published levels of acetaminophen (Tylenol) in milk vary enormously but are generally less than 6.4% of the maternal dose. Acetaminophen is cleared for use in infancy anyway, so there is little or no concern about the use of this product by breastfeeding mothers.

Nonsteroidal Anti-inflammatory Drugs (NSAIDs)

Numerous NSAIDs exist, and many of them have been studied in breastfeeding mothers. However, ibuprofen (Advil)

Table 38-2 Relative Infant Doses of Various Analgesic and Anti-inflammatory Drugs in Human Milk

Drug Generic (Brand)	Relative Infant Dose (%)	Clinical Considerations
Common Analgesics		
Aspirin	< 0.1–10	Compatible in low doses. Prolonged use could be problematic, so other analgesics are preferred.
Acetaminophen (Tylenol)	1–6.4	Compatible.
Nonsteroidal Anti-inflammatory Drugs		
Celecoxib (Celebrex)	0.2–0.3	Compatible.
Diclofenac (Voltaren)	1.4 or less	Compatible.
Ibuprofen (Advil)	0.001–0.65	Compatible.
Indomethacin (Indocin)	0.3–1.2	Compatible.
Ketorolac (Toradol)	0.2	Compatible.

and ketorolac (Toradol) are perhaps the two most preferred in this drug family. Ibuprofen is an ideal analgesic for breastfeeding mothers as its milk levels are incredibly low. Less than 0.65% of the maternal dose is transferred daily to the infant.[46] Ketorolac (Toradol) is another popular NSAID that is very controversial. While ketorolac (Toradol) may cause bleeding problems in some postpartum women via its ability to inhibit platelet aggregation, its documented milk levels are all but insignificant. In a study of 10 lactating women who received 10 mg of ketorolac orally four times daily, milk levels of ketorolac were not detectable in four of the subjects.[47] In the six remaining, the concentration of ketorolac in milk 2 hours after a dose ranged from 5.2 to 7.3 mcg/L on day 1 to 5.9 to 7.9 mcg/L on day 2. For most women, the milk level was never above 5 mcg/L. The relative infant dose would only be 0.2% of the daily maternal dose. This study used oral administration rather than intramuscular administration, which would bypass some of the first-pass effect, but even so, ketorolac should still be considered a safe analgesic for breastfeeding mothers.

Recent studies of celecoxib (Celebrex) suggest it is a safe analgesic for breastfeeding mothers. Knoppert estimates that the daily intake in an infant is approximately 20 mcg/kg/day.[48] Data from studies at Texas Tech University of women receiving 200 mg daily suggest a 66 mcg/L average concentration (AUC) of celecoxib in milk.[30] Using these data, the relative infant dose was 0.34% of the maternal dose. Plasma levels of celecoxib in two infants studied were undetectable (< 10 ng/mL).

Morphine and Congeners

The data on morphine and breast milk levels are highly variable. Some studies show morphine levels are relatively high, and others have found them to be relatively low. But a more important factor about morphine is its poor oral bioavailability—less than 25% is orally absorbed due to a high first-pass effect in the liver. In a more recent study, the concentration of morphine in breast milk was only 82 mcg/L following two 4-mg epidural injections,[49] and produced no sedation in breastfed infants. Combined with its rather limited levels in milk and its poor oral bioavailability, morphine is considered compatible with breastfeeding so long as the maternal doses are low to moderate and the infant is stable.

Codeine and hydrocodone are the most common opioid analgesics used to treat pain in breastfeeding mothers. Codeine is a prodrug that is metabolized into morphine, which is the active ingredient. Thus, the rate of metabolism

in an individual affects the efficacy of pain relief. In addition, codeine is metabolized by CYP2D6, which is expressed in varying degrees secondary to several different polymorphisms.[50] In a study following twelve 60-mg doses, the estimated concentration of codeine in milk was 0.35 mg/L or 0.1% of the maternal dose.[51] Two studies reported apnea, bradycardia, or cyanosis in breastfed infants after repeated 4–6 hourly maternal doses of 60 mg codeine,[52,53] but a third that evaluated codeine levels in 17 samples of breast milk found no neonatal effects.[54] Based on this work, the American Academy of Pediatrics has historically recommended codeine for lactating women if indicated because the levels of codeine in breast milk are quite low. However, one infant death has been reported following the maternal use of codeine (60 mg every 12 hours, subsequently reduced to 30 mg every 12 hours from day 2 to 14).[55] Morphine levels in the mother were apparently elevated, as CYP2D6 genotyping of the mother suggested that she was an ultrarapid genotype. In 2007, the FDA issued a Public Health Advisory that reviewed the rare but potentially fatal side effect of neonatal death from morphine overdose obtained via breast milk.[56] This, however, is a rare and unusual finding, and in most cases, codeine taken in short courses and at low doses should be safe for the breastfed infant. The FDA advisory recommends that if codeine is prescribed for a breastfeeding woman, the lowest dose possible be used, and the woman should be counseled to watch for signs of excessive sleepiness and/or difficulty nursing or rousing the infant.

While codeine is still probably compatible in most situations, hydrocodone (Vicodin, Vicoprofen, Norco, Lorcet, Lortab) is probably a safer alternative because hydrocodone does not have an active metabolite; it is already active, and thus it avoids the problem encountered with rapid metabolizers who need large doses to get an analgesic effect. Ultimately, each infant should be closely monitored for symptoms of exposure to include oversomnolence, apnea, and poor feeding.

▍Antibiotics and Antifungals

Aside from analgesics, the second most commonly used class of medications by breastfeeding mothers is the antibiotics. Levels and relative infant doses are provided in Table 38-3. There are numerous reviews of the transfer of antibiotics into human milk available for the interested reader.[57-59]

Table 38-3 Relative Infant Doses of Various Antibiotics in Human Milk

Drug Generic (Brand)	Relative Infant Dose (%)	Clinical Considerations
Amoxicillin (Amoxil)	1.5	Compatible. Observe infant for diarrhea or thrush.
Cephalexin (Keflex)	0.53	Compatible. Observe infant for diarrhea or thrush.
Cefotaxime (Claforan)	0.34	Compatible. Observe infant for diarrhea or thrush.
Dicloxacillin (Dynapen)	1.26	Compatible. Observe infant for diarrhea or candida diaper rash.
Azithromycin (Zithromax)	5.8	Compatible. Observe infant for diarrhea or thrush.
Clarithromycin (Biaxin)	2	Compatible. Observe infant for diarrhea or diaper rash.
Erythromycin (E-mycin)	< 2.3	Compatible. Use postnatally associated with infantile hypertrophic pyloric stenosis. Observe for diarrhea or thrush.
Ciprofloxacin (Cipro)	2.6	Compatible. One case of pseudomembranous colitis reported. Observe for diarrhea or candida overgrowth.
Doxycycline (Adoxa, Vibramycin)	4–5.8	Compatible for short-term use (< 3 weeks). Avoid chronic dosing. Observe infant for diarrhea or candida overgrowth.
Tetracycline (Achromycin, Sumycin)	0.8–1.3	Compatible for short-term use. Oral absorption low. Observe infant for diarrhea or candida overgrowth.
Clindamycin (Cleocin)	1.4–2.8	Compatible. One case of pseudomembranous colitis reported. Observe infant for diarrhea or candida overgrowth.
Metronidazole (Flagyl)	10.5–13	Moderate transfer. No adverse effects reported in exposed infants. Dose via milk less than therapeutic dose. May impose bitter taste to milk. For 2-g single oral dose, discard milk for 12–24 h.
Vancomycin (Vanocin)	6.6	Compatible. Poor oral bioavailability. Dose via milk subclinical.

Penicillins

Virtually all of the penicillins and cephalosporins have been studied and are known to produce only trace levels in milk.[60-66]

Tetracyclines

The transfer of the tetracycline antibiotics, such as tetracycline (Sumycin), oxytetracycline (Terramycin), and others into human milk is very low. When mixed with calcium salts, the bioavailability of these tetracyclines is significantly reduced, and it is unlikely the infant would absorb the small levels present in milk. However, doxycycline (Vibramycin, Adoxa) absorption is delayed, but not blocked, and its absorption may be significant over time. Short-term use of these compounds for up to 3 weeks is permissible, and is suitable for treatment of many syndromes. Long-term use, such as for acne, is not recommended for breastfeeding mothers due to the possibility of dental staining in the infant and reduced growth rate in the epiphyseal growth plates.

Fluoroquinolones

Use of fluoroquinolones during lactation is somewhat controversial. Although the dose received via milk is low, pseudomembranous colitis has been reported in one case, although this can occur with any antibiotic.[67] In one group of infants exposed for up to 20 days, a greenish discoloration of the infants' teeth was noted at 12–23 months of age.[68] However, ciprofloxacin (Cipro) use in pediatrics has increased in recent years,[69] and there are now numerous studies indicating that there is little risk from ciprofloxacin exposure. Calcium reputedly may compromise the bioavailability of ciprofloxacin, hence milk calcium may suppress the oral bioavailability in an infant.

In one study of 10 women who received 750 mg of ciprofloxacin (Cipro) every 12 hours, breast milk levels ranged from 3.79 mg/L at 2 hours postdose to 0.02 mg/L at 24 hours.[70] Ciprofloxacin has recently been approved for use in breastfeeding mothers by the Academy of Pediatrics.[5] Ciprofloxacin ophthalmic products are poorly absorbed and the dose is low, so these products may be used by breastfeeding mothers.

Metronidazole (Flagyl)

The use of the antiprotozoal metronidazole (Flagyl) among breastfeeding women is not clear (Box 38-2). Older data suggested it was potentially mutagenic in rodents, although this has never been documented in humans.[71] However, concerns remain, even though it is commonly used by pediatricians. Topical and vaginal preparations of metronidazole (Flagyl) are of no concern to a

> ### ■ **Box 38-2**　A Case of a Mother's Concerns
>
> A 23-year-old woman is successfully breastfeeding her 12-week-old daughter. She seeks care for a vaginal discomfort and subsequently is diagnosed with bacterial vaginosis. This mother has been scrupulous about her diet and avoidance of any medications because of concern about untoward effects on her child.
>
> Bacterial vaginosis is the most frequently reported vaginal condition and is discussed in more detail in Chapter 31. The first choice for treatment of the symptomatic condition is metronidazole (Flagyl) 500 mg taken twice daily for 7 days. Some clinicians are hesitant to prescribe metronidazole because of unproven myths about mutagenicity. Other providers note that the relative infant dose is 9–13%, which is a moderate RID level. In addition, no untoward effects have been reported among breastfeeding infants at the recommended dose. Thus, the usual treatment offered to nonpregnant individuals is reasonable for this breastfeeding dyad.
>
> Since this woman has expressed concerns about drugs and breastfeeding, it may be best to prescribe an alternative treatment—that is, metronidazole gel (MetroGel). This topical treatment is effective for bacterial vaginosis, and essentially there is no transfer of the drug into milk following vaginal application of the topical gel.
>
> Regardless of the route of metronidazole, breastfeeding should not be discontinued. For women with conditions (e.g., trichomonas vaginalis) for which metronidazole is usually indicated in a large oral dose (2 gram single dose), it is commonly suggested that there is a brief interruption of breastfeeding of 12–24 hours, especially because metallic taste of the milk may occur, causing the infant to reject the taste.

breastfeeding mother simply due to limited absorption via these routes of administration. Following oral doses of 1200 mg/d, the maximum concentration in breast milk was 15.5 mg/L on average.[72] Although the relative infant dose of metronidazole is moderate, approximating 9–13% of the maternal dose, metronidazole (Flagyl) is virtually nontoxic, and no untoward effects have been reported in infants. A slight metallic taste of the milk has been reported, and some infants may reject the breast milk due to this taste. Large oral doses (2 g oral dose administered as one dose), which are commonly prescribed for treatment of vaginal trichomoniasis, should be followed by a brief interruption of breastfeeding for perhaps 12–24 hours. In those instances where the 2-g dose cannot be used, a regimen of 500 mg twice daily for 5 days is suitable. Following the use of intravenous metronidazole (Flagyl), a short withholding period of a few hours (2–3 h) to avoid the peak is advised to avoid even higher breast milk levels of the drug.

Macrolides

Erythromycin, a macrolide commonly used to treat chlamydia and other syndromes early postnatally, is problematic. Extensive data now suggest that its use early postnatally may increase the risk of hypertropic pyloric stenosis.[73,74]

Erythromycin and azithromycin (Zithromax) levels in milk are quite low. Following a dose of 2 g erythromycin daily, milk levels varied from 1.6–3.2 mg/L of milk.[75] Azithromycin transfer to milk is minimal and produces a clinical dose of approximately 0.4 mg/kg/day.[76] If given a choice, azithromycin or even clarithromycin (Biaxin) is usually preferred in the early postnatal period.

Antifungals

Nystatin (Mycostatin) is virtually unabsorbed orally, thus its transfer into breast milk is almost nil. Fluconazole (Diflucan) transfers significantly into human milk with a relative infant dose of 16%,[77-79] although this is still subclinical in infants, and though this is higher than the 10% notional safety range, it has proven quite safe in many cases and is far less than clinical doses commonly prescribed directly for infants.

Sulfonamides

Sulfamethoxazole, an older drug, is still commonly used in combination with trimethoprim (sulfamethoxazole/trimethoprim [Bactrim]) for various infections. The relative infant doses of sulfamethoxazole and trimethoprim are 2.3–6%[80,81] and 9%,[81] respectively. These doses are still lower than typical clinical doses used to treat infants. However, sulfonamides should not be used by mothers of infants with hyperbilirubinemia or who have glucose-6-phosphate dehydrogenase deficiency.

Antihypertensives

Antihypertensives are commonly used postnatally. Fortunately, only the beta-blocker family presents a significant risk to breastfed infants, and then only specific agents within this family. Two beta-blockers, atenolol (Tenormin) and acebutolol (Sectral), have been associated with dangerous cyanosis, bradycardia, and hypotension in several reported cases in breastfed infants, although these cases are relatively rare.[82,33] Preferred beta-blockers include propranolol (Inderal) and metoprolol (Lopressor), both of which produce minimal levels in breast milk and have no untoward effects yet reported in breastfeeding infants. Hydralazine (Apresoline) and methyldopa (Aldomet) have been used for years by breastfeeding mothers, virtually without complications. Present studies suggest levels in breast milk are low. The calcium channel blockers have been studied extensively and tend to produce low levels in breast milk, particularly verapamil (Isoptin, Covera-HS) and nifedipine (Procardia). Both of these calcium channel blockers have been used extensively without complications. Nifedipine (Procardia) levels in breast milk are < 8 mcg/kg/d, a particularly low level.[84]

Angiotensin converting enzyme inhibitors (ACE inhibitors) have been extensively studied in breastfeeding mothers. Captopril (Capoten) and enalapril (Vasotec) (but not nadolol [Corgard]) are preferred as breast milk levels are quite low following use of these two agents.[85-87] However, some caution is recommended early postnatally as these agents are potent hypotensives. Since these drugs can cause severe nephrotoxicity when used in the last trimester of pregnancy, they should be used cautiously by mothers with premature infants, at least until the infant is at the gestational age of a full-term infant.

Thyroid and Antithyroid Medications

The transfer of levothyroxine into human milk is negligible, thus treatment of hypothyroidism with oral thyroid supplement is suitable.[88] Liothyronine (Synthroid, L-Thyroxine) levels in breast milk are reportedly slightly higher than levothyroxine, but are still too low to affect thyroid function in the neonate.[89]

In hyperthyroid states, both propylthiouracil (PTU) and methimazole (Tapazole) have been extensively studied in breastfeeding mothers. Propylthiouracil levels in milk are generally the lowest, with milk levels at least tenfold less than the maternal plasma levels. The absolute infant dose would be approximately 0.1 mg/kg/d or 1.8% of the maternal dose. In at least two studies thus far, no changes in infant thyroid function have been reported, and PTU should be considered the agent of choice.[90,91] In another study using radiolabeled PTU, only 0.08% of the maternal dose transferred into human milk over 24 hours.[92]

Psychotherapeutic Agents

The postnatal period is associated with numerous psychiatric disorders. These include depression, generalized anxiety disorders, and psychosis. The risk of postpartum depression is being reported at alarming rates. At present, approximately 10–15% of postpartum women report clinical depression, although almost 80% experience postpartum blues.[93]

Using medications in the early postpartum period has always been controversial. However, recent information suggests that depression itself significantly interferes with optimal parenting that results in neurobehavioral delay in infants.[94-96] In the early postpartum period, all mothers will suffer to some degree from sleep deprivation, pain, and stress. Thus, it becomes important to distinguish between postpartum blues and postpartum depression (Chapter 37). In those women with clear and significant depression, the risk is simply too high to withhold treatment. Therefore, pharmacotherapy of depression diagnosed in the postpartum period is currently recommended.

Sedatives and Hypnotics

The transfer of the benzodiazepines has been studied in breastfeeding mothers. Breast milk levels of diazepam (Valium), lorazepam (Ativan), midazolam (Versed), and others are not excessive. The relative infant dose of diazepam is less than 9% of the maternal dose.[97] While some reports of lethargy, sedation, and poor suckling have been reported, these are rare. If a sedative is required, the shorter half-life analogs, such as lorazepam (Ativan) and midazolam (Versed), are preferred, but long-term exposure is not recommended.[98] The relative infant doses of lorazepam (2.5%) and midazolam (0.6%) are quite low, and sedation in breastfeeding infants is unlikely.

The use of phenothiazine analogs for treating nausea and vomiting should be avoided if possible. Chlorpromazine (Thorazine) and promethazine (Phenergan) may increase the risk of sleep apnea of the baby,[99] increase the risk of sudden infant death syndrome (SIDS),[100] and should probably be avoided in breastfeeding mothers. While the level of these drugs in breast milk is low, other more suitable alternatives such as ondansetron (Zofran) are available for treating nausea.

Tricyclic Antidepressants

Almost all of the current antidepressants have been studied in breastfeeding mothers. More than 40 studies of the tricyclic antidepressants are available and suggest that levels of these agents in milk are low and that they are compatible with breastfeeding. But compliance is often poor with the tricyclics due to side effects such as anticholinergic symptoms, xerostomia, blurred vision, and sedation. The relative infant dose of amitriptyline (Elavil) is less than 1.5% of the maternal dose.[101] Studies thus far have been unable to detect it in the infant's plasma. Doxepin (Sinequan) should be avoided due to reported hypotonia, poor suckling, vomiting, and jaundice.[102] Desipramine (Norpramin) levels in breast milk are minimal. One study of desipramine suggests that a 30 mg/d results in a relative infant dose of approximately 1%.[103]

Selective Serotonin Reuptake Inhibitors

The selective serotonin reuptake inhibitors (SSRIs) are presently the mainstay of depressive therapy, primarily because they are incredibly effective and have minimal toxicity in overdoses. The most often studied drug in breastfeeding mothers in the beginning of the 21st century has been the SSRI antidepressants. Table 38-4 lists the various antidepressants and their relative infant doses.

Neonatal withdrawal symptoms have been commonly reported in infants exposed to SSRIs during pregnancy. These symptoms, which occur early postnatally, consist of poor adaptation, irritability, jitteriness, and poor gaze control in neonates exposed to fluoxetine (Prozac)[104,105] or sertraline (Zoloft) and paroxetine (Paxil).[106]

Clinical studies of breastfeeding patients taking sertraline (Zoloft), fluvoxamine (Luvox), and paroxetine (Paxil) clearly indicate that the transfer of these medications into human milk is low and uptake by the infant is even lower. Thus far, no untoward effects have been reported following the use of these three agents in breastfeeding mothers. Sertraline (Zoloft) appears to be the overwhelming favorite as more than 50 infants have been evaluated in numerous studies and milk and infant plasma levels are quite low to undetectable.

Fluoxetine (Prozac) has been studied in at least 29 breastfeeding infants. Fluoxetine transfers into human milk in relatively higher concentrations, ranging to as high as 9% of the maternal dose.[107] Because of its long half-life active metabolite, clinically relevant plasma levels in infants have been reported. In several, severe untoward symptoms, such as colic, sedation, seizure, or coma have been reported.[108-111] Therefore, fluoxetine is perhaps less preferred unless lower doses are used during pregnancy and early postpartum. However, in reality, the incidence of untoward effects are probably remote, and mothers who cannot tolerate other SSRIs should be maintained on fluoxetine (Prozac) while breastfeeding (Box 38-3).

Citalopram (Celexa) and its new congener, escitalopram (Lexapro), transfer into milk moderately. In a study of seven women receiving an average of 0.41 mg/kg/d of

Table 38-4 Relative Infant Doses of Various Antidepressants in Human Milk

Drug Generic (Brand)	Relative Infant Dose (%)	Clinical Considerations
Amitriptyline (Elavil)	1.5	Compatible; observe for sedation in infant.
Bupropion (Wellbutrin)	0.7–2	Compatible; do not use in patients subject to seizures. Observe for possible milk suppression.
Citalopram (Celexa), escitalopram (Lexapro)	0.4–3.7	Caution; somnolence reported in some newborns.
Desipramine (Norpramin)	1	Compatible; observe for sedation in infant.
Doxepin (Sinequan)	1.2	Unsafe; respiratory arrest and sedation reported.
Fluoxetine (Prozac)	2.6–6.81	Compatible; avoid high maternal dose early postpartum.
Paroxetine (Paxil)	< 2.9	Compatible for infant; avoid use in adolescents.
Sertraline (Zoloft)	0.3–2.2	Compatible; preferred SSRI.
St. John's wort	No data	Compatible; recent data suggest transfer to milk is minimal. No untoward effects noted.
Venlafaxine (Effexor)	6.4	Probably safe; no side effects noted in one study; however, RID is somewhat high.

Box 38-3 A Case of Postpartum Depression

FL had her first baby 5 weeks ago and is breastfeeding her son. FL is feeling increasingly anxious about caring for her baby alone since her parents are returning to their home out of state soon. FL now is unable to sleep because "my thoughts just keep running in my head all night." She presents for a visit requesting "sleeping medicine that will not hurt the baby."

FL has a history of depression for which she took fluoxetine (Prozac) until a year ago. FL weaned herself from the fluoxetine slowly over a few months prior to trying to get pregnant. The rest of her medical history is negative. She has never been hospitalized for a psychiatric disorder. She is not taking any other medications.

FL's speech is quite rapid and she sounds very anxious. She does not want to take an antidepressant medication and continues to suggest she "just needs something to help me sleep when I am not nursing the baby." She denies suicidal ideation or abnormal thoughts about the baby and exhibits appropriate concern for her baby during the visit.

FL's anxiety and insomnia may be symptoms of either postpartum depression or bipolar disorder. The serotonin reuptake inhibitors (SSRIs), which include fluoxetine (Prozac), have been studied in breastfeeding mothers and infants, and although they all transfer into breast milk to a small extent, there are no reports of harm to the breastfeeding infant. Because postpartum depression can be harmful to the mother, infant, and family, treatment is recommended. However, acute anxiety can also be a symptom of bipolar disorder, which can be made worse if the woman is taking an SSRI medication, so an accurate diagnosis is essential.

FL agrees to an acute visit with a psychiatrist who specializes in women's health, and an appointment is made for her in 2 days. After consultation with the psychiatrist, FL is prescribed lorazepam (Ativan) for the next 2 nights with the caveat that FL's partner can be with her and the baby at all times. The psychiatrist also recommends initiating sertraline (Zoloft) as FL does not have a history of bipolar disorder or manic episodes that could be symptomatic of bipolar disorder. FL agrees to return for future care, but requests fluoxetine (Prozac) because she is familiar with it.

The clinician tells FL that fluoxetine is not recommended for breastfeeding because it has a long half-life and clinically effective doses have been detected in infants of breastfeeding mothers. Additional health education includes the fact that sertraline (Zoloft) takes several days to weeks to become completely effective, and therefore, medications that help her deal with the symptoms in the short term may be a good idea. FL is told that the drugs in the sedative/hypnotic family that are used to aid sleep such as lorazepam (Ativan) are safe for use for a short time, because although the medication transfers to breast milk, the dose is slightly less than 9% and sedation has rarely been noted in newborns exposed to these drugs.

Finally, the clinician recommends that FL get 5–7 hours of uninterrupted sleep each night to help ameliorate her symptoms. She is encouraged to pump her milk in the day so the infant can be fed by her partner at night for at least a few nights.

citalopram (Celexa), the average milk level was 97 mcg/L for citalopram (Celexa) and 36 mcg/L for its metabolite (RID = 3.7%).[112] Low concentrations of citalopram were noted in the infants' plasma (2 and 2.3 mcg/L). While no untoward effects have been noted in the published studies, two cases of somnolence have been reported to the manufacturer and at least four other anecdotal cases have been reported to this author. At this time, citalopram (Celexa) should be used cautiously by mothers with premature infants or those subject to apnea. In a recent study of eight breastfeeding women taking an average

of 10 mg/day of escitalopram (Lexapro), the total relative infant dose of escitalopram and its metabolite was reported to be 5.3%.[113] The drug and its metabolite were undetectable in most of the infants tested. No adverse events in the infants have been reported.

Serotonin Norepinephrine Reuptake Inhibitors

The serotonin norepinephrine reuptake inhibitors (SNRIs) inhibit reuptake of both serotonin and norepinephrine in contrast to the SSRIs, which inhibit the reuptake of serotonin only. Although there are fewer studies of SNRIs than of SSRIs in breastfeeding dyads, those that have been done have similar findings. These agents do transfer to breast milk in differing amounts, there are case reports of mild side effects in infants, the neurodevelopmental effects following long-term use are unknown, and it is recommended that they be used for the shortest period of time possible if needed.

Antipsychotics

The literature on the older antipsychotics and their transfer into human milk is poor. These data seem to suggest that low levels of the phenothiazines, such as chlorpromazine (Thorazine), transfer into milk, with some moderate sedation reported.[114,115] Because of their association with neonatal apnea and sedation, the older phenothiazines should be avoided in breastfeeding mothers. The transfer of haloperidol (Haldol) into breast milk is reported to be minimal (RID $\leq$ 11.2%).[116,117]

A number of new reports suggest that the newer atypical antipsychotics may be the better choice of therapy for breastfeeding mothers. Risperidone (Risperdal) levels are reportedly quite low with an estimated relative infant dose of 0.6–6.5% and without any reported sedation in the breastfed infants.[118,119] In several studies of olanzapine (Zyprexa), the relative infant dose ranged from 0.9 to 1.12%.[120-122] No untoward effects were noted in any of the infants.

Clinical Implications

The reader may wonder where to find a simple rating scale to use as a guide to identify drugs that are safe for breastfeeding women. Although no single source exists, several rating scales have been proposed. In 1984, Berglund and colleagues proposed four categories for drugs used during pregnancy and during lactation. This scale is not commonly used today. However, Box 38-4 lists some basic principles that may aid clinicians. Several detailed texts are available, which help the reader in the selection.[6,123-125] Each of these texts has a slightly different set of recommendation categories, but cross-comparisons for specific drugs reveal no significant differences in the actual recommendations as all of them use peer-reviewed research for the basis of these recommendations. In addition, the Specialized Information Services of the National Institutes of Health sponsors

---

Box 38-4 Major Concepts in Using Drugs in Breastfeeding Mothers

Avoid the unnecessary use of medications. This includes most herbal drugs.

Some radioisotopes may require brief interruptions and discarding of the milk.

Select drugs with the lowest relative infant dose.

Select drugs with shorter half-lives and avoid long half-life drugs if possible.

Select drugs with poor oral bioavailability to reduced absorption in infants.

Select drugs for which there are published milk studies.

Check the infant's medications for drug–drug interactions.

Evaluate the age, stability, and condition of the infant in order to determine if the infant can handle exposure to the medication.

Premature infants may be more susceptible to adverse effects of medications. Their clearance mechanisms have not matured.

CNS-active drugs always penetrate breast milk to some degree; an increased level of concern is recommended.

Most drugs can be safely used in breastfeeding mothers, but a risk-versus-benefit assessment is always required prior to use.

A relative infant dose of less than 10% is generally considered compatible with breastfeeding.

a searchable peer-reviewed referenced database that summarizes the fetal and infant risks for most if not all commonly prescribed medications.[126]

Food and Drug Administration (FDA) Categories

At the time of this writing, the FDA is considering a change to the current FDA pregnancy categories for labeling of drugs. If the proposed changes are adopted, the drug label will include a new section on lactation that discusses the risk of the drug to a newborn or infant if the drug is taken by a breastfeeding mother. The proposed labeling is discussed in more detail in Chapter 1.

American Academy of Pediatrics

The American Academy of Pediatrics (AAP), through its Committee on Drugs, has issued several iterations of a list of drugs with potential effects on the breastfeeding dyad. In 2005, the most recent edition was published, presenting the following seven discrete categories: (1) cytotoxic dugs that may interfere with cellular metabolism of the nursing infant; (2) drugs of abuse for which adverse effects on the infant during breastfeeding have been reported; (3) radioactive compounds that require temporary cessation of breastfeeding; (4) drugs for which the effect on nursing infants is unknown but may be of concern; (5) drugs that have been associated with significant effects on some nursing infants and should be given to nursing mothers with caution; (6) maternal medication usually compatible with breastfeeding; and (7) food and environmental agents' effects on breastfeeding.[5] Although the AAP has noted that this document is now outdated, it has not yet been revised. This document does not address some medications such as codeine, but the drugs that are placed in specific categories are likely to continue to belong in those categories.

Lactation Risk Categories

Perhaps the most commonly used scale is a relatively simple one, progressing from a category of drugs that are contraindicated, to a category that is termed *safest*. The elegance of a simple scale enables clinicians to use the system easily. However, any system is limited because new studies are constantly emerging, as are new drugs that have not been well studied for use by the breastfeeding woman and her infant. Table 38-5 shows the lactation risk categories.[6]

Finally, when information about the transfer of a specific drug into breast milk is not available, a reasonable assessment can be made by assessing the molecular size, solubility, pH, protein binding, peak plasma time, half-life, and activity of metabolites.

▌Conclusion

All medications transfer into human milk to some degree. However, few agents actually produce clinically relevant levels in infants. Ultimately, the most important information about a drug is its relative infant dose. These data give

Table 38-5 Lactation Risk Categories

Category	Description
L1—safest	Drugs that have been taken by a large number of breastfeeding mothers without any observed increase in adverse effects in the infant. Controlled studies in breastfeeding women fail to demonstrate a risk to the infant, and the possibility of harm to the breastfeeding infant is remote, or the product is not orally available to an infant.
L2—safer	Drugs that have been studied in a limited number of breastfeeding women without an increase in adverse effects in the infant; and/or the evidence of a demonstrated risk that is likely to follow use of this medication in a breastfeeding woman is remote.
L3—moderately safe	Drugs for which there are no controlled studies in breastfeeding women; however, the risk of untoward effects to a breastfed infant is possible; or controlled studies show only minimal, nonthreatening adverse effects. Drugs should be given only if the potential benefit justifies the potential risk to the infant.
L4—possibly hazardous	Drugs for which there is positive evidence of risk to a breastfed infant or to breast milk production, but the benefits from use in breastfeeding mothers may be acceptable despite the risk to the infant (e.g., if the drug is needed in a life-threatening situation or for a serious disease for which safer drugs cannot be used or are ineffective).
L5—contraindicated	Drugs for which studies in breastfeeding mothers have demonstrated significant and documented risk to the infant based on human experience; or a medication that has a high risk of causing significant damage to an infant. The risk of using the drug in breastfeeding women clearly outweighs any possible benefit from breastfeeding. The drug is contraindicated in women who are breastfeeding an infant.

Source: Hale TW 2008.[6]

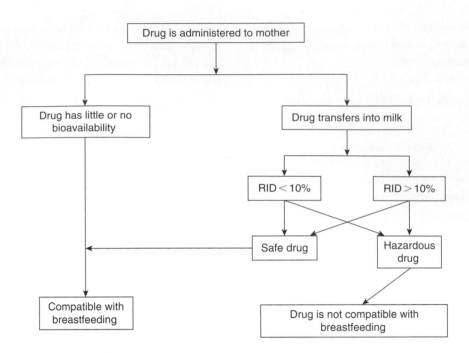

Figure 38-7 Algorithm for risk–benefit analysis in assessing drug use in breastfeeding mothers.

the prescriber an accurate estimate of just how much medication the infant will receive daily. If this is low, relative to the normal infant dose, then the medication is probably safe to use. Figure 38-7 provides an algorithm for risk–benefit analysis in assessing drug use in breastfeeding mothers.

However, in each case, the clinician must first determine a relative risk–benefit analysis for the individual infant. Infant factors that must be assessed are prematurity, weakness, apnea, contraindicated medications, and other factors that would reduce the ability of the infant to tolerate even low levels of maternal medications. The infant has nothing to gain from exposure to medications via mother's milk. Reducing or eliminating exposure should be the desired outcome. However, in most instances, the exposure to medication is generally subclinical. In these instances, the relative risk of avoiding breast milk far exceeds the risk of the medication. Formula-fed infants are known to have higher rates of gastrointestinal syndromes, upper respiratory tract infections, and numerous other syndromes. Thus, it is sometimes riskier to use formula than a mother's own milk.

Often the amount of medication delivered to the infant via milk is substantially less than 4% of the maternal dose, and the amount the infant actually absorbs orally is even less. In healthy infants, this amount is often easily tolerated without untoward effects in most infants. However, as the relative infant dose rises above 7–10% and the toxicity of the medication increases, clinicians should be more cautious in recommending continued breastfeeding if the medication is required.

In most situations, there are numerous medications that can be safely used for specific syndromes. Ultimately the choice of the medication is extremely important. All healthcare providers are advised to carefully choose those medications with lower relative infant doses and fewer side effects in infants. Almost invariably, a suitable drug can be chosen so that a mother can continue to breastfeed her infant safely.

References

1. Shantakumar S, Terry MB, Teitelbaum SL, Britton JA, Millikan RC, Moorman PG, et al. Reproductive factors and breast cancer risk among older women. Breast Cancer Res Treat 2007;102(3):365–74.
2. KimY, Choi JY, Lee KM, Park SK, Ahn SH, Noh DY, et al. Dose-dependent protective effect of breastfeeding against breast cancer among ever-lactated women in Korea. Eur J Cancer Prev 2007;16(2):124–9.
3. Bennett PN. Use of the monographs on drugs. In drugs and human lactation. Amsterdam, Netherlands: Elsevier, 1996:67–74.

4. Matheson I. Drugs taken by mothers in the puerperium. Br Med J (Clin Res Ed) 1985;290(6481):1588–9.

5. Academy of Pediatrics. Transfer of drugs and other chemicals into human milk. Pediatrics 2001;108(3): 776–89.

6. Hale TW. Medications and mothers' milk. Amarillo, TX: Hale Publishing, LP, 2008.

7. Treffers PE. Breastfeeding and contraception *Dutch*. Ned Tijdschr Geneeskd 1999;143(38):1900–4.

8. Booker DE, Pahl IR. Control of postpartum breast engorgement with oral contraceptives. Am J Obstet Gynecol 1967;98(8):1099–101.

9. World Health Organization. Contraception during breastfeeding, 1998. Available from: *www.contraception online.org/contrareport/article01.cfm?art=131* [Accessed June 26, 2009].

10. Dutt S, Wong F, Spurway JH. Fatal myocardial infarction associated with bromocriptine for postpartum lactation suppression. Aust N Z J Obstet Gynaecol 1998;38(1):116–7.

11. Iffy L, O'Donnell J, Correia J, Hopp L. Severe cardiac dysrhythmia in patients using bromocriptine postpartum. Am J Ther 1998;5(2):111–5.

12. Pop C, Metz D, Matei M, Wagner E, Tassan S, Elaerts J. Postpartum myocardial infarction induced by Parlodel *French*. Arch Mal Coeur Vaiss 1998;91(9):1171–4.

13. Webster J, Piscitelli G, Polli A, D'Alberton A, Falsetti L, Ferrari C, et al. Dose-dependent suppression of serum prolactin by cabergoline in hyperprolactinaemia: a placebo controlled, double blind, multicentre study. European Multicentre Cabergoline Dose-finding Study Group. Clin Endocrinol (Oxf) 1992;37(6): 534–41.

14. Ferrari C, Piscitelli G, Crosignani PG. Cabergoline: a new drug for the treatment of hyperprolactinaemia. Hum Reprod 1995;10(7):1647–52.

15. Webster J. A comparative review of the tolerability profiles of dopamine agonists in the treatment of hyperprolactinaemia and inhibition of lactation [published erratum appears in Drug Saf 1996 May;14(5):342]. Drug Saf 1996;14(4):228–38.

16. Anonymous. Single dose cabergoline versus bromocriptine in inhibition of puerperal lactation: randomised, double blind, multicentre study. European Multicentre Study Group for Cabergoline in Lactation Inhibition [see comments]. BMJ 1991;302(6789):1367–71.

17. Caballero-Gordo A, Lopez-Nazareno N, Calderay M, Caballero JL, Mancheno E, Sghedoni D. Oral cabergoline. Single-dose inhibition of puerperal lactation. J Reprod Med 1991;36(10):717–21.

18. Aljazaf K, Hale TW, Ilett KF, Hartmann PE, Mitoulas LR, Kristensen JH, et al. Pseudoephedrine: effects on milk production in women and estimation of infant exposure via breastmilk. Br J Clin Pharmacol 2003;56(1):18–24.

19. Chatterton RT Jr, Hill PD, Aldag JC, Hodges KR, Belknap SM, Zinaman MJ. Relation of plasma oxytocin and prolactin concentrations to milk production in mothers of preterm infants: influence of stress. J Clin Endocrinol Metab 2000;85(10):3661–8.

20. Cox DB, Owens RA, Hartmann PE. Blood and milk prolactin and the rate of milk synthesis in women. Exp Physiol 1996;81(6):1007–20.

21. Ehrenkranz RA, Ackerman BA. Metoclopramide effect on faltering milk production by mothers of premature infants. Pediatrics 1986;78(4):614–20.

22. Kauppila A, Arvela P, Koivisto M, Kivinen S, Ylikorkala O, Pelkonen O. Metoclopramide and breast feeding: transfer into milk and the newborn. Eur J Clin Pharmacol 1983;25(6):819–23.

23. Kauppila A, Kivinen S, Ylikorkala O. A dose response relation between improved lactation and metoclopramide. Lancet 1981;1(8231):1175–7.

24. Hofmeyr GJ, Van Iddekinge B. Domperidone and lactation. Lancet 1983;1(8325):647.

25. Hofmeyr GJ, Van Iddekinge B, Blott JA. Domperidone: secretion in breast milk and effect on puerperal prolactin levels. Br J Obstet Gynaecol 1985;92(2): 141–4.

26. Betzold C. Galactogogues. J Midwifery Womens Health 2004;49:151–4.

27. Brouwers JR, Assies J, Wiersinga WM, Huizing G, Tytgat GN. Plasma prolactin levels after acute and subchronic oral administration of domperidone and of metoclopramide: a cross-over study in healthy volunteers. Clin Endocrinol (Oxf) 1980;12(5):435–40.

28. da Silva OP, Knoppert DC, Angelini MM, Forret PA. Effect of domperidone on milk production in mothers of premature newborns: a randomized, double-blind, placebo-controlled trial. Canadian Med J 2001; 164(1):17–21.

29. Hale TW, Ilett KF. Drug therapy and breastfeeding. From theory to clinical practice. London: Parthenon Press, 2002.

30. Hale TW, McDonald R, Boger J. Transfer of celecoxib into human milk. J Hum Lact 2004;20(4):397–403.

31. Alcorn J, McNamara PJ. Pharmacokinetics in the newborn. Adv Drug Deliv Rev 2003;55(5):667–86.

32. Besunder JB, Reed MD, Blumer JL. Principles of drug biodisposition in the neonate. A critical evaluation of the pharmacokinetic-pharmacodynamic interface (Part I). Clin Pharmacokinet 1988;14(4): 189–216.

33. Gerk PM, Kuhn RJ, Desai NS, McNamara PJ. Active transport of nitrofurantoin into human milk. Pharmacotherapy 2001;21(6):669–75.

34. Lau RJ, Emery MG, Galinsky RE. Unexpected accumulation of acyclovir in breast milk with estimation of infant exposure. Obstet Gynecol 1987;69 (3, pt 2):468–71.

35. Kearns GL, McConnell RF Jr, Trang JM, Kluza RB. Appearance of ranitidine in breast milk following multiple dosing. Clin Pharm 1985;4(3):322–4.

36. Delange F, Chanoine JP, Abrassart C, Bourdoux P. Topical iodine, breastfeeding, and neonatal hypothyroidism. Arch Dis Child 1988;63(1):106–7.

37. Postellon DC, Aronow R. Iodine in mother's milk. JAMA 1982;247(4):463.

38. Raub TJ. P-glycoprotein recognition of substrates and circumvention through rational drug design. Mol Pharmacol 2006;3(1):3–25.

39. Hale TW, Kristensen JH, Hackett LP, Kohan R, Ilett KF. Transfer of metformin into human milk. Diabetologia 2002;45(11):1509–14.

40. Gardiner SJ, Kirkpatrick CMJ, Begg EJ, Zhang M, Moore MP, Saville DJ. Transfer of metformin into human milk. Clin Pharmacol Ther 2003;73(1): 71–7.

41. Briggs GG, Ambrose PJ, Nageotte MP, Padilla G, Wan S. Excretion of metformin into breast milk and the effect on nursing infants. Obstet Gynecol 2005;105(6):1437–41.

42. Alcorn J, Lu X, Moscow JA, McNamara PJ. Transporter gene expression in lactating and nonlactating human mammary epithelial cells using real-time reverse transcription-polymerase chain reaction. J Pharmacol Exp Ther 2002;303(2):487–96.

43. Ilett KF, Kristensen JH. Drug use and breastfeeding. Expert Opin Drug Saf 2005;4(4):745–68.

44. Begg EJ, Duffull SB, Hackett LP, Ilett KF. Studying drugs in human milk: time to unify the approach. J Hum Lact 2002;18:323–32.

45. Bennett PN. Drugs and human lactation. Amsterdam, Netherlands: Elsevier, 1996.

46. Weibert RT, Townsend RJ, Kaiser DG, Naylor, AJ. Lack of ibuprofen secretion into human milk. Clin Pharm 1982;1(5):457–8.

47. Wischnik A, Manth SM, Lloyd J, Bullingham R, Thompson JS. The excretion of ketorolac tromethamine into breast milk after multiple oral dosing. Eur J Clin Pharmacol 1989;36(5):521–4.

48. Knoppert DC, Stempak D, Baruchel S, Koren G. Celecoxib in human milk: a case report. Pharmacotherapy 2003;23(1):97–100.

49. Wittels B, Scott DT, Sinatra RS. Exogenous opioids in human breast milk and acute neonatal neurobehavior: a preliminary study. Anesthesiology 1990;73(5):864–9.

50. Madidi P, Ross CJD, Hayden MR, Carleton BC, Gaedigk A, Leeder JS, Koren G. Pharmacogenetics of neonatal opioid toxicity following maternal use of codeine during breastfeeding: a case control study. Clin Pharmacol Ther 2009;85:31–5.

51. Findlay JW, DeAngelis RL, Kearney MF, Welch RM, Findlay JM. Analgesic drugs in breast milk and plasma. Clin Pharmacol Ther 1981;29(5):625–33.

52. Davis JM, Bhutari VK. Neonatal apnea and maternal codeine use. Pediatr Res 2005;19(4):170A.

53. Naumburg EG, Meny RG, Alger LS. Codeine and morphine levels in breast milk and neonatal plasma. Pediatr Res 1987;21:240A.

54. Meny RG, Naumburg EG, Alger LS, Brill-Miller JL, Brown S. Codeine and the breastfed neonate. J Hum Lact 1993;9(4):237–40.

55. Koren G, Cairns J, Chitayat D, Gaedigk A, Leeder SJ. Pharmacogenetics of morphine poisoning in a breastfed neonate of a codeine-prescribed mother. Lancet 2006;368(9536):704.

56. FDA Public Health Advisory. Use of codeine by some breastfeeding mothers may lead to life-threatening side effects in nursing babies. May 7, 2007. Available from: *www.fda.gov/cder/drug/advisory/codeine.htm* [Accessed January 20, 2009].

57. Kristensen JH, Ilett K. Antibiotic, antifungal, antiviral and antiretroviral drugs. In Hale TW and Hartmann PE, eds. Textbook of human lactation. Amarillo, TX: Hale Publishing LP, 2007:513–21.

58. Nahum GG, Uhl K, Kennedy DL. Antibiotic use in pregnancy and lactation: what is and is not known about teratogenic and toxic risks. Obstet Gynecol 2006;107(5):1120–38.

59. Ben-Ari J, Samra Z, Nahum E, Levy I, Ashkenazi S, Schonfeld TM. Oral amphotericin B for the prevention

of *Candida* bloodstream infection in critically ill children. Pediatr Crit Care Med 2006;7(2):115–8.

60. Blanco JD, Jorgensen JH, Castaneda YS, Crawford SA. Ceftazidime levels in human breast milk. Antimicrob Agents Chemother 1983;23(3):479–80.

61. Kafetzis DA, Lazarides CV, Siafas CA, Georgakopoulos PA, Papadatos CJ. Transfer of cefotaxime in human milk and from mother to foetus. J Antimicrob Chemother 1980;6(suppl A):135–41.

62. Kafetzis DA, Siafas CA, Georgakopoulos PA, Papadatos CJ. Passage of cephalosporins and amoxicillin into the breast milk. Acta Paediatr Scand 1981;70(3):285–8.

63. Matsuda S. Transfer of antibiotics into maternal milk. Biol Res Pregnancy Perinatol 1984;5(2):57–60.

64. Shyu WC, Shah VR, Campbell DA, Venitz J, Jaganathan V, Pittman KA, et al. Excretion of cefprozil into human breast milk. Antimicrob Agents Chemother 1992;36(5):938–41.

65. Yoshioka H, Cho K, Takimoto M, Maruyama S, Shimizu T. Transfer of cefazolin into human milk. J Pediatr 1979;94(1):151–2.

66. Bourget P, Quinquis-Desmaris V, Fernandez H. Ceftriaxone distribution and protein binding between maternal blood and milk postpartum. Ann Pharmacother 1993;27(3):294–7.

67. Harmon T, Burkhart G, Applebaum H. Perforated pseudomembranous colitis in the breast-fed infant. J Pediatr Surg 1992;27(6):744–6.

68. Lumbiganon P, Pengsaa K, Sookpranee T. Ciprofloxacin in neonates and its possible adverse effect on the teeth. Pediatr Infect Dis J 1991;10(8):619–20.

69. Ghaffer F, McCraken GH. Quinolones in pediatrics. In Hoper DC, Rubenstein E, eds. Quinolone antimicrobial agents. Washington, DC: ASM Press, 2003:343–54.

70. Giamarellou H, Kolokythas E, Petrikkos G, Gazis J, Aravantinos D, Sfikakis P. Pharmacokinetics of three newer quinolones in pregnant and lactating women. Am J Med 1989;87(5A):49S–51S.

71. Schwebke JR. Metronidazole: utilization in the obstetric and gynecologic patient. Sex Transm Dis 1995;22(6):370–6.

72. Passmore CM, McElnay JC, Rainey EA, D'Arcy PF. Metronidazole excretion in human milk and its effect on the suckling neonate. Br J Clin Pharmacol 1988;26(1):45–51.

73. Sorensen HT, Skriver MV, Pedersen L, Larsen H, Ebbesen F, Schonheyder HC. Risk of infantile hypertrophic pyloric stenosis after maternal postnatal use of macrolides. Scand J Infect Dis 2003;35(2):104–6.

74. Stang H. Pyloric stenosis associated with erythromycin ingested through breastmilk. Minn Med 1986;69(11):669–70, 682.

75. Knowles JA. Drugs in milk. Pediatric Currents 1972;21:28–32.

76. Kelsey JJ, Moser LR, Jennings JC, Munger MA. Presence of azithromycin breast milk concentrations: a case report. Am J Obstet Gynecol 1994;170(5, pt 1):1375–6.

77. Force RW. Fluconazole concentrations in breast milk. Pediatr Infect Dis J 1995;14(3):235–6.

78. Schilling CG, Sea RE, Larson TA. Excretion of fluconazole in human breast milk [abstract No 130]. Pharmacotherapy 1993;13:287.

79. Kaufman D, Boyle R, Hazen KC, Patrie JT, Robinson M, Donowitz LG. Fluconazole prophylaxis against fungal colonization and infection in preterm infants. N Engl J Med 2001;345(23):1660–6.

80. Chung AM, Reed MD, Blumer JL. Antibiotics and breast-feeding: a critical review of the literature. Paediatr Drugs 2002;4(12):817–37.

81. Miller RD, Salter AJ. The passage of trimethoprim/sulphamethoxazole into breast milk and its significance. In Daikos GK, ed. Progress in chemotherapy: proceedings of the eighth International Congress of Chemotherapy, Athens, 1973. Athens, Greece: Hellenic Society for Chemotherapy, 1974.

82. Boutroy MJ, Bianchetti G, Dubruc C, Vert P, Morselli PL. To nurse when receiving acebutolol: is it dangerous for the neonate? Eur J Clin Pharmacol 1986;30(6):737–9.

83. Schimmel MS, Eidelman AI, Wilschanski MA, Shaw D Jr, Ogilvie RJ, Koren G, et al. Toxic effects of atenolol consumed during breast feeding. J Pediatr 1989;114(3):476–8.

84. Penny WJ, Lewis MJ. Nifedipine is excreted in human milk. Eur J Clin Pharmacol 1989;36(4):427–8.

85. Devlin RG, Duchin KL, Fleiss PM. Nadolol in human serum and breast milk. Br J Clin Pharmacol 1981;12(3):393–6.

86. Devlin RG, Fleiss PM. Captopril in human blood and breast milk. J Clin Pharmacol 1981;21(2):110–3.

87. Redman CW, Kelly JG, Cooper WD. The excretion of enalapril and enalaprilat in human breast milk. Eur J Clin Pharmacol 1990;38(1):99.

88. Mizuta H, Amino N, Ichihara K, Harada T, Nose O, Tanizawa O, et al. Thyroid hormones in human milk and their influence on thyroid function of breast-fed babies. Pediatr Res 1983;17(6):468–71.

89. Varma SK, Collins M, Row A, Haller WS, Varma K. Thyroxine, tri-iodothyronine, and reverse tri-iodothyronine concentrations in human milk. J Pediatr 1978; 93(5):803–6.

90. Cooper DS. Antithyroid drugs: to breast-feed or not to breast-feed. Am J Obstet Gynecol 1987;157(2): 234–5.

91. Kampmann JP, Johansen K, Hansen JM, Helweg J. Propylthiouracil in human milk. Revision of a dogma. Lancet 1980;1(8171):736–7.

92. Low LC, Lang J, Alexander WD. Excretion of carbimazole and propylthiouracil in breast milk [letter]. Lancet 1979;2(8150):1011.

93. O'Hara M, Swain M. Rates and risk of postnatal depression: a meta-analysis. Int Rev Psychiat 1996; 837–54.

94. Lee CM, Gotlib IH. Adjustment of children of depressed mothers: a 10-month follow-up. J Abnorm Psychol 1991;100(4):473–7.

95. Sinclair D, Murray L. Effects of postnatal depression on children's adjustment to school: teacher's reports. Br J Psychiatry 1998;172:58–63.

96. Zekoski EM, O'Hara MW, Wills KE. The effects of maternal mood on mother-infant interaction. J Abnorm Child Psychol 1987;15(3):361–78.

97. Wesson DR, Camber S, Harkey M, Smith DE. Diazepam and desmethyldiazepam in breast milk. J Psychoactive Drugs 1985;17(1):55–6.

98. Kanto JH. Use of benzodiazepines during pregnancy, labour and lactation, with particular reference to pharmacokinetic considerations. Drugs 1982;23(5): 354–80.

99. Kahn A, Hasaerts D, Blum D. Phenothiazine-induced sleep apneas in normal infants. Pediatrics 1985;75(5): 844–7.

100. Cantu TG. Phenothiazines and sudden infant death syndrome. DICP 1989;23(10):795–796.

101. Bader TF, Newman K. Amitriptyline in human breast milk and the nursing infant's serum. Am J Psychiatry 1980;137(7):855–6.

102. Frey OR, Scheidt P, von Brenndorff AI. Adverse effects in a newborn infant breast-fed by a mother treated with doxepin. Ann Pharmacother 1999; 33(6):690–3.

103. Stancer HC, Reed KL. Desipramine and 2-hydroxydesipramine in human breast milk and the nursing infant's serum. Am J Psychiatry 1986;143(12):1597–600.

104. Chambers CD, Johnson KA, Dick LM, Felix RJ, Jones KL. Birth outcomes in pregnant women taking fluoxetine [see comments]. NEJM 1996; 335(14):1010–5.

105. Spencer MJ, Escondido, CA. Fluoxetine hydrochloride (Prozac) toxicity in a neonate. Pediatrics 1993; 92(5):721–2.

106. Stiskal JA, Kulin N, Koren G, Ho T, Ito S. Neonatal paroxetine withdrawal syndrome. Arch Dis Child Fetal Neonatal Ed 2001;84(2):F134–F135.

107. Kristensen JH, Ilett KF, Hackett LP, Yapp P, Paech M, Begg EJ. Distribution and excretion of fluoxetine and norfluoxetine in human milk. Br J Clin Pharmacol 1999;48(4):521–7.

108. Brent NB, Wisner, KL. Fluoxetine and carbamazepine concentrations in a nursing mother/infant pair. Clin Pediatr (Phila) 1998;37(1):41–4.

109. Hale TW, Shum S, Grossberg M. Fluoxetine toxicity in a breastfed infant. Clin Pediatr (Phila) 2001;40(12): 681–4.

110. Lester BM, Cucca J, Andreozzi L, Flanagan P, Oh W. Possible association between fluoxetine hydrochloride and colic in an infant. J Am Acad Child Adolesc Psychiatry 1993;32(6):1253–5.

111. Taddio A, Ito S, Koren G. Excretion of fluoxetine and its metabolite, norfluoxetine, in human breast milk. J Clin Pharmacol 1996;36(1):42–7.

112. Rampono J, Kristensen JH, Hackett LP, Paech M, Kohan R, Ilett KF. Citalopram and demethylcitalopram in human milk; distribution, excretion and effects in breast fed infants. Br J Clin Pharmacol 2000;50(10):263–8.

113. Rampono J, Hackett LP, Kristensen JH, Kohan R, Page-Sharp M, Ilett KF. Transfer of escitalopram and its metabolite demethylescitalopram into breastmilk. Br J Clin Pharmacol 2006;62(3):316–22.

114. Blacker KH, Weinstein BJ, Ellman GL. Mother's milk and chlorpromazine. Am J Psychiatry 1962; 119:178–9.

115. Wiles DH, Orr MW, Kolakowska T. Chlorpromazine levels in plasma and milk of nursing mothers. Br J Clin Pharmacol 1978;5(3):272–3.

116. Ohkubo T, Shimoyama R, Sugawara K. Measurement of haloperidol in human breast milk by high-performance liquid chromatography. J Pharm Sci 1992;81(9):947–9.

117. Whalley LJ, Blain PG, Prime JK. Haloperidol secreted in breast milk. Br Med J (Clin Res Ed) 1981; 282(6278):1746–7.

118. Hill RC, McIvor RJ, Wojnar-Horton RE, Hackett LP, Ilett KF. Risperidone distribution and excretion into human milk: case report and estimated infant

exposure during breast-feeding [letter]. J Clin Psychopharmacol 2000;20(2):285–6.

119. Ilett KF, Hackett LP, Kristensen JH, Vaddadi KS, Gardiner SJ, Begg EJ. Transfer of risperidone and 9-hydroxyrisperidone into human milk. Ann Pharmacother 2004;38(2):273–6.

120. Croke S, Buist A, Hackett LP, Ilett KF, Norman TR, Burrows GD. Olanzapine excretion in human breast milk: estimation of infant exposure. Int J Neuropsychopharmacol 2002;5(3):243–7.

121. Gardiner SJ, Kristensen JH, Begg EJ, Hackett LP, Wilson DA, Ilett KF, et al. Transfer of olanzapine into breast milk, calculation of infant drug dose, and effect on breast-fed infants. Am J Psychiatry 2003;160(8):1428–31.

122. Kirchheiner J, Berghofer A, Bolk-Weischedel D. Healthy outcome under olanzapine treatment in a pregnant woman. Pharmacopsychiatry 2000;33(2):78–80.

123. Hale TW, Hartmann PE (eds). Textbook of human lactation. Amarillo, TX: Hale Publishing, LP, 2007.

124. Briggs GG, Freeman RK, Yaffee SJ. Drugs in pregnancy and lactation, 8th ed. Philadelphia, PA: Lippincott Williams & Wilkins, 2008.

125. Lawrence RA, Lawrence R. Breastfeeding: a guide for the medical profession, 6th ed. St. Louis, MO: Mosby, 2005.

126. Drugs and Lactation Database (LactMed). A peer-reviewed and fully referenced database of drugs to which breastfeeding mothers may be exposed. [Among the data included are maternal and infant levels of drugs, possible effects on breastfed infants and on lactation, and alternate drugs to consider.] Available from: *http://toxnet.nlm.nih.gov/cgi-bin/sis/htmlgen?LACT* [Accessed June 26, 2009].

39

The Newborn

Judy Wright Lott

Chapter Glossary

Classic hemorrhagic disease of the newborn The most common of the three types of newborn bleeding disorders within the general family of vitamin K deficiency bleeding. Occurs within the first 5 days following birth.

Clearance The rate at which a drug is cleared from the circulation per unit of time. Clearance in newborns is affected by renal immaturity and renal disease.

Early-onset hemorrhagic disease Rare form of vitamin K deficiency hemorrhagic disease. Often associated with a mother who is taking drugs that interfere with vitamin K, such as anticonvulsants, anticoagulants, or antibiotics.

Early-onset neonatal sepsis (EONS) Newborn sepsis that develops within the first 7 days following birth. Approximately 85% of newborns with EONS develop the disease within the first 48 hours after birth; it is most often acquired via vertical transmission during labor and birth.

Half-life The time it takes a drug to lose half of its pharmacologic activity.

Late-onset hemorrhagic disease Rare form of vitamin K deficiency hemorrhagic disease that occurs after 14 days of life. Associated with liver disease, celiac disease, and diarrhea. Most often seen in breastfed babies who did not receive vitamin K prophylaxis at birth.

Late-onset neonatal sepsis (LONS) Neonatal sepsis that develops after the first week of life. Commonly attributed to infection acquired in the hospital or home.

Loading dose A first dose that is higher than subsequent doses. Frequently used when administering drugs that have a long half-life.

Ophthalmia neonatorum Neonatal conjunctivitis that is due to gonococcal or chlamydial infection. Can cause blindness if left untreated.

Peak level The highest serum concentration that can be measured following a specific dose of a drug.

Steady state The point in time when the drug concentration in the circulation equals the concentration that is excreted.

Therapeutic range The range of plasma concentration values between the lowest dose that is efficacious and the dose that causes toxicity.

Trough level The lowest detectable or measurable concentration in serum that can be measured following a specific dose of a drug.

Vitamin K deficiency bleeding The most common etiology of hemorrhage; it is associated with a deficiency of clotting factors during the neonatal period.

Volume of distribution (Vd) The relationship between the dose of a drug and the serum concentration. The Vd is affected by fluid balance and properties of the drug itself.

Introduction

This chapter provides an overview of the pharmacologic principles that underlie safe and effective drug therapy for term newborns including routine prophylaxis, health maintenance, and recognition and initial treatment for common newborn problems.

Pharmacologic Prinicples for Newborns

Principles that govern medication—selection, administration, and monitoring—are generally the same for newborns as for other ages; however, the relative immaturity of the neonate's organ systems has a significant impact on the way the newborn body responds to drugs. The neonate is physiologically different than older persons, and these differences affect the specific dosage forms and dosing regimens used. Variables that influence the action of a specific drug include gestational and postnatal age, size, overall condition, presence of disease, development and function of targeted organs, and administration of other drugs.

Pharmacokinetic and pharmacodynamic variables change with increasing maturity.[1,2] The immaturity of the newborn's physiology results in certain drugs having a narrow therapeutic index when administered. Each medication regimen needs to be designed with a monitoring plan that will identify successful and adverse outcomes. This plan should include which indices need to be monitored to determine if the prescribed medication is achieving the desired outcome as well as what needs to be monitored to prevent toxic levels. Most medications marketed in the United States have not been studied in pediatric or neonatal individuals; thus, many commonly used medications are used off label.[3]

Pharmacokinetics and Pharmacodynamics of Import in Newborn Care

Prior to discussing the specific differences in newborn physiology, a brief review of the specific pharmacokinetic and pharmacodynamic processes of import is in order. First, the **volume of distribution** (Vd), which is the relationship between the dose of the drug administered and the serum concentration after administration, can be affected by fluid balance, binding capacity of plasma proteins, and nutritional deficiencies in the newborn, as well as the physical properties of the drug. A second important variable is **half-life** (t 1/2), the time it takes for a drug to lose half of its pharmacologic activity. Half-life can be influenced by renal function, liver function, tissue perfusion, and other concurrent medications. The **steady state** is the point in time at which drug concentration in the body equals the concentration of drug excreted by the body.[1,2,4]

Clearance is the rate at which the drug is cleared from the circulation per unit of time. Clearance is influenced by many factors, including organ maturity and/or function. Organ function is especially important if most of the elimination of the medication is the responsibility of one organ system. For example, a neonate in renal failure will have decreased clearance of gentamicin because gentamicin is primarily excreted from the body through the kidneys.[1,5]

Monitoring Drug Dosing

A **loading dose** is given for medications that have long half-lives wherein the time to reach steady state and therapeutic effectiveness may be unacceptably delayed. An example is a newborn having seizures who needs an antiseizure medication. In this situation, the medication is often administered with an initial loading dose that is greater than the maintenance dose. The **therapeutic range** is the range of concentrations between the lowest level that demonstrates efficacy and the high level above which toxicity is more prevalent. The therapeutic range can be calculated as the therapeutic index.[1,2,4]

In order for the therapeutic range to be useful in clinical practice, an assay must be available for measurement of serum concentrations. Therapeutic drug monitoring includes three types of measurements: **peak levels**, **trough levels**, and therapeutic range. In clinical practice, it is essential to know where in the dosing interval the measurement of a serum concentration is obtained. Peak levels reflect the time of peak drug concentration after the administration of the dose. If one is evaluating peaks, it may be necessary to adjust the subsequent dose in response to the level obtained. If the peak is too high, decrease the dose; if the peak is too low, increase the dose. The trough level reflects elimination of the drug. If one is monitoring troughs, the dosing interval is also adjusted in response to the level obtained. It is imperative that the clinician be aware of which value he or she is interpreting so the most appropriate adjustment can be made. In addition to serum drug levels, the individual response is always taken into consideration when interpreting the serum concentration of a specific drug.

Pharmacokinetics in the Newborn

The uniqueness of the neonate's physiology in light of absorption, protein binding, distribution, metabolism, and excretion must also be taken into consideration in the design of drug regimens. Intramuscular, oral, topical, and rectal routes of administration require absorption from the site to be effective.

Absorption

Absorption is affected by many unique physiologic characteristics of the neonate. Intramuscular administration is not as efficient as intravenous administration. Intramuscular absorption is influenced by muscle tone, muscle mass, and regional blood flow. Neonates have decreased muscle mass and tone, which may lead to unpredictable and incomplete absorption from the intramuscular route. In addition, in many disease states that affect neonates, decreased blood flow to specific organs can decrease absorption of drugs administered intramuscularly. Decreased or erratic absorption can delay the therapeutic response, cause a delay in peak concentration, and result in a longer duration of action.

Topical administration depends on skin integrity, blood flow, and subcutaneous fat for absorption. Premature infants have multiple physiologic characteristics that can influence topical absorption of medications. Increased skin-to-body surface area and decreased integrity of the skin barrier can predispose the neonate to toxicity from topical medications that are typically considered benign in adults. Drugs such as hydrocortisone and antifungal creams may be absorbed through the skin in levels that lead to adverse systemic effects. Conversely, the diminished skin barrier may allow for unique dosing of some medications that takes advantage of this physiologic difference to allow increased drug absorption. This method has been used successfully in adults for hormones and anesthetics. A topical anesthetic, eutectic mixture of local anesthetic (EMLA), has been used for local pain relief in term newborns, although it has been associated with methemoglobinemia in preterm infants; and pharmokinetic studies of drugs such as theophylline have been reported. Further research is needed to determine specific drug regimens for neonates.[1,2,4,6-8]

Gastrointestinal absorption is affected by multiple factors. Gastrointestinal pH is higher in the newborn compared to adult values, and this affects ionization of drugs in the stomach. Newborns also have slower gastric emptying time, less microbial colonization, longer intestinal transit time, decreased pancreatic enzyme activity, and immature biliary function. The clinical status of an individual newborn will also affect drug absorption.[1,2,6,7] These differences make the delivery of oral drugs more variable from neonate to neonate. Thus, oral medications are not recommended for use in the newborn when a rapid response is needed.

Protein Binding

Once absorbed, medications may bind to a variety of plasma proteins, although the majority bind to albumin. In neonates and infants, serum albumin concentrations are lower; therefore, fewer protein binding sites are available. In addition, newborns have higher levels of maternal estrogen and bilirubin in their circulation, which can compete with medications for albumin binding sites. Thus, for a given serum concentration, there is more free or active drug available for pharmacologic action in the newborn.

The clinical condition of the newborn can further affect protein binding; hepatic or renal failure results in altered protein binding. It is especially important to consider albumin levels in the newborn when establishing dosage and monitoring regimens. For example, a newborn with hyperbilirubinemia may have an altered response to a medication because of the excess bilirubin bound to albumin, lowering the availability of albumin binding sites for the medication. Conversely, administration of medications that bind to albumin may increase the bilirubin levels of an icteric newborn.[1,2,4,6,7]

Metabolism

Most medications require metabolism prior to excretion, and the liver is the site of metabolism for most medications that undergo transformation before they are excreted from the body. Liver pathways for metabolism include oxidation, methylation, sulfation, reduction, demethylation, hydroxylation, glucuronidation, and conjugation. These metabolic pathways mature at different times. The function of these pathways is a rate-limiting factor for elimination of drugs. Delayed maturation affects metabolism and the neonate's response to some medications, such as morphine. For example, in an adult, morphine is rapidly metabolized to morphine-6-glucuronide, which is an active metabolite and a more potent compound than morphine. However, in the newborn, this metabolism of morphine does not occur, thus the newborn may need a higher dose (mg/kg) of morphine than adults to provide adequate analgesia. Methylation, reduction, and sulfation are well developed at birth, but the other pathways do not develop fully until 1 to 3 months postbirth.[1,2,4,6,7]

Excretion

Finally, the rate of excretion of drugs may vary based upon the relative immaturity of the neonatal kidney. The neonatal kidney has a high resistance to blood flow, incomplete glomerular and tubular development, and a short loop of Henle. In addition, the kidney receives a low fraction of cardiac output. These variables can result in higher peak concentrations or longer duration of action of some medications by decreasing the rate of elimination of the drug.

Exposure to Drugs via the Placenta and via Breast Milk

There are two other important variables that must be considered in the pharmacology of the neonate—the effects of fetal exposure to drugs and newborn exposure through human milk. Any medication or substance given to the mother can cross the placenta. The consequence of fetal exposure may result in harmful effects, no adverse effect, or minimal adverse effect, depending upon several factors. The molecular weight of the substance, protein binding, lipid solubility, ionization of the drug, maternal serum concentrations, and the integrity of the placental barrier will all play a role in determining the actual concentration of drug that ends up in the fetal compartment when taken during pregnancy. Narcotic administration to the mother near delivery may be seen in the neonate as central nervous system sedation, lethargy, or difficulty nursing. Other hepatically active medications, such as phenobarbital (Luminal), can increase liver enzyme activity in the neonate and cause increased clearance of other drugs that are metabolized by the liver, such as narcotics. Conversely, medications that inhibit liver enzymes may result in slower clearance of hepatically metabolized medications.[1,2,4,6,7]

Transfer of substances from human milk to the neonate is an often-overlooked source of exposure to chemical substances. Variables that influence the amount of drug that will reach the neonate through human milk include protein binding, degree of ionization, and the concentration of the drug in the maternal circulation. Other factors include the time of medication administration versus time period of nursing, the dose of the medication, the length of nursing, and the total volume of human milk ingested[9] (See Chapter 38).

These physiologic differences must be taken into consideration when developing a therapeutic drug plan for the newborn. Following a term birth, the newborn is generally in one of the healthiest periods of life, and thus does not require drug therapy. However, it is incumbent upon the healthcare provider to adequately and appropriately assess the newborn, provide appropriate prophylactic medications, and diagnose and initiate drug therapy as needed. For example, healthcare professionals who routinely provide care for neonates must be knowledgeable and skillful in neonatal resuscitation, including resuscitation drugs. The drugs used for emergency resuscitation of the neonate are beyond the scope of this chapter; the reader is referred to the Neonatal Resuscitation Program developed by the American Academy of Pediatrics and the American Heart Association for a comprehensive review of resuscitation medications and procedures. The remainder of this chapter describes the common newborn conditions requiring pharmacologic intervention.

Routine Medications Used in the Neonatal Period

Routine Prophylaxis for Eyes

Ophthalmia neonatorum or gonorrheal conjunctivitis can occur when a neonate passes through the birth canal of a mother infected with *Neisseria gonorrhea* or *Chlamydia trachomatis* and is the most common cause of acute ophthalmic disease in newborns.[10] Ophthalmia neonatorum can cause corneal ulceration, endophthalmitis, and blindness. Since the introduction of routine eye prophylaxis for all newborns, the incidence of neonatal conjunctivitis and blindness has dramatically decreased.

The first drug used for prophylactic eye treatment was 1% silver nitrate solution. Side effects of the silver nitrate solution included chemical conjunctivitis with edema, redness, and watery discharge. In addition, silver nitrate is ineffective against chlamydia trachomatis, so it has largely been replaced due to the availability of agents that have a broader spectrum and fewer side effects.[11] Acceptable agents for eye prophylaxis include 0.5% erythromycin (EES) ointment, 1% tetracycline ointment, or 1.5–2.5% povidone-iodine solution.[5,10-12] Although eye prophylaxis is done routinely in the United States, these agents are not effective against every type of microorganism. It is important that newborns with conjunctivitis be promptly evaluated to determine the cause and most appropriate therapy.

Hemostasis

Hemostasis is dependent upon adequate supply of clotting factors that are primarily produced by the liver. The prothrombin complex specifically requires the action of vitamin K, which is synthesized by bacteria in the human colon. Vitamin K-dependent clotting factor levels in cord blood of the term fetus are 30–70% those of adults; however, there is a significant drop at birth, due to poor placental transfer of maternal vitamin K, immature liver function, and delayed synthesis of vitamin K by bacteria in the neonatal bowel. Levels of vitamin K-dependent clotting factors gradually rise but do not reach adult levels until about 9 months of age.

Hemorrhage due to a deficiency of vitamin K-dependent clotting factors during the neonatal period is classified as **vitamin K deficiency bleeding**. There are three types of hemorrhagic disease, based upon timing. They include **early-onset hemorrhagic disease**, **classic hemorrhagic disease of the newborn**, and **late-onset hemorrhagic disease**.

Classic vitamin K deficiency bleeding of the newborn is the most common type; it occurs within the first 2 to 5 days postbirth and presents as generalized bleeding. The American Academy of Pediatrics (AAP) recommends administering a single intramuscular dose of vitamin K_1 (0.5 to 1 mg) to all newborns in the first few hours after birth to protect the newborn from this bleeding disorder.[13] The policy recommended that there be further research on the efficacy, safety, and bioavailability of oral formulations, as well as optimal dosing regimens. This policy was reaffirmed in 2006.[14]

Controversy About Treatments for Vitamin K Deficiency

Despite the current vitamin K prophylaxis policy, there continues to be some controversy about the necessity for an intramuscular dose and some parents request that vitamin K be given orally. Full-term newborns have approximately 30–60% of the adult function of vitamin K-dependent coagulation activities.[15]

Early vitamin K deficiency hemorrhage develops in the first 24 hours of life and usually presents as a cephalohematoma, intracranial bleeding, or intraabdominal bleeding. Classic vitamin K deficiency hemorrhage occurs between 1 and 7 days of life and usually presents as gastrointestinal bleeding. The incidence of these two forms of vitamin K deficiency bleeding is between 0.25% and 1% in term newborns.[13] Late vitamin K deficiency bleeding occurs in breastfed infants between 8 days and 12 weeks of life, and 50% of these cases are theorized to be secondary to hepatic dysfunction in the infant. Bottle-fed infants get vitamin K in formula and are effectively protected against vitamin K deficiency bleeding disorders. One intramuscular injection of 0.5 mg or 1 mg vitamin K in the first day of life

effectively prevents classic vitamin K deficiency bleeding and late vitamin K deficiency bleeding.[13-15]

However, a controversy exists regarding dose and route.[16] Plasma concentrations of vitamin K following the intramuscular dose exceed endogenous levels by a factor of 10,000.[17] Studies on adverse effects of intramuscular vitamin K have noted a very small increased risk for developing leukemia in children who received intramuscular dose of vitamin K at birth. These studies are not conclusive, but neither has the relationship between vitamin K and a subsequent cancer risk been disproven to date.[17] However, as more is learned about the etiology of leukemia, it appears less and less likely that vitamin K injections play a role.

Oral administration of 2 mg of vitamin K with the first feeding followed by a second 2-mg oral dose between day 2 and 7 is an alternative to the intramuscular dose. Studies that have compared the oral versus intramuscular doses found that both improve biochemical indices of coagulation status at 1–7 days after birth, but there have not been any randomized trials that compared the two routes with regard to the development of hemorrhagic disease of the newborn.[18] In large observational series, the intramuscular dose is more effective, although the absolute numbers are small. No infants out of 100,000 newborns develop bleeding if intramuscular vitamin K is administered at birth, whereas infants given one oral dose develop bleeding in 1.42 per 100,000 births.[18] At this time, the American Academy of Pediatrics strongly recommends use of the intramuscular dose for all newborns in the United States. In Europe, several different regimens that include oral or intramuscular routes of administration and different doses based on risk status are available.

Early-onset hemorrhagic disease (≤ 24 hours) and late-onset hemorrhagic disease require frequent and prolonged vitamin K therapy, rather than one single dose. Late-onset hemorrhagic disease of the newborn can occur in the absence of prophylaxis at birth, or as a consequence of an underlying disorder, such as cystic fibrosis, biliary atresia, or galactosemia.[19]

Immunizations

The immune system begins developing in early gestation; however, the immune system of the newborn is both immature and inexperienced. The fetus receives benefit from transplacental diffusion of maternal antibodies during gestation, but after birth, circulating antibodies from the mother are no longer available; thus the newborn is more susceptible to communicable infections. Vaccines that protect against communicable diseases have resulted in reductions in the incidence of once common diseases such as diphtheria, polio, varicella (chicken pox), rubella (German measles), and pertussis (whooping cough).[20-22] Currently there are 15 diseases that can be prevented through the administration of vaccinations in children from birth through 6 years of age.[20,22] Table 39-1 summarizes the recommended vaccination schedule for birth through 6 years of age.

There are two vaccines recommended for newborns in the first few days after birth. The first dose of the hepatitis B vaccination series (HepB) is recommended for all newborns prior to discharge from the hospital postbirth. Palivizumab (Synagis) may be given to newborns at risk for developing respiratory syncytial virus.

Hepatitis B virus (HBV), a small, double-shelled virus in the family Hepadnaviridae, is the most common cause of chronic viremia. There are potentially more than 350 million people with chronic HBV worldwide. HBV infection causes acute and chronic hepatitis, cirrhosis of the liver, and approximately 80% of hepatocellular carcinomas. Hepatitis B can be transmitted through the placenta to the fetus from infected mothers; in some cases, the mother may not know she has HBV (Box 39-1). Infants who become infected with hepatitis B virus have a 90% chance of developing chronic hepatitis B virus infection with all its serious potential sequelae, including up to a 25% risk of death from cirrhosis or liver cancer. Thus, the high prevalence of HBV in women of childbearing age, the high transmission rate, and the severe consequences of HBV make the HepB vaccine cost effective.

HepB vaccine is administered intramuscularly in three doses of 0.5 mL of vaccine (10 mcg) each in a series of three injections. This vaccine has been given routinely in the United States since 1991, and the reported incidence of HBV has decreased by 95% in children and by 75% in all age groups. The second and third doses are given at age 1–2 months and age 6 months, respectively. Healthcare providers must be aware that thimerosal-free HepB vaccine has been available since 1999; there is no need to delay vaccination for any newborn.[23] (See Chapter 6 for a description of thimerosal.) Delayed administration of the first dose by even a few weeks puts the newborn at significant risk for developing HBV infection later in infancy.[24,25]

Newborns born to mothers who have chronic hepatitis B (HBsAg-positive) should receive hepatitis B immunoglobulin (0.5 mL) intramuscularly in addition to the HepB vaccine after physiologic stabilization of the infant and preferably within 12 hours of birth. Approximately 19,000 women with chronic hepatitis B virus infection give birth in the United States each year. Postexposure prophylaxis administered

within 12 hours postbirth will prevent HBV infection in 90% of these infants.[26] The hepatitis immune globulin can be administered at the same time as the HepB vaccine but at a separate site.[27]

One additional vaccination, palivizumab (Synagis), is recommended for newborns who have a high risk for developing respiratory syncytial virus. Preterm infants who have bronchopulmonary dysplasia or congenital heart defects are the groups evaluated for appropriateness of this vaccine.[28-31]

Recognition and Treatment of Common Neonatal Disorders

Infection

The incidence of infection in the term newborn in the United States has remained stable at approximately 2–4% since the 1980s.[32] Infection in the newborn period is associated with serious morbidity and mortality. Fifty percent of neonatal deaths in the first 24 hours postbirth are caused by infection. Early recognition and implementation of appropriate antimicrobial agents can significantly improve the prognosis.

Omphalitis or Umbilical Cord Infections

Omphalitis, which is infection of the umbilical cord, is rare in developed countries, although the exact incidence is not known because this infection typically occurs after discharge from the hospital. Omphalitis is generally localized but can spread directly into the bloodstream due to delayed obliteration of the umbilical vessels, causing severe systemic infection. Signs of omphalitis include erythema, edema, discharge, foul smell, bleeding from the cord, and/or failure of the cord to dry out. Omphalitis should be treated with systemic antimicrobial agents based upon the most likely causative microorganism. First-line agents include intravenous treatment with ampicillin and gentamicin.

There is no real evidence that application of topical agents such as isopropyl alcohol, povidone-iodine, chlorhexidine, or dyes prevents the incidence of omphalitis. Alternatively, there is evidence that application of these agents and routine daily care with isopropyl alcohol prolongs the timing for cord drying and separation. Therefore, prophylactic treatment of the umbilical stump with topical agents is not recommended.[32,33]

Table 39-1 Recommended Immunization Schedule for Persons Aged 0–6 Years—United States • 2008

For those who fall behind or start late, see the catch-up schedule

Vaccine ▼ Age ►	Birth	1 month	2 months	4 months	6 months	12 months	15 months	18 months	19–23 months	2–3 years	4–6 years
Hepatitis B[1]	HepB	HepB	*see footnote 1*		HepB						
Rotavirus[2]			Rota	Rota	Rota						
Diphtheria, Tetanus, Pertussis[3]			DTaP	DTaP	DTaP	*see footnote 3*	DTaP				DTaP
Haemophilus influenzae type b[4]			Hib	Hib	*Hib*[4]	Hib					
Pneumococcal[5]			PCV	PCV	PCV	PCV				PPV	
Inactivated Poliovirus			IPV	IPV		IPV					IPV
Influenza[6]						Influenza (Yearly)					
Measles, Mumps, Rubella[7]						MMR					MMR
Varicella[8]						Varicella					Varicella
Hepatitis A[9]						HepA (2 doses)				HepA Series	
Meningococcal[10]										MCV4	

Range of recommended ages

Certain high-risk groups

This schedule indicates the recommended ages for routine administration of currently licensed childhood vaccines, as of December 1, 2007, for children aged 0 through 6 years. Additional information is available at **www.cdc.gov/vaccines/recs/schedules**. Any dose not administered at the recommended age should be administered at any subsequent visit, when indicated and feasible. Additional vaccines may be licensed and recommended during the year. Licensed combination vaccines may be used whenever any components of the combination are indicated and other components of the vaccine are not contraindicated and if approved by the Food and Drug Administration for that dose of the series. Providers should consult the respective Advisory Committee on Immunization Practices statement for detailed recommendations, including for **high-risk conditions: http://www.cdc.gov/vaccines/pubs/ACIP-list.htm**. Clinically significant adverse events that follow immunization should be reported to the Vaccine Adverse Event Reporting System (VAERS). Guidance about how to obtain and complete a VAERS form is available at **www.vaers.hhs.gov** or by telephone, 800-822-7967.

1. **Hepatitis B vaccine (HepB).** *(Minimum age: birth)*
   At birth:
   - Administer monovalent HepB to all newborns prior to hospital discharge.
   - If mother is hepatitis B surface antigen (HBsAg) positive, administer HepB and 0.5 mL of hepatitis B immune globulin (HBIG) within 12 hours of birth.
   - If mother's HBsAg status is unknown, administer HepB within 12 hours of birth. Determine the HBsAg status as soon as possible and if HBsAg positive, administer HBIG (no later than age 1 week).
   - If mother is HBsAg negative, the birth dose can be delayed, in rare cases, with a provider's order and a copy of the mother's negative HBsAg laboratory report in the infant's medical record.

   After the birth dose:
   - The HepB series should be completed with either monovalent HepB or a combination vaccine containing HepB. The second dose should be administered at age 1–2 months. The final dose should be administered no earlier than age 24 months. Infants born to HBsAg-positive mothers should be tested for HBsAg and antibody to HBsAg after completion of at least 3 doses of a licensed HepB series, at age 9–18 months (generally at the next well-child visit).

   4-month dose:
   - It is permissible to administer 4 doses of HepB when combination vaccines are administered after the birth dose. If monovalent HepB is used for doses after the birth dose, a dose at age 4 months is not needed.

2. **Rotavirus vaccine (Rota).** *(Minimum age: 6 weeks)*
   - Administer the first dose at age 6–12 weeks.
   - Do not start the series later than age 12 weeks.
   - Administer the final dose in the series by age 32 weeks. Do not administer any dose later than age 32 weeks.
   - Data on safety and efficacy outside of these age ranges are insufficient.

3. **Diphtheria and tetanus toxoids and acellular pertussis vaccine (DTaP).** *(Minimum age: 6 weeks)*
   - The fourth dose of DTaP may be administered as early as age 12 months, provided 6 months have elapsed since the third dose.
   - Administer the final dose in the series at age 4–6 years.

4. ***Haemophilus influenzae* type b conjugate vaccine (Hib).** *(Minimum age: 6 weeks)*
   - If PRP-OMP (PedvaxHIB® or ComVax® [Merck]) is administered at ages 2 and 4 months, a dose at age 6 months is not required.
   - TriHIBit® (DTaP/Hib) combination products should not be used for primary immunization but can be used as boosters following any Hib vaccine in children age 12 months or older.

5. **Pneumococcal vaccine.** *(Minimum age: 6 weeks for pneumococcal conjugate vaccine [PCV]; 2 years for pneumococcal polysaccharide vaccine [PPV])*
   - Administer one dose of PCV to all healthy children aged 24–59 months having any incomplete schedule.
   - Administer PPV to children aged 2 years and older with underlying medical conditions.

6. **Influenza vaccine.** *(Minimum age: 6 months for trivalent inactivated influenza vaccine [TIV]; 2 years for live, attenuated influenza vaccine [LAIV])*
   - Administer annually to children aged 6–59 months and to all eligible close contacts of children aged 0–59 months.
   - Administer annually to children 5 years of age and older with certain risk factors, to other persons (including household members) in close contact with persons in groups at higher risk, and to any child whose parents request vaccination.
   - For healthy persons (those who do not have underlying medical conditions that predispose them to influenza complications) ages 2–49 years, either LAIV or TIV may be used.
   - Children receiving TIV should receive 0.25 mL if age 6–35 months or 0.5 mL if age 3 years or older.
   - Administer 2 doses (separated by 4 weeks or longer) to children younger than 9 years who are receiving influenza vaccine for the first time or who were vaccinated for the first time last season but only received one dose.

7. **Measles, mumps, and rubella vaccine (MMR).** *(Minimum age: 12 months)*
   - Administer the second dose of MMR at age 4–6 years. MMR may be administered before age 4–6 years, provided 4 weeks or more have elapsed since the first dose.

8. **Varicella vaccine.** *(Minimum age: 12 months)*
   - Administer second dose at age 4–6 years; may be administered 3 months or more after first dose.
   - Do not repeat second dose if administered 28 days or more after first dose.

9. **Hepatitis A vaccine (HepA).** *(Minimum age: 12 months)*
   - Administer to all children aged 1 year (i.e., aged 12–23 months). Administer the 2 doses in the series at least 6 months apart.
   - Children not fully vaccinated by age 2 years can be vaccinated at subsequent visits.
   - HepA is recommended for certain other groups of children, including in areas where vaccination programs target older children.

10. **Meningococcal vaccine.** *(Minimum age: 2 years for meningococcal conjugate vaccine (MCV4) and for meningococcal polysaccharide vaccine (MPSV4))*
    - Administer MCV4 to children aged 2–10 years with terminal complement deficiencies or anatomic or functional asplenia and certain other high-risk groups. MPSV4 is also acceptable.
    - Administer MCV4 to persons who received MPSV4 3 or more years previously and remain at increased risk for meningococcal disease.

The Recommended Immunization Schedules for Persons Aged 0–18 Years are approved by the Advisory Committee on Immunization Practices (www.cdc.gov/vaccines/recs/acip), the American Academy of Pediatrics (http://www.aap.org), and the American Academy of Family Physicians (http://www.aafp.org).

DEPARTMENT OF HEALTH AND HUMAN SERVICES • CENTERS FOR DISEASE CONTROL AND PREVENTION • SAFER • HEALTHIER • PEOPLE™

Source: Centers for Disease Control and Prevention, at www.cdc.gov

---

Box 39-1 Case: Why Does My Newborn Need a Vaccine for Hepatitis?

KM is 24 hours postpartum and worried about how well her baby is breastfeeding. The pediatric staff at the hospital where she gave birth has asked for permission to give her baby the first vaccine to protect against hepatitis B. KM understands that hepatitis B is a sexually transmitted disease and she knows she is not a chronic carrier of the hepatitis antigen. Therefore, she doesn't think her baby needs this vaccine as a newborn. In addition, she is worried about preservatives in the vaccine that might harm her baby.

Hepatitis B can be transmitted across the placenta as well as through contact with body fluids. If the mother has acquired hepatitis B since her initial prenatal labs were drawn, she and her baby might be at risk for developing serious complications because infants who do get infected with hepatitis B have a 90% chance of developing chronic infection. The healthcare provider should provide this information to KM so she can make an informed consent or informed refusal.

Additionally, the healthcare provider can tell KM that the three-shot series, which is given in the first 6 months, will protect the baby if the infant is exposed to body fluids of a person, for example a family member, who knowingly or unknowingly has hepatitis B and that the vaccines used for newborns do not contain thimerosal, the preservative that has mercury in it. Protection against hepatitis B appears to be lifelong after vaccination, and booster doses are not necessary. Approximately 3–9% of newborns or children have some signs of pain at the injection site for a day or two after the injection, and 0.4–6% of newborns and/or children who receive the vaccine will get a slight fever (≤ 37.7°C). The incidence of anaphylaxis is less than 1 in 600,000, and the incidence of hypersensitivity reaction is theoretic, but no cases have been reported.

Sepsis

The incidence of culture-proven neonatal sepsis in the United States is 1–2 per 1000 live births. Newborn sepsis is categorized as **early-onset neonatal sepsis** or **late-onset neonatal sepsis**. Early-onset neonatal sepsis is usually secondary to ascending infection from organisms that are in the vagina. The microorganisms most commonly implicated are *Escherichia coli* and *Group B streptococcus*. Late-onset neonatal sepsis is usually attributed to infection acquired in the hospital or home.

The selection of antimicrobial agents for newborns with suspected sepsis is based on identification of the microorganism and the infant's response to therapy. Gram-positive organisms generally respond to broad-spectrum antibiotics, such as beta-lactamase penicillins, penicillin analogues, and first-generation cephalosporins (beta-lactamases). Gram-negative microorganisms are treated with aminoglycosides and cephalosporins.[32,34-37] Tests must be conducted to determine the specific sensitivity of a microorganism to the antimicrobial agent selected to assure that the appropriate agent is prescribed.

Gram-positive cocci generally respond to penicillin, unless the microorganism produces beta-lactamase (or penicillinase). *Staphylococcus aureus* is a beta-lactamase–producing microorganism and is therefore not responsive to penicillin. A group of semisynthetic penicillins with added side chains are used to treat *S aureus* sepsis. These include methicillin, nafcillin, oxacillin (Bactocill), dicloxacillin (Dynapen), and cloxacillin. First-generation cephalosporins, such as cefazolin (Ancef), cephalexin (Keflex), and cephalothin (Keflin) are also resistant to beta-lactamase.[21,38,39]

Staphylococcus epidermidis and *S aureus* strains may be resistant to penicillin, semisynthetic penicillins, and cephalosporins. Methicillin-resistant *S aureus* (MRSA) is unresponsive to the semisynthetic penicillins, and therefore, vancomycin (Vanocin) is the drug of choice.[40] Vancomycin may also be used for *S epidermidis* infection and infection related to foreign bodies or invasive procedures. The emergence of resistant strains to available antimicrobial agents is an increasing problem.[32,41]

Third-generation cephalosporins treat gram-negative cocci that are penicillin and methicillin resistant. Aminoglycosides or third-generation cephalosporins are the drugs of choice for gram-negative enteric rods. Some gram-negative rods are classified according to their lactose fermentation ability. The lactose-fermenters, *E. coli* and *Klebsiella*, are sensitive to aminoglycosides and third-generation cephalosporins. *Shigella* and *Salmonella* are nonlactose fermenters that respond well to ampicillin and third-generation cephalosporins.[32,34,42-45]

Haemophilus influenzae is usually sensitive to ampicillin and third-generation cephalosporins, although some strains are ampicillin resistant.[32,46] *Pseudomonas* requires combination therapy of an aminoglycoside and an anti-*Pseudomonas* penicillin such as azlocillin (Securopen), carbenicillin (Geocillin), imipenem, mezlocillin (Mezlin), piperacillin (Pipracil), or ticarcillin (Ticar).[32]

Two anaerobic microorganisms, *Bacteroides fragilis* (gram-negative) and *Clostridium* (gram-positive), are sometimes the cause of newborn infection. *B fragilis* is susceptible to metronidazole (Flagyl), clindamycin (Cleocin), and some of the newer beta-lactamases, such as imipenem and ampicillin with sulbactam (Unasyn). *Clostridium* is usually susceptible to penicillin.[32]

A combination of ampicillin or penicillin and gentamicin is useful for antibacterial action against *Streptococci*, *Listeria monocytogenes*, and gram-negative enteric rods. This combination of antimicrobial agents has a synergistic effect (in vitro), increasing the efficacy of either drug if used alone. Additional therapy or selection of other agents is necessary if staphylococcal infection is suspected, if *Pseudomonas* or *Bacteroides* (most often iatrogenically acquired) is present, if there is an outbreak of resistant organisms, or if prolonged ampicillin and gentamicin therapy has been used.

Candida Infections

Oral thrush or monilia is caused by an overgrowth of *Candida albicans* in the mouth. It most often occurs in infants whose mothers have infections secondary to a *Candida* organism or in infants who received antimicrobial

---

▮ Box 39-2 A Case of Thrush

CT is being seen for a 6-week postpartum visit and asks her provider to check for a yeast infection on her nipples. She is breastfeeding her daughter and has developed pain during breastfeeding. She is also worried about the baby's diaper rash. CT had an uncomplicated normal vaginal delivery and has not had any problems breastfeeding. She says the baby latches well, nurses for an average of 20–30 minutes each nursing episode, and is gaining weight. This is her third child; she breastfed her first two children for several months each. She does not have stabbing pain in her breasts; the pain is localized to the nipples and areolae.

Infection with *Candida albicans* is common in infants and can also colonize the nipples and areolae of breastfeeding women; therefore examination of both the mother and infant in this breastfeeding dyad will be important. Interestingly, there is little correlation between the strains of *Candida* found in the oral cavity of an infant and the vagina of that child's mother. Infants can develop thrush without known exposure, but cross-contamination between an infant and a mother's breast does occur.

On exam, CT is afebrile. She has bright red areolae that look shiny and have some flaking. There are no cracks. The rest of the breast exam is benign. Her daughter has white patches inside both cheeks that can not be wiped away, and she has a diaper rash that is distinctive for a bright shiny red appearance without cracking or bleeding.

The presumptive diagnosis is *C albicans* of the nipple and corresponding *C albicans* infection in the infant's mouth (thrush) and perianal area. CT asks her provider if there is a natural treatment she can use so she doesn't have to give the baby any drugs.

CT's provider describes the use of gentian violet, which is painted on the inside of the baby's mouth and on her nipples. Gentian violet is effective but stains clothing, and there are no studies of its use for treating diaper rash. The provider suggests nystatin (Mycostatin) and CT agrees to use it. CT is given the following prescriptions:

1. Nystatin oral suspension 100,000 units; 1 mL is to be placed in each cheek inside the baby's mouth four times per day for 5 days, and do not feed the infant for 5–10 minutes after dose is administered.

2. Nystatin ointment 100,000 units/gram; a 30-gram tube was ordered and CT was instructed to apply a small amount to the infant's diaper area and to her nipples twice a day for 7–10 days as needed.

In addition, the provider advises CT to wash pacifiers, keep diapers off so the baby's bottom is exposed to the air when sleeping, and similarly to avoid bras and nipple pads so all areas that are infected are exposed to dry air whenever possible. She is also advised to wash her hands well after applying the nystatin ointment to her nipples and/or to her baby.

agents that can result in destruction of normal flora. Thrush appears as white or yellowish raised spots on the tongue or sides of the mouth. Thrush is treated with an oral antifungal agent such as nystatin suspension (Mycostatin) or fluconazole (Diflucan)[32] (Box 39-2). Gentian violet is an old-fashioned remedy that is effective but not as effective as nystatin; it stains clothing and can rarely cause mucosal ulcerations, so it is not often recommended unless a family desires to avoid antifungal medications.

C albicans may also present as a diaper rash, particularly in infants with oral thrush. The diaper rash appears as superficial blisters that are usually nontender. The lesions may group together and coalesce to form a large area with smaller satellite blisters at the edges. These satellite lesions are characteristic of candidal infection. Treatment includes topical application of nystatin ointment (Mycostatin), which may be combined with oral administration of fluconazole (Diflucan) to reduce the intestinal content of candida albicans, which may lower the risk of invasive candidiasis in the neonate.[47]

Systemic *C albicans* is becoming more prevalent in the neonatal intensive care unit and is currently the third most common cause of late-onset sepsis.[27] Factors that increase the risk include indwelling intravenous or arterial catheters, prolonged or indiscriminate use of antibacterial agents, third-generation cephalosporins, total parenteral nutrition, mechanical ventilation, long hospitalization, and previous colonization with *Candida*.[48] The treatment of a systemic infection requires intravenous therapy with an antifungal agent, such as amphotericin B, for a prolonged period of time.[48] New drugs are under development for treatment of fungal infections in neonates; however, there is still a lack of sufficient data of the efficacy of these agents in neonates and children.[49,50]

Seizures

Seizures are the most common sign of a neurologic disorder during the neonatal period; the incidence ranges from 1 to 5 per 1000 live births.[51,52] The first month of life is one of the highest risk periods for seizures. Seizures in the newborn are generally triggered by an acute disorder, such as hypoxic-ischemic encephalopathy, stroke, or infection. Seizures are not a disease; they are a sign of acute disturbance within the brain. A seizure is caused by excessive, synchronous electrical discharges or depolarization in the brain, producing stereotypic, repetitive behaviors. Uncontrolled seizures can increase the damage to the central nervous system.[51,52]

Newborn seizures can be classified as subtle, tonic, clonic, or myoclonic, with the subtle being the most common.

Expression of seizures in the newborn include abnormal movement or alterations in tone in the trunk and extremities; abnormal facial, oral, and tongue movements; abnormal eye movements; and changes in respiratory effort.

A prolonged generalized seizure that causes cyanosis, significant changes in heart rate, or apnea that does not respond to adequate ventilation and perfusion therapy should be treated with anticonvulsant medication. The first-line anticonvulsant used in the newborn period is phenobarbital, at a dosage of 20 mg/kg given intravenously for a maximum of 40 mg/kg as a loading dose followed by 3–4 mg/kg per day administered in a divided dose given once every 12 hours. Intravenous phenobarbital reaches the brain rapidly and has a rapid onset of action. Phenobarbital is metabolized by the liver and eliminated by the kidneys. Therapeutic levels vary but generally are in the range of 40 to 60 mcg/mL.[52] Subsequent management will be directed by the pediatric neurologist.

Conclusion

The relative immaturity of the neonatal organ systems affects medication selection, administration, and follow-up. The selection and administration of drugs in the newborn should be based upon a thorough physical examination, careful maternal and neonatal history, and knowledge of the unique physiologic function of the newborn organ systems. In addition, a plan to monitor the effects of the medication, identify adverse or side effects, and appropriately measure drug levels if warranted should be made when any medication is prescribed for a neonate.

References

1. Ohning BL. Neonatal pharmacodynamics—basic principles. I: drug delivery. Neonatal Netw 1995;14:7–12.
2. Ohning BL. Neonatal pharmacodynamics—basic principles. II: drug action and elimination. Neonatal Netw 1995;14:15–9.
3. Conroy S, McIntyre J, Choonara I. Unlicensed and off label drug use in neonates. Arch Dis Child Fetal Neonatal Ed 1999;80:F142, 4; discussion F144–5.
4. Slikker W Jr, Young JF, Corley RA, Dorman DC, Conolly RB, Knudsen TB, et al. Improving predictive modeling in pediatric drug development: pharmacokinetics, pharmacodynamics, and mechanistic modeling. Ann N Y Acad Sci 2005;1053:505–18.

5. Richter R, Below H, Kadow I, Kramer A, Muller C, Fusch C. Effect of topical 1.25% povidone-iodine eye-drops used for prophylaxis of ophthalmia neonatorum on renal iodine excretion and thyroid-stimulating hormone level. J Pediatr 2006;148:401–3.

6. Besunder JB, Reed MD, Blumer JL. Principles of drug biodisposition in the neonate. A critical evaluation of the pharmacokinetic-pharmacodynamic interface (Part II). Clin Pharmacokinet 1988;14:261–86.

7. Milsap RL, Jusko WJ. Pharmacokinetics in the infant. Environ Health Perspect 1994;102(suppl 11): 107–10.

8. Alternative routes of drug administration—advantages and disadvantages (subject review). American Academy of Pediatrics. Committee on Drugs. Pediatrics 1997;100:143–52.

9. Schirm E, Tobi H, de Jong-van den Berg LT. Identifying parents in pharmacy data: a tool for the continuous monitoring of drug exposure to unborn children. J Clin Epidemiol 2004;57:737–41.

10. Matinzadeh ZK, Beiragdar F, Kavemanesh Z, Abolgasemi H, Amirsalari S. Efficacy of topical ophthalmic prophylaxis in prevention of ophthalmia neonatorum. Trop Doct 2007;37:47–9.

11. Chen CJ, Starr CE. Epidemiology of gram-negative conjunctivitis in neonatal intensive care unit patients. Am J Ophthalmol 2008;145:966–70.

12. Simon JW. Povidone-iodine prophylaxis of ophthalmia neonatorum. Br J Ophthalmol 2003;87:1437.

13. American Academy of Pediatrics Committee on Fetus and Newborn. Controversies concerning vitamin K and the newborn. American Academy of Pediatrics Committee on Fetus and Newborn. Pediatrics 2003; 112:191–2.

14. American Academy of Pediatrics Committee on Fetus and Newborn. Policy statement: controversies concerning vitamin K and the newborn. Pediatrics 2006; 118:1266.

15. Autret-Leca E, Jonville-Bera AP. Vitamin K in neonates: how to administer, when and to whom. Paediatr Drugs 2001;3:1–8.

16. Draper G, McNinch A. Vitamin K for neonates: the controversy. BMJ 1994;308:867–8.

17. Huysman MW, Sauer PJ. The vitamin K controversy. Curr Opin Pediatr 1994;6:129–34.

18. Sutor AH. New aspects of vitamin K prophylaxis. Semin Thromb Hemost 2003;29:373–6.

19. Zengin E, Sarper N, Turker G, Corapcioglu F, Etus V. Late hemorrhagic disease of the newborn. Ann Trop Paediatr 2006;26:225–31.

20. Hviid A. Postlicensure epidemiology of childhood vaccination: the Danish experience. Expert Rev Vaccines 2006;5:641–9.

21. Marschall J, Muhlemann K. Duration of methicillin-resistant *Staphylococcus aureus* carriage, according to risk factors for acquisition. Infect Control Hosp Epidemiol 2006;27:1206–12.

22. Marshall GS, Happe LE, Lunacsek OE, Szymanski MD, Woods CR, Zahn M, et al. Use of combination vaccines is associated with improved coverage rates. Pediatr Infect Dis J 2007;26:496–500.

23. Marques RC, Dorea JG, Manzatto AG, Bastos WR, Bernardi JV, Malm O. Time of perinatal immunization, thimerosal exposure and neurodevelopment at 6 months in breastfed infants. Acta Paediatr 2007; 96:864–8.

24. Chang MH. Hepatitis B virus infection. Semin Fetal Neonatal Med 2007;12:160–7.

25. Cohn AC, Broder KR, Pickering LK. Immunizations in the United States: a rite of passage. Pediatr Clin North Am 2005;52:669, 93, v.

26. Lee C, Gong Y, Brok J, Boxall EH, Gluud C. Hepatitis B immunisation for newborn infants of hepatitis B surface antigen-positive mothers. Cochrane Database Syst Rev 2006;(2):CD004790.

27. Chapman RL. Prevention and treatment of *Candida* infections in neonates. Semin Perinatol 2007;31:39–46.

28. Elhassan NO, Sorbero ME, Hall CB, Stevens TP, Dick AW. Cost-effectiveness analysis of palivizumab in premature infants without chronic lung disease. Arch Pediatr Adolesc Med 2006;160:1070–6.

29. Grimaldi M, Gouyon B, Sagot P, Quantin C, Huet F, Gouyon JB, et al. Palivizumab efficacy in preterm infants with gestational age < or = 30 weeks without bronchopulmonary dysplasia. Pediatr Pulmonol 2007; 42:189–92.

30. Simoes EA, Groothuis JR, Carbonell-Estrany X, Rieger CH, Mitchell I, Fredrick LM, et al. Palivizumab prophylaxis, respiratory syncytial virus, and subsequent recurrent wheezing. J Pediatr 2007;151:34–42.

31. Ventre K, Randolph AG. Ribavirin for respiratory syncytial virus infection of the lower respiratory tract in infants and young children. Cochrane Database Syst Rev 2007;(1):CD000181.

32. Lott JW. State of the science: neonatal bacterial infection in the early 21st century. J Perinat Neonatal Nurs 2006;20:62–70.

33. Zupan J, Garner P, Omari AA. Topical umbilical cord care at birth. Cochrane Database Syst Rev 2004;(3): CD001057.

34. Lima-Rogel V, Medina-Rojas EL, Del Carmen Milan-Segovia R, Noyola DE, Nieto-Aguirre K, López-Delarosa A, et al. Population pharmacokinetics of cefepime in neonates with severe nosocomial infections. J Clin Pharm Ther 2008;33:295–306.

35. Murphy JE. Prediction of gentamicin peak and trough concentrations from six extended-interval dosing protocols for neonates. Am J Health Syst Pharm 2005; 62:823–7.

36. Pong AL, Bradley JS. Guidelines for the selection of antibacterial therapy in children. Pediatr Clin North Am 2005;52:869, 94, viii.

37. Pullen J, Driessen M, Stolk LM, Degraeuwe PL, van Tiel FH, Neef C, et al. Amoxicillin pharmacokinetics in (preterm) infants aged 10 to 52 days: effect of postnatal age. Ther Drug Monit 2007;29:376–80.

38. Baltimore RS. Consequences of prophylaxis for group B streptococcal infections of the neonate. Semin Perinatol 2007;31:33–8.

39. Tzialla C, Borghesi A, Stronati M. Neonatal antibiotic prophylaxis for the prevention of early- and late-onset Group B streptococcal sepsis. J Perinat Med 2007;35:252, 253; author reply 254.

40. Bond CA, Raehl CL. Clinical and economic outcomes of pharmacist-managed aminoglycoside or vancomycin therapy. Am J Health Syst Pharm 2005;62: 1596–605.

41. Fanos V, Cuzzolin L, Atzei A, Testa M. Antibiotics and antifungals in neonatal intensive care units: a review. J Chemother 2007;19:5–20.

42. Boyle EM, Brookes I, Nye K, Watkinson M, Riordan FA. "Random" gentamicin concentrations do not predict trough levels in neonates receiving once daily fixed dose regimens. BMC Pediatr 2006;6:8.

43. Clark RH, Bloom BT, Spitzer AR, Gerstmann DR. Empiric use of ampicillin and cefotaxime, compared with ampicillin and gentamicin, for neonates at risk for sepsis is associated with an increased risk of neonatal death. Pediatrics 2006;117:67–74.

44. Dellagrammaticas HD, Christodoulou C, Megaloyanni E, Papadimitriou M, Kapetanakis J, Kourakis G. Treatment of gram-negative bacterial meningitis in term neonates with third generation cephalosporins plus amikacin. Biol Neonate 2000;77:139–46.

45. Schrag SJ, Hadler JL, Arnold KE, Martell-Cleary P, Reingold A, Schuchat A. Risk factors for invasive, early-onset *Escherichia coli* infections in the era of widespread intrapartum antibiotic use. Pediatrics 2006; 118:570–6.

46. Chandran A, Watt JP, Santosham M. Prevention of *Haemophilus influenzae* type b disease: past success and future challenges. Expert Rev Vaccines 2005;4: 819–27.

47. Ozturk MA, Gunes T, Koklu E, Cetin N, Koc N. Oral nystatin prophylaxis to prevent invasive candidiasis in neonatal intensive care unit. Mycoses 2006;49: 484–92.

48. Cetin H, Yalaz M, Akisu M, Hilmioglu S, Metin D, Kultursay N. The efficacy of two different lipid-based amphotericin B in neonatal *Candida* septicemia. Pediatr Int 2005;47:676–80.

49. Steinbach WJ, Benjamin DK. New antifungal agents under development in children and neonates. Curr Opin Infect Dis 2005;18:484–9.

50. Smolinski KN, Shah SS, Honig PJ, Yan AC. Neonatal cutaneous fungal infections. Curr Opin Pediatr 2005; 17:486–93.

51. Clancy RR. Summary proceedings from the neurology group on neonatal seizures. Pediatrics 2006; 117:S23–7.

52. Riviello JJ. Pharmacology review drug therapy for neonatal seizures: part 2. Neo Rev 2004;5(6):262–8.

APPENDIX
Glossary of Abbreviations

Abbreviation	Expanded Form
ac	before meals
ad lib	use freely
AM	morning, before noon
amt	amount
bid	twice daily
bol	bolus (usually intravenously)
cap, caps	capsule
cc	cubic centimeter
cf	with food
CR	controlled release
d/c	discontinue
disp	dispense
DS	double strength
dL	deciliter
elix	elixir
ER	extended release
et	and
g	gram
gr	grain
gtt(s)	drop, drops
h, hr, hrs	hour, hours
hgb	hemoglobin
hs	at bedtime
IM	intramuscular injection
inj	injection

Abbreviation	Expanded Form
IP	intraperitoneal
IU	International Units
IV	intravenous
LA	long acting
L	liter
m	meter (often reported as squared)
max	maximum
mcg	microgram (also abbreviated in some sources as μg)
mEq	milliequivalent
mg	milligram
mL	milliliter
ng	nanogram
od	once per day (rarely used—should use qd)
oz	ounce
per	by or through
pc	after meals
pH	hydrogen ion concentration
PM	evening or afternoon
PO	by mouth or orally
PR	by rectum
prn	as needed; from Latin *pro re nata*
q	every

Abbreviation	Expanded Form
qd	every day
qhs	every night at bedtime
qid	four times daily
SQ	subcutaneous (may also be abbreviated as subc, subq, or SC)
Sig	write on label
SL	sublingually, under the tongue
SR	slow release
sol	solution
supp	suppository
susp	suspension
syr	syrup
tab	tablet
tbsp	tablespoon
troche	lozenge
tsp	teaspoon
tid	three times a day
U	units
U.S.P.	United States Pharmacopeia
vag	vaginally
XL, XT	extended release

Drug Index

Page numbers in **bold** indicate in-depth discussion or dosage information for specific drugs. Brand names are capitalized; generic names are lowercase.

A

A&D ointment, 1123, 1135
abacavir, 70, 689, 691
abatacept, 468, 485
ABC (abacavir), 70, 689, 691
abciximab, 74
Abelcet (amphotericin B), 293
Abilify (aripiprazole), 769, 781, 786, 1016
acamprosate, 218, **219–220**
acarbose, 507, **518**, 520, 524, 529, 535, 1140
Accolate (zafirlukast), 579, 589, 591, 1071
AccuNeb (albuterol), 60
Accupril (quinapril), 274, 399, 425
Accutane (isotretinoin), 274, 807, 809,
        812–813, 825, 968, 975, 1048
acebutolol, **396**, 1159
Aceon (perindopril), 399
Acetadote (acetylcysteine), 75, 78
acetaminophen, 36, 45, 62, 63, 64, 69, 70,
        74–75, 78, 79, 232, 290, 315, 316,
        318, **320**, 323, **327–328**, 337, 338,
        352, 454, 683, 733, 734, **735**, 736,
        821, 849, 972, 978, 1060, 1061, 1063,
        1119, **1155**
    with codeine, 12, **338**, 339, **1119**,
        1124, 1125
    with hydrocodone, **338**, **1119**
    with oxycodone, **338**, **1119**
    with propoxyphene, **339**, 1125
acetazolamide, 220, 480, 713, **837**, 840
acetic acid (vinegar), 961, 965
acetylcysteine, 75, 78, 79
acetylsalicylic acid. *See* aspirin

Achletin (trichlormethiazide), 393
Achromycin (tetracycline), 260, 272, 1157
Aci-Jel (acetic acid), 961
AcipHex (rabeprazole), 610, 617–618
acitretin, 806, **809**
Aclovate (prednicarbate), 802
Acomplia (rimonabant), 165, 169, 173
acorus, 221
ACTH, 976
Actifed (triprolidine/pseudoephedrine),
        74, 1061
Actigall (ursodiol), 1016
Actigall (ursodeoxycholic acid), 1077
actinomycin D, 861, 865
Actisite (tetracycline), 808
Activase (alteplase), 457–458
activated charcoal, **78**, 213, 627
Activella (estradiol/norethindrone), 1013, 1016
Actonel (risedronate), 1032, 1033, 1034
ACTOplus Met (metformin/pioglitazone), 520
Actos (pioglitazone), 167, 518, 520, 522, 523,
        939–940, 1140
Acular (ketorolac), 846, 847
acyclovir, 35, 71, **300–302**, **695–696**, 754, 825,
        978, **1064**, 1151, 1153
Aczone (dapsone), 284
Adacel (Tdap vaccine), 133, 1138
Adalat CC (nifedipine), 404
adalimumab, 467, 468, 473, 474, 482, 484,
        485, 807
adapalene, 808, **809**
Adderall (dextroamphetamine), 210, 555,
        739, 740
adefovir, 310, 527, **684**
Adipex-P (phentermine), 165, 169, 170–171,
        182, 392
Adora (calcium-fortified chocolate), 102
Adoxa (doxycycline), 815, 975, 1157
Adriamycin (doxorubicin), 858, 861, 869
Advair (fluticasone/salmeterol), 575, 589,
        590, 1071

Advicor (niacin/lovastatin), 417
Advil (ibuprofen), 38, 60, 72, 110, 318, 320, 323,
        325, 492, 825, 844, 849, 918, 919,
        926, 929, 1025, 1061, 1119, 1155
AeroBid (flunisolide), 588
African chilies. *See* capsaicin
Afrin (oxymetazoline), 565, 569, 1061
Aggrenox (aspirin/dipyridamole), 419, 420
Agoral (senna), 629
AHAs (alpha hydroxy acids), 826
AH-CHEW D (phenylephrine), 1061
AK Tracin (bacitracin), 846
Akne-Mycin (erythromycin), 808
AK-Pentolate (cyclopentolate), 842
Alamast (pemirolast), 846, 847
Alavert (loratadine), 353, 356
Alba form HC (clioquinol), 555
albuterol, 32, 60, 582–583, **584–585**, 590, 593,
        710, 844, 1070, **1153**
Alcloxa (aluminum chlorhydroxy
        allantoinate), 635
alcohol (ethanol), 39, 40, 75, 110, 188, 205, 209,
        213, **217–221**, 222–228, 232, 264,
        274, 280, 319, 320, 322, 327–328,
        333, 354, 454, 644, 683, 710, 764,
        766, 923, 930, 972, 978, 999, 1025,
        1031, 1046, 1048, **1091**
Aldactone (spironolactone), 174, 322, 394, 395,
        426, 428, 454, 825, 923, 929, 931
Aldara (imiquimod), 693, 798, 978–979
Aldomet (methyldopa), 73, 397, 398, 408, 409,
        428, 491, 776, 825, 923, 981, 1023,
        1071, 1159
alefacept, 807
alendronate, 34, 103, 613, 1032, 1033, **1034**
Alepam (oxazepam), 268
Alesse (oral contraceptive), 814, 886, 906
Aleve (naproxen), 60, 62, 72, 76, 110, 318, 320,
        325–326, 465, 515, 520, 825, 918,
        919, 926, 1005, 1061
alfalfa (*Medicago sativa*), **1079**

1183

D

Subject Index

A

α_1-receptor antagonists, 390
abacavir, 689
abatacept, 468–469, 485
abbreviated new drug applications
    (ANDAs), 3, 18
abnormal uterine bleeding (AUB). *See also*
    dysmenorrhea; menorrhagia
    characteristics, 916, 1003
    diagnosis, 923, 1020–1021
    postmenopause, 924
    during pregnancy, 924
    treatment, 924–928, 1021
abortifacients, 238, 376, 899–910, 943
absence seizures, 706
absolute infant dose (AID), 1146, 1154
absorbent agents, 627–628
absorption. *See* drug absorption
abstinence syndrome, 199. *See also*
    withdrawal syndrome
acamprosate, 218–220, 223
acarbose, 507, 524, 1140
ACE inhibitors. *See* angiotensin-converting
    enzyme (ACE) inhibitors
acetaminophen
    branding, 352
    hepatotoxicity, 65, 70, 74–75
    overdoses, 64–65
    in over-the-counter drugs, 64–65
    pharmacokinetics, 320
    for postpartum pain, 1119
    relative infant dose, 1155
    side effects/adverse effects, 327–328.
        See also hepatotoxicity, drug-induced
acetic acid, 850
acetylcholine receptors
    mental disorder role, 757
    muscarinic, 562, 647, 706, 744, 834, 841
    nicotinic, 184, 562

acetylsalicylic acid. *See* aspirin
acetylureas, 713
acitretin, 806, 809
acne
    inversa, 964, 973–976
    rosacea, 814
    from testosterone use, 1027
    vulgaris, 272, 792, 807, 895
acquired immune deficiency syndrome (AIDS),
    37, 671, 685, 687. *See also* human
    immunodeficiency virus
actin, 1086, 1087, 1089–1090
actinic keratosis, 792, 796, 797–799
actinomycin D, 861, 865
activated charcoal, 78
activated partial thromboplastin time
    (aPPT), 450
active diffusion, 28–29
active immunity, 125, 128–129, 149
active transport, 28
active tubular secretion, 40
acupuncture
    for dysmenorrhea, 922–923
    for fibroid treatment, 944
    history, 229
    for inflammatory bowel disease, 475
    for nausea/vomiting, 620
    for rheumatoid arthritis, 486
    for urinary tract disorders, 652, 662
    for weight loss, 176
acute bacterial rhinosinusitis, 560,
    577–578
acute bronchitis, 570
acute cutaneous lupus erythematosus, 489
acute cystitis, 643, 657, 661
acute external otitis, 850
acute idiosyncratic hypersensitivity reactions,
    71–72. *See also* Stevens-Johnson
    syndrome
acute otitis media, 832, 849, 850
acute pain, 310, 311

acute respiratory distress syndrome
    (ARDS), 868
acute retroviral syndrome, 671, 687
acute salpingitis, 671
acute stress disorder, 750, 772, 774
acute tubulointerstitial nephritis, 76
acyclovir, 299–301, 695–696, 1064
adalimumab, 467–468, 474, 485, 807
adapalene, 808–809
adaptive immunity, 125, 127
addiction. *See also* alcoholism; *specific drugs*;
    substance abuse
    characteristics, 199
    illicit drugs, 199, 204–205, 221–224
    nicotine, 181–195
    opioid, 205–209, 337
    physiology/neurobiology of, 200–204
    polypharmacy, 210
    pseudo-addiction, 337
    in special populations, 200, 221, 224
    treatment, 203–205
    vaccine protection, 151–152
adefovir, 684
adenocarcinoma, 982
adenomyosis, 917, 940
adenosine diphosphate (ADP) receptors,
    419–421, 445, 455–457
adenosine triphosphate (ATP), 1089
adequate intake (AI), 89, 90
adjuvant therapy, 854
adolescents
    asthma classification/control assessment,
        581–582
    attention-deficit hyperactivity disorder, 740
    diabetes incidence, 534–535
    drug addiction risks, 200, 216
    iodine supplementation, 540
    menarche, 991
    menstrual problems, 919–920, 924. *See also*
        specific menstrual problems
    nutrition, 540